# Major Drug Classes and Their Prototypes

**Central Nervous System Stimulants**
*Amphetamines*
Amphetamine sulfate
*Amphetamine-like Drugs*
Methylphenidate
*Methylxanthines*
Caffeine

## Diuretics

**High-Ceiling (Loop) Diuretics**
Furosemide
**Thiazide Diuretics**
Hydrochlorothiazide
**Potassium-Sparing Diuretics**
Spironolactone
Triamterene

## Cardiovascular Drugs

**Drugs That Affect the Renin-Angiotensin System**
*Angiotensin-Converting Enzyme (ACE) Inhibitors*
Captopril
*Angiotensin II Receptor Antagonists*
Losartan
**Calcium Channel Blockers**
*Agents That Affect the Heart and Blood Vessels*
Verapamil
*Agents That Affect Blood Vessels Primarily*
Nifedipine
**Drugs for Hypertension**
*Diuretics*
Hydrochlorothiazide
Furosemide
Spironolactone
*Beta-Adrenergic Blockers*
Propranolol
Metoprolol
*Alpha-Adrenergic Blockers*
Prazosin
*Combined Alpha/Beta Blockers*
Labetalol
*Centrally Acting Antiadrenergics*
Clonidine
*ACE Inhibitors*
Captopril
Enalapril
*Angiotensin II Receptor Antagonists*
Losartan
*Calcium Channel Blockers*
Verapamil
Nifedipine

**Drugs for Angina Pectoris**
*Organic Nitrates*
Nitroglycerin
*Beta Blockers*
Propranolol
Metoprolol
*Calcium Channel Blockers*
Verapamil
Nifedipine
**Drugs for Heart Failure**
*Diuretics*
Hydrochlorothiazide
Furosemide
Spironolactone
*Vasodilators*
Captopril (ACE inhibitor)
*Inotropic Agents*
Digoxin (a cardiac glycoside)
Dopamine (a sympathomimetic)
*Beta Blockers*
Carvedilol
**Antidysrhythmic Drugs**
*Class I: Sodium Channel Blockers*
Quinidine (Class IA)
Lidocaine (Class IB)
*Class II: Beta Blockers*
Propranolol
*Class III: Potassium Channel Blockers*
Bretylium
*Class IV: Calcium Channel Blockers*
Verapamil
*Others*
Adenosine
Digoxin
**Drugs Used to Lower Blood Cholesterol**
*HMG CoA Reductase Inhibitors*
Lovastatin
*Bile Acid–Binding Resins*
Cholestyramine
*Others*
Nicotinic acid
**Anticoagulant, Antiplatelet, and Thrombolytic Drugs**
*Anticoagulants*
Heparin (parenteral)
Enoxaparin (a low molecular weight heparin)
Warfarin (oral)
*Antiplatelet Drugs*
Aspirin
*Thrombolytic Drugs*
Streptokinase
Alteplase (tPA)

*Continued*

# Pharmacology *for* Nursing Care

## THIRD EDITION

# Pharmacology for Nursing Care

## THIRD EDITION

# Richard A. Lehne, Ph.D

*formerly*
*Lecturer, University of Arizona College of Nursing*
*Lecturer, University of Virginia School of Nursing*
*Research Assistant Professor, Department of Pharmacology*
*University of Virginia School of Medicine*

*in consultation with*

*Linda A. Moore, EdD, RN*
*Associate Professor*
*College of Nursing and Health Professions*
*University of North Carolina at Charlotte*
*Charlotte, North Carolina*

*Leanna J. Crosby, DNSc, RN, GNP–C*
*Adjunct Associate Professor*
*Director of Research Laboratories*
*College of Nursing*
*University of Arizona*
*Tucson, Arizona*

*Diane B. Hamilton, PhD, RN*
*Associate Professor*
*School of Nursing*
*Western Michigan University*
*Kalamazoo, Michigan*

## W. B. SAUNDERS COMPANY

*A Division of Harcourt Brace & Company*

PHILADELPHIA  LONDON  TORONTO  MONTREAL  SYDNEY  TOKYO

**W.B. SAUNDERS COMPANY**
*A Division of Harcourt Brace & Company*

The Curtis Center
Independence Square West
Philadelphia, Pennsylvania 19106

**Library of Congress Cataloging-in-Publication Data**

Lehne, Richard A.
    Pharmacology for nursing care / Richard A. Lehne; in consultation
with Linda A. Moore, Leanna J. Crosby, Diane B. Hamilton.—3rd ed.
       p.    cm.
    Includes bibliographical references and index.
    ISBN 0-7216-7150-0
    1. Pharmacology.   2. Nursing.   I. Title.
    [DNLM:   1. Pharmacology—nurses' instruction.   2. Drug Therapy—nurses'
instruction. QV 4 L523p 1998]
    RM301.P457 1998
    615'.1—dc21
    DNLM/DLC                               97-39758

PHARMACOLOGY FOR NURSING CARE            ISBN 0–7216–7150–0

Printed in the United States of America

Last digit is the print number:    9   8   7   6   5   4   3   2   1

Dedicated to the memory of
Elmer and Rellen Perry

# Biographic Information

**Richard A. Lehne, PhD,** received his BA from Drew University and his doctorate in pharmacology from George Washington University. His involvement in nursing education began 19 years ago at the University of Virginia School of Nursing, where he taught undergraduate and graduate courses and was voted best teacher by his students. He has also taught at the University of Arizona in both the School of Nursing and School of Pharmacy. Today, Dr. Lehne lives in Charlottesville, VA, where he is occupied with writing, giving the occasional guest lecture, and dancing as often as possible.

**Linda A. Moore, EdD, RN,** is an Associate Professor at the University of North Carolina at Charlotte. She received her BSN from Duke University and her MSN and EdD from the University of Virginia. Her teaching responsibilities encompass courses for undergraduate (RN to BSN) and graduate students. Her major clinical and research interests are cardiovascular nursing and gerontologic nursing. Dr. Moore is a member of the North Carolina Nurses' Association and Sigma Theta Tau.

**Leanna J. Crosby, DNSc, RN, GNP-C,** received her diploma in nursing from St. Luke's Hospital School of Nursing, her baccalaureate and master's degrees from the University of Virginia, and her doctorate in nursing science from Catholic University of America. Also, she completed the adult nurse practitioner program at the University of Virginia and the gerontologic nurse practitioner program at the University of Arizona. Dr. Crosby has done extensive research in chronic rheumatoid disease, and has taught physiology and pathophysiology to a generation of appreciative graduate and undergraduate students. Currently, she is working as a nurse practitioner within the Department of Veteran Affairs, Tucson VA Medical Center, and is an Adjunct Associate Professor at the University of Arizona College of Nursing.

Dr. Crosby is a member of the American Nurses Association, Sigma Theta Tau, and the Arizona Nurses' Association, and serves on the Arizona State Board of Nursing Advanced Practice Committee. In addition, she is chair of the Advanced Practice Nursing Council at the Tucson VA and serves as the VISN 18 (Arizona, Texas, and New Mexico) coordinator for the Advanced Practice Nursing Network. At the local level, she is chairperson for the Tucson VA IACUC Animal Research Committee and serves on the Research and Development Committee, Research Panel, of the Nurse Professional Standards Board, and the Pharmacy and Therapeutics Committee.

**Diane B. Hamilton, PhD, RN,** received her BA from Northwestern University, her BSN from West Texas State University, her MA in Community Mental Health and Gerontologic Nursing from the University of Iowa, and her PhD in Psychosocial Nursing and Nursing History from the University of Virginia. She has extensive experience in psychiatric nursing, including serving as attending nurse at the Institute of Psychiatry of the Medical University of South Carolina. She has taught psychiatry and behavioral science to medical students, and gerontology, community health, psychiatric nursing, and nursing history to nursing students. Currently, she is an Associate Professor in the School of Nursing at Western Michigan University, where she teaches psychiatric nursing and nursing history and does nursing history research.

Dr. Hamilton is a member of the American Nurses Association, the American Association of the History of Nursing, the American Association for the History of Medicine, the American Association of University Women, and Sigma Theta Tau. In addition, she is an Associate of the Susan B. Anthony Center. Dr. Hamilton is a recipient of the Best of *Image* Award in nursing history, the Lavinia Dock Award for historical scholarship, the Best Investigator Award from the University of Rochester, and the Golden Apple Teaching Award from the Medical University of South Carolina.

# Preface to the Third Edition

## Overview of the Book

Welcome to the third edition of *Pharmacology for Nursing Care*, the pharmacology text that students *like* to read. This edition, like the first and second, was written to be a true textbook—that is, a book that focuses on essentials and downplays secondary details. To give the book its focus, three principal techniques are employed: (1) teaching through prototypes, (2) use of large print for essential information and small print for secondary information, and (3) limiting discussion of adverse effects and drug interactions to ones that are of particular clinical significance. To reinforce the relationship between pharmacologic knowledge and nursing practice, nursing implications are integrated into the body of each chapter. In addition, to provide rapid access to nursing content, nursing implications are summarized at the end of most chapters, using a nursing process format. As in the prior two editions, this edition emphasizes conceptual material, thereby reducing rote memorization, promoting comprehension, and increasing reader friendliness. For a more detailed description of the book's distinguishing features, please refer to the preface to the first edition, which is reprinted herein.

## New in This Edition

All chapters have been revised, some extensively. Topics with significantly expanded coverage include asthma, osteoporosis, hormone replacement therapy, attention-deficit/hyperactivity disorder, Alzheimer's disease, and HIV infection.

Over 100 new drugs have been added. These include angiotensin II receptor antagonists (for hypertension), protease inhibitors (for HIV infection), bisphosphonates (for osteoporosis), low-molecular-weight heparins (for thrombosis), 6 new drugs for diabetes, and 10 new drugs for cancer.

In addition to undergoing general revision, the book contains seven new chapters, two new appendices, a new unit on life span issues, a summary of key points for each chapter, and computer software for students. Also, we will offer updates on the World Wide Web.

## New Chapters

In response to developments in pharmacotherapy and suggestions from students and teachers, I have added seven new chapters:

- *Drug Therapy During Pregnancy and Breast Feeding*
- *Drugs for Other Psychologic Disorders* (drugs for panic disorder, obsessive-compulsive disorder, and Alzheimer's disease)
- *Review of Hemodynamics*
- *Review of the Immune System*
- *Pediatric Immunization*
- *Drugs for HIV Infection and Related Opportunistic Infections*
- *Miscellaneous Noteworthy Drugs* (drugs for obesity, respiratory distress syndrome, benign prostatic hyperplasia, cystic fibrosis, and amyotrophic lateral sclerosis [Lou Gehrig's disease])

## New Unit: Drug Therapy Across the Life Span

In prior editions, information on life span issues was spread throughout the introductory chapters. In this edition, life span–related content has been consolidated into its own unit. In addition, discussion of several life span topics (e.g., teratogenesis) has been greatly expanded. The new unit has three chapters:

- *Drug Therapy During Pregnancy and Breast-Feeding*
- *Drug Therapy in Pediatric Patients*
- *Drug Therapy in Geriatric Patients*

## New Appendices

This edition contains two new appendices. One addresses gender-related content and one addresses drug-related information on the Internet.

- *Guide to Gender-Related Drugs.* Because this book is structured largely on the basis of pharmacologic drug classes, information on drugs employed for gender-related therapy is scattered throughout the book. This guide is intended as a quick reference to these drugs. Topics addressed in the guide include eclampsia, suppression of preterm labor, hormone replacement therapy, emergency postcoital contraception, impotence, and benign prostatic hyperplasia.

- *Drug-Related Information on the Internet.* The Internet offers a vast amount of information on pharmacology and therapeutics. This appendix provides a directory of selected Internet sites where you can find reliable drug-related information.

## Key Points

A list of key points has been added to each chapter, providing a concise summary of chapter content. The list is intended to give additional guidance regarding content to focus on.

## Computer Software

The enclosed software consists of (1) NCLEX-style review questions plus (2) a data base of the 200 most commonly used drugs, from which students can generate their own drug cards. The information on the software comes from *Saunders Nursing Drug Handbook.*

## Updates on the Web

Pharmacology undergoes steady and sometimes rapid evolution. Important new drugs are introduced every year; uses for older drugs change; and previously unknown toxicities of available drugs may be revealed. As a result, a pharmacology text can quickly become outdated. Accordingly, in order to keep this text current, we will provide periodic updates on the World Wide Web. For details on these updates, please contact your W.B. Saunders Educational Sales Representative or our sales support staff (1-800-544-0292).

## Ancillaries

### Teaching Aids: Transparencies, Instructor's Manual, Test Bank

A Transparency Set, Instructor's Manual, and Test Bank are available at no charge to teachers using this text. The Transparency Set (ISBN no. 0-7216-7152-7) contains 100 color transparencies of figures from the text. The Instructor's Manual (0-7216-7151-9) contains suggestions for setting up a pharmacology course, case studies, lecture notes, and more. The Test Bank consists of NCLEX-style questions and is available in two formats: computerized ExaMaster (0-7216-7153-5) and print (0-7216-7404-6). To obtain these teaching aids, contact your W.B. Saunders Educational Sales Representative. If you don't know who your representative is, you can find out by calling W.B. Saunders sales support at 1-800-544-0292.

### Student Study Guide

The Study Guide (ISBN no. 0-7216-7069-5) is new with this edition and features critical thinking exercises along with various review and learning activities.

## Your Comments are Welcome

I would like to hear from you. All feedback is welcome. Suggestions for improving the book are especially helpful, as are reports of mistakes (small or large) that you may spot. Of course, I also like to hear from readers who simply have something nice to say. You can reach me via the Internet at *lehne@adelphia.net* or *ral4f@virginia.edu* or via U.S. mail care of W.B. Saunders Company.

RICHARD A. LEHNE

# Preface to the First Edition

Pharmacology pervades all phases of nursing practice and relates directly to patient care and patient education. Despite its pervasiveness and importance, pharmacology remains an area in which students, practitioners, and teachers are often uneasy. Much of this uneasiness stems from traditional approaches to the subject, in which memorization of details takes precedence over understanding. In this text, the opposite approach is taken. Here, the guiding principle is to establish a basic understanding of drugs, after which secondary details can be learned as needed.

This text was written with two major objectives. The first is to help nursing students establish a knowledge base in the basic science of drugs. The second is to demonstrate how that knowledge can be directly applied in providing patient care and patient education. To achieve these goals, several innovative techniques are employed. These are described below.

***Laying Foundations in Basic Principles.*** Understanding drugs requires a strong foundation in basic pharmacologic principles. To establish this foundation, major chapters are dedicated to the following topics: basic principles that apply to all drugs (Chapters 5 through 9), basic principles of neuropharmacology (Chapter 13), basic principles of antimicrobial chemotherapy (Chapter 77), and basic principles of cancer chemotherapy (Chapter 95).

***Reviewing Physiology and Pathophysiology.*** To understand the actions of a drug, we must first understand the biologic systems that the drug influences. For all major drug families, relevant physiology and pathophysiology are reviewed. Reviews are presented at the beginning of each chapter, rather than in a systems review at the beginning of a unit. For example, in the unit on cardiovascular drugs, which includes separate chapters on hypertension, angina pectoris, heart failure, myocardial infarction, and dysrhythmias, reviews of relevant physiology and pathophysiology begin *each chapter.* This juxtaposition of pharmacology, physiology, and pathophysiology is designed to facilitate understanding of the interrelationships among these subjects.

***Teaching Through Prototypes.*** Within each drug family, we can usually identify one agent that embodies the features that characterize all members of the group. Such a drug can be viewed as a prototype. Since other family members are generally very similar to the prototype, to know the prototype is to know the basic properties of all group members.

The benefits of teaching through prototypes can best be appreciated with an example. Let's consider the non-steroidal anti-imflammatory drugs (NSAIDs), a family that includes aspirin, ibuprofen [Motrin, others], naproxen [Naprosyn, Anaprox], indomethacin [Indocin], and more than 20 other drugs. Traditionally, information on these drugs is presented in a series of paragraphs describing each drug in turn. When attempting to study from such a list, students are likely to learn many drug names and little else; the important concept of similarity among family members is easily lost. In this text, the family prototype—aspirin—is discussed first and in depth. After this, instruction is completed by pointing out the relatively minor ways in which individual NSAIDs differ from aspirin. Not only is this approach more efficient than the traditional approach, it is also more effective in that similarities among family members are emphasized.

***Large Print and Small Print: A Way to Focus on Essentials.*** Pharmacology is exceptionally rich in detail. There are many drug families, each with multiple members and each member with its own catalogue of indications, contraindications, adverse effects, and drug interactions. This abundance of detail confronts the teacher with the difficult question of what to teach, and confronts the student with the equally difficult question of what to study. Attempts to answer these questions can frustrate teacher and student alike. Even worse, in the presence of myriad details, basic concepts can become obscured.

To help establish a focus on essentials, this text employs two type sizes. Large print is intended to say, "On your first exposure to this topic, this is the core of information that you should learn." Small print is intended to say, "Here is additional information that you may want to learn after mastering the material in large print." As a rule, large print is reserved for prototypes, basic principles of pharmacology, and reviews of physiology and pathophysiology. Small print is used for secondary information about the prototypes and for discussion of drugs that are not prototypes. By employing this technique, we have been able to incorporate a large body of detail into this book without having that detail cloud the big picture. Furthermore, because the technique highlights essentials, it minimizes questions about what to teach and what to study.

The use of large and small print is especially valuable for discussing adverse effects and drug interactions. Most drugs are associated with many adverse effects and interactions. As a rule, however, only a few of these are noteworthy. In traditional texts, practically all adverse effects and interactions are presented, creating long and tedious lists. In this text, those few adverse effects and interactions that are especially characteristic are highlighted through presentation in large print; the remainder are noted briefly in small print. As a result, rather than overwhelming students with a long and forbidding list, which can impede comprehension, the approach employed here, by delineating a moderate body of important information, serves to promote comprehension.

***Nursing Implications: Demonstrating the Application of Pharmacology to Nursing Practice.*** The principal reason for asking a nursing student to learn pharmacology is to enhance his or her ability to care for and educate patients. To show students how they can apply pharmacologic knowledge to nursing practice, nursing implications are *integrated into the body of each chapter.* That is, as specific drugs and drug families are discussed, the nursing implications inherent in the pharmacologic information are discussed side-by-side with the basic science. To facilitate access to nursing information, nursing implications are also *summarized at the end of most chapters.* These summaries should serve to reinforce the information presented in the main text.

In chapters that are especially brief or that address drugs that are infrequently used, summaries of nursing implications have been omitted. However, even in these chapters, nursing implications are incorporated into the chapter body.

***A Note About Drug Therapy.*** Throughout this text, as we discuss specific drug families (e.g., beta-adrenergic blockers), we discuss the clinical applications of those drugs. Similarly, in chapters that focus on specific diseases (e.g., Parkinson's disease, hypertension), we indicate which drugs are generally considered most appropriate for treatment. However, it is important to note that clinical applications of individual drugs may change over time: a drug may acquire new indications that are not discussed here, or it may cease to be used for indications that *are* discussed here. Likewise, drug therapy of specific diseases is continually evolving: as superior drugs are developed, they tend to replace older, less desirable agents. Accordingly, although the drug therapies presented in this text reflect a general consensus on what is considered best *today,* these therapies may not be considered best a few years from now—and, in therapeutic areas where there is controversy or where change is especially rapid, the treatments discussed here may be considered inappropriate by some clinicians right now.

***About Dosage Calculations.*** Unlike many nursing pharmacology texts, this one has no section on dosage calculation. The reasons for this departure from tradition are twofold. First, adequate presentation of this important subject simply isn't feasible in a text dedicated to the basic science of drugs; the amount of space that can be allotted is too small. Second, thanks to the availability of several excellent publications on the subject (e.g., *Clinical Calculations,* W.B. Saunders Company), the need to include this information in pharmacology texts has been obviated.

***Ways to Use This Textbook.*** Because of its focus on essentials, this text is especially well suited to serve as the primary text for courses dedicated specifically to pharmacology. In addition, the book's focused approach makes it a valuable resource for pharmacologic instruction within integrated curriculums and for self-directed learning by students and practitioners.

RICHARD A. LEHNE

# Acknowledgments

I want to begin by thanking everyone involved at W.B. Saunders Company for the unconditional support they've given this book over the past 12 years—despite having to deal with an occasionally (some might say notoriously) cantankerous author. For this edition, it has been my good fortune to work with Maura Connor, my editor at Saunders. Maura brought to the project a refreshing blend of warmth, energy, enthusiasm, and attention to detail, along with an exemplary work ethic and remarkable ability to jump start the procrastinating soul (usually). In addition, I would like to express long-overdue public appreciation to the Educational Sales Representatives at Saunders, whose professionalism and hard work have contributed immeasurably to the success of this book.

In writing this edition, as in the first and second, I have enjoyed the wise counsel, good humor, and warm friendship of Drs. Linda A. Moore, Diane B. Hamilton, and Leanna J. Crosby. Special appreciation is due Dr. Moore for updating the Instructor's Manual and creating the new Study Guide that accompanies this edition.

It has been my pleasure to work closely with Boris Starosta, the artist who rendered the elegant new illustrations for this edition. Boris routinely made adjustments to my rough sketches that greatly improved both their visual appeal and power of communication.

I want to thank two contributors: Dr. Theodore G. Tong, who produced the new appendix on drug-related Internet resources, and Dr. Alfred J. Rémillard, who updated the appendix on Canadian drug information, which he wrote originally for the first edition of this text.

I am grateful to Dr. David Benjamin, whose careful review and detailed comments greatly improved Chapter 62 (*Review of the Immune System*). Likewise, I am grateful to Dr. Denis O'Brien for both his critique of Chapter 88 (*Drugs for HIV Infection and Related Opportunistic Infections*) as well as years of friendship and enthusiastic support.

Once the writing is done, a manuscript must be made into a book—a process that can be an author's worst nightmare. However, for this edition, the process was a dream—thanks to the all-star team assembled by Berta Steiner. In addition to Berta herself, I have the highest praise and gratitude for my copy editor—Megan Westerfeld—who did the painstaking job of transmuting the manuscript into its final form, and for Bob Elliott and his colleagues who did a flawless job of transforming the copy-edited manuscript into the book you hold in your hands.

I am deeply grateful to Dr. Alan Agins, friend and colleague, who adopted this text for his class at the University of Virginia and has since shamelessly promoted it while teaching updates in pharmacology to advanced practice nurses throughout the country. Apparently, association with me has not convinced Alan that writing is a hard way to earn a living, given that he has just completed a book of his own.

To conclude, I want to thank the friends and associates who have provided comfort, encouragement, and diversion over the past 20 months as this revision took form. Heading the list are Jean Gratz and Bill Curtis, two long-time friends whose love and humor have buoyed my spirits through three editions of this book. As in the past, Bill continues to find time for frequent and prolonged commiserations, despite the demands of maintaining the formularies at his two dispensaries—C.S.T. and Tastings—where members of his amiable staff, notably Tom Bjornsen and Gordon Maxwell, have catered to my pharmacologic needs for years. At the same venue, I have enjoyed the camaraderie of the LB Club, whose distinguished members include Petie and the Bobs (Sorry. Club rules prohibit disclosing surnames.) as well as Dr. Christopher Perry, our astute, albeit absentee, club physician. Finally, I want to thank my friends in the Charlottesville dance community—most especially my new and very dear partner.

RAL

# CONTENTS

## Unit XV  Chemotherapy of Parasitic Diseases

## Unit XVI  Cancer Chemotherapy

## Unit XVII  Additional Important Drugs

## Unit XVIII  Toxicology

## Appendices

# DETAILED CONTENTS

## Unit III  Drug Therapy Across the Life Span

## Unit IV  Peripheral Nervous System Drugs

**Introduction**

## Unit V Central Nervous System Drugs

# Unit VII Cardiovascular Drugs

## Unit VIII  Drugs That Affect the Blood

# Unit IX Endocrine Drugs

## Unit XI  Respiratory Tract Drugs

## Unit XII  Gastrointestinal Drugs

## Unit XIII  Metabolic Drugs

## Unit XIV  Chemotherapy of Infectious Diseases

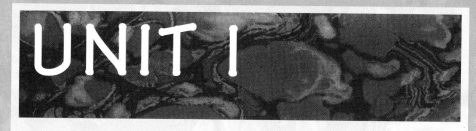

# UNIT I

# Introduction

# CHAPTER 1

# Orientation to Pharmacology

**Four Basic Terms**
**Properties of an Ideal Drug**
    The Big Three: Effectiveness, Safety, and
      Selectivity
    Additional Properties of an Ideal Drug
**The Therapeutic Objective**

**Factors That Determine the Intensity of**
   **Drug Responses**
    Administration
    Pharmacokinetics
    Pharmacodynamics
    Sources of Individual Variation

f you are like most students reading this text, by this time in your life you've been hitting the books for 15 or more years and have probably asked yourself, "What's the purpose of all this education?" In the past your question may have lacked a satisfying answer. Happily, now you have one: The reason you've spent most of your life in school was to get ready to study pharmacology!

There is good reason why you haven't approached pharmacology before now. Pharmacology is a science that draws on information from multiple disciplines, including anatomy, physiology, psychology, chemistry, and microbiology. Consequently, before you could begin your study of pharmacology, you had to become familiar with these other sciences. Now that you've established the requisite knowledge base, you're finally ready to learn about drugs.

## Four Basic Terms

At this point it will be helpful to define four basic terms: *drug, pharmacology, clinical pharmacology,* and *therapeutics.* As we go through these definitions, we will also discuss what the focus of this text will be.

**Drug.** A drug is defined as *any chemical that can affect living processes.* By this definition, virtually all chemicals can be considered drugs, since, when given in large enough amounts, all chemicals will have some effect on life. Clearly, it is beyond the scope of this text to consider all compounds that fit the definition of a drug. Accordingly, rather than studying all drugs, we will limit discussion to those drugs that have therapeutic applications.

**Pharmacology.** Pharmacology can be defined as *the study of drugs and their interactions with living systems.* Given this definition, the science of pharmacology can claim a large body of knowledge as its own. Under our

definition, pharmacology encompasses the study of the physical and chemical properties of drugs as well as their biochemical and physiologic effects. In addition, pharmacology includes knowledge of the history, sources, and uses of drugs and knowledge of drug absorption, distribution, metabolism, and excretion. Since pharmacology encompasses such a broad spectrum of information, it would be inappropriate (not to mention impossible) to address the entire scope of pharmacology in this text. Consequently, we will restrict consideration to information relevant to the clinical setting.

**Clinical Pharmacology.** Clinical pharmacology is defined as *the study of drugs in humans.* This discipline includes the study of drugs in *patients* as well as in *healthy volunteers* (during new drug development). Since clinical pharmacology encompasses all aspects of the interaction between drugs and people, and since our primary interest is the use of drugs to treat patients, clinical pharmacology includes some information that will be outside the scope of this text.

**Therapeutics.** Therapeutics, also known as *pharmacotherapeutics,* is defined as *the use of drugs to diagnose, prevent, or treat disease or to prevent pregnancy.* Alternatively, therapeutics can be defined simply as the medical use of drugs.

Therapeutics will provide the focus of this book. That is, our discussions will focus on the basic science information needed to understand the use of drugs as therapeutic agents. This information should help you understand how drugs produce their effects—both therapeutic and adverse; the reasons for giving a particular drug to a particular patient; and the rationale underlying selection of dosage, route, and schedule of administration. In addition, knowledge of pharmacology will help you understand the strategies employed to promote beneficial drug effects and to minimize undesired effects. It is my hope that by applying this knowledge you will improve patient care and education. It is also my hope that knowledge of pharmacology will render working with medications a less mysterious and therefore more gratifying activity for you.

## Properties of an Ideal Drug

If we were developing a new drug, we would want that drug to be as good as possible. In order to approach perfection, our new drug should have certain properties, such as effectiveness and safety. In the discussion below, we will consider the characteristics that an ideal drug might possess. I must stress, however, that the ideal medication exists in theory only; in reality, *there is no such thing as a perfect drug*. The truth of this statement will become apparent as we consider the properties that an ideal drug should have.

### The Big Three: Effectiveness, Safety, and Selectivity

The three most important characteristics that any drug can have are effectiveness, safety, and selectivity.

**Effectiveness.** An effective drug is one that elicits the responses for which it has been administered. *Effectiveness is the most important property that a drug can have.* Regardless of its other virtues, if a drug is not effective—that is, if it doesn't do anything useful—there is no justification for giving it. Current United States law requires that all new drugs be proved effective prior to release for marketing.

**Safety.** A safe drug is defined as one that cannot produce harmful effects—even if administered in very high doses and for a very long time. *There is no such thing as a safe drug.* All drugs have the ability to cause injury. The chances of producing adverse effects can be reduced by proper drug selection and proper administration. However, the risk of adverse effects can never be eliminated. Certain anticancer drugs, for example, are always associated with an increased risk of serious infection. With other drugs (e.g., opioid analgesics), excessive dosage always carries a risk of fatal respiratory depression. Clearly, drugs are not safe. The fact that drugs are dangerous may explain why the Greeks chose the word pharmakon, which can be translated as *poison*, as a name for these compounds.

**Selectivity.** A selective drug is defined as one that elicits only those responses for which it is given. A selective drug would not produce side effects. *There is no such thing as a selective drug: all medications cause side effects.* Common examples of side effects include the drowsiness that can be caused by antihistamines; the morning sickness, cramps, and depression that can be caused by oral contraceptives; and the constipation, urinary hesitancy, and respiratory depression that can be caused by morphine.

## Additional Properties of an Ideal Drug

**Reversible Action.** For most drugs, it is important that effects be reversible. That is, in most cases, we want drug actions to subside within some appropriate period of time. General anesthetics, for example, would be useless if patients never woke up. Likewise, it is unlikely that oral contraceptives would find widespread acceptance if their use resulted in permanent sterility. For a few drugs, most notably antibiotics and anticancer agents, reversibility is not a desirable characteristic; when using these compounds, we want their toxicity to target cells to endure.

**Predictability.** It would be very helpful if, prior to drug administration, we could know with certainty just how a given patient will respond. Unfortunately, since each patient is unique, the accuracy of such predictions cannot be guaranteed. Accordingly, in order to maximize the chances of eliciting desired responses, we must tailor therapy to the individual.

**Ease of Administration.** An ideal drug should be simple to administer: the route should be convenient, and the number of doses per day should be low. The diabetic patient who faces a lifetime of multiple daily injections is not likely to judge insulin ideal. Likewise, drugs that require intravenous infusion are rarely considered ideal by the nurse who must set up the infusion apparatus and monitor its function.

In addition to convenience, ease of administration has two additional benefits: (1) it can enhance patient compliance, and (2) it can decrease errors in drug administration. Patients are more likely to comply with a dosing schedule that consists of once-a-day administration than with one that requires multiple daily doses. Similarly, hospital personnel are less likely to commit medication errors when administering oral drugs than when preparing and administering intravenous formulations.

**Freedom from Drug Interactions.** When a patient is taking two or more drugs, those drugs can interact with one another. These interactions may either augment or reduce drug responses. For example, the degree of respiratory depression caused by diazepam [Valium], which is normally minimal, can be greatly *intensified* in the presence of alcohol. On the other hand, the antibacterial effects of tetracycline can be substantially *reduced* if this drug is taken concurrently with iron or calcium supplements. Because of the potential for interactions among drugs, when a patient is taking more than one agent, the possible impact of drug interactions must be considered. An ideal drug would not interact with other agents. Unfortunately, few medicines are devoid of significant interactions.

**Low Cost.** An ideal drug would be readily affordable. The cost of drugs can be a substantial financial burden. As an extreme example, 1 year of therapy with human growth hormone (somatrem) can cost between $10,000 and $20,000. More commonly, expense becomes a significant factor for patients who must take drugs chronically.

People with diseases such as hypertension, arthritis, or diabetes, for example, require drug therapy for life. The cumulative expense of such treatment can be huge—even for drugs of moderate price.

**Chemical Stability.** Some drugs lose effectiveness during storage. Others, which may be stable on the shelf, can rapidly lose effectiveness when put into solution (e.g., in preparation for injection). These losses in efficacy result from chemical instability. Because of chemical instability, stocks of certain drugs must be periodically discarded and replaced with fresh supplies. An ideal drug would retain its activity indefinitely, both on the shelf and in solution.

**Possession of a Simple Generic Name.** Generic names of drugs are usually complex, and therefore difficult to remember and pronounce. As a rule, the trade name for a drug is simpler than its generic name. Examples of drugs that have simple trade names and complex generic names include chlordiazepoxide [Librium], acetaminophen [Tylenol], and cephalexin [Keflex]. Since generic names are preferable to trade names (for reasons discussed in Chapter 3), an ideal drug should have a generic name that is easy to recall and pronounce.

## Summary of Properties of an Ideal Drug

From the preceding discussion, you can see that available medications are far from ideal. No drug has all of the properties discussed above: no drug is safe; all drugs produce side effects; drug responses may be difficult to predict and may be altered as a result of drug interactions; and drugs may be expensive, unstable, and difficult to administer. Because medications are not ideal, all members of the health care team must exercise care to promote therapeutic effects and minimize the potential for drug-induced injury.

## The Therapeutic Objective

*The objective of drug therapy is to provide the maximum benefit with minimum harm.* If drugs were ideal, we could achieve this objective with relative ease. However, since drugs are not ideal, we must exercise skill and care if treatment is to result in more good than harm.

As detailed in Chapter 2, you, as a nurse, have a critical responsibility in achieving the therapeutic objective. In order to meet this responsibility, you must understand drugs. The primary purpose of this text is to help you establish that understanding.

## Factors That Determine the Intensity of Drug Responses

Multiple factors determine how an individual will respond to a prescribed dose of a particular drug (Fig. 1-1).

Knowledge of these factors is needed in order to think rationally about how a drug interacts with the patient to produce its effects. In addition, knowledge of these factors is needed if you are to contribute maximally to efforts at achieving the therapeutic objective.

Our ultimate concern when administering a drug is the intensity of the responses that the drug produces. Working our way up from the bottom of Figure 1-1, we can see that the intensity of the response is determined ultimately by the concentration of a drug at its sites of action. As the figure suggests, the prime determinant of this concentration is the administered dose. When administration is performed correctly, the dose that was given will bear a close relationship to the dose that was prescribed. The steps leading from prescribed dose to intensity of drug response are considered below.

### Administration

Dosage size and the route and timing of administration are important determinants of drug responses. Accordingly, the prescribing clinician will consider these variables with care. Unfortunately, drugs are not always administered as prescribed: poor patient compliance and medication errors by hospital staff can result in major discrepancies between the dose that was prescribed and the dose that is actually administered. Such discrepancies can significantly alter the outcome of treatment. To help minimize errors caused by poor compliance, you should give patients complete instruction about their medication and how to take it.

Medication errors made by hospital staff may result in a drug being administered by the wrong route, in the wrong dose, or at the wrong time; the patient may even be given the wrong drug. These errors can be made by pharmacists, physicians, and nurses. Any of these errors will detract from achieving the therapeutic objective.

### Pharmacokinetics

Pharmacokinetic processes determine how much of an administered dose will reach its sites of action. There are four major pharmacokinetic processes: (1) drug absorption, (2) drug distribution, (3) drug metabolism, and (4) drug excretion. Collectively, these processes can be thought of as *the impact of the body on drugs*. The pharmacokinetic processes are discussed at length in Chapter 5.

### Pharmacodynamics

Once a drug has reached its site of action, pharmacodynamic processes determine the nature and intensity of the response. Pharmacodynamics can be thought of as *the impact of drugs on the body*. In most cases, the initial step leading to a response is the binding of a drug to its receptor. This drug-receptor interaction is followed by a se-

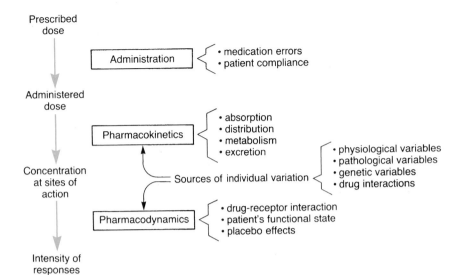

**Figure 1–1. Factors that determine the intensity of drug responses.** (Adapted from Koch-Weser, J. Drug therapy. Serum drug concentrations as therapeutic guides. N. Engl. J. Med. 287:227, 1972.)

quence of events that ultimately results in a response. As indicated in Figure 1-1, the patient's "functional state" can influence pharmacodynamic processes. For example, a patient who has developed tolerance to morphine will respond less to a particular dose than will a patient who lacks tolerance. Placebo (psychologic) effects also help determine the responses that a drug will elicit. Pharmacodynamics is discussed at length in Chapter 6.

### Sources of Individual Variation

Characteristics unique to each patient can influence pharmacokinetic and pharmacodynamic processes and, by doing so, can help determine the patient's responses to drugs. As indicated in Figure 1-1, sources of individual variation include drug interactions; physiologic variables (e.g., age, sex, weight); pathophysiologic variables (especially diminished function of the kidneys and liver, the major organs of drug elimination); and genetic variables. Genetic factors can alter the metabolism of drugs and can predispose the patient to unique drug reactions. Because individuals differ from one another, no two patients will respond identically to the same drug regimen. Accordingly, if the therapeutic objective is to be achieved, it is essential that drug therapy be matched to the individual. Individual variation in drug responses is discussed at length in Chapter 9.

## Summary

Whenever medicines are used, our goal is to promote desired effects and minimize adverse effects. In order to achieve this objective, we need to understand pharmacokinetics and pharmacodynamics, the principal determinants of drug responses. In addition, it is essential that we account for potential sources of individual variation in drug responses. When all these considerations are made, the resulting regimen will be tailored to the individual, and therefore should produce maximum benefit with minimum harm.

## KEY POINTS

- The most important properties of an ideal drug are effectiveness, safety, and selectivity.
- If a drug is not effective, it should not be used.
- There is no such thing as a safe drug: all drugs can cause harm.
- There is no such thing as a selective drug: all drugs can cause side effects.
- The objective of drug therapy is to provide maximum benefit with minimum harm.
- Because all patients are unique, drug therapy must be tailored to each individual.

# CHAPTER 2

# Application of Pharmacology in Nursing Practice

Our objective in this chapter is to answer the following question: "Why should a nursing student learn pharmacology?" To answer this question, we will examine the ways in which a nurse can put knowledge of pharmacology to practical use. Hopefully, when you complete this chapter you will be convinced that an understanding of drugs is necessary for the practice of nursing, and therefore that putting time and energy into learning about drugs will constitute a worthwhile investment.

## Evolution of Nursing Responsibilities Regarding Drugs

At one time the nurse's responsibility regarding medications was limited to the *Five Rights of Drug Administration*, namely, give the *right drug* to the *right patient* in the *right dose* by the *right route* at the *right time*. Clearly, the Five Rights are important. However, although these basics are essential, much more is required if the therapeutic objective is to be achieved. The Five Rights guarantee only that a drug will be administered as prescribed. Correct administration, without additional interventions, cannot ensure that treatment will result in maximum benefit and minimum harm.

The limitations of the Five Rights can be illustrated with this analogy: The nurse who sees his or her responsibility as being over as soon as he or she has administered a patient's medicine would be like a baseball pitcher who felt that his responsibility was over once he had thrown the ball toward the batter. As the pitcher must be ready to re-spond to the consequences of the interaction between ball and bat, the nurse must be ready to respond to the consequences of the interaction between drug and patient. Put another way, although both the nurse and the pitcher have a clear obligation to deliver their respective "pills" in the most appropriate fashion, proper delivery is only the beginning of their responsibilities: *important events will take place after the "pill" is delivered, and these must be responded to.* Like the pitcher, the nurse can respond rapidly and effectively only by anticipating (knowing in advance) what the possible reactions to the pill might be. In order to anticipate possible reactions, both the nurse and the pitcher require certain kinds of knowledge. Just as the pitcher must understand the abilities of the opposing batter, the nurse must understand the patient and the disorder for which he or she is being treated. As the pitcher must know the most appropriate pitch (e.g., fast ball, curve) to deliver in specific circumstances, the nurse must know what medications are appropriate for the patient and must check to ensure that the medication ordered is one of them. Conversely, as the pitcher must know what pitches *not* to throw at a particular batter, the nurse must know what drugs are *contraindicated* for the patient. As the pitcher must know the most likely outcome after the ball and bat interact, the nurse must know the probable consequences of the interaction between drug and patient. Although this analogy is not perfect (the nurse and patient are on the same team, whereas the pitcher and batter are not), it does help us appreciate that the nurse's responsibility extends well beyond the Five Rights. Consequently, in addition to the limited information needed to administer drugs in accordance with the Five Rights, you need to acquire a broad base of pharmacologic knowledge so as to contribute fully to achieving the therapeutic objective.

In drug therapy today, nurses, together with physicians and pharmacists, participate in a system of checks and balances designed to promote beneficial effects and minimize harm. Nurses are especially important within this system because it is the nurse—not the physician—who follows the patient's status most closely. As a result, you are likely to be the first member of the health care team to observe and evaluate drug responses, and to intervene if required. In order to observe and evaluate drug responses, and in order to intervene rapidly and appropriately, you must know *in advance* the responses that a medication is likely to elicit. Put another way, in order to provide professional care, you must understand drugs; the stronger your knowledge of pharmacology, the more you will be able to *anticipate* drug responses and not simply *react* to them after the fact.

Within our system of checks and balances, the nurse has an important role as patient advocate. It is your responsibility to detect errors made by pharmacists and physicians—and mistakes will be made. For example, the physician may overlook potential drug interactions, or may be unaware of alterations in the patient's status that would preclude use of a particular drug, or may select the correct drug but may order an inappropriate dosage or route of administration. Since it is the nurse who actually administers drugs, the nurse is the last person to check medications prior to administration. Consequently, *you are the patient's last line of defense against errors.* It is ethically and legally unacceptable for you to administer a drug that is harmful to the patient—even though the medication has been prescribed by a licensed physician and dispensed by a licensed pharmacist: In your role as patient advocate, you must protect the patient against medication errors made by other members of the health care team. *In serving as patient advocate, it is impossible for you to know too much about drugs.*

## Application of Pharmacology in Patient Care

The two major areas in which you can apply pharmacologic knowledge are patient care and patient education. Patient care is considered in this section. Patient education is considered in the next section. In discussing the applications of pharmacology in patient care, we will focus on seven aspects of drug therapy: (1) preadministration assessment, (2) dosage and administration, (3) evaluating and promoting therapeutic effects, (4) minimizing adverse effects, (5) minimizing adverse interactions, (6) making PRN decisions, and (7) managing toxicity.

### Preadministration Assessment

All drug therapy begins with assessment of the patient. Assessment has three basic goals: (1) collecting base-line data needed to evaluate therapeutic and adverse responses, (2) identifying high-risk patients, and (3) assessing the patient's capacity for self-care. The first two goals are highly specific for each drug. Accordingly, we cannot achieve these goals without understanding pharmacology. The third goal applies generally to all drugs; hence, it does not usually require specific knowledge of the drug to be used. Preadministration assessment is discussed further in Chapter 3 (Pharmacology and the Nursing Process).

***Collecting Baseline Data.*** Baseline data are needed to evaluate drug responses, both therapeutic and adverse. For example, if we plan to give a drug to lower blood pressure, we must know the patient's blood pressure prior to treatment. Without this baseline data, we would have no way of determining the effectiveness of our drug. Similarly, if we are planning to give a drug that can decrease blood cell counts as a side effect, we need to know baseline counts in order to evaluate this potential adverse effect of treatment. Obviously, in order to collect appropriate baseline data, we must first know the effects that our drug is likely to produce.

***Identifying High-Risk Patients.*** Multiple factors can predispose an individual patient to adverse reactions from specific drugs. Important predisposing factors are pathophysiology (especially liver and kidney dysfunction), genetic factors, drug allergies, pregnancy, old age, and extreme youth.

Patients with penicillin allergy provide a dramatic example of those at risk: Giving penicillin to these people can kill them. Accordingly, whenever treatment with penicillin is under consideration, we must determine if the patient has had an allergic reaction to a penicillin in the past. If the patient has a history of penicillin allergy, an alternative antibiotic should be employed. If there is no effective alternative, facilities for managing a severe reaction should be in place before the drug is given.

From the preceding example, we can see that, when drug therapy is being planned, patients at high risk of reacting adversely must be identified. The tools for identification are the patient history, physical examination, and laboratory tests. Of course, if identification is to be successful, you must know what to look for (i.e., you must know the factors that can increase the risk of severe reactions to the drug in question). Once the high-risk patient has been identified, we can take steps to reduce the risk. We might select an alternative drug, or, if no alternative is available, we can at least prepare in advance to manage a possible reaction.

### Dosage and Administration

Earlier, we noted the Five Rights of Drug Administration and agreed on their importance. Although you can implement the Five Rights without a detailed knowledge of pharmacology, having such knowledge can help reduce your contribution to medication errors. Some examples will illustrate this point:

- Certain drugs have more than one indication, and dosage may vary depending upon which indication the drug is being used for. Aspirin, for example, is given in low doses to relieve pain and in higher doses to suppress inflammation (e.g., in patients with arthritis). If you didn't know about these differences, you might administer too much aspirin to the patient with pain or too little to the patient with inflammation.

- Many drugs can be administered by more than one route, and dosage may vary depending upon the route selected. Morphine, for example, may be administered by mouth or by injection (subcutaneous, intramuscular, intravenous). Oral doses are generally much larger than injected doses. Accordingly, if a large dose intended for oral use were to be mistakenly administered by injection, the result could prove fatal. The nurse who understands the pharmacology of morphine is unlikely to make this medication error.
- Certain intravenous agents can cause severe local injury if the line through which they are being administered becomes extravasated. Accordingly, when such drugs are given, special care must be taken to prevent extravasation. The infusion must be monitored closely, and, if extravasation occurs, corrective steps must be taken immediately to minimize harm. The nurse who doesn't understand these drugs will be unprepared to work with them safely.

The following basic guidelines can help ensure correct administration:

- Read the medication order carefully. If the order is unclear, verify it with the prescribing physician.
- Verify the identity of the patient by comparing the name on the wristband with the name on the drug order or administration record.
- Read the medication label carefully. Verify the identity of the drug, the amount of drug (per tablet, volume of liquid, etc.), and its suitability for administration by the intended route.
- Verify dosage calculations.
- Implement any special handling that the drug may require.
- Do not administer any drug if you do not understand the reason for its use.

## Evaluating and Promoting Therapeutic Effects

***Evaluating Therapeutic Responses.*** Evaluation is one of the most important aspects of drug therapy. After all, this is the process that tells us whether or not our drug is doing anything useful. Because the nurse follows the patient's status most closely, the nurse is in the best position to evaluate therapeutic responses.

In order to make an evaluation, you must know the rationale for treatment and the nature and time course of the desired response. If you lack this knowledge, you will be unable to evaluate the patient's progress. When beneficial responses develop as hoped for, ignorance of expected effects might not be so bad. However, when desired responses do not occur, it may be essential to identify this failure quickly, since timely implementation of alternative therapy may be needed.

When evaluating responses to a drug that has more than one application, you can do so only if you know the specific indication for which the medication is being used. Nifedipine, for example, is given for two cardiovascular disorders: hypertension and angina pectoris. When the drug is used to treat hypertension, you should monitor for a reduction in blood pressure. In contrast, when this drug is used to treat angina, you should monitor for a reduction in chest pain. Clearly, if you are to make the proper evaluation, you must understand the reason for drug use.

***Promoting Compliance.*** Drugs can be of great value to patients, but only if they are taken correctly. Drugs that are self-administered in the wrong dose, by the wrong route, or at the wrong time cannot produce maximum benefit—and may even prove harmful. Obviously, successful therapy requires active and informed participation by the patient. By educating patients about the drugs they are taking, you can help elicit the required level of participation.

***Implementing Nondrug Measures.*** The benefits of drug therapy can often be enhanced by nonpharmacologic measures. Examples include (1) enhancing drug therapy of asthma through breathing exercises, biofeedback, and emotional support; (2) enhancing drug therapy of arthritis through exercise, physical therapy, and rest; and (3) enhancing drug therapy of hypertension through weight reduction, smoking cessation, and sodium restriction. As a nurse, you may provide these supportive measures directly, or through patient education, or by coordinating the activities of other health care providers.

## Minimizing Adverse Effects

All drugs have the potential to produce undesired effects. Common examples include gastric erosion caused by aspirin, sedation caused by antihistamines, hypoglycemia caused by insulin, and excessive fluid loss caused by diuretics. When drugs are employed properly, the incidence and severity of such effects can be reduced. Measures to reduce adverse effects include identifying high-risk patients through the patient history, ensuring proper administration through patient education, and forewarning patients about activities that might precipitate an adverse reaction.

When untoward effects cannot be avoided, discomfort and injury can often be minimized by appropriate intervention. For example, timely administration of glucose will prevent brain damage from insulin-induced hypoglycemia. In order to help reduce adverse effects, you must know the following about the drugs you are working with: (1) the major adverse effects that the drug can produce, (2) the time when these reactions are likely to occur, (3) early signs that an adverse reaction is developing, and (4) the interventions that can minimize discomfort and harm.

## Minimizing Adverse Interactions

When a patient is taking two or more drugs, those drugs may interact with one another to diminish therapeutic effects or intensify adverse effects. For example, the ability of oral contraceptives to protect against pregnancy can be reduced by concurrent therapy with phenobarbital (an antiseizure drug), and the risk of thromboembolism from oral contraceptives can be increased by smoking cigarettes.

As a nurse, you can help reduce the incidence and intensity of adverse interactions in several ways. These include taking a thorough drug history, advising the patient to avoid over-the-counter drugs that can interact with the prescribed medication, monitoring for adverse interactions *known* to occur between the drugs the patient is taking, and being alert for as yet *unknown* interactions.

## Making PRN Decisions

A PRN medication order is one in which the nurse has discretion regarding how much drug to give and when to give it. (PRN is an abbreviation that stands for *pro re nata*, a Latin phrase meaning *as needed* or *as the occasion arises*.) PRN orders are most common for hypnotics (sleeping pills). In order to implement a PRN order rationally, you must know the reason for drug use and be able to assess the patient's medication needs. Clearly, the better your knowledge of pharmacology, the better your PRN decisions are likely to be.

## Managing Toxicity

Some adverse drug reactions are extremely dangerous; if toxicity is not diagnosed early and responded to quickly, irreversible injury or death can result. In order to minimize harm, you must know the early signs of toxicity and the procedure for toxicity management.

---

# Application of Pharmacology in Patient Education

---

In most cases, it is the responsibility of the nurse to educate patients about medications. In your role as educator, you must provide the patient with the following information:

- Drug name and therapeutic category (e.g., penicillin: antibiotic)
- Dosage size and dosing schedule
- Route and technique of administration
- Expected therapeutic response and when it should develop
- Nondrug measures to enhance therapeutic responses
- Duration of treatment
- Method of drug storage
- Symptoms of major adverse effects, and measures to minimize discomfort and harm
- Major adverse drug-drug and drug-food interactions
- Whom to contact in the event of therapeutic failure, severe adverse reactions, or severe adverse interactions

In order to communicate this information effectively and accurately, you must first understand it. That is, to be a good educator, you must know pharmacology.

In the discussion below, we will consider the relationship between patient education and the following aspects of drug therapy: dosage and administration, promoting therapeutic effects, minimizing adverse effects, and minimizing adverse interactions.

## Dosage and Administration

***Drug Name.*** The patient should know the name of the medication he or she is taking. If the drug has been prescribed by a trade name, the patient should be given the drug's generic name in addition to the trade name. This information will reduce the risk of overdosage that can result when a patient fails to realize that two prescriptions that bear different names actually contain the same medication.

***Dosage Size and Schedule of Administration.*** Patients must be told how much drug to take and when to take it. For some medications, dosage must be adjusted by the patient. Insulin provides a good example. For insulin therapy to be successful, the patient must adjust the dosage to accommodate alterations in caloric intake. How to make this adjustment is taught by the nurse.

With PRN medications, the schedule of administration is not fixed. Rather, these drugs are taken as conditions require. For example, some people with asthma experience exercise-related respiratory distress. To minimize such attacks, these individuals can take supplementary medication prior to anticipated exertion. It is your responsibility to teach patients when PRN drugs should be taken.

The patient should know what to do if a dose is missed. With oral contraceptives, for example, if one dose is missed, the omitted dose should be taken together with the next scheduled dose. However, if three or more doses are missed, a new cycle of administration must be initiated.

Some patients have difficulty remembering whether or not they have taken their medication. Possible causes include mental illness, advanced age, and complex regimens. To facilitate accurate dosing, you can provide the patient with a pill box that has separate compartments for each day of the week, and then teach him or her to load the compartments weekly. To determine if they have taken their medicine, patients can simply examine the box.

***Technique of Administration.*** Patients must be taught how to administer their drugs. This is especially important for routes that may be unfamiliar (e.g., sublingual for nitroglycerin) and for techniques that are difficult (e.g., subcutaneous injection of insulin). Patients taking oral medications may require special instructions. For example, some oral preparations must not be chewed or crushed; some should be taken with fluids; and some should be taken with meals, whereas others should not. Careful attention must be paid to the patient who, because of disability (e.g., visual or intellectual impairment, limited manual dexterity), may find self-medication difficult.

***Duration of Drug Use.*** Just as patients must know when to take their medicine, they must know when to stop. In some cases (e.g., treatment of acute pain), patients should discontinue drug use as soon as symptoms subside. In other cases (e.g., treatment of hypertension), patients should know that therapy will probably continue lifelong. For other conditions (e.g., gastric ulcers), medication may be prescribed for a specific time interval, after which the patient should return for re-evaluation.

*Drug Storage.* Certain medications are chemically unstable and deteriorate rapidly if stored improperly. Patients who are using unstable drugs must be taught how to store them correctly (e.g., under refrigeration, in light-proof containers). All drugs should be stored where children can't reach them.

## Promoting Therapeutic Effects

In order to participate fully in achieving the therapeutic objective, patients must know the nature and time course of expected beneficial effects. With this knowledge, patients can help evaluate the success or failure of treatment. By recognizing treatment failure, the informed patient will be able to seek timely implementation of alternative therapy.

With some drugs, such as those used to treat depression and schizophrenia, beneficial effects are delayed, taking weeks or months to develop. Awareness that treatment may not produce immediate results will allow the patient to have realistic expectations and will help reduce anxiety about therapeutic failure.

As noted above, nondrug measures can complement drug therapy. For example, although drugs are useful in managing adult-onset diabetes, exercise and caloric restriction are at least as important. Teaching the patient about nondrug measures can greatly increase the chances of success.

## Minimizing Adverse Effects

Knowledge of adverse drug effects will enable the patient to avoid some adverse effects and reduce others through early detection. The following examples should underscore the value of educating patients about the undesired effects of drugs:

- Insulin overdose can cause blood glucose levels to drop precipitously. Early signs of hypoglycemia include sweating and increased heart rate. The patient who has been taught to recognize these early signs can respond by ingesting glucose-rich foods, thereby restoring blood sugar to a safe level. In contrast, the patient who fails to recognize evolving hypoglycemia and does not ingest glucose may become comatose, and may even die.
- Many anticancer drugs predispose patients to acquiring serious infections. The patient who is aware of this possibility can take steps to avoid contagion (e.g., avoiding contact with people who have an infection; avoiding foods likely to contain pathogens). In addition, the informed patient is in a position to notify the physician at the first sign that an infection is developing, thereby allowing rapid treatment. In contrast, the patient who has not received adequate education is at increased risk of death from an infectious disease.
- Some side effects, although benign, can be disturbing if they occur without warning. For example, rifampin (a drug for tuberculosis) imparts a harmless red-orange color to urine, sweat, saliva, and tears. Patients will appreciate knowing about this effect *before* it occurs.

## Minimizing Adverse Interactions

Patient education can help avoid hazardous drug-drug and drug-food interactions. For example, phenelzine (an antidepressant) can cause dangerous elevations in blood pressure if taken in combination with certain drugs (e.g., amphetamines) or certain foods (e.g., most cheeses, figs, avocados). Accordingly, it is essential that patients taking phenelzine be given explicit and emphatic instruction regarding the drugs and foods they must avoid.

## Summary

We began this chapter by asking, "Why should a nursing student learn pharmacology?" To answer the question, we explored the applications of pharmacology in nursing practice. We observed that nursing responsibilities regarding drugs go far beyond the Five Rights of Drug Administration. We observed also that the nurse has a critical role as patient advocate, serving as the patient's last line of defense against medication errors. We then discussed the many ways in which pharmacologic knowledge can be put to practical use in patient care and patient education. We saw that, by applying knowledge of pharmacology, you can have a positive influence on virtually all aspects of drug therapy, thereby helping to maximize benefits and minimize harm. Hopefully your appreciation of the importance of pharmacology in nursing practice, coupled with your desire to provide the best patient care, will provide the motivation you will need to develop an in-depth understanding of drugs.

## KEY POINTS

- Nursing responsibilities with regard to drugs extend far beyond the Five Rights of Drug Administration.
- You are the patient's last line of defense against medication errors.
- Your knowledge of pharmacology has a wide variety of practical applications in patient care and patient education.
- By applying your knowledge of pharmacology, you will make a great contribution to achieving the therapeutic objective of maximum benefit with minimum harm.

# CHAPTER 3

# Pharmacology and the Nursing Process

The nursing process is a conceptual framework that nurses employ to guide health care delivery. In this chapter we will consider how the nursing process can be applied in drug therapy.

## Review of the Nursing Process

Before discussing the nursing process as it applies to drug therapy, we need to review the process itself. Since you are probably familiar with the process already, the review will be brief.

In its simplest form, the nursing process can be viewed as a cyclic procedure that has five basic steps: (1) assessment, (2) analysis (including nursing diagnoses), (3) planning, (4) implementation, and (5) evaluation. These steps are shown schematically in Figure 3–1.

**Assessment.** Assessment consists of collecting data about the patient. These data are used to identify actual and potential health problems. The data base established during assessment provides a foundation for subsequent steps in the process. Important methods of data collection are the patient interview, medical and drug-use histories, the physical examination, observation of the patient, and laboratory tests.

**Analysis: Nursing Diagnoses.** In this step, the nurse analyzes the data base to determine actual and potential health problems. These problems may be physiologic, psychologic, or sociologic. Each problem is stated in the form of a *nursing diagnosis*, which can be defined as an actual or potential health problem that nurses are qualified and licensed to treat.

A complete nursing diagnosis consists of two statements: (1) a statement of the patient's actual or potential health problem, followed by (2) a statement of the problem's probable cause or risk factors. Typically, the statements are separated by the phrase *related to*, as in this example of a drug-associated nursing diagnosis: noncompliance with the prescribed regimen [the problem] related to inability to self-administer medication [the cause].

**Planning.** In the planning step, the nurse delineates specific interventions directed at solving or preventing the problems identified in analysis. The plan must be individualized for each patient. When creating a care plan, the nurse must define goals, set priorities, identify nursing interventions, and establish criteria for evaluating success. In addition to nursing interventions, the plan should include interventions performed by other health care providers. Planning is an ongoing process that must be modified as new data are gathered.

**Implementation (Intervention).** Implementation begins with carrying out the interventions identified during planning. Some interventions are collaborative and others are independent. Collaborative interventions require a physician's order, whereas independent nursing interventions do not. In addition to carrying out interventions, implementation involves coordinating actions of other members of the health care team. Implementation is completed by observing and recording the outcomes of treatment. Records should be thorough and precise.

**Evaluation.** This step is performed to determine the degree to which treatment has been successful. Evaluation is accomplished by analyzing the data collected during implementation. Evaluation should identify those interventions that should be continued, those that should be discontinued, and potential new interventions that should be implemented. Evaluation completes the initial cycle of the nursing process and provides the basis for beginning the cycle anew.

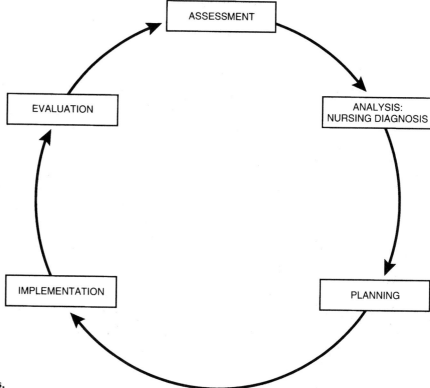

**Figure 3–1. Steps of the nursing process.**

# Application of the Nursing Process in Drug Therapy

Having reviewed the nursing process itself, we can now discuss the process as it pertains to drug therapy. As you will recall from Chapter 1, the overall objective in drug therapy is to produce maximum benefit with minimum harm. To accomplish this objective, we must take into account the unique characteristics of each patient. That is, we must individualize therapy. The nursing process is well suited to help us do this. As the discussion below indicates, in order to apply the nursing process in drug therapy, you must first have a solid knowledge base in pharmacology. You will also see from the discussion that applying the nursing process to drug therapy is, in large part, an exercise in common sense.

## Preadministration Assessment

Preadministration assessment establishes the baseline data needed to tailor drug therapy to the individual. By identifying the variables that can affect an individual's responses to drugs, we can adapt treatment so as to maximize benefits and minimize harm. Preadministration assessment has four basic goals:

- Collection of baseline data needed to evaluate therapeutic responses

- Collection of baseline data needed to evaluate adverse effects
- Identification of high-risk patients
- Assessment of the patient's capacity for self-care

The first three goals are specific to the particular drug being used. Accordingly, in order to achieve these goals, you must know the pharmacology of the drug under consideration. The fourth goal applies more or less equally to all drugs—although this goal may be more critical for some drugs than others.

Important methods of data collection include interviews with the patient and family, observation of the patient, physical examination, laboratory tests, the patient's medical history, and the patient's drug history. The drug history should include prescription drugs, over-the-counter drugs, and drugs taken for nonmedical purposes (alcohol, nicotine, caffeine, illicit drugs). Prior adverse drug reactions should be noted, including drug allergies and idiosyncratic reactions.

**Baseline Data Needed to Evaluate Therapeutic Effects.** Drugs are administered to achieve a desired response. In order to know if we have produced that response, we need to establish baseline measurements of the parameter that therapy is directed at changing. For example, if we are giving a drug to lower blood pressure, we need to know what the patient's blood pressure was prior to treatment. Without this information, we have no basis for determining the effect of our drug. And if we can't determine whether or not a drug is working, there's little justification for giving it. From the above example, it should be obvious that in order to know what baseline measurements to make, you must first know the reason for drug use. This knowledge comes in large part from studying pharmacology.

***Baseline Data Needed to Evaluate Adverse Effects.*** All drugs have the ability to produce undesired effects. In practically all cases, the adverse effects that a particular drug can produce are known. In many cases, development of an adverse effect will be completely obvious in the absence of any baseline data. For example, we don't need special baseline data to know that hair loss following cancer chemotherapy was caused by the drug. However, in other cases, baseline data are needed to determine whether or not an adverse effect has occurred. For example, some drugs can impair liver function. In order to know if a drug has disrupted liver function, we need to know the state of liver function prior to drug use. Without this information, we can't tell from later measurements whether apparent liver dysfunction was pre-existing or caused by the drug. Clearly, in cases like this, baseline data are needed. As noted earlier, knowing what data to collect comes directly from your knowledge of the drug under consideration.

***Identification of High-Risk Patients.*** Because of his or her individual characteristics, a particular patient may be at high risk of experiencing adverse responses to a particular drug. Just which individual characteristics will predispose a patient to adverse reactions depends on the drug under consideration. For example, if a drug is eliminated from the body primarily by renal excretion, an individual with impaired kidney function will be at risk of having this drug accumulate to toxic levels. Similarly, if a drug is eliminated by the liver, an individual with impaired liver function will be at risk of having that drug accumulate to toxic levels. The message here is that, in order to identify the patient at risk, you must know the pharmacology of the drug to be administered.

Multiple factors can increase the patient's risk of adverse reactions to a particular drug. Impaired liver and kidney function were just mentioned. Other characteristics that can predispose the patient to adverse responses include age, body composition, pregnancy, diet, genetic heritage, other drugs being used concurrently, and practically any pathophysiologic condition. These factors are discussed at length in Chapter 7 (Drug-Drug and Drug-Food Interactions), Chapter 8 (Adverse Drug Reactions), Chapter 9 (Individual Variation in Drug Responses), Chapter 10 (Drug Therapy during Pregnancy and Breast Feeding), Chapter 11 (Drug Therapy in Pediatric Patients), and Chapter 12 (Drug Therapy in Geriatric Patients).

When identifying factors that put the patient at risk, you should distinguish between factors that put the patient at extremely high risk versus factors that put the patient at moderate or low risk. The terms *contraindication* and *precaution* can be used for this distinction. A contraindication is defined as a pre-existing condition that precludes use of a particular drug under all but the most desperate circumstances. For example, a previous severe allergic reaction to penicillin (which can be life threatening) would be a contraindication to using penicillin again—unless the patient had a life-threatening infection that could not be controlled with other antibiotics. A precaution, by contrast, can be defined as a pre-existing condition that significantly increases the risk of an adverse reaction to a particular drug, but not to a degree that is life threatening. For example, a previous mild allergic reaction to penicillin would constitute a precaution to using this drug again. That is, the drug may be used, but greater than normal caution must be exercised. Preferably, an alternative drug would be selected.

***Assessment of the Patient's Capacity for Self-Care.*** If drug therapy is to succeed, the outpatient must be willing and able to self-administer medication as prescribed. Accordingly, his or her capacity for self-care must be assessed. If assessment reveals that the patient is incapable of self-medication, alternative care must be arranged.

Multiple factors can affect the capacity for self-care and the probability of adhering to the prescribed regimen. The patient with reduced visual acuity or limited manual dexterity may be unable to self-medicate, especially if the technique of administration is complex. The patient with limited intellectual ability may be incapable of understanding or remembering what he or she is supposed to do. The patient with severe mental illness (e.g., depression, schizophrenia) may lack the understanding or motivation needed to self-medicate. Some patients may lack the money to pay for drugs. Others may fail to take medications as prescribed because of individual or cultural attitudes toward drugs. Among geriatric patients, the most common cause for failed self-medication is a conviction that the drug was simply not needed in the dosage prescribed. A thorough assessment will identify all of these factors, thereby enabling you to account for them when formulating nursing diagnoses and the patient care plan.

## Analysis and Nursing Diagnoses

With respect to drug therapy, the analysis phase of the nursing process has three objectives. First, you must judge the appropriateness of the prescribed regimen. Second, you must identify potential health problems that the drug might cause. Third, you must determine the patient's capacity for self-care.

As the last link in the patient's chain of defense against inappropriate drug therapy, the nurse must analyze the data collected during assessment to determine if the proposed treatment has a reasonable likelihood of being effective and safe. This judgment is made by considering the medical diagnosis, the known actions of the prescribed drug, the patient's prior responses to the drug, and the presence of contraindications to the drug. You should question the drug's appropriateness if (1) the drug has no actions that are known to benefit individuals with the patient's medical diagnosis, (2) the patient failed to respond to the drug in the past, (3) the patient had a serious adverse reaction to the drug in the past, or (4) the patient has a condition or is using a drug that contraindicates the prescribed drug. If any of these conditions apply, you

## TABLE 3-1. EXAMPLES OF NURSING DIAGNOSIS THAT CAN BE DERIVED FROM KNOWLEDGE OF ADVERSE DRUG EFFECTS

| Drug | Adverse Effect | Related Nursing Diagnosis |
|---|---|---|
| Amphetamine | CNS stimulation | Altered sleep pattern related to drug-induced CNS excitation |
| Aspirin | Gastric erosion | Pain related to aspirin-induced gastric erosion |
| Atropine | Urinary retention | Urinary retention related to drug therapy |
| Bethanechol | Stimulation of GI smooth muscle | Bowel incontinence related to drug-induced increase in bowel motility |
| Clonidine | Impotence | Sexual dysfunction related to drug-induced impotence |
| Cyclophosphamide | Reduction in white blood cell counts | Potential for infection related to drug-induced neutropenia |
| Digoxin | Dysrhythmias | Reduced tissue perfusion related to drug-induced cardiac dysrhythmias |
| Furosemide | Excessive urine production | Fluid volume deficit related to drug-induced diuresis |
| Gentamicin | Damage to the eighth cranial nerve | Perceptual/sensory alteration: hearing impairment related to drug therapy |
| Glucocorticoids | Thinning of the skin | Impaired skin integrity related to drug therapy |
| Haloperidol | Involuntary movements | Disturbance in self-esteem related to drug-induced involuntary movements |
| Nitroglycerin | Hypotension | Potential for injury related to dizziness caused by drug-induced hypotension |
| Propranolol | Bradycardia | Decreased cardiac output related to drug-induced bradycardia |
| Warfarin | Spontaneous bleeding | Potential for injury related to drug-induced bleeding |

CNS = central nervous system, GI = gastrointestinal.

should consult with the prescribing physician to determine if the drug should be given.

Analysis must identify potential adverse effects and drug interactions. This is accomplished by synthesizing knowledge of the drug under consideration and the data collected during assessment. Knowledge of the drug itself will indicate adverse effects that practically all patients are likely to experience. Data on the individual patient will indicate additional adverse effects and interactions to which the particular patient is predisposed. Once potential adverse effects and interactions have been identified, pertinent nursing diagnoses can be easily formulated. For example, if treatment is likely to cause respiratory depression, an appropriate nursing diagnosis would be: impaired gas exchange related to drug therapy. Table 3-1 presents additional examples of nursing diagnoses that can be readily derived from knowledge of the adverse effects and interactions that treatment may cause.

Analysis must characterize the patient's capacity for self-care. The analysis should indicate potential impediments to self-care (e.g., visual impairment, reduced manual dexterity, impaired cognitive function, insufficient understanding of the prescribed regimen) so that these factors can be addressed in the care plan. To varying degrees, nearly all patients will be unfamiliar with self-medication and the drug regimen. Accordingly, a nursing diagnosis applicable to almost every patient is: knowledge deficit related to the drug regimen.

## Planning

Planning consists of defining goals, establishing priorities, identifying specific interventions, and establishing criteria for evaluating success. Good planning will allow you to

promote beneficial drug effects. Of equal or greater importance, good planning will allow you to anticipate adverse effects—rather than react to them after the fact.

**Defining Goals.** In all cases, the goal of drug therapy is to produce maximum benefits with minimum harm. That is, we want to employ drugs in such a way as to maximize therapeutic responses while preventing or minimizing adverse reactions and interactions. The objective of planning is to formulate ways to achieve this goal.

**Setting Priorities.** This requires knowledge of the drug under consideration and the patient's unique characteristics—and even then, setting priorities can be difficult. Highest priority is given to life-threatening conditions (e.g., anaphylactic shock, ventricular fibrillation). These may be drug induced or the result of disease. High priority is also given to reactions that cause severe, acute discomfort and to reactions that can result in long-term harm. Since we cannot manage all problems simultaneously, less severe problems must wait until the patient and care provider have the time and resources to address them.

**Identifying Interventions.** The heart of planning is identification of nursing interventions. These interventions can be divided into four major groups: (1) drug administration, (2) interventions to enhance therapeutic effects, (3) interventions to minimize adverse effects and interactions, and (4) patient education (which encompasses information in the first three groups).

When planning drug administration, you must consider dosage size, route of administration, and less obvious factors, including timing of administration with respect to meals and to administration of other drugs. Timing with respect to side effects is also important. For example, if a drug causes sedation, it may be desirable to give the drug at bedtime, rather than in the morning or during the day.

Nondrug measures can help promote therapeutic effects and should be included in the plan. For example, drug therapy of hypertension can be combined with weight loss (in obese patients), salt restriction, and cessation of smoking.

Interventions to prevent or minimize adverse effects are of obvious importance. When planning these interventions, you should distinguish between reactions that develop quickly and those that are delayed. A few drugs can cause severe adverse reactions (e.g., anaphylactic shock) shortly after administration. When planning to administer such a drug, you should ensure that facilities for managing possible reactions are immediately available. Delayed reactions can often be minimized, if not avoided entirely. The plan should include interventions to do so.

Well-planned patient education is central to success. The plan should account for the patient's capacity to learn, and it should address the following: technique of administration, dosage size and timing, duration of treatment, method of drug storage, measures to promote therapeutic effects, and measures to minimize adverse effects. Patient education is discussed at length in Chapter 2.

***Establishing Criteria for Evaluation.*** The need for objective criteria by which to measure desired drug responses is obvious: without such criteria we could not determine if our drug was doing anything useful. As a result, we would have no rational basis for making dosage adjustments and for deciding how long treatment should continue. If the drug is to be used on an outpatient basis, follow-up visits for evaluation should be planned.

## Implementation

Implementation of the care plan in drug therapy has four major components: (1) drug administration, (2) patient education, (3) interventions to promote therapeutic effects, and (4) interventions to minimize adverse effects. These critical nursing activities are discussed at length in Chapter 2.

## Evaluation

Over the course of drug therapy, the patient must be evaluated for (1) therapeutic responses, (2) adverse drug reactions and interactions, (3) compliance (adherence to the prescribed regimen), and (4) satisfaction with treatment. How frequently evaluations are performed depends on the expected time course of therapeutic and adverse effects. Like assessment, evaluation is based on laboratory tests, observation of the patient, physical examination, and patient interviews. The conclusions drawn during evaluation provide the basis for modifying nursing interventions and the drug regimen.

Therapeutic responses are evaluated by comparing the patient's current health status with the baseline data. In order to evaluate treatment, you must know the reason for drug use, the criteria for success (as defined during planning), and the expected time course of responses (some drugs act within minutes, whereas others may take weeks or even months to produce beneficial effects).

The need to anticipate and evaluate adverse effects is self-evident. To make these evaluations, you must know which adverse effects are likely to occur, how they are manifested, and their probable time course. The method of monitoring is determined by the expected effect. For example, if hypotension is expected, blood pressure is monitored; if constipation is expected, bowel function is monitored; and so on. Since some adverse effects can be fatal in the absence of timely detection, it is impossible to overemphasize the importance of monitoring and preparedness for rapid intervention.

Evaluation of compliance is desirable in all patients—and is especially valuable when therapeutic failure occurs or when adverse effects are unexpectedly severe. Methods of evaluating compliance include measurement of plasma drug levels, interviewing the patient, and counting pills. The evaluation should determine if the patient understands when to take medication, what dosage to take, and the technique of administration.

Patient satisfaction with drug therapy increases quality of life and promotes compliance. If the patient is dissatisfied, an otherwise effective regimen may not be taken as prescribed. Factors that can cause dissatisfaction include unacceptable side effects, an inconvenient dosing schedule, difficulty of administration, and high cost. When evaluation reveals dissatisfaction, an attempt should be made to alter the drug regimen to make it more acceptable.

## Use of a Modified Nursing Process Format to Summarize Nursing Implications in This Text

Throughout this text, nursing implications are *integrated into the body of each chapter.* The reason for integrating nursing information with basic science information is to reinforce the relationship between pharmacologic knowledge and nursing practice. In addition to being integrated, nursing implications are *summarized at the end of most chapters.* The purpose of the summaries is to provide a concise and readily accessible reference on patient care and patient education related to specific drugs and drug families.

The format employed for the summaries of nursing implications reflects the nursing process (Table 3–2). However, as you can see, we have modified the headings somewhat. This was done to accommodate the needs of pharmacology instruction and to keep the summaries concise. The components of the format are discussed below.

***Preadministration Assessment.*** This section summarizes the information you should have before giving a drug. Each section begins by stating the reason for drug use. This is followed by a summary of the baseline data needed to evaluate therapeutic and adverse effects. After

## TABLE 3-2. MODIFIED NURSING PROCESS FORMAT FOR SUMMARIES OF NURSING IMPLICATIONS

Preadministration Assessment
    Therapeutic Goal
    Baseline Data
    Identifying High-Risk Patients
Implementation: Administration
    Routes
    Administration
Implementation: Measures to Enhance Therapeutic Effects
Ongoing Evaluation and Interventions
    Summary of Monitoring
    Evaluating Therapeutic Effects
    Minimizing Adverse Effects
    Minimizing Adverse Interactions

this, contraindications and precautions are summarized under the heading *Identifying High-Risk Patients.*

***Implementation: Administration.*** This section summarizes routes of administration, guidelines for dosage adjustment, and special considerations in administration, such as timing with respect to meals, preparation of intravenous solutions, and unusual techniques of administration.

***Implementation: Measures to Enhance Therapeutic Effects.*** This section addresses issues such as diet modification, measures to increase comfort, and ways to promote adherence to the prescribed regimen.

***Ongoing Evaluation and Interventions.*** This section summarizes nursing implications that relate to drug responses, both therapeutic and undesired. As indicated in Table 3-2, the section has four subsections: (1) summary of monitoring, (2) evaluating therapeutic effects, (3) minimizing adverse effects, and (4) minimizing adverse interactions. The monitoring section summarizes the physiologic and psychologic parameters that must be monitored in order to evaluate therapeutic and adverse responses. The section on therapeutic effects summarizes criteria and procedures for evaluating therapeutic responses. The section on adverse effects summarizes the major adverse reactions that should be monitored for and presents interventions to minimize them. The section on adverse interactions summarizes the major drug interactions to be alert for and gives interventions to minimize them.

***Patient Education.*** This topic does not have a section of its own. Rather, patient education is integrated into the other sections. That is, as we summarize the nursing implications that relate to a particular topic, such as drug administration or a specific adverse effect, patient education related to that topic is discussed concurrently. This integration is done to promote clarity and efficiency of com-

munication. In order to make this important information stand out, it appears in color.

***What about Diagnosis and Planning?*** These headings are not used in the summaries. There are several reasons for the omission, the dominant one being efficiency of communication.

Nursing diagnoses have been left out because they are extremely numerous and largely self-evident. Yes, we could have included a list of diagnoses for each drug. However, since nursing diagnoses derive from drug effects, and since all drugs cause many effects (primarily adverse), the list of diagnoses for each drug would be very long. Accordingly, since nursing diagnoses can be readily formulated from one's knowledge of pharmacology, and since a long list of diagnoses would dilute the impact of other important information, we decided to omit nursing diagnoses from the summaries.

Planning has not been used as a heading for three reasons. First, planning applies primarily to the overall management of the disorder for which a particular drug is being used—and much less to the drug itself. Second, since planning is discussed at length and more appropriately in nonpharmacology nursing texts, such as those on medical-surgical nursing, there is no need to repeat this information here. Third, most planning is done with the aid of standardized nursing care plans—either computerized or in print format. These standardized plans are sufficient for most drug-related planning. Please note, however, that although we don't have a separate heading for planning, critical issues in planning are included nonetheless.

## KEY POINTS

- Application of the nursing process in drug therapy is directed at individualizing treatment, which is critical to achieving the therapeutic objective: maximum benefit with minimum harm.
- The goal of preadministration assessment is to gather data needed for (1) evaluation of therapeutic and adverse effects, (2) identification of high-risk patients, and (3) assessment of the patient's capacity for self-care.
- The analysis and diagnosis phase of treatment is directed at (1) judging the appropriateness of the prescribed therapy, (2) identification of potential health problems treatment might cause, and (3) characterization of the patient's capacity for self-care.
- Planning is directed at (1) defining goals, (2) establishing priorities, and (3) establishing criteria for evaluating success.
- In the evaluation stage, the objective is to evaluate (1) therapeutic responses, (2) adverse reactions and interactions, (3) patient compliance, and (4) patient satisfaction with treatment.

# CHAPTER 4

# Drug Legislation, Development, Names, and Information

n this chapter we complete our introduction to pharmacology by considering four diverse but important topics. These are (1) drug regulation, (2) new drug development, (3) the annoying problem of drug names, and (4) sources of drug information.

## Drug Regulation

The history of drug legislation in the United States reflects an evolution in our national posture toward regulating the pharmaceutical industry. That posture has changed from one of minimal control to one of extensive control. For the most part, increased regulation has been beneficial, resulting in safer and more effective drugs.

The first American law to regulate drugs was the *Federal Pure Food and Drug Act of 1906.* This law was very weak: Its only requirement was that drugs be *free of adulterants.* The law said nothing about drug safety and effectiveness.

*The Food, Drug and Cosmetic Act,* passed in 1938, was much stronger than the Pure Food and Drug Act and was the first legislation to regulate drug *safety.* The motivation for the 1938 law was a tragedy in which more than 100 people died following use of a new medication. The lethal preparation contained an antibiotic (sulfanilamide) plus a solubilizing agent (diethylene glycol). Tests revealed that the solvent was the cause of death. (Diethylene glycol is commonly used as automotive antifreeze.) To reduce the chances that such a tragedy might recur, Congress required that all new drugs undergo testing for toxicity. The results of these tests were to be reviewed by the *Food and Drug Administration* (FDA), and only those drugs judged to be safe would receive FDA approval for marketing.

The next major development in drug regulation came in 1962 with the passage of the *Kefauver-Harris Amendments* to the Food, Drug and Cosmetic Act, passed in 1962. This law was created in response to the thalidomide tragedy, which occurred in Europe in the early 1960s. Thalidomide is a sedative now known to cause birth defects. Because the drug was used widely by pregnant women, over 10,000 infants were born with phocomelia, a rare birth defect characterized by the gross malformation or complete absence of arms or legs. This tragedy was especially poignant in that it resulted from nonessential drug use: The women who took thalidomide could have done very well without it. Thalidomide was not a problem in the United States because the drug had been withheld by the FDA.

Because of the European experience with thalidomide, the Kefauver-Harris Amendments sought to strengthen all aspects of drug regulation. One of the bill's major provisions was to require proof of *effectiveness* before a new drug could be marketed. Remarkably, this was the first law to demand that drugs actually be of some benefit. The new act also required that all old drugs that had been introduced between 1932 and 1962 undergo testing for effectiveness; those drugs that could not be proved useful would be withdrawn. Lastly, the Kefauver-Harris Act established rigorous procedures for testing new drugs. These procedures are discussed below under *New Drug Development.*

In 1970, Congress passed the *Controlled Substances Act* (Title II of the Comprehensive Drug Abuse Prevention and Control Act). This legislation set rules for the manufacture and distribution of drugs considered to have potential for abuse. One provision of the law defines categories into which controlled substances are placed. These categories are labeled Schedules I, II, III, IV, and V. Drugs in Schedule I have no accepted medical use in the

United States and are deemed to have a high potential for abuse. Examples include heroin, mescaline, and lysergic acid diethylamide (LSD). Drugs in Schedules II through V have accepted medical applications but also have the potential for abuse. The abuse potential of these agents becomes progressively less as we proceed from Schedule II to Schedule V. The Controlled Substances Act is discussed further in Chapter 35 (Drug Abuse: General Considerations).

In 1992, FDA regulations were changed to permit accelerated approval of drugs for life-threatening or severely debilitating disease, such as acquired immunodeficiency syndrome and cancer. Under the new guidelines, a drug could be approved for marketing prior to completion of phase III trials (see below), provided that rigorous follow-up studies were performed. The rationale for this change was that the unknown risks associated with early approval are balanced by the need for effective drugs.

# New Drug Development

The development and testing of new drugs is an expensive and lengthy process, requiring from 6 to 12 years for completion. It is estimated that for every 5000 compounds that enter testing, only one emerges as a new product.

Rigorous procedures for testing have been established so that newly released drugs might be both safe and effective. Unfortunately, although testing can determine effectiveness, it cannot guarantee that a new drug will be safe: Significant adverse effects may evade detection during testing only to become apparent once a new drug has been released for general use.

## Stages of New Drug Development

The testing of new drugs has two principal steps: *preclinical testing* and *clinical testing*. Preclinical tests are performed in animals. Clinical tests are done in humans. The steps in drug development are outlined in Table 4-1.

### Preclinical Testing

Preclinical testing is required before a new drug may be tested in humans. During preclinical testing, drugs are evaluated for *toxicities, pharmacokinetic properties,* and *potentially useful biologic effects.* Preclinical tests may take 1 to 5 years. When sufficient preclinical data have been gathered, the drug developer may apply to the FDA for permission to begin testing in humans. If the application is approved, the drug is awarded *Investigational New Drug* status and clinical trials may commence.

### Clinical Testing

Clinical trials occur in four phases and may take 2 to 10 years for completion. The first three phases are done before a new drug is marketed. The fourth phase is done after marketing has begun.

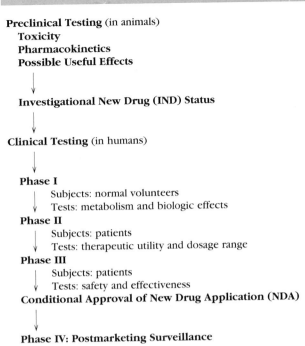

**TABLE 4-1. STEPS IN NEW DRUG DEVELOPMENT**

**Preclinical Testing** (in animals)
   **Toxicity**
   **Pharmacokinetics**
   **Possible Useful Effects**

**Investigational New Drug (IND) Status**

**Clinical Testing** (in humans)

**Phase I**
   Subjects: normal volunteers
   Tests: metabolism and biologic effects
**Phase II**
   Subjects: patients
   Tests: therapeutic utility and dosage range
**Phase III**
   Subjects: patients
   Tests: safety and effectiveness
**Conditional Approval of New Drug Application (NDA)**

**Phase IV: Postmarketing Surveillance**

***Phase I.*** Phase I trials are usually conducted in normal volunteers. However, if a drug is likely to have severe side effects, as many anticancer drugs do, the trial is done in volunteer patients who have the disease under consideration, rather than in normal volunteers. The goal of phase I testing is twofold: evaluation of drug metabolism and determination of effects in humans.

***Phases II and III.*** In these phases, drugs are tested in *patients.* The objective is to determine therapeutic effects, dosage range, and safety. The total number of patients who receive the drug in phases II and III is only 500 to 3000; of these, only a few hundred take the drug for more than 3 to 6 months. Upon completing phase III, the drug developer applies to the FDA for conditional approval of a New Drug Application. If conditional approval is granted, phase IV may begin.

***Phase IV: Postmarketing Surveillance.*** In phase IV, the new drug is released for general use, permitting observation of its effects in a large population. Frequently, new adverse effects are revealed. The success of phase IV depends on voluntary reporting by prescribing physicians.

## Limitations of the Testing Procedure

It is important for nurses and other health care professionals to appreciate the limitations of the drug development process. Two problems are of particular concern. First, information on beneficial and adverse effects in women is very limited. Second, new drugs are likely to have adverse effects that were not detected during clinical trials.

## Limited Information in Women

Very little drug testing is done in women. In practically all cases, women of child-bearing potential are excluded from early clinical trials. The rationale for this exclusion is concern for fetal safety. Unfortunately, FDA policy has taken this concern to an extreme, effectively barring all women of child-bearing age from phase I and phase II trials—whether or not they are actually pregnant or using adequate contraception. At this time, the only women allowed to participate in early clinical trials are those who have life-threatening illnesses that might respond to the drugs under study.

Because of limited drug testing in women, we don't know with precision how women will respond to drugs. We don't know if beneficial effects in women will be equivalent to those seen in men. Nor do we know if adverse effects will be equivalent to those in men. We don't know how timing of drug administration with respect to the menstrual cycle will affect beneficial and adverse responses. We don't know if drug disposition (absorption, distribution, metabolism, excretion) will be the same in women as in men. Furthermore, of the various drugs that might be used to treat a particular illness, we don't know if the ones that are most effective in men will also be most effective in women. Lastly, we don't know about the safety of drug use during pregnancy.

The FDA indicated that it will revise its guidelines to remove some of the restrictions that now bar women of child-bearing age from early trials. However, even if this is done, it will take a long time to close the gender gap in our knowledge of drugs.

## Failure to Detect All Adverse Effects

The testing procedure cannot detect all adverse effects before a new drug is released. There are three reasons for this problem: (1) during clinical trials a relatively small number of patients are given the drug; (2) because these patients are carefully selected, they do not represent the variety of individuals who will eventually take the drug; and (3) patients in trials take the drug for a relatively short time. Because of these unavoidable limitations in the testing process, effects that occur infrequently and effects that take a long time to develop may go undetected. Hence, despite our best efforts, when a new drug is released, it may well have adverse effects of which we are as yet unaware.

Consequently, when working with a new drug, you should be especially watchful for previously unreported drug reactions. If a patient taking a new drug begins to show unusual symptoms, it is prudent to suspect that the new drug may be the cause—even though the symptoms are not yet mentioned in the literature.

## Exercising Discretion Regarding New Drugs

When thinking about prescribing a new drug, the clinician would do well to follow this guideline: *Be neither the first to adopt the new nor the last to abandon the old.*

Recall that the therapeutic objective is to produce maximum benefit with minimum harm. To achieve this objective, we must balance the inherent risks in giving a drug against its potential benefits. As a rule, new drugs have actions very similar to those of older agents. That is, it is rare for a new drug to be able to do something that an older drug can't do already. Consequently, the need to treat a particular disorder seldom constitutes a compelling reason to select a new drug over an agent that has been available for years. Furthermore, new drugs generally present greater risks than the old ones. As noted above, at the time of its introduction, a new drug is likely to have adverse effects that have not yet been reported, and these effects may prove very bad for some patients. In contrast, older, more familiar drugs are less likely to cause unpleasant surprises. Consequently, when we weigh the benefits of a new drug against the risks, it is likely that the benefits will be insufficient to justify the risks—especially when an older drug whose properties are well known would probably provide adequate treatment. Accordingly, when it comes to the use of new drugs, it is usually better to adopt a wait-and-see policy, letting more adventurous clinicians discover the hidden dangers that a new drug may present.

## Drug Names

The topic of drug names is important and can be confusing. The topic is important because the names we employ affect our ability to communicate about medicines. The subject is confusing because we have evolved a system in which any drug can have a large number of names.

In approaching the discussion of drug names, we begin by defining the types of names that drugs have. After that we consider (1) the complications that arise from assigning multiple names to a drug, and (2) the benefits of using just one name: the generic (nonproprietary) name.

### The Three Types of Drug Names

Drugs have three types of names: (1) a chemical name, (2) a generic or nonproprietary name, and (3) a trade or proprietary name. Examples of these names appear in Table 4-2. All of the names in the table are for the same drug, a compound most familiar to us under the trade name Tylenol.

***Chemical Name.*** The chemical name constitutes a description of a drug using the nomenclature of chemistry. As you can see from the example in Table 4-2, a drug's chemical name can be long and complex. Because of their complexity, chemical names are inappropriate for everyday use. For example, few people would communicate using the chemical term *N-acetyl-para-aminophenol* when a more simple generic name (acetaminophen) or trade name (e.g., Tylenol) could be used.

***Generic Name.*** The generic name of a drug is assigned by the United States Adopted Names Council. Each drug has only one generic name. The generic name is also

## TABLE 4–2. THE THREE TYPES OF DRUG NAMES

$$H_3C-\overset{\overset{\displaystyle O}{\|}}{C}-\overset{\overset{\displaystyle H}{|}}{N}-\underset{}{\bigcirc}-OH$$

| Type of Drug Name | Examples |
|---|---|
| *Chemical Name* | *N*-Acetyl-*para*-aminophenol |
| *Generic Name* (nonproprietary name) | Acetaminophen |
| *Trade Name* (proprietary name) | Acephen, Aceta, Anacin-3, Apacet, Arthritis Pain Formula Aspirin Free, Aspirin Free Pain Relief, Banesin, Bromo Seltzer, Dapa, Datril, Dolanex, Dorcol Children's Fever and Pain Reducer, Feverall, Genapap, Genebs, Halenol, Liquiprin Elixir, Meda Tab, Myapap, Neopap, Oraphen-PD, Panadol, Panex, Panex 500, Phenaphen Caplets, Snaplets-FR Granules, St. Joseph Aspirin-Free for Children, Suppap-325, Tapanol Extra Strength, Tempra, Tylenol |

The chemical, generic, and trade names listed are all names for the drug whose structure is pictured in this table. This drug is most familiar to us as Tylenol, one of its trade names.

## TABLE 4–3. GENERIC NAMES AND TRADE NAMES OF SOME COMMONLY USED DRUGS

| Generic Name | Trade Name |
|---|---|
| Chlordiazepoxide | Librium |
| Ibuprofen | Motrin |
| Furosemide | Lasix |
| Fluoxetine | Prozac |
| Acetaminophen | Tylenol |
| Cephalexin | Keflex |

known as the *nonproprietary* name. Generic names are less complex than chemical names but usually more complex than trade names. For reasons presented below, generic names are preferable to trade names for general use.

**Trade Name.** Trade names, also known as *proprietary* or *brand* names, are the names under which a drug is marketed. These names are created by drug companies with the intention that they be easy for nurses, physicians, and consumers to recall and pronounce. Since any drug can be marketed in different formulations and by multiple companies, the number of trade names that a drug can have is large. By way of illustration, Table 4–2 gives the 31 trade names, including Tylenol, that exist for the drug whose generic name is *acetaminophen.*

Trade names must be approved by the FDA. The review process tries to ensure that no two trade names are too similar. In addition, trade names cannot imply unlikely efficacy—which may explain why dexfenfluramine (a new diet pill) is named *Redux* rather than something more suggestive, like *Fat-B-Gone* or *PoundsOff.*

## Which Name To Use, Generic or Trade?

We employ drug names in two ways: (1) for written and verbal communication about medicines and (2) to put on labels to identify medications in containers. In both cases, accurate communication is imperative. For communica-

tion to be accurate, when we read or hear a drug name, we must know what compound that name is referring to. We can't know what's in a pill if we don't know what the name on its bottle means. Likewise, we can't communicate verbally about drugs if the names we employ go unrecognized. Clearly, if we are to communicate accurately, name recognition is essential. As discussed below, name recognition would be enhanced through universal use of generic names.

### The Little Problems with Generic Names

In almost all cases, the generic name for a drug is longer and more complicated than the trade name. This fact is illustrated in Table 4–3, which compares the generic and trade names for six common drugs. A simple analysis reveals that the average generic name in the table has 4.8 syllables. In contrast, the average trade name has only 2.5 syllables. That is, the generic names are nearly twice as long as the trade names.

Because generic names are more complex than trade names, generic names can be more difficult to remember and pronounce. As an exercise, try pronouncing the names in Table 4–3. While trade names like Motrin and Prozac roll off the tongue with ease, their generic counterparts—ibuprofen and fluoxetine—tend to tie the tongue in knots.

Why is it that generic names are more complicated than trade names? One reason is that the pharmaceutical industry has an important role in establishing generic names. When a pharmaceutical company has developed a new drug, that company submits a suggested generic name to the United States Adopted Names Council, the body responsible for assigning a drug its generic name. As a rule, the Council adopts the name the company suggests. Since, from a marketing perspective, it's to the company's advantage to have a product whose trade name is more easily recognized than its generic name, it seems unlikely that a company will suggest a simple, euphonious generic name. Also contributing to the complexity of generic names are the guidelines established by the Council for naming drugs.

### The Big Problems with Trade Names

*The Problem of Multiple Names for the Same Medication.* The principal objection to trade names is their vast number. Although a drug can have only one generic name, the number of trade names it can have is unlimited. As the number of trade names for a single drug increases, the burden of name recognition becomes progressively larger. By way of illustration, the drug whose generic name is acetaminophen has trade names that number in excess of 30 (see Table 4-2). Although most clinicians will recognize this drug's generic name, few are familiar with all of the trade names. As we can see, even though a generic name may be complex, to recall a single generic name for a particular drug remains an easier task than to recall a multitude of trade names for that same drug. Accordingly, if generic names were to be employed universally, accurate communication would be facilitated. Conversely, the use of multiple trade names can do nothing but create confusion.

By clouding communication about drugs, use of trade names can result in "double medication," with potentially disastrous results. Because a patient frequently sees more than one physician, it is possible for a patient to be given prescriptions for the same drug by two different doctors. If those prescriptions are written for different brand names, then the two bottles the patient receives will be labeled with different names. Consequently, although both bottles contain the same drug, the patient may be unaware of this fact. If both medications are taken as prescribed, excessive dosing will result. However, if generic names had been used, both labels would bear the same name, thereby informing the patient that both bottles contain the same drug. Given this information, the patient is likely to consult with the prescribing physicians to determine if both prescriptions should be honored.

**The Problem of Using Trade Names for Combination Products.** Many pharmaceutical preparations are composed of more than one drug. When such combination products are referred to by trade name, the name is unlikely to indicate either the number of drugs present or their identity. Referring to Table 4-4, there is nothing about the trade name *Excedrin Tablets* to suggest that the product bearing this name consists of three different drugs: aspirin, acetaminophen, and caffeine. By discarding the trade name and labeling this product *aspirin plus acetaminophen plus caffeine*, we could eliminate confusion about its composition.

The two *4-Way* products listed in Table 4-4 illustrate the potential for trade names to be misleading, resulting in in-

accurate communication. If nothing else, the name *4-Way* suggests that the product contains more than one drug. In fact, the name seems to imply the presence of *four* drugs. However, as can be seen from the table, this implication is not correct: neither 4-Way preparation is composed of four drugs. One preparation—4-Way Long-Lasting Nasal Spray—contains only one drug. The other preparation—4-Way Fast-Acting Nasal Spray—contains three drugs. Furthermore, please note that these similarly named products are, in fact, completely different from each other; they have no ingredients in common. Hence, in the case of these 4-Way products, we can see that the trade name cannot be taken to mean either (1) the presence of four different drugs, or (2) that these preparations that bear similar names have the same composition. Had generic names been employed to label these products, there could be no confusion about their makeup.

## What If Peas Were Marketed Like Drugs?

Given the problems that trade names create, why do we use trade names at all? We use trade names because the pharmaceutical industry wants them. Why? Because trade names give this industry a unique and powerful tool with which to market its products. As we shall see, the extent to which trade names are exploited to promote drug sales is without parallel in the marketing of any other product.

To understand the immense marketing value that trade names have for the drug companies, it will be helpful to consider the marketing of a product that is not a drug. Take peas, for example. All companies that sell peas use the same name—peas—to identify their product. When we buy peas, no matter whose, all pea packages say PEAS in big letters on the label. Pea packages even have a picture of peas to help us properly identify what's inside. Consequently, when we choose a package of peas, we know with certainty what we're buying.

When we want to compare different brands of peas, the task is easy. Company A's peas are easily distinguished from those of company B or company C by the presence of a company name on the label. Consequently, thanks to the way peas are marketed, we have no trouble understanding (1) just what we are buying, and (2) who made it. As a result, we can easily select the product we want from the manufacturer we like best.

Now let's consider what we could expect if peas were marketed like drugs. Under the new system, pea packages would have no pictures of peas on them. Nor would pea packages proclaim PEAS in big letters to help us identify their contents. Instead, pea packages would be emblazoned with trade names—names like *Vegi-P* or *Producin* or *NuPod-500's*. If peas were marketed using trade names, when we went shopping for peas we'd be obliged to read a lot of fine print to find the product we wanted. And once we finally did turn up a package with peas in it—for example, the one labeled *NuPod-500's*—we'd probably buy *NuPod-500's* for life, it being too much trouble to figure out which of the other packages with meaningless names on them also contain peas. From the point of view of the people who sell *NuPod-500's*, this technique of marketing

| TABLE 4-4. COMPOSITION OF SOME COMMON PREPARATIONS THAT CONTAIN A COMBINATION OF DRUGS | |
|---|---|
| **Product Name** | **Drugs in the Preparation** |
| Excedrin Tablets | Acetaminophen + aspirin + caffeine |
| Excedrin P.M. | Acetaminophen + diphenhydramine |
| 4-Way Long-Lasting Nasal Spray | Oxymetazoline |
| 4-Way Fast-Acting Nasal Spray | Phenylephrine + naphazoline + pyrilamine |

by trade names is a terrific arrangement. Consumers will be loyal to their product not because that product is better or cheaper than someone else's, but because product labeling with trade names makes it very difficult to identify the competition so that comparisons can be made. Fortunately, we don't allow this kind of marketing for peas. When we shop for peas, we demand that all pea packages bear the word PEAS—not *Vegi-P* or *NuPod-500's* or any other trade name. Why we permit medicines to be marketed in any less informative a manner is a disturbing question.

When we consider that drugs, unlike peas, cannot be identified by simple observation, the use of trade names for marketing becomes especially unsettling. With peas, once we open the package, we no longer need the label to identify the contents. We know what peas look like. Hence, even if peas were marketed like drugs, we would not be completely dependent upon labeling to identify the product. With drugs we have no options: since we cannot identify a drug by looking at it, we cannot escape reliance on package labeling to inform us about the medicine inside. It is ironic that a product whose label is so essential for identification can be marketed under a system that employs multiple trade names, thereby making product identification needlessly and dangerously difficult.

## Generic Products versus Brand Name Products

To complete our discussion of drug names, we need to address two questions: (1) Do significant differences exist between different brands of the same drug? (2) If such differences do exist, do they justify the use of trade names?

The answer to our first question is a qualified *Yes.* Yes, examples can be found in which different brands of the same drug are not therapeutically equivalent. However, these examples are rare. In most cases, there is no significant difference among preparations of a drug made by company A, company B, and company Z. Furthermore, it should be noted that drugs marketed under generic names are chemically identical to those marketed under trade names. For example, the medication present in tablets available generically as *diazepam* is identical to the chemical in tablets marketed under the trade name *Valium.*

In those cases in which drug preparations do differ from one another, the differences are not in the chemical composition of the drugs themselves. Rather, differences concern either the rate or extent of absorption. Differences in absorption can occur because of differences in the way that drug formulations (e.g., tablets, capsules, sustained-release preparations) are manufactured. Hence, even though brand A and brand B contain the same amount of the same drug, these preparations may be absorbed differently and, as a result, may produce quantitatively different effects. Occasionally, such differences are large enough to be of therapeutic significance.

Since, in some cases, variations in absorption between different brands of the same drug can be large enough to affect the outcome of therapy, do such variations justify the use of trade names in order to identify a preferred product? The answer to this question is a resounding NO!

If physicians want to prescribe a drug made by a particular company, they needn't resort to trade names to do so; their preference can be indicated simply by including the manufacturer's name on the prescription. As with peas, if we prefer a particular brand (e.g., Bird's Eye), that's what we ask for. We haven't found it necessary to create a complicated system of alternative names for peas in order to distinguish one brand from another. On the contrary, common sense tells us that such a system of trade names would make it more difficult, not easier, for us to clearly communicate our needs. Perhaps some day we will market medicines with as much common sense as we use for vegetables.

## Conclusion Regarding Generic Names and Trade Names

In the preceding discussion, we considered the advantages and disadvantages associated with trade names and generic names. We noted that, although generic names may be long, this disadvantage is more than offset by the fact that each drug has only one generic name. In contrast, the sole virtue of trade names—ease of recall and pronunciation—is far outweighed by the problems that stem from the existence of multiple trade names for a single drug. Multiple trade names can impede name recognition and can thereby promote medication errors and miscommunication about drugs. With generic names, the opposite is achieved: facilitation of communication and promotion of safe and effective drug use. Clearly, generic names are preferable to trade names. Accordingly, until such time as trade names are outlawed, the least we can do is actively discourage their use. In this text, generic names are employed for routine discussion. Although trade names are presented, they are not emphasized. We may eventually see the day when trade names are abandoned and generic names are employed universally. On that day, efforts to achieve the therapeutic objective will receive a significant boost.

## Sources of Drug Information

There is much more to pharmacology than we can address in this text. When you need additional information, the sources discussed below should be helpful.

### People

*Clinicians and Pharmacists.* Nurses and other clinicians can be invaluable sources of information about medicines. Pharmacists know a great deal about drugs and are usually eager to share their expertise.

*Poison Control Centers.* Poison control centers are present throughout the country. These centers are accessible by telephone, permitting rapid access to information about medicines and toxic compounds. Appendix F lists the names, addresses, and telephone numbers of the certified regional poison centers in the United States.

*Pharmaceutical Sales Representatives.* Pharmaceutical sales representatives (drug representatives) can be useful sources of drug information. These people know their own products very well, and they can provide detailed, authoritative information about them. Keep in mind, however, that the ultimate job of the drug representative is *sales—not education.* Because the objective is sales, drug representatives may fail to volunteer negative information about their product. Likewise, they are unlikely to point out superior qualities in a competing drug. (Is a Chevrolet salesperson going to extol the virtues of a Ford?) Such a lack of complete candor does not mean that drug representatives are unethical; they are simply doing their job. However, since full disclosure may be inconsistent with success, the drug representative may not be your best source of information—especially if you are trying to establish an unbiased comparison between the representative's product and a drug from a competing manufacturer.

## Published Information

The publications described below are general references. These works cover a broad range of topics but in limited depth. Accordingly, these references are most useful as initial sources of information. If more detail is needed, specialty publications should be consulted. Some important drug references, including the ones described below, are listed in Table 4-5.

## TABLE 4–5. SOME IMPORTANT DRUG REFERENCES

**General Information on Drug Actions, Pharmacokinetics, Therapeutics, Adverse Effects, and Drug Interactions**

*Drug Evaluations.* American Medical Association, Chicago (updated annually)
*Goodman and Gilman's The Pharmacological Basis of Therapeutics*, 9th ed. Hardman, J.G., et al. (eds.) McGraw-Hill, New York, 1996
*Pharmacotherapy: A Pathophysiologic Approach*, 2nd ed. DiPiro, J.T., et al. (eds.). Elsevier Science Publishing, New York, 1992
*Applied Therapeutics: The Clinical Use of Drugs*, 6th ed. Young, L.Y. and Koda-Kimble, M.A. (eds.). Applied Therapeutics, Inc., Vancouver, WA, 1995

**Detailed Information on Specific Drugs and Drug Families**

*AHFS Drug Information.* McEvoy, G.K. (ed.). American Society of Hospital Pharmacists, Bethesda, MD (updated annually)
*Drug Facts and Comparisons*, Loose-leaf ed. Facts and Comparisons, St. Louis (updated monthly)
*Physicians' Desk Reference.* Medical Economics Data Production Co., Montvale, NJ (updated annually)
*United States Pharmacopeia Drug Information (USP DI): Drug Information for the Health Care Professional.* The United States Pharmacopeial Convention, Inc., Rockville, MD (updated bimonthly)

**Very Current Information**

*The Medical Letter.* The Medical Letter, Inc., New Rochelle, NY (published biweekly)

## Text-Like Books

*Goodman and Gilman's The Pharmacological Basis of Therapeutics* is the classic text/reference on pharmacology used by medical students and practicing physicians. As its name implies, this book focuses on the basic science information that underlies drug use—and not on therapeutics per se. New editions are released about every 5 years.

*Drug Evaluations*, a comprehensive reference prepared by the American Medical Association, discusses drugs from the perspective of therapeutics. Hence, in contrast to the text originated by Goodman and Gilman, this book emphasizes clinical aspects of pharmacology rather than basic science. The book is especially helpful for obtaining comparative information on the various agents that might be employed to manage a specific disorder. The book is updated annually.

*Pharmacotherapy: A Pathophysiologic Approach* is a comprehensive text on drug therapy. As in *Drug Evaluations*, each chapter focuses on the treatment of a specific disorder. To facilitate understanding of drug therapy, the book presents thorough reviews of pathophysiology.

*Applied Therapeutics: The Clinical Use of Drugs* is another comprehensive text on drug therapy, with each chapter focusing on a specific disorder. However, this book is different from the others in that it employs a case study approach to presenting content on pharmacology and therapeutics.

## Newsletter

*The Medical Letter* is a bimonthly publication that gives very current information on drugs. A typical issue discusses two or three agents. Discussions consist of a summary of data from clinical trials plus a conclusion regarding the drug's therapeutic utility. The conclusions can be a valuable guide when deciding whether or not to use a new drug.

## Reference Books

*The Physicians' Desk Reference*, also known as the PDR, is a reference work financed by the pharmaceutical industry. The information on each drug is identical to the information on its package insert. In addition to textual content, the PDR has a pictorial section for product identification. The PDR is updated annually.

*Drug Facts and Comparisons* is a comprehensive reference that contains monographs on virtually every drug marketed in the United States. Information is provided on drug actions, indications, warnings, precautions, adverse reactions, dosage, and administration. In addition to describing the properties of single medications, the book lists the contents of all combination products sold in this country. Indexing is by generic name and by trade name. Revised editions are published annually.

A number of drug references have been compiled expressly for nurses. All of these address topics of special interest to the nurse, including information on administration, assessment, evaluation, and patient education. Representative nursing drug references include *Nurse's Drug Handbook, Drugs and Nursing Implications,* and *Nurses' Drug Reference.*

**Internet**

The Internet can be a valuable source of drug information. However, since anyone, regardless of qualifications, can post information, not everything you find will be accurate. Accordingly, you need to exercise discretion when searching for information. A list of reliable drug-related Internet sites is given in Appendix H.

## KEY POINTS

* The Food, Drug and Cosmetic Act of 1938 was the first legislation to regulate drug safety.
* The Kefauver-Harris Amendments, passed in 1962, were the first legislation to demand that drugs actually be of some benefit.
* The Controlled Substances Act, passed in 1970, set rules for the manufacture and distribution of drugs considered to have potential for abuse.
* Development of a new drug is an extremely expensive process that takes years to complete.
* Drug testing in phase II and phase III clinical trials is limited to a relatively small number of patients, most of whom take the drug for a relatively short time.
* Since women are generally excluded from trials of new drugs, our understanding of drugs in women is limited.
* When a new drug is released for general use, it may well have adverse effects that have not yet been detected. Consequently, when working with a new drug, you should be especially watchful for previously unreported drug reactions.
* Drugs have three types of names: a chemical name, a generic or nonproprietary name, and a trade or proprietary name.
* Each drug has only one generic name but can have many trade names.
* Generic names facilitate communication and therefore are good. In contrast, trade names confuse communication and should be outlawed. (Note: even science authors are allowed to voice an opinion now and then.)
* Since the job of the drug representative is sales and not education, this person may not be your best source of drug information—especially if you are trying to establish an unbiased comparison between the representative's product and a drug from a competing manufacturer.
* As pharmacology students, you should know that *Goodman and Gilman's The Pharmacological Basis of Therapeutics* (aka G & G) is the classic text/reference on pharmacology.

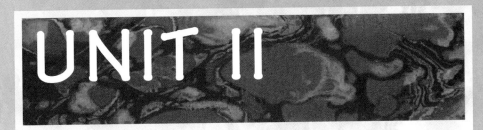

# UNIT II

# Basic Principles of Pharmacology

Pharmacokinetics
Pharmacodynamics
Drug-Drug and Drug-Food Interactions
Adverse Drug Reactions
Individual Variation in Drug Responses

# Pharmacokinetics

The term *pharmacokinetics* is derived from two Greek words: *pharmakon* (drug or poison) and *kinesis* (motion). As this derivation implies, pharmacokinetics is the study of drug movement throughout the body. Pharmacokinetics also includes drug metabolism and drug excretion.

There are four basic pharmacokinetic processes: absorption, distribution, metabolism, and excretion (Fig. 5–1). Absorption is defined as the movement of a drug from its site of administration into the blood. Distribution is defined as drug movement from the blood to the interstitial space of tissues and from there into cells. Metabolism (biotransformation) is defined as enzymatically mediated alteration of drug structure. Excretion is the movement of drugs and their metabolites out of the body. (The combination of drug metabolism plus excretion is called elimination.) The four pharmacokinetic processes, acting in concert, determine the concentration of a drug at its sites of action.

## Application of Pharmacokinetics in Therapeutics

By applying knowledge of pharmacokinetics to drug therapy, we can help maximize desirable effects and minimize harm. Recall that the intensity of a drug response is directly related to the concentration of a drug at its site of action. To maximize beneficial effects, we must achieve concentrations that are high enough to elicit desired responses; to minimize harm, we must avoid unnecessarily high concentrations. This balance is achieved by selecting the most appropriate route, dosage, and schedule of drug administration. The only means by which we can rationally choose the most effective route, dosage, and schedule is by considering pharmacokinetic factors.

As a nurse, you will have ample opportunity to apply knowledge of pharmacokinetics in clinical practice. For example, by understanding the reasons behind selection of route, dosage, and timing of drug administration, you will be less likely to commit medication errors than will the nurse who, through lack of this knowledge, administers medications by blindly following physicians' orders. Also, as noted in Chapter 2, physicians do make mistakes. Accordingly, you will have occasion to question or even challenge physicians regarding their selection of dosage, route, or schedule of drug administration. In order to alter a physician's decision, you will need a rational argument to support your position. To present the argument, you will need to understand pharmacokinetics.

Knowledge of pharmacokinetics can increase job satisfaction. Working with medications is usually a significant component of nursing practice. For the nurse who lacks

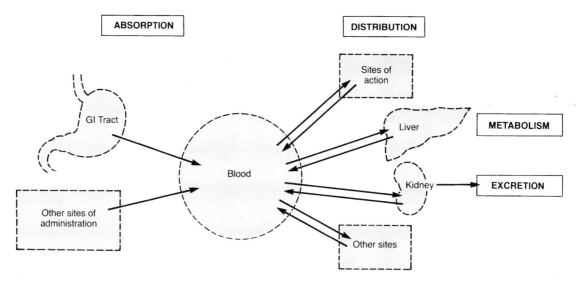

**Figure 5–1. The four basic pharmacokinetic processes.** Dotted lines represent membranes that must be crossed as drugs move throughout the body.

knowledge of pharmacokinetics, drugs will always be somewhat mysterious and, as a result, will be a potential source of ill ease. By helping to demystify drug therapy, knowledge of pharmacokinetics can decrease some of the stress of nursing practice and can increase intellectual and professional satisfaction.

## A Note to Chemophobes

Before we proceed to the heart of this chapter, some advance notice (and encouragement) are in order for the chemophobes (students who fear chemistry) who are reading this text. Since drugs are chemicals, we cannot discuss pharmacology meaningfully without occasionally talking about chemistry. This chapter has some chemistry in it. In fact, the chemistry presented here is the most difficult in the book. Accordingly, once you've worked your way through this chapter, the chapters that follow will be a relative breeze. Since the concepts addressed here are fundamental, and since they reappear frequently, all students, including chemophobes, are encouraged to learn this material now—regardless of the effort required.

I also want to comment on the chemical structures that appear in the book. Structures are presented only to illustrate and emphasize concepts. They are not intended for memorization. And they are certainly not intended for exams. So, relax, look at the pictures, and focus on the concepts they are trying to help you grasp.

## Passage of Drugs Across Membranes

All four phases of pharmacokinetics—absorption, distribution, metabolism, and excretion—involve drug move-

ment. To move throughout the body, drugs must cross membranes. Drugs must cross membranes to enter the blood from their site of administration. Once in the blood, drugs must cross membranes to reach their sites of action. In addition, drugs must cross membranes to undergo metabolism and excretion. Accordingly, the factors that determine the passage of drugs across biologic membranes have a profound influence on all aspects of pharmacokinetics.

## Membrane Structure

Biologic membranes are composed of layers of individual cells. The cells composing most membranes are very close to one another—so close, in fact, that drugs must usually pass *through* cells, rather than between them, in order to cross the membrane. Hence, the ability of a drug to cross a biologic membrane is determined primarily by its ability to pass through single cells. The major barrier to passage through a cell is the cytoplasmic membrane (the membrane that surrounds every cell).

The basic structure of the cell membrane is depicted in Figure 5-2. As indicated, the basic membrane structure consists of a double layer of molecules known as *phospholipids*. Phospholipids are simply lipids (fats) that contain an atom of phosphate.

In Figure 5-2, the phospholipid molecules are depicted as having a round head (the phosphate-containing component) and two tails (long-chain hydrocarbons). The large objects embedded in the membrane represent protein molecules. These proteins serve a variety of functions.

## Three Ways to Cross a Cell Membrane

The three most important ways by which drugs cross cell membranes are (1) passage through channels or pores, (2) passage with the aid of a transport system, and (3) direct penetration of the membrane itself. Of these three, direct penetration of the membrane is most common.

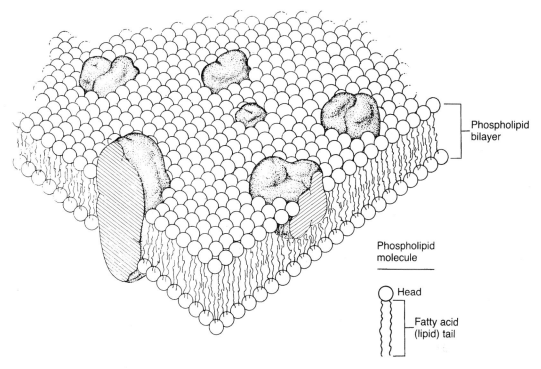

**Figure 5–2. Structure of the cell membrane.** The cell membrane consists primarily of a double layer of phospholipid molecules. The large globular structures represent protein molecules imbedded in the lipid bilayer. (Modified from Singer, S.J., and Nicolson, G.L. The fluid mosaic model of the structure of cell membranes. Science 175:720, 1972. Copyright 1972 by AAAS.)

## Channels and Pores

Very few drugs cross membranes via channels or pores. The channels in membranes are extremely small (approximately 4 angstroms). Consequently, only the smallest of compounds (molecular weight less than 200) can use these holes as a route of transit. Agents with the ability to cross membranes via channels include small ions, such as potassium and sodium.

## Transport Systems

Transport systems are carriers that can move drugs from one side of the cell membrane to the other. Some transport systems require the expenditure of energy; others do not. All transport systems are selective: they will not carry just any drug. Whether or not a transporter will carry a particular drug depends upon the drug's structure.

Transport systems are an important means of drug transit. For example, certain orally administered drugs could not be absorbed unless there were transport systems to move them across the membranes that separate the lumen of the intestine from the blood. A number of drugs could not reach intracellular sites of action without a transport system to move them across the cell membrane. Renal excretion of many drugs would be extremely slow were it not for transport systems in the kidney that can pump drugs from the blood into the renal tubules.

## Direct Penetration of the Membrane

For most drugs, movement throughout the body is dependent on their ability to penetrate membranes directly. This is because most drugs are too large to pass through channels or pores, and because most drugs lack transport systems to help them cross all the membranes that separate them from sites of action, metabolism, and excretion.

In order to directly penetrate membranes, a drug must be *lipid* soluble (lipophilic). Recall that membranes are composed primarily of lipids. Consequently, if a drug is to penetrate membranes, it must be able to dissolve into the lipids that compose the membrane.

Certain kinds of molecules are *not* lipid soluble and therefore cannot penetrate membranes. This category consists of *polar molecules* and *ions*.

## Polar Molecules

Polar molecules are molecules with uneven distribution of electrical charge. That is, positive and negative charges within the molecule tend to congregate separately from one another. Water is the classic example of a polar molecule. As depicted in Figure 5-3A, the electrons (negative charges) in the water molecule spend more time in the vicinity of the oxygen atom than in the vicinity of the two hydrogen atoms. As a result, the area around the oxygen atom tends to be negatively charged, whereas the area around the hydrogen atoms tends to be positively charged.

Kanamycin (Fig. 5-3B), an antibiotic, is an example of a polar *drug*. The hydroxyl groups, which attract electrons, give kanamycin its polar nature.

Although polar molecules have an uneven *distribution of charge*, they have no *net charge*. Polar molecules have an equal number of protons (which bear a single positive

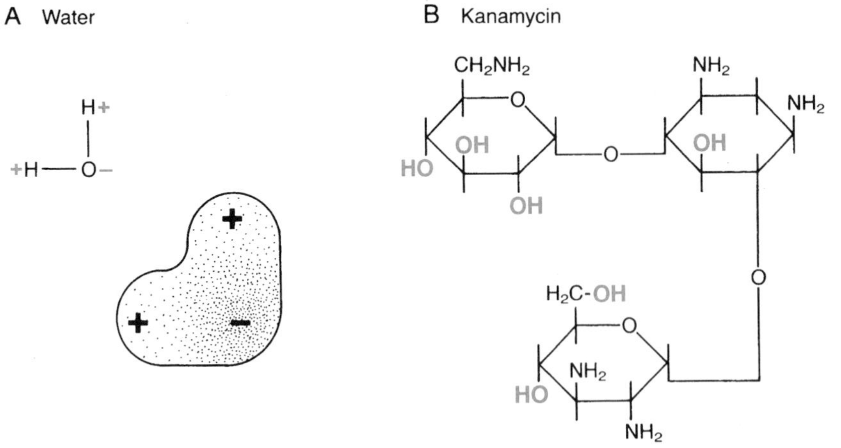

A  Water

B  Kanamycin

**Figure 5–3. Polar molecules.** *A*, Stippling shows the distribution of electrons within the water molecule. As indicated, water's electrons spend more time near the oxygen atom than near the hydrogen atoms, making the area near the oxygen atom somewhat negative and the area near the hydrogen atoms more positive. *B*, Kanamycin is a polar drug. The –OH groups of kanamycin attract electrons, thereby causing the area around these groups to be more negative than the rest of the molecule.

charge) and electrons (which bear a single negative charge). As a result, the positive and negative charges balance each other exactly, and the molecule as a whole has neither a net positive nor a net negative charge. (Molecules that *do* bear a net charge are called *ions.* These are discussed below.)

There is a general rule in chemistry that states: "like dissolves like." In accord with this rule, polar molecules will dissolve in *polar* solvents (such as water) but will not dissolve in *nonpolar* solvents (such as oil). Table sugar provides a common example. As I'm sure you've observed, sugar, which is a polar compound, readily dissolves in water but does not dissolve in salad oil, butter, and other lipids, which are nonpolar compounds. Just as sugar is unable to dissolve in lipids, polar drugs are unable to dissolve in the lipid bilayer of the cell membrane.

### Ions

Ions are defined as molecules that have a *net electrical charge* (either positive or negative). With rare exceptions, *ions are unable to cross membranes.*

#### Quaternary Ammonium Compounds

Quaternary ammonium compounds are molecules that contain at least one atom of nitrogen and *carry a positive charge at all times.* The constant charge on these compounds results from atypical bonding to the nitrogen. In most nitrogen-containing compounds, the nitrogen atom bears only three chemical bonds. In contrast, the nitrogen atoms of quaternary ammonium compounds have four chemical bonds (Fig. 5–4A). It is because of the fourth bond that quaternary ammonium compounds always carry a positive charge. Because of the charge, these compounds are unable to cross most membranes.

Tubocurarine (Fig. 5–4B) is a representative quaternary ammonium compound. In purified form, tubocurarine is employed as a muscle relaxant during surgery and other procedures. A crude preparation—curare—is used by South American Indians as an arrow poison. When employed for hunting, tubocurarine (curare) produces paralysis of the diaphragm and other skeletal muscles, causing death by asphyxiation. Interestingly, even though meat

from animals killed with curare is laden with poison, it can be eaten without ill effect. The reason this poison can be ingested safely is that tubocurarine, being a quaternary ammonium compound, cannot cross membranes and therefore cannot be absorbed from the intestine; as long as it remains in the intestine, curare can do no harm. As you might gather, when tubocurarine is used clinically, it cannot be administered by mouth; instead, it must be injected. Once in the bloodstream, tubocurarine has ready access to its sites of action on muscles.

### pH-Dependent Ionization

Unlike quaternary ammonium compounds, which always carry a charge, certain drugs can exist in either a charged or an uncharged form. Many drugs are either weak organic acids or weak organic bases. Weak acids and bases can exist in charged and uncharged forms. Whether a weak acid or base will carry a charge is determined by the pH of the surrounding medium.

A review of acid-base chemistry will be helpful. An acid is defined as a compound that can give up a hydrogen ion (proton). Put another way, *an acid is a proton donor.* A

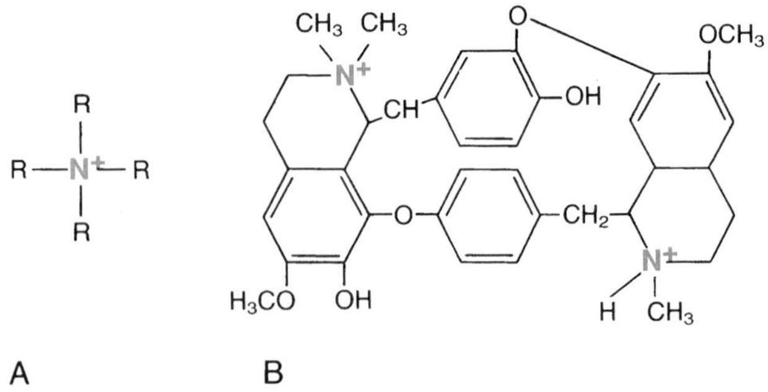

A                    B

**Figure 5–4. Quaternary ammonium compounds.** *A*, The basic structure of quaternary ammonium compounds. Because the nitrogen atom has bonds to four organic radicals, the quaternary ammonium compound always carries a positive charge. Because of this charge, quaternary ammonium compounds are not lipid soluble and cannot cross most membranes. *B*, Tubocurarine is a representative quaternary ammonium compound. Note that tubocurarine contains two "quaternized" nitrogen atoms.

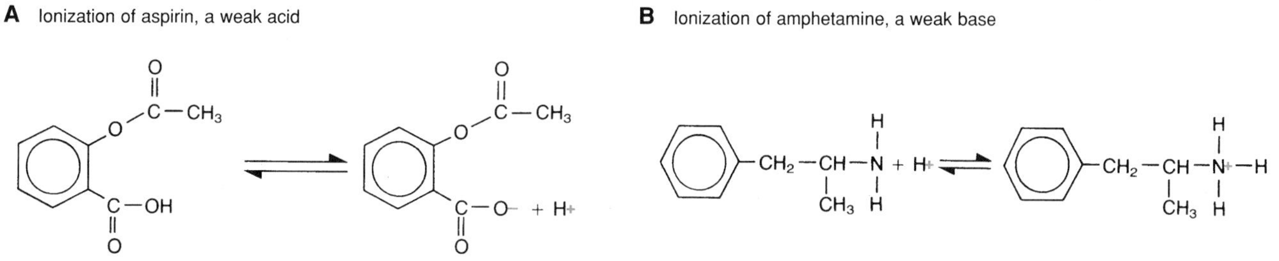

**A** Ionization of aspirin, a weak acid

**B** Ionization of amphetamine, a weak base

**Figure 5–5. Ionization of weak acids and weak bases.** The extent of ionization of weak acids (*A*) and weak bases (*B*) depends upon the pH of their surroundings. The ionized (charged) forms of acids and bases are not lipid soluble and do not readily cross membranes. Note that *acids* ionize by giving up a proton and that *bases* ionize by taking on a proton.

base is defined as a compound that can take on a hydrogen ion. That is, *a base is a proton acceptor.* When an acid gives up its proton, which is positively charged, the acid itself becomes negatively charged. Conversely, when a base accepts a proton, the base becomes positively charged. These reactions are depicted in Figure 5-5, which uses aspirin as an example of an acid and amphetamine as an example of a base. Because the process of an acid giving up a proton or a base accepting a proton converts the acid or base into a charged particle (ion), the process for either an acid or a base is termed *ionization.*

The extent to which a weak acid or weak base becomes ionized is determined by the pH of its environment. The following rules apply:

- *Acids tend to ionize in basic (alkaline) media.*
- *Bases tend to ionize in acidic media.*

An example of the pH-dependent ionization of a drug will illustrate the significance of this phenomenon. We will use aspirin for our example. Being an acid, aspirin tends to give up its proton (become ionized) in basic media. Conversely, aspirin will keep its proton and remain nonionized in acidic media. Hence, when aspirin is in the stomach (an acidic medium) most of the aspirin molecules will remain nonionized. Because aspirin molecules are nonionized in the stomach, they are able to be absorbed across the membranes that separate the stomach from the bloodstream. When aspirin molecules pass from the stomach into the small intestine, where the environment is relatively alkaline, they will change to their ionized form. As a result, absorption of aspirin from the intestine is impeded.

### Ion Trapping (pH Partitioning)

Because the ionization of drugs is pH dependent, when the pH of the fluid on one side of a membrane differs from the pH of the fluid on the other side, drug molecules will tend to accumulate on the side where the pH most favors their ionization. Accordingly, since acidic drugs tend to ionize in basic media, and since basic drugs tend to ionize in acidic media, *when there is a pH gradient between two sides of a membrane,*

- *Acidic drugs will accumulate on the alkaline side.*
- *Basic drugs will accumulate on the acidic side.*

The process whereby a drug accumulates on the side of a membrane where the pH most favors its ionization is referred to as *ion trapping* or *pH partitioning.* Figure 5-6 shows the steps of ion trapping using aspirin as an example.

Since ion trapping can influence the movement of drugs throughout the body, the process is not simply of academic interest. Rather, ion trapping has practical clinical implications. Knowledge of ion trapping helps us understand drug absorption as well as the movement of drugs to sites of action, metabolism, and excretion. Understanding of ion trapping can be put to practical use on those occasions when it is necessary to actively influence drug movements. Management of poisoning is such an occasion: By manipulating urinary pH, we can employ ion trapping to draw toxic substances from the blood into the urine, thereby accelerating their removal from the body.

## Absorption

Absorption is defined as *the movement of a drug from its site of administration into the blood.* The *rate* of absorption determines how *soon* effects will begin. The *amount* of absorption helps determine how *intense* the effects will be.

### Factors Affecting Drug Absorption

The rate at which a drug is absorbed is influenced by the physical and chemical properties of the drug itself and by physiologic and anatomic factors at the site of absorption.

*Rate of Dissolution.* Before a drug can be absorbed it must first dissolve. Hence, the rate of dissolution helps determine the rate of absorption. Drugs in formulations that allow rapid dissolution have a faster onset than drugs formulated for slow dissolution.

*Surface Area.* The surface area available for absorption is a major determinant of the rate of absorption. The larger the surface area, the faster absorption will be. For this reason, orally administered drugs are usually absorbed from the small intestine rather than from the stomach. (Recall

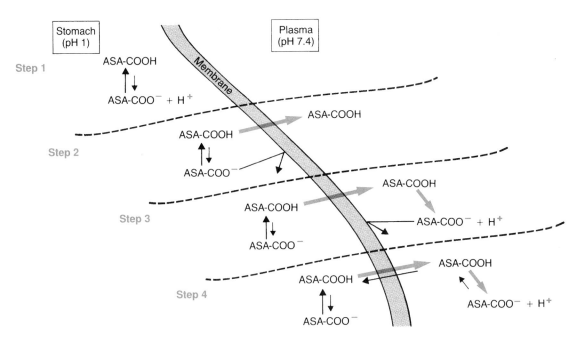

**Figure 5–6. Ion trapping of drugs.** This figure demonstrates ion trapping using aspirin as an example. Because it is an acidic drug, aspirin will be nonionized in acid media and ionized in alkaline media. This figure demonstrates how the process of ion trapping will cause molecules of orally administered aspirin to move from the acidic (pH 1) environment of the stomach to the more alkaline (pH 7.4) environment of the plasma, thereby causing aspirin to accumulate in the blood. In the figure, aspirin (acetylsalicylic acid) is depicted as ASA with its COOH (carboxylic acid) group attached. **Step 1**, Once ingested, ASA dissolves in the stomach contents. After dissolving, some of the ASA molecules will give up a proton and become ionized. However, most of the ASA in the stomach will remain nonionized. (Most of the aspirin molecules in the stomach will be nonionized because the stomach is acidic, and acidic drugs don't ionize in acidic media.) **Step 2**, Since most of the ASA molecules in the stomach are nonionized (and therefore lipid soluble), most ASA molecules in the stomach can readily cross the membranes that separate the stomach lumen from the plasma. Because of the concentration gradient that exists between the stomach and the plasma, nonionized ASA molecules will begin moving into the plasma. (Note that because of their charge, ionized ASA molecules cannot leave the stomach.) **Step 3**, As the nonionized ASA molecules enter the relatively alkaline environment of the plasma, most of these molecules will give up an $H^+$ and become negatively charged ions. Those ASA molecules that become ionized in the plasma cannot diffuse back into the stomach. **Step 4**, As the nonionized ASA molecules in the plasma become ionized, more nonionized molecules will pass from the stomach to the plasma to replace them. This passage will occur because the laws of diffusion demand equal concentrations of diffusible substances on both sides of the membrane. Since only the nonionized form of the ASA is able to diffuse across the membrane, it is this form that the laws of diffusion will attempt to equilibrate. Nonionized ASA will continue to move from the stomach to the plasma until the amount of ionized ASA in plasma has become large enough to prevent conversion of newly arrived nonionized molecules into the ionized form. Equilibrium will then be established between the plasma and the stomach. At equilibrium, there will be equal amounts of nonionized ASA in stomach and plasma. However, on the plasma side, the amount of ionized ASA will be much larger than on the stomach side. Since there are equal amounts of nonionized ASA on both sides of the membrane but much more ionized ASA in the plasma, the total amount of ASA in plasma will be much higher than in the stomach.

that the small intestine, because of its lining of microvilli, has an extremely large surface area, whereas the surface area of the stomach is relatively small.)

**Blood Flow.** Drugs are absorbed most rapidly from sites where blood flow is high. This is because blood containing newly absorbed drug will be replaced rapidly by drug-free blood, thereby maintaining a large gradient between the concentration of drug outside the blood and the concentration of drug in the blood. The greater this concentration gradient, the more rapid absorption will be.

**Lipid Solubility.** As a rule, highly lipid-soluble drugs are absorbed more rapidly than drugs whose lipid solubility is low. This is because lipid-soluble drugs can readily cross

the membranes that separate them from the blood, whereas drugs of low lipid solubility cannot.

**pH Partitioning.** pH partitioning can influence drug absorption. Absorption will be enhanced when the difference between the pH of plasma and the pH at the site of administration is such that drug molecules will have a greater tendency to be ionized in the plasma.

## Characteristics of Commonly Used Routes of Administration

The routes of administration that are used most commonly fall into two major groups: *enteral* (via the gastrointestinal tract) and *parenteral.* The literal definition of *parenteral* is *outside the gastrointestinal tract.* However, in common parlance, the term *parenteral* is used to mean *by injection.* The principal parenteral routes are *intravenous, subcutaneous,* and *intramuscular.*

For each of the major routes of administration—oral (PO), intravenous (IV), intramuscular (IM), and subcutaneous (SC)—the pattern of drug absorption (i.e., the rate and extent of absorption) is unique. Consequently, the route by which a drug is administered will significantly affect both the time of onset and the intensity of effects. Why do patterns of absorption differ between routes? Because the barriers to absorption associated with each route are different. In the discussion below, we will examine these barriers and their influence on absorption pattern. In addition, as we discuss each major route, we will consider its clinical advantages and disadvantages.

## Intravenous

***Barriers to Absorption.*** When a drug is administered intravenously, there are no barriers to absorption. Recall that absorption is defined as the movement of a drug from its site of administration into the blood. Since IV administration puts a drug directly into the blood, all barriers to absorption are bypassed.

***Absorption Pattern.*** Intravenous administration results in "absorption" that is both instantaneous and complete. Intravenous "absorption" is instantaneous in that drug enters the blood directly. "Absorption" is complete in that virtually all of the administered dose reaches the blood.

***Advantages.*** *Rapid Onset.* Intravenous administration results in rapid onset of drug action. Although rapid onset is not always important, it is clearly beneficial in emergencies.

*Control.* Since the entire dose is administered directly into the blood, we have precise control over levels of drug in the blood. This contrasts with the other major routes of administration, and especially with oral administration (see below).

*Use of Large Fluid Volumes.* The intravenous route is the only parenteral route that permits the use of large volumes of fluid. Some drugs that require parenteral administration are poorly soluble in water and therefore must be dissolved in a large volume. Because of the physical limitations presented by soft tissues (e.g., muscle, subcutaneous tissue), injection of large volumes at these sites is not possible. In contrast, the amount of fluid that can be infused into a vein, although limited, is nonetheless relatively large.

*Use of Irritant Drugs.* Certain drugs, because of their irritant properties, can be administered only by the intravenous route. A number of anticancer drugs, for example, are very chemically reactive. If present in high concentrations, these agents can cause severe local injury. However, when administered through a freely flowing IV line, these drugs are rapidly diluted in the blood, thereby minimizing the risk of injury.

***Disadvantages.*** *High Cost, Difficulty, and Inconvenience.* Intravenous administration is expensive, difficult, and in-

convenient. The cost of IV administration sets and their set-up charges can be substantial. Setting up an IV line takes time and special training. Because of the difficulty involved, most patients are unable to self-administer IV drugs, and therefore must depend on a health care professional. Because patients are tethered to lines and bottles, their mobility is limited (unless a portable infusion pump is being employed). In sharp contrast to this picture, oral administration is easy, convenient, and cheap.

*Irreversibility.* More important than cost or convenience, IV administration can be *dangerous.* Once a drug has been injected, there is no turning back: the drug is in the body and cannot be retrieved. Hence, if dosage is excessive, avoiding toxicity may be impossible.

To minimize risk, intravenous drugs should be injected slowly (over 1 minute or more). Since all of the blood in the body is circulated about once every minute, by injecting a drug over a 1-minute interval, we cause it to be diluted in the largest volume of blood possible. By doing so, we can avoid drug concentrations that are unnecessarily—or even dangerously—high.

Performing IV injections slowly has the additional advantage of reducing the risk of toxicity to the central nervous system (CNS). When a drug is injected into the antecubital vein of the arm, about 15 seconds is required for the drug to reach the brain. Consequently, if the dosage is sufficient to cause CNS toxicity, signs of toxicity may become apparent 15 seconds after starting the injection. If the injection is being done slowly (e.g., over a 1-minute interval), only 25% of the total dose will have been administered when signs of toxicity appear. If administration is discontinued immediately, adverse effects will be much less than they would have been had the entire dose been injected.

*Fluid Overload.* When drugs are administered in a large volume, fluid overload can occur. This can be a significant problem for patients with hypertension, kidney disease, or heart failure.

*Infection.* Infection can occur from injecting a contaminated drug. Fortunately, the risk of infection is much lower today than it was before the development of modern techniques for sterilizing drugs intended for IV use.

*Embolism.* Intravenous administration carries a risk of embolism (blood vessel blockage at a site distant from the point of administration). Embolism can be caused in several ways. First, insertion of an IV needle can injure the venous wall, leading to formation of a thrombus (clot); embolism can result if the clot breaks loose and becomes lodged in another vessel. Second, injection of hypotonic or hypertonic fluids can destroy red blood cells; the debris from these cells can produce embolism.

Lastly, injection of drugs that are not fully dissolved can lead to embolism. Particles of undissolved drug are like small grains of sand, which can become embedded in blood vessels and cause blockage. Because of the risk of embolism, you should check intravenous solutions prior to administration to ensure that drugs are completely dissolved. If the fluid is cloudy or contains particulate matter, the drug is not dissolved and the fluid must not be administered.

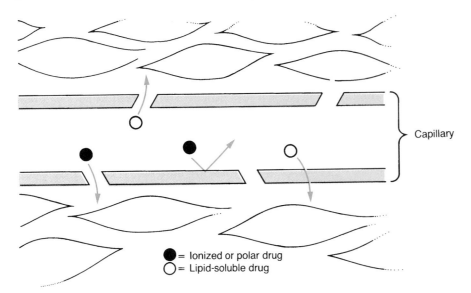

= Ionized or polar drug
◯ = Lipid-soluble drug

**Figure 5–7. Drug movement at typical capillary beds.** In most capillary beds, "large" gaps exist between the cells that compose the capillary wall. Drugs and other molecules can pass freely into and out of the bloodstream through these gaps. (As illustrated, lipid-soluble compounds can also pass directly through the cells of the capillary wall.)

*The Importance of Reading Labels.* Not all formulations of the same drug are appropriate for IV administration. Accordingly, it is essential to read the label before giving a drug intravenously. Two examples will illustrate the importance of this admonition. Our first example is insulin. Only one preparation of insulin can be administered safely IV. That preparation, which is usually labeled *insulin injection*, consists of insulin in *solution*. In all other preparations, insulin is present as a particulate suspension. These preparations are intended for subcutaneous administration only. Because of their particulate nature, these preparations could prove fatal if administered IV. By checking the label, inadvertent intravenous administration of particulate insulin can be avoided.

Epinephrine provides our second example of the importance of reading the label before giving an IV drug. Epinephrine, which stimulates the cardiovascular system, can be injected by several routes (intramuscular, intravenous, subcutaneous, intracardiac, intraspinal). It must be noted, however, that a solution prepared for use by one route will differ in concentration from a solution prepared for use by other routes. For example, whereas solutions intended for *subcutaneous* administration are *concentrated,* solutions intended for *intravenous* use are *dilute.* If a solution prepared for subcutaneous use were to be inadvertently administered intravenously, the result could prove *fatal.* (Intravenous administration of concentrated epinephrine could overstimulate the heart and blood vessels, causing severe hypertension, cerebral hemorrhage, stroke, and death.) The message here is that it is not sufficient to simply administer the *right drug;* you must also be sure that the formulation and concentration are *appropriate for the intended route.*

### Intramuscular

*Barriers to Absorption.* When a drug is injected intramuscularly, the only barrier to absorption is the *capillary wall.* In capillary beds that serve muscles and most other tissues, there are "large" spaces between the cells that compose the capillary wall (Fig. 5–7). Drugs can pass through these spaces with ease; no cell membranes need to be crossed in order to enter the bloodstream. Hence, like intravenous administration, intramuscular administration presents no significant barriers to absorption.

*Absorption Pattern.* Drugs administered intramuscularly may be absorbed rapidly or slowly. The rate of absorption is determined largely by two factors: (1) water solubility of the drug and (2) blood flow to the site of injection. Drugs that are highly soluble in water will be absorbed rapidly (within 10 to 30 minutes), whereas drugs that are poorly soluble will be absorbed slowly. Similarly, absorption will be rapid from sites where blood flow is high, and slow where blood flow is low.

*Advantages.* The intramuscular route can be used for parenteral administration of *poorly soluble drugs.* Recall that drugs must be dissolved if they are to be administered intravenously. Consequently, the IV route cannot be used for poorly soluble compounds. In contrast, since little harm will come from depositing a suspension of undissolved drug in the interstitial space of muscle tissue, the IM route is acceptable for drugs whose water solubility is poor.

A second advantage of the IM route is that we can use it to administer *depot preparations* (preparations from which the drug is absorbed gradually over an extended time). Depending on the depot formulation, the effects of a single injection may persist for days, weeks, or even months. For example, *benzathine penicillin G*, a depot preparation of penicillin, can release therapeutically effective amounts of penicillin for a month or more following a single IM injection. In contrast, a single IM injection of penicillin G itself would be absorbed and excreted in less than 1 day. The obvious advantage of depot preparations is that they can greatly reduce the number of injections required during long-term therapy.

*Disadvantages.* The major drawbacks of IM administration are *discomfort* and *inconvenience.* Intramuscular injection of some preparations can be painful. Also, IM injections can cause local tissue injury and possibly nerve damage (if the injection is done improperly). Like all other forms of parenteral administration, IM injections are less convenient than oral administration.

## Subcutaneous

From a pharmacokinetics perspective, SC administration is nearly identical to IM administration. As with IM administration, there are no significant barriers to absorption: once a drug has been injected SC, it readily enters the blood by passing through the spaces between cells of the capillary wall. As with IM administration, blood flow and drug solubility are the major determinants of how fast absorption takes place. Because of the above similarities between SC and IM administration, these routes have similar advantages (suitability for poorly soluble drugs and depot preparations) and drawbacks (discomfort, inconvenience, potential for injury).

## Oral

In the discussion below, the abbreviation PO is used in reference to oral administration. This abbreviation stands for *per os*, a Latin phrase meaning *by way of the mouth*.

*Barriers to Absorption.* Following oral administration, drugs may be absorbed from the stomach or from the intestine. In either case, there are two barriers to cross: (1) the layer of *epithelial cells* that lines the gastrointestinal (GI) tract, and (2) the *capillary wall*. Since the walls of the capillaries that serve the GI tract offer no significant resistance to absorption, the major barrier to absorption is the gastrointestinal epithelium. To cross this layer of tightly packed cells, drugs must pass *through* the cells rather than *between* them.

*Absorption Pattern.* Because of multiple factors, the rate and extent of drug absorption following oral administration can be *highly variable*. Factors that can influence absorption include (1) solubility and stability of the drug, (2) gastric and intestinal pH, (3) gastric emptying time, (4) food in the gut, (5) coadministration of other drugs, and (6) special coatings on the drug preparation.

*Advantages.* Oral administration is easy, convenient, and inexpensive. (By inexpensive, we don't mean that oral drugs themselves are inexpensive, but rather that there is no cost for the process of administration.) Because of its relative ease, oral administration is the preferred route for self-medication.

Although absorption of orally administered drugs can be highly variable, this route is still *safer than parenteral injection.* With oral administration, there is no risk of fluid overload, infection, or embolism. Furthermore, since oral administration is potentially reversible, whereas injections are not, oral administration is much safer than injections. Recall that with parenteral administration there is no turning back: Once a drug has been injected, there is very little that we can do to prevent its absorption and subsequent effects. Therefore, when giving drugs parenterally, we must live with the consequences of our mistakes. In contrast, if need be, there are steps we can take to prevent

absorption following inappropriate oral administration. For example, by inducing either emesis (vomiting) or catharsis (rapid emptying of the small intestine and bowel) or both, we can move orally administered drugs out of the body before there has been sufficient time for absorption. In addition, we can prevent harm from orally administered drugs by giving activated charcoal, a compound that adsorbs drugs while they are still in the GI tract; once drugs are adsorbed onto the charcoal, they cannot be absorbed into the bloodstream. Our ability to prevent the absorption of orally administered drugs gives PO medications a safety factor that is unavailable with drugs injected parenterally.

*Disadvantages. Variability.* The major disadvantage of PO therapy is that absorption can be highly variable. That is, a drug administered to patient A may be absorbed rapidly and completely, whereas the same drug may be absorbed slowly and incompletely when administered to patient B. This variability makes it difficult to control the concentration of a drug at its sites of action, and therefore makes it difficult to control the onset, intensity, and duration of responses.

*Inactivation.* Oral administration can lead to inactivation of certain drugs. Penicillin G, for example, can't be taken orally because it would be destroyed by stomach acid. Similarly, insulin can't be taken orally because it would be destroyed by digestive enzymes.

Some drugs can't be taken orally because they would undergo rapid inactivation by hepatic enzymes as they pass through the liver on their way from the GI tract to the general circulation. This phenomenon, known as the "first-pass effect," is discussed later in the chapter.

*Patient Requirements.* Oral drug administration requires a conscious, cooperative patient. Drugs cannot be administered PO to comatose individuals or to individuals who, for whatever reason (e.g., psychosis, seizure, obstinacy, nausea), are unable or unwilling to swallow oral medications.

*Local Irritation.* Some oral preparations cause local irritation of the GI tract, which can result in discomfort, nausea, and vomiting.

## Comparing Oral Administration with Parenteral Administration

Because of ease, convenience, and relative safety, *oral administration is generally preferred to parenteral administration.* However, there are situations in which parenteral administration is clearly superior. Parenteral administration may be indicated in emergencies when rapid onset is required. Parenteral administration is desirable when plasma drug levels must be tightly controlled. (Because of variable absorption, oral administration does not permit tight control of plasma drug levels.) Parenteral administration is preferred for those drugs that would be destroyed by gastric acidity or digestive enzymes if given orally (e.g., insulin, penicillin G). Drugs such as the quaternary ammonium compounds, which cannot cross membranes, require parenteral administration to produce systemic effects. Parenteral administration is also required for those drugs that would cause severe local injury if administered by mouth (e.g., certain anticancer agents). In addition, parenteral administration is indicated when the prolonged effects of a depot preparation are desired. Lastly, parenteral therapy is superior to oral therapy for those patients who cannot or will not take drugs orally.

## Pharmaceutical Preparations for Oral Administration

There are several kinds of "packages" (formulations) into which a drug can be put for oral administration. Three such formulations—*tablets, enteric coatings,* and *sustained-release preparations*—are discussed below.

Before we discuss drug formulations, it will be helpful to define two terms: *chemical equivalence* and *bioavailability*. Two drug preparations would be considered *chemically equivalent* if they contained the same amount of the identical chemical compound (drug). Two preparations would be considered equal in *bioavailability* if the drug they contained were absorbed at the same rate and to the same extent. Please note that it is possible for two formulations of the same drug to be chemically equivalent while differing in bioavailability.

**Tablets.**  A tablet is a mixture of a drug plus binders and fillers, all of which have been compressed together. Tablets made by different manufacturers can differ in their rates of disintegration and dissolution, causing differences in their bioavailability. As a result, two tablets that contain the same amount of the same drug can have quantitative differences in therapeutic effects.

**Enteric-Coated Preparations.**  Enteric-coated preparations consist of drugs that have been covered with a material designed to dissolve in the intestine but not in the stomach. Materials used for enteric coatings include fatty acids, waxes, and shellac. Since enteric-coated preparations release their contents into the intestine and not into the stomach, these preparations are employed for two general purposes: (1) to protect drugs from acid and pepsin in the stomach and (2) to protect the stomach from drugs that can cause gastric discomfort.

The primary disadvantage of enteric-coated preparations is that absorption can be even more variable than with tablets. Since gastric emptying time can vary from minutes up to 12 hours, and since enteric-coated preparations cannot be absorbed until they leave the stomach, variations in gastric emptying time can alter the time of onset of these drugs. Furthermore, there are occasions when enteric coatings fail to dissolve, thereby allowing medication to pass through the GI tract without being absorbed at all.

**Sustained-Release Preparations.**  Sustained-release formulations are capsules filled with tiny spheres that contain the actual drug; the spheres have coatings that are designed to dissolve at variable rates. Since some spheres dissolve more slowly than others, drug is released steadily throughout the day. The primary advantage of sustained-release preparations is that they permit a reduction in the number of daily doses. These formulations have the additional advantage of producing relatively steady drug levels for an extended time (much like giving a drug by infusion). The major disadvantages of sustained-release formulations are high cost and the potential for variable absorption.

## Additional Routes of Administration

Drugs can be administered by a number of routes in addition to those discussed above. Drugs can be applied *topically* for local therapy of the skin, eyes, ears, nose, mouth, and vagina. In a few cases, topical agents (e.g., nitroglycerin, nicotine) are formulated for *transdermal* absorption into the systemic circulation. Some drugs are *inhaled* to elicit local effects in the lung, especially in the treatment of asthma. Other inhalational agents (e.g., volatile anesthetics, oxygen) are used for their systemic effects. *Rectal suppositories* may be employed for local effects or for effects throughout the body. *Vaginal suppositories* may be employed to treat local disorders. For management of some conditions, drugs must be injected directly into a specific tissue or organ (e.g., heart, joints, nerves, central nervous system). The unique characteristics of these routes are addressed throughout the book as we discuss specific drugs that employ them.

# Distribution

Distribution is defined as *the movement of drugs throughout the body.* Drug distribution is determined by three major factors: blood flow to tissues, the ability of a drug to exit the vascular system, and, to a lesser extent, the ability of a drug to enter cells.

## Blood Flow to Tissues

In the first phase of distribution, drugs are carried in the blood to the tissues and organs of the body. The rate at which drugs are delivered to a particular tissue is determined by the blood flow to that tissue. Since most tissues are well perfused, regional blood flow is rarely a limiting factor in drug distribution.

There are two pathologic conditions—abscesses and tumors—in which low regional blood flow can affect drug therapy. An abscess is a pus-filled pocket of infection that has no internal blood vessels. Because abscesses lack a blood supply, antibiotics cannot reach the bacteria within. Accordingly, if drug therapy of an abscess is to be effective, the abscess must first be surgically drained.

Solid tumors have a restricted blood supply. Although blood flow to the outer regions of tumors is relatively high, blood flow becomes progressively lower toward the core. As a result, we cannot achieve high drug levels deep within solid tumors. Limited blood flow is a major reason why solid tumors are so resistant to drug therapy.

## Exiting the Vascular System

Once a drug has been delivered to an organ or tissue via the blood, the next phase of distribution is to exit the vasculature. Leaving the blood occurs at capillary beds. Since most drugs do not produce their effects within the blood, the ability to leave the vascular system is an important determinant of drug actions. Exiting the vascular system is also necessary for drugs to undergo metabolism and excretion.

### Typical Capillary Beds

Most capillary beds offer no resistance to the departure of drugs. That is, in most tissues, drugs can leave the vasculature by passing through pores in the capillary wall. Since drugs pass *between* capillary cells rather than *through* them, movement into the interstitial space is not impeded. The exit of drugs from a typical capillary bed is illustrated in Figure 5–7.

### The Blood-Brain Barrier

The term *blood-brain barrier* refers to the unique anatomy of the capillaries that serve the CNS. As shown in Figure 5–8, there are *tight junctions* between the cells that compose the walls of most capillaries in the CNS. These junctions are so tight that they prevent drug passage. Consequently, in order to leave the blood and reach sites of action within the brain, a drug must be able to pass *through* cells of the capillary wall. Only drugs that are *lipid soluble* or have a *transport system* can cross the blood-brain barrier to a significant degree.

The presence of the blood-brain barrier is a mixed blessing. The good news is that the barrier protects the brain from being injured by potentially toxic substances. The bad news is that the barrier can be a significant obstacle to therapy of CNS disorders. The barrier can, for example, impede access of antibiotics to CNS infections.

The blood-brain barrier is not fully developed at birth. As a result, newborns are much more sensitive than older children or adults to medicines that act on the brain. Likewise, neonates are especially vulnerable to CNS poisons.

### Placental Drug Transfer

The membranes of the placenta separate the maternal circulation from the fetal circulation (Fig. 5–9). *The membranes of the placenta do NOT constitute an absolute barrier to the passage of drugs.* The same factors that determine the movement of drugs across other membranes determine the movement of drugs across the placenta. Accordingly, lipid-soluble, nonionized compounds readily pass from the maternal bloodstream into the blood of the fetus. In contrast, compounds that are ionized, highly polar, or protein bound (see below) are excluded.

Drugs that have the ability to cross the placenta can cause serious harm. Many compounds can cause birth defects, ranging from low birth weight to mental retardation to gross malformations. (Recall the thalidomide experience.) If a pregnant woman is a habitual user of opioids (e.g., heroin), her child will be born drug dependent and will need treatment with a heroin substitute to prevent withdrawal. The use of respiratory depressants (anesthetics and analgesics) during delivery can depress respiration in the neonate; infants exposed to respiratory depressants must be monitored closely until breathing has normalized.

### Protein Binding

Drugs can form reversible bonds with various proteins in the body. Of all the proteins to which drugs can bind, *plasma albumin* is the most important.

Albumin is the most abundant protein in plasma. Like other proteins, albumin is a large molecule (molecular

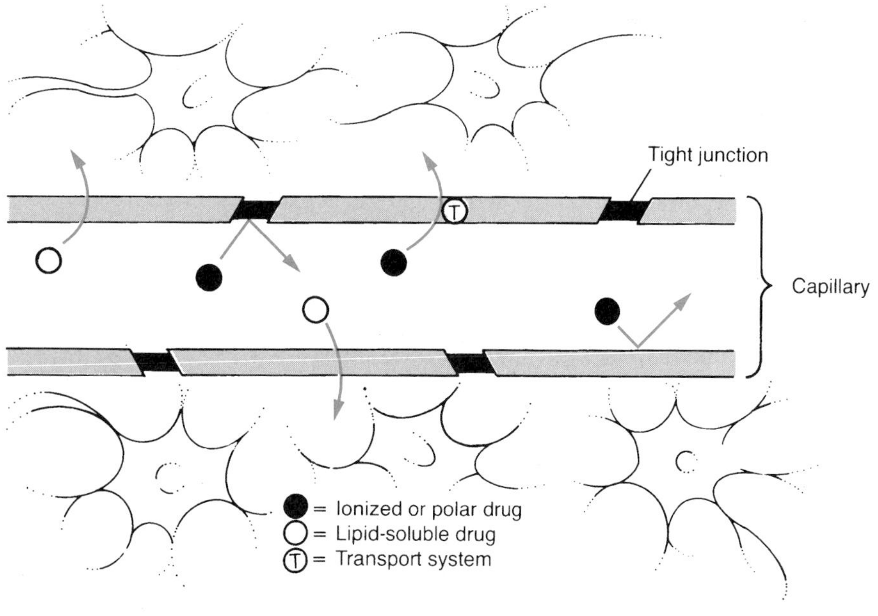

**Figure 5–8. Drug movement across the blood-brain barrier.** Tight junctions between the cells that compose the walls of the capillaries that serve the CNS prevent drugs from passing between cells to exit the vascular system. Conse-quently, in order to reach sites of action within the brain, a drug must pass directly through the cells of the capillary wall. To do this, the drug must be lipid soluble or be able to use an existing transport system.

● = Ionized or polar drug
○ = Lipid-soluble drug
Ⓣ = Transport system

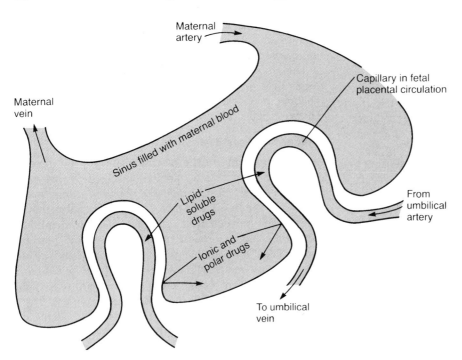

**Figure 5–9. Placental drug transfer.** To enter the fetal circulation, drugs must cross membranes of the maternal and fetal vascular systems. Lipid-soluble drugs can readily cross these membranes and enter the fetal blood. In contrast, ions and polar molecules are retained in the maternal blood.

weight = 69,000). Because of its size, *albumin always remains within the bloodstream;* albumin is too large to squeeze through pores in the capillary wall, and no transport system exists by which it might leave.

Figure 5-10A depicts the binding of drug molecules to albumin. Note that the drug molecules are much smaller than albumin. (The molecular mass of the average drug is about 300 to 500 compared with 69,000 for albumin.) As indicated by the two-way arrows, binding between albumin and drugs is *reversible.* As a result, a drug may exist either *bound* or *unbound* (free).

For drugs with the ability to bind to plasma albumin, only some molecules will be bound at any moment. The percentage of drug molecules that will be bound is determined by the strength of the attraction between albumin and the drug. For example, the attraction between albumin and warfarin (an anticoagulant) is strong, causing nearly all (99%) of the warfarin molecules in plasma to be bound, leaving only 1% free. For gentamicin (an antibiotic), the ratio of bound to free is quite different; since the attraction between gentamicin and albumin is relatively weak, less than 10% of the gentamicin molecules in plasma will be bound, leaving more than 90% free.

An important consequence of protein binding is restriction of drug distribution. Because albumin is too large to leave the bloodstream, drug molecules that are bound to albumin cannot leave either (Fig. 5-10B). Only those drug molecules that are free (not protein bound) can exit capillaries and become distributed to spaces outside the vasculature. However, drug molecules that are protein bound cannot leave the bloodstream to reach sites of action, metabolism, or excretion.

In addition to restricting the distribution of drugs, protein binding can be a source of drug interactions. As suggested by Figure 5-10A, each molecule of albumin has only a few sites to which drug molecules can bind.

Because the number of binding sites is limited, drugs that bind to albumin will compete with one another for those sites. As a result, one drug can displace another from albumin, causing the free concentration of the displaced drug to rise. By increasing levels of free drug, competition for binding can increase the intensity of drug responses. If the intensity increases excessively, toxicity can result.

## Entering Cells

Some drugs must enter cells to reach their sites of action, and practically all drugs must enter cells to undergo

**A**   Reversible Binding of a Drug to Albumin

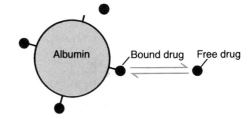

**B**   Retention of Protein-Bound Drug Within the Vasculature

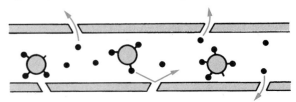

**Figure 5–10. Protein binding of drugs.** *A*, Albumin is the most prevalent protein in plasma and the most important of the proteins to which drugs can become bound. *B*, Only unbound (free) drugs can leave the vascular system. Bound drugs are too large to fit through the gaps between cells in the capillary wall.

metabolism and excretion. The factors that determine the ability of a drug to cross cell membranes are the same factors that determine the passage of drugs across all other membranes, namely, lipid solubility, the presence of a transport system, or both.

As we will discuss in Chapter 6, many drugs produce their effects by binding to receptors located on the external surface of the cell membrane. Obviously, these drugs do not need to cross the cell membrane in order to act.

# Metabolism

Drug metabolism, also known as *biotransformation,* is defined as *the enzymatic alteration of drug structure.* Practically all drug metabolism takes place in the liver.

## Hepatic Drug-Metabolizing Enzymes

Most of the drug metabolism that takes place in the liver is performed by the *hepatic microsomal enzyme system,* also known as the *P-450 system.* The term *P-450* refers to cytochrome P-450, a key component of this enzyme system. (Note: cytochrome P-450 is not a single compound, but rather a large family of compounds with similar structures.)

Hepatic microsomal enzymes are capable of catalyzing a wide variety of reactions that employ drugs as substrates. Some of these reactions are illustrated in Figure 5–11. As these examples indicate, drug metabolism doesn't always result in the breakdown of drugs into smaller molecules; drug metabolism can also result in the synthesis of a molecule that is larger than the parent drug.

## Therapeutic Consequences of Drug Metabolism

Drug metabolism has five possible consequences of therapeutic significance: (1) accelerated renal excretion of drugs, (2) drug inactivation, (3) increased therapeutic action, (4) activation of prodrugs, and (5) increased or decreased toxicity. Figure 5–11 depicts reactions that illustrate these consequences of metabolism.

*Accelerated Renal Drug Excretion. The most important consequence of drug metabolism is the promotion of renal drug excretion.* As discussed in the next section, the kidney, which is the major organ of drug excretion, is unable to excrete drugs that are highly lipid soluble. By converting lipid-soluble drugs into more polar (less lipid-soluble) compounds, drug metabolism makes it possible for the kidney to excrete many drugs. In the case of certain highly lipid-soluble drugs (e.g., thiopental), renal excretion would require years for completion were it not for conversion of these agents into more polar compounds by drug-metabolizing enzymes.

*Drug Inactivation.* Drug metabolism can convert pharmacologically active compounds to inactive forms. This

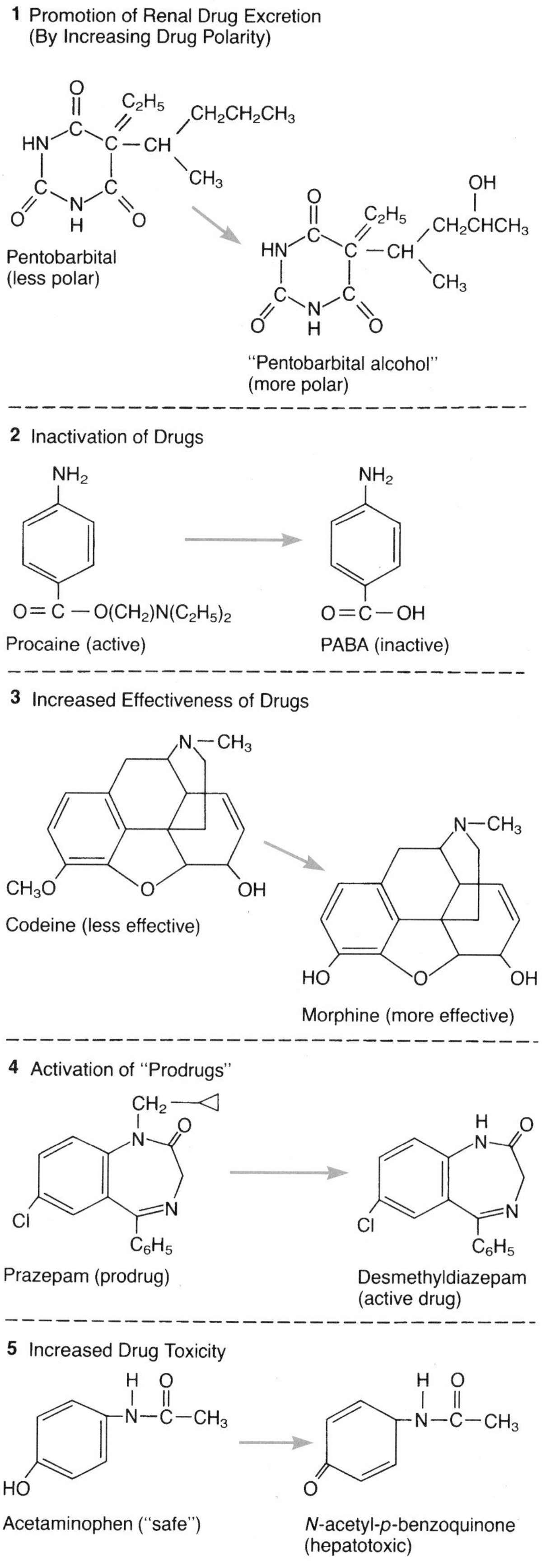

**Figure 5–11. Therapeutic consequences of drug metabolism.**

phenomenon is illustrated by the conversion of procaine (a local anesthetic) into PABA (*para*-aminobenzoic acid), an inactive metabolite (see Fig. 5-11).

**Increased Therapeutic Action.** Metabolism can increase the effectiveness of some drugs. This consequence of metabolism is illustrated by the conversion of codeine into morphine (see Fig. 5-11). The analgesic activity of morphine is so much greater than that of codeine that formation of morphine may account for virtually all the pain relief that occurs following codeine administration.

**Activation of Prodrugs.** A *prodrug* is a compound that is pharmacologically inactive as administered and then undergoes conversion to its active form within the body. Activation of a prodrug is illustrated by the metabolic conversion of prazepam into desmethyldiazepam (see Fig. 5-11). (Prazepam is a close relative of diazepam, a drug familiar to us under the trade name Valium.)

**Increased or Decreased Toxicity.** By converting drugs into inactive forms, metabolism can decrease toxicity. Conversely, metabolism can increase the potential for harm by converting relatively safe compounds into forms that are toxic. Increased toxicity is illustrated by the conversion of acetaminophen into a hepatotoxic metabolite (see Fig. 5-11). It is this product of metabolism, and not acetaminophen itself, that causes injury when acetaminophen is taken in overdose.

## Special Considerations in Drug Metabolism

Several factors can influence the rate at which drugs are metabolized. These factors must be accounted for in drug therapy.

**Age.** The drug-metabolizing capacity of infants is limited. The liver does not develop its full capacity to metabolize drugs until about 1 year after birth. *During the time prior to hepatic maturation, infants are especially sensitive to drugs, and care must be taken to avoid injury.*

**Induction of Drug-Metabolizing Enzymes.** Some drugs act on the liver to increase rates of drug metabolism. For example, when phenobarbital is administered for a few days, it can cause the drug-metabolizing capacity of the liver to double. Phenobarbital increases metabolism by causing the liver to synthesize drug-metabolizing enzymes. This process of stimulating enzyme synthesis is referred to as *induction.*

Induction of drug-metabolizing enzymes can have two therapeutic consequences. First, by stimulating the liver to produce more drug-metabolizing enzymes, a drug can increase the rate of its own metabolism, thereby necessitating an increase in its dosage to maintain therapeutic effects. Second, induction of drug-metabolizing enzymes can accelerate the metabolism of other drugs used concurrently, necessitating an increase in *their* dosages.

**First-Pass Effect.** The term *first-pass effect* refers to the rapid hepatic inactivation of certain oral drugs. When drugs are administered orally, they are absorbed from the GI tract and carried directly to the liver by way of the hepatic portal circulation. If the capacity of the liver to metabolize a drug is extremely high, that drug can be completely inactivated on its first pass through the liver; hence, no therapeutic effects will occur. To circumvent the first-pass effect, drugs that undergo rapid hepatic metabolism are often administered parenterally. This permits the drug to temporarily bypass the liver, thereby allowing it to reach therapeutic levels in the systemic blood.

Nitroglycerin is the classic example of a drug that undergoes such rapid hepatic metabolism that it is largely without effect following oral administration. However, when administered sublingually (under the tongue), nitroglycerin is very active. Sublingual administration is effective because it permits nitroglycerin to be absorbed through the oral mucosa directly into the systemic circulation. Once in circulation, the drug is carried to its sites of action prior to passage through the liver. Hence, therapeutic action can be exerted before the drug is exposed to hepatic enzymes.

**Nutritional Status.** Hepatic drug-metabolizing enzymes require a number of co-factors to function. In the malnourished patient, these co-factors may be deficient, causing drug metabolism to be compromised.

**Competition between Drugs.** When two drugs are metabolized by the same metabolic pathway, they may compete with each other for metabolism, and thereby decrease the rate at which one or both agents are metabolized. If metabolism is depressed enough, a drug can accumulate to dangerous levels. As discussed in Chapter 63, this kind of interaction can lead to toxic accumulation of terfenadine and astemizole, two popular antihistamines.

# Excretion

Drug excretion is defined as *the removal of drugs from the body.* Drugs and their metabolites can exit the body in urine, bile, sweat, saliva, breast milk, and expired air. The most important organ for drug excretion is the kidney.

## Renal Drug Excretion

The kidneys account for the majority of drug excretion. When the kidneys are healthy, they serve to limit the duration of action of many drugs. Conversely, if renal failure occurs, both the duration and intensity of drug responses may increase.

### Steps in Renal Drug Excretion

Urinary excretion of drugs is the net result of three processes: (1) glomerular filtration, (2) passive tubular reabsorption, and (3) active tubular secretion. These processes are depicted in Figure 5-12.

**Glomerular Filtration.** Renal excretion begins at the glomerulus of the kidney tubule. The glomerulus consists of a capillary network surrounded by Bowman's capsule; small pores perforate the capillary walls. As blood flows through the glomerular capillaries, fluids and small molecules—including drugs—are forced through the pores of the capillary wall. This process, called glomerular filtration, moves drugs from the blood into the tubular urine. Blood cells and large molecules (e.g., proteins) are too big to pass through the capillary pores and therefore do not undergo filtration. Because large molecules are not filtered, drugs bound to albumin remain behind in the blood.

***Passive Tubular Reabsorption.*** As depicted in Figure 5-12, the vessels that deliver blood to the glomerulus return to proximity with the renal tubule at a point distal to the glomerulus. At this distal site, drug concentrations in the blood are lower than drug concentrations in the tubule. This concentration gradient acts as a driving force to move drugs from the lumen of the tubule back into the blood. Since lipid-soluble drugs can readily cross the membranes that compose the tubular and vascular walls, *drugs that are lipid soluble undergo passive reabsorption from the tubule back into the blood.* In contrast, drugs that are not lipid soluble (ions and polar compounds) remain in the urine to be excreted. By converting lipid-soluble drugs into more polar forms, drug metabolism reduces the passive reabsorption of drugs and thereby accelerates their excretion.

***Active Tubular Secretion.*** There are active transport systems in the kidney tubules that pump drugs from the blood to the tubular urine. The tubules have two classes of pumps, one for organic acids and one for organic bases. These pumps have a relatively high capacity and play a significant role in the excretion of certain compounds.

## Factors That Modify Renal Drug Excretion

***pH-Dependent Ionization.*** The phenomenon of pH-dependent ionization can be used to accelerate renal excretion of drugs. Recall that passive tubular reabsorption is limited to lipid-soluble compounds. Since ions are not lipid soluble, drugs that are ionized at the pH of tubular urine will remain in the tubule and be excreted. Consequently, by manipulating urinary pH in such a way as to promote the ionization of a drug, we can decrease passive reabsorption and thereby hasten its excretion. This principle has been employed to promote the excretion of poisons as well as medications that have been taken in toxic doses.

The treatment of aspirin poisoning provides an example of how manipulation of urinary pH can be put to therapeutic advantage. When children have been exposed to toxic doses of aspirin, they can be treated, in part, by giving an agent that elevates urinary pH (i.e., makes the urine more basic). Since aspirin is an acidic drug, and since acids tend to ionize in basic media, elevation of urinary pH causes more of the aspirin molecules present in urine to become ionized. As a result, less drug is passively reabsorbed and therefore more is excreted.

***Competition for Active Tubular Transport.*** Competition between drugs for active tubular transport can delay their renal excretion, thereby prolonging their effects. The active transport systems of the renal tubules can be

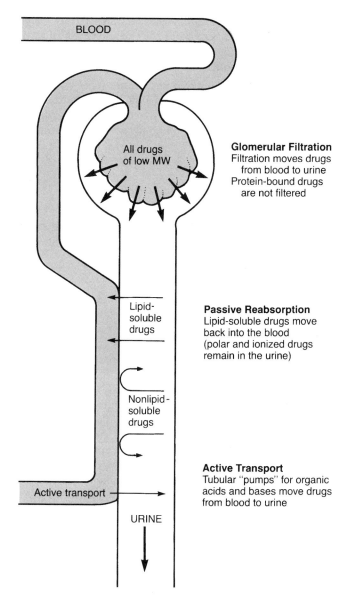

**Figure 5–12. Renal drug excretion.** (Redrawn from Binns, T.B. [ed.]. Absorption and Distribution of Drugs. Edinburgh, Churchill Livingstone, 1964.)

envisioned as motor-driven revolving doors that carry drugs from the plasma into the renal tubules. These "revolving doors" can carry only a limited number of drug molecules per unit time. Accordingly, if there are too many molecules present, some must wait their turn. Because of competition, if we administer two drugs at the same time, and if both drugs use the same system of transport, the excretion of each will be delayed by the presence of the other.

Competition for transport has been employed clinically to prolong the effects of drugs that normally undergo very rapid renal excretion. For example, when administered alone, penicillin is rapidly cleared from the blood by active tubular transport. Excretion of penicillin can be delayed by concurrent administration of probenecid, an agent that is removed from the blood by the same tubular transport system that pumps penicillin. Hence, if a large dose of probenecid is administered, renal excretion of penicillin will be delayed while the transport system is occupied with moving the probenecid. By delaying penicillin excretion, probenecid prolongs antibacterial effects.

**Age.** The kidneys of newborns are not fully developed. Until their kidneys reach full capacity (a few months after birth), infants have a limited capacity to excrete drugs. This limitation must be accounted for when medicating an infant.

## Nonrenal Routes of Drug Excretion

In most cases, excretion of drugs by nonrenal routes has minimal clinical significance. However, in certain situations, nonrenal excretion can have important therapeutic and toxicologic consequences.

### Breast Milk

Drugs taken by breast-feeding women can undergo excretion into the milk. As a result, breast-feeding can expose the nursing infant to drugs. The factors that influence the appearance of drugs in milk are the same factors that determine the passage of drugs across membranes. Accordingly, lipid-soluble drugs will have ready access to breast milk, whereas drugs that are polar, ionized, or protein bound will not enter the milk in significant amounts. Because infants may be harmed by compounds excreted in breast milk, it is recommended that nursing mothers avoid all drugs. If a woman must take medication, she should consult with her physician to ensure that it will not appear in her milk in concentrations high enough to harm her baby. If toxic amounts will be excreted in milk, breast-feeding must cease.

### Other Nonrenal Routes of Excretion

The *bile* is an important route of excretion for certain drugs. Recall that bile is secreted into the intestine and then leaves the body in the feces. In some cases, drugs entering the intestine in bile may undergo reabsorption back into the portal blood. This reabsorption, referred to as *enterohepatic recirculation*, can substantially prolong a drug's sojourn in the body.

The *lungs* are the major route by which volatile anesthetics are excreted.

Small amounts of drugs can appear in *sweat* and *saliva*. These routes have little therapeutic or toxicologic significance.

## Time Course of Drug Responses

To achieve the therapeutic objective, we must control the time course of drug responses. We need to regulate the time at which drug responses start, the time they are most intense, and the time they cease. Since the four pharmacokinetic processes—absorption, distribution, metabolism, and excretion—determine how much drug will be at its sites of action at any given time, these processes are the major determinants of the time course over which drug responses will take place. Having discussed the individual processes that contribute to determining the time course of drug action, we are now prepared to discuss the time course itself.

## Plasma Drug Levels

In most cases, the time course of drug action bears a direct relationship to the concentration of drug in the blood. Hence, before discussing the time course per se, it will be helpful to review several important concepts related to plasma drug levels.

### Clinical Significance of Plasma Drug Levels

Clinicians frequently monitor plasma drug levels in efforts to regulate drug responses. When measurements indicate that drug levels are inappropriate, these levels can be adjusted up or down by changing dosage or the timing of administration.

The practice of regulating plasma drug levels in order to control drug responses should seem a bit odd given that (1) drug responses are related to drug concentrations at *sites of action* and that (2) the site of action of most drugs is not in the plasma. The question arises, "Why adjust plasma levels of a drug when what really matters is the concentration of that drug at its sites of action?" The answer to this question begins with the following observation: more often than not, it is a practical impossibility to measure drug concentrations at sites of action. For example, when a patient with epilepsy takes phenytoin (an anticonvulsant), we cannot routinely draw samples from inside the skull to see if brain levels of the medication are adequate for seizure control. Fortunately, in the case of phenytoin and most other drugs, it is not necessary to measure drug concentrations at actual sites of action in order to have an objective basis for adjusting dosage. Experience has shown that for most drugs *there is a direct correlation between therapeutic and toxic responses and the amount of drug present in plasma*. Therefore, although we can't usually measure drug concentrations at sites of action, we can determine plasma drug concentrations that, in turn, are highly predictive of therapeutic and toxic responses. Accordingly, the dosing objective is commonly spoken of in terms of achieving a specific plasma level of a drug.

### Two Plasma Drug Levels Defined

Two plasma drug levels are of special importance: (1) the minimum effective concentration, and (2) the toxic concentration. These levels are depicted in Figure 5-13 and defined below.

**Minimum Effective Concentration.** The minimum effective concentration (MEC) is defined as *the plasma drug level below which therapeutic effects will not occur*. Hence, to be of benefit, a drug must be present in concentrations at or above the MEC.

**Toxic Concentration.** Toxicity occurs when plasma drug levels climb too high. The plasma level at which

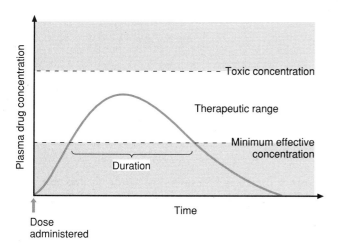

**Figure 5–13. Single-dose time course.**

toxic effects begin to appear is termed the toxic concentration. Doses must be kept small enough so that the toxic concentration is not reached.

### Therapeutic Range

As indicated in Figure 5-13, there is a range of plasma drug levels, falling between the MEC and the toxic concentration, that is termed the therapeutic range. When plasma levels are within the therapeutic range, there is enough drug present to produce therapeutic responses but not so much that toxicity results. *The objective of drug dosing is to maintain plasma drug levels within the therapeutic range.*

The width of the therapeutic range is a major determinant of the ease with which a drug can be used safely. Drugs that have a narrow therapeutic range are difficult to administer safely. Conversely, drugs that have a wide therapeutic range can be administered safely with relative ease. Acetaminophen, for example, has a relatively wide therapeutic range: the toxic concentration is about 30 times greater than the MEC. Because of this wide therapeutic range, the dosage does not need to be highly precise: a broad range of doses can be employed to produce plasma levels that will be above the MEC but that will not reach the toxic concentration. In contrast, lithium (used for manic-depressive illness) has a very narrow therapeutic range: the toxic concentration is only three times greater than the MEC. Since toxicity can result from lithium levels that are not much greater than those needed to produce therapeutic effects, lithium dosing must be done carefully if therapeutic effects are to be achieved without causing toxicity. If lithium had a wider therapeutic range, the drug would be much easier to use.

Understanding the concept of therapeutic range can facilitate patient care. Because drugs with a narrow therapeutic range are more dangerous than drugs with a wide therapeutic range, patients taking drugs with a narrow therapeutic range are the most likely to require nursing intervention for drug-related complications. The nurse who is aware of this fact can focus attention on these patients. In contrast, the nurse who has no basis for predicting which drugs are most likely to produce toxicity has no basis for allocating attention, and therefore is obliged to monitor all patients with equal diligence—a process that is both stressful and inefficient.

However, lest you get the wrong impression, the above advice should not be construed as an invitation to be lax about patients taking drugs that have a wide therapeutic range. Even these drugs can cause harm. Hence, although patients receiving drugs with a narrow therapeutic range should be monitored most closely, common sense dictates that patients receiving safer drugs must not be neglected.

### Single-Dose Time Course

Figure 5-13 shows how plasma drug levels change over time after a single dose of an oral medication. The rise in drug levels occurs as the medicine undergoes absorption. Drug levels then decline as metabolism and excretion eliminate the drug from the body.

Because responses cannot occur until plasma drug levels have reached the MEC, there is a period of latency between drug administration and onset of effects. The extent of this delay is determined by the rate of absorption.

The duration of effects is determined largely by the combination of metabolism and excretion. As long as plasma levels remain above the MEC, therapeutic responses will be maintained; when plasma levels fall below the MEC, responses will cease. Since metabolism and excretion are the processes most responsible for causing plasma drug levels to fall, these processes are the primary determinants of how long drug effects will persist.

### Drug Half-Life

Before proceeding to the topic of multiple dosing, we need to discuss the concept of half-life. When a patient ceases drug use, the combination of metabolism and excretion will cause the amount of drug in the body to decline. The half-life of a drug is an index of just how rapidly that decline will occur.

Drug half-life is defined as *the time required for the amount of drug in the body to decrease by 50%.* A few drugs have half-lives that are extremely short—on the order of minutes. In contrast, the half-lives of some drugs exceed 1 week. Drugs with short half-lives leave the body quickly. Drugs with long half-lives leave slowly.

Note that, in our definition of half-life, a *percentage*—not a specific *amount*—of drug is lost during one half-life. That is, the half-life does not specify, for example, that 2 gm or 18 mg will leave the body in a given time. Rather, the half-life tells us that, no matter what the amount of drug in the body may be, half (50%) will leave during a specified period of time (the half-life). The actual amount of drug that is lost during one half-life will depend upon just how much drug is present: the more drug that is in the body, the larger the amount lost during one half-life.

The concept of half-life is best understood through an example. Morphine provides a good illustration. The half-life of morphine is approximately 3 hours. By definition, this means that body stores of morphine will decrease by 50% every 3 hours—regardless of how much morphine is in the body. If there is 50 mg of morphine in the body, 50% (25 mg) will be lost in 3 hours; if there is only 2 mg of morphine in the body, only 1 mg (50% of 2 mg) will be lost in 3 hours. Note that in both cases, morphine levels drop by 50% during an interval of one half-life. However, the actual *amount* lost is larger when total body stores of the drug are higher.

The half-life of a drug determines the dosing interval (i.e., how much time separates each dose). For drugs with a short half-life, the dosing interval must be correspondingly short; if a long interval were used, drug levels would fall below the MEC between doses, and therapeutic effects would be lost. Conversely, if a drug has a long half-life, a long time can separate doses without loss of effects.

## Drug Levels Produced with Repeated Doses

Multiple dosing leads to drug accumulation. When a patient takes a single dose of a drug, plasma levels simply go up and then come down. In contrast, when a patient takes repeated doses of a drug, the process is more complex and results in drug accumulation. The factors that determine the rate and extent of accumulation are considered below.

### The Process by Which Plateau Drug Levels Are Achieved

Administering repeated doses of a drug will cause that drug to build up in the body until a *plateau* (steady level) has been achieved. What causes drug levels to reach plateau? To begin with, common sense tells us that if a second dose of a drug is administered before all of the prior dose has been eliminated, total body stores of that drug will be higher after the second dose than after the initial dose. As succeeding doses are administered, drug levels will climb even higher. The drug will continue to accumulate until a state has been achieved in which the amount of drug eliminated between doses equals the amount administered. *When the amount of drug eliminated between doses equals the dose administered, average drug levels will remain constant and plateau will have been reached.*

The process by which multiple dosing produces a plateau is illustrated in Figure 5–14. The drug in this figure is a hypothetical agent with a half-life of exactly 1 day. The regimen consists of a 2-gm dose administered once daily. For the purpose of illustration, we will assume that absorption takes place instantly. Upon administration of the first 2-gm dose (day 1 in the figure), total body stores go from zero to 2 gm. Within one half-life (1 day), body stores drop by 50%—from 2 gm down to 1 gm. At the beginning of day 2, the second 2-gm dose is given, causing body stores to rise from 1 gm up to 3 gm. Over the next 1-day half-life, body stores again drop by 50%, this time from 3 gm down to 1.5 gm. When the third dose is given, body stores go from 1.5 gm up to 3.5 gm. Over the next half-life, stores drop by 50% down to 1.75 gm. When the fourth

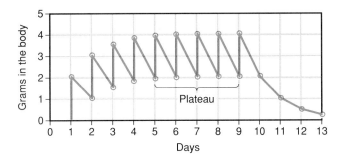

**Figure 5–14. Drug accumulation with repeated administration.** This figure illustrates the accumulation of a hypothetical drug during repeated administration. The drug has a half-life of 1 day. The dosing schedule is 2 gm once a day on days 1 through 9. Note that plateau is reached at about the beginning of day 5 (i.e., after four half-lives). Note also that, when administration is discontinued, it takes about 4 days (four half-lives) for most (94%) of the drug to leave the body.

dose is given, drug levels climb to 3.75 gm and, between doses, levels again drop by 50%, this time to approximately 1.9 gm. When the fifth dose is given (at the beginning of day 5), drug levels go up to about 3.9 gm. This process of accumulation continues until body stores reach 4 gm. When total body stores of this drug are 4 gm, 2 gm will be lost each day (i.e., over one half-life). Since a 2-gm dose is being administered each day, when body stores reach 4 gm, the amount lost between doses will equal the dose administered. At this point, body stores will simply alternate between 4 gm and 2 gm; average body stores will be stable; and plateau will have been reached. Note that the reason that plateau is finally reached is that the actual amount of drug lost between doses gets larger each day. That is, although 50% of total body stores are lost each day, the amount in grams grows progressively larger because total body stores are getting larger day by day. Plateau is reached when the amount lost between doses grows to be as large as the amount administered.

### Time to Plateau

When a drug is administered repeatedly in the same dose, *plateau will be reached in approximately four half-lives.* For the hypothetical agent illustrated in Figure 5–14, total body stores approached their peak near the beginning of day 5, or approximately 4 full days after treatment began. Since the half-life of this drug is 1 day, reaching plateau in 4 days is equivalent to reaching plateau in four half-lives.

*As long as dosage remains constant, the time required to reach plateau is independent of dosage size.* Put another way, the time required to reach plateau employing a large dose of a particular drug is identical to the time required to reach plateau employing a small dose of that drug. Referring to the drug in Figure 5–14, just as it took four half-lives (4 days) to reach plateau when a dose of 2 gm was administered daily, it would also take four half-lives to reach plateau if a dose of 4 gm were administered each day. It is true that the *height* of the plateau would be greater if a 4-gm dose were given, but the time required to reach plateau would not be altered by the increase in dosage. To confirm this statement, substitute a dose of 4 gm in the exercise we went through to demonstrate accumulation to plateau with a dose of 2 gm.

## Techniques for Reducing Fluctuations in Drug Levels

As can be seen from Figure 5-14, when drugs are administered repeatedly, drug levels will fluctuate between doses. The degree of fluctuation that can be tolerated will depend upon a drug's therapeutic range: if there is not much difference between the toxic concentration and the MEC, then fluctuations must be kept to a minimum.

Two procedures can be employed to reduce fluctuations in drug levels. One technique is to administer drugs by *continuous infusion*. With this procedure, plasma levels can be kept nearly constant. The second procedure is to *reduce the dosage size and reduce the dosing interval* (keeping the total daily dose constant). For example, rather than giving the drug from Figure 5-14 in 2-gm doses once every 24 hours, we could give this drug in 1-gm doses every 12 hours. With this altered dosing schedule, the total daily dose would remain unchanged, as would total body stores at plateau. However, instead of fluctuating over a range of 2 gm between doses, levels would fluctuate over a range of 1 gm.

## Loading Doses Versus Maintenance Doses

As discussed above, if we were to administer a drug in repeated doses of equal size, an interval equivalent to four half-lives would be required to achieve plateau. For drugs whose half-lives are long, achieving plateau could take days or even weeks. When plateau must be achieved more quickly, a large initial dose can be administered. This large initial dose is called a *loading dose*. After high drug levels have been established with a loading dose, plateau can be maintained by giving smaller doses. These smaller doses are referred to as *maintenance doses*.

The claim that use of a loading dose will shorten the time to plateau may appear to contradict an earlier statement, which said that the time to plateau is not affected by dosage size. However, there is no contradiction. For any *specified* dosage, it will always take four half-lives to reach plateau. When a loading dose is administered followed by maintenance doses, we have not reached plateau *for the loading dose*. Rather, we have simply used the loading dose to rapidly produce a drug level equivalent to the plateau level for a smaller dose. If we wished to achieve plateau level for the loading dose, we would be obliged to either administer repeated doses equivalent to the loading dose for a period of four half-lives or administer a dose even larger than the original loading dose. Think about it.

## Decline from Plateau

*When drug administration is discontinued, most (94%) of the drug in the body will be eliminated over an interval equal to four half-lives.* This statement can be validated with simple arithmetic. Let's consider a patient who has been taking morphine. In addition, let's assume that, at the time dosing ceased, the total body store of mor-

phine was 40 mg. Within one half-life after drug withdrawal, morphine stores will decline by 50%—down to 20 mg. During the second half-life, stores will again decline by 50%, dropping from 20 mg to 10 mg. During the third half-life, the level will decline once more by 50%—from 10 mg down to 5 mg. During the fourth half-life, the level will again decline by 50%—from 5 mg down to 2.5 mg. Hence, over a period of four half-lives, total body stores of morphine will drop from an initial level of 40 mg down to 2.5 mg, an overall decline of 94%. Most of the drug in the body will be cleared within four half-lives.

The time required for drugs to leave the body is important when toxicity develops. Let's consider the elimination of digitoxin (a drug used to treat heart failure) as an example. Digitoxin, true to its name, is a potentially dangerous drug with a narrow therapeutic range. In addition, the half-life of digitoxin is very long—about 7 days. What will be the consequence of digitoxin overdose? Toxic levels of the drug will remain in the body for a long time: Since digitoxin has a half-life of 7 days, and since four half-lives are required for most of the drug to be cleared from the body, it could take weeks for digitoxin stores to fall to a safe level. During the time that excess drug remains in the body, significant effort will be required to keep the patient alive. If digitoxin had a shorter half-life, body stores would decline more rapidly, thereby making management of overdose less difficult.

It is important to note that the concept of half-life does not apply to the elimination of all drugs. A few agents, most notably ethanol (alcohol), leave the body at a *constant rate*, regardless of how much is present. The implications of this kind of decline for ethanol are discussed in Chapter 36.

## KEY POINTS

- Pharmacokinetics consists of four basic processes: absorption, distribution, metabolism, and excretion.
- Pharmacokinetic processes determine the concentration of a drug at its sites of action, and thereby determine the intensity and time course of responses.
- To cross membranes, most drugs must dissolve directly into the lipid bilayer of the membrane. Accordingly, lipid-soluble drugs can cross membranes easily, whereas drugs that are polar or ionized cannot.
- Acidic drugs ionize in basic (alkaline) media, whereas basic drugs ionize in acidic media.
- Absorption is defined as the movement of a drug from its site of administration into the blood.
- Absorption is enhanced by rapid drug dissolution, high lipid solubility of the drug, a large surface area for absorption, and high blood flow to the site of administration.
- Intravenous administration has several advantages: rapid onset, precise control over the amount of drug entering the blood, suitability for use with large volumes of fluid, and suitability for irritant drugs.
- Intravenous administration has several disadvantages: high cost, difficulty, inconvenience, danger because of

- irreversibility, and the potential for fluid overload, infection, and embolism.
- Intramuscular administration has two advantages: suitability for insoluble drugs and suitability for depot preparations.
- Intramuscular administration has two disadvantages: inconvenience and the potential for discomfort.
- Subcutaneous administration has the same advantages and disadvantages as intramuscular administration.
- Oral administration has the advantages of ease, convenience, economy, and safety.
- The principal disadvantage of oral administration is high variability.
- Enteric-coated oral formulations are designed to release their contents in the small intestine, and not in the stomach.
- Sustained-release oral formulations are designed to release their contents slowly, thereby permitting a longer interval between doses.
- Distribution is defined as the movement of drugs throughout the body.
- In most tissues, drugs can easily leave the vasculature through spaces between the cells that compose the capillary wall.
- The term *blood-brain barrier* refers to the presence of tight junctions between the cells that compose capillary walls in the CNS. Because of this barrier, drugs must pass *through* the cells of the capillary wall (rather than between them) in order to reach the CNS.
- The membranes of the placenta do *not* constitute an absolute barrier to the passage of drugs. The same factors that determine drug movements across all other membranes determine the movement of drugs across the placenta.
- Many drugs bind reversibly to plasma albumin. While bound to albumin, drug molecules cannot leave the vascular system.
- Drug metabolism (biotransformation) is defined as the enzymatic alteration of drug structure.
- Most drug metabolism takes place in the liver and is catalyzed by the cytochrome P-450 system of enzymes.
- The most important consequence of drug metabolism is promotion of renal drug excretion (by converting lipid-soluble drugs into more polar [less lipid-soluble] forms).
- Other consequences of drug metabolism are conversion of drugs to less active or inactive forms, conversion of drugs to more active forms, conversion of prodrugs to their active forms, and conversion of drugs to more toxic or less toxic forms.

- Some drugs can induce (stimulate) synthesis of hepatic drug-metabolizing enzymes, and can thereby accelerate their own metabolism and the metabolism of other drugs.
- The term *first-pass effect* refers to the rapid inactivation of some oral drugs on their first pass through the liver following absorption from the intestine.
- Most drugs are excreted by the kidney.
- Renal drug excretion has three steps: glomerular filtration, passive tubular reabsorption, and active tubular secretion.
- Drugs that are highly lipid soluble undergo extensive passive reabsorption back into the blood, and therefore cannot be excreted by the kidney (until they are converted to more polar forms by the liver).
- Drugs can be excreted into breast milk, thereby posing a threat to the nursing infant.
- For most drugs, there is a direct correlation between the level of drug in plasma and the intensity of therapeutic and toxic effects.
- The minimum effective concentration (MEC) of a drug is defined as the plasma drug level below which therapeutic effects will not occur.
- The therapeutic range of a drug lies between the MEC and the toxic concentration.
- Drugs with a wide therapeutic range are relatively easy to use safely, whereas drugs with a narrow therapeutic range are difficult to use safely.
- The half-life of a drug is defined as the time required for the amount of drug in the body to decline by 50%.
- Drugs that have a short half-life must be administered more frequently than drugs that have a long half-life.
- When drugs are administered repeatedly, drug levels will gradually rise and then reach a steady plateau.
- The time required to reach plateau is equivalent to about four half-lives.
- The time required to reach plateau is independent of dosage size, although the *height* of the plateau will be higher with larger doses.
- If plasma drug levels fluctuate too much between doses, the fluctuations could be reduced by (1) giving smaller doses at shorter intervals (keeping the total daily dose the same) or (2) using a continuous infusion.
- For a drug with a long half-life, it may be necessary to use a loading dose to achieve plateau quickly.
- When drug administration is discontinued, most (94%) of the drug in the body will be eliminated over four half-lives.

# CHAPTER 6

# Pharmacodynamics

Pharmacodynamics is defined as the study of the biochemical and physiologic effects of drugs and the molecular mechanisms by which those effects are produced. In short, pharmacodynamics is the study of what drugs do to the body and how they do it.

In order to participate rationally in achieving the therapeutic objective, nurses need a basic understanding of pharmacodynamics. You must know about drug actions in order to educate patients about their medication. Knowledge of drug effects is also needed in order to make informed decisions on PRN orders. In addition, knowledge of pharmacodynamics is applied when evaluating patients for drug responses, both beneficial and harmful. You will also need to understand drug actions when conferring with the physician about drug therapy; the nurse who believes that a patient is receiving inappropriate medication or is being denied a required drug will need to support that conviction with arguments based at least in part on knowledge of pharmacodynamics.

## Dose-Response Relationships

The dose-response relationship (i.e., the relationship between the size of an administered dose and the intensity of the response produced) is a fundamental concern in therapeutics. Dose-response relationships determine the minimum amount of drug that we can use, the maximum response that a drug can elicit, and how much we need to increase the dosage to produce the desired increase in response.

### Basic Features of the Dose-Response Relationship

The basic characteristics of dose-response relationships are illustrated in Figure 6-1. Part A of the figure shows

dose-response data plotted on *linear* coordinates. Part B shows the same data plotted on *semilogarithmic* coordinates (i.e., the scale on which dosage is plotted is logarithmic rather than linear). The most obvious and important characteristic revealed by these curves is that the dose-response relationship is *graded.* That is, as dosage is increased, the response becomes progressively larger. Because drug responses are graded, therapeutic effects can be adjusted to fit the needs of each patient. To tailor treatment to a particular patient, all we need do is raise or lower the dosage until a response of the desired intensity is achieved. If drug responses were *all-or-nothing* instead of graded, drugs could produce only one intensity of response. If that response were too strong or too weak for a particular patient, there would be nothing we could do to adjust its intensity to better suit the patient. Clearly, the graded nature of the dose-response relationship is essential for successful drug therapy.

As indicated in Figure 6-1, the dose-response relationship can be viewed as having three phases. Phase 1 (see Fig. 6-1B) occurs at low doses; the curve is flat during this phase because doses are too low to elicit a measurable response. During phase 2, an increase in dose elicits a corresponding increase in the response; it is during this phase that the dose-response relationship is graded. As the dose is raised higher, we eventually reach a point where an increase in dose is unable to elicit a further increase in response; at this point, the curve flattens out into phase 3.

### Maximal Efficacy and Relative Potency

Dose-response curves reveal two characteristic properties of drugs: *maximal efficacy* and *relative potency.* Curves that reflect these properties are shown in Figure 6-2.

#### Maximal Efficacy

Maximal efficacy is defined as *the largest effect that a drug can produce.* Maximal efficacy is indicated by the height of the dose-response curve.

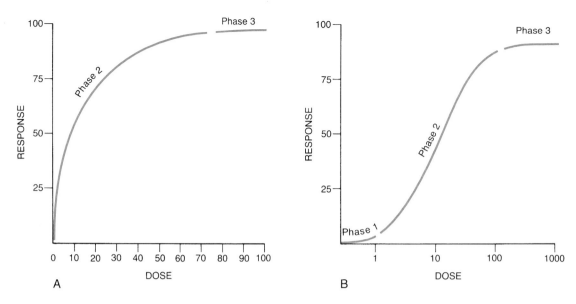

**Figure 6–1. Basic components of the dose-response curve.** *A,* A dose-response curve with dose plotted on a linear scale. *B,* The same dose-response relationship shown in *A* but with the dose plotted on a logarithmic scale. Note the three phases of the dose-response curve. *Phase 1,* The curve is relatively flat; doses are too low to elicit a significant response. *Phase 2,* The curve climbs upward as increases in dose elicit a corresponding increase in response. *Phase 3,* The curve levels off; increases in dose are unable to elicit further increases in response. (Phase 1 is not indicated in *A* because very low doses cannot be shown on a linear scale.)

The concept of maximal efficacy is illustrated by the dose-response curves for meperidine [Demerol] and pentazocine [Talwin], two morphine-like pain relievers (Fig. 6–2A). As we can see, the curve for pentazocine levels off at a maximum height below that of the curve for meperidine. This tells us that the maximum degree of pain relief we can achieve with pentazocine is less than the maximum degree of pain relief we can achieve with meperidine. Put another way, no matter how much pentazocine we administer, we can never produce the degree of pain relief that we can with meperidine. Accordingly, we would say that meperidine has greater maximal efficacy than pentazocine.

Despite what intuition might tell us, a drug with very high maximal efficacy is not always more desirable than a drug with lower efficacy. Recall that we want to match the intensity of the response to the patient's needs. This may be difficult to do with a drug that produces extremely intense responses. For example, certain diuretics (e.g., furosemide) have such high maximal efficacy that they can pose a danger of causing severe dehydration. If we only want to mobilize a modest volume of water, a diuretic with lower maximal efficacy (e.g., hydrochlorothiazide) would be preferred. Similarly, if a patient had a headache, we would not select a powerful analgesic (e.g., morphine) for relief; rather, we would select an analgesic with lower maximal efficacy, such as aspirin. Put another way, it is neither appropriate nor desirable to hunt squirrels with an atomic cannon.

## Relative Potency

The term *potency* refers to the amount of drug that must be given to elicit an effect. Potency is indicated by the relative position of the dose-response curve along the *X* (dosage) axis.

The concept of potency is illustrated by the curves in Figure 6–2B. These curves plot doses for two analgesics—morphine and meperidine—versus the degree of pain relief achieved. As we can see, for any particular degree of pain relief, the required dose of meperidine is larger than the required dose of morphine. Since morphine produces pain relief at lower doses than meperidine, we would say that morphine is more potent than meperidine. That is, a potent drug is one that produces its effects at low doses.

*Potency is rarely an important characteristic of a drug.* The fact that morphine is more potent than meperidine does not mean that morphine is a superior medicine. In fact, the only consequence of morphine's greater potency is that morphine can be given in smaller amounts. The difference between providing pain relief with morphine versus meperidine is much like the difference between purchasing candy with a dime instead of two nickels; although the dime is smaller (more potent) than the two nickels, the purchasing power of the dime and the two nickels is identical.

Although potency is usually of no clinical concern, it can be important if a drug is so lacking in potency that doses become inconveniently large. For example, if a drug were of extremely low potency, we might need to administer that drug in huge doses multiple times a day to achieve beneficial effects. In a case such as this, an alternative drug with higher potency would be desirable. Fortunately, it is rare for a drug to be so lacking in potency that doses of inconvenient magnitude need be given.

*It is important to note that the potency of a drug implies nothing about its maximal efficacy!* Potency and ef-

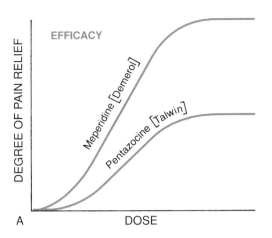

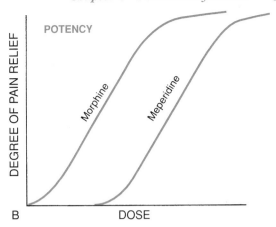

**Figure 6–2. Dose-response curves demonstrating efficacy and potency.** *A,* Efficacy, or "maximal efficacy," is an index of the maximal response that a drug can produce. The efficacy of a drug is indicated by the height of its dose-response curve. In this example, meperidine has greater efficacy than pentazocine. Efficacy is an important quality in a drug. *B,* Potency is an index of how much drug must be administered to elicit a desired response. In this example, pain relief with meperidine requires higher doses than pain relief with morphine. We would say that morphine is more potent than meperidine. Note that, if administered in sufficiently high doses, meperidine can produce just as much pain relief as morphine. Potency is usually not an important quality in a drug.

ficacy are completely independent qualities. Drug A can be more effective than drug B even though drug B may be more potent. Also, drugs A and B can be equally effective even though one may be more potent. As we saw in Figure 6-2B, although meperidine happens to be less potent than morphine, the maximal degree of pain relief that we can achieve with these drugs is identical.

A final comment on the word *potency* is in order. In everyday parlance, we tend to use the word potent to express the pharmacologic concept of effectiveness. That is, when most people say, "This drug is very potent," what they mean is, "This drug produces powerful effects." They do not mean, "This drug produces its effects at low doses." In pharmacology, we use the words potent and potency with the specific meanings given above. These words will be used with those specific meanings throughout this text. We will use potency only in reference to the dosage needed to produce effects; we will not use the term to imply anything about the maximal effects that a drug can produce.

# Drug-Receptor Interactions

## Introduction to Drug Receptors

Drugs are not "magic bullets"; they are simply chemicals. Being chemicals, all that drugs can do to produce their effects is interact with other chemicals. Receptors are the special "chemicals" in the body that drugs interact with to produce their effects.

We can define a receptor as *any functional macromolecule in a cell to which a drug binds to produce its effects.* Under this broad definition, many cellular components could be considered drug receptors, since drugs bind to many cellular components (e.g., enzymes, ribosomes, tubulin) to produce their effects. However, although the formal definition of a receptor encompasses all functional macromolecules, *the term* receptor *is generally reserved for what is arguably the most important group of macromolecules through which drugs act: the body's own receptors for hormones, neurotransmitters, and other regulatory molecules.* The other macromolecules to which drugs bind, such as enzymes and ribosomes, can be thought of simply as target molecules, rather than as true receptors.

The general equation for the interaction between drugs and their receptors is as follows (where D = drug and R = receptor):

$$D + R \rightleftharpoons D\text{-}R \text{ COMPLEX} \rightarrow RESPONSE$$

As suggested by the equation, binding of drugs to their receptors is almost always reversible.

A receptor is analogous to a light switch: like the switch, a receptor must be in the ON configuration to influence cellular function. Receptors are activated ("turned on") by interaction with other molecules. Under normal circumstances, receptor activity is regulated by endogenous compounds (neurotransmitters, hormones, other regulatory molecules). When a drug binds to a receptor, all that it can do is mimic or block the actions of endogenous regulatory molecules. By doing so, the drug will either increase or decrease the rate of the physiologic activity normally controlled by that receptor.

An illustration will help clarify the receptor concept. Let's consider receptors for norepinephrine (NE) in the heart. Cardiac output is controlled in part by NE acting at specific receptors in the heart. Norepinephrine is supplied to those receptors by neurons of the autonomic nervous system (Fig. 6-3). When the need to increase cardiac output arises, the following events take place: (1) the firing rate of autonomic neurons to the heart is increased, causing increased release of NE; (2) NE then binds to receptors on the heart; and (3) as a consequence of the interaction between NE and its receptors, both the rate and force of cardiac contractions are increased, thereby increasing cardiac output. When the demand for cardiac output subsides, the autonomic neurons reduce their firing rate, binding of NE to its receptors diminishes, and cardiac output returns to resting levels.

The same cardiac receptors whose function is regulated by endogenous NE can also serve as receptors for drugs. That is, just as endogenous molecules can bind to these receptors, so can compounds that enter the body as drugs. The binding of drugs to these receptors can have one of two effects: (1) drugs can *mimic* the action of endogenous NE (and thereby increase cardiac output), or (2) drugs can *block* the action of endogenous NE (and thereby prevent stimulation of the heart).

Several important properties of receptors and drug-receptor interactions are illustrated by this example:

- The receptors through which drugs act are normal points of control of physiologic processes.
- Under physiologic conditions, receptor function is regulated by molecules supplied by the body.
- All that drugs can do at receptors is mimic or block the action of the body's own regulatory molecules.
- Because drug action is limited to mimicking or blocking the body's own regulatory molecules, drugs cannot give cells new functions. Rather, drugs can only alter the rate of pre-existing processes. In other words, drugs cannot make the body do anything that it is not already capable of doing.*
- Drugs produce their therapeutic effects by helping the body use its pre-existing capacities to the patient's best advantage. Put another way, medications simply help the body help itself.
- In theory, it should be possible to synthesize drugs that can alter the rate of any biologic process for which receptors exist.

## Receptors and Selectivity of Drug Action

In Chapter 1 we noted that selectivity is a highly desirable characteristic of a drug, since the more selective a drug is, the fewer side effects it will produce. Selective drug action is possible, in large part, because drugs act through specific receptors.

The body employs many different kinds of receptors to regulate its sundry physiologic activities. There are receptors for each neurotransmitter (e.g., norepinephrine, acetylcholine, dopamine); there are receptors for each hormone (e.g., progesterone, insulin, thyrotropin); and there are receptors for all of the other molecules that the body uses to regulate physiologic processes (e.g., histamine, prostaglandins, leukotrienes). As a rule, each type of receptor participates in the regulation of just a few processes.

---

*The only exception to this rule is gene therapy. By inserting genes into cells, we actually *can* make them do something that they were previously incapable of doing.

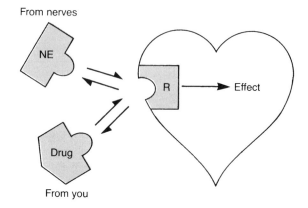

From nerves

NE

R → Effect

Drug

From you

**Figure 6–3. Interaction of drugs with receptors for norepinephrine.** Under physiologic conditions, cardiac output can be increased by the binding of norepinephrine (NE) to receptors (R) on the heart. NE is supplied to these receptors by nerves. These same receptors can be acted upon by drugs. Drugs can act at these receptors to *mimic* endogenous NE (and thereby increase cardiac output), or drugs can *block* the actions of endogenous NE (and thereby reduce cardiac output).

Selective drug action is made possible by the existence of many types of receptors, each regulating just a few processes. Common sense tells us that if a drug interacts with only one kind of receptor, and if that receptor type regulates just a few processes, then the effects of the drug will be limited. Conversely, intuition also tells us that if a drug interacts with several different receptor types, then that drug is likely to elicit a wide variety of responses.

How can a drug interact with one receptor type and not with others? In some important ways, a receptor is analogous to a lock and a drug is analogous to a key for that lock: just as only those keys with the proper profile can fit a particular lock, only those drugs with the proper size, shape, and physical properties can bind to a particular receptor.

The binding of acetylcholine (a neurotransmitter) to its receptor illustrates the lock-and-key analogy (Fig. 6–4). To bind with its receptor, acetylcholine must have a shape that is complementary to the shape of the receptor; in addition, acetylcholine must possess positive charges that are positioned so as to permit their interaction with corresponding negative sites on the receptor. If acetylcholine lacked these properties, it would be unable to interact with the receptor.

Like the acetylcholine receptor, all other receptors impose specific requirements on the molecules with which they will interact. Because receptors have such specific requirements, it is possible to synthesize drugs that interact with just one receptor type to the exclusion of all others. Such medications tend to elicit selective responses.

Even though a drug is selective for only one type of receptor, it is possible for that drug to produce nonselective effects. How can this be? If a single receptor type is responsible for regulating several physiologic processes, then drugs that interact with that receptor will also influ-

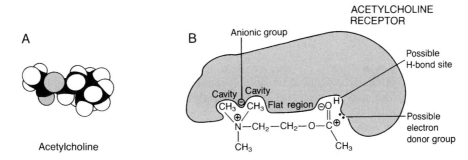

**Figure 6–4. Interaction of acetylcholine with its receptor.** *A,* Three-dimensional model of the acetylcholine molecule. *B,* Binding of acetylcholine to its receptor. Note how the shape of the acetylcholine molecule closely matches the shape of the receptor. Note also how the positive charges on acetylcholine align with the negative sites on the receptor. (Modified from Goldstein, A., Aronow, L., and Sumner, M. K. Principles of Drug Action: The Basis of Pharmacology, 2nd ed. New York, John Wiley & Sons, 1974. Copyright © 1974. Reprinted by permission of John Wiley & Sons, Inc.)

ence a variety of processes. For example, in addition to modulating perception of pain, morphine receptors help regulate other processes, including respiration and motility of the bowel. Consequently, although morphine is selective for one class of receptor, the drug can still produce a variety of effects. In clinical practice, it is common for morphine to cause respiratory depression and constipation along with reduction of pain. Note that morphine produces these varied effects not because it lacks receptor selectivity, but because the receptor for which morphine is selective helps regulate a variety of physiologic processes.

One final comment on selectivity: *Selectivity does not guarantee safety.* A compound can be highly selective for a particular receptor and yet still be extremely dangerous. For example, although botulinus toxin is highly selective for one type of receptor, the compound is anything but safe: This toxin can cause paralysis of the muscles of respiration, resulting in death from respiratory arrest.

## Theories of Drug-Receptor Interaction

In the discussion below, we consider two theories of drug-receptor interaction: (1) the simple occupancy theory and (2) the modified occupancy theory. These theories help explain dose-response relationships and the ability of drugs to mimic or block the actions of endogenous regulatory molecules.

### Simple Occupancy Theory

The simple occupancy theory of drug-receptor interaction states that (1) the intensity of the response to a drug is proportional to the number of receptors occupied by that drug and that (2) a maximal response will occur when *all* available receptors have been occupied. This relationship between receptor occupancy and the intensity of the response is shown graphically in Figure 6–5.

Although certain aspects of dose-response relationships can be explained by the simple occupancy theory, other important phenomena cannot. Specifically, there is noth-

ing in this theory to explain why one drug should be more potent than another. In addition, this theory cannot explain how one drug can have higher maximal efficacy than another. That is, according to this theory, two drugs acting at the same receptor should produce the same maximal effect, providing that their dosages were high enough to produce 100% receptor occupancy. We have already seen, however, that this is not true. As illustrated in Figure 6–2A, there is a dose of pentazocine above which no further increase in response can be elicited. Presumably, all receptors are occupied when the dose-response curve levels off. However, at 100% receptor occupancy, the response elicited by pentazocine is less than that elicited by

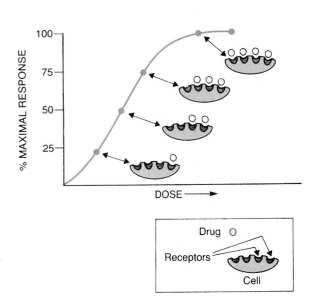

**Figure 6–5. Model of simple occupancy theory.** The simple occupancy theory states that the intensity of response to a drug is proportional to the number of receptors occupied; maximal response is reached with 100% receptor occupancy. Since the hypothetical cell in this figure has only four receptors, maximal response is achieved when all four receptors are occupied. (Please note: real cells have thousands of receptors.)

morphine. Simple occupancy theory cannot account for this difference.

## Modified Occupancy Theory

The modified occupancy theory of drug-receptor interaction explains certain observations that cannot be accounted for with the simple occupancy theory. The simple occupancy theory assumes that all drugs acting at a particular receptor are identical with respect to (1) the ability to bind to the receptor and (2) the ability to influence receptor function once binding has taken place. The modified occupancy theory is based on different assumptions.

The modified theory ascribes two qualities to drugs: *affinity* and *intrinsic activity*. The term *affinity* refers to the strength of the attraction between a drug and its receptor. *Intrinsic activity* refers to the ability of a drug to activate the receptor following binding. *Affinity and intrinsic activity are independent properties.*

**Affinity.** As noted, the term *affinity* refers to the strength of the attraction between a drug and its receptor. Drugs with high affinity are strongly attracted to their receptors. Conversely, drugs with low affinity are weakly attracted.

The affinity of a drug for its receptors is reflected in its *potency*. Because they are strongly attracted to their receptors, drugs with high affinity can bind to their receptors when present in low concentrations. Because they bind to receptors at low concentrations, drugs with high affinity are effective in low doses. That is, *drugs with high affinity are very potent.* Conversely, drugs with low affinity must be present in high concentrations to bind to their receptors. Accordingly, these drugs are not very potent.

**Intrinsic Activity.** The term *intrinsic activity* refers to the ability of a drug to activate a receptor following binding. Drugs with high intrinsic activity cause intense receptor activation. Conversely, drugs with low intrinsic activity cause only slight activation.

The intrinsic activity of a drug is reflected in its *maximal efficacy*. Drugs with high intrinsic activity have high maximal efficacy. That is, by causing intense receptor activation, they are able to cause intense responses. Conversely, if intrinsic activity is low, maximal efficacy will be low as well.

It should be noted that, under the modified occupancy theory, the intensity of the response to a drug is still related to the number of receptors occupied. The wrinkle added by the modified theory is that intensity is also related to the ability of the drug to activate receptors once binding has occurred. Under the modified theory, two drugs can occupy the same number of receptors but produce effects of different intensity; the drug with greater intrinsic activity will produce the more intense response.

## Agonists, Antagonists, and Partial Agonists

As noted above, when drugs bind to receptors they can do one of two things: they can either *mimic* the action of endogenous regulatory molecules or they can *block* the action of endogenous regulators. Drugs that mimic the body's own regulatory molecules are called *agonists*. Drugs that block the actions of endogenous regulators are called *antagonists*. Like full agonists, *partial agonists* also mimic the actions of endogenous regulatory molecules, but they produce responses of reduced intensity.

### Agonists

*Agonists are molecules that activate receptors.* Since neurotransmitters, hormones, and all other endogenous regulators of receptor function activate the receptors to which they bind, all of these compounds are considered agonists. When drugs act as agonists, they simply bind to receptors and mimic the actions of the body's own regulatory molecules.

In terms of the modified occupancy theory, an agonist is a drug that has both *affinity* and *high intrinsic activity*. Affinity allows the agonist to bind to receptors, while intrinsic activity allows the bound agonist to "activate" or "turn on" receptor function.

Many therapeutic agents produce their effects by functioning as agonists. Dobutamine, for example, is a drug that mimics the action of norepinephrine at receptors on the heart, thereby causing heart rate and force of contraction to increase. The insulin that we administer as a drug mimics the actions of endogenous insulin at receptors. Norethindrone, a component of many oral contraceptives, acts by "turning on" receptors for progesterone.

It is important to note that agonists do not necessarily make physiologic processes go faster; receptor activation can also slow down a particular process. For example, there are receptors on the heart that, when activated by acetylcholine (the body's own agonist for these receptors), will cause heart rate to decrease. Drugs that mimic the action of acetylcholine at these receptors will also decrease heart rate. Since such drugs produce their effects by causing receptor activation, they would be called agonists—despite the fact that their effect is to slow heart rate down.

### Antagonists

*Antagonists produce their effects by preventing receptor activation by endogenous regulatory molecules and drugs.* Antagonists have virtually no effects of their own on receptor function.

In terms of the modified occupancy theory, an antagonist is a drug with affinity for a receptor but with no intrinsic activity. Affinity allows the antagonist to bind to receptors, but lack of intrinsic activity prevents the bound antagonist from causing receptor activation.

Although antagonists do not cause receptor activation, they most certainly *do* produce pharmacologic effects. Antagonists produce their effects *by preventing the activation of receptors by agonists*. Antagonists can produce beneficial effects by blocking the actions of endogenous regulatory molecules or by blocking the actions of drugs. (The ability of antagonists to block the actions of drugs is employed most commonly in the treatment of poisoning.)

It is important to note that the response to an antagonist is determined by how much *agonist* is present. Since antagonists act by preventing receptor activation, *if there is no agonist present, administration of an antagonist will have no observable effect*; the drug will bind to its receptors but nothing will happen. On the other hand, if receptors are undergoing activation by agonists, administration of an antagonist will shut the process down, resulting in an observable response. This is an important concept; please think about it.

Many therapeutic agents produce their effects by acting as receptor antagonists. Antihistamines, for example, suppress allergy symptoms by binding to receptors for histamine, thereby preventing activation of these receptors by histamine released in response to allergens. The use of antagonists to treat drug toxicity is illustrated by naloxone, an agent that blocks receptors for morphine and related opioids; by preventing activation of opioid receptors, naloxone can completely reverse all symptoms of opioid overdose.

**Noncompetitive versus Competitive Antagonists.** Antagonists can be subdivided into two major classes: (1) noncompetitive antagonists and (2) competitive antagonists. Most antagonists are competitive.

*Noncompetitive (Insurmountable) Antagonists.* Noncompetitive antagonists bind irreversibly to receptors. The effect of irreversible binding is equivalent to reducing the total number of receptors available for activation by an agonist. Since the intensity of the response to an agonist is proportional to the total number of receptors occupied, and since noncompetitive antagonists decrease the number of receptors available for activation, noncompetitive antagonists *reduce the maximal response* that an agonist can elicit. If sufficient antagonist is present, agonist effects will be blocked completely. Dose-response curves illustrating inhibition by a noncompetitive antagonist are shown in Figure 6-6A.

Since the binding of noncompetitive antagonists is irreversible, inhibition by these agents cannot be overcome—no matter how much agonist may be available. Because inhibition by noncompetitive antagonists cannot be reversed, these agents are rarely used therapeutically. (Recall from Chapter 1 that reversibility is one of the properties of an ideal drug.)

The fact that noncompetitive antagonists bind irreversibly to receptors does not mean that their effects last forever. Cells are constantly breaking down "old" receptors and synthesizing new ones. Consequently, the effects of noncompetitive antagonists wear off as the receptors to which they are bound are replaced. Since the life cycle of a receptor can be relatively short, the effects of noncompetitive antagonists may subside in a few days.

*Competitive (Surmountable) Antagonists.* Competitive antagonists bind *reversibly* to receptors. As their name implies, competitive antagonists produce receptor blockade by competing with agonists for receptor binding. If an agonist and a competitive antagonist have equal affinity for a particular receptor, that receptor will be occupied by whichever agent—agonist or antagonist—is present in the highest concentration. If there are more antagonist molecules present than agonist molecules, antagonist molecules will occupy the receptors and receptor activation will be blocked. Conversely, if agonist molecules outnumber the antagonists, receptors will be occupied mainly by the agonist and little inhibition will occur.

Because competitive antagonists bind reversibly to receptors, the inhibition they cause is surmountable. In the presence of sufficiently high amounts of agonist, agonist molecules will occupy all receptors and inhibition will be completely overcome. The dose-response curves shown in Figure 6-6B illustrate the process of overcoming the effects of a competitive antagonist with large doses of an agonist.

## Partial Agonists

A partial agonist is an agonist that has only *moderate intrinsic activity*. As a result, *the maximal effect that a partial agonist can produce is lower than that of a full agonist.* Pentazocine is an example of a partial agonist. As the curves in Figure 6-2A indicate, the degree of pain relief that can be achieved with pentazocine is much lower than the relief that can be achieved with meperidine (a full agonist).

Partial agonists are interesting in that they can act as *antagonists* as well as *agonists*. For example, when pentazocine is administered by itself, it occupies opioid receptors and produces moderate relief of pain. In this situation, the drug is acting as an agonist. However, if a pa-

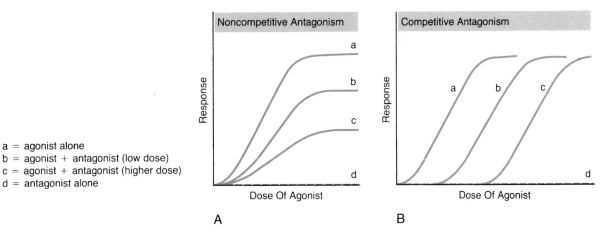

a = agonist alone
b = agonist + antagonist (low dose)
c = agonist + antagonist (higher dose)
d = antagonist alone

**A**                    **B**

**Figure 6–6. Dose-response curves in the presence of competitive and noncompetitive antagonists.** *A,* Effect of a noncompetitive antagonist on the dose-response curve of an agonist. Note that noncompetitive antagonists decrease the maximal response achievable with an agonist. *B,* Effect of a competitive antagonist on the dose-response curve of an agonist. Note that the maximal response achievable with the agonist is not reduced. Competitive antagonists simply increase the amount of agonist required to produce any given intensity of response.

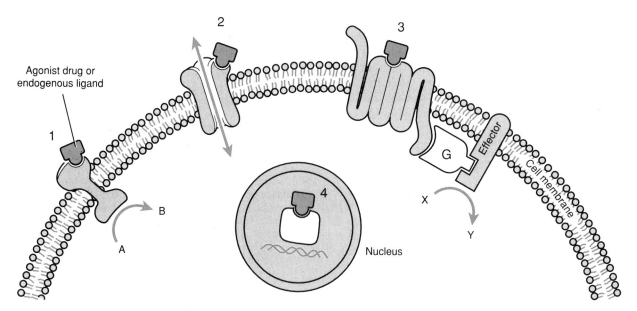

**Figure 6–7. The four primary receptor families.** *1,* Cell membrane-embedded enzyme. *2,* Ligand-gated ion channel. *3,* G protein–coupled receptor system (G = G protein). *4,* Transcription factor.

tient is already taking meperidine (a full agonist at opioid receptors) and is then given a large dose of pentazocine, pentazocine will occupy the opioid receptors and prevent their activation by meperidine. As a result, rather than experiencing the high degree of pain relief that meperidine can produce, the patient will experience only the limited relief that pentazocine can produce. In this situation, pentazocine is acting as both an *agonist* (producing moderate pain relief) and an *antagonist* (blocking the higher degree of relief that could have been achieved with meperidine by itself).

## The Four Primary Receptor Families

Although the body has many different receptors, they compose only four primary families: cell membrane-embedded enzymes, ligand-gated ion channels, G protein-coupled receptor systems, and transcription factors. These families are depicted in Figure 6-7. In the discussion below, the term *ligand-binding domain* refers to the specific region of the receptor where binding of drugs and endogenous regulatory molecules takes place.

***Cell Membrane–Embedded Enzymes.*** As shown in Figure 6-7, receptors of this type span the cell membrane. The ligand-binding domain is located on the cell surface, and the enzyme's catalytic site is inside. Binding of an endogenous regulatory molecule or agonist drug activates the enzyme, thereby increasing its catalytic activity. Responses to activation of these receptors occur in seconds. Insulin is representative of the endogenous ligands that act through this type of receptor.

***Ligand-Gated Ion Channels.*** Like membrane-embedded enzymes, ligand-gated ion channels span the cell membrane. The function of these receptors is to regulate flow of ions into and out of cells. Each ligand-gated channel is specific for a particular ion (e.g., Na+, Ca++). As shown in

Figure 6-7, the ligand-binding domain is on the cell surface. When an endogenous ligand or agonist drug binds the receptor, the channel opens, allowing ions to flow inward or outward. (The direction of flow is determined by the concentration gradient of the ion across the membrane.) Responses to activation of a ligand-gated ion channel are extremely fast, often occurring in milliseconds. Several neurotransmitters, including acetylcholine and GABA, act through this type of receptor.

***G Protein–Coupled Receptor Systems.*** G protein-coupled receptor systems have three components: the receptor itself, G protein (so named because it binds GTP), and an effector (typically an ion channel or an enzyme). These systems work as follows: binding of an endogenous ligand or agonist drug activates the receptor, which in turn activates G protein, which in turn activates the effector. Responses to activation of this type of system develop rapidly. Numerous endogenous ligands, including norepinephrine, serotonin, histamine, and many peptide hormones, act through G protein-coupled receptor systems.

As shown in Figure 6-7, the receptors that couple to G proteins are serpentine structures that traverse the cell membrane seven times. For some of these receptors, the ligand-binding domain is found on the cell surface. For others, the ligand-binding domain is located in a pocket accessible from the cell surface.

***Transcription Factors.*** Transcription factors differ from the receptors discussed thus far in two ways: (1) transcription factors are found within the cell rather than on the surface and (2) responses to activation of these receptors are delayed. Transcription factors are situated on DNA in the cell nucleus. Their function is to regulate protein synthesis. Activation of these receptors by endogenous ligands or by agonist drugs stimulates transcription of messenger RNA molecules, which then act as templates for synthesis of specific proteins. The entire process—from activation of the transcription factor through completion of protein synthesis—may take hours or even days. Because transcription factors are intracellular, they can be activated only by ligands that are sufficiently lipid soluble to cross the cell membrane. Endogenous ligands that act through transcription factors include thyroid hormone and all of the steroid hormones (e.g., progesterone, testosterone, cortisol).

## Regulation of Receptor Sensitivity

Receptors are dynamic components of the cell. In response to continuous activation (or inhibition), the number of receptors on the cell surface can change, as can their sensitivity to agonist molecules (drugs and endogenous ligands). For example, when the receptors of a cell are continually exposed to an *agonist,* the cell usually becomes less responsive. When this occurs, the cell is said to be *desensitized* or *refractory,* or to have undergone *downregulation.* Several mechanisms may be responsible, including destruction of receptors by the cell and modification of receptors such that they respond less fully. Continuous exposure to *antagonists* has the opposite effect, causing the cell to become *hypersensitive* (also referred to as *supersensitive*). One mechanism that can cause hypersensitivity is synthesis of more receptors.

## Drug Responses That Do Not Involve Receptors

Although the effects of most drugs result from drug-receptor interactions, some drugs do not act through receptors. Rather, they act through simple physical or chemical interactions with other small molecules.

Common examples of "receptorless drugs" include antacids, antiseptics, saline laxatives, and chelating agents. Antacids reduce gastric acidity by direct chemical interaction with stomach acid. The antiseptic action of ethyl alcohol results from precipitating bacterial proteins. Magnesium hydroxide, a powerful laxative, acts by retaining water in the intestinal lumen through an osmotic effect. Dimercaprol, a chelating agent, prevents toxicity from heavy metals (e.g., arsenic, mercury) by forming complexes with these compounds. All of these pharmacologic effects are the result of simple physical or chemical interactions, and not the result of interactions with cellular receptors.

## Interpatient Variability in Drug Responses

The dose required to produce a therapeutic response can vary substantially among patients. The reason for this variability is that people differ from one another. In this section we consider interpatient variation as a general issue.

The specific kinds of differences that underlie variability in drug responses are discussed in Chapter 9.

In order to promote the therapeutic objective, you must be alert to interpatient variation in drug responses. Because of interpatient variation, it is not possible to predict exactly how an individual patient will respond to medication. Hence, each patient must be evaluated to determine his or her actual response to treatment. The nurse who appreciates the reality of interpatient variability will be better prepared to anticipate, evaluate, and respond appropriately to each patient's therapeutic needs.

### Measurement of Interpatient Variability

An example of how interpatient variability is measured will facilitate our discussion. Let's assume that we've just developed a new antacid and wish to evaluate variability in patient responses. To make this evaluation, we must first define a specific *therapeutic objective* or *endpoint.* For our antacid, an appropriate endpoint is elevation of gastric pH to a value of 5.

Having defined a therapeutic endpoint, we can now perform our study. Subjects for this study are 100 people with gastric ulcers. We begin our experiment by giving each subject a low initial dose (100 mg) of our drug. We then measure gastric pH to determine how many individuals achieved the therapeutic goal of pH 5. Let's assume that only two people responded to the initial dose. To the remaining 98 subjects, we give an additional 20-mg dose and again determine whose gastric pH rose to 5. Let's assume that six more subjects responded to this dose (120 mg total). We continue the experiment, administering doses in 20-mg increments, until all 100 subjects have responded with the desired elevation in gastric pH.

The data from our hypothetical experiment are plotted in Figure 6-8. The plot is called a *frequency distribution curve.* We can see from the curve that a wide range of doses was required to produce the desired response in all subjects. For some subjects, a dose of only 100 mg was sufficient to produce the target response. For other subjects, the therapeutic endpoint was not achieved until a total dose of 240 mg had been given.

### The ED50

The dose at the middle of the frequency distribution curve is termed the ED50 (see Fig. 6-8). (*ED* is an abbreviation for *effective dose.*) The ED50 is defined as *the dose that is required to produce a defined therapeutic response in 50% of the population.* In the case of our antacid, the ED50 was 170 mg—the dose needed to elevate gastric pH to a value of 5 in 50 of the 100 people tested.

The ED50 can be considered a "standard" dose and, as such, is frequently the dose selected for initial treatment. After evaluating the patient's response to this "standard" dose, we can then adjust subsequent doses up or down in accordance with the patient's need.

### Clinical Implications of Interpatient Variability

Interpatient variation has four important clinical consequences. As a nurse you should be aware of these implications:

| Dose of Drug (mg) | Number of Subjects Responding at Each Dose |
|:---:|:---:|
| 100 | 2 |
| 120 | 6 |
| 140 | 17 |
| 160 | 25 |
| 180 | 25 |
| 200 | 17 |
| 220 | 6 |
| 240 | 2 |

A

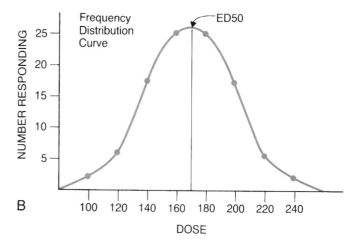

B

**Figure 6–8. Interpatient variation in drug responses.** *A,* Data from clinical testing of a hypothetical ant-acid in 100 patients. The goal of the study was to determine the dosage of antacid required by each patient to elevate gastric pH to 5. Note the wide variability in doses needed to produce the target response for the 100 subjects. *B,* Frequency distribution curve for the data in *A.* The dose at the middle of the curve is termed the ED50—the dose that will produce a predefined intensity of response in 50% of the population.

- *The initial dose of a drug is necessarily an approximation. Subsequent doses must be "fine tuned" based on the patient's response.* Because initial doses are approximations, it would be wise not to challenge the physician if the prescribed initial dose differs by a small amount (e.g., 10% to 20%) from recommended doses in a published drug reference. Rather, you should administer the medication as prescribed and evaluate the response; dosage adjustments can then be made as needed. Of course, if the physician's order calls for a dose that differs from the recommended dose by a large amount, that order should be challenged.
- *When given an average effective dose (ED50), some patients will be undertreated, whereas others will have received more drug than they need.* Accordingly, when therapy is initiated with a dose equivalent to the ED50, it is especially important to evaluate the patient's response. Patients who fail to respond will need an increase in dosage. Conversely, patients who show signs of toxicity will need to have their dosage reduced.
- *Since drug responses are not completely predictable, you must look at the patient (and not the* Physicians' Desk Reference*) to determine if too much or too little medication has been administered.* In other words, doses should be adjusted on the basis of the patient's response and not just on the basis of what some reference says is supposed to work. For example, although many postoperative patients receive adequate pain relief with an "average" dose of morphine, this dose is not appropriate for everyone: An average dose may be effective for some patients, ineffective for others, and toxic for still others. Clearly, dosage must be adjusted on the basis of the patient's response, and must not be given in blind compliance with the dosage recommended in a book.

- *Because of variability in responses, nurses, patients, and other concerned individuals must evaluate actual responses and be prepared to inform the prescribing physician about these responses so that proper adjustments in dosage can be made.*

## The Therapeutic Index

The therapeutic index is a measure of a drug's safety. The therapeutic index is determined using laboratory animals and is defined as *the ratio of a drug's LD50 to its ED50.* (The *LD50* is the dose that is lethal to 50% of the animals treated.) A large therapeutic index indicates that a drug is relatively safe. Conversely, a small therapeutic index indicates that a drug is relatively unsafe.

The concept of therapeutic index is illustrated by the frequency distribution curves in Figure 6-9. Part A of the figure shows curves for therapeutic and lethal responses to drug "X." Part B shows equivalent curves for drug "Y." We can see in Figure 6-9A that the average lethal dose (100 mg) for drug X is much larger than the average therapeutic dose (10 mg). Since this drug's lethal dose is much larger than its therapeutic dose, common sense tells us that the drug should be relatively safe. The safety of this drug is reflected in its large therapeutic index, which is 10. In contrast, drug Y is unsafe. As shown in Figure 6-9B, the average lethal dose for drug Y (20 mg) is only twice the average therapeutic dose (10 mg). Hence, for drug Y, a dose only twice the ED50 could be lethal to 50% of those treated. Clearly, drug Y is not safe. This lack of safety is reflected in its small therapeutic index.

The curves for drug Y illustrate a phenomenon that is even more important than the therapeutic index. As we can see, there is *overlap* between the curve for therapeu-

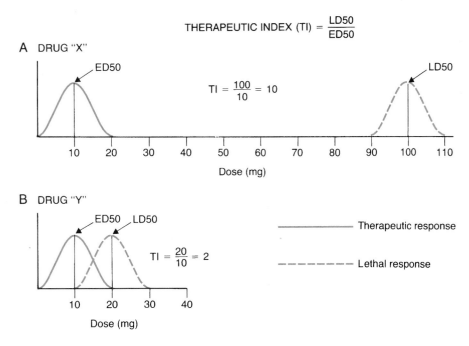

**Figure 6–9. The therapeutic index.** *A,* Frequency distribution curves indicating the ED50 and LD50 for drug "X." Because its LD50 is much greater than its ED50, drug X is relatively safe. *B,* Frequency distribution curves indicating the ED50 and LD50 for drug "Y." Because its LD50 is very close to its ED50, drug Y is not very safe. Also note the *overlap* between the effective-dose curve and the lethal-dose curve.

tic effects and the curve for lethal effects. This overlap tells us that the high doses needed to produce therapeutic effects in some people may be large enough to cause death. The message here is that, if a drug is to be truly safe, the highest dose required to produce therapeutic effects must be substantially lower than the lowest dose capable of causing death.

# KEY POINTS

- Pharmacodynamics is the study of the biochemical and physiologic effects of drugs and the molecular mechanisms by which those effects are produced.
- For most drugs, the dose-response relationship is graded. That is, the response gets more intense with increasing dosage.
- Maximal efficacy is defined as the biggest effect a drug can produce.
- Although efficacy is important, there are many situations in which a drug with relatively low efficacy is preferable to a drug with very high efficacy.
- A potent drug is simply a drug that produces its effects at low doses. As a rule, potency is not important.
- Potency and efficacy are independent qualities. Drug *A* can be more effective than drug *B* even though drug *B* may be more potent. Also, drugs *A* and *B* can be equally effective, although one may be more potent than the other.
- A receptor can be defined as any functional macromolecule in a cell to which a drug binds to produce its effects.

- Binding of drugs to their receptors is almost always reversible.
- The receptors through which drugs act are normal points of control for physiologic processes.
- Under physiologic conditions, receptor function is regulated by molecules supplied by the body.
- All that drugs can do at receptors is mimic or block the action of the body's own regulatory molecules.
- Because drug action is limited to mimicking or blocking the body's own regulatory molecules, drugs cannot give cells new functions. Rather, drugs can only alter the rate of pre-existing processes.
- Receptors make selectivity of drug action possible.
- If a drug interacts with only one type of receptor, and if that receptor type regulates just a few processes, then the effects of the drug will be relatively selective.
- If a drug interacts with only one type of receptor, but that receptor type regulates multiple processes, then the effects of the drug will be nonselective.
- If a drug interacts with multiple receptors, its effects will be nonselective.
- Selectivity does not guarantee safety.
- The term *affinity* refers to the strength of the attraction between a drug and its receptor.
- Drugs with high affinity have high relative potency.
- The term *intrinsic activity* refers to the ability of a drug to activate receptors.
- Drugs with high intrinsic activity have high maximal efficacy.
- Agonists are molecules that activate receptors.
- In terms of the modified occupancy theory, agonists have both affinity and high intrinsic activity. Affinity

allows them to bind to receptors, while intrinsic activity allows them to "activate" the receptor after binding.

- Antagonists are drugs that prevent receptor activation by endogenous regulatory molecules and drugs.
- In terms of the modified occupancy theory, antagonists have affinity for receptors but no intrinsic activity. Affinity allows the antagonist to bind to receptors, but lack of intrinsic activity prevents the bound antagonist from causing receptor activation.
- Antagonists have observable effects in the absence of agonists.
- Partial agonists have only moderate intrinsic activity. Hence their maximal efficacy is lower than that of full agonists.
- Partial agonists can act as *agonists* (if there is no full agonist present) and as *antagonists* (in a full agonist *is* present).
- There are four primary families of receptors: cell membrane-embedded enzymes, ligand-gated ion channels, G protein-coupled receptor systems, and transcription factors.

- Continuous exposure of cells to agonists can result in receptor desensitization (aka refractoriness or downregulation), whereas continuous exposure to antagonists can result in hypersensitivity (aka supersensitivity).
- Some drugs act through simple physical or chemical interactions with other small molecules rather than through receptors.
- The ED50 is defined as the dose required to produce a defined therapeutic response in 50% of the population.
- The initial dose of a drug is necessarily an approximation. Subsequent doses must be "fine tuned" based on the patient's response.
- An average effective dose (ED50) is perfect for some people, insufficient for others, and excessive for still others.
- Since drug responses are not completely predictable, you must look at the patient (and not some drug reference book) to determine if dosage is appropriate.
- The therapeutic index—defined as the LD50:ED50 ratio—is a measure of a drug's safety. Drugs with a high therapeutic index are safe; drugs with a low therapeutic index are not.

# CHAPTER 7

# Drug-Drug and Drug-Food Interactions

## Drug-Drug Interactions

Drug-drug interactions can occur whenever a patient takes two or more drugs. Some interactions are both intended and desired, as when we combine drugs to treat hypertension. In contrast, some interactions are both unintended and undesired, as when we precipitate malignant hyperthermia in the patient receiving halothane and succinylcholine. Some adverse interactions are well known, and hence generally avoidable. Many others are yet to be documented.

Drug interactions occur because patients frequently take more than one drug. They may be taking multiple drugs to treat a single disorder. They may have multiple disorders that require treatment with different drugs. They may be taking over-the-counter drugs in addition to their prescription medicines. And they may be taking caffeine, nicotine, alcohol, and other drugs that have nothing to do with their illness.

Our objective in this chapter is to establish an overview of drug interactions, emphasizing the basic mechanisms by which drugs can interact. We will not attempt to catalogue the huge number of specific interactions that are known. For information on interactions of specific drugs, please refer to the chapters in which those drugs are discussed.

### Consequences of Drug-Drug Interactions

When drug A acts on drug B, there are three possible outcomes: drug A may intensify the effects of drug B, drug A may reduce the effects of drug B, or the combination may produce a new response not seen with either drug alone.

### Intensification of Effects

When a patient is taking two medications, one drug may intensify the effects of the other. This type of interaction is often termed *potentiative*. Potentiative interactions may be beneficial or detrimental. A potentiative interaction that enhances therapeutic effects is clearly beneficial. Conversely, a potentiative interaction that intensifies adverse effects is clearly detrimental. Examples of beneficial and detrimental potentiative interactions follow.

*Increased Therapeutic Effects.* The interaction between ampicillin and sulbactam represents a beneficial potentiative interaction. When administered alone, ampicillin undergoes rapid inactivation by bacterial enzymes. By inhibiting these enzymes, sulbactam prolongs and intensifies ampicillin's therapeutic effects.

*Increased Adverse Effects.* The interaction between aspirin and warfarin represents a detrimental potentiative interaction. Warfarin is an anticoagulant used to suppress formation of blood clots. Unfortunately, if the dosage of warfarin is too high, the patient is at risk of spontaneous bleeding. Accordingly, for therapy to be safe and effective, the dosage must be high enough to suppress clot formation but not so high that spontaneous bleeding occurs. Like warfarin, aspirin also suppresses clot formation. As a result, if aspirin and warfarin are taken concurrently, the risk of spontaneous bleeding is significantly increased. Clearly, potentiative interactions such as this are undesirable.

### Reduction of Effects

Interactions that result in reduced drug effects are often termed *inhibitory*. As with potentiative interactions, inhibitory interactions can be beneficial or detrimental. Inhibitory interactions that result in reduced toxicity are beneficial. Conversely, inhibitory interactions that result in reduced therapeutic effects are detrimental. Examples of these interactions follow.

***Reduced Therapeutic Effects.*** The interaction between propranolol and terbutaline represents a detrimental inhibitory interaction. Terbutaline is taken by people with asthma to produce bronchial dilation. Propranolol, a drug used for cardiovascular disorders, can act in the lung to block the effects of terbutaline. Hence, if propranolol and terbutaline are taken together, propranolol can reduce terbutaline's therapeutic effects. Inhibitory actions such as this, which can result in therapeutic failure, are clearly detrimental.

***Reduced Adverse Effects.*** The use of naloxone to treat morphine overdose is an excellent example of a beneficial inhibitory interaction. When administered in excessive dosage, morphine can produce coma and profound respiratory depression. Naloxone, a drug that blocks morphine's actions, can completely reverse all symptoms of toxicity. The benefits of such an inhibitory interaction are obvious.

### Creation of a Unique Response

Rarely, the combination of two drugs produces a new response not seen with either agent alone. To illustrate, let's consider the combination of alcohol with disulfiram [Antabuse], a drug used to treat alcoholism. When alcohol and disulfiram are combined, a host of unpleasant and dangerous responses can result. These effects do not occur when disulfiram or alcohol is used alone.

## Basic Mechanisms of Drug-Drug Interactions

Drugs can interact by way of four basic mechanisms: (1) direct chemical or physical interaction, (2) pharmacokinetic interaction, (3) pharmacodynamic interaction, and (4) combined toxicity.

### Direct Chemical or Physical Interaction

Some drugs, because of their physical or chemical properties, can undergo direct interaction with other drugs. Direct physical and chemical interactions usually render both drugs inactive.

Direct interactions occur most commonly when drugs are combined in IV solutions. Frequently, but not always, such interactions cause formation of a precipitate. If a precipitate appears when drugs are mixed together in an IV solution, that solution should be discarded. Remember, however, that direct drug interactions may not always leave visible evidence. Hence simple inspection of the solution cannot be relied upon to reveal all direct interactions. Because drugs can interact in solution, you should *never combine two or more drugs in the same container unless it has been established that a direct interaction will not occur.*

The same kinds of interactions that can take place when drugs are mixed together in bottles can also occur when drugs are mixed together in the patient. However, since drugs are diluted in body water following administration, and since dilution decreases chemical interactions, significant interactions within the patient are much less likely than in a bottle.

### Pharmacokinetic Interactions

Drug interactions can affect all four of the basic pharmacokinetic processes. That is, when two drugs are taken together, one may alter the absorption, distribution, metabolism, or excretion of the other.

***Altered Absorption.*** Drug absorption may be enhanced or reduced as a result of drug interactions. The impact of drug interactions on absorption can be of considerable clinical significance.

There are several mechanisms by which one drug can alter the absorption of another:

- By elevating gastric pH, antacids can decrease the ionization of basic drugs in the stomach, thereby increasing the ability of these agents to cross membranes and be absorbed. Antacids have the opposite effect on weak acids.
- Laxatives can reduce absorption of other drugs by accelerating their passage through the intestine.
- Drugs that depress peristalsis (e.g., morphine, atropine) prolong drug transit time in the intestine, thereby increasing the time for absorption.
- Drugs that induce vomiting can decrease absorption of orally administered drugs.
- Cholestyramine and certain other adsorbent drugs, which are administered orally but do not undergo absorption, can adsorb other drugs onto themselves and thereby prevent their absorption into the body.
- Drugs that reduce regional blood flow can reduce absorption of other drugs from that region. For example, when epinephrine is injected together with a local anesthetic (as is often done), the epinephrine causes local vasoconstriction, thereby reducing regional blood flow and delaying absorption of the anesthetic.

***Altered Distribution.*** There are two principal mechanisms by which one drug can alter the distribution of another: (1) competition for protein binding and (2) alteration of extracellular pH.

*Competition for Protein Binding.* When two drugs bind to the same site on plasma albumin, coadministration of those drugs produces competition for binding. As a result, binding of one or both agents is reduced, causing plasma levels of free drug to rise. In theory, the increase in free drug can intensify effects. However, since the newly freed drug usually undergoes rapid elimination, the increase in plasma levels of free drug is rarely sustained or significant.

*Alteration of Extracellular pH.* Because of the pH partitioning effect (see Chapter 5), a drug with the ability to change extracellular pH can alter the distribution of other drugs. For example, if a drug were to increase extracellular pH, that drug would increase the ionization of acidic drugs present in extracellular fluids (i.e., plasma and interstitial fluid). As a result, acidic drugs would be drawn from within cells (where the pH was below that of the extracellular fluid) into the extracellular space. Hence the alteration in pH would change drug distribution.

The ability of drugs to alter pH and thereby alter the distribution of other drugs can be put to practical use in the management of poisoning. For example, symptoms of aspirin toxicity can be reduced with sodium bicarbonate, a drug that elevates extracellular pH. By increasing the pH outside cells, bicarbonate causes aspirin to move from intracellular sites into the interstitial fluid and plasma, thereby minimizing injury to cells.

***Altered Metabolism.*** Drug metabolism may be increased or decreased as a result of interactions between drugs. As a rule, drugs that increase the metabolism of other drugs do so through induction of liver enzymes. Drugs that decrease the metabolism of other drugs do so by either inhibiting liver enzymes or competing for the same metabolic pathway.

*Induction of Drug-Metabolizing Enzymes.* As discussed in Chapter 5, some drugs can act in the liver to induce synthesis of hepatic drug-metabolizing enzymes. Drugs that promote induction are referred to as *inducing agents*. The classic example of an inducing agent is phenobarbital, a member of the barbiturate family. Inducing agents can stimulate their own metabolism as well as that of other drugs.

Inducing agents can increase the rate of drug metabolism by as much as two- to threefold. This increase develops over 7 to 10 days. Rates of metabolism return to normal 7 to 10 days after the inducing agent has been withdrawn.

When an inducing agent is taken concurrently with another medicine, dosage of the other medicine may require adjustment. For example, if a woman taking oral contraceptives were to begin taking phenobarbital, induction of drug metabolism by phenobarbital could accelerate metabolism of the contraceptive to such an extent that protection against pregnancy would be lost. To maintain contraceptive efficacy, dosage of the contraceptive should be increased. Conversely, when a patient *discontinues* an inducing agent, dosages of other drugs may need to be *lowered*. If dosage is not reduced, drug levels may climb dangerously high as rates of hepatic metabolism decline to noninduced values.

*Inhibition of Metabolism.* If drug A inhibits the metabolism of drug B, then levels of drug B will rise (unless the dosage of drug B is lowered). The results may be beneficial or harmful. Inhibition of metabolism by ketoconazole (an antifungal drug) provides an interesting case in point. If ketoconazole is combined with terfenadine [Seldane], a very popular antihistamine, the ability of ketoconazole to inhibit terfenadine metabolism may result in cardiac arrest—a clearly undesirable outcome. In contrast, if we combine ketoconazole with cyclosporine, an expensive immunosuppressant, therapeutic levels of cyclosporine can be achieved with lower doses, thereby greatly reducing the cost of treatment—a clearly beneficial result.

*Competition for Metabolism.* One drug may decrease the rate of metabolism of another by competing with that drug for the same metabolic pathway. Although such interactions have been reported, they are rarely of clinical significance.

***Altered Renal Excretion.*** Drugs can alter all three phases of renal excretion (filtration, reabsorption, and secretion). By doing so, one drug can alter the renal excretion of another. Glomerular filtration can be decreased by drugs that reduce cardiac output: a reduction in cardiac output decreases renal blood flow, which in turn decreases glomerular filtration; the decrease in filtration results in delayed drug excretion. By altering urinary pH, one drug can alter the ionization of another, thereby increasing or decreasing the extent to which that drug undergoes passive tubular reabsorption. Lastly, competition between two drugs for active tubular secretion can decrease the renal excretion of both agents.

## Pharmacodynamic Interactions

By influencing pharmacodynamic processes, one drug can alter the effects of another. Pharmacodynamic interactions are of two basic types: (1) interactions in which the interacting drugs act at the *same* site and (2) interactions in which the interacting drugs act at *separate* sites. Pharmacodynamic interactions may be potentiative or inhibitory, and are of great clinical significance.

***Interactions at the Same Receptor.*** Interactions that occur at the same receptor are almost always *inhibitory*. Inhibition occurs when an antagonist drug blocks access of an agonist drug to its receptor. These agonist-antagonist interactions are described in Chapter 6. There are many agonist-antagonist interactions of clinical importance. Some reduce therapeutic effects and are therefore undesirable. Others reduce toxicity and are of obvious benefit. The interaction between naloxone and morphine noted above is an example of a beneficial inhibitory interaction: by blocking access of morphine to its receptors, naloxone can reverse all effects of morphine overdose.

***Interactions Resulting from Actions at Separate Sites.*** Even though two drugs have different mechanisms of action and act at separate sites, if both drugs influence the same physiologic process, then one drug can alter responses produced by the other. Interactions resulting from effects produced at different sites may be potentiative or inhibitory.

The interaction between morphine and diazepam [Valium] illustrates a potentiative interaction resulting from concurrent use of drugs that act at separate sites. Morphine and diazepam are central nervous system (CNS) depressants, but these drugs do not share the same mechanism of action. Hence, when these agents are administered together, the ability of each to depress CNS function reinforces the depressant effects of the other. This potentiative interaction can result in profound CNS depression.

The interaction between two diuretics—hydrochlorothiazide and spironolactone—illustrates how the effects of a drug acting at one site can *counteract* the effects of a second drug acting at a different site. Hydrochlorothiazide acts on the distal convoluted tubule of the nephron to *increase* excretion of potassium. Acting at a different site in the kidney, spironolactone works to *decrease* renal excretion of potassium. Consequently, when these two drugs are administered together, the potassium-sparing effects of spironolactone tend to balance the potassium-wasting effects of hydrochlorothiazide, leaving renal excretion of potassium at about the same level it would have been had no drugs been given at all.

## Combined Toxicity

Common sense tells us that if drug A and drug B are both toxic to the same organ, then using them together will cause more injury to that organ than if they were not combined. For example, when we treat tuberculosis with isoniazid and rifampin, both of which are hepatotoxic, we cause more liver injury than if we used just one of the drugs. (Unfortunately, this is an unusual situation in which both drugs are essential for therapy; hence, the combination can't be avoided.) However, in most cases we *can* avoid combining drugs that have overlapping toxicities—which is what we should do whenever possible.

## Clinical Significance of Drug-Drug Interactions

From the foregoing it should be clear that drug interactions have the potential to significantly affect the outcome of therapy. As a result of drug-drug interactions, the intensity of responses may be increased or reduced. Interactions that increase therapeutic effects or reduce toxicity are desirable. Conversely, interactions that reduce therapeutic effects or increase toxicity are detrimental.

Common sense tells us that the risk of a serious drug interaction is proportional to the number of drugs that a patient is taking. That is, the more drugs the patient receives, the greater the risk of a detrimental interaction. Since the average hospitalized patient receives 6 to 10 drugs, interactions are common. Accordingly, you should always be alert for them.

Interactions are especially important for drugs that have a low therapeutic index. For these agents, an interaction that produces a modest increase in drug levels can result in toxicity. Conversely, an interaction that produces a modest decrease in drug levels can result in therapeutic failure.

Although a large number of important interactions have been documented, many more are yet to be discovered. Therefore, if a patient develops unusual symptoms, it is wise to suspect that a drug interaction may be the cause—especially since yet another drug might be given to control the new symptoms.

We can minimize adverse interactions in several ways. The most obvious is to minimize the number of drugs a patient receives. Indiscriminate use of multiple-drug therapy does not constitute good treatment—and increases the risk of undesired interactions. A second and equally important means of avoiding detrimental interactions is to take a thorough drug history. A history that identifies all drugs the patient is taking allows the prescriber to adjust the regimen accordingly. Please note, however, that patients who are taking illicit drugs or over-the-counter preparations may fail to report such drug use. You should be aware of this possibility and make a special effort to ensure that the patient's drug use profile is complete. Additional measures for reducing adverse interactions include adjusting the dosage when an inducer of metabolism is added to or deleted from the regimen, adjusting the timing of administration to minimize interference with absorption, and monitoring for early signs of toxicity when combinations of toxic agents cannot be avoided.

## Drug-Food Interactions

Drug-food interactions are both important and poorly understood. They are important because they can result in toxicity or therapeutic failure. They are poorly understood because research has been sorely lacking.

### Impact of Food on Drug Absorption

Food frequently decreases the *rate* of drug absorption, and occasionally decreases the *extent* of absorption. Reducing the rate of absorption merely delays the onset of effects; peak effects are not lowered. In contrast, reducing the extent of absorption reduces the intensity of peak responses.

The interaction between calcium-containing foods and tetracycline antibiotics is perhaps the classic example of food reducing drug absorption. Tetracyclines bind with calcium to form an insoluble and nonabsorbable complex. Hence, if tetracyclines are administered with milk products or calcium supplements, absorption is reduced and antibacterial effects may be lost.

High-fiber foods can reduce absorption of some drugs. For example, absorption of digoxin [Lanoxin], a drug used for cardiac disorders, is reduced significantly by wheat bran, rolled oats, and sunflower seeds. Since digoxin has a low therapeutic index, reduced absorption can result in therapeutic failure.

Very rarely, food *increases* the extent of drug absorption. When this occurs, peak effects are heightened. For example, a high-calorie meal more than doubles the absorption of saquinavir [Invirase], a new drug for HIV infection. Conversely, if saquinavir is taken without food, absorption may be insufficient for antiviral activity.

### Impact of Food on Drug Metabolism: The Grapefruit Juice Effect

Researchers recently discovered that grapefruit juice can inhibit the metabolism of certain drugs. The effect is quite remarkable. For example, coadministration of grapefruit juice produced a 406% increase in blood levels of felodipine, a calcium-channel blocker used for hypertension. In addition to felodipine and other calcium-channel blockers, grapefruit juice has been shown to increase blood levels of terfenadine [Seldane], cyclosporine [Sandimmune], midazolam [Versed], and caffeine.

Grapefruit juice raises drug levels by inhibiting drug metabolism. The actual inhibitor is naringenin, a human metabolite of naringen, which is a compound found in grapefruit. Naringenin acts by inhibiting an isozyme of cytochrome P-450, a key component of the body's drug metabolizing system (see Chapter 5). Since inhibition of cytochrome P-450 by naringenin persists for some time, drugs needn't be administered concurrently with grapefruit juice for an interaction to occur. That is, metabolism can still be inhibited to some extent even if the patient drinks grapefruit juice in the morning but waits until later in the day to take his or her medicine. Since inhibition of metabolism is dose dependent, the more grapefruit juice the patient drinks, the greater the inhibition will be.

At this time, the clinical significance of the grapefruit juice effect has not been established. Nonetheless, given the dramatic increases in drug levels that can result, it would seem imprudent to ignore the effect when a patient is taking a medicine whose metabolism is known to be inhibited by grapefruit juice.

## Impact of Food on Drug Toxicity

Drug-food interactions sometimes result in increased toxicity. The most dramatic example is the interaction between MAO inhibitors (a family of antidepressants) and foods rich in tyramine (e.g., aged cheeses, yeast extracts, Chianti wine); the combination can cause blood pressure to rise to a life-threatening level. To avoid disaster, patients taking MAO inhibitors must be warned about the consequences of consuming tyramine-rich foods, and they must be given a list of foods to strictly avoid (see Chapter 30). Other drug-food combinations that can increase toxicity include the following: theophylline (an asthma medicine) plus caffeine, which can result in excessive CNS excitation; potassium-sparing diuretics (e.g., spironolactone) plus salt substitutes, which can result in dangerously high potassium levels; and aluminum-containing antacids (e.g., Maalox) plus citrus beverages (e.g., orange juice), which can result in excessive absorption of aluminum.

## Impact of Food on Drug Action

Although most drug-food interactions concern drug absorption and drug metabolism, food may also (rarely) have a direct impact on drug action. For example, foods rich in vitamin K (e.g., broccoli, Brussels sprouts, cabbage) can reduce the effects of warfarin, an anticoagulant. How? As discussed in Chapter 50, warfarin acts by inhibiting vitamin K–dependent clotting factors; when vitamin K is more abundant, warfarin is less able to inhibit the clotting factors, and therapeutic effects are reduced.

## Timing of Drug Administration with Respect to Meals

Administration of drugs at the appropriate time with regard to meals is an important facet of drug therapy. As discussed above, the absorption of some drugs can be significantly decreased by food; hence they should be administered on an empty stomach. Conversely, the absorption of other drugs can be increased by food; hence they should be administered with meals.

Many drugs cause stomach upset when taken without food. If food does not reduce their absorption, then these drugs should definitely be administered with meals. However, if food *does* reduce their absorption, then we have a difficult choice: we can administer them with food and thereby reduce stomach upset (good news), but re-

duce absorption (bad news)—or we can administer them without food and thereby improve absorption (good news), but increase stomach upset (bad news). Unfortunately, the correct choice is obvious. (The best solution may be to select an alternative drug that doesn't upset the stomach.)

When the medication order says to administer a drug with food or on an empty stomach, just what does this mean? To administer a drug with food means to administer it with or shortly after a meal. To administer a drug on an empty stomach means to administer it either 1 hour before a meal or 2 hours after.

Medication orders frequently fail to indicate when a drug should be administered with respect to meals. As a result, inappropriate administration may occur. If you are uncertain about when a drug should be administered, ask the prescriber if it should be taken on an empty stomach or with food, and if there are any foods or beverages to avoid.

## KEY POINTS

- Some drug-drug interactions are intended and beneficial; others are detrimental.
- Drug-drug interactions may result in intensified effects, diminished effects, or an entirely new effect.
- Potentiative interactions are beneficial when they increase therapeutic effects and detrimental when they increase adverse effects.
- Inhibitory interactions are beneficial when they decrease adverse effects and detrimental when they decrease beneficial effects.
- Because drugs can interact in solution, you should never combine two or more drugs in the same container unless you are certain that a direct interaction will not occur.
- Drug interactions can result in increased or decreased absorption.
- Competition for protein binding rarely results in a sustained or significant increase in plasma levels of free drug.
- Drugs that induce hepatic drug-metabolizing enzymes can accelerate the metabolism of other drugs.
- When an inducing agent is added to the regimen, it may be necessary to increase the dosages of other drugs. Conversely, when an inducing agent is discontinued, dosages of other drugs may need to be reduced.
- A drug that inhibits the metabolism of other drugs will increase their levels. The result may be beneficial or detrimental.
- Drugs that act as antagonists at a particular receptor will diminish the effects of drugs that act as agonists at that receptor. The result may be beneficial (if the antagonist prevents toxic effects of the agonist), or it may be detrimental (if the antagonist prevents therapeutic effects of the agonist).
- Drugs that are toxic to the same organ should not be combined (if at all possible).

- We can help reduce the risk of adverse interactions by minimizing the number of drugs the patient is given and by taking a thorough drug history.
- Food may reduce the rate or extent of drug absorption. Reducing the extent of absorption reduces peak therapeutic responses; reducing the rate of absorption merely delays onset of effects.
- Very rarely, food may *increase* the rate of drug absorption.

- A component of grapefruit juice can inhibit the metabolism of certain drugs, thereby causing their blood levels to rise.
- Foods may increase drug toxicity. The combination of an MAO inhibitor with tyramine-rich food is the classic example.
- When the medication order says to administer a drug on an empty stomach, this means administer it either 1 hour before a meal or 2 hours after.

# CHAPTER 8

# Adverse Drug Reactions

An adverse drug reaction is broadly defined as any undesired response to a drug. Adverse reactions can range in intensity from annoying to life threatening.

Recall that *safety* is one of the most important characteristics of an ideal drug. A safe drug would be one that is unable to cause severe adverse effects. There is no such thing as a safe drug: severe adverse reactions can occur with *all* medications. Fortunately, when drugs are used properly, many adverse reactions can be avoided, or at least kept to a minimum.

## Scope of the Problem

Drugs can adversely affect all body systems and in varying degrees of intensity. Among the more mild reactions are drowsiness, nausea, itching, and rash. Severe reactions include respiratory depression, neutropenia, hepatocellular injury, anaphylaxis, and hemorrhage—all of which can result in death.

Although adverse reactions can occur in all patients, some are more vulnerable than others. Adverse events are most common in the elderly and the very young. (Patients over 60 account for nearly 50% of all cases of adverse effects.) Severe illness also increases the risk of an adverse reaction. Likewise, adverse events are more common in patients receiving multiple drugs than in patients taking just one.

Some data on adverse drug reactions will underscore the clinical significance of the problem. In North America, the annual expense associated with adverse drug reactions may range as high as $5 billion. Of all hospital admissions, about 5% are for adverse reactions to drugs. Moreover, adverse drug reactions account for approximately 1 of 7 hospital days. A large fraction (10% to 20%) of hospitalized patients experience one or more adverse drug reactions during their stay. About 0.8% of hospitalized patients re-

ceive drug-induced injuries that are disabling. A significant number of drug-induced deaths occur annually.

## Definitions

### Side Effect

A side effect is formally defined as *a nearly unavoidable secondary drug effect produced at therapeutic doses.* Common examples include drowsiness caused by antihistamines and gastric irritation caused by aspirin. Side effects are generally predictable and their intensity is dose dependent. Some side effects develop soon after the onset of drug use, whereas others may not appear until a drug has been taken for weeks or months.

### Toxicity

The formal definition of toxicity is *an adverse drug reaction caused by excessive dosing.* Examples include coma from an overdose of morphine and severe hypoglycemia from an overdose of insulin. Although the formal definition of toxicity includes only those severe reactions that occur when dosage is excessive, in everyday parlance the term *toxicity* has come to mean any severe adverse reaction, regardless of the dose that caused it. For example, when administered in therapeutic doses, many anticancer drugs cause neutropenia (profound loss of neutrophilic white blood cells), thereby putting the patient at high risk of infection. This neutropenia would be called a toxicity even though it was produced when dosage was therapeutic.

### Allergic Reaction

An allergic reaction is an immune response. For an allergic reaction to occur there must be prior sensitization of the immune system. Once the immune system has been sensitized to a drug, re-exposure to that drug can trigger an allergic response. The intensity of allergic reactions can range from mild itching to severe rash to anaphylaxis. (Anaphylaxis is a life-threatening response characterized by bronchospasm, laryngeal edema, and a precipitous drop in blood pressure.) Estimates suggest that less than 10% of adverse drug reactions are of the allergic type.

The intensity of an allergic reaction is determined primarily by the degree of sensitization of the immune system—not by drug dosage. That is, *the intensity of allergic reactions is largely independent of drug dosage*. As a result, a dose that elicits a very strong reaction in one allergic patient may elicit a very mild reaction in another. Furthermore, since a patient's sensitivity to a drug can change over time, a dose that elicits a mild reaction early in treatment may produce an intense response later on.

Very few medications cause severe allergic reactions. The drug family responsible for the majority of serious reactions is the *penicillins*. Penicillin allergy is discussed at length in Chapter 78.

## Idiosyncratic Effect

An idiosyncratic effect is defined as *an uncommon drug response resulting from a genetic predisposition*. To illustrate this concept, let's consider responses to succinylcholine, a drug used to produce flaccid paralysis of skeletal muscle. In most patients, succinylcholine-induced paralysis is brief, lasting only a few minutes. In contrast, genetically predisposed patients may become paralyzed for hours. Why the prolonged effect? In all patients, the effects of succinylcholine are terminated through enzymatic inactivation of the drug. Since most people have very high levels of the inactivating enzyme, paralysis is short lived. However, in a small percentage of patients, the genes that code for succinylcholine-metabolizing enzymes are abnormal, producing enzymes that inactivate the drug very slowly. As a result, paralysis is greatly prolonged.

## Iatrogenic Disease

The word *iatrogenic* is derived from two words: *iatros*, the Greek word for physician and *-genic*, a combining form meaning *to produce*. Hence, an iatrogenic disease is *a disease produced by a physician*. The term iatrogenic disease is also used to denote *a disease produced by drugs*.

Iatrogenic diseases are nearly identical to idiopathic (naturally occurring) diseases. For example, patients taking certain antipsychotic drugs may develop a syndrome whose symptoms closely resemble those of Parkinson's disease. Because this syndrome is (1) drug induced and (2) essentially identical to a naturally occurring pathology, we would call the syndrome an iatrogenic disease.

## Physical Dependence

Physical dependence develops during long-term use of certain drugs, such as opioids, alcohol, barbiturates, and amphetamines. We can define physical dependence as a state in which the body has adapted to prolonged drug exposure in such a way that an abstinence syndrome will result if drug use is discontinued. The precise nature of the abstinence syndrome is determined by the drug upon which the individual is dependent.

Although physical dependence is usually associated with "narcotics" (heroin, morphine, other opioids), these are not the only dependence-inducing drugs. In addition to the opioids, a variety of other centrally acting drugs (e.g., ethanol, barbiturates, amphetamines) can promote dependence. Furthermore, some drugs that work outside the central nervous system (CNS) can cause physical dependence of a sort. Because a variety of drugs can cause physical dependence of one type or another, and because withdrawal reactions have the potential for harm, *patients should be warned against abrupt discontinuation of any medication without first consulting a knowledgeable health professional.*

## Carcinogenic Effect

The term *carcinogenic effect* refers to the ability of certain medications and environmental chemicals to cause cancers. Fortunately, only a few therapeutic agents cause cancer. Ironically, several of the drugs used to *treat* cancer are among the drugs with the greatest carcinogenic potential.

Evaluating drugs for the ability to cause cancer is extremely difficult. Evidence of neoplastic disease may not appear until 20 or more years after initial exposure to a cancer-causing compound. Consequently, it is unlikely that carcinogenic potential will be detected during preclinical and clinical trials of a new drug. Accordingly, when a new drug is released for general marketing, we cannot know with certainty that the drug will not eventually prove carcinogenic.

Diethylstilbestrol (DES) illustrates the problem posed by the delayed appearance of cancer following exposure to a carcinogenic drug. DES is a synthetic hormone with actions similar to those of estrogen. At one time DES was used to prevent spontaneous abortion during high-risk pregnancies. It was not until years later, when vaginal and uterine cancers developed in females who had been exposed to this drug *in utero*, that the carcinogenic actions of DES became known.

## Teratogenic Effect

A *teratogenic effect* can be defined as a drug-induced birth defect. Medicines and other chemicals capable of causing birth defects are called teratogens. Teratogenesis is discussed at length in Chapter 10.

# Identifying Adverse Drug Reactions

It can be very difficult to determine whether a specific drug is responsible for an observed adverse event. This is because other factors—especially the underlying illness and other drugs being taken—could be the actual cause.

# MED**W**ATCH

THE FDA MEDICAL PRODUCTS REPORTING PROGRAM

For VOLUNTARY reporting
by health professionals of adverse
events and product problems

Page ____ of ____

Form Approved: OMB No. 0910-0291 Expires: 1/31/96
See OMB statement on reverse

FDA Use Only (MB)

Triage unit
sequence #

PLEASE TYPE OR USE BLACK INK

## A. Patient information

1. Patient identifier

In confidence

2. Age at time of event:
or _____
Date of birth:

3. Sex
☐ female
☐ male

4. Weight
_____ lbs
or
_____ kgs

## B. Adverse event or product problem

1. ☐ Adverse event   and/or   ☐ Product problem (e.g., defects/malfunctions)

2. Outcomes attributed to adverse event (check all that apply)
☐ death _____ (mo/day/yr)
☐ life-threatening
☐ hospitalization – initial or prolonged
☐ disability
☐ congenital anomaly
☐ required intervention to prevent permanent impairment/damage
☐ other: _____

3. Date of event (mo/day/yr)

4. Date of this report (mo/day/yr)

5. Describe event or problem

6. Relevant tests/laboratory data, including dates

7. Other relevant history, including preexisting medical conditions (e.g., allergies, race, pregnancy, smoking and alcohol use, hepatic/renal dysfunction, etc.)

## C. Suspect medication(s)

1. Name (give labeled strength & mfr/labeler, if known)
#1
#2

2. Dose, frequency & route used
#1
#2

3. Therapy dates (if unknown, give duration) from/to (or best estimate)
#1
#2

4. Diagnosis for use (indication)
#1
#2

5. Event abated after use stopped or dose reduced
#1 ☐ yes ☐ no ☐ doesn't apply
#2 ☐ yes ☐ no ☐ doesn't apply

6. Lot # (if known)
#1
#2

7. Exp. date (if known)
#1
#2

8. Event reappeared after reintroduction
#1 ☐ yes ☐ no ☐ doesn't apply
#2 ☐ yes ☐ no ☐ doesn't apply

9. NDC # (for product problems only)
____ — ____ — ____

10. Concomitant medical products and therapy dates (exclude treatment of event)

## D. Suspect medical device

1. Brand name

2. Type of device

3. Manufacturer name & address

4. Operator of device
☐ health professional
☐ lay user/patient
☐ other: _____

5. Expiration date (mo/day/yr)

6.
model # _____
catalog # _____
serial # _____
lot # _____
other # _____

7. If implanted, give date (mo/day/yr)

8. If explanted, give date (mo/day/yr)

9. Device available for evaluation? (Do not send to FDA)
☐ yes   ☐ no   ☐ returned to manufacturer on _____ (mo/day/yr)

10. Concomitant medical products and therapy dates (exclude treatment of event)

## E. Reporter (see confidentiality section on back)

1. Name & address          phone #

2. Health professional?
☐ yes ☐ no

3. Occupation

4. Also reported to
☐ manufacturer
☐ user facility
☐ distributor

5. If you do NOT want your identity disclosed to the manufacturer, place an " X " in this box. ☐

Mail to: MED**W**ATCH
5600 Fishers Lane
Rockville, MD 20852-9787

*or* FAX to:
1-800-FDA-0178

FDA

FDA Form 3500 (6/93)   Submission of a report does not constitute an admission that medical personnel or the product caused or contributed to the event.

**Figure 8–1. FDA form for reporting adverse drug events.**

To help determine if a particular drug is responsible, the following questions should be asked:

- Did symptoms appear shortly after the drug was first used?
- Did symptoms abate when the drug was discontinued?
- Did symptoms reappear when the drug was reinstituted?
- Is the illness itself sufficient to explain the event?
- Are other drugs in the regimen sufficient to explain the event?

If the answers reveal a temporal relationship between the presence of the drug and the adverse event, and if the event cannot be explained by the illness itself or by other drugs in the regimen, then there is a high probability that the drug under suspicion is indeed the culprit.

## Adverse Reactions to New Drugs

As we discussed in Chapter 4, preclinical and clinical trials of new drugs cannot detect all of the adverse reactions that a new drug might be capable of causing. Consequently, when a new drug is released for general marketing, information regarding its adverse reactions is incomplete.

Because newly released drugs may have as-yet unreported adverse effects, you should be alert for unusual responses when giving these agents. If the patient develops new symptoms, it is wise to suspect that the drug may be responsible—even if the symptoms are not described in the literature. If the drug is especially new, you may be the first clinician to have observed this particular effect.

When a drug is suspected of causing a previously unknown adverse effect, that effect should be reported to the FDA. It is only through voluntary reporting by alert clinicians that a drug's potential for harm can be made widely known. Accordingly, all suspected adverse effects should be reported, even if absolute proof of the drug's complicity has not been established. The form used for reporting adverse reactions is reproduced in Figure 8–1.

## Ways to Minimize Adverse Drug Reactions

The responsibility for reducing adverse drug reactions lies with everyone associated with drug manufacture and use. The pharmaceutical industry must strive to produce the safest possible medicinal agents; the physician must select the least harmful medication for a particular patient; the nurse must evaluate patients for adverse drug reactions and must educate patients in ways to avoid or minimize harm; and patients and their families must watch for signs that an adverse reaction may be developing, and should alert the physician if they appear.

Anticipation of adverse reactions can help minimize them. Both the nurse and the patient should know the major adverse reactions that a drug can produce. This knowledge will allow early identification of adverse effects, thereby permitting timely implementation of measures to minimize harm.

Certain drugs are toxic to specific organs. When patients are using these drugs, function of the target organ should be monitored. The liver, kidneys, and bone marrow are important sites of drug toxicity. For drugs that are toxic to the liver, the patient should be monitored for signs and symptoms of liver damage (malaise, abdominal discomfort, jaundice, dark urine) and periodic tests of liver function should be performed. For drugs that are toxic to the kidneys, the patient should undergo routine urinalysis and measurement of serum creatinine; in addition, periodic tests of creatinine clearance should be performed. For drugs that are toxic to bone marrow, periodic blood cell counts are required.

Adverse effects can be reduced through individualization of therapy. When prescribing a drug for a particular patient, the physician must balance the risks of that drug versus its probable benefits. Drugs that are likely to cause ill effects for a specific patient should be avoided. For example, if a patient has a history of penicillin allergy, we can avoid a potentially severe reaction by withholding penicillin and administering a suitable substitute. Similarly, when treating pregnant patients, we must withhold drugs that can harm the developing fetus (see Chapter 10).

Lastly, we must be aware that patients being treated for chronic disorders are especially prone to developing adverse reactions. Included in this group are patients with hypertension, epilepsy, heart disease, and psychoses. When drugs must be used on a long-term basis, the patient should be informed about the adverse effects that may develop over time and should be monitored periodically for their appearance.

## KEY POINTS

- All drugs can cause adverse effects. There is no such thing as a safe drug.
- Patients at increased risk of adverse drug events include the very young, the elderly, the very ill, and those taking multiple drugs.
- An iatrogenic disease is defined as a drug- or physician-induced disease.
- An idiosyncratic effect is defined as an adverse drug reaction based on a genetic predisposition.
- A carcinogenic effect is defined as drug-induced cancer.
- A teratogenic effect is defined as a drug-induced birth defect.
- The intensity of an allergic drug reaction is based on the degree of immune system sensitization—not on drug dosage.
- At the time a new drug is released, it well may have the ability to cause adverse effects that are as yet unknown.
- Measures to minimize adverse drug events include avoiding drugs that are likely to harm a particular patient, monitoring the patient for signs and symptoms of likely adverse effects, educating the patient about possible adverse effects, and testing organs that are vulnerable to a particular drug.

# CHAPTER 9

# Individual Variation in Drug Responses

**Body Weight and Composition**
**Age**
**Pathophysiology**
   Kidney Disease
   Liver Disease
   Acid-Base Imbalance
   Altered Electrolyte Status
**Tolerance**
   Pharmacodynamic Tolerance
   Metabolic Tolerance
   Tachyphylaxis

**Placebo Effect**
**Genetics**
**Variability in Absorption**
   Bioavailability
   Other Causes of Variable Absorption
**Failure to Take Medicine as Prescribed**
**Drug Interactions**
**Diet**

ndividual variation in drug responses has been a recurrent theme throughout the early chapters of this text. We noted that, because of individual variation, we must tailor drug therapy to each patient. In this chapter we discuss the major factors that can cause one patient to respond to drugs differently from another. With this information you will be better prepared to reduce individual variation in drug responses, thereby maximizing the benefits of treatment and reducing the potential for harm. As we discuss sources of individual variation, we will review and integrate much of the information presented in previous chapters.

## Body Weight and Composition

In the absence of adjustments in dosage, body size can be a significant determinant of drug effects. Recall that the intensity of the response to a drug is determined in large part by the concentration of the drug at its sites of action—the higher the concentration, the more intense the response. Common sense tells us that if a small person and a large person are given the same amount of the same drug, the drug will achieve a higher concentration in the small person, and therefore will produce more intense effects. To compensate for this potential source of individual variation, dosages must be adapted to the size of the patient.

When adjusting dosage to account for patient size, the clinician may base the adjustment on *body surface area* rather than on body weight per se. The reason for this practice is that surface area determinations account not

only for the patient's weight but also for how fat or lean the patient may be. Since percentage body fat can change drug distribution, and since altered distribution can change the concentration of a drug at its sites of action, dosage adjustments based on body surface area provide a more precise means of controlling drug responses than do adjustments based on weight alone.

## Age

Drug sensitivity varies with age. Infants are especially sensitive to drugs, as are the elderly. In the very young, heightened drug sensitivity is the result of organ system immaturity. In the elderly, heightened sensitivity results largely from progressive organ system degeneration. Other factors that affect sensitivity in the elderly are increased severity of illness, the presence of multiple pathologies, and treatment with multiple drugs. The clinical challenge created by heightened drug sensitivity in the very young and the elderly is discussed at length in Chapters 11 and 12.

## Pathophysiology

Abnormal physiology can alter responses to drugs. In this section we examine the impact on drug responses produced by four pathophysiologic states: (1) kidney disease, (2) liver disease, (3) acid-base imbalance, and (4) altered electrolyte status.

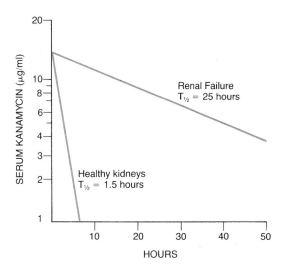

**Figure 9–1. Effect of renal failure on kanamycin half-life.** Kanamycin was administered at time "0" to two patients, one with healthy kidneys and one with renal failure. Note that drug levels decline very rapidly in the patient with healthy kidneys and extremely slowly in the patient with renal failure, indicating that renal failure greatly reduces the capacity to remove this drug from the body.

## Kidney Disease

Kidney disease can reduce drug excretion, causing drugs to accumulate in the body. If dosage is not lowered, drugs may accumulate to toxic levels. Consequently, if a patient is taking a drug whose elimination is dependent upon the kidneys, and if renal failure begins to develop, dosage must be decreased so that drug levels will remain within the therapeutic range.

The impact of renal disease on plasma drug levels is illustrated in Figure 9–1. The figure shows the decline in plasma levels of kanamycin (an antibiotic) following injection of the drug into two patients, one with healthy kidneys and one with renal failure. Elimination of kanamycin is exclusively renal. As shown in the figure, kanamycin levels fall off rapidly in the patient with good kidney function; the half-life of kanamycin in this patient is brief—only 1.5 hours. In contrast, drug levels decline very slowly in the patient with renal failure. Because of kidney disease, the half-life of kanamycin has increased by nearly 17-fold—from 1.5 hours to 25 hours. Under these conditions, if dosage is not reduced, kanamycin will quickly accumulate to toxic levels.

## Liver Disease

Like kidney disease, liver disease can cause drugs to accumulate. Recall that the liver is the major site of drug metabolism. Hence, if the liver ceases to function, rates of metabolism will fall and drug levels will climb. To prevent accumulation to toxic levels, patients with liver disease should have their dosages reduced. Of course, this guideline applies only to those drugs that are eliminated primarily by the liver; liver dysfunction will not affect plasma levels of drugs that are eliminated largely by nonhepatic mechanisms (e.g., renal excretion).

### Acid-Base Imbalance

By altering pH partitioning (see Chapter 5), changes in acid-base status can alter the absorption, distribution, metabolism, and excretion of drugs.

Figure 9–2 illustrates the impact of altered acid-base status on drug distribution. This figure summarizes the results of an experiment examining the effects of altered acid-base status on the distribution of phenobarbital (a weak acid). The experiment was performed in a dog. The upper curve shows plasma levels of phenobarbital. The lower curve shows plasma pH. Acid-base status was altered by having the dog inhale a mixture of gas rich in carbon dioxide ($CO_2$), thereby causing respiratory acidosis. In the figure, acidosis is indicated by the drop in plasma pH. Note that the decline in pH is associated with a parallel drop in levels of phenobarbital. Upon discontinuation of $CO_2$ administration, plasma pH returned to normal and phenobarbital levels moved upward.

Why did acidosis alter plasma levels of phenobarbital? Recall that because of pH partitioning, if there is a difference in pH on two sides of a membrane, a drug will accumulate on the side where the pH most favors that drug's ionization; acidic drugs will accumulate on the alkaline side, whereas basic drugs will accumulate on the acidic side. Since phenobarbital is a weak acid, it tends to accumulate in alkaline environments. Accordingly, when the dog inhaled $CO_2$, causing extracellular pH to decline, phenobarbital left the plasma and entered cells, where the environment was less acidic (more alkaline) than in plasma. When $CO_2$ administration ceased and plasma pH returned to normal, the pH partitioning effect caused phenobarbital to leave cells and re-enter the blood; hence, the increase in plasma drug levels seen after $CO_2$ withdrawal.

### Altered Electrolyte Status

Electrolytes (e.g., potassium, sodium, calcium, magnesium) have important roles in cell physiology. Consequently, when electrolyte levels become disturbed, multiple cellular processes can be disrupted. Excitable tissues (nerves and muscles) are especially sensitive to alterations in electrolyte status. Given that disturbances in electrolyte balance can have widespread effects on cell physiology, we might expect that electrolyte imbalances would cause profound and widespread effects on responses to drugs. However, this does not seem to be the case; examples in which electrolyte changes have a significant impact on drug responses are rare.

Perhaps the most important example of an altered drug effect occurring in response to electrolyte imbalance involves digoxin, a drug used to treat heart disease. The most serious toxicity of digoxin is production of potentially fatal cardiac dysrhythmias.

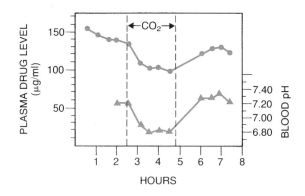

**Figure 9–2. Altered drug distribution in response to altered plasma pH.** *Lower curve,* Plasma (extracellular) pH. Note the decline in pH in response to inhalation of $CO_2$. *Upper curve,* Plasma levels of phenobarbital. Note the decline in plasma drug levels during the period of extracellular acidosis. This decline results from the redistribution of phenobarbital into cells. (See text for details.) (Redrawn from Waddell, W.J., and Butler, T.C. The distribution and excretion of phenobarbital. J. Clin. Invest. 36:1217, 1957, by copyright permission of the American Society for Clinical Investigation.)

The tendency of digoxin to disturb cardiac rhythm is related to levels of potassium: when potassium levels are depressed, the ability of digoxin to induce dysrhythmias is greatly increased. Accordingly, all patients receiving digoxin must undergo regular measurement of serum potassium to ensure that levels remain within a safe range. Digoxin toxicity and its relationship to potassium levels are discussed at length in Chapter 46.

## Tolerance

Tolerance can be defined as *decreased responsiveness to a drug as a result of repeated drug administration.* Patients who are tolerant to a drug require higher doses to produce the same effects that could be achieved with smaller doses before the tolerance developed. There are three categories of drug tolerance: (1) pharmacodynamic tolerance, (2) metabolic tolerance, and (3) tachyphylaxis.

### Pharmacodynamic Tolerance

The term *pharmacodynamic tolerance* refers to the familiar type of tolerance associated with long-term administration of drugs such as morphine and heroin. The person who is pharmacodynamically tolerant requires increased drug levels to produce effects that could formerly be elicited at lower drug levels. Put another way, in the presence of pharmacodynamic tolerance, the minimum effective concentration (MEC) of a drug is abnormally high. Although the molecular mechanisms for pharmacodynamic tolerance are not fully understood, this form of tolerance is thought to result from an adaptive process that occurs in response to chronic receptor stimulation.

### Metabolic Tolerance

Metabolic tolerance is defined as tolerance resulting from accelerated drug metabolism. This form of tolerance is brought about by the ability of certain drugs (e.g., barbiturates) to induce synthesis of hepatic drug-metabolizing enzymes, thereby causing rates of drug metabolism to increase. Because of increased metabolism, dosage must be increased to maintain therapeutic drug levels. Unlike pharmacodynamic tolerance, which causes the MEC to increase, metabolic tolerance does not influence the level of drug required to elicit a response: in the person with metabolic tolerance, dosage is increased so that plasma drug levels can be maintained at pretolerance levels; the increase in dosage is not employed to produce drug levels that are above normal.

The experiment summarized in Table 9-1 demonstrates the development of metabolic tolerance in response to repeated administration of pentobarbital, a central nervous system (CNS) depressant. The experiment used two groups of rabbits, a control group and an experimental group. Rabbits in the experimental group were pretreated with pentobarbital for 3 days (60 mg/kg/day, SC) and then given an IV challenging dose (30 mg/kg) of this same drug; drug effect (sleeping time) and plasma

**TABLE 9-1. DEVELOPMENT OF METABOLIC TOLERANCE AS A RESULT OF REPEATED PENTOBARBITAL ADMINISTRATION**

| | Type of Pretreatment | |
|---|---|---|
| **Results** | None | Pentobarbital |
| Sleeping time (minutes) | 67 ± 4 | 30 ± 7 |
| Pentobarbital half-life in plasma (minutes) | 79 ± 3 | 26 ± 2 |
| Plasma level of pentobarbital upon awakening (μg/ml) | 9.9 ± 1.4 | 7.9 ± 0.6 |

Data from Remmer, H. Drugs as activators of drug enzymes. *In* Brodie, B.B., and Erdos, E.G. (eds.). Metabolic Factors Controlling Duration of Drug Action (Proceedings of First International Pharmacological Meeting, Vol. 6). New York, Macmillan, 1962, p. 235.

drug levels were then measured. The control rabbits received the challenging dose of pentobarbital but did not receive any pretreatment. As indicated in Table 9-1, the challenging dose of pentobarbital had less effect on the pretreated rabbits than on the control animals. Specifically, whereas the control rabbits slept for an average of 67 minutes, the average sleeping time for the pretreated animals was only 30 minutes, an effect less than half that produced in the controls.

Why was pentobarbital less effective in the pretreated animals? The data on the plasma half-life of pentobarbital suggest an answer. As shown in the table, the half-life of pentobarbital was much shorter in the experimental animals than in the control group. Since elimination of pentobarbital depends primarily on metabolic conversion, the reduced half-life seen in the experimental animals indicates accelerated metabolism. This increase in metabolism, which was brought on by pentobarbital pretreatment, explains why the experimental rabbits were more tolerant than the control animals.

You might ask, "How do we know that the experimental rabbits had not developed *pharmacodynamic* tolerance?" The absence of pharmacodynamic tolerance is indicated by the plasma drug levels measured at the time the rabbits awoke. In the pretreated rabbits, the waking drug levels were slightly below the waking drug levels in the control group. Had the experimental animals developed pharmacodynamic tolerance, they would have required an increase in drug concentration to maintain sleep; hence, if pharmacodynamic tolerance were present, drug levels would have been abnormally high at the time of awakening rather than reduced.

### Tachyphylaxis

Tachyphylaxis is a form of tolerance that can be defined as a reduction in drug responsiveness brought on by repeated dosing *over a short time.* Hence, unlike pharmacodynamic and metabolic tolerance, which takes days or longer to develop, tachyphylaxis occurs quickly. Tachyphylaxis is not a common mechanism of drug tolerance.

Transdermal nitroglycerin provides a good example of tachyphylaxis. When nitroglycerin is administered using a transdermal patch, effects are lost rapidly (in less than 24 hours) if the patch is left in place around the clock. As discussed in Chapter 45, this loss of effect results from depletion of a co-factor that nitroglycerin needs to act. When nitroglycerin is administered on an intermittent schedule, rather than continuously, the co-factor can be replenished and no loss of effect occurs.

## Placebo Effect

A *placebo* is a preparation that is devoid of intrinsic pharmacologic activity. Any response that a patient may have to a placebo is based solely on the patient's psychologic reaction to the idea of taking a medication and not to any direct physiologic or biochemical action of the placebo itself. The primary use of the placebo is as a control preparation during the testing of new medications.

The *placebo effect* is defined as that component of a drug response that is caused by psychologic factors and not by the biochemical or physiologic properties of the drug. Although it is impossible to assess with precision the contribution that psychologic factors make to the overall response to any particular drug, it is probably correct to say that with practically all medications some fraction of the total response results from a placebo effect.

Although placebo effects are determined by psychologic factors and not physiologic ones, the presence of a placebo response does not imply that a patient's original pathology was "all in the head." Placebo responses are real. Not only are placebo responses real, they can be of great therapeutic significance. For example, there is little doubt that some fraction of the pain relief experienced by patients taking nitroglycerin for angina pectoris is due to placebo effects. The fact that relief of anginal pain may be due in part to placebo effects and not entirely to the pharmacologic properties of nitroglycerin does not make the pain relief less real or less beneficial.

Not all placebo responses are beneficial; placebo responses can also be negative. If a patient believes that a medication is going to be effective, then placebo responses are likely to help promote recovery. Conversely, if a patient is convinced that a particular medication is ineffective or perhaps even harmful, then placebo effects are likely to detract from his or her progress.

Because the placebo effect depends on the patient's attitude toward medicine, fostering a positive attitude can help promote beneficial effects. In this regard, it is desirable that all members of the health care team present the patient with an optimistic (but realistic) assessment of the effects that therapy is likely to produce. It is also important that members of the team be consistent with one another; the beneficial placebo responses may well be decreased if, for example, nurses on the day shift repeatedly reassure a patient about the likely benefits of his or her regimen, while nurses on the night shift express pessimism about those same drugs.

## Genetics

A patient's unique genetic makeup can lead to drug responses that are qualitatively and quantitatively different from those of the population at large. Unique drug responses based on genetic heritage are often referred to as *idiosyncratic effects* (see Chapter 8).

The most common mechanism by which genetic differences modify drug responses is alteration of drug metabolism: genetic variations can result in increased or decreased metabolism of certain drugs. Some people, for example, have a genetically determined insufficiency in their ability to metabolize succinylcholine (a muscle relaxant). Hence, if succinylcholine is administered to these individuals, muscle relaxation is prolonged. Other drugs whose rate of metabolism is genetically determined include isoniazid (a drug for tuberculosis) and tolbutamide (a drug for diabetes). If genetically determined abnormalities in rates of drug metabolism are not too great, they can be compensated for by adjustments in dosage. However, when the alteration in metabolic rate is extremely large (as is the case with succinylcholine), then the drug should not be administered.

Some genetically determined drug responses are based on factors other than altered rates of metabolism. For example, some individuals have red blood cells that are deficient in an enzyme called glucose-6-phosphate dehydrogenase. This deficiency renders the individual susceptible to hemolysis (red blood cell destruction) if given certain drugs, including aspirin, sulfanilamide (an antibiotic), and primaquine (an antimalarial agent). About 10% of African American males and many Near Eastern and Mediterranean males are subject to this idiosyncratic reaction.

## Variability in Absorption

Both the rate and extent of drug absorption can vary from one patient to another. These variations in absorption can contribute to individual variation in drug responses. Differences in manufacturing processes are a major source of variability in drug absorption, although absorption may also be altered by other factors. Several causes of variable absorption have been addressed previously, primarily in Chapter 5 (Pharmacokinetics) and Chapter 7 (Drug-Drug and Drug-Food Interactions); hence, their discussion here will be brief.

### Bioavailability

The term *bioavailability* refers to the ability of a drug to reach the systemic circulation from its site of administration. Different preparations of the same drug can vary in their bioavailability. As discussed in Chapter 5, such factors as tablet disintegration time, enteric coatings, and sustained-release formulations can alter bioavailability, and can thereby make drug responses variable.

Differences in bioavailability occur primarily with oral administration and not with parenteral administration. Fortunately, even with oral agents, when differences in bioavailability do exist between preparations of the same drug, those differences are usually so small that they lack clinical significance.

Differences in bioavailability are of greatest concern for drugs with a narrow therapeutic range. When the thera-

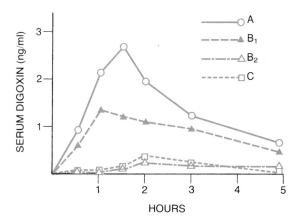

**Figure 9–3. Variations in bioavailability among preparations of digoxin.** On four separate occasions, the subject in this study was given two digoxin tablets (0.25 mg each) following an overnight fast. The tablets were from different sources (A, $B_1$, $B_2$, C). Blood levels of digoxin reveal clear differences in bioavailability among the different digoxin preparations. (See text for details.) (Redrawn from Lindenbaum, J., Mellow, M.H., Blackstone, M.O., and Butler, V.P., Jr. Variation in biologic availability of digoxin from four preparations. N. Engl. J. Med. 285:1344, 1971.)

peutic range is narrow, a relatively small change in drug level can produce a significant change in response: a small decline in drug level may cause therapeutic failure, whereas a small increase in drug level may cause toxicity. Under these conditions, differences in bioavailability can have a significant impact. Because drugs produced by different manufacturers can vary in bioavailability, it is strongly recommended that patients taking drugs that have a narrow therapeutic range never switch from one brand to another without first consulting their physician.

The experiment summarized in Figure 9-3 illustrates the extent to which bioavailability can vary between different preparations of the same drug. In this experiment, a volunteer was given four different preparations of digoxin, a drug that has a narrow therapeutic range and that is used to treat cardiac disorders. For each of the four digoxin preparations (A, $B_1$, $B_2$, and C), bioavailability was determined by measuring levels of digoxin in blood following ingestion of two 0.25-mg tablets. As Figure 9-3 indicates, levels of digoxin varied widely. Although the dosage of all four preparations was identical, digoxin levels achieved with preparation A were twice as high as those achieved with preparation $B_1$; preparations $B_2$ and C were absorbed so poorly that blood levels were barely measurable. These data offer a dramatic demonstration of the differences in bioavailability that can exist between different preparations of the same drug.

## Other Causes of Variable Absorption

Several factors in addition to bioavailability can alter drug absorption, and thereby lead to individual variations in drug responses. Alterations in gastric pH can affect absorption by altering the pH partitioning effect. Prolongation of gastric emptying time can delay absorption of drugs that need to reach the intestine before they are absorbed. Diarrhea can reduce absorption by accelerating transport of drugs through the intestine. Conversely, con-

stipation can enhance absorption by prolonging the time available for absorption. The presence of food in the stomach tends to *delay* absorption of most drugs; in some cases, food can decrease the *extent* of absorption as well. For example, absorption of tetracycline will be reduced substantially if this drug is ingested together with milk and other dairy products that contain calcium. Lastly, there are multiple mechanisms by which drug interactions can result in decreased or increased drug absorption (see Chapter 7).

## Failure to Take Medicine as Prescribed

Medications are not always administered as prescribed: dosage size and timing may be altered, doses may be omitted, and extra doses may be taken. Failure to administer medication as prescribed is a common explanation for variability in the response to a prescribed dose of a drug. As a rule, such failure results from either poor patient compliance or medication errors made by hospital staff.

Patient compliance can be defined as cooperative and accurate participation in one's own drug therapy. Multiple factors can influence compliance. These include manual dexterity, visual acuity, intellectual capacity, psychologic state, attitude toward drugs, and ability to pay for medication.

Patient education is an important means of promoting compliance. Instruction must be convincing and clear. In most cases, it is the responsibility of the nurse to provide this instruction. By succeeding in promoting compliance, you can contribute greatly to reducing variability.

Medication errors are an obvious source of individual variation. Medication errors can originate with physicians, nurses, and pharmacists. However, since the nurse is usually the last member of the health care team to check medications prior to administration, it is ultimately the nurse's responsibility to ensure that medication errors are avoided.

## Drug Interactions

By definition, a drug interaction is a process in which one drug alters the effects of another. Drug interactions can be an important source of variability in drug responses. The mechanisms by which one drug can alter the effects of another and the clinical consequences of drug interactions are discussed at length in Chapter 7.

## Diet

Diet can affect responses to drugs, primarily by affecting the patient's general health status. A diet that promotes good health will enable drugs to elicit therapeutic responses and will increase the patient's capacity to tolerate adverse effects. Poor nutrition will have the opposite effect.

Starvation can affect responses by reducing protein binding. Starvation causes plasma levels of albumin to fall. As a result, binding of drugs to albumin declines, causing levels of free drug to rise, which in turn causes drug responses to become more intense. For certain drugs (e.g., warfarin, an anticoagulant), the resultant increase in effects could be disastrous.

Although nutrition can affect drug responses by the general mechanisms noted, there are only a few examples of a specific nutritional factor affecting the response to a specific drug.

One important and well-documented illustration of the impact that diet can have on drug responses involves a drug family known as monoamine oxidase (MAO) inhibitors, which are used to treat depression. The most serious adverse effect of these drugs is malignant hypertension, a reaction that can be triggered by foods that contain tyramine (a breakdown product of the amino acid tyrosine). Accordingly, patients taking MAO inhibitors must rigidly avoid all tyramine-rich foods (e.g., beef liver, ripe cheeses, yeast products, Chianti wine). The interaction of tyramine-containing foods with MAO inhibitors is discussed at length in Chapter 30.

## KEY POINTS

- In order to maximize beneficial drug responses and minimize harm, we must adjust therapy to account for sources of individual variation.
- As a rule, small patients need smaller doses than large patients.
- Dosage adjustments made to account for size are often based on body surface area, rather than simply on body weight.
- Infants and the elderly are more sensitive to drugs than are older children and younger adults.
- Kidney disease can decrease drug excretion, and thereby cause drug levels to rise. To prevent toxicity, dosage should be reduced.
- Liver disease can decrease drug metabolism, and thereby cause drug levels to rise. To prevent toxicity, dosage should be reduced.
- When a patient becomes tolerant to a drug, the dosage must be increased to maintain beneficial effects.
- Pharmacodynamic tolerance results from adaptive changes that occur in response to prolonged drug exposure. Pharmacodynamic tolerance increases the MEC of a drug.
- Pharmacokinetic tolerance results from accelerated drug metabolism. Pharmacokinetic tolerance does not change the MEC.
- A placebo effect is the component of a drug response that can be attributed to psychologic factors, and not to direct physiologic or biochemical actions of the drug.
- Placebo responses are very real, and can contribute to the success or failure of treatment.
- Genetic factors—especially genetically determined rates of drug metabolism—can be a source of individual variation.
- Bioavailability refers to the ability of a drug to reach the systemic circulation from its site of administration.
- Differences in bioavailability matter most for drugs that have a narrow therapeutic range.
- Poor patient compliance is a major source of individual variation.

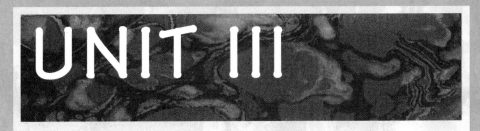

# UNIT III

# Drug Therapy across the Life Span

Drug Therapy during Pregnancy and Breast-Feeding

Drug Therapy in Pediatric Patients

Drug Therapy in Geriatric Patients

# CHAPTER 10

# Drug Therapy during Pregnancy and Breast-Feeding

Our topic for this chapter is drug therapy in women who are pregnant or breast-feeding. The challenge is to provide effective treatment for the mother while avoiding harm to the fetus or nursing infant. Unfortunately, meeting the challenge is confounded by a lack of reliable data on pregnancy-related drug toxicity.

## Drug Therapy during Pregnancy: Basic Considerations

Drug use during pregnancy is common: between one-half and two-thirds of pregnant women take at least one medication, and the majority take more. Some drugs are used to treat pregnancy-related conditions, such as constipation and pre-eclampsia. Some are used to treat chronic disorders, such as hypertension, diabetes, and epilepsy. And some are used for infectious diseases or cancer. In addition to taking these therapeutic agents, pregnant women frequently take drugs of abuse, such as alcohol, cocaine, and heroin.

Drug therapy in pregnancy presents a vexing dilemma. In pregnant patients, as in all other patients, the benefits of treatment must balance the risks. Of course, when drugs are used during pregnancy, risks apply to the fetus as well as the mother. Unfortunately, the risks for most drugs used in pregnancy have not been established—hence the dilemma: the clinician is obliged to balance risks versus benefits, without knowing what the risks really are. The reasons that underlie our lack of knowledge are discussed below under *Identification of Teratogens*.

Despite the imposing challenge of balancing risks versus benefits, drug therapy during pregnancy cannot and should not be avoided. The health of the fetus depends on the health of the mother. Hence, conditions that threaten the mother's health must be addressed—for the sake of the baby as well as the mother. Chronic asthma provides a good example. Uncontrolled asthma is far more dangerous to the fetus than the drugs used for its treatment. Among asthmatic women who fail to take medication, the incidence of stillbirths is doubled. If all women with asthma took medication, an estimated 2000 babies would be saved annually.

## Physiologic Changes during Pregnancy and Their Impact on Drug Disposition and Dosing

Pregnancy brings on physiologic changes that can alter drug disposition. Changes in the kidney, liver, and gastrointestinal tract are of particular interest. Because of these changes, a compensatory change in dosage may be needed.

By the third trimester, renal blood flow is doubled, causing a large increase in glomerular filtration rate. As a result, there is accelerated clearance of drugs that are eliminated by glomerular filtration. Elimination of lithium, for example, is increased by 100%. To compensate for accelerated excretion, dosage must be increased.

For some drugs, hepatic metabolism increases during pregnancy. Three anticonvulsants—phenytoin, carbamazepine, and valproic acid—provide examples. As with drugs whose renal clearance is increased, these drugs will require an increase in dosage.

Tone and motility of the bowel decrease in pregnancy, causing intestinal transit time to increase. Because of prolonged transit, there is more time for drugs to be absorbed. In theory, this could increase levels of drugs whose absorption is normally poor. Similarly, there is more time for reabsorption of drugs that undergo enterohepatic recirculation; hence, effects of these drugs could be prolonged. In both cases, a reduction in dosage might be needed.

## Placental Drug Transfer

Essentially all drugs can cross the placenta, although some cross more readily than others. The factors that determine drug passage across the membranes of the placenta are the same factors that determine drug passage across all other membranes. Accordingly, drugs that are lipid soluble cross the placenta easily, whereas drugs that are ionized, highly polar, or protein bound cross with difficulty. Nonetheless, for practical purposes, the clinician should assume that any drug taken during pregnancy will reach the fetus.

## Adverse Reactions during Pregnancy

Drugs taken during pregnancy can adversely affect both the mother and fetus. The effect of greatest concern is *teratogenesis* (production of birth defects). This topic is discussed separately below. Not only are pregnant women subject to the same adverse effects as everyone else, they may also suffer effects unique to pregnancy. For example, when heparin (an anticoagulant) is taken by pregnant women, it can cause osteoporosis, which in turn causes compression fractures of the spine. Use of prostaglandins (e.g., misoprostol), which stimulate uterine contraction, can cause abortion. Conversely, use of aspirin near term can suppress contractions in labor. In addition, aspirin increases the risk of serious bleeding.

Regular use of dependence-producing drugs (e.g., heroin, barbiturates, alcohol) during pregnancy can result in the birth of a drug-dependent infant. If the infant is not supplied with a drug that can support its dependence, a withdrawal syndrome will ensue. Symptoms include shrill crying, vomiting, and extreme irritability. The neonate should be weaned from dependence by giving progressively smaller doses of the drug on which it is dependent.

Certain pain relievers used during delivery can depress respiration in the neonate. The infant should be closely monitored until respiration becomes normal.

## Drug Therapy during Pregnancy: Teratogenesis

The term *teratogenesis* is derived from *teras*, the Greek word for *monster*. Translated literally, *teratogenesis* means to *produce a monster*. Consistent with this derivation, we usually think of birth defects in terms of gross malformations, such as cleft palate, clubfoot, and hydrocephalus. However, birth defects are not limited to distortions of gross anatomy; birth defects also include behavioral and biochemical anomalies.

### Incidence and Causes of Congenital Anomalies

The incidence of *major* structural abnormalities (i.e., abnormalities that are life threatening or require surgical correction) is about 6%. Half of these are obvious and are reported at birth. The other half involve internal organs (e.g., heart, liver, gastrointestinal tract) and are not dis-

covered until later in life or at autopsy. The incidence of minor structural abnormalities is unknown, as is the incidence of functional abnormalities (e.g., growth retardation, mental retardation).

Congenital anomalies have multiple causes, including genetic heritage, environmental chemicals, and drugs. Genetic factors account for about 25% of all birth defects. Of the genetically based anomalies, Down's syndrome is the most common. Only 3% of all birth defects are caused by drugs. For the majority of congenital anomalies, the cause is unknown.

### Teratogenesis and Stage of Development

Fetal sensitivity to teratogens changes during development; hence, the effect of a teratogen is highly dependent upon when the drug is given. As shown in Figure 10-1, development occurs in three major stages: the *preimplantation/presomite period* (conception through week 2), the *embryonic period* (weeks 3 through 8), and the *fetal period* (week 9 through term). During the preimplantation/presomite period, teratogens act in an "all or nothing" fashion: if the dose is sufficiently high, the result is death of the conceptus; however, if the dose is sublethal, the conceptus is likely to recover fully.

*Gross malformations* are produced by exposure to teratogens during the *embryonic period* (roughly the first trimester). This is the time when the basic shape of internal organs and other structures is being established. Hence it is not surprising that interference at this stage results in conspicuous anatomic distortions. Because the fetus is especially vulnerable during the embryonic period, expectant mothers must take special care to avoid exposure to teratogens during this time.

Teratogen exposure during the *fetal period* (i.e., the second and third trimesters) disrupts *function* rather than gross anatomy. Of the developmental processes that occur in the fetal period, growth and development of the brain are especially important. Disruption of brain development can result in learning deficits and behavioral abnormalities.

### Identification of Teratogens

For the following reasons, human teratogens are extremely difficult to identify: the incidence of congenital anomalies is generally low; animal tests may not be applicable; prolonged exposure may be required; teratogenic effects may be delayed; behavioral effects are difficult to document; and controlled experiments can't be done in humans. As a result, only a few drugs are considered *proven* teratogens. Drugs whose teratogenicity has been documented (or at least is highly suspected) are listed in Table 10-1. It is important to note, however, that *lack of proof of teratogenicity does not mean that a drug is safe*; it only means that the available information is insufficient to make a definitive judgment. Conversely, *proof of teratogenicity does not mean that every exposure will result in a birth defect*; with most teratogens, the risk of malformation is only about 10%.

To prove that a drug is a teratogen, three criteria must be met: (1) the drug must cause a characteristic set of malformations; (2) it must act only during a specific window

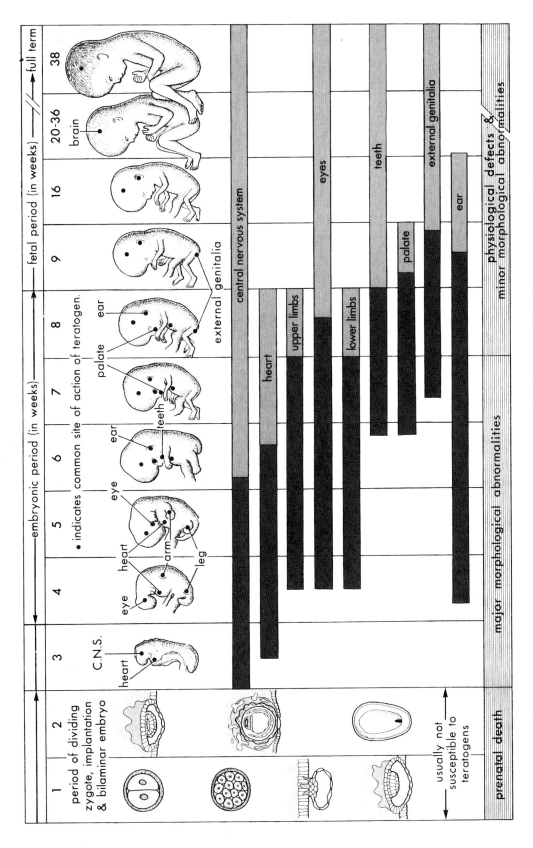

**Figure 10–1. Effects of teratogens at various stages of development of the fetus.** (From Moore, K.L. The Developing Human: Clinically Oriented Embryology, 5th ed. Philadelphia, W.B. Saunders Company, 1993.)

*ACE[†] Inhibitors*

All ACE inhibitors are teratogens

*Anticancer Drugs/Immunosuppressants*

Aminopterin
Busulfan
Cyclophosphamide
Methotrexate

*Antiseizure Drugs*

Carbamazepine
Phenytoin
Trimethadione
Valproic acid

*Vitamin A Derivatives*

Etretinate
Isotretinoin
Vitamin A (>18,000 IU/day)

*Other Drugs*

Alcohol (high doses)
Cocaine (high doses)
Lithium
Tetracycline
Thalidomide
Warfarin

*Sex Hormones*

Estrogens
Progestins
Androgens

---

*The absence of a drug from this table does not mean that the drug is not a teratogen; it only means that teratogenicity has not been proved. For most proven teratogens, the risk of a congenital anomaly is only 10%.

[†]ACE = angiotensin-converting enzyme.

---

of vulnerability (e.g., weeks 4 through 7 of gestation); and (3) the incidence of malformations should increase with increasing dosage and duration of exposure. Obviously, we can't do experiments in humans to see if a drug meets these criteria. The best we can do is systematically collect and analyze data on drugs taken during pregnancy in the hope that useful information on teratogenicity will be revealed.

Studies in animals are of limited value, in part because teratogenicity often depends on species. That is, drugs that are teratogens in laboratory animals may nonetheless be safe in humans. Conversely, and more importantly, drugs that fail to cause anomalies in animals may later prove teratogenic in humans. The most notorious example is thalidomide. In studies with pregnant animals, thalidomide was harmless. However, when thalidomide was taken by pregnant women, about 30% had babies with severe malformations. The take-home message is this: lack of teratogenicity in animals is not proof of safety in humans. Accordingly, we cannot assume that a new drug is safe for use in human pregnancy just because it has met

FDA requirements, which are based on tests done in pregnant animals.

Some teratogens act quickly, whereas others require prolonged exposure. Thalidomide represents the fast-acting teratogens; a single dose can cause malformation. In contrast, alcohol (ethanol) must be taken repeatedly in high doses if gross malformation is to result. (Lower doses of alcohol may produce subtle anomalies.) Because a single exposure to a rapid-acting teratogen can produce obvious malformation, rapid-acting teratogens are easier to identify than slow-acting teratogens.

Teratogens that produce delayed effects are among the hardest to identify. The best example is diethylstilbestrol, an estrogenic substance that causes vaginal cancer in female offspring 18 or so years after birth.

Teratogens that affect behavior may be nearly impossible to identify. Behavioral changes are often delayed, and therefore may not be apparent until the child goes to school. By this time, it may be difficult to establish a correlation between drug use during pregnancy and the behavioral deficit. Furthermore, if the deficit is subtle, it may not even be recognized.

## FDA Risk Categories

In 1983, the Food and Drug Administration (FDA) established a system for classifying drugs according to their probable risks to the fetus. According to this system, drugs can be put into one of five categories: A, B, C, D, and X (Table 10-2). Drugs in Risk Category A are the least dangerous; controlled studies have been done in pregnant women and have failed to demonstrate a risk of fetal harm. In contrast, drugs in Category X are the most dangerous; these drugs are known to cause human fetal harm, and their risk to the fetus outweighs any possible therapeutic benefit. Drugs in Categories B, C, and D are progressively more dangerous than drugs in category A and less dangerous than drugs in Category X. The law does not require classification of drugs that were in use before 1983; hence most drugs are not classified.

## Minimizing the Risk of Teratogenesis

Common sense tells us that the best way to minimize teratogenesis is to minimize use of drugs. If at all possible, pregnant women should avoid drugs entirely. At the least, all unnecessary drug use should be eliminated. Alcohol and cocaine, for example, which are known to harm the developing fetus, have no valid indications and their use cannot be justified. Nurses and other health professionals should warn pregnant women against use of all nonessential drugs.

As noted above, some disease states (e.g., epilepsy, asthma, diabetes) pose a greater risk to fetal health than the drugs used for their treatment. However, even in these disorders, in which drug therapy reduces the risk of disease-induced fetal harm, we must still take steps to minimize harm from drugs. Accordingly, drugs that pose a high risk of teratogenesis should be discontinued and safer alternatives should be used in their place.

Rarely, a pregnant woman has a disease that requires use of drugs that have a high probability of causing teratogenesis. Many anticancer drugs, for example, are

## TABLE 10-2. FDA PREGNANCY CATEGORIES

| Category | Category Description |
|---|---|
| A | *Remote Risk of Fetal Harm*: Controlled studies in women have been done and have failed to demonstrate a risk of fetal harm during the first trimester, and there is no evidence of risk in later trimesters. |
| B | *Slightly More Risk Than A*: Animal studies show no fetal risk, but controlled studies have not been done in women *or* animal studies do show a risk of fetal harm, but controlled studies in women have failed to demonstrate a risk during the first trimester, and there is no evidence of risk in later trimesters. |
| C | *Greater Risk Than B*: Animal studies show a risk of fetal harm, but no controlled studies have been done in women *or* no studies have been done in women or animals. |
| D | *Proven Risk of Fetal Harm*: Studies in women show proof of fetal damage, but the potential benefits of use during pregnancy may be acceptable despite the risks (e.g., treatment of life-threatening disease for which safer drugs are ineffective). A statement on risk will appear in the "WARNINGS" section of drug labeling. |
| X | *Proven Risk of Fetal Harm*: Studies in women or animals show definite risk of fetal abnormality *or* adverse reaction reports indicate evidence of fetal risk. The risks clearly outweigh any possible benefit. A statement on risk will appear in the "CONTRAINDICATIONS" section of drug labeling. |

highly toxic to the developing fetus, yet cannot be ethically withheld from the pregnant patient. If the patient elects to use such drugs, termination of pregnancy should be considered.

Reducing the risk of teratogenesis also applies to the patient who is *not* pregnant but is taking a teratogenic drug. If she is of reproductive age, she should be educated about the teratogenic risk as well as the necessity of using a reliable form of birth control.

### Responding to Teratogen Exposure

When a pregnant woman has been exposed to a known teratogen, the first step is to determine exactly when the drug was taken, and exactly when the pregnancy began. If drug exposure was not during the period of organogenesis (i.e., during weeks 2 through 8), the patient should be reassured that the risk of drug-induced malformation is minimal. In addition, the patient should be reminded that

3% of all babies have some kind of conspicuous malformation, independent of teratogen exposure. This is important because otherwise the drug is sure to be blamed if the baby should turn out abnormal.

What should be done if the exposure *did* occur during organogenesis? First, a reference (e.g., Briggs et al.'s *Drugs in Pregnancy and Lactation*) should be consulted to determine the type of malformation expected. Next, at least two ultrasound scans should be done to assess the extent of injury. If the malformation is severe, termination of pregnancy should be considered. If the malformation is minor (e.g., cleft palate), it may be correctable by surgery, either shortly after birth or later in childhood.

## Drug Therapy during Breast-Feeding

Drugs taken by lactating women can be excreted in breast milk. If drug concentrations in milk rise high enough, a pharmacologic effect can occur in the infant, raising the question of possible harm. Unfortunately, there has been very little systematic research on this issue. As a result, although a few drugs are known to be hazardous (Table 10-3), the possible danger posed by many others remains undetermined.

Although nearly all drugs can enter breast milk, the extent of entry varies greatly. The factors that determine entry into breast milk are the same factors that determine drug passage across membranes. Accordingly, drugs that are lipid soluble enter breast milk readily, whereas drugs that are ionized, highly polar, or protein bound tend to be excluded.

Most drugs can be detected in milk, but concentrations are generally too low to be harmful. Hence breast-feeding is usually safe, even though drugs are being taken. Nonetheless, prudence is always in order: if the nursing

## TABLE 10-3. DRUGS THAT ARE CONTRAINDICATED DURING BREAST-FEEDING

*Controlled Substances*
    Amphetamine
    Cocaine
    Heroin
    Marijuana
    Phencyclidine

*Anticancer Agents/Immunosuppressants*
    Cyclophosphamide
    Cyclosporine
    Doxorubicin

*Others*
    Bromocriptine
    Ergotamine
    Lithium
    Methotrexate
    Nicotine

mother can avoid drugs, she certainly should. Moreover, when drugs must be taken, steps should be taken to minimize risk. These steps include

- Dosing immediately after breast-feeding (to minimize drug concentrations in milk at the next feeding)
- Avoiding drugs that have a long half-life
- Choosing drugs that tend to be excluded from milk
- Choosing drugs that are least likely to affect the infant (when such information is available)
- Avoiding drugs that are known to be hazardous (Table 10-3)

## KEY POINTS

- Because hepatic metabolism and glomerular filtration increase during pregnancy, dosages of some drugs may need to be increased.
- Lipid-soluble drugs cross the placenta readily, whereas drugs that are ionized, polar, or protein bound cross with difficulty. Nonetheless, essentially all drugs cross to some degree.
- When prescribing drugs during pregnancy, the clinician must try to balance the benefits of treatment versus the risks—without knowing what the risks really are.
- About 6% of all babies are born with gross structural malformations.
- Only 3% of birth defects are caused by drugs.

- *Gross malformations* result from exposure to teratogens *early* in pregnancy (i.e., during weeks 3 through 8 of gestation)—the time of organogenesis.
- *Functional impairments* (e.g., mental retardation) result from exposure to teratogens *later* in pregnancy.
- For most drugs, we lack reliable data on the risks of use during pregnancy.
- Lack of teratogenicity in animals is not proof of safety in humans.
- Some drugs (e.g., thalidomide) are teratogenic with a single exposure, whereas teratogenesis from others (e.g., alcohol) requires prolonged exposure.
- FDA Pregnancy Categories indicate the relative risks of drug use. Drugs in Category X pose the highest risk of fetal harm and are contraindicated during pregnancy.
- Any woman of reproductive age who is taking a known teratogen must be counseled about the teratogenic risk and the necessity of using a reliable form of birth control.
- Drugs that are lipid soluble readily enter breast milk, whereas drugs that are ionized, polar, or protein bound tend to be excluded. Nonetheless, essentially all drugs enter to some degree.
- Although most drugs can be detected in breast milk, concentrations are usually too low to harm the nursing infant.
- Certain drugs are known to reach dangerous levels in breast milk and must be avoided during breast-feeding.

# CHAPTER 11

# Drug Therapy in Pediatric Patients

The very young and the very old respond differently to drugs than the rest of the population. Most differences are *quantitative*. That is, patients in both age groups are more sensitive to drugs than are other patients, and they show greater individual variation. Drug sensitivity in the very young results largely from *organ system immaturity*. Drug sensitivity in the elderly results largely from *organ system degeneration*. Because of heightened drug sensitivity, patients in both age groups are at increased risk of adverse drug reactions. In this chapter we discuss the physiologic factors that underlie heightened drug sensitivity in pediatric patients, as well as ways to promote safe and effective drug use. Drug therapy regarding geriatric patients is the topic of Chapter 12.

Pediatrics covers all patients under the age of 16. Because of ongoing growth and development, pediatric patients of different ages present different therapeutic challenges. Traditionally, the pediatric population is subdivided into six groups:

- premature infants (less than 36 weeks' gestational age)
- full-term infants (36 to 40 weeks' gestational age)
- neonates (first 4 postnatal weeks)
- infants (weeks 5 to 52 postnatal)
- children (1 to 12 years)
- adolescents (12 to 16 years)

Not surprisingly, as young patients grow older, they become more like adults with respect to drug therapy. Conversely, the very young—those less than 1 year old, and especially those less than 1 month old—are very different from adults. If drug therapy in these patients is to be safe and effective, we must account for these differences.

Pediatric drug therapy is made even more difficult by insufficient drug information. The Food and Drug Administration does not require drug trials in children. As a result, for most drugs given to young patients, we lack good information on pharmacokinetics and effects, both therapeutic and adverse. In fact, of the drugs represented in the 1990 *Physicians' Desk Reference* (PDR), less than 10% have been approved for use in children. Despite lack of approval, and despite lack of good information, the clinician must nonetheless use these drugs to treat pediatric patients. Hence, similar to drug therapy during pregnancy, the clinician must try to balance benefits versus risks, without knowing with precision what the benefits and risks really are.

## Pharmacokinetics: Neonates and Infants

As discussed in Chapter 5, pharmacokinetic factors determine the concentration of a drug at its sites of action, and hence the intensity and duration of responses. If drug levels are elevated, responses will be more intense. If drug elimination is delayed, responses will be prolonged. Because the organ systems that regulate drug levels are not fully developed in the very young, these patients are at risk of both possibilities: drug effects that are unusually intense *and* prolonged. By accounting for pharmacokinetic differences in the very young, we can increase the chances that drug therapy will be both effective and safe.

Figure 11-1 illustrates how drug levels differ between infants and adults following administration of equivalent doses (i.e., doses adjusted for body weight). When a drug is administered *intravenously* (Fig. 11-1A), levels decline more slowly in the infant than in the adult. As a result, drug levels in the infant remain above the minimum effective concentration (MEC) longer than in the adult, thereby causing effects to be prolonged. When a drug is administered *subcutaneously* (Fig. 11-1B), not only do levels in the infant remain above the MEC *longer* than in the adult, these levels also rise *higher*, causing effects to be more intense as well as more prolonged. From these illustrations,

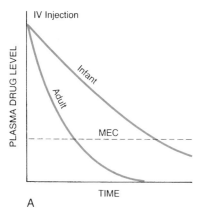
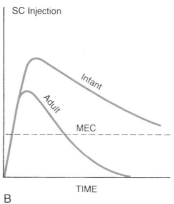

**Figure 11–1. Comparison of plasma drug levels in adults and infants.** *A*, Plasma drug levels following intravenous injection. Dosage was adjusted for body weight. Note that plasma levels remain above the minimum effective concentration (MEC) much longer in the infant. *B*, Plasma drug levels following subcutaneous injection. Dosage was adjusted for body weight. Note that both the maximum drug level and the duration of action are greater in the infant. (Redrawn from Levine, R.R. Pharmacology: Drug Actions and Reactions. Boston, Little, Brown, 1973.)

it is clear that adjustment of dosage for infants on the basis of body size alone is not sufficient to achieve safe results.

If small body size is not the major reason for heightened drug sensitivity in infants, what is? The increased sensitivity of infants is due largely to the immature state of five pharmacokinetic processes: (1) drug absorption, (2) renal drug excretion, (3) hepatic drug metabolism, (4) protein binding of drugs, and (5) exclusion of drugs from the central nervous system (CNS) by the blood-brain barrier.

## Absorption

*Oral Administration.* Gastrointestinal physiology in the infant is very different from that in the adult. Because of these differences, drug absorption may be enhanced or impeded, depending on the physicochemical properties of the drug involved.

Gastric emptying time is both prolonged and irregular in early infancy, and then gradually reaches adult values by 6 to 8 months. For drugs that are absorbed primarily from the stomach, delayed gastric emptying enhances absorption. On the other hand, for drugs that are absorbed primarily from the intestine, absorption is delayed. Because gastric emptying time is irregular, the precise impact on absorption is not predictable.

Gastric acidity is very low 24 hours after birth and does not reach adult values for 2 years. Because of low acidity, absorption of acid-labile drugs is increased.

*Intramuscular Administration.* Drug absorption following IM injection in the *neonate* is *slow* and *erratic.* Delayed absorption is due in part to low blood flow through muscle during the first days of postnatal life. By early *infancy*, absorption of IM drugs becomes more rapid than in neonates and adults.

*Percutaneous Absorption.* Because the skin of the very young is thin, percutaneous drug absorption is significantly greater than in older children and adults. This increases the risk of toxicity from topical drugs.

## Distribution

*Protein Binding.* Binding of drugs to albumin and other plasma proteins is limited in the infant. This is because (1) the amount of albumin is relatively low, and (2) endoge-

nous compounds (e.g., fatty acids, bilirubin) compete with drugs for available binding sites. Consequently, drugs that ordinarily undergo extensive protein binding in adults undergo much less binding in infants. As a result, the concentration of *free* levels of such drugs is relatively high in the infant, thereby intensifying effects. To ensure that effects are not too intense, dosages in infants should be reduced. Protein-binding capacity reaches adult values within 10 to 12 months.

*Blood-Brain Barrier.* The blood-brain barrier is not fully developed at birth. As a result, drugs and other chemicals have relatively easy access to the CNS, making the infant especially sensitive to drugs that can affect CNS function. Accordingly, all medicines employed for their CNS effects (e.g., morphine, phenobarbital) should be given in reduced dosage. Dosage should also be reduced for drugs used for actions *outside* the CNS if those drugs are capable of producing CNS toxicity as a side effect.

## Hepatic Metabolism

The drug-metabolizing capacity of newborns is low. As a result, neonates are especially sensitive to drugs that are eliminated primarily by hepatic metabolism. When these drugs are used, dosages must be reduced. The capacity of the liver to metabolize many drugs increases rapidly about 1 month after birth, and approaches adult levels a few months later. Complete maturation of the liver develops by 1 year.

The minimal drug-metabolizing capacity of newborns is illustrated by the data in Table 11–1. These data are from experiments on the metabolism and effects of hexobarbital (a CNS depressant) in newborn and adult animals. *Metabolism* was measured in microsomal enzyme preparations made from the livers of *guinea pigs.* The effect of hexobarbital—CNS depression—was assessed in *mice.* Duration of sleeping time following hexobarbital injection was used as the index of CNS depression.

As indicated in Table 11–1, the drug-metabolizing capacity of the adult liver is much greater than the drug-metabolizing capacity of the newborn liver: whereas the adult liver preparation metabolized an average of 33% of the hexobarbital presented to it, there was virtually no measurable metabolism by the newborn preparation.

The physiologic impact of limited drug-metabolizing capacity is indicated by observing sleeping time in newborns versus

## TABLE 11-1. COMPARISON OF THE METABOLISM AND EFFECTS OF HEXOBARBITAL IN ADULT VERSUS NEWBORN ANIMALS

| Age | Percentage of Hexobarbital Metabolized (in 1 hr) | Duration of Drug-Induced Sleep | |
|---|---|---|---|
| | | 10-mg/kg Dose | 50-mg/kg Dose |
| Newborn | "0" | 6 hours | Eternal* |
| Adult | 28 to 39 | <5 minutes | 12 to 22 minutes |

Data from Jondorf, W.R., Maickel, R.P., and Brodie, B.B. Inability of newborn mice and guinea pigs to metabolize drugs. Biochem. Pharmacol. 1:352, 1958.
*The 50-mg/kg dose was lethal to newborn animals.

## TABLE 11-2. RENAL FUNCTION IN ADULTS VERSUS INFANTS

| | Average Infant | Average Adult |
|---|---|---|
| *Body Weight* | | |
| kilograms | 3.5 | 70 |
| *Inulin Clearance* | | |
| ml/minute | 3 (approximate) | 130 |
| T ½ (minutes) | 630 | 120 |
| *Para-aminohippuric Acid (PAH) Clearance* | | |
| ml/minute | 12 (approximate) | 650 |
| T ½ (minutes) | 160 | 43 |

Adapted from Goldstein, A., Aronow, L., and Kalman, S.M. Principles of Drug Action: The Basis of Pharmacology, 2nd ed. New York, John Wiley & Sons, 1974. Copyright © 1974. Reprinted by permission of John Wiley & Sons, Inc.

adults following injection of hexobarbital. As shown in Table 11-1, a low dose (10 mg/kg) of hexobarbital caused adult mice to sleep less than 5 minutes. In contrast, the same dose caused newborns to sleep for *6 hours*. The differential effects on adults and newborns are much more dramatic at a higher dose (50 mg/kg): whereas the adults merely slept for 20 minutes, this dose was *lethal* to newborns.

## Renal Excretion

Renal drug excretion is significantly reduced at birth. Renal blood flow, glomerular filtration, and active tubular secretion are all low during infancy. Because the drug-excreting capacity of infants is limited, drugs that are eliminated primarily by renal excretion must be given in reduced dosage. Adult levels of renal function are achieved by 1 year.

The relative inability of the infant kidney to excrete foreign compounds is illustrated by the data in Table 11-2. These data show rates of renal excretion for two compounds: inulin and *para*-aminohippuric acid (PAH). Inulin is excreted entirely by glomerular filtration. PAH is excreted by a combination of glomerular filtration and active tubular secretion. Note that the half-life for inulin is 630 minutes in infants but only 120 minutes in adults. Since inulin is eliminated by glomerular filtration alone, these data tell us that the glomerular filtration rate in the infant is much slower than in the adult. From the data for clearance of PAH, taken together with the data for clearance of inulin, we can conclude that tubular secretion in infants is also much slower than in adults.

## Pharmacokinetics: Children 1 Year and Older

By the age of 1 year, most pharmacokinetic parameters are similar to those in adults. Hence drug sensitivity in children over the age of 1 is more like that of adults than of the very young. Although pharmacokinetically similar to adults, children do differ in one important way: they me-

tabolize drugs *faster* than adults. Drug-metabolizing capacity is markedly elevated until the age of 2 years, and then gradually declines. A further sharp reduction takes place at puberty, when adult values are reached. Because of enhanced drug metabolism in children, an increase in dosage or a reduction in dosing interval may be needed for drugs that are eliminated by hepatic metabolism.

## Adverse Drug Reactions

Like adults, pediatric patients are subject to adverse reactions when drug levels rise too high. In addition to these dose-related reactions, pediatric patients are vulnerable to unique adverse effects related to the immature state of organ systems and to ongoing growth and development. Among these age-related effects are growth suppression (caused by glucocorticoids), discoloration of developing teeth (caused by tetracyclines), and kernicterus (caused by sulfonamides). Table 11-3 presents a list of drugs that can cause unique adverse effects in the pediatric patient. Care should be taken to avoid these drugs in patients vulnerable to their actions.

## Dosage Determination

Because of the pharmacokinetic factors discussed above, dosage selection for pediatric patients is difficult. Selecting a dosage is a particular problem in the very young, since pharmacokinetic factors are undergoing rapid change.

Pediatric doses have been established for some drugs but not for others. For drugs that do not have an established pediatric dose, dosage can be extrapolated from

## TABLE 11-3. ADVERSE DRUG REACTIONS UNIQUE TO PEDIATRIC PATIENTS

| Drug | Adverse Effect |
|---|---|
| Androgens | Premature puberty in males; reduced adult height from premature epiphyseal closure |
| Aspirin and other salicylates | Severe intoxication from acute overdose (acidosis, hyperthermia respiratory depression); Reye's syndrome in children with chickenpox or influenza |
| Chloramphenicol | Gray syndrome (neonates and infants) |
| Glucocorticoids | Growth suppression with prolonged use |
| Fluoroquinolones | Tendon rupture |
| Hexachlorophene | CNS toxicity (infants) |
| Nalidixic acid | Cartilage erosion |
| Phenothiazines | Sudden infant death syndrome |
| Sulfonamides | Kernicterus (neonates) |
| Tetracyclines | Staining of developing teeth |

adult doses. The method of conversion employed most commonly is based on *body surface area*:

Approximate child's dose =

$$\frac{\text{Body surface area of the child} \times \text{Adult dose}}{1.73 \ m^2}$$

Please note that initial pediatric doses—whether based on established pediatric doses or extrapolated from adult doses—are at best an *approximation*. Subsequent doses must be adjusted on the basis of clinical outcome and plasma drug concentrations. These adjustments are especially important in neonates and younger infants. Clearly, if dosage adjustments are to be optimal, it is essential that we monitor the patient for therapeutic and adverse responses.

## Promoting Compliance

Achieving accurate and timely dosing requires informed participation of the child's parents or guardian and, to the extent possible, active involvement of the child as well. Effective education is critical. The following issues should be addressed:

- Dosage size and timing
- Route and technique of administration
- Duration of treatment
- Proper drug storage
- The nature and time course of desired responses
- The nature and time course of adverse responses

Written instructions should be provided. For techniques of administration that are difficult, a demonstration should be made, after which the parents should repeat the procedure to show their understanding. With young children, spills and spitting out are common causes of inaccurate dosing; parents should be taught to estimate the amount of drug lost and to readminister that amount, being careful not to overcompensate. When more than one person is helping medicate a child, all participants should be warned against multiple dosing. Multiple dosing can be avoided by maintaining a drug administration chart. With some disorders—especially infections—symptoms may resolve before the prescribed course of treatment has been completed. Parents should be instructed to complete the full treatment nonetheless. Additional ways to promote compliance include (1) selecting the most convenient dosage form and dosing schedule, (2) suggesting mixing oral drugs with food or juice (when allowed) to improve palatability, (3) providing a calibrated medicine spoon or syringe for measuring doses of liquid pediatric formulations, and (4) taking extra time with young or disadvantaged parents to help ensure conscientious and skilled participation.

## KEY POINTS

- Because of organ system immaturity, very young patients are highly sensitive to drugs.
- In neonates and young infants, drug responses may be unusually intense and prolonged.
- Absorption of IM drugs in *neonates* is slower than in adults. In contrast, absorption of IM drugs in *infants* is more rapid than in adults.
- Protein binding capacity is limited early in life. Hence free concentrations of some drugs may be especially high.
- The blood-brain barrier is not fully developed at birth. Hence neonates are especially sensitive to drugs that affect the CNS.
- The drug-metabolizing capacity of neonates is low. Hence neonates are especially sensitive to drugs that are eliminated primarily by hepatic metabolism.
- Renal excretion of drugs is low in neonates. Hence drugs that are eliminated primarily by the kidney must be given in reduced dosage.
- In children 1 year and older, most pharmacokinetic parameters are similar to those in adults. Hence drug sensitivity is more like that of adults than of the very young.
- Children differ pharmacokinetically from adults in that children metabolize drugs faster.
- Initial pediatric doses are at best an approximation. Hence subsequent doses must be adjusted on the basis of clinical outcome and plasma drug levels.

# CHAPTER 12

# Drug Therapy in Geriatric Patients

**Pharmacokinetic Changes in the Elderly**
**Pharmacodynamic Changes in the Elderly**
**Adverse Drug Reactions and Drug Interactions**
**Promoting Compliance**

D rug use among the elderly is disproportionately high. Whereas the elderly (those over the age of 65) constitute only 12% of the U.S. population, they consume 31% of the nation's prescribed drugs. Reasons for this intensive use of drugs include increased severity of illness, the presence of multiple pathologies, and excessive prescribing.

Drug therapy in the elderly represents a special therapeutic challenge. As a rule, older patients are more sensitive to drugs than are younger adults, and they show wider individual variation. In addition, the elderly experience more adverse drug reactions and drug-drug interactions. The principal factors underlying these complications of therapy are (1) altered pharmacokinetics (secondary to organ system degeneration), (2) multiple and severe illnesses, (3) multiple drug therapy, and (4) poor compliance. To help ensure that drug therapy is as safe and effective as possible, *individualization of treatment is essential: each patient must be monitored for desired and adverse responses, and the regimen must be adjusted accordingly.* Since the elderly typically suffer from chronic illnesses, the usual objective is to reduce symptoms and improve quality of life, since cure is generally impossible.

## Pharmacokinetic Changes in the Elderly

The aging process can affect all phases of pharmacokinetics. From early adulthood on, there is a gradual, progressive decline in organ function. This decline can alter the absorption, distribution, metabolism, and excretion of drugs. As a rule, these pharmacokinetic changes result in increased drug sensitivity (largely from reduced hepatic and renal drug elimination). It should be noted, however, that the extent of change varies greatly among patients: pharmacokinetic changes may be minimal in patients who

have remained physically fit, whereas they may be dramatic in patients who have aged less gracefully. Accordingly, you should keep in mind that age-related changes in pharmacokinetics are not only a potential source of increased sensitivity to drugs, they are also a potential source of increased variability. The physiologic changes that underlie alterations in pharmacokinetics are summarized in Table 12–1.

### Absorption

Altered gastrointestinal absorption is not a major factor in drug sensitivity in the elderly. As a rule, the *percentage* of an oral dose that becomes absorbed does not change with age. However, the *rate* of absorption may be slowed (because of delayed gastric emptying and reduced splanchnic blood flow). As a result, drug responses may be somewhat delayed. Gastric acidity is reduced in the elderly and may alter the absorption of certain drugs. For example, some drug formulations require high acidity to dissolve. Absorption of these formulations may be reduced.

### Distribution

Four factors can alter drug distribution in the elderly: increased percent body fat, decreased percent lean body mass, decreased total body water, and reduced concentration of serum albumin. The increase in body fat seen in the elderly provides a storage depot for *lipid-soluble* drugs (e.g., thiopental). As a result, plasma levels of these drugs are reduced, causing a reduction in drug effects. Because of the decline in lean body mass and total body water, *water-soluble* drugs (e.g., ethanol) become distributed in a smaller volume than in younger adults. As a result, the concentration of these drugs is increased, causing their effects to be more intense. Although albumin levels are only slightly reduced in healthy adults, these levels can be significantly reduced in adults who are malnourished. Because of reduced albumin levels, protein binding of drugs decreases, causing levels of free drug to rise. As a result, drug effects may be more intense.

## TABLE 12-1. PHYSIOLOGIC CHANGES THAT CAN AFFECT PHARMACOKINETICS IN THE ELDERLY

*Absorption of Drugs*
  Increased gastric pH
  Decreased absorptive surface area
  Decreased splanchnic blood flow
  Decreased GI motility
  Delayed gastric emptying

*Distribution of Drugs*
  Increased body fat
  Decreased lean body mass
  Decreased total body water
  Decreased serum albumin
  Decreased cardiac output

*Metabolism of Drugs*
  Decreased hepatic blood flow
  Decreased hepatic mass
  Decreased activity of hepatic enzymes

*Excretion of Drugs*
  Decreased renal blood flow
  Decreased glomerular filtration rate
  Decreased tubular secretion
  Decreased number of nephrons

### Metabolism

Rates of hepatic drug metabolism tend to decline with age. Principal factors underlying the decline are reduced hepatic blood flow, reduced liver size, and decreased activity of some hepatic enzymes. Because liver function is diminished, the half-lives of certain drugs may be increased, thereby prolonging responses. Responses to oral drugs that ordinarily undergo extensive first-pass metabolism may be enhanced. It must be noted, however, that the degree of decline in drug metabolism varies greatly among individuals. As a result, we cannot predict whether drug responses will be significantly changed in any particular patient.

### Excretion

Renal drug function, and hence drug excretion, undergo progressive decline beginning in early adulthood. Drug accumulation secondary to reduced renal excretion is the most important cause of adverse drug reactions in the elderly. The decline in renal function is the result of reductions in renal blood flow, glomerular filtration rate, tubular secretion, and number of nephrons. Co-existence of renal pathology can further compromise kidney function. The degree of decline in renal function varies greatly among individuals. Accordingly, when patients are taking drugs that are eliminated primarily by the kidneys, renal function should be assessed. In the elderly, the proper index of renal function is *creatinine clearance*—not serum *creatinine levels*. Creatinine levels do not reflect kidney function in the elderly because the source of serum creatinine—lean muscle mass—declines in parallel with the decline in kidney function. As a result, creatinine levels may be normal even though renal function is greatly reduced.

## Pharmacodynamic Changes in the Elderly

Alterations in receptor properties may underlie altered sensitivity to some drugs. However, information on such pharmacodynamic changes is very limited. In support of the possibility of altered pharmacodynamics is the observation that beta-adrenergic blocking agents (drugs used for cardiac disorders) are *less* effective in the elderly than in younger adults when present at equivalent concentrations. Possible explanations for this observation include (1) a reduction in the number of available beta receptors and (2) a reduction in the affinity of beta receptors for beta-receptor blocking agents. Other drugs (certain CNS depressants, warfarin) produce effects that are more intense in the elderly than in younger adults when present at equivalent plasma concentrations, suggesting a possible increase in receptor number, receptor affinity, or both. Unfortunately, our knowledge of pharmacodynamic changes in the elderly is restricted to a few families of drugs.

## Adverse Drug Reactions and Drug Interactions

Adverse drug reactions (ADRs) are seven times more common in the elderly than in younger adults, accounting for about 16% of hospital admissions among older individuals, and 50% of all medication-related deaths. The vast majority of these reactions are dose related—not idiosyncratic. Symptoms in the elderly are often nonspecific (e.g., dizziness, cognitive impairment), making identification of ADRs difficult.

Perhaps surprisingly, the increase in ADRs seen in the elderly is not the direct result of aging per se; rather, multiple factors predispose the older patient to ADRs. The most important factors are

- Drug accumulation secondary to reduced renal function
- Polypharmacy (treatment with multiple drugs)
- Greater severity of illness
- The presence of multiple pathologies
- Greater use of drugs that have a low therapeutic index (e.g., digoxin, a drug for heart failure)
- Increased individual variation secondary to altered pharmacokinetics
- Inadequate supervision of long-term therapy
- Poor patient compliance

The majority of ADRs in the elderly are avoidable. Measures that can reduce the incidence of ADRs include

- Taking a thorough drug history, including over-the-counter medications
- Accounting for the pharmacokinetic and pharmacodynamic changes that occur with aging
- Initiating therapy with low doses

- Monitoring clinical responses and plasma drug levels to provide a rational basis for dosage adjustment
- Employing the simplest regimen possible
- Monitoring for drug-drug interactions and iatrogenic illness
- Periodically reviewing the need for continued drug therapy, and discontinuing medications as appropriate
- Encouraging the patient to dispose of old medications
- Taking steps to promote compliance (see below)

## Promoting Compliance

As many as 40% or more of elderly patients fail to take their medicines as prescribed. Some patients never fill their prescriptions, some fail to refill their prescriptions, and some don't follow the prescribed dosing schedule. Noncompliance can result in either therapeutic failure (from underdosing or erratic dosing) or toxicity (from overdosing). Of the two possibilities, underdosing with resulting therapeutic failure is by far (90%) the more common.

Multiple factors underlie nonadherence to the prescribed regimen (Table 12-2). Among these factors are forgetfulness; failure to comprehend instructions (because of intellectual, visual, or auditory impairment); inability to pay for medications; and use of complex regimens (several drugs taken several times a day). All of these factors can contribute to *unintentional* noncompliance. However, in the majority of cases (about 75%), noncompliance among the elderly is *intentional*. The principal reason given for intentional noncompliance is the patient's conviction that the drug was simply not needed in the dosage prescribed. Unpleasant side effects and expense also contribute to intentional noncompliance.

A number of steps can be taken to promote adherence to the prescribed regimen. These include

- Simplifying the regimen so that the number of drugs and doses per day is the smallest possible
- Explaining the treatment plan using clear, concise verbal and written instructions
- Choosing an appropriate dosage form (e.g., a liquid formulation if the patient has difficulty swallowing)
- Labeling drug containers clearly, and avoiding containers that are difficult to open by patients with impaired dexterity (e.g., those with arthritis)
- Suggesting the use of a calendar, diary, or pill counter to record drug administration
- Asking the patient if he or she has access to a pharmacy and can afford the medication
- Enlisting the aid of a friend, relative, or visiting health care professional
- Monitoring for therapeutic responses, adverse reactions, and plasma drug levels

It must be noted, however, that the benefits of these measures will be restricted primarily to patients whose nonadherence is *unintentional*. Unfortunately, these measures are generally inapplicable to the patient whose

### TABLE 12-2. FACTORS THAT CONTRIBUTE TO POOR COMPLIANCE IN THE ELDERLY

Multiple chronic disorders
Multiple prescription medications
Multiple doses/day for each medication
Multiple prescribers
Changes in the regimen (addition of drugs, changes in dosage size or timing)
Cognitive or physical impairment (reduction in memory, hearing, visual acuity, color discrimination, or manual dexterity)
Living alone
Recent discharge from hospital
Low literacy
Inability to pay for drugs
Personal conviction that a drug is unnecessary or the dosage is too high
Presence of side effects

nonadherence is *intentional*. For these patients, intensive education may help.

## KEY POINTS

- Older patients are generally more sensitive to drugs than younger adults, and they show wider individual variation.
- Individualization of therapy for the elderly is essential: each patient must be monitored for desired and adverse responses, and the regimen adjusted accordingly.
- Aging-related organ system decline can change drug absorption, distribution, metabolism, and (especially) excretion.
- The *rate* of drug absorption may be slowed in the elderly, although the *extent* of absorption is usually unchanged.
- Concentrations of lipid-soluble drug may be low in the elderly, and concentrations of water-soluble drugs may be high.
- Reduced liver function may prolong drug effects.
- Reduced renal function, with resultant drug accumulation, is the most important cause of adverse drug reactions in the elderly.
- Because the degree of renal impairment among the elderly varies, creatinine clearance (a test of renal function) should be determined for all patients taking drugs that are eliminated primarily by the kidneys.
- Adverse drug reactions are much more common in the elderly than in younger adults.
- Factors underlying the increase in adverse reactions include polypharmacy, severe illness, multiple pathologies, and treatment with dangerous drugs.
- Noncompliance is common among the elderly.
- Reasons for noncompliance include forgetfulness, side effects, low income, complex regimens, and failure to comprehend instructions.
- Most (90%) cases of noncompliance among the elderly are intentional. Reasons include expense, side effects, and the patient's conviction that the drug is unnecessary or the dosage too high.

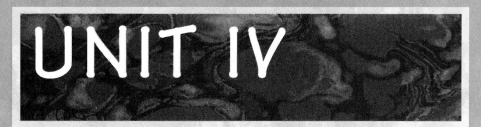

# UNIT IV

# Peripheral Nervous System Drugs

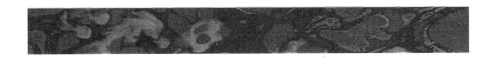

# Introduction

# Basic Principles of Neuropharmacology

Neuropharmacology can be defined as *the study of drugs that alter processes controlled by the nervous system.* Neuropharmacologic drugs produce effects equivalent to those produced by excitation or suppression of neuronal activity. Neuropharmacologic agents can be divided into two broad categories: (1) peripheral nervous system drugs and (2) central nervous system (CNS) drugs.

The neuropharmacologic drugs constitute a large and important family of therapeutic agents. These drugs are used to treat conditions that range from depression to epilepsy to hypertension to asthma. The clinical significance of neuropharmacologic agents is reflected in the fact that over 25% of the chapters in this text are dedicated to them.

Why do we have so many neuropharmacologic drugs? The answer can be found in a concept discussed in Chapter 6: most therapeutic agents act by helping the body help itself. That is, most drugs produce their therapeutic effects by coaxing the body to perform normal processes in a fashion that benefits the patient. Since the nervous system participates in the regulation of practically all bodily processes, practically all bodily processes can be influenced by drugs that alter neuronal regulation. By mimicking or blocking neuronal regulation, neuropharmacologic drugs can modify such diverse processes as skeletal muscle contraction, cardiac output, vascular tone, respiration, gastrointestinal function, uterine motility, glandular secretion, and functions unique to the CNS, such as pain perception, ideation, and mood. Given the broad spectrum of processes that neuropharmacologic drugs can alter, and given the potential benefits to be gained by manipulating those processes, it should be no surprise that neuropharmacologic drugs have widespread clinical applications.

We will begin our study of neuropharmacology by discussing peripheral nervous system drugs (Chapters 15 through 20), after which we will discuss central nervous system drugs (Chapters 22 through 37). The principal rationale for this order of presentation is that our understanding of peripheral nervous system pharmacology is much clearer than our understanding of central nervous system pharmacology. Why is this so? Because the peripheral nervous system is much less complex than the CNS, and also more accessible to experimentation. By placing our initial focus on the peripheral nervous system, we can establish a firm knowledge base in neuropharmacology before proceeding to the less definitive and vastly more complex realm of the CNS.

## How Neurons Regulate Physiologic Processes

As a rule, if we want to understand the effects of a drug on a particular physiologic process, we must first understand the process itself. Accordingly, if we wish to understand the impact of drugs on neuronal regulation of bodily function, we must first understand how neurons regulate bodily function when drugs are absent.

The primary steps in the process through which a neuron elicits a response from another cell are illustrated in Figure 13-1. This figure depicts two cells: a neuron and a postsynaptic cell. The postsynaptic cell might be another neuron, a muscle cell, or a cell within a secretory gland. There are three basic steps in the process by which the neuron influences the behavior of the postsynaptic cell: (1) conduction of an action potential along the axon of the neuron, (2) release of neurotransmitter from the axon terminal, and (3) binding of transmitter molecules to receptors on the postsynaptic cell. As a result of transmitter-receptor binding, a series of events is initiated in the postsynaptic cell, leading to a change in that cell's behavior. The precise nature of the change depends on the identity of the neurotransmitter and the type of cell involved. If

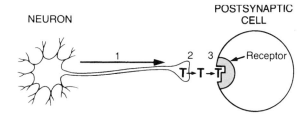

**Figure 13–1. How neurons regulate other cells.** The steps in the process by which neurons elicit responses from other cells are (1) action potential, (2) release of neurotransmitter (T), and (3) interaction of T with receptor.

the postsynaptic cell is another neuron, it may increase or decrease its firing rate; if the cell is part of a muscle, it may contract or relax; and if the cell is glandular, it may increase or decrease its rate of secretion.

The three steps discussed above can be viewed as constituting two primary processes: *axonal conduction* and *synaptic transmission*. Axonal conduction is simply the process of conducting an action potential down the axon of the neuron. Synaptic transmission refers to steps 2 and 3 above—the steps by which information is carried across the gap between the neuron and the postsynaptic cell.

# Basic Mechanisms by Which Neuropharmacologic Agents Act

## Sites of Action: Axons versus Synapses

In order to influence a process under neuronal control, a drug can alter one of two basic neuronal activities: axonal conduction or synaptic transmission. *The vast majority of neuropharmacologic agents produce their effects by altering synaptic transmission*; axonal conduction is rarely a target for drugs. Why do most neuropharmacologic agents act by altering synaptic transmission? Because drugs that affect this process can produce effects that are much more *selective* than those produced by drugs that alter axonal conduction.

### Axonal Conduction

Drugs that act by altering axonal conduction are not very selective. Recall that the process of conducting an impulse along an axon is essentially the same in all neurons. As a consequence, a drug that alters axonal conduction can affect conduction in all nerves to which it has access. Such a drug cannot produce selective effects.

*Local anesthetics*, and possibly *general anesthetics*, are the only drugs whose therapeutic effects are the result of altered (decreased) axonal conduction. Since these agents produce nonselective inhibition of axonal conduction, they will suppress transmission in any nerve that they reach. Hence, although the anesthetics are certainly valuable, their indications are limited.

## Synaptic Transmission

In contrast to drugs that alter axonal conduction, drugs that alter synaptic transmission can produce effects that are highly selective. These drugs can elicit selective responses because synapses, unlike axons, are not all the same. Synapses at different sites employ different transmitters. In addition, for many transmitters, the body employs more than one type of receptor. Hence, by using a drug that selectively influences a specific neurotransmitter or a specific type of receptor, we can alter one neuronally regulated process while leaving the majority of other neuronally regulated processes unaffected. Because of their ability to produce selective effects, drugs that act by altering synaptic transmission have numerous applications.

### Receptors

The ability of a neuron to influence the behavior of another cell depends ultimately upon the ability of that neuron to alter receptor activity on the target cell. As discussed above, neurons alter receptor activity through release of transmitter molecules, which diffuse across the synaptic gap and bind to appropriate receptors on the postsynaptic cell. If the target cell lacked receptors for the type of transmitter that a particular neuron released, that neuron would have virtually no means by which to alter function in the target cell.

The effects of neuropharmacologic drugs, like those of neurons, are dependent upon altering receptor activity. That is, no matter what its precise mechanism of action, a neuropharmacologic drug ultimately produces its effects through influencing receptor activity on its target cells. Without altering receptor function, neuropharmacologic agents cannot produce effects. This commonsense concept is central to understanding the actions of neuropharmacologic drugs. In fact, this concept is so critical to our understanding of neuropharmacologic agents that I will repeat it: *the impact of a drug on a neuronally regulated process is dependent upon the ability of that drug to directly or indirectly influence receptor activity on target cells.*

### Steps in Synaptic Transmission

To understand how drugs alter receptor activity, we must first understand the steps by which synaptic transmission takes place, since it is by modifying these steps that neuropharmacologic drugs influence receptor function. The steps in synaptic transmission are summarized in Figure 13–2.

*Step 1: Synthesis.* For synaptic transmission to take place, molecules of transmitter must be present within the nerve terminal. Hence, we can look upon synthesis of transmitter as being the first step in transmission. In the figure, the letters Q, R, and S represent the precursor molecules from which the transmitter (T) is made.

*Step 2: Storage.* Once transmitter is synthesized, it must be stored until the time of its release. Storage of transmitter molecules takes place within vesicles—tiny packets present in the axon terminal. Each nerve terminal contains a large number of transmitter-filled vesicles.

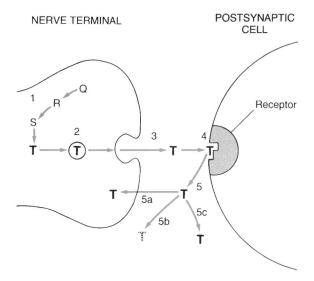

NERVE TERMINAL      POSTSYNAPTIC CELL

**Figure 13–2. Steps in synaptic transmission. Step 1,** Synthesis of transmitter (T) from precursor molecules (Q, R, and S). **Step 2,** Storage of transmitter in vesicles. **Step 3,** Release of transmitter. In response to an action potential, vesicles fuse with the terminal membrane and discharge their contents into the synaptic gap. **Step 4,** Action at receptor. Transmitter binds (reversibly) to its receptor on the postsynaptic cell, causing a response in that cell. **Step 5,** Termination of transmission. Transmitter dissociates from its receptor and is then removed from the synaptic gap by (a) reuptake into the nerve terminal, (b) enzymatic degradation, or (c) diffusion away from the gap.

**Step 3: Release.** Release of transmitter is triggered by the arrival of an action potential at the axon terminal. The action potential initiates a process in which vesicles undergo fusion with the terminal membrane, causing release of their contents into the synaptic gap. With each action potential, only a small fraction of all vesicles present in the axon terminal are caused to discharge their contents.

**Step 4: Receptor Binding.** Following their release, transmitter molecules diffuse across the synaptic gap and then undergo *reversible* binding to receptors on the postsynaptic cell. This binding initiates a cascade of events that result in altered behavior of the postsynaptic cell.

**Step 5: Termination.** Transmission is terminated by dissociation of transmitter from its receptors, followed by removal of free transmitter from the synaptic gap. Transmitter can be cleared from the synaptic gap by three processes: (1) reuptake, (2) enzymatic degradation, and (3) diffusion. In those synapses where transmission is terminated by reuptake, axon terminals contain "pumps" for the active transport of transmitter molecules back into the neuron (step 5a in Fig. 13–2). Following reuptake, molecules of transmitter may be degraded, or they may be repackaged in vesicles for reuse. In synapses where transmitter is cleared by enzymatic degradation (step 5b), the synapse contains large quantities of transmitter-inactivating enzymes. Although simple diffusion away from the synaptic gap (step 5c) is a potential means of terminating transmitter action, this process is very slow and generally of little significance.

## Effects of Drugs on the Steps of Synaptic Transmission

As noted above, all neuropharmacologic agents (except for anesthetics) produce their effects by directly or indirectly altering receptor activity. We also noted that the way in which drugs alter receptor activity is by interfering with synaptic transmission. Because synaptic transmission has multiple steps, the process offers a number of opportunities for intervention with drugs. In this section, we will look at the specific ways in which drugs can alter the steps of synaptic transmission. By way of encouragement, although this information may appear complex, it isn't. In fact, it's largely self-evident.

Before discussing specific mechanisms by which drugs can alter receptor activity, we need to understand what drugs are capable of doing to receptors in general terms. From the broadest perspective, when a drug influences receptor function, that drug can do just one of two things: it can enhance receptor activation or it can reduce receptor activation. What do we mean by receptor activation? For our purposes, we can define *activation* as *an effect on receptor function equivalent to that produced by the natural neurotransmitter at a particular synapse.* Hence, a drug whose effects mimic the effects of a natural transmitter would be said to *increase* receptor activation. Conversely, a drug whose effects were equivalent to reducing the amount of natural transmitter available for receptor binding would be said to *decrease* receptor activation.

It should be noted that activation of a receptor does not necessarily mean that a physiologic process will go faster; receptor activation by drugs can also result in a process going slower. For example, a drug that mimicked the effects of acetylcholine at receptors on the heart would cause heart rate to decrease. Since the effect of this drug on receptor function mimicked that of the natural neurotransmitter, the drug would be said to activate acetylcholine receptors, despite the fact that this activation caused heart rate to decline.

Having defined what we mean by receptor activation, we are ready to consider how drugs can influence receptor activity by altering the steps of synaptic transmission. As we discussed, a drug can have one of two effects on a receptor: increased activation or decreased activation. Table 13–1 summarizes the mechanisms by which drugs, acting on the various steps of synaptic transmission, can increase or decrease the activation of receptors. As we consider these mechanisms one by one, their common-sense nature should become apparent.

**Transmitter Synthesis.** There are three different effects that drugs are known to have on transmitter synthesis. They can (1) increase transmitter synthesis, (2) decrease transmitter synthesis, or (3) cause the synthesis of transmitter molecules that are more effective than the natural transmitter.

The impact of increased or decreased transmitter synthesis on receptor activity should be obvious. A drug that increases transmitter synthesis will cause receptor activation to be increased. That is, as a result of increased transmitter synthesis, storage vesicles will contain transmitter

**TABLE 13-1. EFFECTS OF DRUGS ON SYNAPTIC TRANSMISSION AND THE RESULTING IMPACT ON RECEPTOR ACTIVATION**

| Step of Junctional Transmission | Drug Action | Impact on Receptor Activation* |
|---|---|---|
| Synthesis of transmitter | Increased synthesis of T | Increase |
| | Decreased synthesis of T | Decrease |
| | Synthesis of "super" T | Increase |
| Storage of transmitter | Reduced storage of T | Decrease |
| Release of transmitter | Promotion of T release | Increase |
| | Inhibition of T release | Decrease |
| Binding to receptor | Direct receptor stimulation | Increase |
| | Enhanced response to T | Increase |
| | Blockade of T binding | Decrease |
| Termination of transmission | Blockade of T reuptake | Increase |
| | Prevention of T breakdown | Increase |

*Receptor activation is defined as production of an effect equivalent to that produced by the natural transmitter that acts on a particular receptor.
T = transmitter.

in abnormally high amounts. Hence, when an action potential reaches the axon terminal, more transmitter will be released, and therefore more transmitter will be available to receptors on the postsynaptic cell, causing activation of those receptors to increase. Conversely, a drug that decreases transmitter synthesis will cause the transmitter content of vesicles to decline, resulting in reduced transmitter release and decreased activation of receptors.

Some drugs can cause neurons to synthesize transmitter molecules whose structure is different from that of normal transmitter molecules. For example, by acting as substrates for enzymes in the axon terminal, drugs can be converted into "super" transmitters (molecules whose ability to activate receptors is greater than that of the naturally occurring transmitter at a particular site). Release of these supertransmitters will obviously cause receptor activation to increase. In theory, it should be possible to cause the synthesis of *faulty* transmitter molecules (i.e., molecules with a reduced ability to activate a particular receptor). However, we have no drugs that are known to act by this mechanism.

***Transmitter Storage.*** Drugs that interfere with transmitter storage will cause receptor activation to decrease. This is because disruption of storage depletes vesicles of their transmitter content, thereby decreasing the amount of transmitter available for release.

***Transmitter Release.*** Drugs either can *promote* release or they can *inhibit* release. Drugs that promote release will increase receptor activation; drugs that inhibit release will reduce receptor activation. The amphetamines (CNS stimulants) are examples of drugs that act by pro-

moting transmitter release. Botulinus toxin, in contrast, acts by inhibiting transmitter release.*

***Receptor Binding.*** Many neuropharmacologic drugs act directly at receptors. Drugs in this category can either (1) bind to receptors and cause activation, (2) bind to receptors and thereby prevent receptor activation by other agents, or (3) bind to receptor components and thereby enhance receptor activation by the natural transmitter at the site.

In the terminology introduced in Chapter 6, drugs that directly activate receptors are called *agonists*, whereas drugs that prevent receptor activation are called *antagonists*. We have no special name for drugs that bind to receptors and thereby enhance the effects of the natural transmitter. The direct-acting receptor agonists and antagonists constitute the largest and most important groups of neuropharmacologic drugs.

Examples of drugs that act directly at receptors are numerous. Drugs that bind to receptors and cause *activation* include morphine (used for its effects on the CNS), epinephrine (used mainly for its effects on the cardiovascular system), and bethanechol (used for its effects on the gastrointestinal system). Drugs that bind to receptors and *prevent* their activation include naloxone (used to treat overdose with morphine-like drugs), succinylcholine (used to relax skeletal muscles), and haloperidol (used to treat schizophrenia). The principal examples of drugs that bind to receptors and thereby enhance the actions of a natural transmitter are the benzodiazepines. This drug family, which includes diazepam [Valium] and related drugs, is used to treat anxiety, seizure disorders, and muscle spasm.

***Termination of Transmitter Action.*** Drugs can interfere with the termination of transmitter action by two mechanisms: (1) blockade of transmitter reuptake and (2) inhibition of transmitter degradation. Drugs that act by either mechanism will cause the concentration of transmitter in the synaptic gap to rise, thereby causing receptor activation to increase.

## Multiple Receptor Types and Selectivity of Drug Action

As we discussed in Chapter 1, selectivity is one of the most desirable qualities a drug can have, since a selective drug is able to alter a disease process while leaving other physiologic processes largely unaffected.

Many neuropharmacologic agents display a high degree of selectivity. This selectivity is possible because the nervous system works through multiple types of receptors to regulate the organs under its control. If neurons

*Botulinus toxin blocks release of acetylcholine from the neurons that control skeletal muscles, including the muscles of respiration. The potential for disaster is obvious.

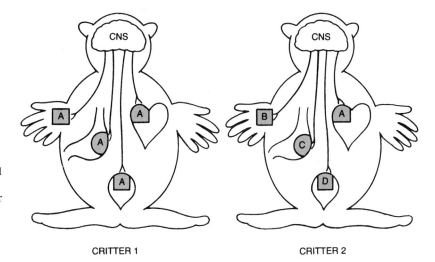

**Figure 13–3. Multiple drug receptors and selective drug action. Critter 1,** All organs are regulated through stimulation of type A receptors. Drugs that affect type A receptors on one organ will affect type A receptors on all other organs. Hence, selective drug action is impossible. **Critter 2,** This critter employs four types of receptors (A, B, C, and D) to regulate his four organs. A drug that acts at one type of receptor will not affect the others. Hence, selective drug action can be achieved.

CRITTER 1                                    CRITTER 2

had only one or two types of receptors through which to act, selective effects by neuropharmacologic drugs could not be achieved.

The relationship between multiple receptor types and selective drug action is illustrated by the somewhat whimsical characters in Figure 13-3. Let's begin by considering Critter 1. This critter can perform four functions: he can pump blood, digest food, shake hands, and empty his bladder. As indicated in the figure, all four functions are under neuronal control, and, in all cases, that control is exerted by activation of the same type of receptor (designated A).

As long as Critter 1 remains healthy, having use of only one receptor type to regulate his various functions presents no problem. Selective physiologic regulation can be achieved simply by sending impulses down the appropriate nerves. When there is a need to increase cardiac output, impulses are sent down the nerve to his heart; when digestion is needed, impulses are sent down the nerve to his stomach; and so forth.

Although having only one receptor type is no disadvantage when all is well, if Critter 1 gets sick, having only one receptor type creates a difficult therapeutic problem. Let's assume he develops heart disease and we need to give a drug that will help increase cardiac output. To stimulate cardiac function, we need to administer a drug that will activate receptors on his heart. Unfortunately, since the receptors on his heart are the same as the receptors on his other organs, a drug that stimulates cardiac function will stimulate all of his other organs as well. Consequently, any attempt to improve cardiac output with drugs will necessarily be accompanied by side effects. These effects will range from silly (compulsive handshaking) to embarrassing (enuresis) to hazardous (gastric ulcers). Such side effects are not likely to elicit either gratitude or compliance. Please note that all of these undesirable effects are the direct result of the fact that this critter's nervous system works through only one type of receptor to regulate all of his organs. That is, the presence of only one receptor type has made selective drug action impossible.

Now let's consider Critter 2. Although this critter might be the twin of Critter 1, he differs in one important way: whereas all functions in Critter 1 are regulated through just one type of receptor, Critter 2 employs different receptors to control each of his four functions. Because of this simple but important difference, the selective drug action that was impossible with Critter 1 can be achieved easily with Critter 2. We can, for example, selectively enhance cardiac function in Critter 2 without risking the side effects to which Critter 1 was predisposed. This can be done simply by administering an agonist agent that binds selectively to receptors on the heart (type A receptors). If this medication is sufficiently selective for type A receptors, it will not interact with receptor types B, C, or D. Hence, function in structures regulated by those receptors will be unaffected. Note that our ability to produce selective drug action in Critter 2 is made possible because his nervous system works through different types of receptors to regulate function in his various organs. The message from this example is: *the more types of receptors we have to work with, the greater our chances of producing selective drug effects.*

## An Approach to Learning about Peripheral Nervous System Drugs

As noted above, to understand the ways in which drugs can alter a process under neuronal control, we must first understand how the nervous system itself regulates that process. Accordingly, when preparing to study peripheral nervous system pharmacology, you must first establish a working knowledge of the peripheral nervous system itself. In particular, you need to know two basic types of information about peripheral nervous system function. First, you need to know the types of receptors through which the peripheral nervous system works when influencing the function of a specific organ. Second, you need to know what the normal response to activation of those receptors is. All of the information you will need about peripheral nervous system function is reviewed in Chapter 14.

Once you understand the peripheral nervous system itself, you can go on to learn about peripheral nervous system drugs. Although learning about these drugs will require significant effort, the learning process itself is straightforward. To understand any particular peripheral nervous system drug, you need three types of information: (1) the type (or types) of receptor through which the drug acts, (2) the normal response to activation of those receptors, and (3) what the drug in question does to receptor function (i.e., does the drug increase or decrease receptor activation?). Armed with these three types of information, you can readily predict the major effects of any peripheral nervous system drug.

An example will serve to illustrate this learning process. Let's consider a drug named *isoproterenol* for our example. The first information we need is the identity of the receptors at which isoproterenol acts. Isoproterenol acts at two types of receptors, named beta$_1$ and beta$_2$. Next, we need to know the normal responses to activation of these receptors. The most prominent responses to activation of beta$_1$ receptors are *increased heart rate* and *increased force of cardiac contraction*. The primary responses to activation of beta$_2$ receptors are *bronchial dilation* and *elevation of glucose levels in blood*. Lastly, we need to know whether isoproterenol increases or decreases the activation of beta$_1$ and beta$_2$ receptors. At both types of receptor, isoproterenol causes *activation*. Armed with these three primary pieces of information about isoproterenol, we can now predict the principal effects of this drug. By *activating* beta$_1$ and beta$_2$ receptors, isoproterenol can elicit three major responses: (1) increased cardiac output (by increasing heart rate and force of contraction), (2) dilation of the bronchi, and (3) elevation of blood glucose levels. Depending on the patient to whom this drug is given, these responses may be beneficial or they may be detrimental.

From this example, you can see how easy it is to predict the effects of a peripheral nervous system drug once you've mastered just three kinds of information. Accordingly, I strongly encourage you to take the approach suggested when studying peripheral nervous system agents. That is, for each peripheral nervous system drug, you should learn (1) the identity of the receptors at which that drug acts, (2) the normal responses to activation of those receptors, and (3) whether the drug in-creases or decreases receptor activation. With this information, you can predict most of the important effects of any peripheral nervous system drug.

## KEY POINTS

- Except for local anesthetics, which suppress axonal conduction, all neuropharmacologic drugs act by altering synaptic transmission.
- Ultimately, the impact of a drug on a neuronally regulated process is dependent upon the drug's ability to directly or indirectly alter receptor activity on target cells.
- Synaptic transmission consists of five basic steps: transmitter synthesis, transmitter storage, transmitter release, binding of transmitter to its receptor, and termination of transmission by dissociation of transmitter from the receptor followed by transmitter reuptake or degradation.
- Drugs can do one of two things to receptor function: they can increase receptor activation or they can decrease receptor activation.
- Drugs that increase transmitter synthesis will increase receptor activation.
- Drugs that decrease transmitter synthesis will decrease receptor activation.
- Drugs that promote synthesis of "super" transmitters will increase receptor activation.
- Drugs that impede transmitter storage will decrease receptor activation.
- Drugs that promote transmitter release will increase receptor activation.
- Drugs that suppress transmitter release will decrease receptor activation.
- Agonist drugs will increase receptor activation.
- Antagonist drugs will decrease receptor activation.
- Drugs that bind to receptors and enhance the actions of the natural transmitter at the receptor will increase receptor activation.
- Drugs that block transmitter reuptake will increase receptor activation.
- Drugs that inhibit transmitter degradation will increase receptor activation.
- The presence of multiple receptor types increases our ability to produce selective drug effects.
- For each peripheral nervous system drug that you study, you should learn the identity of the receptors at which the drug acts, the normal responses to activation of those receptors, and whether the drug increases or decreases receptor activation.

# CHAPTER 14

# Physiology of the Peripheral Nervous System

To understand peripheral nervous system drugs, we must first understand the peripheral nervous system itself. The objective of this chapter is to help you develop that understanding.

It is not uncommon for students to be at least slightly apprehensive about studying the peripheral nervous system—especially the autonomic component. In fact, it is not uncommon for students who have studied this subject before to be thoroughly convinced that they will never, ever really understand it. This reaction is unfortunate in that, although there is a lot to know about the peripheral nervous system, the information is not terribly difficult to grasp. In this chapter, information on the peripheral nervous system is presented in a fashion that differs from traditional methods of teaching this material. Hopefully, this approach will facilitate learning.

Since our ultimate goal concerns pharmacology—and not physiology—we will not attempt to discuss everything there is to know about the peripheral nervous system. Rather, we will limit discussion to those aspects of peripheral nervous system physiology that have a direct bearing on our ability to understand drugs.

## Divisions of the Nervous System

The nervous system has two main divisions, the *central nervous system* and the *peripheral nervous system*. The central nervous system is subdivided into the brain and the spinal cord.

The peripheral nervous system has two major subdivisions: (1) *the somatic motor system* and (2) *the auto-nomic nervous system*. The autonomic nervous system is further subdivided into the *parasympathetic nervous system* and the *sympathetic nervous system*. The somatic motor system controls movement of voluntary muscles, whereas the two subdivisions of the autonomic nervous system regulate many "involuntary" processes.

The autonomic nervous system is the principal focus of this chapter. The somatic motor system is also considered, but discussion is limited.

## Overview of Autonomic Nervous System Functions

The autonomic nervous system has three principal functions: (1) regulation of the heart, (2) regulation of secretory glands (salivary, gastric, sweat, and bronchial glands), and (3) regulation of smooth muscles (muscles of the bronchi, blood vessels, urogenital system, and gastrointestinal tract). These regulatory activities are shared between the sympathetic and parasympathetic divisions of the autonomic nervous system.

## Principal Functions of the Parasympathetic Nervous System

The parasympathetic nervous system performs seven regulatory functions that have particular relevance to the actions of peripheral nervous system drugs. Specifically, stimulation of appropriate parasympathetic nerves causes (1) slowing of heart rate, (2) increased gastric secretion, (3) emptying of the bladder, (4) emptying of the bowel, (5) focusing of the eye for near vision, (6) constriction of the pupil, and (7) contraction of bronchial smooth muscle. Just how the parasympathetic nervous system elicits these responses is discussed later under *Functions of Cholinergic Receptor Subtypes.*

From the above we can see that the parasympathetic nervous system is concerned primarily with what might be called the "housekeeping" chores of the body (digestion of food and excretion of wastes). In addition, the system helps control vision and conserve energy (by reducing cardiac work).

As you might guess, therapeutic agents that work by altering parasympathetic nervous system function are used primarily for their effects on the gastrointestinal tract, the bladder, and the eye. Occasionally, these drugs are also used for their effects on the heart and lungs.

A variety of poisons act by mimicking or blocking effects of parasympathetic stimulation. Among these poisons are nerve gases, insecticides, and toxic compounds found in certain mushrooms and plants.

## Principal Functions of the Sympathetic Nervous System

The main functions of the sympathetic nervous system are (1) regulation of the cardiovascular system, (2) regulation of body temperature, and (3) implementation of the "fight-or-flight" reaction.

The sympathetic nervous system exerts multiple influences on the heart and blood vessels. Stimulation of sympathetic nerves to the heart increases cardiac output. Stimulation of sympathetic nerves to arterioles and veins causes vasoconstriction. Release of epinephrine from the adrenal gland results in vasoconstriction in most vascular beds and vasodilation in certain others. By exerting its influence over blood vessels and the heart, the sympathetic nervous system can achieve three homeostatic objectives: (1) maintenance of blood flow to the brain, (2) redistribution of blood flow during exercise, and (3) compensation for blood loss (primarily by causing vasoconstriction).

The sympathetic nervous system helps regulate body temperature in three ways: (1) By regulating blood flow to the skin, sympathetic nerves can increase or decrease heat loss. By *dilating* surface vessels, sympathetic nerves increase blood flow to the skin and thereby accelerate heat loss. Conversely, *constriction* of cutaneous vessels conserves heat. (2) Sympathetic nerves to sweat glands promote secretion of sweat, thereby helping the body cool. (3) By inducing piloerection (erection of hair), sympathetic nerves can increase heat conservation.

When we are faced with adversity, the sympathetic nervous system mobilizes various components of the body in preparation for fight-or-flight. The fight-or-flight response has several features. These are (1) increased heart rate and blood pressure, (2) shunting of blood away from the skin and viscera and into skeletal muscles, (3) dilation of the bronchi to improve oxygenation, (4) dilation of the pupils (perhaps to promote visual acuity), and (5) mobilization of stored energy, an action that provides glucose for the brain and fatty acids for muscle activity. The sensation of

being "cold with fear" is brought on by the shunting of blood away from the skin. The phrase "wide-eyed with fear" may be based on pupillary dilation.

Many therapeutic agents produce their effects by altering functions under sympathetic control. These drugs are used primarily for their effects on the heart, vascular system, and lungs. Agents that alter cardiovascular function are used to treat hypertension, heart failure, angina pectoris, and other disorders. Drugs affecting the lungs are used primarily for asthma.

## Basic Mechanisms by Which the Autonomic Nervous System Regulates Physiologic Processes

To understand how drugs influence processes under autonomic nervous system control, we must first understand how the autonomic nervous system itself regulates those activities. The basic mechanisms by which the autonomic nervous system regulates physiologic processes are discussed below.

### Patterns of Innervation and Control

Most structures under autonomic nervous system control are innervated by sympathetic nerves and by parasympathetic nerves. The relative influence of the sympathetic nervous system versus that of the parasympathetic nervous system depends on the organ under consideration.

In many of the organs that receive dual innervation, the influence of sympathetic nerves *opposes* that of parasympathetic nerves. For example, in the heart, *sympathetic* nerves *increase* heart rate, whereas *parasympathetic* nerves *slow* heart rate (Fig. 14–1).

In some organs that receive nerves from both divisions of the autonomic nervous system, the effects of sympathetic and parasympathetic nerves are *complementary,* rather than opposite. For example, in the male reproductive system, erection is regulated by parasympathetic nerves while ejaculation is controlled by sympathetic nerves; if attempts at reproduction are to succeed, cooperative interaction of both systems is needed.

A few structures under autonomic control receive innervation from only one division of the system. The principal examples of such structures are the blood vessels, which are innervated exclusively by sympathetic nerves.

In summary, there are three basic patterns of autonomic innervation and regulation: (1) innervation by *both* divi-

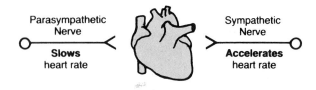

**Figure 14–1. Opposing effects of parasympathetic and sympathetic nerves.**

sions of the autonomic nervous system in which the effects of the two divisions are *opposed,* (2) innervation by *both* divisions of the autonomic nervous system in which the effects of the two divisions are *complementary,* and (3) innervation and regulation by *only one* division of the autonomic nervous system.

## Feedback Regulation

Feedback regulation is a process that allows a system to adjust itself by responding to incoming information. Practically all physiologic processes are regulated at least in part by feedback control.

Figure 14-2 depicts a feedback control loop typical of those used by the autonomic nervous system. The main elements of this loop are (1) a *sensor,* (2) an *effector,* and (3) neurons connecting the sensor to the effector. The purpose of the sensor is to monitor the status of a physiologic process. Information picked up by the sensor is sent to the central nervous system (spinal cord and brain), where it is integrated with other relevant information. Signals (instructions for change) are then sent from the central nervous system along nerves of the autonomic system to the effector. In response to these instructions, the effector then makes appropriate adjustments in the process. The entire procedure is termed a *reflex.*

***Baroreceptor Reflex.*** From a pharmacologic perspective, the most important feedback loop of the autonomic nervous system is one that helps regulate *blood pressure.* This system is referred to as the *baroreceptor reflex.* (Baroreceptors are receptors that sense blood pressure.) You should be familiar with this feedback system because the reflexes that control blood pressure often oppose our attempts to modify blood pressure with drugs.

Feedback (reflex) control of blood pressure is achieved as follows: (1) Baroreceptors located in the carotid sinus and aortic arch monitor changes in blood pressure and send this information to the brain. (2) In response to alterations in blood pressure, the brain sends impulses along nerves of the autonomic nervous system, instructing the heart and blood vessels to behave in such a way as to restore blood pressure to normalcy. Accordingly, when blood pressure *falls,* the baroreceptor reflex causes vasoconstriction and elevation of cardiac output so as to bring blood pressure back up. Conversely, when blood pressure *rises*

too high, the baroreceptor reflex causes vasodilation and a reduction in cardiac output, thereby causing blood pressure to decline. The baroreceptor reflex is discussed in greater detail in Chapter 40 (Review of Hemodynamics).

## Autonomic Tone

The term *autonomic* tone refers to the steady, day-to-day influence exerted by the autonomic nervous system on a particular organ or organ system. Autonomic tone provides a basal level of control over which reflex regulation is superimposed.

When an organ is innervated by both divisions of the autonomic nervous system, one division—either sympathetic or parasympathetic—provides most of the basal control, thereby obviating conflicting instruction. Recall that when an organ receives nerves from both divisions of the autonomic nervous system, it is common for those divisions to exert opposing influences. If both divisions were to send impulses simultaneously, the resultant conflicting instructions would not be productive. By having only one division of the autonomic nervous system provide the basal control to an organ, this possible source of counterproductivity is avoided.

The branch of the autonomic nervous system that controls organ function most of the time is said to provide the *predominant tone* to that organ. *In most organs, the parasympathetic nervous system provides the predominant tone.* The vascular system, which is regulated almost exclusively by the *sympathetic* nervous system, is the principal exception to this general rule.

## Anatomic Considerations

Although a great deal is known about the anatomy of the peripheral nervous system, very little of this information bears any meaningful relationship to our ability to understand peripheral nervous system drugs. The few details of peripheral nervous system anatomy that *do* pertain to pharmacology are summarized in Figure 14-3.

## Parasympathetic Nervous System

Pharmacologically relevant aspects of parasympathetic anatomy are shown in Figure 14-3. Note that there are *two* neurons in the pathway leading from the spinal cord to the organs innervated by parasympathetic nerves. The junction (synapse) between these two neurons occurs within a structure called a *ganglion.* (A ganglion is simply a lump created by a group of nerve cell bodies.) Not surprisingly, the neurons that go from the spinal cord to the parasympathetic ganglia are called *preganglionic neurons,* whereas the neurons that go from the ganglia to effector organs are called *postganglionic neurons.*

The anatomy of the parasympathetic nervous system offers two general sites at which drugs can act. These are (1) the synapses between preganglionic neurons and postganglionic neurons and (2) the junctions between postganglionic neurons and their effector organs.

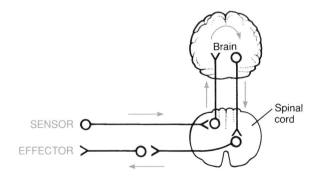

**Figure 14–2. Feedback loop of the autonomic nervous system.**

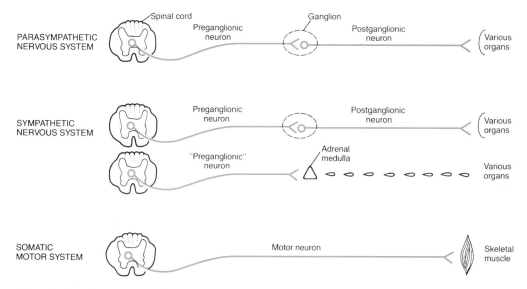

**Figure 14–3. The basic anatomy of the parasympathetic and sympathetic nervous systems and the somatic motor system.**

## Sympathetic Nervous System

Pharmacologically relevant aspects of sympathetic nervous system anatomy are illustrated in Figure 14-3. As you can see, these features are nearly identical to those of the parasympathetic nervous system. Like the parasympathetic nervous system, the sympathetic nervous system employs *two* neurons in the pathways leading from the spinal cord to the organs under its control. As with the parasympathetic nervous system, the junctions between those neurons are located in *ganglia*. Neurons leading from the spinal cord to the sympathetic ganglia are termed *preganglionic neurons*, and neurons leading from ganglia to effector organs are termed *postganglionic neurons*.

The *medulla of the adrenal* gland is a feature of the sympathetic nervous system that requires comment. Although not a neuron per se, the adrenal medulla can be looked on as the functional equivalent of a postganglionic neuron of the sympathetic nervous system. (The adrenal medulla influences the body by releasing epinephrine into the bloodstream, which then produces effects much like those that occur in response to stimulation of postganglionic sympathetic nerves.) Since the adrenal medulla is very similar in function to a postganglionic neuron, it is appropriate to refer to the nerve leading from the spinal cord to the adrenal as *preganglionic*, even though there is no ganglion, as such, in this pathway.

As with the parasympathetic nervous system, drugs that affect the sympathetic nervous system have two general sites of action: (1) the synapses between preganglionic and postganglionic neurons (including the adrenal medulla), and (2) the junctions between postganglionic neurons and their effector organs.

## Somatic Motor System

Pharmacologically relevant anatomy of the somatic motor system is depicted in Figure 14-3. Note that there is *only one* neuron in the pathway from the spinal cord to the muscles innervated by somatic motor nerves. Because this pathway contains only one neuron, peripherally acting drugs that affect somatic motor system function have only one site of action: the *neuromuscular junction* (i.e., the junction between the somatic motor nerve and the muscle).

## Introduction to Transmitters of the Peripheral Nervous System

The peripheral nervous system employs three neurotransmitters: *acetylcholine, norepinephrine,* and *epinephrine.* Any given junction in the peripheral nervous system uses only one of these transmitter substances. A fourth compound—*dopamine*—may also serve as a peripheral nervous system transmitter, but this role has not been demonstrated conclusively.

To understand peripheral nervous system pharmacology, it is necessary to know the identity of the transmitter employed at each of the junctions of the peripheral nervous system. This information is summarized in Figure 14-4.

As the figure indicates, *acetylcholine* is the transmitter employed at most junctions of the peripheral nervous system. Acetylcholine is the transmitter released by (1) all preganglionic neurons of the parasympathetic nervous system, (2) all preganglionic neurons of the sympathetic nervous system, (3) all postganglionic neurons of the parasympathetic nervous system, (4) all motor neurons to skeletal muscles, and (5) most postganglionic neurons of the sympathetic nervous system that go to sweat glands.

*Norepinephrine* is the transmitter released by practically all postganglionic neurons of the sympathetic nervous system. The only exceptions to this rule are the postganglionic sympathetic neurons that go to sweat glands, which employ acetylcholine as their transmitter.

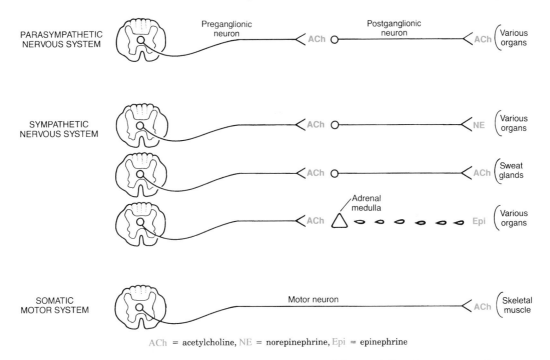

ACh = acetylcholine, NE = norepinephrine, Epi = epinephrine

**Figure 14–4. Transmitters employed at specific junctions of the peripheral nervous system.**
Summary
1. *All preganglionic* neurons of the *parasympathetic* and *sympathetic* nervous systems release *acetylcholine* as their transmitter.
2. *All postganglionic* neurons of the *parasympathetic* nervous system release *acetylcholine* as their transmitter.
3. *Most postganglionic* neurons of the *sympathetic* nervous system release *norepinephrine* as their transmitter.
4. *Postganglionic* neurons of the sympathetic nervous system that innervate *sweat glands* release *acetylcholine* as their transmitter.
5. The principal transmitter released by the *adrenal medulla* is *epinephrine*.
6. *All motor neurons* to *skeletal muscles* release *acetylcholine* as their transmitter.

*Epinephrine* is the major transmitter released by the adrenal medulla. (The adrenal medulla also releases some norepinephrine.)

Much of what follows in this chapter is based on the information summarized in Figure 14-4. Accordingly, I strongly urge you to learn (memorize) this information now.

## Introduction to Receptors of the Peripheral Nervous System

The peripheral nervous system works through several different types of receptors. An understanding of these receptors is central to an understanding of peripheral nervous system pharmacology. All effort that you invest in learning about these receptors now will be richly rewarded as we discuss peripheral nervous system drugs in the chapters that follow.

### Primary Receptor Types: Cholinergic Receptors and Adrenergic Receptors

There are two basic categories of receptors associated with the peripheral nervous system: *cholinergic receptors* and *adrenergic receptors*. Cholinergic receptors are de-fined as receptors that mediate responses to acetyl-choline. These receptors mediate responses at all junctions where acetylcholine is the transmitter. Adrenergic receptors are defined as receptors that mediate responses to epinephrine (adrenaline) and norepinephrine. These receptors mediate responses at all junctions where nor-epinephrine or epinephrine is the transmitter.

### Subtypes of Cholinergic and Adrenergic Receptors

Not all cholinergic receptors are the same; likewise, not all adrenergic receptors are the same. For each of these two major receptor categories there are receptor subtypes. There are three major subtypes of cholinergic receptors, referred to as nicotinic$_N$, nicotinic$_M$, and muscarinic.* There are four major subtypes of adrenergic receptors, referred to as alpha$_1$, alpha$_2$, beta$_1$, and beta$_2$.

In addition to the four major subtypes of adrenergic receptors, there is another adrenergic receptor type, re-

*Evidence gathered in recent years indicates that not all muscarinic receptors are the same. That is, like nicotinic receptors, muscarinic receptors come in subtypes. At least three subtypes have been identified. However, since our understanding of these receptors is relatively new, and since drugs that can selectively alter their function are few, we will defer discussion of muscarinic subtypes to a future edition of this text.

ferred to as the *dopamine* receptor. Although dopamine receptors are classified as adrenergic, these receptors do not respond to epinephrine or norepinephrine. Rather, they respond only to dopamine, a neurotransmitter found primarily in the central nervous system.

# Exploring the Concept of Receptor Subtypes

The concept of receptor subtypes is important and potentially confusing. This section discusses what a receptor subtype is and why receptor subtypes matter to us as students of pharmacology.

## What Do We Mean by the Term Receptor Subtype?

Receptors that respond to the same transmitter but nonetheless are different from one another would be called receptor subtypes. For example, receptors that respond to acetylcholine can be found (1) within ganglia of the autonomic nervous system, (2) at neuromuscular junctions, and (3) on organs regulated by the parasympathetic nervous system. However, even though all of these receptors can be activated by acetylcholine, there is clear evidence that the receptors at these three sites are different from one another. Hence, although all of these receptors belong to the same major receptor category (cholinergic), they are sufficiently unlike one another as to constitute distinct receptor subtypes.

## How Do We Know that Receptor Subtypes Exist?

Historically, our knowledge of receptor subtypes came from observing responses to drugs. In fact, were it not for drugs, receptor subtypes might never have been discovered.

The data in Table 14-1 illustrate the types of drug responses that led to the realization that receptor subtypes exist. These data summarize the results of an experiment designed to study the effects of a natural transmitter (acetylcholine) and a series of drugs (nicotine, muscarine,

### TABLE 14-1. RESPONSES OF SKELETAL MUSCLE AND CILIARY MUSCLE TO A SERIES OF DRUGS

| | Response | |
| --- | --- | --- |
| **Drug** | Skeletal Muscle | Ciliary Muscle |
| Acetylcholine | Contraction | Contraction |
| Nicotine | Contraction | No response |
| Muscarine | No response | Contraction |
| Acetylcholine: after *d*-tubocurarine | No response | Contraction |
| Acetylcholine: after atropine | Contraction | No response |

*d*-tubocurarine, and atropine) on two tissues: skeletal muscle and ciliary muscle. (The ciliary muscle is the muscle responsible for focusing the eye for near vision.) As these data indicate, although skeletal muscle and ciliary muscle both contract in response to acetylcholine, these tissues respond differently from each other to drugs. In the discussion below, we will examine the selective responses of these tissues to drugs and see how those responses point to the existence of receptor subtypes.

At synapses on skeletal muscle and ciliary muscle, acetylcholine is the transmitter employed by neurons to elicit contraction. Since both types of muscle respond to acetylcholine, it is safe to conclude that both muscles have receptors for this substance. Since acetylcholine is the natural transmitter for these receptors, we would classify these receptors as *cholinergic*.

What do the effects of nicotine on skeletal muscle and ciliary muscle suggest? The effects of nicotine on these muscles suggest four possible conclusions: (1) Since skeletal muscle contracts when nicotine is applied, we can conclude that skeletal muscle has receptors at which nicotine can act. (2) Since ciliary muscle does *not* respond to nicotine, we can tentatively conclude that ciliary muscle does not have receptors for nicotine. (3) Since nicotine mimics the effects of acetylcholine on skeletal muscle, we can conclude that nicotine may act at the same receptors on skeletal muscle at which acetylcholine acts. (4) Since both types of muscle have receptors for acetylcholine, and since nicotine appears to act only at the acetylcholine receptors on skeletal muscle, we can tentatively conclude that the acetylcholine receptors on skeletal muscle are different from the acetylcholine receptors on ciliary muscle.

What do the responses to muscarine suggest? The conclusions that can be drawn regarding responses to muscarine are exactly parallel to those drawn for nicotine. These conclusions are: (1) ciliary muscle has receptors that respond to muscarine, (2) skeletal muscle may not have receptors for muscarine, (3) muscarine may be acting at the same receptors on ciliary muscle as does acetylcholine, and (4) the receptors for acetylcholine on ciliary muscle may be different from the receptors for acetylcholine on skeletal muscle.

The responses of skeletal muscle and ciliary muscle to nicotine and muscarine suggest, but do not prove, that the cholinergic receptors on these two tissues are different; the responses of these two tissues to *d*-tubocurarine and *atropine,* both of which are receptor blocking agents, eliminate any doubts as to the presence of cholinergic receptor subtypes. When both types of muscle are *pretreated* with *d*-tubocurarine and then exposed to acetylcholine, the response to acetylcholine is blocked—*but only in skeletal muscle.* Tubocurarine pretreatment does not reduce the ability of acetylcholine to stimulate ciliary muscle. Conversely, pretreatment with atropine selectively blocks the response to acetylcholine in ciliary muscle; however, atropine does nothing to prevent acetylcholine from stimulating receptors on skeletal muscle. Since tubocurarine can selectively block cholinergic receptors in skeletal muscle, whereas atropine can selectively block cholinergic receptors in ciliary muscle, we can conclude with certainty that the receptors for acetylcholine in these two types of muscle must be different from each other.

The data just discussed illustrate the essential role of drugs in revealing the presence of receptor subtypes. If acetylcholine were the only probe that we had, all that we would have been able to observe is that both skeletal muscle and ciliary muscle can respond to this agent. This simple observation would provide no basis for suspecting that the receptors for acetylcholine in these two tissues are different. It is only through the use of selectively acting drugs that the presence of receptor subtypes was initially revealed.

Today, the technology for identifying receptors and their subtypes is extremely sophisticated—not that studies like the one just discussed are no longer of value. In addition to performing traditional drug-based studies, scientists are now cloning receptors using DNA hybridization technology. As you can imagine, this allows us to understand receptors in ways that were unthinkable in the past.[†]

### How Can Drugs Be More Selective than Transmitters at Receptor Subtypes?

Drugs achieve their selectivity for receptor subtypes by having structures that are different from those of natural transmitters. The relationship between structure and receptor selectivity is illustrated in Figure 14-5. In this figure, cartoon drawings are used to represent drugs (nicotine and muscarine), receptor subtypes (nicotinic and muscarinic), and acetylcholine (the natural transmitter at nicotinic and muscarinic receptors). From the structures shown, we can easily imagine how acetylcholine is able to interact with both kinds of receptor subtypes, whereas nicotine and muscarine can interact only with the receptor subtypes whose structure is complementary to their own. It is by synthesizing chemicals of varied structure that pharmaceutical scientists have been able to produce drugs that are more selective for specific receptor subtypes than the natural transmitters that act at those sites.

### Why Do Receptor Subtypes Exist?

It is not unreasonable for us to wonder why Mother Nature has bothered to create more than one type of receptor for any given transmitter. Unfortunately, definitive answers to questions along this line will have to come from Mother Nature herself. That is to say, the physiologic benefits of having multiple receptor subtypes for the same transmitter are not immediately obvious. In fact, as noted earlier, were it not for drugs, we probably wouldn't know that receptor subtypes existed at all.

[†]In addition to revealing exciting new information about receptors previously identified, this spiffy technology is so powerful that new receptors and receptor subtypes are being discovered at a dizzying rate. Which means, of course, that students in the future will have many more receptors to contend with than you do. So, when it seems like you're working awfully hard to master the information on receptors in this chapter and the ones that follow, look on the bright side—you could be studying pharmacology 10 years from now.

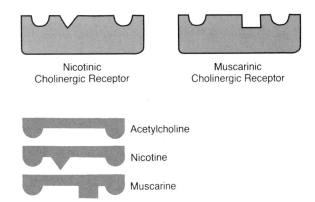

**Figure 14–5. Drug structure and receptor selectivity.** These cartoon figures illustrate the relationship between structure and receptor selectivity. The structure of acetylcholine allows this transmitter to interact with both receptor subtypes. In contrast, because of their unique configurations, nicotine and muscarine are selective for the cholinergic receptor subtypes whose structure complements their own.

### Do Receptor Subtypes Matter to Us? You Bet!

Although receptor subtypes are of uncertain physiologic relevance, from the viewpoint of therapeutics, receptor subtypes are invaluable. The presence of receptor subtypes makes possible a dramatic increase in the selectivity of drug actions. For example, thanks to the existence of subtypes of cholinergic receptors (and the development of drugs selective for those receptor subtypes), it is possible to influence the activity of selected cholinergic receptors (e.g., receptors of the neuromuscular junction) without altering the activity of all other cholinergic receptors (i.e., the cholinergic receptors found in all autonomic ganglia and all target organs of the parasympathetic nervous system). Were it not for the existence of receptor subtypes, a drug that acted on cholinergic receptors at one site would alter the activity of cholinergic receptors at all other sites. Clearly, the existence of receptor subtypes for a particular transmitter makes possible drug actions that are much more selective than could be achieved if all of the receptors for that transmitter were the same.

## Locations of Receptor Subtypes

Since many of the drugs that we will be discussing are selective for specific receptor subtypes, knowledge of the sites at which specific receptor subtypes are located will help us predict which organs a drug will affect. Accordingly, in laying our foundation for the study of peripheral nervous system drugs, it is important to learn the sites at which the subtypes of adrenergic and cholinergic receptors are located. This information is summarized in Figure 14-6. You will find it very helpful to master the contents of this figure before proceeding much further. (In the interest of minimizing confusion, subtypes of adrenergic receptors in Figure 14-6 are listed simply as

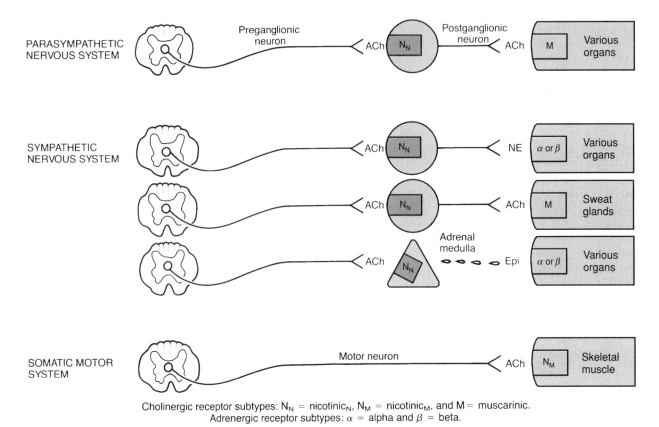

Cholinergic receptor subtypes: $N_N$ = nicotinic$_N$, $N_M$ = nicotinic$_M$, and M = muscarinic.
Adrenergic receptor subtypes: $\alpha$ = alpha and $\beta$ = beta.

**Figure 14–6. Locations of cholinergic and adrenergic receptor subtypes.**
Summary
1. *Nicotinic$_N$ receptors are located on the cell bodies of all postganglionic neurons* of the *parasympathetic* and *sympathetic* nervous systems. *Nicotinic$_N$* receptors are also located on cells of the adrenal medulla.
2. *Nicotinic$_M$ receptors are located on skeletal muscle.*
3. *Muscarinic receptors are located on all organs* regulated by the *parasympathetic* nervous system (i.e., organs innervated by postganglionic parasympathetic nerves). *Muscarinic receptors are also located on sweat glands.*
4. *Adrenergic receptors—alpha, beta,* or both—are located on *all organs* (except sweat glands) regulated by the *sympathetic* nervous system (i.e., organs innervated by postganglionic sympathetic nerves). *Adrenergic receptors are also located on organs regulated by epinephrine released from the adrenal medulla.*

alpha and beta rather than as alpha$_1$, alpha$_2$, beta$_1$, and beta$_2$. The locations of all four subtypes of adrenergic receptors are discussed in the section that follows.)

## Functions of Cholinergic and Adrenergic Receptor Subtypes

Knowledge of receptor function is an absolute requirement for understanding peripheral nervous system drugs. By knowing the receptors at which a drug acts, and by knowing what those receptors do, we can predict the major effects of any peripheral nervous system drug.

Tables 14-2 and 14-3 summarize the pharmacologically relevant functions of peripheral nervous system receptors. Table 14-2 summarizes responses elicited by activation of cholinergic receptor subtypes. Table 14-3 summarizes responses to activation of adrenergic receptor subtypes. Before attempting to study specific peripheral

nervous system drugs, you should master the contents of the appropriate table. Table 14-2 should be mastered before studying cholinergic drugs (Chapters 15, 16, and 17). Table 14-3 should be mastered before studying adrenergic drugs (Chapters 18, 19, and 20). Students who study these tables in preparation for learning about peripheral nervous system drugs will find the process of learning the pharmacology relatively simple (and perhaps even enjoyable). Conversely, students who attempt to study the pharmacology without first mastering the appropriate table are likely to meet with frustration.

## Functions of Cholinergic Receptor Subtypes

Table 14-2 summarizes the pharmacologically relevant responses to activation of the three subtypes of cholinergic receptors: nicotinic$_N$, nicotinic$_M$, and muscarinic. The information in this table should be committed to memory.

**TABLE 14–2. FUNCTIONS OF PERIPHERAL CHOLINERGIC RECEPTOR SUBTYPES**

| Receptor Subtype | Location | Response to Receptor Activation |
|---|---|---|
| *Nicotinic$_N$* | All autonomic nervous system ganglia and the adrenal medulla | Stimulation of parasympathetic and sympathetic postganglionic nerves and release of epinephrine from the adrenal medulla |
| *Nicotinic$_M$* | Neuromuscular junction | Contraction of skeletal muscle |
| *Muscarinic* | All parasympathetic target organs: | |
| | Eye | Contraction of the ciliary muscle focuses the lens for near vision<br>Contraction of the iris sphincter muscle causes miosis (decreased pupil diameter) |
| | Heart | Decreased rate |
| | Lung | Constriction of bronchi<br>Promotion of secretions |
| | Bladder | Voiding |
| | GI tract | Salivation<br>Increased gastric secretions<br>Increased intestinal tone and motility<br>Defecation |
| | Sweat glands* | Generalized sweating |
| | Sex organs | Erection |
| | Blood vessels† | Vasodilation |

Radial muscle — Sphincter muscle — Pupil — Miosis

* Although sweating is due primarily to stimulation of muscarinic receptors by acetylcholine, the nerves that supply acetylcholine to sweat glands belong to the sympathetic nervous system rather than the parasympathetic nervous system.
†Cholinergic receptors on blood vessels are not associated with the nervous system.

We can group responses to cholinergic receptor activation into three major categories based on the subtype of receptor involved:

- Activation of *nicotinic$_N$* (neuronal) receptors promotes *ganglionic transmission* at all ganglia of the sympathetic and parasympathetic nervous systems. In addition, activation of nicotinic$_N$ receptors promotes *release of epinephrine from the adrenal medulla.*
- Activation of *nicotinic$_M$* (muscle) receptors causes *contraction of skeletal muscle.*
- Activation of *muscarinic* receptors, which are located on target organs of the parasympathetic nervous system, elicits an appropriate response from the organ involved. Specifically, muscarinic activation causes (1) increased glandular secretions (from pulmonary, gastric, intestinal, and sweat glands); (2) contraction of smooth muscle in the bronchi, bladder, and gastrointestinal tract; (3) slowing of heart rate; (4) contraction of the sphincter muscle of

the iris, resulting in miosis (reduction in pupillary diameter); and (5) contraction of the ciliary muscle of the eye, causing the lens to focus for near vision.

Muscarinic cholinergic receptors on blood vessels require additional comment. These receptors are not associated with the nervous system in any way. That is, no nerves terminate at vascular muscarinic receptors. It is not at all clear as to how, or even if, these receptors are activated physiologically. However, regardless of their physiologic relevance, the cholinergic receptors on blood vessels do have pharmacologic significance, in that drugs that are able to activate these receptors will cause vasodilation, which in turn will cause blood pressure to fall.

## Functions of Adrenergic Receptor Subtypes

Adrenergic receptor subtypes and their functions are summarized in Table 14-3. You should commit this information to memory.

## TABLE 14–3. FUNCTIONS OF PERIPHERAL ADRENERGIC RECEPTOR SUBTYPES

| Receptor Subtype | Location | Response to Receptor Activation | |
|---|---|---|---|
| *Alpha₁* | Eye | Contraction of the radial muscle of the iris causes mydriasis (increased pupil size) | Radial muscle — Sphincter muscle Pupil Mydriasis |
| | Arterioles<br>  Skin<br>  Viscera<br>  Mucous membranes | Constriction | |
| | Veins | Constriction | |
| | Sex organs, male | Ejaculation | |
| | Bladder neck and prostatic capsule | Contraction | |
| *Alpha₂\** | Presynaptic nerve terminals | Inhibition of transmitter release | α₂ NE NE NE NE R |
| *Beta₁* | Heart | Increased rate<br>Increased force of contraction<br>Increased A V conduction velocity | |
| | Kidney | Renin release | |
| *Beta₂* | Arterioles<br>  Heart<br>  Lung<br>  Skeletal muscle | Dilation | |
| | Bronchi | Dilation | |
| | Uterus | Relaxation | |
| | Liver | Glycogenolysis | |
| | Skeletal muscle | Enhanced contraction, glycogenolysis | |
| *Dopamine* | Kidney | Dilation of kidney vasculature | |

\*Note: Alpha₂ receptors in the central nervous system are postsynaptic. NE = norepinephrine, R = receptor.

## Alpha₁ Receptors

Alpha₁ receptors are located in the eyes, blood vessels, male sex organs, bladder, and prostatic capsule.

*Ocular* alpha₁ receptors are present on the *radial muscle* of the iris. Activation of these receptors leads to mydriasis (dilation of the pupil). As depicted in Table 14-3, the fibers of the radial muscle are arranged like the spokes of a wheel. Because of this configuration, contraction of the radial muscle causes the pupil to enlarge. (If you have difficulty remembering that *mydriasis* means pupillary enlargement, whereas *miosis* means pupillary constriction, just remember that mydriasis [enlargement] is a larger word than miosis.)

Activation of alpha₁ receptors in *blood vessels* produces *vasoconstriction*. Alpha₁ receptors are present on veins and on arterioles in many capillary beds.

Activation of alpha₁ receptors in the sexual apparatus of males causes *ejaculation.*

Activation of alpha₁ receptors in smooth muscle of the *bladder neck* and *prostatic capsule* causes contraction.

## Alpha₂ Receptors

Alpha₂ receptors of the peripheral nervous system are located on *nerve terminals* (see Table 14-3) and not on the organs innervated by the autonomic nervous system. Because alpha₂ receptors are located on nerve terminals, these receptors are referred to as *presynaptic* or *prejunctional.* The function of these receptors is to regulate transmitter release. As depicted in Table 14-3, norepinephrine can bind to alpha₂ receptors on the same neuron from which it was released. The consequence of this norepinephrine-receptor interaction is suppression of further norepinephrine release. Hence, presynaptic alpha$_2$ receptors can help reduce transmitter release when too much transmitter has accumulated in the synaptic gap. Drug effects resulting from activation of peripheral alpha$_2$ receptors are of minimal clinical significance.

Alpha$_2$ receptors are also present in the central nervous system. In contrast to peripheral alpha$_2$ receptors, central alpha$_2$ receptors are therapeutically relevant. We will consider these receptors in later chapters.

## Beta$_1$ Receptors

Beta$_1$ receptors are located in the heart and kidney. *Cardiac* beta$_1$ receptors have great therapeutic significance. Activation of these receptors *increases heart rate, force of contraction,* and *velocity of impulse conduction through the atrioventricular (AV) node.*

Activation of beta$_1$ receptors in the *kidney* causes *release of renin* into the blood. Since renin promotes synthesis of angiotensin, a powerful vasoconstrictor, activation of renal beta$_1$ receptors is a means by which the nervous system helps elevate blood pressure. (The role of renin in the regulation of blood pressure is discussed in depth in Chapter 41.)

## Beta$_2$ Receptors

Beta$_2$ receptors mediate several important processes. Activation of beta$_2$ receptors in the lung leads to *bronchial dilation.* Activation of beta$_2$ receptors in the uterus causes *relaxation of uterine smooth muscle.* Activation of beta$_2$ receptors in arterioles of the heart, lungs, and skeletal muscles causes *vasodilation* (an effect opposite to that of alpha$_1$ activation). Activation of beta$_2$ receptors in the liver and skeletal muscle promotes *glycogenolysis* (breakdown of glycogen into glucose), thereby increasing blood levels of glucose.

## Dopamine Receptors

In the periphery, the only dopamine receptors of clinical significance are located in the vasculature of the kidney. Activation of these receptors *dilates renal blood vessels*, thereby enhancing renal perfusion.

In the central nervous system, receptors for dopamine are of great therapeutic significance. The functions of these receptors are discussed in Chapter 22 (Drugs for Parkinson's Disease) and Chapter 29 (Antipsychotic Agents).

# Receptor Specificity of the Adrenergic Transmitters

The receptor specificity of adrenergic transmitters is more complex than the receptor specificity of acetylcholine. Whereas acetylcholine can activate all three subtypes of cholinergic receptors, not every adrenergic transmitter (epinephrine, norepinephrine, dopamine) can interact with each of the five subtypes of adrenergic receptors.

Receptor specificity of adrenergic transmitters is as follows: (1) *epinephrine* can activate all alpha and beta receptors, but not dopamine receptors; (2) *norepinephrine*

**TABLE 14–4. RECEPTOR SPECIFICITY OF ADRENERGIC TRANSMITTERS**

| Transmitter | Adrenergic Receptor Subtype | | | | |
|---|---|---|---|---|---|
| | Alpha$_1$ | Alpha$_2$ | Beta$_1$ | Beta$_2$ | Dopamine |
| Epinephrine | ← | | | → | |
| Norepinephrine | ← | | → | | |
| Dopamine | ← → | | ← | → | ← → |

can activate alpha$_1$, alpha$_2$, and beta$_1$ receptors, but not beta$_2$ or dopamine receptors; and (3) *dopamine* can activate alpha$_1$, beta$_1$, and dopamine receptors. (Note that dopamine itself is the only transmitter capable of activating dopamine receptors.) Receptor specificity of the adrenergic transmitters is summarized in Table 14–4.

Knowing that epinephrine is the only transmitter that acts at beta$_2$ receptors can serve as an aid to remembering the functions of this receptor subtype. Recall that epinephrine is released from the adrenal medulla (and not from neurons) and that the function of epinephrine is to prepare the body for fight or flight. Accordingly, since epinephrine is the only transmitter that activates beta$_2$ receptors, and since epinephrine is released only in preparation for fight or flight, times of fight or flight will be the only occasions on which beta$_2$ receptors will undergo significant activation. As it turns out, the physiologic changes elicited by beta$_2$ activation are precisely those needed for success in the fight-or-flight response. Specifically, activation of beta$_2$ receptors will cause (1) dilation of blood vessels in the heart, lungs, and skeletal muscles, thereby increasing blood flow to these organs; (2) dilation of the bronchi, thereby increasing oxygenation; (3) glycogenolysis, thereby increasing available energy; and (4) relaxation of uterine muscle, thereby preventing delivery, a process that would be inconvenient for anyone preparing for fight or flight. Hence, if you think of the physiologic requirements for success during fight or flight, you will have a good picture of the responses that beta$_2$ activation can bring about.

# Transmitter Life Cycles

In this section we consider the life cycles of acetylcholine, norepinephrine, and epinephrine. Since a number of drugs produce their effects by interfering with specific phases of the transmitter life cycle, knowledge of these cycles will help us understand drug actions.

## Life Cycle of Acetylcholine

The life cycle of acetylcholine (ACh) is depicted in Figure 14–7. This cycle begins with the synthesis of ACh from two precursors: choline and acetyl-coenzyme A. Following synthesis, ACh is stored in vesicles and is later

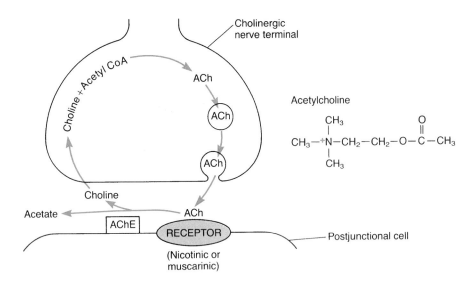

**Figure 14–7. Life cycle of acetylcholine.** Note that transmission is terminated by enzymatic degradation of ACh and not by uptake of intact ACh back into the nerve terminal. (ACh = acetylcholine, AChE = acetylcholinesterase, Acetyl CoA = acetyl coenzyme A.)

released in response to an action potential. Following release, ACh binds to receptors (nicotinic$_N$, nicotinic$_M$, or muscarinic) located on the postjunctional cell. Upon dissociating from its receptors, ACh is destroyed almost instantaneously by *acetylcholinesterase* (AChE), an enzyme present in abundance on the surface of the postjunctional cell. AChE degrades ACh into two inactive products—acetate and choline. Uptake of choline into the cholinergic nerve terminal completes the life cycle of ACh. Note that an inactive substance (choline), and not the active transmitter (acetylcholine), is taken back up for reuse.

Therapeutic and toxic agents can interfere with the ACh life cycle at several points. Botulinus toxin inhibits ACh release. A number of medicines and poisons act at cholinergic receptors to mimic or block the actions of ACh. Several therapeutic and toxic agents act by inhibiting AChE, thereby causing ACh to accumulate in the junctional gap.

### Life Cycle of Norepinephrine

The life cycle of norepinephrine is depicted in Figure 14-8. As indicated, this cycle begins with the synthesis of norepinephrine from a series of precursors. The final step of synthesis takes place within vesicles, where norepinephrine is stored prior to its release. Following release, norepinephrine binds to adrenergic receptors. As shown in the figure, norepinephrine can interact with *postsynaptic* alpha$_1$ and beta receptors and with *presynaptic* alpha$_2$ receptors. Transmission is terminated by *reuptake* of norepinephrine back into the nerve terminal. (Note that the termination process for norepinephrine differs from that for acetylcholine, whose effects are terminated by enzymatic degradation and not by reuptake.) Following reuptake, norepinephrine can undergo one of two fates: (1) uptake into vesicles for reuse, or (2) inactivation by monoamine oxidase (MAO), an enzyme found in the nerve terminal.

Practically every step in the life cycle of norepinephrine can be altered by therapeutic agents: we have drugs that alter the synthesis, storage, and release of norepinephrine; we have drugs that act at adrenergic receptors to mimic or block the effects of norepinephrine; we have drugs, such as cocaine and tricyclic antidepressants, that inhibit the reuptake of norepinephrine (and thereby intensify transmission); and we have drugs that inhibit the breakdown of norepinephrine by MAO, causing an increase in the amount of transmitter available for release.

### Life Cycle of Epinephrine

The life cycle of epinephrine is much like that of norepinephrine—although there are some significant differences. This cycle begins with the synthesis of epinephrine within chromaffin cells of the adrenal medulla. These cells produce epinephrine by first making norepinephrine, which is then converted enzymatically to epinephrine. (Since sympathetic neurons lack the enzyme needed to convert norepinephrine to epinephrine, epinephrine is not produced in sympathetic nerves.) Following synthesis, epinephrine is stored in vesicles until the time of its release. Once released from the adrenal medulla, epinephrine travels via the bloodstream to target organs throughout the body. Termination of epinephrine's actions is accomplished primarily via hepatic metabolism, and not by uptake into nerves.

## KEY POINTS

- The peripheral nervous system has two major divisions: the autonomic nervous system and the somatic motor system.
- The autonomic nervous system has two major divisions: the sympathetic nervous system and the parasympathetic nervous system.
- The parasympathetic nervous system has several functions of relevance to pharmacology: it slows heart rate, increases gastric secretion, empties the bladder and bowel, focuses the eye for near vision, constricts the pupil, and contracts bronchial smooth muscle.
- Principal functions of the sympathetic nervous system are regulation of the cardiovascular system, regulation of body temperature, and implementation of the fight-or-flight response.
- In some organs (e.g., the heart), the sympathetic and parasympathetic nervous systems have opposing ef-

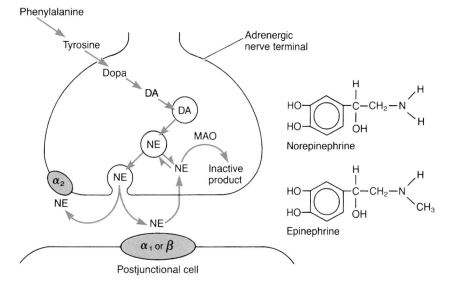

**Figure 14–8. Life cycle of norepinephrine.** Note that transmission is terminated by reuptake of NE into the nerve terminal and not by enzymatic degradation. Note also the structural similarity between epinephrine and norepinephrine. (DA = dopamine, NE = norepinephrine, MAO = monoamine oxidase.)

fects; in other organs (e.g., male sex organs), the sympathetic and parasympathetic nervous systems have complementary effects; in still other organs (most notably the blood vessels), function is regulated by only one branch of the autonomic nervous system.

- The baroreceptor reflex helps regulate blood pressure.
- In most organs regulated by the autonomic nervous system, the parasympathetic nervous system provides the dominant tone.
- In blood vessels, the sympathetic nervous system provides the dominant tone.
- Pathways from the spinal cord to organs under sympathetic and parasympathetic control consist of two neurons: a preganglionic neuron and a postganglionic neuron.
- The adrenal medulla is the functional equivalent of a postganglionic sympathetic neuron.
- Somatic motor pathways from the spinal cord to skeletal muscles have only one neuron.
- The peripheral nervous system employs three transmitters: acetylcholine, norepinephrine, and epinephrine.
- Acetylcholine is the transmitter released by all preganglionic neurons of the sympathetic nervous system, all preganglionic neurons of the parasympathetic nervous system, all postganglionic neurons of the parasympathetic nervous system, postganglionic neurons of the sympathetic nervous system that go to sweat glands, and all motor neurons.
- Norepinephrine is the transmitter released by all postganglionic neurons of the sympathetic nervous system, except those that go to sweat glands.
- Epinephrine is the major transmitter released by the adrenal medulla.
- There are three subtypes of cholinergic receptors: nicotinic$_N$, nicotinic$_M$, and muscarinic.
- There are four major subtypes of adrenergic receptors: alpha$_1$, alpha$_2$, beta$_1$, and beta$_2$.
- Although receptor subtypes are of uncertain physiologic significance, they are of great pharmacologic significance.

- Activation of nicotinic$_N$ receptors promotes transmission at all autonomic ganglia, and promotes release of epinephrine from the adrenal medulla.
- Activation of nicotinic$_M$ receptors causes contraction of skeletal muscle.
- Activation of muscarinic receptors increases glandular secretion (from pulmonary, gastric, intestinal, and sweat glands); contracts smooth muscle in the bronchi, bladder, and gastrointestinal tract; slows heart rate; contracts the iris sphincter; contracts the ciliary muscle (thereby focusing the lens for near vision); and dilates blood vessels.
- Activation of alpha$_1$ receptors contracts the radial muscle of the eye (causing mydriasis), constricts veins and arterioles, promotes ejaculation, and contracts smooth muscle in the bladder neck and prostatic capsule.
- Activation of *peripheral* alpha$_2$ receptors is of minimal pharmacologic significance.
- Activation of beta$_1$ receptors increases heart rate, force of myocardial contraction, and conduction through the AV node, and promotes release of renin by the kidney.
- Activation of beta$_2$ receptors dilates the bronchi, relaxes uterine smooth muscle, increases glycogenolysis, enhances contraction of skeletal muscle, and dilates arterioles (in the heart, lungs, and skeletal muscle).
- Activation of dopamine receptors dilates blood vessels in the kidney.
- Neurotransmission at cholinergic junctions is terminated by degradation of acetylcholine by acetylcholinesterase.
- Neurotransmission at adrenergic junctions is terminated by reuptake of intact norepinephrine into nerve terminals.
- Following reuptake, norepinephrine may be stored in vesicles for reuse or destroyed by monoamine oxidase.

I know it's a lot of work, but there's really no way around it: You've got to incorporate this information into your personal data base.

# Cholinergic Drugs

The cholinergic drugs are agents that influence the activity of cholinergic receptors. Most of these drugs act directly at cholinergic receptors, where they mimic or block the actions of acetylcholine. Some of these drugs—the cholinesterase inhibitors—influence cholinergic receptors indirectly by preventing the breakdown of acetylcholine.

The cholinergic drugs have both therapeutic and toxicologic significance. Therapeutic applications of cholinergic drugs are limited but valuable. The toxicology of cholinergic drugs is extensive, encompassing such agents as nicotine, insecticides, and compounds designed for chemical warfare.

There are six categories of cholinergic drugs. These categories, along with representative agents, are summarized in Table 1. The *muscarinic agonists*, represented by bethanechol, are drugs that selectively mimic the effects of acetylcholine at muscarinic receptors. The *muscarinic antagonists*, represented by atropine, selectively block the effects of acetylcholine at muscarinic receptors. *Ganglionic stimulating agents*, of which nicotine is the major representative, selectively mimic the effects of acetylcholine at nicotinic$_N$ receptors of autonomic ganglia. *Ganglionic blocking agents*, represented by trimethaphan, selectively block ganglionic nicotinic$_N$ receptors. *Neuromuscular blocking agents*, represented by *d*-tubocurarine and succinylcholine, selectively block the effects of acetylcholine at nicotinic$_M$ receptors of the neuromuscular junction. The *cholinesterase inhibitors*, represented by neostigmine and physostigmine, prevent the breakdown of acetylcholine by acetylcholinesterase, and can thereby increase the stimulation of all cholinergic receptors in the body.

## TABLE 1. CATEGORIES OF CHOLINERGIC DRUGS

| Category | Representative Drugs |
|---|---|
| **Muscarinic agonists** | Bethanechol |
| **Muscarinic antagonists** | Atropine |
| **Ganglionic stimulating agents** | Nicotine |
| **Ganglionic blocking agents** | Trimethaphan |
| **Neuromuscular blocking agents** | *d*-Tubocurarine, succinylcholine |
| **Cholinesterase inhibitors** | Neostigmine, physostigmine |

Table 2 is your master key to understanding the cholinergic drugs. This table lists the three subtypes of cholinergic receptors (muscarinic, nicotinic$_N$, and nicotinic$_M$) and indicates for each receptor type: (1) location, (2) responses to activation, (3) drugs that produce activation (agonists), and (4) drugs that prevent activation (antagonists). This information, along with the detailed information on cholinergic receptor function summarized in Table 14-2, is just about all you need in order to predict the actions of cholinergic drugs.

An example will demonstrate the combined value of Table 2 and Table 14-2. Let's consider *bethanechol* for our example. As indicated in Table 2, bethanechol is a selective *agonist* at *muscarinic* cholinergic receptors. Referring to Table 14-2, we see that activation of muscarinic receptors can produce the following: ocular effects (miosis and ciliary muscle contraction), slowing of heart rate, bronchial constriction, urination, glandular secretion, stimulation of

## TABLE 2. SUMMARY OF CHOLINERGIC DRUGS AND THEIR RECEPTORS

| | Receptor Subtype | | |
|---|---|---|---|
| | Muscarinic | Nicotinic$_N$ | Nicotinic$_M$ |
| *Receptor Location* | Sweat glands<br>Blood vessels<br>All organs regulated by the parasympathetic nervous system | All ganglia of the autonomic nervous system | Neuromuscular junctions (NMJ) |
| *Effects of Receptor Activation* | Many, including:<br>↓ Heart rate<br>↑ Gland secretion<br>Smooth muscle contraction | Promotes ganglionic transmission | Skeletal muscle contraction |
| *Receptor Agonists* | Bethanechol<br>Cholinesterase inhibitors: physostigmine, neostigmine (these drugs indirectly stimulate all cholinergic receptors) | Nicotine | (Nicotine*) |
| *Receptor Antagonists* | Atropine | Trimethaphan | d-Tubocurarine, succinylcholine |

*The doses of nicotine needed to stimulate nicotinic$_M$ receptors of the NMJ are much higher than the doses needed to stimulate nicotinic$_N$ receptors in autonomic ganglia.

the gastrointestinal tract, penile erection, and vasodilation. Since bethanechol *activates* muscarinic receptors, the drug is capable of eliciting all of these responses. Hence, by knowing which receptors bethanechol stimulates (from Table 2), and by knowing what those receptors do (from Table 14-2), you can predict the kinds of responses we might expect bethanechol to produce.

In the chapters that follow, we will employ the approach just described for understanding peripheral nervous system drugs. That is, for each drug discussed, you will want to know (1) the receptors that the drug affects, (2) the normal responses to activation of those receptors, and (3) whether the drug in question increases or decreases receptor activation. All of this information is contained in Table 2 and Table 14-2. Accordingly, if you master the information in these tables now, you will be prepared to follow discussions in succeeding chapters with relative ease—and perhaps even pleasure. In contrast, if you postpone mastery of these tables, you are likely to find it both difficult and dissatisfying to proceed.

# CHAPTER 15

# Muscarinic Agonists and Antagonists

**Muscarinic Agonists**
  Bethanechol
  Other Muscarinic Agonists
  Toxicology of Muscarinic Agonists

**Muscarinic Antagonists**
  Atropine
  Other Muscarinic Antagonists
  Toxicology of Muscarinic Antagonists

The muscarinic agonists and antagonists produce their effects through direct interaction with muscarinic receptors. The muscarinic agonists cause receptor activation, whereas the antagonists prevent receptor activation.

## Muscarinic Agonists

The muscarinic agonists are drugs that bind to muscarinic receptors and thereby cause their activation. Since nearly all muscarinic receptors are associated with the parasympathetic nervous system, the responses to muscarinic agonists closely resemble those produced by stimulation of parasympathetic nerves. Because their effects resemble those of parasympathetic stimulation, muscarinic agonists are known alternatively as *parasympathomimetic agents.*

### Bethanechol

Bethanechol embodies the characteristics that typify all muscarinic agonists and will serve as our prototype for the group.

#### Mechanism of Action

Bethanechol is a direct-acting muscarinic agonist. The drug binds reversibly to muscarinic cholinergic receptors and causes their activation. At therapeutic doses, bethanechol acts selectively at muscarinic receptors, having little or no effect on nicotinic cholinergic receptors.

#### Pharmacologic Effects

Bethanechol can elicit all of the responses typical of muscarinic receptor activation. Accordingly, we can readily predict the effects of bethanechol by knowing the information on muscarinic responses summarized in Table 14–2.

The major structures affected by muscarinic activation are the *heart, exocrine glands, smooth muscles,* and *eye.*

Muscarinic agonists act on the heart to cause *bradycardia* (decreased heart rate) and on exocrine glands to increase *sweating, salivation, bronchial secretions,* and *secretion of gastric acid.* In most smooth muscles, muscarinic agonists promote *contraction,* causing *constriction of the bronchi, increased tone and motility of gastrointestinal smooth muscle,* and *contraction of the bladder.* In vascular smooth muscle, these drugs cause *relaxation;* the resultant vasodilation can produce hypotension. Activation of muscarinic receptors in the eye has two effects: (1) *miosis* (pupillary constriction), and (2) *contraction of the ciliary muscle,* resulting in accommodation for near vision. (The ciliary muscle, which is attached to the lens, focuses the eye for near vision by altering lens curvature.)

#### Pharmacokinetics

Bethanechol is administered orally and by SC injection. Following oral drug administration, effects begin in 30 to 60 minutes and persist for approximately 1 hour. With SC injection, effects begin more rapidly (in 5 to 15 minutes).

To produce an equivalent therapeutic response, oral doses of bethanechol must be about 40 times larger than SC doses. As indicated in Figure 15–1, bethanechol is a *quaternary ammonium compound,* and hence always carries a positive charge. This charge greatly impedes absorption across the membranes of the gastrointestinal tract. As a result, only a small fraction of oral bethanechol is absorbed. In contrast, since the barriers to absorption of subcutaneously administered drugs are minimal, bethanechol is readily absorbed following SC injection. These differences in absorption underlie the differences in dosage for the two routes.

#### Therapeutic Uses

Although bethanechol can produce a broad range of pharmacologic effects, its therapeutic uses are limited. The principal indication is urinary retention.

*Urinary Retention.* Bethanechol relieves urinary retention by activating muscarinic receptors of the urinary tract. Muscarinic stimulation increases voiding pressure

121

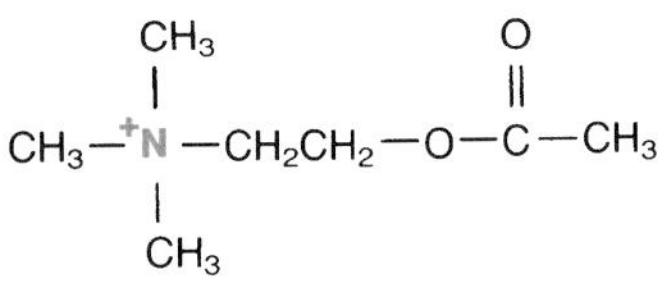

Acetylcholine

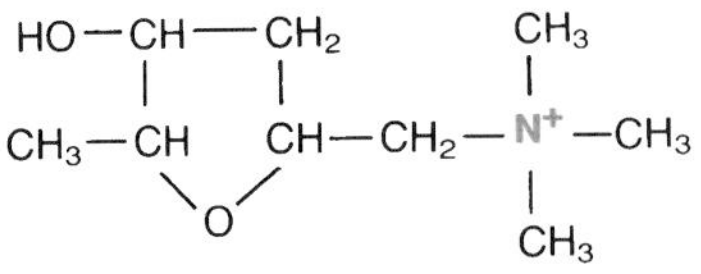

Muscarine

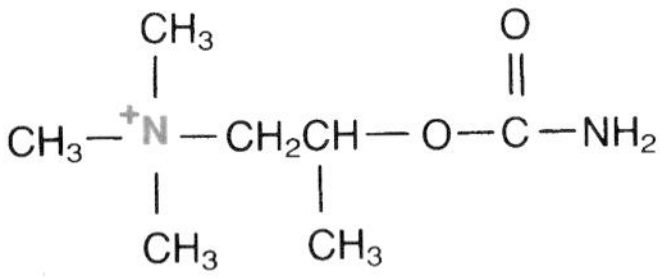

Bethanechol

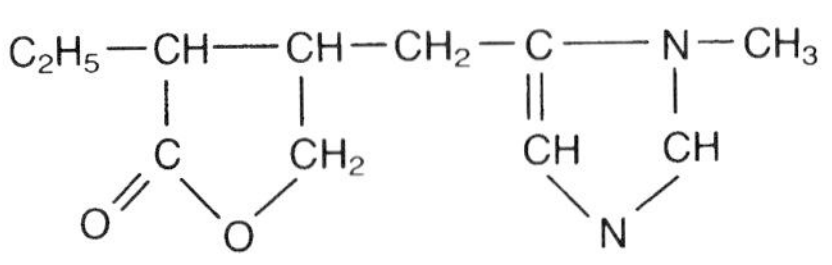

Pilocarpine

**Figure 15–1. Structures of muscarinic agonists.** Note that, with the exception of pilocarpine, all of these agents are quaternary ammonium compounds, and therefore always carry a positive charge. Because of this charge, these compounds cross membranes poorly.

(by contracting the detrusor muscle of the bladder) and relaxes the urinary sphincters. Bethanechol is used to treat urinary retention in postoperative and postpartum patients. The drug should not be used to treat urinary retention caused by physical obstruction of the urinary tract, since increased pressure in the tract in the presence of blockage could cause injury. When patients are treated with bethanechol, a bedpan or urinal should be readily available.

*Gastrointestinal Uses.* Bethanechol has been used on an investigational basis to treat *gastroesophageal reflux.* Benefits may result from increased esophageal motility and increased pressure in the lower esophageal sphincter.

Bethanechol can help treat disorders associated with gastrointestinal paralysis. Benefits derive from increased tone and motility of gastrointestinal smooth muscle. Specific applications are *adynamic ileus, gastric atony,* and *postoperative abdominal distention.* Bethanechol should not be given if physical obstruction of the gastrointestinal tract is present, since, in the presence of blockage, increased propulsive contractions might result in damage to the intestinal wall.

## Adverse Effects

In theory, bethanechol can produce the full range of muscarinic responses as side effects. However, in actual practice, side effects are relatively rare, and their incidence depends on the route of administration. With oral administration, side effects are uncommon. In contrast, when bethanechol is given *subcutaneously,* the incidence of side effects is relatively high.

*Cardiovascular System.* Bethanechol can cause *hypotension* (secondary to vasodilation) and *bradycardia.* Accordingly, the drug is contraindicated for patients with low blood pressure or low cardiac output.

*Alimentary System.* At usual therapeutic doses, bethanechol can cause *excessive salivation, increased secretion of gastric acid, abdominal cramps,* and *diarrhea.* Higher doses can cause *involuntary defecation.* Bethanechol is contraindicated in patients with gastric ulcers, since stimulation of acid secretion could intensify gastric erosion, causing bleeding and possibly perforation. The drug is also contraindicated for patients with *intestinal obstruction* and for those recovering from *recent surgery of the bowel.* In both cases, the ability of bethanechol to increase the tone and motility of intestinal smooth muscle could result in rupture of the bowel wall.

*Urinary Tract.* Because of its ability to contract the bladder, and thereby increase pressure within the urinary tract, bethanechol can be hazardous to patients with *urinary tract obstruction* or *weakness of the bladder wall.* In both groups of patients, elevation of pressure within the urinary tract could rupture the bladder. Accordingly, bethanechol is contraindicated for patients with either disorder.

*Exacerbation of Asthma.* By stimulating muscarinic receptors in the lungs, bethanechol can cause bronchoconstriction. Accordingly, *the drug is contraindicated for patients with latent or active asthma.*

*Dysrhythmias in Hyperthyroid Patients.* Bethanechol can cause *dysrhythmias* in hyperthyroid patients. Accordingly, the drug is contraindicated for these people. The mechanism of dysrhythmia induction is explained below.

If given to hyperthyroid patients, bethanechol may increase heart rate to the point of initiating a dysrhythmia. (Note that increased heart rate is opposite to the effect that muscarinic agonists have on most patients.) When hyperthyroid patients are given bethanechol, their initial cardiovascular responses are like those of anyone else: bradycardia and hypotension. In reaction to hypotension, the baroreceptor reflex attempts to return blood pressure to normal. Part of this reflex involves the release of increased amounts of norepinephrine from the sympathetic nerves that regulate heart rate. In patients who are not hyperthyroid, this increase in norepinephrine release serves to increase cardiac output, and thereby helps restore blood pressure. However, in hyperthyroid patients, increased amounts of norepinephrine can induce cardiac dysrhythmias. The reason for this unusual response is that in hyperthyroid patients the heart is exquisitely sensitive to the effects of norepinephrine; hence, relatively small amounts of norepinephrine can cause stimulation sufficient to elicit a dysrhythmia.

### Preparations, Dosage, and Administration

*Preparations.* Bethanechol [Urecholine, Duvoid, Myotonachol] is available in tablets (5, 10, 25, and 50 mg) and as an injection (5 mg/ml).

*Dosage and Administration.* Oral. Adult dosages range from 10 to 50 mg 3 to 4 times a day. Administration with meals can cause nausea and vomiting. To avoid this problem, oral doses should be administered 1 hour before meals or 2 hours after.

Subcutaneous. The usual adult dosing schedule is 5 mg administered up to 4 times a day. (Note that this dosage is significantly lower than the oral dosage.) The injectable form of bethanechol is intended for *subcutaneous* administration only. *Bethanechol must never be injected intramuscularly or intravenously,* since the resulting high drug levels can cause severe toxicity (bloody diarrhea, bradycardia, profound hypotension, cardiovascular collapse).

### Other Muscarinic Agonists

#### Pilocarpine

Pilocarpine is a muscarinic agonist used only for glaucoma, an ophthalmic disorder characterized by elevated intraocular pressure with subsequent injury to the optic nerve. The basic pharmacology of pilocarpine and its use in glaucoma are discussed in Chapter 97 (Drugs for the Eye).

#### Acetylcholine

Clinical use of acetylcholine is restricted to dilation of the pupil in ophthalmic surgery. Two factors explain the limited utility of this drug. First, acetylcholine lacks selectivity: in addition to stimulating muscarinic cholinergic receptors, acetylcholine can also stimulate all nicotinic cholinergic receptors. Second, because of rapid destruction by cholinesterases, acetylcholine has a half-life that is extremely short—too short for most clinical applications.

#### Muscarine

Although muscarine is not used clinically, this agent has historic and toxicologic significance. Muscarine is of historic interest because of the role it played in the discovery of cholinergic receptor subtypes. The drug has toxicologic significance because of its presence in certain poisonous mushrooms.

## Toxicology of Muscarinic Agonists

*Sources of Muscarinic Poisoning.* Muscarinic poisoning can result from ingestion of certain mushrooms and from overdosage with two kinds of medications: (1) direct-acting muscarinic agonists (bethanechol, pilocarpine), and (2) cholinesterase inhibitors (see Chapter 16).

Of the mushrooms that cause poisoning, only a few do so through muscarinic stimulation. Mushrooms of the *Inocybe* and *Clitocybe* species have especially high concentrations of muscarine, and ingestion of these mushrooms can produce typical signs of muscarinic toxicity. Interestingly, *Amanita muscaria*, the mushroom from which muscarine was originally extracted, actually contains very little muscarine; poisoning by this mushroom is due to toxins other than muscarinic agonists.

*Symptoms.* Manifestations of muscarinic poisoning result from excessive stimulation of muscarinic receptors. Prominent symptoms are profuse salivation, lacrimation (tearing), visual disturbances, bronchospasm, diarrhea, bradycardia, and hypotension. Severe poisoning can produce cardiovascular collapse.

*Treatment.* Management is direct and specific: administer *atropine* (a selective muscarinic blocking agent) and provide supportive therapy. By blocking access of muscarinic agonists to their receptors, atropine can reverse most signs of toxicity.

## Muscarinic Antagonists

Muscarinic antagonists are drugs that competitively block the actions of acetylcholine at muscarinic receptors. Because the majority of muscarinic receptors are located on structures innervated by parasympathetic nerves, the muscarinic antagonists are also known as *parasympatholytic drugs.* Additional names for these agents are *antimuscarinic drugs, muscarinic blockers,* and *anticholinergic drugs.*

The term *anticholinergic* can be a source of confusion and requires comment. This term is unfortunate in that it implies blockade at *all* cholinergic receptors. However, as normally used, the term anticholinergic only indicates blockade of *muscarinic* receptors. Therefore, when a drug is described as being anticholinergic, you can take this to mean that the drug produces selective muscarinic blockade—and not blockade of all other cholinergic receptors.

## Atropine

Atropine is the best known muscarinic antagonist and will serve as our prototype for the group. The actions of all other muscarinic antagonists are qualitatively similar to those of this drug.

Atropine is found naturally in a variety of plants, including *Atropa belladonna* (deadly nightshade) and *Datura stramonium* (also known as Jimson weed, stinkweed, and devil's apple). Because of its presence in *A. belladonna,* atropine is referred to as a *belladonna alkaloid.*

### Mechanism of Action

Atropine produces its effects through competitive blockade at muscarinic receptors. Like all other receptor antagonists, atropine has no *direct* effects of its own. Rather, all responses to atropine result from *preventing receptor activation* by endogenous acetylcholine (or by drugs that act as muscarinic agonists).

At therapeutic doses, atropine produces selective blockade of muscarinic cholinergic receptors. However, if the dosage is sufficiently high, the drug will produce some blockade of nicotinic receptors as well.

### Pharmacologic Effects

Since atropine acts by causing muscarinic receptor blockade, its effects are opposite to those caused by muscarinic activation. Accordingly, we can readily predict the effects of atropine by knowing the normal responses to muscarinic receptor activation (see Table 14-2) and by knowing that atropine will reverse those responses. Like the muscarinic agonists, the muscarinic antagonists exert their influence primarily on the *heart, exocrine glands, smooth muscles,* and *eye.*

*Heart.* Atropine *increases heart rate.* Since stimulation of cardiac muscarinic receptors decreases heart rate, *blockade* of these receptors with atropine will cause heart rate to increase.

*Exocrine Glands.* Atropine *decreases secretion* from salivary glands, bronchial glands, sweat glands, and the acid-secreting cells of the stomach. Note that these effects are opposite to those of muscarinic agonists, which increase secretion from exocrine glands.

*Smooth Muscle.* By preventing activation of muscarinic receptors on smooth muscle, atropine causes re-

*laxation of the bronchi, decreased tone of the urinary bladder,* and *decreased tone and motility of the gastrointestinal tract.* In the absence of an exogenous muscarinic agonist (e.g., bethanechol), muscarinic blockade has no effect on vascular smooth muscle tone; this is because there is no parasympathetic innervation of these receptors.

**Eye.** Blockade of muscarinic receptors on the iris sphincter causes *mydriasis* (dilation of the pupil). Blockade of muscarinic receptors on the ciliary muscle produces *cycloplegia* (relaxation of the ciliary muscle), thereby focusing the lens for far vision.

**Central Nervous System (CNS).** At therapeutic doses, atropine can cause mild CNS *excitation.* Toxic doses can cause *hallucinations* and *delirium,* which can resemble psychosis. Extremely high doses can result in coma, respiratory arrest, and death.

**Dose Dependency of Muscarinic Blockade.** It is important to note that not all muscarinic receptors are equally sensitive to blockade by atropine and most other muscarinic antagonists: at some sites, muscarinic receptors can be blocked with relatively low doses, whereas at other sites much higher doses are needed. Table 15–1 indicates the order in which specific muscarinic receptors will be blocked as the dose of atropine is increased.

Differences in receptor sensitivity to muscarinic blockers are of clinical significance. As indicated in Table 15–1, the doses needed to block muscarinic receptors in the stomach and bronchial smooth muscle are higher than the doses needed to block muscarinic receptors at all other locations. Accordingly, if we want to use atropine to treat peptic ulcer disease (by suppressing gastric acid secretion) or asthma (by dilating the bronchi), we cannot do so without also affecting the heart, exocrine glands, many smooth muscles, and the eye. Because of these obligatory side effects, atropine and most other muscarinic antagonists are not preferred drugs for treating peptic ulcers or asthma.

## TABLE 15-1. RELATIONSHIP BETWEEN DOSAGE AND RESPONSES TO ATROPINE

| Dosage of Atropine | Response Produced |
| --- | --- |
| Low Doses | Salivary glands—decreased secretion<br>Sweat glands—decreased secretion<br>Bronchial glands—decreased secretion |
| | Heart—increased rate<br>Eye—mydriasis, blurred vision |
| | Urinary tract—interference with voiding<br>Intestine—decreased tone and motility<br>Lung—dilation of bronchi |
| High Doses | Stomach—decreased acid secretion |

Note that doses of atropine that are high enough to decrease gastric acid secretion or dilate the bronchi will also affect all other structures under muscarinic control. As a result, atropine and most other muscarinic antagonists are not very desirable for treating peptic ulcer disease or asthma.

## Pharmacokinetics

Atropine may be administered orally, topically (to the eye), and by injection (IM, SC, and IV). The drug is rapidly absorbed following oral administration and distributes to all tissues, including the CNS. Elimination is by a combination of hepatic metabolism and urinary excretion. Atropine has a half-life of approximately 3 hours.

## Therapeutic Uses

**Preanesthetic Medication.** The cardiac effects of atropine can be helpful during surgery. Procedures that stimulate baroreceptors of the carotid body can initiate reflex slowing of the heart, resulting in profound bradycardia. Since this reflex is mediated by muscarinic receptors on the heart, pretreatment with atropine can prevent dangerous reductions in heart rate.

Certain anesthetics—especially ether, which is obsolete—irritate the respiratory tract, and thereby stimulate secretion from salivary, nasal, pharyngeal, and bronchial glands. If these secretions are sufficiently profuse, they can interfere with respiration. By blocking muscarinic receptors on secretory glands, atropine can help prevent excessive secretions. Fortunately, modern anesthetics are much less irritating than ether. The availability of these new anesthetics has greatly reduced the use of atropine as an antisecretagogue during anesthesia.

**Disorders of the Eye.** By blocking muscarinic receptors in the eye, atropine can cause mydriasis and paralysis of the ciliary muscle. Both actions can be helpful during eye examinations and ocular surgery. The ophthalmic uses of atropine and other muscarinic antagonists are discussed in Chapter 97.

**Bradycardia.** Atropine can accelerate heart rate in certain patients with bradycardia. Heart rate is increased because blockade of cardiac muscarinic receptors prevents the parasympathetic nervous system from slowing the heart.

**Biliary Colic.** Biliary colic is characterized by intense abdominal pain brought on by passage of a gallstone through the bile duct. This pain is usually treated with morphine. In some cases, atropine may be combined with morphine to relax biliary tract smooth muscle, thereby helping alleviate discomfort.

**Intestinal Hypertonicity and Hypermotility.** By blocking muscarinic receptors in the intestine, atropine can decrease both the tone and motility of intestinal smooth muscle. This action can be beneficial in conditions characterized by excessive intestinal motility, such as mild dysentery and diverticulitis. When taken for these disorders, atropine can reduce both the frequency of bowel movements and associated abdominal cramps.

**Muscarinic Agonist Poisoning.** Atropine is a specific antidote to poisoning by agents that activate muscarinic receptors. By blocking muscarinic receptors, atropine can reverse all signs of muscarinic poisoning. As discussed above, muscarinic poisoning can result from an overdose with medications that promote muscarinic activation (e.g., bethanechol, cholinesterase inhibitors) and from ingestion of certain mushrooms.

**Peptic Ulcer Disease.** Because it can suppress secretion of gastric acid, atropine has been used to treat peptic ulcer disease. Unfortunately, when administered in doses that are strong enough to block the muscarinic receptors that regulate secretion of gastric acid, atropine also blocks most other muscarinic receptors. Hence, treatment of ulcers is necessarily associated with a broad range of antimuscarinic side effects (dry mouth, blurred vision, urinary retention, constipation, and so forth). Because of these side effects, atropine is not a first-choice drug for ulcer therapy. Rather, atropine is reserved for those cases in which symptoms cannot be relieved with preferred medications (e.g., antibiotics, histamine$_2$ receptor antagonists, sucralfate).

*Asthma.* By blocking bronchial muscarinic receptors, atropine can promote bronchial dilation, thereby improving respiration in patients with asthma. Unfortunately, in addition to dilating the bronchi, atropine also causes drying and thickening of bronchial secretions, effects that can be harmful to the patient. Furthermore, when given in the doses needed to dilate the bronchi, atropine causes a variety of antimuscarinic side effects. Because of the potential for harm, and because superior medicines are available, atropine has a very limited role in asthma therapy.

## Adverse Effects

Most side effects of atropine and other muscarinic antagonists are the direct result of muscarinic receptor blockade. Accordingly, they can be predicted from your knowledge of muscarinic receptor function.

*Dry Mouth (Xerostomia).* Blockade of muscarinic receptors on salivary glands can inhibit salivation to such an extent that the mouth becomes dry. Not only is this uncomfortable, it can impede swallowing. Patients should be informed that dryness can be alleviated by chewing gum, sucking on hard candy, and sipping fluids.

*Blurred Vision and Photophobia.* Blockade of muscarinic receptors on the ciliary muscle and the sphincter of the iris can paralyze both muscles. Paralysis of the ciliary muscle focuses the eye for far vision, causing nearby objects to appear blurred. Patients should be forewarned about this effect and advised to avoid hazardous activities if their vision is significantly impaired.

Paralysis of the iris sphincter prevents constriction of the pupil, thereby rendering the eye unable to adapt to bright light. Patients should be advised to wear dark glasses if photophobia (intolerance to light) is a problem. Room lighting for hospitalized patients should be kept low.

*Elevation of Intraocular Pressure.* Paralysis of the iris sphincter can cause intraocular pressure (IOP) to rise. The mechanism of this effect is discussed in Chapter 97 (Drugs for the Eye). Because they can raise IOP, muscarinic blockers are contraindicated for patients with glaucoma, a disease characterized by abnormally high IOP. In addition, antimuscarinic drugs should be used with caution in patients who may not have glaucoma per se but for whom a predisposition to glaucoma may be present; included in this group are all individuals older than 40.

*Urinary Retention.* Blockade of muscarinic receptors in the urinary tract reduces pressure within the bladder and increases the tone of the urinary sphincter. These effects can produce urinary hesitancy or urinary retention. In the event of severe urinary retention, catheterization or treatment with a muscarinic agonist (e.g., bethanechol) may be required. Patients should be advised that urinary retention can be minimized by voiding just prior to taking their medication.

*Constipation.* Muscarinic blockade decreases the tone and motility of intestinal smooth muscle. The resultant delay in transit through the intestine can produce constipation. Patients should be informed that constipation can be minimized by increasing dietary fluids and fiber. A laxative may be needed if constipation is severe. Because of their ability to decrease smooth muscle tone, muscarinic antagonists are contraindicated for patients with intestinal atony, a condition in which intestinal tone is already low.

*Anhidrosis.* Blockade of muscarinic receptors on sweat glands can produce anhidrosis (a deficiency or absence of sweat). Since sweating is necessary for cooling the body, patients who cannot sweat are at risk of hyperthermia. Patients should be warned of this possibility and advised to avoid activities that might lead to overheating (e.g., exercising on a hot day).

*Tachycardia.* Blockade of cardiac muscarinic receptors eliminates the parasympathetic influence on the heart. By removing the "braking" influence of parasympathetic nerves, muscarinic antagonists can cause tachycardia (excessive heart rate). Caution must be exercised in patients with preexisting tachycardia.

*Asthma.* Administration of antimuscarinic drugs to patients with asthma can cause thickening and drying of bronchial secretions, which can result in bronchial plugging. Consequently, although muscarinic antagonists can be used to treat asthma, they can also be harmful.

## Drug Interactions

A number of drugs that are not classified as muscarinic antagonists can nonetheless produce significant muscarinic blockade. These drugs include *antihistamines, phenothiazine antipsychotics,* and *tricyclic antidepressants.* Because of their prominent antimuscarinic actions, these drugs can greatly enhance the antimuscarinic effects of atropine and related agents. Accordingly, it is wise to avoid combined use of atropine with other drugs capable of causing muscarinic blockade.

### Preparations, Dosage, and Administration

Atropine sulfate is dispensed in oral tablets (0.4 and 0.6 mg); as an ointment or solution for ophthalmic use; and in solution for SC, IM, and IV injection. The average systemic dose for adults is 0.5 mg.

## Other Muscarinic Antagonists

*Scopolamine.* Scopolamine is a muscarinic antagonist with actions much like those of atropine, but with two exceptions: (1) whereas therapeutic doses of atropine produce mild CNS excitation, therapeutic doses of scopolamine produce sedation, and (2) scopolamine *suppresses emesis and motion sickness,* whereas atropine does not. Principal uses for scopolamine are motion sickness (see Chapter 73), production of cycloplegia and mydriasis for ophthalmic procedures (see Chapter 97), and production of preanesthetic sedation and obstetric amnesia.

*Ipratropium Bromide.* Ipratropium [Atrovent] is an antimuscarinic drug used to treat asthma and chronic obstructive pulmonary disease. The drug is administered by inhalation, and systemic absorption is minimal. As a result, therapy is not associated with typical antimuscarinic side effects (dry mouth, blurred vision, urinary hesitancy, constipation, and so forth). The pharmacology and applications of ipratropium are discussed fully in Chapter 69.

**Pirenzepine and Telenzepine.** These drugs produce selective blockade of $M_1$-muscarinic receptors—the subtype of muscarinic receptor involved in regulating the secretion of gastric acid. Both drugs can effectively suppress acid secretion in patients with peptic ulcer disease, but neither is currently available in the United States. Because these drugs are selective blockers of $M_1$-muscarinic receptors, the incidence of dry mouth, blurred vision, and other typical antimuscarinic side effects is minimal.

**Dicyclomine.** This drug is indicated for irritable bowel syndrome (spastic colon, mucous colitis) and functional bowel disorders (diarrhea, hypermotility). Administration may be oral (40 mg 4 times a day) or by IM injection (20 mg 4 times a day). Dicyclomine has many trade names, including Bentyl, Byclomine, Di-Spaz, and Antispas.

**Centrally Acting Anticholinergics.** Several anticholinergic drugs, including *trihexyphenidyl* [Artane] and *benzatropine* [Cogentin], are employed to treat Parkinson's disease and drug-induced parkinsonism. Benefits derive from blockade of muscarinic receptors in the CNS. The centrally acting anticholinergics and their use in parkinsonism are discussed in Chapter 22.

**Mydriatic Cycloplegics.** Five muscarinic antagonists—*atropine, homatropine, scopolamine, cyclopentolate,* and *tropicamide*—are employed to produce mydriasis and cycloplegia in ophthalmic procedures. These applications are discussed in Chapter 97.

**Antisecretory Anticholinergics.** A number of muscarinic blockers are available for suppressing gastric acid secretion in patients with peptic ulcer disease. However, since superior antiulcer drugs are available, and since the anticholinergic agents produce significant side effects (dry mouth, blurred vision, urinary retention, and so forth), these drugs are used only rarely. Trade names and dosages for the antisecretory anticholinergics are summarized in Table 15-2. All of these agents are administered orally, and one—glycopyrrolate—may also be administered IM and IV.

## Toxicology of Muscarinic Antagonists

**Sources of Antimuscarinic Poisoning.** Sources of poisoning include natural products (e.g., *Atropa belladonna, Datura stramonium*); selective antimuscarinic drugs (e.g., atropine, scopolamine); and other drugs with pronounced antimuscarinic properties (e.g., antihistamines, phenothiazines, tricyclic antidepressants).

### TABLE 15-2. ANTISECRETORY ANTICHOLINERGICS

| Generic Names | Trade Names | Usual Adult Dose (mg) |
|---|---|---|
| Anisotropine | Valpin 50 | 50 |
| Clidinium | Quarzan | 2.5-5 |
| Glycopyrrolate | Robinul | 1-2 |
| Hexocyclium | Tral Filmtabs | 25 |
| Isopropamide | Darbid | 5-10 |
| Mepenzolate | Cantil | 25-50 |
| Methantheline | Banthine | 1-2 |
| Methscopolamine | Pamine | 2.5-5 |
| Oxyphencyclimine | Daricon | 1-2 |
| Propantheline | Pro-Banthine | 7.5-15 |
| Tridihexethyl chloride | Pathilon | 25-50 |

**Symptoms.** Symptoms of antimuscarinic poisoning, which are the direct result of excessive muscarinic blockade, include dry mouth, blurred vision, photophobia, hyperthermia, CNS effects (hallucinations, delirium), and skin that is hot, dry, and flushed. Death results from respiratory depression secondary to blockade of cholinergic receptors in the brain.

**Treatment.** Treatment consists of (1) minimizing absorption of the antimuscarinic agent and (2) administering an antidote. Absorption can be reduced by giving syrup of ipecac followed by activated charcoal. The ipecac induces vomiting, thereby removing unabsorbed poison from the stomach. The charcoal adsorbs poison within the intestine, thereby preventing its absorption into the blood.

The most effective antidote to antimuscarinic poisoning is *physostigmine,* an inhibitor of acetylcholinesterase. By inhibiting cholinesterase, physostigmine causes acetylcholine to accumulate at all cholinergic junctions. As acetylcholine builds up, it competes with the antimuscarinic agent for receptor binding, thereby reversing excessive muscarinic blockade. The pharmacology of physostigmine is discussed in Chapter 16 (Cholinesterase Inhibitors).

**Warning.** It is important to differentiate between antimuscarinic poisoning, which often resembles psychosis (hallucinations, delirium), and an actual psychotic episode. Since a true psychotic episode is not ordinarily associated with signs of excessive muscarinic blockade (dry mouth, hyperthermia, dry skin, and so forth), differentiating is not usually difficult. We need to make the differential diagnosis because antipsychotic drugs, which have antimuscarinic properties of their own, will intensify symptoms if given to a victim of antimuscarinic poisoning.

## KEY POINTS

- Muscarinic agonists work through direct activation of muscarinic cholinergic receptors, thereby causing bradycardia; increased secretion from sweat, salivary, bronchial, and gastric glands; contraction of intestinal, bronchial, and urinary tract smooth muscle; and, in the eye, miosis and accommodation for near vision.
- Bethanechol, the prototype of the muscarinic agonists, is used primarily to relieve urinary retention.
- Subcutaneous doses of bethanechol are 40 times smaller than oral doses.
- Muscarinic agonist poisoning is characterized by profuse salivation, tearing, visual disturbances, bronchospasm, diarrhea, bradycardia, and hypotension.
- Muscarinic agonist poisoning is treated with atropine.
- Atropine, the prototype of the muscarinic antagonists, blocks the actions of acetylcholine at muscarinic cholinergic receptors, and thereby (1) increases heart rate; (2) reduces secretion from sweat, salivary, bronchial, and gastric glands; (3) relaxes intestinal, bronchial, and urinary tract smooth muscle; (4) acts in the eye to cause mydriasis and cycloplegia; and (5) acts in the CNS to produce excitation (at low doses) and delirium and hallucinations (at toxic doses).

- Important uses of muscarinic antagonists include preanesthetic medication, ophthalmic examinations, reversal of bradycardia, and treatment of muscarinic agonist poisoning.
- Classic adverse effects of muscarinic antagonists are dry mouth, blurred vision, photophobia, tachycardia, urinary retention, constipation, and suppression of sweating.
- Certain drugs—especially antihistamines, tricyclic antidepressants, and phenothiazine antipsychotics—have prominent antimuscarinic actions. These should be used cautiously, if at all, in patients taking atropine and other muscarinic antagonists.
- Muscarinic antagonist poisoning is characterized by dry mouth, blurred vision, photophobia, hyperthermia, hallucinations and delirium, and skin that is hot, dry, and flushed.
- The best antidote for muscarinic antagonist poisoning is physostigmine, an inhibitor of acetylcholinesterase.

# Summary of Major Nursing Implications*

## Bethanechol

### Preadministration Assessment

#### Therapeutic Goal
Treatment of nonobstructive urinary retention.

#### Baseline Data
Record fluid intake and output.

#### Identifying High-Risk Patients
Bethanechol is *contraindicated* for patients with *peptic ulcer disease, urinary tract obstruction, intestinal obstruction, coronary insufficiency, hypotension, asthma,* and *hyperthyroidism.*

### Implementation: Administration

#### Routes
Oral, SC
*Never administer IM or IV!*

#### Administration
**Oral.** Advise patients to take 1 hour before meals or 2 hours after to reduce gastric upset.

**Subcutaneous.** Subcutaneous doses are much smaller than oral doses. Check SC doses carefully.

**Both Routes.** Since effects on the intestine and urinary tract can be rapid and dramatic, ensure that a bedpan or bathroom is readily accessible.

### Ongoing Evaluation and Interventions

#### Evaluating Therapeutic Effects
Monitor fluid intake and output to evaluate treatment of urinary retention.

#### Minimizing Adverse Effects
Excessive muscarinic stimulation can cause salivation, sweating, urinary urgency, bradycardia, and hypotension. Monitor blood pressure and pulse rate. Observe for signs of muscarinic excess and report these to the physician.

Inform patients about manifestations of muscarinic excess and advise them to notify the nurse or physician if these occur.

### Management of Acute Toxicity
Overdose produces manifestations of excessive muscarinic stimulation (salivation, sweating, involuntary urination and defecation, bradycardia, severe hypotension). Treat with supportive measures and atropine (SC or IV).

## Atropine and Other Muscarinic Antagonists

### Preadministration Assessment

#### Therapeutic Goal
*Atropine* has many applications, including *preanesthetic medication* and treatment of *bradycardia, biliary colic, intestinal hypertonicity and hypermotility,* and *muscarinic agonist poisoning.*

#### Identifying High-Risk Patients
Atropine and other muscarinic antagonists are *contraindicated* for patients with *glaucoma, intestinal atony, urinary tract obstruction,* and *tachycardia.* Use with *caution* in patients with *asthma.*

### Implementation: Administration

#### Routes
*Atropine* is administered PO, IV, IM, and SC.

#### Administration
Dry mouth from muscarinic blockade may interfere with swallowing. Advise the patient to moisten the mouth by sipping water prior to oral administration.

### Ongoing Evaluation and Interventions

#### Minimizing Adverse Effects
**Dry Mouth (Xerostomia).** Decreased salivation can dry the mouth. Teach the patient that xerostomia can be relieved by chewing gum, sucking on hard candy, and sipping fluids.

---

*Patient education information is highlighted in color.

**Blurred Vision.** Paralysis of the ciliary muscle may reduce visual acuity. Warn the patient against participation in hazardous activities if vision is impaired.

**Photophobia.** Muscarinic blockade prevents the pupil from constricting in response to bright light. Keep hospital room lighting low to reduce visual discomfort. Advise the patient to wear sunglasses outdoors.

**Urinary Retention.** Muscarinic blockade in the bladder and urinary sphincter can cause urinary hesitancy or retention. Advise the patient that urinary retention can be minimized by voiding just prior to taking anticholinergic medication. If urinary retention is severe, catheterization or treatment with bethanechol (a muscarinic agonist) may be required.

**Constipation.** Reduced tone and motility of the gut may cause constipation. Advise the patient that constipation can be reduced by increasing dietary fiber and fluids. A laxative may be needed if constipation is severe.

**Hyperthermia.** Suppression of sweating may result in hyperthermia. Advise the patient to avoid vigorous exercise in warm environments.

**Tachycardia.** Blockade of cardiac muscarinic receptors can accelerate heart rate. Monitor pulse rate and report significant increases.

## Minimizing Adverse Interactions

*Antihistamines, tricyclic antidepressants,* and *phenothiazines* have prominent antimuscarinic actions. Coadministration of these agents with atropine and other muscarinic antagonists can lead to excessive muscarinic blockade.

## Management of Acute Toxicity

**Symptoms.** Overdose produces dry mouth, blurred vision, photophobia, hyperthermia, hallucinations, and delirium; the skin becomes hot, dry, and flushed. Differentiate muscarinic antagonist poisoning from psychosis!

**Treatment.** Treatment centers on removing ingested poison (with syrup of ipecac); adsorbing ingested poison onto activated charcoal; and administering *physostigmine,* an inhibitor of acetylcholinesterase.

# CHAPTER 16

# Cholinesterase Inhibitors

Reversible Cholinesterase Inhibitors
Neostigmine
Physostigmine
Other Reversible Cholinesterase Inhibitors
Treatment of Myasthenia Gravis

"Irreversible" Cholinesterase Inhibitors
Basic Pharmacology
Toxicology

Cholinesterase inhibitors are drugs that prevent the degradation of acetylcholine (ACh) by acetylcholinesterase (cholinesterase). By preventing the inactivation of ACh, the cholinesterase inhibitors enhance the actions of ACh released from cholinergic nerves. Hence, the cholinesterase inhibitors can be looked upon as indirect-acting cholinergic agonists. Since cholinesterase inhibitors can intensify transmission at all cholinergic junctions (muscarinic, ganglionic, and neuromuscular), these drugs can elicit a wide variety of responses. Because of this relative lack of selectivity, the cholinesterase inhibitors have limited therapeutic applications. An alternative name for the cholinesterase inhibitors is *anticholinesterase agents*.

There are two basic categories of cholinesterase inhibitors: (1) *reversible inhibitors* and (2) *"irreversible" inhibitors*. The reversible inhibitors produce effects of moderate duration. In contrast, the irreversible inhibitors produce effects that are prolonged.

## Reversible Cholinesterase Inhibitors

### Neostigmine

Neostigmine [Prostigmin] typifies the reversible cholinesterase inhibitors and will serve as our prototype for the group. The principal indication for neostigmine is *myasthenia gravis*.

#### Chemistry

As indicated in Figure 16–1, neostigmine contains a quaternary nitrogen atom, and therefore always carries a positive charge. Because of this charge, neostigmine cannot readily cross membranes, including those of the gastrointestinal tract, the blood-brain barrier, and the placenta. Consequently, neostigmine is absorbed poorly following oral administration and has minimal effects on the brain and the developing fetus.

#### Mechanism of Action

Neostigmine and the other reversible cholinesterase inhibitors can be envisioned as poor substrates for cholinesterase (ChE). As indicated in Figure 16–2, the normal function of ChE is to break down acetylcholine into choline and acetic acid. This process is termed a *hydrolysis* reaction because of the water molecule involved. As depicted in Figure 16–3A, hydrolysis of ACh takes place in two steps: (1) binding of ACh to the active center of ChE, followed by (2) splitting of ACh, which regenerates free ChE. The overall reaction between ACh and ChE is extremely fast. As a result, one molecule of ChE can break down a huge amount of ACh in a very short time.

As depicted in Figure 16–3B, the reaction between neostigmine and ChE is very similar to the reaction between ACh and ChE. The difference between the two reactions is simply that the splitting of neostigmine by ChE occurs more *slowly* than the splitting of ACh. Hence, once neostigmine becomes bound to the active center of ChE, the drug remains in place for a relatively long time, thereby preventing ChE from catalyzing the breakdown of ACh. ChE remains inhibited until it finally succeeds in splitting off neostigmine.

#### Pharmacologic Effects

By preventing inactivation of ACh, neostigmine and the other cholinesterase inhibitors can intensify transmission at virtually all junctions where ACh is the transmitter. In sufficient doses, the cholinesterase inhibitors can produce skeletal muscle stimulation, activation of muscarinic receptors, ganglionic stimulation, and activation of cholinergic receptors in the central nervous system (CNS). However, when used *therapeutically*, the cholinesterase inhibitors usually affect only muscarinic receptors and nicotinic receptors of the neuromuscular junction. Ganglionic transmission and CNS function are usually unaltered.

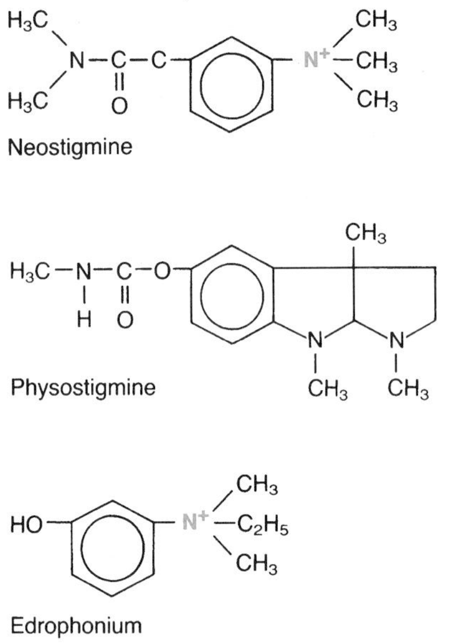

**Figure 16–1. Structural formulas of reversible cholinesterase inhibitors.** Note that neostigmine and edrophonium are quaternary ammonium compounds, but physostigmine is not. What does this difference imply about the relative abilities of these drugs to cross membranes, including the blood-brain barrier?

*Muscarinic Responses.* Muscarinic effects of the cholinesterase inhibitors are identical to those of the direct-acting muscarinic agonists. By preventing breakdown of ACh, cholinesterase inhibitors can cause increased glandular secretions, increased tone and motility of gastrointestinal smooth muscle, bradycardia, urinary urgency, bronchial constriction, miosis, and focusing of the lens for near vision.

*Neuromuscular Effects.* The effects of cholinesterase inhibitors on skeletal muscle are dose dependent. At *therapeutic* doses, these drugs *increase* force of contraction. In contrast, *toxic* doses *reduce* force of contraction. Contractile force is reduced because excessive amounts of ACh at the neuromuscular junction (NMJ) keep the motor end-plate in a state of constant depolarization, thereby causing depolarizing neuromuscular blockade (see Chapter 17).

*Central Nervous System.* Effects on the CNS vary with drug concentration. Therapeutic drug levels can produce mild *stimulation*, whereas toxic levels *depress* the CNS, including the areas that regulate respiration. However, it must be noted that, for CNS effects to occur, the inhibitor must first penetrate the blood-brain barrier; some cholinesterase inhibitors can do this only when present in very high concentrations.

## Pharmacokinetics

Neostigmine may be administered orally or by injection (SC, IM, or IV). Because neostigmine carries a positive charge, the drug is poorly absorbed following oral administration. Hence, oral doses must be much greater than parenteral doses to produce equivalent effects. Once absorbed, neostigmine can reach sites of action at the NMJ and at peripheral muscarinic receptors, but cannot cross the blood-brain barrier to produce effects within the CNS. Duration of action is 2 to 4 hours. Neostigmine is eliminated by enzymatic degradation: cholinesterase, the enzyme that neostigmine inhibits, eventually converts neostigmine itself into an inactive product.

## Therapeutic Uses

*Myasthenia Gravis.* Myasthenia gravis is a major indication for neostigmine and several other reversible cholinesterase inhibitors. Treatment of myasthenia is discussed separately later.

*Reversal of Nondepolarizing Neuromuscular Blockade.* By causing accumulation of ACh at the NMJ, cholinesterase inhibitors can reverse the effects of nondepolarizing neuromuscular blocking agents (e.g., tubocurarine). This ability has two clinical applications: (1) reversal of neuromuscular blockade in postoperative patients and (2) treatment of overdosage with nondepolarizing neuromuscular blockers. When neostigmine is used to treat neuromuscular blocker overdosage, artificial respiration must be maintained until muscle function has fully recovered. At the doses employed to reverse neuromuscular blockade, neostigmine is likely to elicit substantial muscarinic responses; symptoms of excessive muscarinic stimulation can be reduced with atropine. It is important to note that cholinesterase inhibitors cannot be employed to counteract the effects of succinylcholine, a *depolarizing* neuromuscular blocker.

## Adverse Effects

*Excessive Muscarinic Stimulation.* Accumulation of ACh at muscarinic receptors can result in excessive salivation, increased gastric secretions, increased tone and motility of the gastrointestinal tract, urinary urgency, bradycardia, sweating, miosis, and spasm of accommodation (focusing of the lens for near vision). If necessary, these responses can be suppressed with atropine.

*Neuromuscular Blockade.* If administered in toxic doses, cholinesterase inhibitors can cause accumulation of ACh in amounts sufficient to produce depolarizing neuromuscular blockade. Paralysis of respiratory muscles can be fatal.

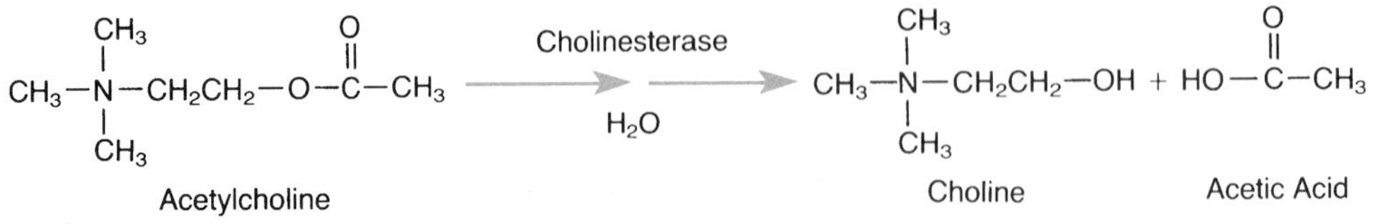

**Figure 16–2. Hydrolysis of acetylcholine by cholinesterase.**

A  REACTION BETWEEN ACh and ChE

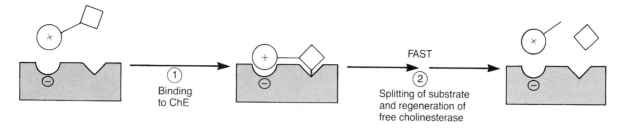

B  REVERSIBLE INHIBITION OF ChE (BY NEOSTIGMINE)

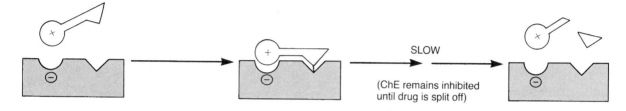

C  "IRREVERSIBLE" INHIBITION OF ChE (BY DFP)

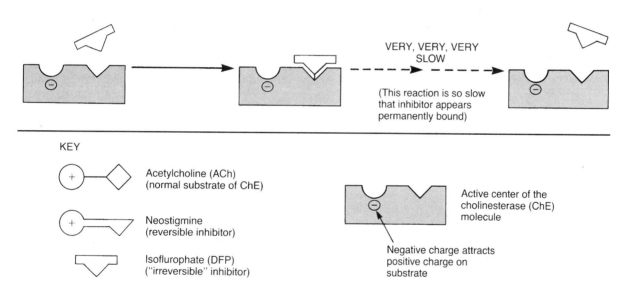

**Figure 16–3. Inhibition of cholinesterase by reversible and "irreversible" inhibitors.**

## Precautions and Contraindications

Most of the precautions and contraindications regarding the cholinesterase inhibitors are the same as those for the direct-acting muscarinic agonists. These include (1) obstruction of the gastrointestinal tract, (2) obstruction of the urinary tract, (3) peptic ulcer disease, (4) asthma, (5) coronary insufficiency, and (6) hyperthyroidism. The rationales underlying these precautions are discussed in Chapter 15. In addition to precautions related to muscarinic stimulation, cholinesterase inhibitors are contraindicated for patients receiving succinylcholine.

## Drug Interactions

***Muscarinic Antagonists.*** The effects of cholinesterase inhibitors at muscarinic receptors are opposite to those of atropine and other muscarinic antagonists. Consequently, cholinesterase inhibitors can be used to overcome excessive muscarinic blockade caused by atropine. Conversely, atropine can be used to reduce excessive muscarinic stimulation caused by cholinesterase inhibitors.

***Nondepolarizing Neuromuscular Blockers.*** By causing accumulation of ACh at the NMJ, cholinesterase inhibitors can reverse muscle relaxation brought on by tubocurarine and other nondepolarizing neuromuscular blocking agents.

***Depolarizing Neuromuscular Blockers.*** Cholinesterase inhibitors do not reverse the muscle-relaxant effects of succinylcholine, a depolarizing neuromuscular blocker. In fact, since cholinesterase inhibitors will decrease the breakdown of succinylcholine by cholinesterase, cholinesterase inhibitors will actually *intensify* neuromuscular blockade caused by succinylcholine.

## Acute Toxicity

*Symptoms.* Overdose with cholinesterase inhibitors causes *excessive muscarinic stimulation* and *respiratory depression*. (Respiratory depression results from a combination of depolarizing neuromuscular blockade and CNS depression.) The state produced by cholinesterase inhibitor poisoning is sometimes referred to as *cholinergic crisis*.

*Treatment.* Intravenous *atropine* will alleviate the muscarinic effects of cholinesterase inhibition. Since respiratory depression from cholinesterase inhibitors cannot be managed with drugs, treatment consists of mechanical ventilation with oxygen. Suctioning may be necessary if atropine fails to suppress bronchial secretions.

### Preparations, Dosage, and Administration

*Preparations.* Neostigmine [Prostigmin] is available as two salts: *neostigmine bromide* (for oral use) and *neostigmine methylsulfate* (for IM, SC, and IV injection). Neostigmine bromide is dispensed in 15-mg tablets. Neostigmine methylsulfate is available in solutions containing 0.25, 0.5, and 1.0 mg/ml.

*Dosage and Administration.* Dosages for *myasthenia gravis* are highly individualized. Oral therapy ranges from 15 to 375 mg/day administered in divided doses every 3 to 4 hours. *It is important to note that oral doses of neostigmine are about 30 times greater than parenteral doses.*

To treat *poisoning by nondepolarizing neuromuscular blockers*, the initial dose is 0.5 to 2.0 mg administered by slow IV injection. Additional doses totaling a maximum of 5 mg may be administered as required.

## Physostigmine

The pharmacology of physostigmine is like that of neostigmine—except for differences related to their ability to cross membranes. As indicated in Figure 16-1, neostigmine is a quaternary ammonium compound and always carries a positive charge. In contrast, physostigmine is not a quaternary ammonium compound and does not carry a charge. Because physostigmine is uncharged, the drug crosses membranes more readily than neostigmine. This ability makes physostigmine superior to neostigmine for some applications.

## Therapeutic Uses

*Treatment of Muscarinic Antagonist Poisoning.* Physostigmine is the drug of choice for treating poisoning by atropine and other drugs that cause muscarinic blockade (e.g., antihistamines, tricyclic antidepressants, phenothiazine antipsychotics). Physostigmine counteracts antimuscarinic poisoning by causing ACh to build up at muscarinic junctions. The accumulated ACh competes with the muscarinic blocker for receptor binding, and thereby reverses the blockade. Physostigmine is preferred to neostigmine for antimuscarinic poisoning because, lacking a charge, physostigmine is able to cross the blood-brain barrier to reverse muscarinic blockade in the CNS.

The usual dosage to reverse antimuscarinic poisoning is 2 mg given by IM or slow IV injection.

*Glaucoma.* Physostigmine and several other cholinesterase inhibitors can lower intraocular pressure in patients with glaucoma. However, superior drugs are available. The role of anticholinesterase agents in treating glaucoma is discussed in Chapter 67 (Drugs for the Eye).

### Other Reversible Cholinesterase Inhibitors

Four cholinesterase inhibitors—*ambenonium*, *demecarium*, *edrophonium*, and *pyridostigmine*—have pharmacologic effects much like those of neostigmine, our prototype for the family. One of these drugs—edrophonium—is noteworthy for its very brief duration of action. Routes of administration and indications for these drugs are summarized in Table 16-1.

Tacrine [Cognex] is a relatively new drug used for Alzheimer's disease. Benefits derive from inhibiting cholinesterase in the CNS. Tacrine is discussed fully in Chapter 34.

## Treatment of Myasthenia Gravis

*Pathophysiology.* Myasthenia gravis is a disease characterized by muscle weakness and a predisposition to rapid fatigue. Common symptoms include ptosis (drooping eyelids) and difficulty with swallowing. Patients with severe myasthenia may have difficulty breathing due to weakness of the muscles of respiration.

The symptoms of myasthenia gravis are caused by an autoimmune process in which the patient's immune system produces antibodies directed against nicotinic$_M$ receptors on skeletal muscle. As a result of attack by these antibodies, the number of receptors at the neuromuscular junction is reduced by 70% to 90%, resulting in the muscle weakness that characterizes myasthenia.

*Treatment.* Reversible cholinesterase inhibitors (e.g., neostigmine) are the mainstay of myasthenia therapy. By preventing ACh inactivation, anticholinesterase agents can intensify the effects of ACh released from motor neurons, and can thereby increase muscle strength. Cholinesterase inhibitors do not cure myasthenia; these drugs only produce symptomatic relief. Consequently, patients are likely to need therapy lifelong.

When working with the hospitalized myasthenic patient, keep in mind that muscle strength may be insufficient to permit swallowing. Accordingly, you should assess the patient's ability to swallow before giving oral medications. Assessment can be accomplished by determining if the patient can swallow a few sips of water. If the patient is unable to swallow, a parenteral drug will be needed.

*Side Effects of Treatment.* Since cholinesterase inhibitors can inhibit acetylcholinesterase at any location, these drugs will cause ACh to accumulate at muscarinic junctions as well as at the neuromuscular junction. If muscarinic responses are excessive, atropine may be given to suppress them. However, atropine should not be employed *routinely* since this drug can mask the early signs (e.g., excessive salivation) of overdose with anticholinesterase agents.

## TABLE 16–1. CLINICAL APPLICATIONS OF CHOLINESTERASE INHIBITORS

| Generic Name [Trade Name] | Routes | Myasthenia Gravis | | Glaucoma | Reversal of Nondepolarizing Neuromuscular Blockade | Antidote to Poisoning by Muscarinic Antagonists | Alzheimer's Disease |
|---|---|---|---|---|---|---|---|
| | | Diagnosis | Treatment | | | | |
| *Reversible Inhibitors* | | | | | | | |
| Ambenonium [Mytelase Caplets] | PO | | ✔ | | | | |
| Demecarium [Humorsol] | Topical | | | ✔ | | | |
| Edrophonium [Tensilon, Enlon, Reversol] | IM,IV | ✔ | | | ✔ | | |
| Neostigmine [Prostigmin] | PO,IM, IV,SC | ✔ | ✔ | | ✔ | | |
| Physostigmine [Eserine, Antilirium] | Topical, IM, IV | | | ✔ | | ✔ | |
| Pyridostigmine [Mestinon, Regonol] | PO,IM,IV | | ✔ | | ✔ | | |
| Tacrine [Cognex] | PO | | | | | | ✔ |
| *Irreversible Inhibitors* | | | | | | | |
| Echothiophate [Phospholine Iodide] | Topical | | | ✔ | | | |

***Dosage Adjustment.*** In the treatment of myasthenia gravis, establishing an optimal dosage for cholinesterase inhibitors can be a challenge. Dosage determination is accomplished by administering a small initial dose followed by additional small doses until an optimal level of muscle function has been produced. Important signs of improvement include increased ease of swallowing and increased ability to raise the eyelids. You can contribute to the process of dosage determination by keeping records of (1) times of drug administration, (2) times at which fatigue occurs, (3) the state of muscle strength before and after drug administration, and (4) signs of excessive muscarinic stimulation.

To maintain optimal responses, patients must occasionally modify dosage themselves. To do this, patients must be taught to recognize signs of undermedication (difficulty in swallowing, ptosis) and signs of overmedication (excessive salivation, other muscarinic responses). Patients may also need to modify dosage in anticipation of exertion. For example, patients may find it necessary to take supplementary medication 30 to 60 minutes prior to such activities as eating and shopping.

***Myasthenic Crisis.*** Patients who are inadequately medicated may experience *myasthenic crisis*, a state characterized by extreme muscle weakness (caused by insufficient ACh at the neuromuscular junction). Left untreated, myasthenic crisis can result in death owing to paralysis of the muscles of respiration. A cholinesterase inhibitor (e.g., neostigmine) is used to relieve the crisis.

***Cholinergic Crisis.*** As noted above, overdose with a cholinesterase inhibitor can produce cholinergic crisis. Like myasthenic crisis, cholinergic crisis is characterized by extreme muscle weakness or frank paralysis. In addition, cholinergic crisis is accompanied by signs of excessive muscarinic stimulation. Treatment consists of respiratory support plus atropine. The offending cholinesterase inhibitor should be withheld until muscle strength has returned.

***Distinguishing Myasthenic Crisis from Cholinergic Crisis.*** Since myasthenic crisis and cholinergic crisis share similar symptoms (muscle weakness or paralysis), but are treated very differently, it is essential to distinguish between them. A history of medication use or signs of excessive muscarinic stimulation are usually sufficient to permit a differential diagnosis. If these clues are inadequate, the differential diagnosis can be made by administering a challenging dose of *edrophonium*, an ultrashort-acting cholinesterase inhibitor. If edrophonium-induced elevation of ACh levels alleviates symptoms, the crisis is myasthenic. Conversely, if edrophonium intensifies symptoms, the crisis is cholinergic. Since the symptoms of cholinergic crisis will be made even worse by edrophonium, atropine and oxygen should be immediately available whenever edrophonium is used to distinguish myasthenic crisis from cholinergic crisis.

***Use of Identification by the Patient.*** Because of the possibility of experiencing either myasthenic crisis or cholinergic crisis, and because both of these crises can be fatal, myasthenic patients should be encouraged to wear a Medic Alert bracelet or some other form of identification to inform emergency medical personnel of their condition.

# "Irreversible" Cholinesterase Inhibitors

The "irreversible" cholinesterase inhibitors are highly toxic. These agents are employed primarily as *insecticides*. During World War II, huge quantities of irreversible cholinesterase inhibitors were produced for possible use as *nerve gases*. Fortunately, these deadly weapons were never deployed. The only clinical indication for the irreversible inhibitors is *glaucoma*.

## Basic Pharmacology

### Chemistry

All irreversible cholinesterase inhibitors contain an atom of *phosphorus* (Fig. 16–4). Because of this phosphorus atom, the irreversible inhibitors are known as *organophosphate* cholinesterase inhibitors.

All of the irreversible cholinesterase inhibitors are *highly lipid soluble*. As a result, these drugs are readily absorbed from all routes of administration. They can even be absorbed directly through the skin. This ease of absorption, along with the toxicity of these drugs, forms the basis for their use as insecticides and their potential use as agents of chemical warfare. Once absorbed, the organophosphate inhibitors have ready access to all tissues and organs, including the CNS.

### Mechanism of Action

The irreversible cholinesterase inhibitors bind to the active center of cholinesterase, thereby preventing the enzyme from hydrolyzing ACh. Although these drugs can be split from ChE, the splitting reaction takes place *extremely* slowly (see Fig. 16–3C). Hence, under normal conditions, their binding to ChE can be considered irreversible. Because binding is permanent, effects per-

sist until new molecules of cholinesterase can be synthesized.

Although we normally consider the bond between the irreversible inhibitors and cholinesterase to be permanent, this bond can, in fact, be broken. To break the bond, and thereby reverse the inhibition of cholinesterase, we must administer *pralidoxime* (see below).

### Pharmacologic Effects

The irreversible cholinesterase inhibitors produce essentially the same spectrum of effects as the reversible inhibitors. The principal difference is that responses to the irreversible inhibitors last a long time, whereas responses to the reversible inhibitors are short lived.

### Therapeutic Uses

The irreversible cholinesterase inhibitors have only one indication: treatment of *glaucoma*—and for that indication, only one drug (echothiophate) is available. This limited clinical use of these agents should not be surprising given their potential for toxicity. The use of echothiophate for glaucoma is discussed in Chapter 97 (Drugs for the Eye).

## Toxicology

*Sources of Poisoning.* Poisoning by the organophosphate cholinesterase inhibitors is not uncommon. Agricultural workers have been poisoned by accidental ingestion of organophosphate insecticides and by absorption of these lipid-soluble compounds directly through the skin. In addition, because organophosphate insecticides are readily available to the general public, poisoning may occur accidentally or from homicide and suicide attempts.

*Symptoms.* Toxic doses of irreversible cholinesterase inhibitors produce a state of *cholinergic crisis*, a condition characterized by *excessive muscarinic stimulation* and *depolarizing neuromuscular blockade*. Overstimulation of muscarinic receptors results in profuse secretions from salivary and bronchial glands, involuntary urination and defecation, laryngospasm, and bronchoconstriction. Neuromuscular blockade can result in paralysis, followed by death from apnea. Convulsions of CNS origin precede paralysis and apnea.

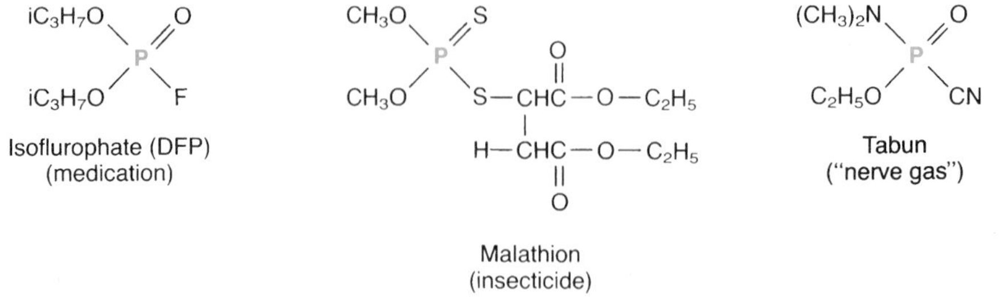

**Figure 16–4. Structural formulas of "irreversible" cholinesterase inhibitors.** Note that the irreversible cholinesterase inhibitors contain an atom of phosphorus. Because of this atom, these drugs are known as organophosphate cholinesterase inhibitors. All of the organophosphate inhibitors are highly lipid soluble, and therefore move throughout the body with ease.

**Treatment.** Treatment involves the following: (1) instituting mechanical ventilation using oxygen, (2) giving *atropine* to reduce muscarinic stimulation, (3) giving *pralidoxime* to reverse inhibition of cholinesterase (primarily at the NMJ), and (4) giving *diazepam* to suppress convulsions.

**Pralidoxime.** Pralidoxime [Protopam] is a specific antidote to poisoning by the *irreversible* (organophosphate) cholinesterase inhibitors. This drug is *not* effective against poisoning by *reversible* cholinesterase inhibitors. Pralidoxime reverses poisoning by causing organophosphate inhibitors to dissociate from the active center of cholinesterase. Reversal is most effective at the neuromuscular junction; the drug is much less effective at reversing cholinesterase inhibition at muscarinic and ganglionic sites. Furthermore, since pralidoxime is a quaternary ammonium compound, it cannot cross the blood-brain barrier, and therefore cannot reverse cholinesterase inhibition in the CNS.

To be effective, pralidoxime must be administered soon after organophosphate poisoning has occurred. If too much time is allowed to elapse, a process called *aging* takes place. In this process, the bond between the organophosphate inhibitor and cholinesterase increases in strength. Once aging has occurred, pralidoxime is unable to cause the inhibitor to dissociate from the enzyme.

## KEY POINTS

- Cholinesterase inhibitors prevent breakdown of ACh by acetylcholinesterase, causing ACh to accumulate in synapses, which in turn causes stimulation of muscarinic receptors, nicotinic receptors in ganglia and the NMJ, and cholinergic receptors in the CNS.
- The major use of reversible cholinesterase inhibitors is

treatment of myasthenia gravis. Benefits derive from accumulation of ACh at the NMJ.
- Secondary uses for reversible cholinesterase inhibitors are reversal of nondepolarizing neuromuscular blockade, and treatment of glaucoma, Alzheimer's disease, and poisoning by muscarinic antagonists.
- Because neostigmine (a quaternary ammonium compound) does not cross membranes easily, and hence is poorly absorbed from the GI tract, oral doses are much larger than parenteral doses.
- Because physostigmine crosses membranes easily, this drug is preferred for treating poisoning by muscarinic antagonists.
- Irreversible cholinesterase inhibitors, also known as organophosphate cholinesterase inhibitors, are used primarily as insecticides. The only indication for these potentially toxic drugs is glaucoma.
- Because they are highly lipid soluble, the organophosphate cholinesterase inhibitors can be absorbed directly through the skin and can distribute easily to all tissues and organs.
- Overdose with cholinesterase inhibitors produces cholinergic crisis, a state characterized by depolarizing neuromuscular blockade plus signs of excessive muscarinic stimulation (hypersalivation, tearing, sweating, bradycardia, involuntary urination and defecation, miosis, and spasm of accommodation). Death results from respiratory depression.
- Poisoning by reversible inhibitors is treated with atropine (to reverse muscarinic stimulation) plus mechanical ventilation.
- Poisoning by organophosphate cholinesterase inhibitors is treated with atropine, mechanical ventilation, pralidoxime (to reverse inhibition of cholinesterase, primarily at the NMJ), and diazepam (to suppress seizures).

# Summary of Major Nursing Implications*

## Reversible Cholinesterase Inhibitors

| | |
|---|---|
| Neostigmine | Edrophonium |
| Physostigmine | Pyridostigmine |
| Ambenonium | Tacrine |
| Demecarium | |

## Preadministration Assessment

### Therapeutic Goal

These drugs are used to *treat myasthenia gravis, glaucoma,* and *Alzheimer's disease*; to *reverse nondepolarizing neuromuscular blockade*; and to *treat muscarinic*

*antagonist poisoning.* Applications of individual agents are summarized in Table 16–1.

### Baseline Data

**Myasthenia Gravis.** Determine the extent of neuromuscular dysfunction by assessing muscle strength, fatigue, ptosis, and ability to swallow.

### Identifying High-Risk Patients

Cholinesterase inhibitors are *contraindicated* for patients with *mechanical obstruction of the intestine or urinary tract*. Exercise *caution* in patients with *peptic ulcer disease, bradycardia, asthma*, or *hyperthyroidism*.

## Implementation: Administration

### Routes

These drugs are given orally, topically, and by IM, IV,

and SC injection. Routes for individual agents are summarized in Table 16–1.

## Administration and Dosage in Myasthenia Gravis

*Administration.* Assess the patient's ability to swallow before giving oral medication. If swallowing is impaired, parenteral medication is required.

*Optimizing Dosage.* Monitor for therapeutic responses (see below) and adjust the dosage accordingly. Teach patients to distinguish between insufficient and excessive dosing so that they can participate effectively in dosage adjustment.

*Oral versus Parenteral Doses.* Oral doses of *neostigmine* are about 30 times greater than parenteral doses. If a patient is switched from oral to parenteral medication, the dosage must be greatly reduced.

## Reversing Nondepolarizing Neuromuscular Blockade

To reverse toxicity from overdosage with tubocurarine and other nondepolarizing neuromuscular blocking agents, administer neostigmine by slow IV infusion. Support respiration until muscle strength has recovered fully.

## Treating Muscarinic Antagonist Poisoning

*Physostigmine* is the drug of choice for this indication. The usual dose is 2 mg administered by IM or slow IV injection.

## Implementation: Measures to Enhance Therapeutic Effects

### Myasthenia Gravis

*Promoting Compliance.* Inform patients that myasthenia gravis is not curable, and hence treatment will be lifelong. Encourage patients to take their medication as prescribed.

*Using Identification.* Since myasthenic patients are at risk of fatal complications (cholinergic crisis, myasthenic crisis), encourage them to wear a Medic Alert bracelet or similar identification to inform emergency medical personnel of their condition.

## Ongoing Evaluation and Interventions

### Evaluating Therapeutic Effects

*Myasthenia Gravis.* Monitor and record (1) times of drug administration; (2) times at which fatigue occurs; (3) state of muscle strength, ptosis, and ability to swallow; and (4) signs of excessive muscarinic stimulation. Dosage is increased or decreased based on these observations.

Monitor for *myasthenic crisis* (extreme muscle weakness, paralysis of respiratory muscles), which can occur when cholinesterase inhibitor dosage is insufficient. Manage with respiratory support and increased dosage.

Be certain to distinguish myasthenic crisis from cholinergic crisis. Do this by observing for signs of excessive muscarinic stimulation, which will accompany cholinergic crisis but not myasthenic crisis. If necessary, these crises can be distinguished by administering *edrophonium*, which will reduce symptoms of myasthenic crisis and intensify symptoms of cholinergic crisis.

### Minimizing Adverse Effects

*Excessive Muscarinic Stimulation.* Accumulation of ACh at muscarinic receptors can cause profuse salivation, increased tone and motility of the gut, urinary urgency, sweating, miosis, spasm of accommodation, bronchoconstriction, and bradycardia. Inform patients about signs of excessive muscarinic stimulation and advise them to notify the physician if these occur. Excessive muscarinic responses can be reduced with *atropine*.

*Cholinergic Crisis.* This condition results from cholinesterase inhibitor overdose. Manifestations are skeletal muscle paralysis (from depolarizing neuromuscular blockade) and signs of excessive muscarinic stimulation (e.g., salivation, sweating, miosis, bradycardia).

Manage with mechanical ventilation and atropine. Cholinergic crisis must be distinguished from myasthenic crisis.

# CHAPTER 17

# Neuromuscular Blocking Agents and Ganglionic Blocking Agents

The drugs discussed in this chapter act through blockade of nicotinic cholinergic receptors. The *neuromuscular* blocking agents block nicotinic$_M$ receptors at the neuromuscular junction. The *ganglionic* blocking agents block nicotinic$_N$ receptors in autonomic ganglia. The neuromuscular blockers have important clinical applications. In contrast, the ganglionic blockers, once used widely for hypertension, have been largely supplanted by newer drugs.

# Neuromuscular Blocking Agents

Neuromuscular blocking agents prevent acetylcholine from activating nicotinic$_N$ receptors on skeletal muscles, and thereby cause muscle relaxation. These drugs are given to produce muscle relaxation during surgery, endotracheal intubation, mechanical ventilation, and other procedures.

## Control of Muscle Contraction

Before we discuss the neuromuscular blockers themselves, it will be helpful to review physiologic control of muscle contraction. In particular, we need to understand *excitation-contraction coupling*, the process by which an action potential in a motor neuron leads to contraction of a muscle.

### Basic Concepts: Polarization, Depolarization, and Repolarization

The concepts of *polarization*, *depolarization*, and *repolarization* are important to our understanding of muscle contraction, as well as our understanding of neuro-

muscular blockers. In *resting* muscle there is uneven distribution of electrical charge between the inner and outer surfaces of the cell membrane. As shown in Figure 17-1, positive charges cover the outer surface of the membrane and negative charges cover the inner surface. Because of this uneven charge distribution, the resting membrane is said to be *polarized*.

When the membrane *depolarizes*, positive charges move from outside the membrane to the inside. So many positive charges move inward that the inside of the membrane becomes more positive than the outside (see Fig. 17-1).

Under physiologic conditions, depolarization of the muscle membrane is followed almost instantaneously by *repolarization*. Repolarization is accomplished by pumping positively charged ions out of the cell. Repolarization restores the original resting membrane state, with positive charges on the outer surface and negative charges on the inner surface.

### Steps in Muscle Contraction

The steps leading to muscle contraction are summarized in Figure 17-2. The process begins with the arrival of an action potential at the terminal of a motor neuron, causing acetylcholine (ACh) to be released into the subneural space. Acetylcholine then binds reversibly to nicotinic$_M$ receptors on the motor end-plate (a specialized region of the muscle membrane that contains the receptors for ACh) and causes the end-plate to *depolarize*. This depolarization initiates a muscle action potential (i.e., a wave of depolarization that spreads rapidly over the entire muscle membrane), which in turn triggers the release of calcium from the sarcoplasmic reticulum (SR) of the muscle. This calcium permits the interaction of actin and myosin, thereby causing contraction. Very rapidly, ACh dissociates from the motor end-plate, the motor end-plate

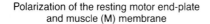

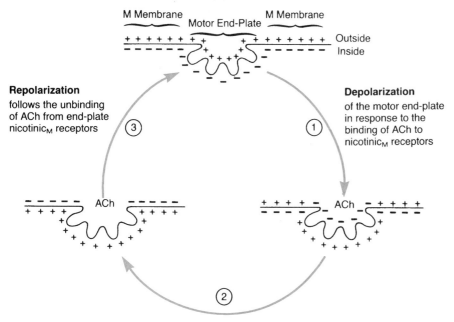

Polarization of the resting motor end-plate and muscle (M) membrane

M Membrane — Motor End-Plate — M Membrane
Outside
Inside

**Repolarization**
follows the unbinding of ACh from end-plate nicotinic$_M$ receptors

③

**Depolarization**
of the motor end-plate in response to the binding of ACh to nicotinic$_M$ receptors

①

ACh

ACh

②

Depolarization of the end-plate triggers a wave of depolarization (action potential) to move down the entire muscle membrane

**Figure 17–1. The depolarization-repolarization cycle of the motor end-plate and muscle membrane.**

repolarizes, the muscle membrane repolarizes, and calcium is taken back up into the SR. Because there is no longer any calcium available to support the interaction of actin and myosin, the muscle relaxes.

*Sustained* muscle contraction requires a continuous series of motor neuron action potentials. These action potentials cause repeated release of ACh, which causes repeated activation of nicotinic receptors on the motor end-plate. As a result, the end-plate goes through repeating cycles of depolarization and repolarization, which results in sufficient release of calcium to sustain contraction. If for some reason the motor end-plate fails to repolarize—that is, if the end-plate remains in a *depolarized* state—the signal for calcium release will stop, calcium will undergo immediate reuptake into the SR, and contraction will cease.

## Classification of Neuromuscular Blockers

The neuromuscular blockers can be classified according to *mechanism of action* and *time course of action*. When classified by mechanism of action, these drugs fall into two categories: nondepolarizing agents and depolarizing agents. When classified by time course of action, these drugs fall into four categories: long acting, intermediate acting, short acting, and ultrashort acting.

## Nondepolarizing Neuromuscular Blockers: Tubocurarine

Tubocurarine is the oldest nondepolarizing neuromuscular blocker and will serve as our prototype for the group.

The pharmacologic powers of tubocurarine were known to primitive hunters long before coming to the attention of modern scientists. Tubocurarine is one of several active principles found in *curare*, an arrow poison used for hunting by South American Indians. When shot into a monkey or other small animal, curare-tipped arrows cause relaxation (paralysis) of skeletal muscles. Death results from paralyzing the muscles of respiration.

The clinical utility of tubocurarine is based on the same action that is useful in hunting: production of skeletal muscle relaxation. Relaxation of skeletal muscles is helpful in patients undergoing surgery, endotracheal intubation, mechanical ventilation, and other procedures.

### Chemistry

Tubocurarine and all other neuromuscular blocking agents contain a *quaternary nitrogen* atom (Fig. 17–3). As a result, these drugs always carry a positive charge, and therefore cannot readily cross membranes.

The inability to cross membranes has three clinical consequences. First, neuromuscular blockers cannot be administered orally. Instead, they must all be administered parenterally (almost always IV). Second, these drugs cannot cross the blood-brain barrier, and hence have no effect on the central nervous system (CNS). Third, neuromuscular blockers cannot readily cross the placenta. Thus, effects on the fetus are minimal.

### Mechanism of Action

Tubocurarine acts by competing with ACh for binding to nicotinic$_M$ receptors on the motor end-plate (Fig. 17–4). Since tubocurarine does not activate these receptors,

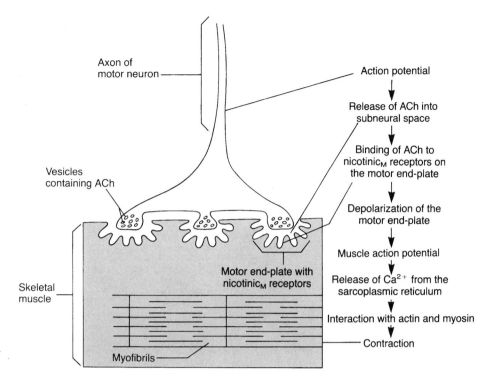

**Figure 17–2. Steps in excitation-contraction coupling.**

binding does not result in contraction. Muscle relaxation persists as long as the amount of tubocurarine at the neuromuscular junction (NMJ) is sufficient to prevent receptor occupation by ACh. Muscle function can be restored by eliminating tubocurarine from the body or by increasing the amount of ACh at the NMJ.

## Pharmacologic Effects

*Muscle Relaxation.* The primary effect of tubocurarine is relaxation of skeletal muscles. Muscle relaxation produces a state of *flaccid paralysis.*

Although tubocurarine can paralyze all skeletal muscles, not all muscles are affected at once. The first muscles to become paralyzed are the levator muscle of the eyelid and the muscles of mastication. Paralysis occurs next in muscles of the limbs, abdomen, and glottis. The last muscles affected are the muscles of respiration—the intercostals and the diaphragm.

*Hypotension.* Tubocurarine can lower blood pressure by two mechanisms: (1) release of histamine and (2) partial ganglionic blockade. Histamine lowers blood pressure by promoting vasodilation. Ganglionic blockade lowers blood pressure by decreasing sympathetic tone to arterioles and veins. Tubocurarine suppresses ganglionic transmission by causing partial blockade of nicotinic$_N$ receptors in autonomic ganglia.

*Central Nervous System.* As noted above, tubocurarine and the other neuromuscular blocking agents are unable to cross the blood-brain barrier. Consequently, these drugs have no effect on the CNS. Please note: *neuromuscular blockers do not diminish consciousness or perception of pain—even when administered in doses that produce complete paralysis.*

## Pharmacokinetics

Paralysis develops rapidly (in minutes) following IV injection. Peak effects persist for 35 to 60 minutes and then decline. Complete recovery may take several hours. Tubocurarine is eliminated by a combination of hepatic metabolism and renal excretion.

## Therapeutic Uses

Tubocurarine can be used for muscle relaxation during surgery, mechanical ventilation, endotracheal intubation, and electroconvulsive therapy. These applications are discussed later under *Therapeutic Uses of Neuromuscular Blockers.*

## Adverse Effects

The principal adverse effects of tubocurarine concern the respiratory and cardiovascular systems.

*Respiratory Depression.* Paralysis of respiratory muscles can produce respiratory arrest. Because of this risk, facilities for artificial ventilation must be immediately available. Patients must be monitored closely and continuously. When tubocurarine is withdrawn, vital signs must be monitored until muscle function has fully recovered.

*Cardiovascular Effects.* As noted above, tubocurarine can cause *hypotension* secondary to histamine release and partial ganglionic blockade. In addition, the drug can cause *bradycardia, dysrhythmias,* and *cardiac arrest.* The mechanism underlying these latter effects is not clear.

## Precautions and Contraindications

*Myasthenia Gravis.* Neuromuscular blocking agents must be used with special care in patients with myasthenia gravis, a condition characterized by skeletal muscle

NONDEPOLARIZING BLOCKERS

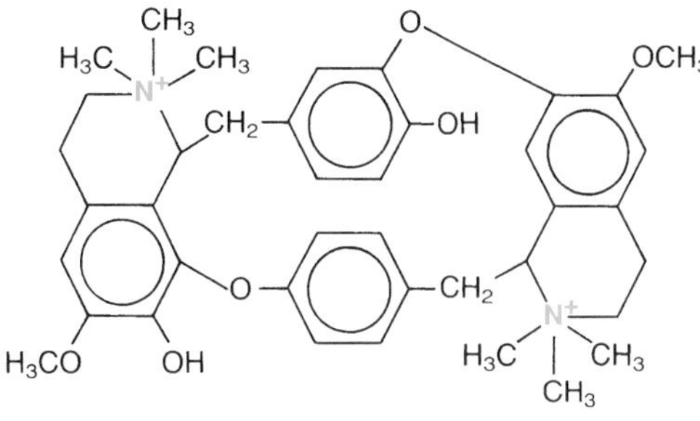

Tubocurarine

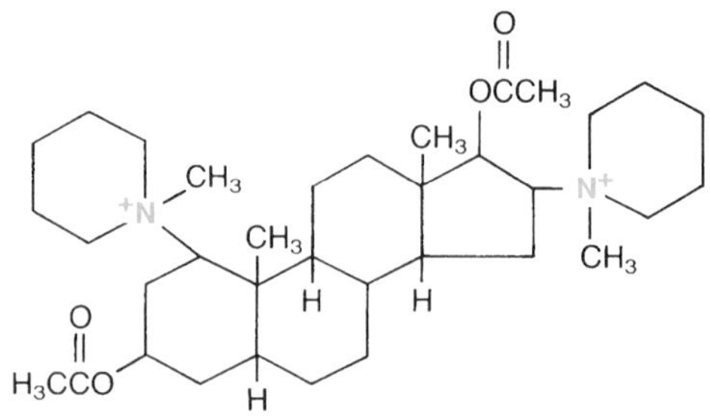

Pancuronium

DEPOLARIZING BLOCKER

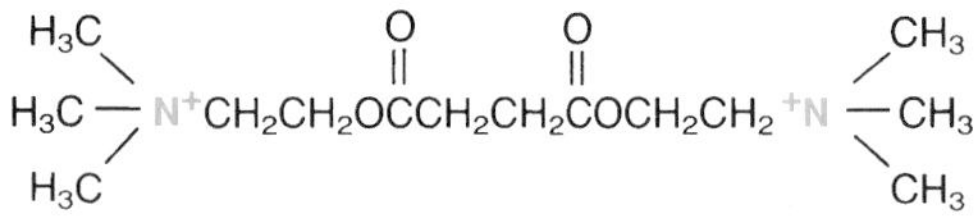

Succinylcholine

**Figure 17–3. Structural formulas of representative neuromuscular blocking agents.** Note that all of these agents contain quaternary nitrogen atoms and therefore cross membranes poorly. Consequently, these drugs must be administered parenterally and have little effect on the central nervous system or the developing fetus.

weakness. The cause of weakness is a reduction in the number of nicotinic$_M$ receptors on the motor end-plate. Because receptor number is reduced, neuromuscular blockade occurs very readily in these patients; doses that would have a minimal effect on other patients can produce complete paralysis in patients with myasthenia. Accordingly, dosing must be done with great care. Myasthenia gravis and its treatment are discussed in Chapter 16.

**Electrolyte Disturbances.** Responses to tubocurarine can be altered by electrolyte abnormalities. For example, low potassium levels can enhance paralysis, whereas high potassium levels can reduce paralysis. Because electrolyte status can influence the depth of neuromuscular blockade, it is important to maintain normal electrolyte balance.

## Drug Interactions

Tubocurarine can interact with many other drugs. Interactions of primary interest are discussed below.

**General Anesthetics.** All inhalation anesthetics produce some degree of skeletal muscle relaxation, and can thereby enhance the actions of tubocurarine and the other neuromuscular blockers. Consequently, when general anesthetics and neuromuscular blockers are combined (as they often are), the dosage of the neuromuscular blocker should be reduced to avoid excessive neuromuscular blockade.

**Antibiotics.** Several antibiotics can intensify responses to neuromuscular blockers. Among them are *aminoglycosides* (e.g., gentamicin), *tetracyclines*, and certain other nonpenicillin antibiotics.

**Cholinesterase Inhibitors.** Cholinesterase inhibitors can *decrease* the effects of tubocurarine and other *nondepolarizing* neuromuscular blockers. (As discussed later in the chapter, cholinesterase inhibitors have the opposite effect on responses to succinylcholine, a *depolarizing* neuromuscular blocker.)

How do cholinesterase inhibitors decrease the effects of tubocurarine? Recall that nondepolarizing blockers compete with ACh for binding to nicotinic$_M$ receptors. By decreasing the degradation of ACh, cholinesterase inhibitors increase the amount of ACh available to compete with tubocurarine for receptor binding. As more ACh (and less tubocurarine) occupies nicotinic$_M$ receptors, the degree of neuromuscular blockade declines.

The ability of cholinesterase inhibitors to decrease responses to nondepolarizing neuromuscular blockers has two clinical applications: (1) management of overdose with a nondepolarizing neuromuscular blocker and (2) reversal of neuromuscular blockade following surgery and other procedures.

## Toxicology

Overdose with tubocurarine has three major effects: (1) prolonged apnea, (2) massive histamine release, and (3) cardiovascular collapse. Apnea is managed with respiratory support plus a cholinesterase inhibitor (e.g., neostigmine) to reverse neuromuscular blockade. Antihistamines are given to counteract released histamine. Cardiovascular toxicity must be assessed and treated as indicated.

## Preparations, Dosage, and Administration

Tubocurarine is always administered parenterally. The usual route is intravenous. Intramuscular injections are employed occasionally.

Because of their potential for harm, tubocurarine and other neuromuscular blockers are administered only by clinicians specially trained in their use. Whenever these

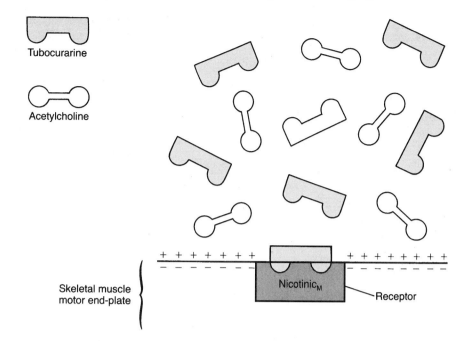

**Figure 17–4. Mechanism of nondepolarizing neuromuscular blockade.** Tubocurarine competes with ACh for binding to nicotinic$_M$ receptors on the motor end-plate. Binding of tubocurarine does not depolarize the endplate, and therefore causes no contraction. At the same time, the presence of tubocurarine prevents ACh from binding to the receptor to produce contraction.

drugs are given, facilities for artificial respiration and management of cardiovascular complications must be at hand.

Tubocurarine is dispensed in solution (20 units/ml) for IM and IV injection. The dosage depends on the indication. A typical dosage for the adult surgical patient is 40 to 60 units IV at the time of the initial incision, followed by 20 to 30 units a few minutes later. During long operations, additional doses of 20 to 30 units may be administered as needed.

## Nondepolarizing Neuromuscular Blockers: Others

In addition to tubocurarine, 10 other nondepolarizing blockers are approved for use in the United States. Like tubocurarine, they all act by competing with acetylcholine at nicotinic$_M$ receptors on the motor end-plate. Differences among them relate primarily to time course of action (Table 17–1) and cardiovascular effects. With all of these drugs, respiratory depression secondary to neuromuscular blockade is the major concern. Respiratory depression can be reversed by giving a cholinesterase inhibitor.

### Long-Acting Agents

**Metocurine.** Metocurine [Metubine] is a semisynthetic derivative of tubocurarine with a similar time course of action. The drug is used primarily for muscle relaxation during surgery. Metocurine causes less histamine release than tubocurarine and less ganglionic blockade. As a result, the risk of hypotension is low.

**Doxacurium.** Doxacurium [Nuromax] is a long-acting neuromuscular blocker used for muscle relaxation during general anesthesia and intubation. The drug is eliminated by the kidneys; hence muscle relaxation will be prolonged in patients with renal failure. Doxacurium is devoid of adverse cardiovascular effects.

**Pipercuronium.** Pipercuronium [Arduan] is indicated for muscle relaxation during surgery and intubation. Because its effects are long lasting, this drug is not recommended for procedures of less than 90 minutes' duration. Pipercuronium does not release histamine, does not cause vagal block, and is generally free of ad-

verse cardiovascular effects. Duration of paralysis may be prolonged and unpredictable in obese patients and in patients with renal failure.

**Rocuronium.** Rocuronium [Zemuron] has a rapid onset and long duration of action. The only neuromuscular blocker with a faster onset is succinylcholine, a *depolarizing* neuromuscular blocker. In contrast to succinylcholine, whose effects fade rapidly, rocuronium has effects that persist for 30 to 70 minutes. Rocuronium does not cause histamine release. Elimination is by hepatic metabolism. The drug is approved for muscle relaxation during intubation, surgery, and mechanical ventilation.

### Intermediate-Acting Agents

**Atracurium.** Atracurium [Tracrium] is approved for muscle relaxation during surgery, intubation, and mechanical ventilation. The drug can cause hypotension secondary to histamine release. Like succinylcholine, atracurium is eliminated by plasma cholinesterases, not by the liver or kidneys. Hence, atracurium may be desirable for patients with renal or hepatic dysfunction since these disorders will not prolong the drug's effects.

**Cisatracurium.** Cisatracurium [Nimbex], a close relative of atracurium, is approved for muscle relaxation during surgery, intubation, and mechanical ventilation. Elimination is by spontaneous degradation, not by the hepatic metabolism or renal excretion. Hence, like atracurium, cisatracurium would seem desirable for patients with kidney or liver dysfunction. Histamine release with the drug is minimal.

**Gallamine.** Gallamine [Flaxedil] is used for muscle relaxation during general anesthesia and mechanical ventilation. The drug does not cause histamine release or ganglionic blockade, and therefore does not induce hypotension. Gallamine can cause tachycardia by blocking vagal input to the heart. The drug is excreted entirely by the kidneys; hence effects will be prolonged in patients with renal failure.

**Pancuronium.** Pancuronium [Pavulon] is approved for muscle relaxation during general anesthesia, intubation, and mechanical ventilation. The drug does not cause histamine release, ganglionic blockade, or hypotension. Vagolytic effects may produce tachycardia. Elimination is primarily renal.

**Vecuronium.** Vecuronium [Norcuron], an analog of pancuronium, is used for muscle relaxation during general anesthesia and intubation. The drug does not produce ganglionic or vagal

## TABLE 17-1. NEUROMUSCULAR BLOCKERS: TIME COURSE OF ACTION*

| Generic Name | Route | Time to Maximum Paralysis (min) | Duration of Effective Paralysis (min) | Time to Nearly Full Spontaneous Recovery† |
|---|---|---|---|---|
| *Long Acting* | | | | |
| Doxacurium [Nuromax] | IV | 4-10 | 100 | Hours |
| Metocurine [Metubine] | IV | 3-5 | 25-90 | Hours |
| Pipercuronium [Arduan] | IV | 3-5 | 90-120 | Hours |
| Rocuronium [Zemuron] | IV | 1-3 | 30-70 | — |
| Tubocurarine | IV, IM‡ | 2-5 | 35-60 | Hours |
| *Intermediate Acting* | | | | |
| Atracurium [Tracrium] | IV | 2-5 | 20-35 | 60-70 min |
| Cisatracurium [Nimbex] | IV | 2-5 | 20-35 | — |
| Gallamine [Flaxedil] | IV | 2-5 | 15-30 | — |
| Pancuronium [Pavulon] | IV | 3-4 | 35-45 | 60-70 min |
| Vecuronium [Norcuron] | IV | 3-5 | 25-30 | 45-60 min |
| *Short Acting* | | | | |
| Mivacurium [Mivacron] | IV | 2-5 | 10-15 | 21-34 min |
| *Ultrashort Acting* | | | | |
| Succinylcholine [Anectine, others] | IV, IM‡ | 1 | 4-6 | — |

*Time course of action can vary widely with dosage and route of administration. The values presented are for an average adult dose administered as a single IV injection.
†Because spontaneous recovery can take a long time, recovery from the *nondepolarizing* agents (all of the drugs listed except succinylcholine) is often accelerated by giving a cholinesterase inhibitor.
‡Intramuscular administration is rare.

block and does not release histamine. Consequently, cardiovascular effects are minimal. Vecuronium is excreted primarily in the bile; hence paralysis may be prolonged in patients with liver dysfunction. Paralysis may also be prolonged in obese patients.

### Short-Acting Agent

**Mivacurium.** Mivacurium [Mivacron] is the shortest-acting *nondepolarizing* neuromuscular blocker. The only neuromuscular blocker with a shorter duration is succinylcholine, a *depolarizing* neuromuscular blocker. Paralysis is maximal 2 to 5 minutes after IV injection and persists for only 10 to 17 minutes. Like succinylcholine, mivacurium is metabolized by plasma cholinesterase. As a result, effects are prolonged in patients with low levels of that enzyme. Mivacurium can cause facial flushing secondary to histamine release. Other cardiovascular effects are minimal.

## Depolarizing Neuromuscular Blockers: Succinylcholine

Succinylcholine, an ultrashort-acting drug, is the only depolarizing neuromuscular blocker in clinical use. This drug differs from the nondepolarizing blockers with regard to mechanism of action, mode of elimination, interaction with cholinesterase inhibitors, and management of toxicity.

### Mechanism of Action

Succinylcholine produces a state known as depolarizing neuromuscular blockade. Like acetylcholine, succinylcholine binds to nicotinic$_M$ receptors on the motor endplate and thereby causes depolarization. This depolarization produces transient muscle contractions (fascicula-

tions). Then, instead of dissociating rapidly from the receptor, succinylcholine remains bound. By remaining bound, the drug prevents the end-plate from repolarizing. That is, succinylcholine maintains the end-plate in a state of *constant depolarization*. Since the end-plate must repeatedly depolarize and repolarize to maintain muscle contraction, succinylcholine's ability to keep the end-plate depolarized causes paralysis (following the brief initial period of contraction). Paralysis persists until plasma levels of succinylcholine decline, thereby allowing the drug to dissociate from its receptors.

### Pharmacologic Effects

**Muscle Relaxation.** The muscle-relaxant effects of succinylcholine are much like those of tubocurarine; both drugs produce a state of flaccid paralysis. However, despite this similarity, it should be noted that the effects of succinylcholine differ from those of tubocurarine in two ways: (1) paralysis from succinylcholine is preceded by transient contractions and (2) the paralysis abates much more rapidly.

**Central Nervous System.** Like tubocurarine, succinylcholine has no effect on the CNS. The drug can produce complete paralysis without decreasing consciousness or the ability to feel pain.

### Pharmacokinetics

Succinylcholine has an extremely short duration of action. Paralysis peaks about 1 minute after IV injection and fades completely 4 to 10 minutes later.

Paralysis is brief because succinylcholine is rapidly degraded by *pseudocholinesterase*, an enzyme present in plasma. (This enzyme is called pseudocholinesterase to distinguish it from "true" cholinesterase, the enzyme found at synapses where ACh is the transmitter.) Because of its presence in plasma, pseudocholinesterase is also known as *plasma cholinesterase*. In most individuals, pseudocholinesterase is highly active and can eliminate succinylcholine in minutes.

## Therapeutic Uses

Succinylcholine is used primarily for muscle relaxation during endotracheal intubation, electroconvulsive therapy, endoscopy, and other short procedures. Because of its brief duration of action, succinylcholine is less desirable than tubocurarine and other nondepolarizing blockers for use during surgery and mechanical ventilation. Clinical applications are discussed further under *Therapeutic Uses of Neuromuscular Blockers.*

## Adverse Effects

*Prolonged Apnea in Patients with Low Pseudocholinesterase Activity.* A few people, because of their genetic heritage, produce a form of pseudocholinesterase that has extremely low activity. As a result, they are unable to degrade succinylcholine rapidly. If succinylcholine is given to these people, paralysis can persist for hours, instead of just a few minutes. Not surprisingly, succinylcholine is contraindicated for these individuals.

Patients suspected of having low pseudocholinesterase activity should be tested for this possibility before receiving full succinylcholine doses. Pseudocholinesterase activity can be assessed by direct measurement of a blood sample or by administering a tiny test dose of succinylcholine. If the test dose produces muscle relaxation that is unexpectedly intense and prolonged, pseudocholinesterase activity is probably low.

*Malignant Hyperthermia.* Malignant hyperthermia is a rare and potentially fatal condition that can be triggered by succinylcholine, and by all inhalation anesthetics as well. The condition is characterized by muscle rigidity associated with a profound elevation of temperature—sometimes to as high as 43°C. Temperature becomes elevated because of excessive and uncontrolled metabolic activity in muscle. Left untreated, the condition can rapidly prove fatal. Malignant hyperthermia is a genetically determined reaction that has an incidence of about 1 in 25,000. Individuals with a family history of the reaction should not receive succinylcholine.

Treatment of malignant hyperthermia includes (1) immediate discontinuation of succinylcholine and the accompanying anesthetic, (2) cooling of the patient with ice or an infusion of iced saline, and (3) administering *dantrolene*, a drug that stops heat generation by acting directly on skeletal muscle to reduce its metabolic activity. The pharmacology of dantrolene is discussed in Chapter 24.

*Postoperative Muscle Pain.* Between 10% and 70% of patients receiving succinylcholine experience postoperative muscle pain, most commonly in the neck, shoulder,

and back. Pain develops 12 to 24 hours after surgery and may persist for several hours or days. The cause of pain may be the muscle contractions that occur during the initial phase of succinylcholine action.

*Hyperkalemia.* Succinylcholine promotes release of potassium from tissues. Rarely, potassium release is sufficient to cause severe hyperkalemia. Death from cardiac arrest has occurred. Significant hyperkalemia is most likely in patients with burns, nerve damage, or neuromuscular disease.

## Drug Interactions

*Cholinesterase Inhibitors.* These drugs *potentiate* the effects of succinylcholine. Potentiation occurs because cholinesterase inhibitors decrease the activity of pseudocholinesterase, the enzyme that inactivates succinylcholine. Note that the effect of cholinesterase inhibitors on succinylcholine is opposite to their effect on *nondepolarizing* neuromuscular blockers.

*Antibiotics.* The effects of succinylcholine, like those of tubocurarine, can be potentiated by certain antibiotics, including *aminoglycosides*, *tetracyclines*, and certain other nonpenicillin antibiotics.

## Toxicology

Overdose can produce prolonged apnea. Since there is no specific antidote to succinylcholine poisoning, management is purely supportive. Recall that with tubocurarine overdose, paralysis can be reversed with a cholinesterase inhibitor. Since cholinesterase inhibitors delay the degradation of succinylcholine, use of these agents would prolong—not reverse—succinylcholine toxicity.

### Preparations, Dosage, and Administration

Succinylcholine chloride [Anectine, Quelicin, Sucostrin] is available in solution and as a powder. The drug is usually administered IV but can also be injected IM. Solutions of succinylcholine are unstable and should be used within 24 hours. Multidose vials are stable for up to 2 weeks.

Dosage must be individualized and depends on the specific application. A typical adult dose for brief procedures is 25 to 75 mg administered as a single IV injection. For prolonged procedures, succinylcholine may be administered by infusion at a rate of 2.5 to 4.3 mg/min.

## Therapeutic Uses of Neuromuscular Blockers

The primary applications of the neuromuscular blocking agents are discussed below. No one agent is used for all of these applications.

## Muscle Relaxation During Surgery

Production of muscle relaxation during surgery offers two benefits. First, relaxation of skeletal muscles, especially those of the abdominal wall, makes the surgeon's work easier. Second, muscle relaxants allow us to decrease the dosage of the general anesthetic, thereby decreasing the risks associated with anesthesia. Before neuromuscular blockers became available, surgical muscle relaxation had to be achieved with the general anesthetic alone, often requiring high levels of anesthetic. (As noted above, inhalation anesthetics have muscle relaxant properties of their own.) By combining a neuromuscular blocker with the general anesthetic, we can achieve adequate surgical muscle relaxation with less anesthetic than was possible when paralysis had to be achieved with an anesthetic alone. By allowing a reduction in anesthetic levels, neuromuscular blockers have decreased the risk of respiratory depression from anesthesia. In addition, since less anesthetic is administered, recovery from anesthesia occurs more rapidly.

Whenever neuromuscular blockers are employed during surgery, it is extremely important that anesthesia be maintained at a level sufficient to produce unconsciousness. Recall that neuromuscular blockers do not enter the CNS, and therefore have no effect on hearing, thinking, or the ability to feel pain; all that these drugs do is produce paralysis. Neuromuscular blockers are obviously and definitely not a substitute for anesthesia. It does not require a great deal of imagination to appreciate the horror of the surgical patient who is completely paralyzed from neuromuscular blockade yet fully awake thanks to inadequate anesthesia. Clearly, full anesthesia must be provided whenever surgery is performed on a patient who is under neuromuscular blockade.

Full recovery from neuromuscular blockade may take from one to several hours. During the recovery period, patients must be monitored closely to ensure adequate ventilation. A patent airway should be maintained until the patient can swallow or speak. Recovery from the effects of *nondepolarizing* neuromuscular blockers (e.g., tubocurarine) can be accelerated with a cholinesterase inhibitor.

### Facilitation of Mechanical Ventilation

Some patients who require mechanical ventilation still have some spontaneous respiratory movements—movements that can fight the rhythm of the respirator. By suppressing these movements, neuromuscular blocking agents can reduce resistance to ventilation.

When neuromuscular blockers are used to facilitate mechanical ventilation, patients should be treated as if they were awake—even though they will appear to be sleeping. (Remember that the patient is paralyzed, and hence there is no way to assess state of consciousness.) Because the patient may be fully awake, steps should be taken to ensure comfort at all times. Furthermore, since neuromuscular blockade does not affect hearing, nothing should be said in the patient's presence that might be inappropriate for him or her to hear.

Being fully awake but completely paralyzed can be a stressful and generally horrific experience. (Think about it.) Accordingly, many clinicians do not recommend routine use of neuromuscular blockers during prolonged mechanical ventilation in intensive care units.

### Adjunct to Electroconvulsive Therapy

Electroconvulsive therapy is an effective treatment for severe depression (see Chapter 30). Benefits derive strictly from the effects of electroshock on the brain; the convulsive movements that can accompany electroshock

do not help relieve depression. Since convulsions per se serve no useful purpose, and since electroshock—induced convulsions can be harmful, neuromuscular blockers are now used to prevent convulsive movements during electroshock therapy. Because of its short duration of action, *succinylcholine* is the preferred neuromuscular blocker for this application.

### Endotracheal Intubation

An endotracheal tube is a large catheter that is inserted past the glottis and into the trachea to facilitate ventilation. Gag reflexes can fight tube insertion. By suppressing these reflexes, neuromuscular blockers can make intubation easier. Because of its short duration of action, succinylcholine is the preferred neuromuscular blocker for this use.

#### Diagnosis of Myasthenia Gravis

Tubocurarine can be used to diagnose myasthenia gravis when safer diagnostic procedures have been inconclusive. To diagnose myasthenia, a small test dose of tubocurarine is administered. Since the dose is too small to affect individuals who do not have myasthenia, a significant reduction in muscle strength would be diagnostic of myasthenia. If the test dose does decrease strength, neostigmine (a cholinesterase inhibitor) should be administered immediately; the resultant elevation in ACh at the NMJ will reverse neuromuscular blockade. It must be stressed that use of tubocurarine to diagnose myasthenia gravis is not without risk: if the patient does have myasthenia, the challenging dose may be sufficient to cause pronounced respiratory depression. Consequently, facilities for artificial ventilation must be immediately available.

## Ganglionic Blocking Agents

Ganglionic blocking agents produce a broad spectrum of pharmacologic effects. Because they lack selectivity, the ganglionic blockers have limited applications. These drugs are used only to lower blood pressure—and then only in special circumstances. In the United States, two ganglionic blockers are available: *trimethaphan* and *mecamylamine*. Trimethaphan will serve as our prototype.

### Trimethaphan

#### Mechanism of Action

Trimethaphan [Arfonad] interrupts impulse transmission through ganglia of the autonomic nervous system. The drug blocks transmission by competitive antagonism with acetylcholine at ganglionic nicotinic receptors. Since the nicotinic receptors of sympathetic and parasympathetic ganglia are the same, trimethaphan blocks transmission at all autonomic ganglia. By blocking all ganglionic transmission, the drug can, in effect, shut down the entire autonomic nervous system, thereby depriving organs of all autonomic regulation.

In addition to blocking ganglionic transmission, trimethaphan has two other actions: (1) vasodilation (from a direct effect on blood vessels) and (2) release of histamine. Both actions can reduce blood pressure.

#### Pharmacologic Effects

Since trimethaphan acts by depriving organs of autonomic regulation, to predict the drug's effects, we need to know how the autonomic nervous system is affecting specific organs at the time of drug administration. That is, we need to know which branch of the autonomic nervous system is providing the pre-

## TABLE 17-2. PREDOMINANT AUTONOMIC TONE AND RESPONSES TO GANGLIONIC BLOCKADE

| Location | Predominant Tone | Response to Ganglionic Blockade |
|---|---|---|
| Salivary glands | Parasympathetic | Dry mouth |
| Ciliary muscle | Parasympathetic | Blurred vision |
| Iris sphincter | Parasympathetic | Photophobia (from mydriasis) |
| Urinary bladder | Parasympathetic | Urinary retention |
| Gastrointestinal tract | Parasympathetic | Constipation |
| Heart | Parasympathetic | Tachycardia |
| Sweat glands | Sympathetic* | Anhidrosis |
| Arterioles | Sympathetic | Hypotension (from vasodilation) |
| Veins | Sympathetic | Orthostatic hypotension (from pooling of blood in veins secondary to venous dilation) |

*Sympathetic nerves to sweat glands release acetylcholine as their transmitter, which acts at muscarinic receptors on the sweat glands.

dominant tone to specific organs. By knowing the source of predominant tone to an organ, and by knowing that ganglionic blockade will remove that tone, we can predict the effects that ganglionic blockade will produce.

Table 17-2 indicates (1) the major structures innervated by autonomic nerves, (2) the branch of the autonomic nervous system that provides the predominant tone to those structures, and (3) the responses to ganglionic blockade. As the table shows, *the predominant autonomic tone to most organs is provided by the parasympathetic nervous system.* The sympathetic branch provides the predominant tone only to *sweat glands, arterioles,* and *veins.*

Since the parasympathetic nervous system provides the predominant tone to most organs, and since the parasympathetic nervous system works through muscarinic receptors to influence organ function, *most responses to ganglionic blockade resemble those produced by muscarinic antagonists.* These responses include dry mouth, blurred vision, photophobia, urinary retention, constipation, tachycardia, and anhidrosis.

In addition to their parasympatholytic effects, ganglionic blockers produce *hypotension.* These drugs lower blood pressure by causing dilation of arterioles and veins. Vasodilation results primarily from blocking sympathetic nerve traffic to vascular smooth muscle.

### Pharmacokinetics

Trimethaphan is a quaternary ammonium compound and therefore always carries a positive charge. As a result, this drug cannot readily cross membranes. Accordingly, trimethaphan must be administered parenterally. The drug has a brief duration of action and is eliminated by renal excretion.

### Therapeutic Uses

***Controlled Hypotension in Surgery.*** Trimethaphan can produce controlled hypotension during surgery. Controlled reductions in blood pressure can (1) reduce blood loss and (2) facilitate surgery by decreasing the amount of blood in the surgical field.

***Hypertensive Crisis.*** A hypertensive crisis is a condition in which blood pressure has risen so high as to constitute an immediate danger. Trimethaphan is one of several drugs that can be used to reduce blood pressure in patients with acute, severe hypertension.

### Adverse Effects

Trimethaphan produces a broad spectrum of undesired effects, all of which are the predictable consequence of generalized inhibition of the autonomic nervous system. Side effects fall into two groups: (1) antimuscarinic effects (caused by parasympathetic blockade), and (2) hypotension (caused largely by sympathetic blockade).

***Antimuscarinic Effects.*** Blockade of parasympathetic ganglia produces typical antimuscarinic responses: dry mouth, blurred vision, photophobia, urinary retention, constipation, tachycardia, and anhidrosis. Antimuscarinic responses are discussed in detail in Chapter 15.

***Hypotension.*** By causing arteriolar dilation, ganglionic blockers can produce a profound reduction in blood pressure. Excessive hypotension can be the most serious adverse effect of ganglionic blockade. If blood pressure drops too low, it may be necessary to administer a vasoconstrictor (e.g., norepinephrine) to restore pressure to a safe level.

***Orthostatic Hypotension.*** Orthostatic hypotension is defined as a drop in blood pressure that occurs upon assuming an upright posture. Ganglionic blockers promote orthostatic hypotension by dilating veins. Venous dilation causes blood to "pool" in veins when the patient moves from a recumbent to an upright posture. As a result, return of blood to the heart is significantly reduced, causing a reduction in cardiac output and a subsequent fall in blood pressure.

Since much of the hypotension that results from ganglionic blockade is dependent upon posture, patients who are supine or in Trendelenburg's position (head down) experience less hypotension than patients in reverse Trendelenburg's position (head up). Consequently, the blood pressure of patients receiving trimethaphan can be raised or lowered by the simple expedient of changing body position: if blood pressure is too low, lower the head and raise the feet; if blood pressure is too high, raise the head and lower the feet.

### Preparations, Dosage, and Administration

Trimethaphan camsylate [Arfonad] is available in solution (50 mg/ml) for IV infusion. The drug must be diluted to 1 mg/ml with 5% dextrose prior to use. The average infusion rate is 3 to 4 ml/min (3 to 4 mg/min). The rate is adjusted to achieve the desired reduction in blood pressure. No other drugs should be added to the infusion fluid.

### Mecamylamine

Mecamylamine is a ganglionic blocking agent with pharmacologic properties much like those of trimethaphan. The principal difference between the two drugs is pharmacokinetic: mecamylamine can cross membranes with ease, whereas trimethaphan cannot. As a result, mecamylamine can be administered orally. In addition, the drug can cross the blood-brain barrier to produce CNS effects (mental aberrations, weakness, fatigue, and sedation).

**Therapeutic Use.** Mecamylamine is indicated for *essential hypertension* in selected patients. The drug is reserved for those rare cases in which blood pressure cannot be reduced with more desirable medications.

**Adverse Effects.** The principal concern is *orthostatic hypotension*. Inform patients that hypotension can be minimized by moving slowly when assuming an upright posture. Also, warn patients that hypotension can cause fainting and, consequently, they should sit or lie down if they become dizzy or lightheaded. In addition to hypotension, mecamylamine can cause typical antimuscarinic effects (dry mouth, blurred vision, photophobia, urinary retention, tachycardia, constipation, anhidrosis).

**Preparations, Dosage, and Administration.** Mecamylamine hydrochloride [Inversine] is available in 2.5-mg tablets for oral use. The dosage is 2.5 mg twice daily initially and then gradually increased until the target blood pressure has been achieved. The average daily maintenance dose is 25 mg.

## KEY POINTS

All of these key points apply to the *neuromuscular blocking* agents.

- Sustained contraction of skeletal muscle results from repetitive stimulation of nicotinic$_M$ receptors on the motor end-plate, which causes the end-plate to go through repeating cycles of depolarization and repolarization.
- Neuromuscular blockers interfere with nicotinic$_M$ receptor activation, and thereby cause muscle relaxation.
- Nondepolarizing neuromuscular blockers act by competing with ACh for binding to nicotinic$_M$ receptors.
- Succinylcholine, the only depolarizing neuromuscular blocker in use, binds to nicotinic$_M$ receptors, causing the end-plate to depolarize; the drug then remains bound, which keeps the end-plate from repolarizing.
- The neuromuscular blockers are used to produce muscle relaxation during surgery, endotracheal intubation, and mechanical ventilation.
- Neuromuscular blockers do not reduce consciousness or pain.
- The major adverse effect of neuromuscular blockers is respiratory depression.
- Cholinesterase inhibitors can reverse the effects of nondepolarizing neuromuscular blockers but will intensify the effects of succinylcholine.
- Succinylcholine can cause malignant hyperthermia, a life-threatening condition.
- Succinylcholine is eliminated by plasma cholinesterases. Effects are greatly prolonged in patients with low plasma cholinesterase activity.
- All of the neuromuscular blockers are quaternary ammonium compounds and therefore must be administered parenterally (almost always IV).

## Summary of Major Nursing Implications

### Neuromuscular Blocking Agents

| | |
|---|---|
| Atracurium | Pancuronium |
| Cisatracurium | Pipercuronium |
| Doxacurium | Rocuronium |
| Gallamine | Succinylcholine |
| Metocurine | Tubocurarine |
| Mivacurium | Vecuronium |

Except where noted otherwise, the implications summarized below apply to all of the neuromuscular blocking agents.

### Preadministration Assessment

#### Therapeutic Goal

Provision of muscle relaxation during surgery, endotracheal intubation, mechanical ventilation, electroconvulsive therapy, and other procedures.

#### Identifying High-Risk Patients

Use all neuromuscular blockers with *caution* in patients with *myasthenia gravis*.

*Succinylcholine* is *contraindicated* for patients with *low pseudocholinesterase activity* or a *personal or familial history of malignant hyperthermia*.

### Implementation: Administration

#### Routes

**Intravenous.** *All* neuromuscular blockers.

**Intramuscular.** *Tubocurarine* and *succinylcholine*.

#### Administration

Neuromuscular blockers are dangerous drugs that should be administered only by clinicians skilled in their use.

### Implementation: Measures to Enhance Therapeutic Effects

Neuromuscular blockers do not affect consciousness or perception of pain. When used during surgery, these drugs must be accompanied by adequate anesthesia. When neuromuscular blockers are used for prolonged paralysis during mechanical ventilation, care should be taken to ensure comfort (e.g., positioning the patient comfortably, moistening the mouth periodically). Since patients may be awake (but won't appear to be), conversations held in their presence should convey only information that is appropriate for them to hear.

## Ongoing Evaluation and Interventions

### Minimizing Adverse Effects

***Apnea.*** All neuromuscular blockers can cause respiratory arrest. Facilities for intubation and mechanical ventilation should be immediately available.

Monitor respiration constantly during the period of peak drug action. When drug administration is discontinued, take vital signs at least every 17 minutes until recovery is complete.

Cholinesterase inhibitors can be used to reverse respiratory depression caused by *nondepolarizing* neuromuscular blockers—but not by succinylcholine, a *depolarizing* blocker.

***Malignant Hyperthermia.*** *Succinylcholine* can trigger malignant hyperthermia. Predisposition to this reaction is genetic. Assess for a family history of the reaction.

***Muscle Pain.*** *Succinylcholine* may cause muscle pain. Reassure the patient that this response, although unpleasant, is not unusual.

***Hypotension.*** Several neuromuscular blockers can cause hypotension secondary to ganglionic blockade or release of histamine. Antihistamines may help counteract this effect.

### Minimizing Adverse Interactions

***Antibiotics.*** Certain antibiotics, including *aminoglycosides* and *tetracyclines*, can intensify neuromuscular blockade. Use these antibiotics with caution.

***Cholinesterase Inhibitors.*** These drugs delay inactivation of *succinylcholine*, thereby greatly prolonging paralysis. Accordingly, cholinesterase inhibitors are contraindicated for patients receiving succinylcholine.

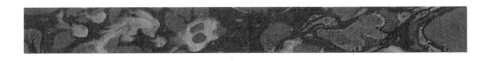

# Adrenergic Drugs

# CHAPTER 18

# Adrenergic Agonists

A drenergic agonists produce their effects by causing activation of adrenergic receptors. Since the sympathetic nervous system acts through these same receptors, responses to adrenergic agonists and responses to stimulation by the sympathetic nervous system are very similar. Because of this similarity, adrenergic agonists are often referred to as *sympathomimetics*. Adrenergic agonists have a broad spectrum of clinical applications, ranging from treatment of heart failure to relief of asthma to delay of preterm labor.

Learning about adrenergic agonists can be a challenge. To facilitate learning, we will approach these drugs in four stages. First we will discuss the general mechanisms by which drugs can activate adrenergic receptors. Next we will establish an overview of the major adrenergic agonists, focusing on their receptor specificity and chemical classification. After that we will address the adrenergic receptors themselves; for each receptor type—alpha$_1$, alpha$_2$, beta$_1$, beta$_2$, and dopamine—we will discuss the beneficial and harmful effects that can result from receptor activation. Lastly, we will integrate all of this information by discussing the characteristic properties of representative individual sympathomimetic drugs.

It should be noted that this chapter is intended only as an *introduction* to the adrenergic agonists. Our objective here is to discuss the basic properties of the sympathomimetic drugs and establish an overview of their applications and adverse effects. Virtually all the drugs addressed in this chapter are discussed again in later chapters. In those subsequent chapters, the clinical applications of the adrenergic agonists are considered in greater depth than they are here.

## Mechanisms of Adrenergic Receptor Activation

Drugs can activate adrenergic receptors by four basic mechanisms: (1) direct receptor binding, (2) promotion of norepinephrine (NE) release, (3) blockade of NE reuptake, and (4) inhibition of NE inactivation. Note that only the first mechanism is *direct*. With the other three mechanisms, receptor activation occurs by an *indirect* process. Examples of drugs that act by these four mechanisms are presented in Table 18–1.

*Direct Receptor Binding.* Direct interaction with receptors is the most common mechanism by which drugs activate peripheral adrenergic receptors. The direct-acting receptor stimulants produce their effects by binding to adrenergic receptors and mimicking the actions of natural transmitters (NE, epinephrine, dopamine). In this chapter, all of the drugs discussed activate adrenergic receptors directly.

*Promotion of NE Release.* By acting on terminals of sympathetic nerves to cause release of NE, drugs can

## TABLE 18-1. MECHANISMS OF ADRENERGIC RECEPTOR ACTIVATION

| Mechanism of Stimulation | Examples |
| --- | --- |
| *Direct Mechanism* | |
| Binding to receptor to cause activation | Epinephrine |
| | Isoproterenol |
| | Ephedrine* |
| *Indirect Mechanisms* | |
| Promotion of NE release | Ephedrine* |
| | Amphetamines |
| Inhibition of NE reuptake | Cocaine |
| | Tricyclic antidepressants |
| Inhibition of MAO | MAO inhibitors |

NE = norepinephrine, MAO = monamine oxidase.
*Ephedrine is a mixed-acting drug that activates receptors directly and also promotes release of norepinephrine.

bring about activation of adrenergic receptors. Agents that promote receptor activation by this indirect mechanism include the amphetamines and ephedrine. (Ephedrine can also stimulate adrenergic receptors directly.)

**Inhibition of NE Reuptake.** Recall that reuptake of NE into terminals of sympathetic nerves is the major mechanism by which adrenergic transmission is terminated. By blocking NE reuptake, drugs can cause NE to accumulate within the synaptic gap, and can thereby increase receptor activation. Agents that act by blocking NE reuptake include cocaine and the tricyclic antidepressants.

**Inhibition of NE Inactivation.** As discussed in Chapter 14, some of the NE in terminals of adrenergic neurons is subject to inactivation by monoamine oxidase (MAO). Hence, drugs that inhibit MAO will increase the amount of NE available for release, and will thereby enhance receptor activation. (It should be noted that, in addition to being present in sympathetic nerves, MAO is present in the liver and the intestinal wall. The significance of MAO at these other sites is considered later in the chapter.)

In this chapter, which is dedicated to *peripherally* acting sympathomimetics, practically all of the drugs discussed act exclusively by *direct* receptor activation. The only exception is *ephedrine*, an agent that works by a combination of direct receptor activation and promotion of NE release.

Most of the *indirect-acting* adrenergic agonists are used for their ability to activate adrenergic receptors in the *central nervous system* (CNS)—not for their effects in the periphery. The indirect-acting sympathomimetics (e.g., amphetamine, cocaine) are mentioned here to emphasize that, although these agents are employed for their effects on the brain, they can and will cause activation of adrenergic receptors in the periphery. Peripheral activation is responsible for certain toxicities of these drugs (e.g., cardiac dysrhythmias, hypertension).

# Overview of the Adrenergic Agonists

## Chemical Classification: Catecholamines versus Noncatecholamines

The adrenergic agonists fall into two major chemical classes: catecholamines and noncatecholamines. As we shall see, the catecholamines and noncatecholamines differ from each other in three important respects: (1) oral usability, (2) duration of action, and (3) ability to act in the CNS. Accordingly, if we know which category a particular adrenergic agonist belongs to, we will know three of that drug's prominent characteristics.

### Catecholamines

The catecholamines are so named because they contain a *catechol* group and an *amine* group. A catechol group is simply a benzene ring that has hydroxyl groups on two adjacent carbons (Fig. 18-1). The amine component of the catecholamines is *ethylamine*. Structural formulas for each of the major catecholamines—epinephrine, norepinephrine, isoproterenol, dopamine, and dobutamine—are presented in Figure 18-1. Because of their chemistry, all of the catecholamines have three characteristics in common: (1) they cannot be taken orally, (2) they have a brief duration of action, and (3) they cannot cross the blood-brain barrier.

The actions of two enzymes—*monoamine oxidase* and *catechol-o-methyltransferase* (COMT)—explain why the catecholamines have short half-lives and cannot be used orally. MAO and COMT are located in the liver and the intestinal wall. Both enzymes are very active and quickly destroy catecholamines administered by any route. Because these enzymes are located in the liver and intestinal wall, catecholamines that are administered orally become inactivated before they can reach the systemic circulation. Hence, catecholamines are ineffective if given by mouth. Because of rapid inactivation by MAO and COMT, three catecholamines—norepinephrine, dopamine, and dobutamine—are effective only if administered by continuous infusion. Administration by other parenteral routes (e.g., SC, IM) will not permit adequate blood levels to be achieved.

The catecholamines cannot cross the blood-brain barrier because they are polar. (Recall from Chapter 5 that polar compounds penetrate membranes poorly.) The polar nature of the catecholamines is due to the hydroxyl groups on the catechol portion of the molecule. Because they cannot cross the blood-brain barrier, catecholamines have minimal effects on the CNS.

You should be aware that catecholamine-containing solutions, which are normally colorless when first prepared, will turn pink or brown over time. This pigmentation is caused by oxidation of the catecholamine molecule. As a

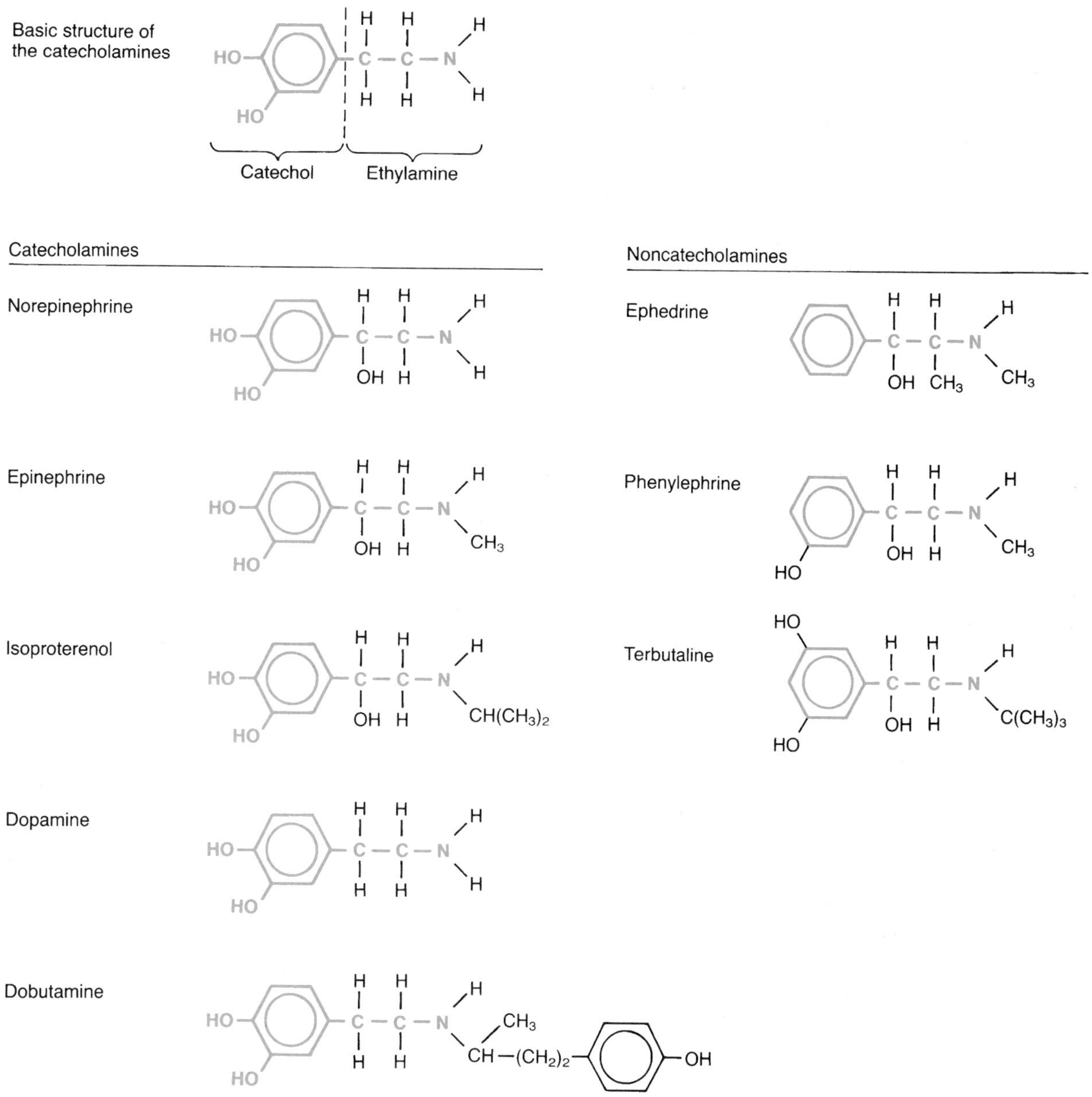

**Figure 18–1. Structures of catecholamines and noncatecholamines.** *Catecholamines:* Note that all of the catecholamines share the same basic chemical formula. Because of their biochemical properties, the catecholamines cannot be used orally, cannot cross the blood-brain barrier, and have short half-lives (owing to rapid inactivation by MAO and COMT).

*Noncatecholamines:* Although structurally similar to catecholamines, noncatecholamines differ from catecholamines in three important ways: (1) noncatecholamines are usable orally; (2) they can cross the blood-brain barrier; and (3) since they are not rapidly metabolized by MAO or COMT, they have much longer half-lives than the catecholamines.

rule, *catecholamine solutions should be discarded as soon as discoloration appears.* The only exception to this rule applies to *dobutamine,* which can be used up to 24 hours after the solution was made, even if discoloration has developed.

## Noncatecholamines

The noncatecholamines have ethylamine in their structure (see Fig. 18-1) but do not contain the catechol portion that characterizes the catecholamines. The noncate-

cholamines considered in this chapter are ephedrine, phenylephrine, and terbutaline.

The noncatecholamines differ from the catecholamines in several important respects. First, because they lack a catechol group, noncatecholamines are not substrates for COMT and are metabolized slowly by MAO. As a result, the noncatecholamines have half-lives that are much longer than those of the catecholamines. Furthermore, since they do not undergo rapid degradation by MAO and COMT, the noncatecholamines can be given orally, whereas the catecholamines cannot. Lastly, the noncatecholamines are considerably less polar than the catecholamines. As a result, the noncatecholamines are more able to penetrate the blood-brain barrier and influence the CNS.

## Receptor Specificity

To understand the actions of individual adrenergic agonists, we need to know their receptor specificity. Since the sympathomimetic drugs differ widely from one another with respect to the receptors they can activate, learning the receptor specificity of these drugs will take some effort.

Variability in receptor specificity among the adrenergic agonists can be illustrated with three drugs: terbutaline, isoproterenol, and epinephrine. Terbutaline is highly selective, acting at beta$_2$ receptors only. Isoproterenol is less selective, acting at beta$_1$ receptors as well as beta$_2$ receptors. Epinephrine is less selective yet, acting at all four subtypes (alpha$_1$, alpha$_2$, beta$_1$, and beta$_2$) of adrenergic receptors.

The receptor specificities of the major adrenergic agonists are summarized in Table 18-2. In the upper part of the table, receptor specificity is presented in tabular format. In the lower part, the same information is presented schematically. By learning (memorizing) the content of Table 18-2, you will have taken a major step toward understanding the pharmacology of the sympathomimetic drugs.

Please note that the concept of receptor specificity is *relative*—not absolute. The ability of a drug to selectively activate certain receptors to the exclusion of others is dependent upon dosage: at low doses, selectivity is maximal; as dosage increases, selectivity declines. For example, when terbutaline is administered in low to moderate doses, the drug is highly selective for beta$_2$-adrenergic receptors. However, if the dosage is high, terbutaline will activate beta$_1$ receptors as well. The information on receptor specificity in Table 18-2 refers to usual therapeutic doses. So-called selective agents will activate additional adrenergic receptors if the dosage is abnormally high.

# Therapeutic Applications and Adverse Effects of Adrenergic Receptor Activation

In this section we discuss the responses—both therapeutic and adverse—that can be elicited with sympathomimetic drugs. Since many adrenergic agonists activate more than one type of receptor (see Table 18-2), it could be quite confusing if we were to talk about the effects of the sympathomimetics employing specific drugs as examples. Consequently, rather than attempting to structure this presentation around representative drugs, we will discuss the actions of the adrenergic agonists one receptor at

## TABLE 18-2. RECEPTOR SPECIFICITY OF REPRESENTATIVE ADRENERGIC AGONISTS

| Catecholamines | | Noncatecholamines | |
| --- | --- | --- | --- |
| Drug | Receptors Activated | Drug | Receptors Activated |
| Epinephrine | $\alpha_1$, $\alpha_2$, $\beta_1$, $\beta_2$ | Ephedrine* | $\alpha_1$, $\alpha_2$, $\beta_1$, $\beta_2$ |
| Norepinephrine | $\alpha_1$, $\alpha_2$, $\beta_1$ | Phenylephrine | $\alpha_1$ |
| Isoproterenol | $\beta_1$, $\beta_2$ | Terbutaline | $\beta_2$ |
| Dobutamine | $\beta_1$ | | |
| Dopamine† | $\alpha_1$, $\beta_1$, dopamine | | |

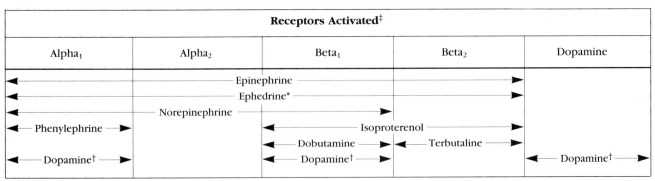

| Receptors Activated‡ | | | | |
| --- | --- | --- | --- | --- |
| Alpha$_1$ | Alpha$_2$ | Beta$_1$ | Beta$_2$ | Dopamine |

$\alpha$ = alpha, $\beta$ = Beta.
*Ephedrine is a mixed-acting agent that causes NE release and also activates alpha and beta receptors directly.
†Receptor activation by dopamine is dose dependent.
‡This chart represents in tabular form the same information on receptor specificity given above. Arrows indicate the range of receptors that the drugs can stimulate (at usual therapeutic doses).

a time. Our discussion begins with alpha$_1$ receptors, and then moves sequentially to alpha$_2$ receptors, beta$_1$ receptors, beta$_2$ receptors, and dopamine receptors. For each receptor type, we will discuss both the therapeutic and the adverse responses that can result from receptor activation.

To understand the effects of any specific adrenergic agonist, all that you need is two types of information: (1) the identity of the receptor type at which the drug acts and (2) the effects produced by activating those receptors. Combining these two types of information will reveal a profile of drug action. This is the same approach to understanding neuropharmacologic agents that we discussed in Chapter 13.

Before you go into the rest of this chapter, I encourage you (strongly advise you) to review Table 14-3. Since we are about to discuss the clinical consequences of adrenergic receptor activation, and since Table 14-3 summarizes the responses to activation of these receptors, the benefits of being familiar with Table 14-3 are obvious. If you choose not to memorize Table 14-3 now, at least be prepared to refer to the table as we discuss the consequences of receptor activation.

## Clinical Consequences of Alpha$_1$ Activation

In this section we discuss the therapeutic and adverse effects that can result from activation of alpha$_1$-adrenergic receptors. As indicated in Table 18-2, drugs capable of activating alpha$_1$ receptors include epinephrine, norepinephrine, phenylephrine, ephedrine, and dopamine.

### Therapeutic Applications of Alpha$_1$ Activation

Activation of alpha$_1$ receptors elicits two responses that can be of therapeutic use: (1) *vasoconstriction* (in blood vessels of the skin, viscera, and mucous membranes), and (2) *mydriasis*. Of these two responses, vasoconstriction is the one for which alpha$_1$ activation is most often employed. Use of alpha$_1$-activating agents to produce mydriasis is relatively rare.

*Hemostasis.* Hemostasis is defined as the arrest of bleeding. Drugs capable of alpha$_1$ activation produce hemostasis by causing vasoconstriction. Alpha$_1$ stimulants are given to stop bleeding primarily in the skin and mucous membranes. Epinephrine, applied topically, is the alpha$_1$-activating agent used most for this purpose.

*Nasal Decongestion.* Nasal congestion results from dilation and engorgement of blood vessels in the nasal mucosa. Drugs can relieve congestion by causing alpha$_1$-mediated vasoconstriction. Specific alpha$_1$-activating agents employed as nasal decongestants include phenylephrine (applied topically) and ephedrine (taken orally).

*Adjunct to Local Anesthesia.* Alpha$_1$ agonists are frequently combined with local anesthetics to delay anesthetic absorption. Absorption is delayed because alpha$_1$-mediated vasoconstriction reduces blood flow to the site of anesthetic administration. Delay of anesthetic absorp-

tion has three benefits: (1) it prolongs anesthesia, (2) it allows a reduction in anesthetic dosage, and (3) it reduces the systemic effects that a local anesthetic might produce. The drug used most frequently to delay anesthetic absorption is epinephrine.

*Elevation of Blood Pressure.* Because of their ability to cause vasoconstriction, alpha$_1$ agonists can be used to elevate blood pressure in hypotensive states. Please note, however, that alpha$_1$ agonists are not the primary therapy for hypotension; rather, these drugs are reserved for situations in which other measures, including fluid replacement, have failed to restore blood pressure to a satisfactory level.

*Mydriasis.* Activation of alpha$_1$ receptors on the radial muscle of the iris causes mydriasis (dilation of the pupil). Production of mydriasis can facilitate eye examinations and ocular surgery. Note that the ophthalmic applications of alpha$_1$ activation are the only applications that are not based on vasoconstriction.

### Adverse Effects of Alpha$_1$ Activation

All of the adverse effects associated with alpha$_1$ activation result directly or indirectly from vasoconstriction.

*Hypertension.* Alpha$_1$ agonists can produce hypertension by causing widespread vasoconstriction. Severe hypertension is most likely with parenteral administration. Accordingly, when an alpha$_1$ agonist is given parenterally, cardiovascular status must be monitored continuously; never leave the patient unattended.

*Necrosis.* If the intravenous line employed to administer an alpha$_1$ agonist becomes extravasated, local seepage of the drug may result in necrosis (tissue death). The cause of necrosis is lack of blood flow secondary to excessive local vasoconstriction. If extravasation occurs, the area should be infiltrated with an alpha$_1$-blocking agent (e.g., phentolamine). By counteracting alpha$_1$-mediated vasoconstriction, the antagonist will help minimize injury.

*Bradycardia.* Alpha$_1$ agonists can cause reflex slowing of the heart. The mechanism is this: alpha$_1$-mediated vasoconstriction elevates blood pressure, which triggers the baroreceptor reflex, causing heart rate to decline. In patients with marginal cardiac reserve, the decrease in cardiac output may compromise tissue perfusion.

## Clinical Consequences of Alpha$_2$ Activation

As discussed in Chapter 14, alpha$_2$ receptors in the periphery are located *presynaptically*, and their activation inhibits norepinephrine release. Several adrenergic agonists (e.g., epinephrine, norepinephrine, ephedrine) are capable of causing alpha$_2$ activation. However, the ability of drugs to activate alpha$_2$ receptors in the periphery has only minimal clinical significance. There are no therapeutic applications related to activation of peripheral alpha$_2$ receptors. Furthermore, activation of these receptors rarely causes adverse effects of any consequence.

In contrast to alpha$_2$ receptors in the periphery, alpha$_2$ receptors in the CNS are of great clinical significance. The principal response to stimulation of central alpha$_2$ receptors is a reduction of sympathetic outflow to the heart and blood vessels. By decreasing sympathetic outflow, drugs that stimulate central alpha$_2$ receptors act to *reduce* stimulation of adrenergic receptors in the periphery. The drugs that stimulate alpha$_2$ receptors in the CNS are discussed in Chapter 20 (Indirect-Acting Antiadrenergic Agents).

## Clinical Consequences of Beta$_1$ Activation

All of the clinically relevant responses to activation of beta$_1$ receptors result from activating beta$_1$ receptors in the *heart*; activation of renal beta$_1$ receptors is not associated with either beneficial or adverse effects. As indicated in Table 18-2, beta$_1$ receptors can be activated by epinephrine, norepinephrine, isoproterenol, dopamine, dobutamine, and ephedrine.

### Therapeutic Applications of Beta$_1$ Activation

*Cardiac Arrest.* By activating cardiac beta$_1$ receptors, drugs can initiate contraction in a heart that has stopped beating. It should be noted, however, that drugs are not the preferred treatment for cardiac arrest; rather, drugs should be used only after more desirable procedures (mechanical thumping, DC cardioversion) have failed to restart the heart. When a beta$_1$ agonist is indicated, epinephrine—injected directly into the heart—is the preferred drug.

*Heart Failure.* Heart failure is characterized by a reduction in the force of myocardial contraction, resulting in insufficient cardiac output. Since activation of beta$_1$ receptors in the heart has a positive inotropic effect (i.e., increases the force of contraction), drugs that activate these receptors can improve cardiac performance.

*Shock.* This condition is characterized by profound hypotension and greatly reduced tissue perfusion. The primary goal of treatment is to maintain blood flow to vital organs. By increasing heart rate and force of contraction, beta$_1$ stimulants can increase cardiac output and can thereby improve tissue perfusion.

*Atrioventricular Heart Block.* Atrioventricular (AV) heart block is a condition in which impulse conduction from the atria to the ventricles is impeded or blocked entirely. As a consequence, the ventricles are no longer driven at an appropriate rate. Since activation of cardiac beta$_1$ receptors can enhance impulse conduction through the AV node, beta$_1$ stimulants can help overcome AV block. It should be noted, however, that drugs are only a temporary form of treatment; for long-term management, a pacemaker is implanted.

### Adverse Effects of Beta$_1$ Activation

All of the adverse effects of beta$_1$ activation result from activating beta$_1$ receptors in the *heart*; activating renal beta$_1$ receptors is not associated with untoward effects.

*Altered Heart Rate or Rhythm.* Overstimulation of cardiac beta$_1$ receptors can produce *tachycardia* (excessive heart rate) and *dysrhythmias* (irregular heart beat).

*Angina Pectoris.* In some patients, drugs that activate beta$_1$ receptors can precipitate an attack of angina pectoris, a condition characterized by substernal pain in the region of the heart. Anginal pain occurs when oxygen supply (blood flow) to the heart is insufficient to meet the heart's oxygen needs. The most common cause of angina is coronary atherosclerosis (accumulation of lipids and other substances in coronary arteries). Since beta$_1$ agonists increase cardiac oxygen demand (by increasing heart rate and force of contraction), patients with compromised coronary blood flow are at risk of an anginal attack.

## Clinical Consequences of Beta$_2$ Activation

### Therapeutic Applications of Beta$_2$ Activation

Therapeutic applications of beta$_2$ activation are limited to the lung and the uterus. Drugs used for their beta$_2$-activating ability include epinephrine, isoproterenol, and terbutaline.

*Asthma.* Asthma is a chronic condition characterized by bronchoconstriction occurring in response to a variety of stimuli. During a severe attack, airflow can be reduced so greatly as to threaten life. Since drugs that activate beta$_2$ receptors in the lung promote *bronchodilation*, these agents can help relieve or prevent asthma attacks.

For therapy of asthma, adrenergic agonists that are *selective for beta$_2$ receptors* (e.g., terbutaline) are preferred to less selective agents (e.g., epinephrine, isoproterenol). This is especially true for patients who suffer from *angina pectoris* or *tachycardia* in addition to asthma; we do not want to give these patients drugs that can activate beta$_1$ receptors since the drugs would aggravate the cardiac disorder.

Several of the beta$_2$ agonists used to treat asthma are administered by *inhalation*. This route is desirable in that it helps minimize adverse systemic effects. It should be noted, however, that inhalation does not guarantee safety: serious systemic toxicity can result from overdosage with inhaled sympathomimetics. Accordingly, patients must be warned against inhaling too much medication.

*Delay of Preterm Labor.* Activation of beta$_2$ receptors in the uterus relaxes uterine smooth muscle. This action can be exploited to delay preterm labor.

### Adverse Effects of Beta$_2$ Activation

*Hyperglycemia.* The most noteworthy adverse response to beta$_2$ activation is *hyperglycemia* (elevation of blood glucose). Beta$_2$ agonists can cause hyperglycemia by acting on the liver and skeletal muscles to promote breakdown of glycogen into glucose. As a rule, these drugs produce hyperglycemia only in patients with *diabetes*; in patients with normal pancreatic function, insulin will be released in response to glucose elevation, thereby reducing blood glucose to an appropriate level. If hyperglycemia develops in the diabetic patient, insulin dosage should be increased.

**Tremor.** Tremor is the most common side effect of beta$_2$ agonists. It occurs because activation of beta$_2$ receptors in skeletal muscle enhances contraction. Tremor generally fades over time and can be minimized by initiating therapy with low doses.

## Clinical Consequences of Dopamine Receptor Activation

Activation of peripheral dopamine receptors causes dilation of the vasculature of the kidneys. This effect is exploited in the treatment of *shock*: by dilating renal blood vessels, we can improve renal perfusion and can thereby reduce the risk of kidney failure. *Dopamine* itself is the only drug available that can activate dopamine receptors. It should be noted that, when dopamine is given to treat shock, the drug also enhances cardiac performance (by virtue of its ability to activate beta$_1$ receptors in the heart).

## Multiple Receptor Activation: Treatment of Anaphylactic Shock

*Pathophysiology of Anaphylaxis.* Anaphylactic shock is a manifestation of severe allergy. The reaction is characterized by *hypotension* (from widespread vasodilation), *bronchoconstriction*, and *edema of the glottis.* Although histamine contributes to these responses, symptoms are due largely to release of other mediators (e.g., leukotrienes). Anaphylaxis can be triggered by a variety of substances, including bee venom, wasp venom, and certain drugs (e.g., penicillins).

*Treatment.* *Epinephrine*, injected subcutaneously, is the treatment of choice for anaphylactic shock. Beneficial responses derive from the ability of epinephrine to activate three types of adrenergic receptors: alpha$_1$, beta$_1$, and beta$_2$. By activating these receptors, epinephrine can reverse the most severe manifestations of the anaphylactic reaction. Activation of beta$_1$ receptors increases cardiac output, thereby helping to elevate blood pressure. Blood pressure is also increased because of epinephrine's ability to promote alpha$_1$-mediated vasoconstriction. In addition to increasing blood pressure, vasoconstriction helps suppress glottal edema. By activating beta$_2$ receptors, epinephrine can counteract bronchoconstriction. Individuals who are prone to severe allergic responses should be advised to carry a syringe of epinephrine at all times. (Antihistamines are not especially useful against anaphylaxis because histamine is only a minor contributor to the overall reaction.)

## Properties of Representative Adrenergic Agonists

Our objective in this section is to establish an overview of the adrenergic agonists. This overview is presented in the form of "drug digests" that highlight characteristic features of representative sympathomimetic agents.

As noted above, there are two major keys to understanding individual adrenergic agonists: (1) knowledge of the receptors that the drug can activate and (2) knowledge of the therapeutic and adverse effects that receptor activation can elicit. Integrating these two types of information will reveal the spectrum of effects that a particular drug can produce.

Unfortunately, knowing the effects that a drug is capable of producing does not always allow us to predict the *actual clinical applications* of that drug. Why? Because some adrenergic agonists are not used for all of the effects that they are able to produce. Norepinephrine, for example, can activate alpha$_1$ receptors and can therefore produce mydriasis; however, although norepinephrine can produce mydriasis, the drug is not actually used for this purpose. Similarly, although isoproterenol is capable of producing uterine relaxation (through beta$_2$ activation), isoproterenol is not employed clinically for this effect. Because receptor specificity is not always a predictor of the therapeutic applications of a particular adrenergic agonist, for each of the drugs discussed below, approved clinical applications are indicated.

### Epinephrine

- *Receptor specificity*: Alpha$_1$, alpha$_2$, beta$_1$, beta$_2$
- *Chemical classification*: Catecholamine

Epinephrine [Adrenalin, others] was among the first adrenergic agonists employed clinically and can be considered the prototype of the sympathomimetic drugs. Because of its prototypic status, epinephrine is discussed in detail.

#### Therapeutic Uses

Epinephrine can activate all four subtypes of adrenergic receptors. As a consequence, the drug can produce a broad spectrum of beneficial sympathomimetic effects:

- Because of its ability to cause alpha$_1$-mediated vasoconstriction, epinephrine is used to (1) delay absorption of local anesthetics, (2) control superficial bleeding, (3) reduce nasal congestion, and (4) elevate blood pressure.
- Activation of alpha$_1$ receptors on the iris is employed to produce mydriasis during ophthalmologic procedures.
- Because of its ability to activate beta$_1$ receptors, epinephrine is used to (1) overcome AV heart block and (2) restore cardiac function in patients with cardiac arrest.
- Activation of beta$_2$ receptors in the lung promotes bronchodilation in patients with asthma.
- Because of its ability to activate a combination of alpha and beta receptors, epinephrine is the treatment of choice for anaphylactic shock.

#### Pharmacokinetics

*Absorption.* Epinephrine may be administered topically, by injection, and by inhalation. The drug cannot be given orally; as discussed above, epinephrine and other catecholamines cannot be given orally because they undergo destruction by MAO and COMT before reaching the systemic circulation. With subcutaneous injection, absorption is slow because of epinephrine-induced local vasoconstriction. Absorption is more rapid following intramuscular injection. When epinephrine is inhaled (to treat asthma), systemic absorption is usually minimal; however, if dosing is excessive, systemic absorption can be sufficient to cause serious toxicity.

*Inactivation.* Epinephrine has a short plasma half-life because of two processes: enzymatic inactivation and uptake into adrenergic nerves. The enzymes that inactivate epinephrine and other catecholamines are MAO and COMT.

## Adverse Effects

Because of its ability to activate the four major adrenergic receptor subtypes, epinephrine can produce multiple adverse effects.

*Hypertensive Crisis.* Vasoconstriction secondary to excessive alpha$_1$ activation can produce a dramatic and dangerous increase in blood pressure. Cerebral hemorrhage can occur. Because of the potential for severe hypertension, patients receiving *parenteral* epinephrine must undergo continuous monitoring of cardiovascular status.

*Dysrhythmias.* Excessive activation of beta$_1$ receptors in the heart can produce dysrhythmias. Because of their sensitivity to catecholamines, hyperthyroid patients are at high risk for epinephrine-induced dysrhythmias.

*Angina Pectoris.* By activating beta$_1$ receptors in the heart, epinephrine can increase both the work and the oxygen demand of the heart. If the increase in oxygen demand is big enough, an anginal attack may ensue. Precipitation of angina is especially likely in patients with coronary atherosclerosis.

*Necrosis Following Extravasation.* If an IV line containing epinephrine becomes extravasated, the resultant localized vasoconstriction may cause necrosis. Because of this possibility, patients receiving IV epinephrine should be monitored closely. If extravasation occurs, injury can be minimized by local injection of phentolamine, an alpha-adrenergic antagonist.

*Hyperglycemia.* In diabetics, epinephrine can cause hyperglycemia. Hyperglycemia results from breakdown of glycogen in response to activation of beta$_2$ receptors in liver and skeletal muscle. If hyperglycemia develops, insulin dosage should be increased.

## Drug Interactions

*Monoamine Oxidase Inhibitors.* The MAO inhibitors are drugs that suppress the activity of MAO. These agents are used primarily to treat depression (see Chapter 30). Since MAO is one of the enzymes that inactivate epinephrine and other catecholamines, inhibition of MAO will prolong and intensify epinephrine's effects. As a rule, patients receiving an MAO inhibitor should not be given epinephrine.

*Tricyclic Antidepressants.* As discussed in Chapter 30, tricyclic antidepressants block the uptake of catecholamines into adrenergic neurons. Since neuronal uptake is one mechanism by which the actions of norepinephrine and other catecholamines are terminated, blockade of uptake can intensify and prolong epinephrine's effects. Accordingly, patients receiving a tricyclic antidepressant may require a reduction in epinephrine dosage.

*General Anesthetics.* Several inhalation anesthetics render the myocardium hypersensitive to activation by beta$_1$ agonists. When the heart is in this hypersensitive state, exposure to epinephrine and other beta$_1$ agonists can cause dysrhythmias. These dysrhythmias may respond to a beta-adrenergic blocker (e.g., propranolol).

*Alpha-Adrenergic Blocking Agents.* Drugs that block alpha-adrenergic receptors can prevent their activation by epinephrine. Alpha blockers (e.g., phentolamine) can be used to treat toxicity (e.g., hypertension, local vasoconstriction) caused by excessive epinephrine-induced alpha activation.

*Beta-Adrenergic Blocking Agents.* Drugs that block beta-adrenergic receptors can prevent their activation by epinephrine. Beta-blocking agents (e.g., propranolol) can reduce adverse effects (e.g., dysrhythmias, anginal pain) caused by epinephrine and other beta$_1$ agonists.

## Preparations, Dosage, and Administration

Epinephrine [Adrenalin, others] is dispensed in solution for administration by several routes: intravenous, subcutaneous, intramuscular, intracardiac, intraspinal, inhalation, and topical. As indicated in Table 18–3, the strength of the epinephrine solution employed depends in large part on the route of administration. Note that solutions intended for *intravenous* administration are *less concentrated* than solutions intended for administration by most other routes. The reason that epinephrine must be diluted for intravenous use is that *intravenous administration of a concentrated epinephrine solution can produce potentially fatal reactions* (severe dysrhythmias and hyperten-

| TABLE 18–3. EPINEPHRINE SOLUTIONS: CONCENTRATIONS FOR DIFFERENT ROUTES OF ADMINISTRATION | |
|---|---|
| **Concentration of Epinephrine Solution** | **Route of Administration** |
| 1% (1:100) | Oral Inhalation |
| 0.1% (1:1,000) | Subcutaneous Intramuscular Intraspinal |
| 0.01% (1:10,000) | Intravenous Intracardiac |
| 0.001% (1:100,000) | In combination with local anesthetics |

sion). Therefore, *before epinephrine is administered intravenously, the solution should be carefully checked to ensure that its concentration is appropriate for intravenous use!* Aspirate prior to IM or SC injection to avoid inadvertent injection into a vein.

Patients receiving intravenous epinephrine should be monitored constantly. They should be observed for signs of excessive cardiovascular activation (e.g., dysrhythmias, hypertension) and for possible extravasation of the IV line. If systemic toxicity develops, epinephrine should be discontinued; if indicated, an alpha-adrenergic blocker, a beta-adrenergic blocker, or both should be given to suppress symptoms. If an epinephrine-containing IV line becomes extravasated, administration should be discontinued and the region of extravasation infiltrated with an alpha-adrenergic blocker.

### Norepinephrine

- *Receptor specificity:* Alpha$_1$, alpha$_2$, beta$_1$
- *Chemical classification:* Catecholamine

Norepinephrine is similar to epinephrine in many respects. With regard to receptor specificity, NE differs from epinephrine only in that NE does not activate beta$_2$ receptors. Accordingly, NE can elicit all of the responses that epinephrine can, except those that are beta$_2$ mediated. Because NE is a catecholamine, the drug cannot be given orally and is subject to rapid inactivation by MAO and COMT. Adverse effects are nearly identical to those of epinephrine: dysrhythmias, angina, hypertension, and local necrosis upon extravasation. In contrast to epinephrine, NE does not promote hyperglycemia, a response that is mediated by beta$_2$ receptors. As with epinephrine, responses to NE can be modified by MAO inhibitors, tricyclic antidepressants, general anesthetics, and adrenergic blocking agents.

Despite its similarities with epinephrine, NE has limited clinical applications. The only recognized indications are *hypotensive states* and *cardiac arrest.*

Norepinephrine [Levophed] is dispensed in solution (1 mg/ml) for administration by intravenous infusion only. Patients should never be left unattended. Cardiovascular status should be monitored continuously. Care must be taken to avoid extravasation.

## Isoproterenol

- *Receptor specificity:* Beta$_1$ and beta$_2$
- *Chemical classification:* Catecholamine

Isoproterenol [Isuprel] differs significantly from NE and epinephrine in that isoproterenol acts only at beta-adrenergic receptors. Isoproterenol was the first beta-selective agent employed clinically and will serve as our prototype of the beta-selective adrenergic agonists.

### Therapeutic Uses

***Cardiovascular.*** By activating beta$_1$ receptors on the heart, isoproterenol can benefit patients with several cardiovascular disorders. The drug can help overcome AV heart block, it can restart the heart following cardiac arrest, and it can increase cardiac output during shock.

***Asthma.*** By activating beta$_2$ receptors in the lung, isoproterenol can cause bronchodilation, thereby decreasing airway resistance. Following its introduction, isopro-

terenol became a mainstay of asthma therapy. However, because of the development of more selective beta-adrenergic agonists (i.e., drugs that activate beta$_2$ receptors only), use of isoproterenol for asthma has declined.

### Adverse Effects

Since isoproterenol does not activate alpha-adrenergic receptors, the drug produces fewer adverse effects than norepinephrine or epinephrine. The major undesired responses are cardiac. Excessive activation of beta$_1$ receptors in the heart can cause *dysrhythmias* and *angina pectoris.* In addition to its cardiac effects, isoproterenol can cause *hyperglycemia in diabetics* by promoting beta$_2$-mediated glycogenolysis.

### Drug Interactions

The major drug interactions of isoproterenol are nearly identical to those of epinephrine. Effects are *enhanced by MAO inhibitors* and *tricyclic antidepressants* and *reduced* by *beta-adrenergic blocking agents.* Like epinephrine, isoproterenol can cause dysrhythmias in patients receiving certain *inhalation anesthetics.*

### Receptor Specificity

Isoproterenol activates beta$_1$ and beta$_2$ receptors but not alpha-adrenergic receptors. Because it can activate beta$_1$ as well as beta$_2$ receptors, when used to treat asthma, isoproterenol will cause beta$_1$ activation of the heart as a side effect. Accordingly, isoproterenol should not be used to treat asthma in patients who also have angina, tachycardia, or any other cardiac disorder that might be aggravated by beta$_1$ activation. Because isoproterenol is unable to distinguish between beta$_1$ and beta$_2$ receptors, and because beta$_2$-selective adrenergic agonists (e.g., terbutaline) are now available, use of isoproterenol to treat asthma has greatly declined.

### Preparations and Administration

***Preparations.*** Isoproterenol hydrochloride [Isuprel] is available in solution (0.2 mg/ml) for parenteral administration and in glossets (10 and 15 mg) for sublingual administration. In addition, the drug is available in a metered-dose aerosol device [Isuprel Mistometer, Medihaler-Iso] for treatment of asthma.

***Administration.*** For therapy of *asthma,* isoproterenol can be administered by oral inhalation, sublingually, and intravenously. For routine therapy, oral inhalation is preferred.

When used to *stimulate the heart,* isoproterenol can be administered IV, IM, and by intracardiac injection. The dosage for intramuscular administration is about 10 times greater than the dosage employed by the other two routes.

## Dopamine

- *Receptor specificity:* Dopamine, beta$_1$, and, at high doses, alpha$_1$
- *Chemical classification:* Catecholamine

### Receptor Specificity

The degree of receptor specificity displayed by dopamine is dose dependent. When administered in low therapeutic doses, dopamine acts on dopamine receptors only. At moderate therapeutic doses, dopamine activates beta$_1$ receptors in addition to dopamine receptors. At very high doses, dopamine activates alpha$_1$ receptors along with beta$_1$ and dopamine receptors.

## Therapeutic Uses

*Shock.* The major indication for dopamine is shock. Benefits derive from effects on the heart and the renal vasculature. By activating beta$_1$ receptors in the heart, dopamine can increase cardiac output, thereby improving tissue perfusion. By activating dopamine receptors in the kidney, dopamine can dilate renal blood vessels, thereby improving renal perfusion, which in turn reduces the risk of renal failure. Treatment can be evaluated by monitoring output of urine.

*Heart Failure.* Heart failure is characterized by reduced tissue perfusion secondary to reduced cardiac output. Dopamine can help alleviate symptoms by activating beta$_1$ receptors on the heart, which increases cardiac output by increasing myocardial contractility.

## Adverse Effects

The most common adverse effects of dopamine—*tachycardia*, *dysrhythmias*, and *anginal pain*—result from activation of beta$_1$ receptors in the heart. Because of its cardiac actions, dopamine is contraindicated for patients with tachydysrhythmias or ventricular fibrillation. Since high concentrations of dopamine cause alpha$_1$ activation, extravasation may result in *necrosis* from localized vasoconstriction; tissue injury can be minimized by local administration of phentolamine, an alpha-adrenergic blocking agent.

## Drug Interactions

*MAO inhibitors* can intensify the effects of dopamine on the heart and blood vessels. If a patient is receiving an MAO inhibitor, the dosage of dopamine must be reduced by at least 90%. *Tricyclic antidepressants* can also intensify dopamine's actions, but not to the extent seen with MAO inhibitors. Certain *general anesthetics* can sensitize the myocardium to the stimulant actions of dopamine and other catecholamines, thereby creating a risk of dysrhythmias. *Diuretics* can complement the beneficial effects of dopamine on the kidney.

### Preparations, Dosage, and Administration

*Preparations.* Dopamine hydrochloride [Intropin] is dispensed in aqueous solutions that range in concentration from 40 to 160 mg/ml.

*Dosage.* Dopamine must be diluted prior to infusion. For treatment of *shock*, a dilution of 400 µg/ml can be used. The recommended initial rate of infusion is 2 to 5 µg/kg/min. If needed, the infusion rate can be gradually increased to a maximum of 20 to 50 µg/kg/min.

*Administration.* Administration is intravenous. Because of extremely rapid inactivation by MAO and COMT, dopamine must be given by *continuous infusion*. A metering device is needed to control the flow rate. Cardiovascular status must be closely monitored. If extravasation occurs, the infusion should be stopped and the region of extravasation infiltrated with an alpha-adrenergic antagonist.

### Dobutamine

- *Receptor specificity:* Beta$_1$
- *Chemical classification:* Catecholamine

*Actions and Uses.* At therapeutic doses, dobutamine causes selective activation of beta$_1$-adrenergic receptors. The only indication for the drug is *heart failure*.

*Adverse Effects.* The major adverse effect is tachycardia. Blood pressure and the electrocardiogram (EKG) should be monitored closely.

*Drug Interactions.* Effects of dobutamine on the heart and blood vessels are intensified greatly by *MAO inhibitors*. In patients receiving an MAO inhibitor, the dosage of dobutamine must be reduced by at least 90%. Concurrent use of *tricyclic antidepressants* may cause a moderate increase in the cardiovascular effects of dobutamine. Certain *general anesthetics* can sensitize the myocardium to the stimulant actions of dobutamine, thereby increasing the risk of dysrhythmias.

*Preparations, Dosage, and Administration.* Dobutamine hydrochloride [Dobutrex] is dispensed in solution (12.5 mg/ml) in 20-mg vials. This concentrated solution must be diluted to at least 50 ml prior to use. Because of rapid inactivation by MAO and COMT, dobutamine is administered by IV infusion only. Rates of infusion usually range from 2.5 to 10 µg/kg/min.

### Phenylephrine

- *Receptor specificity:* Alpha$_1$
- *Chemical classification:* Noncatecholamine

Phenylephrine is a selective alpha$_1$ agonist. The drug can be administered locally to reduce nasal congestion and parenterally to elevate blood pressure. In addition, phenylephrine can be applied to the eye to dilate the pupil. Lastly, phenylephrine can be coadministered with local anesthetics to retard absorption of the anesthetic.

## Terbutaline

- *Receptor specificity:* Beta$_2$
- *Chemical classification:* Noncatecholamine

## Therapeutic Uses

*Asthma.* Terbutaline can reduce airway resistance in asthma by causing beta$_2$-mediated bronchodilation. Since terbutaline is "selective" for beta$_2$ receptors, it produces much less activation of the heart than does isoproterenol. Accordingly, terbutaline is preferred to isoproterenol and related drugs for therapy of asthma. It must be remembered, however, that receptor selectivity is only relative: if administered in large doses, terbutaline will lose selectivity and activate beta$_1$ receptors as well as beta$_2$ receptors. Accordingly, patients should be warned not to exceed recommended doses, since doing so may cause undesired cardiac stimulation.

*Delay of Preterm Labor.* By activating beta$_2$ receptors in the uterus, terbutaline can relax uterine smooth muscle, thereby delaying labor. However, although terbutaline can be employed to delay labor, a different beta$_2$ agonist—ritodrine—is the drug of choice for this indication.

ample, the use of alpha$_1$ agonists to relieve nasal congestion is discussed in Chapter 70. Table 18-4 summarizes the chapters in which adrenergic agonists are discussed again.

## Adverse Effects

Adverse effects are minimal at therapeutic doses. Tremor is most common. If the dosage is excessive, terbutaline can cause tachycardia by activating beta$_1$ receptors in the heart.

### Ephedrine

- *Receptor specificity:* Alpha$_1$, alpha$_2$, beta$_1$, beta$_2$
- *Chemical classification:* Noncatecholamine

Ephedrine is referred to as a *mixed-acting drug* because it activates adrenergic receptors by *direct* and *indirect* mechanisms. Direct activation results from binding of the drug to alpha and beta receptors. Indirect activation results from release of NE from adrenergic neurons.

#### Therapeutic Uses

*Nasal Congestion.* Ephedrine can reduce nasal congestion by causing alpha$_1$-mediated vasoconstriction. When used for this indication, the drug can be administered topically or orally. As a rule, topical administration is preferred. This is because systemic reactions to topical administration are minimal, whereas oral administration results in activation of adrenergic receptors throughout the body.

*Narcolepsy.* Narcolepsy is a CNS disorder characterized by sudden and irresistible "attacks" of sleep. Ephedrine is one of several medications employed for treatment. Benefits are thought to result from activation of adrenergic receptors in the brain. Ephedrine has access to CNS receptors because, being a noncatecholamine, the drug is able to cross the blood-brain barrier.

#### Adverse Effects

Since ephedrine activates the same receptors as epinephrine, these drugs share the same adverse effects: *hypertension, dysrhythmias, angina,* and *hyperglycemia.* In addition to these shared effects, ephedrine can act in the CNS to cause *insomnia.*

## Discussion of Adrenergic Agonists in Other Chapters

All of the drugs presented in this chapter are discussed again in chapters that address specific applications. For ex-

## KEY POINTS

- Adrenergic agonists are also known as sympathomimetics because their effects mimic those caused by the sympathetic nervous system.
- Most adrenergic agonists act by direct stimulation of adrenergic receptors. A few act by indirect mechanisms: promotion of norepinephrine release, blockade of norepinephrine uptake, and inhibition of norepinephrine degradation.
- Adrenergic agonists in the catecholamine family cannot be taken orally (because of destruction by MAO and COMT), have a brief duration of action (because of destruction by MAO and COMT), and cannot cross the blood-brain barrier (because they are polar molecules).
- Adrenergic agonists that are not catecholamines can be taken orally, have a longer duration than the catecholamines, and can cross the blood-brain barrier.
- Activation of alpha$_1$ receptors causes vasoconstriction and mydriasis.
- Alpha$_1$ agonists are used primarily for hemostasis, nasal decongestion, and elevation of blood pressure, and as adjuncts to local anesthetics.
- Major adverse effects that can result from alpha$_1$ activation are hypertension and local necrosis (if extravasation occurs).
- Activation of alpha$_2$ receptors in the *periphery* is of minimal clinical significance. In contrast, drugs that activate alpha$_2$ receptors in the *CNS* produce useful effects (see Chapter 20).
- All of the clinically relevant responses to activation of beta$_1$ receptors result from activating beta$_1$ receptors in the *heart.*
- Activation of cardiac beta$_1$ receptors increases heart rate, force of contraction, and conduction through the AV node.
- Drugs that activate beta$_1$ receptors can be used to treat heart failure, AV block, and cardiac arrest.
- Potential adverse effects from beta$_1$ activation are tachycardia, dysrhythmias, and angina.
- Drugs that activate beta$_2$ receptors are used to treat asthma and to delay preterm labor.
- Principal adverse effects from beta$_2$ activation are hyperglycemia (in diabetic patients) and tremor.
- Activation of dopamine receptors dilates renal blood vessels, which is useful in shock.
- Epinephrine is a catecholamine that activates alpha$_1$, alpha$_2$, beta$_1$, and beta$_2$ receptors.
- Epinephrine is the drug of choice for treating anaphylactic shock: by activating alpha$_1$, beta$_1$, and beta$_2$ receptors, the drug can elevate blood pressure, suppress glottal edema, and counteract bronchoconstriction.

- Epinephrine can also be used to control superficial bleeding, restart the heart after cardiac arrest, and delay absorption of local anesthetics.
- Epinephrine should not be combined with MAO inhibitors, and should be used cautiously in patients taking tricyclic antidepressants.
- Dopamine is a catecholamine whose receptor specificity is highly dose dependent: at low therapeutic doses, dopamine acts on dopamine receptors only; at moderate doses, dopamine activates beta$_1$ receptors in addition to dopamine receptors; at high doses, dopamine activates alpha$_1$ receptors along with beta$_1$ receptors and dopamine receptors.

- Isoproterenol is a catecholamine that activates beta$_1$ and beta$_2$ receptors.
- Isoproterenol can be used to enhance cardiac performance (by activating beta$_1$ receptors) and to treat asthma (by activating beta$_2$ receptors).
- Terbutaline is a noncatecholamine that produces selective activation of beta$_2$ receptors.
- Terbutaline can be used to treat asthma and to delay preterm labor.
- Because terbutaline is "selective" for beta$_2$ receptors, it produces much less activation of the heart than does isoproterenol. Accordingly, terbutaline is preferred to isoproterenol and related drugs for therapy of asthma.

# Summary of Major Nursing Implications

## Epinephrine

### Preadministration Assessment

#### Therapeutic Goal
Epinephrine has multiple uses. Major applications include treatment of *anaphylaxis* and *cardiac arrest*. Other uses include *control of superficial bleeding, delay of local anesthetic absorption*, and *nasal decongestion*.

#### Identifying High-Risk Patients
Epinephrine must be used with *great caution* in patients with *hyperthyroidism, cardiac dysrhythmias, organic heart disease*, or *hypertension. Caution* is also needed in patients with *angina pectoris* or *diabetes* and in those receiving *MAO inhibitors, tricyclic antidepressants*, or *general anesthetics*.

### Implementation: Administration

#### Routes
Topical, oral inhalation, and parenteral (IV, IM, SC, intracardiac, intraspinal). Rapid inactivation by MAO and COMT prohibits oral use.

#### Administration
The concentration of epinephrine solutions varies with the route of administration (see Table 18-3). To avoid serious injury, check solutions carefully to ensure that their concentration is appropriate for the intended route. Aspirate prior to SC and IM administration to avoid inadvertent injection into a vein.

Epinephrine solutions oxidize over time, causing them to turn pink or brown. Discard discolored solutions.

### Ongoing Evaluation and Interventions

#### Evaluating Therapeutic Effects
In patients receiving intravenous epinephrine, monitor cardiovascular status continuously.

#### Minimizing Adverse Effects
*Cardiovascular Effects.* By stimulating the heart, epinephrine can cause *anginal pain, tachycardia*, and *dysrhythmias*. These reactions can be decreased with a beta-adrenergic blocking agent (e.g., propranolol).

By stimulating alpha$_1$ receptors on blood vessels, epinephrine can cause intense vasoconstriction, which can result in *severe hypertension*. Blood pressure can be lowered with an alpha-adrenergic blocking agent (e.g., phentolamine).

*Necrosis.* If an IV line delivering epinephrine becomes extravasated, necrosis may result. Exercise care to avoid extravasation. If extravasation occurs, infiltrate the region with phentolamine to minimize injury.

*Hyperglycemia.* Epinephrine may cause hyperglycemia in diabetics. If hyperglycemia develops, insulin dosage should be increased.

#### Minimizing Adverse Interactions
*MAO Inhibitors and Tricyclic Antidepressants.* These drugs prolong and intensify the actions of epinephrine. Patients taking these antidepressants require a reduction in epinephrine dosage.

*General Anesthetics.* When combined with certain general anesthetics, epinephrine can induce cardiac dysrhythmias. These may respond to a beta$_1$-adrenergic blocker.

## Dopamine

### Preadministration Assessment

#### Therapeutic Goal
Improvement of hemodynamic status in patients with shock or heart failure. Benefits derive from enhanced cardiac performance and increased renal perfusion.

#### Baseline Data
Full assessment of cardiac, hemodynamic, and renal status is needed.

## Identifying High-Risk Patients

Dopamine is *contraindicated* for patients with *tachydysrhythmias* or *ventricular fibrillation*. Use with *extreme caution* in patients with *organic heart disease*, *hyperthyroidism*, or *hypertension* and in patients receiving *MAO inhibitors*. *Caution* is also needed in patients with *angina pectoris* and in those receiving *tricyclic antidepressants* or *general anesthetics*.

## Implementation: Administration

### Route

Intravenous.

### Administration

Administer by continuous infusion, employing a metering device to control the flow rate.

If extravasation occurs, stop the infusion immediately and infiltrate the region with an alpha-adrenergic antagonist.

## Ongoing Evaluation and Interventions

### Evaluating Therapeutic Effects

Monitor cardiovascular status continuously. Increased urine output is one index of success. Diuretics may complement the beneficial effects of dopamine on the kidney.

### Minimizing Adverse Effects

*Cardiovascular Effects.* By stimulating the heart, dopamine may cause *anginal pain*, *tachycardia*, or *dysrhythmias*. These reactions can be decreased with a beta-adrenergic blocking agent (e.g., propranolol).

*Necrosis.* If the IV line delivering dopamine becomes extravasated, necrosis may result. Exercise care to avoid extravasation. If extravasation occurs, infiltrate the region with phentolamine.

### Minimizing Adverse Interactions

*MAO Inhibitors.* Concurrent use of MAO inhibitors and dopamine can result in severe cardiovascular toxicity. If a patient is taking an MAO inhibitor, dopamine dosage must be reduced by at least 90%.

*Tricyclic Antidepressants.* These drugs prolong and intensify the actions of dopamine. Patients receiving them may require a reduction in dopamine dosage.

*General Anesthetics.* When combined with certain general anesthetics, dopamine can induce dysrhythmias. These may respond to a beta$_1$-adrenergic blocker.

# Dobutamine

## Preadministration Assessment

### Therapeutic Goal

Improvement of hemodynamic status in patients with heart failure.

### Baseline Data

Full assessment of cardiac, renal, and hemodynamic status is needed.

## Identifying High-Risk Patients

Use with *great caution* in patients with *organic heart disease*, *hyperthyroidism*, *tachydysrhythmias*, or *hypertension* and in those taking an *MAO inhibitor*. *Caution* is also needed in patients with *angina pectoris* and in those receiving *tricyclic antidepressants* and *general anesthetics*.

## Implementation: Administration

### Route

Intravenous.

### Administration

Administer by continuous infusion. Dilute concentrated solutions prior to use. Infusion rates usually range from 2.5 to 10 µg/kg/min. Adjust the infusion rate on the basis of the cardiovascular response.

## Ongoing Evaluation and Interventions

### Evaluating Therapeutic Effects

Monitor cardiac function (heart rate, EKG), blood pressure, and urine output. When possible, monitor central venous pressure and pulmonary wedge pressure as well.

### Minimizing Adverse Effects

Major adverse effects are *tachycardia* and *dysrhythmias*. Monitor the EKG and blood pressure closely. Adverse cardiac effects can be reduced with a beta-adrenergic antagonist.

### Minimizing Adverse Interactions

*MAO Inhibitors.* Concurrent use of an MAO inhibitor with dobutamine can cause severe cardiovascular toxicity. If a patient is taking an MAO inhibitor, dobutamine dosage must be reduced by at least 90%.

*Tricyclic Antidepressants.* These drugs can prolong and intensify the actions of dobutamine. Patients receiving them may require a reduction in dobutamine dosage.

*General Anesthetics.* When combined with certain general anesthetics, dobutamine can cause cardiac dysrhythmias. These may respond to a beta$_1$-adrenergic antagonist.

# CHAPTER 19

# Adrenergic Antagonists

The adrenergic antagonists cause direct blockade of adrenergic receptors. With only one exception, all of the adrenergic antagonists produce *reversible* (competitive) receptor blockade.

In contrast to some adrenergic agonists (e.g., epinephrine), the adrenergic antagonists display a high degree of receptor specificity. Because of this specificity, the adrenergic-blocking agents can be neatly divided into two major groups: (1) *alpha-adrenergic blocking agents* (drugs that produce selective blockade of alpha-adrenergic receptors) and (2) *beta-adrenergic blocking agents* (drugs that produce selective blockade of beta receptors). The drugs that belong to these two groups are listed in Table 19–1.

Our approach to the adrenergic antagonists mirrors the approach we took to the adrenergic agonists. That is, we will begin by discussing the therapeutic and adverse effects that can result from blocking alpha- and beta-adrenergic receptors, after which we will discuss the individual drugs that produce receptor blockade.

I remind you that it is much easier to understand responses to the adrenergic drugs if you first understand the responses to activation of adrenergic receptors. Accordingly, if you have not yet mastered (memorized) Table 14–3, you should do so now (or at least be prepared to consult the table as we proceed).

## Alpha-Adrenergic Antagonists I: Therapeutic and Adverse Responses to Alpha Blockade

In this section we discuss the beneficial and adverse responses that can result from blockade of alpha-adrenergic receptors. Properties of individual blocking agents are discussed later.

### Therapeutic Applications of Alpha Blockade

*Practically all of the clinically useful responses to alpha-adrenergic antagonists result from blockade of alpha$_1$ receptors on blood vessels.* For patients with benign prostatic hyperplasia (BPH), blockade of alpha$_1$ receptors in the bladder and prostate can be beneficial. Blockade of alpha$_1$ receptors in the eye and blockade of alpha$_2$ receptors have no recognized therapeutic applications.

***Essential Hypertension.*** Hypertension (high blood pressure) can be treated with a variety of drugs, including the alpha-adrenergic antagonists. Alpha antagonists lower blood pressure by blocking alpha$_1$ receptors on arterioles

## TABLE 19-1. RECEPTOR SPECIFICITY OF ADRENERGIC ANTAGONISTS

| Category | Drugs | Receptors Blocked |
|---|---|---|
| *Alpha-adrenergic blocking agents* | Phentolamine | alpha₁, alpha₂ |
| | Phenoxybenzamine | alpha₁, alpha₂ |
| | Doxazosin | alpha₁, |
| | Prazosin | alpha₁, |
| | Terazosin | alpha₁, |
| *Beta-adrenergic blocking agents* | Carteolol | beta₁, beta₂ |
| | Carvedilol* | beta₁, beta₂ |
| | Labetalol* | beta₁, beta₂ |
| | Nadolol | beta₁, beta₂ |
| | Penbutolol | beta₁, beta₂ |
| | Pindolol | beta₁, beta₂ |
| | Propranolol | beta₁, beta₂ |
| | Sotalol | beta₁, beta₂ |
| | Timolol | beta₁, beta₂ |
| | Acebutolol | beta₁ |
| | Atenolol | beta₁ |
| | Betaxolol | beta₁ |
| | Bisoprolol | beta₁ |
| | Esmolol | beta₁ |
| | Metoprolol | beta₁ |

*Also blocks alpha₁-adrenergic receptors.

and veins, causing vasodilation. Dilation of arterioles reduces arterial pressure directly. Dilation of veins lowers arterial pressure by an indirect process: in response to venous dilation, return of blood to the heart decreases, thereby decreasing cardiac output, which in turn reduces arterial pressure. The role of alpha-adrenergic blockers in essential hypertension is discussed further in Chapter 44 (Drugs for Hypertension).

**Reversal of Toxicity from Alpha₁ Agonists.** Overdose with an alpha-adrenergic agonist (e.g., epinephrine) can produce *hypertension* secondary to excessive stimulation of alpha₁ receptors on blood vessels. When this occurs, blood pressure can be lowered by reversing the vasoconstriction with an alpha-adrenergic antagonist.

If an IV line containing an alpha agonist becomes extravasated, necrosis can occur secondary to intense local vasoconstriction. By infiltrating the region with phentolamine (an alpha-adrenergic antagonist), we can block the vasoconstriction and thereby prevent injury.

**Benign Prostatic Hyperplasia.** BPH results from proliferation of cells in the prostate gland. Symptoms include dysuria, increased frequency of daytime urination, nocturia, urinary hesitance and intermittence, urinary urgency, a sensation of incomplete voiding, and a reduction in the size and force of the urinary stream. All of these symptoms can be improved with drugs that block alpha₁ receptors; benefits result from reduced contraction of smooth muscle in the bladder neck and prostatic capsule. BPH is discussed further in Chapter 99.

**Pheochromocytoma.** A pheochromocytoma is a catecholamine-secreting tumor derived from cells of the sympathetic nervous system. These tumors are usually located in the adrenal medulla. If secretion of catecholamines (epinephrine, norepinephrine) is sufficiently great, persistent hypertension can result. The principal cause of hypertension is activation of alpha₁ receptors on blood vessels, although activation of beta₁ receptors on the heart can also contribute. The preferred treatment is surgical removal of the tumor, but alpha-adrenergic blockers can also be employed.

Alpha-blocking agents have two roles in managing pheochromocytoma. First, in patients with inoperable tumors, alpha blockers are given chronically to suppress hypertension. Second, when surgery is indicated, alpha blockers are administered preoperatively to reduce the risk of acute hypertension during the procedure. (The surgical patient is at risk of acute hypertension because manipulation of the tumor can cause massive release of catecholamines.)

**Raynaud's Disease.** Raynaud's disease is a peripheral vascular disorder characterized by vasospasm in the toes and fingers. Prominent symptoms are local sensations of pain and cold. Alpha-adrenergic blocking agents can suppress symptoms by preventing alpha-mediated vasoconstriction. It should be noted, however, that although alpha blockers can relieve symptoms of Raynaud's disease, these drugs are generally ineffective against other peripheral vascular disorders that involve inappropriate vasoconstriction.

## Adverse Effects of Alpha Blockade

The most significant adverse effects of the alpha-adrenergic antagonists result from blockade of alpha₁ receptors. Detrimental effects associated with alpha₂ blockade are minor.

### Adverse Effects of Alpha₁ Blockade

**Orthostatic Hypotension.** This is the most serious adverse response to alpha-adrenergic blockade. Orthostatic hypotension can reduce blood flow to the brain, thereby causing dizziness, lightheadedness, and even syncope (fainting).

The cause of orthostatic hypotension is blockade of alpha receptors on *veins*, which reduces muscle tone in the venous wall. Because of reduced venous tone, blood tends to pool (accumulate) in veins when the patient assumes an erect posture. (This redistribution of blood is analogous to the movement of water within a long, skinny balloon. When the balloon is horizontal, the water distributes evenly. However, when the balloon is suspended by one end, fluid pressure stretches the balloon, causing water to pool at the low end.) Because of venous pooling, return of blood to the heart is reduced. This reduction in venous return decreases cardiac output, which in turn causes blood pressure to fall.

Patients should be informed about symptoms of hypotension (lightheadedness, dizziness) and advised to sit or lie down if these occur. In addition, patients should be informed that orthostatic hypotension can be minimized by avoiding abrupt transitions from a supine or sitting position to an erect posture.

**Reflex Tachycardia.** Alpha-adrenergic antagonists can increase heart rate by triggering the baroreceptor reflex. Activation of the reflex occurs as follows: (1) blockade of vascular alpha₁ receptors causes vasodilation; (2) vasodilation reduces blood pressure; (3) baroreceptors sense the reduction in blood pressure and, in an attempt to restore normal pressure, initiate a reflexive increase in heart rate via the autonomic nervous system. If necessary, reflex tachycardia can be suppressed with a beta-adrenergic blocking agent.

**Nasal Congestion.**  Alpha blockade can dilate the blood vessels of the nasal mucosa, producing nasal congestion.

**Inhibition of Ejaculation.**  Since activation of alpha$_1$ receptors is required for ejaculation (see Table 14–3), blockade of these receptors can cause impotence. This form of drug-induced impotence is reversible and resolves when the alpha blocker is withdrawn.

The ability of alpha blockers to inhibit ejaculation can be a major reason for noncompliance. If a patient deems the adverse sexual effects of alpha blockade unacceptable, a change in medication will be required. Since males may be reluctant to discuss such concerns, a tactful interview will be needed to discern if drug-induced impotence is discouraging drug use.

**Sodium Retention and Increased Blood Volume.**  By reducing blood pressure, alpha blockers can promote renal retention of sodium and water, thereby causing blood volume to increase. The steps in this process are as follows: (1) by reducing blood pressure, alpha$_1$ blockers decrease renal blood flow; (2) in response to reduced perfusion, the kidney excretes less sodium and water; and (3) the resultant retention of sodium and water increases blood volume. As a result of these events, blood pressure is elevated, blood flow to the kidney is increased, and, as far as the kidney is concerned, all is well. Unfortunately, this compensatory elevation in blood pressure tends to negate the effects for which alpha-blocking drugs are often given. That is, alpha antagonists are often used to treat hypertension; by increasing blood volume and blood pressure, the kidney effectively counteracts the blood pressure-lowering action of alpha blockade. In order to prevent the kidney from "neutralizing" the hypotensive actions of alpha-blocking agents, these drugs are usually combined with a diuretic when employed to treat hypertension.

### Adverse Effects of Alpha$_2$ Blockade

The most significant adverse effect associated with alpha$_2$ blockade is *potentiation of the reflex tachycardia that can occur in response to blockade of alpha$_1$ receptors.* Why does alpha$_2$ blockade intensify reflex tachycardia? Recall that peripheral alpha$_2$ receptors are located presynaptically and that activation of these receptors inhibits norepinephrine release. Hence, if alpha$_2$ receptors are blocked, release of norepinephrine will increase. Since the reflex tachycardia caused by alpha$_1$ blockade is ultimately the result of increased firing of the sympathetic nerves to the heart, and since alpha$_2$ blockade will cause each nerve impulse to release a greater amount of norepinephrine, alpha$_2$ blockade will potentiate reflex tachycardia initiated by blockade of alpha$_1$ receptors. Accordingly, drugs such as phentolamine, which block alpha$_2$ as well as alpha$_1$ receptors, cause greater reflex tachycardia than do drugs that block alpha$_1$ receptors only.

# Alpha-Adrenergic Antagonists II: Properties of Individual Alpha Blockers

Only five alpha-adrenergic antagonists are employed clinically. Because the alpha blockers often cause postural hypotension, therapeutic uses for these drugs are limited.

As can be seen from Table 19–1, the alpha-adrenergic blocking agents can be subdivided into two groups. One subgroup—the *nonselective* alpha-blocking agents—contains drugs that block alpha$_1$ *and* alpha$_2$ receptors. *Phentolamine* is the prototype for this group. The second subgroup, represented by *prazosin*, contains drugs that produce *selective alpha$_1$ blockade.*

## Prazosin

**Actions and Uses.**  Prazosin [Minipress] is a competitive antagonist that produces selective blockade of alpha$_1$-adrenergic receptors. By blocking alpha$_1$ receptors, prazosin can cause dilation of arterioles and veins. The principal indication for prazosin is *hypertension*. The drug can also decrease symptoms of BPH, although it is not approved for this use.

**Pharmacokinetics.**  Prazosin is administered orally. Antihypertensive effects peak in 1 to 3 hours and persist for 10 hours. The drug undergoes extensive hepatic metabolism followed by excretion in the bile. Only about 10% is eliminated in the urine. The half-life is 2 to 3 hours.

**Adverse Effects.**  Blockade of alpha$_1$ receptors can cause *orthostatic hypotension, reflex tachycardia, inhibition of ejaculation*, and *nasal congestion*. The most serious of these is postural hypotension. Patients should be educated about the symptoms of hypotension (dizziness, lightheadedness) and advised to sit or lie down if they occur. Patients should also be informed that orthostatic hypotension can be minimized by moving slowly when making the transition from a supine or sitting position to an upright position.

About 1% of patients lose consciousness 30 to 60 minutes after receiving their first prazosin dose. This "first-dose" effect is the result of severe postural hypotension. To minimize the first-dose effect, the initial dose should be small (1 mg or less). After this low initial dose, the dosage can be gradually increased with little risk of the patient fainting. Patients who are beginning treatment should be forewarned about the first-dose effect and advised to avoid driving and other hazardous activities for 12 to 24 hours. Administering the initial dose at bedtime eliminates the risk of a first-dose effect.

**Preparations, Dosage, and Administration.**  Prazosin hydrochloride [Minipress] is available in capsules (1, 2, and 5 mg) for oral use. The initial adult dosage for essential hypertension is 1 mg taken 2 or 3 times a day. For maintenance therapy, the dosage is 6 to 15 mg/day administered in divided doses.

## Terazosin

**Actions and Uses.**  Like prazosin, terazosin [Hytrin] is a selective and competitive antagonist at alpha$_1$ adrenergic receptors. The drug is approved for hypertension and BPH.

**Pharmacokinetics.**  Terazosin is administered orally, and peak effects develop in 1 to 2 hours. The drug's half-life is 9 to 12 hours, which allows beneficial effects to be maintained with once-a-day dosing. Terazosin undergoes hepatic metabolism followed by excretion in the bile and urine.

**Adverse Effects.**  Like other alpha-blocking agents, terazosin can cause *orthostatic hypotension, reflex tachycardia, nasal congestion*, and *inhibition of ejaculation*. In addition, terazosin is associated with a high incidence (16%) of *headache*. As with prazosin, the first dose can cause profound hypotension. To minimize this first-dose effect, the initial dose should be administered at bedtime.

***Preparations, Dosage, and Administration.*** Terazosin [Hytrin] is available in tablets and capsules (1, 2, 5, and 10 mg) for oral use. Antihypertensive therapy is initiated with a 1-mg dose, administered at bedtime to minimize the first-dose effect. The dosage can be gradually increased as needed and tolerated. The recommended dosage range for maintenance therapy is 1 to 5 mg once daily. Dosing for BPH is similar to that for hypertension.

### Doxazosin

***Actions and Uses.*** Doxazosin [Cardura] is a selective and competitive inhibitor of alpha1-adrenergic receptors. The drug is indicated for hypertension and BPH.

***Pharmacokinetics.*** Doxazosin is administered orally, and peak effects develop in 2 to 3 hours. The drug has a prolonged half-life (22 hours); hence treatment can be accomplished with once-a-day dosing. Most (98%) of the drug in blood is protein bound. Doxazosin undergoes extensive hepatic metabolism followed by biliary excretion.

***Adverse Effects.*** Like prazosin and terazosin, doxazosin can cause *orthostatic hypotension, reflex tachycardia, nasal congestion,* and *inhibition of ejaculation.* As with prazosin, the first dose can cause profound hypotension. First-dose hypotension can be minimized by giving the initial dose at bedtime.

***Preparations, Dosage, and Administration.*** Doxazosin [Cardura] is dispensed in tablets (1, 2, 4, and 8 mg) for oral administration. The initial dosage for hypertension or BPH is 1 mg once a day. The dosage may be gradually increased as needed, up to a maximum of 16 mg once daily for hypertension or 8 mg once daily for BPH.

### Phentolamine

***Actions and Uses.*** Like prazosin, phentolamine [Regitine] is a competitive adrenergic antagonist. However, in contrast to prazosin, phentolamine blocks alpha2 as well as alpha1 receptors. Phentolamine has two applications: (1) treatment of pheochromocytoma and (2) prevention of tissue necrosis following extravasation of drugs that produce alpha1-mediated vasoconstriction (e.g., norepinephrine).

***Adverse Effects.*** Like prazosin, phentolamine can produce the typical adverse effects associated with alpha-adrenergic blockade: *orthostatic hypotension, reflex tachycardia, nasal congestion,* and *inhibition of ejaculation.* Because of its ability to block alpha2 receptors, *phentolamine produces greater reflex tachycardia than prazosin.* If reflex tachycardia is especially severe, heart rate can be reduced with a beta-adrenergic blocker. Since tachycardia can aggravate angina pectoris and myocardial infarction, phentolamine is contraindicated for patients with either disorder.

Overdose can produce profound hypotension. If necessary, blood pressure can be elevated with *norepinephrine. Epinephrine* should *not* be used, because the drug can cause blood pressure to drop even further! Why? Because in the presence of alpha1 blockade, the ability of epinephrine to promote vasodilation (via activation of vascular beta2 receptors) may outweigh the ability of epinephrine to cause vasoconstriction (via activation of vascular alpha1 receptors). Further lowering of blood pressure is not a problem with norepinephrine because norepinephrine does not activate beta2 receptors.

***Preparations, Dosage, and Administration.*** Phentolamine [Regitine] is dispensed in solution (5 mg/25 ml) for IM and IV administration. The dosage for preventing hypertension during surgical excision of a pheochromocytoma is 5 mg (IM or IV). For preventing necrosis following extravasation of IV norepinephrine, the region should be infiltrated with 5 to 10 mg of phentolamine diluted in 10 ml of saline.

### Phenoxybenzamine

***Actions and Uses.*** Like phentolamine, phenoxybenzamine [Dibenzyline] blocks alpha1 and alpha2 receptors. However, unlike all of the other alpha-adrenergic antagonists, phenoxybenzamine is a *noncompetitive* receptor antagonist. Hence, receptor blockade is *not reversible.* As a result, the effects of phenoxybenzamine are long lasting. (Responses to a single dose can persist for several days.) Effects subside as newly synthesized receptors replace the ones that have been irreversibly blocked. Phenoxybenzamine is approved only for pheochromocytoma.

***Adverse Effects.*** Like the other alpha-adrenergic antagonists, phenoxybenzamine can produce *orthostatic hypotension, reflex tachycardia, nasal congestion,* and *inhibition of ejaculation.* Reflex tachycardia is greater than that caused by prazosin and about equal to that caused by phentolamine.

If administered in excessive amounts, phenoxybenzamine, like phentolamine, will cause profound hypotension. Furthermore, since hypotension is the result of *irreversible* alpha1 blockade, phenoxybenzamine-induced hypotension cannot be corrected with an alpha1 agonist. To restore blood pressure, patients must be given IV fluids, which elevate blood pressure by increasing blood volume.

***Preparations, Dosage, and Administration.*** Phenoxybenzamine hydrochloride [Dibenzyline] is available in 10-mg capsules for oral use. The initial adult dosage is 10 mg per day. The dosage can be increased every 4 days until the desired level of alpha blockade has been achieved. Daily maintenance dosages for adults range from 20 to 60 mg.

# Beta-Adrenergic Antagonists I: Therapeutic and Adverse Responses to Beta Blockade

In this section we consider the beneficial and adverse responses that can result from blockade of beta-adrenergic receptors. Properties of individual beta-blocking agents are discussed later.

## Therapeutic Applications of Beta Blockade

*Practically all of the therapeutic effects of the beta-adrenergic antagonists result from blockade of beta1 receptors in the heart.* The major consequences of blocking these receptors are (1) reduced heart rate, (2) reduced force of contraction, and (3) reduced velocity of impulse conduction through the atrioventricular (AV) node. Because of these effects, beta blockers are useful in a variety of pathologic states.

***Hypertension.*** Beta-adrenergic blocking agents are drugs of choice for many patients with hypertension. Because of their use in this common disorder, the beta blockers are one of our most widely prescribed families of drugs.

The exact mechanism by which beta blockers reduce blood pressure is not known. Older proposed mechanisms include reduction of cardiac output through blockade of beta1 receptors in the heart and suppression of renin release through blockade of beta1 receptors in the kidney (see Chapter 41 for a discussion of the role of renin in blood pressure control). More recently, we have learned that long-term use of beta blockers reduces peripheral vascular resistance, an action that could account for most of the antihypertensive response to these drugs. The mechanism of this important but unexpected action is not known. The role of beta-adrenergic blocking agents in hypertension is discussed further in Chapter 44.

**Angina Pectoris.** Angina pectoris (paroxysmal pain in the region of the heart) occurs when oxygen sup-ply (blood flow) to the heart is insufficient to meet cardiac oxygen demand. Anginal attacks can be precipitated by exertion, intense emotion, and other factors. Beta-adrenergic blockers are a mainstay of antianginal therapy. By blocking beta$_1$ receptors in the heart, these drugs decrease cardiac work. This brings oxygen demand back into balance with oxygen supply, and thereby prevents pain. Angina pectoris and its treatment are the subject of Chapter 45.

**Cardiac Dysrhythmias.** Beta-adrenergic blocking agents are especially useful for treating dysrhythmias that involve excessive electrical activity in the sinus node and atria. By blocking cardiac beta$_1$ receptors, these drugs can (1) decrease the rate of sinus nodal discharge, and (2) suppress conduction of atrial impulses through the AV node, thereby preventing the ventricles from being driven at an excessive rate. The use of beta-adrenergic blockers to treat dysrhythmias is discussed at length in Chapter 48.

**Myocardial Infarction.** A myocardial infarction (MI) is a region of myocardial necrosis caused by localized interruption of blood flow to the heart wall. Treatment with a beta blocker can reduce pain, infarct size, mortality, and the risk of reinfarction. To be effective, therapy with a beta-blocker must commence soon after an MI has occurred, and should be continued for several years. The role of beta blockers in treating MI is discussed further in Chapter 47.

**Hyperthyroidism.** Hyperthyroidism (excessive production of thyroid hormone) is associated with an increase in the sensitivity of the heart to catecholamines (e.g., norepinephrine, epinephrine). As a result, normal levels of sympathetic activity to the heart can generate tachydysrhythmias and angina pectoris. Blockade of cardiac beta$_1$ receptors suppresses these responses.

**Migraine.** When taken prophylactically, beta-adrenergic blocking agents can reduce the frequency of migraine attacks. However, although beta blockers are effective as prophylaxis, these drugs are not able to abort a migraine headache once it has begun. The mechanism by which beta blockers prevent migraine is not known. Treatment of migraine and other headaches is the subject of Chapter 28.

**Stage Fright.** Public speakers and other performers sometimes experience "stage fright." Prominent symptoms are tachycardia and sweating brought on by generalized discharge of the sympathetic nervous system. Beta blockers help by preventing the beta$_1$-mediated tachycardia.

**Pheochromocytoma.** As discussed earlier, a pheochromocytoma secretes large amounts of catecholamines, which can cause excessive stimulation of the heart. Cardiac stimulation can be counteracted by beta$_1$ blockade.

**Glaucoma.** Beta blockers are important drugs for treating glaucoma, a condition characterized by elevated intraocular pressure with subsequent injury to the optic nerve. The group of beta blockers used in glaucoma (see Table 97–2) is different from the group of beta blockers discussed in this chapter. Glaucoma and its treatment are addressed in Chapter 97 (Drugs for the Eye).

## Adverse Effects of Beta Blockade

Although therapeutic responses to beta blockers are due almost entirely to blockade of beta$_1$ receptors, adverse effects involve both beta$_1$ and beta$_2$ blockade. Consequently, the nonselective beta-adrenergic blocking agents (drugs that block beta$_1$ and beta$_2$ receptors) produce a broader spectrum of adverse effects than do the "cardioselective" beta-adrenergic antagonists (drugs that selectively block beta$_1$ receptors at usual therapeutic doses).

### Adverse Effects of Beta$_1$ Blockade

All of the adverse effects of beta$_1$ blockade are the result of blocking beta$_1$ receptors in the heart. Blockade of renal beta$_1$ receptors does not produce adverse effects of clinical significance.

**Bradycardia.** Blockade of cardiac beta$_1$ receptors can produce bradycardia (excessively slow heart rate). If necessary, heart rate can be increased using a combination of isoproterenol (a beta-adrenergic agonist) and atropine (a muscarinic antagonist). Isoproterenol competes with the beta blocker for cardiac beta$_1$ receptors, thereby promoting cardiac stimulation. By blocking muscarinic receptors on the heart, atropine prevents slowing of the heart by the parasympathetic nervous system.

**Reduced Cardiac Output.** Beta$_1$ blockade can reduce cardiac output by decreasing heart rate and the force of myocardial contraction. Because they can decrease cardiac output, *beta blockers are contraindicated for most patients with heart failure and should be used with great caution in patients with reduced cardiac reserve.* In both cases, any further decrease in cardiac output could result in insufficient tissue perfusion.

**Precipitation of Heart Failure.** In some patients, suppression of cardiac function with a beta blocker can be so great as to cause outright heart failure, a condition in which the heart is unable to pump a sufficient amount of blood to maintain adequate perfusion of tissues. Patients should be informed about the early signs of heart failure (shortness of breath, night coughs, swelling of the extremities) and instructed to notify the physician if these occur. As noted above, beta-adrenergic blocking agents are contraindicated for most patients who already have heart failure.

**AV Heart Block.** AV heart block is defined as suppression of impulse conduction through the AV node. In its most severe form, AV block prevents *all* atrial impulses from reaching the ventricles. Since blockade of cardiac beta$_1$ receptors can suppress AV conduction, production of AV block is a potential complication of beta-blocker therapy. These drugs are contraindicated for patients with pre-existing AV block.

**Rebound Cardiac Excitation.** Long-term use of beta blockers can sensitize the heart to catecholamines. As a result, if a beta blocker is withdrawn *abruptly*, anginal pain or ventricular dysrhythmias may develop. This phenomenon of increased cardiac activity in response to abrupt cessation of beta-blocker therapy is referred to as *rebound excitation*. The risk of rebound excitation can be minimized by the simple expedient of withdrawing these drugs gradually (e.g., by tapering the dosage over a period of 1 to 2 weeks). If rebound excitation occurs, dosing should be temporarily resumed. Patients should be warned against abrupt cessation of treatment. Also, they should be advised to carry an adequate supply of their beta blocker when traveling.

## Adverse Effects of Beta$_2$ Blockade

***Bronchoconstriction.*** Blockade of beta$_2$ receptors in the lung can cause constriction of the bronchi. (Recall that activation of these receptors promotes bronchodilation.) For most people, the degree of bronchoconstriction is insignificant. However, when bronchial beta$_2$ receptors are blocked in patients with asthma, the resulting increase in airway resistance can be life threatening. Accordingly, *drugs that block beta$_2$ receptors are contraindicated for people with asthma*. If these individuals must use a beta blocker, they should use only those agents that are beta$_1$ selective (e.g., metoprolol).

***Inhibition of Glycogenolysis.*** As noted in Chapter 14, epinephrine, acting at beta$_2$ receptors in skeletal muscle and the liver, can stimulate glycogenolysis (breakdown of glycogen into glucose). Beta$_2$ blockade will inhibit this process. Although suppression of beta$_2$-mediated glycogenolysis is inconsequential for most people, interference with this process can be detrimental to patients with *diabetes*. This is because diabetics are especially dependent on beta$_2$-mediated glycogenolysis as a way to overcome severe reductions in blood glucose levels. If the diabetic patient requires a beta blocker, a beta$_1$-selective agent should be chosen.

# Beta-Adrenergic Antagonists II: Properties of Individual Beta Blockers

The beta-adrenergic antagonists can be subdivided into two groups: *nonselective* beta blockers and *cardioselective* beta blockers. The nonselective agents, represented by propranolol, block beta$_1$ *and* beta$_2$ receptors. The cardioselective agents, represented by metoprolol, produce selective blockade of beta$_1$ receptors (at usual therapeutic doses). Our discussion of the individual beta blockers focuses on the two prototypes: propranolol and metoprolol.

## Propranolol

Propranolol [Inderal] was the first beta-adrenergic blocker to receive widespread clinical use and remains one of our most important beta-blocking agents. Propranolol blocks beta$_1$ and beta$_2$ receptors, and is the prototype of the nonselective beta-adrenergic antagonists.

### Pharmacologic Effects

By blocking cardiac beta$_1$ receptors, propranolol can *reduce heart rate, decrease the force of ventricular contraction*, and *suppress impulse conduction through the AV node*. The net response to these effects is a reduction in cardiac output.

By blocking beta$_1$ receptors in the kidney, propranolol can *suppress secretion of renin*.

Blockade of beta$_2$ receptors has three major effects: (1) blockade of beta$_2$ receptors in the lung can cause *bronchoconstriction*, (2) blockade of beta$_2$ receptors on certain blood vessels can produce *vasoconstriction*, and (3) blockade of beta$_2$ receptors in skeletal muscle and the liver can cause *inhibition of glycogenolysis*.

### Pharmacokinetics

Propranolol is *highly lipid soluble* and therefore can readily cross membranes. The drug is well absorbed following oral administration, but, because of extensive metabolism on its first pass through the liver, less than 30% of each dose reaches the systemic circulation. Because of its ability to cross membranes, propranolol is widely distributed to all tissues and organs, including the central nervous system (CNS). Propranolol is inactivated by hepatic metabolism, and the metabolites are excreted in the urine.

### Therapeutic Uses

Practically all of the applications of propranolol are based on blockade of beta$_1$ receptors in the heart. The drug's most important indications are *hypertension*, *angina pectoris*, and *cardiac dysrhythmias*. The role of propranolol and other beta blockers in these disorders is discussed in Chapter 44 (Drugs for Hypertension), Chapter 45 (Drugs for Angina Pectoris), and Chapter 48 (Antidysrhythmic Drugs). Additional indications include *myocardial infarction*, *migraine headache*, and "*stage fright*."

### Adverse Effects

The most serious adverse effects of propranolol result from blockade of beta$_1$ receptors in the heart and blockade of beta$_2$ receptors in the lung.

***Bradycardia.*** Beta$_1$ blockade in the heart can cause bradycardia. Heart rate should be assessed before each dose. If necessary, heart rate can be increased by administering atropine and isoproterenol.

***AV Heart Block.*** By slowing conduction of impulses through the AV node, propranolol can cause AV heart block. The drug is contraindicated for patients with preexisting AV block (if the block is greater than first degree).

***Heart Failure.*** In patients with cardiac disease, suppression of myocardial contractility by propranolol can result in heart failure. Patients should be informed about the early signs of heart failure (shortness of breath, night coughs, swelling of the extremities) and instructed to notify the physician if these occur. Propranolol is generally contraindicated for patients with pre-existing heart failure.

***Rebound Cardiac Excitation.*** Abrupt withdrawal of propranolol can cause rebound excitation of the heart, resulting in tachycardia or ventricular dysrhythmias. To avoid rebound excitation, propranolol should be withdrawn slowly by giving progressively smaller doses over 1 to 2 weeks. Patients should be warned against abrupt cessation of drug use. In addition, they should be advised to carry an adequate supply of the drug when traveling.

***Bronchoconstriction.*** Blockade of beta$_2$ receptors in the lung can cause bronchoconstriction. As a rule, increased airway resistance is hazardous only to patients with asthma and other obstructive pulmonary disorders.

***Inhibition of Glycogenolysis.*** Blockade of beta$_2$ receptors in skeletal muscle and the liver can inhibit glycogenolysis. This effect can be dangerous for people with diabetes (see below).

***CNS Effects.*** Because of its lipid solubility, propranolol can readily cross the blood-brain barrier to reach sites in the CNS. Primary neuropsychiatric responses are *depression* and *insomnia*. The drug may also cause *nightmares* and *hallucinations*. Propranolol should be used with caution in patients with a history of major depression.

## Precautions, Warnings, and Contraindications

***Severe Allergy.*** Propranolol should be avoided in patients with a history of severe allergic reactions (anaphylaxis). Recall that epinephrine, the drug of choice for anaphylaxis, relieves symptoms in large part by activating beta$_1$ receptors in the heart and beta$_2$ receptors in the lung. If these receptors are blocked by propranolol, the ability of epinephrine to act will be dangerously impaired.

***Diabetes.*** Propranolol can be detrimental to the diabetic in two ways. First, by blocking beta$_2$ receptors in muscle and the liver, propranolol can suppress glycogenolysis, thereby eliminating an important mecha-nism for correcting hypoglycemia (which can occur when insulin dosage is excessive). Second, by blocking beta$_1$ receptors, propranolol can suppress tachycardia, which normally serves as an early warning signal that blood glucose levels are falling too low. (When blood glucose drops below a safe level, the sympathetic nervous system is activated, causing an increase in heart rate.) By "masking" tachycardia, propranolol can delay awareness of hypoglycemia, thereby compromising the diabetic's ability to correct the problem in a timely fashion. Diabetic patients who are taking propranolol should be warned that tachycardia may no longer be a reliable indicator of hypoglycemia. In addition, they should be taught to recognize alternative signs (sweating, hunger, fatigue, poor concentration) that blood glucose is falling perilously low. Because of its ability to suppress glycogenolysis and mask tachycardia, propranolol must be used with caution by di-

abetic patients. Also, patients may need to reduce their dosage of insulin.

***Cardiac, Respiratory, and Psychiatric Disorders.*** Propranolol can exacerbate *heart failure*, *AV heart block*, *sinus bradycardia*, *asthma*, and *bronchospasm*. The drug is contraindicated for patients with these disorders. In addition, propranolol should be used with caution in patients with a history of *depression*.

## Drug Interactions

***Calcium Channel Blockers.*** The cardiac effects of certain calcium channel blockers (e.g., verapamil) are identical to those of propranolol: reduction of heart rate, suppression of AV conduction, and suppression of myocardial contractility. When propranolol and calcium channel blockers are used concurrently, there is a risk of excessive cardiac suppression.

***Insulin.*** As discussed above, propranolol can impede early recognition of insulin-induced hypoglycemia. In addition, propranolol can block glycogenolysis, the body's mechanism for correcting hypoglycemia.

## Preparations, Dosage, and Administration

***General Dosing Considerations.*** Establishing an effective propranolol dosage is difficult for two reasons: (1) patients vary widely in their requirements for propranolol and (2) there is a poor correlation between blood levels of propranolol and the response produced. The explanation for these observations is that responses to propranolol are dependent on the activity of the sympathetic nervous system. If sympathetic activity is high, then the dose needed to reduce receptor activation will be high as well. Conversely, if sympathetic activity is low, then low doses will be sufficient to produce receptor blockade. Since sympathetic activity varies among patients, propranolol requirements vary also. Accordingly, the dosage must be adjusted by monitoring the patient's response, and not by relying on dosing information in a drug reference.

***Preparations.*** Propranolol hydrochloride [Inderal] is available in three oral formulations: (1) tablets (10 to 90 mg); (2) sustained-release capsules (60 to 160 mg); and (3) oral solutions (4, 8, and 80 mg/ml). The drug is also available in solution (1 mg/ml) for IV administration.

***Dosage.*** For treatment of *hypertension*, the initial dosage is 40 mg twice a day. Daily maintenance dosages usually range from 120 to 240 mg (in divided doses), although some patients may need as much as 640 mg/day. The usual adult dosage for *angina pectoris* is 160 mg/day.

## Metoprolol

Metoprolol [Lopressor, Toprol XL] is the prototype of the "cardioselective" beta-adrenergic antagonists. At usual therapeutic doses, metoprolol blocks beta$_1$ receptors only. Please note, however, that selectivity for beta$_1$ receptors is not absolute: at higher doses, metoprolol and the other "cardioselective" agents will block beta$_2$ receptors as well as beta$_1$ receptors. Because their effects on beta$_2$ receptors are normally minimal, the cardioselective agents are not likely to cause bronchoconstriction or suppression of glycogenolysis. As a result, these drugs are preferred to the nonselective beta blockers for patients with asthma and diabetes.

***Pharmacologic Effects.*** By blocking cardiac beta₁ re-ceptors, metoprolol has the same impact on the heart as propranolol: the drug reduces heart rate, force of con-traction, and impulse conduction through the AV node. Also like propranolol, metoprolol reduces secretion of renin by the kidney. In contrast to propranolol, metopro-lol does not block bronchial beta₂ receptors (at usual ther-apeutic doses), and therefore does not increase airway resistance.

***Pharmacokinetics.*** Metoprolol is moderately lipid soluble and is well absorbed following oral administration. Like propranolol, metoprolol undergoes extensive metabolism on its first pass through the liver. As a result, only about 40% of an oral dose reaches the systemic circulation. Elimination is by hepatic metabolism and renal excretion.

***Therapeutic Uses.*** The primary indication for meto-prolol is *hypertension*. The drug is also approved for *angina pectoris* and *myocardial infarction*.

***Adverse Effects.*** The major adverse effects of meto-prolol involve the heart. Like propranolol, metoprolol can cause *bradycardia, reduction of cardiac output, AV heart block, heart failure,* and *rebound cardiac excita-tion following abrupt withdrawal*. In contrast to propra-nolol, metoprolol causes minimal bronchoconstriction and does not interfere with beta₂-mediated glycogenolysis.

***Precautions, Warnings, and Contraindications.*** Like propranolol, metoprolol is contraindicated for patients with *heart failure, sinus bradycardia,* and *AV heart block that is greater than first degree*. Because metopro-lol produces only minimal blockade of beta₂ receptors, the drug is safer than propranolol for use by patients with asthma or a history of severe allergic reactions. In addi-tion, since metoprolol does not suppress beta₂-mediated glycogenolysis, the drug can be used more safely than pro-pranolol by diabetics. It should be noted, however, that metoprolol, like propranolol, will "mask" tachycardia, thereby depriving the diabetic of an early indication that hypoglycemia is developing.

***Preparations, Dosage, and Administration.*** Metoprolol is available in standard oral tablets (50 and 100 mg) under the trade name Lopressor and in sustained-release oral tablets (50, 100, and 200 mg) under the trade name Toprol XL. The drug is also available in solution (1 mg/ml) for IV administration. The initial dosage for hypertension is 100 mg/day in single or divided doses. The dosage for maintenance therapy ranges from 100 to 400 mg/day in divided doses. Intravenous administration is reserved for myocardial infarction.

## Other Beta-Adrenergic Blockers

In the United States, 15 beta blockers are approved for treatment of cardiovascular disorders (hypertension, angina pectoris, cardiac dysrhythmias, myocardial infarc-tion). Principal differences among these drugs concern re-ceptor specificity, pharmacokinetics, indications, and side effects.

In addition to the agents used for cardiovascular disor-ders, there is a group of beta blockers used to treat glau-coma. These drugs are discussed in Chapter 97 (Drugs for the Eye).

Pharmacologic properties of the beta blockers em-ployed for cardiovascular disorders are discussed below.

***Receptor Specificity.*** As noted above, the beta block-ers fall into two major groups: *nonselective* agents and *cardioselective* agents. The nonselective agents block beta₁ and beta₂ receptors, whereas the cardioselective agents block beta₁ receptors only (at usual therapeutic doses). Because of their limited side effects, the cardiose-lective agents are preferred for patients with asthma or diabetes. Two beta blockers—*labetalol* and *carvedilol*—differ from all the others in that they block *alpha* adren-ergic receptors in addition to beta receptors. The receptor specificity of individual beta blockers is indicated in Tables 19–1 and 19–2.

***Pharmacokinetics.*** Pharmacokinetic properties of the beta blockers are summarized in Table 19–2. The relative *lipid solubility* of these agents is of particular importance. The drugs with the highest lipid solubility—propranolol and penbutolol—have two prominent features: they pen-etrate the blood-brain barrier with ease, and they are elim-inated primarily by hepatic metabolism. The drugs with low lipid solubility (e.g., acebutolol, atenolol) penetrate the blood-brain barrier poorly, and are eliminated primar-ily by renal excretion. The drugs with moderate lipid sol-ubility—metoprolol, labetalol, and pindolol—are able to penetrate the blood-brain barrier, and are eliminated by a combination of hepatic metabolism and renal excretion.

***Therapeutic Uses.*** Principal indications for the beta-adrenergic blockers are *hypertension, angina pectoris,* and *cardiac dysrhythmias*. Other uses include prophy-laxis of migraine headache, treatment of myocardial in-farction, and suppression of symptoms in individuals with situational anxiety (e.g., stage fright). Approved and in-vestigational uses of the beta blockers are summarized in Table 19–3.

*Esmolol* and *sotalol* differ from the other beta blockers in that they are not used for hypertension. Because of its very short half-life (15 minutes), *esmolol* is clearly un-suited for treating hypertension, which requires that blood levels be maintained throughout the day, every day, for an indefinite time. The only approved indication for es-molol is emergency intravenous therapy of *supraventric-ular tachycardia*. *Sotalol* is approved only for *ventricular dysrhythmias*. Esmolol and sotalol are discussed further in Chapter 48 (Antidysrhythmic Drugs).

***Adverse Effects.*** By blocking cardiac beta₁ receptors, all of the beta blockers can cause *bradycardia, AV heart block,* and, rarely, *heart failure*. By blocking beta₂ recep-tors in the lung, the *nonselective* agents can cause signifi-cant *bronchoconstriction* in patients with asthma and chronic obstructive pulmonary disease. In addition, by blocking beta₂ receptors in the liver and skeletal muscle, the *nonselective* agents can *inhibit glycogenolysis*, thereby compromising the ability of diabetic patients to

## TABLE 19–2. CLINICAL PHARMACOLOGY OF THE BETA-ADRENERGIC BLOCKING AGENTS

| Generic Name | Trade Name | Receptors Blocked | ISA | Lipid Solubility | Half-Life (hr) | Route* | Maintenance Dosage in Hypertension† |
|---|---|---|---|---|---|---|---|
| Acebutolol | Sectral | | + | Low | 3–4 | PO | 400 mg once/day |
| Atenolol | Tenormin | | 0 | Low | 6–9 | PO, IV | 50 mg once/day |
| Betaxolol | Kerlone | | 0 | Low | 14–22 | PO | 10 mg once/day |
| Bisoprolol | Zebeta | Beta₁ | 0 | Low | 9–12 | PO | 5 mg once/day |
| Esmolol | Brevibloc | | 0 | Low | 0.15 | IV | Not for hypertension |
| Metoprolol | Lopressor | | 0 | Moderate | 3–7 | PO, IV | 100 mg once/day |
| slow release | Toprol XL | | | | | PO | 100 mg once/day |
| Carteolol | Cartrol | | ++ | Low | 6 | PO | 2.5 mg once/day |
| Carvedilol‡ | Coreg | | 0 | — | 5–11 | PO | 12.5 mg twice/day |
| Labetalol‡ | Normodyne, Trandate | | 0 | Moderate | 6–8 | PO, IV | 300 mg twice/day |
| Nadolol | Corgard | Beta₁ | 0 | Low | 20–24 | PO | 40 mg once/day |
| Penbutolol | Levatol | and | + | High | 5 | PO | 20 mg once/day |
| Pindolol | Visken | Beta₂ | +++ | Moderate | 3–4 | PO | 10 mg twice/day |
| Propranolol | Inderal | | 0 | High | 3–5 | PO, IV | 60 mg twice/day |
| slow release | Inderal LA | | 0 | High | 3–5 | PO | 120 mg once/day |
| Sotalol | Betapace | | 0 | Low | 12 | PO | Not for hypertension |
| Timolol | Blocadren | | 0 | Low | 4 | PO | 20 mg twice/day |

ISA = intrinsic sympathomimetic activity (partial agonist activity).
*Oral administration is used for essential hypertension. Intravenous administration is reserved for acute myocardial infarction (atenolol, metoprolol), cardiac dysrhythmias (esmolol, propranolol), and severe hypertension (labetalol).
†These are the lowest doses normally used for maintenance in hypertension.
‡Blocks alpha₁-adrenergic receptors in addition to beta receptors.

compensate for insulin-induced hypoglycemia. Because of their ability to block alpha-adrenergic receptors, *carvedilol* and *labetalol* can cause *postural hypotension*. Although *CNS effects* (insomnia, depression) can occur with all beta blockers, these effects may be more prominent with the highly lipid-soluble agents. Abrupt discontinuation of any beta blocker can produce *rebound cardiac excitation*. Accordingly, all beta blockers should be withdrawn slowly (by tapering the dosage over 1 to 2 weeks).

**Intrinsic Sympathomimetic Activity (Partial Agonist Activity).** The term *intrinsic sympathomimetic activity* (ISA) refers to the ability of certain beta blockers—especially *pindolol*—to act as *partial agonists* at beta-adrenergic receptors. (As discussed in Chapter 6, a partial agonist is a drug whose binding to a receptor produces a limited degree of receptor activation, while at the same time preventing strong agonists from binding to the receptor to cause full activation.)

In contrast to other beta blockers, agents with ISA have very little effect on resting heart rate and cardiac output. When patients are at rest, stimulation of the heart by the sympathetic nervous system is low. If an ordinary beta blocker is given, it will block sympathetic stimulation, causing heart rate and cardiac output to decline. However, if a beta blocker has ISA, its own ability to cause limited receptor activation will compensate for blocking receptor

activation by the sympathetic nervous system; consequently, resting heart rate and cardiac output are not reduced.

Because of their ability to provide a low level of cardiac stimulation, beta blockers with ISA are preferred to other beta blockers for use in patients with bradycardia or borderline heart failure. Conversely, these agents should not be given to patients with myocardial infarction, since their ability to cause even limited cardiac stimulation can be detrimental.

**Dosage and Administration.** With the exception of esmolol, all of the beta blockers discussed in this chapter can be administered *orally*. Three drugs—*atenolol, labetalol*, and *propranolol*—may be given *intravenously* as well. *Esmolol* is administered only by IV injection.

Maintenance dosages for hypertension are summarized in Table 19–2. For most beta blockers, dosing can be done just once a day. For the drugs with especially short half-lives, twice-a-day dosing is required (unless an extended-release formulation is available).

## KEY POINTS

- Most of the beneficial responses to alpha blockers, including reduction of blood pressure in patients with hypertension, result from blockade of alpha₁ receptors on blood vessels.

## TABLE 19-3. BETA-ADRENERGIC BLOCKING AGENTS: SUMMARY OF THERAPEUTIC USES*

| | Hypertension | Angina Pectoris | Cardiac Dysrhythmias | Myocardial Infarction | Migraine Prophylaxis | Stage Fright |
|---|---|---|---|---|---|---|
| Acebutolol | A | | A | | | |
| Atenolol | A | A | I | A | I | I |
| Betaxolol | A | | | | | |
| Bisoprolol | A | I | I | | | |
| Carteolol | A | I | | | | |
| Carvedilol | A | I | | | | |
| Esmolol | | I | A | | | |
| Labetalol | A | | | | | |
| Metoprolol | A | A | I | A | I | |
| Nadolol | A | A | I | | I | I |
| Penbutolol | A | | | | | |
| Pindolol | A | | I | | | I |
| Propranolol | A | A | A | A | A | I |
| Sotalol | | | A | | | |
| Timolol | A | | I | A | A | I |

A = FDA-approved use, I = investigational use.
* A group of beta blockers not discussed in this chapter is used to treat glaucoma. These beta blockers are discussed in Chapter 97 (Drugs for the Eye).

- Alpha blockers reduce symptoms of BPH by blocking alpha$_1$ receptors in the bladder neck and prostatic capsule, which causes the smooth muscle at those sites to relax.
- The major adverse effects of alpha blockers are *orthostatic hypotension* (caused by blocking alpha$_1$ receptors on veins); *reflex tachycardia* (caused by blocking alpha$_1$ receptors on arterioles); *nasal congestion* (caused by blocking alpha$_1$ receptors in blood vessels of the nasal mucosa); and *inhibition of ejaculation* (caused by blocking alpha$_1$ receptors in male sex organs).
- The first dose of an alpha blocker can cause fainting from profound orthostatic hypotension, the so-called first-dose effect.
- The alpha blockers used most frequently—prazosin, doxazosin, and terazosin—produce selective blockade of alpha$_1$ receptors.
- Beta blockers produce most of their beneficial effects by blocking beta$_1$ receptors in the heart, thereby reducing heart rate, force of contraction, and AV conduction.
- Principal indications for beta blockers are hypertension, angina pectoris, and supraventricular tachydysrhythmias.
- Potential adverse effects from beta$_1$ blockade are bradycardia, reduced cardiac output, AV block, and precipitation of heart failure.

- Potential adverse effects from beta$_2$ blockade are bronchoconstriction (a concern for people with asthma) and reduced glycogenolysis (a concern for people with diabetes).
- In addition to adverse effects caused by blockade of receptors in the periphery, beta blockers can cause depression and insomnia (from actions in the CNS).
- The beta blockers can be subdivided into two groups: (1) *nonselective* beta blockers (e.g., propranolol), which block beta$_1$ *and* beta$_2$ receptors, and (2) *cardioselective* beta blockers (e.g., metoprolol), which block beta$_1$ receptors only (at usual therapeutic doses).
- Beta blockers can be hazardous to patients with severe allergies because they can block the beneficial actions of epinephrine, the drug of choice for treating anaphylactic shock.
- Beta blockers can be detrimental to diabetics because they suppress glycogenolysis (an important mechanism for correcting insulin-induced hypoglycemia), and they suppress tachycardia (an early warning signal that blood glucose levels are falling too low).
- Combining a beta blocker with a calcium channel blocker can produce excessive cardiosuppression.
- Cardioselective beta blockers are preferred to nonselective beta blockers for patients with asthma or diabetes.

# Summary of Major Nursing Implications*

## Alpha₁-Adrenergic Antagonists

Doxazosin
Prazosin
Terazosin

### Preadministration Assessment

#### Therapeutic Goal
Reduction of blood pressure in patients with *essential hypertension* and reduction of symptoms in patients with *benign prostatic hyperplasia*.

#### Baseline Data
*Essential Hypertension.* Determine blood pressure.

*Benign Prostatic Hyperplasia.* Determine the degree of nocturia, daytime frequency, hesitance, intermittency, terminal dribbling (at the end of voiding), urgency, impairment of size and force of urinary stream, dysuria, and sensation of incomplete voiding.

#### Identifying High-Risk Patients
The only contraindication is hypersensitivity to these drugs.

### Implementation: Administration

#### Route
Oral.

#### Administration
Instruct patients to take the initial dose at bedtime to minimize the "first-dose" effect. All three drugs may be taken with food.

### Ongoing Evaluation and Interventions

#### Evaluating Therapeutic Effects
*Essential Hypertension.* Evaluate by monitoring blood pressure.

*Benign Prostatic Hyperplasia.* Evaluate for improvement in the symptoms listed above under *Baseline Data*.

#### Minimizing Adverse Effects
*Orthostatic Hypotension.* Alpha₁ blockade can cause postural hypotension. Inform patients about the symptoms of hypotension (dizziness, lightheadedness), and advise them to sit or lie down if these occur. Advise patients to move slowly when changing from a supine or sitting position to an upright posture.

*First-Dose Effect.* The first dose of prazosin, terazosin, or doxazosin may cause fainting from severe orthostatic hypotension. Forewarn patients about this effect, and advise them to avoid driving and other hazardous activities for 12 to 24 hours after receiving the initial dose. To minimize risk, advise patients to take the first dose at bedtime.

## Beta-Adrenergic Antagonists

| | |
|---|---|
| Acebutolol | Metoprolol |
| Atenolol | Nadolol |
| Labetalol | Penbutolol |
| Betaxolol | Pindolol |
| Bisoprolol | Propranolol |
| Carteolol | Timolol |
| Carvedilol | |

Except where noted, the implications summarized here apply to all beta-adrenergic blocking agents.

### Preadministration Assessment

#### Therapeutic Goal
Principal indications are *hypertension*, *angina pectoris*, and *cardiac dysrhythmias*. Indications for individual agents are summarized in Table 19-3.

#### Baseline Data
*Hypertension.* Determine standing and supine blood pressure.

*Angina Pectoris.* Determine the incidence, severity, and circumstances of anginal attacks.

*Cardiac Dysrhythmias.* Obtain a baseline electrocardiogram (EKG).

#### Identifying High-Risk Patients
*All* beta blockers are *contraindicated* for patients with *sinus bradycardia* and *AV heart block* (greater than first degree); also, they are *generally contraindicated* for patients with *heart failure*. Use with *caution* (especially the nonselective agents) in patients with *asthma, bronchospasm, diabetes,* and *history of severe allergic reactions.* Use *all* beta blockers with caution in patients with a *history of depression* and in those taking *calcium channel blockers.*

### Implementation: Administration

#### Routes
*Oral.* All beta blockers except esmolol.

*Intravenous. Atenolol, labetalol, metoprolol, propranolol.*

---

## Administration

For maintenance therapy of hypertension, administer once or twice daily (see Table 19-2).

Warn patients against abrupt discontinuation of treatment.

## Ongoing Evaluation and Interventions

### Evaluating Therapeutic Effects

*Hypertension.* Monitor blood pressure and heart rate prior to each dose. Advise outpatients to monitor blood pressure and heart rate daily.

*Angina Pectoris.* Advise patients to record the incidence, circumstances, and severity of anginal attacks.

*Cardiac Dysrhythmias.* Monitor for improvement in the EKG.

### Minimizing Adverse Effects

*Bradycardia.* Beta$_1$ blockade can reduce heart rate. If bradycardia is severe, withhold medication and notify the physician. If necessary, administer atropine and isoproterenol to restore heart rate.

*AV Heart Block.* Beta$_1$ blockade can decrease AV conduction. Do not give beta blockers to patients with AV block greater than first degree.

*Heart Failure.* Suppression of myocardial contractility can cause heart failure. Inform patients about early signs of heart failure (shortness of breath, night coughs, swelling of the extremities), and instruct them to notify the physician if these occur.

*Rebound Cardiac Excitation.* Abrupt withdrawal of beta blockers can cause tachycardia and ventricular dysrhythmias. Warn patients against abrupt discontinuation of drug use. Advise patients to carry an adequate supply of medication when traveling.

*Postural Hypotension.* By blocking alpha-adrenergic receptors, *carvedilol* and *labetalol* can cause postural hypotension. Inform patients about signs of hypotension (lightheadedness, dizziness), and advise them to sit or lie down if these develop. Advise patients to move slowly when changing from a supine or sitting position to an upright posture.

*Bronchoconstriction.* Beta$_2$ blockade can cause substantial airway constriction in patients with asthma. The risk of bronchoconstriction is much lower with the cardioselective agents than with the nonselective agents.

*Effects in Diabetics.* Beta$_1$ blockade can "mask" tachycardia, an early sign of hypoglycemia. Warn patients that tachycardia cannot be relied on as an indicator of impending hypoglycemia, and teach them to recognize other indicators (sweating, hunger, fatigue, poor concentration) that blood glucose is becoming dangerously low. Beta$_2$ blockade can prevent glycogenolysis, an emergency means of increasing blood glucose. Patients may need to reduce their insulin dosage. Cardioselective beta blockers are preferred to nonselective agents in patients with diabetes.

*CNS Effects.* Beta blockers can cause depression, insomnia, and nightmares. If these effects occur, it may be helpful to switch to a beta blocker with low lipid solubility (see Table 19-2).

### Minimizing Adverse Interactions

*Calcium Channel Blockers.* Two calcium channel blockers—verapamil and diltiazem—can intensify the cardiosuppressant effects of the beta blockers. Use the combination with caution.

*Insulin.* Beta blockers can prevent the compensatory glycogenolysis that normally occurs in response to insulin-induced hypoglycemia. Diabetic patients may need to reduce their insulin dosage.

# CHAPTER 20

# Indirect-Acting Antiadrenergic Agents

**Adrenergic Neuron Blocking Agents**
  Reserpine
  Guanethidine
  Guanadrel

**Centrally Acting Alpha$_2$ Agonists**
  Clonidine
  Guanabenz and Guanfacine
  Methyldopa

The indirect-acting antiadrenergic agents are drugs that prevent stimulation of peripheral adrenergic receptors, but they do so by mechanisms that do not involve direct receptor interaction. There are two categories of indirect-acting antiadrenergic drugs. The first group—*adrenergic neuron-blocking agents*—consists of drugs that act within the terminals of sympathetic neurons to decrease norepinephrine release. The second group—the *centrally acting alpha$_2$ agonists*—consists of drugs that act within the central nervous system (CNS) to reduce the outflow of impulses along sympathetic nerves. With both groups, the net result of drug actions is a reduction in the stimulation of peripheral adrenergic receptors. Hence, the pharmacologic effects of the indirect-acting adrenergic blocking agents are similar to those of drugs that block adrenergic receptors directly.

## Adrenergic Neuron Blocking Agents

The adrenergic neuron blocking agents are drugs that act presynaptically to reduce the release of norepinephrine from sympathetic neurons. (These drugs have very little effect on the release of epinephrine from the adrenal medulla.) Our discussion of the adrenergic neuron blockers focuses on two agents: reserpine and guanethidine.

### Reserpine

Reserpine is a naturally occurring compound prepared from the root of *Rauwolfia serpentina*, a shrub indigenous to India. Because of its source, reserpine is classified as a *Rauwolfia alkaloid*. The primary indication for reserpine is hypertension. When employed clinically, the drug can produce several serious side effects, the most important being severe mental depression.

### Mechanism of Action

Reserpine produces its pharmacologic effects by causing *depletion of norepinephrine (NE) from postganglionic sympathetic neurons*. By doing so, the drug can decrease the stimulation of practically all adrenergic receptors. Hence, the effects of reserpine closely resemble those produced by a combination of alpha- and beta-adrenergic blockade.

There are two mechanisms by which reserpine depletes NE from neurons. First, reserpine acts on vesicles within the nerve terminal to cause displacement of stored NE, thereby exposing the transmitter to destruction by monoamine oxidase (MAO). Second, reserpine suppresses norepinephrine synthesis. As depicted in Figure 20–1, reserpine decreases NE synthesis by blocking the uptake of dopamine (the immediate precursor of NE) into presynaptic vesicles, the structures that contain the enzymes needed to convert dopamine into NE. A week or two may be required for maximal transmitter depletion to develop.

In addition to its peripheral effects, reserpine can cause depletion of transmitters (serotonin, catecholamines) from neurons within the CNS. Depletion of these CNS transmitters underlies the most serious side effect of reserpine—deep emotional depression—and also explains the occasional use of reserpine in psychiatry.

### Pharmacologic Effects

*Peripheral Effects.* By depleting sympathetic neurons of norepinephrine, reserpine decreases the activation of alpha- and beta-adrenergic receptors. Decreased activation of beta receptors slows heart rate and reduces cardiac output. Decreased alpha activation promotes vasodilation. All three effects cause a *decrease in blood pressure*.

*Effects on the CNS.* Reserpine produces sedation and a state of indifference to the environment. In addition, the drug can cause severe depression. These effects are thought to result from depletion of certain neurotransmitters (catecholamines, serotonin) from neurons in the brain.

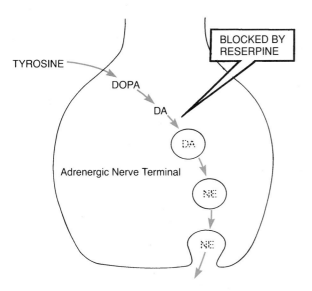

**Figure 20–1. Mechanism of reserpine action.** Reserpine depletes neurons of norepinephrine (NE) by two mechanisms. (1) As indicated in this figure, reserpine blocks the uptake of dopamine (DA) into vesicles, thereby preventing NE synthesis. (2) Reserpine displaces NE from vesicles, thereby allowing degradation of NE by monoamine oxidase present in the nerve terminal (not shown).

## Therapeutic Uses

*Hypertension.* The principal indication for reserpine is hypertension. Antihypertensive effects result from vasodilation and reduced cardiac output. Since these effects occur secondary to depletion of NE, and since transmitter depletion occurs slowly, full antihypertensive responses can take a week or more to develop. Conversely, when reserpine is discontinued, effects may persist for several weeks as the NE content of sympathetic neurons becomes replenished. Because its side effects can be severe, and because more desirable drugs are available (see Chapter 44), reserpine is not a preferred drug for hypertension.

*Psychotic States.* Reserpine can be used to treat agitated psychotic patients, such as those suffering from certain forms of schizophrenia. However, since superior drugs are available (e.g., phenothiazine antipsychotics), reserpine is rarely employed in psychotherapy.

## Adverse Effects

*Depression.* Reserpine can produce severe depression that may persist for months after the drug is withdrawn. Suicide has occurred. All patients should be informed about the risk of depression. Also, they should be educated about signs of depression (e.g., early morning insomnia, loss of appetite, change in mood) and instructed to notify the physician immediately if these develop. Because of the risk of suicide, patients who develop depression may require hospitalization. *Reserpine is contraindicated for patients with a history of depressive disorders.*

*Cardiovascular Effects.* Depletion of norepinephrine from sympathetic neurons can result in *bradycardia, or-*

*thostatic hypotension*, and *nasal congestion*. Bradycardia is caused by decreased activation of beta$_1$ receptors in the heart. Hypotension and nasal congestion are caused by reduced activation of alpha receptors on blood vessels. Patients should be informed that orthostatic hypotension, the most serious cardiovascular effect, can be minimized by moving slowly when changing from a supine to an upright posture. In addition, patients should be advised to sit or lie down if lightheadedness or dizziness occurs.

*Gastrointestinal Effects.* By mechanisms that are not understood, reserpine can stimulate several aspects of gastrointestinal function. The drug can increase secretion of gastric acid, which may result in ulcer formation. In addition, reserpine can increase the tone and motility of intestinal smooth muscle, thereby causing cramps and diarrhea.

### Preparations, Dosage, and Administration

Reserpine is available in tablets (0.1 and 0.25 mg) for oral use. The drug may be administered with food if gastrointestinal upset occurs. The initial dosage for hypertension in adults is 0.5 mg/day. For maintenance therapy, the dosage should be reduced to 0.1 to 0.25 mg/day.

## Guanethidine

Guanethidine [Ismelin] is an adrenergic neuron blocking agent with hypotensive actions similar to those of reserpine. However, in contrast to reserpine, guanethidine cannot cross the blood-brain barrier, and hence does not adversely affect the CNS. The drug's most prominent adverse effects are diarrhea and profound orthostatic hypotension. Because of these effects, guanethidine has been largely replaced by more desirable drugs.

### Mechanism of Action

*Primary Action: Inhibition of Norepinephrine Release.* Guanethidine acts presynaptically to inhibit release of NE from sympathetic neurons. In order to inhibit NE release, guanethidine must first be taken up into nerve terminals. Uptake takes place via the same transport system employed for reuptake of NE. Once inside the sympathetic nerve terminal, guanethidine acts to prevent NE release. The precise mechanism by which the drug inhibits release is not known.

*Secondary Actions.* In addition to blocking NE release, guanethidine has two other actions. First, during *initial* use, guanethidine can *promote NE release*. As a result, the early phase of therapy may be associated with transient *sympathomimetic effects*, rather than sympathetic blockade. Second, with chronic use, guanethidine, like reserpine, *depletes NE from sympathetic nerves.*

### Pharmacologic Effects

The pharmacologic effects of guanethidine, like those of reserpine, result from decreased activation of alpha- and beta-adrenergic receptors. The most pronounced cardiovascular effects are *bradycardia, decreased cardiac output*, and a *great reduction in venous smooth muscle tone.* As a result of these effects, systolic blood pressure falls, especially when the patient is standing.

## Therapeutic Use

The only indication for guanethidine is *hypertension.* Because of its tendency to cause diarrhea and severe orthostatic hypotension, guanethidine is not used routinely. Rather, the drug is reserved for patients whose blood pressure cannot be controlled with more desirable drugs.

## Adverse Effects

*Diarrhea.* Like reserpine, guanethidine stimulates the gastrointestinal system; diarrhea is the most common result. In most cases, diarrhea can be managed with antidiarrheal drugs (e.g., diphenoxylate, loperamide, anticholinergic agents). The mechanism underlying diarrhea is in dispute.

*Orthostatic Hypotension.* Guanethidine-induced orthostatic hypotension can be severe. Blood pressure may fall so low that perfusion of the heart and brain is seriously compromised. Supine and standing blood pressure should be monitored. If standing blood pressure drops too low, guanethidine should be withheld and the physician notified. Patients should be warned about orthostatic hypotension and informed that it can be minimized by moving slowly when assuming an erect posture. Also, patients should be informed that factors that promote vasodilation (e.g., alcohol consumption, warm environments, strenuous exercise) can intensify orthostatic hypotension and should be avoided.

*Hypertension.* Although used to *treat* hypertension, guanethidine can *cause* hypertension in the patient with a pheochromocytoma (a catecholamine-secreting tumor). Recall that guanethidine stimulates NE release during the initial phase of treatment. Since pheochromocytomas contain massive amounts of NE, guanethidine-induced NE release can result in a dramatic rise in blood pressure.

## Drug Interactions

*Tricyclic antidepressants* and other drugs that block the reuptake of NE into adrenergic neurons will also block the uptake of guanethidine, thereby keeping guanethidine from its site action. Hence, reuptake blockers will reduce guanethidine's effects.

### Preparations, Dosage, and Administration

Guanethidine monosulfate [Ismelin] is available in 10- and 25-mg tablets for oral use. The initial dosage for hypertension in adults is 10 mg administered once daily. The dosage can be increased every 5 to 7 days to a maintenance level of 25 to 50 mg administered once daily. Dosage should be reduced in patients who develop orthostatic hypotension or severe diarrhea.

### Guanadrel

Guanadrel [Hylorel] is a close relative of guanethidine. Both drugs share the same mechanism of action, therapeutic use, drug interactions, and adverse effects (although diarrhea is less troubling with guanadrel). Guanadrel has a shorter half-life than guanethidine, and hence must be administered twice daily (rather than once daily). The usual initial dosage for adults is 10 mg/day. Maintenance dosages range from 20 to 75 mg/day.

# Centrally Acting Alpha₂ Agonists

The drugs discussed in this section act within the CNS to reduce the firing of sympathetic neurons. These drugs are used primarily for hypertension.

Why are we discussing centrally acting drugs in a unit on peripheral nervous system pharmacology? Because the effects of these drugs are ultimately the result of decreased activation of alpha- and beta-adrenergic receptors in the periphery. That is, by inhibiting the firing of sympathetic neurons, the centrally acting agents decrease the release of NE from sympathetic nerves, thereby reducing activation of peripheral adrenergic receptors. Hence, although these drugs act within the CNS, their effects are like those of the direct-acting adrenergic receptor blockers. Accordingly, it seems appropriate to discuss these agents in the context of peripheral nervous system pharmacology—rather than presenting them in the context of CNS drugs.

## Clonidine

Clonidine [Catapres] is an antihypertensive agent that acts within the CNS. Except for rare instances of rebound hypertension, the drug is generally free of serious adverse effects. Because it is both effective and safe, clonidine is widely used.

### Mechanism of Action

Clonidine is an alpha₂-adrenergic agonist that causes "selective" stimulation of alpha₂ receptors in the CNS—specifically, in brainstem areas associated with autonomic regulation of the cardiovascular system. By stimulating central alpha₂ receptors, clonidine reduces sympathetic outflow to blood vessels and the heart.

### Pharmacologic Effects

The most significant effects of clonidine occur in the heart and the vascular system. By suppressing the firing of sympathetic nerves to the heart, clonidine can cause *bradycardia* and a *decrease in cardiac output.* By suppressing sympathetic regulation of blood vessels, the drug promotes vasodilation. The net result of cardiac suppression and vasodilation is a *decrease in blood pressure.* Blood pressure is reduced in both supine and standing subjects. (Note that the effect of clonidine on blood pressure is unlike that of the peripheral alpha-adrenergic blockers, which tend to decrease blood pressure only when the patient is standing.) Since the hypotensive effects of clonidine are not posture dependent, orthostatic hypotension with this drug is minimal.

### Pharmacokinetics

Clonidine is very lipid soluble. As a result, the drug is readily absorbed following oral administration and undergoes wide distribution throughout the body, including the

CNS. Hypotensive responses begin 30 to 60 minutes after administration and peak in 4 hours. Effects of a single dose may persist for as long as 1 day. Clonidine is eliminated by a combination of hepatic metabolism and renal excretion.

## Therapeutic Uses

Clonidine is approved only for *hypertension*. However, the drug has been used on an investigational basis to treat various other conditions, including menopausal flushing; migraine; withdrawal from opioids, alcohol, and tobacco; and Tourette's syndrome (a CNS disease characterized by uncontrollable jerking and verbal outbursts that are frequently obscene).

## Adverse Effects

***Drowsiness.*** CNS depression is very common. About 35% of patients experience drowsiness; an additional 8% experience outright sedation. These responses become less intense with continued drug use. Patients in their early weeks of treatment should be advised to avoid hazardous activities if alertness is impaired.

***Xerostomia.*** Xerostomia (dry mouth) is common, occurring in about 40% of patients. The reaction usually diminishes over the first 2 to 4 weeks of clonidine therapy. Although not dangerous, xerostomia can be annoying enough to discourage drug use. Patients should be advised that discomfort can be reduced by chewing gum, sucking on hard candy, and taking frequent sips of fluids.

***Rebound Hypertension.*** Rebound hypertension is defined as a large increase in blood pressure occurring in response to abrupt clonidine withdrawal. This rare but serious reaction is caused by overactivity of the sympathetic nervous system, and can be accompanied by nervousness, tachycardia, and sweating. Left untreated, the reaction may persist for a week or more. If blood pressure climbs dangerously high, it should be lowered with a combination of alpha- and beta-adrenergic blocking agents. Rebound effects can be avoided by withdrawing clonidine slowly (over 2 to 4 days). Patients should be informed about rebound hypertension and warned not to discontinue clonidine without consulting the physician.

***Use in Pregnancy.*** Clonidine is embryotoxic in animals. Because of the possibility of fetal harm, clonidine is not recommended for use by pregnant women. Pregnancy should be ruled out before therapy is instituted.

***Other Adverse Effects.*** Clonidine can cause a variety of adverse effects, including *constipation, impotence, gynecomastia,* and adverse *CNS effects* (e.g., vivid dreams, nightmares, anxiety, depression). *Localized skin reactions* are common with transdermal clonidine patches.

### Preparations, Dosage, and Administration

***Preparations.*** Clonidine hydrochloride [Catapres] is available in tablets (0.1, 0.2, and 0.3 mg) for oral use and in transdermal systems [Catapres-TTS] that contain 2.5, 5, or 7.5 mg of drug.

***Dosage and Administration. Oral.*** For treatment of hypertension, the initial adult dosage is 0.1 mg twice a day. The usual maintenance dosage is 0.2 to 0.8 mg/day administered in divided doses. By taking the majority of the daily dose at bedtime, adverse consequences of sedation can be minimized.

***Transdermal.*** Transdermal patches are applied to a region of hairless, intact skin on the upper arm or torso. A new patch is applied every 7 days.

### Guanabenz and Guanfacine

The pharmacology of guanabenz [Wytensin] and guanfacine [Tenex] is very similar to that of clonidine. Like clonidine, both drugs stimulate brainstem alpha$_2$-adrenergic receptors, and thereby reduce sympathetic outflow to the heart and blood vessels. The result is a reduction in cardiac output and blood pressure. Both drugs also share the major adverse effects of clonidine: sedation and dry mouth. In addition, both can cause rebound hypertension following abrupt withdrawal.

## Methyldopa

Methyldopa [Aldomet, Amodopa] is a widely used antihypertensive agent. Like clonidine, the drug lowers blood pressure by acting at sites within the CNS. Certain side effects (hemolytic anemia, hepatic necrosis) can be severe. Given the potential hazards of the drug, its frequent usage is difficult to understand.

### Mechanism of Action

The mechanism of action of methyldopa is similar to that of clonidine. Like clonidine, methyldopa inhibits sympathetic outflow from the CNS by causing alpha$_2$ stimulation in the brain. Methyldopa differs from clonidine in that methyldopa itself is not an alpha$_2$ agonist. Before it can act, methyldopa must first be taken up into brainstem neurons, where it is then converted to methylnorepinephrine, a compound that *is* an effective alpha$_2$ agonist. Release of methylnorepinephrine results in alpha$_2$ stimulation.

### Pharmacologic Effects

The most prominent response to methyldopa is a drop in blood pressure. The drug reduces blood pressure primarily by causing vasodilation—and not by effects on the heart. Vasodilation occurs because of reduced sympathetic traffic to blood vessels. At usual therapeutic doses, methyldopa does not decrease heart rate or cardiac output. Hence, hypotensive actions cannot be ascribed to cardiac depression. The hemodynamic effects of methyldopa are very much like those of clonidine: both drugs lower blood pressure in supine and standing subjects, and both produce relatively little orthostatic hypotension.

### Therapeutic Use

The only indication for methyldopa is *hypertension*. Methyldopa was one of the earliest antihypertensive agents available and remains in wide use.

### Adverse Effects

***Positive Coombs' Test and Hemolytic Anemia.*** A positive Coombs' test* develops in 10% to 20% of patients taking methyldopa chronically. The test usually turns positive

---

*The Coombs' test detects the presence of antibodies directed against the patient's own red blood cells. These antibodies can cause hemolysis (i.e., red cell lysis).

between the 6th and 12th month of treatment. Of those patients with a positive test result, only a few (about 5%) develop hemolytic anemia. Coombs'-positive patients who do not have hemolytic anemia may continue methyldopa treatment. However, if hemolytic anemia develops, methyldopa should be withdrawn immediately. For most patients, hemolytic anemia resolves soon after drug withdrawal—although the Coombs' test may remain positive for months. A Coombs' test should be performed prior to treatment and 6 to 12 months later. Blood counts (hematocrit, hemoglobin or red cell count) should be obtained prior to treatment and periodically thereafter.

**Hepatotoxicity.** Methyldopa has been associated with hepatitis, jaundice, and, rarely, fatal hepatic necrosis. All patients should undergo periodic assessment of liver function. If signs of hepatotoxicity appear, methyldopa should be discontinued immediately. Liver function usually normalizes following drug withdrawal.

**Other Adverse Effects.** Methyldopa can cause *xerostomia*, *sexual dysfunction*, *orthostatic hypotension*, and a variety of *CNS effects*, including drowsiness, reduced mental acuity, nightmares, and depression. These responses are not usually dangerous, but they can detract from compliance.

### Preparations, Dosage, and Administration

**Preparations.** *Methyldopa* [Aldomet, Amodopa] is available in tablets (125, 250, and 500 mg) and in a suspension (50 mg/ml) for oral use. In addition, a derivative of methyldopa, named *methyldopate* [Aldomet], is available as an injection (50 mg/ml in 5-ml vials) for IV use.

**Oral Therapy.** For treatment of hypertension, the initial adult dosage is 250 mg 2 to 3 times a day. Daily maintenance dosages usually range from 0.5 to 2 gm administered in two to four divided doses.

**Intravenous Therapy.** Methyldopa, administered by slow IV infusion, is indicated for hypertensive emergencies. However, since faster-acting drugs are available, use of methyldopa is rare. Methyldopa for infusion should be diluted in 5% dextrose to a concentration of 10 mg/ml. The usual adult dose is 250 to 500 mg infused over 30 to 60 minutes. Dosing may be repeated every 6 hours as required.

## KEY POINTS

- All the drugs discussed in this chapter reduce stimulation of peripheral alpha- and beta-adrenergic receptors, but they do so by mechanisms other than direct receptor blockade.
- The principal indication for all the drugs discussed in this chapter is hypertension.
- Reserpine acts by depleting NE from adrenergic neurons.
- Guanethidine is taken up by adrenergic neurons, where it blocks NE release and, eventually, depletes NE from storage vesicles.
- Clonidine and methyldopa reduce sympathetic outflow to the heart and blood vessels by causing stimulation of alpha$_2$-adrenergic receptors in the brainstem.
- The principal adverse effect of reserpine is depression.
- The principal adverse effects of guanethidine are orthostatic hypotension and diarrhea.
- The principal adverse effects of clonidine are drowsiness, dry mouth, and rebound hypertension following abrupt drug withdrawal.
- The principal adverse effects of methyldopa are hemolytic anemia and hepatic toxicity.

# Summary of Major Nursing Implications*

## Reserpine

### Preadministration Assessment

#### Therapeutic Goal
Reduction of blood pressure in hypertensive patients.

#### Baseline Data
Determine blood pressure.

#### Identifying High-Risk Patients
Reserpine is *contraindicated* for patients with *active peptic ulcer disease* or a *history of depression*.

### Implementation: Administration

#### Route
Oral.

### Administration
Administer with food to reduce gastric upset.

## Ongoing Evaluation and Interventions

### Evaluating Therapeutic Effects
Full antihypertensive effects may take a week or more to develop. Monitor blood pressure to evaluate treatment.

### Minimizing Adverse Effects
**Depression.** Reserpine can cause profound depression. Inform patients about signs of depression (e.g., early morning insomnia, loss of appetite, change in mood) and instruct them to notify the physician if these develop. Hospitalization may be required. Avoid reserpine in patients with a history of depression.

**Orthostatic Hypotension.** Inform patients that orthostatic hypotension can be minimized by moving slowly when changing from a seated or supine position to an upright posture. Advise patients to sit or lie down if dizziness or lightheadedness occurs.

*Patient education information is highlighted in color.

# Guanethidine

## Preadministration Assessment

### Therapeutic Goal
Reduction of blood pressure in hypertensive patients.

### Baseline Data
Determine blood pressure in supine position, standing position, and, if possible, immediately after exercise.

### Identifying High-Risk Patients
Guanethidine is *contraindicated* for patients with *pheochromocytoma.*

## Implementation: Administration

### Route
Oral.

### Administration
For ambulatory patients, the entire daily dose is usually taken at one time.

## Ongoing Evaluation and Interventions

### Evaluating Therapeutic Effects
Monitor supine and standing blood pressure. Dosage is adjusted on the basis of the therapeutic response.

### Minimizing Adverse Effects
*Orthostatic Hypotension.* Orthostatic hypotension can be severe. Monitor supine and standing blood pressure. If standing blood pressure falls too low, withhold medication and notify the physician. Educate patients about the signs of hypotension (dizziness, lightheadedness) and advise them to sit or lie down if these occur. Advise patients to move slowly when changing from a supine or sitting position to an upright posture. Warn patients to avoid factors that can promote hypotension (e.g., alcohol, warm environments, strenuous exercise).

*Diarrhea.* Diarrhea is common. If necessary, manage with antidiarrheal drugs.

*Hypertension.* Guanethidine can cause severe hypertension in patients with *pheochromocytoma.* The drug is contraindicated for these patients.

### Minimizing Adverse Interactions
*Tricyclic antidepressants* and other drugs that block the NE uptake pump can decrease the effects of guanethidine and should be avoided.

# Clonidine

## Preadministration Assessment

### Therapeutic Goal
Reduction of blood pressure in hypertensive patients.

### Baseline Data
Determine blood pressure.

### Identifying High-Risk Patients
Clonidine is embryotoxic to animals and should not be used during *pregnancy.* Rule out pregnancy before initiating treatment.

## Implementation: Administration

### Routes
Oral, transdermal.

### Administration
*Oral.* Advise the patient to take the major portion of the daily dose at bedtime to minimize the adverse consequences of sedation.

*Transdermal.* Instruct the patient to apply transdermal patches to hairless, intact skin on the upper arm or torso. A new patch is applied every 7 days.

## Ongoing Evaluation and Interventions

### Evaluating Therapeutic Effects
Monitor blood pressure.

### Minimizing Adverse Effects
*Drowsiness and Sedation.* Inform patients about possible CNS depression and warn them to avoid hazardous activities if alertness is impaired.

*Xerostomia.* Dry mouth is very common. Inform patients that discomfort can be reduced by chewing gum, sucking on hard candy, and taking frequent sips of fluids.

*Rebound Hypertension.* Severe hypertension occurs rarely following abrupt clonidine withdrawal. Treat with a combination of alpha- and beta-adrenergic blockers. To avoid rebound hypertension, withdraw clonidine slowly (over 2 to 4 days). Inform patients about rebound hypertension and warn them against abrupt discontinuation of treatment.

# Methyldopa

## Preadministration Assessment

### Therapeutic Goal
Reduction of blood pressure in hypertensive patients.

### Baseline Data
Obtain baseline values for blood pressure, blood counts (hematocrit, hemoglobin or red cell count), Coombs' test, and liver function tests.

### Identifying High-Risk Patients
Methyldopa is *contraindicated* for patients with active *liver disease* and for those with a *history of methyldopa-induced liver dysfunction.*

## Implementation: Administration

### Routes

Oral (for routine management of hypertension).
Intravenous (for hypertensive emergencies).

### Administration

Most patients on oral therapy require divided (two to four) daily doses. For some patients, blood pressure can be controlled with a single daily dose at bedtime.

## Ongoing Evaluation and Interventions

### Evaluating Therapeutic Effects

Monitor blood pressure.

## Minimizing Adverse Effects

*Hemolytic Anemia.* If hemolysis occurs, withdraw methyldopa immediately; hemolytic anemia usually resolves soon thereafter. Obtain a Coombs' test prior to treatment and 6 to 12 months later. Obtain blood counts (hematocrit, hemoglobin or red cell count) prior to treatment and periodically thereafter.

*Hepatotoxicity.* Methyldopa can cause hepatitis, jaundice, and fatal hepatic necrosis. Assess liver function prior to treatment and periodically thereafter. If liver dysfunction develops, discontinue methyldopa immediately. In most cases, liver function will then return to normal.

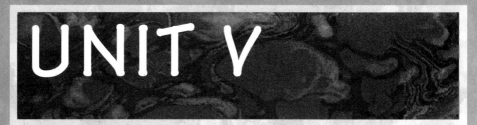

# UNIT V

# Central Nervous System Drugs

*UNIT V Continues*

# Introduction

# CHAPTER 21

# Introduction to Central Nervous System Pharmacology

Transmitters of the CNS
The Blood-Brain Barrier
How Do CNS Drugs Produce Therapeutic Effects?
Adaptation of the CNS to Prolonged Drug Exposure
Development of New Psychotherapeutic Drugs
Approaching the Study of CNS Drugs

The central nervous system (CNS) drugs—agents that act on the brain and spinal cord—are used widely for medical and nonmedical purposes. Medical applications include treatment of mental illnesses, suppression of seizures, relief of pain, and production of anesthesia. CNS drugs are used nonmedically for their stimulant, depressant, euphoriant, and other "mind-altering" abilities.

Despite the widespread use of CNS drugs, knowledge of these agents is limited. Much of our ignorance stems from the anatomic and neurochemical complexity of the brain and spinal cord. (There are more than 50 billion neurons in the cerebral hemispheres alone.) Because of this complexity, we are a long way from fully understanding both the CNS itself and the drugs used to influence its function.

Although much is known about the actions of CNS transmitters at various sites in the brain and spinal cord, it is not usually possible to relate these known actions in a precise way to behavioral or psychologic processes. For example, although we know the locations of specific CNS sites at which norepinephrine appears to act as a transmitter, and although we know the effect of norepinephrine at most of these sites (suppression of neuronal excitability), we do not know the precise relationship between suppression of neuronal excitability at each of these sites and the impact of that suppression on the overt function of the organism. This example illustrates the general state of our knowledge of CNS transmitter function: we have a great deal of detailed information about the biochemistry and electrophysiology of CNS transmitters, but we are as yet unable to assemble those details into a completely meaningful picture.

## Transmitters of the CNS

In contrast to the peripheral nervous system, in which only three compounds—acetylcholine, norepinephrine, and epinephrine—serve as neurotransmitters, the CNS contains more than a dozen compounds that appear to serve as neurotransmitters (Table 21-1). Furthermore, since there are numerous sites within the CNS for which no transmitter has been identified, it is clear that additional compounds, yet to be discovered, also mediate neurotransmission in the brain and spinal cord.

It is important to note that none of the compounds that are thought to be CNS neurotransmitters has actually been proved to serve this function. The reason for uncertainty lies with the technical difficulties involved in CNS research. However, although absolute proof may be lacking, the evidence supporting a neurotransmitter role for several compounds (e.g., dopamine, norepinephrine, serotonin, enkephalins) is completely convincing.

## The Blood-Brain Barrier

As discussed in Chapter 5, the blood-brain barrier impedes the entry of drugs into the brain. Passage across the barrier is limited to lipid-soluble agents and to drugs that are able to cross by way of specific transport systems. Drugs that are protein bound and drugs that are highly ionized cannot cross.

The presence of the blood-brain barrier is a mixed blessing. On the positive side, the barrier protects the brain from injury by potentially toxic substances. On the negative side, the barrier can be a significant obstacle in therapeutics.

The blood-brain barrier is not fully developed at birth. Accordingly, newborn infants are much more sensitive to CNS drugs than are older children and adults.

## TABLE 21–1. NEUROTRANSMITTERS OF THE CNS

*Monoamines*

Norepinephrine
Epinephrine
Dopamine
Serotonin

*Amino Acids*

Aspartate
Glutamate
GABA
Glycine

*Peptides*

Dynorphins
Endorphins
Enkephalins
Neurotensin
Somatostatin
Substance P
Oxytocin
Vasopressin

*Others*

Acetylcholine
Histamine

# How Do CNS Drugs Produce Therapeutic Effects?

Although much is known about the biochemical and electrophysiologic effects of CNS drugs, in most cases we cannot state with certainty the relationship between these effects and production of beneficial responses. Why is this so? In order to fully understand how a drug alters symptoms, we need to understand, at a biochemical and physiologic level, the pathophysiology of the disorder being treated. In the case of most CNS disorders, this knowledge is deficient. That is, we do not fully understand the brain in either health or disease. Given our incomplete understanding of the CNS itself, we must exercise caution when attempting to assign a precise mechanism for a drug's therapeutic effects.

Although we can't state with certainty how CNS drugs act, we do have sufficient data to permit the formulation of plausible hypotheses. Consequently, as we study the CNS drugs, proposed mechanisms of action will be presented. However, keep in mind that these mechanisms are tentative, representing our best guesses based upon data available today. As we learn more, it is almost certain that these concepts will need to be modified, if not discarded entirely.

# Adaptation of the CNS to Prolonged Drug Exposure

When CNS drugs are taken chronically, effects may differ from those observed during initial use. These altered effects are the result of adaptive changes that occur in the brain in response to prolonged drug exposure. The brain's ability to adapt to drugs can produce alterations in therapeutic effects and in side effects. Adaptive changes are often beneficial, although they can also be detrimental.

***Increased Therapeutic Effects.*** Certain drugs used in psychiatry—antipsychotics and antidepressants—must be taken for several weeks before full therapeutic effects develop. It has been suggested that beneficial responses are delayed because these responses result from adaptive changes and not from the direct effects of drugs on synaptic function. Hence, full therapeutic effects are not seen until the CNS has had time to modify itself in response to prolonged drug exposure.

***Decreased Side Effects.*** When CNS drugs are taken chronically, the intensity of side effects may decrease (while therapeutic effects remain undiminished). For example, phenobarbital (an anticonvulsant) produces sedation during the initial phase of therapy; however, with continued treatment, sedation declines while full protection from seizures is retained. Similarly, when morphine is given to control pain, nausea is a common side effect early on; however, as treatment continues, nausea diminishes while analgesic effects persist. Adaptations within the brain may explain these phenomena.

***Tolerance and Physical Dependence.*** Tolerance and physical dependence are special manifestations of CNS adaptation. (Tolerance is defined as a decreased response occurring in the course of prolonged drug use. Physical dependence is defined as a state in which abrupt discontinuation of drug use will precipitate a withdrawal syndrome.) Research indicates that the kinds of adaptive changes that underlie tolerance and dependence are such that, once they have taken place, continued drug use is required for the brain to function "normally." If drug use is stopped, the drug-adapted brain can no longer function properly and a withdrawal syndrome ensues. The withdrawal reaction continues until the adaptive changes have had time to revert, thereby restoring the CNS to its original state.

# Development of New Psychotherapeutic Drugs

Because of deficiencies in our knowledge of the neurochemical and physiologic changes that underlie mental disease, it is impossible to take a rational approach to the development of truly new (nonderivative) psychotherapeutic agents. History bears this out: virtually all of the major advances in psychopharmacology have been happy accidents.

In addition to our relative ignorance about the neurochemical and physiologic correlates of mental illness, two other factors contribute to the difficulty in generating truly new psychotherapeutic agents. (1) In contrast to many other diseases, we have no adequate animal models of mental illness. Accordingly, animal research is not likely to reveal new types of psychotherapeutic agents. (2) Mentally healthy individuals cannot be used as subjects to assess potential psychotherapeutic agents; this is because most psychotherapeutic drugs either have no effect on healthy individuals or produce paradoxical effects.

Once a new drug has been stumbled upon, variations on that agent can be developed systematically. The following process is employed: (1) structural analogs of the new agent are synthesized, (2) these analogs are run through biochemical and physiologic screening tests to determine whether or not they possess activity similar to that of the parent compound, and (3) after serious toxicity has been ruled out, promising agents are tested in humans for possible psychotherapeutic activity. By following this procedure, it is possible to develop drugs that have fewer side effects than the original drug and perhaps even superior therapeutic effects. However, although this procedure may produce small advances, it is not likely to yield a major therapeutic breakthrough.

# Approaching the Study of CNS Drugs

Because our understanding of the CNS is less complete than our understanding of the peripheral nervous system, our approach to studying CNS drugs will differ from the approach we took with peripheral nervous system agents. When we studied the pharmacology of the peripheral nervous system, we emphasized the importance of understanding transmitters and their receptors prior to embarking on a study of drugs. Since our knowledge of CNS transmitters is insufficient to allow this approach, rather than making a detailed examination of CNS transmitters before we study CNS drugs, we will discuss drugs and transmitters concurrently. Hence, for now, all that you need to know about CNS transmitters is that (1) there are a lot of them, (2) their precise functional roles are not clear, and (3) their complexity makes it difficult for us to know with any certainty just how CNS drugs produce their effects.

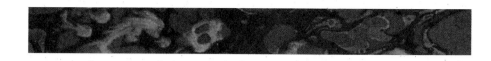

# Neurologic Drugs

# CHAPTER 22

# Drugs for Parkinson's Disease

Parkinson's disease is a neurologic disorder characterized by disturbance of movement. The primary pathology is loss of dopaminergic neurons in the substantia nigra, and the most effective therapy is replacement of dopamine using levodopa.

## Pathophysiology of Parkinson's Disease

Parkinson's disease is a disorder of the *extrapyramidal system*, a complex neuronal network that helps regulate movement. When extrapyramidal function is disrupted, *dyskinesias* (disorders of movement) result. The dyskinesias that characterize Parkinson's disease are *tremor at rest*, *rigidity*, *postural instability*, and *bradykinesia* (slowed movement); in severe disease bradykinesia may progress to *akinesia* (complete absence of movement). In addition to these movement disorders, patients frequently experience *psychologic disturbances*, including dementia, depression, and impaired memory. As a rule, symptoms first appear in middle age and progress steadily.

The symptoms of Parkinson's disease result from disruption of neurotransmission within the *striatum*, an important component of the extrapyramidal system. A highly simplified model of striatal neurotransmission is depicted in Figure 22–1A. As indicated, proper functioning of the striatum requires a balance between two neurotransmitters: *dopamine* (DA) and *acetylcholine* (ACh). Dopamine is an *inhibitory* transmitter; ACh is *excitatory*. According to the model, the neurons that release DA inhibit neurons that release GABA (another inhibitory transmitter). In contrast, the neurons that release ACh excite the neurons that release GABA. Movement is normal when the inhibitory influence of DA and the excitatory influence of ACh are in balance.

In Parkinson's disease, there is an imbalance between DA and ACh in the striatum (Fig. 22–1B). The cause of the imbalance is *degeneration of the neurons that supply DA to the striatum*. (Why these neurons degenerate is not known.) In the absence of DA, the excitatory influence of ACh becomes unopposed, causing excessive stimulation of the neurons that release GABA. Overactivity of these GABAergic neurons contributes to the movement disorders seen in Parkinson's disease.

As discussed in Chapter 24, movement disorders similar to those of Parkinson's disease can occur as side effects of therapy with antipsychotic agents. These dyskinesias, which are referred to as *extrapyramidal side effects*, result from blockade of dopamine receptors in the striatum. This drug-induced parkinsonism can be managed with some of the drugs used to treat Parkinson's disease.

## Overview of Drug Therapy

### Therapeutic Goal

The goal of treatment is to improve the patient's ability to carry out activities of daily life. Drug selection and dosage are determined by the extent to which Parkinson's disease interferes with such activities as work, walking, dressing, eating, bathing, and rising from a bed or a chair. Improving the capacity for these activities is primarily a function of decreasing bradykinesia, gait disturbance, and postural instability. Tremor and rigidity, although disturbing, are less disabling.

It is important to note that drug therapy of Parkinson's disease provides only symptomatic relief, not cure.

A   Normal

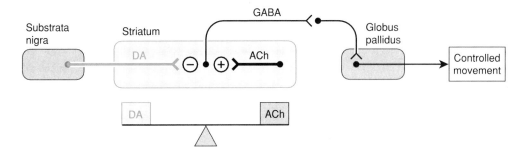

B   Parkinson's Disease

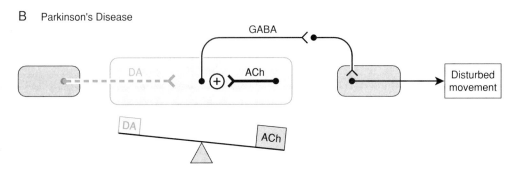

**Figure 22–1. A model of neurotransmission in the healthy striatum and parkinsonian striatum.** *A*, In the healthy striatum, dopamine (DA) released from neurons originating in the substantia nigra inhibits the firing of neurons in the striatum that release gamma-aminobutyric acid (GABA) as their transmitter. Conversely, neurons located within the striatum, which release acetylcholine (ACh) as their transmitter, excite the GABAergic neurons. Hence, under normal conditions, the inhibitory actions of DA are balanced by the excitatory actions of ACh, and controlled movement results.

*B*, In Parkinson's disease, the neurons that supply DA to the striatum degenerate. In the absence of DA, the excitatory effects of ACh go unopposed, and disturbed movement results.

Furthermore, with only one possible exception—selegiline—the drugs employed do not alter the progression of the disease.

### Treatment Strategy

Given the neurochemical basis of parkinsonism—too little striatal DA and too much ACh—the strategy for treatment is self-evident: therapy must be directed at restoring the functional balance between DA and ACh. To restore this balance, two types of drugs are used: (1) agents that directly or indirectly activate DA receptors and (2) agents that block ACh receptors.

### Overview of Drugs Employed

Table 22–1 presents an overview of the drugs used to treat Parkinson's disease. As indicated, these drugs fall into two major categories: (1) *dopaminergic drugs* (drugs that promote activation of dopamine receptors), and (2) *anticholinergic drugs* (drugs that prevent activation of cholinergic receptors). The dopaminergic agents act by a variety of mechanisms, including promotion of dopamine synthesis, direct activation of dopamine receptors, and prevention of dopamine degradation. In contrast, all of the anticholinergic agents act by the same mechanism: blockade of muscarinic cholinergic receptors in the striatum.

## Basic Pharmacology of the Drugs Used to Treat Parkinson's Disease

### Levodopa

#### Use in Parkinson's Disease

***Beneficial Effects.*** Levodopa [Dopar, Larodopa] is the drug of choice for Parkinson's disease. With initial treatment, about 75% of patients experience a 50% reduction in severity of symptoms. Levodopa is so effective, in fact, that a diagnosis of Parkinson's disease should be questioned if the patient fails to respond.

Full therapeutic responses may take several months to develop. Consequently, although the effects of levodopa can be significant, patients should not expect improvement immediately. Rather, they should be informed that beneficial effects are likely to increase steadily over the first few months of treatment.

In contrast to the dramatic improvements seen during initial therapy, long-term therapy with levodopa has been disappointing. Although symptoms may be well controlled during the first 2 years of treatment, by the end of

## TABLE 22–1. OVERVIEW OF DRUGS FOR PARKINSON'S DISEASE

| Drug Class | Drug | Mechanism of Action |
|---|---|---|
| *Dopaminergic drugs* | Levodopa | Increases synthesis of dopamine |
| | Carbidopa | Used with levodopa to prevent destruction of levodopa in the periphery |
| | Selegiline | Used with levodopa to prevent destruction of dopamine in the CNS; may retard progression of disease |
| | Amantadine | Promotes release of dopamine |
| | Bromocriptine | Activates dopamine receptors directly |
| | Pergolide | Activates dopamine receptors directly |
| *Anticholinergic drugs* | Benztropine | All of these drugs act by blocking receptors for acetylcholine in the CNS |
| | Biperidin | |
| | Diphenhydramine | |
| | Ethopropazine | |
| | Procyclidine | |
| | Trihexyphenidyl | |

5 years the patient's ability to function may deteriorate to pretreatment levels. This probably reflects progression of the disease and not development of tolerance to levodopa.

***Acute Loss of Effect.*** Acute loss of effect occurs in two patterns: gradual loss and abrupt loss. Gradual loss ("wearing off") develops near the end of the dosing interval, and simply indicates that plasma drug levels have declined to a subtherapeutic value. Wearing off can be minimized by shortening the dosing interval and by adjunctive use of a direct-acting dopamine agonist (see below). Wearing off can also be reduced by using the controlled-release formulation of levodopa [Sinemet CR].

Abrupt loss of effect, often referred to as the "on-off" phenomenon, can occur at any time during the dosing interval—even while drug levels are high. "Off" times may last from minutes to hours. Over time, "off" periods are likely to increase in both intensity and frequency. The "on-off" phenomenon is difficult to correct. As discussed below, avoidance of high-protein meals may help.

### Mechanism of Action

Levodopa reduces symptoms of Parkinson's disease by promoting synthesis of dopamine in the striatum (Fig. 22–2). Once in the bloodstream, levodopa is transported across the blood-brain barrier and taken up by the few dopaminergic nerve terminals that remain in the striatum. Following uptake, levodopa, which has no direct effects of its own, is converted to dopamine (DA), its active form. By promoting synthesis of DA, levodopa helps restore a proper balance between DA and ACh.

The enzymatic conversion of levodopa to dopamine is depicted in Figure 22–3. As indicated, the enzyme that catalyzes this reaction is called a *decarboxylase* (because it removes a carboxyl group from levodopa). The activity of decarboxylases is enhanced by *pyridoxine* (vitamin $B_6$).

Why is Parkinson's disease treated with levodopa and not dopamine itself? Dopamine cannot be employed for two reasons. First, dopamine cannot cross the blood-brain barrier (see Fig. 22–2). As noted, levodopa crosses the barrier by means of an active transport system; this system will not transport dopamine. Second, dopamine has such a short half-life in the blood that it would be impractical to use even if it could cross the blood-brain barrier.

### Pharmacokinetics

Levodopa is administered orally and undergoes rapid absorption from the small intestine. Food delays absorption by slowing gastric emptying. Furthermore, since neutral amino acids compete with levodopa for intestinal absorption (and also transport across the blood-brain barrier), high-protein foods will reduce therapeutic effects.

Only a small fraction of an administered dose of levodopa reaches the brain. The majority of each dose is converted to dopamine in the periphery by decarboxylases present in the liver and intestine; about 2% escapes peripheral decarboxylation and enters the brain. Like the enzymes that decarboxylate levodopa within the brain, peripheral decarboxylases work faster in the presence of pyridoxine.

### Adverse Effects

Most untoward effects of levodopa are dose dependent. The elderly are especially sensitive to adverse effects.

***Nausea and Vomiting.*** Most patients experience nausea and vomiting early in treatment. These effects result from activation of dopamine receptors in the chemoreceptor trigger zone (CTZ) of the medulla. Nausea and vomiting can be reduced by administering levodopa in low initial doses and with meals. (The presence of food retards levodopa absorption, causing a decrease in peak plasma drug levels and a corresponding decrease in stimulation of the CTZ.) However, since administration with food can reduce therapeutic effects (by decreasing levodopa absorption), administration with meals should be avoided if possible.

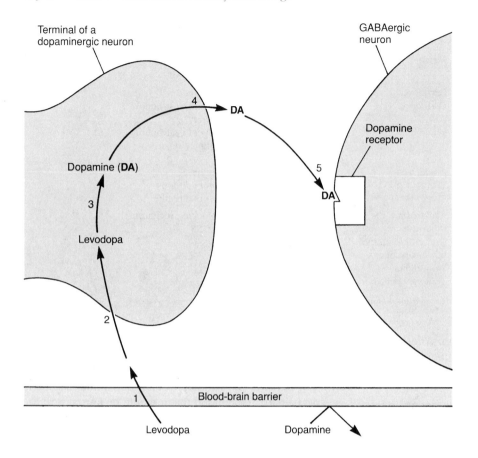

**Figure 22–2. Steps leading to alteration of CNS function by levodopa.** To produce its beneficial effects in parkinsonism, levodopa must be (1) transported across the blood-brain barrier; (2) taken up by a dopaminergic nerve terminal in the striatum; (3) converted into dopamine; (4) released into the synaptic space; and (5) bound to a dopamine receptor on a striatal GABAergic neuron, causing that neuron to decrease its firing rate. Note that dopamine itself is unable to cross the blood-brain barrier, and hence cannot be used to treat parkinsonism.

**Dyskinesias.** Ironically, levodopa, a drug given to *alleviate* movement disorders, causes movement disorders in many patients. About 80% of those treated develop involuntary movements (head bobbing, tics, grimacing) within the first year of therapy. These dyskinesias develop just before or soon after optimal levodopa dosage has been achieved. The only treatment is to reduce levodopa dosage. Unfortunately, dosage reduction may lead to re-emergence of parkinsonian symptoms.

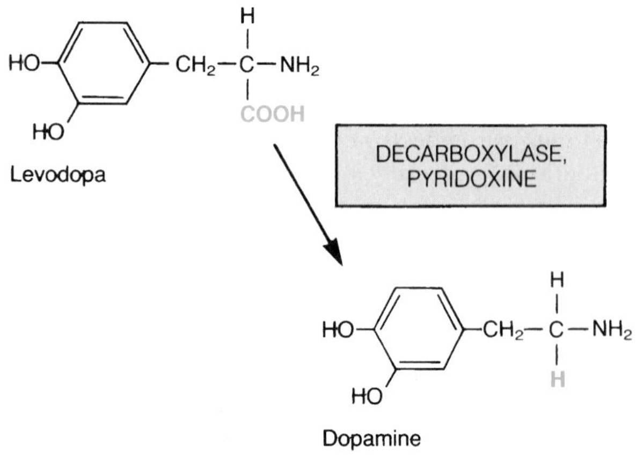

**Figure 22–3. Conversion of levodopa to dopamine.** Decarboxylases present in the brain, liver, and intestine convert levodopa into dopamine. Pyridoxine (vitamin $B_6$) accelerates the reaction.

**Cardiovascular Effects.** *Postural hypotension* is common early in treatment. The mechanism of this paradoxical effect is not known. Hypotension can be reduced by increasing intake of salt and water. An alpha-adrenergic agonist can also help.

Conversion of levodopa to dopamine in the periphery can result in excessive activation of beta$_1$ receptors in the heart. Activation of these receptors can cause *dysrhythmias*, particularly in patients with cardiac disease.

**Psychiatric Effects.** Psychologic disturbances (confusion, paranoia, visual hallucinations, vivid dreams, nightmares) are common. These reactions are seen most frequently in elderly patients who are taking levodopa along with other drugs that have psychologic effects (e.g., anticholinergic drugs, amantadine, dopamine agonists). Adverse psychologic effects may respond to a reduction in levodopa dosage or to a reduction in the dosage of other drugs. As a rule, antipsychotic drugs cannot be used to treat psychotic symptoms; since antipsychotic agents block dopamine receptors, they would nullify the beneficial effects of levodopa.

**Other Adverse Effects.** Levodopa may *darken sweat and urine*; patients should be forewarned of this harmless effect. The drug can *activate malignant melanoma* and consequently should be avoided in patients with undiagnosed skin lesions.

## Drug Holidays

With long-term use of levodopa, adverse effects tend to increase and therapeutic effects tend to diminish. For some patients, the situation may improve following a

## TABLE 22-2. MAJOR DRUG INTERACTIONS OF LEVODOPA

| Drug Category | Drug | Mechanism of Interaction |
|---|---|---|
| Drugs that decrease beneficial effects of levodopa | Pyridoxine (vitamin B$_6$) | Enhanced destruction of levodopa |
| | Antipsychotics | Blockade of dopamine receptors |
| Drugs that increase beneficial effects of levodopa | Carbidopa | Inhibition of the peripheral decarboxylation of levodopa |
| | Anticholinergics | Blockade of cholinergic receptors in the CNS |
| | Amantadine | Promotion of dopamine release |
| | Bromocriptine | Stimulation of dopamine receptors |
| | Pergolide | Stimulation of dopamine receptors |
| | Selegiline | Inhibition of dopamine breakdown |
| Drugs that increase levodopa toxicity | MAO inhibitors | Inhibition of MAO increases the risk of severe levodopa-induced hypertension |

"drug holiday," defined as a brief (e.g., 10-day) interruption of treatment. When the holiday is successful, beneficial effects are achieved with lower doses. Because doses are lower, the incidence of dyskinesias and adverse psychologic effects is lowered as well. Unfortunately, drug holidays do not correct the "on-off" phenomenon.

Drug holidays are not without risk. Since drug withdrawal will immobilize the patient, the holiday must take place in a hospital. In addition to severe psychologic distress, immobilization presents a risk of deep vein thrombosis, aspiration pneumonitis, and decubitus ulcers.

### Drug Interactions

Interactions between levodopa and other drugs can (1) decrease beneficial effects of levodopa, (2) increase beneficial effects of levodopa, and (3) increase toxicity from levodopa. Major interactions are summarized in Table 22-2. Several interactions are discussed immediately below; others are discussed later in the chapter.

***Antipsychotic Drugs.*** All of the antipsychotic drugs in current use (e.g., chlorpromazine, haloperidol) block receptors for dopamine. By blocking dopamine receptors in the striatum, antipsychotic agents will decrease therapeutic effects of levodopa. Accordingly, concurrent use of antipsychotic agents with levodopa should be avoided.*

***Monoamine Oxidase Inhibitors.*** Levodopa can cause a hypertensive crisis if administered to an individual taking a nonselective inhibitor of monoamine oxidase (MAO). The mechanism of this interaction is as follows: (1) Levodopa elevates neuronal stores of DA and norepinephrine (NE) by promoting synthesis of both compounds. (2) Since intraneuronal MAO serves to inactivate DA and NE, inhibition of MAO allows elevated neuronal stores of these transmitters to grow even larger. (3) Since both DA and NE promote vasoconstriction, release of these agents in supranormal amounts can lead to massive vasoconstriction, thereby causing blood pressure to rise

dangerously high. To avoid hypertensive crisis, MAO inhibitors should be withdrawn at least 2 weeks prior to initiating levodopa.

***Anticholinergic Drugs.*** Since excessive stimulation of cholinergic receptors contributes to the dyskinesias of Parkinson's disease, drugs that block cholinergic receptors can help reduce symptoms. Hence, anticholinergic agents may enhance the therapeutic effects of levodopa.

***Pyridoxine.*** Pyridoxine (vitamin B$_6$) stimulates decarboxylase activity. By accelerating decarboxylation of levodopa in the periphery, pyridoxine can decrease the amount of levodopa that reaches the central nervous system (CNS). As a result, therapeutic effects of levodopa are reduced. Patients should be informed about this interaction and instructed to avoid multivitamin preparations that contain pyridoxine.

### Food Interactions

Meals with a high protein content can reduce therapeutic responses to levodopa. Why? Because neutral amino acids compete with levodopa for absorption from the intestine and for transport across the blood-brain barrier. Hence, a high-protein meal can significantly reduce both the amount of levodopa that gets absorbed and the amount that gets transported into the brain. It has been suggested that a high-protein meal could trigger an abrupt loss of effect (i.e., an "off" episode). Accordingly, patients should be advised to spread their protein consumption evenly throughout the day's meals.

### Preparations, Dosage, and Administration

Levodopa [Dopar, Larodopa] is dispensed in tablets and capsules (100, 250, and 500 mg) for oral administration. To minimize adverse effects, especially drug-induced movement disorders, dosage must be individualized. The usual initial dosage is 0.5 to 1.0 gm/day administered in two or more divided doses. The total daily dosage can be increased gradually to a maximum of 8 gm. Full therapeutic responses may take 6 months to develop.

## Carbidopa Plus Levodopa

The combination of carbidopa plus levodopa, marketed as Sinemet, is our most effective therapy for Parkinson's disease. The combination is much more effective than levodopa alone.

---

*A new antipsychotic, olanzepine [Zyprexa], does not reverse beneficial effects of levodopa, and hence may be used to treat psychosis in patients with Parkinson's disease.

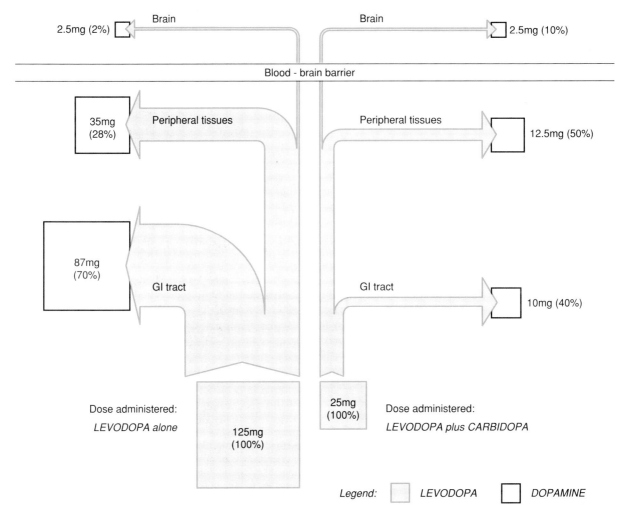

**Figure 22–4. Fate of levodopa in the presence and absence of carbidopa.** In the absence of carbidopa, 98% of an administered dose of levodopa is converted to dopamine by decarboxylases in the intestine and peripheral tissues, leaving only 2% for actions in the brain. Hence, in order to deliver 2.5 mg of levodopa to the brain, the dose of levodopa must be large (125 mg). By inhibiting intestinal and peripheral decarboxylases, carbidopa increases the percentage of levodopa available to the brain. Hence, the dose needed to deliver 2.5 mg is greatly reduced (to 25 mg in this example). Since carbidopa cannot cross the blood-brain barrier, it does not interfere with conversion of levodopa to dopamine by decarboxylases in the brain. Furthermore, since carbidopa reduces peripheral production of dopamine (from 35 mg to 12.5 mg in this example), peripheral toxicity (nausea, cardiovascular effects) is much less. (Data in the figure are extrapolated from data of Nutt, J.G., and Fellman, J.H. Pharmacokinetics of levodopa. Clin. Neuropharmacol. 7:35, 1984.)

## Mechanism of Action

Carbidopa is used to enhance the effects of levodopa. Carbidopa has no therapeutic effects of its own, and is always used in conjunction with levodopa. Carbidopa enhances the actions of levodopa by inhibiting decarboxylases in the *periphery*, and thereby makes more levodopa available to the CNS. Carbidopa does not prevent the conversion of levodopa to dopamine by decarboxylases within the brain because carbidopa is unable to cross the blood-brain barrier.

The impact of carbidopa is shown schematically in Figure 22-4, which compares the fate of levodopa in the presence and absence of carbidopa. In the absence of carbidopa, about 98% of levodopa is converted to dopamine by decarboxylases in the GI tract and peripheral tissues, leaving only 2% for entry into the brain. In contrast, when decarboxylases are inhibited by carbidopa, only 90% of levodopa is decarboxylated in the GI tract and periphery, leaving 10% for actions in the brain.

## Advantages of Carbidopa

The combination of carbidopa plus levodopa is superior to levodopa alone in three ways:

- By increasing the fraction of levodopa available for actions within the CNS, carbidopa allows the dosage of levodopa to be reduced by about 75%. (In the example in Figure 22–4, in order to provide 2.5 mg of dopamine to the brain, we must administer 125 mg of levodopa if carbidopa is absent, but only 25 mg if carbidopa is present.)

- By reducing production of dopamine in the periphery, carbidopa reduces cardiovascular responses to levodopa and also reduces nausea and vomiting.
- By causing direct inhibition of decarboxylase, carbidopa obviates stimulation of decarboxylase by pyridoxine. As a result, carbidopa eliminates concern about decreasing the effects of levodopa through inadvertent use of vitamin preparations that contain pyridoxine.

### Disadvantages of Carbidopa

Carbidopa has no adverse effects of its own; any adverse responses associated with the drug are due to potentiation of levodopa's effects. When levodopa is combined with carbidopa, abnormal movements and psychiatric disturbances may occur sooner and may be more intense than when levodopa is employed alone.

### Preparations, Dosage, and Administration

Carbidopa is almost always administered with levodopa in a formulation that contains both drugs. These combination products (tablets and sustained-release capsules) are marketed under the trade name Sinemet. Sinemet tablets are available in three strengths: (1) 10 mg carbidopa/100 mg levodopa, (2) 25 mg carbidopa/100 mg levodopa, and (3) 25 mg carbidopa/250 mg levodopa. The sustained-release capsules [Sinemet CR] contain 50 mg carbidopa and 200 mg levodopa.

Carbidopa without levodopa, dispensed under the trade name Lodosyn, is available by special request for investigational use. This preparation is employed when dosages of levodopa and carbidopa must be titrated separately.

When patients who have been taking levodopa alone are switched over to the combination of carbidopa plus levodopa, at least 8 hours should elapse between the last dose of levodopa and the first dose of the combination. The delay is needed to prevent excessive potentiation of residual levodopa by carbidopa. Also, when switching from therapy with levodopa alone to the combination, the total daily dose of levodopa must be reduced substantially: the dose of levodopa within the combination regimen should be only 25% of the dose employed when levodopa was being administered alone. For patients who are not currently receiving levodopa, therapy can be initiated with either 10 mg carbidopa/100 mg levodopa or 25 mg carbidopa/100 mg levodopa, each taken 3 times a day.

## Amantadine

***Actions and Uses.*** Originally developed as an antiviral agent (see Chapter 87), amantadine [Symmetrel, Symadine] is also effective in Parkinson's disease. The drug relieves symptoms by promoting release of dopamine from remaining dopaminergic terminals in the striatum. Responses develop rapidly (often within 2 to 3 days) but are less profound than those seen with levodopa. Furthermore, responses may begin to diminish within 3 to 6 months. Amantadine may be employed alone in the early stages of Parkinson's disease and in combination with other drugs (levodopa/carbidopa, anticholinergic agents) later on.

***Adverse Effects.*** Amantadine can cause adverse *CNS effects* (confusion, lightheadedness, anxiety) and effects that resemble those caused by *muscarinic blockade* (blurred vision, urinary retention, dry mouth, constipation). These responses are generally mild when amantadine is used alone. However, if amantadine is combined with an anticholinergic agent, both the CNS and peripheral responses will be intensified.

Patients taking amantadine for 1 month or longer often develop *livedo reticularis*, a condition characterized by mottled discoloration of the skin. Livedo reticularis is a benign condition that gradually subsides following amantadine withdrawal.

***Preparations, Dosage, and Administration.*** Amantadine [Symmetrel, Symadine] is dispensed in 100-mg capsules and in a syrup (10 mg/ml) for oral use. The usual dosage is 100 mg twice daily. Since amantadine is eliminated primarily by the kidneys, dosage must be reduced in patients with renal impairment.

Amantadine often loses effectiveness after several months. If effects diminish, they can be restored by increasing the dosage or by interrupting treatment for several weeks.

Amantadine can enhance responses to levodopa and anticholinergic agents. When combined with these drugs, amantadine is administered in the same doses employed when taken alone.

## Dopamine Receptor Agonists: Bromocriptine and Pergolide

### Bromocriptine

***Actions and Uses.*** Bromocriptine [Parlodel] is a direct-acting dopamine agonist. Beneficial effects result from *activation of dopamine receptors in the striatum*. Responses are superior to those of amantadine and the centrally acting anticholinergic drugs, but are inferior to those of levodopa. Although bromocriptine can be used as monotherapy, the drug is usually employed as an adjunct to levodopa. When combined with levodopa, bromocriptine can prolong therapeutic responses and reduce motor fluctuations. In addition, since bromocriptine allows the dosage of levodopa to be reduced, the incidence of levodopa-induced dyskinesias may be reduced.

***Adverse Effects.*** Adverse effects are dose dependent and occur in 30% to 50% of patients. *Nausea* is most common, occurring in over 50% of those treated. The most common dose-limiting effects are *psychologic reactions* (confusion, nightmares, agitation, hallucinations, paranoid delusions). These reactions occur in about 30% of patients and are most likely when the dosage is high. Like levodopa, bromocriptine can cause *dyskinesias* and *postural hypotension*.

***Preparations, Dosage, and Administration.*** Bromocriptine mesylate is available in 5-mg capsules [Parlodel] and 2.5-mg tablets [Parlodel Snap Tabs] for oral use. The initial dosage is 1.25 mg twice daily, administered with meals. Dosage is gradually increased until the desired response has been achieved. Maintenance dosages range from 30 to 100 mg/day.

### Pergolide

***Actions, Uses, and Adverse Effects.*** Pergolide [Permax] is similar to bromocriptine with respect to actions, uses, and adverse effects. Like bromocriptine, pergolide reduces symptoms of Parkinson's disease by causing direct activation of dopamine receptors in the striatum. When used as an adjunct to levodopa, pergolide can prolong symptomatic control, reduce fluctuations in motor responses, and reduce the incidence of levodopa-induced dyskinesias. Like bromocriptine, pergolide can cause nausea, postural hypotension, and adverse psychologic reactions (hallucinations, confusion, sedation, paranoid delusions).

**Preparations, Dosage, and Administration.** Pergolide mesylate [Permax] is dispensed in tablets (0.05, 0.25, and 1 mg) for oral administration. The recommended initial dosage is 0.05 mg once daily. Dosage is gradually increased to a maximum of 5 mg/day (in three divided doses).

## Selegiline

### Actions and Uses

Selegiline [Eldepryl, Carbex] is a *selective inhibitor of type B monoamine oxidase* (MAO-B), the enzyme that inactivates dopamine in the striatum. Another form of MAO, known as MAO-A, inactivates norepinephrine and serotonin. As discussed in Chapter 30, nonselective inhibitors of MAO (i.e., drugs that inhibit MAO-A *and* MAO-B) are used to treat depression—and pose a risk of hypertensive crisis as a side effect. Since selegiline is a selective inhibitor of MAO-B, the drug is not an antidepressant and, at recommended doses, does not present a risk of hypertensive crisis.

Selegiline appears to benefit patients with Parkinson's disease in two ways. First, when used as an adjunct to levodopa, *selegiline can suppress destruction of dopamine derived from levodopa.* The mechanism is inhibition of MAO-B. By helping preserve dopamine, selegiline can prolong the effects of levodopa, and can thereby decrease fluctuations in motor control. Unfortunately, these benefits decline dramatically within 12 to 24 months.

In addition to preserving dopamine, selegiline may delay the progression of Parkinson's disease. When used early in the disease, selegiline can delay the need for levodopa. This may reflect a delay in the progression of the disease, or it may simply reflect direct symptomatic relief from selegiline itself.

If selegiline does slow the progression of Parkinson's disease, what might be the mechanism? In experimental animals, selegiline can prevent development of parkinsonism following exposure to MPTP, a neurotoxin that causes selective degeneration of dopaminergic neurons. (Humans accidentally exposed to MPTP develop severe parkinsonism.) Neuronal degeneration is caused not by MPTP itself but rather by a *toxic metabolite* of MPTP. Formation of this metabolite is catalyzed by MAO-B. By inhibiting MAO-B, selegiline prevents formation of the toxic metabolite, and thereby protects against neuronal injury. If selegiline does retard progression of Parkinson's disease, this mechanism could explain the effect. That is, just as selegiline protects animals by suppressing formation of a neurotoxic metabolite of MPTP, the drug may retard progression of Parkinson's disease by suppressing formation of a neurotoxic metabolite of an as-yet unidentified compound.

A recent study raises serious doubts about the benefits of selegiline—and indicates the drug may actually be harmful. In the study, patients were treated either with levodopa alone or with levodopa plus selegiline. After 5 years, the degree of disability in both groups was the same, indicating that selegiline had no long-term effect on the progression of the disease. Even more striking, however, were the data on mortality: the death rate for the group receiving dopamine plus selegiline was nearly double the death rate for the group receiving levodopa alone. Most of the difference could be accounted for by deaths directly due to Parkinson's disease.

### Pharmacokinetics

Selegiline is rapidly absorbed following oral administration and readily penetrates the blood-brain barrier. Irreversible inhibition of MAO-B follows. Selegiline undergoes hepatic metabolism followed by renal excretion. Two metabolites—*L-amphetamine* and *L-methamphetamine*—are *CNS stimulants*. These metabolites do not appear to contribute to the drug's therapeutic effects but *can* contribute to toxicity.

### Adverse Effects

When selegiline is used alone, the principal adverse effect is *insomnia*, presumably because of CNS excitation by amphetamine and methamphetamine. Insomnia can be minimized by administering the last daily dose at noon.

#### Drug Interactions

**Levodopa.** When used with *levodopa*, selegiline can intensify adverse responses to levodopa-derived dopamine. These reactions—orthostatic hypotension, dyskinesias, and psychologic disturbances (hallucinations, confusion)—can be reduced by decreasing the dosage of levodopa.

**Meperidine.** Like the nonselective MAO inhibitors, selegiline can cause a dangerous interaction with *meperidine* [Demerol]. Symptoms include stupor, rigidity, agitation, and hyperthermia. The combination should be avoided.

**Fluoxetine.** Selegiline should not be combined with *fluoxetine* [Prozac]. The combination of a nonselective MAO inhibitor plus fluoxetine has been fatal. Although this interaction has not been reported with selegiline, prudence dictates caution. Accordingly, fluoxetine should be withdrawn at least 14 days before giving selegiline.

#### Preparations, Dosage, and Administration

Selegiline [Eldepryl, Carbex] is available in 5-mg tablets and capsules for oral administration. The usual dosage is 5 mg taken with breakfast and lunch. Since a total daily dose of 10 mg is sufficient to produce complete inhibition of MAO-B, larger doses are unnecessary.

## Centrally Acting Anticholinergic Drugs

The classic anticholinergic agents (e.g., atropine) were the first anticholinergic drugs employed to treat Parkinson's disease. Although these drugs were effective, they also caused intense anticholinergic effects in the periphery (dry mouth, blurred vision, photophobia, constipation, urinary retention, tachycardia). With the advent of newer cholinergic blockers, referred to as *centrally act-*

*ing anticholinergic agents*, use of the classic cholinergic blockers for parkinsonism has become obsolete. The centrally acting agents are just as effective as the older agents and have the advantage of producing fewer anticholinergic effects in the periphery.

## Mechanism of Action

As discussed earlier, excessive stimulation of striatal cholinergic receptors contributes to the symptoms of Parkinson's disease. The centrally acting anticholinergic drugs help control symptoms by blocking access of acetylcholine to these receptors.

## Therapeutic Use

When used to treat Parkinson's disease, the centrally acting anticholinergics are less effective than levodopa but also produce fewer serious adverse effects. These drugs may be employed alone or in combination with levodopa.

The anticholinergic drugs are often preferred agents for treating mild parkinsonism in *younger* patients. These drugs are effective enough to control mild symptoms, and their use avoids exposing the patient to the more serious adverse effects of levodopa. Anticholinergic drugs are generally avoided in the *elderly* because of the risk of severe CNS effects.

## Adverse Effects

*Peripheral Effects.* Like the classic anticholinergic drugs, the centrally acting agents are able to block cholinergic receptors in the periphery. As a result, these drugs can cause *dry mouth, blurred vision, photophobia, urinary retention, constipation,* and *tachycardia.* These effects are usually dose limiting. Blockade of cholinergic receptors in the eye may precipitate or aggravate *glaucoma.* Accordingly, intraocular pressure should be determined periodically. For a more complete discussion of peripheral anticholinergic responses, refer to Chapter 15 (Muscarinic Agonists and Antagonists).

*CNS Effects.* Anticholinergic agents may cause confusion, delusions, depression, and hallucinations. These responses are most likely in the elderly.

*Withdrawal.* If anticholinergic agents are discontinued abruptly, symptoms of parkinsonism may be intensified. Accordingly, these drugs should be withdrawn gradually.

### TABLE 22-3. DOSAGES OF CENTRALLY ACTING ANTICHOLINERGIC DRUGS

| Generic Name | Trade Name | Dosage Range (mg/day) |
|---|---|---|
| Benztropine | Cogentin | 0.5-6 |
| Biperidin | Akineton | 2-16 |
| Diphenhydramine | Benadryl, others | 25-100 |
| Ethopropazine | Parsidol | 50-600 |
| Procyclidine | Kemadrin | 2.5-20 |
| Trihexyphenidyl | Artane, others | 1-15 |

### Preparations, Dosage, and Administration

The anticholinergic drugs used in parkinsonism are listed in Table 22-3. Trade names and dosage ranges are given. Dosing is initiated with the lower value in the table and then gradually increased until the desired therapeutic response has been achieved or until side effects have become intolerable. These drugs are administered in two or three divided daily doses.

# Drug Selection

Drug selection is based on the severity of symptoms and the patient's ability to tolerate the side effects of specific drugs.

For patients with *mild* symptoms, an *anticholinergic* agent or *amantadine* is indicated. (Anticholinergic drugs should be used only in younger patients because CNS effects can be severe in the elderly.) *Selegiline* is an option—although recent findings question the benefits of the drug, and suggest it may be dangerous.

For patients with advanced disease, *levodopa/carbidopa* is the treatment of choice. If levodopa/carbidopa is inadequate, selegiline, amantadine, or a dopamine agonist (bromocriptine, pergolide) may be added to the regimen. In addition, levodopa/carbidopa may be combined with an anticholinergic agent (except in elderly patients and those with a history of psychosis, since the risk of adverse psychologic reactions is high).

# Surgical Treatments for Parkinson's Disease

## Pallidotomy

Pallidotomy is a neurosurgical procedure directed at destroying the globus pallidus. As indicated in Figure 22-1, the globus pallidus, which helps regulate movement, receives its input from the striatum. In Parkinson's disease, striatal input to the globus pallidus is disrupted, causing the globus pallidus itself to malfunction. It has been argued that altered output from the globus pallidus underlies most of the symptoms of Parkinson's disease, including tremor, rigidity, and bradykinesia. The results of pallidotomy offer great support to this argument: for many patients, the procedure yields a substantial—sometimes miraculous—reduction of symptoms.

## Fetal Tissue Transplants

In 1995, researchers finally obtained definitive proof that transplanting fetal dopaminergic neurons into the brain can benefit a patient with Parkinson's disease. In this case study, the patient had severe parkinsonism that would no longer respond to drug therapy. Following the transplant, symptoms steadily improved over 3 months, eventually allowing the patient to perform all activities of daily living without assistance. The improvements were sustained for 15 months, at which time the patient died of a massive pulmonary embolism unrelated to the procedure. Autopsy revealed that the grafts not only took but had become seamlessly integrated into the surrounding tissue. This was the first clear demonstration of a correlation between graft survival and improvement of symptoms.

In prior studies, some patients improved and some didn't. However, since direct observation of the grafts was not possible, there was no definitive way to tell if the clinical successes were due to successful implants, or if the clinical failures were due to failed implants. In this new study, all doubt was removed.

## KEY POINTS

- Parkinson's disease is a neurologic disorder characterized by tremor at rest, rigidity, postural instability, and bradykinesia.
- The primary pathology of Parkinson's disease is degeneration of neurons that supply dopamine to the striatum, thereby causing an imbalance between dopamine and acetylcholine.
- Parkinson's disease is treated with two kinds of drugs: agents that directly or indirectly activate dopamine receptors and agents that block cholinergic receptors.
- Levodopa (combined with carbidopa) is the most effective treatment for Parkinson's disease.
- Levodopa relieves symptoms by promoting the synthesis of dopamine in the striatum.
- The enzyme that converts levodopa to dopamine is called a decarboxylase.

- Acute loss of response to levodopa occurs in two patterns: gradual "wearing off," which develops at the end of the dosing interval, and abrupt loss of effect ("on-off" phenomenon), which can occur at any time during the dosing interval.
- The principal adverse effects of levodopa are nausea, dyskinesias, hypotension, and psychiatric disturbances.
- Antipsychotic drugs block dopamine receptors, and can thereby negate the effects of levodopa.
- Combining levodopa with a nonselective monoamine oxidase inhibitor can result in hypertensive crisis.
- Because amino acids compete with levodopa for absorption from the intestine and transport across the blood-brain barrier, high-protein meals can reduce the effects of levodopa.
- Carbidopa enhances the effects of levodopa by preventing decarboxylation of levodopa in the periphery. Since carbidopa cannot cross the blood-brain barrier, it does not prevent conversion of levodopa to dopamine in the brain.
- Amantadine relieves symptoms of early Parkinson's disease by promoting release of dopamine from remaining dopaminergic neurons in the striatum.
- Bromocriptine relieves symptoms of Parkinson's disease by causing direct stimulation of dopamine receptors in the striatum.
- Selegiline relieves symptoms of Parkinson's disease by inhibiting MAO-B, the brain enzyme that inactivates dopamine.
- Centrally acting anticholinergic drugs relieve symptoms of Parkinson's disease by blocking cholinergic receptors in the striatum.

## Summary of Major Nursing Implications*

### Levodopa/Carbidopa [Sinemet]

## Preadministration Assessment

### Therapeutic Goal
Treatment is directed at improving the patient's ability to carry out activities of daily living. Levodopa does not cure Parkinson's disease.

### Baseline Data
Assess overt manifestations of Parkinson's disease (bradykinesia, akinesia, postural instability, tremor, rigidity) and the extent to which these manifestations interfere with activities of daily living (ability to work, dress, bathe, walk, etc.).

### Identifying High-Risk Patients
Levodopa is *contraindicated* for patients with *malignant melanoma* (the drug can activate this neoplasm)

and for patients taking *MAO inhibitors*. Exercise *caution* in patients with *cardiac disease* and *psychiatric disorders*.

## Implementation: Administration

### Route
Oral.

### Administration
Inform the patient that levodopa may be taken with food to reduce nausea and vomiting. However, high-protein meals should be avoided.

Parkinsonism may render self-medication impossible. Assist the patient with dosing when needed. If appropriate, involve family members in medicating the outpatient.

If the patient has been taking levodopa alone, allow at least 8 hours to elapse between the last dose of levodopa and the first dose of levodopa/carbidopa. The dosage of levodopa in the combination should be reduced to no more than 25% of the dosage employed when levodopa was being taken alone.

*Patient education information is highlighted in color.

So that expectations may be realistic, inform the patient that effects of levodopa may be delayed for weeks to months. This knowledge will facilitate compliance.

## Ongoing Evaluation and Interventions

### Evaluating Therapeutic Effects

Evaluate for improvements in activities of daily living and for reductions in bradykinesia, postural instability, tremor, and rigidity.

### Managing Acute Loss of Effect

Gradual "wearing off" at the end of the dosing interval can be reduced by using a controlled-release formulation of levodopa/carbidopa or by adjunctive therapy with a direct-acting dopamine agonist.

Forewarn patients about possible abrupt loss of therapeutic effects ("on-off" phenomenon) and instruct them to notify the physician if this occurs. Avoiding high-protein meals may help.

### Minimizing Adverse Effects

*Nausea and Vomiting.* Inform the patient that nausea and vomiting can be reduced by taking levodopa with food. Instruct the patient to notify the physician if nausea and vomiting persist or become severe.

*Dyskinesias.* Inform patients about possible levodopa-induced movement disorders (tremor, dystonic movements, twitching) and instruct them to notify the physician if these develop.

If the hospitalized patient develops dyskinesias, withhold levodopa and consult with the physician about a possible reduction in dosage.

*Dysrhythmias.* Inform patients about signs of excessive cardiac stimulation (palpitations, tachycardia, irregular heartbeat) and instruct them to notify the physician if these occur.

*Orthostatic Hypotension.* Inform patients about symptoms of hypotension (dizziness, lightheadedness) and advise them to sit or lie down if these occur. Advise patients to move slowly when assuming an erect posture.

*Psychiatric Disturbances.* Inform patients about possible adverse psychiatric effects (confusion, paranoia, visual hallucinations, vivid dreams, nightmares) and instruct them to notify the physician if these develop.

### Minimizing Adverse Interactions

*Antipsychotic Drugs.* These drugs can block responses to levodopa and should be avoided.

*MAO Inhibitors.* Concurrent use of levodopa and an MAO inhibitor can produce severe hypertension. Withdraw MAO inhibitors at least 2 weeks before initiating levodopa.

*Anticholinergic Drugs.* These agents can enhance therapeutic responses to levodopa, but they also increase the risk of adverse psychiatric effects.

*High-Protein Meals.* Amino acids compete with levodopa for absorption from the intestine and for transport across the blood-brain barrier. Instruct the patient to avoid high-protein meals.

## Centrally Acting Anticholinergic Drugs

### General Implications

Centrally acting anticholinergic drugs have the same pharmacologic properties as the "classic" anticholinergic agents. Relevant nursing implications are summarized in Chapter 15.

### Implications Specific to Parkinson's Disease

#### Therapeutic Goal

Treatment is directed at improving the patient's ability to carry out activities of daily life. Anticholinergic drugs do not cure Parkinson's disease.

#### Baseline Data

Assess overt manifestations of Parkinson's disease (bradykinesia, akinesia, postural instability, tremor, rigidity) and the extent to which these manifestations interfere with activities of daily living.

#### Minimizing Adverse Effects

Many patients with Parkinson's disease are elderly, and therefore highly susceptible to the ability of anticholinergic drugs to induce *glaucoma* and *psychologic disturbances*. Intraocular pressure should be monitored periodically. Observe the patient for altered intellectual or emotional status.

#### Discontinuation of Treatment

Abrupt withdrawal of anticholinergics can intensify symptoms of parkinsonism. Warn the patient against abrupt discontinuation of treatment.

# CHAPTER 23

# Drugs for Epilepsy

The term *epilepsy* refers to a group of disorders characterized by excessive excitability of neurons within the central nervous system (CNS). This abnormal neuronal activity can produce a variety of symptoms, ranging from brief periods of unconsciousness to violent convulsions. In the United States, about 2.5 million people have epilepsy. Approximately 50% of them can be rendered seizure free with drugs; another 25% can expect significant improvement.

The terms *seizure* and *convulsion* are not synonymous. *Seizure* is a general term that applies to all types of epileptic events. In contrast, the term *convulsion* has a more limited meaning, applying only to abnormal motor phenomena, for example, the jerking muscle movements that occur during a grand mal attack. Accordingly, although all convulsions may be called seizures, it is not correct to call all seizures convulsions. Absence seizures, for example, manifest as brief periods of unconsciousness, which may or may not be accompanied by involuntary movements. Since not all epileptic seizures involve convulsions, we will refer to the agents used to treat epilepsy as *antiseizure drugs*, rather than anticonvulsants. An alternative name is *antiepileptic drug*.

## Seizure Generation

Seizures are initiated by synchronous, high-frequency discharge from a group of hyperexcitable neurons, called a *focus*. A focus may result from several causes, including congenital defects, hypoxia at birth, head trauma, and cancer. Seizures result when discharge from a focus spreads to other brain areas, thereby recruiting normal neurons to discharge abnormally along with the focus.

The overt manifestations of a particular seizure disorder depend upon the location of the seizure focus and the neuronal connections to that focus. (The connections to the focus determine the brain areas to which seizure activity can spread.) If seizure activity invades a very limited part of the brain, a partial or local seizure occurs. In contrast, if seizure activity spreads to a large portion of the brain, a generalized seizure develops.

An experimental procedure referred to as *kindling* may explain how a focal discharge is eventually able to generate a seizure. Experimental kindling is performed by implanting a small electrode into the brain of an experimental animal. The electrode is used to deliver localized stimuli for a brief interval once each day. When stimuli are first administered, no seizures result. However, after repeated once-a-day delivery, these stimuli eventually elicit a seizure. If the procedure of brief, daily stimulation is continued for long enough, spontaneous seizures will begin to occur.

The process of kindling may be telling us something about seizure development in humans. For example, kindling may account for the delay that can take place between injury to the head and eventual development of seizures. Furthermore, kindling may explain why the seizures associated with some forms of epilepsy become more frequent as time passes. Also, the progressive nature of kindling suggests that early treatment might prevent seizure disorders from becoming more severe over time.

# Types of Seizures

Seizure can be divided into two broad categories: (1) *partial (focal) seizures* and (2) *generalized seizures*. In partial seizures, seizure activity begins focally in the cerebral cortex and undergoes limited spread to adjacent cortical areas. In generalized seizures, focal seizure activity is conducted widely throughout both hemispheres of the brain. Drugs used to treat partial and generalized seizures are summarized in Table 23-1.

## Partial Seizures

Partial seizures fall into two major groups: (1) *simple partial seizures* and (2) *complex partial seizures*. Complex partial seizures involve *impairment of consciousness*, whereas simple partial seizures do not. Simple partial seizures may appear as convulsions in a single limb or muscle group, but with no effect on consciousness. Complex partial seizures may manifest as an attack of confused or bizarre behavior during which consciousness is impaired. In some patients, partial seizures may evolve secondarily into generalized seizures.

## Generalized Seizures

Generalized seizures may be convulsive or nonconvulsive. As a rule, generalized seizures produce immediate loss of consciousness. Characteristics of specific generalized seizures are discussed briefly below.

***Tonic-Clonic Seizures (Grand Mal).*** In tonic-clonic seizures, neuronal discharge spreads throughout the entire cerebral cortex. These seizures manifest as major convulsions, characterized by a period of muscle rigidity (tonic phase) followed by synchronous muscle jerks (clonic phase). Tonic-clonic seizures are accompanied by marked impairment of consciousness and are followed by a period of CNS depression, referred to as the postictal state.

***Absence Seizures (Petit Mal).*** Absence seizures are characterized by loss of consciousness for a brief time (10 to 30 seconds). Seizures usually involve mild, symmetric motor activity (e.g., eye blinking) but may occur with no motor activity at all. The patient may experience hundreds of absence attacks per day. Absence seizures occur primarily in children and usually cease during the early teens.

***Atonic Seizures.*** These seizures are characterized by sudden loss of muscle tone. If seizure activity is limited to the muscles of the neck, "head drop" occurs. However, if the muscles of the limbs and trunk are involved, a "drop attack" can occur, causing the patient to suddenly collapse.

***Myoclonic Seizures.*** These seizures consist of sudden rapid muscle contractions. Seizure activity may be limited to just one limb (focal myoclonus) or it may involve the entire body (massive myoclonus).

***Status Epilepticus.*** Status epilepticus (SE) is defined as a seizure that persists for 30 minutes or more. There are several types of SE, including generalized convulsive SE, absence SE, and myoclonic SE. Generalized convulsive SE, which can be life threatening, is discussed further later in the chapter.

***Febrile Seizures.*** Fever-associated seizures are common among children ages 6 months to 5 years. Febrile seizures typically manifest as generalized tonic-clonic convulsions of short duration. Children who experience these seizures are not at high risk of developing epilepsy later in life.

# How Antiseizure Drugs Work

We have long known that antiseizure drugs can (1) suppress discharge of neurons within a seizure focus and (2) suppress propagation of seizure activity from the focus to other areas of the brain. However, until recently we did not know how these effects were achieved. It now appears that antiseizure drugs act through three basic mechanisms: suppression of sodium influx, suppression of calcium influx, and potentiation of gamma-aminobutyric acid (GABA).

***Suppression of Sodium Influx.*** Before discussing drug actions, we need to review sodium channel physiology. Neuronal action potentials are propagated by influx of sodium through sodium channels, which are gated pores in the cell membrane that control sodium entry. For sodium influx to occur, the channel must be in an *activated state*. Immediately following sodium entry, the channel goes into an *inactivated state*, during which further sodium entry is prevented. Under normal circumstances, the inactive channel very quickly returns to the activated state, thereby permitting more sodium entry and propagation of another action potential.

**TABLE 23-1. SEIZURE TYPES AND THEIR TREATMENT**

| Seizure Type | Drugs of Choice | Alternatives |
| --- | --- | --- |
| *Partial Seizures* | | |
| Simple partial, complex, partial, and secondarily generalized | Valproate Carbamazepine Phenytoin | Phenobarbital Primidone Lamotrigine Gabapentin |
| *Generalized Seizures* | | |
| Tonic-clonic (grand mal) | Valproate Carbamazepine Phenytoin | Phenobarbital Primidone Lamotrigine |
| Absence (petit mal) | Valproate Ethosuximide | Clonazepam Lamotrigine |
| Atonic, myoclonic | Valproate | Clonazepam |
| Status epilepticus | Lorazepam Diazepam Phenytoin | Phenobarbital Pentobarbital Lidocaine |

At least four antiseizure drugs—phenytoin, carbamazepine, valproic acid, and lamotrigine—reversibly bind to sodium channels while they are in the inactivated state, and thereby prolong channel inactivation. By delaying return to the active state, these drugs decrease the ability of neurons to fire at high frequency. As a result, seizures that depend on high-frequency discharge are suppressed.

***Suppression of Calcium Influx.*** Valproic acid and ethosuximide, which are used to treat absence seizures, act by inhibiting influx of calcium ions through a special class of calcium channels, known as *T-type calcium channels*. In most neurons, T currents (the electric currents generated by influx of calcium ions through T-type channels) play a minimal role in action potential generation. However, in certain neurons of the hypothalamus, T currents are large enough to cause an action potential to fire. This is significant because these same hypothalamic neurons are responsible for generating absence seizures. Hence, by blocking calcium inflow through T-type channels, valproate and ethosuximide are able to suppress generation of absence seizures.

***Potentiation of GABA.*** Several antiseizure medications potentiate the actions of GABA, an inhibitory neurotransmitter that is widely distributed throughout the brain. By augmenting the inhibitory influence of GABA, these drugs decrease neuronal excitability and thereby suppress seizure activity. Drugs increase the influence of GABA by several mechanisms. Benzodiazepines and barbiturates enhance the effects of GABA by mechanisms that involve direct binding to GABA receptors. Gabapentin, a new drug, acts by promoting GABA release. Vigabatrin, another new drug, inhibits the enzyme that degrades GABA, and thereby increases GABA availability.

# General Therapeutic Considerations

## Therapeutic Goal

The goal in treating epilepsy is to reduce seizures to an extent that enables the patient to live a normal or near-normal life. Ideally, treatment should eliminate seizures entirely. However, this may not be possible without causing intolerable side effects. Hence, we must balance the desire for complete seizure control against the acceptability of undesired drug effects.

## Diagnosis and Drug Selection

Control of seizures requires proper drug selection. As indicated in Table 23–1, most antiseizure medications are selective for specific seizure disorders. Phenytoin, for example, is useful for treating tonic-clonic and partial seizures but not absence seizures. Conversely, ethosuximide is active against absence seizures but does not work against tonic-clonic or partial seizures. The only drug that appears effective against practically all forms of epilepsy is

valproic acid. Since most antiseizure drugs are selective for specific seizure disorders, effective treatment requires a proper match between the drug and the seizure. This match can be made only if the seizure type has been accurately diagnosed.

Making a diagnosis requires physical, neurologic, and laboratory evaluations along with a thorough history. The history should determine the age of onset of seizure activity, the frequency and duration of seizure events, precipitating factors, and times when seizures occur. Physical and neurologic evaluations may reveal signs of head injury or other disorders that could underlie seizure activity, although in many patients the physical and neurologic evaluations may be normal. An electroencephalogram (EEG) is essential for diagnosis of seizure type. Other diagnostic tests that may be employed include computerized axial tomography (CAT), positron emission tomography (PET), and magnetic resonance imaging (MRI).

## Drug Evaluation

Once an antiseizure drug has been selected, a trial period is needed to determine its effectiveness. During this time there is no guarantee that seizures will not occur. Accordingly, until seizure control is certain, the patient should be warned not to participate in activities that could be hazardous if a seizure were to occur (e.g., driving, operating dangerous machinery).

During the process of drug evaluation, adjustments in dosage are often needed. No drug should be considered ineffective until it has been tested in sufficiently high dosage and for a reasonable period of time. Measurement of plasma drug levels can be a valuable tool for establishing dosage and evaluating the effectiveness of a specific drug.

Maintenance of a seizure frequency chart is essential for evaluating treatment. The chart should be maintained by the patient or a family member and should contain a complete record of all seizure events. This record will enable the physician to determine if treatment has been effective. The nurse should teach the patient how to create and use a seizure frequency chart.

## Monitoring Plasma Drug Levels

Monitoring plasma drug levels is a common practice in epilepsy therapy. For most antiseizure drugs, the plasma drug levels that produce therapeutic and toxic effects have been established. Hence, knowledge of drug levels can serve as a useful guide for adjusting dosage. Table 23–2 gives the plasma drug levels that define the therapeutic range for the major antiseizure drugs.

Monitoring plasma drug levels is especially helpful when treating major convulsive disorders (e.g., tonic-clonic seizures). Since these seizures can be dangerous, and since delay of therapy may allow the condition to worsen, rapid control of seizures is desirable. However, since these seizures occur infrequently, a long time may be needed to establish control if clinical outcome is relied on as the only means of determining an effective dosage.

## TABLE 23-2. CLINICAL PHARMACOLOGY OF MAJOR ANTISEIZURE MEDICATIONS

| Generic Name | Trade Name | Daily Maintenance Dosage | | Therapeutic Serum Concentration (µg/ml) |
| --- | --- | --- | --- | --- |
| | | Adults (mg) | Children (mg/kg) | |
| Carbamazepine | Tegretol, others | 600-1200 | 15-30 | 4-12 |
| Clonazepam | Klonopin | 1.5-20 | 0.1-0.2 | 0.02-0.08 |
| Ethosuximide | Zarontin | 750-2000 | 20-40 | 40-100 |
| Gabapentin | Neurontin | 900-1800 | NA | ND |
| Lamotrigine | Lamictal | 100-500 | NA | ND |
| Phenobarbital | Many names | 120-250 | 3-5 | 15-40 |
| Phenytoin | Dilantin | 300-400 | 4-7 | 10-20 |
| Primidone | Mysoline | 750-1500 | 10-25 | 5-12 |
| Valproic acid | Depakene | 1000-3000 | 15-60 | 50-150 |

NA = not approved, ND = not determined.

By adjusting initial doses on the basis of plasma drug levels (rather than on the basis of seizure control), we can readily achieve drug levels that are likely to be effective, thereby increasing our chances of establishing control quickly.

Measurements of plasma drug levels are not especially important for determining effective dosages for *absence* seizures. Because absence seizures occur very frequently (up to several hundred a day), simple observation of the patient is the best means for establishing an effective dosage: if seizures stop, dosage is sufficient; if seizures continue, more drug is probably needed.

In addition to serving as a guide for dosage adjustment, knowledge of plasma drug levels can serve as an aid to (1) monitoring compliance, (2) determining the cause of lost seizure control, and (3) identifying the causes of toxicity, especially in patients receiving multidrug therapy.

### Promoting Compliance

Epilepsy is a chronic condition that requires regular and continuous therapy. As a result, seizure control is highly dependent on patient compliance. In fact, it is estimated that noncompliance accounts for about 50% of all treatment failures. Accordingly, promoting compliance should be a priority for all members of the health care team.

Several measures can help promote compliance. These are (1) educating the patient and family about the chronic nature of epilepsy and the importance of adhering to the prescribed regimen, (2) monitoring plasma drug levels as a means of encouraging and evaluating compliance, and (3) deepening patient and family involvement by having them maintain a seizure frequency chart.

### Withdrawing Antiseizure Medication

Some forms of epilepsy undergo spontaneous remission; hence discontinuation of medication may at some time be appropriate. Unfortunately, there are no firm guidelines to indicate the most appropriate time to withdraw treatment. However, once the decision to discontinue treatment has been made, agreement does exist on how drug withdrawal should be accomplished. *The most important rule governing discontinuation of antiseizure medication is that withdrawal be done slowly (over a period of 6 weeks to several months).* Failure to gradually reduce dosage is a frequent cause of status epilepticus. If the patient is taking two drugs to control seizures, the drugs should be withdrawn sequentially, not simultaneously.

## Basic Pharmacology of the Major Antiseizure Drugs

The drugs used most frequently for seizure control are *phenytoin, phenobarbital, carbamazepine,* and *valproic acid*. Most of the discussion below focuses on these four agents. Applications of the antiseizure drugs are summarized in Table 23-1. Therapeutic blood levels are summarized in Table 23-2. Chemical classification of antiseizure agents is summarized in Table 23-3.

### Phenytoin

Phenytoin [Dilantin] is a broad-spectrum antiseizure agent. This drug is active against partial and tonic-clonic seizures but not absence seizures. Phenytoin is of historic note in that it was the first drug to suppress seizure activity without producing generalized depression of the entire CNS. Hence phenytoin heralded the development of selective medications that could treat epilepsy while leaving most CNS functions undiminished.

#### Mechanism of Action

At the concentrations achieved clinically, phenytoin causes selective inhibition of sodium channels. Specifically, the drug delays recovery of inactive sodium channels back into the active

TABLE 23-3. CHEMICAL CLASSIFICATION OF ANTISEIZURE DRUGS

| Hydantoins | Benzodiazepines |
|---|---|
| Phenytoin | Diazepam |
| Mephenytoin | Clonazepam |
| Fosphenytoin | Clorazepate |
| Ethotoin | Lorazepam |
| **Barbiturates** | **Others** |
| Phenobarbital | Valproate |
| Mephobarbital | Carbamazepine |
| **Succinimides** | Primidone |
| Ethosuximide | Gabapentin |
| Methsuximide | Lamotrigine |
| Phensuximide | Felbamate |
| | Phenacemide |
| **Oxazolidinediones** | Acetazolamide |
| Trimethadione | Magnesium sulfate |
| Paramethadione | |

state. As a result, entry of sodium into neurons is inhibited, and therefore action potentials are suppressed. Blockade of sodium entry is limited to neurons that are hyperactive. Therefore, the drug suppresses activity of seizure-generating neurons while leaving healthy neurons unaffected.

## Pharmacokinetics

Phenytoin has unusual pharmacokinetic properties that must be accounted for in therapy. Both the absorption and metabolism of the drug vary substantially among patients. In addition, small changes in dosage can produce disproportionately large changes in plasma drug levels. Because of these kinetic characteristics, a dosage that is both effective and safe is difficult to establish and, once determined, must be adhered to rigidly.

**Absorption.** Absorption of oral phenytoin is variable. Variability exists between *different formulations* of phenytoin (e.g., tablets versus extended-release capsules) and between preparations made by *different manufacturers.*

**Metabolism.** Individuals differ widely in the rate at which they metabolize phenytoin. As a result, the half-life of phenytoin varies substantially among patients, ranging from 8 to 60 hours.

The capacity of the liver to metabolize phenytoin is very limited. As a result, the relationship between dosage and plasma levels of phenytoin is unusual. Therapeutic doses of phenytoin are only slightly smaller than the doses needed to saturate the hepatic enzymes that metabolize the drug. Consequently, if phenytoin is administered in doses only slightly greater than those needed for therapeutic effects, the liver's capacity to metabolize the drug will be overwhelmed, causing plasma levels of phenytoin to rise dramatically. This unusual relationship between dosage and plasma levels is illustrated in Figure 23-1A. As can be seen, once plasma levels of phenytoin have reached the therapeutic range, small changes in dosage produce large changes in drug levels. As a result, small in-

creases in dosage can cause toxicity, and small decreases can cause therapeutic failure. This relationship makes it difficult to establish and maintain a dosage that is both safe and effective.

Figure 23-1B indicates the relationship between dosage and plasma drug levels that exists for most drugs. As can be seen, this relationship is *linear*, in contrast to the non-linear relationship that exists for phenytoin. Accordingly, for most drugs, if the patient is taking doses that produce plasma drug levels that are within the therapeutic range, small deviations from that dosage produce only small deviations in plasma drug levels. Because of this relationship, it is relatively easy to maintain drug levels that are safe and effective.

## Therapeutic Uses

**Epilepsy.** Phenytoin can be used to treat all major forms of epilepsy except absence seizures. The drug is especially effective against tonic-clonic seizures, and is a drug of choice for treating these seizures in adults and older children. (Carbamazepine is preferred to phenytoin for treating tonic-clonic seizures in young children.) Although phenytoin can be used to treat simple and complex partial seizures, the drug is less effective against these seizures than against tonic-clonic seizures. Phenytoin can be administered intravenously to treat generalized convulsive status epilepticus.

**Cardiac Dysrhythmias.** Phenytoin is active against certain types of dysrhythmias. Antidysrhythmic applications are discussed in Chapter 48.

## Adverse Effects

**Effects on the CNS.** Although phenytoin acts on the CNS in a relatively selective fashion to suppress seizures, the drug is not completely devoid of CNS side effects—especially when dosage is excessive. At therapeutic drug levels, sedation and other CNS effects are mild. At plasma levels above 20 µg/ml, toxic effects can occur. *Nystagmus* (continuous back-and-forth movements of the eyes) is relatively common. Other manifestations of excessive dosage include *sedation*, *ataxia* (staggering gait), *diplopia* (double vision), and *cognitive impairment*.

**Gingival Hyperplasia.** Gingival hyperplasia (excessive growth of gum tissue) is characterized by swelling, tenderness, and bleeding of the gums. This effect occurs in about 20% of patients. Gingival hyperplasia can be minimized by good oral hygiene, including dental flossing and gum massage. Patients should be given instruction in these techniques and encouraged to practice them. In some cases, gingival hyperplasia is so great as to require gingivectomy (surgical removal of excess gum tissue).

**Skin Rash.** Between 2% and 5% of patients develop a *morbilliform (measles-like) rash*. Rarely, morbilliform rash progresses to exfoliative dermatitis or Stevens-Johnson syndrome (an inflammatory skin disease characterized by red macules, papules, and tubercles). If a rash develops, phenytoin should be discontinued.

**Cardiovascular Effects.** When phenytoin is administered by IV injection (to treat status epilepticus), cardiac dysrhythmias

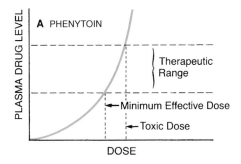
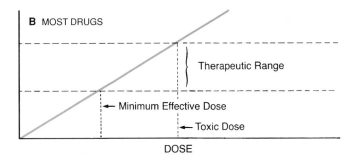

**Figure 23–1. Relationship between dose and plasma level for phenytoin versus most other drugs.**
*A*, Within the therapeutic range, small increments in phenytoin dosage produce sharp increases in plasma drug levels. This relationship makes it difficult to maintain plasma phenytoin levels within the therapeutic range.

*B*, Within the therapeutic range, small increments in dosage produce small increases in drug levels. With this relationship, moderate fluctuations in dosage are unlikely to result in either toxicity or loss of therapeutic effects.

and hypotension may result. These dangerous responses can be minimized by injecting phenytoin slowly and in dilute solution.

**Other Adverse Effects.** *Hirsutism* (overgrowth of hair in unusual places) can be a disturbing response, especially in young women. Interference with vitamin D metabolism may cause *rickets* and *osteomalacia* (softening of the bones). Interference with vitamin K metabolism can lower prothrombin levels, thereby causing *bleeding tendencies in newborns* whose mothers took phenytoin during pregnancy.

### Drug Interactions

Phenytoin interacts with a large number of drugs. The more important interactions are discussed below.

***Interactions Resulting from Induction of Hepatic Drug-Metabolizing Enzymes.*** Phenytoin stimulates synthesis of hepatic drug-metabolizing enzymes. By increasing drug metabolism, phenytoin can decrease the effects of other drugs, including *oral contraceptives*, *warfarin* (an anticoagulant), and *glucocorticoids* (anti-inflammatory/immunosuppressive drugs). Because it is desirable to avoid pregnancy while taking antiseizure medication, and because phenytoin can decrease the effectiveness of oral contraceptives, women who are taking these drugs should increase the dosage of the contraceptive.

***Drugs That Increase Plasma Levels of Phenytoin.*** Since the therapeutic range of phenytoin is narrow, slight increases in phenytoin levels can cause toxicity. Consequently, caution must be exercised when phenytoin is used concurrently with drugs that can increase phenytoin levels. Drugs known to elevate phenytoin levels include *diazepam* (an antianxiety agent and antiseizure drug), *isoniazid* (a drug used to treat tuberculosis), *cimetidine* (a drug used to treat gastric ulcers), and *alcohol* (when taken acutely). These agents increase phenytoin levels by reducing the rate at which phenytoin is metabolized. *Valproic acid* (an antiseizure drug) elevates levels of free phenytoin by displacing phenytoin from binding sites on plasma proteins.

***Drugs That Decrease Plasma Levels of Phenytoin.*** Drugs known to decrease phenytoin levels include *folic acid*, *carbamazepine* and *phenobarbital* (antiseizure drugs), and alcohol (when used chronically). These agents reduce phenytoin levels by accelerating phenytoin metabolism. By lowering phenytoin levels, these drugs can increase the risk of seizures.

***CNS Depressants.*** The depressant effects of *alcohol*, *barbiturates*, and *other CNS depressants* will add to those of phenytoin. Patients should be advised to avoid alcohol and other drugs with CNS-depressant properties.

### Preparations, Dosage, and Administration

***Preparations.*** Phenytoin [Dilantin] is available in an injectable form and in four *oral* formulations: chewable tablets [Dilantin Infatab], oral suspension [Dilantin-125], prompt-acting capsules, and extended-release capsules [Dilantin Kapseals].

As noted above, phenytoin products differ significantly in bioavailability. *Differences in bioavailability exist among different formulations of phenytoin (e.g., tablets versus capsules) and among the same formulations produced by different manufacturers.* Because of differences in bioavailability, and because small changes in phenytoin absorption can produce large changes in plasma drug levels, *patients should not switch from one formulation of phenytoin to another or from one brand of phenytoin to another without the physician's approval and supervision.* (It should be noted that phenytoin is one of the rare examples of a drug for which there are significant differences among preparations produced by different manufacturers.)

***Dosage.*** Because patients vary widely in their ability to metabolize phenytoin, *dosing is highly individualized.* Initial doses are usually given twice daily. Once a maintenance dosage has been established, once-a-day dosing is often possible (using extended-release capsules). For *adults*, a typical *initial* dosage is 150 mg twice a day; *maintenance* dosages usually range between 300 and 400 mg/day. For *children*, a typical *initial* dosage is 2.5 mg/kg twice a day; *maintenance* dosages usually range between 4 and 7 mg/kg/day.

Plasma drug levels are often monitored as an aid to dosage determination. *The dosing objective is to produce phenytoin levels between 10 and 20 μg/ml.* Levels below

10 µg/ml are too low to control seizures; at levels above 20 µg/ml, signs of toxicity begin to appear. Because phenytoin has a relatively narrow therapeutic range (between 10 and 20 µg/ml), and because of the nonlinear relationship between phenytoin dosage and phenytoin plasma levels, *once a safe and effective dosage has been established, the patient should adhere to it rigidly, because small deviations from the established dosage can cause toxicity or therapeutic failure.*

*When treatment with phenytoin is discontinued, dosage should be reduced gradually. Abrupt withdrawal may precipitate seizures.*

**Administration.** *Oral* preparations may cause gastric discomfort. The patient should be informed that gastric upset can be reduced by administering phenytoin with meals or immediately after meals. Patients using the oral suspension of phenytoin should be instructed to shake the preparation well before dispensing, since failure to do so may result in uneven dosing.

*Intravenous* administration is used to treat generalized convulsive status epilepticus. *It is imperative that infusions be performed slowly* (no faster than 50 mg/min), since rapid administration can cause cardiovascular collapse. Phenytoin should not be added to an existing IV infusion, since mixing phenytoin with other solutions is likely to produce a precipitate. Solutions of phenytoin are highly alkaline and can cause local venous irritation; irritation can be reduced by flushing the IV needle or catheter with sterile saline immediately after completing the phenytoin infusion.

## Phenobarbital

Phenobarbital is one of our oldest antiseizure medications. The drug is effective and inexpensive, and has few serious side effects. Because of these qualities, phenobarbital remains one of our most commonly used antiseizure drugs.

Phenobarbital belongs to the barbiturate family. However, in contrast to most barbiturates, which produce generalized depression of the CNS, phenobarbital is able to suppress seizures at doses that produce minimal disruption of CNS function. Because it can reduce seizures without causing sedation, phenobarbital is classified as an *anticonvulsant barbiturate* (to distinguish it from most other barbiturates, which are employed as daytime sedatives or as "sleeping pills").

The basic pharmacology of the barbiturates is discussed in Chapter 32. Discussion here is limited to the use of phenobarbital for seizures.

### Mechanism of Antiseizure Action

Phenobarbital suppresses seizures by potentiating the effects of GABA. Specifically, the drug binds to GABA receptors, causing the receptor to respond more intensely to GABA itself.

### Pharmacokinetics

Phenobarbital is absorbed completely following oral administration. The drug's half-life is approximately 4 days. Because of this prolonged half-life, 2 to 3 weeks are required for plasma levels of phenobarbital to reach a plateau. (Recall that, in the absence of a loading dose, an interval equivalent to four half-lives is required for plateau to be achieved.) Phenobarbital is eliminated by a combination of hepatic metabolism and renal excretion.

## Therapeutic Uses

*Epilepsy.* Phenobarbital is effective against partial seizures and generalized tonic-clonic seizures but not against absence seizures. Until recently, phenobarbital had been a drug of choice for tonic-clonic seizures and partial seizures in older children and adults. However, most clinicians now prefer to treat these epilepsies with carbamazepine, phenytoin, or valproic acid—drugs that cause fewer neuropsychologic effects than phenobarbital. Intravenous phenobarbital can be used for generalized convulsive status epilepticus, but lorazepam and diazepam are preferred.

*Sedation and Induction of Sleep.* Like other barbiturates, phenobarbital can be used to produce daytime sedation and to promote sleep at night. These applications are discussed in Chapter 32.

## Adverse Effects

*Neuropsychologic Effects.* Drowsiness is the most common CNS effect. During the initial phase of therapy, sedation develops in practically all patients. With continued drug use, tolerance to sedation develops. Some children experience *paradoxical responses*: instead of becoming sedated, they may become *irritable* and *hyperactive*. *Depression* may occur in adults. Elderly patients may experience *agitation* and *confusion*.

*Physical Dependence.* Like all other barbiturates, phenobarbital can cause physical dependence. However, at the doses employed to treat epilepsy, significant dependence is unlikely.

*Exacerbation of Intermittent Porphyria.* Phenobarbital and other barbiturates can increase the risk of acute intermittent porphyria. Accordingly, barbiturates are absolutely contraindicated for patients with a history of this disorder. The relationship of barbiturates to intermittent porphyria is discussed further in Chapter 32.

*Adverse Effects in Pregnancy.* Use of barbiturates during pregnancy has been associated with congenital abnormalities. Women who take phenobarbital during pregnancy or become pregnant while taking the drug should be informed of the potential risk to the fetus.

*Other Adverse Effects.* Like phenytoin, phenobarbital can interfere with the metabolism of vitamins D and K. Disruption of vitamin D metabolism can cause *rickets* and *osteomalacia*. Disruption of vitamin K metabolism can cause *bleeding tendencies in neonates* whose mothers took phenytoin during pregnancy.

### Toxicity

When taken in moderately excessive doses, phenobarbital causes *nystagmus* and *ataxia*. Severe overdosage produces generalized *CNS depression*; death results from depression of respiration. Barbiturate toxicity and its treatment are discussed at length in Chapter 32.

## Drug Interactions

*Induction of Drug-Metabolizing Enzymes.* Phenobarbital acts on the liver to induce (stimulate) the synthesis of drug-metabolizing enzymes. By doing so, phenobarbital can increase the rate at which many drugs are inactivated, thereby decreasing their effects. Of particular concern are reduced effects of *oral contraceptives* and *warfarin.*

***CNS Depressants.*** Being a CNS depressant itself, phenobarbital will intensify CNS depression caused by other drugs (e.g., alcohol, benzodiazepines, opioids), possibly causing severe respiratory depression and coma. Patients should be warned against combining phenobarbital with other drugs that have CNS-depressant properties.

***Valproic Acid.*** Valproic acid is an anticonvulsant that has been used in combination with phenobarbital. By competing with phenobarbital for drug-metabolizing enzymes, valproic acid can increase plasma levels of phenobarbital by approximately 40%. Hence, when this combination is used, the dosage of phenobarbital must be reduced.

### Drug Withdrawal

When phenobarbital is withdrawn, *dosage should be reduced gradually*, since abrupt withdrawal can precipitate status epilepticus. Patients should be warned of this danger and instructed not to discontinue phenobarbital too quickly.

#### Preparations, Dosage, and Administration

***Preparations.*** Phenobarbital is dispensed in three oral formulations: tablets, capsules, and elixir. The drug is also available in formulations for IM and IV administration.

***Dosage.*** *Maintenance dosages* for *adults* range from 50 to 100 mg/day administered in two or three divided doses. Maintenance dosages for *children* range from 3 to 5 mg/kg/day administered in two or three divided doses. When dosage is being established, plasma drug levels may be used as a guide; target levels are 15 to 40 μg/ml.

*Loading doses* may sometimes be needed. Because phenobarbital has a long half-life, several weeks are required for drug levels to reach plateau. If plateau must be reached sooner, a loading schedule can be employed. For example, doses that are twice normal can be given for 4 days. Unfortunately, these large doses are likely to produce substantial CNS depression.

***Administration.*** Phenobarbital may be administered orally, IV, and IM. Oral administration is employed for routine therapy of epilepsy. Intravenous administration is needed for status epilepticus.

Intravenous injection must be done slowly. If administration is too rapid, excessive CNS depression may result. Phenobarbital is highly alkaline and may cause local tissue injury if extravasation occurs.

## Carbamazepine

Carbamazepine [Tegretol, others] is a mainstay of antiseizure therapy. The drug is active against partial seizures and tonic-clonic seizures but not absence seizures.

### Mechanism of Action

Carbamazepine suppresses high-frequency neuronal discharge in and around seizure foci. The mechanism appears to be the same as that of phenytoin: delayed recovery of sodium channels from their inactivated state.

### Pharmacokinetics

Absorption of oral carbamazepine is delayed and variable. Peak levels are achieved in 4 to 12 hours. Overall bioavailability is about 80%. The drug distributes well to tissues.

Elimination is by hepatic metabolism. Carbamazepine is unusual in that its half-life decreases as therapy progresses. During the initial phase of treatment, the drug's half-life is approximately 40 hours. The half-life decreases to about 15 hours with continued treatment. The explanation is that carbamazepine, like phenytoin and phenobarbital, is an inducer of hepatic drug-metabolizing enzymes; by increasing the rate of its own metabolism, carbamazepine causes its own half-life to diminish.

### Therapeutic Uses

***Epilepsy.*** Carbamazepine is effective against tonic-clonic, simple partial, and complex partial seizures. Because the drug causes fewer adverse effects than phenytoin and phenobarbital, it is often preferred to these agents. Many clinicians consider carbamazepine the drug of first choice for partial seizures. Carbamazepine is not effective against absence, myoclonic, or atonic seizures.

***Bipolar Disorder (Manic-Depressive Illness).*** Carbamazepine can provide symptomatic control in patients with bipolar disorder, and is often effective in patients refractory to lithium. The role of carbamazepine in bipolar disorder is discussed in Chapter 31.

***Trigeminal and Glossopharyngeal Neuralgias.*** A neuralgia is a severe, stabbing pain that occurs along the course of a nerve. Carbamazepine can reduce neuralgia associated with the trigeminal and glossopharyngeal nerves. The mechanism of this analgesic effect is unknown. It should be noted that although carbamazepine can reduce pain in these specific neuralgias, the drug is not generally effective as an analgesic, and is not indicated for other kinds of pain.

### Adverse Effects

***CNS Effects.*** In contrast to phenytoin and phenobarbital, carbamazepine has minimal effects on cognitive function. This is a primary reason for selecting carbamazepine over these other drugs.

Carbamazepine can cause a variety of *neurologic effects*, including visual disturbances (nystagmus, blurred vision, diplopia), ataxia, vertigo, unsteadiness, and headache. These reactions are common during the first weeks of treatment, affecting between 35% and 50% of patients. Fortunately, tolerance usually develops with continued drug use. These effects can be minimized by initiating therapy at low doses and by giving the largest portion of the daily dose at bedtime.

***Hematologic Effects.*** Carbamazepine-induced bone marrow suppression can cause *leukopenia, anemia,* and *thrombocytopenia.* However, serious reactions are rare. Thrombocytopenia and anemia, which have an incidence of 5%, respond to discontinuation of drug use. Leukopenia, which has an incidence of 10%, is usually transient and subsides even with continued drug use; accordingly, carbamazepine should not be withdrawn unless the white blood cell count drops below 2500/mm³.

Fatal *aplastic anemia* has occurred during carbamazepine therapy. This reaction is extremely rare, having an incidence of 1 in 200,000. Very few cases have been reported since 1964, and in many of these a direct cause-and-effect relationship could not be established.

To reduce the risk of serious hematologic effects, complete blood counts should be performed before treatment and periodically thereafter. Patients with pre-existing hematologic abnormalities should not be given carbamazepine. Patients should be informed about manifestations of hematologic abnormalities (fever, sore throat, pallor, weakness, infection, easy bruising, petechiae) and instructed to notify the physician if these occur.

*Hypo-osmolarity.* Carbamazepine can inhibit renal excretion of water, apparently by promoting secretion of antidiuretic hormone. Water retention can reduce the osmolarity of blood and other body fluids, thereby posing a threat to patients with heart failure. Periodic monitoring of serum sodium content is recommended.

*Dermatologic Effects.* Carbamazepine has been associated with a number of dermatologic effects, including morbilliform rash (10% incidence), photosensitivity reactions, Stevens-Johnson syndrome, and exfoliative dermatitis. Mild reactions can often be treated with prednisone (an anti-inflammatory agent) or with an antihistamine. Severe reactions necessitate drug withdrawal.

### Drug Interactions

*Induction of Drug-Metabolizing Enzymes.* Carbamazepine is an effective inducer of hepatic drug-metabolizing enzymes. By promoting synthesis of these enzymes, carbamazepine can increase the rate at which it and other drugs are inactivated. Accelerated inactivation of *oral contraceptives* and *warfarin* is of particular concern.

*Phenytoin and Phenobarbital.* Both phenytoin and phenobarbital are effective inducers of hepatic drug metabolism. Hence, if either drug is taken with carbamazepine, induction of metabolism is likely to be greater than with carbamazepine alone. Accordingly, phenytoin and phenobarbital can further accelerate the metabolism of carbamazepine, thereby decreasing its effects.

### Preparations, Dosage, and Administration

Carbamazepine [Tegretol, others] is available in standard tablets (200 mg), chewable tablets (100 mg), and an oral suspension (100 mg/5 ml). The drug should be administered with meals to reduce gastric upset. Administering the largest portion of the daily dose at bedtime can help reduce adverse CNS effects.

Therapy is initiated with small doses (100 to 200 mg twice a day) to minimize side effects. The dosage is then increased gradually (every 1 to 3 weeks) until control of seizures is achieved. Maintenance dosages for *adults* range from 600 to 1200 mg/day, administered in divided doses. Maintenance dosages for *children* range from 15 to 30 mg/kg/day, administered in divided doses.

## Valproic Acid

Valproic acid [Depakene, Depakote] is approved by the Food and Drug Administration (FDA) only for treatment of absence seizures. However, the drug is also active against tonic-clonic, atonic, and myoclonic seizures, and is used widely to treat these disorders. In addition, valproic acid provides protection against partial seizures. The drug is generally devoid of serious side effects, but death from liver toxicity has occurred rarely.

### Mechanism of Action

Valproic acid appears to act by two mechanisms. First, the drug shares the same mechanism as phenytoin and carbam-

azepine: suppression of high-frequency neuronal firing through blockade of sodium channels. Second, the drug suppresses calcium influx through T-type calcium channels. In addition, the drug may augment the inhibitory influence of GABA.

### Pharmacokinetics

Valproic acid is readily absorbed following oral administration and is widely distributed throughout the body. The drug undergoes extensive hepatic metabolism followed by renal excretion.

Therapeutic responses are often seen at plasma drug levels of 50 to 150 μg/ml. However, the correlation between plasma levels and therapeutic effects is not very tight.

### Therapeutic Uses

*Absence Seizures.* Absence seizures are the only FDA-approved indication for valproic acid. For these seizures, valproic acid provides the same degree of control as ethosuximide. Some clinicians consider valproic acid to be the drug of first choice for absence seizures. Others believe that valproic acid, because of its ability to cause liver injury (see below), should be reserved for patients who have failed to respond to ethosuximide.

*Other Seizures.* Although labeled only for absence seizures, valproic acid can provide effective control of most other seizures. The drug can suppress tonic-clonic seizures, partial seizures, myoclonic seizures, and atonic seizures. Because valproic acid causes fewer serious adverse effects than phenobarbital and phenytoin, the drug is increasingly preferred.

*Bipolar Disorder.* Like carbamazepine, valproic acid can provide symptomatic control in patients with bipolar disorder. This application is discussed in Chapter 31.

### Adverse Effects

Valproic acid is generally well tolerated and causes minimal sedation and cognitive impairment. Gastrointestinal effects are most common. Hepatotoxicity is rare but serious.

*Gastrointestinal Effects.* Nausea, vomiting, and indigestion are common, occurring in 16% of those treated. These effects are transient and rarely require drug withdrawal. Gastrointestinal effects can be minimized by administering valproic acid with food and by using an enteric-coated formulation.

*Hepatotoxicity.* Rarely, valproic acid has been associated with fatal liver failure. Most deaths have occurred within the first few months of therapy. The overall incidence of fatal hepatotoxicity is about 1 in 30,000. However, in high-risk patients—children under the age of 2 years who are receiving multidrug therapy—the incidence is 1 in 500. To minimize the risk of fatal liver injury, the following guidelines have been established.

- Don't use valproic acid in conjunction with other drugs in children under the age of 3 years.
- Don't use valproic acid in patients with pre-existing liver dysfunction.
- Evaluate liver function before initiating treatment and periodically thereafter. (Unfortunately, monitoring liver function may fail to provide advance warning of

severe hepatotoxicity. In some patients, fatal liver failure developed so rapidly that it was not preceded by abnormal test results.)

• Inform patients about signs and symptoms of liver injury (reduced appetite, malaise, nausea, abdominal pain, jaundice) and instruct them to notify the physician if these develop.

• Use valproic acid in the lowest effective dosage.

*Teratogenic Effects.* Valproic acid can adversely affect the developing fetus. In laboratory animals the drug has caused intrauterine growth retardation, fetal resorption, and major developmental abnormalities. Available data suggest, but do not prove, that the drug may also be teratogenic in humans. Valproic acid is classified in FDA Pregnancy Category D: there is evidence of human fetal risk, but the drug may be used during pregnancy if the potential benefits are considered to outweigh the potential risks.

*Other Adverse Effects.* Valproic acid may cause *rash, weight gain, hair loss,* and *blood dyscrasias* (leukopenia, thrombocytopenia, red blood cell aplasia). Significant CNS effects are uncommon.

### Drug Interactions

*Phenobarbital.* Valproic acid decreases the rate at which phenobarbital is metabolized. Blood levels of phenobarbital may rise by 40%, resulting in significant CNS depression. When the combination is used, levels of phenobarbital should be monitored. If levels rise too high, phenobarbital dosage should be reduced.

*Phenytoin.* Valproic acid can displace phenytoin from binding sites on plasma proteins. The resultant increase in the concentration of free phenytoin may lead to toxicity. Phenytoin levels and clinical status should be monitored.

### Preparations, Dosage, and Administration

*Preparations.* Valproic acid is available in three closely related chemical forms: (1) valproic acid itself, (2) the sodium salt of valproic acid, and (3) divalproex sodium, which is a combination of valproic acid plus its sodium salt. All three forms have identical antiseizure actions.

Valproic acid [Depakene] is available in 250-mg capsules. The sodium salt of valproic acid [Depakene] is available in a syrup (50 mg/ml). Divalproex sodium [Depakote] is available in delayed-release tablets (125, 250, and 500 mg).

*Dosage and Administration.* Daily doses are small initially and then gradually increased to a maintenance level. For *adults,* the initial dosage is 5 to 15 mg/kg/day, usually administered in two divided doses. The usual adult maintenance dosage is 10 to 20 mg/kg/day. For *children* ages 1 to 12 years, the initial dosage is 10 to 30 mg/kg/day, usually administered in divided doses. The usual pediatric maintenance dosage is 20 to 30 mg/kg/day. For both adults and children, the dosage should be increased if phenobarbital or another inducer of hepatic drug metabolism is taken concurrently.

Patients should be instructed to swallow the tablets and capsules intact, without chewing or crushing. Gastric discomfort can be decreased by administering valproic acid with meals.

### Ethosuximide

*Therapeutic Use.* Ethosuximide [Zarontin] is a drug of choice for absence seizures, the only seizures for which it is indicated. Absence seizures are abolished in 60% of patients, and, in newly diagnosed patients, practical control is achieved in 80% to 90%. Ethosuximide is inactive against tonic-clonic, simple partial, and complex partial seizures.

*Mechanism of Action.* Ethosuximide suppresses neurons in the thalamus that are responsible for generating absence seizures. The specific mechanism is inhibition of low-threshold calcium currents, known as T currents. Ethosuximide does not block sodium channels, and does not enhance GABA-mediated neuronal inhibition.

*Pharmacokinetics.* Ethosuximide is well absorbed following oral administration. Therapeutic effects occur at plasma levels of 40 to 100 µg/ml. The drug is eliminated by a combination of hepatic metabolism and renal excretion. Ethosuximide does not induce hepatic drug-metabolizing enzymes.

*Adverse Effects and Drug Interactions.* Ethosuximide is generally devoid of significant adverse effects and interactions. During the initial phase of treatment, the drug may cause *drowsiness, dizziness,* and *lethargy.* These responses diminish with continued use. *Nausea* and *vomiting* may occur and can be reduced by administering ethosuximide with food. Rare but serious reactions include *systemic lupus erythematosus, leukopenia,* and *aplastic anemia.*

*Preparations, Dosage, and Administration.* Ethosuximide [Zarontin] is available in capsules (250 mg) and in a syrup (250 mg/5 ml) for oral use. For children ages 3 to 6 years, the initial dosage is 250 mg/day. For older children and adults, the initial dosage is 500 mg/day. Dosage should be gradually increased until control of seizures is obtained. Maintenance dosages range from 750 to 2000 mg/day for adults, and from 20 to 40 mg/kg/day for children.

Since absence seizures occur many times each day, monitoring the clinical response (rather than plasma drug levels) is the preferred method for determining dosage. Dosage should be increased until seizures have been controlled or until adverse effects become too great.

When withdrawal of ethosuximide is indicated, dosage should be reduced gradually.

### Clonazepam

Clonazepam [Klonopin] belongs to the benzodiazepine family of drugs. The basic pharmacology of the benzodiazepines is discussed in Chapter 32. Consideration here is limited to the use of clonazepam in epilepsy.

*Actions and Uses.* Clonazepam is indicated for absence, myoclonic, and atonic seizures. (Atonic seizures are characterized by a loss of all muscle tone.) The drug is not used to treat tonic-clonic or partial seizures. For therapy of absence seizures, ethosuximide and valproic acid are preferred to clonazepam. Some patients develop tolerance to clonazepam within months, causing loss of seizure control. Furthermore, exacerbation of symptoms is common when the drug is withdrawn. Accordingly, use of clonazepam is limited. Clonazepam and other benzodiazepines appear to suppress seizures by enhancing the inhibitory effects of GABA on CNS neurons.

*Adverse Effects.* Like other benzodiazepines, clonazepam is generally devoid of serious adverse effects. *CNS depression* (drowsiness, lethargy, fatigue) is common early in therapy but diminishes with continued drug use. Like phenobarbital, clonazepam can cause *paradoxical excitement* (hyperactivity, aggression, decreased ability to concentrate) in children. Clonazepam may stimulate secretion from salivary glands and glands of the upper respiratory tract; these secretions may compromise breathing in patients with respiratory diseases.

*Drug Interactions.* Depressant effects of clonazepam add with those of other *CNS depressants* (e.g., alcohol, opioids, barbiturates, antihistamines). Accordingly, concurrent use of these drugs should be avoided.

Combined treatment with clonazepam and *valproic acid* has caused tonic seizures and should be avoided. The mechanism of this interaction is not known.

***Preparations, Dosage, and Administration.*** Clonazepam [Klonopin] is dispensed in tablets (0.5, 1, and 2 mg) for oral administration. The initial dosage for *adults* is 0.5 mg 3 times a day. The maximum dosage is 20 mg/day. The initial dosage for *infants* and *children* is 0.01 to 0.03 mg/kg/day. Dosage may be gradually increased to a maximum of 0.2 mg/kg/day.

As with other drugs used to treat epilepsy, abrupt discontinuation may trigger seizures. Accordingly, withdrawal of clonazepam should be done slowly.

## Primidone

Primidone [Mysoline] is active against all major seizure disorders except absence seizures. The drug is nearly identical in structure to phenobarbital. As a result, the pharmacology of both agents is very similar.

***Pharmacokinetics.*** Primidone is readily absorbed following oral administration. In the liver, much of the drug undergoes conversion to two active metabolites: phenobarbital and phenylethylmalonamide. Seizure control is produced by primidone itself and by these metabolites.

***Therapeutic Uses.*** Primidone is effective against tonic-clonic, simple partial, and complex partial seizures. The drug is not active against absence seizures.

As a rule, primidone is employed in combination with another antiseizure drug, usually phenytoin or carbamazepine. Primidone is never taken together with phenobarbital; since phenobarbital is one of the active metabolites of primidone, concurrent use of these drugs would be irrational.

***Adverse Effects.*** Sedation, ataxia, and dizziness are common during the initial phase of treatment but diminish with continued drug use. Like phenobarbital, primidone can cause confusion in the elderly and paradoxical hyperexcitability in children. A sense of acute intoxication can occur shortly after administration. As with phenobarbital, primidone is absolutely contraindicated for patients with acute intermittent porphyria. Serious adverse reactions (acute psychosis, leukopenia, thrombocytopenia, systemic lupus erythematosus) have occurred but are rare.

***Drug Interactions.*** Drug interactions for primidone are similar to those for phenobarbital. Primidone can induce hepatic drug-metabolizing enzymes and can thereby reduce the effects of oral contraceptives, oral anticoagulants, and other drugs. In addition, primidone can intensify responses to other CNS depressants.

***Preparations, Dosage, and Administration.*** Primidone [Mysoline] is available in tablets (50 and 250 mg) and in suspension (250 mg/5 ml) for oral use. Therapy in adults is initiated with a dose of 100 to 125 mg at bedtime. Dosage is gradually increased over the next 10 days to a maintenance amount of 250 mg 3 or 4 times a day. The maximum dosage is 500 mg 4 times a day.

## Newer Drugs

### Gabapentin

***Actions and Uses.*** Gabapentin [Neurontin], a new drug with a broad spectrum of anticonvulsant activity, is approved for adjunctive therapy of partial seizures (with or without secondary generalization). The drug is an analog of GABA, but does not directly affect GABA receptors. Rather, it appears to act by enhancing GABA release, thereby increasing GABA-mediated inhibition of neuronal firing.

***Pharmacokinetics.*** Gabapentin is rapidly absorbed following oral administration, and reaches peak plasma levels in 2 to 3 hours. Absorption is not affected by food. However, as the dosage gets larger, the percent absorbed gets smaller (because the intestinal transport system for uptake of the drug becomes saturated). Gabapentin is not metabolized and is excreted intact in the urine. The half-life is 5 to 7 hours.

***Drug Interactions.*** Unlike most antiseizure drugs, gabapentin is devoid of significant drug interactions. Gabapentin neither induces nor inhibits hepatic drug metabolizing enzymes, and does not affect the metabolism of other anticonvulsants. As a result, gabapentin is well suited for combined therapy with other agents.

***Adverse Reactions.*** The most common effects are somnolence, dizziness, ataxia, fatigue, and nystagmus. These are usually mild to moderate and often diminish with continued drug use. Patients should avoid driving and other hazardous activities until they are confident that the degree of impairment is not significant. Safety in pregnancy and breast-feeding has not been established.

***Preparations, Dosage, and Administration.*** Gabapentin [Neurontin] is dispensed in capsules (100, 300, and 400 mg) for oral administration. The usual maintenance dosage is 900 to 1800 mg/day in three divided doses. Dosing is begun with a 300-mg dose at bedtime, followed the next day by 600 mg (in two divided doses), and the next day by 900 mg (in three divided doses). Thereafter, the dosage can be raised rapidly to maintenance levels. Dosage should be reduced in patients with renal impairment. Gabapentin is not approved for children under 12 years.

### Lamotrigine

***Actions and Uses.*** Lamotrigine [Lamictal] has a broad spectrum of antiseizure activity, but is approved only for adjunctive therapy of partial seizures in adults. However, the drug may also benefit infants and children with Lennox-Gastaut syndrome, as well as adults with absence, myoclonic, or generalized tonic-clonic seizures. Benefits appear to derive from blockade of sodium channels.

***Pharmacokinetics.*** Administration is oral and absorption is nearly complete, both in the presence and absence of food. Blood levels peak in 1.5 to 5 hours and decline with a half-life of 24 hours. The drug undergoes hepatic metabolism followed by renal excretion.

***Drug Interactions.*** The half-life is affected by drugs that induce or inhibit hepatic drug-metabolizing enzymes. Enzyme inducers (e.g., carbamazepine, phenytoin, phenobarbital) decrease the half-life of lamotrigine to 10 hours, whereas valproate (an enzyme inhibitor) increases the half-life to about 60 hours.

***Adverse Effects.*** Rash occurs in 10% of patients, and is most likely in those who are also taking valproate. Although rash is usually benign, it can be an early sign of two life-threatening skin reactions: Stevens-Johnson syndrome and toxic epidermal necrolysis. Deaths have occurred. *Accordingly, lamotrigine should be withdrawn immediately if a rash develops.* Other common side effects include dizziness, diplopia (double vision), blurred vision, nausea, vomiting, and headache. Safety in pregnancy and breast-feeding has not been established.

***Preparations, Dosage, and Administration.*** Lamotrigine [Lamictal] is dispensed in tablets (25, 100, 150, and 200 mg) for oral administration. The dosage depends on what other drugs are being taken. For patients taking an *inducer* of drug metabolism (e.g., carbamazepine, phenytoin, phenobarbital), dosing is begun at 50 mg/day, and then gradually increased to between 150 and 250 mg twice a day for maintenance. For patients taking *valproate* (an enzyme inhibitor), dosing is begun at 25 mg every other day, and then gradually increased to between 50 and 75 mg twice daily for maintenance.

### Felbamate

Felbamate [Felbatol] is a relatively new drug with a broad spectrum of antiseizure activity. Unfortunately, felbamate has been associated with aplastic anemia and liver failure, and hence is not recommended.

***Mechanism of Action.*** Felbamate increases seizure threshold and suppresses seizure spread. The mechanism underlying these effects is not known. Unlike some antiseizure drugs (e.g., phenobarbital, benzodiazepines), felbamate does not interact with GABA receptors and does not enhance the inhibitory actions of GABA.

***Pharmacokinetics.*** Felbamate is well absorbed following oral administration, even in the presence of food. Peak plasma levels are achieved in 1 to 4 hours. The drug readily penetrates to the CNS. Although therapeutic plasma levels have not been established, levels of 20 to 120 μg/ml have been measured during clinical trials. Felbamate is eliminated in the urine, primarily unchanged. The drug's half-life is 14 to 23 hours.

***Therapeutic Uses.*** Felbamate is approved for (1) adjunctive or monotherapy in adults with partial seizures (with or without generalization), and (2) adjunctive therapy in children with Lennox-Gastaut syndrome. However, because of toxicity concerns, the manufacturer and the FDA have recommended that patients suspend use of the drug, except when the physician feels the benefits outweigh the risks.

***Adverse Effects.*** Felbamate appears to cause *aplastic anemia* and *liver damage*. Aplastic anemia has occurred in 21 patients, 3 of whom died. Acute liver failure occurred in eight patients, four of whom died. Because of the risk of liver failure, felbamate should not be used by patients with pre-existing liver dysfunction. In addition, patients taking the drug should be monitored for indications of liver injury.

The most common adverse effects are gastrointestinal disturbances (anorexia, nausea, vomiting) and CNS effects (insomnia, somnolence, dizziness, headache, diplopia). These effects occur more frequently when felbamate is combined with other drugs than when used alone.

***Drug Interactions.*** Felbamate can alter plasma levels of other antiseizure drugs and vice versa. Felbamate increases levels of phenytoin and valproic acid. Levels of felbamate are increased by valproic acid and reduced by phenytoin and carbamazepine. Increased levels of phenytoin and valproic acid (and possibly felbamate) could lead to toxicity; reduced levels of felbamate could lead to therapeutic failure. Therefore, to keep levels of these drugs within the therapeutic range, drug levels should be monitored and dosages should be adjusted accordingly.

***Preparations, Dosage, and Administration.*** Felbamate [Felbatol] is available in tablets (400 and 600 mg) and an oral suspension (600 mg/5 ml). For *older children* (over 14 years old) and *adults*, the initial dosage is 1200 mg/day in divided doses; the maximum dosage is 3600 mg/day. For *younger children* (2 to 14 years old), the initial dosage is 15 mg/kg/day in divided doses; the maximum dosage is 45 mg/kg/day or 3600 mg/day, whichever is less.

### Vigabatrin

Vigabatrin [Sabril] can suppress partial and secondarily generalized seizures, but may exacerbate absence and myoclonic seizures. The drug acts by inhibiting GABA transaminase, the enzyme that degrades GABA. By preventing GABA degradation, vigabatrin increases GABA availability in the CNS, and thereby enhances GABA-mediated inhibition of neuronal activity. Common adverse effects are depression, sedation, dizziness, and fatigue. Severe psychosis has occurred rarely. The maintenance dosage is 2 to 4 gm once a day. Vigabatrin is currently available in Europe and Australia but not in the United States.

### Topiramate

Topiramate [Topamax] is approved for adjunctive therapy of partial seizures in adults. The drug is administered orally and bioavailability is about 80%. Elimination is by renal excretion. Side effects include difficulty concentrating, drowsiness, dizziness, and incoordination. Kidney stones have occurred in 1.5% of patients, but most have continued using the drug. No drug interactions have been reported. Topiramate is available in tablets (50, 100, and 200 mg) for oral use. Dosing is begun at 50 mg/day and then gradually increased to 200 mg twice daily for maintenance.

# Antiseizure Therapy during Pregnancy

## Treatment of Epilepsy

Although most pregnant women who take antiseizure medication give birth to normal babies, *in utero* exposure to these drugs does carry some risk, especially during the first trimester. The dilemma, therefore, is to balance the risk of drug-induced fetal injury against the risk of injury from convulsions that might occur if antiseizure medication were withdrawn. Most clinicians agree that the risk to the fetus from uncontrolled convulsions is greater than the risk from antiseizure medications. Hence, as a general rule, women with major seizure disorders should continue to take antiseizure drugs throughout pregnancy. To minimize fetal risk, the lowest effective dosage should be determined and maintained. In addition, since the risk of fetal malformation is proportional to the number of drugs being taken, just one drug should be used whenever possible.

As discussed in Chapter 10, drug disposition changes during pregnancy. In particular, renal excretion of drugs increases, as does hepatic metabolism. As a result, an increase in dosage may be needed. To determine dosing requirements during pregnancy, drug levels should be measured at least once a month.

Valproic acid and carbamazepine are associated with an increased incidence of neural tube defects. Treatment with folic acid prior to conception and throughout pregnancy may reduce this risk. A dose of 5 mg/day has been recommended.

Four drugs—phenobarbital, phenytoin, carbamazepine, and primidone—reduce levels of vitamin K-dependent clotting factors (by inducing hepatic enzymes). As a result, there is an increased risk of bleeding. To reduce this risk, women taking these drugs should be given 20 mg of vitamin K daily during the last few weeks of pregnancy, and the baby should be given a 1-mg IM injection of vitamin K at birth.

In addition to their influence on clotting, inducers of hepatic metabolism can decrease blood levels of oral contraceptives, thereby rendering them ineffective. All women of child-bearing age should be informed of this drug interaction, and dosages of oral contraceptives should be increased as required.

## Pre-eclampsia and Eclampsia

*Pre-eclampsia* is a hypertensive disorder that develops after the 20th week of pregnancy. The condition is characterized by hypertension, proteinuria, and generalized edema. Patients with pre-eclampsia are at risk of developing seizures. If seizures occur, the condition is then termed *eclampsia*. Although the cause of seizures is not clear, possibilities include cerebral edema, vasospasm, ischemia, and hypertensive encephalopathy.

*Magnesium sulfate* is the drug of choice both for prophylaxis of seizures in women with pre-eclampsia and for treatment of seizures in women with eclampsia. For prophylaxis, a 10-gm IM loading dose is given, followed by 5 gm IM every 4 hours for maintenance. To treat eclamptic seizures, a 4-gm intravenous loading dose is given, followed by 5 gm IM every 4 hours for maintenance. As an alternative, maintenance can be achieved with an IV fusion. To ensure therapeutic effects and prevent toxicity, blood levels of magnesium should be monitored. The target range is 4 to 7 mEq/L (the normal range for magnesium is 1.5 to 2 mEq/L).

Management of pre-eclamptic and eclamptic hypertension is discussed in Chapter 44 under *Drugs for Hypertensive Disorders of Pregnancy*.

# Generalized Convulsive Status Epilepticus

Generalized convulsive SE is characterized by an unrelenting series of tonic-clonic seizures that lasts for 30 minutes or longer. Consciousness is lost during the entire attack. Tachycardia, elevation of blood pressure, and hyperthermia are typical. Metabolic sequelae include hypoglycemia and acidosis. Attacks pose a risk of permanent neurologic injury (cognitive impairment, memory loss, worsening of the underlying seizure disorder) and even death. A common cause of SE is failure to take antiseizure medication as prescribed.

Generalized convulsive SE is a medical emergency that requires immediate treatment. The goal is to maintain ventilation, correct hypoglycemia, and terminate the seizure. An IV line is established to draw blood for analysis of glucose levels, electrolyte levels, and drug levels. The line is also used to administer glucose and antiseizure drugs.

An intravenous benzodiazepine—either *diazepam* [Valium] or *lorazepam* [Ativan]—is used initially. Both drugs can terminate seizures quickly. Diazepam has a short duration of action, and hence must be administered repeatedly. In contrast, antiseizure effects of lorazepam last up to 72 hours. Because of its prolonged effects, lorazepam is preferred to diazepam by many specialists. The initial dose for lorazepam is 4 mg, administered by a 2-minute IV push. The initial dose for diazepam is 10 mg, administered no faster than 2 mg/min. Dosing with either drug is repeated if seizures are not controlled in 5 to 10 minutes. Although both drugs can be administered IM, this route is not effective for treating SE.

Once seizures have been stopped with a benzodiazepine, either *phenytoin* [Dilantin] or *fosphenytoin* [Cerebyx] is given for long-term suppression. Because the effects of diazepam are short lived, follow-up treatment with a long-acting drug is essential when diazepam is used for initial control. However, when lorazepam is used for initial control, follow-up therapy may be unnecessary, because the effects of lorazepam are prolonged. *Phenobarbital* may be used as an alternative to phenytoin or fosphenytoin for long-term control.

## KEY POINTS

- Seizures are initiated by discharge from a group of hyperexcitable neurons, called a focus.
- In partial seizures, excitation undergoes limited spread from the focus to adjacent cortical areas.
- In generalized seizure, excitation spreads widely throughout both hemispheres of the brain.
- Antiseizure drugs act through three basic mechanisms: suppression of sodium influx, suppression of calcium influx, and potentiation of the inhibitory effects of GABA.
- The goal in treating epilepsy is to reduce seizures to an extent that enables the patient to live a normal or near-normal life; complete elimination of seizures may not be possible without causing intolerable side effects.
- Most antiseizure drugs are selective for particular seizures; hence successful treatment depends on choosing the correct drug.
- Monitoring plasma drug levels is valuable for adjusting dosage, monitoring compliance, determining the cause of lost seizure control, and identifying the cause of toxicity, especially in patients taking more than one drug.
- Noncompliance accounts for nearly half of all treatment failures. Hence promoting compliance is a treatment priority.
- Withdrawal of antiseizure drugs must be done very gradually, since abrupt withdrawal can trigger status epilepticus.
- Most antiseizure drugs cause CNS depression, which can be deepened by concurrent use of other CNS depressants (e.g., alcohol, antihistamines, opioids, other antiseizure drugs).
- Phenytoin is active against partial seizures and tonic-clonic seizures but not absence seizures.
- The capacity of the liver to metabolize phenytoin is limited. As a result, doses only slightly greater than those needed for therapeutic effects can push phenytoin levels into the toxic range.
- The therapeutic range for phenytoin is 10 to 20 μg/ml.
- When phenytoin levels rise above 20 μg/ml, CNS toxicity develops. Signs include nystagmus, sedation, ataxia, diplopia, and cognitive impairment.
- Phenytoin causes gingival hyperplasia in 20% of patients.
- Because phenytoin products differ in bioavailability, and because small changes in absorption can produce large changes in plasma drug levels, patients should not switch from one formulation of phenytoin to another or from one brand of phenytoin to another without the physician's approval and supervision.
- Like phenytoin, phenobarbital is active against partial and tonic-clonic seizures but not absence seizures.

- Unlike other barbiturates, phenobarbital is able to suppress seizures without causing generalized CNS depression.
- Like phenytoin and phenobarbital, carbamazepine is active against partial seizures and tonic-clonic seizures.
- Because carbamazepine causes less cognitive impairment than phenytoin or phenobarbital, it is often preferred to these drugs.
- Carbamazepine can cause leukopenia, anemia, and thrombocytopenia—and very rarely, fatal aplastic anemia. To reduce the risk of serious hematologic effects, complete blood counts should be performed before treatment and periodically thereafter.
- Valproic acid is a very-broad-spectrum antiseizure drug, being active against partial seizures and most generalized seizures, including tonic-clonic, absence, atonic, and myoclonic seizures.
- Valproic acid can cause serious liver injury, especially in children under 2 years of age who are taking other antiseizure drugs.
- Phenytoin, phenobarbital, and carbamazepine induce synthesis of hepatic drug-metabolizing enzymes, and can thereby accelerate inactivation of other drugs. Inactivation of oral contraceptives and warfarin is of particular concern.
- Antiseizure drugs can interact with one another in complex ways, causing their blood levels to change. Dosages must be adjusted to compensate for these interactions.
- Antiseizure drugs can harm the developing fetus, especially during the first trimester. However, the fetus is at greater risk from uncontrolled seizures than from antiseizure drugs. Accordingly, women with major seizure disorders should continue taking medication throughout pregnancy.
- Fetal risk can be minimized by using just one antiseizure drug (if possible) and in the lowest effective dosage.
- Magnesium sulfate is the drug of choice both for prophylaxis of seizures in women with pre-eclampsia and for treatment of seizures in women with eclampsia.
- Initial control of generalized convulsive status epilepticus is accomplished with an IV benzodiazepine—either diazepam or lorazepam. When diazepam is used, follow-up treatment with phenytoin is essential for prolonged suppression.

# Summary of Major Nursing Implications*

## Nursing Implications That Apply to All Antiseizure Medications

### Preadministration Assessment

#### Therapeutic Goal
The goal of treatment is to minimize or eliminate seizure events, thereby allowing the patient to live a normal or near-normal life.

#### Baseline Data
Before initiating treatment, it is essential to know the type of seizure involved (e.g., absence, tonic-clonic) and the frequency of seizure events.

### Implementation: Administration

#### Dosage Determination
Dosages are often highly individualized and difficult to establish. Clinical evaluation of therapeutic and adverse effects is essential to establish a dosage that is both safe and effective. For several antiseizure drugs (especially those used to treat tonic-clonic seizures), knowledge of plasma drug levels can be a significant aid to dosage determination.

#### Promoting Compliance
Seizure control requires rigid adherence to the prescribed regimen; noncompliance is a major cause of therapeutic failure. To promote compliance, educate the patient about the importance of taking antiseizure medication exactly as prescribed. Monitoring plasma drug levels can motivate compliance and facilitate assessment of noncompliance.

### Ongoing Evaluation and Interventions

#### Evaluating Therapeutic Effects
Teach the patient (or a family member) to maintain a seizure frequency chart, indicating the date, time, and nature of all seizure events. The prescriber can use this record to evaluate treatment, make dosage adjustments, and alter drug selections.

#### Minimizing Danger from Uncontrolled Seizures
Advise the patient to avoid potentially hazardous activities (e.g., driving, operating dangerous machinery) until seizure control has been achieved. Also, since seizures may recur after they are largely under control, advise the patient to carry some form of identification (e.g., Medic-Alert bracelet) to aid in diagnosis and treatment if a seizure occurs.

#### Minimizing Adverse Effects
*CNS Depression.* Practically all antiseizure medications depress the CNS. Signs of CNS depression (sedation, drowsiness, lethargy) are most prominent during the initial phase of treatment and decline with continued drug use. Forewarn patients about CNS depression, and advise them to avoid driving and other hazardous activities if CNS depression is significant.

**Withdrawal Seizures.** Abrupt discontinuation of anti-seizure medication can lead to status epilepticus. Consequently, withdrawal of medication should be done slowly (over 6 weeks to several months). Forewarn patients about the dangers of abrupt drug withdrawal, and instruct them never to discontinue drug use without consulting the physician. Advise patients who are planning to travel to carry extra medication to ensure a continued supply in the event they become stranded where medication is unavailable.

**Usage in Pregnancy.** In most cases, the risk from uncontrolled seizures exceeds the risk from medication, hence women with major seizure disorders should continue to take antiseizure drugs during pregnancy. However, the lowest effective dosage should be employed and, if possible, only one drug should be used.

### Minimizing Adverse Interactions

**CNS Depressants.** Drugs with CNS-depressant actions (e.g., alcohol, antihistamines, barbiturates, opioids) will intensify the depressant effects of antiseizure drugs, thereby posing a risk of excessive CNS depression. Warn the patient against using alcohol and other CNS depressants.

# Phenytoin

Nursing implications for phenytoin include those presented below as well as those presented above for all antiseizure drugs.

## Preadministration Assessment

### Therapeutic Goal
Oral phenytoin is used to treat partial seizures (simple and complex) and tonic-clonic seizures. Intravenous phenytoin is used to treat convulsive status epilepticus.

### Identifying High-Risk Patients
Intravenous phenytoin is *contraindicated* for patients with *sinus bradycardia, SA block, second- or third-degree AV block, and Stokes-Adams syndrome.*

## Implementation: Administration

### Routes
Oral, IV, and (rarely) IM.

### Administration
**Oral.** Instruct the patient to take phenytoin exactly as prescribed. Inform the patient that, once a safe and effective dosage has been established, small deviations in dosage can lead to toxicity or to loss of seizure control.

Advise the patient to take phenytoin with meals to reduce gastric discomfort.

Instruct the patient to shake the phenytoin oral suspension before dispensing in order to provide consistent dosing.

Warn the patient not to switch formulations or brands of phenytoin without the physician's approval and oversight.

**Intravenous.** To minimize the risk of severe reactions (e.g., cardiovascular collapse) infuse phenytoin slowly (no faster than 50 mg/min).

Do not mix phenytoin solutions with other drugs.

To minimize venous inflammation at the site of injection, flush the needle or catheter employed for phenytoin administration with saline immediately after completing the infusion.

## Ongoing Evaluation and Interventions

### Minimizing Adverse Reactions
**CNS Effects.** Inform the patient that excessive doses can produce sedation, ataxia, diplopia, and interference with cognitive function. Instruct the patient to notify the physician if these occur.

**Gingival Hyperplasia.** Inform the patient that phenytoin often promotes overgrowth of gum tissue. To minimize harm and discomfort, instruct the patient in proper techniques of brushing, flossing, and gum massage.

**Skin Rash.** Inform the patient that phenytoin can cause a morbilliform (measles-like) rash that may progress to a more serious reaction. Instruct the patient to notify the physician immediately if a rash develops. Use of phenytoin should stop.

**Withdrawal Seizures.** Abrupt discontinuation of phenytoin can trigger convulsive status epilepticus. Warn the patient against abrupt cessation of treatment.

### Minimizing Adverse Interactions
Phenytoin is subject to a large number of significant interactions with other drugs; some are summarized below. Warn the patient against use of any drugs not specifically approved by the physician.

**CNS Depressants.** Warn the patient against use of alcohol and all other drugs with CNS-depressant properties, including opioids, barbiturates, and antihistamines.

**Warfarin and Oral Contraceptives.** Phenytoin can decrease the effects of these agents (and other drugs) by inducing hepatic drug-metabolizing enzymes. Dosages of warfarin and oral contraceptives may need to be increased.

# Phenobarbital

Nursing implications that apply to the antiseizure applications of phenobarbital include those presented below and those presented above for all antiseizure drugs. Nursing implications that apply to the barbiturates as a group are summarized in Chapter 32.

## Preadministration Assessment

### Therapeutic Goal
Oral phenobarbital is used to treat partial seizures (simple and complex) and tonic-clonic seizures. Intravenous therapy is used for convulsive status epilepticus.

### Identifying High-Risk Patients

Phenobarbital is *contraindicated* for patients with a *history of acute intermittent porphyria*. The drug should be used with extreme *caution* during *pregnancy*.

## Implementation: Administration

### Routes

Oral and IV.

### Administration

*Oral.* A loading schedule using larger than normal doses may be employed to initiate treatment. Monitor the patient for excessive CNS depression while these large doses are used.

*Intravenous.* Rapid IV infusion can cause severe adverse effects. Perform infusions slowly.

## Ongoing Evaluation and Interventions

### Minimizing Adverse Effects

*Neuropsychologic Effects.* Warn the patient that sedation may occur during the initial phase of treatment. Advise the patient to avoid hazardous activities if sedation is significant.

Inform parents that children may become irritable and hyperactive. Instruct parents to notify the physician if these behaviors occur.

*Exacerbation of Intermittent Porphyria.* Phenobarbital can exacerbate acute intermittent porphyria. Accordingly, the drug is absolutely contraindicated for patients with a history of this disorder.

*Use in Pregnancy.* Warn women of child-bearing age that barbiturates may cause birth defects.

*Withdrawal Seizures.* Abrupt withdrawal of phenobarbital can trigger seizures. Warn the patient against abrupt discontinuation of treatment.

### Minimizing Adverse Interactions

*Interactions Due to Induction of Drug Metabolism.* Phenobarbital can decrease responses to other drugs by inducing hepatic drug-metabolizing enzymes. Effects on *oral contraceptives* and *warfarin* are of particular concern. Patients using these drugs require increased dosages to maintain therapeutic responses.

*CNS Depressants.* Warn the patient against use of alcohol and all other drugs with CNS-depressant properties (e.g., opioids, benzodiazepines).

*Valproic Acid.* Valproic acid increases blood levels of phenobarbital. To avoid toxicity, the dosage of phenobarbital should be reduced.

## Carbamazepine

Nursing implications for carbamazepine include those presented below as well as those presented above for all antiseizure drugs.

## Preadministration Assessment

### Therapeutic Goal

Carbamazepine is used to treat partial seizures (simple and complex) and tonic-clonic seizures.

### Baseline Data

Obtain complete blood counts prior to treatment.

### Identifying High-Risk Patients

Carbamazepine is *contraindicated* for patients with a *history of bone marrow depression or adverse hematologic reactions to other drugs.*

## Implementation: Administration

### Route

Oral.

### Administration

Advise the patient to administer carbamazepine with meals to decrease gastric upset.

Use of low initial doses and administering the largest portion of the daily dose at bedtime can minimize adverse CNS effects.

## Ongoing Evaluation and Interventions

### Minimizing Adverse Effects

*CNS Effects.* Carbamazepine can cause headache, visual disturbances (nystagmus, blurred vision, diplopia), ataxia, vertigo, and unsteadiness. To minimize these effects, initiate therapy with low doses and have the patient take the largest portion of the daily dose at bedtime.

*Hematologic Effects.* Carbamazepine can cause leukopenia, anemia, thrombocytopenia, and, very rarely, fatal aplastic anemia. To reduce the risk of serious hematologic effects, (1) obtain complete blood counts prior to treatment and periodically thereafter; (2) avoid carbamazepine in patients with pre-existing hematologic abnormalities; and (3) inform patients about manifestations of hematologic abnormalities (fever, sore throat, pallor, weakness, infection, easy bruising, petechiae), and instruct them to notify the physician if these occur.

### Minimizing Adverse Interactions

*Interactions Due to Induction of Drug Metabolism.* Carbamazepine can decrease responses to other drugs by inducing hepatic drug-metabolizing enzymes. Effects on oral contraceptives and oral anticoagulants are of particular concern. Patients using these drugs will require increased dosages to maintain therapeutic responses.

*Phenytoin and Phenobarbital.* These drugs can decrease responses to carbamazepine by inducing drug-metabolizing enzymes (beyond the degree of induction caused by carbamazepine itself). Dosage of carbamazepine may need to be increased.

# Valproic Acid

Nursing implications for valproic acid include those presented below as well as those presented above for all antiseizure drugs.

## Preadministration Assessment

### Therapeutic Goal
Valproic acid is labeled only for treatment of absence seizures. However, the drug is also used widely to treat tonic-clonic seizures, myoclonic seizures, atonic seizures, and partial seizures (simple and complex).

### Baseline Data
Obtain baseline tests of liver function.

### Identifying High-Risk Patients
Valproic acid is *contraindicated* for patients with *significant hepatic dysfunction* and for *children under the age of 3 years who are taking other antiseizure drugs.*

## Implementation: Administration

### Route
Oral.

### Administration
Advise patients to take valproic acid with meals to reduce gastric upset.

Instruct patients to ingest tablets and capsules intact, without crushing or chewing.

## Ongoing Evaluation and Interventions

### Minimizing Adverse Effects
*Hepatotoxicity.* Rarely, valproic acid has caused fatal liver injury. To minimize the risk of hepatotoxicity, (1) don't use valproic acid in conjunction with other drugs in children under the age of 3 years; (2) don't use valproic acid in patients with pre-existing liver dysfunction; (3) evaluate liver function before initiating treatment and periodically thereafter; (4) inform patients about signs and symptoms of liver injury (reduced appetite, malaise, nausea, abdominal pain, jaundice), and instruct them to notify the physician if these develop; and (5) use valproic acid in the lowest effective dosage.

*Teratogenesis.* Valproic acid may cause birth defects. Advise women of child-bearing age to avoid pregnancy. If pregnancy occurs, the risks to the fetus must be weighed against the benefits of continued drug use.

### Minimizing Adverse Interactions
*Anticonvulsants.* Valproic acid can elevate plasma levels of phenytoin and phenobarbital. Levels of phenobarbital and phenytoin should be monitored and their dosages adjusted accordingly.

# CHAPTER 24

# Drugs for Muscle Spasm and Spasticity

**Drug Therapy of Muscle Spasm: Centrally Acting
    Muscle Relaxants**
**Drugs for Spasticity**
    Baclofen
    Diazepam
    Dantrolene

I n this chapter we consider two groups of drugs that promote skeletal muscle relaxation. One group is used to treat localized muscle spasm. The other is used to treat spasticity. With only one exception (dantrolene), these drugs produce their therapeutic effects through actions in the central nervous system (CNS). As a rule, the drugs used to treat spasticity do not relieve acute muscle spasm and vice versa. Hence, the two groups are not interchangeable.

## Drug Therapy of Muscle Spasm: Centrally Acting Muscle Relaxants

Muscle spasm is defined as an involuntary contraction of a muscle or muscle group. Muscle spasm is often painful and decreases the patient's level of functioning. Spasm can result from a variety of causes, including epilepsy, hypocalcemia, acute and chronic pain syndromes, and trauma (localized skeletal muscle injury). Discussion in this chapter is limited to spasm resulting from muscle injury.

Treatment of spasm involves physical measures as well as pharmacologic therapy. Physical measures include immobilization of the affected muscle, application of cold compresses, whirlpool baths, and physical therapy. For drug therapy, two groups of medicines are used: (1) analgesic anti-inflammatory agents (e.g., aspirin), and (2) centrally acting skeletal muscle relaxants. The analgesic anti-inflammatory agents are discussed in Chapter 64 (Aspirin-like Drugs). The centrally acting skeletal muscle relaxants are discussed below.

The family of centrally acting muscle relaxants consists of nine drugs (Table 24–1). All share similar pharmacologic properties. Hence, we will consider these drugs as a group.

## Mechanism of Action

The mechanism by which the centrally acting muscle relaxants relieve spasm is not clear. In laboratory animals, high doses can depress spinal reflexes. However, these doses are much higher than those used to relieve spasm in humans. Hence, many investigators believe that relaxation of spasm results from the sedative properties of these drugs, and not from specific actions exerted on CNS pathways involved in the control of muscle tone.

## Therapeutic Use

The centrally acting muscle relaxants are used to treat localized spasm resulting from muscle injury. These agents can decrease local pain and tenderness and can increase range of motion. Treatment is almost always associated with sedation. The ability of central muscle relaxants to relieve discomfort of muscle spasm appears about equal to that of aspirin and the other analgesic anti-inflammatory drugs. Since there are no studies to indicate the superiority of one centrally acting muscle relaxant over another, drug selection is based largely on the physician's preference and the patient's response. With the exception of diazepam, the central muscle relaxants are not useful for spasticity or other muscle disorders resulting from CNS pathology.

## Adverse Effects

*CNS Depression.* All of the centrally acting muscle relaxants can produce generalized depression of the CNS. Drowsiness, dizziness, and lightheadedness are common. Patients should be warned not to participate in hazardous activities (e.g., driving) if CNS depression is significant.

Depression of the CNS caused by central muscle relaxants can be additive with that caused by other drugs. Hence the patient should be warned against concurrent use of other CNS depressants (e.g., opioids, antihistamines, alcohol, barbiturates).

*Physical Dependence.* Chronic, high-dose therapy can cause physical dependence, manifesting as an abstinence

## TABLE 24–1. DRUGS FOR MUSCLE SPASM: CENTRALLY ACTING MUSCLE RELAXANTS

| Generic Name | Trade Names | Usual Adult Oral Maintenance Dosage |
| --- | --- | --- |
| Baclofen | Lioresal | 15 to 20 mg 3 to 4 times/day |
| Carisoprodol | Soma | 350 mg 4 times/day |
| Chlorphenesin | Maolate | 400 to 800 mg 4 times/day |
| Chlorzoxazone | Paraflex, Parafon Forte, Remular-S | 250 mg 3 to 4 times/day |
| Cyclobenzaprine | Flexeril | 10 mg 3 times/day |
| Diazepam | Valium, Valrelease, Zetran | 2 to 10 mg 3 to 4 times/day |
| Metaxalone | Skelaxin | 800 mg 3 to 4 times/day |
| Methocarbamol | Robaxin | 1000 mg 4 times/day |
| Orphenadrine | Norflex, Banflex, others | 100 mg morning and evening |

syndrome if these drugs are abruptly withdrawn. Accordingly, withdrawal should always be done slowly.

**Hepatic Toxicity.** *Chlorzoxazone* [Maolate] can cause hepatitis and potentially fatal hepatic necrosis. Because of this potential for harm, and because the benefits of chlorzoxazone are questionable, the drug should not be used.

**Other Adverse Effects.** *Carisoprodol* can be hazardous to patients predisposed to intermittent porphyria, and therefore is contraindicated for these people. *Cyclobenzaprine* has significant anticholinergic (atropine-like) properties; possible effects include dry mouth, blurred vision, photophobia, urinary retention, and constipation.

### Dosage and Administration

All centrally acting skeletal muscle relaxants can be administered orally. In addition, two agents—methocarbamol and diazepam—can be administered by injection (IM and IV). Average oral maintenance dosages for adults are listed in Table 24–1.

# Drugs for Spasticity

The term *spasticity* refers to a group of movement disorders of CNS origin. These disorders are characterized by heightened muscle tone, spasm, and loss of dexterity. The most common causes of spasticity are multiple sclerosis and cerebral palsy. Other causes include traumatic spinal cord lesions and stroke. Spasticity is managed with a combination of drugs and physical therapy.

Three drugs—baclofen, diazepam, and dantrolene—are effective in treating spasticity. Two of these agents—baclofen and diazepam—act in the CNS to relieve spasticity. The third drug—dantrolene—acts directly on skeletal muscle. With the exception of diazepam, the drugs employed to treat muscle spasm (i.e., the centrally acting muscle relaxants) are ineffective against spasticity.

## Baclofen

### Mechanism of Action

Baclofen acts within the spinal cord to suppress hyper-

active reflexes involved in regulation of muscle movement. The precise mechanism of reflex attenuation is not known. Since baclofen is a structural analog of the inhibitory neurotransmitter gamma-aminobutyric acid (GABA) (Fig. 24–1), the drug may act by mimicking the actions of GABA on spinal neurons. Baclofen has no direct effects on skeletal muscle.

### Therapeutic Use

Baclofen can reduce spasticity associated with multiple sclerosis, spinal cord injury, and cerebral palsy but not with stroke. The drug decreases flexor and extensor spasms and suppresses resistance to passive movement. These actions reduce the discomfort of spasticity and allow increased performance. Since baclofen has no direct muscle-relaxant action, and hence does not decrease muscle strength, baclofen is preferred to dantrolene in patients whose spasticity is associated with significant muscle weakness. Baclofen does not relieve the spasticity of Parkinson's disease or Huntington's chorea.

### Adverse Effects

The most common side effects involve the CNS and GI tract. Serious adverse effects are rare.

**CNS Effects.** Baclofen is a CNS depressant and frequently causes drowsiness, dizziness, weakness, and fatigue. These responses are most intense during the early phase of therapy and diminish with continued drug use.

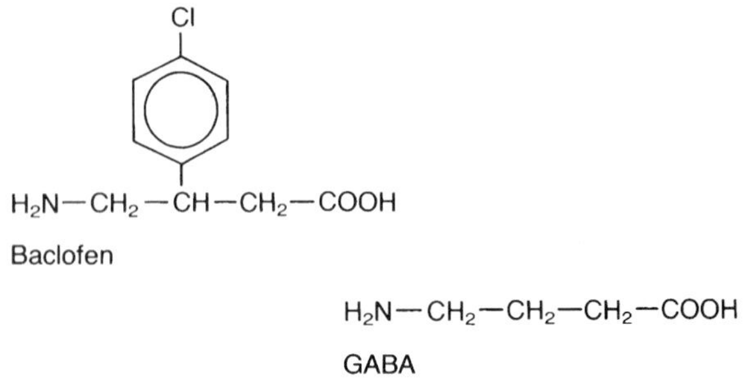

Figure 24–1. Structural similarity between baclofen and gamma-aminobutyric acid (GABA).

CNS depression can be minimized with doses that are small initially and then gradually increased. Patients should be cautioned against use of alcohol and other CNS depressants, since baclofen potentiates the depressant actions of these drugs.

Overdose with baclofen can produce coma and respiratory depression. Since there is no antidote to baclofen poisoning, treatment is supportive.

Although baclofen does not appear to cause physical dependence, abrupt discontinuation of the drug has been associated with adverse reactions, including visual hallucinations, paranoid ideation, and seizures. Accordingly, drug withdrawal should be done slowly (over 1 to 2 weeks).

***Other Adverse Effects.*** Baclofen frequently causes *nausea*, *constipation*, and *urinary retention*. Patients should be warned about these possible reactions.

#### Preparations, Dosage, and Administration

***Oral.*** Baclofen [Lioresal] is dispensed in tablets (10 and 20 mg) for oral use. Dosages are low initially (e.g., 5 mg 3 times a day) and then gradually increased. Maintenance dosages range from 15 to 20 mg administered 3 to 4 times a day.

***Intrathecal.*** Baclofen can be administered by intrathecal infusion using an implantable pump. The average maintenance dosage is 300 to 800 µg/day.

## Diazepam

Diazepam is a member of the benzodiazepine family. Although diazepam is the only benzodiazepine labeled for treating spasticity, other benzodiazepines would probably be effective as well. The basic pharmacology of the benzodiazepines is discussed in Chapter 32. The use of diazepam in spasticity is considered below.

***Actions.*** Like baclofen, diazepam acts within the CNS to suppress spasticity. Beneficial effects appear to result from mimicking the actions of GABA at receptors in the spinal cord and brain. Diazepam does not affect skeletal muscle directly. Since diazepam has no direct effects on muscle strength, the drug is preferred to dantrolene in patients whose strength is marginal.

***Adverse Effects.*** *Sedation* is common when treating spasticity. To minimize sedation, initiate therapy with low doses. Other adverse effects are discussed in Chapter 32.

***Preparations, Dosage, and Administration.*** For oral use, diazepam [Valium, Valrelease, Zetran] is dispensed in tablets (2, 5, and 10 mg), sustained-release capsules (15 mg), and solution (1 and 5 mg/ml). The drug is also available as an injection (5 mg/ml) for IM and IV administration. The usual oral dosage for adults is 2 to 10 mg 3 to 4 times a day.

## Dantrolene

### Mechanism of Action

Unlike baclofen and diazepam, which act within the CNS, dantrolene acts directly on skeletal muscle to relieve spasticity. The drug's primary action is suppression of calcium release from the sarcoplasmic reticulum (SR). This, in turn, decreases the ability of skeletal muscle to contract. Fortunately, therapeutic doses have only minimal effects on smooth muscle and cardiac muscle.

### Therapeutic Uses

***Spasticity.*** Dantrolene can relieve spasticity associated with multiple sclerosis, cerebral palsy, and spinal cord injury. Unfortunately, since dantrolene suppresses spasticity by causing a generalized reduction in the ability of skeletal muscle to contract, treatment may be associated with a significant decrease in strength. As a result, for some patients, overall function may be reduced rather than improved. Accordingly, care must be taken to ensure that the benefits of therapy (reduced spasticity) outweigh the harm (reduced strength).

***Malignant Hyperthermia.*** Malignant hyperthermia is a rare, life-threatening syndrome that can be triggered by any general anesthetic and by succinylcholine, a neuromuscular blocking agent. Onset of symptoms is most abrupt with succinylcholine (when used alone or in combination with an anesthetic). Prominent symptoms are muscle rigidity and profound elevation of temperature. The heat of malignant hyperthermia is generated by muscle contraction occurring secondary to massive release of calcium from the SR. Dantrolene relieves symptoms by acting on the SR to block calcium release. Malignant hyperthermia is discussed further in Chapter 17.

### Adverse Effects

***Hepatic Toxicity.*** Dose-related liver damage is dantrolene's most serious adverse effect. Liver injury has an incidence of 1 in 1000. Death has occurred. Hepatotoxicity is most common in women over 35. In contrast, liver injury in children under 10 years is rare. To reduce the risk of liver damage, tests of liver function should be performed prior to treatment and throughout the treatment interval. Because of the potential for liver damage, dantrolene should be administered in the lowest effective dosage and for the shortest time necessary.

***Other Adverse Effects.*** *Muscle weakness, drowsiness,* and *diarrhea* are the most common side effects. Muscle weakness is a direct extension of dantrolene's pharmacologic action. Other disturbing reactions include *anorexia, nausea, vomiting,* and *acne-like rash.*

#### Preparations, Dosage, and Administration

***Preparations.*** Dantrolene sodium [Dantrium] is dispensed in capsules (25, 50, and 100 mg) for oral use and as a powder to be reconstituted for IV injection.

***Use in Spasticity.*** For treatment of spasticity, the drug is administered orally. The initial dosage in adults is 25 mg once daily. The usual maintenance dosage is 100 mg 2 to 4 times a day. If beneficial effects do not develop within 45 days, dantrolene therapy should cease.

***Use in Malignant Hyperthermia.*** *Preoperative Prophylaxis.* Patients with a history of malignant hyperthermia can be given dantrolene for prophylaxis prior to elective surgery. The dosage is 4 to 8 mg/kg/day in four divided doses for 1 to 2 days preceding surgery.

*Treatment of an Ongoing Crisis.* For treatment of malignant hyperthermia, dantrolene is administered by IV push. The initial dose is 2 mg/kg. Administration is repeated until symptoms are controlled or until a total dose of 10 mg/kg has been given. Other management measures are discussed in Chapter 17.

## KEY POINTS

- Localized muscle spasm is treated with centrally acting muscle relaxants and aspirin-like drugs.
- Spasticity is treated with three drugs: baclofen, diazepam, and dantrolene.
- All centrally acting muscle relaxants produce generalized CNS depression.
- Chlorzoxazone, a central muscle relaxant, is marginally effective and can cause fatal hepatic necrosis. The drug should not be used.
- Baclofen and diazepam relieve spasticity by mimicking the inhibitory actions of GABA in the CNS.
- Like the centrally acting muscle relaxants, baclofen and diazepam cause generalized CNS depression.
- In contrast to the other drugs in this chapter, dantrolene acts directly on muscle to promote relaxation.
- With prolonged use, dantrolene can cause potentially fatal liver damage. Monitor liver function and minimize dosage and duration of treatment.
- In addition to relief of spasticity, dantrolene is used to treat malignant hyperthermia, a potentially fatal condition caused by succinylcholine and general anesthetics.

## Summary of Major Nursing Implications*

### Drugs Used to Treat Muscle Spasm: Centrally Acting Skeletal Muscle Relaxants

| | |
|---|---|
| Baclofen | Diazepam |
| Carisoprodol | Metaxalone |
| Chlorphenesin | Methocarbamol |
| Chlorzoxazone | Orphenadrine |
| Cyclobenzaprine | |

The nursing implications summarized below apply to all centrally acting muscle relaxants used to treat muscle spasm.

### Preadministration Assessment

#### Therapeutic Goal
Relief of signs and symptoms of muscle spasm.

### Implementation: Administration

#### Routes
*Oral.* Used for all central skeletal muscle relaxants.

*Parenteral. Methocarbamol* and *diazepam* may be given IM and IV as well as PO.

#### Dosage
See Table 24-1.

### Implementation: Measures to Enhance Therapeutic Effects

The treatment plan should include appropriate physical measures (e.g., immobilization of the affected muscle, application of cold compresses, whirlpool baths, and physical therapy).

### Ongoing Evaluation and Interventions

#### Minimizing Adverse Effects
*CNS Depression.* All central muscle relaxants cause CNS depression. Inform patients about possible effects (drowsiness, dizziness, lightheadedness, fatigue) and advise them to avoid hazardous activities (e.g., driving) if significant impairment occurs.

*Hepatic Toxicity. Chlorzoxazone* can cause hepatitis and potentially fatal hepatic necrosis. The drug should not be used.

#### Minimizing Adverse Interactions
*CNS Depressants.* Caution the patient against use of CNS depressants (e.g., alcohol, benzodiazepines, opioids, antihistamines) since these will intensify depressant effects of the muscle relaxants.

#### Avoiding Withdrawal Reactions
Central muscle relaxants can cause physical dependence. To avoid an abstinence syndrome, withdraw gradually. Warn the patient against abrupt discontinuation of treatment.

### Baclofen

### Preadministration Assessment

#### Therapeutic Goal
Relief of signs and symptoms of spasticity.

#### Baseline Data
Assess for muscle rigidity, muscle spasm, pain, range of motion, and dexterity.

### Implementation: Administration

#### Route
Oral.

#### Administration
The spastic patient may be unable to self-medicate. Provide assistance if needed.

---

*Patient education information is highlighted in color.

## Ongoing Evaluation and Interventions

### Evaluating Therapeutic Effects

Monitor for reductions in rigidity, muscle spasm, and pain and for improvements in dexterity and range of motion.

### Minimizing Adverse Effects

*CNS Depression.* Baclofen is a CNS depressant. Inform patients about possible depressant effects (drowsiness, dizziness, lightheadedness, fatigue) and advise them to avoid hazardous activities (e.g., driving) if significant impairment occurs.

### Minimizing Adverse Interactions

*CNS Depressants.* Caution the patient against use of CNS depressants (e.g., alcohol, benzodiazepines, opioids, antihistamines) since these will intensify depressant effects of baclofen.

### Avoiding Withdrawal Reactions

Abrupt withdrawal can cause visual hallucinations, paranoid ideation, and seizures. Caution the patient against abrupt discontinuation of treatment.

## Dantrolene

The nursing implications summarized here apply only to the use of dantrolene for spasticity.

## Preadministration Assessment

### Therapeutic Goal

Relief of signs and symptoms of spasticity.

### Baseline Data

Assess for muscle rigidity, muscle spasm, pain, range of motion, and dexterity. Obtain laboratory tests of liver function.

### Identifying High-Risk Patients

Dantrolene is *contraindicated* for patients with *active hepatic disease* (e.g., cirrhosis, hepatitis).

## Implementation: Administration

### Route

Oral.

### Administration

The spastic patient may be unable to self-medicate. Provide assistance if needed.

## Ongoing Evaluation and Interventions

### Summary of Monitoring

*Therapeutic Effects.* Monitor for reductions in rigidity, muscle spasm, and pain and for improvements in dexterity and range of motion.

*Adverse Effects.* Monitor liver function tests and for reductions in muscle strength.

### Minimizing Adverse Effects

*CNS Depression.* Dantrolene is a CNS depressant. Inform patients about possible depressant effects (drowsiness, dizziness, lightheadedness, fatigue) and advise them to avoid hazardous activities (e.g., driving) if significant impairment occurs.

*Hepatic Toxicity.* Dantrolene is hepatotoxic. Assess liver function prior to treatment and periodically thereafter. If signs of liver dysfunction develop, withdraw dantrolene. Inform patients about signs of liver dysfunction (e.g., jaundice, abdominal pain, malaise) and instruct them to notify the physician if these develop.

*Muscle Weakness.* Dantrolene can decrease muscle strength. Evaluate muscle function to ensure that benefits of therapy (decreased spasticity) are not outweighed by reductions in strength.

### Minimizing Adverse Interactions

*CNS Depressants.* Caution the patient against use of CNS depressants (e.g., alcohol, benzodiazepines, opioids, antihistamines), since these will intensify depressant effects of dantrolene.

## Diazepam

Nursing implications for diazepam and the other benzodiazepines are summarized in Chapter 32.

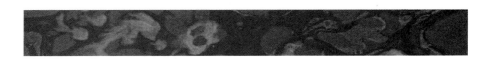

# Analgesics and Anesthetics

# CHAPTER 25

# Opioid (Narcotic) Analgesics

nalgesics are drugs that relieve pain without causing loss of consciousness. As a group, the opioids are the most effective analgesics available. The opioid family, whose name derives from opium, includes such widely used agents as morphine, codeine, meperidine [Demerol], and propoxyphene [Darvon].

## Introduction to the Opioids

### Terminology

*Opioid* is a general term defined as any drug, natural or synthetic, that has actions similar to those of morphine. The term *opiate* is more specific and applies only to compounds present in opium (e.g., morphine, codeine).

The term *narcotic* has had so many definitions that it can no longer be used with precision. Narcotic has been used to mean analgesic, central nervous system (CNS) depressant, and any drug capable of causing physical dependence. Narcotic has also been employed in a legal context to designate not only the opioids but also such diverse drugs as cocaine, marijuana, and lysergic acid diethylamide (LSD). Because of its more precise definition, *opioid* is clearly preferable to *narcotic* as a label for a discrete family of pharmacologic agents.

### Endogenous Opioid Peptides

The body has three families of peptides that have opioid-like properties. These families are named *enkephalins*, *endorphins*, and *dynorphins*. Although we know that endogenous opioid peptides serve as neurotransmitters, neurohormones, and neuromodulators, the precise physiologic role of these compounds is not fully understood. Endogenous opioid peptides are found in the CNS and in peripheral tissues.

### Opioid Receptors

There are three main classes of opioid receptors, designated *mu*, *kappa*, and *delta*. From a pharmacologic perspective, mu receptors are most important. This is because opioid analgesics act primarily through activation of mu receptors, although they also produce weak activation of kappa receptors. As a rule, opioid analgesics do not interact with delta receptors. In contrast to opioid analgesics, endogenous opioid peptides act through all three types of opioid receptors, including delta receptors. Important responses to activation of mu and kappa receptors are summarized in Table 25–1.

**Mu Receptors.** Responses to activation of mu receptors include analgesia, respiratory depression, euphoria, and sedation. In addition, mu activation is related to development of physical dependence.

A recent study in genetically engineered mice underscores the importance of mu receptors in drug action. In this study, researchers employed mice from which the gene for mu receptors had been deleted. When these mice were given morphine, the drug had no effect. It did not produce analgesia; it did not produce physical dependence; and it did not reinforce social behaviors that are thought to indicate subjective effects. Hence, at least in mice, mu receptors appear both necessary and sufficient to mediate the major actions of opioid drugs.

**Kappa Receptors.** As with mu receptors, activation of kappa receptors can produce analgesia and sedation. In addition, kappa activation may underlie psychotomimetic effects seen with certain opioids.

## TABLE 25-1. IMPORTANT RESPONSES TO ACTIVATION OF MU AND KAPPA RECEPTORS

| | Receptor Type | |
|---|---|---|
| Response | Mu | Kappa |
| Analgesia | ✔ | ✔ |
| Respiratory depression | ✔ | |
| Sedation | ✔ | ✔ |
| Euphoria | ✔ | |
| Physical dependence | ✔ | |
| Decreased GI motility | ✔ | ✔ |

## TABLE 25-2. DRUG ACTIONS AT MU AND KAPPA RECEPTORS

| | Receptor Type | |
|---|---|---|
| Drugs | Mu | Kappa |
| *Pure Opioid Agonists* | | |
| Morphine, codeine, meperidine, and other morphine-like drugs | Agonist | Agonist |
| *Agonist-Antagonists Opioids* | | |
| Pentazocine, nalbuphine, and butorphanol | Antagonist | Agonist |
| Buprenorphine | Partial agonist | Antagonist |
| *Pure Opioid Antagonists* | | |
| Naloxone, naltrexone, and nalmefene | Antagonist | Antagonist |

## Classification of Drugs That Act at Opioid Receptors

Drugs that act at opioid receptors are classified on the basis of how they affect receptor function. At each type of receptor, a drug can act in one of three ways: as an *agonist*, *partial agonist*, or *antagonist*. (Recall from Chapter 6 that a partial agonist is a drug that produces low to moderate receptor activation when administered alone, but will block the actions of a full agonist if the two drugs are given concurrently.) Based on these actions, drugs that bind opioid receptors fall into three major groups: (1) pure opioid agonists, (2) agonist-antagonist opioids, and (3) pure opioid antagonists. The actions of drugs in these groups at mu and kappa receptors are summarized in Table 25-2.

**Pure Opioid Agonists.** The pure opioid agonists activate mu and kappa receptors. By activating these receptors, the pure agonists can produce analgesia, euphoria, sedation, respiratory depression, physical dependence, constipation, and other effects. As indicated in Table 25-3, the pure agonists can be subdivided into two groups: *strong opioid agonists* and *moderate-to-strong opioid agonists*. Morphine is the prototype of the strong agonists. Codeine is the prototype of the moderate-to-strong agonists.

**Agonist-Antagonist Opioids.** Five agonist-antagonist opioids are available: pentazocine, nalbuphine, butorphanol, dezocine, and buprenorphine. The actions of these drugs at mu and kappa receptors are summarized in Table 25-2. When administered alone, the agonist-antagonist opioids produce analgesia. However, if given to a patient who is taking a pure opioid agonist, these drugs can *antagonize* analgesia caused by the pure agonist. Pentazocine [Talwin] is the prototype of the agonist-antagonists.

**Pure Opioid Antagonists.** The pure opioid antagonists act as antagonists at mu and kappa receptors. These drugs do not produce analgesia or any of the other effects caused by opioid agonists. The principal use for these agents is reversal of respiratory and CNS depression caused by overdose with opioid agonists. Naloxone [Narcan] is the prototype of the pure antagonists.

# Basic Pharmacology of the Opioids

## Morphine

Morphine is the prototype of the strong opioid analgesics and remains the standard by which newer opioids are measured. Morphine has multiple pharmacologic effects, including analgesia, sedation, euphoria, respiratory depression, cough suppression, and suppression of bowel motility. The drug is named after Morpheus, the Greek god of dreams.

### Source

Morphine is found in the seed pod of the poppy plant, *Papaver somniferum*. The drug is prepared by extraction from opium, which is the dried juice of the poppy seed pod. In addition to morphine, opium contains two other medicinal compounds: codeine (an analgesic) and papaverine (a smooth muscle relaxant).

### Overview of Pharmacologic Actions

Morphine has multiple pharmacologic actions. In addition to relieving pain, the drug causes drowsiness, mental clouding, reduction of anxiety, and a sense of well-being. Through actions in the CNS and periphery, morphine can cause respiratory depression, constipation, urinary retention, orthostatic hypotension, emesis, miosis, cough suppression, and biliary colic. With prolonged treatment, the drug produces tolerance and physical dependence.

Individual effects of morphine may be beneficial, detrimental, or both. For example, analgesia is clearly beneficial, whereas respiratory depression and urinary reten-

## TABLE 25-3. OPIOID ANALGESICS: ABUSE LIABILITY AND MAXIMAL PAIN RELIEF

| Drug and Category | Controlled Substances Act Schedule | Abuse Liability | Maximal Pain Relief |
|---|---|---|---|
| *Strong Opioid Agonists* | | | |
| Alfentanil | II | High | High |
| Fentanyl | II | High | High |
| Hydromorphone | II | High | High |
| Levomethadyl | II | High | NA* |
| Levorphanol | II | High | High |
| Meperidine | II | High | High |
| Methadone | II | High | High |
| Morphine | II | High | High |
| Oxymorphone | II | High | High |
| Remifentanil | NR | — | High |
| Sufentanil | II | High | High |
| *Moderate-to-Strong Opioid Agonists* | | | |
| Codeine | II | Moderate | Moderate to high |
| Hydrocodone | III † | Moderate | Moderate to high |
| Oxycodone | II | Moderate | Moderate to high |
| Propoxyphene | IV | Low | Moderate |
| *Agonist-Antagonist Opioids* | | | |
| Buprenorphine | V | Low | Moderate |
| Dezocine | NR ‡ | Low | Moderate |
| Butorphanol | NR ‡ | Low | Moderate to high |
| Nalbuphine | NR ‡ | Low | Moderate to high |
| Pentazocine | IV | Low | Moderate to high |

*NA = not applicable. Levomethadyl is used only for treating opioid addicts. The drug is not used for pain relief.

†In the United States, hydrocodone is available only in combination with aspirin or acetaminophen. These combination products are classified under Schedule III.

‡NR = not regulated under the Controlled Substances Act.

tion are clearly detrimental. Certain other effects, such as sedation and reduced bowel motility, may be beneficial or detrimental, depending on the circumstances of drug use.

### Therapeutic Use: Relief of Pain

The principal indication for morphine is relief of moderate to severe pain. The drug can relieve postoperative pain, chronic pain of cancer, and pain associated with labor and delivery. In addition, morphine is the drug of choice for relieving pain of myocardial infarction (MI) and dyspnea associated with left ventricular failure and pulmonary edema. Morphine may also be administered preoperatively for sedation and reduction of anxiety.

Morphine relieves pain without affecting other senses (e.g., sight, touch, smell, hearing) and without causing loss of consciousness. The drug is more effective against constant, dull pain than against sharp, intermittent pain. However, even sharp pain can be relieved by sufficiently large doses. The ability of morphine to cause mental

clouding, sedation, euphoria, and anxiety reduction can contribute to relief of pain.

To understand morphine-induced analgesia, we need to understand pain itself. Pain has two components: *sensation* and *suffering* (emotional reaction to the sensation of pain). Morphine decreases both the sensation of pain and the suffering that pain elicits. For some patients, the suffering component may be reduced even though perception of pain remains relatively undiminished. Hence, morphine may make the patient feel better without actually decreasing pain sensation. Accordingly, patients should not be told that morphine will make their pain go away, because it may not. Rather, patients should be told that morphine will make them feel more comfortable.

The use of morphine and other opioids to relieve pain is discussed in depth later in the chapter under *Clinical Use of Opioids*.

***Mechanism of Analgesic Action.*** Morphine and other opioid agonists relieve pain by mimicking the actions of endogenous opioid peptides, primarily at mu receptors. This hypothesis is based on the following observations:

- Opioid peptides and morphine-like drugs both produce analgesia when administered to experimental subjects.
- Opioid peptides and morphine-like drugs share structural similarities (Fig. 25-1).
- Opioid peptides and morphine-like drugs bind to the same receptors in the CNS.
- The receptors to which opioid peptides and morphine-like drugs bind are located in regions of the brain and spinal cord that are associated with perception of pain.
- Subjects rendered tolerant to analgesia from morphine-like drugs show cross-tolerance to analgesia from opioid peptides.
- The analgesic effects of opioid peptides and morphine-like drugs can both be blocked by the same antagonist (naloxone).

From these data it is postulated that (1) opioid peptides serve a physiologic role as modulators of pain perception, and (2) morphine-like drugs produce analgesia by mimicking the actions of endogenous opioid peptides.

## Adverse Effects

*Respiratory Depression.* Respiratory depression is the most serious adverse effect of the opioids. At equianalgesic doses, all of the pure opioid agonists depress respiration to the same degree. Death following overdose is almost always due to respiratory arrest. Opioids depress respiration primarily through activation of mu receptors, although activation of kappa receptors also contributes.

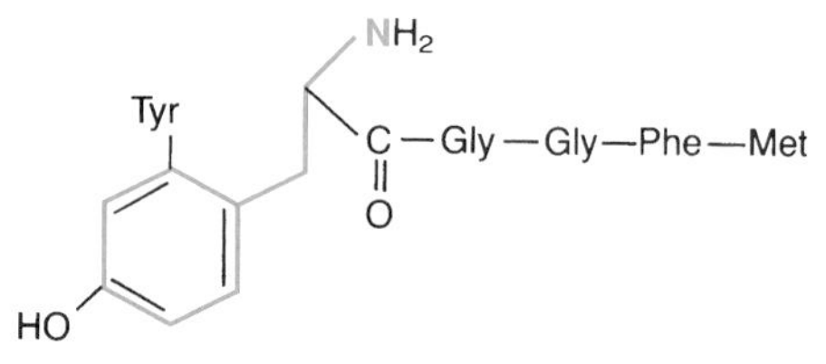

Met-Enkephalin

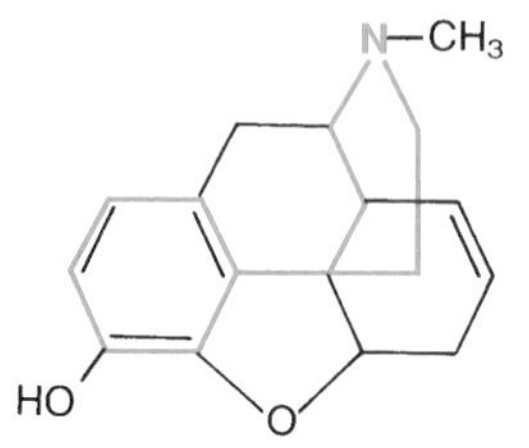

Morphine

**Figure 25-1. Structural similarity between morphine and met-enkephalin.** In the morphine structural formula, highlighting indicates the part of the molecule thought responsible for interaction with opioid receptors. In the met-enkephalin structural formula, highlighting indicates the region of structural similarity with morphine.

The time course of respiratory depression varies with route of administration. Depressant effects begin about 7 minutes after IV injection, 30 minutes after IM injection, and up to 90 minutes after SC injection. With all of these routes, significant depression may persist for 4 to 5 hours. When morphine is administered by spinal injection, onset of respiratory depression may be *delayed for hours*; you should be alert to this possibility.

With prolonged use of opioids, tolerance develops to respiratory depression. Huge doses that would be lethal to nontolerant individuals have been taken by opioid addicts without noticeable effect. Similarly, tolerance to respiratory depression develops during long-term clinical use of opioids (e.g., in patients with cancer).

When administered at usual therapeutic doses, opioids rarely cause significant respiratory depression. However, although uncommon, substantial respiratory depression can occur. Accordingly, respiratory rate should be determined prior to opioid administration. If the rate is 12 per minute or less, the opioid should be withheld and the physician notified. Certain patients, including the very young, the elderly, and those with respiratory disease (e.g., asthma, emphysema) are especially sensitive to respiratory depression and must be monitored closely. Outpatients should be informed about the risk of respiratory depression and instructed to notify the physician if respiratory distress occurs.

Respiratory depression is increased by concurrent use of other drugs with CNS-depressant actions (e.g., alcohol, barbiturates, benzodiazepines). Accordingly, these drugs should be avoided. Outpatients should be warned against use of alcohol and all other CNS depressants.

*Constipation.* Opioids promote constipation through a combination of effects on the gastrointestinal tract. Through actions exerted in the CNS and locally, these drugs suppress propulsive intestinal contractions, intensify nonpropulsive contractions, increase the tone of the anal sphincter, and inhibit secretion of fluids into the intestinal lumen. Bowel function should be monitored. A diet high in fiber and fluids will minimize disruption of bowel function. A laxative may be needed if constipation cannot be managed with diet alone.

Because of their effects on the intestine, opioids are highly effective for managing diarrhea. In fact, antidiarrheal use of these drugs preceded their analgesic use by centuries. The effect of opioids on intestinal function is an interesting example of how a drug response can be viewed as detrimental (constipation) or beneficial (relief of diarrhea) depending on who is taking the medication. Opioids employed specifically to treat diarrhea are discussed in Chapter 73.

*Orthostatic Hypotension.* Morphine-like drugs lower blood pressure by blunting the baroreceptor reflex and by dilating peripheral arterioles and veins. Peripheral vasodilation results primarily from morphine-induced release of histamine. Hypotension is mild in the recumbent patient but can be substantial when the patient assumes an erect posture. Patients should be informed about symptoms of hypotension (lightheadedness, dizziness) and instructed to sit or lie down if these occur. Also, patients should be informed that hypotension can be minimized by moving slowly when changing from a supine or seated position to an upright position. Patients should be warned against ambulation if hypotension is significant. Hospitalized patients may require ambulatory assistance. Hypotensive drugs can exacerbate opioid-induced hypotension.

*Urinary Retention.* Morphine can cause urinary hesitancy and urinary retention by increasing tone in the sphincter of the bladder. Also, by increasing tone in the detrusor muscle, the drug can elevate pressure within the bladder, causing urinary urgency. In addition to its direct effects on the urinary tract, morphine may interfere with voiding by suppressing awareness of bladder stimuli. Accordingly, patients should be encouraged to void every 4 hours. Urinary hesitancy or retention is especially likely in patients with prostatic hypertrophy.

Urinary retention should be assessed by monitoring intake and output and by palpating the lower abdomen every 4 to 6 hours for bladder distention. If a change in intake-output ratio develops, or if bladder distention is detected, or if the patient reports difficulty in voiding, the physician should be notified. Catheterization may be required.

In addition to causing urinary retention, morphine may decrease urine production. The drug reduces urine formation largely by decreasing renal blood flow, and partly by promoting release of antidiuretic hormone.

*Cough Suppression.* Morphine-like drugs act at opioid receptors in the medulla to suppress cough. Suppression of spontaneous cough may lead to accumulation of secretions in the airway. Accordingly, patients should be instructed to actively cough at regular intervals. Lung status should be assessed by auscultation for rales. The ability of opioids to suppress cough is put to clinical use in the form of codeine- and hydrocodone-based cough remedies.

*Biliary Colic.* Morphine can induce spasm of the common bile duct, causing pressure within the biliary tract to rise. Symptoms range from epigastric distress to biliary colic. In patients with pre-existing biliary colic, morphine may intensify pain rather than relieve it. Certain opioids (e.g., meperidine) cause less smooth muscle spasm than morphine, and hence are less likely to exacerbate biliary colic.

*Emesis.* Morphine promotes nausea and vomiting through direct stimulation of the chemoreceptor trigger zone (CTZ) of the medulla. These reactions are greatest with the initial dose and diminish with subsequent doses. Nausea and vomiting are uncommon in recumbent patients, but occur in 15% to 40% of ambulatory patients, suggesting a vestibular component to these effects. Nausea and vomiting can be reduced by pretreatment with an antiemetic (e.g., metoclopramide) and by having the patient remain still.

*Elevation of Intracranial Pressure.* Morphine can elevate intracranial pressure (ICP). The mechanism of this effect is indirect: by suppressing respiration, morphine increases the $CO_2$ content of blood, which dilates the cerebral vasculature, causing ICP to rise. Accordingly, if respiration is maintained at a normal rate, ICP will remain normal as well.

*Euphoria/Dysphoria.* *Euphoria* is defined as a sense of well-being. Morphine often produces euphoria when administered to patients in pain. Although euphoria can enhance pain relief, it also contributes to the drug's potential for abuse. Euphoria is caused by activation of mu receptors.

In some individuals, morphine causes *dysphoria* (a sense of anxiety and being ill at ease). Dysphoria is uncommon among patients in pain, but may occur when morphine is taken in the absence of pain.

*Sedation.* When administered to relieve pain, morphine is likely to cause drowsiness and some mental clouding. Although these effects can complement the drug's analgesic actions, they can also be detrimental. Outpatients should be warned about CNS depression and advised to avoid hazardous activities (e.g., driving) if sedation is significant. Sedation can be minimized by (1) reducing the size of each dose and the dosing interval, (2) using opioids that have short half-lives, and (3) giving small doses of a CNS stimulant (methylphenidate or dextroamphetamine) in the morning and early afternoon.

*Miosis.* Morphine and other opioids cause pupillary constriction (miosis). In response to toxic doses, the pupil may constrict to "pinpoint" size. Since miosis can impair vision in dim light, room light should be kept bright during waking hours.

## Pharmacokinetics

Morphine is administered by several routes: oral, intramuscular, intravenous, subcutaneous, epidural, and intrathecal. Onset of effects is slower with oral administration than with parenteral administration. With four routes—oral, IM, IV, and SC—analgesia lasts 4 to 5 hours. With two routes—epidural and intrathecal—analgesia may persist up to 24 hours.

In order to relieve pain, morphine must cross the blood-brain barrier and enter the CNS. Since the drug is not very lipid soluble, it does not cross the barrier easily. Consequently, only a small fraction of an administered dose reaches sites of analgesic action. Since the blood-brain barrier is not well developed in infants, these patients generally require lower doses than older children and adults.

Morphine is inactivated by hepatic metabolism. When taken by mouth, the drug must pass through the liver on its way to the systemic circulation. Much of an oral dose is inactivated during this first pass through the liver. Consequently, oral doses need to be substantially larger than parenteral doses to produce equivalent analgesic effects. Analgesia and other effects may be intensified and prolonged in patients with liver disease; hence it may be necessary to reduce the dosage or lengthen the dosing interval.

## Tolerance and Physical Dependence

With continuous use, morphine can cause tolerance and physical dependence. These phenomena, which are generally inseparable, reflect cellular adaptations that occur in response to prolonged opioid exposure.

*Tolerance.* Tolerance can be defined as a state in which a large dose is required to produce the same response that could formerly be elicited by a smaller dose. Alternatively, tolerance can be defined as a condition in which a particular dose produces a smaller response than it could when treatment began. Because of tolerance, dosage must be increased to maintain analgesic effects.

Tolerance develops to many—but not all—of morphine's actions. With prolonged treatment, tolerance develops to *analgesia, euphoria,* and *sedation.* As a result, with long-term therapy, an increase in dosage may be required to maintain these desirable effects. Fortunately, as tolerance develops to these therapeutic effects, tolerance also develops to *respiratory depression.* As a result, the high doses needed to control pain in the tolerant individual are not associated with increased respiratory depression.

Very little tolerance develops to *constipation* and *miosis.* Even in highly tolerant addicts, constipation remains a chronic problem, and constricted pupils are characteristic.

*Cross-tolerance* exists among the opioid agonists (e.g., meperidine, methadone, codeine, heroin). Accordingly, individuals tolerant to one of these agents will be tolerant to the others. No cross-tolerance exists between opioids and general CNS depressants (e.g., barbiturates, ethanol, benzodiazepines, general anesthetics).

*Physical Dependence.* Physical dependence is defined as a state in which an abstinence syndrome will occur if drug use is abruptly discontinued. Opioid dependence results from adaptive cellular changes that occur in response to the continuous presence of these drugs. Although the exact nature of these changes is unknown, it is clear that, once these compensatory changes have taken place, the body requires the continued presence of opioids to function normally. If opioids are withdrawn, an abstinence syndrome will result.

The intensity and duration of the opioid abstinence syndrome depends on the half-life of the drug being used and the degree of physical dependence. With opioids that have relatively short half-lives (e.g., morphine), symptoms of abstinence are intense but brief. In contrast, with opioids that have long half-lives (e.g., methadone), symptoms are less intense but more prolonged. With any opioid, the intensity of withdrawal symptoms parallels the degree of physical dependence.

For individuals who are highly dependent, the abstinence syndrome can be extremely unpleasant. Initial reactions include yawning, rhinorrhea, and sweating. Onset occurs about 10 hours after the last dose. These early responses are followed by anorexia, irritability, tremor, and "gooseflesh"—hence the term *cold turkey.* At its peak, the syndrome manifests as violent sneezing, weakness, nausea, vomiting, diarrhea, abdominal cramps, bone and muscle pain, muscle spasm, and kicking movements— hence, "kicking the habit." Administration of opioids at any time during withdrawal will rapidly reverse all signs

and symptoms. Left untreated, the morphine withdrawal syndrome runs its course in 7 to 10 days. It should be emphasized that, although withdrawal from opioids is unpleasant, the syndrome is rarely dangerous. In contrast, withdrawal from general CNS depressants (e.g., barbiturates, alcohol) can be lethal (see Chapter 32).

To minimize the abstinence syndrome, opioids should be withdrawn gradually. When the degree of dependence is moderate, symptoms can be avoided by administering progressively smaller doses over 3 days. When the patient is highly dependent, dosage should be tapered more slowly—over 7 to 10 days. With a proper withdrawal procedure, symptoms of abstinence will resemble those of a mild case of influenza—even when the degree of dependence is high.

It is important to note that physical dependence is rarely a complication when opioids are taken acutely to treat pain. Hospitalized patients receiving morphine 2 to 3 times a day for up to 2 weeks show no significant signs of dependence. If morphine is withheld from these patients, no significant signs of withdrawal can be detected. The issue of physical dependence as a clinical concern is discussed further later in the chapter.

Infants exposed to opioids *in utero* may be born drug dependent. If the infant is not provided with opioids, an abstinence syndrome will occur. Signs of withdrawal include excessive crying, sneezing, tremor, hyperreflexia, fever, and diarrhea. The infant can be weaned from drug dependence by administering dilute opium tincture in progressively smaller doses.

Cross-dependence exists among pure opioid agonists. As a result, any pure agonist will prevent withdrawal in a patient who is physically dependent on any other pure agonist.

## Abuse Liability

Morphine and the other opioids are subject to abuse, largely because of their ability to cause pleasurable experience (e.g., euphoria, sedation, a sensation in the lower abdomen resembling orgasm). Physical dependence contributes to abuse: once dependence exists, the ability of opioids to ward off withdrawal serves to reinforce their desirability in the mind of the abuser.

The abuse liability of the opioids is reflected in their classification under the Controlled Substances Act. (The provisions of this act are discussed in Chapter 35.) As shown in Table 25-3, morphine and practically all other strong opioid agonists are classified under Schedule II of the act. This classification reflects a moderate to high abuse liability. The agonist-antagonist opioids have a lower abuse liability and are classified under Schedule IV (pentazocine) or Schedule V (buprenorphine), or have no classification at all (dezocine, butorphanol, nalbuphine). Members of the health care team who prescribe, dispense, and administer opioids must adhere to the procedures set forth in the Controlled Substances Act.

Fortunately, abuse is rare when opioids are employed to treat pain. The issue of abuse as a clinical concern is discussed further later in the chapter.

## Precautions

Some patients are more likely than others to experience adverse reactions to opioids. Common sense dictates that opioids be used with special caution in these people. Conditions that can predispose patients to adverse reactions are discussed below.

**Decreased Respiratory Reserve.** Because of its respiratory depressant action, morphine can further compromise respiration in patients with impaired pulmonary function. Accordingly, the drug should be used with caution in patients with asthma, emphysema, kyphoscoliosis, chronic cor pulmonale, and extreme obesity. Caution must also be exercised in patients taking other drugs that can depress respiration (e.g., barbiturates, benzodiazepines, general anesthetics).

**Pregnancy.** Morphine does not cause birth defects in humans. However, regular use of opioids during pregnancy can cause physical dependence in the fetus. Accordingly, prolonged use by pregnant women should be avoided if possible.

**Labor and Delivery.** Use of morphine during delivery can suppress uterine contractions and cause respiratory depression in the neonate. Following delivery, respiration in the neonate should be monitored closely. Respiratory depression can be reversed with naloxone. The use of opioids in obstetrics is discussed further later in the chapter.

**Head Injury.** In patients with head injury, morphine can exacerbate elevation of ICP and can complicate diagnosis. Use of opioids in patients with head injury is discussed further later in the chapter.

**Other Precautions.** *Infants* and *elderly patients* are especially sensitive to the respiratory depressant action of morphine. In patients with *inflammatory bowel disease*, morphine may cause toxic megacolon or paralytic ileus. Since morphine and all other opioids are inactivated by the liver, effects of these agents may be intensified and prolonged in patients with *liver impairment*. Severe hypotension may occur in patients with pre-existing *hypotension* or *reduced blood volume*. In patients with *prostatic hypertrophy*, opioids may cause acute urinary retention; repeated catheterization may be required.

## Drug Interactions

The major interactions between morphine and other drugs are summarized in Table 25–4. Some of these interactions are adverse; others are beneficial.

**CNS Depressants.** All drugs with CNS-depressant actions (e.g., barbiturates, benzodiazepines, alcohol) can intensify sedation and respiratory depression caused by morphine and other opioids. Outpatients should be warned against use of alcohol and all other CNS depressants.

**Anticholinergic Drugs.** These agents (e.g., antihistamines, tricyclic antidepressants, atropine-like drugs) can exacerbate morphine-induced constipation and urinary retention.

**Hypotensive Drugs.** Antihypertensive drugs and other drugs that lower blood pressure can exacerbate morphine-induced hypotension.

**Monoamine Oxidase Inhibitors.** The combination of meperidine (a morphine-like drug) with a monoamine

### TABLE 25–4. INTERACTIONS OF MORPHINE-LIKE DRUGS WITH OTHER DRUGS

| Interacting Drugs | Outcome of the Interaction |
|---|---|
| *Adverse Interactions* | |
| CNS depressants | Increased respiratory depression and sedation |
|   Barbiturates | |
|   Benzodiazepines | |
|   Alcohol | |
|   General anesthetics | |
|   Antihistamines | |
|   Phenothiazines | |
| Agonist-antagonist opioids | Precipitation of a withdrawal reaction |
| Anticholinergic drugs | Increased constipation and urinary retention |
|   Atropine-like drugs | |
|   Antihistamines | |
|   Phenothiazines | |
|   Tricyclic antidepressants | |
| Hypotensive agents | Increased hypotension |
| Monoamine oxidase inhibitors | Hyperpyrexic coma |
| *Beneficial Interactions* | |
| Amphetamines | Increased analgesia and decreased sedation |
| Antiemetics | Suppression of nausea and vomiting |
| Naloxone | Suppression of symptoms of opioid overdose |

oxidase (MAO) inhibitor has produced a syndrome characterized by excitation, delirium, hyperpyrexia, convulsions, and severe respiratory depression. Death has occurred. Although this reaction has not been reported with combined use of an MAO inhibitor and morphine, prudence suggests that the combination nonetheless be avoided.

**Agonist-Antagonist Opioids.** These drugs (e.g., pentazocine, buprenorphine) can precipitate a withdrawal syndrome if administered to an individual who is physically dependent on a pure opioid agonist. The basis of this reaction is considered later in the chapter. Patients taking pure opioid agonists should be weaned from these drugs before beginning treatment with an agonist-antagonist.

**Opioid Antagonists.** Opioid antagonists (e.g., naloxone) can counteract most actions of morphine and other pure opioid agonists. Opioid antagonists are employed primarily to treat opioid overdose. The actions and uses of the opioid antagonists are discussed in detail later in the chapter.

**Other Interactions.** *Antiemetics* of the phenothiazine type (e.g., promethazine [Phenergan]) may be combined with opioids to reduce nausea and vomiting. *Amphetamines* and *clonidine* can enhance opioid-induced analgesia. *Amphetamines* can also offset sedation.

## Toxicity

**Clinical Manifestations.** Opioid overdose produces a classic triad of signs: *coma, respiratory depression,* and *pinpoint pupils.* Coma is profound, and the patient cannot be aroused. Respiratory rate may be as low as 2 to 4 per minute. Although the pupils are constricted initially, they may dilate as hypoxia sets in secondary to respiratory depression. Hypoxia may cause blood pressure to fall. Prolonged hypoxia may result in shock. When death occurs, respiratory arrest is almost always the immediate cause.

**Treatment.** Treatment consists primarily of *ventilatory support* and giving an *opioid antagonist.* Traditionally, naloxone [Narcan] has been the antagonist of choice. However, nalmefene [Revex], a new and longer acting antagonist, may be preferred for many patients. The pharmacology of the opioid antagonists is discussed later in the chapter.

## Preparations, Dosage, and Administration

**General Guidelines on Dosage and Administration.** Dosage must be individualized. High doses are required for patients with a low tolerance to pain or with extremely painful disorders. Patients with sharp, stabbing pain need higher doses than patients with dull pain. Elderly adults generally require lower doses than younger adults. Neonates require relatively low doses because of their poorly developed blood-brain barriers. For all patients, dosage should be reduced as pain subsides. Outpatients should be warned not to increase dosage without consulting the physician.

Before an opioid is administered, respiratory rate, blood pressure, and pulse rate should be determined. The drug should be withheld and the physician notified if respiratory rate is at or below 12 per minute, if blood pressure is significantly below the pretreatment value, or if pulse rate is significantly above or below the pretreatment value.

As a rule, opioids should be administered on a fixed schedule—not on a PRN basis. With a fixed schedule, medication is given before intense pain returns. As a result, the patient is spared needless discomfort; furthermore, anxiety about recurrence of pain is reduced. If breakthrough pain occurs, supplemental doses should be given.

Morphine and practically all other opioid agonists are classified under Schedule II of the Controlled Substances Act and must be dispensed accordingly.

**Preparations.** Morphine sulfate is available in seven formulations: *standard tablets* [MSIR] (15 and 30 mg); *soluble tablets* (10, 15, and 30 mg); *controlled-release tablets* [MS Contin, Roxanol SR] (30 and 60 mg); *sustained-release capsules* [Kadian] (20, 50, and 100 mg); *oral solution* [MSIR, Roxanol] (2, 4, and 20 mg/ml); *rectal suppositories* [RMS] (5, 10, 20, and 30 mg); and *solution for injection* [Astramorph PF, Duramorph] (concentrations range from 0.5 to 15 mg/ml).

**Dosage and Routes of Administration.** *Oral.* Oral administration is generally reserved for treating chronic, severe pain, such as that associated with cancer. Because oral morphine undergoes extensive metabolism on its first pass through the liver, oral doses are usually higher than parenteral doses. A typical dosage is 10 to 30 mg repeated every 4 hours as needed. However, oral dosing is highly individualized; hence, some patients may require 75 mg or more. Controlled-release tablets may be administered every 8 to 12 hours. Patient should be instructed to swallow these tablets intact, without crushing or chewing.

*Intramuscular and Subcutaneous.* Both routes are painful and unreliable. For adults, dosing is initiated at 5 to 10 mg every 4 hours, and then adjusted up or down as needed. The usual dosage for children is 0.1 to 0.2 mg/kg repeated every 4 hours as needed.

*Intravenous.* Intravenous morphine should be injected slowly (over 4 to 5 minutes). Rapid IV injection can cause severe adverse effects (profound hypotension, cardiac arrest, respiratory arrest) and should be avoided. When IV injections are made, an opioid antagonist (e.g., naloxone) and facilities for respiratory support should be available. Injections should be given with the patient lying down to minimize hypotension. The usual dose for adults is 4 to 10 mg (diluted in 4 to 5 ml of water for injection). The usual pediatric dose is 0.05 to 0.1 mg/kg.

*Epidural and Intrathecal.* When morphine is employed for spinal analgesia, epidural injection is preferred to intrathecal. With either route, onset of analgesia is rapid and the duration prolonged (up to 24 hours). The most troubling side effects of spinal morphine are delayed respiratory depression and delayed cardiac depression. Be alert for possible late reactions. The usual adult epidural dose is 5 mg. Intrathecal doses are much smaller—about one-tenth the epidural dose.

## Other Strong Opioid Agonists

In an effort to produce a strong analgesic with a low potential for abuse and respiratory depression, pharmaceutical scientists have created many new opioid analgesics. However, none of the newer pure opioid agonists can be considered truly superior to morphine: the newer pure opioids are essentially equal to morphine with respect to analgesic action, abuse liability, and the ability to cause respiratory depression. Also, to varying degrees, all of these drugs cause sedation, euphoria, constipation, urinary retention, cough suppression, hypotension, and miosis. However, despite their similarities to morphine, the newer drugs do have unique qualities. These special characteristics may render one agent more desirable than another in a particular clinical situation. With all of the newer pure opioid agonists, toxicity can be reversed with an opioid antagonist (e.g., naloxone). Important differences between morphine and the newer strong opioid analgesics are discussed below. Tables 25-5 and 25-6 summarize dosages, routes, and time courses for morphine and the newer opioid agonists.

## TABLE 25-5. CLINICAL PHARMACOLOGY OF PURE OPIOID AGONISTS*

| Drug and Route | Equivalent Dose (mg)† | Time Course of Analgesic Effects | | |
| --- | --- | --- | --- | --- |
| | | Onset (min) | Peak (min) | Duration (hr) |
| Codeine | | | | |
| PO | 200 | 30-45 | 60-120 | 4 |
| IM | 120 | 10-30 | 30-60 | 4 |
| SC | 120 | 10-30 | 30-60 | 4 |
| Hydrocodone | | | | |
| PO | 10 | 10-30 | 30-60 | 4-6 |
| Hydromorphone | | | | |
| PO | 7.5 | 30 | 90-120 | 4 |
| IM | 1.5 | 15 | 30-60 | 4-5 |
| IV | 1.5 | 10-15 | 15-30 | 2-3 |
| SC | 1.5 | 15 | 30-90 | 4 |
| Levorphanol | | | | |
| PO | 4 | 10-60 | 90-120 | 4-5 |
| IM | 2 | — | 60 | 4-5 |
| IV | 2 | — | Within 20 | 4-5 |
| SC | 2 | — | 60-90 | 4-5 |
| Meperidine | | | | |
| PO | 300 | 15 | 60-90 | 2-4 |
| IM | 75 | 10-15 | 30-50 | 2-4 |
| IV | 75 | 1 | 5-7 | 2-4 |
| SC | 75 | 10-15 | 30-50 | 2-4 |
| Methadone | | | | |
| PO | 20 | 30-60 | 90-120 | 4-6‡ |
| IM | 10 | 10-20 | 60-120 | 4-5‡ |
| IV | 10 | — | 15-30 | 3-4‡ |
| Morphine | | | | |
| PO | 60 | — | 60-120 | 4-5§ |
| IM | 10 | 10-30 | 30-60 | 4-5 |
| IV | 10 | — | 20 | 4-5 |
| SC | 10 | 10-30 | 50-90 | 4-5 |
| Epidural | 10 | 15-60 | — | Up to 24 |
| Intrathecal | 10 | 15-60 | — | Up to 24 |
| Oxycodone | | | | |
| PO | 30 | 15-30 | 60 | 3-4 |
| Oxymorphone | | | | |
| IM | 1 | 10-15 | 30-90 | 3-6 |
| IV | 1 | 5-10 | 15-30 | 3-4 |
| SC | 1 | 10-20 | — | 3-6 |
| Rectal | 10 | 15-30 | 120 | 3-6 |
| Propoxyphene | | | | |
| PO | —‖ | 15-60 | 120 | 4-6 |

*Pure agonists used primarily for general anesthesia are listed in Table 25-6.
†Dose in milligrams that produces a degree of analgesia equivalent to that produced by a 10-mg intramuscular dose of morphine.
‡With repeated doses, methadone's duration of action may increase up to 48 hours.
§Effects of extended-release tablets may persist for 8 to 12 hours.
‖A dose of propoxyphene equivalent to 10 mg of morphine would be too toxic to administer.

## TABLE 25-6. CLINICAL PHARMACOLOGY OF OPIOIDS USED PRIMARILY FOR GENERAL ANESTHESIA

| Drug and Route | Equivalent Dose (mg)* | Time Course | | |
|---|---|---|---|---|
| | | Onset (min) | Peak (min) | Duration (min) |
| Alfentanil | | | | |
|   IV | 0.3-1 | 1 | 2 | 20-40 |
| Fentanyl† | | | | |
|   IV | 0.1 | 1-2 | 3-5 | 30-60 |
|   IM | 0.1 | 7-8 | 20-30 | 60-120 |
| Remifentanil | | | | |
|   IV | — | rapid | rapid | 5-10 |
| Sufentanil | | | | |
|   IV | 0.02 | 1-3 | 20 | 40-180 |

*Dose in milligrams that produces a degree of analgesia equivalent to that produced by a 10 mg of morphine IM.
†Also given transdermally for prolonged analgesia and transmucosally as a preanesthetic medication and to induce conscious sedation (see text).

## Meperidine

Meperidine [Demerol] shares the major pharmacologic properties of morphine. The drug is employed primarily to relieve pain. For obstetric analgesia, meperidine is preferred to morphine; the drug does not delay or diminish uterine contractions, and neonatal respiratory depression is less pronounced.

Meperidine causes less smooth muscle spasm than morphine. As a result, meperidine is less likely to cause constipation, urinary retention, and biliary colic. Meperidine may interact with MAO inhibitors to cause excitation, delirium, hyperpyrexia, and convulsions. Repeated dosing in patients with renal disease results in accumulation of normeperidine, a toxic metabolite that can cause dysphoria and seizures.

Meperidine is available in tablets (50 and 100 mg) and a syrup formulation (10 mg/ml) for oral use, and in solution (50 and 100 mg/ml) for injection (IV, IM, or SC). In addition, the drug is available in single-dose vials, ampules, and syringes. The usual adult dosage is 50 to 150 mg (IM, SC, or PO) repeated every 3 to 4 hours as needed. The usual dosage for children is 1 to 1.8 mg/kg (IM, SC, or PO) repeated every 3 or 4 hours as needed.

## Methadone

Methadone [Dolophine] has pharmacologic properties very similar to those of morphine. The drug is effective orally and has a long duration of action. Repeated dosing can result in accumulation. Methadone is used for pain relief and treatment of opioid addicts. The use of methadone in drug-abuse treatment programs is discussed in Chapter 37.

Methadone is dispensed in standard tablets (5 and 10 mg) and solution (1 and 2 mg/ml) for oral use, and in solution (10 mg/ml) for IM and SC administration. In addition, the drug is available in dispersible 40-mg tablets; this formulation is used only for detoxification and maintenance of opioid addicts. Usual oral analgesic doses for adults range from 2.5 to 20 mg repeated every 3 to 4 hours as needed.

## Levomethadyl

Levomethadyl [ORLAAM] is a long-acting analog of methadone approved only for treating opioid addicts. The rationale for using this strong opioid is discussed in Chapter 37. The drug is available only through programs for addiction treatment.

Levomethadyl is administered orally and effects last up to 72 hours. The initial dose is 20 to 40 mg (or 1.2 to 1.3 times the existing dose of methadone for patients being switched from that drug). The maintenance dosage, which is achieved gradually, ranges between 70 and 100 mg taken 3 times a week. The most common adverse effects are excessive sweating, constipation, abdominal pain, decreased libido, and delayed or absent ejaculation. Some patients being switched from methadone experience mood fluctuations and anxiety.

## Heroin

Heroin is a strong opioid agonist that is very similar to morphine in structure and actions. Heroin is an effective analgesic and is employed legally in Europe to relieve pain. In the United States, federal legislation prohibits the medical use of this drug. Heroin has been banned from American medicine because of its high abuse liability and because it does not appear to offer any benefits over opioids with a lower abuse potential.

Heroin is preferred to other opioids as a drug of abuse largely because of its pharmacokinetic properties. Heroin has greater lipid solubility than morphine, and therefore crosses the blood-brain barrier more readily. As a result, when heroin is injected IV, the drug accumulates in the brain more rapidly and to a higher level than would an equivalent dose of IV morphine. Once in the brain, heroin (diacetylmorphine) is rapidly converted into monoacetylmorphine and then into morphine (Fig. 25-2). It is these metabolites, and not heroin itself, that produce the subjective effects that follow heroin injection. In this regard, heroin can be viewed as a vehicle for facilitating transport of morphine into the brain.

## Fentanyl

Fentanyl [Sublimaze, Duragesic, Fentanyl Oralet] is a strong opioid analgesic with a high milligram potency. The drug is available for parenteral, transdermal, and transmucosal administration.

*Parenteral.* Parenteral fentanyl [Sublimaze] is employed primarily for induction and maintenance of surgical anesthesia. The drug is well suited for these applications because of its rapid onset and relatively short duration of action (see Table 25-6). Most effects are like those of morphine. In addition, fentanyl can

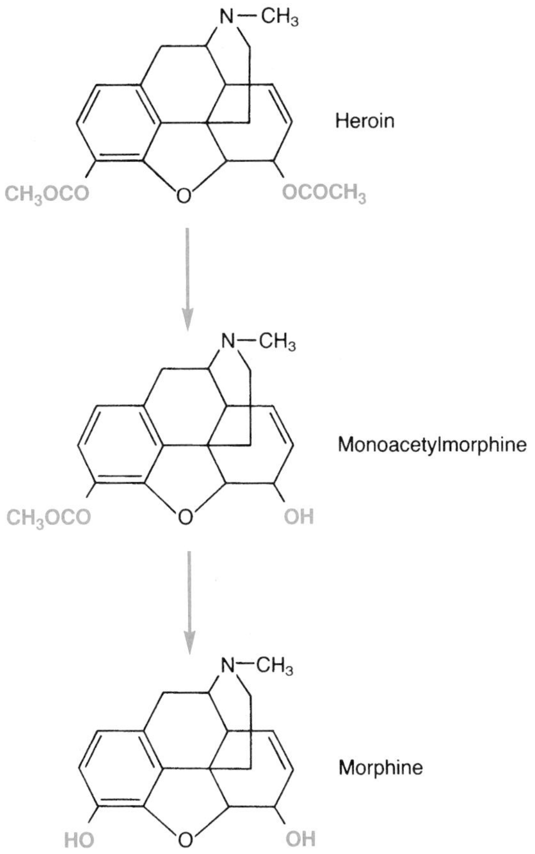

**Figure 25–2. Biotransformation of heroin into morphine.** Heroin, as such, is biologically inactive. Once in the body, heroin is converted to monoacetylmorphine (MAM) and then into morphine itself. MAM and morphine are responsible for the effects elicited by injection of heroin.

cause muscle rigidity, which can interfere with induction of anesthesia. As discussed in Chapter 27 (General Anesthetics), the combination of fentanyl plus droperidol, available commercially as Innovar, is used to produce a state known as "neurolept analgesia." Parenteral fentanyl is a Schedule II preparation.

***Transdermal.*** The fentanyl transdermal system [Duragesic] consists of a fentanyl-containing "patch" that is applied to the skin of the upper torso. The drug is slowly released from the patch and absorbed through the skin, reaching effective levels in 24 hours. Levels remain steady for another 48 hours, after which the patch should be removed and a new one applied. If a new patch is not applied, effects will nonetheless persist for several hours because of continued absorption of residual fentanyl that remained in the skin after the old patch was removed.

Transdermal fentanyl is indicated for chronic severe pain, such as that associated with cancer. Because analgesia is delayed, fentanyl patches are not suited for acute or postoperative pain. The patches should not be used in children under 12 years old, or in anyone under 18 who weighs less than 110 pounds. Also, patches should not be used for mild pain that responds to less powerful analgesics.

Transdermal fentanyl has the same adverse effects as other opioids (respiratory depression, sedation, constipation, urinary retention, nausea, and so forth). Adverse effects may persist for hours following patch removal because of continued drug absorption from the skin. Signs of toxicity can be reversed with an opioid antagonist (e.g., naloxone). Used patches should be

flushed down the toilet. Unused patches should be stored out of reach of children.

Fentanyl patches are available in four sizes, which deliver fentanyl to the systemic circulation at rates of 25, 50, 75, and 100 µg/hr. If the patient is not already tolerant to opioids, therapy should begin with the smallest patch. If a dosage greater than 100 µg/hr is required, a combination of patches can be applied. Since full analgesic effects can take up to 24 hours to develop, PRN therapy with a short-acting opioid may be required until the patch takes effect. For the majority of patients, patches can be replaced every 72 hours, although some patients may require a new patch every 48 hours. Fentanyl patches are regulated under Schedule II of the Controlled Substances Act.

***Transmucosal.*** The transmucosal fentanyl system [Fentanyl Oralet] looks like a lollipop, consisting of a raspberry-colored lozenge on a plastic handle. The drug is approved for preanesthetic medication before surgery and for inducing conscious sedation prior to painful diagnostic or therapeutic procedures.

Despite its benign appearance, transmucosal fentanyl is a powerful and dangerous analgesic approved for use only in a hospital setting. Administration should be done by someone trained in the use of anesthetic drugs. Because of the risk of hypoventilation, continuous direct monitoring is required. Facilities for respiratory and cardiac resuscitation must be immediately available. The drug is contraindicated for children who weigh less than 10 kg (22 lb) and for treatment of acute or chronic pain in any patient.

When patients suck on a Fentanyl Oralet, some of the drug is absorbed directly and rapidly through the oral mucosa, and some is swallowed and absorbed slowly from the GI tract. Total bioavailability is about 50%. Analgesia begins in 5 to 15 minutes, peaks in 20 minutes, and persists for 1 to 2 hours.

Adverse effects are like those of other opioids. Preoperative itching of the nose and eyes is common, as are postoperative nausea and vomiting. However, the biggest danger is profound respiratory depression.

Fentanyl Oralets are supplied in three sizes: 200, 300, and 400 µg. The recommended dosage for adults is 5 µg/kg, up to a maximum of 400 µg. Pediatric dosages range from 5 to 15 µg/kg. Patients should be instructed to suck the lozenge, not chew it. Consumption of the entire lozenge takes 10 to 20 minutes. Because onset of analgesia is delayed, dosing should begin 20 to 40 minutes prior to anticipated need. If the desired effect is achieved before the entire lozenge is consumed, the remainder should be flushed down a toilet. Fentanyl Oralets are regulated under Schedule II of the Controlled Substances Act.

### Alfentanil and Sufentanil

Alfentanil [Alfenta] and sufentanil [Sufenta] are intravenous opioids related to fentanyl. Both drugs are used for induction of anesthesia, for maintenance of anesthesia (in combination with other agents), and as sole anesthetic agents. Pharmacologic effects are like those of morphine. Sufentanil has an especially high milligram potency (about 1000 times that of morphine). As indicated in Table 25-6, both alfentanil and sufentanil have a rapid onset of action. Alfentanil has an unusually brief duration. Both drugs are Schedule II agents.

### Remifentanil

Remifentanil [Ultiva] is a new intravenous opioid with a rapid onset and brief duration. The brief duration results from rapid metabolism by plasma and tissue esterases, and not hepatic metabolism or renal excretion. Remifentanil is approved for analgesia during surgery and during the immediate postoperative period. Administration is by continuous IV infusion. Effects begin in minutes, and terminate 5 to 10 minutes after the infusion is stopped. For surgical analgesia, the infusion rate is 0.05 to 2 µg/min. For postoperative analgesia, the infusion rate is 0.025 to 0.2 µg/min. Adverse effects during the infusion include respiratory depression, hypotension, bradycardia, and muscular rigidity sufficient to compromise breathing. Postinfusion effects include nausea (44%), vomiting (22%), and headache (18%). Remifentanil is not regulated under the Controlled Substances Act.

### Hydromorphone, Oxymorphone, and Levorphanol

*Basic Pharmacology.* All three drugs are strong opioid agonists with pharmacologic actions like those of morphine. All three are indicated for relief of moderate to severe pain. Dosages and time courses are summarized in Table 25-5. Adverse effects include respiratory depression, sedation, cough suppression, constipation, urinary retention, nausea, and vomiting. Toxicity can be reversed with an opioid antagonist (e.g., naloxone). All three drugs are Schedule II substances.

*Preparations, Dosage, and Administration. Hydromorphone.* Hydromorphone [Dilaudid] is available in oral tablets (1, 2, 3, and 4 mg), rectal suppositories (3 mg), and solution (1, 2, 3, 4, and 10 mg/ml) for IM and SC injection. The usual adult oral dosage is 2 mg every 4 to 6 hours. The adult rectal dosage is 3 mg every 6 to 8 hours. Usual SC and IM dosages are 1 to 4 mg every 4 to 6 hours.

*Oxymorphone.* Oxymorphone [Numorphan] is available in solution (1 and 1.5 mg/ml) for parenteral administration and in 5-mg rectal suppositories. The initial IV dose is 0.5 mg. Usual SC and IM dosages are 1 to 1.5 mg every 4 to 6 hours as needed. The rectal dosage is 5 mg every 4 to 6 hours.

*Levorphanol.* Levorphanol [Levo-Dromoran] is available in 2-mg oral tablets and in solution (2 mg/ml) for SC injection. The usual oral or SC dosage for adults is 2 to 3 mg.

## Moderate-to-Strong Opioid Agonists

The moderate-to-strong opioid agonists are similar to morphine in most respects. Like morphine, these drugs produce analgesia, sedation, and euphoria. In addition, they can cause respiratory depression, constipation, urinary retention, cough suppression, and miosis. Differences between the moderate-to-strong opioids and morphine are primarily quantitative: the moderate-to-strong opioids produce less analgesia and respiratory depression than morphine and have a somewhat lower potential for abuse. As with morphine, toxicity from the moderate-to-strong agonists can be reversed with naloxone.

### Codeine

*Actions and Uses.* Codeine is indicated for relief of mild to moderate pain. The drug is usually administered by mouth. Maximal analgesic effects are less than with morphine. When taken in its usual analgesic dose (30 mg), codeine produces about as much pain relief as 325 mg of aspirin or 325 mg of acetaminophen.

For analgesic use, codeine is dispensed alone and in combination with a nonopioid analgesic, either aspirin or acetaminophen. Since codeine and nonopioid analgesics relieve pain by different mechanisms, the combination of codeine with a nonopioid can produce greater pain relief than either agent alone. Codeine alone is classified under Schedule II of the Controlled Substances Act. The combination preparations are classified under Schedule III. Although codeine is classified along with morphine in Schedule II, the abuse liability of codeine appears to be significantly lower.

Codeine is an extremely effective cough suppressant and is widely used for this action. The antitussive dose (10 mg) is lower than analgesic doses. Codeine is dispensed in combination with various agents for suppression of cough. These mixtures are classified under Schedule V.

*Preparations, Dosage, and Administration.* Codeine is administered orally and parenterally (IV, IM, and SC). For oral therapy, the drug is available in standard and soluble tablets (15, 30, and 60 mg). For parenteral therapy, the drug is dispensed in solution (30 and 60 mg/ml).

The usual analgesic dosage for adults is 15 to 60 mg (PO, IV, IM, or SC) every 3 to 6 hours (to a maximum of 120 mg/24 hr). The usual analgesic dosage for children 1 year and older is 0.5 mg/kg (PO, IM, or SC) every 4 to 6 hours (to a maximum of 60 mg/24 hr).

### Propoxyphene

Propoxyphene [Darvon, Dolene] has analgesic effects about equal to those of aspirin. The drug is frequently prescribed in combination with a nonopioid analgesic, either aspirin or acetaminophen. These combinations can produce greater pain relief than either propoxyphene or the nonopioid alone. Propoxyphene has a low potential for abuse, primarily because large doses cause toxic psychosis. Furthermore, excessive doses often prove fatal; hence the drug should not be dispensed to patients suspected of suicidal tendencies. Physical dependence is minimal. Propoxyphene, alone or in combination with a nonopioid analgesic, is classified under Schedule IV of the Controlled Substances Act.

Propoxyphene is available as two salts: propoxyphene hydrochloride and propoxyphene napsylate. Both are administered orally. Propoxyphene hydrochloride is dispensed in capsules (32 and 65 mg); the usual adult dosage is 65 mg repeated every 4 hours as needed. The napsylate salt is dispensed in 100-mg tablets and in suspension (10 mg/ml); the usual adult dosage is 100 mg repeated every 4 hours as needed.

### Hydrocodone and Oxycodone

Hydrocodone [Vicodin, others] and oxycodone [Roxicodone, Percodan, Percocet] have analgesic actions equivalent to those of codeine. Both drugs are taken orally to relieve pain. The usual dosage for both is 5 mg. Oxycodone is available in 5-mg tablets, in solution (5 and 20 mg/ml), and in combination with aspirin or acetaminophen. Hydrocodone is available only in combination with aspirin or acetaminophen. Oxycodone, alone or combined with aspirin or acetaminophen, is classified under Schedule II. The combination of hydrocodone with aspirin or acetaminophen is classified under Schedule III.

### Tramadol

Tramadol [Ultram] is a moderately strong analgesic with minimal potential for dependence, abuse, or respiratory depression. The drug relieves pain through a combination of opioid and nonopioid mechanisms. Tramadol was approved for use in the United States in 1995, but has been used in Europe for over 10 years.

*Mechanism of Action.* Tramadol is an analog of codeine that relieves pain in part through weak agonist activity at mu opioid receptors. However, the drug seems to work primarily by blocking uptake of norepinephrine and serotonin, thereby activating monoaminergic spinal inhibition of pain. Naloxone (an opioid antagonist) only partially blocks tramadol's effects.

*Therapeutic Use.* Tramadol is approved for moderate to moderately severe pain. The drug is less effective than morphine and no more effective than codeine combined with aspirin or acetaminophen. Analgesia begins 1 hour after oral administration, is maximal at 2 hours, and continues for 6 hours.

*Pharmacokinetics.* Tramadol is administered by mouth and reaches peak plasma levels in 2 hours. Elimination is by hepatic metabolism and renal excretion. The half-life is 5 to 6 hours.

***Adverse Effects and Interactions.*** Tramadol has been used by millions of patients, and serious adverse effects have been rare. The most common effects are sedation, dizziness, headache, dry mouth, and constipation. Respiratory depression is minimal. Seizures have been reported in 83 patients; hence the drug should be avoided in those with epilepsy and other neurologic disorders. Severe allergic reactions have developed rarely.

***Drug Interactions.*** Tramadol can intensify responses to *CNS depressants* (e.g., alcohol, benzodiazepines), and therefore should not be combined with these agents. By inhibiting uptake of norepinephrine, tramadol can precipitate hypertensive crisis if combined with a *monoamine oxidase inhibitor*; accordingly, the combination is absolutely contraindicated.

***Abuse Liability.*** The abuse liability of tramadol is very low and the drug is not regulated under the Controlled Substances Act. Nonetheless, there have been a few reports of abuse, dependence, withdrawal, and intentional overdose, presumably for subjective effects. Consequently, tramadol should not be given to patients with a history of drug abuse, and the recommended dosage should not be exceeded.

***Preparations, Dosage, and Administration.*** Tramadol [Ultram] is dispensed in 50-mg tablets for oral administration. The recommended adult dosage is 50 to 100 mg every 4 to 6 hours as needed, up to a maximum of 400 mg/day. The dosing interval should be increased for patients with hepatic or renal dysfunction.

## Agonist-Antagonist Opioids

Five agonist-antagonist opioids are available: pentazocine, nalbuphine, butorphanol, dezocine, and buprenorphine.

With the exception of buprenorphine, all of these drugs act as antagonists at mu receptors and agonists at kappa receptors (see Table 25-2). Compared with pure opioid agonists, the agonist-antagonists have a low potential for abuse, produce less respiratory depression, and generally have less powerful analgesic effects. If given to a patient who is physically dependent on a pure opioid agonist, these drugs can precipitate a withdrawal reaction. The clinical pharmacology of the agonist-antagonists is summarized in Table 25-7.

### Pentazocine

***Actions and Uses.*** Pentazocine [Talwin] was the first agonist-antagonist opioid available and can be considered the prototype for the group. The drug is indicated for mild to moderate pain. Pentazocine is less effective than morphine against severe pain.

Pentazocine acts as an *agonist* at kappa receptors and an *antagonist* at mu receptors. By activating kappa receptors, the drug produces analgesia, sedation, and respiratory depression. However, unlike the respiratory depression caused by morphine, *respiratory depression caused by pentazocine is limited:* beyond a certain dose, no further depression occurs. Because it lacks agonist actions at mu receptors, pentazocine produces little or no euphoria. In fact, at supratherapeutic doses, pentazocine produces unpleasant reactions (anxiety, strange thoughts, nightmares, hallucinations). These psychotomimetic ef-

## TABLE 25-7. CLINICAL PHARMACOLOGY OF OPIOID AGONIST-ANTAGONISTS

| Drug and Route | Equivalent Dose (mg)* | Time Course of Analgesic Effects | | |
| --- | --- | --- | --- | --- |
| | | Onset (min) | Peak (min) | Duration (hr) |
| Buprenorphine | | | | |
|   IM | 0.3 | 15 | 60 | Up to 6 |
|   IV | 0.3 | <15 | <60 | Up to 6 |
| Butorphanol | | | | |
|   IM | 2-3 | 10 | 30-60 | 3-4 |
|   IV | 2-3 | 2-3 | 30 | 2-4 |
|   Intranasal | 2-3 | Within 15 | 60-120 | 4-5 |
| Dezocine | | | | |
|   IM | 10 | 30 | 30-150 | 2-4 |
|   IV | 10 | 15 | 30-150 | 2-4 |
| Nalbuphine | | | | |
|   IM | 10 | Within 15 | 60 | 3-6 |
|   IV | 10 | 2-3 | 30 | 3-4 |
|   SC | 10 | Within 15 | — | 3-6 |
| Pentazocine | | | | |
|   PO | 180 | 15-30 | 60-90 | 3† |
|   IM | 60 | 15-20 | 30-60 | 2-3† |
|   IV | 60 | 2-3 | 15-30 | 2-3† |
|   SC | 60 | 15-20 | 30-60 | 2-3† |

*Dose in milligrams that produces a degree of analgesia equivalent to that produced by a 10-mg IM dose of morphine.

†Duration may increase greatly in patients with liver disease.

fects may result from stimulation of kappa receptors. Because of its subjective effects, pentazocine has a low potential for abuse and is classified as a Schedule IV substance.

Adverse effects are generally like those of morphine. However, in contrast to the pure opioid agonists, pentazocine increases cardiac work. Accordingly, a pure agonist (e.g., morphine) is preferred to pentazocine for relieving pain in patients with myocardial infarction.

*If administered to a patient who is physically dependent on a pure opioid agonist, pentazocine can precipitate an abstinence syndrome.* Recall that mu receptors mediate physical dependence on pure opioid agonists and that pentazocine acts as an antagonist at these receptors. By blocking access of the pure agonist to mu receptors, pentazocine will prevent receptor activation, thereby triggering withdrawal. Accordingly, *pentazocine and other drugs that block mu receptors should never be administered to a person who is physically dependent on a pure opioid agonist.* If a pentazocine-like agent is to be used, the pure opioid agonist must first be withdrawn.

Physical dependence can occur with pentazocine, but symptoms of withdrawal are generally mild (e.g., cramps, fever, anxiety, restlessness). Treatment is rarely required. As with pure opioid agonists, toxicity from pentazocine can be reversed with naloxone.

***Preparations, Dosage, and Administration.*** For oral therapy, pentazocine [Talwin] is dispensed in 50-mg tablets that also contain 0.5 mg of naloxone (to prevent abuse). The usual adult dosage is 50 mg every 3 to 4 hours as needed.

For parenteral therapy, pentazocine is available in solution (30 mg/ml as the lactate salt). Administration is IV, IM, and SC. The usual adult dosage is 30 mg every 3 to 4 hours as needed.

### Nalbuphine

Nalbuphine [Nubain] has pharmacologic actions similar to those of pentazocine. The drug is an agonist at kappa receptors and an antagonist at mu receptors. Analgesic effects are somewhat less than those of morphine. Like pentazocine, nalbuphine can cause psychotomimetic reactions. Respiratory depression is limited. With prolonged treatment, physical dependence can develop. Symptoms of abstinence are less intense than with morphine but more intense than with pentazocine. Nalbuphine has a low abuse potential and is not regulated under the Controlled Substances Act. As with the pure opioid agonists, toxicity can be reversed with naloxone. Like pentazocine, nalbuphine will precipitate a withdrawal reaction if administered to an individual who is physically dependent on a pure opioid agonist. Nalbuphine is dispensed in solution (10 and 20 mg/ml) for IV, IM, and SC injection. The usual adult dosage is 10 mg repeated every 3 to 6 hours as needed.

### Butorphanol

Butorphanol [Stadol] has actions similar to those of pentazocine. The drug is an agonist at kappa receptors and an antagonist at mu receptors. Analgesic effects are somewhat less than those of morphine. As with pentazocine, there is a "ceiling" to respiratory depression. The drug can cause psychotomimetic reactions, but these are rare. Butorphanol increases cardiac work and should not be given to patients with myocardial infarction. Physical dependence can occur, but symptoms of withdrawal are relatively mild. The drug may induce a withdrawal reaction in patients physically dependent on a pure opioid agonist. Butorphanol has a low potential for abuse and is not regulated under the Controlled Substances Act. Toxicity can be reversed with naloxone.

Butorphanol is administered parenterally (IM and IV) and by nasal spray. The usual adult IV dosage is 1 mg every 3 to 4 hours as needed. The usual IM dosage is 2 mg every 3 to 4 hours as needed. The usual intranasal dosage is 1 mg (one spray from the metered-dose spray device) repeated in 60 to 90 minutes if needed; the two-dose sequence may then be repeated every 3 to 4 hours as needed.

### Dezocine

Dezocine [Dalgan] has analgesic effects equivalent to those of morphine. The drug's adverse effects are like those of the pure opioid agonists, except that there is a ceiling to respiratory depression. Fatal respiratory depression has not been reported. Effects on cardiac performance are modest, but caution should be exercised in patients with coronary artery disease. Dezocine appears to have a low potential for abuse and is not regulated under the Controlled Substances Act. The drug is dispensed in solution (5, 10, and 15 mg/ml) for IM and IV administration. The usual IM dosage is 5 to 20 mg every 3 to 6 hours as needed. The usual IV dosage is 2.5 to 10 mg every 2 to 4 hours.

### Buprenorphine

Buprenorphine [Buprenex] differs significantly from other opioid agonist-antagonists. The drug is a partial agonist at mu receptors and an antagonist at kappa receptors. Analgesic effects are like those of morphine, but significant tolerance has not been observed. Although buprenorphine can depress respiration, severe respiratory depression has not been reported. Like pentazocine, buprenorphine can precipitate a withdrawal reaction in persons physically dependent on pure opioid agonists. Psychotomimetic reactions can occur but are rare. Physical dependence develops but symptoms of abstinence are delayed; peak responses may not occur until 2 weeks after the last dose was taken. Buprenorphine appears to have a low potential for abuse and is classified as a Schedule V substance.

Although pretreatment with naloxone can prevent toxicity from buprenorphine, naloxone cannot readily reverse toxicity that has already developed. It appears that buprenorphine binds very tightly to its receptors, and cannot be readily displaced by naloxone once it is bound.

Buprenorphine is dispensed in solution (0.3 mg/ml) for administration by IM or slow IV injection. The usual dosage for patients age 13 and older is 0.3 mg repeated every 6 hours as needed.

## Clinical Use of Opioids

### General Considerations

#### Assessment of Pain

To maximize relief, you must first assess the patient's pain. Pain status should be evaluated prior to opioid administration and about 1 hour after. Unfortunately, since pain is a subjective experience affected by multiple factors (e.g., cultural influences, patient expectations, associated disease), there is no reliable objective method for determining just how much discomfort the patient is feeling. That is, we cannot measure pain with instruments equivalent to those employed to monitor blood pressure, cardiac performance, and other physiologic parameters.

As a result, assessment must ultimately be based on the patient's description of his or her experience. Accordingly, you should ask the patient where the pain is located, what type of pain is present (e.g., dull, sharp, stabbing), how the pain changes with time, what makes the pain better, and what makes the pain worse. In addition, you should assess for psychologic factors that can reduce pain threshold (anxiety, depression, fear, anger).

When attempting to assess pain, keep in mind that what the patient says about his or her pain may not always be the truth. A few patients who are pain free may claim to feel pain so as to receive medication for its euphoriant effects. Conversely, some patients may claim to feel fine even though they are experiencing considerable discomfort. Such patients may misrepresent their experience for any of several reasons: some may fear addiction, some may fear needles, and some may feel a need to be stoic and bear the pain. Patients like these must be listened to with care if their true pain status is to be evaluated and responded to with appropriate measures for relief.

## Acute Pain Versus Chronic Pain

Opioids are generally reserved for acute pain. With the exception of cancer-caused pain, use of opioids for chronic pain is not usually appropriate. Alternatives to opioids for chronic pain include nonopioid analgesics (acetaminophen and aspirin-like drugs), nerve block, transcutaneous electrical nerve stimulation (TENS), tricyclic antidepressants, and neurosurgery. If disabling pain persists despite these therapies, treatment with an opioid may be indicated.

## Dosing Guidelines

***Dosage Determination.*** Dosage of opioid analgesics must be adjusted to accommodate individual variation. "Standard" doses cannot be relied upon as appropriate for all patients. For example, if a "standard" 10-mg dose of morphine were employed for all adults, only about 70%

would receive adequate relief; the other 30% would be undertreated. Not all patients have the same tolerance for pain; hence some will need larger doses than others for the same disorder. Some conditions hurt more than others. For example, patients recovering from open chest surgery are likely to experience greater pain and need larger doses than patients recovering from an appendectomy. Elderly patients metabolize opioids slowly, and therefore require lower doses than younger adults. Because the blood-brain barrier of newborns is poorly developed, these patients are especially sensitive to opioids; hence they generally require smaller doses than older infants and young children.

***Dosing Schedule.*** As a rule, *opioids should be administered on a fixed schedule* (e.g., every 4 hours) rather than on a PRN basis. With a fixed schedule, each dose is given before pain returns, thereby sparing the patient needless discomfort. In contrast, when PRN dosing is employed, there can be a long delay between onset of pain and production of relief: each time pain returns, the patient must call the nurse; wait for the nurse to respond; wait for the nurse to evaluate the pain; wait for the nurse to sign out medication; wait for the nurse to prepare and administer the injection; and then wait for the drug to undergo absorption and finally produce analgesia. This delay causes unnecessary discomfort and creates anxiety about pain recurrence. Use of a fixed dosing schedule reduces these problems. As discussed below, allowing the patient to self-administer opioids using a patient-controlled analgesia (PCA) device can provide even greater protection against pain recurrence than can be achieved by having the nurse administer opioids on a fixed schedule. The differences between PRN dosing, fixed-schedule dosing, and use of a PCA device are shown graphically in Figure 25–3.

***Avoiding Withdrawal.*** When opioids are administered in high doses for 20 days or more, clinically significant physical dependence may develop. Under these conditions, abrupt withdrawal will precipitate an abstinence

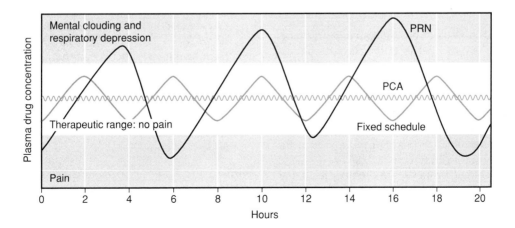

**Figure 25–3. Fluctuations in opioid blood levels seen with three dosing procedures.** Note that, with PRN dosing, opioid levels can fluctuate widely, going from subtherapeutic to excessive and back again. In contrast, when opioids are administered with a PCA device or on a fixed schedule, levels stay within the therapeutic range, allowing continuous pain relief with minimal adverse effects.

syndrome. To minimize symptoms of abstinence, opioids should be withdrawn slowly, tapering off the dosage over 3 days. If the degree of dependence is especially high, as can occur in opioid addicts, dosage should be tapered over 7 to 10 days.

## Physical Dependence, Abuse, and Addiction as Clinical Concerns

Most people in our society, including many health care professionals, harbor strong fears regarding the ability of "narcotics" to cause "addiction." In a clinical setting, such excessive concern is both unwarranted and counterproductive. Because of inappropriate fears, physicians frequently prescribe less pain medication than patients need, and nurses frequently administer less medication than was prescribed. The result, according to one estimate, is that only 25% of patients receive doses of opioids that are sufficient to relieve suffering. One pain specialist described this unacceptable situation as follows: "The excessive and unrealistic concern about the dangers of addiction in the hospitalized medical patient is a significant and potent force for the undertreatment with narcotics."

When treating a patient for pain, you may have to decide how much opioid to give and when to give it. If you are excessively concerned about the ability of opioids to cause physical dependence and addiction, you will be unable to make a rational decision. Furthermore, in your role as patient advocate, it is your responsibility to intervene and request an increase in dosage if the prescribed dosage has proved inadequate. If you fear that dosage escalation may cause addiction, you are less likely to make the request.

The object of the following discussion is to dispel excessive concerns about dependence, abuse, and addiction in the medical patient so that these concerns do not result in undermedication and needless suffering.

### Definitions

Before we can discuss the clinical implications of physical dependence, abuse, and addiction, we need to define these terms.

*Physical Dependence.* As discussed above, physical dependence is a state in which an abstinence syndrome will occur if the dependence-producing drug is abruptly withdrawn. *Physical dependence should NOT be equated with addiction.*

*Abuse.* Abuse can be broadly defined as *drug use that is inconsistent with medical or social norms.* By this definition, abuse is determined primarily by the reason for drug use and by the setting in which that use occurs—and not by the pharmacologic properties of the drug itself. For example, whereas it is not considered abuse to administer 20 mg of morphine in a hospital to relieve pain, it *is* considered abuse to administer the same dose of the same drug on the "street" to produce euphoria. The concept of abuse is discussed at length in Chapter 35.

*Addiction.* Addiction can be defined as a behavior pattern characterized by continued use of a psychoactive substance despite physical, psychologic, or social harm. Note that nowhere in this definition is addiction equated with physical dependence. In fact, physical dependence is not even part of the definition. The concept of addiction is discussed further in Chapter 35.

Although physical dependence is not required for addiction to occur, physical dependence *can* contribute to addictive behavior. If an individual has already established a pattern of compulsive drug use, physical dependence can reinforce that pattern. For the individual with a marginal resolve to discontinue opioid use, the desire to avoid symptoms of withdrawal may be sufficient to promote continued drug use. However, in the presence of a strong desire to discontinue opioids, physical dependence, by itself, is insufficient to motivate continued addictive behavior.

### Minimizing Fears about Physical Dependence

For the following three reasons, there is little to fear regarding physical dependence upon opioids in the hospitalized patient.

- Development of significant physical dependence is extremely rare when opioids are given acutely to relieve pain. For most patients, the doses employed and the duration of treatment are insufficient to cause significant dependence.
- Even when physical dependence does occur, patients rarely develop addictive behavior and continue opioid administration after their pain has subsided. The vast majority of patients who become physically dependent in a clinical setting simply go through gradual withdrawal and never take opioids again. This observation emphasizes the point that physical dependence per se is insufficient to cause addiction.
- Physical dependence as such is not a problem. As long as the dependent person takes opioids, dependence has no symptoms. Addicts participating in methadone treatment programs are highly dependent on methadone, yet they experience no significant ill effects and function normally (as long as they take methadone on a regular schedule). Physical dependence does not prevent methadone-treated addicts from leading productive and fulfilling lives.

From the preceding we can see there is little to fear regarding physical dependence during the therapeutic use of opioids. We can conclude, therefore, that there is no justification for withholding opioids from patients in pain on the basis of concerns about physical dependence.

### Minimizing Fears about Addiction

The principal reason for abandoning fears about opioid addiction in patients is simple: *development of addiction to opioids as a result of clinical exposure to these drugs is extremely rare.* Results of the Boston Collaborative Drug Study showed that, of 12,000 patients taking opioids, only 4 became drug abusers. Furthermore, as discussed below, if abuse or addiction *does* occur, it is probable that these behaviors reflect tendencies that existed before the patient entered the hospital, rather than inappropriate medical use of opioids during the hospital stay.

For the purpose of this discussion, the population can be divided into two groups: individuals who are prone to drug abuse and individuals who are not. One source estimates that about 8% of the population is prone to drug abuse, whereas the other 92% is not. Individuals who are prone to drug abuse have a tendency to abuse drugs in the hospital and outside. Nonabusers, on the other hand, will not abuse drugs in a clinical setting or anywhere else. Withholding analgesics from abuse-prone individuals is not going to reverse their tendency to abuse drugs. Conversely, administering opioids to nonabuse-prone persons will not change their personalities and convert them into "drug fiends."

If a patient who did not formerly abuse opioids does abuse these drugs following therapeutic exposure, you should not feel responsible for having created an addict. That is, if a patient tries to continue opioid use after leaving the hospital, it is probable that the patient is of the abuse-prone personality type. Therefore, the pattern of abuse that emerged during clinical exposure to opioids was the result of tendencies that were established before the patient ever entered the hospital—and not the consequence of therapy. The only action that might have prevented opioid abuse by such a patient would have been to withhold opioids entirely—an action that would not have been feasible.

### Balancing the Need to Provide Pain Relief with the Desire to Minimize Abuse

Although concerns about opioid abuse in the clinical setting are small, they cannot be dismissed entirely. You are still obliged to administer opioids with discretion in an effort to minimize abuse. Some reasonable attempt must be made to determine who is likely to abuse drugs and who is not. As a rule, distinguishing abusers from nonabusers can be done with some confidence. When nonabusers say they need more pain relief, believe them and provide it. In contrast, when an obvious abuser requests more analgesic, some healthy skepticism is in order. When there is doubt as to whether a patient is abuse prone or not, logic dictates giving the patient the benefit of the doubt and providing the medication. If the patient is an abuser, little harm will result from giving unneeded medication. However, if the patient is a nonabuser, failure to provide medication would prolong suffering for no justifiable reason.

In order to minimize physical dependence and abuse, opioid analgesics should be administered in the lowest effective dosages for the shortest time needed. Be aware, however, that larger doses are needed for patients who have more intense pain and for those who have developed tolerance. As pain diminishes, opioid dosage should be reduced. As soon as possible, the patient should be switched to a nonopioid analgesic, such as aspirin or acetaminophen.

In summary, when working with opioids, as with any other drugs, you must balance the risks of therapy against the benefits. The risk of addiction from therapeutic use of opioids is real but very small. Consequently, concerns about addiction should play a real but secondary role in making decisions about giving these drugs. Dosages should be sufficient to relieve pain. Suffering because of insufficient dosage is unacceptable. However, it is also unacceptable to promote possible abuse through failure to exercise good judgment.

## Patient-Controlled Analgesia

Patient-controlled analgesia (PCA) is a method of drug delivery that permits the patient to self-administer parenteral (IV, SC, epidural) opioids on an "as-needed" basis. PCA has been employed primarily for relief of pain in postoperative patients. Other candidates include patients experiencing pain caused by cancer, trauma, myocardial infarction, vaso-occlusive sickle cell crisis, and labor. As discussed below, PCA offers several advantages over opioids administered by the nurse.

***PCA Devices.*** PCA has been made possible by the development of reliable PCA devices. A PCA device consists of an electronically controlled infusion pump that can be activated by the patient to deliver a preset bolus dose of an opioid. The opioid is delivered through an indwelling catheter. In addition to providing bolus doses on demand, some PCA devices can deliver a basal infusion of opioid.

An essential feature of all PCA devices is a timing control. This control limits the total dose that can be administered each hour, thereby reducing the risk of overdose. In addition, the timing control regulates the minimum interval (e.g., 10 minutes) between doses. This interval, referred to as the "lock-out" or "delay" interval, prevents the patient from administering a second dose before the first has had time to produce its full effect.

***Drug Selection and Dosage Regulation.*** The opioids that have been used most extensively for PCA are morphine and meperidine [Demerol]. Other pure opioid agonists (e.g., methadone, hydromorphone, fentanyl) have also been employed, as have agonist-antagonist opioids (e.g., nalbuphine, buprenorphine).

Prior to starting PCA, the postoperative patient should be given an opioid loading dose (e.g., 2 to 10 mg of morphine). Once effective opioid levels have been established with the loading dose, PCA can be initiated, provided the patient has recovered sufficiently from anesthesia. For PCA with morphine, initial bolus doses of 1 mg are typical. The size of the bolus should be increased if analgesia is inadequate, and decreased if excessive sedation occurs. The size of the bolus dose is usually increased during sleeping hours, thereby promoting rest by prolonging the interval between doses.

***Comparison of PCA with Traditional Intramuscular Therapy.*** The objective of therapy with analgesics is to provide comfort while minimizing sedation and other side effects, especially respiratory depression. This objective is best achieved by maintaining plasma levels of opioids that are steady (i.e., that have minimal fluctuations). In this manner, side effects from excessively high levels can be avoided, as can the return of severe pain from low levels.

In the traditional management of postoperative pain, patients are given an IM injection of an opioid every 3 to 4 hours. With this dosing schedule, plasma levels of the opioid can vary widely. Shortly after the injection, plasma levels may rise very high, causing excessive sedation and possibly respiratory depression. Late in the dosing interval, pain may return as plasma levels drop to their lowest point.

In contrast to traditional therapy, PCA is ideally suited to maintain steady levels of opioids. This is because PCA relies on small doses given frequently (e.g., 1 mg of morphine every 10 minutes) rather than on large doses given infrequently (e.g., 20 mg of morphine every 3 hours). Maintenance of steady drug levels can be facilitated further if the PCA device is capable of delivering a basal opioid infusion. Because plasma drug levels remain relatively steady, PCA can provide continuous control of pain while avoiding the adverse effects associated with excessive drug levels.

An additional advantage of PCA is rapid relief of pain. Since the patient can self-administer an IV dose of opioid as soon as pain begins to return, there is a minimal delay between detection of pain and restoration of an adequate drug level. With traditional therapy, the patient must wait for the nurse to respond to a request for more drug; this delay allows pain to grow more intense.

Studies indicate that PCA is associated with accelerated recovery. When compared with patients receiving traditional IM analgesia, postoperative patients receiving PCA show improved early mobilization, greater cooperation during physical therapy, and a shorter hospital stay.

**Patient Education.** Patient education is essential for successful PCA. Surgical patients should be educated preoperatively. Education should include an explanation of what PCA is along with instruction on how to activate the PCA device.

Patients should be told not to fear overdose; the PCA device will not permit self-administration of excessive doses. Patients should be informed that there is a time lag (about 10 minutes) between activation of the device and production of maximal analgesia. To reduce discomfort associated with physical therapy, changing of dressings, ambulation, and other potentially painful activities, patients should be taught to activate the pump prophylactically (e.g., 10 minutes prior to the anticipated activity). Patients should be informed that at night, the PCA device will be adjusted to deliver larger doses than during waking hours; the purpose of this adjustment is to prolong the interval between doses and thereby facilitate sleep.

## Use of Opioids in Specific Settings

**Postoperative Pain.** Opioid analgesics offer several benefits to the postoperative patient. The most obvious is increased comfort through reduction of pain. In addition, by reducing painful sensation, opioids can facilitate early movement and intentional cough. In patients who have undergone thoracic surgery, opioids permit chest movement that would otherwise be too uncomfortable to allow adequate ventilation. By promoting ventilation, opioids can reduce the risk of hypoxia and pneumonitis.

Opioids are not without drawbacks for the postoperative patient. These agents can cause constipation and urinary retention. Suppression of reflex cough can result in respiratory tract complications. In addition, analgesia may delay diagnosis of postoperative complications, since pain will not be present to signal their development.

**Obstetric Analgesia.** When administered to relieve pain during delivery, opioids may depress fetal respiration and uterine contractions. Since these effects are less likely with meperidine than with other strong opioids, meperidine is often the preferred opioid for obstetric use. Dosage should be high enough to reduce maternal discomfort to a tolerable level, but not so high as to cause pronounced respiratory depression in the neonate. Since opioids cross the blood-brain barrier of the infant more readily than that of the mother, doses that have little effect on maternal respiration may nonetheless cause profound respiratory depression in the infant. For meperidine, the usual dosage is 50 to 100 mg every 2 to 3 hours. Administration should be parenteral (IV or IM). Timing of administration is important: if the drug is given too early, it can inhibit or delay the progress of uterine contractions; if given too late, it can cause excessive neonatal sedation and respiratory depression. Following delivery, respiration in the neonate should be monitored closely. Naloxone can reverse respiratory depression and should be on hand.

**Head Injury.** Opioids must be employed with caution in the patient with head injury. Head injury can cause respiratory depression accompanied by elevation of intracranial pressure; opioids can exacerbate these symptoms. In addition, since miosis, mental clouding, and vomiting can be valuable diagnostic signs following head injury, and since opioids can cause these same effects, use of opioids can complicate diagnosis.

**Myocardial Infarction.** Morphine is the opioid of choice for decreasing pain of myocardial infarction. With careful control of dosage, morphine can reduce discomfort without causing excessive respiratory depression and adverse cardiovascular effects. In addition, by lowering blood pressure, morphine can decrease cardiac work. If excessive hypotension or respiratory depression occurs, it can be reversed with naloxone. Since pentazocine and butorphanol increase cardiac work and oxygen demand, these agonist-antagonist opioids should generally be avoided.

**Sickle Cell Vaso-occlusive Crisis.** Sickle cell disease can produce several types of crises: hemolytic crisis, aplastic crisis, splenic sequestration crisis, and vaso-occlusive crisis. Of these, vaso-occlusive crisis is most common. Vaso-occlusion can cause extreme pain in the affected area (e.g., hands and feet, joints and extremities, abdomen). Acute pain generally lasts several days, but may then be followed by dull, aching pain that persists for weeks. The mainstays of treatment are hydration and analgesics.

Studies have shown that patients generally fail to receive adequate analgesia. If the pain is moderate, a non-opioid analgesic (acetaminophen or a nonsteroidal anti-inflammatory agent) may be sufficient. However, if pain is severe, intensive therapy with an opioid is required. Parenteral (IV or IM) morphine and meperidine have been employed. Patient-controlled analgesia may be especially effective.

High doses of intravenous *methylprednisolone* (a glucocorticoid) can shorten the duration of sickle-cell crisis. However, rebound pain may occur when treatment is stopped. For management of sickle-cell crisis, glucocorticoids are used together with opioids, not instead of them. The basic pharmacology of the glucocorticoids is discussed in Chapter 65.

*Hydroxyurea*, a drug traditionally used to treat cancer, was recently shown to decrease the frequency of sickle-cell crises. In patients with sickle-cell disease, the drug increases production of fetal hemoglobin, which in turn decreases sickling of red blood cells. Beneficial effects take several months to develop. Unfortunately, hydroxyurea depresses bone marrow function and can cause leukemia, hence treatment must be monitored carefully. The basic pharmacology of hydroxyurea is discussed in Chapter 95.

**Cancer.** Treating chronic pain of cancer differs substantially from treating acute pain of other disorders. When treating cancer pain, the objective is to maximize comfort. Psychologic and physical dependence are minimal concerns. Patients should be given as much medication as needed to relieve pain. In the words of one pain specialist, "No patient should wish for death because of the physician's reluctance to use adequate amounts of opioids." With proper therapy, cancer pain can be effectively managed in 85% to 95% of patients.

Appropriate management of cancer pain requires appropriate drug selection. Not all patients need a strong opioid. If pain is mild, it can often be relieved with aspirin or another nonopioid analgesic. If pain cannot be relieved with a nonopioid alone, a moderate-to-strong opioid (e.g., codeine) may be added. Only when pain can no longer be controlled with weaker analgesics should a strong opioid be given. Morphine is frequently the drug of choice. Oral therapy is as effective as parenteral therapy and generally preferred. Parenteral opioids should be reserved for patients who cannot take oral drugs because of persistent nausea and vomiting or because of an inability to swallow.

For control of chronic pain, opioids should be given on a fixed schedule (e.g., every 4 hours around the clock) and not on a PRN basis. Use of a fixed schedule ensures continuous suppression of pain, thereby sparing the patient discomfort as well as anxiety about pain returning. If breakthrough pain occurs, fixed dosing can be supplemented with PRN dosing.

Over the course of treatment, escalation of opioid dosage may be required. The need for increased dosage may reflect development of tolerance, or it may reflect progression of the disease. Fortunately, tolerance in cancer patients is rarely so great that adequate analgesia can no longer be achieved. Because analgesic needs may increase, patients should be re-evaluated on a regular basis to determine their drug requirements.

A mixture called *Brompton's cocktail*, named after the British hospital in which it was developed, has been advocated for managing cancer pain. A typical cocktail consists of heroin (in variable amounts), 10 mg of cocaine, 2.5 ml of 98% ethanol, 5 ml of syrup, and chloroform water. Controlled studies indicate that oral morphine solution is as effective as Brompton's cocktail and preferred over the cocktail by most patients.

# Opioid Antagonists

Opioid antagonists are drugs that block the effects of opioid agonists. Principal uses are treatment of opioid overdose, reversal of postoperative opioid effects (e.g., respiratory depression), and management of opioid addiction. Three pure antagonists are available: naloxone [Narcan], nalmefene [Revex], and naltrexone [ReVia, formerly Trexan].

## Naloxone

### Mechanism of Action

Naloxone [Narcan] is a structural analog of morphine that acts as a competitive antagonist at opioid receptors. By blocking access of opioid agonists to these receptors, naloxone prevents the agonists from producing effects. Naloxone can reverse most actions of the opioid agonists, including respiratory depression, coma, and analgesia.

### Pharmacologic Effects

When administered in the absence of opioids, naloxone has no significant effects. If administered prior to giving an opioid, naloxone will block opioid actions. If administered to a patient who is already receiving opioids, naloxone will reverse analgesia, sedation, euphoria, and respiratory depression. If administered to an individual who is physically dependent on opioids, naloxone will precipitate an immediate withdrawal reaction.

### Pharmacokinetics

Naloxone may be administered IV, IM, or SC. Following IV injection, effects begin almost immediately, and persist for about 1 hour. Following IM or SC injection, effects begin within 2 to 5 minutes and persist for several hours. Elimination is by hepatic metabolism. The half-life is approximately 2 hours. Naloxone cannot be used orally because of rapid first-pass inactivation.

### Therapeutic Uses

*Reversal of Opioid Overdose.* Naloxone is the drug of choice for treating overdose with pure opioid agonists. The drug reverses respiratory depression, coma, and other signs of opioid toxicity. Naloxone can also reverse toxicity from agonist-antagonist opioids (e.g., pentazocine, nalbuphine). However, the doses required may be higher than those needed to reverse poisoning by pure agonists.

Dosage must be carefully titrated when treating toxicity in opioid addicts. Because the degree of physical dependence in these individuals is likely to be high, if dosage is excessive, naloxone can transport the patient from a state of poisoning to one of acute withdrawal. Accordingly, treatment should be initiated with a series of small doses rather than a single large dose. Because the half-life of naloxone is shorter than that of most opioids, repeated doses are required until the crisis has passed.

In some cases of accidental poisoning, there may be uncertainty as to whether unconsciousness is due to opioid overdose or to overdose with a general CNS depressant (e.g., barbiturate, alcohol, benzodiazepine). When uncertainty exists, naloxone is nonetheless indicated. If the cause of poisoning is a barbiturate or another general CNS depressant, naloxone will be of no benefit—but neither will it cause any harm. If a cumulative dose of 10 mg fails to elicit a response, it is unlikely that opioids are involved; hence other intoxicants should be suspected.

***Reversal of Postoperative Opioid Effects.*** Following surgery, naloxone may be employed to reverse excessive respiratory and CNS depression caused by opioids given preoperatively or intraoperatively. Dosage should be titrated with care; the objective is to achieve adequate ventilation and alertness without reversing opioid actions to the point of unmasking pain.

***Reversal of Neonatal Respiratory Depression.*** When opioids are given for analgesia during labor and delivery, respiratory depression may occur in the neonate. If respiratory depression is substantial, naloxone should be administered to restore ventilation.

### Preparations, Dosage, and Administration

***Preparations and Routes.*** Naloxone [Narcan] is available in solution (0.4 mg/ml) for IV, IM, and SC injection. A dilute solution (0.02 mg/ml) is available for treating neonates.

***Opioid Overdose.*** The initial dosage is 0.4 mg for adults and 10 μg/kg for children. The preferred route is IV. However, IM or SC injection may be employed if IV administration is not possible. Dosing is repeated at 2- to 3-minute intervals until a satisfactory response has been achieved. Additional doses may be needed at 1- to 2-hour intervals for up to 72 hours, depending on the duration of action of the offending opioid.

***Postoperative Opioid Effects.*** Initial therapy for adults consists of 0.1 to 0.2 mg IV repeated every 2 to 3 minutes until an adequate response has been achieved. Additional doses may be required at 1- to 2-hour intervals.

***Neonatal Respiratory Depression.*** The initial dose is 10 μg/kg (IV, IM, or SC). This dose is repeated every 2 to 3 minutes until respiration is satisfactory.

### Other Opioid Antagonists

#### Naltrexone

Naltrexone [ReVia, formerly Trexan] is a pure opioid antagonist approved for treating opioid abuse and alcohol abuse. In opioid abuse the objective is to prevent euphoria if the abuser should take an opioid. Since naltrexone can precipitate a withdrawal reaction in persons who are physically dependent on opioids, candidates for treatment must be detoxified (rendered opioid-free) before naltrexone is given. Although naltrexone can block opioid-induced euphoria, the drug does not prevent craving for opioids. As a result, many addicts fail to comply with the treatment program. Therapy with naltrexone has been considerably less successful than with methadone, a drug that eliminates craving for opioids while blocking euphoria. Naltrexone is dispensed in 50-mg tablets. A typical dosing schedule consists of 100 mg on Monday and Wednesday and 150 mg on Friday. Alternatively, the drug can be administered daily in 50-mg doses. Use of naltrexone in alcoholism is discussed in Chapter 36.

#### Nalmefene

***Uses.*** Nalmefene [Revex] is a *long-acting* analog of naltrexone. This new drug is approved for reversing postoperative opioid effects and for treating opioid overdose. Nalmefene must be used with caution when treating overdose in patients suspected of being opioid dependent, because too much nalmefene could precipitate prolonged withdrawal.

***Pharmacokinetics.*** Effects begin 2 minutes after IV injection (the usual route) and peak within 5 minutes. The duration of action depends on the dosages: effects may fade within 30 to 60 minutes when a small dose is given, or may last many hours when a large dose is given. Most importantly, when nalmefene is used at effective doses, effects persist longer than those of most opioids. Nalmefene undergoes complete but slow hepatic metabolism, followed by renal excretion. The half-life is 11 hours—considerably longer than that of naloxone.

***Preparations, Dosage, and Administration.*** Nalmefene [Revex] is available in two concentrations. The low concentration (100 μg/ml), dispensed in blue-labeled ampules, is used to reverse postoperative opioid effects. The high concentration (1 mg/ml), dispensed in green-labeled ampules, is used for opioid overdose.

The usual route of administration is IV. However, if IV access is impossible, nalmefene may be given IM or SC. Dosages are the same for all routes, but with IM or SC administration, onset of effects is delayed.

For postoperative use, the initial dose is 0.25 μg/kg. This dose is repeated at 2- to 5-minute intervals (for a maximum of four total doses) until the desired degree of opioid reversal has been achieved.

Treatment of opioid overdose depends on whether the victim is opioid dependent. If the victim is *not* dependent, treatment consists of two doses: 0.5 mg/70 kg initially, followed by 1 mg/70 kg 2 to 5 minutes later. If opioid dependency is suspected, a small (0.1 mg/70 kg) challenge dose is given. If the challenge dose does not precipitate withdrawal, then treatment continues as for patients who are not dependent.

## KEY POINTS

- Analgesics are drugs that relieve pain without causing loss of consciousness.
- Opioids are the most effective analgesics available.
- There are three major classes of opioid receptors, designated mu, kappa, and delta.
- Morphine and other pure opioid agonists relieve pain by mimicking the actions of endogenous opioid peptides primarily at mu receptors (and partly at kappa receptors).
- Opioid-induced sedation and euphoria can complement pain relief.
- Because opioids produce desirable subjective effects (e.g., euphoria), they have a high liability for abuse.
- Respiratory depression is the most serious adverse effect of the opioids.

- Other important adverse effects are constipation, urinary retention, orthostatic hypotension, biliary colic, emesis, and elevation of ICP.
- Because of first-pass metabolism, oral doses of morphine must be larger than parenteral doses to produce equivalent effects.
- Because the blood-brain barrier is poorly developed in infants, these patients need smaller opioid doses (adjusted for body weight) than older children and adults.
- With prolonged opioid use, tolerance develops to analgesia, euphoria, sedation, and respiratory depression, but not to constipation and miosis.
- Cross-tolerance exists among the various opioid agonists, but not between opioid agonists and general CNS depressants.
- With prolonged opioid use, physical dependence develops. An abstinence syndrome will occur if the opioid is abruptly withdrawn.
- In contrast to the withdrawal syndrome associated with general CNS depressants, the opioid withdrawal syndrome, although unpleasant, is not dangerous.
- To minimize the symptoms of abstinence, opioids should be withdrawn gradually.
- Precautions to opioid use include pregnancy, labor and delivery, head injury, and decreased respiratory reserve.
- Patients taking opioids should avoid alcohol and other CNS depressants since these drugs can intensify opioid-induced sedation and respiratory depression.
- Patients taking opioids should avoid anticholinergic drugs (e.g., antihistamines, tricyclic antidepressants, atropine-like drugs) since these drugs can exacerbate opioid-induced constipation and urinary retention.
- Opioid overdose produces a classic triad of signs: coma, respiratory depression, and pinpoint pupils.
- All strong opioid agonists are essentially equal to morphine with regard to analgesia, abuse liability, and respiratory depression.
- Like morphine, codeine and other moderate-to-strong opioid agonists produce analgesia, sedation, euphoria, respiratory depression, constipation, urinary retention, cough suppression, and miosis. These drugs differ from morphine in that they produce less analgesia and respiratory depression and have a lower potential for abuse.
- The combination of codeine with a nonopioid analgesic (e.g., aspirin, acetaminophen) produces greater pain relief than either agent alone.
- Most agonist-antagonist opioids act as agonists at kappa receptors and as antagonists at mu receptors.
- Pentazocine and other agonist-antagonist opioids produce less analgesia than morphine and have a lower potential for abuse.

- With agonist-antagonist opioids, there is a ceiling to respiratory depression.
- If given to a patient who is physically dependent on pure opioid agonists, an agonist-antagonist will precipitate withdrawal.
- Pure opioid antagonists act as antagonists at mu receptors and kappa receptors.
- Naloxone and other pure opioid antagonists can reverse respiratory depression, coma, analgesia, and most other effects of pure opioid agonists.
- Pure opioid antagonists are used primarily to treat opioid overdose.
- If administered in excessive dosage to an individual who is physically dependent on opioid agonists, naloxone will precipitate an immediate withdrawal reaction.
- Opioid dosage must be individualized. Patients with a low tolerance to pain or with extremely painful conditions need high doses. Patients with sharp, stabbing pain need higher doses than patients with dull pain. Elderly adults generally require lower doses than younger adults. Neonates require relatively low doses.
- As a rule, opioids should be administered on a fixed schedule (with supplemental doses for breakthrough pain) rather than PRN.
- A PCA device is an electronically controlled infusion pump that can be activated by the patient to deliver a preset dose of opioid through an indwelling catheter. Some PCA devices also deliver a basal opioid infusion.
- PCA devices provide steady plasma drug levels, thereby maintaining continuous pain control while avoiding unnecessary sedation and respiratory depression.
- Use of parenteral opioids during delivery can suppress uterine contractions and cause respiratory depression in the neonate.
- Cancer patients should be given as much medication as they need to relieve pain. No patient should wish for death because you or the physician is reluctant to provide adequate amounts of opioids.
- Addiction is a behavior pattern characterized by continued use of a psychoactive substance despite physical, psychologic, or social harm. Physical dependence and addiction are not the same.
- Abuse is defined as drug use that is inconsistent with medical or social norms.
- Because of excessive and inappropriate fears about addiction and abuse, physicians frequently prescribe less pain medication than patients need, and nurses frequently administer less medication than was prescribed.
- Please! Dispel your concerns about abuse and addiction and give your patients the medication they need to relieve suffering. That's what opioids are for, after all.

# Summary of Major Nursing Implications*

## Pure Opioid Agonists

| | |
|---|---|
| Alfentanil | Methadone |
| Codeine | Morphine |
| Fentanyl | Oxycodone |
| Hydrocodone | Oxymorphone |
| Hydromorphone | Propoxyphene |
| Levomethadyl | Remifentanil |
| Levorphanol | Sufentanil |
| Meperidine | |

## Preadministration Assessment

### Therapeutic Goal

Relief or prevention of moderate to severe pain while causing minimal respiratory depression, constipation, urinary retention, and other adverse effects.

### Baseline Data

*Pain Assessment.* Assess pain before administration and 1 hour later. Determine the location, time of onset, and quality of pain (e.g., sharp, stabbing, dull). Also, assess for psychologic factors that can lower pain threshold (anxiety, depression, fear, anger). Since pain is subjective and determined by multiple factors (e.g., cultural influences, patient expectations, associated disease), there is no reliable objective method for determining how much discomfort the patient is experiencing. Ultimately, you must rely on your ability to interpret what patients have to say about their pain. When listening to patients, be aware that a few may claim discomfort when their pain is under control, whereas others may claim to feel fine when they are actually in pain.

*Vital Signs.* Prior to administration, determine respiratory rate, blood pressure, and pulse rate.

### Identifying High-Risk Patients

*All opioids* are *contraindicated* for *premature infants* (both during and after delivery). *Morphine* is *contraindicated* following *biliary tract surgery*.

Use opioids with *caution* in patients with *head injury, profound CNS depression, coma, respiratory depression, pulmonary disease* (e.g., emphysema, asthma), *cardiovascular disease, hypotension, reduced blood volume, prostatic hypertrophy, urethral stricture,* and *liver impairment. Caution* is also required when treating *infants, elderly or debilitated patients*, and patients receiving *MAO inhibitors, CNS depressants, anticholinergic drugs, and hypotensive agents*.

## Implementation: Administration

### Routes

Oral, IM, IV, SC, rectal, epidural, intrathecal, transdermal (fentanyl), and transmucosal (fentanyl). Routes for specific opioids are summarized in Tables 25-5 and 25-6.

### Dosage

*General Guidelines.* Adjust dosage to meet individual needs. Higher doses are required for patients with low pain tolerance or with especially painful conditions. Patients with sharp, stabbing pain need higher doses than patients with dull, constant pain. Elderly patients generally require lower doses than younger adults. Neonates require relatively low doses because of their poorly developed blood-brain barriers. For all patients, dosage should be reduced as pain subsides.

Oral doses are larger than parenteral doses. Check to ensure that the dose is appropriate for the intended route.

Tolerance may develop with prolonged treatment, necessitating dosage escalation. Warn outpatients not to increase dosage without consulting the physician.

*Dosage in Patients with Cancer.* Cancer is the principal disease for which opioids are used chronically. The objective is to maximize comfort. Physical dependence is a minor concern. Cancer patients should receive opioids on a fixed schedule around the clock—not PRN. If breakthrough pain occurs, fixed dosing can be supplemented with PRN dosing. Because of tolerance to opioids or intensification of pain, dosage escalation may be required. Hence patients should be re-evaluated on a regular basis to determine if pain control is adequate.

*Discontinuing Opioids.* Although significant dependence in hospitalized patients is rare, it can occur. To minimize symptoms of abstinence, withdraw opioids slowly, tapering the dosage over 3 days. Warn outpatients against abrupt discontinuation of treatment.

### Administration

Prior to administration, determine respiratory rate, blood pressure, and pulse rate. Withhold medication and notify the physician if respiratory rate is at or below 12 per minute, if blood pressure is significantly below the pretreatment value, or if pulse rate is significantly above or below the pretreatment value.

As a rule, opioids should be administered on a fixed schedule, with supplemental doses as needed.

Perform intravenous injections slowly (over 4 to 5 minutes). Rapid injection may produce severe adverse effects (profound hypotension, respiratory arrest, cardiac arrest) and should be avoided. When making an IV injection, have an opioid antagonist (e.g., naloxone) and facilities for respiratory support available.

---

*Patient education information is highlighted in color.

Perform injections (especially IV) with the patient lying down to minimize hypotension.

Opioid agonists are regulated under the Controlled Substances Act and must be dispensed accordingly. All of the pure agonists are Schedule II substances, except for propoxyphene (Schedule IV), hydrocodone (Schedule III), and remifentanil (not regulated).

## Concern for Opioid Abuse as a Factor in Dosage and Administration

Although opioids have a high potential for abuse, abuse is rare in the clinical setting. Consequently, when balancing the risk of abuse against the need to relieve pain, do not give excessive weight to concerns about abuse. The patient must not be allowed to suffer because of your unwarranted fears about abuse and dependence.

Although abuse is rare in the clinical setting, it can occur. To keep abuse to a minimum: (1) exercise clinical judgment when interpreting requests for opioid doses that seem excessive, (2) use opioids in the lowest effective doses for the shortest time required, (3) reserve opioid analgesics for patients with moderate to severe pain, and (4) switch to a nonopioid analgesic when the intensity of pain no longer justifies an opioid.

Responses to analgesics can be reinforced by nondrug measures, such as positioning the patient comfortably, showing concern and interest, and reassuring the patient that the medication will provide relief. Rest, mood elevation, and diversion can raise pain threshold and should be promoted. Conversely, anxiety, depression, fatigue, fear, and anger can lower pain threshold and should be minimized.

## Ongoing Evaluation and Interventions

### Evaluating Therapeutic Effects

Evaluate for pain control 1 hour after opioid administration. If analgesia is insufficient, consult with the physician about an increase in dosage. Patients taking opioids chronically for suppression of cancer pain should be re-evaluated on a regular basis to determine if their dosage is adequate.

### Minimizing Adverse Effects

*Respiratory Depression.* Monitor respiration in all patients. If respiratory rate is 12 per minute or less, withhold medication and notify the physician. Warn outpatients about respiratory depression, and instruct them to notify the physician if respiratory distress occurs.

Certain patients, including the very young, the elderly, and those with respiratory disease (e.g., asthma, emphysema), are especially sensitive to the respiratory depression and must be monitored closely.

Delayed respiratory depression may develop following spinal administration of morphine. Be alert to this possibility.

When employed during labor and delivery, opioids may cause respiratory depression in the neonate. Monitor the infant closely. Have naloxone available to reverse opioid toxicity.

*Sedation.* Inform patients that opioids may cause drowsiness. Warn them against participation in hazardous activities (e.g., driving) if sedation is significant. Sedation can be minimized by (1) using smaller doses given more frequently, (2) using opioids with short half-lives, and (3) giving small doses of a CNS stimulant (methylphenidate or dextroamphetamine) in the morning and early afternoon.

*Orthostatic Hypotension.* Monitor blood pressure and pulse rate. Inform patients about symptoms of hypotension (dizziness, lightheadedness), and advise them to sit or lie down if these occur. Inform patients that hypotension can be minimized by moving slowly when assuming an erect posture. Warn patients against ambulation if hypotension is significant. If appropriate, assist hospitalized patients with ambulation.

*Constipation.* Monitor bowel function and inform the physician if constipation develops. Advise outpatients to increase dietary fiber and fluids. If these measures fail to normalize bowel function, a laxative may be needed.

*Urinary Retention.* To evaluate urinary retention, monitor intake and output, and palpate the lower abdomen for bladder distention every 4 to 6 hours. If there is a change in intake-output ratio, or if bladder distention is detected, or if the patient reports difficulty in voiding, notify the physician. Catheterization may be required. Interference with voiding is especially likely in patients with prostatic hypertrophy.

Since opioids may suppress awareness of bladder stimuli, encourage patients to void every 4 hours.

*Biliary Colic.* By constricting the common bile duct, morphine can increase pressure within the biliary tract, thereby causing severe pain. Biliary colic is much less likely with meperidine.

*Emesis.* Initial doses of opioids may cause nausea and vomiting. These reactions can be minimized by pretreatment with an antiemetic (e.g., promethazine) and by having the patient remain still. Tolerance to emesis develops quickly.

*Cough Suppression.* Cough suppression may result in accumulation of secretions in the airway. Instruct patients to cough at regular intervals. Auscultate the lungs for rales.

*Miosis.* Miosis can impair vision in dim light. Keep hospital room lighting bright during waking hours.

*Opioid Dependence in the Neonate.* The infant whose mother abused opioids during pregnancy may be born drug dependent. Observe the infant for signs of withdrawal (e.g., excessive crying, sneezing, tremor, hyperreflexia, fever, diarrhea) and notify the physician if these develop (usually within a few days after birth). The infant can be weaned from drug dependence by administering dilute opium tincture in progressively smaller doses.

## Minimizing Adverse Interactions

*CNS Depressants.* Opioids can intensify responses to other CNS depressants (e.g., barbiturates, benzodiazepines, alcohol, antihistamines), thereby presenting a risk of profound sedation and respiratory depression. Warn patients against use of alcohol and other CNS depressants.

*Agonist-Antagonist Opioids.* These drugs (e.g., pentazocine, nalbuphine) can precipitate an abstinence syndrome if administered to a patient who is physically dependent on a pure opioid agonist. Before administering an agonist-antagonist, make certain the patient has been withdrawn from opioid agonists.

*Anticholinergic Drugs.* These agents (e.g., atropine-like drugs, tricyclic antidepressants, phenothiazines) can exacerbate opioid-induced constipation and urinary retention.

*Hypotensive Drugs.* Antihypertensive agents and other drugs that lower blood pressure can exacerbate opioid-induced orthostatic hypotension.

*Opioid Antagonists.* Opioid antagonists (e.g., naloxone) can precipitate an abstinence syndrome if administered in excessive dosage to a patient who is physically dependent on opioids. To avoid this reaction, carefully titrate the dosage of the antagonist.

## Agonist-Antagonist Opioids

| | |
|---|---|
| Buprenorphine | Nalbuphine |
| Butorphanol | Pentazocine |
| Dezocine | |

Except for the differences presented below, the nursing implications for these drugs are much like those of the pure opioid agonists.

## Therapeutic Goal

Relief of moderate to severe pain.

## Routes

Oral, IV, IM, SC, and intranasal (butorphanol). Routes for individual agents are summarized in Table 25–7.

## Differences from Pure Opioid Agonists

Maximal pain relief with the agonist-antagonists is generally lower than with pure opioid agonists.

Most agonist-antagonists have a ceiling to respiratory depression, thereby minimizing concerns about insufficient oxygenation.

Agonist-antagonists cause little euphoria. Hence abuse liability is low.

Agonist-antagonists increase cardiac work and should not be given to patients with acute myocardial infarction.

Because of their antagonist properties, agonist-antagonists can precipitate an abstinence syndrome in patients physically dependent on opioid agonists. Accordingly, patients must be withdrawn from pure opioid agonists before receiving an agonist-antagonist.

## Naloxone

### Therapeutic Goal

Reversal of (1) postoperative opioid effects, (2) neonatal respiratory depression, and (3) overdose with pure opioid agonists.

### Routes

Intravenous, IM, and SC. For initial treatment, administer IV. Once opioid-induced CNS and respiratory depression have been reversed, IM or SC administration may be employed.

### Dosage

Titrate dosage carefully. In opioid addicts, excessive doses can precipitate withdrawal. In postoperative patients, excessive doses can bring on pain by reversing opioid-mediated analgesia.

# CHAPTER 26

# Local Anesthetics

L ocal anesthetics are drugs that suppress pain by blocking impulse conduction along axons. Conduction blockade occurs only in neurons located near the site of anesthetic administration. The great advantage of local anesthesia, as compared with inhalation anesthesia, is that pain can be suppressed without causing generalized depression of the entire nervous system. Hence, local anesthetics allow performance of medical and surgical procedures with much less risk than is associated with general anesthetics.

We will begin the chapter by considering the pharmacology of the local anesthetics as a group. Next we will discuss three prototypic agents: procaine, lidocaine, and cocaine. We will conclude by discussing specific routes of anesthetic administration.

## Basic Pharmacology of the Local Anesthetics

### Classification

Most local anesthetics fall into one of two groups: *esters* or *amides*. As shown in Figure 26-1, the ester-type anesthetics, represented by *procaine* [Novocain], contain an ester linkage in their structure; in contrast, the amide-type agents, represented by *lidocaine* [Xylocaine], contain an amide linkage. The ester-type agents and amide-type agents differ in two important ways: mode of inactivation and relative ability to promote allergic responses. These differences are discussed in detail later. Characteristic properties of the esters and amides are summarized in Table 26-1.

### Mechanism of Action

Local anesthetics stop axonal conduction by *blocking sodium channels* in the axonal membrane. Recall that propagation of an action potential requires that sodium ions move from outside the axon to the inside. This influx takes place through sodium channels. Hence, by blocking axonal sodium channels, local anesthetics prevent sodium entry, and thereby bring conduction to a halt.

### Selectivity of Anesthetic Effects

Local anesthetics are nonselective modifiers of neuronal function. That is, these drugs will block action potentials in all neurons to which they have access. The only way that we can achieve selectivity is through delivery of the anesthetic to a limited area.

Although local anesthetics can block traffic in all neurons, blockade develops more rapidly in some than in others. Specifically, small, nonmyelinated neurons undergo blockade more rapidly than large, myelinated neurons. Because of this differential sensitivity, there is a temporal sequence in which sensations are lost: perception of pain is lost first, followed in order by perception of cold, warmth, touch, and deep pressure.

It should be noted that the effects of local anesthetics are not limited to sensory neurons; these drugs also block conduction in *motor neurons*.

### Time Course of Local Anesthesia

Ideally, local anesthesia would begin promptly and would persist no longer (or shorter) than needed. Unfortunately, although onset of anesthesia is usually rapid (see Tables 26-2 and 26-3), duration of anesthesia is often less than ideal: in some cases, anesthesia persists longer than

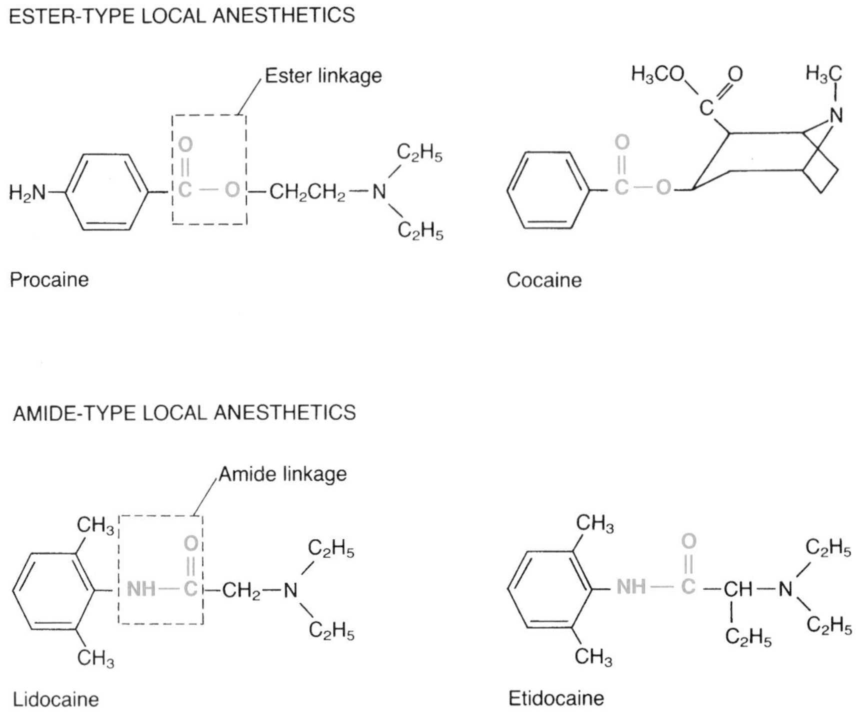

ESTER-TYPE LOCAL ANESTHETICS

Procaine

Cocaine

AMIDE-TYPE LOCAL ANESTHETICS

Lidocaine

Etidocaine

**Figure 26–1. Structural formulas of representative local anesthetics.**

needed; in others, repeated administration is required to maintain anesthesia of sufficient duration.

*Onset* of local anesthesia is determined largely by the molecular properties of the anesthetic. Before anesthesia can occur, the anesthetic must diffuse from its site of administration to its sites of action inside the axonal membrane; anesthesia is delayed until this movement has occurred. The ability of an anesthetic to penetrate the axonal membrane is determined by three properties: *molecular size, lipid solubility,* and *degree of ionization at tissue pH.* Anesthetics of small size, high lipid solubility, and low ionization cross the axonal membrane relatively rapidly. In contrast, anesthetics of large size, low lipid solubility, and high ionization cross more slowly. Obviously, anesthetics that penetrate the axon most rapidly have the fastest onset of action.

*Termination* of local anesthesia occurs as molecules of anesthetic diffuse out of neurons and are carried away in the blood. The same factors that determine onset of anesthesia (molecular size, lipid solubility, degree of ionization) also help determine duration. In addition, *regional blood flow* is an important determinant of how long anesthesia will last. In areas where blood flow is high, anesthetic is carried away quickly, and hence effects terminate with relative haste. In regions where blood flow is low, anesthesia is more prolonged.

## Use with Vasoconstrictors

Local anesthetics are frequently administered in combination with a vasoconstrictor—usually epinephrine. The vasoconstrictor decreases local blood flow and thereby delays systemic absorption of the anesthetic. Delaying absorption offers two benefits: it *prolongs anesthesia* and *reduces the risk of toxicity.* Why is toxicity reduced? First, by delaying absorption, we can use less anesthetic. Second, by delaying absorption, we can establish a more favorable balance between the rate of entry of anesthetic into circulation and the capacity of the body to convert the anesthetic into inactive metabolites.

It should be noted that absorption of the vasoconstrictor itself into the blood can result in systemic toxicity (e.g., palpitations, tachycardia, nervousness, hypertension). If adrenergic stimulation from absorption of epinephrine is excessive, symptoms can be controlled with alpha- and beta-adrenergic antagonists.

## Fate in the Body

***Absorption and Distribution.*** Although administered for local effects, local anesthetics do get absorbed into the

### TABLE 26–1. CONTRASTS BETWEEN ESTER AND AMIDE LOCAL ANESTHETICS

|  | Ester-type Anesthetics | Amide-type Anesthetics |
|---|---|---|
| *Characteristic chemistry* | Ester bond | Amide bond |
| *Representative agents* | Procaine | Lidocaine |
| *Incidence of allergic reactions* | Low | Very low |
| *Method of metabolism* | Plasma esterases | Hepatic enzymes |

### TABLE 26-2. TOPICAL LOCAL ANESTHETICS: TRADE NAMES, INDICATIONS, AND TIME COURSE OF ACTION

| | Generic Name | Trade Name | Indications | | Time Course of Action* | |
|---|---|---|---|---|---|---|
| | | | Skin | Mucous Membranes | Peak Effect (min) | Duration (min) |
| *Amides* | Dibucaine[†] | Nupercainal | ✔ | | <5 | 15-45 |
| | Lidocaine[†] | Xylocaine, others | ✔ | ✔ | 2-5 | 15-45 |
| *Esters* | Benzocaine | Many names | ✔ | ✔ | <5 | 15-45 |
| | Butamben | Butesin | ✔ | | — | — |
| | Cocaine | | | ✔ | 2-5 | 30-60 |
| | Tetracaine[†] | Pontocaine | ✔ | ✔ | 3-8 | 30-60 |
| *Others* | Dyclonine | Dyclone | | ✔ | <10 | <60 |
| | Pramoxine | Tronothane, others | ✔ | | 3-5 | — |

*Based primarily on application to mucous membranes.
[†]Also administered by injection.

bloodstream and become distributed to all parts of the body. The rate of absorption is determined in large part by blood flow to the site of administration.

**Metabolism.** The process by which a local anesthetic is metabolized depends on the category—ester or amide—to which it belongs. *Ester-type* local anesthetics are metabolized in the *blood* by enzymes known as *esterases*. In contrast, *amide-type* agents are metabolized by enzymes in the *liver*. For both types of anesthetic, metabolism results in inactivation.

The balance between rate of absorption and rate of metabolism is of clinical significance. If a local anesthetic is absorbed more slowly than it is metabolized, plasma drug levels will remain low and systemic reactions will be minimal. However, if absorption occurs too swiftly, absorption will outpace metabolism, plasma drug levels will rise, and the risk of systemic toxicity will increase.

## Adverse Effects

Adverse effects can occur locally or distant from the site of administration. Systemic effects are most common.

**Central Nervous System.** When absorbed in sufficient amounts, local anesthetics cause central nervous system

### TABLE 26-3. INJECTABLE LOCAL ANESTHETICS: TRADE NAMES AND TIME COURSE OF ACTION

| | Generic Name | Trade Name | Time Course of Action* | |
|---|---|---|---|---|
| | | | Onset (min) | Duration (hr) |
| *Esters* | Procaine | Novocain | 2-5 | 0.25-1.0 |
| | Chloroprocaine | Nesacaine | 6-12 | 0.25-0.5 |
| | Tetracaine[†] | Pontocaine | ≤15 | 2-3 |
| *Amides* | Lidocaine[†] | Xylocaine, others | <2 | 0.5-1 |
| | Prilocaine | Citanest | <2 | ≥1 |
| | Mepivacaine | Carbocaine, Isocaine, Polocaine | 3-5 | 0.75-1.5 |
| | Bupivacaine | Marcaine, Sensorcaine | 5 | 2-4 |
| | Etidocaine | Duranest | 3-5 | 5-10 |
| | Ropivacaine | Naropin | 1-15 | 2-6 |

*Values are for *infiltration* anesthesia in the absence of epinephrine (epinephrine prolongs duration two- to three-fold).
[†]Also administered topically.

(CNS) excitation followed by depression. During the excitation phase, convulsions may occur. These can be controlled with intravenous diazepam or, if necessary, a neuromuscular blocking agent (e.g., succinylcholine). Depressant effects range from drowsiness to unconsciousness; death can occur secondary to depression of respiration. If respiratory depression is prominent, mechanical ventilation with oxygen is indicated.

**Cardiovascular System.** When absorbed in sufficient amounts, local anesthetics can affect the heart and blood vessels. In the heart, local anesthetics suppress excitability in the myocardium and conducting system, and thereby can cause *bradycardia, heart block, reduced contractile force*, and even *cardiac arrest*. In blood vessels, anesthetics relax vascular smooth muscle; the resultant vasodilation can cause hypotension. As discussed in Chapter 48 (Antidysrhythmic Drugs), the cardiosuppressant actions of one local anesthetic—lidocaine—are exploited to treat dysrhythmias.

**Allergic Reactions.** An array of hypersensitivity reactions, ranging from allergic dermatitis to anaphylaxis, have been triggered by local anesthetics. These reactions, which are relatively uncommon, are much more likely with the *ester-type* anesthetics (e.g., procaine) than with the amides. Patients allergic to one ester-type anesthetic are likely to be allergic to all other ester-type agents. Fortunately, cross-hypersensitivity between the esters and amides has not been observed. Hence, the amides can be used when allergies contraindicate use of ester-type anesthetics.

**Use in Labor and Delivery.** Local anesthetics can depress uterine contractility and maternal expulsion effort. Both actions can prolong labor. Also, local anesthetics can cross the placenta, causing bradycardia and CNS depression in the neonate.

# Properties of Individual Local Anesthetics

## Procaine

Procaine [Novocain] was synthesized in 1905 and is the prototype of the ester-type local anesthetics. The drug is ineffective topically, and hence must be administered by injection. Administration in combination with epinephrine delays absorption. Procaine is readily absorbed but systemic toxicity is rare: plasma esterases rapidly convert the drug to inactive, nontoxic products. Being an ester-type anesthetic, procaine is more likely to cause allergic responses than the amide-type anesthetics. Individuals allergic to procaine are likely to be allergic to all other ester-type anesthetics—but not to the amides.

For many years, procaine was the local anesthetic most preferred for use by injection. However, with the development of newer agents, use of procaine has sharply declined. Once popular in dentistry, procaine is rarely employed in that setting today.

**Preparations.** Procaine hydrochloride [Novocain] is available in solution (1%, 2%, and 10%) for administration by injection. Dilution is required for use by some routes. Epinephrine (at a final concentration of 1:100,000 or 1:200,000) may be combined with procaine to delay absorption.

## Lidocaine

Lidocaine was introduced in 1948 and is the prototype of the amide-type agents. One of today's most widely used local anesthetics, lidocaine can be administered topically and by injection. Anesthesia from lidocaine is more rapid, more intense, and more prolonged than with an equal dose of procaine. Effects can be extended by coadministration of epinephrine. Allergic reactions are rare; individuals allergic to ester-type anesthetics are not cross-allergic to lidocaine. If plasma levels of lidocaine climb too high, CNS and cardiovascular toxicity can result. Inactivation is by hepatic metabolism.

In addition to its use in local anesthesia, lidocaine is employed to treat dysrhythmias (see Chapter 48). Control of dysrhythmias results from suppression of cardiac excitability secondary to blockade of sodium channels.

**Preparations.** Lidocaine hydrochloride [Xylocaine, others] is dispensed in several formulations (cream, ointment, jelly, solution, aerosol) for topical administration. Lidocaine for injection is available in concentrations ranging from 0.5% to 20%; some preparations contain epinephrine (1:50,000, 1:100,000, or 1:200,000).

## Cocaine

Cocaine was the first local anesthetic discovered. Clinical use was initiated in 1884 by Sigmund Freud and Karl Koller. Freud described the physiologic effects of cocaine while Koller focused on the drug's anesthetic actions. As can be seen from its structure (Fig. 26–1), cocaine is an ester-type anesthetic. In addition to causing local anesthesia, cocaine has pronounced effects on the sympathetic and central nervous systems. Sympathetic and CNS effects are due in large part to the drug's ability to block uptake of norepinephrine by adrenergic neurons.

**Anesthetic Use.** Cocaine is an excellent local anesthetic. Administration is topical. The drug is employed for anesthesia of the ear, nose, and throat. Anesthesia develops rapidly and persists for about an hour. Unlike other local anesthetics, cocaine causes intense vasoconstriction (by blocking norepinephrine uptake at sympathetic nerve terminals on blood vessels). Accordingly, the drug should not be given in combination with epinephrine or other vasoconstrictors. Despite its ability to constrict blood vessels, cocaine is readily absorbed following application to mucous membranes; significant effects on the brain and heart can result. The drug is inactivated by plasma esterases and enzymes in the liver.

**CNS Effects.** Cocaine produces generalized CNS stimulation. Moderate doses cause euphoria, loquaciousness, reduced fatigue, and increased sociability and alertness. Excessive doses can cause seizures. Excitation is followed by CNS depression; respiratory arrest and death can result.

Although cocaine does not seem to cause substantial physical dependence, psychologic dependence can be profound. The drug is subject to widespread abuse and is classified under Schedule II of the Controlled Substances Act. Cocaine abuse is discussed in Chapter 37.

***Cardiovascular Effects.*** Cocaine stimulates the heart and causes vasoconstriction. These effects result from (1) central stimulation of the sympathetic nervous system and (2) blockade of norepinephrine uptake in the periphery. Stimulation of the heart can produce tachycardia and potentially fatal dysrhythmias. Vasoconstriction can cause hypertension. Cocaine presents an especially serious risk to individuals with cardiovascular disease (e.g., hypertension, dysrhythmias, angina pectoris).

When used for local anesthesia, cocaine should not be combined with epinephrine, since the combination would increase the risk of cardiovascular toxicity. Furthermore, since a vasoconstrictor would not significantly retard cocaine absorption, the combination would be irrational in addition to dangerous.

***Preparations and Administration.*** Cocaine hydrochloride is available in soluble tablets (135 mg), as a powder (5 and 25 gm), and in solution (40 and 100 mg/ml). Administration is topical. For application to the ear, nose, or throat, a 4% solution is usually employed. The drug must be dispensed in accord with the Controlled Substances Act.

## Other Local Anesthetics

In addition to the drugs discussed above, several other local anesthetics are available. These agents differ from one another with respect to indications, routes of administration, mode of elimination, duration of action, and toxicity.

The local anesthetics can be grouped according to route of administration: topical versus injection. (Very few agents are administered by both routes, largely because the drugs that are suitable for topical application are usually too toxic for parenteral use.) Table 26–2 lists the topically administered local anesthetics along with trade names and time course of action. Table 26–3 presents equivalent information for the injectable agents.

## Clinical Use of Local Anesthetics

## General Precautions

When local anesthetics are administered parenterally, the following precautions apply. Severe reactions can occur with inadvertent injection into arteries and veins. To avoid intravascular injection, aspirate prior to injection. Because serious systemic reactions may occur, parenteral local anesthetics should be given only when equipment for resuscitation is immediately available. An IV line should be

in place prior to administering the anesthetic so as to permit rapid treatment of severe toxicity. Following an injection of anesthetic, the patient should be monitored periodically for cardiovascular status, respiratory function, and state of consciousness. To reduce the risk of toxicity, local anesthetics should be administered in the lowest effective dosage.

## Techniques Employed to Produce Local Anesthesia

Local anesthetics may be administered in two ways: *topically* (for surface anesthesia) and *by injection* (for infiltration anesthesia, nerve block anesthesia, intravenous regional anesthesia, epidural anesthesia, and spinal anesthesia). The characteristics of surface anesthesia and the various types of anesthesia that result from injection are discussed below. It should be noted that injection of local anesthetics requires special skills. Hence administration is usually performed by an anesthesiologist.

### Surface Anesthesia

Surface anesthesia is accomplished by applying a local anesthetic to the skin or a mucous membrane. The agents employed most commonly are *lidocaine*, *tetracaine*, and *cocaine*.

***Systemic Toxicity.*** Topical anesthetics can be absorbed in amounts sufficient to produce systemic toxicity. Cardiovascular reactions and CNS reactions are of principal concern. Since the extent of absorption is proportional to the surface area covered, the risk of toxicity is greatest when the surface area is large. Also, since absorption occurs more readily through mucous membranes than through the skin, toxicity is more likely with application to mucous membranes. If the skin is abraded or otherwise injured, anesthetic absorption will be increased, as will the risk of toxicity.

***Therapeutic Uses.*** Local anesthetics are applied to the skin to relieve pain, itching, and soreness of various causes, including infection, thermal burns, sunburn, diaper rash, wounds, bruises, abrasions, plant poisoning, and insect bites. Application may be made to *mucous membranes* of the nose, mouth, pharynx, larynx, trachea, bronchi, vagina, and urethra. In addition, local anesthetics may be used to relieve discomfort associated with hemorrhoids, anal fissures, and pruritus ani.

### Infiltration Anesthesia

Infiltration anesthesia is achieved by injecting a local anesthetic directly into the immediate area of surgery or manipulation. Anesthesia can be prolonged by combining the anesthetic with epinephrine. However, epinephrine should not be used in areas supplied by end arteries (toes, fingers, nose, ears, penis), since restriction of blood flow at these sites may result in gangrene. The agents employed most frequently for infiltration anesthesia are *procaine*, *lidocaine*, and *bupivacaine*.

### Nerve Block Anesthesia

Nerve block anesthesia is achieved by injecting a local anesthetic into or near the nerves that *supply* the surgical field, but at a site *distant* from the field itself. An advantage of this technique is that anesthesia can be produced using doses that are smaller than those needed for infiltration anesthesia.

Drug selection is based on required duration of anesthesia. For shorter procedures, *lidocaine* or *mepivacaine* might be used. For longer procedures, *bupivacaine* would be appropriate.

### Intravenous Regional Anesthesia

Intravenous regional anesthesia is employed to anesthetize the extremities—hands, feet, arms, lower leg, but not the entire leg (because too much anesthetic would be needed). Anesthesia is produced by injection into a distal vein of an arm or leg. Prior to anesthetic administration, blood is removed from the limb (by gravity or by application of an Esmarch bandage), and a tourniquet is applied to the limb (proximal to the site of anesthetic injection) to prevent anesthetic from entering the general circulation. To ensure complete blockade of arterial flow throughout the procedure, a double tourniquet is used. Following injection, the anesthetic diffuses out of the vasculature and becomes evenly distributed to all areas of the occluded limb. When the tourniquet is loosened at the end of surgery, about 15% to 30% of administered anesthetic is released into the systemic circulation. *Lidocaine—without epinephrine—*is the preferred agent for intravenous regional anesthesia.

### Epidural Anesthesia

Epidural anesthesia is achieved by injecting a local anesthetic into the epidural space (i.e., within the spinal column but outside the dura mater). A catheter placed in the epidural space allows administration by bolus or continuous infusion. Following administration, diffusion of anesthetic across the dura into the subarachnoid space blocks conduction in nerve roots and in the spinal cord itself. Diffusion through intervertebral foramina blocks nerves located in the paravertebral region. With epidural administration, anesthetic can reach the systemic circulation in significant amounts. As a result, when the technique is used during delivery, neonatal depression may result. *Lidocaine* and *bupivacaine* are popular drugs for epidural anesthesia. Because of the risk of cardiac arrest, the 0.75% solution of bupivacaine should not be used for epidural anesthesia in obstetric patients.

### Spinal (Subarachnoid) Anesthesia

*Technique.* Spinal anesthesia is produced by injecting local anesthetic into the subarachnoid space. Injection is made in the lumbar region below the termination of the cord. Spread of anesthetic within the subarachnoid space determines the level of anesthesia achieved. Movement of anesthetic within the subarachnoid space is determined by two factors: (1) the density of the anesthetic solution and (2) the position in which the patient is lying. Anesthetics employed most commonly are *lidocaine*, *tetracaine*, and *bupivacaine*. All must be free of preservatives.

*Adverse Effects.* The most significant adverse effect of spinal anesthesia is *hypotension*. Blood pressure is reduced by venous dilation secondary to blockade of sympathetic nerves. (Loss of venous tone decreases the return of blood to the heart, causing a reduction in cardiac output and a corresponding fall in blood pressure.) Loss of venous tone can be compensated for by placing the patient in a 10- to 15-degree head-down position, which promotes venous return to the heart. If blood pressure cannot be restored through head-down positioning, drugs may be indicated; ephedrine and phenylephrine have been employed to promote vasoconstriction and enhance cardiac performance.

Autonomic blockade may disrupt function of the intestinal and urinary tracts, causing fecal incontinence and either urinary incontinence or urinary retention. The physician should be notified if the patient fails to void within 8 hours of the end of surgery.

Spinal anesthesia frequently causes headache. These "spinal" headaches are posture dependent and can be relieved by having the patient assume a supine position.

## KEY POINTS

- Local anesthetics stop nerve conduction by blocking sodium channels in the axonal membrane.
- Small, unmyelinated neurons are blocked more rapidly than large, myelinated neurons.
- There are two classes of local anesthetics: ester-type anesthetics and amide-type anesthetics.
- Ester-type anesthetics (e.g., procaine) occasionally cause allergic reactions and are inactivated by esterases in the blood.
- Amide-type anesthetics (e.g., lidocaine) rarely cause allergic reactions and are inactivated by enzymes in the liver.
- Onset of anesthesia occurs most rapidly with anesthetics that are small, lipid soluble, and un-ionized at physiologic pH.
- Termination of local anesthesia is determined in large part by regional blood flow. Hence, coadministration of epinephrine, a vasoconstrictor, will prolong anesthesia.
- Local anesthetics can be absorbed in amounts sufficient to cause systemic toxicity. Principal concerns are cardiac depression, vasodilation, and CNS excitation followed by depression.
- Because of the risk of systemic toxicity, an IV line should be in place prior to anesthetic administration (to permit administration of required drugs), and facilities for resuscitation should be immediately available.

## Summary of Major Nursing Implications*

## Injected Local Anesthetics

Bupivacaine    Prilocaine
Chloroprocaine    Procaine
Etidocaine    Ropivacaine
Lidocaine    Tetracaine
Mepivacaine

### Preadministration Assessment

#### Therapeutic Goal

Production of local anesthesia for surgical, dental, and obstetric procedures.

#### Identifying High-Risk Patients

*Ester-type* local anesthetics are *contraindicated* for patients with a *history of serious allergic reactions to these drugs.*

---

*Patient education information is highlighted in color.

## Implementation: Administration

### Preparation of the Patient

The nurse may be responsible for preparing the patient to receive an injectable local anesthetic. Preparation includes cleansing the injection site, shaving the site when indicated, and placing the patient in a position appropriate to receive the injection. Children, elderly patients, and uncooperative patients may require restraint prior to injection by some routes.

### Administration

Injection of local anesthetics is performed by clinicians with special training in their use (physicians, dentists, nurse anesthetists).

## Ongoing Evaluation and Interventions

### Minimizing Adverse Effects

*Systemic Reactions.* Absorption into the general circulation can cause systemic toxicity. Effects on the CNS and heart are of greatest concern. CNS toxicity manifests as a brief period of excitement, possibly including convulsions, followed by CNS depression, which can result in respiratory depression. Cardiotoxicity can manifest as bradycardia, atrioventricular (AV) heart block, and cardiac arrest. Monitor blood pressure, pulse rate, respiratory rate, and state of consciousness. Have facilities for cardiopulmonary resuscitation available. Manage convulsions with IV diazepam or a neuromuscular blocking agent.

*Allergic Reactions.* Severe allergic reactions are rare but can occur. These are most likely with ester-type anesthetics. Avoid ester-type agents in patients with a history of allergy to these drugs.

*Labor and Delivery.* Use of local anesthetics during delivery can cause bradycardia and CNS depression in the newborn. Monitor cardiac status.

*Self-Inflicted Injury.* Since anesthetics eliminate pain, and since pain warns us about injury, the patient recovering from anesthesia must be protected from inadvertent harm until anesthesia wears off. Caution the patient against activities that might result in unintentional harm. Position the patient comfortably.

*Spinal Headache and Urinary Retention.* Patients recovering from spinal anesthesia may experience headache and urinary retention. Headache is posture dependent and can be minimized by having the patient remain supine for about 12 hours. Notify the physician if the patient fails to void within 8 hours.

## Topical Local Anesthetics

| | |
|---|---|
| Benzocaine | Dyclonine |
| Butamben | Lidocaine |
| Cocaine | Pramoxine |
| Dibucaine | Tetracaine |

## Preadministration Assessment

### Therapeutic Goal

Reduction of discomfort associated with local disorders of the skin and mucous membranes.

### Identifying High-Risk Patients

*Ester-type* local anesthetics are *contraindicated* for patients with a *history of serious allergic reactions to these drugs.*

## Implementation: Administration

### Routes

Topical application to skin and mucous membranes.

### Administration

Apply in the lowest effective dosage to the smallest area required. If possible, avoid application to skin that is abraded or otherwise injured.

## Ongoing Evaluation and Interventions

### Minimizing Adverse Effects

*Systemic Toxicity.* Absorption into the general circulation can cause systemic toxicity. Effects on the heart (bradycardia, AV heart block, cardiac arrest) and CNS (excitation, possibly including convulsions, followed by depression) are of greatest concern. Monitor blood pressure, pulse rate, respiratory rate, and state of consciousness. Have facilities for cardiopulmonary resuscitation available.

The risk of systemic toxicity is determined by the extent of absorption. To minimize absorption, apply topical anesthetics to the smallest surface area needed and, when possible, avoid application to injured skin.

*Allergic Reactions.* Severe allergic reactions are rare but can occur; these are most likely with ester-type anesthetics. Avoid ester-type agents in patients with a history of allergy to these drugs.

# General Anesthetics

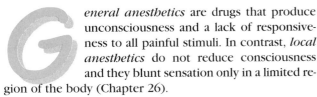

*eneral anesthetics* are drugs that produce unconsciousness and a lack of responsiveness to all painful stimuli. In contrast, *local anesthetics* do not reduce consciousness and they blunt sensation only in a limited region of the body (Chapter 26).

General anesthetics can be divided into two groups: (1) inhalation anesthetics and (2) intravenous anesthetics. The inhalation anesthetics are the main focus of the chapter.

When considering the anesthetics, we need to distinguish between the terms *analgesia* and *anesthesia*. Analgesia refers specifically to loss of sensibility to pain. In contrast, anesthesia refers not only to loss of pain but to loss of all other sensations as well (e.g., touch, temperature, taste). Hence, while analgesics (e.g., aspirin, morphine) can selectively reduce pain without affecting other sensory modalities and without reducing consciousness, the general anesthetics have no such selectivity: during general anesthesia, all sensation is lost, and consciousness is lost as well.

The development of general anesthetics has had an incalculable impact on the surgeon's art. The first general anesthetic (ether) was introduced by Dr. William T. Morton in 1846. Prior to this time, surgery was a brutal and exquisitely painful ordeal, undertaken only under the most desperate circumstances. Immobilization of the surgical field was accomplished with the aid of strong men and straps. Survival of the patient was determined by the surgeon's speed—not by his finesse. With the advent of general anesthesia, all of this changed. General anesthesia

produced a patient who slept through surgery and experienced no pain. These changes allowed surgeons to develop the lengthy and intricate procedures that are routine today. Such procedures were unthinkable before general anesthetics became available.

## Basic Pharmacology of the Inhalation Anesthetics

The information addressed in this section applies to the inhalation anesthetics as a group. We will focus on (1) properties of an ideal anesthetic, (2) pharmacokinetic aspects of inhalation anesthesia, (3) adverse effects of the inhalation anesthetics, and (4) drugs employed as adjuncts to anesthesia.

### Properties of an Ideal Inhalation Anesthetic

An ideal inhalation anesthetic would produce unconsciousness, analgesia, muscle relaxation, and amnesia. Furthermore, induction of anesthesia would be brief and pleasant, as would the process of emergence. Depth of anesthesia could be raised or lowered with ease. Adverse effects would be minimal, and the margin of safety would be large. As one might guess, the ideal inhalation anesthetic does not exist: no single agent has all of these properties.

## Balanced Anesthesia

The term *balanced anesthesia* refers to the use of a combination of drugs to accomplish what we cannot achieve with an inhalation anesthetic alone. Put another way, balanced anesthesia is a technique employed to compensate for the lack of an ideal anesthetic. Drugs are combined in balanced anesthesia to ensure that induction is smooth and rapid, and that analgesia and muscle relaxation are adequate. The agents used most commonly to achieve these goals are (1) short-acting barbiturates (for induction of anesthesia), (2) neuromuscular blocking agents (for muscle relaxation), and (3) opioids and nitrous oxide (for analgesia). The primary benefit of combining drugs to achieve surgical anesthesia is that it permits full general anesthesia at doses of the inhalation anesthetic that are lower (safer) than those that would be required if surgical anesthesia were attempted using an inhalation anesthetic alone.

### Stages of Anesthesia

The state of anesthesia has four stages of increasing depth. These stages were first described for patients undergoing anesthesia with ether, an agent whose effects develop slowly. Because modern anesthetics act much more rapidly than ether, the early stages of anesthesia usually pass so quickly as to be undiscernable. Hence, the stages of anesthesia described below, which are conspicuous during anesthesia with ether, are rarely seen in modern practice.

*I. Stage of Analgesia.* The initial stage of anesthesia begins with the onset of anesthetic administration and extends until consciousness is lost. Stage I is characterized by analgesia and moderate muscle relaxation. Some major surgeries can be performed at this stage.

*II. Stage of Delirium.* Stage II begins with loss of consciousness and extends to the onset of the stage of surgical anesthesia. Stage II is characterized by delirious excitement and reflex muscle activity. Respiration is likely to be irregular. Vomiting and urinary or fecal incontinence may occur. Stage II can be troublesome, and anesthesiologists try to hasten passage through it.

*III. Stage of Surgical Anesthesia.* Stage III extends from the end of stage II to the point where spontaneous respiration ceases. Stage III is characterized by deep unconsciousness, varying degrees of respiratory depression, and suppression of certain reflexes. Muscle relaxation is greater than in stages I and II.

Stage III can be subdivided into four planes of increasing depth. As the patient passes through these planes, respiration becomes progressively weaker.

*IV. Stage of Medullary Paralysis.* Stage IV begins when all spontaneous respiration is lost. Passage into stage IV results from anesthetic overdose. During this stage, vital signs are dangerously depressed; death results from circulatory collapse.

### Molecular Mechanism of Action

Our understanding of how inhalation anesthetics act has changed dramatically in recent years. Attention has shifted from nonspecific effects on neuronal membranes to selective alteration of synaptic transmission. However, despite recent advances, we still don't know with certainty just how these drugs work.

For many years it was postulated that inhalation anesthetics acted by disrupting the lipid bilayer of the neuronal membrane. This longstanding theory was based on the observation that there is a direct correlation between the potency of an anesthetic and its lipid solubility. That is, the more readily an anesthetic could dissolve in the lipid matrix of the neuronal membrane, the more readily that agent could produce anesthesia. Hence, the theory that anesthetics dissolve into neuronal membranes, disrupt their structure, and thereby suppress axonal conduction and possibly synaptic transmission.

New data suggest that anesthetics may act by enhancing the effects of GABA (gamma-aminobutyric acid), the principal inhibitory transmitter in the central nervous system (CNS). Anesthetics appear to enhance GABA's effects by (1) promoting the release of GABA from presynaptic terminals and (2) increasing the binding of GABA to its receptors. Both actions result from the interaction of anesthetics with specific proteins in the neuronal membrane, and not from dissolution of anesthetics into the neuronal membrane, as previously thought. In addition to enhancing the inhibitory actions of GABA, anesthetics may suppress the actions of excitatory neurotransmitters.

## Minimum Alveolar Concentration

The minimum alveolar concentration (MAC) is an index of inhalation anesthetic potency. The MAC is defined as *the minimum concentration of drug in the alveolar air that will produce immobility in 50% of patients exposed to a painful stimulus*. Please note that, by this definition, a *low* MAC indicates high anesthetic potency.

From a clinical perspective, knowledge of the MAC of an anesthetic is of great practical value: the MAC tells us approximately how much anesthetic the inspired air must contain to produce anesthesia. A low MAC indicates that the inspired air need contain only low concentrations of drug to produce anesthesia. Conversely, when a drug has a high MAC, anesthesia can be achieved only when drug concentration in the inspired air is high. Fortunately, most inhalation anesthetics have very low MACs (Table 27–1), and therefore can act at low concentrations. However, one important agent—nitrous oxide—has a very high MAC. The MAC is so high, in fact, that surgical anesthesia cannot be achieved using nitrous oxide alone.

## Pharmacokinetics

### Uptake and Distribution

To produce therapeutic effects, an inhalation anesthetic must reach a concentration in the CNS that is sufficient to suppress neuronal excitability. The principal determinants of anesthetic concentration are (1) uptake from the lungs and (2) distribution to the CNS and other tissues. The kinetics of anesthetic uptake and distribution are complex and will be considered only briefly.

*Uptake.* A major determinant of anesthetic uptake is the concentration of anesthetic in the inspired air: the greater the anesthetic concentration, the more rapid uptake will be. Other factors that contribute to anesthetic uptake are pulmonary ventilation, solubility of the anesthetic in blood, and blood flow through the lungs. An increase in any of these factors will increase the rate of uptake.

*Distribution.* Distribution to specific tissues is determined largely by regional blood flow. Anesthetic levels rise most rapidly in the brain, kidney, heart, and liver—tis-

## TABLE 27-1. PROPERTIES OF THE MAJOR INHALATION ANESTHETICS

| Drug | MAC* (%) | Analgesic Effect | Effect on Blood Pressure | Effect on Respiration | Muscle Relaxant Effect | Extent of Metabolism | Compatible with Epinephrine |
|---|---|---|---|---|---|---|---|
| Nitrous oxide | 105 | ++++ | → | → | 0 | 0 | Yes |
| Halothane | 0.75 | ++ | ↓ | ↓↓ | + | 15% | No |
| Desflurane | 4.58 | ++ | ↓ | ↓↓ | ++ | 2–3% | Yes |
| Enflurane | 1.68 | ++ | ↓ | ↓↓ | ++ | 2–5% | Yes† |
| Isoflurane | 1.15 | ++ | ↓ | ↓↓ | ++ | 1–2% | Yes |
| Methoxyflurane | 0.16 | +++ | ↓ | ↓↓ | + | 50–70% | — |
| Sevoflurane | 1.71 | ++ | ↓ | ↓↓ | ++ | <1% | Yes |

| | | | | |
|---|---|---|---|---|
| 0 | = | No effect | → = | Little or no change |
| + | = | Small effect | | |
| ++ | = | Moderate effect | ↓ = | Moderate decrease |
| +++ | = | Large effect | | |
| ++++ | = | Very large effect | ↓↓ = | Large decrease |

*Minimal alveolar concentration.
†Enflurane sensitizes the myocardium to catecholamines, but less so than halothane.

sues that receive the largest fraction of the cardiac output. Anesthetic levels in these tissues equilibrate with those of blood by 5 to 15 minutes after the onset of drug administration. In skin and skeletal muscles—tissues with an intermediate blood supply—equilibration occurs more slowly. The most poorly perfused tissues—fat, bone, ligaments, and cartilage—are the last to achieve equilibration with anesthetic levels in the blood.

### Elimination

**Export in the Expired Breath.** Inhalation anesthetics are eliminated almost entirely via the lungs; as noted below, hepatic metabolism is only a minor component of elimination. The same factors that determine anesthetic uptake (pulmonary ventilation, blood flow to the lungs, anesthetic solubility in blood and tissues) also determine the rate of anesthetic elimination. Since blood flow to the brain is high, anesthetic levels in the brain drop rapidly upon discontinuation of administration. Anesthetic levels in tissues that have a lower blood flow decline more slowly. Because levels of anesthetic in the CNS decline more rapidly than levels in other tissues, patients can awaken from anesthesia long before all of the anesthetic has left the body.

**Metabolism.** Most inhalation anesthetics undergo very little metabolism. Hence, metabolism does not influence the time course of anesthesia. However, since metabolites of the anesthetics are responsible for some important toxicities (see below), metabolism is nonetheless clinically significant—despite its small extent.

### Adverse Effects

The adverse effects discussed below apply to the inhalation anesthetics as a group. Please note, however, that not all of these effects are seen with every anesthetic.

**Respiratory and Cardiac Depression.** Depression of respiratory and cardiac function is a concern with virtually all inhalation anesthetics. Doses only 2 to 4 times greater than those needed for surgical anesthesia are sufficient to depress pulmonary and cardiac function to the point of lethality. To compensate for respiratory depression, almost all patients require mechanical support of ventilation.

**Sensitization of the Heart to Catecholamines.** Certain inhalation anesthetics can increase the sensitivity of the heart to stimulation by catecholamines (e.g., epinephrine). While in this sensitized state, the heart may develop dysrhythmias in response to catecholamines. Exposure to catecholamines may result from two causes: (1) release of endogenous catecholamines (in response to pain or other stimuli of the sympathetic nervous system), and (2) topical application of catecholamines to control bleeding in the surgical field. Inhalation anesthetics that are especially noted for sensitizing the heart to catecholamines are *halothane* and *methoxyflurane.*

**Malignant Hyperthermia.** Malignant hyperthermia is a rare but potentially fatal reaction that can be triggered by all inhalation anesthetics. Predisposition to the reaction is genetically based. Malignant hyperthermia is characterized by muscle rigidity and a profound elevation of temperature—sometimes to as high as 43°C. Left untreated, the reaction can rapidly prove fatal. The risk of malignant hyperthermia is greatest when an inhalation anesthetic is used in combination with *succinylcholine,* a neuromuscular blocker that also can trigger the reaction. Diagnosis and management of malignant hyperthermia are discussed in Chapter 17.

**Aspiration of Gastric Contents.** During the state of anesthesia, the reflexes that normally prevent aspiration of gastric contents into the lungs are abolished. Aspiration of gastric fluids can cause bronchospasm and pneumonia. Use of an endotracheal tube isolates the trachea and can thereby help prevent these complications.

**Toxicity to Operating Room Personnel.** Chronic exposure to low levels of anesthetics may have adverse effects on operating room personnel. Suspected reactions include headache, reduced alertness, and spontaneous abortion. The risk of these effects can be reduced by the simple expedient of venting anesthetic gases from the operating room.

**Hepatotoxicity.** About 1 in 10,000 patients receiving inhalation anesthesia develops serious liver dysfunction. At one time, it was thought that halothane was more hepatotoxic than other anesthetics. However, it now appears that all inhalation anesthetics are about equal in their ability to injure the liver.

**Renal Toxicity.** Renal injury can occur with *methoxyflurane*. Damage is caused by metabolites of methoxyflurane, and not by the parent compound.

## Drug Interactions

Several classes of drugs—analgesics, CNS depressants, CNS stimulants—can influence the amount of anesthetic required to produce anesthesia. Opioid analgesics allow a reduction in anesthetic dosage, since, with this combination, analgesia needn't be produced by the anesthetic alone. Similarly, since CNS depressants (barbiturates, benzodiazepines, alcohol) have additive depressant effects with anesthetics, acute use of these drugs lowers the required dose of anesthetic. Conversely, acute use of CNS stimulants (amphetamines, cocaine) increases the required dose of anesthetic.

## Adjuncts to Inhalation Anesthesia

Adjuncts to anesthesia are drugs employed to complement the beneficial effects of inhalation anesthetics and to counteract their adverse effects. Some adjunctive agents are administered preoperatively, others are administered intraoperatively, and still others postoperatively.

### Preanesthetic Medications

Preanesthetic medications are administered for three main purposes: (1) reduction of anxiety, (2) production of perioperative amnesia, and (3) relief of preoperative and postoperative pain. In addition, preanesthetic medications are used prophylactically to suppress adverse responses (excessive salivation, excessive bronchial secretion, coughing, bradycardia, vomiting) to certain anesthetics.

**Benzodiazepines.** Benzodiazepines (e.g., diazepam) are given preoperatively to reduce anxiety and promote amnesia. The doses employed produce mild sedation with little or no respiratory depression.

**Barbiturates.** Like the benzodiazepines, barbiturates can relieve anxiety and induce sedation. Respiratory and cardiovascular effects are minimal. Barbiturates with an intermediate duration of action are employed (e.g., pentobarbital, secobarbital).

**Opioids.** Opioids (e.g., morphine) are administered to relieve preoperative and postoperative pain. These drugs may also benefit the patient by suppressing cough.

Opioids can have adverse effects. Because they depress the CNS, opioids can delay awakening after surgery. Effects on the bowel and urinary tract may result in postoperative constipation and urinary retention. Stimulation of the chemoreceptor trigger zone promotes vomiting. Opioid-induced respiratory depression adds with anesthetic-induced respiratory depression, thereby increasing the risk of postoperative respiratory distress.

**Anticholinergic Drugs.** Anticholinergic drugs (e.g., atropine) may be given to decrease the risk of bradycardia during surgery. Surgical manipulations can trigger parasympathetic reflexes, which in turn can produce profound vagal slowing of the heart. Pretreatment with a cholinergic antagonist prevents bradycardia from this cause.

At one time, anticholinergic drugs were needed to prevent excessive bronchial secretions associated with anesthesia. Older anesthetic agents (e.g., ether) irritate the respiratory tract, and thereby cause profuse bronchial secretions. Cholinergic blockers were given to suppress this response. Since the inhalation anesthetics in use today are much less irritating, increases in bronchial secretions are minimal. Consequently, although anticholinergic agents are still employed as adjuncts to anesthesia, their purpose is no longer to suppress secretion.

### Neuromuscular Blocking Agents

Performance of most surgical procedures requires that skeletal muscles be relaxed; neuromuscular blocking agents (e.g., succinylcholine, pancuronium) are given to induce relaxation. By using neuromuscular blockers, we can reduce the dose of general anesthetic. That is, although it is possible to produce surgical muscle relaxation with an anesthetic alone, the required degree of muscle relaxation can be achieved only with deep anesthesia. When skeletal muscles have been relaxed with a neuromuscular blocker, anesthesia need not be so deep.

Muscle relaxants can have adverse effects. Neuromuscular blocking agents prevent contraction of all skeletal muscles, including the diaphragm and other muscles of respiration. Accordingly, patients require mechanical support of ventilation during surgery. Patients recovering from anesthesia may have reduced respiratory capacity owing to residual neuromuscular blockade; hence respiration must be closely monitored until recovery is complete.

It is important to appreciate that neuromuscular blockers produce a state of total flaccid paralysis. In this condition, a patient could be fully awake while appearing to be asleep. Incidents in which paralyzed patients have been awake during surgery, but unable to communicate their agony, are not unheard of. Because neuromuscular blockade can obscure depth of anesthesia, and because failure to maintain adequate anesthesia can result in true horror, the anesthesiologist must be especially watchful to ensure that patients receiving neuromuscular blocking agents also receive adequate amounts of anesthetic.

## Postanesthetic Medications

*Analgesics.* Analgesics are needed to control postoperative pain. If pain is severe, opioids are indicated. For mild pain, aspirin-like drugs may suffice.

*Antiemetics.* Patients recovering from anesthesia often experience nausea and vomiting. This can be suppressed with antiemetics. Among the most effective is ondansetron [Zofran], a drug developed to suppress nausea and vomiting in patients undergoing cancer chemotherapy. Other commonly used antiemetics are promethazine and droperidol.

*Muscarinic Agonists.* Abdominal distention (from atony of the bowel) and urinary retention are potential postoperative complications. Both conditions can be relieved through stimulation of muscarinic receptors. The muscarinic agonist employed most frequently is bethanechol.

## Dosage and Administration

Administration of inhalation anesthetics is performed only by anesthesiologists (physicians) and anesthetists (nurses). Clinicians who lack the training of these specialists have no authority to administer anesthesia. Since knowledge of anesthetic dosage and administration is the responsibility of specialists, and since this text is designed for the beginning student, details on dosage and administration are not presented. If you need this information, consult a textbook of anesthesiology.

## Classification of Inhalation Anesthetics

Inhalation anesthetics fall into two basic categories: *gases* and *volatile liquids*. The gases, as their name implies, exist in a gaseous state at atmospheric pressure. The volatile liquids exist in a liquid state at atmospheric pressure, but can be easily volatilized for administration by inhalation.

The anesthetic gases and volatile liquids in current use are listed in Table 27–2. The volatile liquids—halothane, enflurane, isoflurane, desflurane, methoxyflurane, and sevoflurane—are similar to one another in structure and

### TABLE 27–2. CLASSIFICATION OF THE INHALATION ANESTHETICS

| Class | Anesthetic | |
| | Generic Name | Trade Name |
| --- | --- | --- |
| *Volatile liquids* | Halothane | Fluothane |
| | Enflurane | Ethrane |
| | Isoflurane | Forane |
| | Methoxyflurane | Penthrane |
| | Desflurane | Suprane |
| | Sevoflurane | Ultane |
| *Gases* | Nitrous oxide | |

function. In contrast, the three gases—nitrous oxide, cyclopropane, and ethylene—differ from one another in both structure and pharmacologic properties. Nitrous oxide is the only anesthetic gas used extensively.

# Properties of Individual Inhalation Anesthetics

## Halothane

Halothane [Fluothane] is the prototype of the volatile inhalation anesthetics. Halothane was introduced in 1956 and remains the standard against which the newer volatile liquids are compared.

### Anesthetic Properties

Halothane is an effective anesthetic. For some procedures, anesthesia may be produced with halothane alone. Other procedures require a combination of halothane and other drugs.

*Potency.* Halothane is a high-potency anesthetic. This high potency is reflected in halothane's low MAC (0.75%), which tells us that unconsciousness can be produced when the concentration of halothane in alveolar air is only 0.75%.

*Time Course.* Induction of anesthesia is smooth and relatively rapid. However, although halothane can act quickly, in actual practice, induction is usually produced with thiopental, a rapid-acting barbiturate. Once the patient is unconscious, depth of anesthesia can be raised or lowered with ease. Patients awaken about 1 hour after ceasing halothane inhalation.

*Analgesia.* Halothane is only weakly analgesic. Consequently, when this agent is used for surgical anesthesia, coadministration of a strong analgesic is usually required. The analgesics most commonly employed are opioids (e.g., morphine) and nitrous oxide.

*Muscle Relaxation.* Although halothane has muscle-relaxant actions, the degree of relaxation produced is generally inadequate for surgery. Accordingly, concurrent use of a neuromuscular blocking agent (e.g., pancuronium) is usually required. Although relaxation of *skeletal muscle* is only moderate, halothane does promote significant relaxation of *uterine smooth muscle*. Consequently, when used during parturition, halothane may inhibit uterine contractions, thereby delaying delivery and possibly increasing postpartum bleeding.

### Adverse Effects

*Hypotension.* Halothane causes a dose-dependent reduction in blood pressure. Doses only twice those needed for surgical anesthesia can produce complete circulatory failure and death.

Halothane promotes hypotension by two mechanisms. First, the drug has a direct depressant effect on the myocardium; the resultant decrease in contractility can reduce cardiac output by 20% to 50%. Second, halothane increases vagal tone, thereby slowing heart rate and reducing cardiac output even further.

***Respiratory Depression.*** Halothane produces significant depression of respiration. To ensure adequate oxygenation, two measures are employed: (1) mechanical or manual ventilatory support and (2) enrichment of the inspired gas mixture with additional oxygen.

***Sensitization of the Heart to Catecholamines.*** Halothane sensitizes the heart to catecholamines, thereby increasing the risk of dysrhythmias. Accordingly, caution must be exercised when epinephrine and other catecholamines are employed.

***Malignant Hyperthermia.*** Genetically predisposed patients may experience malignant hyperthermia. Patients with a personal or familial history of malignant hyperthermia should receive halothane only if there is no option—and if halothane *is* employed, it must not be combined with succinylcholine (which would increase the risk of malignant hyperthermia).

***Other Adverse Effects.*** Rarely, halothane produces *hepatitis*, sometimes progressing to massive hepatic necrosis and death. Postoperative *nausea and vomiting* may occur, but these reactions are less common with halothane than with older anesthetics (e.g., ether). By decreasing blood flow to the kidney, halothane can cause a substantial *decrease in urine formation*.

### Elimination

The majority (60% to 80%) of an administered dose is eliminated intact in the exhaled breath. Hepatic metabolism accounts for about 15% of elimination.

## Isoflurane

Isoflurane [Forane] is our most widely used inhalation anesthetic. The drug is potent (MAC = 1.15%) and has properties much like those of halothane. Induction of anesthesia is smooth and rapid, depth of anesthesia can be adjusted with speed and ease, and patients emerge from anesthesia rapidly. Like the other volatile liquids, isoflurane causes respiratory depression and hypotension. With isoflurane, hypotension results from vasodilation rather than reduction of cardiac output. Isoflurane is a more effective muscle relaxant than halothane, but nonetheless is usually employed with a neuromuscular blocker. Like halothane, isoflurane suppresses uterine contraction. Only 0.2% of isoflurane undergoes metabolism; the vast majority of the drug is eliminated unchanged in the expired breath.

It is important to note that the cardiac actions of isoflurane differ significantly from those of halothane. Unlike halothane, isoflurane does not cause myocardial depression. Hence, cardiac output is not decreased. Furthermore, isoflurane does not sensitize the myocardium to catecholamines; hence patients can be given epinephrine and other catecholamines with little fear of precipitating a dysrhythmia.

## Enflurane

Enflurane [Ethrane] has pharmacologic properties very similar to those of halothane. Enflurane was introduced in 1973 and still enjoys widespread use.

Comparison of enflurane with halothane reveals important similarities and a few significant differences. Both anesthetics are very potent: the MAC of enflurane is 1.68%, compared with 0.75% for halothane. As with halothane, induction of anesthesia is smooth and rapid, and depth of anesthesia can be changed quickly and easily. Like halothane, enflurane produces substantial depression of respiration. Accordingly, patients are likely to need ventilatory support; the concentration of inspired oxygen should be at least 35%. Muscle relaxation induced by enflurane is greater than that induced by halothane; however, despite this action, a neuromuscular blocker is usually employed to permit a reduction of enflurane dosage. Like halothane, enflurane can suppress contraction of the uterus, thereby impeding labor. Significantly, sensitization of the myocardium to catecholamines is less with enflurane than with halothane. As a result, patients can be given catecholamines with relative safety. High doses of enflurane can induce seizures, a response not seen with halothane; enflurane should be avoided in patients with a history of seizure disorders. Like halothane, enflurane is eliminated primarily in the exhaled breath as the intact parent compound; about 2% to 5% is eliminated by hepatic metabolism.

## Methoxyflurane

Methoxyflurane [Penthrane] was introduced in 1960 and belongs to the volatile liquid class of inhalation anesthetics. Initial use of the drug was widespread. However, the discovery that methoxyflurane can promote severe renal injury caused a sharp decline in its use.

***Anesthetic Properties.*** With a MAC of only 0.16%, methoxyflurane is our most potent volatile anesthetic. However, despite this potency, induction of anesthesia is slow. Like the other volatile anesthetics, methoxyflurane causes hypotension and respiratory depression. In contrast to other volatile liquids, methoxyflurane produces excellent analgesia without inhibiting uterine contraction.

***Metabolism and Renal Toxicity.*** Methoxyflurane undergoes more metabolism than any other inhalation anesthetic. Between 50% and 70% of the drug is converted to metabolites. Of the metabolites produced, fluoride is the most important. When present in sufficient concentration, fluoride acts directly on renal tubules to cause injury. If renal injury is extensive, death can result. In order to cause renal toxicity, fluoride must achieve blood levels of 40 µM or more. To produce fluoride levels of this magnitude, methoxyflurane must be administered in large amounts. Low-dose, short-term use will not generate enough fluoride to injure the kidneys.

***Therapeutic Use.*** Because of its ability to promote renal injury, methoxyflurane is not used extensively. The drug is employed primarily for analgesia during labor, and even this use is uncommon. Methoxyflurane is acceptable for this application because the doses required are so small that there is no risk of generating fluoride in amounts sufficient to injure the kidneys. Methoxyflurane is preferable to the other volatile anesthetics for use during labor because it does not suppress uterine contractions.

## Desflurane

Desflurane [Suprane] is nearly identical in structure to isoflurane. Induction occurs more rapidly than with any other volatile anesthetic, depth of anesthesia can be changed quickly, and recovery occurs only minutes after ceasing administration. Desflurane is indicated for *maintenance* of anesthesia in adults and children and for *induction* of anesthesia in adults. The drug is not approved for induction in children and infants because of a high incidence of respiratory difficulties (laryngospasm, apnea, increased secretions), which are due to the drug's pungency. Like isoflurane, desflurane can cause respiratory depression and hypotension secondary to vasodilation. During induction, or in response to an abrupt increase in desflurane blood levels, heart rate and blood pressure may increase, causing tachycardia and hypertension. Postoperative nausea and vomiting are possible. Malignant hypertension has occurred in experimental animals. Desflurane undergoes even less metabolism than isoflurane; hence the risk of postperative organ injury is probably low.

### Sevoflurane

Sevoflurane [Ultane] is a new anesthetic similar to desflurane. The drug is approved for induction and maintenance of anesthesia in adults and children. As with desflurane, induction is rapid, depth of anesthesia can be adjusted easily, and recovery occurs minutes after ceasing inhalation. In contrast to desflurane, sevoflurane is neither pungent nor a respiratory irritant; hence, the drug is suitable for mask induction in children. Sevoflurane has a MAC of 1.7% and is eliminated primarily in the exhaled breath.

Adverse effects are minimal. The most common problem is postoperative nausea and vomiting. Although the extent of metabolism is relatively low (3%), it is still sufficient to produce measurable levels of fluoride in plasma and urine; nonetheless, fluoride-related injury to the liver and kidneys is rare. In contrast to desflurane, sevoflurane does not cause tachycardia or hypertension.

## Nitrous Oxide

Nitrous oxide, also known as "laughing gas," differs from the volatile liquid anesthetics in its pharmacologic properties and applications. With respect to pharmacologic properties, nitrous oxide differs from other inhalation anesthetics in two important ways: (1) whereas other inhalation agents have high *anesthetic* potency, the *anesthetic* potency of nitrous oxide is very *low*; and (2) whereas other inhalation agents lack *analgesic* potency, the *analgesic* potency of nitrous oxide is very *high*. These properties have given nitrous oxide a unique pattern of use: because of its low anesthetic potency, nitrous oxide is never employed as a primary anesthetic agent; however, because of its high analgesic potency, nitrous oxide is employed with great regularity as an adjuvant to other inhalation agents to provide supplemental analgesia.

Because nitrous oxide has such low anesthetic potency, *it is virtually impossible to produce surgical anesthesia employing nitrous oxide alone.* The low anesthetic potency of nitrous oxide is reflected in the drug's extremely high MAC, which is greater than 100%. A MAC of this value tells us that, even if it were possible to administer 100% nitrous oxide (i.e., inspired gas that contains only nitrous oxide and no oxygen), this concentration of nitrous oxide would still be insufficient to produce surgical anesthesia. Since practical considerations (i.e., the need to administer at least 30% oxygen) limit the maximum usable concentration of nitrous oxide to 70%, and since much higher concentrations are needed to approach production of surgical anesthesia, it is clear that full anesthesia cannot be achieved with nitrous oxide by itself.

Despite its low anesthetic potency, nitrous oxide may well be our most widely used inhalation agent: *almost all patients undergoing general anesthesia receive nitrous oxide to supplement the analgesic effects of the primary anesthetic.* As indicated in Table 27–1, the analgesic effects of nitrous oxide are substantially greater than those of the other inhalation agents. Reflecting the drug's analgesic potency is the fact that inhalation of 20% nitrous oxide can produce pain relief equivalent to that of morphine. The advantage of providing analgesia with nitrous oxide, rather than relying entirely on the primary anesthetic for pain relief, is that nitrous oxide allows the dosage of the primary anesthetic to be significantly decreased—usually by 50% or more. This reduction in dosage results in decreased respiratory and cardiovascular depression and also leads to faster emergence. When employed in combination with other inhalation anesthetics, nitrous oxide is administered at a concentration of 70%.

When administered at therapeutic concentrations, nitrous oxide has practically no adverse effects. The drug is not toxic to the CNS, nor does it cause cardiovascular or respiratory depression. Furthermore, it is not likely to precipitate malignant hyperthermia.

In certain settings, nitrous oxide can be used alone. When administered by itself, nitrous oxide is employed for *analgesia*—not *anesthesia*. Nitrous oxide alone is used for analgesia in dentistry and during delivery.

### Obsolete Inhalation Anesthetics

Several once-popular anesthetics are now obsolete. These agents include *ethylene, cyclopropane, diethyl ether (ether), vinyl ether,* and *ethyl chloride.* Use of these agents has declined for two reasons: (1) all of these compounds are *explosive* and (2) these drugs offer no advantages over newer, less hazardous anesthetics.

---

# Intravenous Anesthetics

---

Intravenous anesthetics may be used alone or to supplement the effects of inhalation agents. When combined with inhalation anesthetics, intravenous agents offer two potential benefits: (1) they permit dosage of the inhalation agent to be reduced and (2) they produce effects that cannot be achieved with an inhalation agent alone. Several of the drug families discussed in this section—opioids, barbiturates, benzodiazepines—are considered at length in other chapters. Discussion here is limited to their use in anesthesia.

## Short-Acting Barbiturates (Thiobarbiturates)

Short-acting barbiturates, administered intravenously, are employed for *induction of anesthesia.* Three agents are available: (1) *thiopental sodium* [Pentothal], (2) *methohexital sodium* [Brevital], and (3) *thiamylal sodium* [Surital]. Almost every time an inhalation anesthetic is used, one of the short-acting barbiturates is administered first for induction.

***Thiopental.*** Thiopental [Pentothal] was the first short-acting barbiturate and is the prototype for the group. This drug acts rapidly to produce unconsciousness. Analgesic and muscle-relaxant effects are weak.

Thiopental has a rapid onset and short duration of action. Unconsciousness occurs 10 to 20 seconds after IV injection. If thiopental is not followed by inhalation anesthesia, the patient will wake up in approximately 10 minutes.

The time course of thiopental-induced anesthesia is determined by the drug's pattern of distribution. Thiopental is highly lipid soluble, and therefore enters the brain rapidly to begin its effects. Anesthesia is terminated as thiopental undergoes redistribution from the brain and blood to other tissues. Practically no metabolism of the drug takes place between the time of administration and the time of awakening.

Like most of the inhalation anesthetics, thiopental causes cardiovascular and respiratory depression. If administered too rapidly, the drug may cause apnea.

## Benzodiazepines

When administered in large doses, benzodiazepines produce unconsciousness and amnesia. Because of this ability, intravenous benzodiazepines are occasionally given to induce anesthesia; however, the short-acting barbiturates are generally preferred for this purpose. Three benzodiazepines—diazepam, lorazepam, and midazolam—are administered intravenously for induction. Diazepam is the prototype for the group. The basic pharmacology of the benzodiazepines is discussed in Chapter 32.

**Diazepam.** Induction with IV diazepam [Valium] is slower than with barbiturates; unconsciousness develops in about 1 minute. Diazepam is not analgesic and causes very little muscle relaxation. Intravenous diazepam usually produces only moderate cardiovascular and respiratory depression; however, on occasion respiratory depression is severe. Accordingly, whenever diazepam is administered intravenously, facilities for support of respiration must be immediately available.

**Midazolam.** Intravenous midazolam [Versed] may be used for *induction of anesthesia* and to produce *conscious sedation*. When used for induction, midazolam is usually combined with a short-acting barbiturate. Unconsciousness develops in 80 seconds.

Conscious sedation can be produced by combining midazolam with an opioid analgesic (e.g., morphine). The state is characterized by sedation, analgesia, amnesia, and the absence of anxiety. The patient is unperturbed and passive, but responsive to commands, such as "open your eyes." Conscious sedation persists for an hour or so and is suitable for minor surgeries and endoscopic procedures.

Midazolam can cause dangerous cardiorespiratory effects, including respiratory depression and respiratory and cardiac arrest. Accordingly, the drug should be used only in settings that permit constant monitoring of cardiac and respiratory status. Facilities for resuscitation must be immediately available. The risk of adverse effects can be minimized by injecting midazolam slowly (over 2 or more minutes) and by waiting another 2 or more minutes for full effects to develop before giving additional doses.

### Propofol

Propofol [Diprivan] is an intravenous sedative-hypnotic used for induction and maintenance of anesthesia. Like thiopental,

propofol has a rapid onset and short duration of action. Unconsciousness develops within 60 seconds and lasts for 3 to 5 minutes. As with thiopental, redistribution from the brain to other tissues explains the speed of awakening. Although its effects are brief, propofol persists in the body, with a half-life of 3 to 5 hours.

Propofol can cause respiratory depression (including apnea), cardiac depression, hypotension, and pain at the site of injection. Because of the risk of cardiovascular depression, the drug should be used with caution in elderly patients, hypovolemic patients, and patients with compromised myocardial function. Pain at the injection site can be minimized by using a large vein and mixing propofol with a small amount of lidocaine (a local anesthetic) just prior to injection. Because of a high risk of contamination with infectious bacteria, ampules that have been opened should be discarded within 6 hours.

### Etomidate

Etomidate [Amidate] is a potent hypnotic agent used for induction of surgical anesthesia. Unconsciousness develops rapidly and lasts about 5 minutes. The drug has no analgesic actions. Adverse effects associated with single injections include transient apnea, venous pain at the injection site, and suppression of plasma cortisol levels for 6 to 8 hours. Repeated administration can cause hypotension, oliguria, electrolyte disturbances, and a high incidence (50%) of postoperative nausea and vomiting. Cardiovascular effects are less than with barbiturates; hence the drug is preferred to barbiturates for patients with cardiovascular disorders.

## Ketamine

**Anesthetic Effects.** Ketamine [Ketalar] produces a state known as *dissociative anesthesia* in which the patient feels dissociated from his or her environment. In addition, the drug causes sedation, immobility, analgesia, and amnesia; responsiveness to pain is lost. Induction is rapid, and emergence begins within 10 to 15 minutes. Full recovery, however, may take several hours.

**Adverse Psychologic Reactions.** During recovery from ketamine, unpleasant psychologic reactions may occur. Possible reactions include hallucinations, disturbing dreams, and delirium. In some cases, these reactions recur days and even weeks after ketamine had been used. To minimize adverse psychologic effects, the patient should be kept in a soothing, stimulus-free environment until recovery is complete. Premedication with diazepam or midazolam reduces the risk of adverse reactions. Psychologic reactions are *least* likely in children under the age of 15 and in adults over the age of 65.

**Therapeutic Uses.** Ketamine is especially valuable for anesthesia in young children for minor surgical and diagnostic procedures; the drug is frequently used to facilitate changing of burn dressings. Because of its potential for adverse psychologic effects, ketamine should be avoided in patients with a history of psychiatric illness.

## Neuroleptic-Opioid Combination: Droperidol Plus Fentanyl

A unique state, known as *neurolept analgesia*, can be produced with a combination of fentanyl, a potent opioid, plus droperidol, a neuroleptic (antipsychotic) agent. The combination of fentanyl plus droperidol is available pre-mixed under the trade name *Innovar*.

Neurolept analgesia is characterized by quiescence, indifference to surroundings, and insensitivity to pain; the patient appears to be asleep but is not (i.e., complete loss of consciousness does not occur). In large part, neurolept analgesia is similar to the dissociative anesthesia produced by ketamine. Neurolept analgesia is employed for diagnostic and minor surgical procedures (e.g., bronchoscopy, repeated changing of burn dressings).

Adverse effects include hypotension and respiratory depression. Respiratory depression can be severe and may persist for several hours. Respiratory assistance is likely to be required. Like other neuroleptics, droperidol blocks receptors for dopamine and hence should not be given to patients with Parkinson's disease.

For some procedures, the combination of fentanyl plus droperidol is supplemented with nitrous oxide. The state produced by this three-drug regimen is called *neurolept anesthesia*. Neurolept anesthesia produces more analgesia and a greater reduction of consciousness than occurs with neurolept analgesia. Neurolept anesthesia can be used for major surgical procedures.

## KEY POINTS

- *General anesthetics* produce unconsciousness and insensitivity to painful stimuli. In contrast, *analgesics* reduce sensitivity to pain but need not reduce consciousness.
- The term *balanced anesthesia* refers to the use of several drugs to ensure that induction of anesthesia is smooth and rapid and that analgesia and muscle relaxation are adequate.
- The *minimum alveolar concentration (MAC)* of an inhalation anesthetic is defined as the minimum concentration of drug in the alveolar air that will produce immobility in 50% of patients exposed to a painful stimulus. A *low* MAC indicates *high* anesthetic potency!
- Inhalation anesthetics are eliminated almost entirely via the lungs; as a rule, they undergo minimal hepatic metabolism.
- The principal adverse effect of general anesthetics is depression of respiration and cardiac performance.
- *Malignant hyperthermia* is a rare, genetically determined, life-threatening reaction to general anesthetics. Coadministration of succinylcholine, a neuromuscular blocker, increases the risk of the reaction.
- By enhancing analgesia, opioids reduce the required dosage of general anesthetic.
- By enhancing muscle relaxation, neuromuscular blockers reduce the required dosage of general anesthetic.
- Nitrous oxide differs from other general anesthetics in two important ways: (1) the drug has a very high MAC, and therefore cannot be used alone to produce general anesthesia; and (2) the drug has high analgesic potency, and therefore is frequently combined with other general anesthetics to supplement their analgesic effects.
- Induction of anesthesia is usually accomplished with thiopental or another short-acting barbiturate.
- Ketamine is an intravenous anesthetic that produces a state known as *dissociative anesthesia*. Patients recovering from ketamine may experience adverse psychologic reactions.
- The combination of droperidol plus fentanyl, known as Innovar, produces a state called *neurolept analgesia*. Addition of nitrous oxide to the combination produces a state of *neurolept anesthesia*.

# Summary of Major Nursing Implications

## All General Anesthetics

Nursing management of the patient receiving general anesthesia is almost exclusively preoperative and postoperative; intraoperative management is the responsibility of anesthesiologists and anesthetists. Accordingly, our summary of anesthesia-related nursing implications is divided into two sections: (1) implications that pertain to the preoperative patient and (2) implications that pertain to the postoperative patient. Intraoperative implications are not considered.

It should be noted that the nursing implications summarized here are restricted to those that are directly related to anesthesia; nursing implications regarding the overall management of the surgical patient (i.e., implications unrelated to anesthesia) are not presented. (Overall nursing management of the surgical patient is discussed fully—and appropriately—in medical-surgical texts.)

Nursing implications for drugs employed as adjuncts to anesthesia (barbiturates, benzodiazepines, anticholinergic agents, opioids, neuromuscular blocking agents) are summarized in other chapters. Only those implications that apply specifically to the adjunctive use of these agents are addressed here.

## Preoperative Patients: Counseling, Assessment, and Medication

### Counseling

Anxiety is common among patients anticipating surgery; the patient may fear the surgery itself, or may be concerned about the possibility of waking up or experiencing pain during the procedure. Since excessive anxiety can disrupt the smoothness of the surgical course (in addition to being distressing to the patient), you should attempt to dispel preoperative fears. To some extent, fear can be allayed by reassuring the patient that anesthesia will keep him or her asleep for the entire procedure, will prevent pain, and will create amnesia about the experience.

## Assessment

*Medication History.* The patient may be taking drugs that can affect responses to anesthetics. Drugs that act on the respiratory and cardiovascular systems are of particular concern. To decrease the risk of adverse interactions, obtain a thorough history of drug use. *All* drugs—prescription medications, over-the-counter preparations, and illicit agents—should be considered. With illicit drugs, such as alcohol, heroin, or barbiturates, it is important to determine both the duration of use as well as the amount used per day.

*Respiratory and Cardiovascular Function.* Most general anesthetics produce cardiovascular and respiratory depression. In order to evaluate the effects of anesthesia, baseline values for blood pressure, heart rate, and respiration are required. Also, any disease of the cardiovascular and respiratory systems should be noted.

## Preoperative Medication

Preoperative medications (e.g., benzodiazepines, opioids, anticholinergic agents) are employed to (1) calm the patient, (2) provide analgesia, and (3) counteract adverse effects of general anesthetics. As a rule, the nurse is responsible for administering these drugs. Since preoperative medication can have a significant impact on the overall response to anesthesia, it is important that these drugs be administered at an appropriate time—typically 30 to 60 minutes before surgery. Because preoperative medication may produce drowsiness or reduce blood pressure, the patient should remain in bed. A calm environment will complement the effect of sedatives.

## Postoperative Patients: Ongoing Evaluation and Interventions

When receiving a patient for postoperative care, you should know all of the drugs the patient has received in the hospital (anesthetics and adjunctive medications); in addition, you should know what medications the patient was taking at home (especially those for hypertension). With this information, you will be able to anticipate the time course of emergence from anesthesia as well as potential drug-related postoperative complications.

## Evaluations and Interventions That Pertain to Specific Organ Systems

*Cardiovascular and Respiratory Systems.* Anesthetics depress cardiovascular and respiratory function. Monitor vital signs until they return to normal. Determine blood pressure, pulse rate, and respiration immediately upon receipt of the patient, and repeat monitoring at brief intervals until recovery is complete. During the recovery period, observe the patient for respiratory and cardiovascular distress. Be alert for (1) reductions in blood pressure, (2) altered cardiac rhythm, and (3) shallow, slow, or noisy breathing. Have facilities for respiratory support available.

*Central Nervous System.* Return of CNS function is gradual, and precautions must be taken until recovery is complete. When appropriate, employ side rails or straps to avoid accidental falls. Assist ambulation until the patient is able to stand steadily. During the early stage of emergence, the patient may be able to hear, although he or she may appear unconscious; exercise discretion in conversation.

*Gastrointestinal Tract.* Bowel function may be compromised by the surgery itself or by the drugs employed as adjuncts to anesthesia (e.g., opioids, anticholinergics). Constipation or atony of the bowel may occur. Monitor bowel function. A muscarinic agonist (e.g., bethanechol) may be needed to restore peristalsis. Determine bowel sounds before giving oral medications.

Nausea and vomiting are potential postanesthetic reactions. To reduce the risk of aspiration, position the patient with his or her head to the side. Have equipment for suctioning available. Antiemetic medication may be needed.

*Urinary Tract.* Anesthetics and their adjuncts can disrupt urinary tract function. Anesthetics can decrease urine production by reducing renal blood flow; opioids and anticholinergic drugs can cause urinary retention. Monitor urine output. If the patient fails to void, follow hospital protocol. Catheterization or medication (e.g., bethanechol) may be required.

## Management of Postoperative Pain

As anesthesia wears off, the patient may experience postoperative pain. An opioid may be required. Since respiratory depression from opioids will add to residual respiratory depression from anesthesia, use opioids with caution; balance the need to relieve pain against the need to maintain ventilation.

## Implications for Ketamine

Adverse psychologic reactions can develop as the patient emerges from ketamine-induced anesthesia. To minimize these reactions, provide a calm and stimulus-free environment until recovery is complete.

# CHAPTER 28

# Drugs for Headache

Headache is a common symptom that can be triggered by a variety of stimuli, including stress, fatigue, acute illness, and sensitivity to alcohol. Many people experience mild, episodic headaches that can be relieved with over-the-counter medications (aspirin, acetaminophen, ibuprofen). For these individuals, medical intervention is unnecessary. In contrast, some people experience severe, recurrent, debilitating headaches that are frequently unresponsive to aspirin-like drugs. For these individuals, medical attention is merited. In this chapter, our focus is on these severe forms of headache. Specifically, we will discuss drug therapy of migraine, cluster, and tension-type headaches.

When attempting to treat headache, it is essential to differentiate between headaches that have an identifiable underlying cause (e.g., severe hypertension; hyperthyroidism; tumors; infection; disorders of the eye, ear, nose, sinuses, and throat) and headaches that have no identifiable cause (e.g., migraine and cluster headaches). Obviously, if there is a clear cause of the headache, that cause should be treated directly.

As we consider the drugs for headache, three basic principles should be kept in mind. First, antiheadache drugs may be used in two ways: (1) to abort an ongoing attack and (2) to prevent attacks from occurring in the first place. Second, not all patients with a particular type of headache respond to the same drugs; hence, therapy must be individualized. Third, several of the drugs employed to treat severe headaches (e.g., ergotamine, butalbital, opioids) can cause physical dependence. Accordingly, every effort should be made to keep dependence from developing. If dependence does develop, a withdrawal procedure will be needed.

## Migraine Headache: Characteristics and Overview of Treatment

### Characteristics

Migraine headache is characterized by unilateral, throbbing or nonthrobbing head pain, often associated with nausea, vomiting, photophobia, and phonophobia. Precipitating factors include anxiety, fatigue, stress, menstruation, alcohol, and tyramine-containing foods.

Migraine has two primary forms, called *migraine with aura* (formerly known as classic migraine) and *migraine without aura* (formerly known as common migraine). In migraine with aura, the headache is preceded or accompanied by neurologic symptoms, which are typically visual (e.g., flashes of light, a blank area in the field of vision, zigzag patterns). Migraine without aura is the most common form of migraine, affecting 80% to 85% of migraineurs.

In the United States, migraine headache affects nearly 10 million people. Of these, about 60% to 70% are women in their late teens, 20s, or 30s. With some women, migraine attacks are worse during menstruation but subside during pregnancy and cease after menopause, suggesting a hormonal component to the attacks. A family history of the disease is common.

### Pathophysiology

The pathophysiology of migraine is complex and poorly understood. Vascular and hormonal factors are implicated. In the traditional view, the prodromal aura of migraine is caused by constriction of cerebral arteries, whereas the headache itself is caused by subsequent arterial dilation. More recently, attention has focused on serotonin (5-hydroxytryptamine, 5-HT), a neurotransmitter at central and peripheral synapses. Observations that implicate 5-HT include the following: plasma levels of 5-HT drop by 50% during a migraine attack; depletion of 5-HT with reserpine can precipitate an attack in migraine-prone individuals; and administration of 5-HT or sumatriptan, both of which stimulate 5-HT receptors, can abort an ongoing attack.

## Overview of Treatment

Drugs for migraine are employed in two ways: (1) to abort an ongoing attack, and (2) for prophylaxis (i.e., to prevent attacks from occurring). Drugs used to abort an attack include *aspirin-like analgesics*, *opioid analgesics*, *ergot alkaloids*, and *sumatriptan*. Drugs employed for prophylaxis include *beta-adrenergic blockers*, *amitriptyline*, *calcium channel blockers*, *methysergide*, and *valproic acid*.

In addition to drug therapy, nondrug measures should be used. An effort should be made to control or eliminate precipitating factors. Biofeedback and other relaxation techniques can also be helpful.

# Migraine Headache: Abortive Therapy

The objective of abortive therapy is to eliminate headache pain and suppress associated nausea and vomiting. Treatment should commence at the earliest sign of an attack. Because migraine causes nausea, vomiting, and gastric stasis, oral therapy may be ineffective once an attack has begun. Hence, for treatment of an established attack, rectal suppositories, injectable drugs, or an inhalable preparation may be best.

Drug selection depends on the intensity of the attack. For mild to moderate symptoms, an *aspirin-like drug* (e.g., aspirin, ibuprofen, acetaminophen) may be sufficient. If these are inadequate, aspirin combined with codeine may be tried. If these analgesics prove insufficient, the next attack should be treated with *sumatriptan* or an *ergot alkaloid* (ergotamine or dihydroergotamine). If these agents fail to relieve pain, an *opioid analgesic* (e.g., meperidine, butorphanol) may be needed.

*Metoclopramide* [Reglan, others] may be used as an adjunct to other agents for treating an acute migraine attack. This drug suppresses nausea and vomiting caused by the attack itself and by therapy with ergot alkaloids. In addition, metoclopramide can reverse gastric stasis caused by the attack, thereby facilitating absorption of oral medications. Metoclopramide has no direct effect on migraine pain.

## Analgesics

### Aspirin-like Drugs

Aspirin, acetaminophen, ibuprofen, and other aspirin-like analgesics can provide adequate relief of mild-to-moderate migraine attacks. In fact, when combined with metoclopramide (to enhance absorption), aspirin can be as effective as sumatriptan, a powerful new drug for migraine. Moreover, the combination of aspirin plus metoclopramide costs less than sumatriptan and causes fewer side effects. In addition to use in combination with metoclopramide, aspirin is often used in combination with caffeine and butalbital (a barbiturate sedative); the combination is available under the trade name Fiorinal.

Acetaminophen may be used alone or in combination with other drugs. A popular combination, marketed as Midrin, consists of acetaminophen, isometheptene (a sympathomimetic drug), and dichloralphenazone (a sedative).

## Opioid Analgesics

Opioid analgesics are reserved for severe migraine that has not responded to first-line medications. The opioids used most frequently are meperidine [Demerol] and butorphanol nasal spray [Stadol NS]. Meperidine can cause all of the adverse effects associated with other pure opioid agonists (e.g., respiratory depression, sedation) and also has significant abuse potential. These drawbacks are less of a problem with butorphanol.

## Ergotamine

### Mechanism of Antimigraine Action

The actions of ergotamine are complex, and the precise mechanism by which the drug aborts migraine attacks is not known. Ergotamine can alter transmission at serotonergic, dopaminergic, and alpha-adrenergic junctions. Recent evidence suggests that antimigraine effects are related to agonist activity at subtypes of serotonin receptors, specifically 5-HT$_{1B}$ and 5-HT$_{1D}$ receptors.

Relief may also be related to vascular effects. In cranial arteries, ergotamine acts directly to promote constriction and reduce the amplitude of pulsations. In addition, the drug can affect blood flow by depressing the vasomotor center. These vascular effects probably contribute to reduction of migraine pain.

### Therapeutic Uses

Ergotamine is a drug of choice for stopping an ongoing migraine attack. It is also used to treat cluster headaches. Because of the risk of dependence (see below), ergotamine should not be taken daily on a long-term basis.

### Pharmacokinetics

Administration may be oral, sublingual, rectal, or by inhalation. Bioavailability with oral and sublingual administration is low. Bioavailability with rectal and inhalational administration is higher. Although the half-life of ergotamine is only 2 hours, pharmacologic effects can still be observed 24 hours after administration. The drug is eliminated primarily by hepatic metabolism. Metabolites are excreted in the bile.

### Adverse Effects

Ergotamine is well tolerated at usual therapeutic doses. The drug can stimulate the chemoreceptor trigger zone to cause nausea and vomiting in about 10% of patients. This action can augment nausea and vomiting caused by the migraine itself. Concurrent treatment with metoclopramide or a phenothiazine antiemetic can help suppress these responses. Other common side effects include weakness in the legs, myalgia, numbness and tingling in fingers and toes, angina-like pain, and tachycardia or bradycardia.

### Overdose

Acute or chronic overdose can cause serious toxicity (ergotism). Symptoms include the adverse effects seen at therapeutic doses plus signs and symptoms of ischemia caused by constriction of peripheral arteries and arterioles: the extremities become cold, pale, and numb; muscle pain develops; and gangrene may eventually result. Patients should be informed about these responses and instructed to report them immediately. The risk of ergotism is highest in patients with sepsis, peripheral vascular disease, and renal or hepatic impairment. Management consists of discontinuing ergotamine, followed by pharmacologic measures to maintain circulation (treatment with anticoagulants, low-molecular-weight dextran, and/or intravenous nitroprusside as appropriate).

### Physical Dependence

Regular daily use of ergotamine, even in moderate doses, can cause physical dependence. The withdrawal syndrome is characterized by headache, nausea, vomiting, and restlessness (i.e., withdrawal resembles a migraine attack). Patients who begin to experience these symptoms are likely to resume taking the drug, thereby perpetuating the cycle of dependence. Hospitalization may be required to break the cycle. To avoid development of dependence, dosage and duration of treatment must be limited (see dosing guidelines below).

### Contraindications

Ergotamine is contraindicated for patients with hepatic or renal impairment, sepsis (gangrene has resulted), coronary artery disease, and peripheral vascular disease. In addition, the drug should not be taken during pregnancy, since its ability to promote uterine contractions can cause fetal harm or abortion. Because of its effects on the uterus, ergotamine is classified in FDA Pregnancy Category X: the risk of use by pregnant women clearly outweighs any possible benefits. Warn women of child-bearing age to avoid pregnancy while using this drug.

#### Preparations, Dosage, and Administration

Ergotamine by itself is available in tablets for sublingual use and in an aerosol for oral inhalation. In addition, ergotamine is dispensed in combination with other drugs for oral and rectal administration.

*Sublingual.* Ergotamine tartrate [Ergostat] is dispensed in 2-mg tablets for sublingual use. One tablet should be placed under the tongue immediately after onset of aura or headache. If needed, additional tablets can be administered at 30-minute intervals—up to a maximum of 3 tablets/24 hr or 5 tablets/week.

*Inhalation.* Ergotamine tartrate [Medihaler Ergotamine] is dispensed in an aerosol for oral inhalation. Each inhalation delivers 0.36 mg. One inhalation should be done immediately after onset of aura or headache. If pain is not relieved, additional inhalations can be done at 5-minute intervals—up to a maximum of 6/hour or 15/week.

*Oral.* Three oral formulations [Cafergot, Ercaf, Wigraine] contain 1 mg ergotamine tartrate and 100 mg caffeine; a fourth formulation [Cafatine-PB] contains 30 mg pentobarbital and 0.125 mg belladonna alkaloids in addition to the ergotamine and caffeine. The caffeine is present to enhance vasoconstriction and ergotamine absorption. The pentobarbital provides sedation. The belladonna alkaloids suppress emesis. With all four oral formulations, 2 tablets are taken immediately after onset of aura or headache. One additional tablet can be administered every 30 minutes—up to a maximum of 6 per attack or 10/week.

*Rectal.* Ergotamine is available in three rectal formulations [Cafatine Supps, Cafetrate Supps, Wigraine Supps]. Each contains 2 mg ergotamine tartrate and 100 mg caffeine. No more than two suppositories should be administered per attack.

## Dihydroergotamine

### Therapeutic Uses

Parenteral dihydroergotamine is considered a drug of choice for terminating severe, refractory migraine and cluster headaches. Because the drug must be administered parenterally, it is best suited for use in a medical setting (emergency room, physician's office).

### Pharmacologic Effects and Contraindications

The actions of dihydroergotamine are similar to those of ergotamine. Like ergotamine, dihydroergotamine alters transmission at serotonergic, dopaminergic, and alpha-adrenergic junctions. In contrast to ergotamine, dihydroergotamine causes minimal peripheral vasoconstriction, little nausea and vomiting, and no physical dependence. However, diarrhea is a prominent side effect. Contraindications are the same as those for ergotamine: coronary artery disease, peripheral vascular disease, sepsis, pregnancy, and hepatic or renal impairment.

#### Pharmacokinetics

Dihydroergotamine is administered parenterally (SC, IM, IV)—although it may soon be available in an intranasal spray. Because of extensive first-pass metabolism, the drug is not active orally. Elimination is by hepatic metabolism. An active metabolite (8'-hydroxydihydroergotamine) contributes to therapeutic effects. The half-life of dihydroergotamine plus its active metabolite is about 21 hours.

#### Preparations, Dosage, and Administration

Dihydroergotamine mesylate [D.H.E. 45] is dispensed in solution (1 mg/ml) for IM, SC, and IV administration.

*Intramuscular or Subcutaneous.* The initial dose is 1 mg immediately after onset of symptoms. Additional 1-mg doses may be given hourly up to a maximum of 3 mg per attack. Dosage should be adjusted early in therapy to determine a minimal effective dose. This dose should be used for subsequent attacks.

*Intravenous.* One milligram is given initially followed by another 1 mg in 1 hour if needed. Dosage should not exceed 6 mg/week.

*Intranasal.* Administration of 2 mg by nasal spray reduces or eliminates pain in 70% of patients. Intranasal dihydroergotamine is currently investigational.

## Sumatriptan

### Actions and Uses

Sumatriptan [Imitrex] is a relatively new and very effective drug for treating migraine. Both headache and associated symptoms (nausea, photophobia, phonophobia) are relieved. In clinical trials, sumatriptan gave complete relief to more than 90% of patients. Three routes were employed: IV, SC, and PO. Symptoms abated within 10 to 30 minutes after IV administration, within 20 to 60 minutes after SC administration, and within 2 hours after PO administration. Relief was achieved at all stages of the attack. Unfortunately headache returns in about 40% of patients within 24 hours. In comparison, the 24-hour recurrence rate with dihydroergotamine is only 18%. In patients who responded to SC sumatriptan, subsequent administration of oral sumatriptan delayed recurrence but did not prevent it.

Sumatriptan is an analog of serotonin (5-HT), and stimulation of a serotonin receptor subtype (5-HT$_{1B}$ and/or 5-HT$_{1D}$) is thought to underlie the drug's antimigraine effects. Sumatriptan has no affinity for adrenergic, dopaminergic, or muscarinic receptors. The drug has no analgesic actions in animals.

### Pharmacokinetics

In the United States, sumatriptan is available for oral and SC administration. A nasal spray is available in other countries and is under study for use here. With oral administration, absorption is rapid but bioavailability is low (about 15%); hence oral doses are much higher than SC doses. Following subcutaneous injection, peak plasma levels are achieved in 5 to 20 minutes. Sumatriptan is converted to inactive metabolites by the liver, and the metabolites are excreted in the urine. The drug's half-life is short—about 2.6 hours.

### Adverse Effects

Sumatriptan is generally well tolerated. Most side effects are transient and mild. The drug can cause an unpleasant burning sensation in the upper chest and neck and an equally unpleasant sense of constriction or pressure in the neck and throat; however, both sensations are transient. Other mild reactions include vertigo, malaise, fatigue, and feelings of heaviness. Transient pain and redness may occur at sites of SC injection.

*Angina.* Rarely, *angina* has occurred with oral and SC administration. Electrocardiographic changes have been observed in patients with coronary artery disease or Prinzmetal's (vasospastic) angina. To reduce the risk of angina, do not give sumatriptan to patients with risk factors for coronary artery disease (CAD) until CAD has been ruled out. These patients include postmenopausal women, men over 40, smokers, and patients with hypertension, hypercholesterolemia, obesity, diabetes, or a family history of CAD.

*Teratogenesis. Sumatriptan should be avoided during pregnancy.* When given daily to pregnant rabbits, the drug is embryolethal at blood levels only three times higher than those achieved with a 6-mg SC injection in humans (which is a typical dose). Accordingly, unless the physician directs otherwise, women should be instructed to avoid the drug if they are pregnant or think they might be, if they are trying to become pregnant, or if they are not using an adequate form of contraception.

### Drug Interactions

*Ergotamine* and *dihydroergotamine* are vasoconstrictors that may intensify vasoconstriction caused by sumatriptan, possibly resulting in prolonged vasospasm. Accordingly, sumatriptan and the ergotamines should not be used within 24 hours of each other.

#### Preparations, Dosage, and Administration

*Subcutaneous.* Sumatriptan succinate [Imitrex] is available in single-dose vials and prefilled syringes for SC injection. An autoinjector is available for self-administration. The maximum single dose is 6 mg. The maximum that may be given in 24 hours is two 6-mg doses, separated by at least 1 hour. Sumatriptan should be administered no sooner than 24 hours after any ergotamine-containing drug.

*Oral.* Sumatriptan [Imitrex] is available in 25- and 50-mg tablets for oral use. The usual dose is 25 mg, but doses as high as 100 mg may be tried. If the response to the first dose is unsatisfactory after 2 hours, a second dose may be given.

### Zolmitriptan

Zolmitriptan [Zomig] is a new drug similar to sumatriptan. Benefits derive from stimulating 5HT$_{1D}$ receptors. Administration is oral. In clinical trials, zolmitriptan was effective and well tolerated. About 65% of patients responded within 2 hours. Doses ranging from 2.5 to 50 mg were employed. A dose of 2.5 mg produced the most favorable response/tolerability ratio. Headache recurred in 8% to 32% of patients. Adverse effects are generally mild and transient. The most common is a sensation of pressure or tightness in the neck, jaw, or throat. Other adverse effects include nausea, somnolence, and asthenia.

## Migraine Headache: Prophylactic Therapy

Several drugs, when taken prophylactically, can reduce the frequency and intensity of migraine attacks. Prophylactic therapy is indicated for patients who have not responded adequately to abortive therapy, and for patients whose attacks are frequent or especially severe.

### Beta-Adrenergic Blocking Agents

*Propranolol* [Inderal] is the drug of choice for migraine prophylaxis. This agent can reduce the number and intensity of attacks in about 70% of patients. No loss in benefits has occurred over 1 year of continuous treatment. The most common side effects are extreme tiredness and fatigue, which occur in about 10% of patients.

Not all beta blockers are active against migraine. Agents with demonstrated efficacy are *propranolol, atenolol, metoprolol, nadolol,* and *timolol.* Agents shown to be ineffective include *oxprenolol* and *pindolol*. Because only some beta blockers are effective, whereas all of them are able to block beta-adrenergic receptors, it would appear that a mechanism other than beta blockade is responsible for beneficial effects.

The basic pharmacology of the beta-adrenergic blocking agents is discussed in Chapter 19.

### Methysergide

Methysergide [Sansert] was the first effective drug for prophylaxis of migraine. This agent is more effective than propranolol but is also more dangerous. Accordingly, prophylaxis with propranolol is generally preferred. Methysergide is not effective for aborting an ongoing attack. In addition to its utility against migraine, methysergide is a preferred drug for prophylaxis of cluster headaches.

The mechanism by which methysergide provides prophylaxis is not clear. The drug is able to stimulate serotonin receptors in the central nervous system (CNS). Suppression of pain pathways by this mechanism may explain beneficial effects.

Methysergide causes a variety of adverse effects. Fibrotic changes, although rare, are most serious. With long-term therapy, methysergide can cause retroperitoneal, pleuropulmonary, and cardiac fibrosis. Retroperitoneal fibrosis can result in urinary tract obstruction. Pleuropulmonary fibrosis can cause chest pain, dyspnea, and plural effusion. Fibrosis of the aortic and mitral valves can cause heart murmurs and dyspnea. Fibrotic changes may reverse spontaneously upon cessation of drug use; however, surgical correction may be required. Other adverse effects include vascular insufficiency; CNS reactions (insomnia, altered mood, depersonalization, hallucinations, nightmares); and gastrointestinal disturbances (nausea, vomiting, diarrhea).

The usual adult dosage is 2 mg 2 to 4 times a day. Because of its potential for serious toxicity, methysergide should not be taken continuously. Rather, the manufacturer recommends discontinuing the drug for 3 to 4 weeks every 6 months.

### Amitriptyline

Amitriptyline [Elavil, others], a tricyclic antidepressant, provides effective prophylaxis against migraine. In one study, the drug was as effective as methysergide. The mechanism underlying antimigraine actions is not known. Since amitriptyline is effective in patients who are not depressed, it would seem that benefits are *not* dependent on elevation of mood. The basic pharmacology of amitriptyline is discussed in Chapter 30.

### Calcium Channel Blockers

Several calcium channel blockers appear moderately effective at reducing migraine attacks. These include *verapamil, nifedipine, nimodipine,* and *flunarizine* (a drug not yet available in the United States). Curiously, beneficial effects develop slowly, reaching their maximum in 1 to 2 months. Although all of these drugs can relieve vasospasm, it is not clear that vasodilation explains their antimigraine effects. A direct effect on neurons is another possible mechanism.

When used for prophylaxis, calcium channel blockers cause side effects in 20% to 60% of patients. Constipation and orthostatic hypotension are most common. Vascular headache develops in about 25% of patients taking nifedipine.

The basic pharmacology of the calcium channel blockers is discussed in Chapter 42.

### Phenelzine

Phenelzine, a monoamine oxidase inhibitor–type antidepressant, is active against migraine. However, responses are variable, and the drug is potentially dangerous. Accordingly, phenelzine should not be used routinely. Rather, the drug should be re-served for patients who cannot tolerate or who fail to respond to safer drugs. The basic pharmacology of phenelzine is discussed in Chapter 30.

### Valproic Acid

Valproic acid [Depakene], which was used first for epilepsy and more recently for bipolar disorder (manic- depressive illness), is also used for prophylaxis against migraine. The drug reduces the incidence of attacks by 60%. However, when attacks do occur, their intensity and duration are not diminished. In patients with migraine, the most common side effect is nausea. Other side effects include fatigue, tremor, and reversible hair loss. The basic pharmacology of valproic acid is presented in Chapter 23.

## Cluster Headaches

### Characteristics

Cluster headaches occur in a series or "cluster" of attacks. Each attack lasts from 15 minutes to 2 hours and is characterized by severe, nonthrobbing, unilateral pain, usually located in or around the eye. A cluster consists of one or more such attacks every day for 4 to 12 weeks. An attack-free interval of months to years separates each cluster. Although related to migraine, cluster headaches differ in several ways: (1) they are not preceded by an aura, (2) they do not cause nausea and vomiting, (3) they are not associated with a family history of attacks, (4) they occur mostly in males, and (5) treatment is different.

### Treatment

Primary therapy is directed at prophylaxis. Until recently, *methysergide* was the drug of choice for preventing attacks. However, this agent has been replaced by *verapamil* (a calcium channel blocker) as the preferred agent for prophylaxis. Other prophylactic drugs include *lithium* and *glucocorticoids*. When lithium is used, blood levels of the drug must be monitored. Because long-term treatment with glucocorticoids carries a high risk of serious toxicity, use of these drugs should be limited to 3 weeks.

If an attack occurs despite preventative therapy, it can be aborted with sumatriptan or an ergot preparation. The most rapid responses are achieved by injecting *sumatriptan* or *dihydroergotamine*. Slower relief can be achieved with an *ergotamine-caffeine suppository*. Since attacks last less than 2 hours, oral ergotamine, with its slow onset, is less helpful.

An attack may also be terminated by inhalation of *100% oxygen* (for 10 minutes or less). This procedure is effective in up to 93% of patients. The mechanism of relief is unknown.

## Tension-Type Headache

### Characteristics

Tension-type or muscle contraction headaches are the most common form of headache. These headaches are characterized by moderate, nonthrobbing pain, usually located in a "hat band" distribution around the head. Headache is often associated with scalp formication and a sense of tightness or pressure in the head and neck. Precipitating factors include eye strain, aggravation, frustration, and life's daily stresses. Depressive symptoms (sleep disturbances, including early and frequent awakening) are often present.

Tension-type headaches frequently occur together with migraine. In some patients, migraine headaches experienced early in life are later replaced by an unremitting tension-type headache, a condition referred to as chronic headache syndrome.

### Treatment

An acute attack of mild to moderate intensity can be relieved with a nonopioid analgesic, such as acetaminophen or a nonsteroidal anti-inflammatory drug (e.g., aspirin, ibuprofen, naproxen). An analgesic-sedative combination (e.g., aspirin-meprobamate, aspirin-butalbital) may also be used. However, because of their potential for dependence and abuse, these combinations should be reserved for acute therapy of episodic attacks; they are inappropriate for patients with chronic headache syndrome.

For prophylaxis, *amitriptyline* [Elavil, others], a tricyclic antidepressant, is the drug of choice. Administering the drug at bedtime will help relieve any depression-related sleep disturbances in addition to protecting against headache. Amitriptyline can cause anticholinergic side effects (e.g., dry mouth, constipation) and poses a risk of cardiotoxicity at high doses.

## KEY POINTS

- Drugs are used in two ways to treat migraine: abortive therapy and prophylactic therapy.
- The goal of abortive therapy is to eliminate headache pain and associated nausea and vomiting.
- The goal of prophylactic therapy is to reduce the incidence of migraine attacks.
- Aspirin-like analgesics (e.g., aspirin, ibuprofen, acetaminophen) are effective for abortive therapy of mild to moderate migraine.
- Opioid analgesics (e.g., meperidine, butorphanol) are reserved for severe migraine that has not responded to other drugs.
- Ergotamine and sumatriptan are drugs of choice for abortive therapy of severe migraine. Both drugs are thought to act by stimulating receptors for serotonin (5-HT).
- Overdose with ergotamine can cause ergotism, a serious condition in which generalized constriction of peripheral arteries and arterioles causes severe tissue ischemia.
- Ergotamine must not be taken on a routine basis because physical dependence will occur.
- Ergotamine can cause uterine contraction and must not be taken during pregnancy.
- Sumatriptan is teratogenic in animals and should be avoided during pregnancy.
- Sumatriptan can induce angina and should be avoided by patients with coronary artery disease.
- Propranolol is the drug of choice for prophylactic therapy of migraine.

# Summary of Major Nursing Implications*

## ERGOTAMINE

### Preadministration Assessment

#### Therapeutic Goal
Termination of migraine or cluster headache.

#### Baseline Data
Determine the age of onset, frequency, location, intensity, and quality (throbbing or nonthrobbing) of headaches as well as the presence or absence of a prodromal aura. Assess for precipitating factors (e.g., stress, anxiety, fatigue) and for a family history of severe headache.

Assess for possible underlying causes of headache (e.g., severe hypertension; hyperthyroidism; infection; tumors; disorders of the eye, ear, nose, sinuses, or throat). If present, these should be treated directly.

#### Identifying High-Risk Patients
Ergotamine is *contraindicated* in the presence of *hepatic or renal impairment, sepsis, coronary artery disease, peripheral vascular disease,* and *pregnancy.*

### Implementation: Administration

#### Routes
Sublingual, inhalation (ergotamine alone).
Oral, rectal (ergotamine plus caffeine).

### Dosage and Administration
Instruct the patient to commence dosing immediately after onset of symptoms.

Ergotamine can cause physical dependence and serious toxicity if taken in excessive dosage. Inform the patient about the risks of dependence and toxicity and the importance of not exceeding the prescribed dosage.

Nausea and vomiting from the headache and from ergotamine itself may prevent complete absorption of oral ergotamine. Concurrent treatment with metoclopramide or another antiemetic can minimize these effects.

### Implementation: Measures to Enhance Therapeutic Effects
Educate the patient in ways to control, avoid, or eliminate precipitating factors (e.g., stress, fatigue, anxiety, alcohol, tyramine-containing foods).

Teach the patient biofeedback or another relaxation technique. Advise the patient to rest in a quiet, dark room for 2 to 3 hours after drug administration.

### Evaluating Therapeutic Effects
Determine the size and frequency of doses used and the extent to which therapy has reduced the intensity and duration of attacks.

### Ongoing Evaluation and Interventions

#### Minimizing Adverse Effects
*Nausea and Vomiting.* Minimize these by concurrent therapy with metoclopramide or a phenothiazine-type antiemetic.

*Patient education information is highlighted in color.

***Ergotism.*** Toxicity (ergotism) can result from acute or chronic overdosage. Teach patients the early manifestations of ergotism (muscle pain; paresthesias in fingers and toes; extremities become cold, pale, and numb) and instruct them to report these immediately. To treat, (1) withdraw ergotamine and (2) administer drugs (anticoagulants, low-molecular-weight dextran, intravenous nitroprusside) as appropriate to maintain circulation.

***Physical Dependence.*** Warn patients not to overuse ergotamine, since overuse can cause physical dependence. Teach patients the signs and symptoms of withdrawal (headache, nausea, vomiting, restlessness) and instruct them to inform the physician if these develop during a drug-free interval. Patients who become dependent may require hospitalization to bring about withdrawal.

***Abortion.*** Ergotamine is a uterine stimulant that can cause abortion when taken in high doses. Warn women of child-bearing age to avoid pregnancy while using this drug.

# Sumatriptan

## Preadministration Assessment

### Therapeutic Goal
Termination of migraine headache.

### Baseline Data
See implications for ergotamine.

### Identifying High-Risk Patients
Sumatriptan is *contraindicated* in the presence of *coronary artery disease* and *pregnancy*.

## Implementation: Administration

### Routes
Oral, subcutaneous.

## Dosage and Administration
Instruct the patient to administer sumatriptan immediately after onset of symptoms.
Teach the patient how to use the SC autoinjector.

## Implementation: Measures to Enhance Therapeutic Effects

Educate the patient in ways to control, avoid, or eliminate precipitating factors (e.g., stress, fatigue, anxiety, alcohol, tyramine-containing foods).
Teach the patient biofeedback or another relaxation technique.

## Ongoing Evaluation and Interventions

### Evaluating Therapeutic Effects
Determine the size and frequency of doses used and the extent to which therapy has reduced the intensity and duration of attacks.

### Minimizing Adverse Effects
***Angina.*** Sumatriptan can cause anginal pain. Avoid the drug in patients with CAD. In patients with risk factors for CAD, rule out CAD before giving sumatriptan.

***Teratogenesis.*** Sumatriptan can cause birth defects in laboratory animals. Avoid the drug during pregnancy.

### Minimizing Adverse Interactions
***Ergotamine and Dihydroergotamine.*** Combining these drugs with sumatriptan may cause prolonged vasospasm. Do not administer the ergots and sumatriptan within 24 hours of each other.

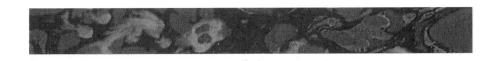

# Psychotherapeutic Drugs

# CHAPTER 29

# Antipsychotic Agents and Their Use in Schizophrenia

The antipsychotic agents are a chemically diverse group of compounds employed to treat a broad spectrum of psychotic disorders. Specific indications include schizophrenia, delusional disorders, acute mania, depressive psychoses, and drug-induced psychoses. In addition to their psychiatric applications, the antipsychotics are used to suppress emesis and to treat Tourette's syndrome and Huntington's chorea.

Since their introduction in the early 1950s, the antipsychotic agents have catalyzed revolutionary change in the management of psychotic illnesses. Before these drugs became available, psychoses were largely untreatable and patients were fated to a life of institutionalization. With the advent of antipsychotic medications, many patients with schizophrenia and other severe psychiatric disorders have been able to leave psychiatric hospitals and return to the community. Others have been spared hospitalization entirely. For those who must remain institutionalized, antipsychotic drugs have at least reduced suffering.

The antipsychotic drugs fall into two major groups: *traditional antipsychotics* and *atypical antipsychotics*. All of the traditional agents block receptors for dopamine in the central nervous system (CNS), and they all can cause serious *movement disorders*, referred to as *extrapyramidal side effects*. Although the atypical agents also block dopamine receptors, the pattern of blockade differs from that of the traditional agents. As a result, the incidence of extrapyramidal reactions with the atypical agents is low.

## Schizophrenia: Clinical Features and Etiology

### Clinical Features

Schizophrenia is a chronic psychotic illness characterized by disordered thinking and a reduced ability to comprehend reality. Symptoms usually emerge during adolescence or early adulthood. The incidence of the disease the United States is about 1%. Diagnostic criteria for schizophrenia are presented in Table 29–1.

*Positive and Negative Symptoms.* Symptoms of schizophrenia can be divided into two groups: positive symptoms and negative symptoms (Table 29–2). Positive symptoms can be viewed as an exaggeration or distortion of normal function, whereas negative symptoms can be viewed as a loss or diminution of normal function. Positive symptoms include hallucinations, delusions, agitation, tension, and paranoia. Negative symptoms include lack of motivation, poverty of speech, blunted affect, poor self-care, and social withdrawal. Traditional antipsychotic agents relieve positive symptoms more effectively than negative symptoms. In contrast, atypical antipsychotic agents relieve both types of symptoms.

*Acute Episodes.* During an acute schizophrenic episode, delusions (fixed false beliefs) and hallucinations are frequently prominent. Delusions are typically religious, grandiose, or persecutory. Auditory hallucinations,

## TABLE 29–1. DSM-IV DIAGNOSTIC CRITERIA FOR SCHIZOPHRENIA

*A. Characteristic Symptoms*

At least two of the following are present for a significant time during a 1-month period (or less if successfully treated):

- Delusions
- Hallucinations
- Disorganized speech (e.g., frequent derailment or incoherence)
- Grossly disorganized or catatonic behavior
- Negative symptoms (affective flattening, alogia, or avolition)

*Note:* Only one symptom is required if delusions are bizarre or if hallucinations consist of either (1) a voice making running comments on the person's behavior or thoughts or (2) voices conversing with each other.

*B. Social/Occupational Dysfunction*

For a significant time since the onset of the disturbance, at least one major area of functioning (e.g., work, interpersonal relations, self-care) is markedly below the preonset level *or*, if the onset occurred in childhood or adolescence, the individual failed to achieve the expected level of interpersonal, academic, or occupational functioning.

*C. Duration*

Continuous signs of the disturbance persist for at least 6 months. This 6-month period must include at least 1 month of symptoms (or less if successfully treated) that meet Criterion A (i.e., active-phase symptoms). It may also include periods of prodromal or residual symptoms; during these times the disturbance is manifested only by negative symptoms or by at least two symptoms from Criterion A that are present in attenuated form (e.g., odd beliefs, unusual perceptual experience).

*D. Schizoaffective and Mood Disorder Exclusion*

Schizoaffective Disorder and Mood Disorder With Psychotic Features have been ruled out because either (1) no Major Depressive, Manic, or Mixed Episodes have occurred concurrently with the active-phase symptoms; or (2) if mood episodes have occurred during active-phase symptoms, their total duration has been brief relative to the duration of the active and residual periods.

*E. Substance/General Medical Condition Exclusion*

The disturbance is not due to the direct physiologic effects of a substance (e.g., drug of abuse, medication) or a general medical condition.

*F. Relationship to a Pervasive Developmental Disorder*

If there is a history of Autistic Disorder or another Pervasive Developmental Disorder, the additional diagnosis of Schizophrenia is made only if prominent delusions or hallucinations are present for at least 1 month (or less if successfully treated).

Adapted from American Psychiatric Association. *Diagnostic and Statistical Manual of Mental Disorders,* 4th ed. Washington, DC, American Psychiatric Press, 1994, pp. 285–286.

which are more common than visual hallucinations, may consist of voices arguing or commenting on one's behavior. The patient may feel controlled by external influences. Disordered thinking and loose association may render rational conversation impossible. Affect may be blunted or labile. Misperception of reality may result in hostility and lack of cooperation. Impaired self-care skills may leave the patient disheveled and dirty. Patterns of sleeping and eating are usually disrupted.

**Residual Symptoms.** After florid symptoms (e.g., hallucinations, delusions) of an acute episode remit, less vivid symptoms may remain. These include suspiciousness, poor anxiety management, and diminished judgment, insight, motivation, and capacity for self-care. As a result of these changes, patients frequently find it difficult to establish close relationships, maintain employment, and function independently in society. Suspiciousness and poor anxiety management contribute to social withdrawal. An inability to appreciate the need for continued drug therapy may cause noncompliance, resulting in relapse and possibly hospital readmission.

**Long-Term Course.** The long-term course of schizophrenia is characterized by episodic acute exacerbations separated by intervals of partial remission. As the years pass, some patients experience progressive decline in mental status and social functioning, whereas others may stabilize. Maintenance therapy with antipsychotic drugs reduces the risk of acute relapse, but may fail to prevent long-term deterioration.

### Etiology

Although there is strong evidence that schizophrenia has a biologic basis, the exact etiology is unknown. Genetic, perinatal, neurodevelopmental, and neuroana-

**TABLE 29-2. POSITIVE AND NEGATIVE SYMPTOMS OF SCHIZOPHRENIA**

| Positive Symptoms | Negative Symptoms |
|---|---|
| Hallucinations | Social withdrawal |
| Delusions | Emotional withdrawal |
| Disordered thinking | Lack of motivation |
| Combativeness | Poverty of speech |
| Agitation | Blunted affect |
| Paranoia | Poor insight |
| | Poor judgment |
| | Poor self-care |

tomic factors may all be involved. Possible primary defects include excessive activation of CNS receptors for dopamine, and insufficient activation of CNS receptors for glutamate. Although psychosocial stressors can precipitate acute exacerbations in susceptible patients, these stressors are not considered causative.

# Traditional Antipsychotic Agents I: Group Properties

In this section we discuss pharmacologic properties shared by all of the traditional agents. Much of our attention focuses on adverse effects. Of these, the extrapyramidal side effects are of particular concern. Because of these neurologic side effects, the traditional antipsychotics are known alternatively as neuroleptics.

## Classification

The traditional antipsychotics can be classified by potency or by chemical structure. From a clinical viewpoint, classification by potency is more informative.

### Classification by Potency

Traditional antipsychotic agents can be classified as *low potency*, *medium potency*, or *high potency* (Table 29-3). The low-potency drugs, represented by chlorpromazine [Thorazine], and the high-potency drugs, represented by haloperidol [Haldol], are of particular interest.

It is important to note that, although the traditional antipsychotics differ from one another in *potency*, all of these drugs are essentially *equal* in their ability to relieve symptoms of psychoses. Recall that the term *potency* refers only to the size of the dose needed to elicit a given response; potency implies nothing about the maximal effect that a drug can produce. Hence, when we say that haloperidol is more potent than chlorpromazine, we mean only that the dose of haloperidol required to relieve psychotic symptoms is smaller than the required dose of chlorpromazine; we do not mean that haloperidol can produce greater effects. When administered in therapeutically equivalent doses, both drugs elicit an equivalent antipsychotic response.

If low-potency and high-potency neuroleptics are equally effective, why should we distinguish between them? The answer is that, although these agents produce identical *antipsychotic* effects, they differ significantly in their *side effects*. Hence, by knowing the potency category to which a particular neuroleptic belongs, we can better predict that drug's undesired responses. This knowledge is useful in drug selection and providing patient care and education.

### Chemical Classification

The traditional antipsychotic agents can be placed into five major groups based on their chemical structures (Table 29-4). One of these groups, the phenothiazines, has three subdivisions. Drugs in all groups are equivalent with respect to antipsychotic actions. Because of this equivalence, chemical classification is not emphasized in this chapter.

Two chemical categories—the *phenothiazines* and the *butyrophenones*—deserve special attention. The phenothiazines were the first of the modern antipsychotic agents. Chlorpromazine, our prototype of the low-potency neuroleptics, is a member of the phenothiazine family. The butyrophenones stand out because they are the family to which haloperidol belongs. Haloperidol is the prototype of the high-potency antipsychotics.

## Mechanism of Action

The traditional antipsychotic drugs block a variety of receptors within and outside the CNS. To varying degrees, these drugs block receptors for dopamine, acetylcholine (muscarinic), histamine, and norepinephrine (alpha$_1$). There is little question that blockade at these receptors is responsible for the major *adverse effects* of the antipsychotics. However, since the etiology of psychotic illness is entirely unknown, the relationship of receptor blockade to *therapeutic effects* can only be guessed. The current dominant theory suggests that traditional antipsychotic drugs suppress symptoms of psychosis by blocking dopamine$_2$ (D$_2$) receptors in the mesolimbic and mesocortical areas of the brain, regions thought to be involved in the expression of psychotic symptoms. In support of this theory is the observation that all of the traditional antipsychotics produce D$_2$ receptor blockade. Furthermore, there is a close correlation between the clinical potency of these drugs and their potency as D$_2$ receptor antagonists.

## Therapeutic Uses

*Schizophrenia.* Schizophrenia is the primary indication for antipsychotic drugs. These agents effectively suppress symptoms during acute psychotic episodes, and, when taken chronically, can greatly decrease the risk of relapse. Initial effects may be seen in 1 to 2 days, but substantial improvement usually takes 2 to 4 weeks, and full effects may not develop for several months. *Positive symptoms* (e.g., delusions, hallucinations) respond better than *negative symptoms* (e.g., social and emotional withdrawal,

## TABLE 29-3. ANTIPSYCHOTIC DRUGS: RELATIVE POTENCY AND INCIDENCE OF SIDE EFFECTS

| Drug | Equivalent Oral Dose (mg)* | Incidence of Side Effects | | | |
|---|---|---|---|---|---|
| | | Sedation | Orthostatic Hypotension | Anticholinergic Effects | Extrapyramidal Effects[†] |
| *Low Potency, Traditional* | | | | | |
| Chlorpromazine | 100 | High | High | Moderate | Moderate |
| Thioridazine | 100 | High | High | High | Low |
| *Medium Potency, Traditional* | | | | | |
| Triflupromazine | 25 | High | Moderate | High | Moderate |
| Acetophenazine | 20 | Moderate | Low | Low | High |
| Loxapine | 15 | Medium | Medium | Low | High |
| Molindone | 10 | Low | Low | Low | High |
| Perphenazine | 8 | Low | Low | Low | High |
| *High Potency, Traditional* | | | | | |
| Trifluoperazine | 5 | Low | Low | Low | High |
| Thiothixene | 4 | Low | Low | Low | High |
| Fluphenazine | 2 | Low | Low | Low | High |
| Haloperidol | 2 | Low | Low | Low | High |
| Pimozide | 0.5 | Low | Low | Low | High |
| *Atypical* | | | | | |
| Clozapine | 50 | High | High | High | Very low |
| Risperidone | 1 | Low | Low | Low | Very low |
| Olanzepine | NA[‡] | High | — | Moderate | Very low |

*Doses listed are the therapeutic equivalent of 100 mg of oral chlorpromazine.
[†]Incidence refers to *early* extrapyramidal reactions (acute dystonia, parkinsonism, akathisia). The incidence of *late* reactions (tardive dyskinesia) is the same for all traditional antipsychotics; tardive dyskinesia has not been reported with atypical antipsychotics.
[‡]NA = not available.

blunted affect, poverty of speech). All of the traditional antipsychotic agents are equally effective, although individual patients may respond better to one drug than another. Consequently, selection among these drugs is based primarily on their side-effect profiles, rather than on their therapeutic effects. It must be noted that antipsychotic drugs do not alter the underlying pathology of schizophrenia. Hence treatment is not curative—it offers only symptomatic relief. Management of schizophrenia is discussed further later in the chapter.

**Bipolar Disorder (Manic-Depressive Illness).** Most patients with bipolar disorder are managed with lithium, the drug of choice for this disease. Neuroleptics may be employed acutely (in combination with lithium) to help manage patients going through a severe manic phase. Bipolar disorder and its treatment are the subject of Chapter 31.

**Tourette's Syndrome.** This rare inherited disorder is characterized by severe motor tics, barking cries, grunts, and outbursts of obscene language, all of which are spontaneous and beyond the control of the patient. At least three antipsychotic drugs—pimozide, fluphenazine, and haloperidol—can help suppress severe symptoms. For mild symptoms, clonidine is the drug of choice.

**Prevention of Emesis.** Neuroleptics suppress emesis by blocking dopamine receptors in the chemoreceptor trigger zone of the medulla. These drugs can be employed to suppress vomiting associated with cancer chemotherapy, gastroenteritis, uremia, and other conditions.

**Other Applications.** Neuroleptics can be used for *dementia and other organic mental syndromes* (psychiatric syndromes resulting from organic causes, such as infection, metabolic disorders, poisoning, and structural injury to the brain), *delusional disorders,* and *schizoaffective disorder.* In addition, these agents can relieve symptoms of *Huntington's chorea.*

## Adverse Effects

Although antipsychotic agents produce a variety of undesired effects, these drugs are, on the whole, very safe; death from overdosage is practically unheard of. Of the many side effects these drugs can produce, the most troubling are the extrapyramidal reactions, especially tardive dyskinesia.

### Extrapyramidal Side Effects

Extrapyramidal side effects (EPSE) are movement disorders resulting from effects of antipsychotic drugs on the extrapyramidal motor system. The extrapyramidal system is the same neuronal network whose malfunction is responsible for the movement disorders of Parkinson's disease. Although the exact cause of EPSE is unclear, blockade of $D_2$ receptors is strongly suspected.

Four types of EPSE occur. These differ from one another with respect to time of onset and management. Three of these reactions—acute dystonia, parkinsonism, and

## TABLE 29–4. ANTIPSYCHOTIC DRUGS: ROUTES AND DOSAGES

| Chemical Class and Generic Name | Trade Name | Route | Total Daily Dose | |
| --- | --- | --- | --- | --- |
| | | | Short-Term | Maintenance |
| TRADITIONAL AGENTS | | | | |
| *Phenothiazine: aliphatic* | | | | |
| Chlorpromazine | Thorazine, Ormazine | PO, IM, R* | 200–1000 | 50–400 |
| Triflupromazine | Vesprin | IM | 30–150 | 20–100 |
| *Pheonthiazine: piperidine* | | | | |
| Mesoridazine | Serentil | PO, IM | 100–400 | 25–200 |
| Thioridazine | Mellaril | PO | 200–800 | 50–400 |
| *Phenothiazine:piperazine* | | | | |
| Acetophenazine | Tindal | PO | 60–150 | 40–80 |
| Fluphenazine | Prolixin, Permitil | PO, IM | 5–50 | 1–15 |
| Perphenazine | Trilafon | PO, IM | 12–64 | 8–24 |
| Trifluoperazine | Stelazine | PO, IM | 10–60 | 4–30 |
| *Thioxanthene* | | | | |
| Thiothixene | Navane | PO, IM | 10–60 | 6–30 |
| *Butyrophenone* | | | | |
| Haloperidol | Haldol | PO, IM | 5–50 | 1–15 |
| *Dihydroindolone* | | | | |
| Molindone | Moban | PO | 40–225 | 15–100 |
| *Dibenzoxazepine* | | | | |
| Loxapine | Loxitane | PO, IM | 20–160 | 10–60 |
| ATYPICAL AGENTS | | | | |
| *Dibenzodiazepine* | | | | |
| Clozapine | Clozaril | PO | 300–900 | 200–400 |
| *Benzisoxazole* | | | | |
| Risperidone | Risperdal | PO | 4–8 | Unknown |
| *Thiobenzodiazepine* | | | | |
| Olanzepine | Zyprexa | PO | 10 | Unknown |

*R = rectal (suppository).

akathisia—occur early in therapy and can be managed with a variety of drugs. The fourth reaction—tardive dyskinesia—occurs late in therapy and has no satisfactory treatment. Characteristics of EPSE are summarized in Table 29-5.

The *early* reactions occur *less frequently* with *low-potency* agents (e.g., chlorpromazine) than with high-potency agents (e.g., haloperidol). In contrast, the risk of *tardive dyskinesia* is equal with *all* antipsychotics.

**Acute Dystonia.** Acute dystonia can be both disturbing and dangerous. The reaction develops within the first few days of therapy, and frequently within hours of the first dose. Typically, the patient develops severe spasm of the muscles of the tongue, face, neck, or back. Oculogyric crisis (involuntary upward deviation of the eyes) and opisthotonus (tetanic spasm of the back muscles causing the trunk to arch forward, while the head and lower limbs are thrust backward) may also occur. Severe cramping can cause joint dislocation. Laryngeal dystonia can impair respiration.

Intense dystonia constitutes a crisis that requires rapid intervention. Initial treatment consists of anticholinergic medication (e.g., benztropine, diphenhydramine) administered IM or IV. As a rule, symptoms resolve within 5 minutes of IV administration and within 15 to 20 minutes of IM administration.

It is important to differentiate between acute dystonia and psychotic hysteria. Misdiagnosis of acute dystonia as hysteria could result in escalation of antipsychotic dosage, thereby causing the acute dystonia to become even worse.

**Parkinsonism.** Antipsychotic-induced parkinsonism is characterized by bradykinesia, mask-like facies, drooling, tremor, rigidity, shuffling gait, cogwheeling, and stooped posture. Symptoms develop within the first month of therapy and are indistinguishable from those of idiopathic Parkinson's disease.

Neuroleptics cause parkinsonism by blocking dopamine receptors in the striatum. Since idiopathic Parkinson's disease is also due to reduced activation of striatal dopamine receptors (see Chapter 22), it is no wonder that

## TABLE 29-5. EXTRAPYRAMIDAL SIDE EFFECTS OF ANTIPSYCHOTIC DRUGS

| Type of Reaction | Time of Onset | Features | Management |
|---|---|---|---|
| *Early Reactions* | | | |
| Acute dystonia | A few hours to 5 days | Spasm of muscles of tongue, face, neck, and back; opisthotonus | Anticholinergic drugs (e.g., benztropine) IM or IV |
| Parkinsonism | 5–30 days | Bradykinesia, mask-like facies, tremor, rigidity, shuffling gait, drooling, cogwheeling, stooped posture | Anticholinergics (e.g., benztropine, diphenhydramine), amantadine, or both |
| Akathisia | 5–60 days | Compulsive, restless movement; symptoms of anxiety, agitation | Reduce dosage or switch to a low-potency antipsychotic. Treat with a benzodiazepine, beta blocker, or anticholinergic drug |
| *Late Reaction* | | | |
| Tardive dyskinesia | Months to years | Oral-facial dyskinesias, choreoathetoid movements | Best approach is prevention; no reliable treatment. Discontinue all anticholinergic drugs. Give benzodiazepines. Reduce antipsychotic dosage. For severe TD, switch to clozapine or possibly another atypical agent |

Parkinson's disease and neuroleptic-induced parkinsonism share the same symptoms.

Neuroleptic-induced parkinsonism is treated with some—but not all—of the drugs used to treat Parkinson's disease. Specifically, centrally acting *anticholinergic drugs* (e.g., benztropine, diphenhydramine) and *amantadine* [Symmetrel] may be employed. Levodopa, however, should be avoided, since this drug promotes activation of dopamine receptors, and might thereby counteract the beneficial effects of antipsychotic treatment.

Use of antiparkinsonism drugs should not continue indefinitely. Antipsychotic-induced parkinsonism tends to resolve spontaneously, usually within months of its appearance. Accordingly, antiparkinsonism drugs should be withdrawn after a few months to determine if they are still required.

**Akathisia.** Akathisia is characterized by pacing and squirming brought on by an uncontrollable need to be in motion. This profound sense of restlessness can be very disturbing. The syndrome usually develops within the first 2 months of treatment. Like other early extrapyramidal reactions, akathisia occurs most frequently with high-potency antipsychotics.

Three types of drugs have been used to suppress symptoms: beta blockers, benzodiazepines, and anticholinergic drugs. Although these can be helpful, a reduction in antipsychotic dosage or switching to a low-potency agent may be more effective.

It is important to differentiate between akathisia and exacerbation of psychosis. If akathisia were to be confused with anxiety or psychotic agitation, it is likely that antipsychotic dosage would be increased, thereby making akathisia more intense.

**Tardive Dyskinesia.** Tardive dyskinesia (TD), the most troubling EPSE, develops in 15% to 20% of patients during long-term therapy. The risk is related to duration of treatment and dosage size. For many patients, symptoms are irreversible.

TD is characterized by involuntary choreoathetoid (twisting, writhing, worm-like) movements of the tongue and face. Patients may also present with lip-smacking movements, and their tongues may flick out in a "fly-catching" motion. One of the earliest manifestations of TD is slow, worm-like movement of the tongue. Involuntary movements that involve the tongue and mouth can interfere with chewing, swallowing, and speaking. Eating difficulties can result in malnutrition and weight loss. Over time, TD produces involuntary movements of the limbs, toes, fingers, and trunk. For some patients, symptoms decline following a dosage reduction or drug withdrawal. For others, TD is irreversible.

The cause of TD is complex and incompletely understood. One theory suggests that symptoms result from excessive *activation* of dopamine receptors. It is postulated that, in response to chronic receptor blockade, dopamine receptors of the extrapyramidal system undergo a functional change such that their sensitivity to activation is increased. Stimulation of these "supersensitive" receptors produces an imbalance in favor of dopamine, and thereby produces abnormal movement. In support of this theory is the observation that symptoms of TD can be reduced (temporarily) by *increasing* antipsychotic dosage, which causes greater dopamine receptor blockade. (Since symptoms eventually return even though antipsychotic dosage is kept at an elevated level, dosage elevation cannot be used to treat TD.)

There is no reliable management for TD. Measures that may be tried include gradual withdrawal of anticholinergic drugs, administration of benzodiazepines, and reducing the dosage of the offending antipsychotic agent. For patients with severe TD, switching to clozapine or risperidone (atypical antipsychotic agents) may be beneficial. These drugs do not seem to cause TD, and may actually suppress symptoms in patients who have developed the disorder.

Since TD has no reliable means of treatment, prevention is the best approach. Antipsychotic drugs should be used in the lowest effective dosage for the shortest time required. After 12 months, the need for continued therapy should be assessed. If drug use must continue, a neurologic evaluation should be done at least every 3 months to detect early signs of TD. For patients with chronic schizophrenia, dosage should be tapered periodically (at least annually) to determine the need for continued treatment.

## Other Adverse Effects

*Neuroleptic Malignant Syndrome.* Neuroleptic malignant syndrome (NMS) is a rare but serious reaction that carries a 4% risk of mortality (down from 30% a decade ago thanks to early diagnosis and intervention). Primary symptoms are "lead-pipe" rigidity, sudden high fever (temperature may exceed 41°C), sweating, and autonomic instability, manifested as dysrhythmias and fluctuations in blood pressure. Level of consciousness may rise and fall, the patient may appear confused or mute, and seizures or coma may develop. Death can result from respiratory failure, cardiovascular collapse, dysrhythmias, and other causes. NMS is more likely with high-potency agents than with low-potency agents.

Treatment consists of supportive measures, drug therapy, and immediate withdrawal of antipsychotic medication. Hyperthermia should be controlled with cooling blankets and antipyretics (e.g., aspirin, acetaminophen). Hydration should be maintained with fluids. Benzodiazepines may relieve anxiety and help reduce blood pressure and tachycardia. Two drugs—*dantrolene* and *bromocriptine*—may be especially helpful. Dantrolene is a direct-acting muscle relaxant (see Chapter 24). In patients with NMS, this drug reduces rigidity and hyperthermia. Bromocriptine is a dopamine receptor agonist (see Chapter 22) that may relieve CNS toxicity.

Resumption of antipsychotic therapy carries a small risk of NMS recurrence. The risk can be minimized by (1) waiting at least 2 weeks before resuming antipsychotic treatment, (2) using the lowest effective dosage, and (3) avoiding high-potency agents. Some clinicians believe that the atypical agent clozapine carries little or no risk of NMS. Hence, if NMS recurs during treatment with a traditional antipsychotic drug, a switch to clozapine may be appropriate.

*Anticholinergic Effects.* Antipsychotic drugs produce varying degrees of muscarinic cholinergic blockade (see Table 29-3). By blocking muscarinic receptors, these drugs can elicit a full spectrum of anticholinergic responses (dry mouth, blurred vision, photophobia, urinary hesitancy, constipation, tachycardia). Patients should be informed about these responses and taught how to minimize danger and discomfort. As indicated in Table 29-3, anticholinergic effects are more likely with low-potency agents than with high-potency agents. Anticholinergic effects and their management are discussed in detail in Chapter 15.

*Orthostatic Hypotension.* Antipsychotic drugs promote orthostatic hypotension by blocking alpha$_1$-adrenergic receptors on blood vessels. Alpha-adrenergic blockade prevents compensatory vasoconstriction when the patient stands; hence, blood pressure falls. Patients should be informed about signs of hypotension (lightheadedness, dizziness) and advised to sit or lie down if these occur. In addition, patients should be informed that hypotension can be minimized by moving slowly when assuming an erect posture. With hospitalized patients, blood pressure and pulses should be checked before drug administration and 1 hour after. Measurements should be made while the patient is lying down and again after the patient has been sitting or standing for 1 to 2 minutes. If blood pressure is low, or if pulse rate is high, the drug should be withheld and the physician consulted. Hypotension is more likely with low-potency antipsychotics than with the high-potency drugs (see Table 29-3). Tolerance to hypotension develops in 2 to 3 months.

*Sedation.* Sedation is common during the early days of treatment but subsides within a week or so. Neuroleptic-induced sedation is thought to result from blockade of histamine receptors in the CNS. Daytime sedation can be minimized by administering the entire daily dose at bedtime. Patients should be warned against participation in hazardous activities (e.g., driving) until sedative effects diminish.

*Neuroendocrine Effects.* Antipsychotics increase levels of circulating prolactin by blocking the inhibitory action of dopamine on prolactin release. Elevation of prolactin levels promotes *gynecomastia* (breast growth) and *galactorrhea* in up to 57% of women. Up to 97% experience menstrual irregularities. Gynecomastia and galactorrhea can also occur in males. Since prolactin can promote growth of prolactin-dependent carcinoma of the breast, neuroleptics should be avoided in patients with this form of cancer. (It should be noted that, although antipsychotic drugs can promote the growth of cancers that already exist, there is no evidence that antipsychotic drugs actually cause cancer.)

*Seizures.* Antipsychotic drugs can reduce seizure threshold, thereby increasing the risk of seizure activity. The risk of seizures is greatest in patients with epilepsy and other seizure disorders. These patients should be monitored, and, if loss of seizure control occurs, the dosage of their antiseizure medication must be increased.

*Sexual Dysfunction.* Antipsychotics can cause sexual dysfunction in women and men. In women, these drugs can suppress libido and impair the ability to achieve orgasm. In men, neuroleptics can suppress libido and cause erectile and ejaculatory dysfunction; the incidence of these effects is 25% to 60%. Drug-induced sexual dysfunction can make treatment unacceptable to sexually active patients, thereby leading to poor compliance. A reduction in dosage or switching to a high-potency antipsychotic may reduce effects on sexual function. Patients should be counseled about possible sexual dysfunction and encouraged to report problems.

***Dermatologic Effects.*** Drugs in the phenothiazine class can sensitize the skin to ultraviolet light, thereby increasing the risk of severe sunburn. Patients should be warned against excessive exposure to sunlight and advised to apply a sunscreen and wear protective clothing. Phenothiazines can also produce pigmentary deposits in the skin, cornea, and lens of the eye.

Handling antipsychotics can cause contact dermatitis in patients and health care personnel. Dermatitis can be prevented by avoiding direct contact with these drugs.

***Agranulocytosis.*** Agranulocytosis is a rare but serious reaction. Among the traditional antipsychotics, the risk is highest with chlorpromazine and certain other phenothiazines. Since agranulocytosis severely compromises the ability to fight infection, white blood cell counts should be done whenever signs of infection (e.g., fever, sore throat) appear. If agranulocytosis is diagnosed, the neuroleptic should be withdrawn. Agranulocytosis reverses upon discontinuation of treatment.

## Physical and Psychologic Dependence

Development of physical and psychologic dependence is rare. Patients should be reassured that addiction and dependence are not likely.

Although physical dependence is minimal, abrupt withdrawal of antipsychotics can precipitate a mild abstinence syndrome. Symptoms result from chronic cholinergic blockade and include restlessness, insomnia, headache, gastric distress, and sweating. This syndrome can be avoided by withdrawing antipsychotic medication gradually.

## Drug Interactions

***Anticholinergic Drugs.*** Drugs with anticholinergic properties will intensify anticholinergic responses to neuroleptics. Patients should be advised to avoid all drugs with anticholinergic actions, including antihistamines and certain over-the-counter sleep aids.

***CNS Depressants.*** Neuroleptics can intensify CNS depression caused by other drugs. Patients should be warned against using alcohol and all other drugs with CNS-depressant actions (e.g., antihistamines, benzodiazepines, barbiturates).

***Levodopa.*** Levodopa (a drug used to treat Parkinson's disease) may counteract the antipsychotic effects of neuroleptics. Conversely, neuroleptics may counteract the therapeutic effects of levodopa. These interactions occur because levodopa and neuroleptics have opposing effects on receptors for dopamine: levodopa activates these receptors, whereas neuroleptics cause blockade.

## Toxicity

The traditional antipsychotic drugs are very safe; death by overdose is extremely rare. With chlorpromazine, for example, the therapeutic index is about 200. That is, the lethal dose is 200 times bigger than the therapeutic dose.

Overdosage produces hypotension, CNS depression, and extrapyramidal reactions. Extrapyramidal reactions can be treated with antiparkinsonism drugs. Hypotension can be treated with IV fluids plus an alpha-adrenergic agonist (e.g., phenylephrine). There is no specific antidote to CNS depression. Excess drug should be removed from the stomach by gastric lavage. (Emetics cannot be used because their effects would be blocked by the antiemetic action of the neuroleptic.)

# Traditional Antipsychotic Agents II: Properties of Individual Agents

All of the traditional antipsychotic drugs are equally effective at suppressing symptoms of schizophrenia, although individual patients may respond better to one drug than another. Hence, differences among these agents relate primarily to their side-effect profiles (see Table 29–3). Because low-potency agents produce more side effects than the high-potency agents, high-potency agents are usually preferred.

## Low-Potency Agents

### Chlorpromazine

Chlorpromazine [Thorazine] was the first modern antipsychotic medication and is the prototype for all that followed. None of the newer agents is superior at relieving symptoms of psychotic illnesses. Chlorpromazine is a low-potency neuroleptic and belongs to the phenothiazine family of compounds.

***Therapeutic Uses.*** Principal indications for chlorpromazine are schizophrenia and other psychotic disorders. Additional psychiatric indications are schizoaffective disorder and the manic phase of bipolar disorder. Other uses include suppression of emesis and relief of intractable hiccoughs.

***Pharmacokinetics.*** Chlorpromazine may be administered orally, IM, and by rectal suppository. Following oral administration, the drug is well absorbed but undergoes extensive first-pass metabolism. As a result, oral bioavailability is only 30%. When chlorpromazine is given by IM injection, peak plasma levels are 10 times those achieved with an equal oral dose. Excretion is renal, almost entirely as metabolites.

***Adverse Effects.*** The most common adverse effects are sedation, orthostatic hypotension, and anticholinergic effects (dry mouth, blurred vision, urinary retention, photophobia, constipation, tachycardia). Neuroendocrine effects—galactorrhea, gynecomastia, and menstrual irregularities—occur occasionally. Photosensitivity reactions are possible, and patients should be warned to minimize unprotected exposure to sunlight. Because chlorpromazine is a low-potency neuroleptic, the risk of early extrapyramidal reactions (dystonia, akathisia, parkinsonism) is relatively low. However, the risk of tardive dyskinesia is the same as with all other traditional agents. Chlorpromazine lowers seizure threshold; hence patients with seizure disorders should be especially diligent about taking antiseizure medication. Agranulocytosis and neuroleptic malignant syndrome occur rarely.

***Drug Interactions.*** Chlorpromazine can intensify responses to CNS depressants (e.g., antihistamines, benzodiazepines, barbiturates) and anticholinergic drugs (e.g., antihistamines, tricyclic antidepressants, atropine-like drugs).

***Preparations, Dosage, and Administration.*** Chlorpromazine [Thorazine, Ormazine] is available in six formulations: *tablets* (10, 25, 50, 100, and 200 mg), *sustained-release capsules* (30, 75, 150, 200, and 300 mg), *syrup* (2 mg/ml), *liquid concentrate* (30 and 100 mg/ml), *rectal suppositories* (25 and 100 mg), and *injection* (25 mg/ml).

*Oral Therapy.* The initial dosage for adults is 25 mg 3 times a day. Dosage should be gradually increased until symptoms are controlled. The usual maintenance dosage is 400 mg/day. Elderly patients require less drug than younger patients.

*Parenteral Therapy.* Parenteral therapy is indicated for the acutely psychotic, hospitalized patient. Intramuscular administration is preferred to intravenous. (Intravenous chlorpromazine is highly irritating and is generally avoided.) The initial dose is 25 to 50 mg. Dosage may be increased gradually to a maximum of 400 mg every 4 to 6 hours. Once symptoms are controlled, oral therapy should be substituted for parenteral.

### Thioridazine

Thioridazine [Mellaril] is a low-potency agent indicated for schizophrenia and other psychotic disorders. The drug belongs to the piperidine subclass of phenothiazines. The most common adverse effects are sedation, orthostatic hypotension, anticholinergic effects, weight gain, and inhibition of ejaculation. Effects seen occasionally include extrapyramidal reactions (dystonia, parkinsonism, akathisia, tardive dyskinesia), galactorrhea, gynecomastia, menstrual irregularities, and photosensitivity reactions. Neuroleptic malignant syndrome, convulsions, agranulocytosis, and pigmentary retinopathy occur rarely. Principal interactions are with anticholinergic drugs and CNS depressants. Thioridazine is dispensed in tablets (10, 15, 25, and 50 mg) for oral use. The initial dosage is 50 to 100 mg 3 times a day. Dosage may be gradually increased until symptoms are controlled, but should not exceed 800 mg/day. The usual maintenance dosage is 200 to 800 mg/day in two to four divided doses.

### Medium-Potency Agents

***Loxapine.*** Loxapine [Loxitane] is a medium-potency agent indicated for schizophrenia and other psychotic disorders. The drug's side-effect profile is similar to that of fluphenazine (see below). Administration is oral and intramuscular. Three formulations are available: capsules (5, 10, 25, and 50 mg), liquid concentrate (25 mg/ml), and injection (50 mg/ml). The initial *oral* dosage is 10 mg twice daily. Dosage is increased until symptoms are controlled, typically with 60 to 100 mg/day in divided doses. The dosage should be reduced for maintenance therapy; the usual range is 20 to 60 mg/day. The *intramuscular* dosage is 12.5 to 50 mg every 4 to 6 hours.

***Molindone.*** Molindone [Moban] is a medium-potency agent used to treat schizophrenia and other psychotic disorders. The most common adverse effects are early extrapyramidal reactions (dystonia, parkinsonism, akathisia) and anticholinergic effects (dry mouth, blurred vision, photophobia, urinary retention, constipation, tachycardia). Effects seen occasionally include sedation, menstrual irregularities, weight loss, and tardive dyskinesia.

Orthostatic hypotension and neuroleptic malignant syndrome occur rarely. Molindone is available in tablets (5, 10, 25, 50, and 100 mg) and an oral concentrate (20 mg/ml). The initial dosage is 50 to 75 mg/day in divided doses. Dosage is then increased until symptoms are controlled. As much as 225 mg/day has been given. Dosage should be reduced to the lowest effective amount for maintenance.

***Perphenazine.*** Perphenazine [Trilafon] is a medium-potency agent used to treat schizophrenia and other psychotic disorders. The drug's side-effect profile is like that of fluphenazine (see below). For therapy of psychotic disorders, perphenazine is given orally and by IM injection. Three formulations are available: tablets (2, 4, 8, and 16 mg), liquid concentrate (16 mg/5 ml), and injection (5 mg/ml). The initial *oral* dosage is 4 to 8 mg 3 times daily. Once symptoms have been controlled, the dosage should be reduced to the lowest effective amount. The initial *intramuscular* dosage is 5 mg every 6 hours. *Parenteral* dosage should not exceed 15 mg/24 hours in ambulatory patients or 30 mg/24 hours in hospitalized patients.

## High-Potency Agents

High-potency agents differ from low-potency agents primarily in that high-potency agents cause more early EPSE but less sedation, orthostatic hypotension, and anticholinergic effects. Because they cause fewer side effects, high-potency agents are generally preferred for initial therapy.

### Haloperidol

***Actions and Uses.*** Haloperidol [Haldol], a member of the *butyrophenone* family, is the prototype of the high-potency neuroleptics. Antipsychotic actions are equivalent to those of chlorpromazine. Principal indications are schizophrenia and acute psychoses. In addition, haloperidol is a preferred drug for Tourette's syndrome.

***Pharmacokinetics.*** Haloperidol may be administered orally and by IM injection. Oral bioavailability is about 60%. Hepatic metabolism is extensive. Parent drug and metabolites are excreted in the urine.

***Adverse Effects.*** As indicated in Table 29–3, early extrapyramidal reactions (dystonia, parkinsonism, akathisia) occur frequently, whereas sedation, hypotension, and anticholinergic effects are uncommon. Note that the incidence of these reactions is exactly opposite to that seen with chlorpromazine and other low-potency agents. The incidence of tardive dyskinesia with haloperidol is the same as with the low-potency drugs. Like chlorpromazine, haloperidol occasionally causes gynecomastia, galactorrhea, and menstrual irregularities. Neuroleptic malignant syndrome, photosensitivity, convulsions, and impotence are rare.

***Preparations, Dosage, and Administration.*** Haloperidol [Haldol] is dispensed in tablets (0.5, 1, 2, 5, 10, and 20 mg) and in a liquid concentrate (2 mg/ml) for oral use. Two injectable forms—*haloperidol lactate* and *haloperidol decanoate*—are available for parenteral (IM) administration. Haloperidol *lactate* is employed for *acute* therapy. Haloperidol *decanoate* is a depot preparation used for *long-term* treatment.

*Oral Therapy.* The initial dosage for adults is 0.5 to 2 mg taken 2 or 3 times a day. For severe illness, daily doses of up to 100 mg have been employed. Once symptoms have been controlled, the dosage should be reduced to the lowest effective amount.

*Intramuscular Therapy.* For acute therapy of severe psychosis, haloperidol lactate is administered IM in doses of 2 to 5 mg. Dosing may be repeated at intervals of 30 minutes to 8 hours. Once symptoms are under control, treatment should be changed to oral therapy. Long-term therapy with haloperidol decanoate is discussed later under *Depot Preparations*.

### Other High-Potency Agents

*Fluphenazine.* Fluphenazine [Prolixin, Permitil] is a high-potency agent indicated for schizophrenia and other psychotic disorders. The drug belongs to the piperazine subclass of phenothiazines. As with other high-potency agents, the most common adverse effects are early extrapyramidal reactions (acute dystonia, parkinsonism, akathisia). The risk of tardive dyskinesia is the same as with all other traditional antipsychotics. Effects seen occasionally include sedation, orthostatic hypotension, anticholinergic effects, gynecomastia, galactorrhea, and menstrual irregularities. Neuroleptic malignant syndrome, convulsions, and agranulocytosis are rare.

Fluphenazine is administered orally and by IM injection. For oral use, the drug is available in tablets (1, 2.5, and 5 mg), an elixir (0.5 mg/ml), and a liquid concentrate (5 mg/ml). The liquid concentrate should be diluted with water, fruit juice, or some other suitable fluid—but not with beverages that contain caffeine, tannins (tea), or pectinates (apple juice) because of physical incompatibilities. The initial *oral dosage* is 2.5 to 10 mg/day given in divided doses every 6 to 8 hours. Daily dosages greater than 3 mg are rarely needed, although some patients may require as much as 30 mg. Once symptoms have been controlled, the dosage should be reduced to the lowest effective amount, typically 1 to 5 mg/day taken as a single dose.

Three injectable preparations are available: *fluphenazine* (2.5 mg/ml), *fluphenazine decanoate* (25 mg/ml), and *fluphenazine enanthate* (25 mg/ml). Fluphenazine itself is used for acute therapy. Fluphenazine enanthate and fluphenazine decanoate are depot preparations used for long-term therapy (see below). *Intramuscular dosages* for acute therapy are usually one-third to one-half the oral dosage.

*Trifluoperazine.* Trifluoperazine [Stelazine] is a high-potency agent used for schizophrenia and other psychotic disorders. The drug belongs to the piperazine subclass of phenothiazines. The most common adverse effects are early extrapyramidal reactions (dystonia, parkinsonism, akathisia). Effects seen occasionally include sedation, orthostatic hypotension, anticholinergic effects, gynecomastia, galactorrhea, menstrual irregularities, and tardive dyskinesia. Neuroleptic malignant syndrome, convulsions, and agranulocytosis are rare.

Trifluoperazine is administered orally and by deep IM injection. Three formulations are available: tablets (1, 2, 5, and 10 mg), liquid concentrate (10 mg/ml), and injection (2 mg/ml). *Oral dosing* is begun at 2 to 5 mg twice daily. Dosage is then increased until an optimal response has been produced, usually with 15 to 20 mg/day. *Intramuscular therapy* is employed acutely. The usual intramuscular dosage is 1 to 2 mg every 4 to 6 hours as needed.

*Thiothixene.* Thiothixene [Navane] is a high-potency agent approved for schizophrenia and other psychotic disorders. The most common adverse effects are early extrapyramidal reactions (dystonia, parkinsonism, akathisia) and anticholinergic responses. Side effects seen occasionally include galactorrhea, gynecomastia, menstrual irregularities, sedation, orthostatic hypotension, and tardive dyskinesia. Agranulocytosis, neuroleptic malignant syndrome, and convulsions are rare.

Thiothixene is administered orally and IM. Three formulations are available: capsules (1, 2, 5, 10, and 20 mg), liquid concentrate (5 mg/ml), and IM solution (2 and 5 mg/ml). The initial *oral* dosage is 2 mg 3 times daily. Dosage is increased until an optimal response has been achieved, usually with 20 to 30 mg/day. The initial *intramuscular* dosage is 4 mg 2 to 4 times daily. Dosage is increased until symptoms are controlled, but should not exceed 30 mg/day.

*Pimozide.* Pimozide [Orap] is a high-potency neuroleptic approved only for suppressing symptoms of *Tourette's syndrome*, a rare disorder characterized by severe motor tics and uncontrollable grunts, barking cries, and outbursts of obscene language. Like other neuroleptics, pimozide can cause sedation, postural hypotension, and extrapyramidal reactions (dystonia, parkinsonism, akathisia, tardive dyskinesia). The drug is available in 2-mg tablets for oral therapy. The initial dosage is 1 to 2 mg/day in divided doses. Dosage should be slowly increased to a maintenance amount of 10 mg/day or 0.2 mg/kg/day (whichever is less).

## Depot Preparations

The depot antipsychotics are long-acting, injectable preparations used for long-term maintenance therapy of schizophrenia. The objective is to prevent relapse and maintain the highest possible level of functioning. The rate of relapse is lower with depot therapy than with oral therapy. Depot preparations are valuable for all patients who need long-term treatment—not just for those who have difficulty with compliance. There is no evidence that depot preparations pose an increased risk of side effects, including neuroleptic malignant syndrome and tardive dyskinesia. In fact, because depot therapy permits a reduction in the total drug burden (the dose per unit time is lower than with oral therapy), the risk of tardive dyskinesia is actually reduced.

The depot preparations used most often are *haloperidol decanoate* and *fluphenazine decanoate*. Following IM or SC injection, active drug (fluphenazine or haloperidol) is slowly absorbed into the blood. Because of this slow, steady absorption, plasma drug levels remain relatively constant between injections. The dosing interval is

### TABLE 29-6. DEPOT ANTIPSYCHOTIC PREPARATIONS

| Generic Name [Trade Name] | Route | Typical Maintenance Dosage |
|---|---|---|
| Haloperidol decanoate [Haldol Decanoate] | IM | 50–200 mg every 4 weeks |
| Fluphenazine decanoate [Prolixin Decanoate] | IM, SC | 2.5–25 mg every 2 weeks |

2 to 4 weeks. Typical maintenance dosages are presented in Table 29-6.

# Atypical Antipsychotic Agents

Atypical antipsychotic agents differ from traditional agents in two important ways. First, atypical agents cause few or no extrapyramidal symptoms, including tardive dyskinesia. Second, atypical agents can relieve positive *and* negative symptoms of schizophrenia, whereas benefits of traditional agents are limited largely to positive symptoms. In the United States, three atypical antipsychotics are available: clozapine, risperidone, and olanzepine.

## Clozapine

Clozapine [Clozaril] is indicated for patients with schizophrenia who have not responded to traditional agents, or who cannot tolerate their extrapyramidal effects. The drug's major adverse effect is agranulocytosis; a few deaths have occurred despite weekly hematologic monitoring.

### Mechanism of Action

Like traditional antipsychotic agents, clozapine blocks receptors for dopamine. However, the pattern of blockade is unique: compared with traditional agents, clozapine produces relatively strong blockade of dopamine$_1$ receptors and relatively weak blockade of dopamine$_2$ receptors. This pattern of receptor blockade may explain the drug's relative lack of extrapyramidal effects, and may also underlie its therapeutic effects. In addition to blocking receptors for dopamine, clozapine blocks receptors for serotonin, norepinephrine (alpha$_1$), histamine, and acetylcholine.

### Therapeutic Use

Because of the risk of fatal agranulocytosis, clozapine should be reserved for patients with severe schizophrenia who have not responded to traditional antipsychotic drugs. In this treatment-resistant group, clozapine has had a 40% to 60% success rate. Furthermore, not only have resistant patients responded, but the quality of the response has been superior: improvement has not been limited to positive symptoms; negative symptoms have improved as well. Patients have become more animated, behavior has been more socially acceptable, and rates of rehospitalization have been low. Because the incidence of EPSE with clozapine is low, the drug is well suited for patients who have experienced severe EPSE with a traditional agent.

### Pharmacokinetics

Clozapine is rapidly absorbed following oral administration. Peak plasma levels develop in 3.2 hours. In blood, about 95% of the drug is bound to plasma proteins. Clozapine undergoes extensive metabolism followed by fecal and urinary excretion. The half-life is approximately 12 hours.

## Adverse Effects and Interactions

In contrast to traditional antipsychotics, clozapine carries a low risk of extrapyramidal effects. Tardive dyskinesia has not been reported. In fact, tardive dyskinesia may improve when patients switch to clozapine from a traditional agent. Neuroendocrine effects (galactorrhea, gynecomastia, amenorrhea) and interference with sexual function are minimal.

***Agranulocytosis.*** Clozapine produces agranulocytosis in 1% to 2% of patients. The overall risk of death is about 1 in 5000, the usual cause being gram-negative septicemia. Agranulocytosis typically occurs during the first 6 months of treatment, and the onset is usually gradual. Why agranulocytosis occurs is unknown.

Because of the risk of fatal agranulocytosis, *weekly* hematologic monitoring is mandatory. If the total white blood cell (WBC) count falls below 3000/mm$^3$ or if the granulocyte count falls below 1500/mm$^3$, treatment should be interrupted. When subsequent *daily* monitoring indicates that counts have risen above these values, clozapine can be resumed. If the total WBC count falls below 2000/mm$^3$ or if the granulocyte count falls below 1000/mm$^3$, clozapine should be permanently discontinued. Blood counts should be monitored for 4 weeks after drug withdrawal.

Patients should be informed about the risk of agranulocytosis and told that clozapine will not be dispensed if the weekly blood test has not been made. Also, patients should be informed about early signs of infection (fever, sore throat, fatigue, mucous membrane ulceration) and instructed to report these immediately.

***Seizures.*** Generalized tonic-clonic convulsions occur in 3% of patients. The risk of seizures is dose related. Patients should be warned not to drive or to participate in other potentially hazardous activities if a seizure has occurred. Patients with a history of seizure disorders should use the drug with great caution.

***Other Adverse Effects.*** The most common side effects are *drowsiness and sedation* (40%), *dizziness* (20%), *hypersalivation* (30%), *tachycardia* (25%), and *constipation* (14%). Additional effects include *postural hypotension* (9%) and elevation of body temperature (5%).

***Drug Interactions.*** Because of its ability to cause agranulocytosis, clozapine is contraindicated for patients taking other drugs that can suppress bone marrow function (e.g., many anticancer drugs).

### Preparations, Dosage, and Administration

Clozapine [Clozaril] is dispensed in tablets (25 and 100 mg) for oral administration. To minimize side effects, treatment should begin with a 12.5-mg dose, followed by 25 mg once or twice daily. Dosage is then increased by 25 mg/day until it reaches 300 to 450 mg/day. Further increases can be made once or twice weekly in increments no larger than 100 mg. The usual maintenance dosage is 300 to 600 mg/day in three divided doses. The maximum dosage is 900 mg/day. If therapy is interrupted, it should resume with a 12.5-mg dose and then follow the original escalation guidelines.

## Risperidone

Risperidone [Risperdal] is a rapid-acting drug that improves positive and negative symptoms of schizophrenia. Like other atypical antipsychotics, risperidone causes fewer extrapyramidal reactions than the traditional agents. Risperidone is structurally unrelated to clozapine.

**Mechanism of Action.** We know that risperidone binds to multiple receptors, but we do not know with certainty how benefits are produced. Risperidone is a powerful antagonist at serotonin$_2$ receptors and a less powerful antagonist at dopamine$_2$ receptors. Antagonism at both sites may underlie therapeutic effects. Weak antagonism at dopamine$_2$ receptors explains why the drug causes few EPSE. Risperidone does not block cholinergic receptors but does block histamine$_1$ receptors as well as alpha-adrenergic receptors.

**Pharmacokinetics.** Absorption of oral risperidone is rapid and not affected by food. Plasma levels peak about 1 hour after oral administration. Much of each dose is metabolized to 9-hydroxyrisperidone, which has activity equivalent to that of risperidone itself. Parent drug and metabolite are excreted primarily in the urine. The effective half life is 24 hours. In patients with hepatic or renal dysfunction, the half-life is prolonged.

**Therapeutic Effects.** Risperidone relieves positive and negative symptoms of schizophrenia. Significant improvement may be seen in 1 week. By contrast, benefits of haloperidol develop more slowly and are limited primarily to positive symptoms. In patients with severe tardive dyskinesia, risperidone may have an antidyskinetic effect. Risperidone has been used for over 1 year without loss of efficacy.

**Adverse Effects.** Side effects are generally infrequent and mild, and only rarely require discontinuation of treatment. The incidence of EPSE is very low at the recommended dosage. However, at dosages above 10 mg/day, there is a dose-related increase in EPSE. Tardive dyskinesia has not been observed. Risperidone increases prolactin levels, but symptoms (gynecomastia, galactorrhea) are uncommon. Adverse effects that have led to discontinuing the drug include agitation, dizziness, somnolence, and fatigue. Excessive doses have caused difficulty concentrating, sedation, and disruption of sleep.

**Preparations, Dosage, and Administration.** Risperidone [Risperdal] is dispensed in tablets (1, 2, 3, and 4 mg) for oral administration. The recommended dosage is 1 mg twice daily the first day, 2 mg twice daily the second day, and 3 mg twice daily thereafter. Dosages above 2 or 3 mg twice daily do not increase therapeutic effects, but do increase the risk of EPSE and other side effects. Dosages should be reduced in patients with renal or hepatic impairment.

## Other Atypical Agents

### Olanzepine

Olanzepine [Zyprexa] is a new drug approved for schizophrenia and other psychotic disorders. This agent is similar to clozapine in structure and actions, but does not cause agranulocytosis.

**Mechanism of Action.** We know that olanzepine binds to multiple receptors, but we don't know with certainty how benefits are produced. Therapeutic effects may result from blockade of receptors for dopamine and serotonin. Adverse effects result in part from blockade of receptors for histamine, acetylcholine, and norepinephrine.

**Pharmacokinetics.** Olanzepine is well absorbed following oral administration. Food does not alter the rate or extent of absorption. Plasma drug levels peak 6 hours after an oral dose and decline with a half-life of 30 hours. Hepatic metabolism of olanzepine is extensive.

**Therapeutic Effects.** In patients with schizophrenia, olanzepine is at least as effective as haloperidol or risperidone, and produces fewer EPSE than either drug. Comparative trials with clozapine have not been done. Interestingly, olanzepine can relieve psychosis induced by drugs for Parkinson's disease without reversing their beneficial effects. Because olanzepine is new, its long-term efficacy in schizophrenia is unknown.

**Adverse Effects.** Olanzepine is generally well tolerated and appears devoid of serious adverse effects. Acute EPSE are minimal when the drug is used at the recommended dosage. Tardive dyskinesia has not been reported. Despite structural similarity with clozapine, olanzepine does not cause agranulocytosis. Following overdosage, the only signs are slurred speech and drowsiness.

Although serious side effects are rare, mild effects are common. Olanzepine causes somnolence in 26% of patients, presumably by blocking histamine$_1$ receptors. Blockade of muscarinic receptors causes constipation and other anticholinergic effects. Alpha$_1$-adrenergic blockade causes orthostatic hypotension. With prolonged use, olanzepine causes weight gain.

**Preparations, Dosage, and Administration.** Olanzepine [Zyprexa] is dispensed in tablets (5, 7.5, and 10 mg) for oral use. The recommended dosage is 5 to 10 mg once daily for the first few days, and 10 mg once daily thereafter. Dosages greater than 10 mg/day do not offer any additional benefits, but do increase the risk of side effects.

### Remoxipride

Remoxipride [Roxiam] produces weak but selective blockade of dopamine$_2$ receptors. This action may underlie the drug's antipsychotic effects. In patients with chronic schizophrenia, remoxipride is as effective as haloperidol. The drug improves positive symptoms (e.g., thought disturbances, hostility, hallucinations, delusions) as well as negative symptoms (e.g., social withdrawal, blunted affect, motor retardation). Administration is oral and absorption is essentially complete. Following partial hepatic metabolism, parent drug and metabolites are excreted in the urine. Like other atypical agents, remoxipride causes fewer EPSE than traditional antipsychotic drugs. There have been no reports of tardive dyskinesia. Postural hypotension is minimal and sedation is less than with haloperidol. An initial therapeutic response occurs at a dosage of 300 to 450 mg/day. Dosage can be reduced to 150 to 300 mg/day for maintenance therapy.

### Sulpiride

Like remoxipride, sulpiride causes selective blockade of dopamine$_2$ receptors. Antipsychotic effects are equivalent to those of chlorpromazine and haloperidol. Extrapyramidal reactions are less common and less severe than with traditional antipsychotics. The incidence of sedation, orthostatic hypotension, and anticholinergic effects is low, but neuroendocrine effects (galactorrhea, gynecomastia, menstrual irregularities) occur frequently.

# Management of Schizophrenia

## Drug Therapy

Drug therapy of schizophrenia has three major objectives: (1) suppression of acute episodes, (2) prevention of acute exacerbations, and (3) maintenance of the highest possible level of functioning.

### Drug Selection

Treatment is usually initiated with a traditional antipsychotic agent. In the absence of specific contraindications, a high-potency agent is employed. Although all traditional agents produce equivalent therapeutic effects, some patients may respond better to one agent than to another. Accordingly, if treatment with one traditional agent is unsuccessful, a trial with a drug from a different chemical class should be made.

Selection among the traditional antipsychotic drugs is based largely on side effects: the patient should not be given a drug that, because of its side-effect profile, is especially likely to cause discomfort, inconvenience, or harm. For example, certain patients (e.g., those with prostatic hypertrophy or glaucoma) are especially sensitive to anticholinergic drugs. Accordingly, these patients should not be treated with low-potency neuroleptics. By similar logic, if the patient has a history of extrapyramidal reactions, high-potency agents should be avoided. By properly matching patients and drugs, side effects can be minimized, comfort can be maximized, and compliance can be promoted. Table 29-7 indicates the antipsychotic agents that should be avoided in specific groups of patients. Note that low-potency agents need to be avoided more frequently than high-potency agents.

Atypical agents (e.g., clozapine, risperidone, olanzepine) represent an alternative to the traditional antipsychotics. Compared with traditional agents, atypical agents have several advantages: they cause far fewer early EPSE, tardive dyskinesia has not been reported, positive and negative symptoms improve, and patients who have been refractory to traditional agents frequently respond to these drugs. Moreover, in patients with TD, these drugs may have an antidyskinetic effect. Because they cause few EPSE (and may actually suppress TD), atypical agents are especially well suited for patients who have experienced severe early EPSE or TD with traditional antipsychotics. Because clozapine can cause fatal agranulocytosis, this drug should be reserved for patients who have failed to respond to trials with at least two traditional antipsychotic agents.

### Dosing

Dosing with neuroleptics is highly individualized. Elderly patients require relatively small doses—typically 30% to 50% of those taken by younger patients. Poorly responsive patients may need larger doses than highly responsive patients. However, very large doses should gen-

## TABLE 29-7. ANTIPSYCHOTIC DRUGS THAT SHOULD BE AVOIDED IN THE PRESENCE OF CERTAIN PREDISPOSING FACTORS

| Predisposing Factor | Antipsychotic Agents to Avoid |
|---|---|
| Glaucome, prostatism, adynamic ileus, urinary hesitancy | Low-potency agents (anticholinergic actions can exacerbate these disorders) |
| Use of anticholinergic drugs (e.g., tricyclic antidepressants) | Low-potency agents (anticholinergic effects will intensify muscarinic blockade) |
| Old age | Low-potency agents (the elderly are especially sensitive to the anticholinergic and sedative effects of these drugs) |
| Active life-style | Low-potency agents (sedative effects can interfere with function) |
| Delirium | Low-potency agents (anticholinergic and hypotensive actions can exacerbate delirium) |
| Cardiovascular disorders | Low-potency agents (anticholinergic and hypotensive actions can exacerbate these disorders) |
| History of extra-pyramidal reactions | High-potency agents (disruption of extrapyramidal function is greatest with these drugs) |
| Active sex life in males | Thioridazine (this agent inhibits ejaculation) |

erally be avoided: huge doses are probably no more effective than moderate doses, whereas they will increase the risk of side effects.

Dosage size and timing are likely to change over the course of therapy. During the initial phase of treatment, antipsychotics should be administered in divided daily doses. Once an effective dosage has been determined, the entire daily dose may be given at bedtime. Since antipsychotics cause sedation, bedtime dosing helps promote sleep while decreasing daytime drowsiness. Doses used early in therapy to gain rapid control of behavior are often very high. For long-term therapy, the dosage should be reduced to the lowest effective amount.

### Routes

*Oral.* Oral administration is preferred for most patients. Antipsychotics are available in tablets, capsules, and liquids for oral use.

The liquid formulations require special handling. These preparations are concentrated and must be diluted prior to use. Dilution may be performed with a variety of fluids, including fruit juices, milk, and carbonated beverages. The oral liquids are light sensitive and must be stored in amber or opaque containers. Liquid formulations of *phenothiazines* can cause contact dermatitis; nurses and patients should take care to avoid skin contact with these preparations.

**Intramuscular.** Intramuscular injection is generally reserved for patients with severe, acute schizophrenia and for long-term maintenance therapy. Depot preparations are given every 2 to 4 weeks (see Table 29–6).

### Initial Therapy

With adequate dosing, symptoms begin to resolve within 1 to 2 days. However, significant improvement takes 1 to 2 weeks, and full response may not be seen for several months.

Some symptoms resolve sooner than others. During the first week, the goal is to reduce agitation, hostility, anxiety, and tension, and to normalize sleeping and eating patterns. Over the next 6 to 8 weeks, symptoms should continue to steadily improve. The goals over this interval are increased socialization, improved self-care and mood, and improved formal thought processes. Of the patients who have not responded within 6 weeks, 50% are likely to respond by the end of 12 weeks.

It is important to note that not all symptoms respond equally. With the traditional antipsychotics, positive symptoms respond much better than negative symptoms. However, with the atypical agents, positive and negative symptoms may both respond well.

### Maintenance Therapy

Schizophrenia is usually chronic, requiring prolonged treatment. The purpose of long-term therapy is to reduce the recurrence of acute florid episodes and to maintain the highest possible level of functioning. Unfortunately, although long-term treatment can be very effective, it also carries a risk of adverse effects, especially tardive dyskinesia.

Following control of an acute episode, antipsychotic therapy should continue for at least 12 months. Withdrawal of medication prior to this time is associated with a 55% incidence of relapse, compared with only 20% in patients who continue drug use. Accordingly, patients must be convinced to continue therapy for the entire 12-month course, even though they may be symptom free and consider themselves "cured."

After 12 months, an attempt should be made to discontinue drug use, provided that symptoms are absent. About 25% of patients do not need drugs beyond this time. To avoid withdrawal reactions, dosage should be tapered gradually. It is important that medication not be withdrawn at a time of stress (e.g., when the patient is being discharged following hospitalization). If relapse occurs in response to withdrawal, treatment should be reinstituted. For many patients, resumption of therapy controls symptoms and prevents further relapse.

When long-term therapy is conducted, dosage should be adjusted with care. To reduce the risk of tardive dys-kinesia and other adverse effects, a minimum effective dosage should be established. Annual attempts should be made to lower the dosage or to discontinue treatment entirely.

Long-acting (depot) antipsychotics are especially well suited for long-term therapy. Depot therapy has three major advantages over oral therapy: (1) the relapse rate is lower, (2) drug levels are more stable between doses, and (3) the total dose per unit time is lower, thereby *reducing* the risk of adverse effects, including TD. In the United States, only 10% of patients receive depot therapy. This low rate is based in large part on the widely held (but incorrect) perception that depot therapy is for "losers"—patients who suffer recurrent relapse because of persistent noncompliance with oral therapy.

### Adjunctive Drugs

*Benzodiazepines* (e.g., lorazepam, alprazolam) can suppress anxiety and promote sleep. Whether these drugs also improve core symptoms of schizophrenia is uncertain. In patients experiencing an acute psychotic episode, benzodiazepines can help suppress anxiety, irritability, and agitation. In addition, the presence of the benzodiazepine may also allow the dosage of antipsychotic medication to be reduced.

*Antidepressants* are appropriate when schizophrenia is associated with depressive symptoms. A tricyclic antidepressant (e.g., imipramine) is usually chosen. Antidepressant dosage is the same as for major depression. The ideal duration of treatment is unknown.

### Promoting Compliance

Poor compliance is a common cause of therapeutic failure, and is responsible for a substantial number of hospital readmissions. Compliance can be difficult to achieve because treatment is prolonged and because patients may fail to appreciate the need for therapy, or they may be unwilling or unable to take medicine as prescribed. In addition, side effects can discourage compliance. Compliance can be enhanced by:

- Ensuring that the medication given to hospitalized patients is actually swallowed and not "cheeked"
- Encouraging family members to oversee medication by outpatients
- Providing patients with written and verbal instructions on dosage size and timing, and encouraging them to take their medicine exactly as prescribed
- Informing patients and their families that antipsychotics must be taken on a regular schedule to be effective, and hence cannot be used on a PRN basis
- Informing patients about side effects of treatment and teaching them how to minimize undesired responses
- Assuring patients that antipsychotic drugs do not cause addiction
- Establishing a good therapeutic relationship with the patient and family
- Using a depot preparation (fluphenazine decanoate, haloperidol decanoate) for long-term therapy

## Nondrug Therapy

Although drugs can be of great benefit in schizophrenia, it is important to appreciate that medication alone does not constitute optimal treatment. The acutely ill patient needs care, support, and protection; a period of hospitalization may be essential. Counseling can offer the patient and family insight into the nature of schizophrenia and can facilitate adjustment and rehabilitation. Although traditional psychotherapy is of little value in reducing symptoms of schizophrenia, establishing a good therapeutic relationship can help promote compliance and can help the physician evaluate the patient, which in turn can facilitate dosage adjustment and drug selection. Behavioral therapy can help reduce stress. Vocational training in a sheltered environment offers the hope of productivity and some measure of independence. Ideally, the patient will be provided with a comprehensive therapeutic program to complement the benefits of medication. Unfortunately, ideal situations don't always exist, leaving many patients to rely on drugs as their sole treatment modality.

## KEY POINTS

- Schizophrenia is the principal indication for antipsychotic drugs.
- Schizophrenia is a chronic illness characterized by disordered thinking and reduced comprehension of reality. Positive symptoms include hallucinations, delusions, and agitation. Negative symptoms include blunted affect, poverty of speech, and social withdrawal.
- Antipsychotic drugs fall into two major groups: traditional agents and atypical agents.
- Traditional antipsychotics are thought to relieve symptoms of schizophrenia by blocking dopamine$_2$ receptors.
- Traditional antipsychotic agents improve positive symptoms of schizophrenia more effectively than negative symptoms.
- Therapeutic responses to antipsychotic drugs develop slowly, often taking several months to become maximal.
- Low-potency traditional agents and high-potency traditional agents produce equal therapeutic effects.
- Traditional antipsychotic drugs produce three types of early EPSE: acute dystonia, parkinsonism, and akathisia.

- Acute dystonia and parkinsonism respond to anticholinergic drugs (e.g., benztropine). Akathisia is harder to treat, but may respond to anticholinergic drugs, benzodiazepines, or beta blockers.
- Tardive dyskinesia, a late EPSE, has no reliable treatment. For patients with severe TD, switching to clozapine or risperidone may be beneficial.
- The risk of early EPSE is much greater with high-potency agents than with low-potency agents, whereas the risk of TD is equal with both groups.
- Neuroleptic malignant syndrome, which can be fatal, is characterized by muscular rigidity, high fever, and autonomic instability. Dantrolene and bromocriptine are used for treatment.
- Low-potency agents produce more sedation, orthostatic hypotension, and anticholinergic effects than high-potency agents.
- Antipsychotic drugs increase levels of circulating prolactin by blocking the inhibitory action of dopamine on prolactin release.
- Levodopa can counteract the beneficial effects of antipsychotic drugs and vice versa. This is because levodopa activates dopamine receptors, whereas antipsychotic drugs cause dopamine-receptor blockade.
- Chlorpromazine [Thorazine] is the prototype of the low-potency agents.
- Haloperidol [Haldol] is the prototype of the high-potency agents.
- Antipsychotic depot preparations—haloperidol decanoate and fluphenazine decanoate—are used for long-term maintenance therapy of schizophrenia.
- Atypical antipsychotic agents (e.g., clozapine, risperidone) differ from traditional antipsychotic agents in that (1) atypical agents cause few or no EPSE, including TD, and (2) atypical agents can relieve positive *and* negative symptoms of schizophrenia, whereas traditional agents relieve primarily positive symptoms.
- Clozapine can cause potentially fatal agranulocytosis. Hence weekly blood tests are mandatory.

## Summary of Major Nursing Implications*

### Traditional Antipsychotic Drugs

| | |
|---|---|
| Acetophenazine | Perphenazine |
| Chlorpromazine | Pimozide |
| Fluphenazine | Thioridazine |
| Haloperidol | Thiothixene |
| Loxapine | Trifluoperazine |
| Molindone | Triflupromazine |

Except where indicated otherwise, these nursing implications apply to all of the traditional antipsychotic drugs.

### Preadministration Assessment

#### Therapeutic Goal

Treatment of schizophrenia has three goals: suppression of acute episodes, prevention of acute exacerbations, and maintenance of the highest possible level of functioning.

#### Baseline Data

Patients should receive a thorough mental status examination and a physical examination.

Observe and record such factors as overt behavior (e.g., gait, pacing, restlessness, volatile outbursts), emotional state (e.g., depression, agitation, mania), intellectual function (e.g., stream of thought, coherence, hallucinations, delusions), and responsiveness to the environment.

*Patient education information is highlighted in color.

Obtain a complete family and social history.

Determine vital signs and obtain complete blood counts, electrolytes, and evaluations of hepatic, renal, and cardiovascular function.

### Identifying High-Risk Patients

Traditional antipsychotic agents are *contraindicated* for patients who are *comatose* or *severely depressed* and for patients with *Parkinson's disease*, *prolactin-dependent carcinoma of the breast*, *bone marrow depression*, and *severe hypotension or hypertension*. Use with *caution* in patients with *glaucoma*, *adynamic ileus*, *prostatic hypertrophy*, *cardiovascular disease*, *hepatic or renal dysfunction*, and *seizure disorders*.

## Implementation: Administration

### Routes

Oral, IM, SC, rectal (suppository). Routes for individual agents are summarized in Tables 29-4 and 29-6.

### Administration

*Dosing.* Divided daily doses are employed initially. Once an effective dosage has been determined, the entire daily dose is usually administered at bedtime, thereby promoting sleep and minimizing daytime sedation. For long-term therapy, the smallest effective dosage should be employed.

*Oral Liquids.* Oral liquid formulations must be protected from light. Concentrated formulations should be diluted just prior to use. Dilution in fruit juice improves palatability.

Oral liquids can cause contact dermatitis. Warn patients against making skin contact with these drugs, and instruct them to flush the affected area if a spill occurs. Take care to avoid skin contact with these preparations yourself.

*Intramuscular.* Make injections into the deltoid or gluteal muscle. Rotate the injection site. Depot preparations are administered every 2 to 4 weeks (see Table 29-6).

## Implementation: Measures to Enhance Therapeutic Effects

### Promoting Compliance

Poor compliance is a common cause of therapeutic failure and rehospitalization. Compliance can be improved by:

- Ensuring that medication is actually swallowed and not "cheeked"
- Encouraging family members to oversee medication by outpatients
- Providing patients with written and verbal instructions on dosage size and timing, and encouraging them to take their medicine as prescribed
- Informing patients and their families that antipsychotic drugs must be taken on a regular schedule to be effective

- Informing patients about side effects of treatment and teaching them how to minimize undesired responses
- Assuring patients that antipsychotic drugs do not cause addiction
- Establishing a good therapeutic relationship with the patient and family
- Using a depot preparation (e.g., fluphenazine decanoate, haloperidol decanoate) for long-term therapy

### Nondrug Therapy

Acutely ill patients need care, support, and protection; hospitalization may be essential. Educate patient and family about the nature of schizophrenia to facilitate adjustment and rehabilitation. Behavioral therapy can help reduce stress. Vocational training in a sheltered environment offers the hope of productivity and some measure of independence.

## Ongoing Evaluation and Interventions

### Evaluating Therapeutic Effects

Success is indicated by improvement in psychotic symptoms. Evaluate for suppression of hallucinations, delusions, agitation, tension, and hostility, and for improvement in judgment, insight, motivation, affect, self-care, social skills, anxiety management, and patterns of sleeping and eating.

### Minimizing Adverse Effects

*Early EPSE: Acute Dystonia, Parkinsonism, and Akathisia.* These reactions develop within hours to months of the onset of treatment. The risk is greatest with high-potency agents. Take care to differentiate these reactions from worsening of psychotic symptoms. Inform patients and their families about symptoms (e.g., muscle spasm of tongue, face, neck, or back; tremor; rigidity; restless movement), and instruct them to notify the physician if these appear. Acute dystonia and parkinsonism respond to anticholinergic drugs (e.g., benztropine). Akathisia may respond to anticholinergic drugs, beta blockers, or benzodiazepines.

*Late EPSE: Tardive Dyskinesia.* TD develops after months or years of continuous therapy. The risk is equal with all traditional antipsychotics. Inform patients and their families about early signs (e.g., fine, worm-like movements of the tongue), and instruct them to notify the physician if these develop. Although there is no reliable treatment, the following measures are recommended: discontinue all anticholinergic drugs; give a benzodiazepine; and discontinue the antipsychotic, or at least reduce the dosage. For severe TD, switch to clozapine or another atypical agent.

*Neuroleptic Malignant Syndrome.* NMS is a rare reaction that carries a 4% risk of mortality. Symptoms include rigidity, fever, sweating, dysrhythmias, and fluctuations in blood pressure. NMS is most likely with high-potency agents.

Treatment consists of supportive measures (use of cooling blankets, rehydration), drug therapy (dantrolene, bromocriptine), and immediate withdrawal of the neuroleptic. If neuroleptic therapy is resumed after symptoms have subsided, the lowest effective dosage of a low-potency drug should be employed. If a second episode occurs, switching to an atypical agent may be helpful.

***Anticholinergic Effects.*** Inform patients about possible anticholinergic reactions (dry mouth, blurred vision, photophobia, urinary hesitancy, constipation, tachycardia, suppression of sweating), and teach them how to minimize discomfort. A complete summary of nursing implications for anticholinergic effects is given in Chapter 15. Anticholinergic effects are most likely with low-potency antipsychotics.

***Orthostatic Hypotension.*** Inform patients about signs of hypotension (lightheadedness, dizziness), and advise them to sit or lie down if these occur. Inform patients that hypotension can be minimized by moving slowly when assuming an erect posture. Orthostatic hypotension is most likely with low-potency antipsychotics.

In hospitalized patients, measure blood pressure and pulses before antipsychotic administration and 1 hour after. Make these measurements while the patient is lying down and again after he or she has been sitting or standing for 1 to 2 minutes. If blood pressure is low, withhold medication and consult the physician.

***Sedation.*** Sedation is most intense during the first weeks of therapy and declines with continued drug use. Warn patients about sedative effects, and advise them to avoid hazardous activity until sedation subsides. Sedation is most likely with low-potency agents.

***Seizures.*** Neuroleptics reduce seizure threshold, thereby increasing the risk of seizures, especially in patients with epilepsy and other seizure disorders. For patients with seizure disorders, adequate doses of antiseizure medication must be employed. Monitor the patient for seizure activity; if loss of seizure control occurs, dosage of antiseizure medication must be increased.

***Sexual Dysfunction.*** In women, antipsychotics can suppress libido and impair the ability to achieve orgasm. In men, antipsychotics can suppress libido and cause erectile and ejaculatory dysfunction. Counsel patients about possible sexual dysfunction and encourage them to report problems. Dosage reduction or switching to a high-potency neuroleptic may be helpful.

***Dermatologic Effects.*** Inform patients that *phenothiazines* can sensitize the skin to ultraviolet light, thereby increasing the risk of sunburn. Advise them to avoid excessive exposure to sunlight, apply a sunscreen, and wear protective clothing.

Oral liquid formulations of antipsychotics can cause contact dermatitis. Warn patients to avoid skin contact with these drugs.

***Neuroendocrine Effects.*** Inform patients that antipsychotics can cause galactorrhea, gynecomastia, and menstrual irregularities.

Antipsychotics can promote growth of prolactin-dependent carcinoma of the breast and must not be used by patients with this cancer.

***Agranulocytosis.*** Agranulocytosis greatly diminishes the ability to fight infection. Inform patients about early signs of infection (fever, sore throat), and instruct them to notify the physician if these develop. If blood tests indicate agranulocytosis, the antipsychotic should be withdrawn.

## Minimizing Adverse Interactions

***Anticholinergics.*** Drugs with anticholinergic properties will intensify anticholinergic responses to antipsychotics. Instruct patients to avoid all drugs with anticholinergic properties, including the antihistamines and certain over-the-counter sleep aids.

***CNS Depressants.*** Antipsychotics will intensify CNS depression caused by other drugs. Warn patients against use of alcohol and all other drugs with CNS-depressant properties (e.g., barbiturates, opioids, antihistamines, benzodiazepines).

***Levodopa.*** Levodopa promotes activation of dopamine receptors and may thereby diminish the therapeutic effects of antipsychotics. These drugs should not be used concurrently.

# Clozapine, an Atypical Agent

## Preadministration Assessment

### Therapeutic Goal and Baseline Data
See *Traditional Antipsychotic Agents.*

### Identifying High-Risk Patients
Clozapine is *contraindicated* for patients with a *history of clozapine-induced agranulocytosis* and for patients with *bone marrow depression* and for those taking *myelosuppressive drugs* (e.g., many anticancer drugs). Use with *caution* in patients with *seizure disorders.*

## Implementation: Administration

### Route
Oral.

### Dosing
To minimize side effects, dosage must be low initially and then gradually increased. If treatment is interrupted, it should resume at the original low dosage.

## Ongoing Evaluation and Interventions

### Evaluating Therapeutic Effects
See *Traditional Antipsychotic Agents.*

### Minimizing Adverse Effects
In contrast to traditional antipsychotic drugs, clozapine carries a low risk of sexual dysfunction, neuroendocrine effects, and extrapyramidal reactions, including tardive dyskinesia.

*Agranulocytosis.* Clozapine produces agranulocytosis in 1% to 2% of patients, typically during the first 6 months of treatment. Deaths have occurred, usually from gram-negative septicemia.

Weekly hematologic monitoring is mandatory. If the total white blood cell (WBC) count falls below 3000/mm$^3$ or if the granulocyte count falls below 1500/mm$^3$, treatment should be interrupted. When subsequent daily monitoring indicates that cell counts have risen above these values, clozapine can be resumed. If the total WBC count falls below 2000/mm$^3$ or if the granulocyte count falls below 1000/mm$^3$, clozapine should be permanently discontinued. Continue monitoring blood counts for 4 weeks.

Warn patients about the risk of agranulocytosis, and inform them that clozapine will not be dispensed without weekly proof of blood counts. Inform patients about early signs of infection (fever, sore throat, fatigue, mucous membrane ulceration), and instruct them to report these immediately.

*Seizures.* Generalized tonic-clonic seizures occur in 3% of patients. Warn patients against driving and other hazardous activities if seizures have occurred.

*Sedation.* Drowsiness and sedation occur in 40%. Warn patients against driving and participation in other hazardous activities if impairment is significant.

## Minimizing Adverse Interactions

*Myelosuppressive Drugs.* Clozapine must not be given to patients taking other drugs that can suppress bone marrow function (e.g., many anticancer agents).

# CHAPTER 30

# Antidepressants

As their name suggests, antidepressants are drugs used to treat depression. These agents fall into four major groups: (1) tricyclic antidepressants, (2) monoamine oxidase inhibitors, (3) selective serotonin reuptake inhibitors, and (4) atypical antidepressants. The principal indication for these drugs is major depression. As a rule, antidepressants are not indicated for uncomplicated bereavement. It should be noted that antidepressants are not merely general psychic stimulants. Rather, these drugs act selectively to alleviate symptoms of depression.

## Major Depression: Clinical Features, Pathogenesis, and Treatment Modalities

Depression is the most common psychiatric illness. Symptoms occur in 13% to 20% of the population. Sadly, only one-third of depressed people seek help. Depression results in more physical and social dysfunction than the vast majority of medical disorders. The estimated annual cost of the disorder in 1990 was over $43 billion. Approximately two-thirds of all suicides are depression related.

### Clinical Features

Diagnostic criteria for a major depressive episode are summarized in Table 30-1. As indicated, the principal symptoms are (1) *depressed mood* and (2) *loss of pleasure or interest in all or nearly all of one's usual activities and pastimes*. Associated symptoms include insomnia (or sometimes hypersomnia); anorexia and weight loss (or sometimes hyperphagia and weight gain); mental slowing and loss of concentration; feelings of guilt, worthlessness, and helplessness; thoughts of death and suicide; and overt suicidal behavior. For a diagnosis to be made, symptoms must be present most of the day, nearly every day, for at least 2 weeks.

Major depression is a frustrating illness in that symptoms may not bear correspondence to external events. That is, rather than occurring in response to life's tragedies, symptoms of major depression may just descend "out of the blue"; otherwise healthy individuals—unexpectedly and without apparent cause—may find themselves feeling profoundly depressed.

It is important to distinguish between major depression and normal grief or sadness. Whereas major depression is an illness, grief or sadness is not. Rather, grief and sadness are appropriate reactions to a major life stressor (e.g., death of a loved one, loss of a job). In most cases, grief and sadness resolve spontaneously over several weeks and do not require medical intervention. However, if symptoms are unusually intense, and if they fail to abate within an appropriate time, a major depressive episode may have been superimposed. If this occurs, treatment is indicated.

### Pathogenesis

The etiology of major depression is undoubtedly complex and not yet known. Since depressive episodes can be triggered by stressful life events in some individuals but not in others, it would appear that, for some individuals, a predisposition to depression exists. Social, developmental, and biologic factors, including genetic heritage, may all contribute to that predisposition.

Clinical observations made in the 1960s led to formulation of the *monoamine hypothesis of depression*, which asserts that depression is caused by a functional insufficiency of monoamine neurotransmitters (norepinephrine, serotonin, or both). This hypothesis is based in large part on two observations: (1) depression can be induced with reserpine, a drug that depletes monoamines from the brain, and (2) the drugs used to treat depression intensify monoamine-mediated neurotransmission. Although these observations lend support to the monoamine hypothesis, it is now clear that the hypothesis is far too simplistic.

**TABLE 30–1. DSM-IV DIAGNOSTIC CRITERIA FOR A MAJOR DEPRESSIVE EPISODE**

A. For a diagnosis of major depression, at least five of the following symptoms must be present for 2 weeks or more, and must represent a change from previous functioning. Furthermore, at least one symptom must be (1) depressed mood or (2) loss of interest or pleasure. (*Note:* Do not include mood-incongruent delusions or hallucinations, or symptoms that are due to a general medical condition.)

- Depressed mood most of the day, nearly every day (*Note:* in children and adolescents, can be irritable mood.)
- Loss of interest or pleasure in all or almost all activities
- Significant weight loss or weight gain without dieting *or* decrease or increase in appetite (*Note:* In children, consider failure to make expected weight gains.)
- Insomnia or hypersomnia
- Psychomotor agitation or retardation
- Fatigue or loss of energy
- Feelings of worthlessness or excessive or inappropriate guilt
- Diminished ability to think or concentrate *or* indecisiveness
- Recurrent thoughts of death, recurrent suicidal ideation, a suicide attempt, or a specific suicide plan

B. The symptoms do not meet the criteria for a Mixed Episode (i.e., an episode in which criteria are met for a Major Depressive Episode *and* a Manic Episode)

C. The symptoms cause clinically significant distress or impairment in social, occupational, or other important areas of functioning.

D. The symptoms are not due to the direct physiologic effects of a substance (e.g., drug of abuse, medication) or a general condition (e.g., hypothyroidism).

E. Major depression should not be diagnosed in the context of bereavement (i.e., after the loss of a loved one), unless the symptoms persist for longer than 2 months, or are characterized by marked functional impairment, morbid preoccupation with worthlessness, suicidal ideation, psychotic symptoms, or psychomotor retardation.

Adapted from American Psychiatric Association. *Diagnostic and Statistical Manual of Mental Disorders*, 4th ed. Washington, DC, American Psychiatric Press, 1994, p. 327.

However, despite its shortcomings, the monoamine hypothesis does provide a useful conceptual framework for understanding antidepressant drugs.

### Treatment Modalities

Depression can be treated with three modalities: (1) drugs, (2) electroconvulsive therapy, and (3) psychotherapy. Each modality has a legitimate role.

Drugs are the primary therapy for major depression. Available antidepressants are listed in Table 30-2. For many patients, the *tricyclic antidepressants* (TCAs) are drugs of first choice. These agents are inexpensive, effective, relatively safe, and easy to administer. *Selective serotonin reuptake inhibitors* (SSRIs) are as effective as the tricyclics and better tolerated. As a result, these drugs have achieved rapid and widespread popularity, even though they cost more than TCAs. *Monoamine oxidase inhibitors* (MAOIs) are generally reserved for patients who have not responded to TCAs or SSRIs. However, for

patients with atypical depression, MAOIs are drugs of choice. *Antianxiety agents* (e.g., diazepam) can be employed in depression, but their use is not routine. As a rule, central nervous system (CNS) stimulants (amphetamines, methylphenidate) are without benefit in depression.

*Electroconvulsive therapy* (ECT) is a valuable tool for treating depression. This procedure is effective, and beneficial responses develop more rapidly than with drugs. Accordingly, ECT is especially appropriate when speed is critical. Candidates for ECT include (1) severely depressed, suicidal patients; (2) elderly patients at risk of starving to death because of depression-induced lack of appetite; and (3) patients who have failed to respond to antidepressant drugs.

The role of psychotherapy in major depression is largely supportive; symptoms do not respond nearly as well to psychotherapy as they do to medication. However, although of less direct benefit than drugs, psychotherapy can help relieve suffering by providing insight, reassurance, and caring.

## Tricyclic Antidepressants

The tricyclic antidepressants (TCAs) are drugs of first choice for many patients with major depression. The first tricyclic agent—imipramine—was introduced to psychiatry in the late 1950s. Since then, the ability of TCAs to relieve depressive symptoms has been firmly established. The most common adverse effects of TCAs are sedation, orthostatic hypotension, and anticholinergic effects. The most hazardous adverse effect is cardiac toxicity. Because all of the TCAs have similar properties, we will discuss these drugs as a group, rather than focusing on a representative prototype.

### Chemistry

The structure of imipramine, a representative TCA, is shown in Figure 30-1. As you can see, the nucleus of this drug has three rings—hence the classification tricyclic antidepressant.

As indicated in Figure 30-1, the three-ringed nucleus of the TCAs is very similar to the three-ringed nucleus of the phenothiazine antipsychotics. Because of this structural similarity, TCAs and phenothiazines have several actions in common. Specifically, both groups of drugs produce varying degrees of *sedation*, *orthostatic hypotension*, and *anticholinergic effects*.

### Mechanism of Action

The proposed mechanism of action of the TCAs is depicted in Figure 30-2. As shown, TCAs block monoamine (norepinephrine and serotonin) reuptake. By blocking reuptake of these neurotransmitters, TCAs can intensify their effects. Such a mechanism would be consistent with the monoamine hypothesis of depression. That is, the

## TABLE 30-2. ANTIDEPRESSANTS: ADVERSE EFFECTS AND EFFECTS ON NEUROTRANSMITTERS

| | Transmitter Reuptake Antagonism | | Anticholinergic Activity | Sedation | Hypotension | Seizure Risk | Cardiac Toxicity | Other Side Effects |
|---|---|---|---|---|---|---|---|---|
| | NE | 5-HT | | | | | | |
| *Tricyclic Antidepressants* | | | | | | | | |
| Amitriptyline | +++ | +++ | ++++ | ++++ | +++ | +++ | ++++ | |
| Clomipramine | ++ | ++++ | ++++ | ++++ | ++ | ++ | ++++ | |
| Desipramine | ++++ | + | ++ | ++ | ++ | ++ | +++ | |
| Doxepin | + | +++ | +++ | ++++ | ++ | ++ | ++ | |
| Imipramine | ++ | +++ | +++ | +++ | +++ | ++ | ++++ | |
| Maprotiline | ++++ | 0 | +++ | +++ | ++ | +++ | +++ | |
| Nortriptyline | +++ | ++ | ++ | +++ | + | ++ | +++ | |
| Protriptyline | ++++ | + | +++ | + | ++ | ++ | ++++ | |
| Trimipramine | ++ | ++ | +++ | ++++ | +++ | ++ | ++++ | |
| *Monoamine Oxidase Inhibitors* | | | | | | | | |
| Phenelzine | * | * | 0 | + | ++ | 0 | 0 | |
| Tranylcypromine | * | * | 0 | † | ++ | 0 | 0 | Hypertensive crisis from tyramine in food |
| *Selective Serotonin Reuptake Inhibitors* | | | | | | | | |
| Fluoxetine | 0 | +++++ | 0 | † | 0 | 0/+ | 0 | Skin rash |
| Fluvoxamine | 0 | +++++ | | ++ | 0 | | | |
| Paroxetine | 0 | +++++ | 0 | 0/+ | 0 | 0 | 0 | |
| Sertraline | 0 | +++++ | 0 | † | 0 | 0 | 0 | |
| *Atypical Antidepressants* | | | | | | | | |
| Amoxapine | +++‡ | +++‡ | +++ | ++ | + | +++ | + | Parkinsonism |
| Bupropion | § | § | ++ | † | + | ++++ | + | Seizures |
| Nefazodone | 0/+ | +++ | + | ++ | + | 0 | 0/+ | |
| Trazodone | 0 | ++ | 0 | +++ | +++ | + | + | Priapism |
| Venlafaxine | ++++ | ++++ | + | + | 0 | + | 0/+ | |

NE = norepinephrine; 5-HT = serotonin; DA = dopamine.
*MAOIs do not block transmitter reuptake. Rather, they increase intraneuronal stores at NE, 5-HT, and DA.
†Produces moderate *stimulation*, not sedation.
‡In addition to blocking NE and 5-HT *reuptake*, amoxapine blocks *receptors* for DA.
§Bupropion primarily inhibits reuptake of DA rather than NE or 5-HT.

monoamine hypothesis, which asserts that depression stems from a *deficiency* in monoamine-mediated neurotransmission, would predict that drugs capable of *increasing* the effects of monoamines would reduce symptoms of depression. This prediction is fulfilled by the tricyclic drugs. The relative abilities of individual tricyclics to block reuptake of norepinephrine and serotonin are summarized in Table 30-2.

We should note that blockade of reuptake, by itself, cannot fully account for the therapeutic effects of the TCAs. This statement is based on the observation that clinical responses to the tricyclics (relief of depressive symptoms) and the biochemical effects of the tricyclics (blockade of transmitter uptake) do not occur in the same time frame. That is, whereas TCAs block transmitter uptake within hours of their administration, relief of depression takes several weeks to develop. Hence, it would appear that, in the interval between the onset of uptake blockade and the onset of a therapeutic response, intermediary neurochemical events must be taking place. Just what these are is not known.

### Pharmacokinetics

Tricyclic antidepressants have half-lives that are long and variable. Because their half-lives are long, TCAs can usually be administered in a single daily dose. Because their half-lives are variable, TCAs require individualization of dosage.

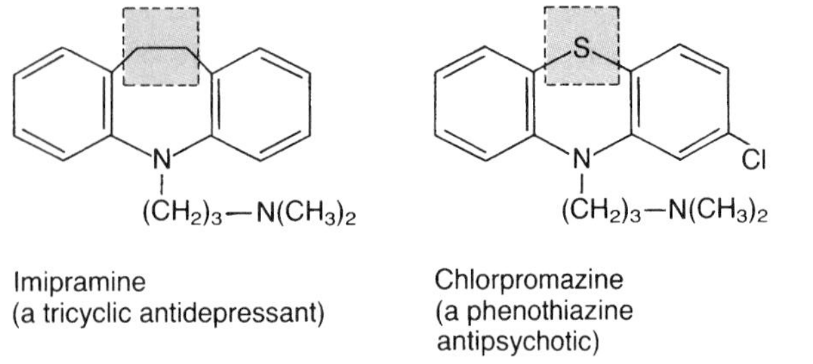

Imipramine
(a tricyclic antidepressant)

Chlorpromazine
(a phenothiazine
antipsychotic)

**Figure 30–1. Structural similarities between tricyclic antidepressants and phenothiazine antipsychotics.** Except for the areas highlighted, the phenothiazine nucleus is nearly identical to that of TCAs. Because of their structural similarities, TCAs and phenothiazines have several pharmacologic properties in common.

## Therapeutic Uses

**Depression.** Tricyclic antidepressants are preferred drugs for treatment of major depression. These medicines can elevate mood, increase activity and alertness, decrease morbid preoccupation, improve appetite, and normalize sleep patterns.

It is important to note that TCAs, and all other antidepressants, do not relieve symptoms immediately. *Initial* responses take from 1 to 3 weeks to develop. One or 2 months may be needed before a *maximal* response is achieved. Because therapeutic effects are delayed, TCAs cannot be used on a PRN basis. Furthermore, a therapeutic trial should not be considered a failure until medication has been administered for at least 1 month without success.

Suicide is always a concern during the treatment of depression. This is because the patient may be so despondent as to perceive suicide as the only means of relief. To reduce the chances of suicide, several precautions can be taken. First, since antidepressants take several weeks to alleviate symptoms, patients with suicidal tendencies should be hospitalized until treatment has had time to substantially reduce suicide risk. In addition, since TCAs

themselves can be vehicles for suicide, the patient should not be given access to a large supply. Accordingly, you should ensure that each dose is actually swallowed and not "cheeked." This precaution will prevent the patient from accumulating multiple doses that might be taken with suicidal intent.

**Bipolar Disorder.** Bipolar disorder (manic-depressive illness) is characterized by alternating episodes of mania and depression (see Chapter 31). Tricyclic antidepressants can be helpful during the depressive phase of this illness. However, there is a risk of inducing mania in some patients.

**Other Uses.** TCAs can benefit patients with *chronic insomnia* (see Chapter 32), *attention-deficit/hyperactivity disorder* (see Chapter 33), and *panic disorder* (see Chapter 32).

## Adverse Effects

The most common undesired responses to TCAs are orthostatic hypotension, sedation, and anticholinergic effects. The most serious adverse effect is cardiac toxicity. Adverse effects of individual agents are summarized in Table 30–2.

**Orthostatic Hypotension.** Orthostatic hypotension is the most serious of the common adverse responses to treatment. Hypotension is due in large part to blockade of alpha$_1$-adrenergic receptors on blood vessels. The patient should be informed that orthostatic hypotension can be minimized by moving slowly when assuming an upright posture. Also, the patient should be instructed to sit or lie down if symptoms of hypotension (dizziness, lightheadedness) occur. For the hospitalized patient, blood pressure and pulse rate should be monitored on a regular schedule (e.g., 4 times daily). These measurements should be taken while the patient is lying down and again after the patient has been sitting or standing for 1 to 2 minutes. If blood pressure is low or pulse rate is high, medication should be withheld and the physician notified.

**Anticholinergic Effects.** The TCAs block muscarinic cholinergic receptors, and can thereby cause an array of

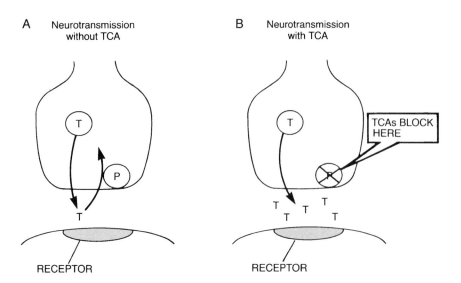

A  Neurotransmission without TCA

B  Neurotransmission with TCA

TCAs BLOCK HERE

RECEPTOR

RECEPTOR

**Figure 30–2. Mechanism of action of tricyclic antidepressants.** *A*, Under drug-free conditions, the actions of norepinephrine and serotonin are terminated by active uptake of these transmitters back into the nerve terminals from which they were released.

*B*, By inhibiting the uptake pumps for norepinephrine and serotonin, tricyclic antidepressants cause these transmitters to accumulate in the synaptic space, thereby intensifying transmission.

(T = transmitter [norepinephrine or serotonin], P = uptake pump, TCA = tricyclic antidepressant.)

anticholinergic effects (dry mouth, blurred vision, photophobia, constipation, urinary hesitancy, and tachycardia). Patients should be informed about possible anticholinergic responses and instructed in ways to minimize discomfort. A detailed discussion of anticholinergic effects and their management is presented in Chapter 15.

*Diaphoresis.* Despite their anticholinergic properties, tricyclic antidepressants often cause diaphoresis (sweating). The mechanism of this paradoxical effect is unknown.

*Sedation.* Sedation is a common response to TCAs. The cause is blockade of histamine receptors in the CNS. Patients should be advised to avoid hazardous activity if sedation is prominent.

*Cardiac Toxicity.* Tricyclics can adversely affect cardiac function. However, in the absence of overdosage or pre-existing cardiac impairment, serious cardiotoxicity is rare. These drugs affect the heart by (1) decreasing vagal influence on the heart (secondary to muscarinic blockade) and (2) acting directly on the bundle of His to slow conduction. Both effects increase the risk of dysrhythmias. To minimize adverse cardiac effects, patients over the age of 40 and those with heart disease should undergo electrocardiographic evaluation prior to treatment and periodically thereafter.

*Seizures.* Tricyclic antidepressants lower seizure threshold. Caution must be exercised in patients with epilepsy and other seizure disorders.

*Hypomania.* On occasion, TCAs produce too much of a good thing, elevating mood from depression all the way to hypomania (mild mania). If hypomania develops, the patient should be evaluated to determine whether elation is drug induced or symptomatic of bipolar disorder.

*Yawngasm.* Rarely, patients taking *clomipramine* [Anafranil] experience yawngasm. Experience what? A spontaneous orgasm while yawning. Honest. This unusual side effect, which affects both males and females, may be considered adverse or beneficial, depending on one's view of such things. In at least one documented case, yawngasms strongly influenced compliance, as evidenced by the patient asking how long she would be "allowed" to continue treatment. Although data are scarce, one might guess that the occasional yawngasm would help dispel depression.

## Drug Interactions

*Monoamine Oxidase Inhibitors.* The combination of a TCA with an MAOI can lead to *severe hypertension* from excessive adrenergic stimulation of the heart and blood vessels. Excessive adrenergic stimulation occurs because (1) inhibition of MAO causes accumulation of norepinephrine in adrenergic neurons and (2) blockade of norepinephrine reuptake by the tricyclics decreases norepinephrine inactivation. Because of the potential for hypertensive crisis, combined therapy with tricyclic antidepressants and MAOIs is generally avoided.

*Direct-Acting Sympathomimetic Drugs.* Tricyclic antidepressants *potentiate* responses to direct-acting sympathomimetics (i.e., drugs such as epinephrine and norepinephrine that produce their effects by direct interaction

with adrenergic receptors). Stimulation by these drugs is increased because TCAs block their uptake into adrenergic terminals, thereby prolonging their presence in the synaptic space.

*Indirect-Acting Sympathomimetic Drugs.* Tricyclic antidepressants *decrease* responses to indirect-acting sympathomimetics (i.e., drugs such as ephedrine and amphetamine that produce their effects by promoting release of transmitter from adrenergic nerves). Effects of indirect-acting sympathomimetics are reduced because TCAs block uptake of these agents into adrenergic nerves, thereby preventing them from reaching their site of action within the nerve terminal.

*Anticholinergic Agents.* Since TCAs exert anticholinergic actions of their own, these drugs will intensify the effects of other medications that have anticholinergic actions. Consequently, patients receiving TCAs should be advised to avoid all other drugs with anticholinergic properties, including antihistamines and certain over-the-counter sleep aids.

*CNS Depressants.* CNS depression caused by TCAs will add with CNS depression caused by other drugs. Accordingly, the patient should be warned against taking all other CNS depressants, such as alcohol, antihistamines, opioids, and barbiturates.

## Toxicity

Overdosage with TCAs can be life threatening. (The lethal dose is only 8 times the average daily dose.) To minimize the risk of death by suicide, the acutely depressed patient should be given no more than a 1-week supply of TCAs at one time.

*Clinical Manifestations.* Symptoms result primarily from *anticholinergic* and *cardiotoxic* actions. The combination of cholinergic blockade and direct cardiotoxicity can produce *dysrhythmias*, including tachycardia, intraventricular blocks, complete atrioventricular block, ventricular tachycardia, and ventricular fibrillation. Responses to peripheral muscarinic blockade include hyperthermia, flushing, dry mouth, and dilation of the pupils.

CNS symptoms are prominent. Early responses are confusion, agitation, and hallucinations. Seizures and coma may follow.

*Treatment.* Absorption of ingested drug can be reduced with gastric lavage followed by administration of activated charcoal. Physostigmine (a cholinesterase inhibitor) is given to counteract anticholinergic actions. Propranolol, lidocaine, or phenytoin can be given to control dysrhythmias. Dysrhythmias should not be treated with procainamide or quinidine, because these drugs will aggravate cardiac depression.

## Dosage and Routes of Administration

*Dosage.* Dosages for individual TCAs are summarized in Table 30–3. General guidelines on dosing are discussed below.

Initial doses of TCAs should be kept low (e.g., 50 mg of imipramine a day for the adult outpatient). Low initial

## TABLE 30-3. ADULT DOSAGE FOR ANTIDEPRESSANTS

| Generic Name | Trade Name | Initial Dose*† (mg/day) | Dose after 4–8 weeks* (mg/day) | Maximum Dose‡ (mg/day) |
|---|---|---|---|---|
| *Tricyclic Antidepressants* | | | | |
| Amitriptyline | Elavil | 50-150 | 100-200 | 300 |
| Clomipramine | Anafranil | 25 | 100-200 | 250 |
| Desipramine | Norpramin | 50-150 | 75-200 | 300 |
| Doxepin | Sinequan | 50-150 | 100-200 | 300 |
| Imipramine | Tofranil | 50-150 | 100-200 | 300 |
| Maprotiline | Ludiomil | 50-100 | 100-150 | 225 |
| Nortriptyline | Aventyl, Pamelor | 25-100 | 75-150 | 150 |
| Protriptyline | Vivactil | 10-40 | 15-40 | 60 |
| Trimipramine | Surmontil | 50-150 | 75-250 | 250 |
| *Monoamine Oxidase Inhibitors* | | | | |
| Phenelzine | Nardil | 45-75 | 45-75 | 75 |
| Tranylcypromine | Parnate | 20-30 | 20-30 | 30 |
| *Selective Serotonin Reuptake Inhibitors* | | | | |
| Fluoxetine | Prozac | 20 | 20-40 | 80 |
| Fluvoxamine | Luvox | 50-100 | 50-300 | 300 |
| Paroxetine | Paxil | 20 | 20-50 | 50 |
| Sertraline | Zoloft | 50 | 50-200 | 200 |
| *Atypical Antidepressants* | | | | |
| Amoxapine | Asendin | 50-150 | 200-300 | 400 |
| Bupropion | Wellbutrin | 200 | 300 | 450 |
| Mirtazepine | Remeron | 15 | — | — |
| Nefazodone | Serzone | 100 | 100-600 | 600 |
| Trazodone | Desyrel | 150 | 150-200 | 400 |
| Venlafaxine | Effexor | 75 | 75-375 | 375 |

*Doses listed are *total daily doses*. Depending on the drug and the patient, the total dose may be given in a single dose or in divided doses.
†Initial doses are employed for 4-8 weeks, the time required for most symptoms to respond. The smaller dose within the range listed is used initially. Dosage is gradually increased as required.
‡Doses higher than these may be needed for some patients with severe depression.

doses minimize adverse reactions and thereby help promote compliance. High initial doses are both undesirable and unnecessary. High initial doses are undesirable in that they pose an increased risk of adverse reactions. They are unnecessary in that onset of therapeutic effects is delayed; hence, aggressive initial dosing offers no benefit.

Because of interpatient variability in metabolism of TCAs, dosing is highly individualized. As a rule, dosage is adjusted on the basis of *clinical response*. However, in the absence of a therapeutic response, *plasma drug levels* can be used as a guide for dosage determination. Levels of imipramine, for example, must be above 225 ng/ml for antidepressant effects to occur. If a patient has not responded to imipramine, measurements should be made to ensure that plasma drug levels are greater than 225 ng/ml. If drug levels are below this value, the dosage should be increased.

Once an effective dosage has been established, most patients can take their entire daily dose at bedtime; the long half-lives of the TCAs make divided daily doses unneces-

sary. Once-a-day dosing at bedtime has several advantages: (1) it is simple to perform, and hence facilitates compliance; (2) it promotes sleep by causing maximal sedation at night; and (3) it reduces the intensity of side effects during the day. If bedtime dosing causes significant sedation in the morning, dosing earlier in the evening can help. Although once-a-day dosing is generally desirable, not all patients can use this schedule. The elderly, for example, can be especially sensitive to the cardiotoxic actions of the tricyclics. As a result, if the entire daily dose were taken at one time, effects on the heart might be intolerable.

Once remission has been produced, therapy should continue for 6 months to a year. Failure to take medication for this period is likely to result in relapse. Patients should be encouraged to continue drug therapy even if they are symptom free and feel that further medication is not needed.

**Routes of Administration.** All TCAs can be administered by mouth, the usual route for these drugs. Two agents—*amitriptyline* and *imipramine*—may be given by IM injection. Intravenous administration is not used; since effects take weeks to develop, there would be no advantage to this route.

## Preparations and Drug Selection

*Preparations.* In the United States, nine TCAs are available (see Tables 30–2 and 30–3). All nine are equally effective. Principal differences among these agents concern side effects (see Table 30–2).

*Drug Selection.* Selection among TCAs is based on side effects. For example, if the patient is experiencing insomnia, a drug with prominent sedative properties (e.g., doxepin) might be selected. Conversely, if daytime sedation is undesirable, a less sedative agent (e.g., desipramine) might be preferred. Elderly patients with glaucoma or constipation and males with prostatic hypertrophy can be especially sensitive to anticholinergic effects; for these patients, a drug with weak anticholinergic properties (e.g., desipramine) would be appropriate.

# Selective Serotonin Reuptake Inhibitors

In recent years, drugs that produce selective blockade of serotonin reuptake have become available. These SSRIs are as effective as the TCAs, but do not cause hypotension, sedation, or anticholinergic effects. Moreover, overdosage does not result in cardiotoxicity. Characteristic side effects of the SSRIs are nausea, insomnia, and sexual dysfunction (especially anorgasmia). SSRIs can interact adversely with MAOIs, hence the combination must be avoided. Fluoxetine, the most popular SSRI, will serve as our prototype for the group.

## Fluoxetine

Fluoxetine [Prozac] is the most widely prescribed antidepressant in the United States. The drug is as effective as the TCAs, causes fewer side effects, and is less dangerous when taken in overdose. Combined use with MAOIs can cause serious adverse effects, and therefore must be avoided.

*Mechanism of Action.* Fluoxetine produces selective inhibition of serotonin reuptake, and thereby intensifies transmission at serotonergic synapses. As with TCAs, blockade of transmitter uptake occurs quickly, whereas therapeutic effects develop slowly. Hence, we can conclude that adaptive cellular changes that take place in response to prolonged uptake blockade must be the actual basis of depression relief. Fluoxetine does not block uptake of dopamine or norepinephrine. In contrast to the TCAs, fluoxetine does not block cholinergic, histaminic, or alpha$_1$-adrenergic receptors. Furthermore, fluoxetine produces CNS excitation rather than sedation.

*Therapeutic Uses.* Fluoxetine is used primarily to treat *major depression*. Antidepressant effects begin in 1 to 3 weeks and are equivalent to those produced by TCAs.

Fluoxetine is also approved for *obsessive-compulsive disorder* (Chapter 34), and is a preferred drug (although not approved) for *panic disorder* (Chapter 34) and *premenstrual syndrome* (Chapter 57). Investigational uses include *bulimia, alcoholism, attention-deficit/hyperactivity disorder, bipolar disorder, migraine, Tourette's syndrome,* and *obesity.*

*Pharmacokinetics.* Fluoxetine is well absorbed following oral administration, even in the presence of food. The drug is widely distributed and highly bound (94%) to plasma proteins. Fluoxetine undergoes extensive hepatic conversion to norfluoxetine, a metabolite with pharmacologic actions like those of fluoxetine itself. Norfluoxetine is eventually converted to inactive metabolites that are excreted in the urine. The half-life of fluoxetine is 2 days and the half-life of norfluoxetine is 7 days. Because the effective half-life is prolonged, about 4 weeks are required to produce steady-state plasma drug levels.

*Adverse Effects.* Fluoxetine is safer and better tolerated than TCAs and MAOIs. In contrast to TCAs, fluoxetine produces little or no cardiotoxicity, hypotension, or muscarinic blockade.

*Sexual dysfunction* (e.g., anorgasmia, delayed ejaculation, decreased libido) is common, occurring in about 70% of men and women. Other common reactions include *nausea* (21%), *headache* (20%), and manifestations of CNS stimulation, including *nervousness* (15%), *insomnia* (14%), and *anxiety* (10%). Fluoxetine can cause *dizziness* and *fatigue*; hence, patients should be warned against participation in hazardous activities (e.g., driving). *Skin rash,* which can be severe, has occurred in 4% of patients; in most cases, rashes readily respond to drug therapy (antihistamines, glucocorticoids) or to withdrawal of fluoxetine. Other common reactions include *diarrhea* (12%), *excessive sweating* (8%), and *anorexia* with associated *weight loss* (11%).

By increasing serotonergic transmission in the brainstem and spinal cord, fluoxetine and other SSRIs can cause *serotonin syndrome.* This syndrome usually begins 2 to 72 hours after initiation of treatment, and is most likely if an SSRI is combined with an MAOI. Signs and symptoms include altered mental status (agitation, confusion, disorientation, anxiety, hallucinations, poor concentration) as well as incoordination, myoclonus, hyperreflexia, excessive sweating, tremor, and fever. Death has occurred. The syndrome resolves spontaneously after discontinuing the drug.

Overdosage causes nausea, vomiting, and signs of CNS stimulation (agitation, restlessness, hypomania, seizures). Because fluoxetine is not cardiotoxic, overdosage is less dangerous than with TCAs.

*Drug Interactions.* Fluoxetine should not be combined with *MAOIs,* since serotonin syndrome can occur. MAOIs should be withdrawn at least 14 days before starting fluoxetine. When fluoxetine is discontinued, at least 5 *weeks* should elapse before giving an MAOI.

Because fluoxetine is highly bound to plasma proteins, it may displace other highly bound drugs. Displacement of *warfarin* (an anticoagulant) is of particular concern. Monitor responses to warfarin closely.

Fluoxetine can elevate plasma levels of *TCAs* and *lithium* (a drug for bipolar disorder). Caution should be exercised if fluoxetine is combined with these agents.

**Preparations, Dosage, and Administration.** Fluoxetine [Prozac] is dispensed in solution (20 mg/5 ml) and pulvules (10 and 20 mg) for oral administration. The drug may be taken with or without food. The recommended initial dosage is 20 mg/day. If needed, the dosage may be increased gradually to a maximum of 80 mg/day; however, some authorities believe that doses greater than 20 mg/day will just increase adverse effects without producing any increase in benefits. If daily doses above 20 mg are used, they should be divided. For elderly patients and patients with impaired liver function, the dosage should be low initially and then cautiously increased if needed. Since fluoxetine often impairs sleep, evening dosing should be avoided for most patients.

## Other Selective Serotonin Reuptake Inhibitors

In addition to fluoxetine, three other SSRIs are available: fluvoxamine [Luvox], sertraline [Zoloft], and paroxetine [Paxil]. All three are similar to fluoxetine. Antidepressant effects equal those of TCAs. Like fluoxetine, the newer SSRIs do not cause hypotension or anticholinergic effects, and, with the exception of fluvoxamine, do not cause sedation. When taken in overdose, these drugs do not cause cardiotoxicity. All three can interact adversely with MAOIs; hence, the combination must be avoided. Characteristic side effects are nausea, insomnia, and sexual dysfunction. Serotonin syndrome is a potential complication with all SSRIs. The principal differences among the SSRIs relate to duration of action. Patients who experience intolerable adverse effects with one SSRI may find a different SSRI more acceptable.

### Sertraline

Sertraline [Zoloft] is much like fluoxetine: both drugs produce selective blockade of serotonin reuptake, both relieve symptoms of major depression, both cause CNS stimulation rather than sedation, and both have minimal effects on seizure threshold or the electrocardiogram (EKG). Sertraline is approved for treating major depression and obsessive-compulsive disorder. Common side effects include headache, tremor, insomnia, agitation, nervousness, nausea, and diarrhea. Sexual dysfunction occurs in 9% to 21% of males. Because of the risk of serotonin syndrome, sertraline must not be combined with MAOIs. Accordingly, MAOIs should be withdrawn at least 14 days before starting sertraline, and sertraline should be withdrawn at least 14 days before starting an MAOI.

Sertraline is slowly absorbed following oral administration. Food increases the extent of absorption. Once in the blood, the drug is highly bound (99%) to plasma proteins. Sertraline undergoes extensive hepatic metabolism followed by elimination in the urine and feces. The plasma half-life is approximately 1 day.

Sertraline is available in 50- and 100-mg tablets. The initial adult dosage is 50 mg/day administered in the morning or evening. After 4 to 8 weeks, the dosage may be increased by 50-mg increments to a maximum of 200 mg/day.

### Fluvoxamine

Like other SSRIs, fluvoxamine [Luvox] produces powerful and selective inhibition of serotonin reuptake. The drug is approved for major depression and obsessive-compulsive disorder. For treatment of depression, fluvoxamine is about equal to TCAs.

Administration is oral, and absorption is rapid and unaffected by food. Fluvoxamine undergoes extensive hepatic metabolism followed by excretion in the urine. The half-life is 15 hours.

Common side effects include nausea and vomiting (37%), dry mouth (26%), headache (22%), and constipation (18%). In contrast to other SSRIs, fluvoxamine has moderate sedative effects, although it nonetheless can cause insomnia. Some patients have developed abnormal liver function tests; liver function should be assessed prior to treatment, and weekly during the first month of therapy. Like other SSRIs, fluvoxamine interacts adversely with MAOIs; hence the combination must be avoided.

Fluvoxamine is available in 50- and 100-mg tablets. Treatment is initiated with daily doses of 50 to 100 mg for 1 week. Dosage is then gradually increased to a maximum of 300 mg/day. Side effects are minimized by giving the entire daily dose at bedtime.

### Paroxetine

Like other SSRIs, paroxetine [Paxil] produces powerful and selective inhibition of serotonin uptake. The drug is approved for treating major depression and is in clinical trials for obsessive-compulsive disorder.

Paroxetine is well absorbed following oral administration, even in the presence of food. The drug is widely distributed and highly bound (95%) to plasma proteins. Concentrations in breast milk equal those in plasma. The drug undergoes hepatic metabolism followed by renal excretion. The half-life is about 20 hours.

Side effects are dose dependent and generally mild. Early reactions include nausea, somnolence, sweating, tremor, and fatigue. These tend to diminish over time. After 5 to 6 weeks, the major complaints are headache and weight gain. Like fluoxetine, paroxetine causes signs of CNS stimulation (increased awakenings, reduced time in REM sleep, insomnia). In contrast to TCAs, paroxetine has no effect on heart rate, blood pressure, or the EKG. Like other SSRIs, paroxetine interacts adversely with MAOIs; hence, the combination must be avoided.

Paroxetine is available in 10- and 20-mg tablets. The recommended initial dosage is 20 mg/day. The entire daily dose is administered in the morning (to minimize sleep disturbance) and with food (to minimize gastrointestinal upset). Dosage may be increased gradually (every 3 to 4 weeks) to a maximum of 50 mg/day.

## Monoamine Oxidase Inhibitors

The MAO inhibitors (MAOIs) are second- or third-choice antidepressants for most patients. Although these drugs are as effective as the tricyclics, they are more dangerous. Of particular concern is the risk of hypertensive crisis in response to foods rich in tyramine. With the advent of SSRIs and other alternatives to TCAs, use of MAOIs continues to decline. At this time, MAOIs are drugs of choice only for atypical depression. Two MAOIs are available: phe-nelzine and tranylcypromine. Others are in development.

### Mechanism of Action

Before discussing the MAOIs, we need to discuss MAO itself. MAO is an enzyme present in the liver, the intestinal wall, and the terminals of monoamine-containing neurons. The function of MAO in neurons is to convert monoamine transmitters—norepinephrine, serotonin, and dopamine—into inactive products. In the liver and intestine, MAO serves to inactivate tyramine and other biogenic amines in food; in addition, these enzymes inactivate biogenic amines administered as drugs.

The body has two forms of MAO, named MAO-A and MAO-B. In the brain, MAO-A inactivates dopamine, whereas MAO-B inactivates norepinephrine and serotonin. In the liver, MAO-A acts on dietary tyramine and other compounds. Currently available antidepressant MAOIs are *nonselective*. That is, they inhibit both MAO-A and MAO-B. Antidepressant agents selective for MAO-A are in development. Selegiline, a selective inhibitor of MAO-B, is used to treat Parkinson's disease (see Chapter 22).

Antidepressant effects of the MAOIs results from inhibiting MAO-A in nerve terminals (Fig. 30–3). By inhibiting intraneuronal MAO-A, these drugs increase the amount of norepinephrine and serotonin available for release, and thereby intensify transmission at noradrenergic and serotonergic junctions.

It should be noted that antidepressant effects of the MAOIs cannot be fully explained by MAO inhibition alone. This statement is based on the fact that the biochemical action of MAOIs (inhibition of MAO) takes place rapidly, whereas the clinical response to MAOIs (relief of depression) develops slowly. In the interval between initial inhibition of MAO and relief of depression, additional neurochemical events must be taking place. It is these as-yet unknown events that are ultimately responsible for the beneficial response to treatment.

The MAOIs can act on MAO in two ways: reversibly and irreversibly. Phenelzine produces irreversible inhibition, whereas tranylcypromine produces reversible inhibition. Recovery from irreversible inhibition requires synthesis of new enzyme, a somewhat slow process. Hence, the effects of phenelzine persist for 2 weeks after drug withdrawal. Recovery from reversible inhibition is more rapid, occurring in 3 to 5 days.

## Therapeutic Uses

*Depression.*  MAOIs are as effective as TCAs for relieving depression. However, because they can be hazardous, MAOIs are generally reserved for patients who have not responded to TCAs, SSRIs, and other safer drugs. However, for one group of patients—those with *atypical depression*—MAOIs are drugs of first choice. As with other antidepressants, beneficial effects do not reach their peak for several weeks.

*Other Uses.*  MAOIs have been used with some success to treat *bulimia* and *obsessive-compulsive disorders*. Like the tricyclics, MAOIs can eliminate spontaneous *panic attacks* in patients with panic disorder.

## Adverse Effects

*CNS Stimulation.*  In contrast to TCAs, MAOIs cause direct CNS stimulation (in addition to exerting antidepressant effects). Excessive stimulation can produce anxiety, agitation, hypomania, and even mania.

*Orthostatic Hypotension.*  Despite their ability to increase the norepinephrine content of peripheral sympathetic neurons, the MAOIs *reduce blood pressure* when administered in usual therapeutic doses. Patients should be informed about signs of hypotension (dizziness, lightheadedness) and advised to sit or lie down if these occur. Also, they should be informed that hypotension can be minimized by moving slowly when assuming an erect posture. For the hospitalized patient, blood pressure and pulse rate should be monitored on a regular schedule (e.g., 4 times daily). These measurements should be taken while the patient is lying down and after the patient has been sitting or standing for 1 to 2 minutes.

MAOIs lower blood pressure through actions in the CNS. The following sequence has been proposed: (1) inhibition of MAO increases the norepinephrine (NE) content of neurons within the vasomotor center; (2) when NE is released, it binds to postsynaptic alpha receptors on neurons within the vasomotor center, thereby decreasing the firing rate of sympathetic nerves that control vascular tone; and (3) this reduction in sympathetic activity results in vasodilation, causing blood pressure to fall.

*Hypertensive Crisis from Dietary Tyramine.*  Although the MAOIs normally produce *hypotension*, these drugs can be the cause of severe *hypertension* if the patient eats

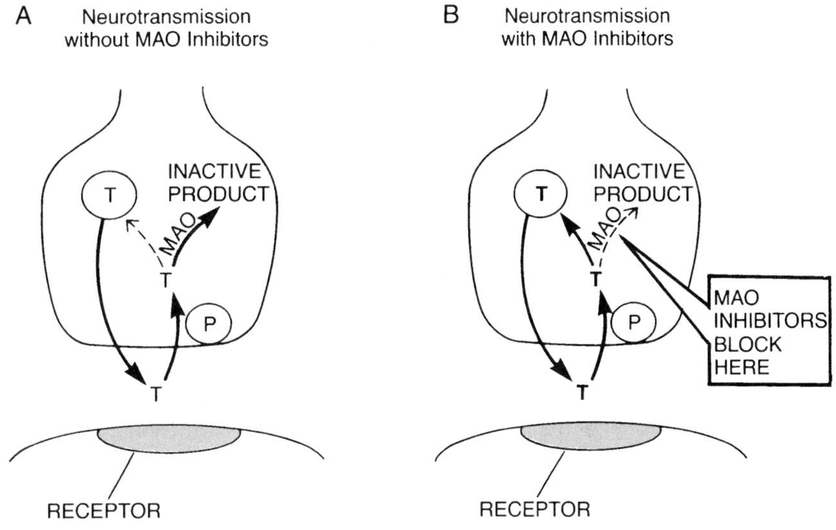

**Figure 30–3. Mechanism of action of monoamine oxidase inhibitors.** *A*, Under drug-free conditions, much of the norepinephrine or serotonin that undergoes reuptake into nerve terminals becomes inactivated by MAO. This inactivation process helps maintain an appropriate concentration of transmitter within the terminal.

*B*, MAO inhibitors prevent inactivation of norepinephrine and serotonin, thereby increasing the amount of transmitter available for release. Release of supranormal amounts of transmitter intensifies transmission.

(T = transmitter [norepinephrine or serotonin], P = uptake pump, MAO = monoamine oxidase.)

A  Neurotransmission without MAO Inhibitors

B  Neurotransmission with MAO Inhibitors

food that is rich in *tyramine*, a substance that promotes the release of norepinephrine from sympathetic neurons. Hypertensive crisis is characterized by headache, tachycardia, hypertension, nausea, and vomiting.

Before considering the mechanism by which hypertensive crisis is produced, let's consider the effect of dietary tyramine under drug-free conditions. In the absence of MAO inhibition, dietary tyramine does not represent a threat. Much of the tyramine in food is metabolized by MAO in the intestinal wall. Furthermore, as shown in Figure 30–4A, any dietary tyramine that does get absorbed passes directly to the liver via the hepatic portal circulation. Once in the liver, tyramine is immediately inactivated by MAO there. Hence, as long as hepatic MAO is functioning, dietary tyramine is prevented from reaching the general circulation, and hence is devoid of adverse effects.

In the presence of MAOIs, the picture is very different: dietary tyramine can produce a life-threatening hypertensive crisis. The mechanism of this reaction has three components (Fig. 30–4B). First, inhibition of *neuronal* MAO augments NE levels within the terminals of sympathetic neurons that regulate cardiac function and vascular tone. Second, inhibition of *hepatic* MAO allows dietary tyramine to pass directly through the liver and enter the systemic circulation intact. Third, upon reaching peripheral sympathetic nerves, tyramine stimulates the release of the accumulated NE, thereby causing massive vasoconstriction and excessive stimulation of the heart; hypertensive crisis results.

To reduce the risk of tyramine-induced hypertensive crisis, the following precautions must be taken:

- MAOIs must not be dispensed to patients considered incapable of rigid adherence to dietary restrictions.
- Before an MAOI is dispensed, the patient must be fully informed about the hazard of ingesting tyramine-rich foods.

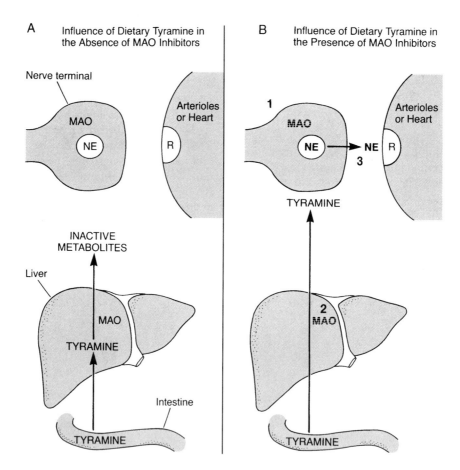

**Figure 30–4. Interaction between dietary tyramine and monoamine oxidase inhibitors.** *A*, In the absence of MAO inhibitors, dietary tyramine is absorbed from the intestine, transported to the liver, and then immediately inactivated by hepatic MAO. No tyramine reaches the general circulation intact.

*B*, Three events occur in the presence of MAO inhibitors. (1) Inhibition of neuronal MAO elevates levels of norepinephrine (NE) in sympathetic nerve terminals. (2) Inhibition of hepatic MAO allows dietary tyramine to pass through the liver and enter the systemic circulation intact. (3) Upon reaching peripheral sympathetic nerve terminals, tyramine promotes the release of accumulated NE stores, thereby causing massive vasoconstriction and excessive stimulation of the heart.

(MAO = monoamine oxidase, R = receptor for norepinephrine.)

- The patient must be provided with a list of specific foods and beverages to avoid. These foods—which include yeast extracts, most cheeses, fermented sausages (e.g., salami, pepperoni, bologna), and aged fish or meat—are listed in Table 30-4.
- The patient should be instructed to avoid all drugs not specifically approved by the physician.

The patient should be informed about the symptoms of hypertensive crisis (headache, tachycardia, palpitations, nausea, vomiting) and instructed to notify the physician immediately if these develop. If the physician is unavailable, the patient should go directly to an emergency department. In the event of hypertensive crisis, blood pressure can be lowered with IV *phentolamine*, a short-acting alpha-adrenergic antagonist; blood pressure declines because of vasodilation secondary to blockade of alpha$_1$ receptors on blood vessels. Sublingual *nifedipine*, a calcium channel blocker, is an alternative; like IV phentolamine, sublingual nifedipine acts rapidly to promote vasodilation.

In addition to tyramine, several other dietary constituents (e.g., caffeine, phenylethylamine) can precipitate hypertension in patients taking MAOIs. Foods that contain these compounds are listed in Table 30-4. The patient should be instructed to avoid them.

## Drug Interactions

*The MAOIs can interact with many drugs to cause potentially disastrous results. Accordingly, the patient should be instructed to avoid all medications—prescription agents and over-the-counter drugs—that have not been specifically approved by the physician.*

***Indirect-Acting Sympathomimetic Agents.*** Indirect-acting sympathomimetics (e.g., ephedrine, amphetamine)

## TABLE 30-4. FOODS THAT CAN INTERACT WITH MAO INHIBITORS

### Foods That Contain Tyramine

| Category | Unsafe Foods (High Tyramine Content) | Safe Foods (Little or No Tyramine) |
|---|---|---|
| Vegetables | Avocados, especially if overripe; fermented bean curd; fermented soybean; soybean paste | Most vegetables |
| Fruits | Figs, especially if overripe; bananas, in large amounts | Most fruits |
| Meats | Meats that are fermented, smoked, or otherwise aged; spoiled meats; liver, unless *very* fresh | Meats that are known to be fresh (exercise caution in restaurants; meat may not be fresh) |
| Sausages | Fermented varieties: bologna, pepperoni, salami, others | Nonfermented varieties |
| Fish | Dried or cured fish; fish that is fermented, smoked, or otherwise aged; spoiled fish | Fish that is known to be fresh; vacuum-packed fish, if eaten promptly or refrigerated only briefly after opening |
| Milk, milk products | Practically all cheeses | Milk, yogurt, cottage cheese, cream cheese |
| Foods with yeast | Yeast extract (e.g., Marmite, Bovril) | Baked goods that contain yeast |
| Beer, wine | Some imported beers; Chianti wine | Major domestic brands of beer; most wines |
| Other foods | Protein dietary supplements; soups (may contain protein extract); shrimp paste; soy sauce | |

### Foods That Contain Other Vasopressors

| Food | Comments |
|---|---|
| Chocolate | Contains phenylethylamine, a pressor agent; large amounts can cause a reaction. |
| Fava beans | Contain dopamine, a pressor agent; reactions are most likely with overripe beans. |
| Ginseng | Headache, tremulousness and manic-like reactions have occurred. |
| Caffeinated beverages | Caffeine is a weak pressor agent; large amounts may cause a reaction. |

are drugs that promote the release of NE from sympathetic nerves. In patients taking MAOIs, these drugs can produce *hypertensive crisis*. The mechanism is the same as that described for tyramine. Patients should be instructed to avoid all sympathomimetic drugs, including ephedrine, methylphenidate, amphetamines, and cocaine. Sympatho-mimetic agents may be present in cold remedies, nasal decongestants, and asthma medications; all of these should be avoided unless approved by the physician.

***Interactions Secondary to Inhibition of Hepatic MAO.*** Inhibition of MAO in the liver can decrease the metabolism of several drugs, including epinephrine, norepinephrine, and dopamine. These drugs must be used with caution since their effects will be intensified and prolonged.

***TCAs and SSRIs.*** The combination of a TCA with an MAOI may produce hypertensive episodes or hypertensive crisis. As a result, this combination is not employed routinely to treat depression. However, although potentially dangerous, the combination can benefit certain patients. If this combination is employed, caution must be exercised.

Combining an MAOI with an SSRI can produce serotonin syndrome. Accordingly, the combination must be avoided.

***Antihypertensive Drugs.*** Combined use of MAOIs and antihypertensive agents may result in excessive lowering of blood pressure. This response should be no surprise considering that MAOIs, by themselves, can cause hypotension.

***Meperidine.*** Meperidine [Demerol] can cause hyperpyrexia (excessive elevation of temperature) in patients receiving MAOIs. Accordingly, if a strong analgesic is required, an agent other than meperidine should be chosen. Furthermore, the analgesic should be administered in its lowest effective dosage.

### Preparations, Dosage, and Administration

MAOIs are dispensed in tablets for oral administration. Dosages are summarized in Table 30–3.

## Atypical Antidepressants

### Amoxapine

Amoxapine [Asendin] is chemically related to the antipsychotic agent loxapine, and has both antidepressant and neuroleptic properties. Antidepressant effects are equivalent to those of the tricyclics. The usual dosage for depression is 200 to 300 mg/day.

Amoxapine is generally well tolerated. Anticholinergic and sedative effects are moderate. Following overdosage, the risk of seizures is greater than with the tricyclics. Caution should be exercised in patients with epilepsy.

Like loxapine and the other antipsychotics, amoxapine can block receptors for dopamine. As a result, the drug can cause extrapyramidal side effects (e.g., parkinsonism, akathisia). Because of the risk of tardive dyskinesia (an extrapyramidal effect that develops with prolonged use of dopamine antagonists), long-term use of amoxapine should be avoided.

### Bupropion

Bupropion [Wellbutrin] is a unique antidepressant similar in structure to amphetamine. Like amphetamine, this agent has stimulant properties and suppresses appetite. Bupropion is devoid of the anticholinergic, antiadrenergic, and cardiotoxic effects associated with tricyclic agents. Antidepressant effects begin in 1 to 3 weeks and are equivalent to those of amitriptyline (a tricyclic antidepressant). The mechanism by which depression is relieved is unknown.

Bupropion is generally well tolerated. The most common adverse effects are weight loss, dry mouth, and dizziness. Other undesired responses include tremor, agitation, and insomnia.

At doses greater than 450 mg/day, bupropion produces seizures in about 0.4% of patients. The risk of seizures is greatly increased in patients with predisposing factors, such as head trauma, pre-existing seizure disorder, CNS tumor, and use of other drugs that lower seizure threshold.

Bupropion [Wellbutrin] is dispensed in 75- and 100-mg tablets for oral use. Dosing must be done carefully to minimize the risk of seizures. Dosage escalation must be done slowly. The initial dosage is 100 mg twice a day. After 4 days, the dosage can be increased to 100 mg 3 times a day. If necessary, the dosage can be increased to a maximum of 150 mg 3 times a day.

### Trazodone

Trazodone [Desyrel] is a second-line agent for treatment of depression. The drug is not very effective when used alone, but, because of its pronounced sedative effects, can be a helpful adjunct for patients with antidepressant-induced insomnia. Trazodone produces selective (but moderate) blockade of serotonin reuptake and may also stimulate serotonin receptors directly. Antidepressant effects take several weeks to develop.

Common side effects are sedation, orthostatic hypotension, nausea, and vomiting. In contrast to the tricyclic agents, trazodone lacks anticholinergic actions and is not cardiotoxic. Accordingly, trazodone may be useful for elderly patients and other individuals for whom the cardiac and anticholinergic effects of the tricyclics may be intolerable.

Trazodone can cause priapism (prolonged, painful erection of the penis). In some cases, surgical intervention has been required. Priapism itself or the procedures required for relief can result in permanent impotence. Patients should be instructed to notify the physician or to go to an emergency room if persistent erection occurs. Prolonged clitoral erection can also occur, but the incidence is extremely low (0.016%).

Overdosage with trazodone is considered safer than with tricyclic agents or MAO inhibitors. Death from overdosage with trazodone alone has not been reported (although death has occurred following overdosage with trazodone in combination with another CNS depressant).

Trazodone is dispensed in tablets (50 to 300 mg) for oral administration. The initial dosage is 150 mg/day in two or three divided doses. Dosage may be gradually increased to a maximum of 400 mg/day (for outpatients) and 600 mg/day (for hospitalized patients).

### Nefazodone

Nefazodone [Serzone] is a relatively new antidepressant whose therapeutic niche has not been determined. Neuropharmacologic actions include inhibition of norepinephrine and serotonin reuptake, and blockade of serotonin$_2$ receptors and alpha$_1$-adrenergic receptors. The contribution of these actions to therapeutic effects is unknown.

Nefazodone is rapidly and completely absorbed following oral administration. Food delays absorption and decreases bioavailability by 20%. Plasma drug levels peak about 1 hour after an oral dose. In the liver, nefazodone undergoes conversion to three active metabolites. The effective half-life of the parent drug and metabolites is 11 to 24 hours.

Nefazodone is generally well tolerated. The most common side effects are headache, somnolence, dry mouth, nausea, dizziness, blurred vision, and other visual disturbances. Sexual dysfunction (impotence, abnormal ejaculation, anorgasmia) has also been reported.

Drugs that block uptake of serotonin, norepinephrine, or both can cause serious reactions if combined with an MAOI. Accordingly, nefazodone and MAOIs must not be combined. If the patient has been taking an MAOI, it should be discontinued at least 2 weeks before starting nefazodone. Conversely, when switching from nefazodone to an MAOI, nefazodone should be discontinued at least 7 days before starting the MAOI.

Nefazodone inhibits hepatic drug-metabolizing enzymes, and can thereby raise levels of other drugs. When present at high levels, terfenadine or astemizole (two nonsedating antihistamines) can cause fatal ventricular dysrhythmias. Accordingly, since nefazodone can raise levels of these drugs, it must not be combined with either agent.

Nefazodone is dispensed in tablets (100, 150, 200, and 250 mg) for oral use. Dosing is begun at 100 mg twice daily. If needed, the dose can be gradually increased to between 150 and 300 mg twice daily. For elderly patients, dosing is begun at 50 mg twice daily; the usual effective range is 50 to 200 mg twice daily.

### Venlafaxine

Venlafaxine [Effexor] is a powerful blocker of norepinephrine and serotonin uptake, and a weak blocker of dopamine uptake. The relationship of these actions to therapeutic effects is uncertain. Venlafaxine does not block cholinergic, histaminergic, or alpha$_1$-adrenergic receptors. In clinical trials, the drug appeared at least as effective as trazodone or imipramine.

Venlafaxine is well absorbed following oral administration, both in the presence and absence of food. Much of each dose is converted to an active metabolite by the liver. The half-life is 5 hours for the parent drug and 11 hours for the major metabolite.

Venlafaxine can cause a variety of adverse effects. The most common are nausea (37%), headache, anorexia, nervousness, sweating, somnolence, and insomnia. Dose-dependent weight loss may occur secondary to anorexia. Venlafaxine also causes dose-related sustained diastolic hypertension; hence blood pressure should be monitored. Sexual dysfunction (e.g., impotence, anorgasmia) may also occur.

Drugs that block uptake of norepinephrine and serotonin can cause serious reactions if combined with an MAOI. Accordingly, MAOIs should be withdrawn at least 14 days before starting venlafaxine. When switching from venlafaxine to an MAOI, venlafaxine should be discontinued 7 days before starting the MAOI.

The recommended initial dosage is 75 mg/day, divided into two or three doses and administered with food. If needed, the dosage may be gradually increased. The usual maximum is 225 mg/day. However, dosages as large as 375 mg/day have been used for severely depressed patients. A dosage reduction is needed for patients with liver dysfunction, and possibly for patients with renal dysfunction.

### Mirtazepine

Mirtazepine [Remeron] is the first representative of a new class of antidepressants. Therapeutic effects appear to result from increased release of serotonin and norepinephrine. Mirtazepine increases release by blocking presynaptic alpha$_2$-adrenergic receptors that serve to inhibit release. In addition to promoting release of serotonin and norepinephrine, mirtazepine is a powerful blocker of two serotonin receptor subtypes: 5HT$_2$ and 5HT$_3$. The contribution of this effect is unclear.

Mirtazepine is well absorbed following oral administration and reaches peak plasma levels in 2 hours. The drug undergoes extensive hepatic metabolism followed by excretion in the urine (75%) and feces (25%). The elimination half-life is 20 to 40 hours.

Mirtazepine is generally well tolerated. Somnolence is the most prominent adverse effect, occurring in 54% of patients. Other side effects include increased appetite (17%), weight gain (8%), cholesterol elevation (15%), and dizziness (7%). Reversible agranulocytosis and neutropenia have occurred rarely. Blockade of muscarinic receptors is moderate; hence, anticholinergic effects are relatively mild. Mirtazepine-induced somnolence can be exacerbated by alcohol, benzodiazepines, and other CNS depressants; hence, these agents should be avoided. Also, mirtazepine should not be combined with MAOIs.

Mirtazepine is available in 15- and 30-mg tablets for oral administration. The initial dosage is 15 mg once a day at bedtime.

## Electroconvulsive Therapy

Although outside the realm of pharmacology, electroconvulsive therapy (ECT) is a valuable treatment for depression and deserves our consideration. ECT has two characteristics that are especially desirable: *effectiveness* and *rapid onset* (relative to antidepressant drugs). Because of these properties, ECT is indicated primarily for two types of patients: (1) those who have failed to respond to pharmacologic treatment for depression (50% will respond to ECT), and (2) severely depressed, suicidal patients who need rapid relief of symptoms.

ECT as practiced today is much less dramatic and traumatic than in the past. Improvements in ECT have resulted in large part from the adjunctive use of drugs. Prior to the delivery of electroshock, patients are treated with a combination of *thiopental* and *succinylcholine*. Thiopental is an injectable, ultrashort-acting anesthetic that prevents conscious awareness of the ECT procedure (without interfering with beneficial actions). Succinylcholine is a short-acting neuromuscular blocking agent that prevents shock-induced convulsive movements, which are both hazardous and unnecessary for a therapeutic response.

ECT can terminate an ongoing episode of depression, but a single treatment cannot prevent recurrence. Accordingly, some patients are now given "maintenance" treatments, at weekly or monthly intervals. In one study, the relapse rate at 6 months in the absence of maintenance was 73%, compared with only 8% when maintenance ECT was employed.

The principal adverse effect of ECT is some loss of memory for events immediately surrounding treatment. Patients do not lose other memories, and their intellectual function is not affected.

## KEY POINTS

- The principal symptoms of major depression are depressed mood and loss of pleasure or interest in one's usual activities and pastimes.

- Therapeutic responses to antidepressants develop slowly. Initial responses develop in 1 to 3 weeks. Maximal responses develop in 1 to 2 months.
- Antidepressant therapy should continue for 6 months to 1 year after symptoms have abated.
- TCAs block reuptake of norepinephrine and serotonin, and thereby intensify transmission at noradrenergic and serotonergic synapses. Over time, this induces adaptive cellular responses that are ultimately responsible for relieving depression.
- The most common adverse effects of TCAs are sedation, orthostatic hypotension, and anticholinergic effects (e.g., dry mouth, constipation).
- The most serious adverse effect of TCAs is cardiotoxicity, which can be lethal when an overdose is taken.
- TCAs can cause hypertensive crisis when combined with an MAOI; hence the combination is generally avoided.
- TCAs intensify responses to direct-acting sympathomimetics (e.g., epinephrine) and diminish responses to indirect-acting sympathomimetics (e.g., amphetamine).
- SSRIs block reuptake of serotonin, and thereby intensify transmission at serotonergic synapses. Over time, this induces adaptive cellular responses that are ultimately responsible for relieving depression.
- SSRIs have two major advantages of TCAs: they cause fewer side effects and are safer when taken in overdose.
- Most SSRIs have stimulant properties, and hence can cause insomnia and nervousness. This contrasts with TCAs, which cause sedation.
- Sexual dysfunction (e.g., anorgasmia) is more common with SSRIs than with other antidepressants.

- SSRIs can cause serotonin syndrome, especially when combined with MAOIs. Symptoms include agitation, confusion, hallucinations, hyperreflexia, tremor, and fever.
- MAOIs increase neuronal stores of norepinephrine and serotonin, and thereby intensify transmission at noradrenergic and serotonergic synapses. Over time, this induces adaptive cellular responses that are ultimately responsible for relieving depression.
- MAOIs are as effective as TCAs and SSRIs, but are much more dangerous.
- MAOIs are first-choice drugs only for patients with atypical depression.
- Like SSRIs (and unlike TCAs) MAOIs cause direct CNS stimulation.
- Like TCAs (and unlike SSRIs) MAOIs cause orthostatic hypotension.
- Patients taking MAOIs must not eat tyramine-rich foods, since hypertensive crisis can result.
- MAOIs must not be combined with indirect-acting sympathomimetics (e.g., ephedrine, amphetamine), since hypertensive crisis can result.
- MAOIs must not be combined with SSRIs, since serotonin syndrome could result.
- ECT relieves depression faster than antidepressant drugs, and often helps in cases where antidepressants have failed.
- ECT has been made safer and less traumatic through adjunctive use of thiopental (which produces unconsciousness) and succinylcholine (which prevents convulsions).

# Summary of Major Nursing Implications*

## Implications That Apply to All Antidepressants

### Psychologic Assessment

Observe and record the patient's behavior. Factors to assess include affect, thought content, interest in the environment, appetite, sleep patterns, and appearance.

### Reducing the Risk of Suicide

Patients who are so depressed that they are a risk to themselves and others should be hospitalized until symptoms are under control. Suicide potential should be evaluated carefully. To prevent patients from accumulating a potentially lethal supply of medication, ensure that each dose is swallowed and not "cheeked." Provide outpatients with no more than a 1-week supply of medication at a time. For patients considered at high risk of suicide, TCAs and MAOIs should be avoided; SSRIs are much safer.

### Promoting Compliance

Inform the patient that antidepressant effects usually develop slowly, over 1 to 3 weeks. This knowledge will make expectations more realistic, and that realism should help promote compliance.

Premature discontinuation of therapy can result in relapse. Educate patients about the importance of taking their medication as prescribed, even though they may be symptom free and therefore feel "cured." In general, treatment should continue for 6 months to a year after symptoms have subsided.

### Nondrug Therapy

Treating depression with drugs alone is not optimal. Emotional support and traditional psychotherapy can complement and reinforce responses to antidepressants. ECT may be indicated for suicidal patients and patients who fail to respond to antidepressant drugs.

### Evaluating Therapeutic Effects

Assess patients for improvement in symptoms, especially depressed mood and loss of interest or pleasure in usual activities.

*Patient education information is highlighted in color.

# Tricyclic Antidepressants

Amitriptyline    Maprotiline
Clomipramine    Nortriptyline
Desipramine    Protriptyline
Doxepin    Trimipramine
Imipramine

In addition to the implications summarized below, see above for implications that apply to all antidepressants.

## Preadministration Assessment

### Therapeutic Goal
Alleviation of symptoms of major depression.

### Baseline Data
Assess psychologic status. Arrange for an EKG for patients with cardiac disease and for patients over 40.

### Identifying High-Risk Patients
TCAs are generally *contraindicated* for patients taking *MAOIs*.

Use all TCAs with *caution* in patients with *cardiac disorders* (e.g., coronary heart disease, progressive heart failure, paroxysmal tachycardia), *elevated intraocular pressure*, *history of urinary retention*, *hyperthyroidism*, *seizure disorders*, and *liver or kidney dysfunction*.

*Doxepin* is *contraindicated* for patients with *glaucoma* or a tendency to *urinary retention*.

*Maprotiline* is *contraindicated* for patients with *seizure disorders*.

## Implementation: Administration

### Routes
Oral (usual).
IM (occasional).

### Administration
Instruct the patient to take medication daily as prescribed and not PRN. Warn the patient not to discontinue treatment once mood has improved, since doing so may result in relapse. Once an effective dosage has been established, the entire daily dose can usually be taken at bedtime.

## Ongoing Evaluation and Interventions

### Minimizing Adverse Effects
***Orthostatic Hypotension.*** Inform patients about symptoms of hypotension (dizziness, lightheadedness), and advise them to sit or lie down if these occur. Inform patients that hypotension can be minimized by moving slowly when assuming an erect posture. For the hospitalized patient, monitor blood pressure and pulse rate on a regular schedule; take measurements while the patient is lying down and again after the patient has been sitting or standing for 1 to 2 minutes. If blood pressure is low or pulse rate is high, withhold medication and inform the physician.

***Anticholinergic Effects.*** Forewarn patients about possible anticholinergic effects (dry mouth, blurred vision, photophobia, urinary hesitancy, constipation, tachycardia), and advise them to notify the physician if these are troublesome. A detailed summary of nursing implications for anticholinergic drugs is presented in Chapter 15.

***Diaphoresis.*** TCAs promote sweating (despite their anticholinergic properties). Excessive sweating may necessitate frequent changes of bedding and clothing.

***Sedation.*** Sedation is most intense during the first weeks of therapy and declines with continued drug use. Advise the patient to avoid hazardous activities (e.g., driving, operating dangerous machinery) if sedation is significant. Administration at bedtime minimizes daytime sedation and promotes sleep.

***Cardiotoxicity.*** TCAs can disrupt cardiac function, but usually only when taken in excessive doses or by patients with heart disease. Elderly patients and those with heart disease should receive an EKG prior to treatment and periodically thereafter.

***Seizures.*** TCAs decrease seizure threshold. Exercise caution in patients with seizure disorders.

***Hypomania.*** TCAs may cause mood to shift from depression to hypomania. If hypomania develops, the patient must be evaluated to determine if elation is drug induced or indicative of bipolar disorder.

### Minimizing Adverse Interactions
***MAO Inhibitors.*** Rarely, the combination of a TCA and an MAO inhibitor has produced hypertensive episodes and hypertensive crisis. Exercise caution if this combination is employed.

***Sympathomimetic Agents.*** TCAs decrease the effects of indirect-acting sympathomimetics (e.g., ephedrine, amphetamine), but potentiate the actions of direct-acting sympathomimetics (e.g., epinephrine, dopamine). If sympathomimetics are to be used, these effects must be accounted for.

***Anticholinergic Agents.*** Drugs capable of blocking muscarinic receptors will enhance the anticholinergic effects of TCAs. Warn the patient against concurrent use of other anticholinergic drugs (e.g., scopolamine, antihistamines, phenothiazines).

***CNS Depressants.*** These drugs will enhance the depressant effects of TCAs. Warn the patient against using alcohol and all other drugs with CNS-depressant properties (e.g., opioids, antihistamines, barbiturates, benzodiazepines).

# Selective Serotonin Reuptake Inhibitors

Fluoxetine        Paroxetine
Fluvoxamine     Sertraline

In addition to the implications summarized below, see above for implications that apply to all antidepressants.

## Preadministration Assessment

### Therapeutic Goal
*All SSRIs.* Relief of symptoms of major depression.

*Fluoxetine, fluvoxamine, sertraline.* Relief of symptoms of obsessive-compulsive disorder.

### Identifying High-Risk Patients
SSRIs are *contraindicated* for patients taking *MAOIs*.

Use with *caution* in patients with *liver disease*, in the *elderly*, and in *women who are pregnant or breastfeeding*.

## Implementation: Administration

### Route
Oral.

### Administration
All SSRIs may be administered with food. Administration in the morning minimizes disruption of sleep.

Warn the patient not to discontinue treatment once mood has improved, since doing so could result in relapse.

## Ongoing Evaluation and Interventions

### Minimizing Adverse Effects
*CNS Stimulation. Fluoxetine, paroxetine,* and *sertraline* can cause nervousness, insomnia, and anxiety. These reactions may respond to a decrease in dosage. (Fluvoxamine causes mild sedation.)

*Serotonin Syndrome.* Symptoms of this potentially fatal syndrome include agitation, confusion, disorientation, anxiety, hallucinations, poor concentration, incoordination, myoclonus, hyperreflexia, excessive sweating, tremor, and fever. The risk is reduced by avoiding concurrent use of SSRIs and MAOIs. Serotonin syndrome resolves spontaneously after discontinuing the SSRI.

*Sexual Dysfunction.* Inform patients about possible sexual dysfunction (e.g., anorgasmia), and encourage them to report problems.

*Dizziness and Fatigue.* Inform patients about possible dizziness and fatigue, and advise them to exercise caution while performing hazardous tasks (e.g., driving).

*Rash. Fluoxetine* may cause rash. Inform patients about the risk of rash and instruct them to notify the physician if rash develops. Treatment consists of drug therapy (antihistamines, glucocorticoids) or withdrawal of fluoxetine.

### Minimizing Adverse Interactions
*Monoamine Oxidase Inhibitors.* MAOIs increase the risk of serotonin syndrome and hence must not be combined with SSRIs. Withdraw MAOIs at least 14 days before starting an SSRI. Withdraw fluoxetine 5 weeks before starting an MAOI; withdraw paroxetine or sertraline at least 2 weeks before starting an MAOI.

*Tricyclic Depressants and Lithium. Fluoxetine* can increase levels of these drugs. Exercise caution.

# Monoamine Oxidase Inhibitors

Phenelzine
Tranylcypromine

## Preadministration Assessment

In addition to the implications summarized below, see above for implications that apply to all antidepressants.

### Therapeutic Goal
Alleviation of symptoms of major depression, especially atypical depression.

### Identifying High-Risk Patients
MAOIs are *contraindicated* for patients taking *SSRIs* and for patients with *pheochromocytoma, congestive heart failure, liver disease, severe renal impairment, cerebrovascular defect* (known or suspected), *cardiovascular disease,* and *hypertension* and for patients *over the age of 60* (because of possible cerebral sclerosis associated with vessel damage).

Use with *caution* in patients taking *TCAs*.

## Implementation: Administration

### Route
Oral.

### Administration
Instruct the patient to take MAOIs every day as prescribed and not PRN. Warn the patient not to discontinue treatment once mood has improved, since doing so may result in relapse.

## Ongoing Evaluation and Interventions

### Minimizing Adverse Effects
*Hypertensive Crisis.* Dietary tyramine, certain other dietary constituents (see Table 30–4), and indirect-acting

sympathomimetics (e.g., amphetamine, methylphenidate, ephedrine, cocaine) can precipitate a hypertensive crisis in patients taking MAOIs.

Inform patients about symptoms of hypertensive crisis (headache, palpitations, tachycardia, nausea, vomiting), and instruct them to notify the physician or report to an emergency department if these develop.

To reduce the risk of hypertensive crisis, the following precautions must be observed: (1) do not give MAOIs to patients who are suicidal or who are considered incapable of rigid adherence to dietary constraints; (2) forewarn the patient about the hazard of hypertensive crisis and the need to avoid tyramine-rich foods and sympathomimetic drugs; (3) provide the patient with a list of specific foods to avoid (see Table 30-4); and (4) instruct the patient to avoid all drugs not approved by the physician.

If hypertensive crisis develops, blood pressure can be lowered with IV phentolamine or sublingual nifedipine.

***Orthostatic Hypotension.*** Inform patients about signs of hypotension (dizziness, lightheadedness), and advise them to sit or lie down if these occur. Inform patients that hypotension can be minimized by moving slowly when assuming an erect posture. For the hospitalized patient, monitor blood pressure and pulse rate on a regular schedule. Take these measurements while the patient is lying down and again after the patient has been sitting or standing for 1 to 2 minutes. If blood pressure is low, withhold medication and inform the physician.

## Minimizing Adverse Interactions

***All Drugs.*** MAOIs can interact adversely with many other drugs. Instruct the patient to avoid all medications—prescription and nonprescription—that have not been specifically approved by the physician.

***Indirect-Acting Sympathomimetics.*** Concurrent use with MAOIs can precipitate a hypertensive crisis. Warn the patient against use of any indirect-acting sympathomimetics (e.g., ephedrine, methylphenidate, amphetamines, cocaine).

***Tricyclic Antidepressants.*** Concurrent use with MAOIs can produce hypertensive episodes and hypertensive crisis. Use this combination with caution.

***SSRIs.*** Concurrent use with MAOIs can cause serotonin syndrome. Avoid the combination.

***Antihypertensive Drugs.*** These drugs will potentiate the hypotensive effects of MAOIs. If these agents are combined, monitor blood pressure periodically.

***Meperidine.*** Meperidine can produce hyperthermia in patients taking MAOIs and should be avoided.

# CHAPTER 31

# Drugs for Bipolar Disorder

**Bipolar Disorder (Manic-Depressive Illness)**
    Clinical Manifestations
    Treatment Strategy
**Lithium**
**Carbamazepine and Valproic Acid**

ur topic in this chapter is drug therapy of bipolar disorder, also known as manic-depressive illness. The mainstay of therapy is lithium, and we will focus largely on this agent.

## Bipolar Disorder (Manic-Depressive Illness)

### Clinical Manifestations

Manic-depressive illness is a cyclic disorder characterized by recurrent fluctuations in mood. Typically, patients experience alternating episodes of mania and depression separated by periods in which mood is normal. The characteristics of manic episodes are described below; the characteristics of depressive episodes are described in Chapter 30 and won't be repeated here.

*Manic episodes* are characterized by persistently heightened, expansive, or irritable mood—typically associated with hyperactivity, excessive enthusiasm, and flight of ideas. Manic individuals display overactivity at work and at play and have a reduced need for sleep. Mania produces excessive sociability and talkativeness. Extreme self-confidence, grandiose ideas, and delusions of importance are common. Manic individuals often indulge in high-risk activities (e.g., questionable business deals, reckless driving, gambling, sexual indiscretions), giving no forethought to the consequences. In severe cases, symptoms may resemble those of paranoid schizophrenia (hallucinations, delusions, bizarre behavior). Specific diagnostic criteria for a manic episode as described in the *Diagnostic and Statistical Manual of Mental Disorders*, fourth edition, are summarized in Table 31–1.

As noted, most individuals with bipolar disorder go through alternating episodes of mania and depression. Untreated episodes of mania or depression generally last from 4 to 13 months. For the majority of patients, periods of normal mood separate the episodes of mania and depression. As time passes, manic and depressive episodes tend to occur more frequently.

### Treatment Strategy

#### Nondrug Therapy

Ideally, bipolar disorder should be treated with a combination of drugs and adjunctive psychotherapy (individual, group, or family); drug therapy alone is not optimal. Bipolar disorder is a chronic illness that requires supportive therapy and education for the patient and family. Counseling can help patients cope with the sequelae of manic episodes, such as strained relationships, reduced self-confidence, and a sense of shame regarding uncontrolled behavior. Certain life stresses (e.g., moving, job loss, bereavement, childbirth) can precipitate a mood change; therapy can help reduce the destabilizing impact of these events. Patients should be taught to recognize early symptoms of mood change, and encouraged to contact the physician immediately if these develop.

#### Drug Therapy

*Overview of Treatment.* Drug therapy of bipolar disorder is summarized in Table 31–2. As indicated, the mainstay of therapy is *lithium*. Lithium can provide symptomatic control during both the manic phase and the depressed phase. In addition, when taken *prophylactically*, lithium can reduce the frequency and severity of recurrent manic and depressive episodes.

When used for initial control of acute mania, lithium is usually combined with a *benzodiazepine* (e.g., lorazepam) or an *antipsychotic* (e.g., haloperidol). These drugs help suppress symptoms until lithium takes effect. Once lithium has taken effect—in about 2 weeks—the benzodiazepine or antipsychotic should be gradually withdrawn.

When used during the depressive phase, lithium can be combined with an antidepressant. Options include a *tri-*

## TABLE 31-1. DSM-IV CRITERIA FOR A MANIC EPISODE*

A. A distinct period of abnormally and persistently elevated, expansive, or irritable mood, lasting at least 1 week (or any duration if hospitalization is necessary).

B. During the period of mood disturbance, three (or more) of the following symptoms have persisted (four if the mood is only irritable) and have been present to a significant degree:

- Inflated self-esteem or grandiosity
- Decreased need for sleep (e.g., feels rested after only 3 hours of sleep)
- More talkative than usual or pressure to keep talking
- Flight of ideas or subjective experience that thoughts are racing
- Distractibility (i.e., attention too easily drawn to unimportant or irrelevant external stimuli)
- Increase in goal-directed activity (either socially, at work or school, or sexually) or psychomotor agitation
- Excessive involvement in pleasurable activities that have a high potential for painful consequences (e.g., engaging in unrestrained buying sprees, sexual indiscretions, or foolish business investments)

C. The mood disturbance is sufficiently severe to cause marked impairment in occupational functioning or in usual social activities or relationships with others, or to necessitate hospitalization to prevent harm to self or others, or there are psychotic features.

D. The symptoms are not due to the direct physiologic effects of a substance (e.g., a drug of abuse, a medication, or other treatment) or a general medical condition (e.g., hyperthyroidism).[†]

---

\* Modified from American Psychiatric Association. *Diagnostic and Statistical Manual of Mental Disorders*, 4th ed. Washington, DC: American Psychiatric Press, 1994, p. 332, reprinted by permission.

[†] Manic-like episodes that are clearly caused by somatic antidepressant treatment (e.g., medication, electroconvulsive therapy, light therapy) should not count toward a diagnosis of bipolar disorder.

---

*cyclic antidepressant* (e.g., imipramine) and *bupropion* [Wellbutrin]. Bupropion may be preferred in that this drug is less likely to transport the patient from depression into hypomania or frank mania.

In recent years, two antiseizure drugs—*carbamazepine* and *valproic acid*—have proved effective for bipolar disorder. Both drugs can control symptoms during manic episodes and depressive episodes, and both can provide prophylaxis against recurrent mania and depression. These agents have been used both as adjuncts to lithium and as alternatives to lithium.

## TABLE 31-2. DRUG THERAPY OF BIPOLAR DISORDER

| Illness Phase | Drug Therapy |
|---|---|
| Manic phase: initial treatment  If hallucinations | Lithium* + a benzodiazepine  Lithium* + an antipsychotic |
| Manic phase: later treatment | Lithium* alone |
| Depressed phase | Lithium* + a tricyclic antidepressant or bupropion |
| Normalized mood | Lithium* (for prophylaxis against recurrence of mania or depression) |

---

*For lithium nonresponders, addition or substitution of valproic acid or carbamazepine may be effective.

**Promoting Compliance.** Poor patient compliance can frustrate attempts to treat acute manic episodes. Patients may resist treatment because they fail to see anything wrong with their thinking or behavior. Furthermore, the experience is not necessarily unpleasant. In fact, individuals going through a manic episode may well enjoy it. As a result, in order to ensure adequate treatment, hospitalization is often needed. To achieve this, collaboration with the patient's family may be required. Since hospitalization per se won't guarantee compliance, lithium administration should be observed to ensure that each dose is actually taken.

After an acute manic episode has been controlled, long-term prophylactic therapy is indicated, making compliance an ongoing concern. To promote compliance, the patient and family should be educated about the nature of manic-depressive illness and the importance of taking medication as prescribed. Family members can help ensure compliance by overseeing medication use, and by urging the patient to visit a physician or psychiatric clinic if a pattern of noncompliance develops.

## Lithium

Lithium can provide symptomatic control in patients with manic-depressive illness. Beneficial effects were first described by John Cade, an Australian, in 1949. However, because of concerns about toxicity, lithium was not approved for use in the United States until 1970. Since lithium has a low therapeutic index, there is a real risk of toxicity. Because significant injury can occur when plasma drug levels are only slightly greater than therapeutic, monitoring lithium levels is mandatory.

## Chemistry

Lithium is a simple inorganic ion that carries a single positive charge. In the periodic table of elements, lithium falls within the same group as potassium and sodium. Accordingly, lithium has properties in common with these two elements. Lithium occurs naturally in animal tissues but has no known physiologic function.

## Pharmacokinetics

*Absorption and Distribution.* Lithium is well absorbed following oral administration. The drug distributes evenly to all tissues and body fluids.

*Excretion.* Lithium has a short half-life, owing to rapid renal excretion. Because of its short half-life (and high toxicity), the drug must be administered in divided daily doses; large, single daily doses cannot be used. Because lithium is excreted by the kidneys, it must be employed with great care in patients with renal impairment.

Sodium depletion will *decrease* renal excretion of lithium, thereby causing the drug to accumulate. Toxicity may result. Accordingly, it is important that sodium levels remain normal. Patients should be instructed to maintain normal sodium intake; a sodium-free diet cannot be used. Since diuretics promote sodium loss, these agents must be employed with caution. Sodium loss secondary to diarrhea can be sufficient to cause lithium accumulation, and the patient should be forewarned of this possibility.

Dehydration will cause lithium retention by the kidneys, posing the risk of accumulation to dangerous levels. Potential causes of dehydration include hot weather and diarrhea. Counsel patients to maintain adequate hydration.

*Plasma Lithium Levels.* Measurement of plasma lithium levels is an essential feature of treatment. *Lithium levels must be kept below 1.5 mEq/L; levels greater than this can produce significant toxicity.* For *initial* therapy of a manic episode, lithium levels should range from 0.8 to 1.4 mEq/L. Once the desired therapeutic effect has been achieved, the dosage should be reduced to produce *maintenance* drug levels of 0.4 to 1.0 mEq/L. Blood for lithium determinations should be drawn in the morning, *12 hours after the evening dose.*

## Therapeutic Uses

*Bipolar Disorder.* Lithium is the drug of choice for controlling manic episodes in patients with bipolar disorder and for long-term prophylaxis against recurrent mania and depression in these patients.

In manic patients, lithium reduces euphoria, hyperactivity, and other symptoms but does not cause sedation. Antimanic effects begin 5 to 7 days after the onset of treatment. However, full effects may not be seen until 2 to 3 weeks. For many patients, adjunctive therapy with a benzodiazepine, an antipsychotic agent, or both can be helpful. Benzodiazepines (e.g., lorazepam) are used to provide sedation in patients with relatively mild symptoms. Antipsychotics (e.g., haloperidol) may be required to provide rapid control in patients with hallucinations and other psychotic symptoms. Once lithium takes effect, the benzodiazepine or antipsychotic should be gradually withdrawn.

Prophylaxis with lithium may not prevent episodes of depression. If depression occurs, adjunctive therapy with an antidepressant is indicated.

*Other Uses.* Although approved only for treatment of manic-depressive illness, lithium has been used with varying degrees of success in other psychiatric disorders, including *alcoholism, bulimia, schizophrenia, premenstrual syndrome,* and *glucocorticoid-induced psychosis.* Nonpsychiatric uses include *hyperthyroidism, cluster headache, migraine,* and *syndrome of inappropriate secretion of antidiuretic hormone.* In addition, lithium can *raise neutrophil counts* in children with chronic neutropenia and in patients receiving anticancer drugs or zidovudine (AZT).

### Mechanism of Action in Manic-Depressive Illness

We do not know the underlying cause of manic-depressive illness, nor do we know how lithium stabilizes mood. Lithium has multiple effects on the nervous system. The drug can modulate synaptic transmission mediated by monoamine neurotransmitters (norepinephrine, serotonin, dopamine). Also, lithium can alter the distribution of neuronally important ions (calcium, sodium, magnesium). In addition, lithium can influence the function of second-messenger systems. Which, if any, of these actions underlies lithium's therapeutic effects is unknown.

## Adverse Effects

Adverse effects of lithium can be divided into two categories: (1) effects that occur at excessive drug levels and (2) effects that occur at therapeutic drug levels. In the discussion that follows, adverse effects produced at excessive lithium levels are considered as a group. Effects produced at therapeutic levels are considered individually.

*Adverse Effects That Occur When Lithium Levels Are Excessive.* Certain toxicities are closely correlated with the concentration of lithium in plasma. As indicated in Table 31–3, mild responses (e.g., fine hand tremor, gastrointestinal upset, thirst, muscle weakness) can develop at lithium levels that are still within the therapeutic range (i.e., below 1.5 mEq/L). When plasma levels exceed 1.5 mEq/L, more serious toxicities begin to appear. At drug levels above 2.5 mEq/L, death has resulted. Patients should be informed about early signs of toxicity and instructed to interrupt lithium use if these appear. The most common cause of lithium accumulation in compliant patients is sodium depletion.

To keep lithium levels within the therapeutic range, plasma drug levels should be monitored routinely. Levels should be measured every 2 to 3 days at the beginning of treatment and every 1 to 3 months during maintenance therapy.

Treatment of acute overdosage is primarily supportive; there is no specific antidote to lithium toxicity. The

## TABLE 31-3. TOXICITIES ASSOCIATED WITH EXCESSIVE PLASMA LEVELS OF LITHIUM

| Plasma Lithium Level | Signs of Toxicity |
|---|---|
| <1.5 mEq/L | Nausea, vomiting, diarrhea, thirst, polyuria, lethargy, slurred speech, muscle weakness, fine hand tremor |
| 1.5–2.0 mEq/L | Persistent GI upset, coarse hand tremor, confusion, hyperirritability of muscles, EKG changes, sedation, incoordination |
| 2.0–2.5 mEq/L | Ataxia, giddiness, high output of dilute urine, serious EKG changes, fasciculations, tinnitus, blurred vision, clonic movements, seizures, stupor, severe hypotension, coma, death (usually secondary to pulmonary complications) |
| >2.5 mEq/L | Symptoms may progress rapidly to generalized convulsions, oliguria, and death |

severely intoxicated patient should be hospitalized. Hemodialysis is an effective means of lithium removal and should be considered whenever drug levels exceed 2.5 mEq/L.

***Tremor.*** Patients may develop a fine hand tremor, especially in the fingers, that can interfere with writing and other motor skills. Lithium-induced tremor can be augmented by stress, fatigue, and certain drugs (antidepressants, antipsychotics, caffeine). Tremor can be reduced with a beta-adrenergic blocking agent (e.g., propranolol) and by measures that reduce peak levels of lithium (i.e., dosage reduction, use of divided doses, or use of a sustained-release formulation).

***Renal Toxicity.*** Chronic administration of lithium has occasionally been associated with degenerative changes in the kidney. The risk of renal injury can be reduced by keeping the dosage low and, when possible, avoiding long-term lithium therapy. Kidney function should be assessed prior to treatment and once a year thereafter.

***Goiter.*** Long-term use of lithium can cause goiter (enlargement of the thyroid gland). Although usually benign, lithium-induced goiter is sometimes associated with hypothyroidism. Treatment with thyroid hormone or withdrawal of lithium will reverse thyroid hypertrophy. Measurement of thyroid hormones ($T_3$ and $T_4$) and thyroid-stimulating hormone (TSH) should be obtained prior to treatment and annually thereafter.

***Teratogenesis.*** Use of lithium during the first trimester of pregnancy is associated with an 11% incidence of birth defects (usually malformations of the heart). Accordingly, *lithium is contraindicated during the first trimester of pregnancy.* Furthermore, unless the benefits of therapy clearly outweigh the potential risk to the fetus, lithium should be avoided during the remainder of pregnancy as

well. Women of child-bearing age should be counseled about the importance of avoiding pregnancy while taking lithium.

***Use in Lactation.*** Lithium readily enters breast milk and can achieve concentrations that are potentially harmful to the nursing infant. Consequently, breast-feeding during lithium therapy should be discouraged.

***Polyuria.*** Polyuria occurs in 50% to 70% of patients taking lithium chronically. In some patients daily urine output may exceed 3 L. Lithium promotes polyuria by antagonizing the effects of antidiuretic hormone. To maintain adequate hydration, patients should be instructed to drink 8 to 12 glasses of fluids daily. Polyuria, nocturia, and excessive thirst can discourage patients from complying with the prescribed regimen.

Lithium-induced polyuria can be *reduced* with a *thiazide diuretic.* The mechanism of this paradoxical effect is not known. Unfortunately, thiazides can increase plasma levels of lithium (perhaps by promoting sodium excretion). Accordingly, a reduction in lithium dosage will be required.

***Early Adverse Effects.*** Several responses occur early in treatment and then usually subside. *Gastrointestinal effects* (e.g., nausea, diarrhea, abdominal bloating, anorexia) are common but transient. About 30% of patients experience transient *fatigue, muscle weakness, headache, confusion,* and *memory impairment. Polyuria* and *thirst* occur in 30% to 50% of those treated, and in many cases these effects persist.

***Other Effects.*** Lithium can cause mild, reversible *leukocytosis* (10,000 to 18,000 WBC/mm$^3$); complete blood counts with a differential should be obtained prior to treatment and annually thereafter. Possible *dermatologic reactions* include psoriasis, acne, folliculitis, and alopecia.

### Drug Interactions

***Diuretics.*** Diuretics promote sodium loss, and can thereby increase the risk of lithium toxicity. Toxicity can occur because, in the presence of low sodium, renal excretion of lithium is reduced, causing lithium levels to rise.

***Anticholinergic Drugs.*** Anticholinergics can cause urinary hesitancy; coupled with lithium-induced polyuria, this can result in considerable discomfort. Unfortunately, the combination of lithium plus an anticholinergic drug cannot always be avoided: patients frequently require concurrent therapy with agents that have prominent anticholinergic properties (antipsychotics, tricyclic antidepressants).

### Preparations, Dosage, and Administration

***Preparations and Administration.*** Lithium is available as two salts: *lithium carbonate* and *lithium citrate.* With either salt, administration is oral. Lithium *carbonate* is dispensed in capsules, standard tablets, and slow-release tablets. Lithium *citrate* is dispensed in a syrup. Lithium formulations and trade names are summarized in Table 31-4.

## TABLE 31–4. LITHIUM PREPARATIONS

| Lithium Salt | Formulation | Lithium Content* | Trade Name |
|---|---|---|---|
| Lithium carbonate ($Li_2CO_3$) | Capsules | 4.06 mEq lithium (150 mg $Li_2CO_3$)<br>8.12 mEq lithium (300 mg $Li_2CO_3$)<br>16.24 mEq lithium (600 mg $Li_2CO_3$) | Eskalith, Lithonate |
| | Tablets | 8.12 mEq lithium (300 mg $Li_2CO_3$) | Eskalith, Lithane, Lithotabs |
| | Tablets: slow-release | 8.12 mEq lithium (300 mg $Li_2CO_3$) | Lithobid |
| | Tablets: controlled release | 12.18 mEq lithium (450 mg $Li_2CO_3$) | Eskalith CR |
| Lithium citrate | Syrup | 8 mEq lithium/5 ml (equivalent to 300 mg $Li_2CO_3$) | Cibalith-S |

*Lithium content is expressed in two ways: (1) mEq of lithium ion and (2) mg of the particular lithium salt of which the preparation is composed.

Lithium can cause gastric upset. This response can be reduced by administering lithium with meals or with milk.

**Dosing.** Dosing with lithium is highly individualized. Dosage adjustments are based on plasma drug levels and clinical response.

Plasma drug levels should be kept within the therapeutic range. Levels between 0.8 and 1.4 mEq/L are generally appropriate for *acute therapy* of manic episodes. For *maintenance therapy*, lithium levels should range from 0.4 to 1.0 mEq/L. (Levels of 0.6 to 0.8 mEq/L are effective for most patients.) To avoid serious toxicity, *lithium levels should not exceed 1.5 mEq/L.*

Knowledge of plasma drug levels is not the only guide to lithium dosing; consideration of the clinical response is at least as important. That is, when evaluating the appropriateness of a lithium dosage, we must not forget to look at the patient. Laboratory tests are all well and good, but they are not a substitute for clinical assessment. If, for example, blood levels of lithium appear proper but clinical evaluation indicates toxicity, there is no question as to the action that should be taken: the dosage should be reduced—despite the apparent acceptability of the dosage as reflected by plasma drug levels.

Because of its short half-life and low therapeutic index, *lithium cannot be administered in a single daily dose*; with once-a-day dosing, peak drug levels would be excessive. Hence, a typical dosage is 300 mg (of lithium carbonate) taken 3 or 4 times a day. A dosage of 600 mg twice daily is acceptable, provided that an extended-release formulation is employed; however, even these preparations cannot be given on a once-daily basis.

# Carbamazepine and Valproic Acid

Carbamazepine [Tegretol, others] and valproic acid [Depakene, Depakote] were originally developed and marketed for treatment of seizure disorders. In recent years, these drugs have been used with success to treat bipolar disorder. At this time, carbamazepine and valproic acid are generally reserved for patients who have failed to respond to lithium or who cannot tolerate lithium's side effects. To initiate therapy, carbamazepine or valproic acid is usually given *in combination with* lithium—not as a substitute for lithium. If the combination works, lithium may be withdrawn later. Valproate is safer than carbamazepine and may be preferred for this reason. The basic pharmacology of carbamazepine and valproate and their use in seizure disorders is discussed in Chapter 23.

## Carbamazepine

Carbamazepine was the first drug to be widely studied as an alternative to lithium for patients with bipolar disorder. Like lithium, carbamazepine reduces symptoms during manic *and* depressive episodes. In addition, the drug appears to provide effective prophylaxis against recurrence of mania and depression. For patients with severe mania, and for those who cycle rapidly, carbamazepine may be superior to lithium. When given to manic patients who have failed to respond to lithium, carbamazepine has had a success rate of about 60%. For treatment of acute manic episodes, the dosage should be low initially (200 to 400 mg/day) and then gradually increased to as much as 1.6 to 2.2 gm/day. Target trough plasma levels are 6 to 12 μg/ml. Side effects that are especially common or troublesome include sedation, gastrointestinal disturbance, tremor, leukopenia, and hepatotoxicity. The mechanism by which carbamazepine stabilizes mood is unknown.

## Valproic Acid

Valproic acid is a promising alternative to lithium for bipolar patients who have failed to respond to lithium or who cannot tolerate its side effects. Clinical studies indicate that valproic acid can control symptoms in acute manic episodes and can provide prophylaxis against recurrent episodes of mania and depression. Like carbamazepine, valproic acid appears especially useful for patients with rapid-cycling bipolar disorder. Therapeutic effects develop over 1 to 2 weeks. Common or troublesome side effects include sedation, nausea, tremor, hepatotoxicity, and hair loss. Nausea can be reduced by using delayed-release tablets or by applying the "sprinkle" formulation to food. The initial dosage for acute mania in adults is 500 to 1000 mg/day in two to four divided doses. Maintenance dosages range from 250 to 500 mg/day. The target plasma drug level is 50 to 125 µg/ml. Valproic acid alters GABA–mediated neurotransmission, and this action may underlie the drug's mood–stabilizing effects.

## KEY POINTS

- Lithium is the principal drug for bipolar disorder.
- To minimize the risk of toxicity, lithium levels must be monitored. The trough level, measured 12 hours after the evening dose, must be kept below 1.5 mEq/L.

- Common side effects that occur at therapeutic lithium levels include tremor, goiter, and polyuria.
- Lithium is teratogenic and must not be used during the first trimester of pregnancy—and should be avoided later in pregnancy if possible.
- A reduction in sodium levels will reduce lithium excretion, causing lithium levels to rise—possibly to toxic concentrations. Patients must maintain normal sodium intake and levels.
- Two anticonvulsants, carbamazepine [Tegretol, others] and valproic acid [Depakene, Depakote], are employed as adjuncts or alternatives to lithium for patients with bipolar disorder.

# Summary of Major Nursing Implications*

## Lithium

### Preadministration Assessment

#### Therapeutic Goal
Control of acute manic episodes in patients with manic-depressive illness, and prophylaxis against recurrent mania and depression in these patients.

#### Baseline Data
Obtain baseline measurements of cardiac status (EKG, blood pressure, pulse), hematologic status (complete blood counts with differential), serum electrolytes, renal function (serum creatinine, creatinine clearance, urinalysis), and thyroid function ($T_3$, $T_4$, and TSH).

#### Identifying High–Risk Patients
Lithium is *contraindicated* during the *first trimester of pregnancy*, and should be avoided later in pregnancy whenever possible. Use with *caution* in the presence of *renal disease, cardiovascular disease, dehydration, sodium depletion,* and *concurrent therapy with diuretics.*

### Implementation: Administration

#### Route
Oral.

#### Administration
Advise the patient to administer lithium with meals or a glass of milk to decrease gastric upset. Instruct the patient to swallow slow-release and controlled-release tablets intact, without crushing or chewing.

#### Promoting Compliance
Rigid adherence to the prescribed regimen is important: deviations in dosage size and timing can cause toxicity, and inadequate dosing may cause relapse.

To promote compliance, educate the patient and his or her family about the nature of manic-depressive illness and the importance of taking lithium as prescribed. Encourage family members to oversee lithium use, and advise them to urge the patient to visit the physician or a psychiatric clinic if a pattern of noncompliance develops.

When medicating inpatients, make certain that each lithium dose is ingested.

### Ongoing Evaluation and Interventions

#### Monitoring Summary
***Lithium Levels.*** Monitor lithium levels to ensure that they remain within the therapeutic range (0.8 to 1.4 mEq/L for initial therapy and 0.4 to 1.0 mEq/L for maintenance therapy). Levels should be measured every 2 to 3 days during initial therapy, and every 1 to 3 months during maintenance. Blood for lithium determination should be drawn in the morning, 12 hours after the evening dose.

***Other Parameters to Monitor.*** Evaluate the patient at least once a year for hematologic status (complete blood count with differential), serum electrolytes, renal function (serum creatinine, creatinine clearance, urinalysis), and thyroid function ($T_3$, $T_4$, and TSH).

#### Evaluating Therapeutic Effects
Evaluate the patient for abatement of manic symptoms (e.g., flight of ideas, pressure of speech, hyperactivity) and for mood stabilization.

#### Minimizing Adverse Effects
***Effects Caused by Excessive Drug Levels.*** Excessive lithium levels can result in serious adverse effects (see Table 31-3). Lithium levels must be monitored (see *Monitoring Summary*) and the dosage adjusted accordingly.

Teach the patient about signs of toxicity, and instruct him or her to withhold medication and notify the physician if these develop.

Renal impairment can cause lithium accumulation. Kidney function should be assessed prior to treatment and once yearly thereafter.

---

*Patient education information is highlighted in color.

Sodium deficiency can cause lithium to accumulate. Instruct the patient to maintain normal sodium intake. Forewarn the patient that diarrhea can cause significant sodium loss. Diuretics promote sodium excretion and must be used with caution.

In the event of severe toxicity, hospitalization may be required. If lithium levels exceed 2.5 mEq/L, hemodialysis should be considered.

**Tremor.** Lithium can cause fine hand tremor that can interfere with motor skills. Tremor can be reduced with a beta-adrenergic blocker (e.g., propranolol) and by measures that reduce peak lithium levels (dosage reduction, use of divided doses or a sustained-release formulation).

**Goiter.** Lithium can promote goiter. Plasma levels of $T_3$, $T_4$, and TSH should be measured prior to treatment and yearly thereafter. Treat hypothyroidism with thyroid hormone.

**Renal Toxicity.** Lithium can cause renal damage. Kidney function should be assessed prior to treatment and once a year thereafter. If renal impairment develops, lithium dosage must be reduced.

**Polyuria.** Lithium increases urine output. Polyuria can be suppressed with a thiazide diuretic; the mechanism of this paradoxical effect is not known. Instruct the patient to drink 8 to 12 glasses of fluid daily to maintain hydration.

**Use in Pregnancy and Lactation.** Lithium is associated with a high incidence of serious birth defects. The drug should be avoided during pregnancy, especially in the first trimester. Counsel women of child-bearing age about the importance of avoiding pregnancy.

Lithium enters breast milk. Advise patients to avoid breast-feeding.

# CHAPTER 32

# Benzodiazepines and Other Drugs for Anxiety and Insomnia

Benzodiazepines
Barbiturates
Nonbenzodiazepine-Nonbarbiturates
    Buspirone
    Zolpidem
    Miscellaneous General CNS Depressants

Management of Anxiety
Management of Insomnia

A nxiety and insomnia are common complaints, and the drugs employed for treatment are prescribed widely. Drugs used to relieve anxiety are called *antianxiety agents* or *anxiolytics*; an older term for these drugs is *tranquilizers*. Drugs that promote sleep are known as *hypnotics*. The distinction between antianxiety effects and hypnotic effects is frequently a matter of dosage: some drugs relieve anxiety in low doses and induce sleep in higher doses. Hence, a single drug may be considered both an antianxiety agent and a hypnotic agent, depending upon the reason for its use and the dosage employed.

Before the benzodiazepines became available, anxiety and insomnia were treated with barbiturates and other *general central nervous system (CNS) depressants*—drugs with multiple undesirable qualities: (1) These drugs are *powerful respiratory depressants* that can readily prove *fatal* in overdose. As a result, they are "drugs of choice" for *suicide*. (2) Because they produce subjective effects that many individuals find desirable, general CNS depressants often have a *high potential for abuse*. (3) With prolonged use, most general CNS depressants produce significant *tolerance and physical dependence*. (4) Barbiturates and certain other CNS depressants *induce synthesis of hepatic drug-metabolizing enzymes*, and can thereby decrease responses to other drugs. Since the benzodiazepines are just as effective as the general CNS depressants, but do not share their undesirable properties, benzodiazepines have largely replaced the general CNS depressants in the management of anxiety and insomnia.

## Benzodiazepines

Benzodiazepines are drugs of first choice for treating anxiety and insomnia. In addition, these agents are used to induce general anesthesia and to manage seizure disorders, muscle spasm, panic disorder, and withdrawal from alcohol.

Benzodiazepines were introduced in the early 1960s and are among the most widely prescribed drugs in the United States. Perhaps the most familiar member of the family is diazepam [Valium]. The most frequently prescribed members are lorazepam [Ativan] and alprazolam [Xanax].

The popularity of the benzodiazepines as sedatives and hypnotics stems from their clear superiority over the alternatives: barbiturates and other general CNS depressants. The benzodiazepines are safer than the general CNS depressants and have a lower potential for abuse. In addition, benzodiazepines produce less tolerance and physical dependence and are subject to fewer drug interactions. Contrasts between the benzodiazepines and barbiturates are summarized in Table 32-1.

Since all of the benzodiazepines produce nearly identical effects, we will consider the family as a group, rather than selecting a representative member as a prototype.

### Overview of Pharmacologic Effects

Practically all responses to benzodiazepines result from actions in the CNS. Benzodiazepines have few direct actions outside the CNS. All of the benzodiazepines produce a similar spectrum of responses. However, because of pharmacokinetic differences, individual benzodiazepines may differ in their clinical applications.

*Central Nervous System.* All beneficial effects of benzodiazepines and most adverse effects result from depressant actions in the CNS. With increasing dosage, effects progress from *sedation* to *hypnosis* to *stupor*.

Benzodiazepines depress neuronal function at multiple sites in the CNS. These drugs *reduce anxiety* through effects on the limbic system, a neuronal network associated

## TABLE 32–1. CONTRASTS BETWEEN BENZODIAZEPINES AND BARBITURATES

| Area of Comparison | Benzodiazepines | Barbiturates |
|---|---|---|
| Relative safety | High | Low |
| Maximal ability to depress CNS function | Low | High |
| Respiratory depressant ability | Low | High |
| Suicide potential | Low | High |
| Ability to cause physical dependence | Low* | High |
| Ability to cause tolerance | Low | High |
| Abuse potential | Low | High |
| Ability to induce drug metabolism | Low | High |

*Although dependence is low in most patients, significant dependence can develop with long-term, high-dose use.

with emotionality. They *promote sleep* through effects on cortical areas and on the sleep-wakefulness clock. They *induce muscle relaxation* through effects on supraspinal motor areas, including the cerebellum. Two important side effects—*confusion* and *anterograde amnesia*—result from effects on the hippocampus and cerebral cortex.

***Cardiovascular System.*** When taken orally, benzodiazepines have negligible effects on the heart and blood vessels. In contrast, when administered *intravenously*—even in therapeutic doses—benzodiazepines can produce profound hypotension and cardiac arrest.

***Respiratory System.*** In contrast to the barbiturates, the benzodiazepines are weak respiratory depressants. When taken alone in therapeutic doses, benzodiazepines produce little or no depression of respiration; and with toxic doses, respiratory depression is moderate at most. With oral therapy, clinically significant respiratory depression occurs only when benzodiazepines are combined with other CNS depressants (e.g., opioids, barbiturates, alcohol).

Although benzodiazepines generally have minimal effects on respiration, they can be a problem for patients with respiratory disorders. In patients with chronic obstructive pulmonary disease (COPD), benzodiazepines may worsen hypoventilation and hypoxemia. In patients with obstructive sleep apnea (OSA), benzodiazepines may exacerbate apneic episodes. In patients who snore, benzodiazepines may convert partial airway obstruction into OSA.

### Molecular Mechanism of Action

Benzodiazepines *potentiate the actions of gamma-aminobutyric acid* (GABA), an inhibitory neurotransmitter found throughout the CNS. These drugs enhance the actions of GABA by binding to specific receptors in a supramolecular structure known as the GABA receptor–chloride channel complex (Fig. 32-1). Please note that benzodiazepines act only by intensifying the effects of GABA; they do not act as direct GABA agonists.

Because benzodiazepines act by amplifying the actions of endogenous GABA, rather than by directly mimicking GABA, there is a limit to how much CNS depression these

drugs can produce. This explains why benzodiazepines are so much safer than the barbiturates—drugs that can directly mimic GABA. Since benzodiazepines simply potentiate the inhibitory effects of endogenous GABA, and since the amount of GABA in the CNS is finite, there is a built-in limit to the depth of CNS depression the benzodiazepines can produce. In contrast, since the barbiturates are direct-acting CNS depressants, maximal effects are limited only by the amount of barbiturate administered.

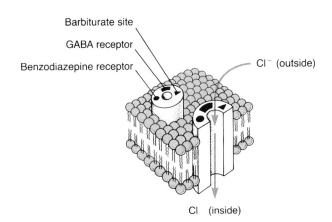

**Figure 32–1. Schematic model of the GABA receptor–chloride channel complex showing binding sites for benzodiazepines and barbiturates.** The GABA receptor-chloride channel complex, which spans the neuronal cell membrane, can exist in an open or closed configuration. Binding of GABA to its receptor causes the chloride channel to *open*. The resulting inward flow of chloride ions hyperpolarizes the neuron (makes the cell highly negative inside) and thereby decreases the cell's ability to fire. Hence GABA is an *inhibitory* neurotransmitter. Binding of a *benzodiazepine* to its receptor on the complex increases the frequency of drainel opening, thereby increasing chloride influx. Hence benzodiazepines enhance the inhibitory effects of GABA. In the absence of GABA, benzodiazepines have no effect on channel opening. Effects of *barbiturates* on the chloride channel are dose dependent: at low doses, barbiturates enhance the actions of GABA (by prolonging the duration of channel opening); at high doses, barbiturates directly mimic the actions of GABA.

## Pharmacokinetics

*Absorption and Distribution.* Most benzodiazepines are well absorbed following oral administration. Because of their high lipid solubility, benzodiazepines readily cross the blood-brain barrier to reach sites within the CNS.

*Metabolism.* Most benzodiazepines undergo extensive metabolic alterations. With few exceptions, the *metabolites are pharmacologically active.* As a result, responses produced by administering a particular benzodiazepine often persist long after the parent drug has disappeared from the plasma. Hence there may be a poor correlation between the plasma half-life of the parent drug and duration of pharmacologic effects. Flurazepam, for example, whose plasma half-life is only 2 to 3 hours, is converted into an active metabolite whose half-life is 50 hours. Hence administration of flurazepam produces long-lasting effects, despite the fact that within 8 to 12 hours of its administration, flurazepam itself can no longer be detected in the blood.

In patients with liver disease, metabolism of benzodiazepines can decline, thereby prolonging and intensifying responses. Because certain benzodiazepines (oxazepam, temazepam, and lorazepam) undergo very little metabolic alteration, these agents may be preferred for patients with hepatic impairment.

*Time Course of Action.* Benzodiazepines differ significantly from one another with regard to time course of action. Specifically, they differ in onset of action, duration of action, and tendency to accumulate with repeated dosing.

Because all of the benzodiazepines have essentially equivalent pharmacologic actions, selection among these drugs is based in large part on differences in time course. For example, if a patient needs medication to accelerate falling asleep, a benzodiazepine with a rapid onset of action (e.g., triazolam) would be indicated. However, if medication is needed to prevent waking later in the night, a benzodiazepine with a slower onset (e.g., estazolam) would be preferred. For treatment of anxiety, a drug with an intermediate duration of action is desirable. For treatment of any benzodiazepine-responsive condition in the elderly, a drug such as lorazepam, which is not likely to accumulate with repeated dosing, is generally preferred.

## Therapeutic Uses

The benzodiazepines have three principal indications: (1) anxiety, (2) insomnia, and (3) seizure disorders. In addition, these drugs are employed as preoperative medication and in the management of muscle spasm, panic disorder, and withdrawal from alcohol. Although all benzodiazepines share the same pharmacologic properties, and therefore might be equally effective for all applications, not every benzodiazepine is actually employed for all potential uses. The principal factors that determine the actual applications of a particular benzodiazepine are (1) the pharmacokinetic properties of the drug itself and (2) research and marketing decisions of pharmaceutical companies. Specific applications of individual benzodiazepines are summarized in Table 32-2.

*Anxiety.* Benzodiazepines are drugs of first choice for treating anxiety. Although all benzodiazepines have anxiolytic properties, only eight are marketed for this indication (see Table 32-3). Anxiolytic effects result from depressing neurotransmission in the limbic system and cortical areas. Guidelines for managing anxiety with benzodiazepines are presented later.

*Insomnia.* Benzodiazepines are drugs of first choice for treating insomnia. These drugs decrease latency time to falling asleep, they reduce awakenings, and they increase total sleeping time. Although all benzodiazepines can relieve insomnia, only five are marketed for this use (see Table 32-4). Management of insomnia with benzodiazepines is discussed later.

*Seizure Disorders.* Four benzodiazepines—diazepam, clonazepam, lorazepam, and clorazepate—are employed to treat seizure disorders. This application is discussed in Chapter 23.

*Muscle Spasm.* One benzodiazepine—diazepam—is used to relieve muscle spasm and spasticity (see Chapter 24). Effects on muscle tone are secondary to actions in the CNS. Diazepam cannot relieve spasm without causing sedation.

*Alcohol Withdrawal.* Diazepam and other benzodiazepines may be administered to facilitate withdrawal from alcohol (see Chapter 36). These drugs are helpful because cross-dependence with alcohol enables them to suppress symptoms of abstinence in individuals physically dependent on alcohol.

*Panic Disorder.* Alprazolam [Xanax], clonazepam [Klonopin], and lorazepam [Ativan] can provide effective treatment of panic disorder. These benzodiazepines and other drugs for panic disorder are discussed in Chapter 34.

*Induction of Anesthesia.* Three benzodiazepines—diazepam [Valium], lorazepam [Ativan], and midazolam [Versed]—can be given IV for induction of anesthesia. In addition, midazolam (in combination with an opioid analgesic) can be used to produce *conscious sedation*, a semiconscious state suitable for endoscopic procedures and minor surgeries. Benzodiazepines are also used for preoperative sedation. All of these anesthetic applications are discussed in Chapter 27.

## Adverse Effects

Benzodiazepines are generally well tolerated, and serious adverse reactions are rare. In contrast to barbiturates and other general CNS depressants, benzodiazepines are remarkably safe drugs.

*CNS Depression.* When taken in sleep-inducing doses, benzodiazepines cause drowsiness, lightheadedness, incoordination, and difficulty in concentrating. When these effects occur at bedtime they are generally inconsequential. However, if sedation and other manifestations of CNS depression persist beyond waking, interference with daytime activities can occur.

*Anterograde Amnesia.* Benzodiazepines can cause anterograde amnesia (impaired recall of events that take place after dosing). Anterograde amnesia has been especially troublesome with *triazolam* [Halcion]. If patients complain of forgetfulness, the possibility of drug-induced amnesia should be evaluated.

*Paradoxical Psychologic Effects.* When employed to treat anxiety, benzodiazepines sometimes cause paradoxi-

## TABLE 32-2. APPLICATIONS OF THE BENZODIAZEPINES

| Generic Name [Trade Name] | Applications | | | | | | |
|---|---|---|---|---|---|---|---|
| | Anxiety | Insomnia | Seizures | Muscle Spasm, Spasticity | Alcohol Withdrawal | Induction of Anesthesia | Panic Disorder |
| Alprazolam [Xanax] | ✔ | | | | | | ✔ |
| Chlordiazepoxide [Librium, others] | ✔ | | | | ✔ | | |
| Clonazepam [Klonopin] | | | ✔ | | | | |
| Clorazepate [Tranxene, Gen-Xene] | ✔ | | ✔ | | ✔ | | |
| Diazepam [Valium, others] | ✔ | | ✔ | ✔ | ✔ | ✔ | |
| Estazolam [ProSom] | | ✔ | | | | | |
| Flurazepam [Dalmane] | | ✔ | | | | | |
| Halazepam [Paxipam] | ✔ | | | | | | |
| Lorazepam [Ativan] | ✔ | | ✔ | | ✔ | ✔ | |
| Midazolam [Versed] | | | | | | ✔* | |
| Oxazepam [Serax] | ✔ | | | | ✔ | | |
| Prazepam [Centrax] | ✔ | | | | | | |
| Quazepam [Doral] | | ✔ | | | | | |
| Temazepam [Restoril] | | ✔ | | | | | |
| Triazolam [Halcion] | | ✔ | | | | | |

*Midazolam, in conjunction with an opioid analgesic, is also used to produce *conscious sedation*, a semiconscious state suitable for minor surgeries and endoscopic procedures.

cal responses, including insomnia, excitation, euphoria, heightened anxiety, and rage. If these occur, benzodiazepines should be withdrawn.

**Respiratory Depression.** Benzodiazepines are only weak respiratory depressants. Death from overdose with *oral* benzodiazepines *alone* has never been documented. Hence, in contrast to the barbiturates, benzodiazepines present little risk as vehicles for suicide. It must be emphasized, however, that although respiratory depression with oral therapy is rare, benzodiazepines can cause severe respiratory depression when administered *intravenously*. In addition, substantial respiratory depression can result from combining oral benzodiazepines with other CNS depressants (e.g., alcohol, barbiturates, opioids).

**Abuse.** The abuse potential of the benzodiazepines is lower than that of barbiturates and most other general CNS depressants. The behavior pattern that constitutes "addiction" is uncommon among patients who take benzodiazepines for therapeutic purposes. When asked about drug-use patterns, individuals who regularly abuse drugs rarely express a preference for benzodiazepines over barbiturates. Because their potential for abuse is low, the benzodiazepines are classified under Schedule IV of the Controlled Substances Act. This contrasts with the barbiturates, most of which are classified under Schedule II or III.

**Use in Pregnancy and Lactation.** Benzodiazepines are highly lipid soluble and can readily cross the placental barrier. Reports based on benzodiazepine use during the first trimester of pregnancy suggest an increased risk of congenital malformations, such as cleft lip, inguinal hernia, and cardiac anomalies. Use near term can cause CNS depression in the neonate. Because they may represent a risk to the fetus, most benzodiazepines are classified in FDA Pregnancy Category D. Four of these drugs—estazolam, quazepam, temazepam, and triazolam—are classified in Category X. Women of child-bearing age should be warned about the potential for fetal harm and instructed to discontinue benzodiazepines if pregnancy occurs.

Benzodiazepines enter breast milk with ease and may accumulate to toxic levels in the breast-fed infant. Accordingly, these drugs should be avoided by nursing mothers.

**Other Adverse Effects.** Occasional reactions include *weakness, headache, blurred vision, vertigo, nausea, vomiting, epigastric distress,* and *diarrhea. Neutropenia* and *jaundice* occur rarely.

## TABLE 32-3. MAJOR DRUGS FOR ANXIETY

| Generic Name | Trade Name | Dosage Forms* | Adult Oral Dosage | | CSA† Schedule |
| --- | --- | --- | --- | --- | --- |
| | | | mg/dose | doses/day | |
| *Benzodiazepines* | | | | | |
| Alprazolam | Xanax | T | 0.25-0.5 | 3 | IV |
| Chlordiazepoxide | Librium, others | C, T, I | 5-25 | 3 or 4 | IV |
| Clorazepate | Tranxene, Gen-Xene | C, T, T-SR | 7.5-15 | 2 to 4‡ | IV |
| Diazepam | Valium, others | C-SR, T, L, I | 2-10 | 2 to 4‡ | IV |
| Halazepam | Paxipam | T | 20-40 | 3 or 4 | IV |
| Lorazepam | Ativan | T, I | 1-3 | 2 or 3 | IV |
| Oxazepam | Serax | C, T | 10-30 | 3 or 4 | IV |
| Prazepam | Centrax | C, T | 10 | 3§ | IV |
| *Nonbenzodiazepine* | | | | | |
| Buspirone | BuSpar | T | 5-10 | 3 | — |

*C = capsule; C-SR = capsule, sustained-release; I = injection; L = oral liquid; T = tablet; T-SR = tablet, sustained-release.
† CSA = Controlled Substances Act.
‡ With the sustained-release formulation, the total daily dose is administered in a single dose.
§ May also be administered in a single 20- to 40-mg dose at bedtime.

## Drug Interactions

Benzodiazepines undergo very few important interactions with other drugs. Unlike barbiturates, benzodiazepines do not induce hepatic drug-metabolizing enzymes. Hence, benzodiazepines do not accelerate the metabolism of other drugs.

**CNS Depressants.** The CNS-depressant actions of benzodiazepines add with those of other CNS depressants (e.g., alcohol, barbiturates, opioids). Hence, although benzodiazepines are very safe when used alone, these drugs can be extremely hazardous in combination with other depressants: *Combined overdose with a benzodiazepine plus another CNS depressant can cause profound respiratory depression, coma, and death. Patients should be warned against use of alcohol and all other CNS depressants.*

## Tolerance and Physical Dependence

**Tolerance.** With prolonged use of benzodiazepines, tolerance develops to some effects but not to others. No tolerance develops to anxiolytic effects, and tolerance to hypnotic effects is generally low. In contrast, significant tolerance develops to antiseizure effects. Patients tolerant to barbiturates, alcohol, and other general CNS depressants show some cross-tolerance to benzodiazepines.

**Physical Dependence.** Benzodiazepines can cause physical dependence—but the incidence of *substantial* dependence is low. When benzodiazepines are discontinued following short-term use at therapeutic doses, the resulting withdrawal syndrome is generally mild and often goes unrecognized. Symptoms include anxiety, insomnia, sweating, tremors, and dizziness. Withdrawal from long-term, high-dose therapy can elicit more serious reactions, such as panic, paranoia, delirium, hypertension, muscle twitches, and outright convulsions. Symptoms of withdrawal are usually more intense with benzodiazepines that have a short duration of action. With one agent—*alprazolam* [Xanax]—dependence may be a greater problem than with other benzodiazepines. Because the benzodiazepine withdrawal syndrome can resemble an anxiety disorder, care must be taken to differentiate withdrawal symptoms from the return of original disease symptoms.

The intensity of withdrawal symptoms can be minimized by discontinuing treatment gradually. Doses should be gradually tapered over several weeks or months. Substituting a benzodiazepine with a long half-life for one with a short half-life is also helpful. Patients should be warned against abrupt cessation of treatment. Following discontinuation of treatment, patients should be monitored for 3 weeks for indications of withdrawal or recurrence of original symptoms.

## Acute Toxicity

**Oral Overdose.** When administered in excessive dosage by mouth, benzodiazepines rarely cause serious toxicity. Symptoms include drowsiness, lethargy, and confusion. Significant cardiovascular and respiratory effects are uncommon. If an individual known to have taken an overdose of benzodiazepines *does* exhibit signs of serious toxicity, it is probable that another drug was taken as well.

**Intravenous Toxicity.** When injected intravenously, even in therapeutic doses, benzodiazepines can cause severe adverse effects. Life-threatening reactions (e.g., profound hypotension, respiratory arrest, cardiac arrest) occur in about 2% of patients.

**General Treatment Measures.** Benzodiazepine-induced toxicity is managed in the same fashion as toxicity from barbiturates and other general CNS depressants.

## TABLE 32–4. DRUGS FOR TRANSIENT INSOMNIA

| Generic Name | Trade Name | Dosage Forms* | Adult Oral Dosage (mg) | CSA[†] Schedule |
|---|---|---|---|---|
| *Benzodiazepines* | | | | |
| Estazolam | ProSom | T | 1–2 | IV |
| Flurazepam | Dalmane | C | 15–30 | IV |
| Quazepam | Doral | T | 7.5–15 | IV |
| Temazepam | Restoril | C | 7.5–30 | IV |
| Triazolam | Halcion | T | 0.125–0.25 | IV |
| *Barbiturates* | | | | |
| Amobarbital | Amytal | C, T, I | 65–200 | II |
| Aprobarbital | Alurate | L | 40–160 | III |
| Butabarbital | Butisol | C, T, L | 50–100 | III |
| Pentobarbital | Nembutal | C, L, I, S | 100 | II |
| Phenobarbital | Luminal, Solfoton | C, T, L, I | 100–320 | IV |
| Secobarbital | Seconal | C, T, RI, I | 100 | II |
| *Nonbenzodiazepine-Nonbarbiturates* | | | | |
| Chloral hydrate | Noctec, others | C, L, S | 500–1000 | IV |
| Ethchlorvynol | Placidyl | C | 500–1000 | IV |
| Glutethimide | Doriden | T | 250–500 | III |
| Methyprylon | Noludar | C, T | 200–400 | III |
| Paraldehyde | Paral | L | 4–8 ml | IV |
| Zolpidem | Ambien | T | 10 | IV |

\*C = capsule; I = injections; L = oral liquid (includes drops, syrups, and elixirs); RI = rectal injection; S = suppository; T = tablet.
[†] CSA = Controlled Substances Act.

Oral benzodiazepines can be removed from the body with gastric lavage followed by ingestion of activated charcoal and a saline cathartic; dialysis may be helpful if symptoms are especially severe. Respiration should be monitored and the airway kept patent. Support of blood pressure with IV fluids and norepinephrine may be required.

**Treatment with Flumazenil.** Flumazenil [Romazicon] is a competitive benzodiazepine receptor antagonist. The drug can reverse the *sedative* effects of benzodiazepines but may not reverse benzodiazepine-induced *respiratory depression*. Flumazenil is approved for treatment of benzodiazepine overdose and for reversing the effects of benzodiazepines following general anesthesia. The principal adverse effect is precipitation of convulsions. This is most likely in patients taking benzodiazepines to treat epilepsy and in patients who are physically dependent on benzodiazepines. Administration of flumazenil is intravenous. Doses are injected slowly (over 30 seconds) and may be repeated every minute as needed. The first dose is 0.2 mg, the second is 0.3 mg, and all subsequent doses are 0.5 mg. Effects of flumazenil fade in about 1 hour; hence additional dosing may be required.

### Preparations, Dosage, and Administration

*Preparations and Dosage.* Preparations and dosages of the benzodiazepines used for anxiety and insomnia are presented in Tables 32–3 and 32–4, respectively. Preparations and dosages of benzodiazepines used to treat other disorders are presented in Chapter 23 (Drugs for Epilepsy), Chapter 24 (Drug Therapy of Muscle Spasm and Spasticity), and Chapter 27 (General Anesthetics).

*Routes.* All benzodiazepines can be administered orally. In addition, three agents—diazepam, chlordiazepoxide, and lorazepam—may also be administered parenterally (IM and IV). When used for sedation or induction of sleep, benzodiazepines are almost always administered by mouth. Intramuscular and intravenous administration are reserved for acute management of alcohol withdrawal, severe anxiety, status epilepticus, and other emergencies.

*Oral.* Patients should be advised to take oral benzodiazepines with food if gastric upset occurs. Also, they should be instructed to swallow sustained-release formulations intact, without crushing or chewing. Patients should be warned not to increase the dosage or discontinue therapy without consulting the physician.

For treatment of insomnia, benzodiazepines should be given on an intermittent schedule (e.g., 3 or 4 days a week) in the lowest effective dosage for the shortest duration required. This will minimize physical dependence and associated drug-dependency insomnia.

*Intravenous.* Intravenous administration is hazardous and must be performed with care. Life-threatening reactions (severe hypotension, respiratory arrest, cardiac arrest) have occurred. In addition, IV administration carries a risk of venous thrombosis, phlebitis, and vascular impairment.

To reduce complications from IV administration, the following precautions should be taken: (1) inject the drug slowly; (2) take care to avoid intra-arterial injection and extravasation; (3) if direct venous injection is impossible, make the injection into infusion tubing as close to the vein as possible; (4) follow the manufacturer's instructions regarding suitable diluents for preparing solutions; and (5) have facilities for resuscitation available.

# Barbiturates

The barbiturates (pronounced bahr-bi-tewr′-ates or bahr-bitch′-oo-rates) have been used since early in the 20th century. These drugs cause relatively nonselective depression of CNS function and are the prototypes of the general CNS depressants. Because they depress multiple aspects of CNS function, barbiturates can be used for daytime sedation, induction of sleep, suppression of seizures, and general anesthesia. Barbiturates cause tolerance and dependence, have a high abuse potential, and are subject to multiple drug interactions. Moreover, these drugs are powerful respiratory depressants that can readily prove fatal in overdose. Because of these undesirable properties, the barbiturates, which were once used widely, have been largely replaced by newer and safer drugs—primarily the benzodiazepines. However, although their use has declined greatly, barbiturates still have important applications in seizure control and anesthesia. Moreover, barbiturates are valuable from an instructional point of view: by understanding these prototypic agents, we gain an understanding of the general CNS depressants as a group, along with an appreciation as to why these drugs are used infrequently for anxiety and insomnia.

## Classification

The barbiturates can be grouped into three classes based on duration of action: (1) ultrashort-acting agents, (2) short- to intermediate-acting agents, and (3) long-acting agents. As indicated in Table 32-5, the duration of action of these drugs is inversely related to their lipid solubility. Barbiturates with the highest lipid solubility have the shortest duration of action. Conversely, barbiturates with the lowest lipid solubility have the longest duration.

Duration of action influences the clinical applications of barbiturates. The ultrashort-acting agents (e.g., thiopental) are used for induction of anesthesia. The short- to intermediate-acting agents (e.g., secobarbital) are used as sedatives and hypnotics. The long-acting agents (e.g., phenobarbital) are used primarily as antiseizure drugs.

## Mechanism of Action

Like benzodiazepines, barbiturates bind to the GABA receptor-chloride channel complex (see Fig. 32-1). As a result of binding, these drugs can (1) enhance the inhibitory actions of GABA and (2) directly mimic the actions of GABA. Since barbiturates can directly mimic GABA, there is no ceiling to the degree of CNS depression they can produce. Hence, in contrast to the benzodiazepines, these drugs can readily cause death when taken in overdose. Although barbiturates can cause general depression of the CNS, they show some selectivity for depressing the *reticular activating system* (RAS), a neuronal network that helps regulate the sleep-wakefulness cycle. By depressing the RAS, barbiturates produce sedation and sleep.

## Pharmacologic Effects

*CNS Depression.* The ability to cause generalized CNS depression underlies the therapeutic effects of the barbiturates as well as many of their adverse effects. As dosage is increased, responses progress from *sedation* to *sleep* to *general anesthesia.*

Most barbiturates can be considered *nonselective* CNS depressants. Exceptions to this rule are phenobarbital and other barbiturates used to control seizures. Seizure control is achieved at doses that have minimal effects on other aspects of CNS function.

*Cardiovascular Effects.* At hypnotic doses, barbiturates produce modest reductions in blood pressure and heart rate. Toxic doses, in contrast, can cause profound hypotension and shock. These reactions result from direct depressant effects on both the myocardium and vascular smooth muscle.

*Induction of Hepatic Drug-Metabolizing Enzymes.* Barbiturates stimulate synthesis of hepatic microsomal enzymes, the principal drug-metabolizing enzymes of the liver. As a result, barbiturates can accelerate their own metabolism as well as the metabolism of many other drugs.

Barbiturates stimulate drug metabolism by promoting the synthesis of porphyrin (Fig. 32-2). Porphyrin is then converted into heme, which in turn is converted into cytochrome P-450, a key component of the hepatic drug-metabolizing enzyme system.

## Tolerance and Physical Dependence

*Tolerance.* Tolerance is defined as reduced drug responsiveness that develops over the course of repeated drug use. When barbiturates are taken regularly, tolerance develops to many—but not all—of their CNS effects. Specifically, tolerance develops to sedative and hypnotic effects and to other effects that underlie barbiturate abuse. However, even with chronic use, *very little tolerance develops to toxic effects.*

In the tolerant user, doses must be increased to elicit the same intensity of response that could formerly be elicited by smaller doses. Hence, individuals who take barbiturates for prolonged

## TABLE 32-5. CHARACTERISTICS OF BARBITURATE SUBGROUPS

| Barbiturate Subgroup | Representative Drug | Lipid Solubility | Time Course | | Applications |
|---|---|---|---|---|---|
| | | | Onset (minutes) | Duration (hours) | |
| Ultrashort-acting | Thiopental | High | 0.5 | 0.2 | Induction of anesthesia; treatment of seizures |
| Short- to intermediate-acting | Secobarbital | Moderate | 10–15 | 3–4 | Treatment of insomnia |
| Long-acting | Phenobarbital | Low | 60 or less | 10–12 | Treatment of seizures and insomnia |

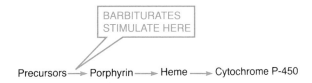

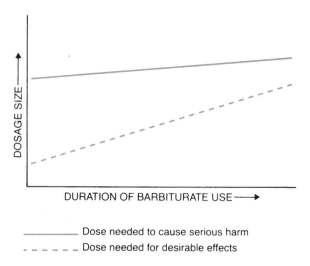

Precursors → Porphyrin → Heme → Cytochrome P-450

**Figure 32–2. Induction of hepatic microsomal enzymes by barbiturates.** By increasing synthesis of porphyrin, barbiturates increase production of cytochrome P-450, a key component of the hepatic drug-metabolizing system.

periods—be it for therapeutic purposes or for purposes of abuse—require steadily increasing doses to achieve the effects they desire.

It is important to note that *very little tolerance develops to respiratory depression.* Because tolerance to respiratory depression is minimal, and because tolerance does develop to therapeutic effects, with continued treatment the lethal (respiratory-depressant) dose remains relatively constant while the therapeutic dose climbs higher and higher (Fig. 32–3). As tolerance to therapeutic effects increases, the therapeutic dose grows steadily closer to the lethal dose—a situation that is clearly hazardous.

As a rule, tolerance to one general CNS depressant bestows tolerance to all other general CNS depressants. Hence, there is cross-tolerance among barbiturates, alcohol, benzodiazepines, general anesthetics, chloral hydrate, and a number of other agents. Tolerance to barbiturates and the other general CNS depressants does not produce significant cross-tolerance with opioids (e.g., morphine).

**Physical Dependence.** Prolonged administration of barbiturates results in physical dependence, a state in which continued drug use is required to avoid an abstinence (withdrawal) syndrome. Physical dependence results from adaptive neurochemical changes that occur in response to chronic drug exposure.

Individuals who are physically dependent on barbiturates exhibit cross-dependence with other general CNS depressants. Because of cross-dependence, a person physically dependent on barbiturates can prevent development of a withdrawal syndrome by taking any other general CNS depressant (e.g., alcohol, benzodiazepines). As a rule, cross-dependence exists among all of the general CNS depressants. However, there is no significant cross-dependence with opioids.

The general CNS depressant abstinence syndrome can be *severe.* Contrary to popular understanding, abrupt withdrawal from general CNS depressants is more dangerous than withdrawal from opioids. Although withdrawal from opioids is certainly unpleasant, the risk of serious injury is low. In contrast, the abstinence syndrome associated with general CNS depressants can be fatal.

The following description illustrates how dangerous withdrawal from general CNS depressants can be. Early reactions include weakness, restlessness, insomnia, hyperthermia, orthostatic hypotension, confusion, and disorientation. By the third day, major convulsive episodes may develop. Approximately 75% of patients experience psychotic delirium (a state similar to alcoholic delirium tremens). In extreme cases, these symptoms may be followed by exhaustion, cardiovascular collapse, and death. The entire abstinence syndrome evolves over approximately 8 days. The intensity of symptoms can be greatly reduced by withdrawing general CNS depressants slowly.

A long-acting barbiturate (e.g., phenobarbital) may be administered to facilitate the withdrawal process. Because of cross-dependence, phenobarbital can substitute for other CNS depressants, and can thereby suppress symptoms of withdrawal.

———————— Dose needed to cause serious harm
– – – – – – Dose needed for desirable effects

**Figure 32–3. Development of tolerance to the toxic and subjective effects of barbiturates.** With prolonged barbiturate use, tolerance develops. However, less tolerance develops to toxic effects than to desired effects. Consequently, as duration of use increases, the difference between the dose producing desirable effects and the dose producing toxicity becomes progressively smaller, thereby increasing the risk of serious harm.

Because of its long half-life, phenobarbital leaves the body slowly, thereby allowing a gradual transition from a drug-dependent state to a drug-free state. When phenobarbital is given to aid withdrawal, its dosage should be reduced gradually over 10 days to 3 weeks.

It is important to note that physical dependence should not be equated with addiction. Addiction is defined as a behavior pattern characterized by continued drug use despite physical, psychologic, or social harm. Although physical dependence can contribute to this behavior pattern, physical dependence, by itself, will neither cause nor sustain addictive behavior. The distinction between addiction and physical dependence is discussed further in Chapter 35 (Drug Abuse: Basic Considerations).

### Pharmacokinetics

Lipid solubility has a significant impact on the pharmacokinetic properties of individual barbiturates. As noted above, barbiturates of high lipid solubility have a rapid onset and brief duration of action. Onset is rapid because lipid solubility allows these drugs to penetrate the blood-brain barrier with ease, thereby reaching their sites of action quickly. As these drugs undergo uptake by tissues other than the brain, their levels in plasma fall, creating a concentration gradient favoring their movement from the brain back into the blood. As a result, highly lipid-soluble barbiturates undergo rapid redistribution from the brain back into the blood and then into other tissues. This redistribution terminates CNS effects.

In comparison to the highly lipid-soluble agents, barbiturates of lower lipid solubility have effects of relatively slow onset but prolonged duration. Onset is delayed because low lipid solubility impedes passage across the blood-brain barrier. Effects are prolonged because their termination is dependent on renal excretion and hepatic metabolism—processes that are slower than simple redistribution of the drug from the brain to other tissues.

With the exception of the highly lipid-soluble agents, all of the barbiturates have long plasma half-lives. These half-lives are so long, in fact, that significant amounts of barbiturate remain in plasma more than 24 hours after giving a single dose. This persistence has two clinical consequences. First, when barbiturates are taken at night to promote sleep, residual drug may cause sedation the following day. Second, since barbiturates are not eliminated entirely in 24 hours, daily administration causes drug accumulation. As a result, the brain undergoes continuous exposure to progressively higher levels of drug—a phenomenon that promotes tolerance.

### Therapeutic Uses

*Insomnia.* By depressing the CNS, barbiturates can promote sleep. However, because they can cause multiple undesired effects, barbiturates have long since been replaced by benzodiazepines as drugs of choice for insomnia.

*Seizure Disorders.* Phenobarbital and certain other barbiturates are employed to treat epilepsy and other seizure disorders (see Chapter 23). These anticonvulsant barbiturates suppress seizures at doses that are essentially nonsedative.

*Induction of Anesthesia.* Thiopental and other highly lipid-soluble barbiturates are given to induce general anesthesia (see Chapter 27). Unconsciousness develops within seconds of IV injection.

*Other Uses.* Barbiturates have been used to treat acute manic states and delirium. In children, these drugs can decrease restlessness secondary to colic, pylorospasm, and whooping cough. In addition, they can help reduce anxiety in children prior to minor dental and medical procedures. Excessive excitation from overdose with CNS stimulants (e.g., amphetamine, theophylline, ephedrine) can be decreased with barbiturates. These drugs can also be employed for emergency treatment of convulsions caused by tetanus, eclampsia, and epilepsy. When administered in anesthetic doses, barbiturates can help reduce mortality from head injury; deep anesthesia reduces the brain's requirements for oxygen and glucose and thereby helps preserve CNS function.

### Adverse Effects

*Respiratory Depression.* Barbiturates reduce ventilation by two mechanisms: (1) depression of brainstem neurogenic respiratory drive and (2) depression of chemoreceptive mechanisms that control respiratory drive. Doses only 3 times greater than those needed to induce sleep can cause complete suppression of the neurogenic respiratory drive. With severe overdose, barbiturates can cause apnea and death.

For most patients, the degree of respiratory depression produced at therapeutic doses is not clinically significant. However, in elderly patients and those with respiratory disease, therapeutic doses can compromise respiration substantially. Combining a barbiturate with another CNS depressant intensifies respiratory depression.

When barbiturates are employed in anesthetic doses during labor and delivery, respiratory depression may occur in the neonate. The infant should be monitored until respiration is normal.

*Suicide.* Barbiturates have a low therapeutic index. Accordingly, overdose can readily result in death. Because of their toxicity, the barbiturates are frequently employed as vehicles for suicide. These drugs should not be dispensed to patients suspected of suicidal tendencies.

*Abuse.* Barbiturates produce subjective effects that many individuals find desirable. As a result, barbiturates have been popular drugs of abuse. The barbiturates that are most prone to abuse are those in the short- to intermediate-acting group (e.g., secobarbital). Individual barbiturates within the group are classified under Schedule II or III of the Controlled Substances Act. These classifications reflect a high potential for abuse. Although barbiturates are frequently abused in nonmedical settings, they are rarely abused during medical use.

*Use in Pregnancy.* Barbiturates readily cross the placenta and can injure the developing fetus. Women of child-bearing age should be informed about the potential for fetal harm and warned against becoming pregnant. Use of barbiturates during the third trimester may cause drug dependence in the infant.

*Exacerbation of Intermittent Porphyria.* Barbiturates can intensify attacks of acute intermittent porphyria, a condition brought on by excessive synthesis of porphyrin. Symptoms include nausea, vomiting, abdominal colic, neuromuscular disturbances, and disturbed behavior. Barbiturates exacerbate porphyria by stimulating porphyrin synthesis (see Fig. 32–2). Because of their ability to intensify porphyria, barbiturates are *absolutely contraindicated* for individuals with a history of the disorder.

*Hangover.* Barbiturates have long half-lives, and therefore can produce residual effects (hangover) when taken to treat insomnia. Hangover can manifest as sedation, impaired judgment, and reduced motor skills. Patients should be forewarned that their ability to perform complex tasks, both manual and intellectual, may be significantly decreased the day after taking a barbiturate to induce sleep.

*Paradoxical Excitement.* In some patients, especially the elderly and debilitated, barbiturates may cause excitation. The mechanism of this paradoxical response is not known.

*Hyperalgesia.* Barbiturates can intensify sensitivity to pain. In addition, these drugs may cause pain directly. Their use has produced muscle pain, joint pain, and pain along nerves.

### Drug Interactions

*CNS Depressants.* Drugs with CNS-depressant properties (e.g., barbiturates, benzodiazepines, alcohol, opioids, antihistamines) intensify each other's effects. If these agents are combined, the degree of CNS depression can be hazardous—perhaps even fatal. Accordingly, patients should be warned emphatically against combining barbiturates with alcohol and other drugs that can depress CNS function.

*Interactions Resulting from Induction of Drug-Metabolizing Enzymes.* As discussed above, barbiturates stimulate synthesis of hepatic drug-metabolizing enzymes, thereby accelerating metabolism of other drugs. Increased metabolism is of particular concern with *warfarin* (an anticoagulant), *oral contraceptives*, and *phenytoin* (an antiseizure agent). When these drugs are taken concurrently with a barbiturate, their dosages should be increased to account for accelerated degradation.

Following barbiturate withdrawal, rates of drug metabolism gradually decline to baseline values. Several weeks are required for this to occur. Drug dosages that had been increased to account for augmented metabolism must now be reduced to their prebarbiturate amount.

### Acute Toxicity

Acute intoxication with barbiturates is a medical emergency; left untreated, overdose can be fatal. Poisoning is often the result of attempted suicide, although it can also occur by accident (usually in children and drug abusers). Since acute toxicity from barbiturates and other general CNS depressants is very similar, the discussion below applies to all of these drugs.

*Symptoms.* Acute barbiturate overdose produces a classic triad of symptoms: *respiratory depression, coma,* and *pinpoint pupils.* (Pupils may later dilate as hypoxia secondary to respiratory depression sets in.) The three classic symptoms are frequently accompanied by *hypotension* and *hypothermia.* Death is likely to be the result of pulmonary complications and renal failure.

*Treatment.* Proper management requires an intensive care unit. With vigorous treatment, most patients recover fully.

Treatment has two principal objectives: (1) removal of barbiturate from the body and (2) maintenance of an adequate oxygen supply to the brain. Oxygenation can be maintained by keeping the airway patent and by administering oxygen.

Several measures can promote barbiturate removal. Unabsorbed drug can be removed from the stomach by gastric lavage and by induction of emesis (e.g., with apomorphine). A saline cathartic can reduce absorption by accelerating drug transit through the intestine. Drug that has already been absorbed can be removed rapidly with hemodialysis. (Peritoneal dialysis is significantly slower.) Forced diuresis and alkalinization of urine may facilitate drug removal via the kidneys.

Steps should be taken to prevent hypotension and loss of body heat. Blood pressure can be supported with fluid replacement and dopamine. Body heat can be maintained with blankets and warming devices.

Barbiturate poisoning has no specific antidote. CNS stimulants should definitely *not* be employed. Not only are stimulants ineffective, they are dangerous: use of these drugs to treat barbiturate poisoning has been associated with a significant increase in mortality. Naloxone, a drug that can reverse poisoning by opioids, is not effective against poisoning by barbiturates.

### Routes

*Oral.* Oral administration is employed for daytime sedation and to treat insomnia. Patients should be warned not to increase their dosage or discontinue treatment without consulting the physician. Dosages should be reduced for elderly patients. When terminating therapy, the dosage should be gradually tapered.

*Intravenous.* Intravenous administration is reserved for general anesthesia and emergency treatment of convulsions. Injections should be made slowly to minimize respiratory depression and hypotension. Blood pressure, pulses, and respiration should be monitored, and facilities for resuscitation should be available. The patient should be under continuous observation. Extravasation may result in local necrosis; hence care must be taken to ensure that extravasation does not occur. Solutions that are cloudy or that contain a precipitate should not be used. Intra-arterial injection should be avoided, since using this route may cause arteriospasm of sufficient duration to cause gangrene.

*Intramuscular.* Barbiturate solutions are highly alkaline and can cause pain and necrosis when injected IM. Consequently, IM injection is generally avoided. Injection in the vicinity of peripheral nerves can cause irreversible neurologic injury.

# Nonbenzodiazepine-Nonbarbiturates

## Buspirone

Buspirone [BuSpar] is quite different from other anxiolytics. Its major advantages are that it does not cause sedation, has no abuse potential, and does not enhance CNS depression caused by benzodiazepines, alcohol, barbiturates, and related drugs. Its major disadvantage is that onset of anxiolytic effects is delayed. Buspirone is said to reduce anxiety while producing even less sedation than the benzodiazepines. The drug is devoid of hypnotic, muscle relaxant, and anticonvulsant actions.

*Mechanism of Action.* The mechanism by which buspirone acts has not been established. The drug binds with high affinity to receptors for serotonin and with lower affinity to receptors for dopamine. Buspirone does not bind to receptors for GABA or benzodiazepines.

*Pharmacokinetics.* Buspirone is well absorbed following oral administration but undergoes extensive metabolism on its first pass through the liver. Administration with food delays absorption but enhances bioavailability (by reducing first-pass metabolism). The drug is excreted in part by the kidneys, primarily as metabolites.

*Therapeutic Use.* Buspirone is labeled only for *short-term* treatment of *anxiety*. However, when taken for as long as 1 year, the drug showed no reduction in antianxiety actions. For treatment of anxiety, the drug appears to be as effective as benzodiazepines. Antianxiety effects take a week or more to develop. Buspirone lacks sedative effects and is not indicated for insomnia. Use of buspirone is discussed further under *Management of Anxiety*.

*Adverse Effects and Interactions.* Buspirone is generally well tolerated. The most common reactions are *dizziness, nausea, headache, nervousness, lightheadedness,* and *excitement*. The drug is nonsedative and does not interfere with daytime activities. Furthermore, the drug poses little or no risk of suicide; huge doses (375 mg/day) have been given to healthy volunteers with only moderate effects (nausea, vomiting, dizziness, drowsiness, miosis). Buspirone does *not* enhance the depressant effects of alcohol, barbiturates, and other general CNS depressants.

*Tolerance, Dependence, and Abuse.* Buspirone has been used for up to 1 year without evidence of tolerance, physical dependence, or psychologic dependence. No withdrawal symptoms have been observed upon termination of treatment. There is no cross-tolerance or cross-dependence between buspirone and other sedative-hypnotics (e.g., benzodiazepines, barbiturates). To date there is no evidence that buspirone has a liability for abuse; hence the drug is not regulated under the Controlled Substances Act.

*Preparations, Dosage, and Administration.* Buspirone [BuSpar] is dispensed in tablets (5 and 10 mg) for oral administration. The usual initial dosage is 5 mg 3 times a day. Daily dosage may be increased to a maximum of 60 mg.

## Zolpidem

*Actions and Uses.* Zolpidem [Ambien] is a relatively new sedative-hypnotic approved for short-term management of *insomnia*. Although structurally unrelated to the benzodiazepines, zolpidem binds to the GABA receptor-chloride channel complex and shares some properties of the benzodiazepines. Like the benzodiazepines, zolpidem can reduce sleep latency and awakenings and can prolong sleep duration. The drug does not significantly reduce time in REM sleep and causes little or no rebound insomnia when therapy is discontinued. In contrast to the benzodiazepines, zolpidem lacks anxiolytic, muscle relaxant, and anticonvulsant actions.

*Pharmacokinetics.* Zolpidem is rapidly absorbed following oral administration. Plasma levels peak in 2 hours. The drug is widely distributed throughout the body, although levels in the brain remain low. Zolpidem is extensively metabolized to inactive compounds that are excreted in the bile, urine, and feces. The drug's half-life is about 2.4 hours.

*Adverse Effects.* Zolpidem has a side effect profile like that of the benzodiazepines. *Daytime drowsiness* and *dizziness* are most common, and these occur in only 1% to 2% of patients. At therapeutic doses, zolpidem causes little or no respiratory depression. Safety in pregnancy has not been established.

***Tolerance, Dependence, and Abuse.*** Short-term treatment is not associated with significant tolerance or physical dependence. Withdrawal symptoms are minimal or absent. Similarly, the abuse liability of zolpidem is low. Accordingly, the drug is classified under Schedule IV of the Controlled Substances Act.

***Drug Interactions.*** Like other sedative-hypnotics, zolpidem can intensify the effects of *CNS depressants.* Accordingly, patients should be warned against combining zolpidem with alcohol and all other drugs that can depress CNS function.

***Preparations, Dosage, and Administration.*** Zolpidem [Ambien] is available in 5- and 10-mg tablets for oral use. The usual dosage is 10 mg. The initial dosage should be reduced to 5 mg for elderly and debilitated patients and for those with hepatic insufficiency. Since zolpidem has a rapid onset of action, it should be taken just prior to bedtime to minimize sedation while awake.

## Miscellaneous General CNS Depressants

### Basic Pharmacologic Profile

The drugs considered in this section have properties very much like those of the barbiturates. All of these agents produce relatively nonselective depression of CNS function.

All of the nonselective CNS depressants are potentially dangerous. These drugs are respiratory depressants and can be lethal in overdose. Accordingly, these drugs should not be given to patients suspected of suicidal tendencies.

At therapeutic doses, the nonselective CNS depressants can cause substantial drowsiness. Patients should be warned to avoid driving and other hazardous activities.

Concurrent use of these drugs with other CNS depressants (e.g., alcohol, barbiturates, benzodiazepines, opioids, antihistamines) can produce profound depression of CNS function. Accordingly, combinations of CNS depressants should be avoided.

Prolonged use can produce tolerance and physical dependence. Consequently, these agents should be reserved for short-term therapy. In patients who have been treated long term, termination should be done gradually to minimize the withdrawal reaction.

Many of the nonselective CNS depressants produce subjective effects that individuals prone to drug abuse consider desirable. Because of this abuse potential, agents in this group are classified under Schedule III or IV of the Controlled Substances Act.

In general, acute overdose resembles poisoning with barbiturates. Characteristic signs are respiratory depression, coma, miosis, and hypotension. Management is the same as with poisoning by barbiturates.

Nonselective CNS depressants should be avoided during pregnancy and lactation. Certain of these agents may cause birth defects if taken during the first trimester. In addition, if these drugs are taken late in pregnancy, the infant may be born drug dependent. The CNS depressants can achieve concentrations in breast milk that are sufficient to cause lethargy in the infant. Nursing mothers should avoid these drugs.

The principal indication for the nonselective CNS depressants is insomnia. Treatment should be short term. Dosages are summarized in Table 32–4.

### Chloral Hydrate

Chloral hydrate [Noctec, Aquachloral Supprettes] is a general CNS depressant with properties similar to those of the barbiturates. Chloral is a prodrug that undergoes rapid conversion to its active form in the liver. The drug's principal application is induction of sleep.

Chloral hydrate is dispensed in capsules, a syrup, and suppositories. Patients should be instructed to swallow the capsules intact, without crushing or chewing. The syrup formulation should be diluted with water, fruit juice, or ginger ale. With oral administration, epigastric distress, nausea, and flatulence are common.

The recommended dosage is 0.5 to 1 gm 30 minutes before bedtime. However, doses in this range are frequently too low to induce sleep. To elicit an adequate response, a dose as large as 2 gm may be needed.

Chloral hydrate is subject to abuse and is classified as a Schedule IV drug. Abuse is similar to that seen in alcoholism. Prolonged consumption of chloral results in substantial tolerance and physical dependence. As a result, chloral addicts may ingest extremely large amounts of the drug. Abrupt withdrawal can cause delirium and seizures. Left untreated, the abstinence syndrome can be fatal.

### Glutethimide

Glutethimide [Doriden] is a general CNS depressant with properties similar to those of the barbiturates. In addition, the drug has prominent anticholinergic actions. Like the barbiturates, glutethimide can intensify episodes of intermittent porphyria and is contraindicated for patients with this disorder. Acute poisoning produces CNS depression together with anticholinergic responses (e.g., dry mouth, visual disturbance, decreased intestinal motility, atony of the urinary bladder, hyperpyrexia). Glutethimide is a Schedule III drug with an abuse liability like that of the barbiturates.

Glutethimide is indicated for short-term (3 to 7 days) management of insomnia. However, because superior agents are available, and because toxicity can be difficult to manage, it would seem that glutethimide has little to recommend its use. The drug is dispensed in 250- and 500-mg tablets. The usual adult dosage is 250 to 500 mg at bedtime.

### Meprobamate

Meprobamate [Miltown, Equanil, others] has pharmacologic properties that lie midway between those of the barbiturates and the benzodiazepines. As a CNS depressant, meprobamate is more selective than the barbiturates but less selective than the benzodiazepines. Meprobamate induces hepatic drug-metabolizing enzymes and can exacerbate intermittent porphyria. Although meprobamate is approved only for treatment of anxiety, the drug is also employed to induce sleep. The usual adult dosage for anxiety is 1.2 to 1.6 gm/day in three or four divided doses. Meprobamate is classified as a Schedule IV drug.

### Paraldehyde

Paraldehyde [Paral] is a CNS depressant with multiple undesirable properties. The drug has a strong odor and unpleasant taste. When administered orally, paraldehyde irritates the throat and stomach; when injected intramuscularly, it can produce local necrosis and nerve injury; when injected intravenously, it can cause cyanosis, pulmonary edema, hypotension, and venous thrombosis.

Solutions of paraldehyde decompose rapidly to acetic acid. Preparations that smell strongly of acetic acid (i.e., that smell like vinegar) should be discarded. Since decomposition occurs rapidly, paraldehyde in containers that have been open for more than 24 hours should not be used.

Poisoning with paraldehyde is quite different from poisoning with other CNS depressants. In addition to causing respiratory depression and hypotension, paraldehyde causes prominent metabolic acidosis. Symptoms of toxicity include rapid, labored breathing; bleeding gastritis; toxic hepatitis; nephrosis; pulmonary hemorrhage; and edema. An oral dose of 25 ml can be fatal.

The principal indications for paraldehyde are induction of sleep and treatment of alcoholic delirium tremens. The drug is employed almost exclusively in hospitals and institutions. Use by outpatients is rare. Despite its undesirable effects, paraldehyde still has some advocates. Given the availability of clearly superior alternatives, the continued use of this drug is mystifying.

The usual oral dosage for adults is 4 to 8 ml diluted in milk or iced fruit juice to mask the drug's taste. Paraldehyde is a Schedule IV drug and must be dispensed accordingly.

### Ethchlorvynol

Ethchlorvynol [Placidyl] is a CNS depressant with a rapid onset and short duration of action. Side effects include dizziness, hypotension, facial numbness, and a mint-like aftertaste. Like the barbiturates, ethchlorvynol can exacerbate acute intermittent porphyria. Ethchlorvynol is classified under Schedule IV and is approved only for short-term management of insomnia. The usual adult dosage is 500 to 1000 mg at bedtime.

# Management of Anxiety

Anxiety is a nearly universal experience that often serves an adaptive function. When anxiety is moderate and situationally appropriate, drug therapy may not be needed or even desirable. In contrast, when anxiety is persistent and disabling, drug therapy is clearly indicated.

In the *Diagnostic and Statistical Manual of Mental Disorders*, fourth edition (DSM-IV), primary anxiety disorders are divided into six classes: generalized anxiety disorder (GAD), panic disorder, phobic disorders, obsessive-compulsive disorder (OCD), post-traumatic stress disorder, and acute stress disorder. In this chapter, discussion is limited to GAD, which is by far the most common anxiety disorder. Panic disorder and OCD are addressed in Chapter 34.

### Situational Anxiety versus Generalized Anxiety Disorder

*Situational Anxiety.* Situational anxiety is a normal response to a stressful situation (e.g., family problems, exams, financial difficulties). Although symptoms may be intense, they are also temporary. If necessary, medication can be used to provide relief, but treatment should be short term. Benzodiazepines are the drugs of choice.

*Generalized Anxiety Disorder.* The hallmark of GAD is unrealistic or excessive anxiety about several events or activities (e.g., work or school performance) that lasts for 6 months or longer. Other psychologic manifestations include vigilance, tension, apprehension, poor concentration, and difficulty falling asleep or staying asleep. Somatic manifestations include trembling, muscle tension, restlessness, and signs of autonomic hyperactivity (e.g., palpitations, tachycardia, sweating, clammy hands). Complete DSM-IV diagnostic criteria for GAD are presented in Table 32-6.

### Treatment of Generalized Anxiety Disorder

GAD can be treated with nondrug therapy and with anxiolytics. Nondrug approaches include supportive ther-apy, cognitive therapy, biofeedback, and relaxation training. These can help relieve symptoms and improve coping skills in anxiety-provoking situations. When symptoms are mild, nondrug therapy may be all that is needed. However, if symptoms are intensely uncomfortable or disabling, antianxiety drugs are indicated. Benzodiazepines and buspirone are chosen most often. Treatment may be prolonged.

**Benzodiazepines.** Benzodiazepines are drugs of first choice for anxiety. Onset of effects is immediate, and the margin of safety is high. Principal side effects are sedation and psychomotor slowing. Patients should be warned about these and informed that they will subside within 7 to 10 days. Because of their abuse potential, benzodiazepines should be used with caution in patients known to abuse alcohol or other psychoactive substances.

Of the 15 benzodiazepines available, 8 are approved for anxiety. The agents prescribed most frequently are diazepam [Valium] and alprazolam [Xanax]. However, since no benzodiazepine has shown any clear superiority over the others, selection among them is largely a matter of physician preference. Dosages for anxiety are summarized in Table 32-3.

---

### TABLE 32–6. DSM-IV DIAGNOSTIC CRITERIA FOR GAD*

A. Excessive anxiety and worry about several events or activities (such as work or school performance) that occur more days than not for at least 6 months.

B. The person finds the worry difficult to control.

C. The anxiety and worry are associated with three (or more) of the following six symptoms (with at least some symptoms present for more days than not for the past 6 months). *Note*: only one item is required in children.

- Restlessness or feeling keyed up or on edge
- Being easily fatigued
- Difficulty concentrating or mind going blank
- Irritability
- Muscle tension
- Sleep disturbance (difficulty falling asleep or staying asleep, or restlessness, unsatisfying sleep)

D. The focus of the anxiety and worry is not related to another psychiatric disorder.

E. The anxiety, worry, or physical symptoms cause clinically significant distress or impairment in social, occupational, or other important areas of functioning.

F. The disturbance is not due to the direct physiologic effects of a substance (e.g., drug of abuse, medication) or a general medical condition (e.g., hyperthyroidism) and does not occur exclusively during a mood disorder, psychotic disorder, or pervasive developmental disorder.

---

* Modified from American Psychiatric Association. *Diagnostic and Statistical Manual of Mental Disorders*, 4th ed. Washington, DC, American Psychiatric Press, 1994, pp. 435–436; reprinted by permission.

Therapy of GAD is generally long term. The relapse rate when benzodiazepines are withdrawn is 60% to 80%. For initial therapy, treatment should last 2 to 4 months, after which drug discontinuation can be tried. Withdrawal should be done very gradually—over a period of several months. If relapse occurs, treatment should resume. Prolonged therapy with benzodiazepines is generally safe and effective—albeit somewhat controversial.

***Buspirone.*** Buspirone [BuSpar] is an alternative to the benzodiazepines for treating anxiety. This drug differs from benzodiazepines in four important ways: (1) it does not cause sedation, (2) it has no abuse potential, (3) it does not intensify the effects of CNS depressants, and (4) its antianxiety effects take a week to begin and several weeks to reach their peak. Because therapeutic effects are delayed, buspirone is not suitable for patients who need immediate relief, nor is it suitable for PRN use. Since buspirone has no abuse potential, the drug may be especially appropriate for patients known to abuse alcohol and other drugs. Because it lacks depressant properties, buspirone is an attractive alternative to benzodiazepines in patients who require long-term therapy but who cannot tolerate benzodiazepine-induced sedation and psychomotor slowing. Buspirone does not display cross-dependence with benzodiazepines. Hence, when patients are switched from a benzodiazepine to buspirone, the benzodiazepine must be tapered off slowly. Furthermore, since the effects of buspirone are delayed, buspirone should be initiated 2 to 4 weeks before beginning benzodiazepine withdrawal.

***Antidepressants.*** Sedating antidepressants, such as imipramine [Tofranil], amitriptyline [Elavil], and trazodone [Desyrel], are effective therapy for GAD. Responses are at least as good as with benzodiazepines, although onset and benefits may be delayed. During the first weeks of treatment, somatic symptoms of anxiety may temporarily increase. Other undesired effects include weight gain, anticholinergic effects, and the potential for death by overdose. Nonetheless, given their efficacy in treating GAD, antidepressants may well be used more in the future.

***Beta Blockers.*** Beta-adrenergic blocking agents (e.g., propranolol) can relieve symptoms caused by autonomic hyperactivity (tachycardia, palpitations, tremor, sweating). These drugs may be most valuable as an aid to coping with situational anxiety, such as that experienced by individuals who are overly apprehensive about public speaking. Beta blockers are not as effective as benzodiazepines for GAD and are not recommended as primary therapy.

# Management of Insomnia

## Sleep Physiology

Sleep is a complex state characterized by a reduced level of consciousness and minimal physical activity. The sleeping state has two primary divisions: *rapid-eye-movement* (REM) sleep and *non-rapid-eye-movement* (NREM) sleep. Sleeping begins with a period of NREM sleep, after which periods of REM sleep and NREM sleep alternate until waking takes place.

REM sleep is the phase during which most recallable dreams occur. A typical night's sleep has four to six REM periods, accounting for approximately 30% of total sleeping time. In males, penile erection is common during REM sleep. This curious phenomenon is independent of dream content. Except for the benzodiazepines, the drugs used to remedy sleep disorders often reduce the total time spent in REM sleep.

The precise physiologic benefits of sleep have not been established. Some studies suggest that deprivation of REM sleep can produce adverse psychologic reactions; other studies do not support this conclusion. A recent study indicated that REM sleep is important for consolidating perceptual learning. Regardless of the value that specific stages of sleep may or may not have, one thing is clear: when we don't get enough sleep, we tend to be drowsy the next day and less able to function. If fatigue or reduced alertness compromises daytime performance, some form of intervention may be needed.

## Causes of Insomnia

Insomnia is defined as an inability to sleep. Some people have difficulty falling asleep, some have difficulty maintaining sleep, and some are troubled by early morning awakening. About 10% of people in the United States feel they have a significant insomnia problem.

Loss of sleep is often the result of a medical disorder. Pain often keeps people awake. Sleep disturbances are common in patients with psychiatric disorders. Sleep is frequently lost because of concern over impending surgery and other procedures.

At one time or another, nearly everyone suffers from *situational insomnia.* Worry about exams may keep students awake. Job-related pressures may deprive workers of sleep. Unfamiliar surroundings may render sleeping difficult for travelers. Major life stressors (bereavement, divorce, loss of job) frequently disrupt sleep. Other factors, such as uncomfortable bedding, excessive noise, and bright light, can deprive most anyone of sound sleep.

## Management Strategy

Treatment is highly dependent on the cause of insomnia. Accordingly, if therapy is to be successful, the underlying reason for sleep loss must be determined. To make this assessment, a thorough history is required.

***Nondrug Management.*** Not everyone with insomnia should be treated with drugs. For some individuals, avoidance of naps and adherence to a regular sleep schedule is sufficient. For others, decreased consumption of caffeine-containing beverages (e.g., coffee, tea, cola drinks) may be all that is needed. Still others may benefit from restful activity as bedtime approaches. If the history reveals that environmental factors are responsible for lack of sleep, the patient should be advised of ways to correct these factors or to compensate for them. All patients should be counseled about sleep fitness (also known as sleep hygiene). Rules for sleep fitness are summarized in Table 32-7.

## TABLE 32-7. RULES FOR SLEEP FITNESS

- Establish a regular time to go to bed and a regular time to rise. This will help reset your biologic clock.
- Sleep only as long as needed to feel refreshed. Too much time in bed causes fragmented and shallow sleep. In contrast, restricting time in bed helps consolidate and deepen sleep.
- Insulate your bedroom against light and sounds that disturb your sleep (e.g., install carpeting and insulated curtains.)
- Keep your bedroom temperature moderate. High temperature may disturb sleep.
- Exercise daily, but not later than 7 PM. Regular exercise helps deepen sleep.
- Avoid daytime naps. Staying awake during the day helps you sleep at night.
- Avoid caffeine, especially in the evening.
- Avoid drinking too much in the evening so as to minimize nighttime trips to the bathroom.
- Avoid alcohol in the evening. Although alcohol can help you fall asleep, it causes sleep to be fragmented.
- Avoid tobacco; it disturbs sleep (and shortens your life, too).
- Try having a light snack near bedtime, since hunger can disturb sleep—but don't eat heavily.
- Relax before bedtime with soft music, mild stretching, yoga, or pleasurable reading.
- Leave your problems outside the bedroom. Reserve time earlier in the evening to work on your problems and to plan tomorrow's activities.
- Reserve your bedroom for sleeping (and sex). This will help condition your brain to see the bedroom as a place where sleep happens. Don't eat, read, or watch TV in bed.
- If you don't fall asleep within 20 minutes or so, get up and do something relaxing (e.g., read, listen to music, watch TV), and then return to bed when you feel drowsy. Repeat as often as required.
- Don't look at the clock if you wake up during the night. If necessary, turn its face away from the bed.

*Cause-Specific Drug Therapy.* When the cause of insomnia is a known medical disorder, primary therapy should be directed at the underlying illness; hypnotics should be employed only as adjuncts. For example, if pain is the reason for lack of sleep, analgesics should be prescribed. If insomnia is secondary to major depression, antidepressants are the appropriate treatment. If anxiety is the cause of insomnia, the patient should be given an anxiolytic.

*Therapy with Hypnotic Drugs.* Hypnotics should be reserved for those patients whose insomnia cannot be managed by other means. If nondrug measures can relieve insomnia, hypnotics should be avoided. Likewise, if insomnia is secondary to an identified and treatable pathology, specific therapies directed at that pathology are clearly preferable to hypnotics.

### Transient Insomnia: Basic Guidelines for Drug Therapy

Drug therapy of transient insomnia should be short term. The patient should be reassessed on a regular basis to determine if drug therapy is still needed. If insomnia persists, an underlying pathology may well be the cause. Every effort should be made to diagnose this pathology rather than cover it up with continued use of hypnotics.

Escalation of dosage should be avoided. A need for increased dosage suggests development of tolerance. If hypnotic effects are lost in the course of treatment, it is preferable to interrupt therapy rather than elevate dosage. Interruption will allow tolerance to decline, thereby restoring responsiveness to treatment.

In certain patients, hypnotics must be employed with special caution. Patients who snore heavily and patients with respiratory disorders have reduced respiratory reserve, which can be further compromised by the respiratory-depressant actions of hypnotics. Hypnotic agents are generally contraindicated for use during pregnancy; these drugs have the potential for causing fetal harm, and their use is never an absolute necessity. Except for the benzodiazepines, most hypnotics can be lethal if taken in overdose. Accordingly, these drugs should not be given to individuals suspected of suicidal tendencies.

Patients taking hypnotics should be forewarned that residual CNS depression may be present the following day. Although CNS depression may not be pronounced, it may nonetheless be sufficient to compromise intellectual or physical performance.

When hypnotics are employed, care must be taken to prevent *drug-dependency insomnia*, a condition that can lead to inappropriate prolongation of therapy. Drug-dependency insomnia is a particular problem with the barbiturates, and develops as follows: (1) Insomnia motivates treatment with hypnotics. (2) With continuous drug use, low-level physical dependence develops. (3) Upon cessation of treatment, a mild withdrawal syndrome occurs and disrupts sleep. (4) Failing to recognize that the inability to sleep is a manifestation of drug withdrawal, the patient becomes convinced that insomnia has returned and resumes drug use. (5) Continued drug use leads to heightened physical dependence, making it even more difficult to withdraw medication without producing another episode of drug-dependency insomnia. To minimize drug-dependency insomnia, hypnotics should be employed judiciously. That is, they should be used in the lowest effective dosage for the shortest time required.

### Transient Insomnia: Specific Drugs Used for Treatment

Prescription drugs employed for transient insomnia include benzodiazepines, barbiturates, and other general CNS depressants (see Table 32-4). In addition, several over-the-counter sleep aids are available.

The various hypnotic drugs have similarities and differences regarding their effects on sleep. Properties shared by all hypnotics are the abilities to accelerate onset of sleep and to maintain sleep. Important differences exist with respect to (1) suppression of REM sleep, (2) tolerance to hypnotic effects, and (3) tendency to promote rebound insomnia (drug-dependency insomnia).

# Melatonin . . . Hypnotic or Hype?

In recent years, melatonin has been the subject of at least four popular books and has received prominent coverage in the media. Proponents claim melatonin can treat insomnia and jet lag, protect against cancer and pregnancy, and prolong life and youthfulness. However, despite the publicity, very little is actually known about melatonin's efficacy or safety. Why? Because only a few clinical trials have been performed—and these were short and involved just a few subjects. What follows is a summary of what we do know.

Melatonin is a hormone produced by the pineal gland. Secretion is suppressed by environmental light and stimulated by darkness. Normally, secretion is low during the day, begins to rise around 9 PM, reaches a peak between 2 AM and 4 AM, and returns to baseline by morning. Signals that control secretion travel along a multineuron pathway that connects the retina to the pineal. Nocturnal secretion is greatest in children and declines with age. In blind people, melatonin secretion has no predictable pattern. Melatonin levels are low in insomniacs.

Although melatonin is a hormone, it is marketed as a dietary supplement—not as a drug. As a result, melatonin is not regulated by the Food and Drug Administration (FDA) and has not been reviewed for safety and efficacy. Because melatonin is not regulated, commercial preparations may contain impurities and may not have the exact amount of melatonin advertised on the package label (typically 0.3, 1.5, or 3 mg). Melatonin is the only hormone that can be purchased without a prescription. It is available in health food stores, vitamin shops, and even airport newsstands.

Several small, short-term trials suggest that melatonin can promote sleep. For example, doses of 0.3 to 1 mg taken at 1 to 2 hours before bedtime hastened onset of sleep and the time to REM sleep, without reducing total time in REM sleep. At a slightly higher dose (2 mg of a controlled-release formulation 2 hours before bedtime), melatonin hastened sleep onset by 14 minutes and decreased total time awake during the night by 24 minutes. When taken in huge doses (80 to 100 mg) at noon, melatonin has caused daytime fatigue. In blind insomniacs, treatment with melatonin for 3 weeks normalized the melatonin production cycle and relieved insomnia. Because small doses of melatonin may fail to elevate melatonin levels throughout the night, maintenance of sleep may be best with larger doses or with sustained-release formulations.

Melatonin appears to have a favorable impact on jet lag. In one study, the severity and duration of jet lag were reduced by taking 5 mg of melatonin once daily for 3 days before the flight and 3 days after. In another study, subjective feelings of fatigue were reduced by taking 8 mg at 10 PM on the evening of the flight and for 3 days after. In general, travelers taking melatonin report improvement in disturbed sleep cycles, mood, daytime fatigue, and recovery time.

When used short term in low doses (e.g., under 2 mg), melatonin has not caused observable adverse effects. In contrast, short-term use of large doses has caused hangover, headache, nightmares, hypothermia, and transient depression. Possible adverse effects of long-term use are unknown.

In conclusion, melatonin is the miracle that awaits definitive proof. Small studies on insomnia and jet lag have been encouraging. However, large-scale, long-term, carefully controlled trials are needed to prove that melatonin is truly safe and effective and to establish optimal dosages and dosing schedules.

---

**Benzodiazepines.** Benzodiazepines are drugs of first choice for short-term treatment of insomnia. These agents are safe and effective and lack the undesirable properties typical of other hypnotics. Benzodiazepines have a low abuse potential, cause minimal tolerance and physical dependence, present a minimal risk of suicide, and undergo few interactions with other drugs. For treatment of transient insomnia, dosing should be intermittent (every two or three nights), and should last only 2 to 3 weeks.

Benzodiazepines have multiple desirable effects related to sleep: they decrease the latency to sleep onset, they decrease the number of awakenings, and they increase total sleeping time. In addition, they impart a sense of deep and refreshing sleep. Tolerance to hypnotic actions develops slowly; benzodiazepines have been taken nightly for several weeks without a noticeable loss in hypnotic effects. Treatment does not significantly reduce the amount of REM sleep, and there is no rebound increase in REM sleep when treatment stops. Furthermore, withdrawal of benzodiazepines is not associated with significant rebound insomnia.

Only five benzodiazepines are marketed specifically for use as hypnotics (see Table 32–4). However, any benzodiazepine with a short to intermediate onset could be employed.

Two agents—*triazolam* [Halcion] and *flurazepam* [Dalmane]—can be considered prototypes of the benzodiazepines used to promote sleep. Triazolam has a rapid onset and short duration of action, making it a good choice for patients who have difficulty falling asleep (as compared with difficulty maintaining sleep). Flurazepam has a delayed onset and more prolonged duration of action, making it a good choice for patients who have difficulty maintaining sleep. With triazolam, daytime sedation is minimal; with flurazepam, daytime sedation may be significant.

**Barbiturates.** The barbiturates are a distant second choice to the benzodiazepines for short-term therapy of insomnia. Barbiturates are hazardous and have a high potential for abuse. Tolerance, dependence, and a host of drug interactions further decrease their desirability. Although several barbiturates are approved for insomnia (see Table 32–4), these agents have been largely abandoned in favor of benzodiazepines.

Several sleep-related effects of the barbiturates differ from those of the benzodiazepines. At the beginning of therapy, barbiturates tend to suppress REM sleep. However, with continued treatment, time spent in REM sleep returns to normal. "Hangover" and residual daytime sedation are relatively common. Tolerance develops rapidly to hypnotic effects; hence, if barbiturates are taken on a routine basis, dosage must be increased periodically to maintain a response. Withdrawal of barbiturates is associated with rebound insomnia and increased REM sleep.

Secobarbital [Seconal], a short- to intermediate-acting barbiturate, can be considered the prototype of the barbiturates employed to promote sleep. The drug has a rapid onset of action, and therefore can benefit patients who have difficulty falling asleep. Elimination of secobarbital is relatively rapid. Hence daytime sedation is less intense than with long-acting barbiturates.

**Other Prescription Sleep Aids.** Nonbenzodiazepine-nonbarbiturate hypnotics are listed in Table 32–4. With the exception of zolpidem, these drugs have pharmacologic effects like those of the barbiturates. Benzodiazepines are almost always preferred.

**Nonprescription Sleep Aids.** Over-the-counter sleep aids (e.g., Compoz, Sominex) contain an *antihistamine* (diphenhydramine, pyrilamine, or doxylamine) as their active ingredient. Although sedation can be a prominent side effect when antihistamines are taken to treat allergies, relief of insomnia is not always impressive. Antihistamines are less effective than benzodiazepines and frequently cause anticholinergic side effects.

### Drugs for Chronic Insomnia

Most cases of chronic insomnia are caused by mental disorders. These include depression, psychosis, dementia, anxiety disorders, and substance abuse. Primary treatment is directed at the underlying illness. However, if this fails to normalize sleep, additional treatment may be indicated. The drugs used most commonly are *trazodone* [Desyrel] and *tricyclic antidepressants* (e.g., amitriptyline [Elavil]). The dosage for trazodone is 25 to 200 mg. The dosage for amitriptyline is 25 to 50 mg. Both agents are administered at bedtime. No tolerance develops to hypnotic effects with prolonged use. For all of these drugs, the abuse potential is minimal. The basic pharmacology of trazodone and the tricyclics is discussed in Chapter 30 (Antidepressants).

## KEY POINTS

- Drugs used to treat anxiety are called antianxiety agents, anxiolytics, or tranquilizers.

- Drugs that promote sleep are called hypnotics.
- Barbiturates and other general CNS depressants are very undesirable in that they can cause fatal respiratory depression, have a high potential for abuse, cause significant tolerance and physical dependence, and often induce hepatic drug-metabolizing enzymes.
- Benzodiazepines are preferred to barbiturates and other general CNS depressants because benzodiazepines are much safer, have a low abuse potential, cause less tolerance and dependence, and don't induce drug-metabolizing enzymes.
- Although benzodiazepines can cause physical dependence, the withdrawal syndrome is usually mild (except in patients who have undergone prolonged, high-dose therapy).
- To minimize withdrawal symptoms, benzodiazepines should be withdrawn gradually, over several weeks or even months.
- Benzodiazepines cause minimal respiratory depression when used alone but can cause profound respiratory depression when combined with other CNS depressants (e.g, opioids, barbiturates, alcohol).
- Benzodiazepines produce their effects by enhancing the actions of GABA, the principal inhibitory neurotransmitter in the CNS.
- Although benzodiazepines undergo extensive metabolism, in most cases the metabolites are pharmacologically active. As a result, responses produced by administering a particular benzodiazepine often persist long after the parent drug has disappeared from the plasma.
- All of the benzodiazepines have essentially equivalent pharmacologic actions; hence, selection among these drugs is based in large part on differences in time course.
- The principal indications for benzodiazepines are anxiety, insomnia, and seizure disorders.
- The principal adverse effects of benzodiazepines are daytime sedation and anterograde amnesia.
- Flumazenil, a benzodiazepine receptor antagonist, can be used to treat benzodiazepine overdose.
- Generalized anxiety disorder is a chronic condition that usually requires prolonged therapy.
- The principal drugs for treating generalized anxiety disorder are benzodiazepines and buspirone.
- When insomnia has a treatable cause (e.g., pain, depression, schizophrenia), primary therapy should be directed at the underlying illness; hypnotics should be used only as adjuncts.
- Benzodiazepines are drugs of choice for treating transient insomnia.
- When benzodiazepines are used for transient insomnia, dosing should be intermittent (every two or three nights) and should last only 2 to 3 weeks.
- Buspirone differs from benzodiazepines in four important ways: (1) it does not cause sedation, (2) it has no abuse potential, (3) it does not intensify the effects of CNS depressants, and (4) its antianxiety effects take a week or more to develop.

# Summary of Major Nursing Implications*

## Benzodiazepines

The nursing implications summarized here apply to the benzodiazepines as a group and to their use in anxiety and insomnia.

## Preadministration Assessment

### Therapeutic Goal

Benzodiazepines are used to promote sleep, relieve symptoms of anxiety, suppress seizure disorders (see Chapter 23), relax muscle spasm (see Chapter 24), and ease withdrawal from alcohol (see Chapter 36). They are also used for preanesthetic medication and to induce general anesthesia (see Chapter 27).

### Baseline Data

**For Insomnia.** Determine the nature of the sleep disturbance (prolonged latency, frequent awakenings, early morning awakening) and how long it has lasted. Assess for a possible underlying cause (e.g., medical illness, psychiatric illness, use of caffeine and other stimulants, poor sleep hygiene, major life stressor).

**For Anxiety.** Determine the nature, duration, and intensity of symptoms. Differentiate situational anxiety from generalized anxiety disorder.

### Identifying High-Risk Patients

Benzodiazepines are *contraindicated* during *pregnancy* and for patients who experience *sleep apnea*. Use with *caution* in patients with *suicidal tendencies* and a *history of substance abuse.*

## Implementation: Administration

### Routes

*Oral. All* benzodiazepines.
**IM and IV.** *Diazepam, chlordiazepoxide,* and *lorazepam.*

### Administration

*Oral.* Advise patients to administer benzodiazepines with food if gastric upset occurs. Instruct patients to swallow sustained-release formulations intact, without crushing or chewing.

Warn patients not to increase the dosage or discontinue treatment without consulting the physician.

To minimize physical dependence when treating insomnia, administer intermittently (three or four nights a week) and use the lowest effective dosage for the shortest duration required.

To minimize the abstinence syndrome, taper the dosage gradually (over several weeks).

*Intravenous.* Perform IV injections with care. Life-threatening reactions (severe hypotension, respiratory arrest, cardiac arrest) have occurred, along with less serious reactions (venous thrombosis, phlebitis, vascular impairment). To reduce complications, follow these guidelines: (1) make injections slowly; (2) take care to avoid intra-arterial injection and extravasation; (3) if direct venous injection is impossible, inject into infusion tubing as close to the vein as possible; (4) follow the manufacturer's instructions regarding suitable diluents for preparing solutions; and (5) have facilities for resuscitation available.

## Implementation: Measures to Enhance Therapeutic Effects

*For Insomnia.* Educate patients about sleep fitness (see Table 32–7). Reassure patients with situational insomnia that sleep patterns will normalize once the precipitating stressor has been eliminated. Ensure that correctable underlying causes of insomnia (psychiatric or medical illness, use of stimulant drugs) are being managed.

*For Anxiety.* Encourage patients with generalized anxiety disorder to take their medicine as prescribed. Reassure them that significant physical dependence on benzodiazepines is rare; hence they should not allow concerns about "addiction" to interfere with compliance.

Ideally, patients will receive psychotherapy, which can provide support, encouragement, and skills for coping with anxiety-provoking situations.

Relaxation therapy (meditation, relaxation exercises, biofeedback) can help reduce tension.

## Ongoing Evaluation and Interventions

### Evaluating Therapeutic Effects

*For Insomnia.* Insomnia is usually self-limiting. Consequently, drug therapy is usually short term. Benzodiazepines should be discontinued periodically to determine if they are still required. If insomnia is long-term, make a special effort to identify possible underlying causes (e.g., psychiatric illness, medical illness, use of caffeine and other stimulants).

*For Anxiety.* For generalized anxiety disorder, benzodiazepines can be discontinued periodically (e.g., every 6 to 8 weeks) to determine if they are still needed.

### Minimizing Adverse Effects

*CNS Depression.* Drowsiness may be present on the day following hypnotic use of benzodiazepines. Warn patients about possible residual CNS depression and advise them to avoid hazardous activities (e.g., driving) if daytime sedation is significant.

*Paradoxical Effects.* Inform patients about possible paradoxical reactions (rage, excitement, heightened anxiety), and instruct them to notify the physician if these

---

*Patient education information is highlighted in color.

occur. If the reaction is verified, benzodiazepines should be withdrawn.

**Physical Dependence.** With most benzodiazepines, significant physical dependence is rare. However, with one agent—*alprazolam* [Xanax]—substantial dependence has been reported. With all benzodiazepines, development of dependence can be minimized by using the lowest effective dosage for the shortest time necessary and by using intermittent dosing when treating insomnia.

When dependence is mild, withdrawal can elicit insomnia and other symptoms that resemble anxiety. These symptoms must be distinguished from a return of the patient's original anxiety state or sleep disorder. Warn patients about possible drug-dependency insomnia during or after benzodiazepine withdrawal.

When dependence is severe, withdrawal reactions may be serious (panic, paranoia, delirium, hypertension, convulsions). To minimize symptoms, withdraw benzodiazepines slowly (over several weeks). Warn patients against abrupt discontinuation of treatment. After drug cessation, patients should be monitored for 3 weeks for signs of withdrawal or recurrence of original symptoms.

**Abuse.** The abuse potential of the benzodiazepines is low. However, these drugs are abused by some individuals. Be alert to requests for increased dosage, since these may reflect an attempt at abuse. Benzodiazepines are classified under Schedule IV of the Controlled Substances Act and must be dispensed accordingly.

**Use in Pregnancy and Lactation.** Benzodiazepines may injure the developing fetus, especially during the first trimester. Inform women of child-bearing age about the potential for fetal harm and warn them against becoming pregnant. If pregnancy occurs, benzodiazepines should be withdrawn.

Benzodiazepines readily enter breast milk and may accumulate to toxic levels in the breast-fed infant. Warn mothers against breast-feeding.

### Minimizing Adverse Interactions

**CNS Depressants.** Combined overdose with a benzodiazepine plus another CNS depressant can cause profound respiratory depression, coma, and death. Warn patients against use of alcohol and all other CNS depressants (e.g., opioids, barbiturates, antihistamines).

## Barbiturates

The nursing implications summarized below pertain to the barbiturates as a group. Implications specific to *phenobarbital* in the treatment of epilepsy are summarized in Chapter 23.

### Preadministration Assessment

#### Therapeutic Goal

Barbiturates are used to promote sleep (see Table 32-4), suppress seizures (see Chapter 23), and induce general anesthesia (see Chapter 27).

#### Baseline Data

For patients with *insomnia*, determine the nature of the sleep disturbance (prolonged latency, frequent awakenings, early morning awakening) and how long it has lasted. Assess for a possible underlying cause (e.g., medical illness, psychiatric illness, use of caffeine and other stimulants, poor sleep hygiene, major life stressor).

### Identifying High-Risk Patients

Barbiturates are *contraindicated* for patients with *severe respiratory disease* and *active or latent porphyria*. Use with *caution* in *elderly patients* and those with *respiratory disease*. Do not dispense to *individuals suspected of suicidal tendencies* or to those with a *history of sedative-hypnotic abuse*.

## Implementation: Administration

### Routes

Oral, IV, IM, and rectal.

### Administration

**Oral.** Warn patients not to increase the dosage or discontinue treatment without consulting the physician. Dosages should be reduced for elderly patients.

**Intravenous.** Make injections slowly to minimize respiratory depression and hypotension. Monitor blood pressure, pulses, and respiration. Have facilities for resuscitation immediately available. Observe the patient continuously. Do not inject solutions that are cloudy or that contain a precipitate. Extravasation may cause local necrosis; take care to ensure that extravasation does not occur. Intra-arterial administration may cause gangrene (secondary to arteriospasm) and must be avoided.

**Intramuscular.** Barbiturate solutions are highly alkaline and can cause pain and necrosis when injected IM. Consequently, IM injection is generally avoided. Avoid injection in the vicinity of peripheral nerves since irreversible nerve damage may result.

## Ongoing Evaluation and Interventions

### Evaluating Therapeutic Effects

Since insomnia is usually self-limiting, drug therapy should be short term. If insomnia is long term, make a special effort to identify a possible underlying cause (e.g., psychiatric illness, medical illness, use of caffeine and other stimulants).

### Minimizing Adverse Effects

**CNS Depression.** Inform patients about symptoms of CNS depression (sedation, lethargy, incoordination) and warn them against participation in hazardous activities (e.g., driving, operating machinery). Hospitalized patients may require ambulatory assistance.

**Respiratory Depression.** Barbiturates are strong respiratory depressants. Use with caution in elderly patients and those with respiratory disease.

When administered in anesthetic doses during labor and delivery, barbiturates can depress respiration in the neonate. Monitor the infant until respiration is normal.

**Tolerance.** Tolerance develops with prolonged treatment, and cross-tolerance exists with other general CNS depressants but not with opioids. If tolerance develops, temporary interruption of treatment is preferable to an increase in dosage. Warn patients against escalation of dosage without consulting the physician. To minimize tolerance, employ the lowest effective dosage for the shortest time necessary.

**Physical Dependence.** Physical dependence develops with prolonged treatment, and cross-dependence exists with other general CNS depressants, but not with opioids. The barbiturate abstinence syndrome can be severe, possibly life threatening. Manifestations can be minimized by withdrawing barbiturates slowly. Warn patients against abrupt discontinuation of treatment.

**Drug-Dependency Insomnia.** When used for insomnia, barbiturates may cause drug-dependency insomnia upon cessation of treatment. This must be distinguished from reemergence of the original sleep disorder. To minimize drug-dependency insomnia, administer barbiturates in the lowest effective dosage for the shortest time necessary.

**Abuse.** Short- to intermediate-acting barbiturates (e.g., secobarbital) have a high potential for abuse. Be alert to escalating requests for medication, since these may reflect attempts at abuse. Barbiturates are regulated under the Controlled Substances Act and must be dispensed accordingly.

**Suicide.** Barbiturates are "drugs of choice" for suicide. Do not dispense to patients suspected of suicidal tendencies.

**Use in Pregnancy.** Barbiturates readily cross the placenta and can injure the developing fetus. Inform women of child-bearing age about the potential for fetal harm and warn them against becoming pregnant.

Infants exposed to barbiturates during the third trimester may be born drug dependent; an abstinence syndrome may develop several days after parturition.

## Minimizing Adverse Interactions

**CNS Depressants.** Combined use of barbiturates and other CNS depressants (e.g., benzodiazepines, alcohol, opioids) can cause profound respiratory depression, coma, and death. Warn patients against use of alcohol and all other CNS depressants.

**Interactions Secondary to Accelerated Drug Metabolism.** Barbiturates induce hepatic drug-metabolizing enzymes, thereby accelerating the degradation of other drugs. Increased metabolism is of particular concern with *warfarin*, *oral contraceptives*, and *phenytoin*. Advise women taking oral contraceptives to consider an alternative form of birth control.

## Managing Toxicity

Overdose can be life threatening. Manifestations include respiratory depression, coma, pinpoint pupils, and hypotension. Death may result from pulmonary complications or renal failure. Treatment requires an intensive care unit. Principal management objectives are removal of the drug and maintenance of oxygenation. There is no specific antidote to barbiturate poisoning; CNS stimulants should not be employed.

# CHAPTER 33

# Central Nervous System Stimulants and Their Use in Attention-Deficit/Hyperactivity Disorder

Central nervous system (CNS) stimulants increase the activity of CNS neurons. Most stimulants act by enhancing neuronal excitation. A few act by suppressing neuronal inhibition. If given in sufficient dosage, all CNS stimulants can cause convulsions.

Clinical applications of the CNS stimulants are limited. Currently these drugs have two principal indications: attention-deficit/hyperactivity disorder and narcolepsy. In addition, CNS stimulants can be used to treat obesity. At one time CNS stimulants were given to counteract poisoning by CNS depressants, but this use has been discredited.

Please note that CNS stimulants are not the same as antidepressants. The antidepressants act selectively to alter mood, and hence can relieve depression while leaving other CNS functions unaffected. In contrast, CNS stimulants cannot elevate mood without producing generalized excitation. Accordingly, the role of CNS stimulants in treating depression is minor.

Our principal focus is on *amphetamines, methylphenidate* [Ritalin], and *methylxanthines* (e.g., caffeine). These agents are by far the most widely used CNS stimulants.

## Amphetamines

The amphetamine family consists of amphetamine, dextroamphetamine, and methamphetamine. All are powerful CNS stimulants. In addition to their central actions, amphetamines have significant actions in the periphery—actions that can cause cardiac stimulation and vasoconstriction. The amphetamines have a high potential for abuse. As a result, therapeutic applications are limited.

### Chemistry

*Dextroamphetamine and Levamphetamine.* The amphetamines are molecules that contain an asymmetric carbon atom. Because of that asymmetric carbon, amphetamines can exist as mirror images of each other. Such compounds are termed optical isomers or enantiomers. Dextroamphetamine and levamphetamine, whose structures are shown in Figure 33-1, illustrate the mirror-image concept. As we can see, dextroamphetamine and levamphetamine both contain the same atomic components—but those components are arranged differently around the asymmetric carbon. Because of this structural difference, these compounds have somewhat different pharmacologic properties. Dextroamphetamine is more selective than levamphetamine for causing CNS stimulation, and hence produces fewer peripheral side effects.

*Amphetamine.* The term *amphetamine* refers not to a single compound but rather to a 50:50 mixture of dextroamphetamine and levamphetamine. (In chemistry, we refer to such equimolar mixtures of enantiomers as racemic.)

*Methamphetamine.* Methamphetamine is simply dextroamphetamine with an extra methyl group (see Figure 33-1).

### Mechanism of Action

The amphetamines act by promoting release of biogenic amines (norepinephrine, dopamine, serotonin) from neurons. Transmitter release occurs in both the CNS and the periphery. Most effects of amphetamines result from release of norepinephrine. However, release of dopamine and serotonin also contribute.

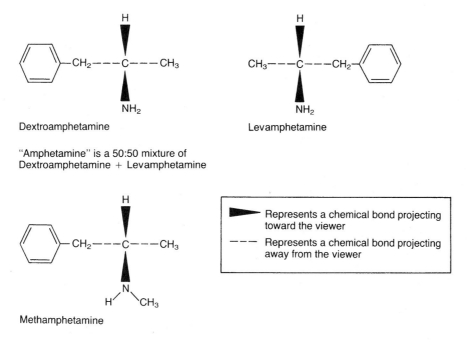

**Figure 33–1. Structural formulas of the amphetamines.** "Amphetamine" is a 50:50 mixture of dextroamphetamine plus levamphetamine. Note that dextroamphetamine and levamphetamine are simply mirror images of each other. Both compounds contain the same atomic components.

## Pharmacologic Effects

**Central Nervous System.** The amphetamines have prominent effects on mood and arousal. At usual doses, these drugs increase wakefulness and alertness, reduce fatigue, elevate mood, and augment self-confidence and initiative. Euphoria, talkativeness, and increased motor activity are likely. Task performance that had been reduced by fatigue or boredom improves.

In addition to their effects on mood and arousal, amphetamines can stimulate respiration and suppress appetite and perception of pain. Stimulation of the medullary respiratory center increases respiration. Effects on the hypothalamic feeding center depress appetite. By a mechanism that is not understood, amphetamines can enhance the analgesic effects of morphine and other opioids.

**Cardiovascular System.** Cardiovascular effects occur secondary to release of norepinephrine from sympathetic nerves. Norepinephrine acts in the heart to increase atrioventricular conduction, heart rate, and force of contraction. Excessive cardiac stimulation can produce dysrhythmias. In blood vessels, norepinephrine promotes constriction. Excessive vasoconstriction can produce hypertension.

## Tolerance

With regular amphetamine use, tolerance develops to elevation of mood, suppression of appetite, and stimulation of the heart and blood vessels. In highly tolerant users, doses up to 1000 mg (IV) every few *hours* may be required to maintain euphoric effects. This compares with *daily* doses of 5 to 30 mg for nontolerant individuals.

## Physical Dependence

Chronic use of amphetamines produces physical dependence. If amphetamines are abruptly withdrawn after prolonged use, an abstinence syndrome will result. Symptoms of withdrawal include exhaustion, depression, prolonged sleep, excessive eating, and a craving for more of the drug. Sleep patterns may take months to normalize.

## Abuse

Because amphetamines can produce euphoria (extreme mood elevation), these compounds have a high potential for abuse. Psychologic dependence can occur. (Users familiar with CNS stimulants find the psychologic effects of amphetamines nearly identical to those of cocaine.) Because of their abuse potential, amphetamines are classified under Schedule II of the Controlled Substances Act and must be dispensed accordingly. Whenever amphetamines are used therapeutically, their potential for abuse must be weighed against any potential benefits.

## Adverse Effects

**CNS Stimulation.** Stimulation of the CNS can cause *insomnia*, *restlessness*, and *extreme loquaciousness*. These effects can occur at therapeutic doses.

**Weight Loss.** By suppressing appetite, amphetamines can cause loss of weight. For people who are lean to start with, weight loss is considered an adverse effect. Conversely, for people who are obese, weight loss is desirable.

**Cardiovascular Effects.** Stimulation of the heart and blood vessels can result in *dysrhythmias*, *anginal pain*, and *hypertension*. Accordingly, amphetamines must be employed with extreme caution in patients with cardiovascular disease.

*Psychosis.* Excessive amphetamine use produces a state of paranoid psychosis, characterized by hallucinations and paranoid delusions (suspiciousness, feelings of being watched). Amphetamine-induced psychosis looks very much like schizophrenia. Symptoms are thought to result from release of dopamine. Consistent with this hypothesis is the observation that symptoms can be alleviated with a dopamine-receptor blocking agent (e.g., haloperidol). Following amphetamine withdrawal, psychosis usually resolves spontaneously within a week.

In some individuals, amphetamines can unmask latent schizophrenia. For these individuals, symptoms of psychosis do not clear spontaneously; hence psychiatric care is needed.

### Acute Toxicity

*Symptoms.* Overdose produces dizziness, confusion, hallucinations, paranoid delusions, palpitations, dysrhythmias, and hypertension. Death is rare. Fatal overdose is associated with convulsions, coma, and cerebral hemorrhage.

*Treatment.* Hallucinations can be controlled with chlorpromazine (an antipsychotic drug). An alpha-adrenergic blocker (e.g., phentolamine) can reduce hypertension (by promoting vasodilation). Because of its ability to block alpha receptors, chlorpromazine contributes to lowering blood pressure. Seizures can be managed with diazepam. Acidification of the urine can accelerate amphetamine excretion.

### Therapeutic Uses

*Attention-Deficit/Hyperactivity Disorder.* Amphetamines are useful drugs for attention-deficit/hyperactivity disorder (ADHD). This disorder and its treatment are discussed later in the chapter.

*Narcolepsy.* Narcolepsy is a disorder characterized by daytime somnolence and uncontrollable attacks of sleep. By stimulating the CNS, amphetamines can promote arousal and thereby alleviate these symptoms.

*Obesity.* Because they suppress appetite, the amphetamines have been employed in programs for weight loss. However, because of their high abuse potential, and because they offer no advantages over less dangerous drugs, amphetamines are not generally recommended for weight reduction. The use of amphetamines and other drugs in the management of obesity is discussed in Chapter 99.

### Preparations, Dosage, and Administration

*Preparations and Administration.* Four amphetamine preparations are available: amphetamine sulfate (racemic amphetamine), dextroamphetamine sulfate [Dexedrine, others], methamphetamine [Desoxyn], and an amphetamine mixture [Adderall]. The route for all four is oral. Amphetamines are regulated under Schedule II of the Controlled Substances Act and must be dispensed accordingly. (Note: Amphetamines are not approved for IV administration. Amphetamines for IV use are available only through illegal sources.)

*Dosage.* The dosage for narcolepsy ranges from 5 to 60 mg/day. Dosages for ADHD are presented later in the chapter. Dosages for obesity are presented in Chapter 99.

## Methylphenidate

Although methylphenidate [Ritalin] is structurally dissimilar from the amphetamines, the pharmacologic effects of methylphenidate and the amphetamines are nearly identical. Consequently, methylphenidate can be considered an amphetamine in all but structure and name. The mechanism of action, adverse effects, and abuse liability of methylphenidate are the same as those of the amphetamines. Methylphenidate has two indications: ADHD and narcolepsy. The dosage for narcolepsy is 10 to 60 mg daily. The dosage for ADHD is discussed later in the chapter. Like the amphetamines, methylphenidate is administered orally. Methylphenidate is classified under Schedule II of the Controlled Substances Act and must be dispensed accordingly.

## Methylxanthines

The methylxanthines are derivatives of xanthine, hence the family name. As indicated in Figure 33–2, these compounds consist of a xanthine nucleus to which one or more methyl groups is attached. Caffeine, the most familiar member of the family, will serve as our prototype.

### Caffeine

Caffeine is consumed worldwide for its stimulant effects. In the United States, per capita consumption is about 200 mg/day—mostly in the form of coffee. Although clinical applications of caffeine are few, caffeine remains of interest because of its widespread ingestion for nonmedical purposes.

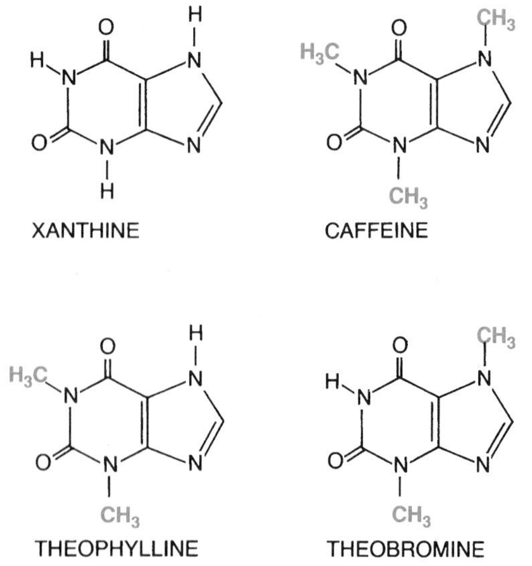

XANTHINE   CAFFEINE

THEOPHYLLINE   THEOBROMINE

**Figure 33–2. Structural formulas of the methylxanthines.**

## TABLE 33–1. DIETARY CAFFEINE

| Source | Caffeine Content |
|---|---|
| Coffee: Regular | |
|   Brewed | 40–180 mg/cup |
|   Instant | 30–120 mg/cup |
| Coffee: Decaffeinated | |
|   Brewed | 2–5 mg/cup |
|   Instant | 1–5 mg/cup |
| Tea | |
|   Brewed | 20–110 mg/cup |
|   Instant | 25–50 mg/cup |
| Cola drinks | 40–60 mg/12 oz |
| Cocoa | 2–50 mg/cup |
| Chocolate milk | 2–7 mg/5 oz |
| Milk chocolate | 1–15 mg/oz |
| Baker's chocolate | 25–35 mg/oz |

## Dietary Sources

Caffeine is present in chocolate and in beverages prepared from various natural products. Common dietary sources are coffee, tea, and cola drinks. The caffeine in cola drinks derives partly from the cola nut and partly from caffeine added by the manufacturer. Caffeine is also present in many noncola soft drinks. The caffeine content of chocolate and caffeine-containing beverages is shown in Table 33–1.

## Mechanism of Action

Several mechanisms of action have been proposed for caffeine and the other methylxanthines. These include (1) reversible blockade of adenosine receptors, (2) enhancement of calcium permeability in the sarcoplasmic reticulum, and (3) inhibition of cyclic nucleotide phosphodiesterase, resulting in accumulation of cyclic adenosine monophosphate (cyclic AMP). Blockade of adenosine receptors appears responsible for most of caffeine's effects.

## Pharmacologic Effects

*Central Nervous System.* In low doses, caffeine decreases drowsiness and fatigue, and increases the capacity for prolonged intellectual exertion. With increasing dosage, caffeine produces nervousness, insomnia, and tremors. When administered in very large amounts, the drug can cause convulsions. Despite popular belief, there is little evidence that caffeine can restore mental function in individuals intoxicated with alcohol.

*Heart.* High doses of caffeine stimulate the heart. When caffeine-containing beverages are consumed in excessive quantities, dysrhythmias may result.

*Blood Vessels.* Caffeine affects blood vessels in the periphery differently from those in the CNS. In the *periphery*, caffeine promotes *vasodilation*, whereas in the *CNS*, caffeine promotes *vasoconstriction*. The ability of caffeine to constrict cerebral blood vessels is thought to underlie the drug's ability to relieve certain types of headache.

*Bronchi.* Caffeine and other methylxanthines cause relaxation of bronchial smooth muscle, and thereby promote bronchodilation. Theophylline is an especially effective bronchodilator and, because of this action, is widely prescribed to treat asthma.

*Kidney.* Caffeine is a diuretic. The mechanism underlying increased urine formation is not fully understood.

*Reproduction.* When applied to cells in culture, caffeine can cause chromosomal damage and mutations. However, the concentrations of caffeine required to elicit these responses are much greater than those that can be achieved by drinking caffeine-containing beverages. Although there has been concern that ingestion of caffeine by pregnant women might cause fetal harm, studies have failed to demonstrate an association between caffeine consumption and birth defects. Nonetheless, the drug has caused birth defects in animals. Accordingly, it would seem prudent to minimize ingestion of caffeine during pregnancy.

## Pharmacokinetics

Caffeine is readily absorbed from the gastrointestinal tract and achieves peak plasma levels within 1 hour. Plasma half-life ranges from 3 to 7 hours. Elimination is by hepatic metabolism.

## Therapeutic Uses

*Neonatal Apnea.* Premature infants may experience prolonged apnea (lasting 15 seconds or more) along with bradycardia. Hypoxemia and neurologic damage may result. Caffeine and other methylxanthines can reduce the number and duration of apnea episodes and can promote a more regular pattern of breathing.

*Promoting Wakefulness.* Caffeine is used commonly as an aid to staying awake. The drug is marketed in various over-the-counter preparations [NoDoz, Vivarin, others] for this purpose. Of course, individuals desiring increased alertness needn't take a pill; they can get just as much caffeine by drinking coffee or some other caffeine-containing beverage.

*Other Applications.* Intravenous caffeine can help relieve headache induced by spinal puncture. The drug is used orally to enhance analgesia induced by opioids and non-narcotic agents (e.g., aspirin).

### Acute Toxicity

Caffeine poisoning is characterized by intensification of the responses seen at low doses. Stimulation of the CNS results in excitement, restlessness, and insomnia; if the dosage is sufficiently high, convulsions may occur. Tachycardia and respiratory stimulation are likely. Sensory phenomena (ringing in the ears, flashing lights) are common. Death from caffeine overdose is rare. When fatalities have occurred, between 5 and 10 gm have been ingested.

### Preparations, Dosage, and Administration

*Oral.* Oral caffeine is dispensed in tablets (100, 150, and 200 mg) and timed-release capsules (200 mg). The usual dosage for promoting alertness is 100 to 200 mg every 3 to 4 hours as needed.

**Parenteral.** Caffeine plus sodium benzoate is dispensed as an injection (250 mg/ml in 2-ml ampuls) for IV and IM administration. The usual adult dose (IM or IV) is 500 mg. The dosage for neonatal apnea is 10 mg/kg for the initial dose and 2.5 mg/kg daily thereafter.

### Theophylline

Theophylline has pharmacologic actions much like those of caffeine. Like caffeine, theophylline is an effective CNS stimulant. However, in contrast to caffeine, theophylline has important applications in the treatment of asthma; benefits derive from the drug's ability to promote bronchodilation. Antiasthmatic applications of theophylline are discussed in Chapter 69.

### Theobromine

Theobromine is a methylxanthine that occurs naturally in the seeds of *Theobroma cacao*, from which cocoa and chocolate are made. The caffeine content of these seeds is relatively low. Although there are similarities between theobromine and caffeine, these compounds do differ. The most distinct difference is that caffeine is a CNS stimulant, whereas theobromine is not. Accordingly, any CNS excitation produced by ingestion of cocoa and chocolate derives from their caffeine content and not from theobromine.

## Miscellaneous CNS Stimulants

### Pemoline

**Actions, Uses, and Adverse Effects.** Pemoline [Cylert] is a CNS stimulant with effects much like those of the amphetamines. The drug differs from the amphetamines primarily in that it causes less cardiac stimulation and vasoconstriction. The only approved indication for pemoline is ADHD (see below). The drug has been used investigationally in narcolepsy but is not approved for this application. The abuse potential of pemoline is less than that of the amphetamines and methylphenidate. As a result, pemoline is classified under Schedule IV of the Controlled Substances Act, whereas the amphetamines and methylphenidate are classified under Schedule II. Adverse effects of pemoline are generally like those of other CNS stimulants.

Rarely, pemoline causes *acute liver failure*. Deaths have occurred. Patients should be taught about signs of liver failure (jaundice, dark urine, nausea, fatigue) and instructed to discontinue the drug if these develop. In addition, patients should undergo periodic tests of liver function. However, since liver failure may develop suddenly, routine testing may not be helpful.

**Preparations, Dosage, and Administration.** Pemoline [Cylert] is dispensed in standard tablets (18.75, 37.5, and 75 mg) and in chewable tablets (37.5 mg) for oral use. The usual dosage for ADHD is 56.25 mg/day, administered as a single dose in the morning.

### Strychnine

Strychnine was introduced in the 16th century as a rat poison. At one time the drug was also employed therapeutically. Although strychnine is no longer used as a medicine, it remains a source of accidental poisoning and is of interest for that reason.

Strychnine is a powerful convulsant that stimulates the CNS at all levels. The drug produces stimulation by blocking receptors for glycine, an inhibitory neurotransmitter.

#### Strychnine Poisoning

**Causes.** A common cause of strychnine poisoning is ingestion of strychnine-based rodenticides by children. Poisoning also occurs through the use of "street drugs" to which strychnine has been added. (Since strychnine does not enhance the effects of illicit drugs, the practice of mixing this agent with street drugs is not only dangerous, it is also devoid of any pharmacologic rationale.) The lethal dose in children is about 15 mg. Doses between 50 and 100 mg are lethal in adults.

**Symptoms.** The first manifestation of strychnine poisoning is stiffness in the muscles of the face and neck. This is followed by a generalized increase in reflex excitability. During the early stages of poisoning, the victim is fully conscious. As poisoning progresses, convulsions occur. Strychnine-induced convulsions are characterized by tonic contraction of all voluntary muscles; contraction of the diaphragm, abdominal muscles, and thoracic muscles stops respiration. Convulsive episodes alternate with periods of depression until the victim dies or until the poisoning is successfully treated. Few patients survive beyond the fifth convulsive episode; some are killed by the first. Death is from respiratory arrest.

**Treatment.** Management is directed primarily at control of convulsions and support of respiration. Intravenous diazepam is the treatment of choice to suppress convulsions. If poisoning is severe, general anesthesia or neuromuscular blockade may be needed to eliminate convulsive activity. If anticonvulsant therapy fails to permit adequate breathing, mechanical support of respiration is indicated.

### Doxapram

Doxapram [Dopram] stimulates the CNS at all levels. The drug is employed clinically for its ability to stimulate respiration. However, since the doses required to increase respiration are close to those that can produce generalized CNS stimulation and convulsions, doxapram must be used with great care. Furthermore, although doxapram is labeled for treatment of general CNS depressant poisoning, its use for this purpose should be discontinued; experience has shown that respiratory depression from CNS depressant poisoning can be managed more safely and effectively with mechanical support of ventilation than with pharmacologic stimulation of respiration.

### Cocaine

Cocaine is a powerful CNS stimulant with a high potential for abuse. The only clinical application of this drug—local anesthesia—is discussed in Chapter 26. The basic pharmacology of cocaine and cocaine abuse are discussed in Chapter 37.

# Attention-Deficit/Hyperactivity Disorder

## ADHD in Children

ADHD is the most common psychiatric disorder of childhood. In the United States, over 2 million school-age children are affected—an average of one child with ADHD for every classroom. The incidence in boys is 4 to 8 times the incidence in girls. Symptoms begin between age 3 and 7, and persist into the teens in the majority of patients. In most cases, symptoms can be managed with drugs. Methylphenidate [Ritalin] is the agent employed most frequently.

### Signs and Symptoms

ADHD is characterized by *inattention*, *hyperactivity*, and *impulsivity*. Affected children are fidgety, unable to concentrate on schoolwork, and unable to wait their turn; switch excessively from one activity to another; call out excessively in class; and never complete tasks. For a diagnosis to be made, symptoms must appear prior to age 7 and must be present for at least 6 months. Since other disorders—especially anxiety and depression—may cause similar symptoms, diagnosis must be done with care. Specific diagnostic criteria for ADHD, as described in the *Diagnostic and Statistical Manual of Mental Disorders*, fourth edition, are summarized in Table 33-2. Depending on the symptom profile, ADHD can be subclassified as predominately inattentive type, predominately hyperactive-impulsive type, or combined type. Former names for ADHD—*hyperkinetic syndrome* and *minimal brain dysfunction*—are misleading and should be abandoned.

## Etiology

Although various theories have been proposed, the underlying pathophysiology of ADHD has not been established. Several theories implicate dysregulation in neuronal pathways that employ monoamine transmitters (norepinephrine, dopamine, serotonin). These theories would be consistent with the beneficial effects of stimulant drugs, which act by promoting monoamine release.

## Management Overview

Multiple strategies may be employed to manage ADHD. In addition to drugs, the treatment program can include family therapy, parent training, and cognitive therapy for the child. Although many experts believe that a combination of cognitive therapy and stimulant drugs constitutes the most effective treatment, there is no proof that this is true. A large trial to test this assumption is in progress.

## Treatment with Stimulant Drugs

Stimulant drugs are the mainstay of therapy. The most effective agents are methylphenidate [Ritalin], dextroamphetamine [Dexedrine], and pemoline [Cylert]. Of these, methylphenidate is by far the most commonly employed: over 70% of children with ADHD receive this drug.

*Methylphenidate.* Children with ADHD respond dramatically to methylphenidate. The drug increases attention span and goal-oriented behavior while decreasing impulsiveness, distractibility, hyperactivity, and restlessness. Overall behavior becomes more tolerable to parents and teachers. Tests of cognitive function (memory, reading, arithmetic) often improve significantly.

Although reduction of impulsiveness and hyperactivity with a stimulant may seem paradoxical—it isn't. Methylphenidate doesn't suppress rowdy behavior directly. Rather, the drug acts to improve attention and focus. Impulsiveness and hyperactivity decline because the child is now able to concentrate on the task at hand. It should be noted that methylphenidate does not create positive behavior; it only reduces negative behavior. Accordingly, methylphenidate cannot give a child good study skills and other appropriate behaviors. Rather, these must be learned once the disruptive behavior is no longer an impediment.

Methylphenidate is available in two formulations: standard tablets and sustained-release tablets. Both formula-

tions act rapidly, and benefits should be apparent within an hour. With the standard tablets, the child may need two or three doses a day. In contrast, the sustained-release tablets are administered just once a day. Not only is once-

### TABLE 33-2. DSM-IV DIAGNOSTIC CRITERIA FOR ADHD*

A. Either (1) or (2)

  (1) **Inattention.** Six (or more) of the following symptoms have persisted for at least 6 months:

- Often fails to give close attention to details or makes careless mistakes in schoolwork, work, or other activities
- Often has difficulty sustaining attention in tasks or play activities
- Often does not seem to listen when spoken to directly
- Often does not follow through on instructions and fails to finish schoolwork, chores, or duties in the workplace
- Often has difficulty organizing tasks and activities
- Often avoids, dislikes, or is reluctant to engage in tasks that require sustained mental effort (e.g., schoolwork, homework)
- Often loses things necessary for tasks or activities (e.g., toys, school assignments, pencils, books, tools)
- Is often easily distracted by extraneous stimuli
- Is often forgetful in daily activities

  (2) **Hyperactivity-impulsivity.** Six (or more) of the following symptoms have persisted for at least 6 months:

*Hyperactivity*

- Often fidgets with hands or feet or squirms in seat
- Often leaves seat in classroom or in other situations in which remaining seated is expected
- Often runs about or climbs excessively in situation in which it is inappropriate (in adolescents or adults, may be limited to subjective feelings of restlessness)
- Often has difficulty playing or engaging in leisure activities quietly
- Is often "on the go" or often acts as if "driven by a motor"
- Often talks excessively

*Impulsivity*

- Often blurts out answers before questions have been completed
- Often has difficulty awaiting turn
- Often interrupts or intrudes on others (e.g., butts into conversations or games)

B. Some hyperactive-impulsive or inattentive symptoms were present before age 7 years.

C. Symptoms are present in two or more settings (e.g., at school [or work] and at home).

D. There must be clear evidence of clinically significant impairment in social, academic, or occupational functioning.

E. The symptoms do not occur exclusively during the course of a pervasive developmental disorder, schizophrenia, or other psychotic disorder, and are not better accounted for by another mental disorder (e.g., mood disorder, anxiety disorder, dissociative disorder, or a personality disorder).

*Modified from American Psychiatric Association. *Diagnostic and Statistical Manual of Mental Disorders*, 4th ed. Washington, DC, American Psychiatric Press, 1994, pp. 83–85; reprinted with permission.

## TABLE 33-3. STIMULANTS USED TO TREAT ADHD

| Drug and Formulation | Trade Name | Dosage |
|---|---|---|
| *Methylphenidate* | | |
| Tablets, standard | Ritalin | 10 mg at 8 AM and noon, 5 mg at 4 PM |
| Tablets, SR* | Ritalin-SR | 20 mg in morning |
| *Dextroamphetamine* | | |
| Tablets | Dexedrine | 5 mg at 8 AM, noon, and 4 PM |
| Capsules, SR* | Dexedrine Spansules | 5-15 mg at 8 AM |
| *Pemoline* | | |
| Tablets | Cylert | 56.25 mg at 8 AM |

*SR = sustained release.

daily dosing more convenient, it also saves the child from the stigma associated with taking medicine at school.

Treatment is initiated with a 5-mg dose administered in the morning. With the standard tablets, a second dose is usually given at noon. If needed, a third dose may be given at 4 PM (if the child's behavior is intolerable at home). The dosage may be gradually increased as needed—but should not exceed 60 mg/day. A typical dosage is shown in Table 33-3. Dosage is assessed by monitoring for improvement in symptoms and appearance of side effects. Blood levels of methylphenidate may also be followed.

Principal adverse effects are *insomnia* and *growth suppression*. Insomnia results from CNS stimulation, and can be minimized by (1) reducing the size of the afternoon dose and (2) taking the afternoon dose no later than 4 PM. Growth suppression occurs secondary to appetite suppression. Growth suppression can be minimized by administering methylphenidate during or after meals, which reduces the impact of appetite suppression, and by taking "drug holidays" on weekends and in the summer, which creates the opportunity for growth to catch up. Once treatment ceases, a rebound increase in growth takes place; as a result, adult height is usually not affected. Other adverse effects include *headache* and *abdominal pain*, which have an incidence of 10%, and *lethargy* and *listlessness*, which can occur when dosage is excessive.

Stimulants should be interrupted periodically. The rationale for this practice is to (1) assess the need for continued treatment and (2) minimize suppression of growth. Many children can reduce or eliminate drug use on weekends and holidays. In no case should treatment continue for more than 1 school year without interruption. The summer school break is often a good opportunity for a prolonged drug holiday, with treatment resuming, if indicated, after school resumes.

**Dextroamphetamine.** Dextroamphetamine [Dexedrine, others] is as effective as methylphenidate for ADHD. In fact, some children who fail to respond to methylphenidate may respond to this drug. Dextroamphetamine acts rapidly, and effects should be apparent an hour after dosing. A typical dosage is 5 mg administered at 8 AM,

noon, and 4 PM. Adverse effects are like those of methylphenidate.

**Pemoline.** Pemoline [Cylert] is somewhat less effective than methylphenidate and dextroamphetamine for children with ADHD. Because of the risk of acute liver failure, pemoline should not be used as a first-line drug. Pemoline has a prolonged half-life, and therefore can be administered once daily. Pemoline has a lower abuse potential than methylphenidate and dextroamphetamine, and consequently is classified as a Schedule IV drug (rather than Schedule II). The usual dosage is 56.25 mg administered in the morning.

### Treatment with Nonstimulant Drugs

*Tricyclic Antidepressants.* Desipramine [Norpramin, Pertofrane] and imipramine [Tofranil] can reduce symptoms in children with ADHD. These drugs decrease hyperactivity but have little effect on impulsivity and inattention. Responses develop slowly; initial effects are seen in 2 to 3 weeks, and peak effects occur around 6 weeks. Tolerance frequently develops within a few months. In contrast to the stimulants, which can be discontinued on weekends, antidepressants must be taken continuously. Adverse effects include sedation and anticholinergic effects. More importantly, sudden death (from cardiotoxicity) has occurred in at least three children. When compared with stimulants, antidepressants have their benefits (no insomnia, no abuse potential, no growth suppression) as well as drawbacks (anticholinergic effects, tolerance, less efficacy, risk of sudden death). Since these agents are less effective and more dangerous than the stimulants, they are considered second-choice drugs for ADHD. The basic pharmacology of these antidepressants is presented in Chapter 30.

*Monoamine Oxidase Inhibitors.* Two monoamine oxidase (MAO) inhibitors—tranylcypromine [Parnate] and clorgyline—can reduce symptoms of ADHD. Effects are nearly identical to those of dextroamphetamine. Common side effects are drowsiness and reduced appetite. As discussed in Chapter 30, the principal concern with MAO inhibitors is hypertensive crisis, which can be precipitated by tyramine-rich foods. Since it is nearly impossible to ensure that children rigidly avoid these foods, it seems unlikely that MAO inhibitors can be used safely.

*Clonidine.* Clonidine [Catapres], which is used primarily for hypertension, may benefit children with ADHD. In small clinical trials the drug has reduced hyperactivity and impulsiveness. Irritability, sedation, and hypotension are the major side effects. The basic pharmacology of clonidine is discussed in Chapter 20.

## ADHD in Adults

Contrary to traditional assumptions, we now know that ADHD can persist into adulthood. Symptoms include poor concentration, stress intolerance, antisocial behavior, outbursts of anger, and inability to maintain a routine. Just how many children with ADHD are likely to exhibit symptoms as adults? The incidence is uncertain; estimates range widely—from just a few percent to as high as 70%. Much of this uncertainty stems from a lack of clearly defined diagnostic criteria.

As in childhood ADHD, stimulants are the principal drugs used in adults. Methylphenidate is prescribed most frequently. Dextroamphetamine and pemoline are alternatives. About 33% of adults fail to respond to stimulants or are unable to tolerate their side effects. For these patients, a trial with a nonstimulant may be appropriate; possible choices include imipramine, bupropion [Wellbutrin], and propranolol [Inderal].

## KEY POINTS

- The amphetamine family consists of dextroamphetamine, amphetamine (a racemic mixture of dextroamphetamine and levamphetamine), and methamphetamine.
- The amphetamines produce most of their effect by causing release of norepinephrine from neurons in the CNS and periphery. Some effects result from release of dopamine and serotonin.

- Through actions in the CNS, the amphetamines can increase wakefulness and alertness, reduce fatigue, elevate mood, stimulate respiration, and suppress appetite.
- By promoting release of norepinephrine from peripheral neurons, amphetamines can cause vasoconstriction and cardiac effects (increased heart rate, increased atrioventricular conduction, and increased force of contraction).
- The most common adverse effects of amphetamines are insomnia and weight loss. Amphetamines may also cause psychosis and adverse cardiovascular effects (dysrhythmias, angina, hypertension).
- The principal indications for amphetamines are ADHD and narcolepsy.
- The pharmacology of methylphenidate is nearly identical to that of the amphetamines.
- Methylphenidate is the drug most frequently prescribed for ADHD.
- Methylphenidate and other CNS stimulants reduce symptoms of ADHD by enhancing the child's ability to focus.
- Caffeine and other methylxanthines act primarily by blocking adenosine receptors.
- Responses to caffeine are dose dependent: low doses decrease drowsiness and fatigue; higher doses cause nervousness, insomnia, and tremors; and huge doses cause convulsions.
- Caffeine has two principal uses: treatment of apnea in premature infants and reversal of drowsiness.

# Summary of Major Nursing Implications*

## Amphetamines and Methylphenidate

## Preadministration Assessment

### Therapeutic Goal

*Amphetamines and Methylphenidate.* Reduction of symptoms in children and adults with ADHD. Reduction of sleep attacks in patients with narcolepsy.

*Amphetamines Only.* Facilitation of weight loss in conjunction with a comprehensive weight loss program.

### Baseline Data

*Children with ADHD.* Document the degree of inattention, impulsivity, hyperactivity, and other symptoms of ADHD. Symptoms must be present for at least 6 months to allow a diagnosis of ADHD. Obtain baseline values of height and weight.

*Narcolepsy.* Document the frequency and circumstances of sleep attacks.

### Identifying High-Risk Patients

*Amphetamines* are *contraindicated* for patients with *symptomatic cardiovascular disease, advanced arteriosclerosis, hypertension, hyperthyroidism, agitated states,* and a *history of drug abuse* and in those who have taken *monoamine oxidase inhibitors* within the previous 2 weeks.

## Implementation: Administration

### Route
Oral.

### Administration
Instruct the patient to swallow sustained-release and long-acting tablets intact, without crushing or chewing.

Children with ADHD should take the morning dose after breakfast and the last daily dose by 4 PM.

Amphetamines and methylphenidate are classified under Schedule II of the Controlled Substances Act and must be dispensed accordingly.

---

*Patient education information is highlighted in color.

## Ongoing Evaluation and Interventions

### Evaluating Therapeutic Effects

***Children with ADHD.*** Monitor for reductions in symptoms (impulsiveness, hyperactivity, inattention) and for improvement in cognitive function. Periodic drug holidays are required to determine if therapy is still needed. Continuous treatment for longer than 1 school year should not be done.

### Minimizing Adverse Effects

***Excessive CNS Stimulation.*** Amphetamines and methylphenidate can cause restlessness and insomnia. Advise patients to use the smallest dose required and to avoid dosing late in the day. Advise patients to minimize or eliminate dietary caffeine (e.g., coffee, tea, caffeine-containing soft drinks).

***Weight Loss.*** Appetite suppression can cause weight loss. Administering the morning dose after breakfast and the last daily dose early in the afternoon will minimize interference with eating.

***Cardiovascular Effects.*** Warn patients about cardiovascular responses (palpitations, hypertension, angina, dysrhythmias) and instruct them to notify the physician if these develop.

***Psychosis.*** If amphetamine-induced psychosis develops, therapy should be discontinued. For most individuals, symptoms resolve within a week. For some patients, drug-induced psychosis may represent unmasking of latent schizophrenia; these patients require psychiatric care.

***Withdrawal Reactions.*** Abrupt discontinuation can produce extreme fatigue and depression. Minimize by withdrawing amphetamines and methylphenidate gradually.

### Minimizing Abuse

If the medical history reveals that the patient is prone to drug abuse, monitor use of amphetamines and methylphenidate closely.

Avoid routine use of amphetamines for weight loss.

## Caffeine

### General Considerations

Caffeine is usually administered to promote wakefulness. Warn patients against habitual caffeine use to compensate for chronic lack of sleep. Advise patients to consult the physician if fatigue is persistent or recurrent.

### Minimizing Adverse Effects

***Cardiovascular Effects.*** Inform patients about cardiovascular responses to caffeine (palpitations, rapid pulse, dizziness) and instruct them to discontinue caffeine if these occur.

***Excessive CNS Stimulation.*** Warn patients that overdose can cause convulsions. Advise them to take no more caffeine than is needed.

# CHAPTER 34

# Other Psychologic Disorders: Panic Disorder, Obsessive-Compulsive Disorder, and Alzheimer's Disease

## Panic Disorder

### Characteristics

Panic disorder is characterized by recurrent, intensely uncomfortable episodes known as panic attacks. As defined in the American Psychiatric Association's *Diagnostic and Statistical Manual of Mental Disorders*, fourth edition (DSM-IV), panic attacks have a sudden onset, reach peak intensity within 10 minutes, and have four (or more) of the following symptoms:

- Palpitations, pounding heart, racing heartbeat
- Chest pain or discomfort
- Sensation of shortness of breath or smothering
- Feeling of choking
- Dizziness, lightheadedness
- Nausea or abdominal discomfort
- Derealization (feelings of unreality) or depersonalization (feeling detached from oneself)
- Fear of losing control or going crazy
- Fear of dying
- Tingling or numbness in the hands
- Flushes or chills

Symptoms typically dissipate within 30 minutes. Many patients go to emergency departments because they think they are having a heart attack. Some patients experience panic attacks daily, whereas others have only one or two a month. Panic disorder is a common condition that affects 1.6% Americans at some time in their lives. The incidence in women is 2 to 3 times the incidence in men. Onset of panic disorder is usually in the late teens or early twenties. Although the underlying cause of panic disorder is not understood, dysregulation of noradrenergic and serotonergic systems is thought to be involved.

Perhaps 50% of patients with panic disorder also experience *agoraphobia*, a condition characterized by anxiety about being in places or situations from which escape might be either difficult or embarrassing, or in which help might be unavailable in the event that a panic attack should occur. Agoraphobia leads to avoidance of certain places (e.g., elevators, bridges, tunnels, movie theaters) and situations (e.g., being outside the home alone; being in a crowd; standing on line; driving in traffic; traveling by bus, train, or plane). In extreme cases, agoraphobics may never set foot outside the home. Because of avoidance behavior, agoraphobia can severely limit occupational and social options.

### Treatment

Between 70% and 90% of patients with panic disorder respond well to treatment. Two modalities may be employed: *drug therapy* and *cognitive-behavioral therapy*. As a rule, patients experience rapid and significant improvement. Drug therapy helps suppress panic attacks, while cognitive-behavioral therapy helps patients become more comfortable with the situations and places that they have been avoiding. Additional benefit can be derived from avoiding caffeine and sympathomimetics (these agents can trigger panic attacks), avoiding sleep deprivation (which can predispose to panic attacks), and doing regular aerobic exercise (which can reduce anxiety).

The principal drugs used for panic disorder—*antidepressants* and *benzodiazepines*—are discussed below. Drug therapy should continue for at least 6 to 9 months.

Stopping sooner than this is associated with a high rate of relapse.

## Antidepressants

Antidepressants are the initial drugs of choice for blocking panic attacks. These agents decrease the frequency and intensity attacks, anticipatory anxiety, and avoidance behavior. All three classes of antidepressants—*selective serotonin reuptake inhibitors* (SSRIs), *tricyclic antidepressants* (TCAs), and *monoamine oxidase inhibitors* (MOAIs)—are equally effective. These drugs decrease panic attacks regardless of whether the patient is actually depressed. However, if the patient *does* have co-existing depression, antidepressants will benefit the depression and panic disorder simultaneously. Dosages should be low initially and then slowly increased. Excessive initial doses can exacerbate anxiety and must be avoided. With all antidepressants, full benefits take 6 to 12 weeks to develop.

Although MAOIs (e.g., phenelzine) are very effective in panic disorder, these drugs are difficult to use. MAOIs can cause significant side effects (orthostatic hypotension, weight gain, sexual dysfunction); in addition, patients must adhere rigidly to a tyramine-free diet (to avoid hypertensive crisis). Because of these drawbacks, MAOIs are generally reserved for patients who fail to respond to safer drugs.

The basic pharmacology of the antidepressants is discussed at length in Chapter 30. Dosages for panic disorder are summarized in Table 34-1.

## Benzodiazepines

Alprazolam [Xanax] and other benzodiazepines provide rapid and effective protection against panic attacks. These drugs also reduce anticipatory anxiety and phobic avoidance. In contrast to antidepressants, which take weeks or even months to work, benzodiazepines often provide relief with the first few doses. The principal side effect of the benzodiazepines is sedation, but some tolerance develops within 7 to 10 days. Benzodiazepines can cause physical dependence, making withdrawal extremely hard for some patients. The difficulty is that withdrawal produces intense anxiety, which people with panic disorder are often unable to tolerate. To minimize withdrawal symptoms, benzodiazepines should be withdrawn very slowly—over a period of several months. The basic pharmacology of the benzodiazepines is discussed in Chapter 32. Dosages for panic disorder are summarized in Table 34-1.

# Obsessive-Compulsive Disorder

## Characteristics

Obsessive-compulsive disorder (OCD) is a potentially disabling condition characterized by persistent obsessions and compulsions that cause marked distress, consume at least 1 hour a day, and significantly interfere with daily living. An *obsession* is defined as a recurrent, persistent thought, impulse, or mental image that is unwanted and distressing, and comes involuntarily to mind despite attempts to ignore or suppress it. Common obsessions include fear of contamination (e.g., acquiring a disease by touching another person), aggressive impulses (e.g., harming a family member), a need for orderliness or symmetry (e.g., personal bathroom items must be arranged in a precise way), and repeated doubts (e.g., did I unplug the iron?). A *compulsion* is a ritualized mental act or behavior that the patient is driven to perform in response to his or her obsessions. In the patient's mind, carrying out the compulsion is essential to prevent some horrible event

## TABLE 34-I. SOME DRUGS FOR PANIC DISORDER

| Drug | Initial Dosage | Maintenance Dose |
|---|---|---|
| *Selective Serotonin Reuptake Inhibitors* | | |
| Fluoxetine [Prozac] | 2.5-5 mg at breakfast | 5-20 mg/day |
| Fluvoxamine [Luvox] | 25 mg at bedtime | 100-300 mg/day |
| Paroxetine [Paxil] | 10 mg at bedtime | 20-40 mg/day |
| Sertraline [Zoloft] | 50 mg once a day | 100-200 mg/day |
| *Tricyclic Antidepressants* | | |
| Imipramine [Tofranil] | 10-25 mg at bedtime | 100-300 mg/day |
| Desipramine [Norpramin] | 10-25 mg at bedtime | 100-300 mg/day |
| *Monoamine Oxidase Inhibitors* | | |
| Phenelzine [Nardil] | 15 mg at breakfast | 30-40 mg bid |
| *Benzodiazepines* | | |
| Alprazolam [Xanax] | 0.25 mg tid-qid | 2-4 mg/day |
| Clonazepam [Klonopin] | 0.25 mg bid | 1-2 mg/day |
| Lorazepam [Ativan] | 0.5 mg tid-qid | 3-8 mg/day |

**TABLE 34–2. DSM-IV DIAGNOSTIC CRITERIA FOR OBSESSIVE-COMPULSIVE DISORDER**

A. The presence of either obsessions or compulsions:

*Obsessions*

1. Recurrent and persistent thoughts, impulses, or images that are experienced, at some time during the disturbance, as intrusive and senseless and that cause marked anxiety and distress.

2. The thoughts, impulses, or images are not simply excessive worries about real-life problems.

3. The person attempts to ignore or suppress the thoughts, impulses, or images, or to neutralize them with some other thought or action.

4. The person recognizes that the obsessions are a product of his or her own mind.

*Compulsions*

1. Repetitive behaviors (e.g., hand washing, putting objects in order) or mental acts (e.g., praying, counting, repeating words silently) that the person feels driven to perform in response to an obsession or according to rigid rules.

2. The behaviors or mental acts are performed to prevent or reduce distress or to prevent some dreaded event; however, these behaviors or mental acts either have no realistic connection with what they are designed to neutralize or prevent, or are clearly excessive.

B. At some time during the disorder, the person recognizes that the obsessions or compulsions are excessive or unreasonable. (This does not apply to children.)

C. The obsessions or compulsions cause marked distress, are time consuming (take >1 hour a day), or significantly interfere with normal routines, occupational or academic functioning, or usual social activities or relationships.

D. The symptoms are not related to another psychiatric disorder, and are not caused by a substance, medication, or general medical illness.

---

*Adapted from American Psychiatric Association. *Diagnostic and Statistical Manual of Mental Disorders*, 4th ed. Washington, DC, American Psychiatric Press, 1994, pp. 422–423.

from occurring (e.g., death of a parent). If performing the compulsion is suppressed or postponed, the patient experiences increased anxiety. Common compulsions include hand-washing, mental counting, arranging objects symmetrically, and hoarding. Patients usually understand that their compulsive behavior is excessive and senseless, but nonetheless are unable to stop. DSM-IV criteria for OCD are presented in Table 34–2.

## Treatment

Patients with OCD respond to drug therapy and behavioral therapy. Optimal treatment consists of both. Behavioral therapy is considered more important in OCD than in any other psychiatric disorder. In the technique employed, patients are exposed to sources of their fears, while being encouraged to refrain from acting out their compulsive rituals. When no dire consequences come to pass, despite the absence of "protective" rituals, patients are able to gradually give up their compulsive behavior. Although this form of therapy causes great anxiety, it is often successful.

The only drugs currently approved for OCD are clomipramine, fluoxetine, and fluvoxamine. All three drugs are antidepressants: clomipramine is a TCA; fluoxetine and fluvoxamine are SSRIs. Benefits with all three re-

sult from enhancing serotonergic transmission. Since responses are delayed, treatment should continue for at least 10 weeks before concluding that an apparent treatment failure is real.

### Clomipramine

Clomipramine [Anafranil] is the only TCA effective in OCD. About 70% of patients experience a significant improvement. Initial effects take 4 weeks to develop, and maximal effects are seen in 12 weeks.

Benefits derive from blockade of serotonin reuptake, which enhances transmission at serotonergic synapses. Among the TCAs, clomipramine is the most effective serotonin uptake inhibitor. The drug differs from the SSRIs in that it blocks uptake of norepinephrine in addition to blocking uptake of serotonin. Like other TCAs, clomipramine also blocks adrenergic, cholinergic, and histaminergic *receptors.*

Doses should be low initially (20 to 25 mg/day) and then gradually increased. Side effects can be minimized by dividing the early doses and taking them with meals. Maintenance doses of 150 to 250 mg/day are achieved in 2 to 4 weeks.

Clomipramine can cause multiple side effects. Sedation, dry mouth, dizziness, and tremor occur in over 50% of patients. Other common effects include weight gain, constipation, blurred vision, insomnia, headache, and nausea. The reaction of greatest concern is induction of *seizures*. Because of the risk of seizures, clomipramine should be avoided in patients with a history of seizures or head injury. Clomipramine greatly increases the risk of hypertensive crisis from MAOIs, and therefore is contraindicated for patients taking these drugs.

The basic pharmacology of clomipramine and other TCAs is discussed in Chapter 30.

### Selective Serotonin Reuptake Inhibitors

Of the SSRIs available, fluoxetine [Prozac], fluvoxamine [Luvox], and sertraline [Zoloft] are currently approved for OCD; trials with paroxetine [Paxil] are in progress. SSRIs reduce symptoms of OCD by enhancing serotonergic transmission. Responses are about equal to those seen with clomipramine. Common side effects of SSRIs are insomnia, anorexia, nausea, dyspepsia, and sexual dysfunction (especially delayed or absent orgasm). Despite this array of side effects, SSRIs are considerably safer than clomipramine. The dosage for fluoxetine is 20 mg/day. Higher doses have been employed, but have not yielded better responses. Dosing with fluvoxamine is begun at 50 mg/day, and can be increased to a maximum of 300 mg/day. The basic pharmacology of SSRIs is discussed in Chapter 30.

# Alzheimer's Disease

Alzheimer's disease (AD) is a devastating illness characterized by progressive memory loss, impaired thinking, personality changes, and inability to perform routine tasks of daily living. AD affects about 4 million Americans and kills about 100,000 each year, making it the fourth leading cause of death among adults. The annual cost of AD—$80 to $90 billion—is exceeded only by the cost of heart disease and cancer. Major pathologic findings in AD are degeneration of cholinergic neurons and the presence of neurotic plaques and neurofibrillary tangles. There is no clearly effective therapy for AD, and no prospect of one in the near future.

## Pathophysiology

The underlying cause of AD is unknown. Scientists have discovered important pieces of the AD puzzle, but still don't know how they fit together. It may well be that AD results from a combination of factors, rather than from a single cause.

### Degeneration of Neurons

Neuronal degeneration occurs in the *hippocampus* early in AD, followed later by degeneration of neurons in the *cerebral cortex*. The hippocampus serves an important role in memory. The cerebral cortex is central to speech, perception, reasoning, and other higher func-

tions. As hippocampal neurons degenerate, short-term memory begins to fail. As cortical neurons degenerate, patients begin having difficulty with language. With advancing cortical degeneration, more severe symptoms appear. These include complete loss of speech, loss of bladder and bowel control, and complete inability for self-care. AD eventually destroys enough brain function to cause death.

### Impact on Neurotransmitters

In patients with AD, levels of *acetylcholine* (ACh) decrease by 90%. This dramatic drop contrasts with the small decline that occurs naturally with age. Loss of ACh is significant for two reasons. First, ACh is an important transmitter in the hippocampus and cerebral cortex, the regions where neuronal degeneration occurs. Second, ACh is critical to forming memories, and its decline has been linked to memory loss in AD. In addition to the large drop in ACh, patients with AD experience small reductions in norepinephrine, serotonin, gamma-aminobutyric acid, and somatostatin.

### Neuritic Plaques and Beta-Amyloid

Neuritic plaques, which form outside of neurons, are a hallmark of AD. These spherical bodies are composed of a central core of beta-amyloid (a protein fragment) surrounded by remnants of axons and dendrites. Neuritic plaques are seen mainly in the hippocampus and cerebral cortex. The relationship of neuritic plaques to the disease process is unknown.

In patients with AD, beta-amyloid is present in high levels and may contribute to neuronal injury. Several lines of evidence support this possibility: beta-amyloid can kill hippocampal cells grown in culture; it can release free radicals, which injure cells; it can disrupt potassium channels; and it may form channels in the cell membrane that permit excessive entry of calcium. Lastly, low doses of beta-amyloid cause vasoconstriction, and high doses cause permanent blood vessel injury (secondary to release of oxygen free radicals). By disrupting blood vessels, beta-amyloid could slowly starve neurons to death.

### Neurofibrillary Tangles and Tau

Like neuritic plaques, neurofibrillary tangles are a prominent feature of AD. These tangles, which form inside neurons, result when the orderly arrangement of microtubules becomes disrupted (Fig. 34–1). The underlying cause is production of an abnormal form of tau, a protein that in healthy neurons forms cross-bridges between microtubules, and thereby keeps them in a stable configuration. In patients with AD, tau twists into paired helical filaments. As a result, the orderly arrangement of microtubules transforms into neurofibrillary tangles.

### Apolipoprotein E4

Apolipoprotein E (apoE), long known for its role in cholesterol transport, has recently been linked to AD. Like some other proteins, apoE has more than one form. In fact, it has three forms, named apoE2, apoE3, and apoE4. (Don't ask what happened to apoE1). Only one form—

A   Normal

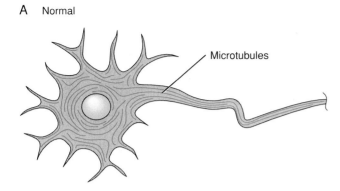

Microtubules

B   Alzheimer's Disease

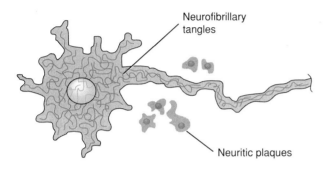

Neurofibrillary
tangles

Neuritic plaques

**Figure 34–1. Histologic changes in Alzheimer's disease.**
*A.* Healthy neuron. *B.* Neuron affected by Alzheimer's disease,
showing characteristic intracellular neurofibrillary tangles.
Note also extracellular neuritic plaques.

apoE4—is associated with AD. Genetic research has
shown that individuals with one or two copies of the gene
that codes for apoE4 are at increased risk for AD. In contrast, apoE2 seems to protect in some way.

What does apoE4 do? One possibility is that it promotes
formation of neuritic plaques. ApoE4 binds quickly and
tightly to beta-amyloid, causing this normally soluble substance to become insoluble, which could promote deposition of beta-amyloid in plaque.

It is important to note that apoE4 is neither necessary
nor sufficient to cause AD. There are many people with
AD who do not have the gene for apoE4. Conversely, in
one study involving people who were 90 years old and ho-
mozygous for apoE4, 50% had not developed AD.

## Risk Factors, Symptoms, and Diagnosis

### Risk Factors

The major known risk factor for AD is advancing age. In
90% of patients, the age of onset is 65 years or older. After
age 65, the risk of AD increases exponentially, doubling
every 10 years. The only other known risk factor is a family history of AD. Being female may be a risk factor; however, the high incidence of AD in women may occur sim-

ply because women live longer than men. *Possible* risk
factors include head injury, low educational level, and
production of apoE4.

### Symptoms

Alzheimer's is a disease in which symptoms progress re-
lentlessly from mild to moderate to severe (Table 34–3).
Symptoms typically begin after age 65, but may appear in
people as young as 40. Early in the disease patients begin
to experience memory loss and confusion. They may be
disoriented and get lost in familiar surroundings.
Judgment becomes impaired and personality may change.
As the disease progresses, patients have increasing difficulty with self-care. Between 70% and 90% eventually develop behavior problems (wandering, pacing, agitation,
screaming). Symptoms may intensify in the evening, a
phenomenon known as "sundowning." In the final stages
of AD, the patient is unable to recognize close family
members or communicate in any way. All sense of identity
is lost and the patient is completely dependent on others
for survival. The time from onset of symptoms to death
may be 20 years or longer, but is usually 4 to 8 years.
Although there is no clearly effective therapy for core
symptoms of AD, other symptoms (e.g., incontinence, depression) can be treated. In addition, resources are available to help families cope with AD and prepare for future
caregiving needs.

### Diagnosis

There is no specific test for AD. Hence, a definitive diagnosis is possible only at autopsy, when the brain can be
examined for characteristic neuritic plaques and neurofibrillary tangles. Prior to autopsy, diagnosis is done largely
by exclusion. That is, when all other possible causes of dementia have been ruled out, a probable diagnosis of AD
can be made. Criteria for a probable diagnosis are summarized in Table 34–4.

**TABLE 34–3. SYMPTOMS OF ALZHEIMER'S DISEASE**

*Mild Symptoms*

   Confusion and memory loss
   Disorientation; getting lost in familiar surroundings
   Problems with routine tasks
   Changes in personality and judgment

*Moderate Symptoms*

   Difficulty with activities of daily living, such as feeding
      and bathing
   Anxiety, suspiciousness, agitation
   Sleep disturbances
   Wandering, pacing
   Difficulty recognizing family and friends

*Severe Symptoms*

   Loss of speech
   Loss of appetite; weight loss
   Loss of bladder and bowel control
   Total dependence on caregiver

## TABLE 34-4. DIAGNOSTIC CRITERIA FOR PROBABLE ALZHEIMER'S DISEASE*

- Dementia established by clinical examination, documented by mental status testing, and confirmed by neuropsychological testing
- Deficits in two or more cognitive areas (e.g., memory, attention, language, personality, visuospatial functions)
- Cognitive deterioration is progressive
- Cognitive deterioration occurs in the presence of a clear sensorium (i.e., in the absence of delirium)
- Age of onset is between 40 and 90 years
- The individual has no systemic or other illnesses that affect the brain and that can produce dementia

*Established by the National Institute of Neurological and Communicative Disorders and Stroke (NINCDS) and by the Alzheimer's Disease and Related Disorders Association (ADRDA).

## Drug Therapy

Only three drugs—tacrine, donepezil, and ergoloid mesylates—are approved by the Food and Drug Administration (FDA) for AD. Tacrine and donepezil, which enhance cholinergic transmission, have modest effects. Ergoloid mesylates has little or no effect, despite its FDA approval.

### Tacrine

*Mechanism of Action.* Tacrine [Cognex] is a reversible inhibitor of acetylcholinesterase (AChE), the enzyme that breaks down acetylcholine (ACh). By inhibiting AChE, tacrine increases availability of ACh at cholinergic synapses. In patients with AD, the result is enhanced transmission by cholinergic neurons in the central nervous system (CNS) that have not been destroyed yet. There is no evidence that tacrine slows the actual disease process.

*Therapeutic Effect.* Tacrine is approved for patients with mild to moderate AD. Unfortunately, only 30% of patients respond, and their improvement is modest and short lasting. In the patients who do respond, improvements in cognition and function are about equal, reversing the degree of decline that normally occurs over 6 to 12 months. Although improvements are neither universal, dramatic, nor long lasting, and although tacrine poses a significant risk of serious liver damage (see below), the benefits seem worth the risk—given the devastating effects of AD and the need for any drug that offers some hope of relief.

*Pharmacokinetics.* Tacrine is administered orally and food decreases absorption. Bioavailability is low because of substantial first-pass metabolism. Blood levels peak in 2 hours, and decline with an elimination half-life of 3 hours. Tacrine crosses the blood-brain barrier with ease, and is retained in the CNS.

*Adverse Effects.* *Hepatotoxicity* is both common and troubling. Liver injury is monitored by assessing serum for elevations in alanine aminotransferase (ALT), an enzyme released from liver cells when they are damaged. In 50%

of patients, ALT levels are greater than 3 times the amount considered normal. Depending on the degree of ALT elevation and other indices of liver damage (e.g., jaundice, elevation of serum bilirubin), tacrine must be given in reduced dosage or discontinued. In most patients, liver damage reverses after tacrine is withdrawn. The recommended schedule for ALT measurement is as follows: every 2 weeks for the first 16 weeks, then monthly for 2 months, and every 3 months thereafter.

By elevating ACh in the periphery, tacrine can cause typical *cholinergic effects.* Gastrointestinal effects are most frequent. These include nausea/vomiting (28%), diarrhea (16%), and dyspepsia (9%). Other common side effects include myalgia, headache, and ataxia.

*Preparations, Dosage, and Administration.* Tacrine [Cognex] is dispensed in capsules (10, 20, 30, and 40 mg) for oral administration. Dosing is begun at 10 mg 4 times a day, and then gradually increased to a maximum of 40 mg 4 times a day. Administration is usually between meals to enhance absorption. However, tacrine can be given with meals if stomach upset occurs.

### Donepezil

Donepezil [Aricept] was recently approved by the FDA for mild to moderate AD. Like tacrine, donepezil inhibits AChE, and thereby enhances transmission at central and peripheral cholinergic synapses. Therapeutic responses appear about equal to those of tacrine. Donepezil does not affect the underlying disease process. Common side effects are nausea and diarrhea. Bradycardia may also develop, especially in patients with predisposing heart disorders. In contrast to tacrine, donepezil does not injure the liver. Donepezil is available in 5- and 10-mg tablets. The dosage is 5 mg/day initially, and can be increased to 10 mg/day.

### Ergoloid Mesylates

Although ergoloid mesylates [Hydergine, Gerimal] is FDA approved for AD, benefits are minimal at most. The drug acts in the CNS to enhance neuronal metabolism, and may also improve cerebral blood flow. The usual dosage is 3 mg 3 times a day. Ergoloid mesylates is contraindicated for patients with acute psychosis.

### Investigational Drugs

*Acetyl-L-Carnitine.* This agent is structurally similar to ACh, and therefore may interact with cholinergic receptors. In addition, it may undergo conversion to ACh in the CNS, thereby increasing ACh levels. In clinical studies, the drug has improved cognition in patients with AD. It may also slow disease progression.

*Nonsteroidal Anti-inflammatory Drugs.* There is mounting evidence of a link between inflammation and AD. Epidemiologic data suggest that regular use of nonsteroidal anti-inflammatory drugs (NSAIDs; e.g., ibuprofen) can decrease the risk of AD. The longer NSAIDs are used, the lower the apparent risk. In a study of elderly twins, the risk of AD was 10 times lower in the twin who used NSAIDs. Acetaminophen, which does not reduce inflammation, does not lower the risk of AD.

*Estrogens.* Estrogens appear to reduce the risk of AD. In a study of postmenopausal women, those who used hormone replacement therapy (HRT) had a 30% to 40% reduction in the risk of AD after 10 years. In those who developed AD despite using HRT, the onset of symptoms was delayed. In women who already have AD, estrogens appear to improve memory. As discussed in Chapter 57, HRT has the important benefits of reducing the risk of osteoporosis and heart disease. The principal concern with HRT is that it may (or may not) produce a small increase in the risk of breast cancer.

### Drugs for Behavioral Symptoms

Patients with AD may need medication for delusions, agitation, depression, or anxiety. Delusions may respond to haloperidol [Haldol], clozapine [Clozaril], or risperidone [Risperdal]. Various drugs may be tried for agitation, including propranolol [Inderal], trazodone [Desyrel], thioridazine [Mellaril], and haloperidol. Anxiety can be lowered with lorazepam [Ativan] or buspirone [BuSpar]. SSRIs, such as fluoxetine [Prozac] can help relieve depression. Tricyclic antidepressants, which have significant anticholinergic actions, should be used with caution, since they may intensify symptoms of AD.

## KEY POINTS

- Patients with panic disorder experience recurrent panic attacks. Symptoms include palpitations, pounding heart, chest pain, derealization or depersonalization, and fear of dying or going crazy.
- Many patients with panic disorder also experience agoraphobia, a condition characterized by anxiety about being in places or situations from which escape might be difficult or embarrassing, or in which help might be unavailable if a panic attack should occur.
- Panic disorder can be treated with antidepressants (SSRIs, TCAs, MAOIs) and benzodiazepines.
- Benzodiazepines reduce panic attacks quickly, whereas antidepressants take weeks or months to act.
- Weaning panic disorder patients from benzodiazepines must be done very gradually, so as to minimize anxiety and other symptoms of withdrawal.
- Obsessive-compulsive disorder (OCD) is characterized by persistent obsessions and compulsions that cause marked distress, consume at least 1 hour a day, and significantly interfere with daily living.
- Optimal treatment for OCD consists of behavior therapy and drug therapy.
- Behavior therapy is more important in OCD than in any other psychiatric disorder.
- Three drugs are approved for OCD: clomipramine, fluoxetine, and fluvoxamine. All three block serotonin reuptake (and thereby enhance serotonergic transmission), and responses to all three are delayed.
- Clomipramine increases the risk of seizures, and therefore must be avoided by patients with a history of head injury or seizure disorders.
- Alzheimer's disease (AD) is a relentless illness characterized by progressive memory loss, impaired thinking, personality changes, and inability to perform routine tasks of daily living.
- The histopathology of AD is characterized by neuritic plaques, neurofibrillary tangles, and degeneration of cholinergic neurons in the hippocampus and cerebral cortex.
- Neuritic plaques are spherical, extracellular bodies that consist of a beta-amyloid core surrounded by remnants of axons and dendrites.
- In patients with AD, beta-amyloid is present in high levels and may contribute to neuronal injury.
- Neurofibrillary tangles result from production of a faulty form of tau, a protein that in healthy neurons serves to maintain the orderly arrangement of neurotubules.
- The major known risk factor for AD is advancing age.
- Tacrine, a cholinesterase inhibitor, increases availability of acetylcholine at cholinergic synapses, and thereby enhances transmission by CNS cholinergic neurons that have not yet been destroyed by AD.
- Tacrine produces a modest improvement in about 30% of patients with AD; the remaining 70% don't respond.
- The major adverse effect of tacrine is liver damage, which is common and requires regular monitoring of serum ALT.

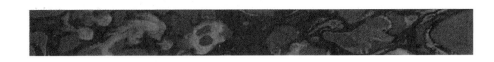

# Drug Abuse

# CHAPTER 35

# Drug Abuse: Basic Considerations

**Definitions**
**Diagnostic Criteria for Substance Abuse and**
   **Substance Dependence**
**Factors Contributing to Drug Abuse**
**Approaches to Modifying Drug-Using Behavior**
**The Controlled Substances Act**

From the dawn of civilization, mind-altering drugs have held a fascination for humankind. Throughout history, people have taken drugs to elevate mood, release inhibitions, distort perceptions, induce hallucinations, and modify thinking. Many of those who use mind-altering drugs restrict usage to socially approved patterns. However, many others self-administer drugs to excess. Excessive drug use is our concern in this chapter and the two that follow.

Drug abuse confronts the clinician in a variety of ways, making knowledge of abuse a necessity. Important areas in which expertise on drug abuse may be applied include (1) diagnosis and treatment of acute toxicity, (2) diagnosis and treatment of secondary medical complications of drug abuse, (3) facilitating drug withdrawal, and (4) educating and counseling drug abusers.

We will approach drug abuse in two stages. In this chapter we discuss basic concepts that apply to drug abuse. In Chapters 36 and 37 we focus on specific abused agents.

## Definitions

### Drug Abuse

Drug abuse can be defined as *using a drug in a fashion inconsistent with medical or social norms*. Traditionally, the term also implies drug usage that is harmful to the individual or society. As we shall see, although we can give abuse a general definition, deciding whether a particular instance of drug use constitutes "abuse" is often difficult.

Whether or not drug use is considered abuse depends, in part, on the purpose for which a drug is taken. Not everyone who takes large doses of psychoactive agents is an abuser. For example, we do not consider it abuse to take opioids in large doses on a long-term basis to relieve pain caused by cancer. However, we do consider it abusive for

an otherwise healthy individual to take those same opioids in the same doses for the purpose of producing euphoria.

When we speak of drug abuse, we should be aware that abuse can have different degrees of severity. Some people, for example, use heroin only occasionally, whereas others use it habitually and compulsively. Although both patterns of drug use are socially condemned, and therefore constitute abuse, there is an obvious quantitative difference between taking heroin once or twice and taking it routinely and compulsively.

Note that by the definition given above, *drug abuse is culturally defined*. Because abuse is culturally defined, and because societies differ from one another and are changeable, there can be wide variations in what is labeled abuse. *What is defined as abuse can vary from one culture to another.* For example, in the United States, moderate consumption of alcohol is not usually considered abuse. In contrast, any ingestion of alcohol would be considered abuse in some Moslem societies. Furthermore, *what is defined as abuse can vary from one time to another within the same culture.* For example, when a few Americans first began to experiment with LSD and other psychedelic drugs, these agents were legal and their use was not generally disapproved. However, when use of psychedelics became widespread, our societal posture changed and legislation was passed to make the manufacture, sale, and use of these drugs illegal.

Within the United States there is divergence of opinion about what constitutes drug abuse. For example, some people would consider *any* use of marijuana to be drug abuse, whereas others would call smoking marijuana abusive only if it were done *habitually*. Similarly, although many Americans do not seem to consider cigarette smoking to be drug abuse (even though the practice is compulsive and clearly harmful to the individual and society), there are others who believe very firmly that cigarette smoking constitutes a blatant form of abuse.

As we can see, distinguishing between culturally acceptable drug use and drug use that is to be called abuse is more in the realm of social science than pharmacology. Accordingly, since this is a pharmacology text and not a sociology text, we will not attempt to define just what patterns of drug use do or do not constitute abuse. Instead, we will focus on the pharmacologic properties of abused drugs—leaving distinctions about what is and is not abuse to sociologists and legislators. Fortunately, we can identify the drugs that tend to be abused and discuss their pharmacology without having to resolve all arguments about what patterns of use should or should not be considered abusive.

As discussed later, the American Psychiatric Association has established diagnostic criteria for *substance abuse*, a specific substance use disorder. These objective criteria are largely independent of cultural bias, and should not be confused with the concept of drug abuse as just presented.

### Addiction

The American Society of Addiction Medicine defines addiction as *a disease process characterized by the continued use of a specific psychoactive substance despite physical, psychologic, or social harm.* Please note that nowhere in this definition is addiction equated with physical dependence. As discussed below, although physical dependence can contribute to addictive behavior, it is neither necessary nor sufficient for addiction to occur. Addiction can be considered essentially equivalent to *substance dependence* as defined in the fourth edition of the *Diagnostic and Statistical Manual of Mental Disorders* (DSM-IV) (see below).

### Other Definitions

*Tolerance* results from regular drug use and can be defined as a state in which a particular dose elicits a smaller response than it formerly did. As tolerance increases, higher and higher doses are needed to elicit desired effects.

*Cross-tolerance* is a state in which tolerance to one drug confers tolerance to another drug. Cross-tolerance generally develops among drugs within a particular class, but not between drugs in different classes. For example, tolerance to one opioid (e.g., heroin) confers cross-tolerance to other opioids (e.g., meperidine), but not to CNS depressants, psychostimulants, psychedelics, or nicotine.

*Psychologic dependence* can be defined as an intense subjective need for a particular psychoactive drug.

*Physical dependence* can be defined as a state in which an abstinence syndrome will occur if drug use is discontinued. Physical dependence is the result of neuroadaptive processes that take place in response to prolonged drug exposure.

*Cross-dependence* refers to the ability of one drug to support physical dependence on another drug. When cross-dependence exists between drug A and drug B, drug A will be able to prevent withdrawal in a patient physically dependent on drug B, and vice versa. As with cross-tolerance, cross-dependence generally exists among drugs

in the same pharmacologic family, but not between drugs in different families.

A *withdrawal syndrome* is a constellation of signs and symptoms that occur in physically dependent individuals when they discontinue drug use. Quite often, the symptoms seen during withdrawal are the opposite of the effects produced by the drug being withdrawn. For example, discontinuation of a CNS depressant can cause CNS excitation.

## Diagnostic Criteria for Substance Abuse and Substance Dependence

Diagnostic criteria for substance abuse and substance dependence are set forth in DSM-IV, published by the American Psychiatric Association. A summary appears in Table 35-1. As defined in DSM-IV, substance dependence, which can be equated with addiction, is a more severe disorder than substance abuse. Accordingly, individuals whose drug problem is not bad enough to meet the criteria for substance dependence might nonetheless meet the criteria for substance abuse.

As indicated in Table 35-1, tolerance and withdrawal are among the criteria for substance dependence. Please note, however, that tolerance and withdrawal, by themselves, are neither necessary nor sufficient for substance dependence (addiction) to exist. Put another way, the pattern of drug use that constitutes substance dependence can exist in persons who are not physically dependent on drugs and who have not developed tolerance. Since this distinction is extremely important, I will express it yet one more way: *being physically dependent on a drug is not the same as being addicted!* Many people are physically dependent but do not meet the criteria for substance dependence. These people are not considered addicts because they do not demonstrate the behavior pattern that constitutes substance dependence. Patients with terminal cancer, for example, are often physically dependent on opioids; however, since their lives are not disrupted by their medication (quite the contrary), their drug use does not meet the criteria for substance dependence (nor substance abuse, for that matter). Similarly, some degree of physical dependence occurs in all patients who take barbiturates to control epilepsy; despite their physical dependence, epileptics do not carry out stereotypic addictive behavior, and therefore cannot be considered substance dependent under DSM-IV criteria.

Having stressed that physical dependence and substance dependence (addiction) are different from each other, we must note that these two phenomena are not entirely unrelated. As discussed below, although physical dependence is not the same as addiction, physical dependence often contributes to addictive behavior.

**TABLE 35–1. DSM-IV DIAGNOSTIC CRITERIA FOR SUBSTANCE ABUSE AND SUBSTANCE DEPENDENCE***

*Substance Abuse*

Substance abuse is a maladaptive pattern of substance use leading to clinically significant impairment or distress, as manifested by one (or more) of the following within a 12-month period:

- Recurrent substance use that results in a failure to fulfill major role obligations at work, school, or home
- Recurrent substance use in situations in which it is physically hazardous
- Recurrent substance-related legal problems
- Continued substance use despite persistent or recurrent social or interpersonal problems caused or exacerbated by the substance

Individuals who display tolerance, withdrawal, and other symptoms of substance dependence would be diagnosed under substance dependence, a more severe disorder, rather than under substance abuse.

*Substance Dependence*

Substance dependence is a maladaptive pattern of substance use, leading to clinically significant impairment or distress, as manifested by three (or more) of the following, occurring at any time in the same 12-month period:

- Tolerance to the substance
- Withdrawal, as manifested by either:
  — the characteristic withdrawal syndrome for the substance, or
  — the same (or closely related) substance is taken to relieve or avoid withdrawal symptoms
- The substance is often taken in larger amounts or over a longer time than intended
- Substance use continues despite a persistent desire or repeated efforts to cut down or control consumption
- A great deal of time is spent in activities necessary to obtain the substance, use the substance, or recover from its effects
- Important social, occupational, or recreational activities are given up or reduced because of substance use
- Substance use continues despite knowledge of a persistent or recurrent physical or psychologic problem that substance use probably caused or exacerbated (e.g., drinking despite knowing that alcohol made an ulcer worse)

*Modified from American Psychiatric Association. *Diagnostic and Statistical Manual of Mental Disorders*, 4th ed. Washington, DC, American Psychiatric Press, 1994, pp. 181–183; reprinted by permission.

# Factors Contributing to Drug Abuse

Drug abuse is the end result of a progressive involvement with drugs. Taking psychoactive drugs is usually initiated out of curiosity. From this initial involvement, the user can progress to occasional use. Occasional use can then evolve into compulsive use. Factors that play a role in the progression from experimental use to compulsive use are discussed below.

## Reinforcing Properties of Drugs

Although there are several reasons for initiating drug use (e.g., curiosity, peer pressure), individuals would not continue drug use unless drugs gave them desirable feelings or experiences. By making people feel "good," drugs reinforce the reasons for their use. Conversely, if drugs did not give people experiences that they found desirable, the reasons for initiating drug use would not be reinforced, and drug use would stop.

Reinforcement by drugs can occur in two ways. First, drugs can give the individual an experience that is pleasurable. Cocaine, for example, produces a state of euphoria. Second, drugs can reduce the intensity of unpleasant experience. For example, drugs can reduce anxiety and stress.

The reinforcing properties of drugs can be clearly demonstrated in experiments with animals. In the laboratory, animals will self-administer most of the drugs that are abused by humans (e.g., opioids, barbiturates, alcohol, cocaine, amphetamines, phencyclidine, nicotine, caffeine). When these drugs are made freely available, animals develop patterns of drug use that are similar to those of humans. Animals will self-administer these drugs (except for nicotine and caffeine) in preference to eating, drinking, and sex. If permitted, these animals often die from lack of food and fluid. These observations strongly suggest that pre-existing psychopathology is not necessary for drug abuse to take place. Rather, these studies suggest that drug abuse results, in large part, from the reinforcing properties of drugs themselves.

## Physical Dependence

As defined above, physical dependence is a state in which an abstinence syndrome will occur if drug use is discontinued. The degree of physical dependence is determined largely by dosage size and duration of use. Physical dependence is greatest in those who use large doses for a long time. The more physically dependent a person is, the more intense the withdrawal syndrome. Substantial physical dependence develops to the opioids (e.g., morphine, heroin) and CNS depressants (e.g., barbiturates, alcohol). Physical dependence tends to be less prominent with other abused drugs (e.g., psychostimulants, psychedelics, marijuana).

Physical dependence can contribute to compulsive drug use. Once dependence has developed, the desire to avoid withdrawal becomes a motivator for continued drug administration. Furthermore, if the drug is administered after the onset of withdrawal, its ability to alleviate the discomfort of withdrawal can reinforce its desirability. It must be noted, however, that although physical dependence plays a role in the abuse of drugs, physical dependence should not be viewed as the primary cause of addictive behavior. Rather, physical dependence is just one of several factors that can contribute to the development and continuation of compulsive use.

## Psychologic Dependence

Psychologic dependence is defined as an intense subjective need for a drug. Individuals who are psychologically dependent feel very strongly that their sense of well-being is dependent upon continued drug use; a sense of "craving" is felt when the drug is unavailable. There is no question that psychologic dependence can be a major factor in addictive behavior. For example, it is psychologic dependence—and not physical dependence—that plays the principal role in causing renewed use of opioids by addicts who had previously gone through withdrawal.

## Social Factors

Social factors can play an important role in the development of drug abuse. The desire for social status and approval is a common reason for initiating drug use. Also, since initial drug experiences are frequently unpleasant, the desire for social approval can be one of the most compelling reasons for repeating drug use after the initial exposure. For example, most people do not especially enjoy their first cigarette; if it were not for peer pressure, many people would quit before reaching the point where they began to experience smoking as pleasurable. Similarly, initial use of heroin, with its accompanying nausea and vomiting, is often deemed unpleasant; peer pressure is a common reason for maintaining heroin use long enough to develop tolerance to these undesirable effects.

## Drug Availability

Drug availability is clearly a factor in the development and maintenance of abuse. Abuse can flourish only in those environments where drugs can be readily obtained. In contrast, where procurement of drugs is difficult, drug abuse is minimal. The ready availability of drugs in hospitals and clinics is a major reason for the unusually high incidence of addiction seen among pharmacists, nurses, and physicians. It is the desire to reduce drug abuse through reducing drug availability that provides much of the rationale for law enforcement efforts directed at the manufacture and distribution of illicit drugs.

## Vulnerability of the Individual

Some individuals are more prone to becoming drug abusers than others. By way of illustration, let's consider three individuals from the same social setting who have equal access to the same psychoactive drug. The first person experiments with the drug briefly and never uses it again. The second person progresses from experimentation to occasional use. The third goes on to take the drug compulsively. Since social factors, drug availability, and the properties of the drug itself are the same for all three individuals, these factors cannot explain the three different patterns of drug use that developed. We must conclude, therefore, that the three patterns developed because of differences in the users themselves: one individual was not prone to drug abuse, one had only moderate tendencies toward abuse, and the third was highly vulnerable to becoming an abuser.

Several psychologic factors have been associated with tendencies toward drug abuse. Drug abusers are frequently individuals who are impulsive, have a low tolerance for frustration, and are rebellious against social norms. Other psychologic factors that seem to predispose individuals to abusing drugs include depressive disorders, anxiety disorders, and antisocial personality. It is also clear that individuals who abuse one type of drug are likely to abuse other drugs.

There is speculation that some instances of drug abuse may actually be attempts at self-medication to relieve emotional discomfort. For example, some people may use alcohol and other depressants as a means of controlling severe anxiety. Although their drug use may appear excessive, it may be no more than is needed to prevent feelings that are deemed intolerable.

Genetics also contribute to drug abuse. Vulnerability to alcoholism, for example, may result from an inherited predisposition.

# Approaches to Modifying Drug-Using Behavior

In the treatment of drug abuse, the *ideal* goal is *complete cessation* of drug use. However, total abstinence is not the only outcome that can be considered successful. Treatment that changes drug use from compulsive to moderate will permit increased productivity, better physical health, and a decrease in socially unacceptable behavior. Clearly, this outcome is beneficial both to the individual and to society—even though some degree of drug use continues. It must be noted, however, that in the treatment of some forms of abuse, nothing short of total abstinence can be considered a true success. Experience has shown that abusers of *cigarettes*, *alcohol*, and *opioids* are rarely capable of sustained moderation. Hence, for many of these individuals, abstinence must be complete if there is to be any hope of avoiding a return to compulsive drug use.

Multiple techniques are employed in hopes of modifying drug-using behavior. Techniques that have shown some degree of success include (1) therapy directed at resolving emotional problems that underlie drug use, (2) substitution of alternative rewards for the rewards of drug use, (3) threats and external pressure to discourage drug use, and (4) use of pharmacologic agents to modify the effects of abused drugs. It is common for a treatment program to incorporate two or more of these behavior modification methods. It is worth noting that at least two approaches to reducing drug abuse have *not* met with much success. These are (1) prolonged hospitalization and (2) traditional individual psychotherapy in the absence of other forms of treatment.

Of the pharmacologic aids for modifying drug-using behavior, *disulfiram* [Antabuse] and *naltrexone* [Trexan] have proved most beneficial—and even these drugs are not employed widely. Disulfiram helps the alcoholic avoid drinking (see Chapter 36). Naltrexone, an opioid antagonist, is employed to treat opioid abuse (see Chapter 37).

# The Controlled Substances Act

The *Comprehensive Drug Abuse Prevention and Control Act of 1970*, known informally as the *Controlled Substances Act*, is the principal federal legislation addressing drug abuse. One objective of the act is to reduce the chances that drugs originating from legitimate sources will become available to drug abusers. To accomplish this goal, the act sets forth regulations for the handling of controlled substances by manufacturers, distributors, pharmacists, nurses, and physicians. Enforcement of the act is the responsibility of the *Drug Enforcement Administration (DEA)*, an arm of the United States Department of Justice.

## Record Keeping

In order to keep track of controlled substances that originate from legitimate sources, a written record must be made of all transactions involving these agents. Every time a controlled substance is purchased or dispensed, the transfer must be recorded. Physicians, pharmacists, and hospitals must keep an inventory of all controlled substances in stock. This inventory must be reported to the DEA every 2 years. Although not specifically obliged to do so by the act, many hospitals require that floor stocks of controlled substances be counted at the beginning and end of each nursing shift.

## Drug Enforcement Administration Schedules

Each drug preparation regulated under the Controlled Substances Act has been assigned to one of five categories: Schedule I, II, III, IV, or V. Drugs in Schedule I have a high potential for abuse and have no approved medical use in the United States. In contrast, drugs in Schedules II through V all have approved applications. Assignment of drugs to Schedules II through V is based on their abuse potential and their potential for causing physical or psychologic dependence. Drugs in Schedule II have the highest potential for abuse and dependence. Drugs in the remaining schedules have decreasing abuse and dependence liabilities. Table 35–2 lists the primary drugs that come under each of the five DEA Schedules.

Scheduling of drugs under the Controlled Substances Act undergoes periodic re-evaluation. With increased understanding of the abuse and dependence liabilities of a drug, the DEA may choose to reassign it to a different Schedule.

## Prescriptions

The Controlled Substances Act places restrictions on prescribing drugs in Schedules II through V. (Drugs in Schedule I have no approved uses, and therefore are not prescribed at all.) Only physicians who have registered with the DEA are authorized to prescribe controlled drugs. Regulations on prescribing controlled substances are summarized below.

*Schedule II.* All prescriptions for Schedule II drugs must be typed or filled out in ink or indelible pencil and signed by the prescribing physician. Oral prescriptions may be made, but only in emergencies, and a written prescription must follow within 72 hours. Prescriptions of Schedule II drugs cannot be refilled. Hence, a new prescription must be written if continued therapy is needed.

*Schedules III and IV.* Prescriptions for drugs in Schedules III and IV may be oral or written. If authorized by the physician, these prescriptions may be refilled up to 5 times. Refills must be made within 6 months of the original order. If additional medication is needed beyond the amount provided for in the original prescription, a new prescription must be written.

*Schedule V.* The same regulations for prescribing drugs in Schedules III and IV apply to drugs in Schedule V. In addition, Schedule V drugs may be dispensed *without* a prescription provided the following conditions are met: (1) the drug is dispensed by a pharmacist; (2) the amount dispensed is very limited; (3) the recipient is at least 18 years old and can prove it; (4) the pharmacist writes and initials a record indicating the date, the name and amount of the drug, and the name and address of the recipient; and (5) state and local laws do not prohibit dispensing Schedule V drugs without a prescription.

## Labeling

When drugs in Schedules II, III, and IV are dispensed, their containers must bear this label: *Caution—Federal law prohibits the transfer of this drug to any person other than the patient for whom it was prescribed*. The label must also indicate whether the drug belongs to Schedule II, III, or IV. The symbols C-II, C-III, and C-IV are used to indicate the Schedule.

## State Laws

All states have their own laws regulating drugs of abuse. In many cases, the provisions of the state law are more stringent than those of the federal law. As a rule, whenever there is a difference between state and federal laws, the more restrictive of the two takes precedence.

## KEY POINTS

- Drug abuse can be defined as drug use that is inconsistent with medical or social norms.
- Drug abuse is a culturally defined term, and hence what is considered abuse can vary from one culture to another and from one time to another within the same culture.
- Addiction can be defined as a disease process characterized by the continued use of a specific psychoactive substance despite physical, psychologic, or social harm.
- Addiction is largely equivalent to substance dependence as defined in DSM-IV.
- Tolerance is a state in which a particular drug dose elicits a smaller response than it formerly did.

## TABLE 35-2. DRUG CLASSIFICATION UNDER THE CONTROLLED SUBSTANCES ACT

| Shedule I Drugs | Schedule II Drugs | Schedule III Drugs | Schedule IV Drugs | Schedule V Drugs |
|---|---|---|---|---|
| *Opioids* | *Opioids* | *Opioids* | *Opioids* | *Opioids* |
| Acetylmethadol | Alfentanil | Hydrocodone syrup | Pentazocine | Buprenorphine |
| Heroin | Codeine | Paregoric | Propoxyphene | Diphenoxylate plus |
| Normethadone | Fentanyl | *Stimulants* | *Stimulants* | atropine |
| Many others | Hydromorphone | Benzphetamine | Diethylpropion | |
| *Psychedelics* | Levorphanol | Phendimetrazine | Fenfluramine | |
| Bufotenin | Meperidine | *Barbiturates* | Mazindol | |
| Diethyltryptamine | Methadone | Aprobarbital | Pemoline | |
| Dimethyltryptamine | Morphine | Butabarbital | Phentermine | |
| Ibogaine | Opium tincture | Metharbital | *Barbiturates* | |
| *d*-Lysergic acid | Oxycodone | Talbutal | Mephobarbital | |
| diethylamide (LSD) | Oxymorphone | Thiamylal | Methohexital | |
| Mescaline | Sufentanil | Thiopental | Phenobarbital | |
| 3,4-Methylenedioxy- | *Psychostimulants* | *Miscellaneous* | *Benzodiazepines* | |
| methamphetamine | Amphetamine | *Depressants* | Alprazolam | |
| (MDMA) | Cocaine | Glutethimide | Chlordiazepoxide | |
| Psilocin | Dextroamphetamine | Methyprylon | Clonazepam | |
| Psilocybin | Methamphetamine | *Anabolic Steroids* | Clorazepate | |
| *Cannabis* | Methylphenidate | Fluoxymesterone | Diazepam | |
| *Derivatives* | Phenmetrazine | Methyltestosterone | Estazolam | |
| Hashish | *Barbiturates* | Nandrolone | Flurazepam | |
| Marijuana | Amobarbital | Oxandrolone | Halazepam | |
| *Others* | Pentobarbital | Stanozolol | Lorazepam | |
| Methaqualone | Secobarbital | Testosterone | Midazolam | |
| Phencyclidine | *Cannabinoids* | | Oxazepam | |
| | Dronabinol (THC) | | Prazepam | |
| | Nabilone | | Quazepam | |
| | | | Temazepam | |
| | | | Triazolam | |
| | | | *Miscellaneous* | |
| | | | *Depressants* | |
| | | | Chloral hydrate | |
| | | | Ethchlorvynol | |
| | | | Ethinamate | |
| | | | Meprobamate | |
| | | | Paraldehyde | |

- Cross-tolerance is a state in which tolerance to one drug confers tolerance to another drug.
- Psychologic dependence is defined as an intense subjective need for a particular psychoactive drug.
- Physical dependence is a state in which an abstinence syndrome will occur if drug use is discontinued. *Note:* physical dependence is not equivalent to addiction.
- Cross-dependence refers to the ability of one drug to support physical dependence on another drug.
- A withdrawal syndrome is a group of signs and symptoms that occur in physically dependent individuals when they discontinue drug use.
- As defined in DSM-IV, substance dependence is a more severe substance use disorder than substance abuse.
- Although tolerance and withdrawal are among the diagnostic criteria for substance dependence, they are neither necessary nor sufficient for a diagnosis.

- Although physical dependence is not the same as addiction (substance dependence), physical dependence can certainly contribute to addictive behavior.
- Drugs can reinforce their own use by providing pleasurable experiences, reducing the intensity of unpleasant experiences, and warding off a withdrawal syndrome.
- Some individuals, because of psychologic or genetic factors, are more prone to drug abuse than others.
- In drug-abuse treatment programs, the ideal goal is complete abstinence. However, treatment that substantially reduces drug use can still be considered successful.
- Under the Controlled Substances Act, drugs in Schedule I have a high potential for abuse and no medically approved use in the United States. Drugs in Schedules II through V have progressively less abuse potential and are all medically approved.

# CHAPTER 36

# Drug Abuse: Alcohol

Alcohol (ethyl alcohol, ethanol) is the most commonly used and abused drug in the United States. Although alcohol does have some therapeutic applications, the drug is of primary interest because of its nonmedical use. When consumed in moderation, alcohol improves coronary health, prolongs life, and, many would strongly argue, contributes to the joy of living. Conversely, when consumed in excess, alcohol does nothing but diminish life both in quality and quantity. These dose-related contrasts between the detrimental and beneficial effects of alcohol were aptly summed up by our 16th president, Abraham Lincoln, when he noted:

> *"None seemed to think the injury arose from use of a bad thing, but from the abuse of a very good thing."*

In approaching our study of alcohol, we will begin by discussing the basic pharmacology of this widely used drug. After that, we will discuss alcohol abuse and the drugs employed in its treatment.

## Basic Pharmacology of Alcohol

### Central Nervous System Effects

*Acute Effects.* Alcohol is a central nervous system (CNS) depressant. Like the barbiturates, alcohol causes general (relatively nonselective) depression of CNS function. Alcohol appears to affect the nervous system primarily by enhancing the actions of gamma-aminobutyric acid (GABA), an inhibitory neurotransmitter.

The effects of alcohol on the CNS are dose dependent. When dosage is low, the higher brain centers (cortical areas) are primarily affected. As dosage is increased, more primitive brain areas (e.g., medulla) become depressed. With depression of cortical function, thought processes and learned behaviors are altered, inhibitions are released, and self-restraint is replaced by increased sociability and expansiveness. Cortical depression also results in significant impairment of motor function. As CNS depression deepens, reflexes diminish greatly and consciousness becomes impaired. At very high doses, alcohol produces a state of general anesthesia. (Alcohol is not actually used for anesthesia because anesthetic doses are very close to lethal doses). Table 36–1 summarizes the effects of alcohol as a function of blood alcohol level and indicates the brain areas involved.

*Chronic Effects.* When consumed chronically and in excess, alcohol can produce severe neurologic and psychiatric disorders. Injury to the CNS is caused by the direct actions of alcohol and by the nutritional deficiencies frequently suffered by chronic heavy drinkers.

Two neuropsychiatric syndromes commonly seen in alcoholics are *Wernicke's encephalopathy* and *Korsakoff's psychosis.* Both disorders are caused by thiamine deficiency, which results from poor diet and alcohol-induced suppression of thiamine absorption. Wernicke's encephalopathy is characterized by confusion, nystagmus, and abnormal ocular movements. This syndrome is readily reversible with thiamine. Korsakoff's psychosis is characterized by polyneuropathy, inability to convert short-term memory to long-term memory, and confabulation. Korsakoff's psychosis is not reversible.

Perhaps the most dramatic effect of long-term excessive alcohol consumption is enlargement of the cerebral ventricles, presumably in response to atrophy of the cerebrum itself. These gross anatomic changes are associated with impairment of intellectual function and memory. With cessation of drinking, ventricular enlargement and cognitive deficits reverse (partially) in some individuals but not in all.

### Other Pharmacologic Effects

*Cardiovascular System.* When alcohol is consumed *acutely* and in moderate doses, cardiovascular effects are

## TABLE 36-1. CENTRAL NERVOUS SYSTEM RESPONSES AT VARIOUS BLOOD ALCOHOL LEVELS

| Blood Alcohol Level (%) | Pharmacologic Response | Brain Area Affected |
|---|---|---|
| -0.50 | | |
| | Peripheral collapse | Medulla |
| -0.45 | | |
| | Respiratory depression | |
| -0.40 | Stupor, coma | |
| | | Diencephalon |
| -0.35 | Apathy, inertia | |
| -0.30 | Altered equilibrium | Cerebellum |
| | Double vision | |
| -0.25 | Altered perception | Occipital lobe |
| -0.20 | ↓ Motor skills | |
| | Slurred speech | Parietal lobe |
| -0.15 | Tremors | |
| | Ataxia | |
| -0.10 | ↓ Attention | |
| | Loquaciousness | |
| | Altered judgment | Frontal lobe |
| -0.05 | Increased confidence | |
| | Euphoria, ↓ inhibitions | |

minor, the most prominent effect being *dilation of cutaneous blood vessels*—an action that increases blood flow to the skin. By increasing blood flow to the body surface, alcohol imparts a sensation of warmth, while at the same time promoting heat loss. Hence, despite images of Saint Bernards with little barrels of whiskey about their necks, alcohol may do more harm than good for the individual stranded in the snow and suffering from hypothermia.

Although the cardiovascular effects of moderate alcohol consumption are unremarkable, chronic and excessive alcohol consumption is clearly harmful. Abuse of alcohol results in *direct damage to the myocardium*, thereby increasing the risk of heart failure. Some investigators believe that alcohol may be the major cause of cardiomyopathy in the Western world.

In addition to damaging the heart, alcohol produces a dose-dependent elevation of blood pressure. The cause is vasoconstriction in vascular beds of skeletal muscle brought on by increased activity of the sympathetic nervous system. It is estimated that heavy drinking may be responsible for 10% of all cases of hypertension.

Not all of the cardiovascular effects of alcohol are deleterious: there is clear evidence that people who drink *moderately** experience less coronary artery disease (CAD) than abstainers. It is important to note, however, that with *heavy* drinking (5 or more drinks/day) the risk

of CAD is greatly increased. Available data suggest that alcohol protects against CAD largely by raising levels of HDL cholesterol. (As discussed in Chapter 49, HDL cholesterol protects against CAD, whereas LDL cholesterol promotes it.) Additional protection may result from activating the body's system for dissolving blood clots. The degree of cardioprotection appears equal for wine, beer, and distilled spirits. That is, protection is determined by the amount of alcohol consumed—not by the particular beverage the alcohol is in.

**Respiration.** Like all other CNS depressants, alcohol depresses respiration. Respiratory depression from moderate drinking is negligible. However, when consumed in excess, alcohol can cause death by respiratory arrest. The respiratory depressant effects of alcohol are potentiated by other CNS depressants (e.g., benzodiazepines, opioids, barbiturates).

**Liver.** Alcohol-induced liver damage can progress from fatty liver, to hepatitis, to cirrhosis—depending on the amount of alcohol consumed. Acute use of alcohol causes reversible accumulation of fat and protein in the liver. With more prolonged consumption, *hepatitis* develops in about 90% of heavy drinkers. In 8% to 20% of chronic alcoholics, hepatitis evolves into *cirrhosis*—a condition characterized by proliferation of fibrous tissue and destruction of liver parenchymal cells. Although various factors can cause cirrhosis, alcohol abuse is unquestionably the major cause of *fatal* cirrhosis.

**Stomach.** Immoderate use of alcohol can cause *erosive gastritis*. About one third of alcoholics have this disorder. Alcohol causes gastritis by two mechanisms. First, alcohol stimulates secretion of gastric acid. Second, when present in high concentrations, alcohol can injure the gastric mucosa directly.

**Kidney.** Alcohol is a diuretic. The drug promotes urine formation by inhibiting the release of antidiuretic hormone (ADH) from the pituitary. Since ADH acts on the kidney to promote water reabsorption, thereby decreasing urine formation, a reduction in circulating ADH will increase urine formation.

**Pancreas.** Approximately 35% of cases of acute pancreatitis can be attributed to alcohol, making alcohol the second most common cause of this disorder. Flare-ups typically occur after a bout of heavy drinking. Only 5% of alcoholics develop pancreatitis, and then only after years of overindulgence.

**Sexual Function.** Alcohol has both psychologic and physiologic effects related to human sexual behavior. Although alcohol is not exactly an aphrodisiac, the ability of alcohol to release people from their inhibitions *has* been known to motivate sexual activity. Ironically, the physiologic effects of alcohol may frustrate attempts at consummating the sexual activity that the psychologic effects of alcohol helped bring about: objective measurements in males and females show that alcohol significantly decreases our physiologic capacity for sexual responsiveness. The opposing psychologic and physiologic effects of alcohol on sexual function were aptly depicted in litera-

*Moderate drinking is defined by the U.S. Health Department as two drinks/day or less for men and one drink/day or less for women.

ture long ago by no less an authority than William Shakespeare. In *Macbeth* (Act 2, Scene 2), Macduff inquires of a porter "What . . . does drink especially provoke?" To which the porter replies,

> *Lechery, sir, it provokes, and unprovokes; it provokes the desire, but it takes away the performance.*

In males, long-term use of alcohol may promote *feminization*. Symptoms include testicular atrophy, impotence, sterility, and breast enlargement.

## Impact on Longevity

The effects of alcohol on life span depend on the amount of alcohol consumed. Heavy drinkers have a higher mortality rate than the population at large. Causes of increased mortality include cirrhosis, respiratory disease, cancer, and fatal accidents. The risk of death associated with alcohol abuse increases markedly in individuals who consume six or more drinks a day.

Interestingly, people who consume *moderate* amounts of alcohol live longer than those who abstain. When compared with nondrinkers, moderate drinkers have a 30% lower mortality rate, and a 50% lower incidence of myocardial infarction. According to a study by the American Medical Association, if all Americans were to give up drinking, deaths from heart disease would increase by 81,000 a year. However, despite the apparent benefits of drinking—and the apparent health disadvantage of abstinence—no one is recommending that abstainers take up drinking. Furthermore, when the risks of alcohol outweigh any possible benefits—as is the case for the people listed in Table 36-2—then alcohol consumption should obviously be avoided.

## Pharmacokinetics

*Absorption.* Alcohol is absorbed from the stomach and small intestine. About 20% of ingested alcohol is absorbed from the stomach. Gastric absorption is relatively slow and is delayed even further by the presence of food. Milk is especially effective at retarding absorption. Absorption from the small intestine is rapid and largely independent of the presence of food; about 80% of ingested alcohol is absorbed from this site. Because most alcohol is absorbed from the small intestine, gastric emptying time (the time required for the contents of the stomach to be released

**TABLE 36-2. PEOPLE WHO SHOULD AVOID ALCOHOL***

- Women who are pregnant or trying to conceive.
- People who plan to drive or perform other activities that require unimpaired attention or muscular coordination.
- People taking antihistamines, sedatives, or other drugs that can intensify alcohol's effects.
- Recovering alcoholics.
- People under age 21.

Caution is indicated for people with a strong family history of alcoholism and for those with diabetes, peptic ulcer disease, and other medical conditions that can be exacerbated by alcohol.

*According to the National Institute on Alcohol Abuse and Alcoholism.

into the small intestine) is a major determinant of individual variation in alcohol absorption.

*Distribution.* Alcohol is distributed to all tissues and body fluids. The drug crosses the blood-brain barrier with ease, allowing alcohol in the brain to equilibrate rapidly with alcohol in the blood. Alcohol also crosses the placenta and can affect the developing fetus.

*Metabolism.* Alcohol is metabolized in both the liver and stomach. The liver is the primary site. The pathway for alcohol metabolism is shown in Figure 36-1. As depicted, the process begins with conversion of alcohol to acetaldehyde, a reaction catalyzed by *alcohol dehydrogenase*. This reaction is slow and puts a limit on the rate at which alcohol can be inactivated. Once formed, acetaldehyde undergoes *rapid* conversion to acetic acid. Through a series of reactions, acetic acid is then used to synthesize cholesterol, fatty acids, and other compounds.

The kinetics of alcohol metabolism differ from those of most other drugs. With most drugs, as plasma drug levels rise, the amount of drug metabolized per unit time increases. This is not true for alcohol: as the alcohol content of blood increases, there is almost no change in the speed of alcohol breakdown. That is, alcohol is metabolized at a relatively *constant rate*—regardless of how much alcohol is in the body. The average rate at which individuals can metabolize alcohol is about *15 ml (0.5 oz) per hour*.

Because alcohol is metabolized at a slow and constant rate, there is a limit to how much alcohol one can consume without having the drug accumulate in the body.

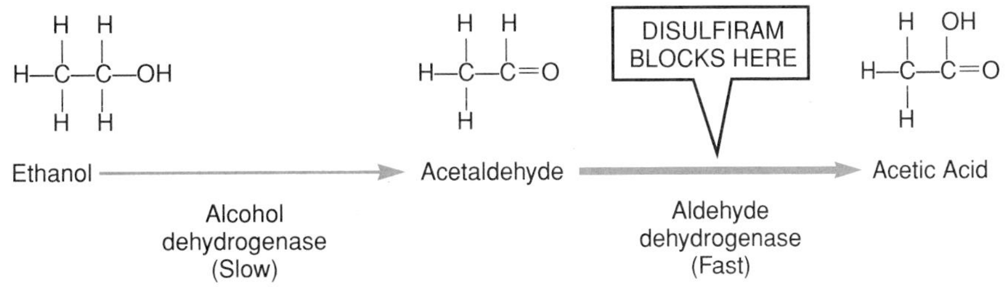

**Figure 36-1. Ethanol metabolism and the effect of disulfiram.** Conversion of ethanol into acetaldehyde takes place slowly (at a rate of about 15 ml/hr). Consumption of more than 15 ml/hr will cause ethanol to accumulate. Effects of disulfiram result from accumulation of acetaldehyde secondary to inhibition of aldehyde dehydrogenase.

## TABLE 36-3. ALCOHOL CONTENT OF BEER, WINE, AND WHISKEY

|  | Wine | Beer | Whiskey |
| --- | --- | --- | --- |
| Usual serving | 1 glass | 1 can or bottle | 1 shot |
| Serving size | 150 ml (5 oz) | 360 ml (12 oz) | 45 ml (1.5 oz) |
| Alcohol concentration | 12%[a] | 5%[c] | 40%[e] |
| Alcohol per serving | 18 ml[b] (0.6 oz) | 18 ml[d] (0.6 oz) | 18 ml[f] (0.6 oz) |

[a]The alcohol content of wine varies from 8% to 20%; typical table wines contain 12%.

[b]The alcohol in a 5-ounce glass of wine varies from 12 to 30 ml, depending on the alcohol concentration in the wine. Wine with 12% alcohol has 18 ml alcohol per 5-ounce glass.

[c]The alcohol content of beer varies: 5% alcohol is typical of American premium beers; cheaper American beers and light beers have less alcohol (2.4% to 5%); and imported beers may have more alcohol (6%). Beer sold in Europe may have 7% to 8% alcohol.

[d]The alcohol in a 12-ounce can of beer varies from 9 to 29 ml, depending on the alcohol concentration in the beer. Beer with 5% alcohol has 18 ml per 12-ounce can.

[e]Whiskeys and other distilled spirits (e.g., rum, vodka, gin) are usually 80 proof (40% alcohol) but may also be 100 proof (50% alcohol).

[f]The alcohol in a 1.5-ounce shot of whiskey can be either 18 or 22.5 ml, depending on the proof of the whiskey. Eighty-proof whiskey has 18 ml alcohol per 1.5-ounce serving.

For practical purposes, that limit is about *one drink per hour*. Consumption of more than one drink per hour—be that drink beer, wine, straight whiskey, or a cocktail—will result in alcohol buildup.

The information in Table 36–3 helps explain why we are unable to metabolize more than one drink's worth of alcohol per hour. As the table indicates, beer, wine, and whiskey differ from one another with respect to alcohol concentration and usual serving size. However, despite these differences, it turns out that *the average can of beer, the average glass of wine, and the average shot of whiskey all contain the same amount of alcohol, namely, 18 ml (0.6 oz)*. Since the liver can metabolize about 15 ml of alcohol per hour, and since the average alcoholic drink contains 18 ml of alcohol, one drink contains just about the amount of alcohol that the liver can comfortably process. Consumption of more than one drink per hour will overwhelm the capacity of the liver for alcohol metabolism, and therefore will cause alcohol to accumulate.

When used on a regular basis, alcohol induces synthesis of hepatic drug-metabolizing enzymes, thereby increasing the rate of its own metabolism and that of other drugs. As a result, individuals who consume alcohol routinely in high amounts can metabolize the drug faster than people who drink occasionally and moderately.

Males and females differ with respect to activity of alcohol dehydrogenase in the stomach. Specifically, women have much lower activity than men. As a result, gastric metabolism of alcohol in women is significantly less than in men. This difference partly explains why women achieve higher blood alcohol levels than men after consuming an equivalent number of drinks.

***Blood Levels of Alcohol.*** Since alcohol in the brain rapidly equilibrates with alcohol in the blood, blood levels of alcohol are predictive of CNS effects. The behavioral effects associated with specific blood levels of alcohol are summarized in Table 36–1. The earliest effects (euphoria, reduced inhibitions, increased confidence) are seen when blood alcohol content is about 0.05%. As blood alcohol rises, intoxication becomes more intense. When blood alcohol exceeds 0.4%, there is a substantial risk of respiratory depression, peripheral collapse, and death.

### Tolerance

Chronic consumption of alcohol produces tolerance. As a result, in order to alter consciousness, people who drink on a regular basis require larger amounts of alcohol than people who drink only on occasion. Tolerance to alcohol confers cross-tolerance to general anesthetics, barbiturates, and other general CNS depressants. However, no cross-tolerance develops to opioids. Tolerance subsides within a few weeks following cessation of alcohol use.

Although tolerance develops to many of the effects of alcohol, *very little tolerance develops to respiratory depression*. Consequently, the lethal dose of alcohol for chronic, heavy drinkers is not much greater than the lethal dose for nondrinkers. Alcoholics may tolerate blood alcohol levels as high as 0.4% (four times the amount normally defined by law as intoxicating) with no marked reduction in consciousness; however, if blood levels rise only slightly above this level, death may result.

### Physical Dependence

Chronic use of alcohol produces physical dependence. If alcohol is withdrawn abruptly, an abstinence syndrome will result. The intensity of the abstinence syndrome is proportional to the degree of physical dependence. Individuals who are physically dependent on alcohol show cross-dependence with other general CNS depressants (e.g., barbiturates, chloral hydrate, benzodiazepines) but not with opioids. The alcohol withdrawal syndrome and its management are discussed in detail below.

### Drug Interactions

***CNS Depressants.*** The CNS effects of alcohol are additive with the effects of other CNS depressants (e.g., barbiturates, benzodiazepines, opioids). Consumption of alcohol with other CNS depressants intensifies the psychologic and physiologic manifestations of CNS depression. Combining alcohol with other CNS depressants greatly increases the risk of death from respiratory depression.

***Aspirin-like Drugs.*** Like alcohol, the aspirin-like drugs can injure the gastrointestinal mucosa. The combined effects of alcohol and aspirin-like drugs can result in significant gastric bleeding. In addition, the combination of alcohol with acetaminophen may pose a risk of potentially fatal liver injury (see Chapter 64).

***Disulfiram.*** The combination of alcohol with disulfiram [Antabuse] can cause a variety of adverse effects, some of which are extremely hazardous. These effects, and the use of disulfiram in the treatment of alcoholism, are discussed later in the chapter.

***Antihypertensive Drugs.*** Since alcohol raises blood pressure, it will tend to counteract the effects of antihypertensive medications. Elevation of blood pressure is most significant when the dosage of alcohol is high.

## Use in Pregnancy and Lactation

***Pregnancy.*** Consumption of alcohol during pregnancy can cause *fetal alcohol syndrome* (FAS). This syndrome is seen in one of three children born to alcoholic mothers. Children with FAS are characterized by mild to moderate mental retardation, slow growth rate, craniofacial malformations, and limb abnormalities. Also, resistance to infection is greatly reduced (apparently secondary to immune system derangement).

In addition to FAS, alcohol use during pregnancy can result in *stillbirth, spontaneous abortion, low birth weight,* and *mental retardation.* (Alcohol may be the greatest teratogenic cause of mental deficiency in the Western world.) Neonates whose mothers consumed large amounts of alcohol during pregnancy may be born with *physical dependence* on alcohol. These infants will need to undergo withdrawal therapy.

From the above, it is clear that pregnancy is a contraindication to use of alcohol. Mild FAS has been caused by consuming as little as 30 ml of alcohol a day. Drinking 30 ml of alcohol twice weekly is associated with an increase in second-trimester spontaneous abortion. Although there may be some small amount of alcohol that can be consumed safely during pregnancy, we do not know what that amount is. Consequently, in the interests of fetal health, pregnant women should be advised to avoid alcohol entirely.

***Lactation.*** Unless alcohol consumption is extremely heavy, alcohol in breast milk is not likely to reach levels that can affect the nursing infant. (Alcohol does enter breast milk, but significant amounts will not be present until maternal blood levels of alcohol reach 0.3%—a level associated with gross intoxication.) Use of alcohol during lactation may inhibit the milk ejection reflex.

## Acute Overdose

Acute overdose with alcohol produces vomiting, coma, pronounced hypotension, and respiratory depression. The combination of vomiting and unconsciousness can result in aspiration, which in turn can result in pulmonary obstruction and pneumonia. Alcohol-induced hypotension results from a direct effect on peripheral blood vessels, and cannot be corrected with vasoconstrictors (e.g., epinephrine). Hypotension can lead to renal failure (secondary to compromised renal blood flow) and to cardiovascular shock, which is a common cause of alcohol-

related death. Although death can also result from respiratory depression, this is not the usual cause.

Since the symptoms of acute alcohol poisoning can mimic symptoms of other pathologies (e.g., diabetic coma, skull fracture), a definitive diagnosis may not be possible without measuring alcohol in the blood, urine, or expired air. The smell of "alcohol" on the breath is not a reliable means of diagnosis, since the breath odors we associate with alcohol consumption are due to impurities in alcoholic beverages—and not to alcohol itself. Hence, these odors may or may not be present.

Alcohol poisoning is treated like poisoning with all other general CNS depressants. Details of management are discussed in Chapter 32. Alcohol can be removed from the body by gastric lavage and dialysis. Stimulants (e.g., caffeine, pentylenetetrazol) should not be administered.

## Summary of Precautions and Contraindications

Alcohol can injure the gastrointestinal mucosa and should not be consumed by persons with *peptic ulcer disease.* Alcohol is harmful to the liver and should not be used by individuals with *liver disease.* Alcohol should be avoided during *pregnancy* because of the risk of fetal alcohol syndrome, mental retardation, reduced birth weight, stillbirth, and spontaneous abortion.

Alcohol must be used with caution by patients with *epilepsy.* During alcohol use, the CNS is depressed. When alcohol consumption ceases, the CNS undergoes rebound excitation, and this excitation can precipitate seizures.

Alcohol can cause serious adverse effects if combined with *CNS depressants, aspirin-like drugs, vasodilators,* and *disulfiram.* These combinations should be avoided.

### Therapeutic Uses

Although our emphasis has been on the nonmedical use of alcohol, it should be remembered that alcohol does have therapeutic applications.

***Topical.*** Alcohol applied to the skin can promote cooling in febrile patients. Topical alcohol is also a popular skin disinfectant. In addition, alcohol application can help prevent decubitus ulcers.

***Oral.*** Because of its ability to promote gastric secretion, alcohol can serve as an aid to digestion in bedridden patients. Oral alcohol is frequently used as self-medication for insomnia.

***Intravenous.*** Solutions of alcohol (5% or 10%) in 5% dextrose are administered by slow IV infusion to provide calories and fluid replacement. Intravenous alcohol is also used to treat poisoning by methanol and ethylene glycol.

***Local Injection.*** Injection of alcohol in the vicinity of nerves produces nerve block. This technique can be used to relieve pain of trigeminal neuralgia, inoperable carcinoma, and other causes.

## Alcohol Abuse

*Alcoholism* is a chronic disorder characterized by impaired control over drinking, preoccupation with alcohol consumption, use of alcohol despite awareness of adverse consequences, and distortions in thinking, especially as evidenced by denial of a drinking problem. The development and manifestations of alcoholism are influenced by genetic, psychosocial, and environmental factors. The disease is progressive and often fatal. In the United States, about 8% of adults are alcoholics.

In the *Diagnostic and Statistical Manual of Mental Disorders*, fourth edition (DSM-IV), the pattern of alcohol use that constitutes alcoholism is termed *alcohol dependence* (if tolerance and withdrawal are present) or *alcohol abuse* (if tolerance and withdrawal are absent). Complete diagnostic criteria from DSM-IV for alcohol dependence and alcohol abuse are given in Table 36–4.

Misuse of alcohol is responsible for 6 million nonfatal injuries each year—and 100,000 deaths. Causes of death range from liver disease to automobile wrecks. Fully 45% of all fatal highway crashes are alcohol related. Among teens, alcohol-related crashes are the leading cause of

death. Alcohol also causes industrial accidents, and is responsible for 40% of industrial fatalities.

Alcohol abuse is a major public health problem, and its consequences are numerous. Alcoholism produces psychologic derangements, including anxiety, depression, and suicidal ideation. Malnutrition, secondary to inadequate diet and malabsorption, is common. Poor work performance and disruption of family life reflect the social deterioration suffered by alcoholics. Alcohol abuse during pregnancy can result in fetal alcohol syndrome, stillbirth, spontaneous abortion, low birth weight, and mental retardation. Lastly, chronic alcohol abuse is harmful to the body; consequences include liver disease, cardiomyopathy, and brain damage—not to mention injury and death from accidents.

Chronic alcohol consumption produces substantial tolerance. Tolerance is both pharmacokinetic (accelerated alcohol metabolism) and pharmacodynamic. Pharmacodynamic tolerance is evidenced by an increase in the blood alcohol level required to produce intoxication. Alcoholics may tolerate blood alcohol levels of 200 to 400 mg/dl—2 to 4 times the level that defines legal intoxication in most states—with no marked reduction in consciousness. It should be noted, however, that very little tolerance develops to respiratory depression. Hence, as the alcoholic consumes increasing amounts in an effort to produce desired psychologic effects, the risk of death from respiratory arrest gets increasingly high. Cross-tolerance exists with general anesthetics and other CNS depressants, but not with opioids.

Chronic use of alcohol produces physical dependence, and abrupt withdrawal produces an abstinence syndrome. When the degree of physical dependence is low, withdrawal symptoms are mild (disturbed sleep, weakness, nausea, anxiety, mild tremors) and last for less than a day. In contrast, the withdrawal syndrome experienced by individuals highly dependent upon alcohol is severe. Symptoms begin 12 to 72 hours after the last drink and continue for 5 to 7 days. Early manifestations include cramps, vomiting, hallucinations, and intense tremors; heart rate, blood pressure, and temperature may rise; and tonic-clonic seizures may develop. As the syndrome progresses, disorientation and loss of insight occur. A few alcoholics (less than 1%) experience *delirium tremens* (severe persecutory hallucinations). These hallucinations can be so vivid and lifelike that alcoholics often cannot distinguish them from reality. In extreme cases, alcohol withdrawal can result in cardiovascular collapse and death. Drugs used to ease withdrawal are discussed below.

## TABLE 36–4. DIAGNOSTIC CRITERIA FOR ALCOHOL DEPENDENCE AND ALCOHOL ABUSE*

### Alcohol Dependence

Alcohol dependence is a maladaptive pattern of alcohol use, leading to clinically significant impairment or distress, as manifested by three (or more) of the following, occurring at any time in the same 12-month period:

- Tolerance to alcohol
- Withdrawal from alcohol
- Consumption of alcohol in larger amounts or over longer periods than intended
- Continued alcohol use despite a persistent desire or repeated efforts to cut down or control consumption
- A great deal of time is spent drinking alcohol or recovering from its effects
- Important social, occupational, or recreational activities are given up or reduced because of alcohol
- Alcohol use continues despite knowledge of a persistent or recurrent physical or psychologic problem that alcohol probably caused or exacerbated (e.g., drinking despite knowing that alcohol made an ulcer worse)

### Alcohol Abuse

Alcohol abuse is a maladaptive pattern of alcohol use leading to clinically significant impairment or distress, as manifested by one (or more) of the following within a 12-month period:

- Recurrent alcohol use that results in a failure to fulfill major role obligations at work, school, or home
- Recurrent alcohol use in situations in which it is physically hazardous
- Recurrent alcohol-related legal problems
- Continued alcohol use despite persistent or recurrent social or interpersonal problems caused or exacerbated by alcohol

Individuals who display tolerance, withdrawal, and other symptoms of alcohol dependence would be diagnosed under alcohol dependence rather than alcohol abuse.

*Adapted from the general diagnostic criteria for substance dependence and substance abuse as presented in American Psychiatric Association. *Diagnostic and Statistical Manual of Mental Disorders*, 4th ed. Washington, DC, American Psychiatric Press, 1994, pp. 181–183.

## Drugs Employed in the Treatment of Alcoholism

About 1 million Americans seek treatment for alcoholism every year. Unfortunately, the success rate is discouraging: nearly 50% relapse during the first few months of treatment. The objective of therapy is to modify drinking patterns (i.e., to reduce or completely eliminate alcohol consumption). Drugs can help in two ways: they can facilitate withdrawal, and they can help maintain abstinence after withdrawal has been accomplished.

## Drugs Used to Facilitate Withdrawal

Management of withdrawal depends on the degree of alcohol dependence. When dependence is mild, withdrawal can be accomplished on an outpatient basis without the use of drugs. However, when dependence is great, withdrawal carries a risk of death. In this case, hospitalization and drug therapy are indicated.

**Benzodiazepines.** The objective of drug therapy is to suppress symptoms of abstinence. In theory, any drug that has cross-dependence with alcohol (i.e., any of the general CNS depressants) should be effective. However, in actual practice, benzodiazepines are the drugs of choice. The benzodiazepines employed most frequently are chlordiazepoxide [Librium, others], diazepam [Valium, Zetran], and lorazepam [Ativan]. Traditionally, benzodiazepines have been administered around the clock on a fixed schedule. However, recent evidence indicates that PRN administration in response to symptoms may be just as effective and results in speedier withdrawal.

**Atenolol.** Use of atenolol (a beta-adrenergic blocking agent) in conjunction with benzodiazepines appears helpful. Combined therapy with atenolol may permit use of lower benzodiazepine doses and may accelerate improvement in vital signs.

## Drugs Used to Maintain Abstinence

Once withdrawal has been accomplished, continued abstinence can be facilitated with disulfiram or naltrexone. Disulfiram discourages alcohol consumption by causing an intense adverse reaction if alcohol is consumed. Naltrexone discourages consumption primarily by decreasing the craving for alcohol.

### Disulfiram Aversion Therapy

**Therapeutic Use.** Disulfiram [Antabuse] is taken by alcoholics to help them refrain from drinking. This drug discourages drinking by causing severe adverse effects if alcohol is ingested. Disulfiram has no applications outside the treatment of alcoholism.

**Mechanism of Action.** As indicated in Figure 36–1, disulfiram acts by disrupting alcohol metabolism. Specifically, disulfiram causes *irreversible inhibition of aldehyde dehydrogenase*, the enzyme that converts acetaldehyde to acetic acid. As a result, if alcohol is ingested, *acetaldehyde* will accumulate to toxic levels, producing unpleasant and potentially harmful effects.

**Pharmacologic Effects.** The constellation of adverse effects caused by alcohol plus disulfiram is referred to as the *acetaldehyde syndrome*. This syndrome can be very dangerous—even fatal. In its "mild" form, the syndrome manifests as nausea, copious vomiting, flushing, palpitations, headache, sweating, thirst, chest pain, weakness, blurred vision, and hypotension; blood pressure may ultimately decline to shock levels. This reaction, which may last from 30 minutes to several hours, can be brought on by consuming as little as 7 ml of alcohol.

In its more severe manifestations, the acetaldehyde syndrome is life threatening. Potential reactions include marked respiratory depression, cardiovascular collapse, cardiac dysrhythmias, myocardial infarction, acute congestive heart failure, convulsions, and death. Clearly, the acetaldehyde syndrome is not simply unpleasant; this syndrome can be extremely hazardous and must be avoided.

In the absence of alcohol, disulfiram rarely causes significant effects. Drowsiness and skin eruptions may occur during initial drug use. These responses diminish with time.

**Patient Selection.** Because of the severity of the acetaldehyde syndrome, candidates for therapy must be carefully chosen. Alcoholics who lack the determination to stop drinking should not be given disulfiram. In other words, disulfiram must not be administered to those alcoholics who are likely to attempt drinking while undergoing treatment.

**Patient Education.** Patient education is an extremely important component of disulfiram therapy. Patients must be thoroughly informed about the potential hazards of treatment. That is, they must be made aware that consumption of *any* alcohol while taking disulfiram may produce a severe, potentially fatal, reaction. Patients must be warned to avoid all forms of alcohol, including alcohol found in sauces and cough syrups, and alcohol applied to the skin in after-shave lotions, colognes, and liniments. Patients should be made aware that the effects of disulfiram will persist for about 2 weeks after the last dose is taken; alcohol must not be consumed until this interval is over. Individuals using disulfiram should be encouraged to carry identification indicating their status.

**Preparations, Dosage, and Administration.** Disulfiram [Antabuse] is dispensed in tablets (250 and 500 mg) for oral use. At least 12 hours must elapse between the patient's last drink and initiation of treatment. The initial dosage is 500 mg once daily for 1 to 2 weeks. Maintenance dosages range from 125 to 500 mg a day, usually taken as a single dose in the morning. Therapy may last for months or even years.

### Naltrexone

Naltrexone [ReVia], formerly named Trexan, is a pure opioid antagonist that decreases craving for alcohol and blocks alcohol's reinforcing effects. The mechanism underlying these effects is not known. In patients undergoing treatment for alcoholism, naltrexone has cut the relapse rate by 50%. When compared with patients taking placebo, those taking naltrexone reported less craving for alcohol, fewer days drinking, fewer drinks per occasion, and reduced severity of alcohol-related problems. Nausea is the most common adverse effect. Of course, since naltrexone is an opioid antagonist, the drug will precipitate withdrawal if given to individuals with opioid dependence. The dosage for alcoholics is 50 mg/day. Naltrexone is best used in combination with counseling.

### Other Drugs Used in the Treatment of Alcoholism

Malnutrition is a common problem in the chronic alcoholic. Poor nutrition results from two factors: (1) poor diet and (2) malabsorption of nutrients and vitamins. Malabsorption is caused by alcohol-induced damage to the gastrointestinal mucosa. Poor diet is due in part to the fact that alcoholics can meet up to 50% of their caloric needs with alcohol, and therefore consumption of foods with greater nutritional value tends to be subnormal. Because of their poor nutritional state, alcoholics are in need of fat, protein, and vitamins. The B vitamins (thiamine, folic acid, cyanocobalamin) are especially needed. To correct nutritional deficiencies, a program of dietary modification and vitamin supplements should be implemented.

Alcoholics frequently require fluid replacement therapy and antibiotics. Fluids are needed to replace fluids lost because of gastritis or because of vomiting associated with withdrawal. Antibiotics may be needed to manage pneumonitis, a common complication of alcoholism.

## KEY POINTS

- Alcohol is beneficial when consumed in moderation and detrimental when consumed in excess.
- As blood levels of alcohol rise, CNS depression progresses from cortical areas to more primitive brain areas (e.g., medulla).
- Long-term, excessive drinking actually reduces the size of the cerebrum.
- Alcohol produces a dose-dependent increase in blood pressure.
- According to the United States Health Department, moderate drinking is defined as two drinks/day or less for men, and one drink/day or less for women.
- Moderate drinking significantly reduces the risk of CAD, primarily by raising HDL cholesterol, and possibly by activating the endogenous thrombolytic system.
- Excessive drinking causes direct damage to the myocardium.
- Like all other CNS depressants, alcohol depresses respiration.

- Chronic, heavy drinking can cause hepatitis and cirrhosis. People with liver disease should avoid the drug.
- Heavy drinking can cause erosive gastritis.
- Alcohol is a diuretic.
- Excessive drinkers die younger than the population at large.
- Because of the cardioprotective effects of alcohol, *moderate* drinkers live longer than those who abstain.
- Alcohol dehydrogenase is the rate-limiting enzyme in alcohol metabolism.
- Alcohol is metabolized at a constant rate, regardless of how high blood levels rise. In contrast, the rate of metabolism of most drugs increases as blood levels rise.
- Most people can metabolize about *one drink per hour*—be it beer, wine, straight whiskey, or a cocktail. Consumption of more than one drink per hour causes alcohol to accumulate.
- Chronic consumption of alcohol produces tolerance to many of its effects—but not to respiratory depression.
- Tolerance to alcohol confers cross-tolerance to general anesthetics, barbiturates, and other general CNS depressants—but not to opioids.
- The CNS-depressant effects of alcohol are additive with the effects of other CNS depressants.
- The combined effects of alcohol and aspirin-like drugs can cause significant gastric bleeding. People with peptic ulcer disease should avoid the drug.
- Alcohol use during pregnancy can result in fetal alcohol syndrome, stillbirth, spontaneous abortion, low birth weight, and mental retardation. Women who are pregnant or trying to conceive should not drink.
- Benzodiazepines (e.g., chlordiazepoxide, diazepam, lorazepam) are drugs of choice for facilitating withdrawal in alcohol-dependent individuals. Benzodiazepines suppress symptoms because of cross-dependence with alcohol.
- Disulfiram is given to help alcoholics refrain from drinking. The drug blocks acetaldehyde dehydrogenase; hence, if alcohol is consumed, acetaldehyde will accumulate, thereby causing a host of unpleasant and potentially dangerous symptoms.
- Naltrexone helps alcoholics refrain from drinking by decreasing their craving for alcohol and by blocking alcohol's reinforcing effects.

## Summary of Major Nursing Implications†

## Disulfiram

### Preadministration Assessment

#### Therapeutic Goal
Facilitation of abstinence from alcohol.

### Patient Selection
Candidates for therapy must be chosen carefully. Disulfiram must not be given to alcoholics who are likely to attempt drinking while taking this drug.

### Identifying High-Risk Patients
Disulfiram is *contraindicated* for patients *suspected of being incapable of abstinence from alcohol*; for patients with *myocardial disease, coronary occlusion,* or *psychosis*; and for patients who have recently received *alco-*

*hol, metronidazole, paraldehyde, or alcohol-containing medications* (e.g., cough syrups, tonics).

## Implementation: Administration

### Route

Oral.

### Administration

Instruct the patient not to administer the first dose until at least 12 hours after his or her last drink.

Dosing is done once daily and may continue for months or even years.

Tablets may be crushed or mixed with liquid.

## Implementation: Measures To Enhance Therapeutic Effects

Patient education is essential for safety. Inform patients about the potential hazards of treatment, and warn them to avoid all forms of alcohol, including alcohol in vinegar, sauces, and cough syrups and alcohol applied to the skin in aftershave lotions, colognes, and liniments. Inform patients that the effects of disulfiram will persist for about 2 weeks after the last dose and that alcohol must not be consumed during this interval. Encourage patients to carry identification to alert emergency health care personnel to their condition.

# CHAPTER 37

# Drug Abuse: Opioids, Depressants, Psychostimulants, Marijuana, Psychedelics, Inhalants, and Nicotine

I n this chapter, we discuss all of the major drugs of abuse except alcohol, which was the topic of the preceding chapter. As indicated in Table 37-1, abused drugs fall into six major pharmacologic categories: (1) opioids, (2) psychostimulants, (3) depressants, (4) psychedelics, (5) anabolic steroids, and (6) miscellaneous drugs of abuse. The basic pharmacology of many of these drugs has been presented in previous chapters; hence, their discussion here is brief. Agents that have *not* been addressed previously (e.g., marijuana, LSD, nicotine) are discussed in greater depth. Structural formulas of representative controlled substances are shown in Figure 37-1. Street names for some abused drugs are listed in Table 37-2.

## Opioids

The opioids (e.g., morphine, heroin) are major drugs of abuse. This fact is underscored by the classification of most opioids as Schedule II substances. The basic pharmacology of the opioids is discussed in Chapter 25.

### Patterns of Use

Opioid abuse is encountered in all segments of American society. Formerly, opioid use was limited almost exclusively to lower socioeconomic groups residing in cities. However, opioids are now used by people outside cities and by people of means—although the urban poor still constitute the majority of abusers.

For most abusers, initial exposure to opioids occurs either socially (i.e., illicitly) or in the context of pain management in a medical setting. The overwhelming majority of individuals who go on to abuse opioids begin their drug use illicitly. Only an exceedingly small percentage of those exposed to opioids therapeutically develop a pattern of compulsive drug use.

Opioid abuse by health care providers deserves special consideration. It is well established that physicians, nurses, and pharmacists, as a group, abuse opioids to a greater extent than all other groups with similar educational backgrounds. The vulnerability of health care professionals to opioid abuse is primarily the result of drug access.

### Subjective and Behavioral Effects

Moments after IV injection, heroin produces a sensation in the lower abdomen similar to sexual orgasm. This initial reaction, known as a "rush" or "kick," persists for about 45 seconds. After this, the user experiences a prolonged sense of euphoria (well-being); there is a feeling that "all is well with the world." It is for these extended effects, rather than the initial rush, that most opioid abuse occurs.

Interestingly, when individuals first use opioids, nausea and vomiting are prominent, and an overall sense of *dys-*

## TABLE 37-1. PHARMACOLOGIC CATEGORIZATION OF ABUSED DRUGS

| Category | Examples |
| --- | --- |
| *Opioids* | Heroin |
| | Morphine |
| | Meperidine |
| | Hydromorphine |
| *Psychostimulants* | Cocaine |
| | Dextroamphetamine |
| | Methamphetamine |
| | Methylphenidate |
| *Depressants* | |
| Barbiturates | Amobarbital |
| | Secobarbital |
| | Pentobarbital |
| | Phenobarbital |
| Benzodiazepines | Diazepam |
| | Chlordiazepoxide |
| | Lorazepam |
| Miscellaneous | Alcohol |
| | Methaqualone |
| | Chloral hydrate |
| | Meprobamate |
| *Psychedelics* | LSD |
| | Mescaline |
| | Psilocybin |
| | Dimethyltryptamine |
| *Anabolic Steroids* | Nandrolone |
| | Oxandrolone |
| | Testosterone |
| *Miscellaneous* | Marijuana |
| | Phencyclidine |
| | Nicotine |
| | Nitrous oxide |
| | Amyl nitrite |

phoria may be felt. In many cases, were it not for peer pressure, individuals would not continue opioid use long enough to allow these unpleasant reactions to be replaced by a more agreeable experience.

### Preferred Drugs and Routes of Administration

Among street users, *heroin* is the opioid of choice. This agent is easy to procure and is taken by about 90% of opioid abusers. The popularity of heroin is related to its high lipid solubility, which allows the drug to readily cross the blood-brain barrier, and thereby produce initial effects that are both immediate and intense. It is this combination of speed and intensity that sets heroin apart from other opioids, and makes it such a desirable drug.

It should be noted that when heroin is administered orally or subcutaneously, as opposed to intravenously, its effects cannot be distinguished from those of morphine and other opioids. This observation is not surprising when you realize that, once in the brain, heroin is rapidly converted into morphine, the active form through which heroin produces its effects.

Nurses and physicians who abuse opioids often select *meperidine* [Demerol] as their drug of choice. This agent has distinct advantages for these users. First, unlike heroin, meperidine is highly effective when administered orally; hence abuse need not be associated with telltale signs of repeated injections. Second, meperidine produces less pupillary constriction than other opioids, thereby minimizing awkward questions about miosis. Lastly, meperidine has minimal effects on smooth muscle function; hence constipation and urinary retention are less problematic than with other opioid preparations.

### Tolerance and Physical Dependence

*Tolerance.* With prolonged opioid use, tolerance develops to many—but not all—pharmacologic effects. Effects to which tolerance does develop include euphoria, respiratory depression, and nausea. In contrast, little or no tolerance develops to constipation and miosis. Because tolerance to respiratory depression develops in parallel with tolerance to euphoria, respiratory depression does not increase as higher doses are taken to produce desired subjective effects. Persons tolerant to one opioid are cross-tolerant to other opioids. However, there is no cross-tolerance between opioids and general central nervous system (CNS) depressants (e.g., barbiturates, benzodiazepines, alcohol).

*Physical Dependence.* Long-term use produces substantial physical dependence. The abstinence syndrome resulting from opioid withdrawal is described in Chapter 25. It is important to note that, although the opioid withdrawal syndrome can be extremely unpleasant, it is rarely dangerous.

Following the acute abstinence syndrome, which takes about 10 days to run its course, opioid addicts may experience a milder but protracted phase of withdrawal. This second phase, which may persist for months, is characterized by insomnia, irritability, and fatigue. Gastrointestinal hyperactivity and premature ejaculation may also be problems.

### Treatment of Acute Toxicity

Treatment of acute opioid toxicity is discussed at length in Chapter 25 and will only be summarized here. Overdose produces a classic triad of symptoms: *respiratory depression, coma,* and *pinpoint pupils. Naloxone,* an opioid antagonist, is the treatment of choice. This agent rapidly reverses all signs of opioid poisoning. However, dosage must be titrated carefully, since, if too much naloxone is given, the addict will swing from a state of intoxication to one of withdrawal. Because of its short half-life, naloxone must be readministered every few hours until opioid concentrations have dropped to nontoxic levels—a process that may require days for completion. Failure to repeat naloxone dosing may result in the death of patients who had earlier been rendered symptom free.

*Nalmefene* [Revex], a long-acting opioid antagonist, is an alternative to naloxone. Because of its long half-life, nalmefene does not require repeated dosing—an obvious advantage. However, if the dose is excessive in an opioid-

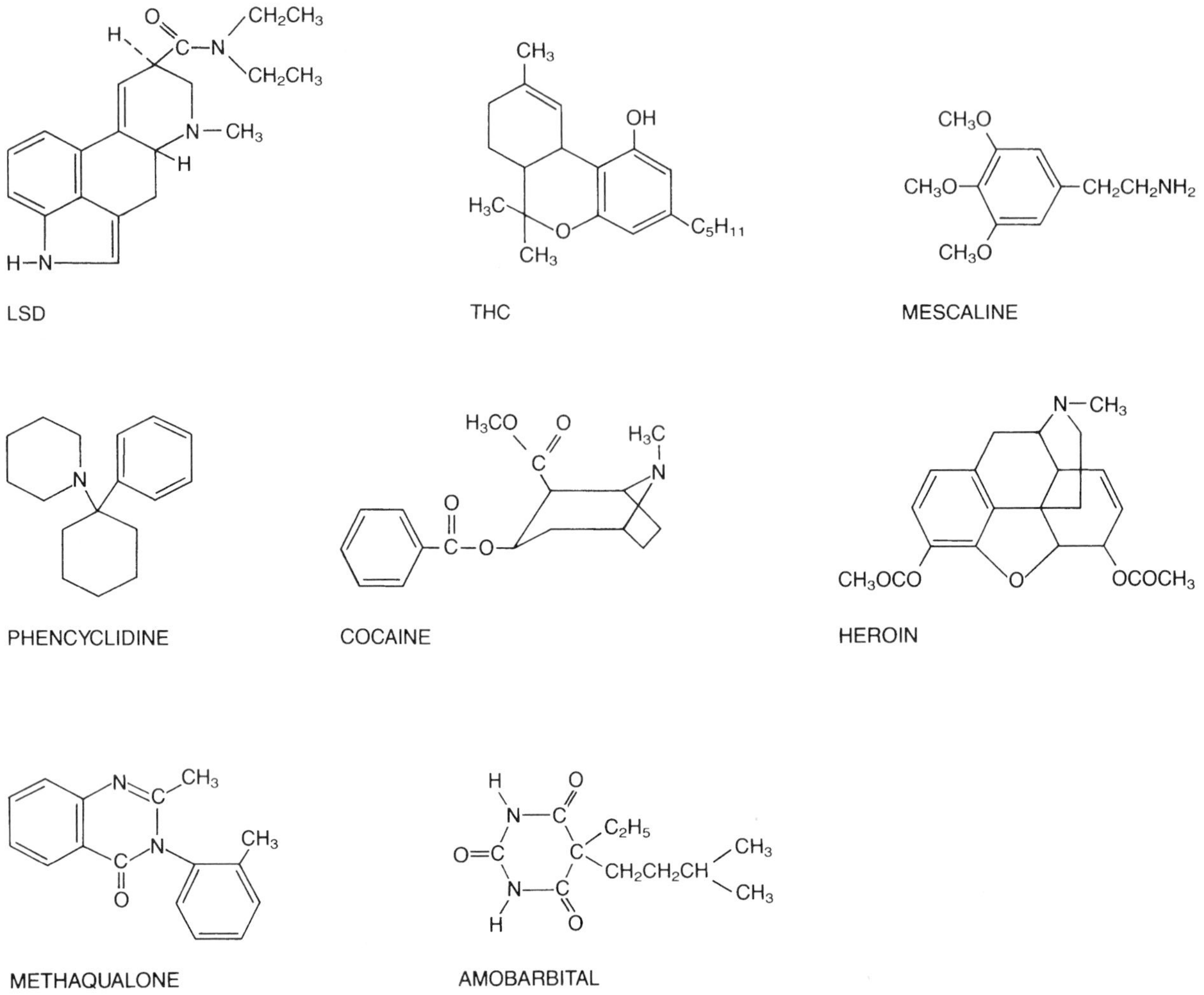

**Figure 37–1. Structural formulas of representative drugs of abuse.** (LSD = *d*-lysergic acid diethylamide; THC = tetrahydrocannabinol.)

dependent person, then nalmefene will put the patient into prolonged withdrawal—an obvious disadvantage.

## Withdrawal Techniques

Persons who are physically dependent on opioids experience unpleasant symptoms if drug use is abruptly discontinued. Techniques for minimizing discomfort are discussed below.

***Use of Methadone.*** Methadone, an oral opioid with a long duration of action, is the agent most commonly employed for easing opioid withdrawal. The first step in methadone-aided withdrawal is to substitute methadone for the opioid upon which the addict is dependent. Because opioids display cross-dependence with one another, methadone will prevent an abstinence syndrome. Once the subject has been stabilized on methadone, withdrawal is accomplished by administering methadone in gradually smaller doses. The resultant abstinence syndrome is mild, with symptoms resembling those of moderate influenza. The entire process of methadone substitution and withdrawal takes about 10 days to complete.

When substituting methadone for another opioid, suppression of the abstinence syndrome requires that methadone dosage be closely matched to the existing degree of physical dependence. Hence, to ensure that methadone dosing is adequate, the extent of physical dependence must be assessed. This can be accomplished by taking a history on the extent of drug use and by observing the patient for symptoms of withdrawal. Of the two approaches, observation is the more reliable. Estimates of drug use based on patient histories may be unreliable because (1) street users don't know the purity of the drugs they have taken, (2) claims of drug use may be inflated in hopes of receiving larger doses of methadone, and (3) addicts from the ranks of the health care professions may report minimal consumption to downplay the extent of abuse. Because information from addicts is not likely to permit accurate assessment of dependence, it is essential to observe the patient to make certain that the methadone dosage is sufficient to suppress withdrawal.

Use of methadone for *maintenance therapy* and *suppressive therapy* is discussed separately below.

***Use of Clonidine.*** Clonidine is a centrally acting alpha$_2$-adrenergic agonist. When administered to an individual who is physically dependent on opioids, clonidine can suppress some—but not all—symptoms of abstinence.

## TABLE 37–2. STREET NAMES FOR ABUSED DRUGS

| Drug | Street Names |
|---|---|
| *Psychedelics* | |
|    *d*-Lysergic acid diethylamide | LSD, LSD-25, acid, blotter, microdot |
|    Dimethyltryptamine | DMT, businessman's trip |
|    Mescaline | Peyote, cactus buttons |
|    3,4-Methylenedioxymethamphetamine | MDMA, ecstasy, XTC |
|    2,5-Dimethoxy-4-methylamphetamine | DOM, STP |
|    Psilocybin | Magic mushrooms |
|    Psilocin | Magic mushrooms |
| *Psychostimulants* | |
|    Amphetamine | Bennies, hearts, whites, cartwheels |
|    Dextroamphetamine | Dexies, oranges, footballs |
|    Methamphetamine | Speed, bombita, crank, crystal meth, ice |
|    Biphetamine | Black beauties |
|    Cocaine | Coke, crack, snow, blow, freebase, pasta, bazooka |
| *General CNS Depressants* | |
|    Pentobarbital | Yellow jackets |
|    Secobarbital | Red devils |
| *Miscellaneous Agents* | |
|    Phencyclidine | PCP, angel dust, dummy dust, hog, peacepill rocket fuel, sheets |
|    Marijuana | Pot, grass, reefer, weed, Panama red, Acapulco gold, many others |
| *Combinations* | |
|    Heroin + cocaine | Speedball |
|    Heroin + crack cocaine | Moon rock |

Clonidine is most effective against symptoms related to autonomic hyperactivity (nausea, vomiting, diarrhea). Modest relief is provided from muscle aches, restlessness, anxiety, and insomnia. Opioid craving is not diminished.

## Use of Opioid Antagonists to Maintain Abstinence

Once a patient has withdrawn from opioids, remaining drug free is often difficult. Use of opioid antagonists is one means of discouraging renewed abuse. Opioid antagonists can decrease abuse by blocking euphoria and all other opioid effects. By preventing pleasurable effects, opioid antagonists eliminate the reinforcing properties of drug use. When the former addict learns that opioid administration will not produce desired responses, drug-using behavior will cease.

Of the opioid antagonists available, *naltrexone* is the agent best suited for treating opioid abuse. Naltrexone is desirable because it is orally usable and because its long half-life permits alternate-day dosing. In contrast to naltrexone, naloxone has low oral efficacy and a half-life that is so short that multiple daily doses would be needed. These properties make naloxone impractical.

## Methadone and Levomethadyl for Maintenance and Suppressive Therapy

In addition to its role in facilitating opioid withdrawal, methadone can be used for *maintenance therapy* and *suppressive therapy*. These strategies are employed to modify drug-using behavior in the addict who is not yet a candidate for withdrawal.

Levomethadyl [ORLAAM] is a long-acting oral congener of methadone. This recently approved drug represents an alternative to methadone for maintenance and suppressive therapy.

*Maintenance Therapy.* Methadone maintenance consists of transferring the addict from the abused opioid to oral methadone. By taking methadone, the addict avoids withdrawal and the need to procure illegal drugs. Methadone maintenance is most effective when done in conjunction with nondrug measures directed at altering patterns of drug use.

*Suppressive Therapy.* The objective of suppressive therapy is to prevent the reinforcing effects of opioid-induced euphoria. Suppression is achieved by giving the addict progressively larger doses of methadone until a very high daily dose (120 mg) is reached. Building up to this dose creates a high degree of tolerance; hence no subjective effects are experienced from the methadone itself. Since cross-tolerance exists between opioids, once the patient is tolerant to methadone, taking street drugs, even in high doses, cannot produce significant psychologic effects. As a result, individuals made tolerant to opioids with methadone will not experience the reinforcing effects of illicit drugs.

Use of methadone to treat opioid addicts is restricted to agencies approved by the FDA and state authorities. These restrictions on the nonanalgesic use of methadone are needed to control methadone abuse, since the drug has about the same abuse liability as morphine and other strong opioids.

## Sequelae of Compulsive Opioid Use

Surprisingly, chronic opioid use has very few direct detrimental effects. Addicts in treatment programs have been maintained on high doses of methadone for years with no significant impairment of health. Furthermore, individuals on methadone maintenance can be successful socially and at work. It appears, then, that opioid use is not necessarily associated with poor health, lack of productivity, or inadequate social interaction.

Although opioids have few *direct* ill effects, there are many *indirect* hazards. These indirect risks stem largely from the lifestyle of the opioid user and from impurities common to street drugs. Infections secondary to sharing nonsterile needles occur frequently. The infections that opioid abusers acquire include septicemia, subcutaneous ulcers, hepatitis, and HIV. Foreign-body emboli have resulted from impurities in opioid preparations. Opioid users suffer an unusually high death rate. Some deaths reflect the violent nature of the subculture in which opioid use often takes place. Many other deaths result from accidental overdose.

# General CNS Depressants

The family of CNS depressants consists of barbiturates, benzodiazepines, alcohol, and a variety of other agents. With the exception of the benzodiazepines, all of these drugs are more alike than different. The benzodiazepines have properties that set them apart. The basic pharmacology of the CNS depressants is discussed in Chapter 32 (except for alcohol, which is the topic of Chapter 36). Discussion here is limited to the abuse of these drugs.

## Barbiturates

The barbiturates embody all of the properties that typify the general CNS depressants, and therefore can be considered the prototypes of the group. Depressant effects are dose dependent and range from mild sedation to sleep to coma to death. With prolonged use, barbiturates produce tolerance and physical dependence.

The abuse liability of the barbiturates stems from their ability to produce subjective effects similar to those of alcohol. The barbiturates with the highest potential for abuse have a short to intermediate duration of action. These agents—amobarbital, pentobarbital, and secobarbital—are classified under Schedule II of the Controlled Substances Act. Other barbiturates appear under Schedules III and IV (see Table 35-2). Despite legal restrictions, barbiturates are available cheaply and in abundance.

*Tolerance.* Regular use of barbiturates produces tolerance to some effects, but not to others. Tolerance to *subjective* effects is significant. As a result, progressively larger doses are needed to produce desired psychologic responses. Unfortunately, very little tolerance develops to *respiratory depression.* Consequently, as barbiturate use continues, the dose needed to produce subjective effects becomes closer and closer to the dose that can cause fatal respiratory depression. (Note that this differs from the pattern seen with opioids, in which tolerance to subjective effects and tolerance to respiratory depression develop in parallel.) Individuals who are tolerant to barbiturates show cross-tolerance with other CNS depressants (e.g., alcohol, benzodiazepines, general anesthetics). However, little or no cross-tolerance develops to opioids.

*Physical Dependence and Withdrawal Techniques.* Chronic barbiturate use can produce substantial physical dependence. Cross-dependence exists between barbiturates and other CNS depressants but not with opioids. When physical dependence is great, the associated abstinence syndrome can be severe—sometimes even fatal (see Chapter 32). In contrast, the opioid abstinence syndrome, although unpleasant, is rarely life threatening.

One technique for easing barbiturate withdrawal employs phenobarbital, a barbiturate with a long duration of action. Because of cross-dependence, substitution of phenobarbital for the abused barbiturate suppresses symptoms of abstinence. Once the patient has been stabilized, the dosage of phenobarbital is gradually tapered off, thereby minimizing symptoms of abstinence.

*Acute Toxicity.* Overdose with barbiturates produces a triad of symptoms: *respiratory depression, coma,* and *pinpoint pupils.* These are the same symptoms that accompany opioid poisoning. Treatment is directed at maintaining respiration and removing the drug from the body; endotracheal intubation and ventilatory assistance may be required. Details of management are presented in Chapter 32. Barbiturate overdose has no specific antidote; naloxone, which reverses poisoning by opioids, is not effective against poisoning by barbiturates.

## Benzodiazepines

Benzodiazepines differ significantly from barbiturates. Benzodiazepines are much safer than the barbiturates, and overdose with *oral* benzodiazepines *alone* is rarely lethal. However, the risk of death is greatly increased when oral benzodiazepines are combined with other CNS depressants (e.g., alcohol, barbiturates) or when benzodiazepines are administered *intravenously.* If severe overdose occurs, signs and symptoms can be reversed with *flumazenil,* a benzodiazepine antagonist. As a rule, tolerance and physical dependence are only moderate when benzodiazepines are taken for legitimate indications but can be substantial when these drugs are abused. In patients who develop physical dependence, the abstinence syndrome can be minimized by withdrawing benzodiazepines very slowly—over a period of months. The abuse liability of the benzodiazepines is much lower than that of the barbiturates. As a result, benzodiazepines are classified as Schedule IV agents. Benzodiazepines are discussed at length in Chapter 32.

### Alcohol and Miscellaneous CNS Depressants

Alcohol is the topic of Chapter 36. Discussion in that chapter focuses on the basic pharmacology of alcohol, alcohol abuse, and drugs used in alcoholism treatment.

In addition to barbiturates, benzodiazepines, and alcohol, other CNS depressants (e.g., paraldehyde, meprobamate, chloral hydrate) are subject to abuse. As noted in Chapter 32, the pharmacologic properties of these drugs are similar to those of the barbiturates.

*Methaqualone* is unique among the CNS depressants and requires special comment. At one time methaqualone [Quaalude] was available legally for use as a sedative. However, because of its high abuse potential and the availability of superior alternatives (i.e., benzodiazepines), methaqualone was withdrawn from the market. This drug differs from other depressants in that overdose is not characterized by obvious signs of CNS depression; rather, poisoning can produce restlessness, hypertonia, and convulsions.

# Psychostimulants

Discussion here focuses on the CNS stimulants with the highest high potential for abuse: amphetamines, cocaine, and related substances. Because of their considerable abuse liability, these drugs are classified as Schedule II agents. In addition to stimulating the CNS, the amphetamines and cocaine can stimulate the heart, blood vessels, and other structures under sympathetic control. Because of these peripheral actions, these agents are also referred to as *sympathomimetics*.

Stimulants that are *not* addressed in this chapter are the ones whose abuse potential is moderate, low, or nonexistent. Included in this group are Schedule III stimulants (e.g., benzphetamine), Schedule IV stimulants (e.g., diethylpropion), and stimulants that are not regulated at all (e.g., caffeine).

## Cocaine

Cocaine is a stimulant with CNS effects similar to those of the amphetamines. In addition, cocaine can produce local anesthesia (see Chapter 26) as well as vasoconstriction and cardiac stimulation. In recent years, use of a form of cocaine known as "crack" has reached epidemic proportions, especially among adolescents. Crack is extremely addictive, and the risk of lethal overdose is high.

In 1992, 4.5 million Americans used cocaine. Of these, 1.3 million used it at least once a month. During the third quarter of 1992, cocaine toxicity resulted in 30,900 visits to emergency departments, primarily for cardiovascular, cerebrovascular, and gastrointestinal problems.

***Forms.*** Cocaine is available in two forms: *cocaine hydrochloride* and *cocaine base* (alkaloidal cocaine, free-base cocaine, "crack"). Cocaine base is heat stabile, whereas cocaine hydrochloride is not. Cocaine hydrochloride is available as a white powder that is frequently diluted ("cut") before sale. Cocaine base is sold in the form of crystals ("rocks") that consist of nearly pure cocaine. Cocaine base is widely known by the street name of "crack," a term inspired by the sound that the crystals make when they are heated.

***Routes of Administration.*** Cocaine *hydrochloride* is usually administered *intranasally*. The drug is "snorted" (inhaled into the nose) and absorbed across the nasal mucosa into the bloodstream. In addition to intranasal administration, cocaine hydrochloride is often injected IV. The hydrochloride form cannot be smoked because of its instability at high temperature.

Cocaine *base* is administered by *smoking*, a process referred to as "freebasing." Smoking delivers large amounts of cocaine to the lungs, and absorption is very rapid. Subjective and physiologic effects are equivalent to those elicited by IV injection.

***Subjective Effects, Patterns of Use, and Addiction.*** The psychologic effects of cocaine appear to result from activation of dopamine receptors secondary to cocaine-induced blockade of dopamine reuptake. At usual doses, cocaine produces euphoria similar that produced by amphetamine. In a laboratory setting, individuals familiar with the effects of cocaine are unable to distinguish between cocaine and amphetamine. Interestingly, lidocaine (a local anesthetic similar to cocaine) produces subjective effects that are indistinguishable from those of cocaine (when both drugs are administered intranasally).

As with many other psychoactive drugs, the intensity of subjective responses depends on the rate at which plasma drug levels rise. Since cocaine levels rise relatively slowly with intranasal administration, this route produces responses of low intensity. In contrast, since intravenous administration and smoking cause nearly instantaneous elevations of plasma drug levels, these routes produce responses that are very intense.

When crack cocaine is smoked, desirable subjective effects begin to fade within minutes and are often replaced by dysphoria. In an attempt to avoid dysphoria and regain euphoria, the cocaine user may administer repeated doses of the drug at short intervals. This pattern of use can rapidly lead to addiction.

***Acute Toxicity: Symptoms and Treatment.*** Overdose is frequent and deaths have occurred. Mild overdose produces agitation, dizziness, tremor, and blurred vision. Severe overdose can produce hyperpyrexia, convulsions, ventricular dysrhythmias, and hemorrhagic stroke. Angina pectoris and myocardial infarction may develop secondary to coronary artery spasm. Psychologic manifestations of overdose include severe anxiety, paranoid ideation, and hallucinations (visual, auditory, or tactile). Because cocaine has a short half-life, symptoms subside in 1 to 2 hours.

Although there is no specific antidote to cocaine toxicity, most symptoms can be controlled with drugs. Intravenous *diazepam* or *lorazepam* can reduce anxiety and suppress seizures. *Diazepam* may also alleviate hypertension and dysrhythmias, since these result from increased central sympathetic activity. If hypertension is severe, it can be corrected with intravenous *nitroprusside* or *phentolamine*. Dysrhythmias associated with prolongation of the QT interval may respond to *hypertonic sodium bicarbonate*. Although beta blockers can suppress dysrhythmias, they can further compromise coronary perfusion (by preventing beta₂-mediated coronary vasodilation); hence their use is controversial. Reduction of thrombus formation with aspirin can reduce the risk of myocardial ischemia. Hyperthermia should be reduced with external cooling.

**Chronic Toxicity.** When administered intranasally on a long-term basis, cocaine can cause atrophy of the nasal mucosa and loss of sense of smell. In extreme cases, necrosis and perforation of the nasal septum have occurred. Nasal pathology results from local ischemia secondary to chronic, cocaine-induced vasoconstriction. Injury to the lungs can occur from smoking cocaine base.

**Toxicity from Use during Pregnancy and Lactation.** Cocaine is highly lipid soluble and readily crosses the placenta, allowing it to accumulate in the fetal circulation. Use of cocaine during pregnancy has been associated with spontaneous abortion, premature delivery, and retardation of intrauterine growth. In addition, congenital abnormalities (e.g., cardiac anomalies, skull malformations) have been reported. Neonates exposed to cocaine during gestation have displayed signs of CNS irritability (increased muscle tone, tremor, electroencephalogram abnormalities) that in some cases have persisted for months. Cerebral infarction has occurred in newborns whose mothers took cocaine just prior to labor. Maternal use of cocaine can produce intoxication in the breast-fed infant.

**Tolerance, Dependence, and Withdrawal.** In animal models, regular administration of cocaine results in *increased* sensitivity to the drug, not tolerance. However, in humans, the opposite occurs. That is, when humans take cocaine on a regular basis, tolerance usually develops; hence dosage must be increased to produce euphoria.

The degree of physical dependence produced by cocaine is in dispute. Some observers report little or no indication of withdrawal following cocaine discontinuation. In contrast, others report symptoms similar to those associated with amphetamines: dysphoria, craving, fatigue, depression, and prolonged sleep.

**Detoxification and Maintenance of Abstinence.** Addiction to crack cocaine is very difficult to treat. The crack addict is typically unresponsive to persuasion and traditional psychotherapeutic techniques. If treatment on an outpatient basis is ineffective, admission to a treatment facility that prevents all access to cocaine may be helpful.

Although various drugs have been given to help maintain abstinence following cocaine withdrawal, none is considered highly effective. Agents that have been tried include antidepressants (e.g., desipramine, bupropion, fluoxetine), dopamine agonists (bromocriptine, amantadine), opioid antagonists (e.g., naltrexone), and mood stabilizers (lithium, carbamazepine).

## Amphetamines

The basic pharmacology of the amphetamines is discussed in Chapter 33. Discussion here is limited to amphetamine abuse.

**Forms and Routes.** The amphetamine family includes dextroamphetamine, methamphetamine, and amphetamine (a racemic mixture of dextroamphetamine and levamphetamine). When taken for purposes of abuse, amphetamines are usually administered orally or IV. In addition, a form of dextroamphetamine known as "ice" or "crystal meth" can be smoked.

**Subjective and Behavioral Effects.** Amphetamines produce arousal and elevation of mood. Euphoria is likely and talkativeness is prominent. A sense of increased physical strength and mental capacity occurs. Self-confidence rises. The amphetamine user feels little or no need for food and sleep. Orgasm is delayed, intensified, and more pleasurable.

**Adverse CNS Effects.** Amphetamines can produce a psychotic state characterized by hallucinations and paranoid ideation. This condition closely resembles paranoid schizophrenia. Although psychosis can be triggered by a single dose, it occurs most commonly in the context of long-term abuse. Amphetamine-induced psychosis usually resolves spontaneously following drug withdrawal. If needed, an antipsychotic agent (e.g., haloperidol) can be given to suppress symptoms.

**Adverse Cardiovascular Effects.** Because of their sympathomimetic actions, amphetamines can cause vasoconstriction and excessive stimulation of the heart. These actions can lead to hypertension, angina pectoris, and dysrhythmias. Overdose may also cause cerebral and systemic vasculitis and renal failure. Vasoconstriction can be relieved with an alpha-adrenergic blocker (e.g., phentolamine). Cardiac stimulation can be reduced with a beta blocker (e.g., labetalol). Drug elimination can be accelerated by giving ammonium chloride to acidify the urine.

**Tolerance, Dependence, and Withdrawal.** Prolonged amphetamine use results in tolerance to mood elevation, appetite suppression, and cardiovascular effects. Although physical dependence is only moderate, psychologic dependence can be intense. Amphetamine withdrawal can produce dysphoria and a strong sense of craving. Other symptoms include fatigue, prolonged sleep, excessive eating, and depression. Depression can persist for months and is a common reason for resuming amphetamine use.

## Marijuana and Related Preparations

### Cannabis sativa, the Source of Marijuana

The source of marijuana is *Cannabis sativa*, the Indian hemp plant—an unusual plant in that it has separate male and female forms. Psychoactive compounds are present in all parts of the male and female plants. However, the greatest concentration of psychoactive substances is found in the flowering tops of the females.

The two most common *Cannabis* derivatives are *marijuana* and *hashish*. Marijuana is a preparation consisting of leaves and flowers of male and female plants. Alternative names for marijuana include *grass, weed, pot,* and *dope*. The terms *joint* and *reefer* apply to marijuana cigarettes. Hashish is a dried preparation of the resinous exudate from female flowers. Hashish is considerably more potent than marijuana.

## Psychoactive Component

The major psychoactive substance in *Cannabis sativa* is *delta-9-tetrahydrocannabinol (THC)*, an oily chemical with high lipid solubility. The structure of THC appears in Figure 37–1.

The THC content of *Cannabis* preparations is variable. The highest concentrations are found in the flowers of the female plant. The lowest concentrations are in the seeds. Depending on growing conditions and the strain of the plant, THC in marijuana preparations may range from 1% to 11%.

## Mechanism of Action

THC has several possible mechanisms. Perhaps the most important of these is activation of specific cannabinoid receptors found in various brain regions. The endogenous ligand for these receptors appears to be *anandamide*, a derivative of arachidonic acid unique to the brain. Other proposed mechanisms are (1) activation of phospholipase $A_2$ in the brain, resulting in increased production of prostaglandin $E_2$, and (2) augmentation of neuronal membrane fluidity through interaction with membrane lipids.

## Pharmacokinetics

*Administration by Smoking.* When marijuana or hashish is smoked, about 60% of the THC content is absorbed. Absorption from the lungs is rapid. Subjective effects begin in minutes and peak in 20 to 30 minutes. Effects from a single marijuana cigarette may persist 2 to 3 hours. Termination of effects results from metabolic conversion of THC to inactive products.

*Oral Administration.* When marijuana or hashish is taken orally, practically all of the THC undergoes absorption. However, the majority of absorbed THC is metabolically inactivated on its first pass through the liver. Hence only 6% to 20% of absorbed drug actually reaches the general circulation. Because of this extensive first-pass metabolism, oral doses must be 3 to 10 times greater than smoked doses to produce equivalent effects. With oral administration, effects are delayed and prolonged; responses begin 30 to 50 minutes after drug ingestion and persist for up to 12 hours.

## Behavioral and Subjective Effects

Marijuana produces three principal subjective effects: *euphoria, sedation,* and *hallucinations*. This set of re-

sponses is unique to marijuana; no other psychoactive drug produces all three. Because of this singular pattern of effects, marijuana is in a class by itself.

*Effects of Low to Moderate Doses.* Responses to low doses of THC are variable and depend on several factors, including dosage size, route of administration, setting of drug use, and expectations and previous experience of the user. The following effects are common: (1) euphoria and relaxation; (2) gaiety and a heightened sense of the humorous; (3) increased sensitivity to visual and auditory stimuli; (4) enhanced sense of touch, taste, and smell; (5) increased appetite and ability to appreciate the flavor of food; and (6) distortion of time perception such that short spans seem much longer than they actually are. In addition to these effects, which might be considered pleasurable (or at least innocuous), moderate doses can produce undesirable responses. These include (1) impairment of short-term memory; (2) decreased capacity to perform multistep tasks; (3) impairment of driving skills (which can be substantially worsened by concurrent use of alcohol); (4) temporal disintegration (inability to distinguish between past, present, and future); (5) depersonalization (a sense of strangeness about the self); (6) decreased ability to perceive the emotions of others; and (7) reduced interpersonal interaction.

*High-Dose Effects.* In high doses, marijuana can have serious adverse psychologic effects. The user may experience hallucinations, delusions, and paranoia. Euphoria may be displaced by intense anxiety, and a dissociative state in which the user feels "outside of himself or herself" may occur. In extremely high doses, marijuana can produce a state resembling toxic psychosis, which may persist for weeks. Because of the widespread use of marijuana, psychiatric emergencies caused by the drug are not uncommon.

Not everyone is equally vulnerable to the adverse psychologic effects of marijuana. Some individuals experience ill effects only at extremely high doses. In contrast, others routinely experience adverse effects at moderate doses. Schizophrenics are at unusually high risk for adverse reactions. In the stabilized schizophrenic, marijuana can precipitate an acute psychotic episode.

*Effects of Chronic Use.* Chronic, excessive use of marijuana has been associated with a behavioral phenomenon known as the *amotivational syndrome*. This syndrome is characterized by apathy, dullness, poor grooming, reduced interest in achievement, and disinterest in the pursuit of conventional goals. The precise relationship between marijuana and development of the syndrome is not known, nor is it certain what other factors may contribute. Available data do not suggest that the amotivational syndrome is due to organic brain damage.

## Physiologic Effects

*Cardiovascular Effects.* Marijuana produces a dose-related increase in heart rate. Increases of 20 to 50 beats/min are typical. However, rates up to 140 beats/min are not uncommon. Pretreatment with propranolol prevents marijuana-induced tachycardia but does not block the drug's subjective effects. Marijuana causes orthostatic hypotension and pronounced reddening of the conjunctivae. These responses apparently result from vasodilation.

**Respiratory Effects.** When used *acutely*, marijuana produces *bronchodilation*. However, when smoked chronically, the drug causes airway constriction. In addition, chronic use is closely associated with development of bronchitis, sinusitis, and asthma. Lung cancer is another possible outcome. Experiments in animals have shown that tar from marijuana smoke is a more potent carcinogen than tar from cigarettes.

**Effects on Reproduction.** Studies in animals have shown multiple effects on reproduction. In males, marijuana decreases spermatogenesis and testosterone levels. In females, the drug reduces levels of follicle-stimulating hormone, luteinizing hormone, and prolactin. In some species, marijuana has caused birth defects. However, teratogenesis has not been proved in humans.

### Tolerance and Dependence

When taken in extremely high doses, marijuana can produce tolerance and physical dependence. Neither effect, however, is remarkable. Some tolerance develops to the cardiovascular, perceptual, and motor effects of marijuana. Little or no tolerance develops to subjective effects.

To demonstrate physical dependence on marijuana, the drug must be given in exceptionally high doses—and even then the degree of dependence is only moderate. Symptoms brought on by abrupt discontinuation of high-dose marijuana include irritability, restlessness, nervousness, insomnia, reduced appetite, and weight loss. Tremor, hyperthermia, and chills may also occur. Symptoms subside in 4 to 5 days. When marijuana use has been moderate, no symptoms of withdrawal are noted.

### Therapeutic Uses

**Suppression of Emesis.** Intense nausea and vomiting are common side effects of cancer chemotherapy. In certain patients these responses can be suppressed more effectively with cannabinoids than with traditional antiemetics (e.g., prochlorperazine, metoclopramide). Two cannabinoid preparations are available: *dronabinol* (THC) and *nabilone* (a synthetic derivative of dronabinol). Dosage forms and dosages are presented in Chapter 73.

**Appetite Stimulation.** Dronabinol (THC) was recently approved for stimulating appetite in patients with AIDS. The goal of treatment is to decrease anorexia, thereby preventing or reversing weight loss.

**Potential Uses.** Proponents of making marijuana available by prescription argue that smoked marijuana can prevent seizures, reduce chronic pain, lower intraocular pressure in patients with glaucoma, improve appetite in patients with AIDS, suppress nausea and vomiting caused by cancer chemotherapy, and suppress spasticity associated with multiple sclerosis and spinal cord injury. In response, the U.S. government argues that we have no proof that marijuana can provide these benefits—and certainly

no proof that smoked marijuana is superior to existing medications for these potential applications. Since clinical trials to demonstrate efficacy of marijuana must be approved by the government, and since the government has been unwilling to approve such trials, it does not appear that the controversy will be resolved soon.

### Comparison of Marijuana with Alcohol

In several important ways, responses to marijuana and alcohol are quite different. Whereas increased hostility and aggression are common sequelae of alcohol consumption, aggressive behavior is rare among marijuana users. Although loss of judgment and control can occur with either drug, such losses are much greater with alcohol. For the marijuana user, increased appetite and food intake are typical. In contrast, heavy drinkers often suffer nutritional deficiencies. Lastly, whereas marijuana can cause toxic psychosis, dissociative phenomena, and paranoia, these severe adverse psychologic reactions rarely occur with alcohol.

## Psychedelics

The psychedelics are a fascinating drug family for which LSD can be considered the prototype. Other family members include mescaline, dimethyltryptamine (DMT), and psilocin. The psychedelics are so named because of their ability to produce what has been termed a *psychedelic state*. Individuals in this state show an increased awareness of sensory stimuli and are likely to perceive the world around them as beautiful and harmonious; the normally insignificant may assume exceptional meaning, the "self" may seem split into an "observer" and a "doer," and boundaries between "self" and "nonself" may fade, producing a sense of unity with the cosmos.

Psychedelic drugs are often referred to as *hallucinogens* or *psychotomimetics*. These names reflect the ability of these agents to produce hallucinations as well as mental states that in many ways resemble psychosis.

It is important to note that although psychedelics are able to cause hallucinations and psychotic-like states, these responses are not the most characteristic effects of these drugs. The characteristic that truly distinguishes the psychedelics from other agents is *their ability to bring on the same types of alterations in thought, perception, and feeling that otherwise occur only in dreams*. In essence, the psychedelics seem able to activate mechanisms for dreaming without causing unconsciousness.

### d-Lysergic Acid Diethylamide (LSD)

**History.** The first person to experience LSD was a Swiss chemist named Albert Hofman. In 1943, 5 years after LSD was first synthesized, Hofman accidentally ingested a minute amount of the drug. The result was a dream-like state accompanied by perceptual distortions and vivid hallucinations. The high potency and unusual actions of LSD led to speculation that the drug might provide a model for studying psychosis. Unfortunately, that speculation did not prove correct: extensive research revealed that the effects of LSD could not be equated with idiopathic psychosis. With the realization that LSD did not produce a "model psychosis," medical interest in the drug declined. Not everyone, however, lost interest in the effects of LSD on the human psyche; during the decade of the 1960s, nonmedical experimentation with the drug flourished. This widespread use caused substantial societal concern, and, by 1970, LSD had been classified as a Schedule I substance. Despite regulatory efforts, street use of LSD continues.

***Mechanism of Action.*** LSD acts at multiple sites in the brain and spinal cord. Effects are thought to result from activation of serotonin$_2$ receptors at these sites. This concept has been reinforced by the observation that ritanserin, a selective blocker of serotonin$_2$ receptors, can prevent the effects of LSD in animal models.

***Pharmacokinetics.*** LSD is usually administered orally but can also be injected or smoked. With oral administration, initial effects can be felt in minutes. Over the next few hours, responses become progressively more intense. Effects subside in 8 to 12 hours.

***Subjective and Behavioral Effects.*** Responses to LSD can be diverse, complex, and changeable. The drug can alter thinking, feeling, perception, sense of self, and sense of relationship to the environment and other people. LSD-induced experiences may be sublime or they may be terrifying. Just what will be experienced during any particular "trip" cannot be predicted.

Perceptual alterations can be dramatic. Colors may appear iridescent or glowing, kaleidoscopic images may appear, and vivid hallucinations may occur. Sensory experiences may merge so that colors seem to be heard and sounds seem to be visible. Afterimages may occur, causing current perceptions to overlap with preceding perceptions. The LSD user may feel a sense of wonderment and awe at the beauty of commonplace things.

LSD can have a profound impact on affect. Emotions may range from elation, good humor, and euphoria to sadness, dysphoria, and fear. The intensity of emotion may be overwhelming.

Thoughts may turn inward. Attitudes may be re-evaluated, and old values assigned new priorities. A sense of new and important insight may be felt. However, despite the intensity of these experiences, enduring changes in beliefs, behavior, and personality are rare.

***Physiologic Effects.*** LSD produces few physiologic effects. Activation of the sympathetic nervous system can produce tachycardia, elevation of blood pressure, mydriasis, piloerection, and hyperthermia. Neuromuscular effects (tremor, incoordination, hyperreflexia, muscular weakness) may also occur.

***Tolerance and Dependence.*** Tolerance to LSD develops rapidly. Substantial tolerance can be seen after just three or four daily doses. Tolerance to subjective and be-

havioral effects develops to a greater extent than to cardiovascular effects. Cross-tolerance exists with LSD, mescaline, and psilocybin, but not with DMT. Since DMT is similar to LSD, the absence of cross-tolerance is surprising. There is no cross-tolerance with amphetamines or THC. Upon cessation of LSD use, tolerance fades rapidly. Abrupt withdrawal of LSD is not associated with an abstinence syndrome; hence, there is no evidence for physical dependence.

***Toxicity.*** Toxic reactions to LSD are primarily psychologic. The drug has never been a direct cause of death, although fatalities have occurred from accidents and suicides.

Acute panic reactions are relatively common and may be associated with a fear of disintegration of the self. Such "bad trips" can usually be managed by a process of "talking down" (providing emotional support and reassurance in a nonthreatening environment). Panic episodes can also be managed with an antianxiety agent (e.g., diazepam). Neuroleptics (e.g., haloperidol, chlorpromazine) may actually intensify the experience; hence their use is questionable.

A small percentage of former LSD users experience episodic visual disturbances, formerly referred to as "flashbacks." These disturbances may manifest as geometric pseudohallucinations, flashes of color, or positive afterimages. Visual disturbances may be precipitated by several factors, including marijuana use, fatigue, stress, and anxiety. Phenothiazines exacerbate these experiences rather than provide relief. In many cases, the disturbances appear to be caused by permanent changes in the visual system.

In addition to panic reactions and visual disturbances, LSD can cause other adverse psychologic effects. Depressive episodes, dissociative reactions, and distortions of body image may occur. When an LSD experience has been intensely terrifying, the user may be left with persistent residual fear. The drug may also cause prolonged psychotic reactions. In contrast to acute effects, which differ substantially from symptoms of schizophrenia, prolonged psychotic reactions mimic schizophrenia faithfully.

***Therapeutic Uses.*** LSD has no recognized therapeutic applications. The drug has been evaluated for possible use in treating alcoholism, opioid addiction, and psychiatric disorders. In addition, LSD has been studied as a possible means of promoting psychologic well-being in patients with terminal cancer. However, for all of these potential uses, LSD proved either ineffective or impractical.

## 3,4-Methylenedioxymethamphetamine (MDMA, Ecstasy)

Use of MDMA ("ecstasy") came to prominence in the mid-1980s, especially among college students. Although originally unregulated, the drug was soon classified as a Schedule I substance. MDMA has mixed properties of a psychedelic and a psychostimulant. Low doses produce

LSD-like psychedelic effects, and higher doses produce amphetamine-like stimulant effects. Moderate doses appear to facilitate interpersonal relationships: users report a sense of closeness with others, lowering of defenses, reduced anxiety, enhanced communication, and increased sociability. Because of these favorable psychologic effects, MDMA was used briefly in psychotherapy. Unfortunately, the drug can cause serious adverse effects. When administered to rats and monkeys in doses only 2 to 4 times greater than those that produce hallucinations in humans, MDMA can cause irreversible destruction of serotonergic neurons, resulting in passivity and insomnia. We do not know if MDMA is neurotoxic in humans. Other adverse effects include tingling and cold sensations as well as neurologic effects (spasmodic jerking, jaw clenching, and teeth grinding).

## Mescaline, Psilocybin, Psilocin, and Dimethyltryptamine

In addition to LSD, the family of psychedelic drugs includes mescaline, psilocin, psilocybin, dimethyltryptamine (DMT), and several related compounds (see Table 35–2). Some psychedelics are synthetic and some are naturally occurring. DMT and LSD represent the synthetic compounds. Mescaline, a constituent of the peyote cactus, and psilocin, a constituent of "magic mushrooms," represent the compounds found in nature.

The subjective and behavioral effects of the miscellaneous psychedelic drugs are similar to those of LSD. Like LSD, these drugs can elicit modes of thought, perception, and feeling that are normally restricted to dreams. In addition, these drugs can cause hallucinations and can induce mental states that resemble psychosis.

The miscellaneous psychedelics differ from LSD with respect to potency and time course of action. LSD is the most potent of the psychedelics, producing its full spectrum of effects at doses as low as 0.5 μg/kg. Psilocin and psilocybin are 100 times less potent than LSD, and mescaline is 4000 times less potent than LSD. Whereas LSD has effects that are prolonged (responses may last 12 or more hours), the effects of mescaline and DMT are shorter: responses to mescaline usually terminate within 8 to 12 hours, and responses to DMT terminate within 1 to 2 hours.

## Phencyclidine

Phencyclidine ("PCP," "angel dust," "peace pill") was originally developed as an anesthetic for animals. The drug was tried briefly as a general anesthetic for humans but was withdrawn because it produced severe emergence delirium. Although rejected for therapeutic use, phencyclidine has become widely used as a drug of abuse. Use has grown in large part because the drug can be synthesized easily by the amateur chemist, making it cheap and abundant. The popularity of phencyclidine is disturbing in

that the drug causes a high incidence of severe adverse effects—effects that make it one of the most dangerous abused substances.

### Chemistry and Pharmacokinetics

*Chemistry.* Phencyclidine is a weak organic base with high lipid solubility. The drug is chemically related to ketamine, an unusual general anesthetic (see Chapter 27). The structural formula of phencyclidine appears in Figure 37–1.

*Pharmacokinetics.* Phencyclidine can be administered orally, intranasally, intravenously, and by smoking. For administration by smoking, the drug is usually sprinkled on plant matter (e.g., oregano, parsley, tobacco, marijuana). Because of its high lipid solubility, phencyclidine is readily absorbed from all sites.

Once absorbed, phencyclidine undergoes substantial gastroenteric recirculation. Because it is a base, phencyclidine in the blood can be drawn into the acidic environment of the stomach (by the pH partitioning effect); from the stomach, the drug re-enters the intestine, from which it then is reabsorbed into the blood. This cycling from the blood to the gastrointestinal tract and back to the blood prolongs the drug's sojourn in the body. Elimination occurs eventually through a combination of hepatic metabolism and renal excretion.

### Mechanism of Action

The mechanism by which phencyclidine affects the CNS is not known with certainty. Studies have demonstrated that the drug binds with high affinity to sites in the cerebral cortex and limbic system, and that it blocks certain glutamate receptors and binds to certain receptors for opioids. However, the relationship between binding activity and psychologic effects has not been established.

### Subjective and Behavioral Effects

Phencyclidine produces a unique set of effects. Hallucinations are prominent. In addition, the drug can produce CNS depression, CNS excitation, and analgesia. This complex response profile is not seen with any other drug of abuse. Because of its singular range of effects, phencyclidine is in a class by itself.

*Effects of Low to Moderate Doses.* At low doses, phencyclidine produces effects like those of alcohol. Low-dose intoxication is characterized by euphoria, release of inhibitions, and emotional lability. Nystagmus, slurred speech, and motor incoordination may also occur.

As dosage is increased, the clinical picture becomes more variable and complex. Symptoms include excitation, disorientation, anxiety, disorganized thoughts, altered body image, and reduced perception of tactile and painful stimuli. Mood may be volatile and hostile. Bizarre behavior may develop. Heart rate and blood pressure are elevated.

*High-Dose (Toxic) Effects.* High doses can cause severe adverse physiologic and psychologic effects. Death may result from a variety of causes.

*Psychologic* effects include hallucinations, confusional states, combativeness, and psychosis. The psychosis closely resembles schizophrenia and may persist for weeks. Individuals with pre-existing psychoses are especially vulnerable to psychotogenic effects. Suicide has been attempted.

The *physiologic* effects of high-dose phencyclidine are varied. Extreme overdose can produce hypertension, coma, seizures, and muscular rigidity associated with severe hyperthermia and rhabdomyolysis (disintegration of muscle tissue).

**Treatment of Toxicity.** Treatment is primarily supportive. Psychotic reactions are best managed by isolation from external stimuli. "Talking down" is not effective, and antipsychotic drugs, such as haloperidol, are of limited help. Physical restraint may be needed to prevent self-inflicted harm and to protect others from assault. If respiration is depressed, mechanical support of ventilation may be needed. Severe hypertension can be managed with diazoxide, a vasodilator. Seizures can be controlled with IV diazepam. If fever is high, external cooling can lower temperature. By promoting muscle relaxation, dantrolene can reduce heat generation and rhabdomyolysis.

Elimination of phencyclidine can be accelerated by continuous gastric lavage and acidification of the urine with ammonium chloride. Continuous lavage is effective because of the gastroenteric recirculation that the drug undergoes. Acidification of urine may promote phencyclidine excretion by reducing tubular reabsorption of this weak base.

# Inhalants

The inhalants are a diverse group of drugs that have only one characteristic in common—administration by inhalation. These drugs can be divided into three classes: anesthetics, volatile nitrites, and organic solvents.

## Anesthetics

Provided that dosage is modest, anesthetics produce subjective effects similar to those of alcohol (euphoria, exhilaration, loss of inhibitions). The anesthetics that have been abused most are *nitrous oxide* ("laughing gas") and *ether*. One reason for the popularity of these drugs is ease of administration: neither agent requires exotic equipment to be used. For nitrous oxide, ready availability also promotes use: small cylinders of the drug, marketed for aerating whipping cream, can be purchased without restriction.

## Volatile Nitrites

Three volatile nitrites—*amyl nitrite, butyl nitrite,* and *isobutyl nitrite*—are subject to abuse. These drugs are abused by homosexual males because of an ability to relax the anal sphincter, and by males in general because of a reputed ability to prolong and intensify sexual orgasm.

The most pronounced pharmacologic effect of volatile nitrites is venodilation, which causes pooling of blood in veins, which in turn causes a profound drop in systolic blood pressure. The result is dizziness, light-headedness, palpitations, and possibly pulsatile headache. Effects begin seconds after inhalation and fade rapidly. The primary toxicity is methemoglobinemia, which can be treated with methylene blue and supplemental oxygen.

In contrast to amyl nitrite, which is manufactured for medical use, butyl nitrite and isobutyl nitrite are produced solely for recreational use. Trade names for butyl nitrite and isobutyl nitrite include Climax, Rush, and Locker Room. On the street, preparations of amyl nitrite are known as "poppers" or "snappers." These terms reflect the fact that amyl nitrite is packaged in glass ampules that make a popping sound when snapped open to allow inhalation.

## Organic Solvents

A wide assortment of solvents have been inhaled to induce intoxication. These compounds include *toluene, gasoline, lighter fluid, paint thinner, nail-polish remover, benzene, acetone, chloroform,* and *model-airplane glue.* These agents are used primarily by children and the very poor—people who, because of age or insufficient funds, lack access to more conventional drugs of abuse.

**Administration.** Solvents are administered by three processes, referred to as "bagging," "huffing," and "sniffing." Bagging is performed by pouring solvent in a plastic bag and inhaling the vapor. Huffing is performed by pouring the solvent on a rag and inhaling the vapor. Sniffing is performed by inhaling the solvent directly from its container.

**Pharmacologic Effects.** The acute effects of organic solvents are somewhat like those of alcohol (euphoria, impaired judgment, slurred speech, flushing, CNS depression). In addition, these compounds can cause visual hallucinations and disorientation with respect to time and place. High doses can cause sudden death. Possible causes include anoxia, respiratory depression, vagal stimulation (which slows heart rate), and dysrhythmias.

Prolonged use is associated with multiple toxicities. Gasoline can cause lead poisoning; chloroform is toxic to the heart, liver, and kidneys; and toluene can cause severe brain damage and bone marrow depression. Many solvents can damage the heart; fatal dysrhythmias have occurred secondary to drug-induced heart block.

**Management.** Management of acute toxicity is strictly supportive. The objective is to stabilize vital signs. We have no antidotes for volatile solvents.

# Nicotine and Smoking

Although tobacco smoke contains many dangerous compounds, nicotine is of greatest concern. Other hazardous components in tobacco smoke include carbon monoxide, hydrogen cyanide, ammonia, nitrosamines, and tar. (Tar is composed of various polycyclic hydrocarbons, some of which are proven carcinogens.)

Cigarette smoking is considered our greatest single cause of preventable illness and premature death. In the United States, smoking contributes to 420,000 deaths a year. The major cause of death is heart disease, which kills 180,000 smokers annually. Smoking is responsible for 120,000 deaths from lung cancer each year—fully 85% of all lung cancer deaths. Another 100,000 deaths result from other cancers, chronic obstructive airway disease, stroke, and miscellaneous disorders. The medical cost of this illness is $50 billion a year. Indirect costs, such as lost time from work and disability, add up to an additional $47 billion annually.

## Basic Pharmacology of Nicotine

### Mechanism of Action

The effects of nicotine result from actions at nicotinic receptors. Whether these receptors will be stimulated or inhibited depends on nicotine dosage. At *low* doses nicotine *stimulates* receptors, whereas *high* doses cause *blockade*. The amount of nicotine received from cigarettes is relatively low. Accordingly, cigarette smoking causes *stimulation* of nicotinic receptors.

Nicotine can stimulate nicotinic receptors at several locations. Most effects result from stimulating nicotinic receptors in autonomic ganglia and the adrenal medulla. In addition, nicotine can stimulate nicotinic receptors in the carotid body, aortic arch, and CNS. As discussed below, actions in the CNS mimic those of cocaine and other highly addictive substances. When present at the levels produced by smoking, nicotine has no significant effect on nicotinic receptors of the neuromuscular junction.

### Pharmacokinetics

Absorption of nicotine depends on whether the delivery system is a cigarette, a cigar, or smokeless tobacco. Nicotine in cigarette smoke is absorbed primarily from the lungs; when cigarette smoke is inhaled, between 90% and 98% of nicotine in the lungs enters the blood. Unlike nicotine in cigarette smoke, nicotine in cigar smoke is absorbed primarily from the mouth, as is nicotine in smokeless tobacco.

Nicotine can cross membranes easily and is widely distributed throughout the body. The drug readily enters breast milk, reaching levels that can be toxic to the nursing infant. It also crosses the placental barrier and can cause fetal harm.

Nicotine is rapidly metabolized to inactive products. Nicotine and its metabolites are excreted by the kidney. The drug's half-life is 1 to 2 hours.

### Pharmacologic Effects

The pharmacologic effects discussed in this section are associated with *low* doses of nicotine. These are the effects caused by smoking cigarettes. Responses to *high* doses of nicotine are discussed under *Acute Poisoning*.

*Cardiovascular Effects.* The cardiovascular effects of nicotine result primarily from stimulating nicotinic receptors in *sympathetic ganglia* and the *adrenal medulla*. Stimulation of these receptors promotes release of norepinephrine from sympathetic nerves and release of epinephrine (and some norepinephrine) from the adrenals. Norepinephrine and epinephrine act on the cardiovascular system to cause vasoconstriction, acceleration of heart rate, and increased force of ventricular contraction. The net result is elevation of blood pressure and increased cardiac work. These effects underlie cardiovascular deaths.

*Gastrointestinal Effects.* Nicotine influences gastrointestinal function primarily by stimulating nicotinic receptors in *parasympathetic* ganglia. This results in increased secretion of gastric acid and increased tone and motility of gastrointestinal smooth muscle. In addition, nicotine can promote vomiting. Nicotine-induced vomiting results from a complex process that involves nicotinic receptors in the aortic arch, the carotid sinus, and the CNS.

*CNS Effects.* Nicotine is a CNS stimulant. The drug stimulates respiration and produces an arousal pattern on the electroencephalogram. Moderate doses can cause tremors, and high doses can cause convulsions.

Nicotine has multiple psychologic effects. The drug increases alertness, facilitates memory, improves cognitive function, reduces aggression, and suppresses appetite. In addition, by promoting release of dopamine, nicotine activates a "pleasure system" located in the mesolimbic system. The effects of nicotine on the pleasure system are identical to those of other highly addictive drugs, including cocaine, amphetamines, and opioids.

*Effects during Pregnancy and Lactation.* Administration of nicotine during pregnancy can cause fetal harm. Nicotine in breast milk can harm the nursing infant. Accordingly, therapeutic formulations of nicotine (nicotine chewing gum, nicotine transdermal patches, nicotine nasal spray) are contraindicated during pregnancy, and their use by nursing mothers is not recommended.

### Tolerance and Dependence

*Tolerance.* Tolerance develops to some effects of nicotine but not to others. Tolerance does develop to nausea and dizziness, which are common in the unseasoned smoker. In contrast, *very little tolerance develops to the cardiovascular actions of nicotine:* Veteran smokers continue to experience increased blood pressure and increased cardiac work whenever they smoke.

*Dependence.* Chronic cigarette smoking results in dependence. By definition, this means that individuals who discontinue smoking will experience an abstinence syndrome. The tobacco withdrawal syndrome is characterized by craving, nervousness, restlessness, irritability, impatience, increased hostility, insomnia, impaired concentration, increased appetite, and weight gain. Symptoms begin about 24 hours after smoking has ceased, and can last for weeks to months. Women report more discomfort than men. Experience has shown that abrupt discontinuation may be preferable to gradual reduction; all that gradual reduction seems to do is prolong suffering.

## Acute Poisoning

Nicotine is highly toxic. Doses as low as 40 mg can be fatal. The drug's toxicity is attested to by its use in insecticides. Common causes of nicotine poisoning include ingestion of tobacco by children and exposure to nicotine-containing insecticides.

*Symptoms.* The most prominent symptoms of nicotine poisoning involve the cardiovascular, gastrointestinal, and central nervous systems. Specific symptoms include nausea, salivation, vomiting, diarrhea, cold sweat, disturbed hearing and vision, confusion, and faintness; pulses may be rapid, weak, and irregular. Death results from respiratory paralysis, which is caused by direct effects of nicotine on the muscles of respiration and by effects exerted within the CNS.

*Treatment.* Management centers on reducing nicotine absorption and supporting respiration; there is no specific antidote to nicotine poisoning. To minimize absorption, patients should be given syrup of ipecac followed by activated charcoal. Ipecac induces vomiting, thereby removing any nicotine remaining in the stomach. Activated charcoal adsorbs nicotine, thereby preventing any nicotine that remains in the GI tract from being absorbed into the blood. If respiration is depressed, ventilatory assistance should be provided. Since nicotine undergoes rapid metabolic inactivation, recovery from the acute phase of poisoning can occur within hours.

## Chronic Toxicity from Smoking

Adverse effects of chronic tobacco smoking range from vascular diseases (coronary artery disease, cerebrovascular disease, peripheral vascular disease) to chronic lung disease to cancers of the larynx, esophagus, oral cavity, lung, bladder, and pancreas. Smoking during pregnancy carries an increased risk of low birth weight, spontaneous abortion, perinatal mortality, and sudden infant death. Quantitatively, cardiovascular disease is the greatest danger of smoking.

Fortunately, many adverse effects of smoking are reversible. Within 5 to 10 years after smoking has ceased, the risks of smoking-related disease for the ex-smoker are only slightly higher than the risks for the person who has never smoked.

## Nicotine Replacement Therapy

Cigarettes are highly addictive, which makes quitting extremely difficult. In fact, the vast majority of people who attempt to quit resume smoking within days. Overall, only 2% to 3% of smokers succeed in quitting each year. Quitting is hard because withdrawal symptoms are unpleasant and because smokers miss the reinforcing effects of nicotine.

As an aid to smoking cessation, smokers can substitute a pharmaceutical source of nicotine for the nicotine in cigarettes—and then gradually withdraw the replacement nicotine. This is analogous to using methadone to wean addicts from heroin. (Of course, this analogy is not completely faithful, in that methadone is essentially harmless when used as prescribed, whereas nicotine, regardless of the delivery system, is still dangerous.)

Three formulations of nicotine are available: chewing gum, transdermal patches, and a nasal spray. With the gum and patches, blood levels of nicotine rise slowly and remain relatively steady. Because nicotine levels rise slowly, these delivery systems produce less pleasure than cigarettes, but nonetheless do relieve withdrawal symptoms. With the nasal spray, blood levels of nicotine rise rapidly, much as they do with smoking. Hence, in addition to suppressing withdrawal, the spray provides some of the subjective pleasure associated with cigarettes.

Long-term quitting rates are significantly greater with replacement therapy than with placebo—although absolute success rates remain low. For example, the 1-year success with nicotine patches is about 25%, compared with 9% for placebo. Success rates are highest when replacement therapy is combined with counseling and behavioral therapy.

## Nicotine Chewing Gum (Nicotine Polacrilex)

*Description.* Nicotine chewing gum [Nicorette] is composed of a gum base plus nicotine polacrilex, an ion exchange resin to which nicotine is bound. The gum must be chewed to release the nicotine. Following its release, nicotine is absorbed across the oral mucosa into the systemic circulation.

*Adverse Effects.* The most common adverse effects are mouth and throat soreness, jaw muscle ache, eructation (belching), and hiccoughs. Use of an optimal chewing technique should minimize all of these effects. Nicotine gum and all other nicotine-containing products should be avoided during pregnancy and lactation.

*Dosage and Administration.* Nicotine gum is available in two dosage strengths: 2 mg/piece and 4 mg/piece. Patients should be advised to chew the gum slowly and intermittently for about 30 minutes. Rapid chewing can release too much nicotine at one time, resulting in effects similar to those of excessive smoking (e.g., nausea, throat irritation, hiccoughs). Since foods and beverages can reduce nicotine absorption, patients should not eat or drink for 15 minutes before chewing and while chewing.

Dosing is individualized and based on the degree of nicotine dependence. For initial therapy, patients with low to moderate nicotine dependence should use the 2-mg strength; highly dependent patients (those who smoke more than 25 cigarettes a day) should use the 4-mg strength. The average adult dosage is 9 to 12 pieces of gum/day. The maximum daily dosage is 30 pieces of the 2-mg strength or 20 pieces of the 4-mg strength. Experience indicates that dosing on a fixed schedule (one piece every 2 to 3 hours) is more effective than PRN dosing for achieving abstinence.

After 3 months without cigarettes, patients should discontinue nicotine use. Withdrawal should be done gradually. Use of nicotine gum beyond 6 months is not recommended.

## Nicotine Transdermal Systems

**Description.** Nicotine transdermal systems are nicotine-containing adhesive patches that, after application to the skin, slowly release their nicotine content. The nicotine is absorbed into the skin and then into the blood, producing steady blood levels of the drug.

Four systems are available: Habitrol, Nicoderm, Nicotrol, and ProStep. As indicated in Table 37–3, each is available in two or three sizes. The larger patches release greater amounts of nicotine.

**Dosage and Administration.** Nicotine transdermal systems are applied once a day to clean, dry, nonhairy skin of the upper body or upper arm. The site should be changed daily and not reused for at least 1 week. With three products (Habitrol, Nicoderm, and ProStep) the patch is left in place for 24 hours and then immediately replaced with a fresh patch. With one product (Nicotrol) the patch is applied in the morning and removed 16 hours later at bedtime. This pattern is intended to simulate nicotine dosing produced by smoking.

Most patients begin treatment with a large patch and then progress to smaller patches over a period of weeks (see Table 37–3). Certain patients (those with cardiovascular disease, those who weigh less than 100 pounds, or those who smoke less than one-half pack of cigarettes a day) should begin treatment with a smaller patch.

**Adverse Effects.** Short-lived erythema, itching, and burning occur under the patch in 35% to 50% of users. In 14% to 17% of users, persistent erythema occurs, lasting up to 24 hours after patch removal. Patients who experience severe, persistent local reactions (e.g., severe erythema, itching, edema) should discontinue the patch and contact the physician. Nicotine patches and all other nicotine-containing products should be avoided during pregnancy and lactation.

## Nicotine Nasal Spray

Nicotine nasal spray [Nicotrol NS] differs from nicotine gum and nicotine patches in that blood levels of nicotine rise rapidly following each administration, thereby more closely simulating smoking. The spray device delivers 0.5 mg of nicotine per activation. Two sprays (one in each nostril) constitute one dose and are equivalent to the amount of nicotine absorbed from one cigarette. Treatment should be started with 1 or 2 doses per hour—and never more than 5 doses per hour, or 40 doses a day. After 4 to 6 weeks, dosing should be gradually reduced and then stopped entirely. Nicotine nasal spray should be avoided by patients with sinus problems, allergies, or asthma.

Quitting success with the spray has been good news and bad news. The good news, as reported in one study, is that nearly 50% of users avoided smoking for 1 year. The bad news is that many of these people continued to use the spray, being unwilling or unable to give it up. Nonetheless, since the spray delivers nicotine without the additional hazards in smoke, using the spray is clearly preferable to smoking.

## Anabolic Steroids

Many athletes take anabolic steroids (androgens) to enhance athletic performance. The principal benefit is increased muscle mass and strength. Because of the massive doses that are employed, the risk of adverse effects is substantial. With long-term use of steroids, an addiction syndrome develops. Because of their abuse potential, most androgens are now classified as Schedule III drugs (see Table 35–2). The basic pharmacology of androgens and their abuse by athletes are discussed at length in Chapter 61.

### TABLE 37–3. NICOTINE TRANSDERMAL SYSTEMS

| Trade Name | Surface Area (cm²) | Nicotine Content (mg) | Dose Absorbed | Duration of Use | |
| --- | --- | --- | --- | --- | --- |
| | | | | For Each Patch | Total |
| Habitrol | 30 | 52.5 | 21 mg/24 hr | First 4–8 wk | 8–12 wk |
| | 20 | 35.0 | 14 mg/24 hr | Next 2–4 wk | |
| | 10 | 17.5 | 7 mg/24 hr | Last 2–4 wk | |
| Nicoderm | 22 | 114.0 | 21 mg/24 hr | First 4–8 wk | 8–12 wk |
| | 15 | 78.0 | 14 mg/24 hr | Next 2–4 wk | |
| | 7 | 36.0 | 7 mg/24 hr | Last 2–4 wk | |
| Nicotrol | 30 | 24.9 | 15 mg/16 hr | First 10–12 wk | 14–20 wk |
| | 20 | 16.6 | 10 mg/16 hr | Next 2–4 wk | |
| | 10 | 8.3 | 5 mg/16 hr | Last 2–4 wk | |
| Prostep | 7 | 30.0 | 22 mg/24 hr | First 4–8 wk | 6–12 wk |
| | 3.5 | 15.0 | 11 mg/24 hr | Next 2–4 wk | |

# KEY POINTS

- Because heroin is very lipid soluble, initial effects are more intense and occur faster than with other opioids. As a result, heroin is the opioid of choice among abusers.
- Among health care providers who abuse opioids, meperidine [Demerol] is a drug of choice. Why? Because meperidine is orally active, causes minimal pupillary constriction, and causes less constipation and urinary retention than other opioids.
- With opioids, tolerance to respiratory depression develops in parallel with tolerance to euphoria. As a result, respiratory depression does not increase as higher doses are taken to produce desired subjective effects.
- Persons tolerant to one opioid are cross-tolerant to other opioids.
- Although the opioid withdrawal syndrome can be extremely unpleasant, it is rarely dangerous.
- Opioid overdose produces a classic triad of symptoms: respiratory depression, coma, and pinpoint pupils. Death can result.
- Naloxone, an opioid antagonist, is the treatment of choice for opioid overdose.
- Naloxone dosage must be titrated carefully, since too much naloxone will transport the patient from a state of intoxication to one of withdrawal. Also, since the half-life of naloxone is shorter than the half-lives of the opioids, naloxone must be administered repeatedly until the crisis is over.
- Because of cross-dependence, methadone can ease withdrawal symptoms in opioid-dependent individuals. To ease withdrawal, methadone is substituted for the abused opioid and then gradually withdrawn.
- In opioid abusers who are not ready for withdrawal, methadone can be used for maintenance therapy or suppressive therapy. In maintenance therapy, the methadone dosage is equivalent to the dosage of the abused opioid, thereby preventing withdrawal. In suppressive therapy, the abuser is rendered opioid tolerant with very high doses of methadone; as a result, use of street opioids can no longer produce subjective effects.
- With barbiturates, tolerance develops to subjective effects but not to respiratory depression. As a result, as increasingly large doses are taken to produce subjective effects, the risk of serious respiratory depression increases. (Note that this differs from the situation with opioids.)
- Individuals who are tolerant to barbiturates show cross-tolerance with other CNS depressants (e.g., alcohol, benzodiazepines, general anesthetics) but not with opioids.
- Individuals who are physically dependent on barbiturates show cross-dependence with other CNS depressants, but not with opioids.
- When physical dependence on barbiturates (and other CNS depressants) is great, the associated abstinence syndrome can be severe—sometimes even fatal. (Note that this differs from the situation with opioids.)
- Overdose with barbiturates produces the same triad of symptoms seen with opioids: respiratory depression, coma, and pinpoint pupils. Death can result.
- In contrast to opioid overdose, barbiturate overdose has no antidote; hence, treatment is only supportive.
- In contrast to overdose with opioids or barbiturates, overdose with benzodiazepines alone is rarely fatal.
- If needed, benzodiazepine overdose can be treated with flumazenil, a benzodiazepine antagonist.
- The psychologic effects of cocaine result from activation of dopamine receptors secondary to cocaine-induced blockade of dopamine reuptake.
- Severe overdose with cocaine can produce hyperpyrexia, convulsions, ventricular dysrhythmias, and hemorrhagic stroke; deaths have occurred. Psychologic effects of overdose include severe anxiety, paranoid ideation, and hallucinations.
- There is no specific antidote to cocaine overdose. Diazepam (IV) can suppress anxiety, seizures, hypertension, and dysrhythmias. Intravenous nitroprusside or phentolamine can treat severe hypertension.
- Regular use of cocaine produces tolerance. Whether significant physical dependence occurs is in dispute.
- Although various drugs have been given to help maintain abstinence following cocaine withdrawal, none is considered highly effective.
- In addition to CNS stimulation, amphetamines cause vasoconstriction and stimulation of the heart. Cardiovascular stimulation may result in hypertension, angina, and dysrhythmias.
- Regular use of amphetamines can produce a state that closely resembles paranoid schizophrenia.
- Although physical dependence on amphetamines is only moderate, psychologic dependence can be intense. Withdrawal can produce dysphoria and a strong sense of craving.
- The major psychoactive substance in marijuana is delta-9-tetrahydrocannabinol (THC).
- THC acts through specific receptors in the brain.
- Marijuana has three principal subjective effects: euphoria, sedation, and hallucinations.
- Physiologic effects of marijuana, as well as tolerance and physical dependence, are minimal.
- Psychedelic drugs produce alterations in thought, perception, and feeling that otherwise occur only in dreams.
- Psychedelic drugs are also known as hallucinogens or psychotomimetics—names that reflect their ability to produce hallucinations and mental states that resemble psychosis.
- Lysergic acid diethylamide (LSD) can be considered the prototype of the psychedelic drugs.
- LSD produces its effects by activating serotonin$_2$ receptors in the brain.
- Although tolerance develops to LSD, physiologic effects and physical dependence are minimal.

- Acute panic reactions to LSD can be managed by "talking down" and by treatment with benzodiazepines. Neuroleptic drugs (e.g., haloperidol) may intensify the reaction.
- LSD users may experience episodic visual disturbances after discontinuing the drug. In many cases, the underlying cause is a permanent change in the visual system.
- Some LSD users experience prolonged psychotic reactions that closely resemble schizophrenia.
- Ecstasy (MDMA) produces psychedelic effects at low doses and amphetamine-like stimulant effects at higher doses.
- When given to laboratory animals in doses only 2 to 4 times greater than those that produce hallucinations in humans, ecstasy causes irreversible destruction of serotonergic neurons.
- Phencyclidine produces alcohol-like effects at low doses and hallucinations and psychotic reactions at higher doses.
- Extreme overdose with phencyclidine can produce hypertension, coma, seizures, and muscular rigidity associated with severe hyperthermia and rhabdomyolysis.
- There is no specific antidote to phencyclidine overdose. "Talking down" is not effective, and antipsychotic drugs are of limited help.
- Cigarette smoking kills 420,000 Americans a year, making smoking the largest preventable cause of premature death.
- The principal cause of death among smokers is heart disease; lung cancer is second.

- Nicotine in cigarette smoke is absorbed from the lung, whereas nicotine in cigar smoke and smokeless tobacco is absorbed from the mouth.
- By stimulating nicotinic receptors in sympathetic ganglia and the adrenal medulla, nicotine promotes vasoconstriction, acceleration of heart rate, and increased force of ventricular contraction, thereby elevating blood pressure and increasing cardiac work. These effects underlie cardiovascular deaths.
- Through actions in the CNS, nicotine increases alertness, facilitates memory, improves cognitive function, reduces aggression, and suppresses appetite. In addition, by promoting release of dopamine, nicotine activates the same mesolimbic pleasure system whose activation underlies addiction to cocaine, amphetamines, and opioids.
- Although tolerance develops to some effects of nicotine, very little tolerance develops to cardiovascular effects: veteran smokers continue to experience an increase in blood pressure and cardiac work whenever they smoke.
- Nicotine causes physical dependence. Withdrawal is characterized by craving, nervousness, restlessness, irritability, impatience, increased hostility, insomnia, impaired concentration, increased appetite, and weight gain.
- Very few people who attempt to quit smoking achieve long-term success, even when quitting is facilitated by nicotine replacement therapy.
- Nicotine for replacement therapy is available in three delivery systems: chewing gum, transdermal patches, and a nasal spray.

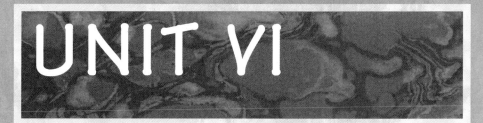

# UNIT VI

# Drugs That Affect Fluid and Electrolyte Balance

Diuretics

Agents Affecting the Volume and Ion
Content of Body Fluids

# Diuretics

iuretics are drugs that increase the output of urine. These agents have two major applications: (1) treatment of hypertension, and (2) mobilization of edematous fluid (associated with heart failure, cirrhosis, and kidney disease). In addition, because of their ability to maintain urine flow, diuretics are used to prevent renal failure.

## Review of Renal Anatomy and Physiology

Understanding the diuretic drugs requires a basic knowledge of the anatomy and physiology of the kidney. Accordingly, we will review these topics before discussing the diuretics themselves.

### Anatomy

The basic functional unit of the kidney is the *nephron.* As indicated in Figure 38-1, the nephron has four functionally distinct regions: (1) the *glomerulus,* (2) the *proximal convoluted tubule,* (3) the *loop of Henle,* and (4) the *distal convoluted tubule.* All nephrons are oriented within the kidney such that the upper portion of Henle's loop is located within the renal cortex and the lower end of the loop descends toward the renal *medulla.* Without this orientation, the kidney would be unable to produce concentrated urine.

In addition to the nephrons, the *collecting ducts* (the tubules into which the nephrons pour their contents) play a critical role in kidney function. As suggested by Figure 38-1, the final segment of the distal convoluted tubule

plus the collecting duct into which it empties can be considered a single functional unit: the *distal nephron.*

### Physiology

#### Overview of Kidney Functions

The kidney serves three basic functions: (1) cleansing of extracellular fluid (ECF) and maintenance of ECF volume and composition; (2) maintenance of acid-base balance; and (3) excretion of metabolic wastes and foreign substances (e.g., drugs, toxins). Of these three functions, maintenance of ECF volume and composition is the one most affected by diuretics.

#### The Three Basic Renal Processes

The effects of the kidney on ECF are the net result of three basic processes: (1) *filtration,* (2) *reabsorption,* and (3) *active secretion.* You should note that, in order to cleanse the entire ECF, huge volumes of plasma must be filtered. Furthermore, in order to maintain homeostasis, practically everything that has been filtered must be reabsorbed—leaving behind only a small volume of urine for excretion.

*Filtration.* Filtration occurs at the *glomerulus* and is the first step in urine formation. Virtually all small molecules (electrolytes, amino acids, glucose, drugs, metabolic wastes) present in plasma undergo filtration. In contrast, cells and large molecules (lipids, proteins) remain behind in the blood. The most prevalent constituents of the filtrate are sodium ions and chloride ions. Bicarbonate ions and potassium ions are also present but in smaller amounts.

The filtration capacity of the kidney is huge. Each minute the kidney produces 125 ml of filtrate, which adds

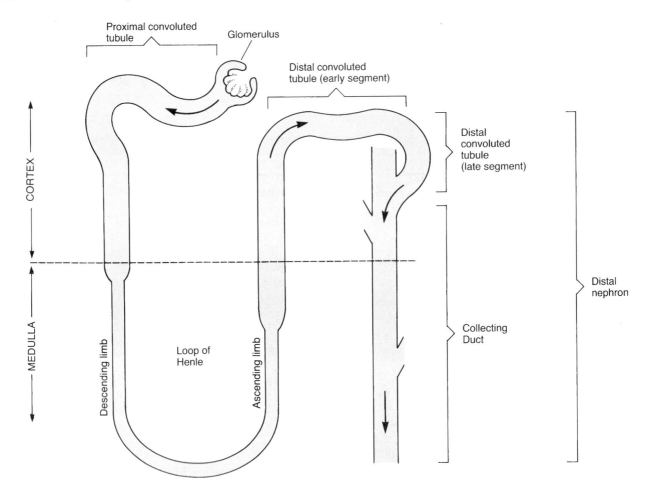

**Figure 38–1. Schematic representation of a nephron and collecting duct.**

up to 180 L/day. Since the total volume of ECF is only 12.5 L, the kidney can process the equivalent of all the ECF in the body every 100 minutes. Hence, the ECF undergoes complete cleansing many times each day.

Please note that filtration is a *nonselective* process, and therefore cannot regulate the composition of urine. Reabsorption and secretion, processes that display a significant degree of selectivity, are the primary determinants of what the urine ultimately contains—and of these two processes, reabsorption is by far the more important.

***Reabsorption.*** Greater than 99% of the water, electrolytes, and nutrients that are filtered at the glomerulus undergo reabsorption. This reabsorption conserves valuable constituents of the filtrate while allowing wastes to be excreted. Reabsorption of solutes (e.g., electrolytes, amino acids, glucose) takes place by way of *active transport*. Water then follows passively along the osmotic gradient created by solute reuptake. Specific sites along the nephron at which reabsorption takes place are discussed below. It is primarily through interference with reabsorption that diuretics produce their effects.

***Active Tubular Secretion.*** The kidney has two kinds of "pumps" for active secretion. These pumps transport compounds from the plasma into the lumen of the nephron. One kind of pump is selective for *organic acids* and the other transports *organic bases*. Together, these pumps can promote the excretion of a wide assortment of molecules, including metabolic wastes, drugs, and toxins. The pumps for active secretion are located in the *proximal convoluted tubule.*

## Processes of Reabsorption That Occur at Specific Sites Along the Nephron

Since most diuretics act by disrupting solute reabsorption, to understand the diuretics, we must first understand the major processes by which nephrons reabsorb filtered solutes. Since sodium and chloride ions are the predominant solutes in the filtrate, reabsorption of these ions is of greatest interest. As we discuss reabsorption, numeric values are given for the percentage of solute reabsorbed at specific sites along the nephron; bear in mind that these values are only approximations. Figure 38–2 gives a summary of the sites of sodium and chloride reabsorption, indicating the amount of reabsorption that occurs at each site.

***Proximal Convoluted Tubule.*** The proximal convoluted tubule (PCT) has a high reabsorptive capacity. As indicated in Figure 38–2, *a large fraction (about 65%) of*

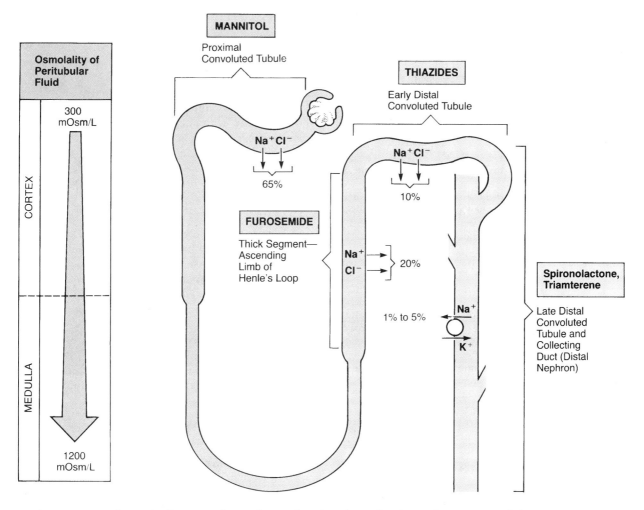

**Figure 38–2. Schematic diagram of a nephron showing sites of sodium absorption and diuretic action.** The percentages indicate how much of the filtered sodium and chloride is reabsorbed at each site.

*filtered sodium and chloride is reabsorbed at the PCT.* In addition, essentially all of the bicarbonate and potassium in the filtrate is reabsorbed here. As sodium, chloride, and other solutes are actively reabsorbed, water follows passively. Since solutes and water are reabsorbed to an equal extent, the tubular urine remains isotonic (i.e., its tonicity is 300 mOsm/L). By the time the filtrate leaves the PCT, sodium and chloride are the only solutes that remain in significant amounts.

**Loop of Henle.** The *descending limb* of the loop of Henle is freely permeable to water. Hence, as tubular urine moves down the loop and passes through the hypertonic environment of the renal medulla, water is drawn from the loop into the interstitial space. This process decreases the volume of the tubular urine and causes the urine to become concentrated (tonicity is increased to about 1200 mOsm/L).

Within the thick segment of the *ascending limb* of the loop of Henle, *about 20% of filtered sodium and chloride is reabsorbed* (see Fig. 38–2). Since, unlike the descending limb, the ascending limb is not permeable to water, water must remain in the loop as reabsorption of

sodium and chloride takes place. This process causes the tonicity of the tubular urine to return to that of the original filtrate (300 mOsm/L).

***Distal Convoluted Tubule (Early Segment).*** *About 10% of filtered sodium and chloride is reabsorbed in the early segment of the distal convoluted tubule.* Water follows passively.

***Late Distal Convoluted Tubule and Collecting Duct (Distal Nephron).*** The distal nephron is the site of two important processes. The first involves the exchange of sodium for potassium and is under the influence of aldosterone. The second determines the final concentration of the urine and is regulated by antidiuretic hormone (ADH).

***Sodium-Potassium Exchange.*** Aldosterone, the principal mineralocorticoid of the adrenal cortex, stimulates reabsorption of sodium from the distal nephron. At the same time, aldosterone causes potassium to be secreted. Although not directly coupled, these two processes—sodium retention and potassium excretion—can be envisioned as an exchange mechanism. This exchange is shown schematically in Figure 38-2. Aldosterone promotes sodium-potassium exchange by stimulating cells of the distal nephron to synthesize more of the pumps responsible for sodium and potassium transport.

***Regulation of Urine Concentration by Antidiuretic Hormone.*** Although of great physiologic significance, ADH has little to do with the actions of diuretics. Hence, discussion of this physiologically important topic is presented in small type.

Antidiuretic hormone acts on the collecting duct to regulate conservation of water. To understand the effects of ADH, we need to know four facts:

- In the absence of ADH, the collecting duct is impermeable to water.
- The collecting duct is oriented such that it begins in the cortex of the kidney and then passes down through the hypertonic renal medulla (see Fig. 38–2).
- Tubular urine entering the collecting duct is isotonic (i.e., 300 mOsm/L).
- Antidiuretic hormone acts on the collecting duct to increase its permeability to water.

By rendering the collecting duct permeable to water, ADH allows water to be drawn from the duct as it passes through the hypertonic renal medulla. Because of this water reabsorption, urine that entered the duct in a relatively dilute state becomes concentrated and reduced in volume.

In the absence of ADH, water cannot be reabsorbed in the collecting duct. As a result, large volumes of dilute urine are produced. The clinical syndrome resulting from ADH deficiency is known as *diabetes insipidus*.

# Introduction to Diuretics

## How Diuretics Work

*Most diuretics share the same basic mechanism of action: blockade of sodium and chloride reabsorption.* By blocking the reabsorption of these prominent solutes, diuretics create osmotic pressure within the nephron that prevents the passive reabsorption of water. Hence, diuretics cause water and solutes to be retained within the nephron, and thereby promote their excretion.

*The increase in urine flow that a diuretic produces is directly related to the amount of sodium and chloride reabsorption that it blocks.* Accordingly, drugs that block solute reabsorption to the greatest degree will produce the most profound diuresis. Since the amount of solute in the nephron becomes progressively smaller as filtrate flows from the proximal tubule to the collecting duct, *drugs whose site of action is early in the nephron have the opportunity to block the greatest amount of solute reabsorption. Accordingly, these agents produce the greatest diuresis.* Conversely, since most of the filtered solute has already been reabsorbed by the time the filtrate reaches the distal parts of the nephron, diuretics that act at these distal sites have very little reabsorption available to block. Consequently, distally acting agents produce relatively scant diuresis.

It is instructive to look at the quantitative relationship between blockade of solute reabsorption and production

of diuresis. Recall that the kidney produces 180 L of filtrate a day, practically all of which normally is reabsorbed. With filtrate production at this volume, a diuretic will increase daily urine output by 1.8 L for each 1% of solute reabsorption that is blocked. A 3% blockade of solute reabsorption will produce 5.4 L of urine a day—a rate of fluid loss that would reduce body weight by 12 pounds in 24 hours. Clearly, with only a small blockade of reabsorption, diuretics can produce a profound effect on the fluid and electrolyte composition of the body.

## Adverse Impact on Extracellular Fluid

In order to promote excretion of water, diuretics must compromise the normal operation of the kidney. By doing so, diuretics can cause *hypovolemia* (from excessive fluid loss), *acid-base imbalance*, and *disturbance of electrolyte levels*. These adverse effects can be minimized by using short-acting diuretics and by timing drug administration such that the kidney is allowed to operate in a drug-free manner between periods of diuresis. Both measures will give the kidney periodic opportunities to readjust the ECF so as to compensate for any undesired alterations produced under the influence of diuretics.

## Classification of Diuretics

There are four major categories of diuretic drugs: (1) *high-ceiling (loop) diuretics* (e.g., furosemide); (2) *thiazide diuretics* (e.g., hydrochlorothiazide); (3) *osmotic diuretics* (e.g., mannitol); and (4) *potassium-sparing diuretics*. The last group, the potassium-sparing agents, can be subdivided into *aldosterone antagonists* (e.g., spironolactone) and *nonaldosterone antagonists* (e.g., triamterene).

In addition to the four major categories of diuretics, there is a fifth group: the *carbonic anhydrase inhibitors*. Although the carbonic anhydrase inhibitors are classified as diuretics, these drugs are employed primarily to lower intraocular pressure and not to increase urine production. Consequently, the carbonic anhydrase inhibitors are discussed in Chapter 97 (Drugs for the Eye) rather than here.

# High-Ceiling (Loop) Diuretics

The high-ceiling agents are the most effective diuretics available. These drugs produce greater loss of fluid and electrolytes than any other diuretics. Because their site of action is in the loop of Henle, the high-ceiling agents are also known as *loop diuretics*.

## Furosemide

Furosemide [Lasix] is the most frequently prescribed loop diuretic and will serve as our prototype for the family.

## Mechanism of Action

Furosemide acts in the thick segment of the ascending limb of Henle's loop to block reabsorption of sodium and chloride (see Fig. 38-2). By blocking solute reabsorption, furosemide prevents passive reabsorption of water. Since a substantial amount (20%) of filtered NaCl is normally reabsorbed in the loop of Henle, interference with reabsorption can produce profound diuresis.

## Pharmacokinetics

Furosemide can be administered orally, IV, and IM. With oral administration, diuresis begins in 60 minutes and persists for 8 hours. Oral therapy is used when rapid onset of effects is not required. Effects of intravenous furosemide begin within 5 minutes and last for 2 hours. Intravenous therapy is used in critical situations (e.g., pulmonary edema) that demand immediate mobilization of fluid. Furosemide undergoes hepatic metabolism followed by renal excretion.

## Therapeutic Uses

Furosemide is a powerful drug that is generally reserved for situations that require rapid or massive mobilization of fluid. This drug should be avoided when less efficacious diuretics (thiazides) will suffice. Conditions that justify use of furosemide include (1) pulmonary edema associated with congestive heart failure; (2) edema of hepatic, cardiac, or renal origin that has been unresponsive to less efficacious diuretics; and (3) hypertension that cannot be controlled with other diuretics. Furosemide is especially useful in patients with severe renal impairment, since, unlike the thiazides (see below), this drug can promote diuresis even when renal blood flow and glomerular filtration rate are low. If treatment with furosemide alone is insufficient, a thiazide diuretic may be added to the regimen. There is no benefit to combining furosemide with another high-ceiling agent.

## Adverse Effects

*Hyponatremia, Hypochloremia, and Dehydration.* Furosemide can produce excessive loss of sodium, chloride, and water. Severe dehydration can result. Signs of developing dehydration include dry mouth, unusual thirst, and oliguria (scanty urine output). Impending dehydration can also be anticipated from excessive loss of weight. If dehydration occurs, furosemide should be withheld.

Dehydration can promote thrombosis and embolism. Symptoms include headache and pain in the chest, calves, or pelvis. The physician should be notified if these develop.

The risk of dehydration and its sequelae can be minimized by initiating therapy with low doses, adjusting the dosage carefully, monitoring weight loss every day, and administering furosemide on an intermittent schedule.

*Hypotension.* Furosemide can cause a substantial drop in blood pressure. At least two mechanisms are involved: (1) loss of volume, and (2) relaxation of venous smooth muscle, which reduces venous return to the heart. Signs

of hypotension include dizziness, lightheadedness, and fainting. If blood pressure falls precipitously, furosemide should be discontinued. Because of the risk of hypotension, blood pressure should be monitored on a routine basis.

Outpatients should be taught to monitor their blood pressure and instructed to notify the physician if it drops substantially. Also, patients should be informed about symptoms of postural hypotension (dizziness, lightheadedness) and advised to sit or lie down if these occur. Patients should be taught that postural hypotension can be minimized by getting up slowly.

*Hypokalemia.* Potassium is lost through increased secretion in the distal nephron. If serum potassium falls below 3.5 mEq/L, fatal dysrhythmias may result. As discussed below under *Drug Interactions*, loss of potassium is of special concern for patients taking digoxin, a drug used for heart failure. Hypokalemia can be minimized by consuming potassium-rich foods (e.g., citrus fruits, potatoes, bananas), taking potassium supplements, or using a potassium-sparing diuretic.

*Ototoxicity.* Rarely, loop diuretics cause hearing impairment. With furosemide, deafness has been transient. With ethacrynic acid (another loop diuretic), irreversible hearing loss has occurred. The ability to impair hearing is unique to the high-ceiling agents; diuretics in other classes are not ototoxic. Because of the risk of hearing loss, caution should be exercised when high-ceiling diuretics are used in combination with other ototoxic drugs (e.g., aminoglycoside antibiotics).

*Hyperglycemia.* Elevation of plasma glucose levels is a potential, albeit uncommon, complication of furosemide therapy. Hyperglycemia appears to result from inhibition of insulin release. Increased glycogenolysis and decreased glycogen synthesis may also contribute. When furosemide is taken by a diabetic, the patient should be especially diligent about monitoring blood glucose content.

*Hyperuricemia.* Elevation of plasma uric acid content is a frequent side effect of treatment. For most patients, furosemide-induced hyperuricemia is asymptomatic. However, for patients predisposed to gout, elevation of uric acid levels may precipitate a gouty attack. Patients should be informed about symptoms of gout (tenderness or swelling in joints) and instructed to notify the physician if these develop.

*Use in Pregnancy.* When administered to pregnant laboratory animals, high-ceiling diuretics have caused maternal death, abortion, fetal resorption, and other adverse effects. There are no definitive studies on the effects of loop diuretics during human pregnancy. However, given the toxicity displayed in animals, prudence dictates that pregnant women use these drugs only if absolutely required.

*Impact on Lipids, Calcium, and Magnesium.* Furosemide reduces HDL cholesterol and raises LDL cholesterol and triglycerides. Although these undesirable effects by themselves can increase the risk of coronary heart disease, they are more than balanced by the beneficial effects of the diuretic therapy on the heart. That is, despite adverse effects on lipids, high-ceiling diuretics reduce the risk of coronary mortality by 25%.

Furosemide increases urinary excretion of magnesium. Magnesium deficiency may result. Symptoms include muscle weakness, tremor, twitching, and dysrhythmias.

**TABLE 38-1. HIGH-CEILING (LOOP) DIURETICS: ROUTES, TIME COURSE, AND DOSAGE**

| Drug | Route | Onset (min) | Duration (hr) | Dosage (mg) | Doses/ day |
|------|-------|-------------|---------------|-------------|------------|
| Furosemide [Lasix] | Oral | Within 60 | 6-8 | 20-80 | 1-2 |
|  | IV or IM | Within 5 | 2 | 20-40 |  |
| Ethacrynic acid [Edecrin] | Oral | Within 30 | 6-8 | 50-100 | 1-2 |
|  | IV | Within 5 | 2 | 50 | 1-2 |
| Bumetanide [Bumex] | Oral | 30-60 | 4-6 | 0.5-2 | 1 |
|  | IV | Within a few | 0.5-1 | 0.5-1 | 1-3 |
| Torsemide [Demadex] | Oral | Within 60 | 6-8 | 5-20 | 1 |
|  | IV | Within 10 | 6-8 | 5-20 | 1 |

Furosemide increases urinary excretion of calcium. This action has been exploited in the treatment of acute hypercalcemia.

## Drug Interactions

**Digoxin.** Digoxin is used to treat heart failure (see Chapter 46) and cardiac dysrhythmias (see Chapter 48). In the presence of low potassium levels, the risk of serious digoxin-induced toxicity (ventricular dysrhythmias) is greatly increased. Since high-ceiling diuretics promote potassium loss, use of these drugs in combination with digoxin can increase the risk of dysrhythmias. This interaction is unfortunate in that most patients who take digoxin for heart failure must also take a diuretic as part of their therapy. To reduce the chances of toxicity, potassium levels should be monitored routinely, and, when indicated, potassium supplements or a potassium-sparing diuretic should be given.

**Ototoxic Drugs.** The risk of furosemide-induced hearing loss is increased by concurrent use of other ototoxic drugs (e.g., aminoglycoside antibiotics). Accordingly, combined use of these drugs should be avoided.

**Potassium-Sparing Diuretics.** The potassium-sparing diuretics (e.g., spironolactone, triamterene) can help counterbalance the potassium-wasting effects of furosemide, thereby reducing the risk of hypokalemia.

**Lithium.** Lithium is used to treat bipolar disorder (see Chapter 31). In the presence of low sodium levels, excretion of lithium is reduced. By lowering sodium levels, furosemide can cause lithium to accumulate to toxic levels. Accordingly, lithium levels should be monitored, and, if they climb too high, lithium dosage should be reduced.

**Antihypertensive Agents.** The hypotensive effects of furosemide add with those of other hypotensive drugs. To avoid excessive reductions in blood pressure, patients may need to reduce or eliminate use of hypotensive medications.

**Nonsteroidal Anti-inflammatory Drugs.** The nonsteroidal anti-inflammatory drugs (NSAIDs; e.g., aspirin) can attenuate the diuretic effects of furosemide. The mechanism appears to be inhibition of prostaglandin synthesis in the kidney. (Part of the diuretic effect of furosemide results from increasing renal blood flow. Furosemide is thought to increase renal blood flow through a prostaglandin-mediated process. By inhibiting prostaglandin

synthesis, NSAIDs prevent the increase in renal blood flow, and thereby partially blunt diuretic effects.)

### Preparations, Dosage, and Administration

**Oral.** Furosemide [Lasix] is available in tablets (20, 40, and 80 mg) and in solution (8 and 10 mg/ml) for oral use. The initial dosage for adults is 20 to 80 mg/day as a single dose. The maximum daily dosage is 600 mg. Twice-daily dosing (8 AM and 2 PM) is common. Administration late in the day produces nocturia and should be avoided.

**Parenteral.** Furosemide is available as an injection (10 mg/ml) for IV and IM administration. The usual parenteral dose for adults is 20 to 40 mg, repeated in 1 or 2 hours if needed. Intravenous administration should be done slowly (over 1 to 2 minutes). For high-dose therapy, furosemide can be administered by continuous infusion at a rate of 4 mg/min or slower.

### Other High-Ceiling Diuretics

In addition to furosemide, three other high-ceiling agents are available: *ethacrynic acid* [Edecrin], *bumetanide* [Bumex], and *torsemide* [Demadex]. All three are very similar to furosemide. They all promote diuresis by inhibiting sodium and chloride reabsorption in the thick ascending limb of the loop of Henle. All are approved for treating edema caused by heart failure, chronic renal disease, and cirrhosis, but only torsemide, like furosemide, is also approved for hypertension. All can cause ototoxicity, hypovolemia, hypotension, hypokalemia, hyperuricemia, hyperglycemia, and disruption of lipid metabolism (i.e., lowering of HDL cholesterol and elevation of LDL cholesterol and triglycerides). Lastly, they all share the same drug interactions: their effects can be blunted by NSAIDs, they can intensify ototoxicity caused by aminoglycosides, they can increase cardiotoxicity caused by digoxin, and they can cause lithium to accumulate to toxic levels. Routes, dosages, and time courses of action are summarized in Table 38-1.

## Thiazides and Related Diuretics

The thiazide diuretics (also known as benzothiadiazides) have effects similar to those of the loop diuretics. Like the loop diuretics, thiazides increase renal excretion of sodium, chloride, potassium, and water. In addition, thiazides elevate plasma levels of uric acid and glucose. The principal difference between the thiazides and the high-ceiling diuretics is that the maximum diuresis produced by the thiazides is considerably lower than the maximum diuresis produced by the high-ceiling agents. In addition, whereas loop diuretics can be effective even when urine flow is scant, the thiazides cannot.

## Hydrochlorothiazide

Hydrochlorothiazide [HydroDIURIL, others] is the most widely used thiazide diuretic and will serve as our prototype for the family. Because of its use in hypertension, a very common disorder, hydrochlorothiazide is one of our most widely used drugs.

### Mechanism of Action

Hydrochlorothiazide promotes urine production by blocking the reabsorption of sodium and chloride in the *early segment of the distal convoluted tubule* (see Fig. 38-2). Retention of sodium and chloride in the nephron causes water to be retained as well, thereby producing an increased flow of urine. Since only 10% of filtered sodium and chloride is normally reabsorbed at the site where thiazides act, the maximum urine flow these drugs can produce is lower that the maximum flow the high-ceiling diuretics produce.

The ability of thiazides to promote diuresis is dependent on adequate kidney function. These drugs are ineffective when glomerular filtration rate (GFR) is low (less than 15 to 20 ml/min). Hence, in contrast to the high-ceiling agents, thiazides cannot be used to promote fluid loss in patients with severe renal impairment.

#### Pharmacokinetics

Diuresis begins about 2 hours after oral administration. Effects peak within 4 to 6 hours, and may persist for up to 12 hours. Most of the drug is excreted unchanged in the urine.

### Therapeutic Uses

*Essential Hypertension.* The primary indication for hydrochlorothiazide is hypertension, a condition for which thiazides are often drugs of first choice. For many hypertensive patients, blood pressure can be controlled with a thiazide alone, although many other patients require multiple-drug therapy. The role of thiazides in hypertension is discussed in Chapter 44.

*Edema.* Thiazides are preferred drugs for mobilizing *edema associated with mild to moderate heart failure.* These drugs are also given to mobilize *edema associated with hepatic or renal disease.*

*Diabetes Insipidus.* Diabetes insipidus is a rare condition characterized by excessive production of urine. In these patients, thiazides reduce urine production by 30% to 50%. The mechanism of this paradoxical effect is unknown.

### Adverse Effects

The adverse effects of the thiazide diuretics are similar to those of the high-ceiling agents. In fact, with the exception that thiazides lack ototoxic actions, the adverse effects of the thiazides and loop diuretics are nearly identical.

*Hyponatremia, Hypochloremia, and Dehydration.* Loss of sodium, chloride, and water can lead to *hyponatremia, hypochloremia,* and *dehydration.* It should be noted, however, that since the diuresis produced by thiazides is moderate, these drugs have a smaller impact on sodium, chloride, and water than the loop diuretics. To evaluate fluid and electrolyte status, electrolyte levels should be determined periodically, and the patient should be weighed on a regular basis.

*Hypokalemia.* Like the high-ceiling diuretics, the thiazides can cause hypokalemia from excessive potassium excretion. As noted previously, potassium loss is of particular concern for patients taking digoxin. Potassium levels should be measured periodically, and, if serum potassium falls below 3.5 mEq/L, treatment with potassium supplements or a potassium-sparing diuretic should be instituted. Hypokalemia can be minimized by eating potassium-rich foods (e.g., citrus fruits, bananas).

*Use in Pregnancy and Lactation.* The thiazides have direct and indirect effects on the developing fetus. By reducing blood volume, thiazides can decrease placental perfusion, and may thereby compromise fetal nutrition and growth. Furthermore, thiazides can cross the placental barrier to produce fetal harm directly; potential effects include electrolyte imbalance, hypoglycemia, jaundice, and hemolytic anemia. Because of the potential for fetal harm, *thiazides should not be used routinely during pregnancy.* Edema of pregnancy is not an indication for diuretic therapy—except when unusually severe. In contrast, edema from pathologic causes (e.g., heart failure, cirrhosis) does constitute a legitimate indication for thiazide use.

Thiazides enter breast milk and can be hazardous to the nursing infant. Women who are taking thiazides should be cautioned against breast-feeding.

*Hyperglycemia.* Like the loop diuretics, the thiazides can elevate plasma levels of glucose. Significant hyperglycemia develops only in diabetics, and these patients should be especially diligent about monitoring blood glucose. To maintain normal glucose levels, the diabetic may require larger doses of insulin or an oral hypoglycemic drug.

*Hyperuricemia.* The thiazides, like the loop diuretics, can cause retention of uric acid, thereby elevating plasma uric acid levels. Although hyperuricemia is usually asymptomatic, it may precipitate gouty arthritis in patients with a history of the disorder. Plasma levels of uric acid should be measured periodically.

*Impact on Lipids, Calcium, and Magnesium.* Thiazides can increase levels of LDL cholesterol, total cholesterol, and triglycerides. In addition, thiazides reduce urinary excretion of calcium; because of this action, thiazides have been used to treat calcium-related kidney stones. Thiazides increase excretion of magnesium, sometimes causing magnesium deficiency; symptoms include muscle weakness, tremor, twitching, and dysrhythmias.

### Drug Interactions

The important drug interactions of the thiazides are nearly identical to those of the loop diuretics. By promoting potassium loss, thiazides can increase the risk of toxicity from *digoxin.* By counterbalancing the potassium-wasting effects of the thiazides, the *potassium-sparing*

**TABLE 38-2. THIAZIDES AND RELATED DIURETICS: DOSAGES AND TIME COURSE OF EFFECTS**

| Generic Name | Trade Name | Time Course of Effects | | Optimal Oral Adult Dosage (mg/day) |
|---|---|---|---|---|
| | | Onset (hr) | Duration (hr) | |
| *Thiazides* | | | | |
| Chlorothiazide | Diuril, Diurigen | 1-2 | 6-12 | 500-2000 |
| Hydrochlorothiazide | Esidrix, Oretic, HydroDIURIL, others | 2 | 6-12 | 25-100 |
| Bendroflumethiazide | Naturetin | 2 | 6-12 | 2.5-15 |
| Benzthiazide | Exna | 2 | 6-12 | 50-200 |
| Hydroflumethiazide | Diucardin, Saluron | 2 | 6-12 | 25-200 |
| Methyclothiazide | Aquatensen, Enduron | 2 | 24 | 2.5-10 |
| Polythiazide | Renese | 2 | 24-48 | 1-4 |
| Trichlormethiazide | Metahydrin, Naqua Diurese | 2 | 24 | 1-4 |
| *Related Drugs* | | | | |
| Chlorthalidone | Hygroton, Thalitone | 2 | 24-72 | 25-200 |
| Indapamide | Lozol | 1-2 | up to 36 | 2.5-5 |
| Metolazone | Zaroxolyn, Mykrox | 1 | 12-24 | 2.5-20 |
| Quinethazone | Hydromox | 2 | 18-24 | 50-100 |

*diuretics* can help prevent excessive potassium loss. By lowering blood pressure, thiazides can augment the effects of other *antihypertensive drugs*. By promoting sodium loss, thiazides can reduce renal excretion of *lithium*, thereby causing the drug to accumulate, possibly to toxic levels. *NSAIDs* may blunt the diuretic effects of thiazides. In contrast to the loop diuretics, the thiazides can be combined with *ototoxic agents* without an increased risk of hearing loss.

### Preparations, Dosage, and Administration

Hydrochlorothiazide [HydroDIURIL, others] is dispensed in tablets (25, 50, and 100 mg) and solution (10 and 100 mg/ml) for oral administration. Like most other thiazides, hydrochlorothiazide is administered only by mouth. The usual adult dosage is 25 to 50 mg once or twice daily. To minimize nocturia, the drug should not be administered late in the day. To minimize electrolyte imbalance, the drug should be administered on an intermittent basis (e.g., every other day). In addition to being marketed alone, hydrochlorothiazide is available in fixed-dose combinations with potassium-sparing diuretics; trade names are Dyazide, Moduretic, Aldactazide, Maxzide, and Spirozide.

### Other Thiazide-Type Diuretics

In addition to hydrochlorothiazide, 12 other thiazides (and related drugs) are approved for use in the United States (Table 38-2). All have pharmacologic properties similar to those of hydrochlorothiazide. With the exception of chlorothiazide, these drugs are administered only by mouth. Chlorothiazide can be administered IV as well as orally. Although the thiazides differ from one another in milligram potency (see Table 38-2), at therapeutically equivalent doses, all can elicit the same degree of diuresis. Although most have the same onset time (1 to 2 hours), these drugs differ significantly with respect to duration. As with hydrochlorothiazide, disturbance of electrolyte balance can be minimized through alternate-day dosing. Nocturia can be minimized by avoiding dosing in the late afternoon.

Table 38-2 lists four drugs—chlorthalidone, indapamide, metolazone, and quinethazone—that are not true thiazides. However, these agents are very similar to thiazides both in structure and function; hence their inclusion in this group.

## Potassium-Sparing Diuretics

The potassium-sparing diuretics can elicit two potentially useful responses. First, these drugs produce a modest increase in urine production. Second, these drugs produce a substantial *decrease in potassium excretion*. Because their diuretic effects are limited, the potassium-sparing drugs are rarely employed alone to promote diuresis. However, because of their marked ability to decrease potassium excretion, these drugs are used with great regularity to counteract potassium loss caused by thiazide and loop diuretics.

There are two subcategories of potassium-sparing diuretics: aldosterone antagonists and nonaldosterone antagonists. Only one aldosterone antagonist—spironolactone—is approved for use in the United States. Two nonaldosterone antagonists—triamterene and amiloride—are currently employed.

### Spironolactone

#### Mechanism of Action

Spironolactone [Aldactone] blocks the actions of aldosterone in the distal nephron. Since aldosterone acts to promote sodium uptake in exchange for potassium secretion (see Fig. 38-2), inhibition of aldosterone by spi-

## TABLE 38-3. POTASSIUM-SPARING DIURETICS: NAMES, DOSAGES AND TIME COURSE OF EFFECTS

| Generic Name | Trade Name | Time Course of Effects | | Usual Adult Dosage (mg/day) |
| | | Onset (hr) | Duration (hr) | |
|---|---|---|---|---|
| Spironolactone | Aldactone | 24-48 | 48-72 | 25-400 |
| Triamterene | Dyrenium | 2-4 | 12-16 | 200-300 |
| Amiloride | Midamor | 2 | 24 | 5-20 |

ronolactone has the opposite effect: *retention of potassium and increased excretion of sodium.* The diuresis caused by spironolactone is scanty because most of the filtered sodium load has already been reabsorbed by the time the filtrate reaches the distal nephron. (Recall that the degree of diuresis a drug produces is directly proportional to the amount of sodium reuptake that it blocks.)

As indicated in Table 38-3, the effects of spironolactone are delayed, taking up to 48 hours to develop. To understand this delay, recall that aldosterone acts by stimulating cells of the distal nephron to synthesize the proteins required for sodium and potassium transport. By preventing aldosterone's action, spironolactone blocks the synthesis of new proteins, but does not stop existing transport proteins from doing their job. Hence the effects of spironolactone are not visible until the existing proteins complete their normal life cycle—a process that takes a day or two to run its course.

### Therapeutic Uses

Spironolactone is indicated primarily for patients with *hypertension* and *edema.* Although it can be employed alone, the drug is used most frequently in combination with a thiazide or loop diuretic. The purpose of spironolactone in these combinations is to counteract the potassium-wasting effects of the more powerful diuretics. Spironolactone also makes a small contribution to diuresis. In addition to its use in hypertension and edema, spironolactone can be given to block the effects of aldosterone in patients with *primary hyperaldosteronism.*

### Adverse Effects

*Hyperkalemia.* The potassium-sparing effects of spironolactone can result in hyperkalemia, a condition that can produce fatal dysrhythmias. Although hyperkalemia is most likely when spironolactone is used alone, hyperkalemia can also develop when spironolactone is used in conjunction with potassium-wasting agents (thiazides and high-ceiling diuretics). If serum potassium rises above 5 mEq/L, or if signs of hyperkalemia develop (e.g., abnormal cardiac rhythm), spironolactone should be discontinued and potassium intake restricted. Injection of insulin can help lower potassium levels by promoting uptake of potassium into cells.

*Endocrine Effects.* Spironolactone is a steroid derivative with a structure similar to that of steroid hormones (e.g., proges-

terone, estradiol, testosterone). As a result, spironolactone can cause a variety of endocrine effects, including *gynecomastia, menstrual irregularities, impotence, hirsutism,* and *deepening of the voice.*

### Drug Interactions

*Thiazide and Loop Diuretics.* Spironolactone is frequently combined with thiazide and loop diuretics. The principal objective is to counteract the potassium-wasting effects of the more powerful diuretic.

*Drugs That Raise Potassium Levels.* Because of the risk of hyperkalemia, *spironolactone must never be combined with potassium supplements or with another potassium-sparing diuretic.* In addition, since *angiotensin-converting enzyme (ACE) inhibitors* can also elevate potassium levels (by suppressing aldosterone secretion), they should be combined with spironolactone only when clearly necessary.

### Preparations, Dosage, and Administration

Spironolactone [Aldactone] is dispensed in tablets (25, 50, and 100 mg) for oral administration. The usual adult dosage is 25 to 100 mg/day. Spironolactone is also marketed in a fixed-dose combination with hydrochlorothiazide under the trade name Aldactazide.

## Triamterene

### Mechanism of Action

Like spironolactone, triamterene [Dyrenium] disrupts sodium-potassium exchange in the distal nephron. However, in contrast to spironolactone, which reduces ion transport indirectly through blockade of aldosterone, triamterene is a *direct inhibitor of the exchange mechanism itself.* The net effect of this inhibition is a decrease in sodium reuptake and a reduction in potassium secretion. Hence, sodium excretion is increased, while potassium is conserved. Because it inhibits ion transport directly, triamterene acts much more quickly than spironolactone. As indicated in Table 38-3, initial responses develop in hours, as compared with days for spironolactone. Like spironolactone, triamterene is unable to cause more than a scant diuresis.

### Therapeutic Uses

Triamterene can be used alone or in combination with other diuretics to treat *hypertension* and *edema.* When used alone, triamterene produces mild diuresis. When combined with other diuretics (e.g., furosemide, hydrochlorothiazide), triamterene augments diuresis and helps counteract the potassium-wasting effects of the more powerful diuretic. It is the latter effect for which triamterene is principally employed.

## Adverse Effects

*Hyperkalemia.* Excessive potassium accumulation is the most significant adverse effect. Hyperkalemia is most likely when triamterene is used alone, but can also occur when the drug is combined with thiazides or high-ceiling agents. Triamterene should never be used in conjunction with another potassium-sparing diuretic or with potassium supplements. In addition, caution is needed if the drug is combined with an ACE inhibitor.

*Other Adverse Effects.* Relatively common side effects include *nausea, vomiting, leg cramps,* and *dizziness. Blood dyscrasias* occur rarely.

### Preparations, Dosage, and Administration

Triamterene [Dyrenium] is available in 50- and 100-mg capsules for oral use. The usual initial dosage is 100 mg twice a day. The maximum daily dosage is 300 mg. Triamterene is also marketed in fixed-dose combinations with hydrochlorothiazide under the trade names Dyazide and Maxzide.

### Amiloride

*Pharmacologic Properties.* Amiloride [Midamor] has actions similar to those of triamterene. Both drugs inhibit potassium loss by direct blockade of sodium-potassium exchange in the distal nephron. Also, both drugs produce only modest diuresis. Although it can be employed alone as a diuretic, amiloride is used primarily to counteract potassium loss caused by more powerful diuretics (thiazides, high-ceiling agents). The major adverse effect of amiloride is hyperkalemia. Accordingly, concurrent use of other potassium-sparing diuretics or potassium supplements must be avoided. Caution is needed if the drug is combined with an ACE inhibitor.

*Preparations, Dosage, and Administration.* Amiloride [Midamor] is dispensed in 5-mg tablets for oral use. Dosing is begun at 5 mg/day and may be increased to a maximum of 20 mg. Amiloride is available in a fixed-dose combination with hydrochlorothiazide under the trade name Moduretic.

## Osmotic Diuretics

Four compounds—mannitol, urea, glycerin, and isosorbide—are classified as osmotic diuretics. However, of the four, only mannitol is used for its diuretic actions. The osmotic agents differ from other diuretics both in mechanism of action and indications.

### Mannitol

Mannitol [Osmitrol] is a simple six-carbon sugar that possesses the four properties characteristic of an osmotic diuretic:

- It is freely filtered at the glomerulus.
- It undergoes minimal reabsorption.
- It is not metabolized to a significant degree.
- It is pharmacologically inert (i.e., it has no direct effects on the biochemistry or physiology of cells).

### Mechanism of Diuretic Action

Mannitol promotes diuresis by creating an osmotic force within the lumen of the nephron. Unlike other solutes, mannitol undergoes minimal reabsorption after filtration. As a result, most of the drug remains within the nephron, creating an osmotic force that inhibits passive reabsorption of water. Hence urine flow increases. The degree of diuresis produced is directly related to the concentration of mannitol in the filtrate; the more mannitol present, the greater the diuresis. Mannitol has no significant effect on the excretion of potassium and other electrolytes.

### Pharmacokinetics

Mannitol does not diffuse across the gastrointestinal epithelium and cannot be transported by the uptake systems that absorb dietary sugars. Accordingly, in order to reach the circulation, the drug must be given parenterally. Following IV injection, mannitol distributes freely to extracellular water. Diuresis begins in 30 to 60 minutes and persists for 6 to 8 hours. Most of the drug is excreted intact in the urine.

### Adverse Effects

*Edema.* Mannitol can leave the vascular system at all capillary beds except those of the brain. When the drug exits capillaries, it draws water along, causing edema. Mannitol must be used with extreme caution in patients with heart disease, since it may precipitate congestive heart failure (CHF) and fulminating pulmonary edema in these patients. If signs of pulmonary congestion or CHF develop, use of the drug must cease immediately. Mannitol must also be discontinued if patients with heart failure or pulmonary edema develop renal failure, since the resultant accumulation of mannitol would increase the risk of cardiac or pulmonary injury.

*Other Adverse Effects.* Common responses include *headache, nausea,* and *vomiting. Fluid and electrolyte imbalance* may also occur.

### Therapeutic Uses

*Prophylaxis of Renal Failure.* Under certain conditions (e.g., dehydration, severe hypotension, hypovolemic shock), blood flow to the kidney is decreased, causing a great reduction in filtrate volume. When the volume of filtrate is this low, the transport mechanisms of the nephron are able to reabsorb virtually all of the sodium and chloride present, causing complete reabsorption of water as well. As a result, urine production ceases, and kidney failure follows. The risk of renal failure can be reduced with mannitol. Since filtered mannitol is not reabsorbed—even when filtrate volume is small—filtered mannitol will remain in the nephron, drawing water with it. Hence, mannitol can preserve urine flow and may thereby prevent renal failure. Thiazides and loop diuretics are not as effective for this application because, under conditions of low filtrate production, there is such an excess of reabsorptive capacity (relative to the amount of filtrate) that these drugs are unable to produce sufficient blockade of reabsorption to promote diuresis.

*Reduction of Intracranial Pressure.* Intracranial pressure (ICP) that has been elevated by cerebral edema can be reduced with mannitol. The drug lowers ICP because its presence in the cerebral vasculature creates an osmotic force that draws edematous fluid out of the brain. There is no risk of increasing cerebral edema because mannitol cannot exit the capillary beds of the brain.

*Reduction of Intraocular Pressure.* Mannitol and other osmotic agents can lower intraocular pressure (IOP). Mannitol reduces IOP by rendering the plasma hyperosmotic with respect to intraocular fluids, thereby creating an osmotic force that draws ocular fluid into the blood. Use of mannitol to lower IOP is reserved for patients who have not responded to more conventional treatment.

### Preparations, Dosage, and Administration

Mannitol [Osmitrol] is administered by IV infusion. Solutions for IV use range in concentration from 5% to 25%. Dosing is complex and varies with the objectives of therapy (prevention of renal failure, lowering of ICP, lowering of IOP). The usual adult dosage for prevention of renal failure is 50 to 100 gm over 24 hours. The rate of infusion should be set to elicit a urine flow of at least 30 to 50 ml/hr. It should be noted that mannitol may crystallize out of solution if exposed to low temperature. Accordingly, preparations should be observed for crystals prior to use. Preparations that contain crystals should be warmed (to redissolve the mannitol) and then cooled to body temperature for administration. A filter needle is employed to withdraw mannitol from the vial; an in-line filter is used to prevent any crystals that may be present from entering the circulation. If urine flow declines to a very low rate or ceases entirely, the infusion should be stopped.

### Urea, Glycerin, and Isosorbide

In addition to mannitol, three other drugs—urea, glycerin, and isosorbide—are classified as osmotic diuretics. Like mannitol, these agents are freely filtered at the glomerulus and undergo limited reabsorption. These properties promote osmotic diuresis. It must be noted, however, that although urea, glycerin, and isosorbide can produce diuresis, none of these drugs is actually used for this purpose. Rather, these agents are used only to reduce intraocular and intracranial pressure. Urea [Ureaphil] is administered intravenously. Glycerin [Osmoglyn] and isosorbide [Ismotic] are administered orally.

## KEY POINTS

- More than 99% of the water, electrolytes, and nutrients that are filtered at the glomerulus undergo reabsorption.
- Most diuretics act by blocking active reabsorption of sodium and chloride, which then prevents passive reabsorption of water.
- The amount of diuresis that a drug produces is directly related to the amount of sodium and chloride reabsorption that it blocks.
- Drugs that act early in the nephron are in a position to block the greatest amount of solute reabsorption; hence these agents produce the most diuresis.

- High-ceiling diuretics (loop diuretics) block sodium and chloride reabsorption in the loop of Henle.
- High-ceiling diuretics produce the greatest diuresis.
- In contrast to thiazide diuretics, high-ceiling diuretics are effective even when the glomerular filtration rate is low.
- High-ceiling diuretics can cause dehydration through excessive fluid loss.
- High-ceiling diuretics can cause hypotension by decreasing blood volume and relaxing venous smooth muscle.
- High-ceiling diuretics can cause hearing loss, which is usually reversible.
- Hypokalemia caused by high-ceiling diuretics is a special problem for patients taking digoxin.
- Thiazide diuretics block sodium and water reabsorption in the early distal convoluted tubule.
- Thiazide diuretics produce less diuresis than high-ceiling diuretics.
- Thiazide diuretics are ineffective when glomerular filtration rate is low.
- Like the high-ceiling diuretics, thiazide diuretics can cause dehydration and hypokalemia; however, thiazides do not cause hearing loss.
- Thiazide-induced hypokalemia is a special problem for patients taking digoxin.
- Potassium-sparing diuretics act by directly or indirectly blocking sodium-potassium "exchange" in the distal convoluted tubule.
- Potassium-sparing diuretics cause only modest diuresis.
- Potassium-sparing diuretics are used primarily to counteract potassium loss in patients taking high-ceiling diuretics or thiazides.
- The principal adverse effect of potassium-sparing diuretics is hyperkalemia.
- Because of the risk of hyperkalemia, potassium-sparing diuretics should not be combined with one another or with potassium supplements, and they should be used cautiously in patients taking ACE inhibitors.
- High-ceiling diuretics and thiazides are used to treat essential hypertension and edema associated with heart failure, cirrhosis, and kidney disease.

## Summary of Major Nursing Implications*

## High-Ceiling (Loop) Diuretics

| | |
|---|---|
| Furosemide | Bumetanide |
| Ethacrynic Acid | Torsemide |

### Preadministration Assessment

#### Therapeutic Goal

High-ceiling diuretics are indicated for patients with (1) pulmonary edema associated with congestive heart failure; (2) edema of hepatic, cardiac, or renal origin that has been unresponsive to less effective diuretics; (3) hypertension that cannot be controlled with thiazide and potassium-sparing diuretics; and (4) patients who need diuretic therapy but have low renal blood flow.

#### Baseline Data

For all patients, obtain baseline values for weight, blood pressure (sitting and supine), pulse, respiration, and electrolytes (sodium, potassium, chloride). For patients with edema, record sites and extent of edema. For patients with ascites, measure abdominal girth.

*Patient education information is highlighted in color.

### Identifying High-Risk Patients

Use with *caution* in patients with *cardiovascular disease, renal impairment, diabetes mellitus,* or a *history of gout* and in patients who are *pregnant* or taking *digoxin, lithium, ototoxic drugs, NSAIDs,* or *antihypertensive drugs.*

## Implementation: Administration

### Routes

*Furosemide and bumetanide.* Oral, IV, IM.

*Ethacrynic acid and torsemide.* Oral, IV.

### Administration

*Oral.* Dosing may be done once daily, twice daily, or on alternate days. Instruct patients who are using once-a-day or alternate-day dosing to take their medication in the morning. Instruct patients using twice-a-day dosing to take their medication at 8 AM and 2 PM (to minimize nocturia).

Advise patients to administer *furosemide* with food if GI upset occurs.

*Parenteral.* Administer IV injections slowly (over 1 to 2 minutes). For high-dose therapy, administer by continuous infusion. Discard discolored solutions.

### Promoting Compliance

Increased frequency of urination is inconvenient and can discourage compliance. To promote compliance, forewarn patients that treatment will increase urine volume and frequency of voiding, and inform them that these effects will subside 6 to 8 hours after dosing. Inform patients that nighttime diuresis can be minimized by avoiding dosing late in the day.

## Ongoing Evaluation and Interventions

### Evaluating Therapeutic Effects

Monitor blood pressure and pulse rate, weigh the patient daily, and evaluate for decreased edema.

Monitor intake and output. Notify the physician if oliguria (urine output less than 25 ml/hr) or anuria (no urine output) develops.

Instruct patients to weigh themselves daily, preferably in the morning before eating, and to maintain a weight record.

### Minimizing Adverse Effects

*Hyponatremia, Hypochloremia, and Dehydration.* Loss of sodium, chloride, and water can cause hyponatremia, hypochloremia, and severe dehydration. Signs of dehydration include dry mouth, unusual thirst, and oliguria. Withhold the drug if these appear.

Dehydration can promote thromboembolism. Monitor the patient for symptoms (headache; pain in the chest, calves, or pelvis), and notify the physician if these develop.

The risk of dehydration and its sequelae can be minimized by (1) initiating therapy with low doses, (2) adjusting the dosage carefully, (3) monitoring weight loss daily, and (4) using an intermittent dosing schedule.

*Hypotension.* Monitor blood pressure. If it falls precipitously, withhold medication and notify the physician.

Teach patients to monitor their blood pressure and instruct them to notify the physician if pressure drops substantially.

Inform patients about signs of postural hypotension (dizziness, lightheadedness), and advise them to sit or lie down if these occur. Inform patients that postural hypotension can be minimized by getting up slowly.

*Hypokalemia.* If serum potassium falls below 3.5 mEq/L, fatal dysrhythmias may result. Hypokalemia can be minimized by consuming potassium-rich foods (e.g., citrus fruits, potatoes, bananas), taking potassium supplements, or using a potassium-sparing diuretic.

*Ototoxicity.* Inform patients about possible hearing loss and instruct them to notify the physician if a hearing deficit develops. Exercise caution when high-ceiling diuretics are used concurrently with other ototoxic drugs (e.g., aminoglycosides).

*Hyperglycemia.* High-ceiling diuretics may elevate blood glucose levels in diabetics. Advise diabetic patients to be especially diligent about monitoring blood glucose.

*Hyperuricemia.* High-ceiling diuretics frequently cause *asymptomatic* hyperuricemia, although gout-prone patients may experience a *gouty attack.* Inform patients about signs of gout (tenderness or swelling in joints), and instruct them to notify the physician if these occur.

### Minimizing Adverse Interactions

*Digoxin.* By lowering potassium levels, high-ceiling diuretics increase the risk of fatal dysrhythmias from digoxin. Serum potassium levels must be monitored and maintained above 3.5 mEq/L.

*Lithium.* High-ceiling diuretics can suppress lithium excretion, thereby causing the drug to accumulate, possibly to toxic levels. Plasma lithium content should be monitored routinely. If drug levels become elevated, lithium dosage should be reduced.

*Ototoxic Drugs.* The risk of hearing loss from high-ceiling diuretics is increased in the presence of other ototoxic drugs (e.g., aminoglycosides). Exercise caution when such combinations are employed.

## Thiazide Diuretics

Thiazide diuretics have actions very similar to those of the high-ceiling diuretics. Hence, nursing implications for the thiazides are nearly identical to those of the high-ceiling agents.

## Preadministration Assessment

### Therapeutic Goal

Thiazide diuretics are used to treat hypertension and edema.

### Baseline Data

For all patients, obtain baseline values for weight, blood pressure (sitting and supine), pulse, respiration, and electrolytes (sodium, chloride, potassium). For patients with edema, record sites and extent of edema.

### Identifying High-Risk Patients

Use with *caution* in patients with *cardiovascular disease, renal impairment, diabetes mellitus,* or a *history of gout* and in patients taking *digoxin, lithium,* or *antihypertensive drugs.*

## Implementation: Administration

### Routes

*Oral.* All thiazide-type diuretics, including chlorothiazide.

**Intravenous.** *Chlorothiazide.*

### Administration

Dosing may be done once daily, twice daily, or on alternate days. When once-a-day dosing is employed, instruct patients to take their medicine early in the day to minimize nocturia. When twice-a-day dosing is employed, instruct patients to take their medicine at 8 AM and 2 PM.

Advise patients to administer thiazides with or after meals if GI upset occurs.

### Promoting Compliance

See implications for *High-Ceiling (Loop) Diuretics.*

## Ongoing Evaluation and Interventions

### Evaluating Therapeutic Effects

See implications for *High-Ceiling (Loop) Diuretics.*

### Minimizing Adverse Effects

Like the high-ceiling diuretics, thiazides can cause *hyponatremia, hypochloremia, dehydration, hypokalemia, hypotension, hyperglycemia,* and *hyperuricemia.* For implications regarding these effects, see implications for *High-Ceiling (Loop) Diuretics.*

*Thiazides can cause fetal harm and can enter breast milk.* These drugs should be avoided during pregnancy unless absolutely required. Caution women not to breastfeed.

### Minimizing Adverse Interactions

Like high-ceiling diuretics, thiazides can interact adversely with *digoxin* and *lithium.* For nursing implications regarding these interactions, see implications for *High-Ceiling (Loop) Diuretics.*

## Potassium-Sparing Diuretics

Spironolactone
Triamterene
Amiloride

## Preadministration Assessment

### Therapeutic Goal

Potassium-sparing diuretics are given primarily to counterbalance the potassium-losing effects of thiazides and high-ceiling diuretics.

### Baseline Data

Obtain baseline values for serum potassium content.

### Identifying High-Risk Patients

Potassium-sparing diuretics are *contraindicated* for patients with *hyperkalemia* and for patients taking *potassium supplements* or *another potassium-sparing diuretic.* Use with *caution* in patients taking *ACE inhibitors.*

## Implementation: Administration

### Route

Oral.

### Administration

Advise patients to take these drugs with or after meals if GI upset occurs.

## Ongoing Evaluation and Interventions

### Evaluating Therapeutic Effects

Monitor serum potassium levels on a regular basis. The objective is to maintain serum potassium levels between 3.5 and 5 mEq/L.

### Minimizing Adverse Effects

*Hyperkalemia.* Hyperkalemia is the principal adverse effect. Instruct patients to restrict intake of potassium-rich foods (e.g., citrus fruits, bananas). If serum potassium levels rise above 5 mEq/L, or if signs of hyperkalemia develop (e.g., abnormal cardiac rhythm), withhold medication and notify the physician. Insulin can be given to drive potassium levels down.

*Endocrine Effects.* Spironolactone may cause *menstrual irregularities* and *impotence.* Inform patients about these effects, and instruct them to notify the physician if they occur.

### Minimizing Adverse Interactions

*Drugs That Raise Potassium Levels.* Because of the risk of hyperkalemia, don't combine a potassium-sparing diuretic with potassium supplements or with another potassium-sparing diuretic. Combine with ACE inhibitors only when clearly indicated.

# CHAPTER 39

# Agents Affecting the Volume and Ion Content of Body Fluids

The drugs discussed in this chapter are used to correct disturbances in the volume and ionic composition of body fluids. Three groups of agents are considered: (1) drugs used to correct disorders of fluid volume and osmolality, (2) drugs used to correct disturbances of hydrogen ion concentration (acid-base status), and (3) drugs used to correct electrolyte imbalances.

## Disorders of Fluid Volume and Osmolality

Good health requires that both the volume and osmolality of extracellular and intracellular fluids remain within a normal range. If a substantial alteration in either the volume or osmolality of these fluids develops, significant harm can result.

Maintenance of fluid volume and osmolality is primarily the job of the kidneys, and even under adverse conditions, renal mechanisms usually succeed in keeping the volume and composition of body fluids within acceptable limits. However, circumstances can arise in which the regulatory power of the kidneys is exceeded. When this occurs, disruption of fluid volume, osmolality, or both can result.

Abnormal states of hydration can be divided into two major categories: *volume contraction* and *volume expansion*. Volume contraction is defined as a *decrease* in total body water; conversely, volume expansion is defined as an *increase* in total body water. States of volume contraction and volume expansion have three subclassifica-

tions based on alterations in extracellular osmolality. For volume contraction, the three subcategories are *isotonic* contraction, *hypertonic* contraction, and *hypotonic* contraction. Volume expansion may also be subclassified as *isotonic*, *hypertonic*, or *hypotonic*. Descriptions and causes of these abnormal states are discussed below.

In the clinical setting, changes in osmolality are described in terms of the sodium content of plasma. Sodium is used as the reference for classification because this ion is the principal extracellular solute. (Recall that plasma sodium content ranges from 135 to 145 mEq/L.) In most cases, the total osmolality of plasma is equal to approximately twice the osmolality of sodium. That is, total plasma osmolality usually ranges from 280 to 300 mOsm/kg water.

## Volume Contraction

### Isotonic Contraction

*Definition and Causes.* Isotonic contraction is defined as volume contraction in which *sodium and water are lost in isotonic proportions*. Hence, although there is a decrease in the total volume of extracellular fluid, there is no change in osmolality. Causes of isotonic contraction include vomiting, diarrhea, kidney disease, and misuse of diuretics. Isotonic contraction is characteristic of cholera, an infection that produces vomiting and severe diarrhea.

*Treatment.* Lost volume should be replaced with fluids that are isotonic to plasma. This can be accomplished by infusion of isotonic (0.9%) sodium chloride in sterile water, a solution in which both sodium and chloride are present at a concentration of 145 mEq/L. Volume should be replenished slowly to avoid pulmonary edema.

## Hypertonic Contraction

***Definition and Causes.*** Hypertonic contraction is defined as volume contraction in which *loss of water exceeds loss of sodium*. Hence, there is a reduction in extracellular fluid volume coupled with an increase in osmolality. Because of extracellular hypertonicity, water is drawn out of cells, thereby producing intracellular dehydration and partial compensation for lost extracellular volume.

Causes of hypertonic contraction include excessive sweating, osmotic diuresis, and feeding excessively concentrated foods to infants. Hypertonic contraction may also develop secondary to extensive burns or to disorders of the central nervous system (CNS) that render the patient unable to experience or report thirst.

***Treatment.*** Volume replacement in hypertonic contraction should be accomplished with hypotonic fluids (e.g., 0.11% sodium chloride) or with fluids that contain no solutes at all. Initial therapy may consist simply of drinking water. Alternatively, 5% dextrose can be infused intravenously; since dextrose is rapidly metabolized to carbon dioxide and water, dextrose solutions can be looked upon as the osmotic equivalent of water alone. Volume replenishment should be done in stages. About 50% of the estimated loss should be replaced during the first few hours of treatment. The remainder should be replenished over 1 to 2 days.

## Hypotonic Contraction

***Definition and Causes.*** Hypotonic contraction is defined as volume contraction in which *loss of sodium exceeds loss of water*. Hence both the volume and osmolality of extracellular fluid are reduced. Since intracellular osmolality now exceeds extracellular osmolality, extracellular volume becomes diminished further by movement of water into cells.

The principal cause of hypotonic contraction is excessive loss of sodium through the kidneys. This may occur because of diuretic therapy, chronic renal insufficiency, or lack of aldosterone (the adrenocortical hormone that promotes renal retention of sodium).

***Treatment.*** If hyponatremia is mild and if renal function is adequate, hypotonic contraction can be corrected by infusion of *isotonic* sodium chloride solution for injection; plasma tonicity will be adjusted by the kidneys. However, if the sodium loss is severe, a *hypertonic* (e.g., 3%) solution of sodium chloride should be infused. Administration should continue until plasma sodium concentration has been raised to about 130 mEq/L. Patients should be monitored for signs of fluid overload (distention of neck veins, peripheral or pulmonary edema). When hypotonic contraction is due to aldosterone insufficiency, patients should receive hormone replacement therapy along with intravenous infusion of isotonic sodium chloride.

## Volume Expansion

Volume expansion is defined as an *increase in the total volume of body fluid*. As with volume contraction, volume expansion may be *isotonic, hypertonic,* or *hypotonic*. Volume expansion may result from an overdose with therapeutic fluids (e.g., sodium chloride infusion) or may be associated with disease states (e.g., heart failure, nephrotic syndrome, cirrhosis of the liver with ascites). The principal drugs employed to correct volume expansion are diuretics and the agents used for heart failure. These drugs are discussed in Chapters 38 and 46, respectively.

# Acid-Base Disturbances

Maintenance of acid-base balance is a complex process, the full discussion of which is beyond the scope of this text. Hence, consideration here is condensed.

Acid-base status is regulated by multiple systems. The most important of these are (1) the bicarbonate–carbonic acid buffer system, (2) the respiratory system, and (3) the kidneys. The respiratory system influences pH through control of $CO_2$ exhalation. Since $CO_2$ represents volatile carbonic acid, exhalation of $CO_2$ tends to elevate pH (reduce acidity), whereas $CO_2$ retention (secondary to respiratory slowing) tends to lower pH. The kidneys influence pH through regulation of bicarbonate excretion. By retaining bicarbonate, the kidneys can raise pH. Conversely, by increasing the excretion of bicarbonate, the kidneys can compensate for alkalosis.

There are four principal types of acid-base imbalance: (1) respiratory alkalosis, (2) respiratory acidosis, (3) metabolic alkalosis, and (4) metabolic acidosis. The causes and treatments of these states are discussed below.

## Respiratory Alkalosis

***Causes.*** Respiratory alkalosis is produced by hyperventilation. Deep and rapid breathing increases loss of $CO_2$, which in turn lowers the $pCO_2$ of blood and increases the pH. Mild hyperventilation may result from a number of causes, including hypoxia, pulmonary disease, and drugs (especially aspirin and other salicylates). Severe hyperventilation can be caused by injury to the CNS and by hysteria.

***Treatment.*** Management of respiratory alkalosis is dictated by the severity of pH elevation. When alkalosis is mild, no specific treatment is indicated. The severe respiratory alkalosis produced by hysteria can be controlled by having the patient rebreathe his or her $CO_2$-laden expired breath. This can be accomplished by holding a paper bag over the nose and mouth. A similar effect can be achieved by having the patient inhale a gas mixture containing 5% $CO_2$. A sedative (e.g., diazepam) can help suppress the hysteria.

## Respiratory Acidosis

***Causes.*** Respiratory acidosis results from retention of $CO_2$ secondary to hypoventilation. Reduced exhalation of

$CO_2$ raises plasma $pCO_2$, which in turn causes plasma pH to fall. Primary causes of impaired ventilation are (1) depression of the medullary respiratory center and (2) pathologic changes in the lungs. With time, the kidneys compensate for respiratory acidosis by excreting less bicarbonate.

*Treatment.* Primary treatment of respiratory acidosis is directed at correcting respiratory impairment. The patient may also need oxygen and ventilatory assistance. Infusion of sodium bicarbonate solution is indicated if acidosis is severe.

## Metabolic Alkalosis

*Causes.* Metabolic alkalosis is characterized by increases in both the pH and bicarbonate content of plasma. Causes include excessive loss of gastric acid (through vomiting or suctioning) and administration of alkalinizing salts (e.g., sodium bicarbonate). The body compensates for metabolic alkalosis by (1) hypoventilation (causing retention of $CO_2$), (2) increased renal excretion of bicarbonate, and (3) accumulation of organic acids.

*Treatment.* In most cases, metabolic alkalosis can be corrected by infusing a solution of *sodium chloride plus potassium chloride*. This facilitates renal excretion of bicarbonate, and thereby promotes normalization of plasma pH. When alkalosis is severe, direct correction of pH is indicated. This can be accomplished by infusing dilute (0.1 N) *hydrochloric acid* through a central venous catheter or by administering an acid-forming salt, such as *ammonium chloride*. Ammonium chloride must not be given to patients with liver failure, since the drug is likely to cause hepatic encephalopathy in these patients.

## Metabolic Acidosis

*Causes.* Principal causes of metabolic acidosis are chronic renal failure, loss of bicarbonate during severe diarrhea, and metabolic disorders that result in overproduction of lactic acid (lactic acidosis) or ketoacids (ketoacidosis). Metabolic acidosis may also result from poisoning by methanol and certain medications (e.g., aspirin and other salicylates).

*Treatment.* Treatment of metabolic acidosis consists of efforts to correct the underlying cause, and, if the acidosis is severe, administration of an alkalinizing salt (e.g., sodium bicarbonate, sodium citrate, sodium lactate).

When an alkalinizing salt is indicated, *sodium bicarbonate* is generally preferred. Administration may be oral or intravenous. If acidosis is mild, oral administration is preferred. Intravenous infusion is usually reserved for severe reductions of pH. When sodium bicarbonate is given IV to treat acute, severe acidosis, caution must be exercised to avoid excessive elevation of plasma pH, since rapid conversion from acidosis to alkalosis can be hazardous. Also, because of the sodium content of sodium bicarbonate, care should be taken to avoid hypernatremia.

# Potassium Imbalances

Potassium is the most abundant *intracellular* cation, having a concentration within cells of about 150 mEq/L. In contrast, *extracellular* concentrations are low (4 to 5 mEq/L). Potassium plays a major role in conducting nerve impulses and maintaining the electrical excitability of muscle. Potassium also helps regulate acid-base balance.

## Regulation of Potassium Levels

Serum levels of potassium are regulated primarily by the kidneys. Under steady-state conditions, urinary output of potassium equals intake. Renal excretion of potassium is increased by aldosterone, an adrenal steroid that promotes conservation of sodium while increasing potassium loss. Potassium excretion is also increased by most diuretics. Potassium-sparing diuretics (e.g., spironolactone) are the exception to this rule.

Potassium levels are influenced by extracellular pH. In the presence of extracellular *alkalosis*, potassium uptake by cells is *enhanced*, causing a *reduction* in extracellular potassium levels. Conversely, extracellular *acidosis* promotes the *exit* of potassium from cells, thereby causing extracellular *hyperkalemia*.

Insulin has a profound effect on potassium: in high doses, insulin stimulates potassium uptake by cells. This ability has been exploited to treat hyperkalemia.

## Hypokalemia

### Causes and Consequences

Hypokalemia is defined as a deficiency of potassium in the blood. By definition, hypokalemia exists when serum potassium levels fall below 3.5 mEq/L. The most common cause of hypokalemia is treatment with thiazide or loop diuretics (see Chapter 38). Other causes include insufficient potassium intake; alkalosis and excessive insulin (both of which decrease extracellular potassium levels by driving potassium into cells); increased renal excretion of potassium (e.g., as caused by aldosterone); and potassium loss associated with vomiting, diarrhea, and abuse of laxatives. Hypokalemia may also occur because of excessive potassium loss in sweat. As a rule, potassium depletion is accompanied by loss of chloride. Insufficiency of both ions produces *hypokalemic alkalosis*.

Hypokalemia has adverse effects on skeletal muscle, smooth muscle, and the heart. Symptoms associated with hypokalemia include weakness or paralysis of skeletal muscle, abnormalities in cardiac impulse conduction, and intestinal dilation and ileus. In patients taking digoxin (a cardiac drug), concurrent hypokalemia is the principal cause of digoxin toxicity.

### Prevention and Treatment

Potassium depletion is treated with a potassium salt. Potassium salts may also be used for *prophylaxis* against insufficiency. For either treatment or prophylaxis, the salt that is generally preferred is *potassium chloride*. The chloride salt of potassium is preferred because chloride deficiency frequently coexists with deficiency of potassium. Other salts (e.g., potassium gluconate, potassium citrate) are also available.

Potassium chloride may be administered orally or IV. Oral administration is preferred for prophylaxis and for treatment of mild deficiency. The intravenous route is employed for severe deficiency and for patients who cannot take potassium orally.

*Oral Potassium Chloride. Uses, Dosage, and Preparations.* Oral potassium chloride may be used for both prevention and treatment of potassium deficiency. Doses for prevention range from 16 to 24 mEq/day. Doses for correction of deficiency range from 40 to 100 mEq/day.

Oral potassium chloride is available in solution and in solid formulations (powder, standard tablets, effervescent tablets, enteric-coated tablets, wax-matrix tablets, microencapsulated particles in capsules). The solution is preferred.

*Adverse Effects.* Potassium chloride *irritates* the *gastrointestinal tract*, frequently causing abdominal discomfort, nausea, vomiting, and diarrhea. Solid forms of potassium chloride (tablets, capsules) can produce high local concentrations of potassium, resulting in severe intestinal injury (ulcerative lesions, bleeding, perforation); death has occurred. These severe effects are less likely with wax-matrix tablets and with capsules that contain microencapsulated particles than with other solid formulations. To minimize gastrointestinal effects, oral potassium chloride should be taken with meals or with a full glass of water. If symptoms of irritation occur, administration should be discontinued. Rarely, oral potassium chloride produces hyperkalemia. This dangerous development is much more likely with intravenous therapy.

*Intravenous Potassium Chloride.* Intravenous potassium chloride is indicated for prevention and treatment of hypokalemia. Intravenous solutions must be diluted (preferably to 40 mEq/L or less) and infused slowly (generally no faster than 10 mEq/hr in adults).

The principal complication of IV therapy is *hyperkalemia*, a condition that can prove fatal. To reduce the risk of hyperkalemia, serum potassium levels should be measured prior to starting the infusion and periodically throughout the treatment interval. In addition, renal function should be assessed before and during treatment to ensure adequate output of urine. If renal failure develops, the infusion should be stopped immediately. Changes in the electrocardiogram (EKG) can provide an early indication that potassium toxicity is developing. Symptoms and treatment of hyperkalemia are discussed in the section that follows.

*Contraindications to Potassium Use.* Potassium should be avoided under conditions that predispose patients to hyperkalemia (e.g., severe renal impairment, use of potassium-sparing diuretics, hypoaldosteronism). Potassium must also be avoided when hyperkalemia already exists.

## Hyperkalemia

### Causes and Consequences

*Causes.* Hyperkalemia (excessive elevation of serum potassium content) can result from a number of causes. These include severe tissue trauma, untreated Addison's disease, acute acidosis (which draws potassium out of cells), misuse of potassium-sparing diuretics, and overdose with intravenous potassium.

*Consequences.* The most serious consequence of hyperkalemia is disruption of the electrical activity of the heart. Because hyperkalemia alters the generation and conduction of cardiac impulses, alterations in the EKG and in cardiac rhythm are usually the earliest signs that potassium levels are climbing dangerously high. With mild elevation of serum potassium (5 to 7 mEq/L), the T wave heightens and the PR interval becomes prolonged. When serum potassium reaches 8 to 9 mEq/L, cardiac arrest occurs, possibly preceded by ventricular tachycardia or ventricular fibrillation.

Effects of hyperkalemia are not limited to the heart. Elevation of serum potassium may cause confusion, anxiety, dyspnea, weakness or heaviness of the legs, and numbness or tingling of the hands, feet, and lips.

### Treatment

Treatment is begun by withholding any foods that contain potassium and any medicines that promote potassium accumulation (e.g., potassium-sparing diuretics, potassium supplements). After this, management consists of measures that (1) counteract potassium-induced cardiotoxicity and (2) lower extracellular levels of potassium. Specific steps include (1) infusion of a *calcium salt* (e.g., calcium gluconate) to offset effects of hyperkalemia on the heart; (2) infusion of *glucose* and *insulin* to promote uptake of potassium by cells and thereby decrease extracellular potassium levels; and (3) if acidosis is present (which is likely), infusion of *sodium bicarbonate* in order to move pH toward alkalinity, and thereby increase cellular uptake of potassium. If the preceding measures prove inadequate, steps can be taken to remove potassium. These include (1) oral or rectal administration of *sodium polystyrene sulfonate*, an exchange resin that absorbs potassium, and (2) peritoneal or extracorporeal dialysis.

## Magnesium Imbalances

Magnesium is required for the activity of many enzymes and for binding of messenger RNA to ribosomes. In addition, magnesium helps regulate neurochemical transmission and the excitability of muscle. The concentration of magnesium within cells is about 40 mEq/L, much higher than its concentration outside cells (about 2 mEq/L).

## Hypomagnesemia

### Causes and Consequences

Low levels of magnesium may result from a variety of causes, including diarrhea, hemodialysis, kidney disease, and prolonged intravenous feeding with magnesium-free solutions. Hypomagnesemia may also be seen in chronic alcoholics and in people with diabetes or pancreatitis. Frequently, patients with magnesium deficiency also present with hypocalcemia and hypokalemia.

Prominent symptoms of hypomagnesemia involve cardiac and skeletal muscle. In the presence of low levels of magnesium, release of acetylcholine at the neuromuscular junction is enhanced. This can increase muscle excitability to the point of tetany. Hypomagnesemia also increases excitability of neurons in the CNS, causing disorientation, psychoses, and seizures.

In the kidneys, hypomagnesemia may lead to nephrocalcinosis (formation of minuscule calcium stones within nephrons). Renal injury occurs when the stones become large enough to block the flow of tubular urine.

### Prevention and Treatment

Frank hypomagnesemia is treated with parenteral magnesium sulfate. For prophylaxis against magnesium deficiency, an oral preparation (magnesium gluconate, magnesium hydroxide) may be used.

***Magnesium Gluconate and Magnesium Hydroxide.*** Tablets of magnesium gluconate or magnesium hydroxide may be taken as supplements to dietary magnesium to help prevent hypomagnesemia. Milk of magnesia (a liquid formulation of magnesium hydroxide) may also be used for prophylaxis. With any of these oral magnesium preparations, excessive doses may cause diarrhea. The adult and pediatric dosage for prevention of deficiency is 5 mg/kg/day.

***Magnesium Sulfate.*** *Uses, Administration, and Dosage.* Magnesium sulfate (IM or IV) is the preferred treatment for severe hypomagnesemia. The IM dosage is 0.5 to 1 gm 4 times a day. For IV therapy, a 10% solution can be used; the infusion rate is 1.5 ml/min or less.

*Adverse Effects.* Excessive levels of magnesium cause *neuromuscular blockade*. Paralysis of the respiratory muscles is of particular concern. By suppressing neuromuscular transmission, magnesium excess can intensify the effects of neuromuscular blocking agents (e.g., tubocurarine, succinylcholine). Hence, caution must be exercised in patients receiving these drugs. The neuromuscular blocking actions of magnesium can be counteracted with calcium. Accordingly, when parenteral magnesium is being employed, an injectable form of calcium (e.g., calcium gluconate) should be immediately available.

In the heart, excessive levels of magnesium can suppress impulse conduction through the atrioventricular (AV) node. Accordingly, magnesium sulfate is contraindicated for patients with AV heart block.

To minimize the risk of toxicity, serum magnesium levels should be monitored. Respiratory paralysis occurs at concentrations of 12 to 15 mEq/L. When magnesium levels exceed 25 mEq/L, cardiac arrest may take place.

## Hypermagnesemia

Toxic elevation of magnesium levels is most common in patients with renal insufficiency, especially when magnesium-containing antacids or cathartics are being used. Symptoms of mild intoxication include muscle weakness (resulting from inhibition of acetylcholine release), hypotension, sedation, and EKG changes. As noted above, respiratory paralysis is likely when plasma levels reach 12 to 15 mEq/L. At higher concentrations of magnesium, there is a risk of cardiac arrest. Muscle weakness and paralysis can be counteracted with an intravenous calcium preparation.

## KEY POINTS

- Treat isotonic volume contraction with isotonic (0.9%) sodium chloride.
- Treat hypertonic volume contraction with hypotonic (e.g., 0.11%) sodium chloride.
- Treat hypotonic volume contraction with hypertonic (e.g., 3%) sodium chloride.
- Treat volume expansion with diuretics.
- Treat respiratory or metabolic acidosis with sodium bicarbonate
- Treat respiratory alkalosis by having the patient inhale 5% carbon dioxide or rebreathe his or her expired air.
- Treat metabolic alkalosis with an infusion of sodium chloride plus potassium chloride. For severe cases, infuse 0.1% hydrochloric acid or ammonium chloride.
- Treat hypokalemia with oral or IV potassium chloride.
- To treat hyperkalemia, begin by withdrawing potassium-containing foods and drugs that promote potassium accumulation (e.g., potassium supplements, potassium-sparing diuretics). Subsequent measures include (1) infusion of a calcium salt to offset the cardiac effects of potassium, (2) infusion of glucose and insulin to promote potassium uptake by cells, and (3) infusion of sodium bicarbonate if acidosis is present.
- Treat hypomagnesemia with IM or IV magnesium sulfate. For prophylaxis, give oral magnesium (e.g., magnesium gluconate).

# UNIT VII

## Cardiovascular Drugs

# Review of Hemodynamics

Hemodynamics is the study of the movement of blood throughout the circulatory system, as well as the regulatory factors and driving forces involved. Concepts introduced here reappear throughout the chapters on cardiovascular drugs. Accordingly, I urge you to review these now. Because this is a pharmacology text, and not a physiology text, discussion is limited to hemodynamic factors that have particular relevance to drugs.

## Overview of the Circulatory System

The circulatory system has two primary functions: (1) delivery of oxygen, nutrients, hormones, electrolytes, and other essentials to cells, and (2) removal of carbon dioxide, metabolic wastes, and other detritus from cells. In addition, the system helps fight infection.

The circulatory system has two divisions: the *pulmonary circulation* and the *systemic circulation*. The pulmonary circulation delivers blood to the lungs. The systemic circulation delivers blood to all tissues except the lungs. The systemic circulation is also known as the *greater circulation or peripheral circulation*.

### Components of the Circulatory System

The circulatory system is composed of the *heart* and *blood vessels*. The heart is the pump that moves blood through the arterial tree. The blood vessels have several functions:

- *Arteries* transport blood under high pressure to tissues.
- *Arterioles* are control valves that regulate local blood flow.
- *Capillaries* are the site for exchange of fluid, oxygen, carbon dioxide, nutrients, hormones, wastes, and so forth.
- *Venules* collect blood from the capillaries.
- *Veins* transport blood back to the heart. In addition, veins serve as a major reservoir for blood.

Arteries and veins differ from each other with respect to distensibility (elasticity). Arteries are very muscular, and hence do not readily stretch. As a result, large increases in arterial pressure cause only small increases in arterial diameter. Veins are much less muscular than arteries, and hence are 6 to 10 times more distensible. As a result, small increases in venous pressure cause large increases in venous diameter, which produces a large increase in venous volume.

### Distribution of Blood

The adult circulatory system contains about 5 liters of blood, which is distributed throughout the system. As indicated in Figure 40-1, 9% is in the pulmonary circulation, 7% is in the heart, and 84% is in the systemic circulation. Within the systemic circulation, however, distribution is uneven: most (64%) of the blood is in veins, venules, and venous sinuses; the remaining 20% is in arteries (13%) and arterioles or capillaries (7%). The large volume of blood in the venous system serves as a reservoir.

### What Makes Blood Flow?

Blood moves within vessels because the force driving flow is greater than the resistance to flow. As indicated in

Pulmonary circulation: **9%**

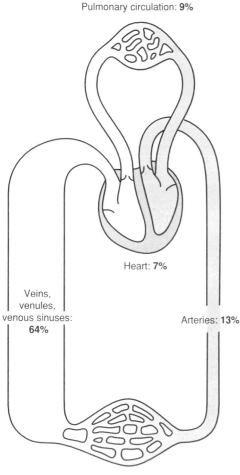

**Figure 40–1. Distribution of blood in the circulatory system.** Note that a large percentage of the blood resides in the venous system.

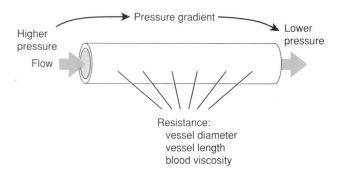

**Figure 40–2. Forces that promote and impede flow of blood.** Blood flows from the point of higher pressure toward the point of lower pressure. Resistance to flow is determined by vessel diameter, vessel length, and blood viscosity.

values (0 to –5 mm Hg) in the right atrium. (Negative atrial pressure is generated by expansion of the chest during respiration.)

Given that pressure is only 18 mm Hg when blood leaves capillaries, we must ask, "How does blood get back to the heart? After all, a pressure of 18 mm Hg does not seem adequate to move blood from the feet all the way up to the thorax." The answer is that, in addition to the small pressure head in venules, three mechanisms help ensure venous return. First, negative pressure in the right atrium helps "suck" blood toward the heart. Second, constriction of smooth muscle in veins increases venous pressure, which helps drive blood toward the heart. Third, and most important, the combination of venous valves and skeletal muscle contraction constitutes an auxiliary "venous pump." As indicated in Figure 40-4A, the venous system is equipped with a system of one-way valves. When skeletal muscles contract (Fig. 40-4B), venous blood is

Figure 40-2, the force that drives blood flow is the pressure gradient between two points in a vessel. Obviously, blood will flow from the point where pressure is higher toward the point where pressure is lower. Resistance to flow is determined by the diameter and length of the vessel, and by blood viscosity. From a pharmacologic viewpoint, the most important determinant of resistance is vessel diameter: the larger the vessel, the smaller the resistance, and vice versa. Accordingly, when vessels dilate, resistance declines, causing blood flow to increase—and when vessels constrict, resistance rises, causing blood flow to decline. In order to maintain adequate flow when resistance rises, blood pressure must rise as well.

## How Does Blood Get Back to the Heart?

As indicated in Figure 40-3, blood pressure falls progressively as blood moves through the systemic circulation. Pressure is 120 mm Hg when blood enters the aorta, 30 mm Hg when blood enters capillaries, only 18 mm Hg when blood leaves capillaries, and then drops to negative

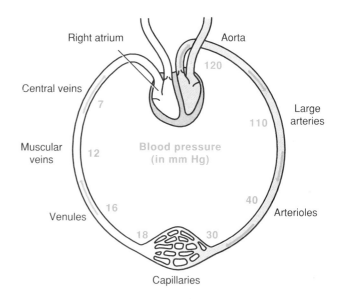

**Figure 40–3. Distribution of pressure within the systemic circulation.** Note that pressure is highest when blood leaves the left ventricle, falls to only 18 mm Hg as blood exits capillaries, and reaches negative values within the right atrium.

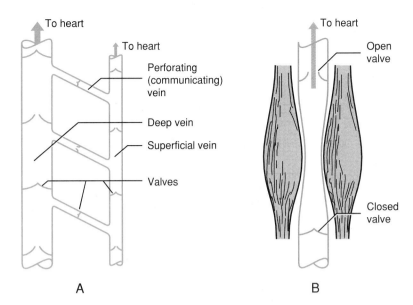

**Figure 40–4. Venous valves and the auxiliary venous "pump."** *A*, Veins and their one-way valves in the leg. Note that the arrangement of valves ensures that blood will move toward the heart. *B*, Contraction of skeletal muscle pumps venous blood toward the heart.

squeezed toward the heart—the only direction permitted by the valves.

## Regulation of Cardiac Output

In the average adult, cardiac output is about 5 L/min. Hence, every minute the heart pumps the equivalent of all the blood in the body. In this section, we consider the major factors that determine how much blood the heart pumps.

### Determinants of Cardiac Output

The basic equation for cardiac output is

$$CO = HR \times SV$$

where CO is cardiac output, HR is heart rate, and SV is stroke volume. According to the equation, an increase in HR or SV will increase CO, whereas a decrease in HR or SV will decrease CO. For the average person, HR is about 70 beats/min and SV is about 70 ml. Multiplying these, we get 4.9 L/min—the average value for cardiac output.

*Heart rate* is controlled primarily by the autonomic nervous system. Rate is increased by the sympathetic branch acting through beta₁-adrenergic receptors in the sinoatrial (SA) node. Rate is decreased by the parasympathetic branch acting through muscarinic receptors in the SA node. Parasympathetic impulses reach the heart via the vagus nerve.

*Stroke volume* is determined largely by three factors: (1) myocardial contractility, (2) cardiac afterload, and (3) cardiac preload. *Myocardial contractility* is defined as the force with which the ventricles contract. Contractility is determined primarily by the degree of cardiac dilation, which in turn is determined by the amount of venous return. The importance of venous return in regulating contractility and stroke volume is discussed separately below. In addition to regulation by venous return, contractility can be increased by the sympathetic nervous system, acting through beta₁-adrenergic receptors in the myocardium.

*Preload* is formally defined as the amount of tension (stretch) applied to a muscle prior to contraction. In the heart, stretch is determined by ventricular filling pressure, that is, the *force of venous return:* the greater filling pressure is, the greater the ventricles will stretch. Cardiac preload can be expressed as either *end-diastolic volume* or *end-diastolic pressure*. As discussed below, an increase in preload will increase stroke volume, whereas a decrease in preload will reduce stroke volume. Frequently, the terms *preload* and *force of venous* return are used interchangeably—although they are not really equivalent.

*Afterload* is formally defined as the load against which a muscle exerts its force (i.e., the load a muscle must overcome in order to contract). For the heart, afterload is the *arterial pressure* that the left ventricle must overcome to eject blood. Common sense tells us that, if afterload increases, stroke volume will decrease. Conversely, if afterload falls, stroke volume will rise. Cardiac afterload is determined primarily by the degree of peripheral resistance, which in turn is determined by constriction and dilation of arterioles: when arterioles constrict, peripheral resistance rises, causing arterial pressure (afterload) to rise as well; conversely, when arterioles dilate, peripheral resistance falls, causing arterial pressure to decline.

### Control of Stroke Volume by Venous Return

Q: How much blood does the heart pump each stroke?
A: Exactly the amount delivered by the veins!

#### Starling's Law of the Heart

*Starling's law* states that the force of ventricular contraction is proportional to muscle fiber length (up to a point). Accordingly, as fiber length (ventricular diameter)

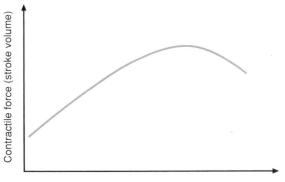

**Figure 40–5. The Starling relationship between myocardial fiber length and contractile force.** Note that an increase in fiber length produces a corresponding increase in contractile force. Fiber length increases as the ventricles enlarge during filling. Increased contractile force is reflected by increased stroke volume.

increases, there is a corresponding increase in contractile force (Figure 40-5). Because of this built-in mechanism, when more blood enters the heart, more is pumped out. As a result, the healthy heart is able to precisely match its output with the volume of blood delivered by the veins: when venous return increases, cardiac output increases correspondingly; conversely, when venous return declines, cardiac output declines to the same extent. Hence, under normal, nonstressed conditions, stroke volume is determined by factors that regulate venous return.

Why does contractile force change as a function of fiber length (ventricular diameter)? Recall that muscle contraction results from the interaction of two proteins: actin and myosin. As the heart stretches in response to increased ventricular filling, actin and myosin are brought into a more optimal alignment with each other, which allows them to interact with greater force.

### Factors That Determine Venous Return

Having established that venous return is the primary determinant of stroke volume (and hence cardiac output), we need to understand the factors that determine venous return. With regard to pharmacology, the most important factor is *systemic filling pressure* (i.e., the force that returns blood to the heart). The normal value for filling pressure is 7 mm Hg. This value can be raised to 17 mm Hg by constriction of veins. Filling pressure can also be raised by an increase in blood volume. Conversely, filling pressure, and hence venous return, can be lowered by venodilation or by reducing blood volume. Blood volume and venous tone can both be altered with drugs.

In addition to systemic filling pressure, three other factors influence venous return: (1) the auxiliary muscle pump discussed above, (2) resistance to flow between peripheral vessels and the right atrium, and (3) right atrial pressure, elevation of which will impede venous return. None of these factors can be directly influenced with drugs.

## Starling's Law and Maintenance of Systemic-Pulmonary Balance

Because the myocardium operates in accord with Starling's law, the right and left ventricles always pump exactly the same amount of blood. When venous return increases, stroke volume of the right ventricle increases, thereby increasing delivery of blood to the pulmonary circulation, which in turn delivers more blood to the left ventricle; this increases filling of the left ventricle, which causes *its* stroke volume to increase. Because an increase in venous return causes the output of *both* ventricles to increase, blood flow through the systemic and pulmonary circulations is always in balance, as long as the heart remains healthy.

In the failing heart, Starling's law breaks down. That is, force of contraction no longer increases in proportion to increased ventricular filling. As a result, blood backs up behind the failing ventricle. The deadly consequences are illustrated in Figure 40-6. In this example, output of the left ventricle is 1% less than the output of the right ventricle, which causes blood to back up in the pulmonary circulation. In only 20 minutes, this small imbalance between left and right ventricular output shifts a liter of blood from the systemic circulation to the pulmonary circulation. In less than 40 minutes, death from pulmonary congestion would ensue. This example underscores the essential nature of systemic-pulmonary balance, and the critical role of Starling's mechanism in maintaining it.

## Regulation of Arterial Pressure

Arterial pressure is the driving force that moves blood through the arterial side of the systemic circulation. The general formula for arterial pressure is

$$AP = PR \times CO$$

where AP is arterial pressure, PR is peripheral resistance, and CO is cardiac output. Accordingly, an increase in PR or CO will increase AP, whereas a decrease in PR or CO will decrease AP. Peripheral resistance is regulated primarily through constriction and dilation of arterioles. Cardiac output is regulated by the mechanisms discussed above. Regulation of arterial pressure through processes that alter PR and CO are discussed below.

### Overview of Control Systems

Arterial pressure is regulated by three systems: the autonomic nervous system (ANS), the renin-angiotensin system (RAS), and the kidneys. These systems differ greatly with regard to time frame of response. The ANS acts in two ways: it responds rapidly (in seconds or minutes) to acute changes in blood pressure, and it also provides steady-state control of AP. The RAS responds more slowly, taking hours or days to influence AP. The kidneys are re-

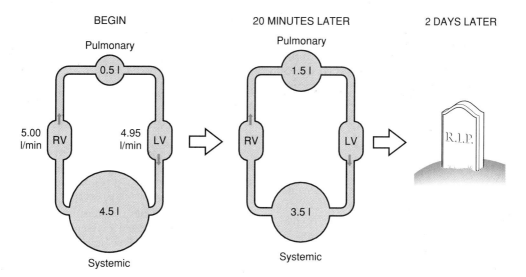

**Figure 40–6. Systemic-pulmonary imbalance that develops when the output of the left and right ventricles is not identical.** In this example, the output of the left ventricle is 1% less than the output of the right ventricle. Hence, while the right ventricle pumps 5000 ml/min, the left pumps only 4950 ml/min—50 ml/min less than the right. This causes blood to back up in the pulmonary circulation. After 20 minutes, 1000 ml of blood has shifted from the systemic circulation to the pulmonary circulation. Death would ensue in less than 40 minutes (the 2 days are an allowance for the undertaker and parson). (Adapted from Burton, A.C. Physiology and Biophysics of the Circulation. Chicago, Year Book Medical Publishers, 1968, p. 144).

sponsible for long-term control, and hence may take days or weeks to adjust AP.

## Steady-State Control by the Autonomic Nervous System

The ANS regulates AP by adjusting cardiac output and peripheral resistance. Sympathetic tone to the heart increases heart rate and contractility, thereby increasing CO. In contrast, parasympathetic tone slows the heart, and thereby reduces CO. As discussed in Chapter 14, blood vessels are regulated by the sympathetic branch of the ANS; they have no parasympathetic innervation. Steady-state sympathetic tone provides a moderate level of vasoconstriction. The resultant resistance to blood flow maintains AP. Complete elimination of sympathetic tone would cause AP to fall by 50%.

## Rapid Control by the Autonomic Nervous System: The Baroreceptor Reflex

The baroreceptor reflex serves to maintain arterial pressure at a predetermined level. When AP changes, the reflex immediately attempts to restore AP to the preset value.

The reflex works as follows. Baroreceptors in the aortic arch and carotid sinus sense AP and relay this information to the vasoconstrictor center of the medulla. When AP changes, the vasoconstrictor center compensates by sending appropriate instructions to arterioles, veins, and the heart. For example, when AP drops, the vasoconstrictor center causes (1) constriction of nearly all arterioles,

thereby increasing peripheral resistance; (2) constriction of veins, thereby increasing venous return; and (3) acceleration of heart rate (by increasing sympathetic impulses to the heart and decreasing parasympathetic impulses). The combined effect of these responses is to restore arterial pressure to the preset level. When AP rises too high, opposite responses occur: the reflex dilates arterioles and veins, and slows the heart.

The baroreceptor reflex is poised for rapid action—but not for prolonged action. When AP falls or rises, the reflex acts within seconds to restore the preset pressure. However, when AP *remains* elevated or lowered, the system resets to the new pressure within 1 to 2 days. After this, the system perceives the new (elevated or reduced) pressure as "normal," and hence ceases to respond.

Drugs that lower AP will trigger the baroreceptor reflex. For example, if we administer a drug that dilates arterioles, the resultant drop in peripheral resistance will reduce AP, causing the baroreceptor reflex to activate. The most noticeable response is *reflex tachycardia*. The baroreceptor reflex can temporarily negate efforts to lower AP with drugs.

## The Renin-Angiotensin System

The RAS supports arterial pressure by causing (1) constriction of arterioles and veins, and (2) retention of water by the kidney. Vasoconstriction is mediated by a hormone named *angiotensin II*; water retention is mediated in part by *aldosterone*. Responses develop in hours (vasoconstriction) to days (water retention). The RAS and its role in controlling blood pressure are discussed at length in Chapter 41.

## Renal Retention of Water

When AP remains low for a long time, the kidney responds by retaining water, which in turn causes AP to rise. Pressure rises because fluid retention increases blood volume, which increases venous pressure, which increases venous return, which increases CO, which increases AP. Water retention is a mechanism for maintaining AP over long periods (weeks, months, years).

Why does a reduction in AP cause the kidney to retain water? First, low AP reduces renal blood flow (RBF), which in turn reduces glomerular filtration rate (GFR). Since less fluid is filtered, less urine is produced, and therefore more water is retained. Second, low AP activates the renin-angiotensin system, causing levels of angiotensin II and aldosterone to rise. Angiotensin II causes constriction of renal blood vessels, and thereby decreases RBF and GFR. Aldosterone promotes renal retention of sodium, which causes water to be retained along with it.

## Postural Hypotension

Postural hypotension, also known as *orthostatic hypotension*, is a reduction in AP that can occur when we move from a supine or seated position to an upright position. The cause of hypotension is pooling of blood in veins, which decreases venous return, which in turn decreases cardiac output. Between 300 and 800 ml of blood can pool in veins when we stand, causing cardiac output to drop by as much as 2 L/min. Why does blood collect in veins? When we stand, gravity increases the pressure that blood exerts on veins. Since veins are not very muscular, they are unable to retain their shape when pressure increases, hence they stretch. The resultant increase in venous volume allows blood to pool.

Two mechanisms help overcome postural hypotension. One is the system of auxiliary venous pumps, which promote venous return. In fact, in healthy individuals, these auxiliary pumps usually prevent postural hypotension from occurring in the first place. When hypotension does occur, the baroreceptor reflex can restore AP by (1) constricting veins and arterioles and (2) increasing heart rate.

What would happen if we gave a drug that promoted dilation of veins (or prevented them from constricting)? In patients taking drugs that interfere with venoconstriction, postural hypotension is more intense and more prolonged. Hypotension is more intense because venous pooling is greater. Hypotension is more prolonged because there is no venoconstriction to help reverse venous pooling. As with drugs that reduce AP by dilating arterioles, drugs that reduce AP by relaxing veins can trigger the baroreceptor reflex, and can thereby cause reflex tachycardia.

## KEY POINTS*

- Arterioles serve as control valves to regulate local blood flow.

*Key points are limited to concepts that might not have been stressed when you studied physiology (e.g., veins serve as a blood reservoir). Important but obvious concepts (e.g., the heart is a pump; arteries deliver blood to tissues under pressure) are not included in this summary.

- Veins are a reservoir for blood.
- Arteries are not very distensible. As a result, large increases in arterial pressure cause only small increases in arterial diameter.
- Veins are highly distensible. As a result, small increases in venous pressure cause large increases in venous diameter.
- The adult circulatory system contains 5 liters of blood, 64% of which is in systemic veins.
- Vasodilation reduces resistance to blood flow, whereas vasoconstriction increases resistance to flow.
- In addition to the small pressure head in venules, three mechanisms help ensure venous return: (1) negative pressure in the right atrium sucks blood toward the heart; (2) constriction of veins increases venous pressure, and thereby drives blood toward the heart; and (3) contraction of skeletal muscles, in conjunction with one-way venous valves, pumps blood toward the heart.
- Heart rate is increased by stimulation of sympathetic nerves and decreased by stimulation of parasympathetic nerves.
- Stroke volume is determined by myocardial contractility, cardiac afterload, and cardiac preload.
- Preload is defined as the amount of tension (stretch) applied to a muscle prior to contraction. In the heart, preload is determined by the force of venous return.
- Afterload is defined as the load against which a muscle exerts its force. For the heart, afterload is the arterial pressure that the left ventricle must overcome to eject blood.
- Cardiac afterload is determined primarily by peripheral resistance, which in turn is determined by constriction or dilation of arterioles.
- Starling's law states that the force of ventricular contraction is proportional to myocardial fiber length. Because of this relationship, when more blood enters the heart, more is pumped out. As a result, the healthy heart is able to precisely match output with venous return.
- The most important determinant of venous return is systemic filling pressure, which can be raised by constriction of veins and by increasing blood volume.
- Because cardiac muscle operates under Starling's law, the right and left ventricles always pump exactly the same amount of blood (assuming the heart is healthy). Hence, balance between the pulmonary and systemic circulations is maintained.
- Arterial pressure is regulated by the autonomic nervous system (ANS), the renin-angiotensin system (RAS), and the kidneys.
- The ANS regulates arterial pressure (1) through tonic control of heart rate and peripheral resistance and (2) through the baroreceptor reflex.
- The baroreceptor reflex is only useful for short-term control of arterial pressure. When pressure *remains* elevated or lowered, the system resets to the new pressure within 1 to 2 days, and hence ceases to respond.
- Drugs that lower arterial pressure trigger the baroreceptor reflex, and thereby cause reflex tachycardia. Hence, the baroreceptor reflex can temporarily negate efforts to lower arterial pressure with drugs.

- The RAS supports arterial pressure by causing (1) constriction of arterioles and veins, and (2) retention of water by the kidney. Vasoconstriction is mediated by angiotensin II; water retention is mediated in part by aldosterone.
- The kidneys provide long-term control of blood pressure by regulating blood volume.

- Postural (orthostatic) hypotension is caused by decreased venous return secondary to pooling of blood in veins when we assume an erect posture.
- Drugs that dilate veins intensify and prolong postural hypotension. As with other drugs that reduce arterial pressure, venodilators can trigger the baroreceptor reflex, and can thereby cause reflex tachycardia.

# CHAPTER 41

# Drugs Acting on the Renin-Angiotensin System

n this chapter we will consider two families of drugs: angiotensin-converting enzyme (ACE) inhibitors and angiotensin II receptor antagonists. Both families produce their effects by interfering with the renin-angiotensin system (RAS). The ACE inhibitors have been available for two decades and have an established role in the treatment of hypertension and heart failure; they are also indicated for myocardial infarction and diabetic nephropathy. The angiotensin II receptor antagonists are new drugs currently approved only for hypertension. We will begin the chapter by reviewing the physiology of the RAS, after which we will discuss the drugs that affect it.

## Physiology of the Renin-Angiotensin System

The RAS has an important role in the regulation of blood pressure, blood volume, and fluid and electrolyte balance. In addition, the system appears to mediate certain pathophysiologic changes associated with hypertension, heart failure, and myocardial infarction. The RAS exerts its effects through the actions of angiotensin II.

### Types of Angiotensin

Before considering the physiology of the RAS, we need to introduce the angiotensin family, which consists of angiotensin I, angiotensin II, and angiotensin III. All three compounds are small polypeptides. Angiotensin I is the precursor of angiotensin II (see Fig. 41–1) and has very little biologic activity. In contrast, angiotensin II has extremely high biologic activity. Angiotensin III, which is

formed by degradation of angiotensin II, has moderate biologic activity.

### Actions of Angiotensin II

Angiotensin II mediates essentially all of the effects of the RAS. The most prominent actions of angiotensin II are vasoconstriction and stimulation of aldosterone release. Both actions serve to raise blood pressure. In addition, angiotensin II can act on the heart and blood vessels to alter their morphology.

*Vasoconstriction.* Angiotensin II is an extremely potent vasoconstrictor. The compound acts directly on vascular smooth muscle to cause contraction. Vasoconstriction is prominent in arterioles and less prominent in veins. As a result of angiotensin-induced vasoconstriction, blood pressure rises. In addition to its direct action on blood vessels, angiotensin II can cause vasoconstriction indirectly by acting in the CNS to increase sympathetic outflow to blood vessels, and by acting on the adrenal medulla to cause release of epinephrine.

*Release of Aldosterone.* Angiotensin II acts on the adrenal cortex to promote synthesis and secretion of aldosterone. Aldosterone, in turn, acts on the kidney to cause retention of sodium and excretion of potassium and hydrogen. Because retention of sodium causes water to be retained as well, aldosterone increases plasma volume, and thereby increases blood pressure. The adrenal cortex is highly sensitive to angiotensin II; as a result, angiotensin II can stimulate aldosterone release even when angiotensin II levels are too low to induce vasoconstriction. Aldosterone secretion is enhanced when sodium levels are low and when potassium levels are high.

*Alteration of Cardiac and Vascular Structure.* Recent data suggest that angiotensin II may cause pathologic

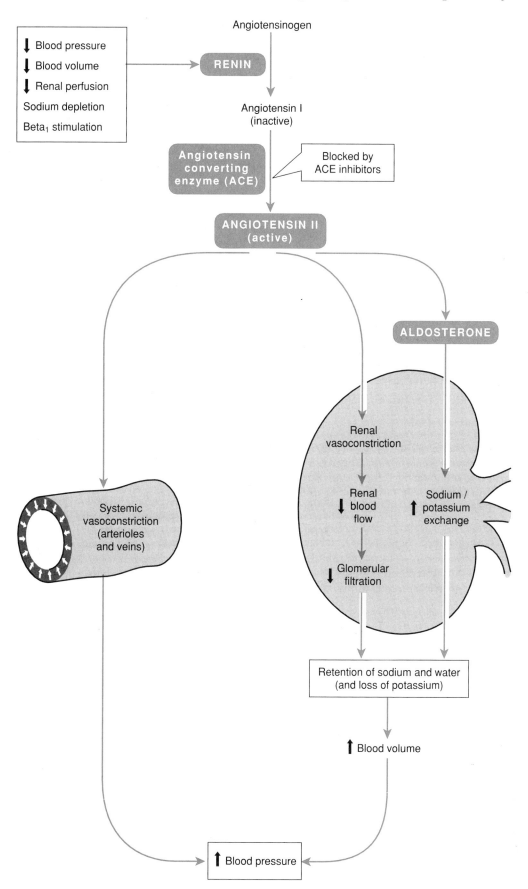

**Figure 41–1. Regulation of blood pressure by the renin-angiotensin system.**

structural changes in the heart and blood vessels. The compound is thought to cause both *hypertrophy* (increased mass of a structure) and *remodeling* (redistribution of mass within a structure). In hypertension, angiotensin II may be responsible for increasing the thickness of blood vessel walls; in atherosclerosis, it may be responsible for thickening the intimal surface of blood vessels; and in heart failure and myocardial infarction, it may be responsible for causing cardiac hypertrophy and fibrosis. Known effects of angiotensin II that could underlie these pathologic changes include:

- Increased migration, proliferation, and hypertrophy of vascular smooth muscle (VSM) cells.
- Increased production of extracellular matrix by VSM cells
- Hypertrophy of cardiac myocytes
- Increased production of extracellular matrix by cardiac fibroblasts

## Formation of Angiotensin II by Renin and Angiotensin-Converting Enzyme

As indicated in Figure 41-1, there are two reactions in the formation of angiotensin II. The first is catalyzed by renin, the second by angiotensin-converting enzyme.

### Renin

Renin (pronounced "ree′nin") catalyzes the formation of *angiotensin I* from *angiotensinogen*. This reaction is the rate-limiting step in angiotensin II formation. Renin is produced by juxtaglomerular cells of the kidney and undergoes controlled release into the bloodstream, where it converts angiotensinogen into angiotensin I.

***Regulation of Renin Release.*** Since renin catalyzes the rate-limiting step in angiotensin II formation, and since renin must be released into the blood in order to act, the factors that regulate renin release regulate the rate of angiotensin II formation.

As indicated in Figure 41-1, release of renin is triggered by multiple factors. Release *increases* in response to a *decline* in blood pressure, blood volume, plasma sodium content, or renal perfusion pressure. Reduced renal perfusion pressure is an especially important stimulant of renin release and can occur in response to (1) stenosis of the renal arteries, (2) reduced systemic blood pressure, and (3) reduced plasma volume (brought on by dehydration, hemorrhage, or chronic sodium depletion). For the most part, these factors increase renin release through effects exerted locally within the kidney. However, some of these factors may also promote renin release through activation of the sympathetic nervous system. Sympathetic nerves increase secretion of renin by causing stimulation of beta₁-adrenergic receptors on juxtaglomerular cells.

Release of renin is *suppressed* by factors opposite to those that cause release. That is, renin secretion is inhibited by elevation of blood pressure, elevation of blood volume, and elevation of plasma sodium content. Hence, as blood pressure, blood volume, and plasma sodium content increase in response to renin release, further release

of renin is suppressed. In this regard we can view release of renin as being regulated by a classic negative feedback loop.

### Angiotensin-Converting Enzyme (Kinase II)

Angiotensin-converting enzyme catalyzes the conversion of angiotensin I (inactive) into angiotensin II (highly active). ACE is located on the luminal surface of all blood vessels; the vasculature of the lungs is especially rich in the enzyme. Since ACE is present in abundance, conversion of angiotensin I into angiotensin II occurs almost instantaneously after angiotensin I has been formed. ACE is a relatively nonspecific enzyme that can act on a variety of substrates in addition to angiotensin I.

Nomenclature regarding ACE can be confusing and requires comment. As just noted, ACE can act on several substrates. When the substrate is angiotensin I, we refer to the enzyme as ACE. However, when the enzyme is acting on other substrates, we refer to it by different names. Of relevance to us, when the substrate is a hormone known as *bradykinin*, we refer to the enzyme as *kinase II*. So, please remember, whether we call it ACE or kinase II, we're talking about the same enzyme.

## Regulation of Blood Pressure by the Renin-Angiotensin System

The RAS is poised to help regulate blood pressure: factors that lower blood pressure turn the system on; factors that raise blood pressure turn the system off. However, although the RAS does indeed contribute to blood pressure control, its role in the *normovolemic, sodium-replete* individual is only modest. In contrast, the system can be a major factor in maintaining blood pressure in the presence of *hemorrhage*, *dehydration*, or *sodium depletion*.

As indicated in Figure 41-1, the RAS, acting through angiotensin II, raises blood pressure through two basic processes: vasoconstriction and renal retention of water and sodium. Vasoconstriction raises blood pressure by increasing total peripheral resistance; retention of water and sodium raises blood pressure by increasing blood volume. Vasoconstriction occurs within minutes to hours of activating the system, and hence can raise blood pressure rapidly. In contrast, days, weeks, or even months are required for the kidney to raise blood pressure by increasing blood volume.

As suggested by Figure 41-1, angiotensin II acts in two ways to promote renal retention of water. First, by constricting renal blood vessels, angiotensin II reduces renal blood flow, and thereby reduces glomerular filtration. Second, angiotensin II stimulates release of aldosterone from the adrenal cortex. Aldosterone then acts on the kidney to promote retention of sodium and water and excretion of potassium.

## Tissue (Local) Renin-Angiotensin Systems

In addition to the traditional RAS that we have been discussing, in which angiotensin II is produced in the blood and then carried to target tissues, it is now evident that angiotensin II can also be produced in individual tissues. This would allow for discrete, local effects of angiotensin II independent of the main system. There is speculation that interference with local production of angiotensin II may underlie some effects of the ACE inhibitors.

# Angiotensin-Converting Enzyme Inhibitors

The ACE inhibitors are important drugs for treating hypertension and heart failure. They are also used for myocardial infarction and kidney disease. Their most prominent adverse effects are cough, first-dose hypotension, and hyperkalemia. Since the introduction of captopril in the early 1970s, eight more ACE inhibitors have become available. For all of these agents, beneficial effects result from suppressing formation of angiotensin II.

## Captopril

Captopril [Capoten] was the first ACE inhibitor to be employed widely and will serve as our prototype for the family. The drug is administered orally to treat hypertension, heart failure, diabetic nephropathy, and myocardial infarction. The most common adverse effects of concern are cough, first-dose hypotension, and hyperkalemia.

### Overview of Pharmacologic Effects

Most beneficial effects of captopril result from inhibition of ACE. By inhibiting ACE, captopril inhibits production of angiotensin II, and thereby removes the influence of this powerful compound. The result is vasodilation (primarily in arterioles and to a lesser extent in veins), reduction of blood volume (through effects on the kidney), and prevention or reversal of possible angiotensin II–mediated pathologic changes in the heart and blood vessels.

Inhibition of kinase II (the name for ACE when the substrate is bradykinin) also contributes to beneficial effects. By inhibiting kinase II, captopril prevents the breakdown of bradykinin, a potent vasodilator. By preserving bradykinin, captopril has a second mechanism for promoting vasodilation.

Certain adverse effects are also related to inhibition of ACE/kinase II. Inhibition of ACE can cause hypotension, hyperkalemia, renal failure, and fetal injury. Inhibition of kinase II, with resultant accumulation of bradykinin, can cause cough and angioedema.

### Pharmacokinetics

Captopril is rapidly absorbed following oral administration. The extent of absorption is about 70%. Absorption can be reduced significantly by food; accordingly, captopril should be administered at least 1 hour before meals. Elimination is rapid: the plasma half-life of the drug is less than 2 hours. Approximately 50% of each dose is excreted unchanged in the urine. Hence, in patients with renal impairment, the drug may accumulate to toxic levels if the dosage is not reduced.

### Therapeutic Uses

*Hypertension.* Captopril has broad applications in hypertension. The drug is especially effective against malignant hypertension and hypertension secondary to renal arterial stenosis. Captopril is also useful against essential hypertension of mild to moderate intensity; in this disorder, maximal benefits may take several weeks to develop.

The mechanism by which captopril lowers blood pressure in essential hypertension is not completely understood. *Initial* responses are proportional to circulating angiotensin II levels and are clearly related to reduced formation of the compound. (By lowering angiotensin II levels, captopril dilates blood vessels and reduces blood volume; both actions help lower blood pressure.) However, with *prolonged* therapy, blood pressure often undergoes an additional decline. During this second phase, there is no correspondence between reductions in blood pressure and reductions in *circulating* angiotensin II levels. It may be that the delayed response is due to reductions in *local* angiotensin II levels—reductions that would not be revealed by measuring angiotensin II in the blood.

Captopril offers several advantages over most other antihypertensive drugs. In contrast to the sympatholytic agents, captopril does not interfere with cardiovascular reflexes. Hence, exercise capacity is not impaired and orthostatic hypotension is minimal. In addition, captopril can be used safely in patients with bronchial asthma, a condition that precludes the use of beta$_2$-adrenergic antagonists. Captopril does not promote hypokalemia, hyperuricemia, or hyperglycemia—side effects seen with thiazide diuretics. Lastly, captopril does not induce lethargy, weakness, or sexual dysfunction—responses that are common with other antihypertensive agents.

The use of ACE inhibitors in hypertension is discussed further in Chapter 44.

*Heart Failure.* Captopril produces multiple benefits in heart failure. By lowering arteriolar tone, captopril improves regional blood flow and, by reducing cardiac afterload, increases cardiac output. By causing venous dilation, the drug reduces pulmonary congestion and peripheral edema. By dilating blood vessels in the kidney, the drug increases renal blood flow, and thereby promotes excretion of sodium and water. This loss of fluid has two beneficial effects: (1) it helps reduce edema, and (2) by lowering blood volume, it decreases venous return to the heart, thereby reducing right-heart size. Lastly, by reducing local production of angiotensin II in the heart, ACE inhibitors may suppress growth of myocytes, and may thereby prevent pathologic thickening of the ventricular wall. The use of ACE inhibitors in heart failure is discussed further in Chapter 46.

*Myocardial Infarction.* In recent years, captopril has been shown to reduce mortality following acute myocardial infarction (heart attack). In addition, the drug decreases the chance of developing overt heart failure. Treatment should begin as soon as possible after infarction and should continue for at least 6 weeks. In patients who develop overt heart failure, treatment should continue long term. As for patients who do not develop heart failure, there are no data to indicate whether continued treatment would be beneficial or not.

**Diabetic and Nondiabetic Nephropathy.** Captopril is approved for treatment of diabetic nephropathy, the leading cause of end-stage renal disease in the United States. In patients with overt nephropathy, as indicated by proteinuria of more than 500 mg/day, captopril can slow progression of renal disease. In patients with less advanced nephropathy (30 to 300 mg proteinuria/day), captopril can delay onset of overt nephropathy. These benefits were first demonstrated in patients with insulin-dependent diabetes mellitus (type I diabetes) and were later demonstrated in patients with non-insulin-dependent diabetes mellitus (type II diabetes). Most recently, ACE inhibitors have been shown to provide similar protection in patients with nephropathy unrelated to diabetes.

The principal protective mechanism appears to be reduction of glomerular filtration pressure. Captopril lowers filtration pressure by reducing levels of angiotensin II, which can raise filtration pressure by two mechanisms. First, angiotensin II raises systemic blood pressure, which raises pressure in the afferent arteriole of the glomerulus (Fig. 41-2). Second, it constricts the efferent arteriole, thereby generating backpressure in the glomerulus. The resultant increase in filtration pressure promotes injury. By reducing levels of angiotensin II, ACE inhibitors lower glomerular filtration pressure, and thereby slow development of renal injury.

### Adverse Effects

Captopril is generally well tolerated. In a group of patients receiving high-dose therapy (about 350 mg/day), less than 12% discontinued treatment because of intolerable reactions. The incidence of adverse effects can be minimized by using low doses (less than 150 mg/day).

**First-Dose Hypotension.** A precipitous drop in blood pressure may occur following the first dose of captopril and other ACE inhibitors. This reaction is caused by widespread vasodilation secondary to abrupt lowering of angiotensin II levels. First-dose hypotension is most likely in patients with severe hypertension, in patients taking diuretics, and in patients who are sodium depleted or volume depleted. To minimize the first-dose effect, initial doses should be low. Also, diuretics should be temporarily discontinued, starting 2 to 3 days before initiating captopril therapy. Blood pressure should be monitored for several hours following the first captopril dose. If hypotension develops, the patient should assume a supine position. If necessary, blood pressure can be raised with an infusion of normal saline.

**Cough.** Persistent, dry, irritating, nonproductive cough can develop with captopril and other ACE inhibitors. This reaction occurs in 5% of patients and is the most common reason for discontinuing therapy. Cough is more troublesome when the patient is supine, and occurs more in women than in men. Cough begins to subside 3 days after discontinuing ACE inhibitors and is gone within 10 days. Cough is caused by accumulation of bradykinin.

**Hyperkalemia.** Inhibition of aldosterone release (secondary to inhibition of angiotensin II production) can cause potassium retention by the kidney. As a rule, significant potassium accumulation is limited to patients taking potassium supplements or a potassium-sparing diuretic. For most other patients, hyperkalemia is rare. Patients should be instructed to avoid potassium supplements and potassium-containing salt substitutes unless they are prescribed by the physician.

**Renal Failure.** ACE inhibitors can cause severe renal insufficiency in patients with bilateral renal artery stenosis or stenosis in the artery to a single remaining kidney. In the presence of renal artery stenosis, the kidneys release large amounts of renin. The resulting high levels of angiotensin II serve to maintain glomerular filtration by two mechanisms: (1) elevation of blood pressure and (2) constriction of efferent glomerular arterioles (Fig. 41-2). When ACE is inhibited in these patients, causing angiotensin II levels to fall, the mechanisms that had been maintaining glomerular filtration fail, causing urine production to drop precipitously. Not surprisingly, *ACE inhibitors are contraindicated for patients with bilateral renal artery stenosis.*

**Fetal Injury.** Use of ACE inhibitors during the *second* and *third* trimesters of pregnancy can injure the developing fetus. Specific effects include hypotension, hyperkalemia, skull hypoplasia, anuria, renal failure (reversible and irreversible), and death. Women who become pregnant while using ACE inhibitors should discontinue treatment as soon as possible. Infants who have been exposed to ACE inhibitors during the second or third trimester should be closely monitored for hypotension, oliguria, and hyperkalemia. Exposure to ACE inhibitors during the first trimester is not associated with fetal injury; pregnant women who have taken ACE inhibitors during the *first* trimester should be told this.

**Angioedema.** Angioedema is a rare and potentially fatal reaction. Symptoms, which result from increased capillary permeability, include giant wheals and edema of the tongue, glottis, and pharynx. Severe reactions should be

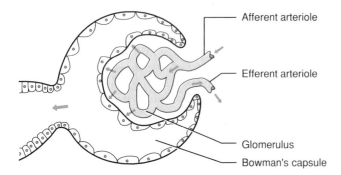

**Figure 41–2. Elevation of glomerular filtration pressure by angiotensin II.** Angiotensin II increases filtration pressure by (1) increasing pressure in the afferent arteriole (secondary to increasing systemic arterial pressure), and (2) constricting the efferent arteriole, thereby generating backpressure in the glomerulus.

Afferent arteriole

Efferent arteriole

Glomerulus

Bowman's capsule

treated with subcutaneous epinephrine. If angioedema develops, captopril should be discontinued and never used again. Angioedema is caused by accumulation of bradykinin.

**Dysgeusia and Rash.** Dysgeusia (impaired or distorted sense of taste) and rash are common. Rashes (maculopapular, morbilliform, others) develop in up to 10% of patients. The incidence of dysgeusia is about 4%. For some patients, dysgeusia may result in anorexia and weight loss. If these complications arise, captopril should be withdrawn. Both reactions resolve following cessation of treatment. At one time, researchers thought that rash and dysgeusia were related to the sulfhydryl group in the captopril molecule. However, this appears to be untrue, since ACE inhibitors that lack a sulfhydryl group also cause these reactions.

**Neutropenia.** Neutropenia, with its associated risk of infection, is a rare but serious complication of therapy. Neutropenia is most likely in patients with renal impairment and in those with collagen vascular diseases (e.g., systemic lupus erythematosus, scleroderma). These patients should be followed closely. Fortunately, neutropenia is reversible if detected early. To promote early detection, a white blood cell count with differential should be obtained every 2 weeks during the first 3 months of therapy and periodically thereafter. If neutropenia develops, captopril should be withdrawn immediately; neutrophil counts should normalize in approximately 2 weeks. In the absence of early detection, neutropenia may progress to fatal agranulocytosis. Patients should be informed about early signs of infection (e.g., fever, sore throat) and instructed to report these immediately.

**Other Adverse Effects.** Captopril can cause a variety of *gastrointestinal disturbances* (e.g., nausea, vomiting, diarrhea, abdominal pain). *Neurologic effects* include headache, dizziness, fatigue, paresthesias, and insomnia.

## Drug Interactions

**Diuretics.** Diuretics may intensify first-dose hypotension. To prevent this interaction, diuretics should be withdrawn 2 to 3 days prior to initiating treatment with captopril. Diuretic therapy can be resumed later if needed.

**Antihypertensive Agents.** The hypotensive effects of captopril are often additive with those of other antihypertensive drugs (e.g., diuretics, sympatholytics, vasodilators, calcium channel blockers). When captopril is added to an antihypertensive regimen, dosages of other drugs may require reduction.

**Drugs That Raise Potassium Levels.** Captopril increases the risk of hyperkalemia caused by *potassium supplements* and *potassium-sparing diuretics*. The risk of hyperkalemia is increased because, by suppressing aldosterone secretion, captopril can reduce excretion of potassium. To minimize the risk of hyperkalemia, potassium supplements and potassium-sparing diuretics should be employed only when clearly indicated.

**Lithium.** ACE inhibitors can make lithium accumulate to toxic levels. Lithium levels should be monitored frequently.

### Preparations, Dosage, and Administration

**Preparations.** Captopril [Capoten] is dispensed in tablets (12.5, 25, 50, and 100 mg) for oral use. Also, the drug is available in fixed-dose combination formulations with hydrochlorothiazide under the trade name Capozide.

**Dosage and Administration.** Captopril should be taken 1 hour before meals. Dosage must be individualized. For adults with *hypertension*, the usual starting dosage is 25 mg 3 times a day. For patients at high risk of first-dose hypotension, a smaller initial dosage should be employed (e.g., 6.25 mg 3 times a day). To achieve an optimum response, the dosage is gradually increased (to a maximum of 450 mg/day). Dosage must be lowered in patients with renal disease.

Dosages for *heart failure*, *myocardial infarction*, and *diabetic nephropathy* are summarized in Table 41-1.

## Enalapril and Enalaprilat

Enalapril [Vasotec] is a prodrug that must be converted into its active form—enalaprilat—by the liver. Enalaprilat is a potent inhibitor of ACE.

**Actions and Uses.** Enalapril has pharmacologic actions and therapeutic uses like those of captopril. Approved indications are hypertension and heart failure.

**Pharmacokinetics.** Enalapril is rapidly absorbed from the GI tract, even in the presence of food. The extent of absorption is about 60%. Conversion to enalaprilat takes several hours. As a result, peak effects are delayed. Enalaprilat has a plasma half-life of 11 hours, considerably longer than that of captopril. Hence, unlike captopril, which must be administered 2 or 3 times a day, enalapril can be administered once or twice a day. Renal insufficiency delays excretion of enalapril, and can thereby promote drug accumulation. To avoid accumulation, dosage should be reduced in the presence of kidney disease.

**Adverse Effects and Interactions.** Enalapril is generally well tolerated. Like captopril, enalapril can cause first-dose hypotension, persistent cough, hyperkalemia, angioedema, and renal failure (in patients with renal artery stenosis). Common but less serious reactions include headache (5%), dizziness (5%), and fatigue (3%). Neutropenia and proteinuria have been reported. Rash and dysgeusia occur, but less frequently than with captopril. Like captopril, enalapril has important interactions with diuretics, antihypertensive agents, potassium supplements, potassium-sparing diuretics, and lithium.

**Preparations, Dosage, and Administration.** *Oral.* Enalapril maleate [Vasotec] is available in tablets (2.5, 5, 10, and 20 mg) for oral use. In contrast to captopril, enalapril may be administered with meals.

For patients with *hypertension*, the initial daily dosage is 2.5 mg for those taking diuretics and for those with kidney disease. An initial dosage of 5 mg/day is appropriate for most other patients. Maintenance dosages range from 10 to 40 mg/day.

For patients with *heart failure*, the usual maintenance dosage is 5 to 20 mg/day administered in two equally divided doses.

*Intravenous.* The active form of enalapril (enalaprilat) [Vasotec I.V.] is available in solution (1.25 mg/ml) for intravenous administration. The initial dose is 1.25 mg administered over 5 minutes. Doses may be increased up to 5 mg and may be repeated every 6 hours for up to 48 hours.

### Newer Ace Inhibitors: Benazepril, Fosinopril, Lisinopril, Moexipril, Quinapril, Ramipril, and Trandolapril

In addition to captopril and enalapril, seven other ACE inhibitors are approved for use in the United States. All are similar to captopril. Their trade names, uses, and dosages are summarized in Table 41-1.

## TABLE 41-1. ACE INHIBITOR DOSAGES

| Drug | Approved Indications | Usual Maintenance Dosages* |
|---|---|---|
| Benazepril [Lotensin] | Hypertension | 20-40 mg/day in 1 or 2 doses |
| Captopril [Capoten] | Hypertension<br>Heart failure<br>LVD after MI†<br>Diabetic nephropathy | 50-150 mg bid or tid<br>50-100 mg bid<br>50 mg tid<br>25 mg tid |
| Enalapril [Vasotec] | Hypertension<br>Heart failure | 10-40 mg/day in 1 or 2 doses<br>5-20 mg/day in 2 doses |
| Enalaprilat [Vasotec I.V.] | Hypertension | 1.25 mg IV every 6 hours |
| Fosinopril [Monopril] | Hypertension<br>Heart failure | 20-80 mg/day in 1 or 2 doses<br>20-40 mg/day |
| Lisinopril [Prinivil, Zestril] | Hypertension<br>Heart failure<br>Acute MI‡ | 20-40 mg once daily<br>5-10 mg once daily<br>10 mg once daily |
| Moexipril [Univasc] | Hypertension | 7.5-30 mg/day in 1 or 2 doses |
| Quinapril [Accupril] | Hypertension<br>Heart failure | 20-40 mg/day in 1 or 2 doses<br>10-20 mg bid |
| Ramipril [Altace] | Hypertension | 2.5-20 mg/day in 1 or 2 doses |
| Trandolapril [Mavik] | Hypertension | 2-4 mg once daily |

*For all ACE inhibitors except fosinopril, dosage must be reduced in patients with significant renal dysfunction.
†Left ventricular dysfunction after myocardial infarction.
‡Acute myocardial infarction.

**Basic Pharmacology.** The newer ACE inhibitors have the same mechanism of action as captopril (inhibition of angiotensin-converting enzyme) and they all produce similar pharmacologic effects. All are approved for hypertension, and some are approved for heart failure. All share the same major adverse effects: persistent cough, first-dose hypotension, hyperkalemia, angioedema, and renal failure (if given to patients with bilateral renal artery stenosis). Furthermore, they all have important interactions with the same drugs: diuretics, antihypertensive agents, potassium supplements, potassium-sparing diuretics, and lithium. Except for lisinopril, all are prodrugs that undergo conversion to their active forms in the small intestine and liver.

**Dosage and Administration.** Like captopril, all of the newer ACE inhibitors are administered orally. However, they all differ from captopril in that (1) they can be administered with food (except moexipril), and (2) they have prolonged half-lives, and therefore can be administered once or twice daily. Dosages are summarized in Table 41-1. With the exception of fosinopril, all require a reduction in dosage for patients with renal insufficiency.

# Angiotensin II Receptor Antagonists

Drugs that block receptors for angiotensin II represent a new way to influence the renin-angiotensin system. At this time, only two such drugs—losartan and valsartan—are approved for clinical use. Other drugs in this class are under development.

## Losartan

Losartan was the first angiotensin II receptor blocker released for general use. The drug is approved only for hypertension. Losartan is available alone under the trade name Cozaar, and in combination with hydrochlorothiazide under the trade name Hyzaar.

**Pharmacologic Effects.** Losartan blocks the actions of angiotensin II at its receptors in blood vessels, the adrenals, and all other tissues. As a result, the effects of losartan are very similar to those of the ACE inhibitors. Like the ACE inhibitors, losartan causes prominent dilation of arterioles and less prominent dilation of veins. Also like the ACE inhibitors, losartan promotes renal excretion of sodium and water. In contrast to the ACE inhibitors, losartan does not cause a clinically significant increase in potassium levels, despite reductions in circulating aldosterone. Also, losartan does not inhibit kinase II, and hence does not increase levels of bradykinin; as a result, the drug does not cause cough or angioedema.

**Pharmacokinetics.** Losartan is rapidly absorbed following oral administration. However, first-pass metabolism limits bioavailability to about 30%. Once in the body, losartan is partially converted to a metabolite that is more active than losartan itself. The half-life of losartan is about 2 hours; the half-life of the metabolite is 6 to 9 hours. Both losartan and the metabolite are highly bound (about 99%) to plasma proteins. Elimination is primarily via the bile.

***Therapeutic Use.*** Losartan is approved only for treatment of hypertension. Blood pressure reductions equal those seen with enalapril. The usual dosage is 50 mg once a day. Possible benefits for patients with heart failure, myocardial infarction, or renal impairment have not been established.

***Adverse Effects.*** Aside from a low incidence of dizziness, losartan appears devoid of significant adverse effects. In contrast to ACE inhibitors, losartan does not cause cough or angioedema, presumably because it does not cause accumulation of bradykinin. Losartan also differs from the ACE inhibitors in that clinically significant hyperkalemia has not occurred.

***Contraindications.*** Like the ACE inhibitors, losartan is contraindicated for pregnant women during the second and third trimesters and for patients with bilateral renal artery stenosis or stenosis in the artery to a single remaining kidney.

### Valsartan

Valsartan [Diovan] is the second angiotensin II receptor blocker to become available in the United States. Like losartan, the drug is approved only for hypertension. The optimal dosage is 80 to 160 mg once a day. Effects of a single dose begin 2 hours after dosing and peak within 6 hours. With repeated doses, antihypertensive effects increase, reaching a maximum after 4 weeks. Valsartan is well tolerated. Side effects are generally mild and transient. Headache and dizziness occur occasionally. Like losartan, and unlike ACE inhibitors, valsartan does not cause cough or angioedema.

## KEY POINTS

- The RAS helps regulate blood pressure, blood volume, and fluid and electrolyte balance.
- The RAS acts through production of angiotensin II.
- Angiotensin II has much greater biologic activity than angiotensin I or angiotensin III.
- Angiotensin II is formed by the actions of two enzymes: renin and ACE.
- Angiotensin II causes vasoconstriction (primarily in arterioles) and release of aldosterone. Angiotensin II may also mediate pathologic changes in the heart and blood vessels.
- The RAS raises blood pressure by causing vasoconstriction and by increasing blood volume (secondary to renal retention of sodium and water).
- In addition to the traditional RAS, in which angiotensin II is produced in the blood and then carried to target tissues, angiotensin II can also be produced locally by tissue-based renin-angiotensin systems.
- Beneficial effects of ACE inhibitors result primarily from inhibition of ACE and partly from inhibition of kinase II.
- By inhibiting ACE, ACE inhibitors decrease production of angiotensin II. The result is vasodilation, decreased blood volume, and, possibly, prevention or reversal of angiotensin II–mediated pathologic changes in the heart and blood vessels.
- ACE inhibitors are used to treat hypertension, heart failure, myocardial infarction, and nephropathy (both diabetic and nondiabetic).
- ACE inhibitors can cause serious first-dose hypotension by causing a sharp drop in circulating angiotensin II.
- Cough, secondary to accumulation of bradykinin, is the most common reason for discontinuing ACE inhibitor therapy.
- By suppressing aldosterone release, ACE inhibitors can cause hyperkalemia. Exercise caution in patients taking potassium supplements or potassium-sparing diuretics.
- ACE inhibitors are dangerous to the fetus during the second and third trimesters but not during the first trimester.
- Losartan acts by blocking receptors for angiotensin II.
- The effects of losartan are much like those of the ACE inhibitors, except that losartan does not cause cough, angioedema, or clinically significant hyperkalemia.

# Summary of Major Nursing Implications*

## Angiotensin-Converting Enzyme Inhibitors

| | |
|---|---|
| Benazepril | Lisinopril |
| Captopril | Moexipril |
| Enalapril | Quinapril |
| Enalaprilat | Ramipril |
| Fosinopril | Trandolapril |

Unless indicated otherwise, the implications summarized below pertain to all of the ACE inhibitors.

## Preadministration Assessment

### Therapeutic Goal

Reduction of blood pressure in patients with hypertension (all ACE inhibitors).

Hemodynamic improvement in patients with heart failure *(captopril, enalapril, fosinopril, lisinopril, quinapril)*.

Slowed progression of diabetic nephropathy *(captopril)*.

Reduction of mortality following acute myocardial infarction *(lisinopril)*.

## Baseline Data

Determine blood pressure and obtain a white blood cell count and differential.

## Identifying High-Risk Patients

ACE inhibitors are *contraindicated* during the *second and third trimesters of pregnancy* and for patients with *bilateral renal artery stenosis* (or stenosis in the artery to a single remaining kidney) or a *history of hypersensitivity reactions* (especially angioedema) *to ACE inhibitors*. Exercise *caution* in patients with *salt or volume depletion*, *renal impairment*, or *collagen disease*, and in those taking *potassium supplements*, *potassium-sparing diuretics*, or *lithium*.

## Implementation: Administration

### Routes

**Oral.** All ACE inhibitors.

**Intravenous.** *Enalaprilat* only.

### Dosage and Administration

Begin therapy with low doses and then gradually increase the dosage. Instruct patients to administer *captopril* and *moexipril* at least 1 hour before meals.

## Ongoing Evaluation and Interventions

### Monitoring Summary

Monitor blood pressure closely for 2 hours after the first dose and periodically thereafter. Obtain a white blood cell count and differential every 2 weeks for the first 3 months of therapy and periodically thereafter.

### Evaluating Therapeutic Effects

**Hypertension.** Monitor for reduced blood pressure. The usual target pressure is systolic/diastolic of 140/90 mm Hg.

**Heart Failure.** Monitor for lessening of signs and symptoms (e.g., dyspnea, cyanosis, jugular vein distention, edema).

**Diabetic Nephropathy.** Monitor for proteinuria.

### Minimizing Adverse Effects

**First-Dose Hypotension.** Severe hypotension can occur with the first dose. Minimize hypotension with low initial doses and by withdrawing diuretics 1 week before treatment. Monitor blood pressure for 2 hours following the first dose. Instruct patients to lie down if hypotension develops. If necessary, infuse normal saline to restore pressure.

**Cough.** Warn patients about the possibility of persistent, dry, irritating, nonproductive cough. Instruct them to consult the physician if cough is bothersome. It may be necessary to discontinue the ACE inhibitor.

**Hyperkalemia.** ACE inhibitors may increase potassium levels. Instruct patients to avoid potassium supplements, potassium-containing salt substitutes, and potassium-sparing diuretics unless they are prescribed by the physician.

**Fetal Injury.** Warn women of child-bearing age that use of ACE inhibitors during the *second* and *third* trimesters of pregnancy can cause fetal injury (hypotension, hyperkalemia, skull hypoplasia, anuria, reversible and irreversible renal failure, death). If the patient becomes pregnant, withdraw ACE inhibitors as soon as possible. Closely monitor infants who have been exposed to ACE inhibitors during the second or third trimester for hypotension, oliguria, and hyperkalemia. Reassure women who took ACE inhibitors during the *first* trimester that this does *not* represent a risk to the fetus.

**Angioedema.** This is a rare and potentially fatal reaction whose symptoms include giant wheals and edema of the tongue, glottis, and pharynx. If angioedema occurs, discontinue the ACE inhibitor and never use it again. Treat severe reactions with subcutaneous epinephrine.

**Renal Failure.** Renal failure is a risk for patients with bilateral renal artery stenosis or stenosis in the artery to a single remaining kidney. ACE inhibitors are contraindicated for these people.

**Rash and Dysgeusia** (mainly with *captopril*). Minimize these reactions by avoiding high doses. Instruct patients to notify the physician if rash or dysgeusia persists. If dysgeusia results in anorexia and weight loss, withdraw the drug. Rash and dysgeusia resolve with cessation of treatment.

**Neutropenia** (mainly with *captopril*). Neutropenia poses a high risk of infection. Inform patients about early signs of infection (fever, sore throat, mouth sores) and instruct them to notify the physician if these occur. Obtain white blood cell counts and differential every 2 weeks during the first 3 months of therapy and periodically thereafter. If neutropenia develops, withdraw the drug immediately; neutrophil counts should normalize in approximately 2 weeks. Neutropenia is most likely in patients with renal impairment and collagen vascular diseases (e.g., systemic lupus erythematosus, scleroderma); monitor these patients closely.

### Minimizing Adverse Interactions

**Diuretics.** Diuretics may intensify first-dose hypotension. Withdraw diuretics 1 week prior to beginning an ACE inhibitor. Diuretics may be resumed later if needed.

**Antihypertensive Agents.** The effects of ACE inhibitors are additive with those of other antihypertensive drugs (e.g., diuretics, sympatholytics, vasodilators, calcium channel blockers). When an ACE inhibitor is added to an antihypertensive regimen, dosages of the other drugs may require reduction.

**Drugs That Elevate Potassium Levels.** ACE inhibitors increase the risk of hyperkalemia associated with *potassium supplements* and *potassium-sparing diuretics*. Risk can be minimized by avoiding potassium supplements and potassium-sparing diuretics except when they are clearly indicated.

**Lithium.** ACE inhibitors can increase serum levels of lithium, causing toxicity. Monitor lithium levels frequently.

# CHAPTER 42

# Calcium Channel Blockers

Calcium channel blockers are drugs that prevent calcium ions from entering cells. These drugs have their greatest effects on the heart and blood vessels. Calcium channel blockers are used widely to treat hypertension, angina pectoris, and cardiac dysrhythmias. Prototypes for the family are nifedipine [Adalat, Procardia] and verapamil [Calan, Isoptin]. Alternative names for the calcium channel blockers are *calcium antagonists* and *slow channel blockers*.

## Calcium Channels: Physiologic Functions and Consequences of Blockade

Calcium channels are gated pores in the cytoplasmic membrane that regulate the entry of calcium ions into cells. Calcium entry plays a critical role in the function of vascular smooth muscle and the heart.

### Vascular Smooth Muscle

The role of calcium channels in vascular smooth muscle (VSM) is to regulate contraction. When an action potential travels down the surface of a smooth muscle cell, calcium channels open and calcium ions flow inward, thereby initiating the contractile process. If calcium channels are blocked, contraction will be prevented and vasodilation will result.

At therapeutic doses, calcium channel blockers act selectively on *peripheral arterioles* and *arteries and arterioles of the heart*. These drugs have no significant effect on veins.

### Heart

In the heart, calcium channels help regulate function of the myocardium, the sinoatrial (SA) node, and the atri-

oventricular (AV) node. Calcium channels at all three sites are coupled to beta$_1$-adrenergic receptors.

**Myocardium.** In cardiac muscle, calcium entry has a positive inotropic effect. That is, calcium increases force of contraction. If calcium channels in atrial and ventricular muscle are blocked, contractile force will diminish.

**SA Node.** Pacemaker activity of the SA node is regulated by calcium influx. When calcium channels are open, spontaneous discharge of the SA node increases. Conversely, when calcium channels close, pacemaker activity declines. Hence, the effect of calcium channel blockade is to reduce heart rate.

**AV Node.** Impulses that originate in the SA node must pass through the AV node on their way to the ventricles. As a result, regulation of AV conduction plays a critical role in coordinating contraction of the ventricles with contraction of the atria.

The excitability of AV nodal cells is regulated by calcium entry. When calcium channels are open, calcium entry increases and cells of the AV node discharge more readily. Conversely, when calcium channels are closed, discharge of AV nodal cells is suppressed. Hence, the effect of calcium channel blockade is to decrease velocity of conduction through the AV node.

***Coupling of Cardiac Calcium Channels to Beta$_1$-Adrenergic Receptors.*** In the heart, calcium channels are coupled to beta$_1$-adrenergic receptors (see Fig. 42-1). As a result, when cardiac beta$_1$ receptors are activated, calcium influx is enhanced. Conversely, when beta$_1$ receptors are blocked, calcium influx is suppressed. Because of this relationship between calcium channels and beta$_1$ receptors, calcium channel blockers and beta blockers have identical effects on the heart. That is, both drug families reduce force of contraction, slow heart rate, and suppress conduction through the AV node.

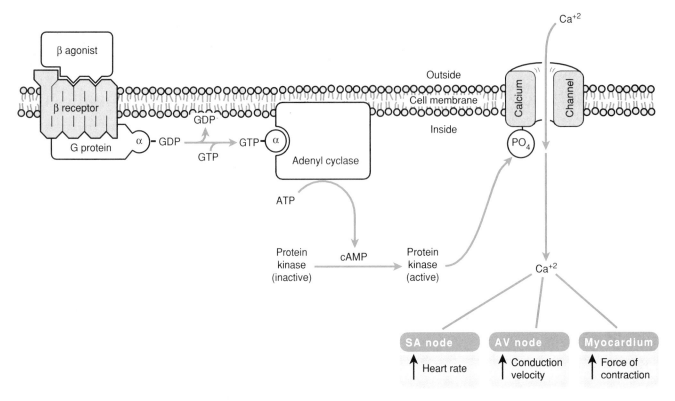

**Figure 42–1. Coupling of cardiac calcium channels with beta₁-adrenergic receptors.** In the heart, beta₁ receptors are coupled to calcium channels. As a result, when cardiac beta₁ receptors are activated, calcium influx is enhanced. The process works as follows. Binding of an agonist (e.g., norepinephrine) causes a conformational change in the beta receptor, which in turn causes a change in G protein, converting it from an inactive state (in which GDP is bound to the alpha subunit) to an active state (in which GTP is bound to the alpha subunit). (G protein is so named because it binds guanine nucleotides: GDP and GTP.) Following activation, the alpha subunit dissociates from the rest of G protein and activates adenylyl cyclase, an enzyme that converts ATP to cyclic AMP (cAMP). Cyclic AMP then activates protein kinase, an enzyme that phosphorylates proteins—in this case, the calcium channel. Phosphorylation changes the channel such that calcium entry is enhanced when the channel opens. (Opening of the channel is triggered by a change in membrane voltage [i.e., by passage of an action potential].)

The effect of calcium entry on cardiac function is determined by the type of cell involved. If the cell is in the SA node, heart rate increases; if the cell is in the AV node, impulse conduction through the node slows; and if the cell is part of the myocardium, force of contraction is increased.

Since binding of a single agonist molecule to a single beta receptor stimulates the synthesis of many cAMP molecules, with the subsequent activation of many protein kinase molecules, causing the phosphorylation of many calcium channels, this system can greatly amplify the signal initiated by the agonist.

## Calcium Channel Blockers: Classification and Sites of Action

### Classification

The calcium channel blockers used in the United States belong to three chemical families (Table 42-1). The largest family is the *dihydropyridines*, for which *nifedipine* is the prototype. This family name is encountered frequently and is worth remembering. The other two families consist of orphans: *verapamil* is the only *phenylalkylamine*, and *diltiazem* is the only *benzothiazepine*. The drug names are important; the family names are not.

### Sites of Action

At therapeutic doses, the dihydropyridines act primarily on arterioles; in contrast, verapamil and diltiazem act on

arterioles *and* the heart (Table 42-1). However, although dihydropyridines don't affect the heart at *therapeutic* doses, *toxic* doses can produce dangerous cardiac suppression (just like verapamil and diltiazem). The differences in selectivity among calcium channel blockers are based on structural differences among the drugs themselves and structural differences among calcium channels.

## Verapamil and Diltiazem: Agents That Act on Vascular Smooth Muscle and the Heart

### Verapamil

Verapamil [Calan, Isoptin, Verelan] blocks calcium channels in blood vessels and the heart. Major indications are angina

## TABLE 42-1. CALCIUM CHANNEL BLOCKERS: CLASSIFICATION AND SITES OF ACTION

| Classification* | Sites of Action |
|---|---|
| *Dihydropyridines* | |
| Nifedipine | Arterioles |
| Amlodipine | Arterioles |
| Felodipine | Arterioles |
| Isradipine | Arterioles |
| Nicardipine | Arterioles |
| Nimodipine | Arterioles |
| Nislodipine | Arterioles |
| *Phenylalkylamines* | |
| Verapamil | Arterioles/Heart |
| *Benzothiazepines* | |
| Diltiazem | Arterioles/Heart |

*A fourth class—diarylaminopropylamine ethers—has one member: *bepridil*. Bepridil can cause serious dysrhythmias and is reserved for patients who don't respond to safer calcium channel blockers.

pectoris, essential hypertension, and cardiac dysrhythmias. Verapamil was the first calcium channel blocker available and will serve as our prototype for the group.

### Hemodynamic Effects

The overall hemodynamic response to verapamil is the net result of (1) direct effects on the heart and blood vessels and (2) reflex responses.

*Direct Effects.* By blocking calcium channels in the heart and blood vessels, verapamil has five direct effects: (1) blockade at peripheral arterioles causes dilation, and thereby reduces arterial pressure; (2) blockade at arteries and arterioles of the heart increases coronary perfusion; (3) blockade at the SA node reduces heart rate; (4) blockade at the AV node decreases AV nodal conduction; and (5) blockade in the myocardium decreases force of contraction. Of the effects on the heart, reduced AV conduction is the most important.

*Indirect (Reflex) Effects.* Verapamil-induced lowering of blood pressure activates the baroreceptor reflex, causing increased firing of sympathetic nerves to the heart. Norepinephrine released from these nerves acts to increase heart rate, AV conduction, and force of contraction. However, since these same three parameters are suppressed by the direct actions of verapamil, the direct and indirect effects tend to negate each other.

*Net Effect.* Since the direct effects of verapamil on the heart are counterbalanced by indirect effects, the drug has little or no net effect on cardiac performance: for most patients, heart rate, AV conduction, and contractility are not noticeably altered. Consequently, the overall cardiovascular effect of verapamil is simply vasodilation accompanied by reduced arterial pressure and increased coronary perfusion.

### Pharmacokinetics

Verapamil may be administered orally and intravenously. The drug is well absorbed following oral ad-

ministration, but undergoes extensive metabolism on its first pass through the liver. Consequently, only about 20% of an oral dose reaches the systemic circulation. Effects begin in 30 minutes and peak within 5 hours. Elimination is primarily by hepatic metabolism. Because the drug is eliminated by the liver, doses must be reduced substantially in patients with liver dysfunction.

### Therapeutic Uses

*Angina Pectoris.* Verapamil is used widely to treat angina pectoris. The drug is approved for vasospastic angina and effort-induced angina. Benefits in both types of angina derive from vasodilation. The role of verapamil in antianginal therapy is discussed further in Chapter 45.

*Essential Hypertension.* Verapamil is a first-line drug for chronic hypertension. The drug lowers blood pressure by promoting dilation of arterioles. The role of verapamil and other calcium channel blockers in hypertension is discussed in Chapter 44.

*Cardiac Dysrhythmias.* Verapamil is used to slow ventricular rate in patients with atrial flutter, atrial fibrillation, and paroxysmal supraventricular tachycardia. Benefits derive from suppressing impulse conduction through the AV node, which prevents the atria from driving the ventricles at an excessive rate. Antidysrhythmic applications are discussed in Chapter 48.

*Migraine.* Verapamil can reduce symptoms of migraine headache. This application is discussed in Chapter 28.

### Adverse Effects

*Common Effects.* Verapamil is generally well tolerated. *Constipation* occurs frequently and is the most common cause of complaints. This problem, which can be especially severe in the elderly, can be minimized by increasing dietary fluids and fiber. Constipation results from blockade of calcium channels in smooth muscle of the intestine. Other common effects—*dizziness, facial flushing, headache,* and *edema of the ankles and feet*—occur secondary to vasodilation. *Gingival hyperplasia* (overgrowth of gum tissue) may also develop.

*Cardiac Effects.* Blockade of calcium channels in the heart can compromise cardiac function. In the SA node, calcium channel blockade can cause bradycardia; in the AV node, blockade can cause partial or complete AV block; and in the myocardium, blockade can decrease contractility. When the heart is healthy, these effects are minimal. However, in patients with certain cardiac diseases, verapamil can seriously exacerbate dysfunction. Accordingly, the drug must be used with special caution in patients with cardiac failure, and must not be used at all in patients with sick sinus syndrome or second-degree or third-degree AV block.

### Drug Interactions

*Digoxin.* Like verapamil, digoxin suppresses impulse conduction through the AV node. Accordingly, when these drugs are used concurrently, the risk of AV block is increased. Patients receiving the combination should be monitored closely.

Verapamil increases plasma levels of digoxin by about 60%, thereby increasing the risk of digoxin toxicity. If toxicity begins to develop, the dosage of digoxin should be reduced.

**Beta-Adrenergic Blocking Agents.** Beta blockers and verapamil blockers have the same effects on the heart: decreased heart rate, decreased AV conduction, and decreased contractility. Hence, when a beta blocker and verapamil are used concurrently, there is a risk of excessive cardiosuppression. To minimize this risk, beta blockers and *intravenous* verapamil should be administered several hours apart from each other.

### Toxicity

*Clinical Manifestations.* Overdose can produce severe hypotension and cardiotoxicity (bradycardia, AV block, ventricular tachydysrhythmias).

*Treatment.* General Measures. Verapamil can be removed from the gastrointestinal tract with an emetic or with gastric lavage followed by a cathartic. Intravenous calcium gluconate can counteract both vasodilation and negative inotropic effects, but will not reverse AV block.

Hypotension. Hypotension can be treated with intravenous norepinephrine, which promotes vasoconstriction (by activating alpha$_1$ receptors on blood vessels) and increases cardiac output (by activating beta$_1$ receptors in the heart). Placing the patient in Trendelenburg's position (inclined with the head down) and administering IV fluids may also help.

Bradycardia and AV Block. Bradycardia and AV block can be treated with isoproterenol (a beta-adrenergic agonist) and with atropine (an anticholinergic drug that will block parasympathetic influences on the heart). If pharmacologic measures are inadequate, electronic pacing may be required.

Ventricular Tachydysrhythmias. The preferred treatment for ventricular dysrhythmias is DC cardioversion. Antidysrhythmic drugs (procainamide, lidocaine) may also be tried.

### Preparations, Dosage, and Administration

*Oral.* Verapamil is available in regular tablets (40, 80, and 120 mg) as Calan and Isoptin; in sustained-release tablets (120, 180, and 240 mg) as Calan SR and Isoptin SR; and in sustained-release capsules (180 and 240 mg) as Verelan. The sustained-release formulations are approved only for essential hypertension. Instruct patients to swallow sustained-release formulations intact, without crushing or chewing.

The usual initial dosage for *angina pectoris* is 80 to 120 mg 3 times a day. The usual initial dosage for *essential hypertension* is 80 mg 3 times a day (using standard tablets) or 240 mg of a sustained-release formulation (administered once a day in the morning with food). Dosages should be reduced for elderly patients and for patients with advanced renal or liver disease. Dosages for dysrhythmias are presented in Chapter 48.

*Intravenous.* Intravenous verapamil [Isoptin] is used for cardiac dysrhythmias. Since IV verapamil can cause severe adverse cardiovascular effects, blood pressure and the electrocardiogram (EKG) should be monitored and equipment for resuscitation should be immediately available. Intravenous dosages for dysrhythmias are presented in Chapter 48.

### Diltiazem

Like verapamil, diltiazem [Cardizem, Dilacor] blocks calcium channels in the heart and blood vessels. As a result, the actions and applications of the two drugs are very similar.

*Hemodynamic Effects.* Diltiazem has the same effects on cardiovascular function as verapamil. Both drugs lower blood pressure through arteriolar dilation and, since their direct suppressant actions are balanced by reflex cardiac stimulation, both have little net effect on the heart.

*Therapeutic Uses.* Like verapamil, diltiazem is used for angina pectoris, essential hypertension, and cardiac dysrhythmias (atrial flutter, atrial fibrillation, paroxysmal supraventricular tachycardia).

*Pharmacokinetics.* Oral diltiazem is well absorbed and then extensively metabolized on its first pass through the liver. As a result, bioavailability is only about 50%. Effects begin rapidly (within a few minutes) and peak within half an hour. The drug undergoes nearly complete metabolism prior to elimination in the urine and feces.

*Adverse Effects.* The adverse effects of diltiazem are like those of verapamil, except that diltiazem causes less constipation. The most common effects are dizziness, flushing, headache, and edema of the ankles and feet. Like verapamil, diltiazem can exacerbate cardiac dysfunction in patients with bradycardia, sick sinus syndrome, heart failure, or second- or third-degree AV block.

*Drug Interactions.* Like verapamil, diltiazem can exacerbate digoxin-induced suppression of AV conduction, and can intensify the cardiosuppressant effects of beta blockers. Patients receiving diltiazem concurrently with digoxin or a beta blocker should be monitored closely for cardiac status.

*Preparations, Dosage, and Administration.* Oral diltiazem is available in standard tablets (30, 60, 90, and 120 mg) as Cardizem and in sustained-release capsules (60, 90, 120, 180, 240, and 300 mg) as Cardizem SR, Cardizem CD, and Dilacor XR. The drug is also available in solution (5 mg/ml) for intravenous administration. The usual initial dosage for hypertension is 180 mg once a day with Cardizem CD or 60 to 120 mg twice a day with Cardizem SR or Dilacor XR. Angina pectoris can be treated with standard tablets (30 mg 4 times a day initially and 60 mg 4 times a day for maintenance).

# Dihydropyridines: Agents That Act Mainly on Vascular Smooth Muscle

All of the drugs discussed in this section belong to the *dihydropyridine* family. At therapeutic doses, these drugs produce significant blockade of calcium channels in blood vessels and minimal blockade of calcium channels in the heart. The dihydropyridines are similar to verapamil in some respects but quite different in others.

## Nifedipine

Nifedipine [Adalat, Procardia] was the first dihydropyridine available and will serve as our prototype for the family. Like verapamil, nifedipine blocks calcium channels in VSM and thereby promotes vasodilation. However, in contrast to verapamil, nifedipine produces very little blockade of calcium channels in the heart. As a result, nifedipine cannot be used to treat dysrhythmias, does not cause adverse cardiac suppression, and is less likely than verapamil to exacerbate pre-existing cardiac disorders. Nifedipine also differs from verapamil in that nifedipine is more likely to cause reflex tachycardia. Contrasts between nifedipine and verapamil are summarized in Table 42–2.

## TABLE 42-2. COMPARISONS AND CONTRASTS BETWEEN NIFEDIPINE AND VERAPAMIL

| Property | Drug | |
|---|---|---|
| | Nifedipine | Verapamil |
| *Direct Effects on the Heart and Arterioles* | | |
| Arteriolar dilation | Yes | Yes |
| Effects on the heart | | |
| Reduced automaticity | No | Yes |
| Reduced AV conduction | No | Yes |
| Reduced contractile force | No | Yes |
| *Major Indications* | | |
| Hypertension | Yes | Yes |
| Angina pectoris (classic and variant) | Yes | Yes |
| Dysrhythmias | No | Yes |
| *Adverse Effects* | | |
| Exacerbation of | | |
| AV block | No | Yes |
| Sick sinus syndrome | No | Yes |
| Heart failure | No | Yes |
| Effects secondary to vasodilation | | |
| Edema (ankles and feet) | Yes | Yes |
| Flushing | Yes | Yes |
| Headaches | Yes | Yes |
| Dizziness | Yes | Yes |
| Reflex tachycardia | Yes | No |
| Constipation | No | Yes |
| *Drug Interactions* | | |
| Intensifies digoxin-induced AV block | No | Yes |
| Intensifies cardiosuppressant effects of beta blockers | No | Yes |
| Often combined with a beta blocker to suppress reflex tachycardia | Yes | No |

## Hemodynamic Effects

**Direct Effects.** The direct effects of nifedipine on the cardiovascular system are limited to blockade of calcium channels in vascular smooth muscle. Blockade of calcium channels in peripheral arterioles causes vasodilation, and thereby lowers arterial pressure. Blockade of calcium channels in arteries and arterioles of the heart increases coronary perfusion. Since nifedipine does not block cardiac calcium channels at usual therapeutic doses, the drug does not significantly reduce automaticity, AV conduction, or contractile force.

**Indirect (Reflex) Effects.** By lowering blood pressure, nifedipine activates the baroreceptor reflex, thereby causing sympathetic stimulation of the heart. Since nifedipine has minimal direct cardiosuppressant actions, cardiac stimulation is unopposed; hence, heart rate and contractile force increase.

It is important to note that reflex effects occur primarily with the *fast-acting* formulation of nifedipine—not with the sustained-release formulation. The reason is this: the baroreceptor reflex is turned on only by a *rapid* fall in blood pressure; a gradual decline will not activate the reflex. With the fast-acting formulation, blood levels of nifedipine rise quickly; hence blood pressure drops quickly and the reflex is activated. Conversely, with the sustained-release formulation, blood levels of nifedipine rise slowly; hence blood pressure falls slowly and the reflex is bypassed.

**Net Effect.** The overall hemodynamic response to nifedipine is simply the sum of its direct effect (vasodilation) and indirect effect (reflex cardiac stimulation). Hence, nifedipine (1) lowers blood pressure, (2) increases heart rate, and (3) increases contractile force. Please note, however, that the reflex increase in heart rate and contractile force are transient and occur primarily with the rapid-acting formulation.

### Pharmacokinetics

Nifedipine is well absorbed following oral administration, but undergoes extensive first-pass metabolism. As a result, only about 50% of an oral dose reaches the systemic circulation. With the fast-acting formulation, effects begin rapidly and peak in 30 minutes; with the sustained-release formulation, effects begin in

20 minutes and peak in 6 hours. The drug is fully metabolized prior to excretion in the urine.

## Therapeutic Uses

*Angina Pectoris.* Nifedipine is indicated for vasospastic angina and angina of effort. The drug is usually combined with a beta blocker to prevent reflex stimulation of the heart, which could intensify anginal pain. The role of nifedipine in angina is discussed further in Chapter 45.

*Hypertension.* Nifedipine is used widely to treat *essential hypertension and hypertensive emergencies.* For therapy of essential hypertension, only the sustained-release formulation is approved. The rapid-acting formulation is used for hypertensive emergencies. The use of calcium channel blockers in hypertensive states is discussed further in Chapter 44.

*Migraine.* Nifedipine has been used on an investigational basis to relieve migraine headache. This application is discussed in Chapter 28.

## Adverse Effects

Some adverse effects of nifedipine are like those of verapamil; others are quite different. Like verapamil, nifedipine can cause *flushing, dizziness, headache, peripheral edema,* and *gingival hyperplasia.* In contrast to verapamil, nifedipine does *not* cause much constipation. Also, since nifedipine causes minimal blockade of calcium channels in the heart, the drug is not likely to exacerbate AV block, heart failure, bradycardia, or sick sinus syndrome. Accordingly, nifedipine is preferred to verapamil for patients with these disorders.

A response that occurs with nifedipine that does not occur with verapamil is *reflex tachycardia.* This response is problematic in that it increases cardiac oxygen demand and can thereby increase pain in patients with angina. To prevent reflex tachycardia, nifedipine can be combined with a beta-adrenergic blocker (e.g., propranolol).

*Rapid-acting nifedipine* has been associated with increased mortality in patients with myocardial infarction and unstable angina. Also, other rapid-acting calcium channel blockers have been associated with an increased risk of myocardial infarction in patients with hypertension. However, in both cases, a cause-and-effect relationship has not been established. Nonetheless, the National Heart, Lung, and Blood Institute has recommended that rapid-acting nifedipine, especially in higher doses, be used with great caution, if at all. It is important to note that these adverse effects have not been associated with *sustained-release* nifedipine or with any other long-acting calcium channel blockers.

## Drug Interactions

*Beta-Adrenergic Blockers.* Beta blockers are combined with nifedipine to prevent reflex tachycardia. It is important to note that whereas beta blockers can *decrease* the adverse cardiac effects of *nifedipine,* they can *intensify* the adverse cardiac effects of *verapamil* and *diltiazem.*

## Toxicity

When taken in excessive dosage, nifedipine loses its selectivity. Hence, toxic doses affect the heart in addition to blood vessels. Consequently, the manifestations and treatment of nifedipine overdose are the same as those described above for verapamil.

### Preparations, Dosage, and Administration

Nifedipine is available in capsules (10 and 20 mg) as Adalat and Procardia and in sustained-release tablets (30, 60, and 90 mg) as Adalat CC and Procardia XL. Instruct patients to swallow sustained-release tablets whole, without crushing or chewing.

For treatment of *angina pectoris,* the usual initial dosage is 10 mg 3 times a day. The usual maintenance dosage is 10 to 20 mg 3 times a day. The maximum recommended dosage is 180 mg/day.

For *essential hypertension,* only the sustained-release tablets are approved. The usual initial dosage is 30 mg once a day.

### Other Dihydropyridines

All of these drugs are similar to nifedipine, the prototype of the dihydropyridines. Like nifedipine, these drugs produce greater blockade of calcium channels in VSM than in the heart.

*Nicardipine.* At therapeutic doses, nicardipine [Cardene, Cardene SR, Cardene I.V.] produces selective blockade of calcium channels in blood vessels and has minimal direct effects on the heart. The drug is indicated for essential hypertension and for effort-induced angina pectoris. The most common adverse effects are flushing, headache, asthenia (weakness), dizziness, palpitations, and edema of the ankles and feet. Gingival hyperplasia (overgrowth of gum tissue) has been reported. Like nifedipine, this drug can be combined safely with a beta-adrenergic blocker to promote therapeutic effects and suppress reflex tachycardia. Nicardipine is available in standard capsules (20 and 30 mg), sustained-release capsules (30, 45, and 60 mg), and an intravenous formulation (2.5 mg/ml). The usual initial dosage for angina pectoris is 20 mg 3 times a day using the standard capsules. The usual initial dosage for essential hypertension is 20 mg 3 times a day (using standard capsules) or 30 mg twice a day (using sustained-release capsules).

*Amlodipine.* At therapeutic doses, amlodipine [Norvasc] produces "selective" blockade of calcium channels in blood vessels, having minimal direct effects on the heart. Approved indications are essential hypertension and angina pectoris (effort induced and vasospastic). Amlodipine is administered orally and absorbed slowly; peak plasma levels develop in 6 to 12 hours. The drug has a long half-life (30 to 50 hours) and therefore is effective with once-a-day dosing. The principal adverse effects are peripheral and facial edema. Flushing, dizziness, and headache may also occur. In contrast to other dihydropyridines, amlodipine causes little reflex tachycardia. The usual initial dosage for hypertension and angina pectoris is 5 mg once a day.

*Isradipine.* Like nifedipine, isradipine [DynaCirc] produces relatively selective blockade of calcium channels in blood vessels. In the United States, the drug is approved only for hypertension. Isradipine is rapidly absorbed following oral administration, but undergoes extensive metabolism on its first pass through the liver. The drug and its metabolites are excreted in the urine. The most common side effects are facial flushing (11%), headache (14%), dizziness (7%), and ankle edema (7%). In contrast to nifedipine, isradipine causes minimal reflex tachycardia. The drug is available in 2.5- and 5-mg capsules. The usual antihypertensive dosage is 2.5 to 5 mg twice a day.

*Felodipine.* Felodipine [Plendil] produces "selective" blockade of calcium channels in blood vessels. In the United States, the drug is approved only for essential hypertension. Felodipine is well absorbed following oral administration but undergoes extensive first-pass metabolism. As a result, bioavailability is only 20%. Plasma levels peak in 2.5 to 5 hours and then decay with a half-life of 24 hours. Because of this prolonged half-life, felodipine is effective with once-a-day dosing. Characteristic adverse effects are reflex tachycardia, peripheral edema, headache, facial flushing, and dizziness. Gingival hyperplasia has been reported. Felodipine is dispensed in extended-release tablets (2.5, 5, and 10 mg). The usual dosage for hypertension is 5 to 10 mg once a day.

**Nimodipine.** Nimodipine [Nimotop] produces selective blockade of calcium channels in *cerebral blood vessels*. The drug's only approved application is prophylaxis of neurologic injury following rupture of an intracranial aneurysm. Benefits derive from preventing the cerebral arterial spasm that follows subarachnoid hemorrhage (SAH) and can result in ischemic neurologic injury. Dosing (60 mg every 4 hours) should begin within 96 hours of SAH and continue for 21 days. As discussed in Chapter 28, nimodipine may also be useful against migraine.

**Nislodipine.** Like nifedipine, nislodipine [Sular] produces selective blockade of calcium channels in blood vessels; the drug has minimal direct effects on the heart. The only approved indication is hypertension. Nislodipine is well absorbed following oral administration, but the first-pass effect limits bioavailability to 5%. Peak plasma levels are reached 6 hours after administration. The most common side effects are dizziness, headache, and peripheral edema. Reflex tachycardia may also occur. Nislodipine is dispensed in extended-release tablets (10, 20, 30, and 40 mg). The dosage for hypertension is 20 to 60 mg once a day.

## KEY POINTS

- Calcium channels are gated pores in the cytoplasmic membrane that regulate entry of calcium into cells.
- In blood vessels, calcium entry causes vasoconstriction; calcium channel blockade causes vasodilation.
- In the heart, calcium entry increases heart rate, AV conduction, and myocardial contractility; calcium channel blockade has the opposite effect.

- In the heart, calcium channels are coupled to $beta_1$ receptors, the activation of which enhances calcium entry. As a result, calcium channel blockade and beta blockade have identical effects on the heart.
- At therapeutic doses, nifedipine and the other dihydropyridines act primarily on VSM; in contrast, verapamil and diltiazem act on VSM *and* the heart.
- *All* calcium channel blockers promote vasodilation, and therefore are useful in hypertension and angina pectoris.
- Because they suppress AV conduction, verapamil and diltiazem are useful against cardiac dysrhythmias, in addition to hypertension and angina pectoris.
- Because of their cardiosuppressant effects, verapamil and diltiazem can cause bradycardia, partial or complete AV block, and exacerbation of heart failure.
- Beta blockers will intensify cardiosuppression caused by verapamil and diltiazem.
- Nifedipine and the other dihydropyridines can cause reflex tachycardia. Tachycardia is most intense with rapid-acting formulations, and much less intense with sustained-release formulations.
- Beta blockers can be used to suppress reflex tachycardia caused by nifedipine and the other dihydropyridines.
- Because they cause vasodilation, all calcium channel blockers can cause dizziness, headache, and peripheral edema.
- In toxic doses, nifedipine and the other dihydropyridines can cause cardiosuppression, just like verapamil and diltiazem.
- *Rapid-acting* nifedipine has been associated with increased mortality in patients with myocardial infarction and unstable angina, although a cause-and-effect relationship has not been established. The National Heart, Lung, and Blood Institute has recommended that rapid-acting nifedipine, especially in higher doses, be used with great caution, if at all.

# Summary of Major Nursing Implications*

## Verapamil and Diltiazem

### Preadministration Assessment

#### Therapeutic Goal
Verapamil and diltiazem are indicated for *hypertension, angina pectoris*, and *cardiac dysrhythmias*.

#### Baseline Data
For *all patients*, determine blood pressure and pulse rate, and obtain laboratory evaluations of liver and kidney function. For patients with *angina pectoris*, obtain baseline data on the frequency and severity of anginal attacks. For baseline data relevant to *hypertension*, refer to Chapter 44.

#### Identifying High-Risk Patients
Verapamil and diltiazem are *contraindicated* for patients with *severe hypotension, sick sinus syndrome* (in the absence of electronic pacing), and *second-* or *third-degree AV block*. Use with *caution* in patients with *heart failure* or *liver dysfunction* and in patients taking *digoxin* or *beta-adrenergic blocking agents*.

### Implementation: Administration

#### Routes
Oral, intravenous.

---

*Patient education information is highlighted in color.

## Administration

**Oral.** *Verapamil* and *diltiazem* may be used for angina pectoris and essential hypertension. *Verapamil* may be used with digoxin to control ventricular rate in patients with atrial fibrillation and atrial flutter.

*Sustained-release formulations* are reserved for essential hypertension. Instruct patients to swallow sustained-release formulation whole, without crushing or chewing.

Prior to administration, measure blood pressure and pulse rate. If hypotension or bradycardia is detected, withhold medication and notify the physician.

**Intravenous.** Intravenous therapy is used for cardiac dysrhythmias. Perform injections slowly (over 2 to 3 minutes). Monitor the EKG for AV block, sudden reduction in heart rate, and prolongation of the PR or QT interval. Have facilities for cardioversion and cardiac pacing immediately available.

## Ongoing Evaluation and Interventions

### Evaluating Therapeutic Effects

**Angina Pectoris.** Keep an ongoing record of anginal attacks, noting the time and intensity of each attack and the likely precipitating event. Teach outpatients to chart the time, intensity, and circumstances of their attacks.

**Essential Hypertension.** Monitor blood pressure periodically. The goal is to reduce systolic/diastolic pressure to 140/90 mm Hg. Teach patients to self-monitor their blood pressure and to maintain a blood pressure record.

### Minimizing Adverse Effects

**Cardiosuppression.** Verapamil and diltiazem can cause bradycardia, AV block, and heart failure. Inform patients about manifestations of cardiac effects (e.g., slow heart beat, shortness of breath, weight gain) and instruct them to notify the physician if these occur. If cardiac impairment is severe, drug use should stop.

**Peripheral Edema.** Inform patients about signs of edema (swelling in ankles or feet) and instruct them to notify the physician if these occur. If necessary, edema can be reduced with a diuretic.

**Constipation.** This response occurs primarily with *verapamil*. Constipation can be minimized by increasing dietary fluids and fiber.

### Minimizing Adverse Interactions

**Digoxin.** The combination of digoxin with verapamil or diltiazem increases the risk of partial or complete AV block. Monitor for indications of impaired AV conduction.

Verapamil (and possibly diltiazem) can increase plasma levels of digoxin. Digoxin dosage should be reduced.

**Beta-Adrenergic Blocking Agents.** Concurrent use of a beta blocker with verapamil or diltiazem can cause bradycardia, AV block, or heart failure. Monitor the patient closely for cardiac suppression. Administer *intravenous verapamil* and beta blockers several hours apart from each other.

## Managing Acute Toxicity

Remove unabsorbed drug with an emetic or with gastric lavage followed by a cathartic. Give intravenous calcium to help counteract excessive vasodilation and reduced myocardial contractility.

To raise blood pressure, give intravenous norepinephrine. Intravenous fluids and placing the patient in Trendelenburg's position can also help.

Bradycardia and AV block can be reversed with isoproterenol and atropine. If these drugs are inadequate, electronic pacing may be required.

Ventricular tachydysrhythmias can be treated with DC cardioversion. Antidysrhythmic drugs (lidocaine or procainamide) may also be used.

# Dihydropyridines

| | |
|---|---|
| Amlodipine | Nicardipine |
| Isradipine | Nimodipine |
| Felodipine | Nislodipine |
| Nifedipine | |

## Preadministration Assessment

### Therapeutic Goal

*Amlodipine*, *nifedipine*, and *nicardipine* are approved for essential hypertension and angina pectoris. *Isradipine*, *felodipine*, and *nislodipine* are approved for hypertension only. *Nimodipine* is used only for subarachnoid hemorrhage.

### Baseline Data

See implications for verapamil and diltiazem.

### Identifying High-Risk Patients

Use dihydropyridines with *caution* in patients with *hypotension*, *sick sinus syndrome* (in the absence of electronic pacing), *angina pectoris* (because of reflex tachycardia), *heart failure*, and *second- or third-degree AV block*.

## Implementation: Administration

### Route

All dihydropyridines are given PO.
*Nicardipine* is administered PO and IV.

### Administration

Instruct patients to swallow sustained-release formulations whole, without crushing or chewing.

## Ongoing Evaluation and Interventions

### Evaluating Therapeutic Effects

See implications for verapamil and diltiazem.

### Minimizing Adverse Effects

*Reflex Tachycardia.* Reflex tachycardia can be suppressed with a beta blocker.

*Peripheral Edema.* Inform patients about signs of edema (swelling in ankles or feet) and instruct them to notify the physician if these occur. If necessary, edema can be reduced with a diuretic.

### Managing Acute Toxicity

See implications for verapamil and diltiazem.

# CHAPTER 43

# Vasodilators

**Basic Concepts in Vasodilator Pharmacology**
    Selectivity of Vasodilatory Effects
    Overview of Therapeutic Uses
    Adverse Effects Related to Vasodilation
**Pharmacology of Individual Vasodilators**
    Hydralazine
    Minoxidil

Diazoxide
Sodium Nitroprusside
Angiotensin-Converting Enzyme Inhibitors
Angiotensin II Receptor Antagonists
Organic Nitrates
Calcium Channel Blockers
Sympatholytics

Vasodilation can be produced with a wide variety of drugs. The major classes of vasodilators, along with representative agents, are shown in Table 43-1. Some of these drugs act primarily on arterioles, some act primarily on veins, and some dilate both types of vessel. The vasodilators are widely used, having indications that range from hypertension to angina pectoris to heart failure. Many of the vasodilators have been discussed in previous chapters. Four agents—hydralazine, minoxidil, diazoxide, and nitroprusside—are introduced here.

In approaching the vasodilators, we will begin by considering concepts that apply to the vasodilators as a group. After that we will discuss the pharmacology of individual agents.

## Basic Concepts in Vasodilator Pharmacology

### Selectivity of Vasodilatory Effects

It is important to appreciate that vasodilators differ from one another with respect to the types of blood vessels they affect. Some agents (e.g., hydralazine) produce selective dilation of arterioles. Others (e.g., nitroglycerin) produce selective dilation of veins. Still others (e.g., prazosin) exert approximately equal effects on arterioles *and* veins. The selectivity of the major vasodilators is summarized in Table 43-2.

The selectivity of a vasodilator determines its hemodynamic effects. For example, dilators of *resistance vessels* (arterioles) cause a decrease in cardiac *afterload* (the force against which the heart must work to pump blood). By decreasing afterload, arteriolar dilators reduce cardiac work while at the same time causing cardiac output and

tissue perfusion to increase. In contrast, dilators of *capacitance vessels* (veins) reduce the force with which blood is returned to the heart, which reduces ventricular filling. This reduction in filling decreases cardiac *preload* (the degree of stretch of the ventricular muscle prior to contraction), which in turn decreases the force of ventricular contraction. Hence, by decreasing preload, venous dilators cause a decrease in cardiac work, along with a decrease in cardiac output and tissue perfusion.

Because hemodynamic responses to arteriolar and venous dilation differ, the selectivity of a vasodilator is a major determinant of its effects, both therapeutic and undesired. Undesired effects related to selective dilation of arterioles and veins are discussed below. Therapeutic implications of selective dilation are discussed in Chapters 44, 45, and 46—the chapters in which the primary uses of the vasodilators are presented.

### Overview of Therapeutic Uses

The vasodilators, as a group, have a broad spectrum of applications. Principal indications are *essential hypertension*, *hypertensive crisis*, *angina pectoris*, and *heart failure*. Additional indications include *pheochromocytoma*, *peripheral vascular disease*, and *production of controlled hypotension during surgery*. The specific applications of any particular agent are determined by its pharmacologic profile. Important facets of that profile are route of administration, site of vasodilation (arterioles, veins, or both), and intensity and duration of effects.

### Adverse Effects Related to Vasodilation

#### Postural Hypotension

Postural (orthostatic) hypotension is defined as a fall in blood pressure brought on by moving from a supine or

## TABLE 43-1. TYPES OF VASODILATORS

| Category | Examples |
|---|---|
| *Angiotensin-Converting Enzyme Inhibitors* | Captopril<br>Enalapril<br>Lisinopril |
| *Angiotensin II Receptor Antagonists* | Losartan<br>Valsartan |
| *Organic Nitrates* | Nitroglycerin<br>Isosorbide dinitrate |
| *Calcium Channel Blockers* | Verapamil<br>Nifedipine<br>Diltiazem |
| *Sympatholytics* | |
| Alpha-adrenergic blockers | Phentolamine<br>Phenoxybenzamine<br>Prazosin<br>Terazosin |
| Ganglionic blockers | Mecamylamine<br>Trimethaphan |
| Adrenergic neuron blockers | Reserpine<br>Guanethidine<br>Guanadrel |
| Centrally acting agents | Clonidine<br>Guanabenz<br>Methyldopa |
| *Other Important Vasodilators* | Hydralazine<br>Minoxidil<br>Nitroprusside<br>Diazoxide |

## TABLE 43-2. VASODILATOR SELECTIVITY

| Vasodilator | Site of Vasodilation | |
|---|---|---|
| | Arterioles | Veins |
| Hydralazine | + | |
| Minoxidil | + | |
| Diltiazem | + | |
| Nifedipine | + | |
| Verapamil | + | |
| Prazosin | + | + |
| Terazosin | + | + |
| Phentolamine | + | + |
| Nitroprusside | + | + |
| Captopril | + | + |
| Enalapril | + | + |
| Lisinopril | + | + |
| Losartan | + | + |
| Nitroglycerin | | + |
| Isosorbide dinitrate | | + |

seated position to an upright position. The underlying cause of orthostatic hypotension is relaxation of smooth muscle in *veins*. Because of venous relaxation, gravity causes blood to "pool" within veins, thereby decreasing venous return to the heart. This reduction in venous return causes a decrease in cardiac output and a corresponding drop in blood pressure. Hypotension from venous dilation is minimal in recumbent subjects because gravity has only a small effect on venous return when we are lying down.

Patients receiving vasodilators should be informed about symptoms of hypotension (lightheadedness, dizziness) and advised to sit or lie down if these occur, since failure to do so may result in fainting. In addition, patients should be informed that they can minimize hypotension by avoiding abrupt transitions from a supine or seated position to an upright position.

### Reflex Tachycardia

Reflex tachycardia can be produced by dilation of *arterioles* or *veins*. The mechanism of reflex tachycardia is as follows: (1a) *arteriolar* dilation causes a direct decrease in arterial pressure or (1b) *venous* dilation reduces cardiac output, which in turn reduces arterial pressure; (2) baroreceptors in the aortic arch and carotid sinus sense the drop in pressure and relay this information to the va-

somotor center of the medulla; and (3) in an attempt to bring blood pressure back up, the medulla sends impulses along sympathetic nerves instructing the heart to beat faster.

Reflex tachycardia is undesirable for two reasons. First, tachycardia can put an unacceptable burden on the heart. Second, if the vasodilator was given to lower blood pressure, tachycardia would raise pressure and thereby counteract beneficial effects.

To help prevent vasodilator-induced reflex tachycardia, patients can be pretreated with a beta-adrenergic blocking agent (e.g., propranolol), which will block sympathetic stimulation of the heart.

### Expansion of Blood Volume

Prolonged use of *arteriolar* or *venous* dilators can cause an increase in blood volume (secondary to prolonged reduction of blood pressure). This increase in blood volume represents an attempt by the body to restore blood pressure to pretreatment levels.

Blood volume is increased by two mechanisms. First, reduced blood pressure triggers secretion of aldosterone by the adrenal glands. Aldosterone then acts on the kidney to promote retention of sodium and water, thereby increasing blood volume. The second mechanism also involves the kidney: by reducing arterial pressure, vasodilators decrease renal blood flow and glomerular filtration rate; because filtrate volume is decreased, the kidney is able to reabsorb an increased amount of sodium and water, which causes blood volume to expand.

Increased plasma volume can negate the beneficial effects of vasodilator therapy. For example, if plasma volume increases during the treatment of hypertension, blood pressure will rise and the benefits of therapy will be canceled. To prevent the kidney from neutralizing the beneficial effects of vasodilation, patients often receive concurrent therapy with a diuretic, which will prevent fluid retention and volume expansion.

# Pharmacology of Individual Vasodilators

Our focus in this section is on four drugs: hydralazine, minoxidil, diazoxide, and sodium nitroprusside. All of the other vasodilators are discussed at length in other chapters; hence, their discussion here is brief.

## Hydralazine

### Cardiovascular Effects

Hydralazine [Apresoline] causes selective dilation of arterioles. The drug has little or no effect on veins. Arteriolar dilation results from a direct action on vascular smooth muscle; the precise mechanism is not known. In response to arteriolar dilation, peripheral resistance and arterial blood pressure fall. In addition, heart rate and myocardial contractility increase, largely by reflex mechanisms. Since hydralazine acts selectively on arterioles, postural hypotension is minimal.

### Pharmacokinetics

*Absorption and Time Course of Action.* Hydralazine is readily absorbed following oral administration. Effects are apparent within 45 minutes and persist for 6 hours or more. When the drug is given parenterally, effects begin rapidly (within 10 minutes) and last for 2 to 4 hours.

*Metabolism.* Hydralazine is inactivated by a metabolic process known as *acetylation*. The ability to acetylate hydralazine and other drugs is genetically determined. Some people are rapid acetylators, whereas others are slow acetylators. The distinction between rapid and slow acetylators can be clinically significant, in that individuals who acetylate hydralazine slowly are likely to have higher blood levels of the drug. These high drug levels can result in excessive vasodilation and other undesired effects. To avoid drug accumulation, hydralazine dosage should be reduced in slow acetylators.

### Adverse Effects

*Reflex Tachycardia.* By lowering arterial blood pressure, hydralazine can trigger reflex stimulation of the heart, thereby causing cardiac work and myocardial oxygen demand to increase. Because hydralazine-induced reflex tachycardia is frequently severe, the drug is almost always used in combination with a beta-adrenergic blocking agent. In fact, the only patients who are not routinely given a beta blocker are those with heart failure. (Beta blockers are generally avoided in heart failure because they can further decrease cardiac output.)

*Increased Blood Volume.* Hydralazine-induced hypotension can cause sodium and water retention and a corresponding increase in blood volume. Expansion of blood volume can be prevented with a diuretic.

*Systemic Lupus Erythematosus–like Syndrome.* Hydralazine can cause an acute rheumatoid syndrome that closely resembles systemic lupus erythematosus (SLE). This syndrome is characterized by muscle pain, joint pain, fever, nephritis, pericarditis, and the presence of antinuclear antibodies. The syndrome occurs most frequently in slow acetylators and is rare when hydralazine dosage is kept below 200 mg/day. If an SLE-like reaction occurs, hydralazine should be discontinued. Symptoms are usually reversible but may take 6 or more months to subside. In some cases, rheumatoid symptoms persist for years.

*Other Adverse Effects.* Common responses include *headache*, *dizziness*, *weakness*, and *fatigue*. These reactions are related to hydralazine-induced hypotension.

### Drug Interactions

Hydralazine is combined with *beta blockers* to protect against reflex tachycardia, and with *diuretics* to prevent sodium and water retention and expansion of blood volume. Drugs that lower blood pressure will intensify hypotensive responses to hydralazine. Accordingly, if hydralazine is used with other *antihypertensive agents*, care must be taken to avoid excessive hypotension.

### Therapeutic Uses

*Essential Hypertension.* Oral hydralazine can be used to lower blood pressure in patients with essential hypertension. The regimen almost always includes a beta blocker, and may also include a diuretic. Although commonly employed in the past, hydralazine has been largely replaced by newer antihypertensive agents (see Chapter 44).

*Hypertensive Crisis.* Parenteral hydralazine is used to lower blood pressure rapidly in severe hypertensive episodes. The drug should be administered in small, incremental doses. If dosage is excessive, severe hypotension may replace the hypertension. Treatment of hypertensive emergencies is discussed further in Chapter 44.

*Heart Failure.* As discussed in Chapter 46, hydralazine can be used on a short-term basis to reduce afterload in patients with heart failure. With prolonged therapy, tolerance to hydralazine develops.

### Preparations, Dosage, and Administration

*Preparations.* Hydralazine [Apresoline] is dispensed in tablets (10, 25, 50, and 100 mg) for oral use and as an injection (20 mg/ml in 1-ml ampules) for parenteral administration. Hydralazine is also available in fixed-dose combinations with hydrochlorothiazide, a diuretic; trade names include Apresoline-Esidrex and Apresodex.

*Oral Therapy.* Dosage should be small initially (10 mg 4 times a day) and then gradually increased. Rapid increases may produce excessive hypotension. Usual maintenance dosages for adults range from 25 to 100 mg 2 times a day. Daily doses greater than 200 mg are associated with an increased incidence of adverse effects and should be avoided.

***Parenteral Therapy.*** Parenteral administration (IV and IM) is reserved for hypertensive crises. The usual dose is 20 to 40 mg, repeated as needed. Blood pressure should be monitored frequently to minimize excessive hypotension. In most cases, patients can be switched from hydralazine injections to oral therapy within 48 hours.

## Minoxidil

Minoxidil [Loniten] produces more intense vasodilation than hydralazine but also causes more severe adverse reactions. Because it is both very effective and very dangerous, minoxidil is reserved for patients with severe hypertension that has been refractory to less dangerous drugs.

### Cardiovascular Effects

Like hydralazine, minoxidil produces selective dilation of *arterioles*. Little or no venous dilation occurs. Arteriolar dilation decreases peripheral resistance and arterial blood pressure. In response to the reduction in blood pressure, reflex mechanisms cause an increase in heart rate and myocardial contractility. These responses can increase cardiac oxygen demand, and can thereby exacerbate angina pectoris.

Vasodilation results from a direct action on vascular smooth muscle (VSM). In order to relax VSM, minoxidil must first be metabolized to minoxidil sulfate. This metabolite then causes potassium channels in VSM to open. The resultant efflux of potassium hyperpolarizes VSM cells, thereby reducing their ability to contract.

### Pharmacokinetics

Minoxidil is rapidly and completely absorbed following oral administration. Vasodilation is maximal within 2 to 3 hours and then gradually declines. Residual effects may persist for 2 days or more. Minoxidil is extensively metabolized; metabolites and parent drug are eliminated in the urine.

### Adverse Effects

***Reflex Tachycardia.*** Blood pressure reduction triggers reflex tachycardia. Tachycardia is a serious side effect and can be minimized by concurrent use of a beta blocker.

***Sodium and Water Retention.*** Fluid retention is both common and serious. Volume expansion may be so severe as to cause cardiac decompensation. Management of fluid retention requires a high-ceiling diuretic (e.g., furosemide) used alone or in combination with a thiazide diuretic. If diuretics are inadequate, dialysis must be employed, or minoxidil must be withdrawn.

***Hypertrichosis.*** About 80% of patients taking minoxidil for 4 weeks or more develop hypertrichosis (excessive growth of hair). Hair growth begins on the face and later develops on the arms, legs, and back. Hypertrichosis appears to result from proliferation of epithelial cells at the base of the hair follicle; vasodilation may also be involved. Overgrowth of hair is a cosmetic problem and can be controlled by shaving or using a depilatory. However, many patients (primarily women) find hypertrichosis both un-

manageable and intolerable and refuse to continue treatment.

***Pericardial Effusion.*** Rarely, minoxidil-induced fluid retention results in pericardial effusion (fluid accumulation beneath the pericardium). In most cases, pericardial effusion is asymptomatic. However, in some cases, fluid accumulation becomes so great as to cause cardiac tamponade (compression of the heart with a resultant decrease in cardiac performance). If tamponade occurs, it must be treated by pericardiocentesis or by surgical drainage.

***Other Adverse Effects.*** Minoxidil may cause *nausea, headache, fatigue, breast tenderness, glucose intolerance, thrombocytopenia,* and *skin reactions* (rashes, Stevens-Johnson syndrome). In addition, the drug has caused *hemorrhagic cardiac lesions* in experimental animals.

### Therapeutic Uses

The only cardiovascular indication for minoxidil is *severe hypertension*. Because of its serious adverse effects, minoxidil is reserved for patients who have failed to respond to safer drugs. To minimize adverse cardiovascular responses (reflex tachycardia, expansion of blood volume, pericardial effusion), minoxidil should be used with a beta blocker and intensive diuretic therapy.

Topical minoxidil [Rogaine] is used to promote hair growth in balding men (see Chapter 98).

### Preparations, Dosage, and Administration

Minoxidil [Loniten] is dispensed in 2.5- and 10-mg tablets for oral administration. The initial dosage is 5 mg once a day; the maximum dosage is 100 mg/day. The usual adult dosage is 10 to 40 mg/day administered in single or divided doses. When a rapid response is needed, a loading dose of 5 to 20 mg is given followed by doses of 2.5 to 10 mg every 4 hours.

## Diazoxide

Diazoxide [Hyperstat IV] is a close relative of the thiazide diuretics but is devoid of diuretic actions. The drug is used for hypertensive emergencies.

### Cardiovascular Effects

Like hydralazine and minoxidil, diazoxide produces selective dilation of *arterioles*; the drug has no significant effect on veins. Intravenous diazoxide causes a rapid drop in diastolic and systolic pressure. Reduced arterial pressure triggers reflex tachycardia along with an increase in myocardial contractility; these effects combine to increase cardiac output. Arteriolar dilation also promotes substantial salt and water retention.

Vasodilation results from a direct effect on vascular smooth muscle. Diazoxide activates potassium channels in VSM, which results in hyperpolarization and a reduced ability to contract.

### Pharmacokinetics

Diazoxide is administered intravenously, either as a bolus injection or by infusion. Bolus injection is generally preferred. Effects begin within minutes and may persist for hours. Most of the drug is eliminated unchanged in the urine.

### Adverse Effects

***Reflex Tachycardia.*** Reflex tachycardia occurs in response to lowering of blood pressure. If necessary, this reaction can be blunted with a beta blocker.

***Salt and Water Retention.*** Diazoxide causes substantial retention of salt and water. This response is due largely to a reduction in glomerular filtration. If fluid retention is severe, edema and even congestive heart failure can result. Edema and expansion of blood volume can be prevented with a diuretic; a high-ceiling agent (e.g., furosemide) is preferred.

*Hyperglycemia.* Like the thiazide diuretics, diazoxide can suppress release of insulin, and can thereby cause blood glucose to rise. For most patients, the degree of hyperglycemia is insignificant. However, for patients with diabetes, hyperglycemia may be substantial. Blood glucose should be monitored daily in diabetic patients, and, if hyperglycemia develops, insulin dosage should be increased.

*Hyperuricemia.* Like the thiazide diuretics, diazoxide can decrease renal excretion of uric acid, thereby raising uric acid levels in blood. For most patients, hyperuricemia is asymptomatic. However, in gout-prone individuals, retention of uric acid may result in a gouty attack.

*Other Adverse Effects.* Diazoxide may cause *gastrointestinal effects* (nausea, vomiting, anorexia), *headache, flushing, hypotension,* and *temporary interruption of labor.* Rapid injection of large doses may produce *severe hypotension, anginal symptoms,* and *myocardial infarction.*

### Drug Interactions

*Diuretics. High-ceiling diuretics* are used to counteract diazoxide-induced retention of salt and water. Since *thiazide diuretics* might potentiate the hyperglycemic and hyperuricemic effects of diazoxide, these diuretics should be avoided.

*Antihypertensive Drugs.* With the exception of high-ceiling diuretics, antihypertensive drugs should not be used routinely in combination with diazoxide. The concurrent use of diazoxide with other hypotensive agents may cause excessive lowering of blood pressure.

### Therapeutic Uses

Parenteral diazoxide is reserved for acute treatment of hypertensive emergencies (e.g., malignant hypertension, hypertensive encephalopathy). Therapy with oral antihypertensive agents should be instituted as soon as possible. In most cases, diazoxide can be discontinued within 4 to 5 days.

### Preparations, Dosage, and Administration

Diazoxide [Hyperstat IV] is dispensed as an injection (15 mg/ml) for IV administration. Until recently, it was common practice to administer diazoxide as a single, large (300-mg) IV bolus. This practice is no longer recommended. Currently, it is considered safer and more effective to use a series of "minibolus" injections, rather than one large injection. Accordingly, treatment should begin with a dose of 1 to 3 mg/kg injected by rapid (30 seconds or less) IV push. Dosing is then repeated every 5 to 15 minutes until the desired reduction in blood pressure has been achieved. Once hypertension has been controlled, injections can be made every 4 to 24 hours. Blood pressure should be monitored closely until an acceptable and stable level has been produced; hourly monitoring should be performed thereafter. The patient should remain recumbent for at least 30 minutes after diazoxide injection. After 4 or 5 days of treatment, the patient can usually be switched to oral antihypertensive therapy.

## Sodium Nitroprusside

Sodium nitroprusside [Nipride, Nitropress] is a potent and efficacious vasodilator. It is also the fastest acting antihypertensive agent available. Because of these qualities, nitroprusside is a drug of choice for treating hypertensive emergencies.

## Cardiovascular Effects

In contrast to hydralazine, minoxidil, and diazoxide, nitroprusside causes *venous* dilation in addition to *arteriolar* dilation. Curiously, although nitroprusside is an effective arteriolar dilator, reflex tachycardia is minimal. Administration is by IV infusion, and onset of effects is immediate. By adjusting the infusion rate, blood pressure can be depressed to almost any level desired. When the infusion is stopped, blood pressure returns to pretreatment levels in minutes. Nitroprusside can trigger retention of sodium and water; furosemide can help offset this effect.

## Mechanism of Action

Once in the body, nitroprusside breaks down to release *nitric oxide* (Figure 43–1), which then activates *guanylate cyclase,* an enzyme present in vascular smooth muscle. Guanylate cyclase catalyzes the production of *cyclic GMP,* which, through a series of reactions, causes vasodilation. This mechanism is similar to that of nitroglycerin.

## Metabolism

As shown in Figure 43–1, nitroprusside contains five *cyanide* groups, which are split free in the first step of nitroprusside metabolism. *Nitric oxide,* the active component of the drug, is released next. Both reactions take place in smooth muscle. Once freed, the cyanide groups are converted to *thiocyanate* in the liver; *thiosulfate* is a required co-factor for this reaction. Thiocyanate is eliminated by the kidneys over several days.

## Adverse Effects

*Excessive Hypotension.* If administered too rapidly, nitroprusside can cause a precipitous fall in blood pressure, resulting in headache, palpitations, nausea, vomiting, and sweating. Blood pressure should be monitored continuously.

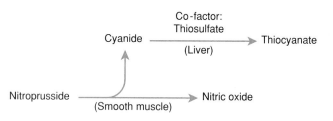

**Figure 43–1. Structure and metabolism of sodium nitroprusside.** Note the five cyanide groups in nitroprusside and their liberation by metabolism. Note also the release of nitric oxide, the active component of nitroprusside.

***Cyanide Poisoning.*** On rare occasions, nitroprusside therapy has resulted in the accumulation of lethal amounts of cyanide. Cyanide buildup is most likely in patients with liver disease and in those with low stores of thiosulfate, the co-factor needed for cyanide detoxification. The chances of cyanide poisoning can be minimized by avoiding rapid infusion (faster than 5 µg/kg/min) for a prolonged time and by coadministration of thiosulfate. If cyanide toxicity occurs, nitroprusside should be discontinued.

***Thiocyanate Toxicity.*** When nitroprusside is given for several days, thiocyanate (a metabolite of nitroprusside) may accumulate. Although much less hazardous than cyanide, thiocyanate can also cause adverse effects. These effects, which involve the central nervous system, include disorientation, psychotic behavior, and delirium. To minimize toxicity, patients receiving nitroprusside for more than 3 days should be monitored for plasma levels of thiocyanate. These levels should not be allowed to exceed 0.1 mg/ml.

### Therapeutic Uses

***Hypertensive Emergencies.*** Nitroprusside is used to lower blood pressure rapidly in hypertensive emergencies. Oral antihypertensive medication should be initiated at the same time that blood pressure is being reduced with nitroprusside. During nitroprusside treatment, furosemide may be needed to prevent excessive retention of fluid.

***Other Uses.*** Nitroprusside is approved for production of controlled hypotension during surgery (to reduce bleeding in the surgical field). In addition, the drug has been employed on an investigational basis to treat severe, refractory congestive heart failure and myocardial infarction.

#### Preparations, Dosage, and Administration

Sodium nitroprusside [Nipride, Nitropress] is dispensed in powdered form (50 mg) to be dissolved and diluted for IV infusion. Fresh solutions may have a faint brown coloration; solutions that are deeply colored (blue, green, dark red) should be discarded. Solutions of nitroprusside can be degraded by light and should be protected with an opaque material.

Blood pressure can be adjusted to practically any level by increasing or decreasing the rate of infusion. The initial infusion rate is 0.3 µg/kg/min. The maximal rate is 10 µg/kg/min. If infusion at the maximal rate for 10 minutes fails to produce an adequate drop in blood pressure, administration should be discontinued. During the infusion, blood pressure should be monitored continuously, either with an arterial line or an electronic monitoring device. No other drugs should be mixed with the infusion solution.

## Angiotensin-Converting Enzyme Inhibitors

Inhibitors of angiotensin-converting enzyme (ACE) promote vasodilation by preventing the conversion of angiotensin I (a weak vasoconstrictor) into angiotensin II (an extremely powerful vasoconstrictor). The primary indication for ACE inhibitors is essential hypertension. These drugs can also benefit patients with heart failure and diabetes. The basic pharmacology of the ACE inhibitors is presented in Chapter 41. The use of these drugs to treat hypertension and heart failure is discussed in Chapters 44 and 46, respectively.

## Angiotensin II Receptor Antagonists

Angiotensin II receptor antagonists (AngIIRAs) are new drugs with actions similar to those of the ACE inhibitors. However, instead of preventing the formation of angiotensin II, these new drugs simply block receptors for angiotensin II. Like the ACE inhibitors, AngIIRAs dilate arterioles and veins. Currently, only two AngIIRAs are available: losartan and valsartan. Their only indication is hypertension. The basic pharmacology of the AngIIRAs is discussed in Chapter 41.

## Organic Nitrates

The organic nitrates (e.g., nitroglycerin, isosorbide dinitrate) produce selective dilation of veins; dilation of arterioles is minimal. The primary indication for these drugs is angina pectoris. In addition, nitroglycerin is given to treat heart failure and myocardial infarction, and to provide controlled hypotension during surgery. The pharmacology of the organic nitrates is discussed in Chapter 45.

## Calcium Channel Blockers

The calcium channel blockers (e.g., verapamil, nifedipine) produce vasodilation by preventing calcium entry into vascular smooth muscle. At therapeutic doses, these drugs produce selective dilation of arterioles; very little venous dilation occurs. The vasodilating ability of these drugs is exploited in the treatment of essential hypertension and angina pectoris. The calcium channel blockers are the subject of Chapter 42.

## Sympatholytics

Sympatholytics are drugs that promote vasodilation by preventing the sympathetic nervous system from causing vasoconstriction. Some of these drugs act by direct blockade of adrenergic receptors on blood vessels. Others act on sympathetic ganglia, on adrenergic neurons, or within the central nervous system.

***Alpha-Adrenergic Blocking Agents.*** The alpha blockers (e.g., phentolamine, prazosin) promote vasodilation by preventing stimulation of alpha-adrenergic receptors on veins and arterioles. In their capacity as vasodilators, these drugs have multiple therapeutic applications, including essential hypertension, peripheral vascular disease, and pheochromocytoma. The alpha blockers are discussed in Chapter 19.

***Ganglionic Blocking Agents.*** The ganglionic blocking agents (mecamylamine, trimethaphan) interrupt impulse transmission through all ganglia of the autonomic nervous system. By doing so, these drugs prevent sympathetic stimulation of arterioles and veins. Ganglionic blockers are used to treat hypertensive emergencies and severe cases of essential hypertension. In addition, these drugs are given to produce hypotension during surgery. The ganglionic blockers are discussed in Chapter 17.

***Adrenergic Neuron Blocking Agents.*** Adrenergic neuron blockers (e.g., reserpine, guanethidine) act within terminals of adrenergic neurons to cause a reduction in norepinephrine release. By decreasing the release of norepinephrine from sympathetic nerves that control vasomotor tone, these drugs promote vasodilation. Their principal indication is essential hypertension. The adrenergic neuron blockers are discussed in Chapter 20.

***Centrally Acting Agents.*** The centrally acting sympatholytics (e.g., clonidine, methyldopa) act within the central nervous system to inhibit outflow of impulses along sympathetic nerves. These agents are used primarily in the treatment of hypertension. Their pharmacology is discussed in Chapter 20.

## KEY POINTS

- Some vasodilators are selective for arterioles, some are selective for veins, and some dilate both types of vessel.
- Drugs that dilate arterioles reduce cardiac afterload, and can thereby reduce cardiac work while increasing cardiac output and tissue perfusion.
- Drugs that dilate veins reduce cardiac preload, and can thereby reduce cardiac work, cardiac output, and tissue perfusion.
- Principal indications for vasodilators are essential hypertension, hypertensive crisis, angina pectoris, and heart failure.
- Drugs that dilate veins can cause orthostatic hypotension.
- Drugs that dilate arterioles or veins can cause reflex tachycardia, which will increase cardiac work and elevate blood pressure. This response can be blunted with a beta blocker.
- Drugs that dilate arterioles or veins can cause fluid retention. This response can be blunted with a diuretic.
- Hydralazine causes selective dilation of arterioles.
- Hydralazine can cause a syndrome that resembles systemic lupus erythematosus.
- Minoxidil causes selective and profound dilation of arterioles.
- Minoxidil can cause hypertrichosis.
- Sodium nitroprusside dilates arterioles *and* veins.
- Prolonged infusion of nitroprusside can result in toxic accumulation of cyanide and thiocyanate.

# CHAPTER 44

# Drugs for Hypertension

ypertension (elevated blood pressure) is a common and chronic disorder that affects about 50 million Americans. Left untreated, hypertension can lead to heart disease, kidney disease, blindness, and stroke. Conversely, a treatment program of lifestyle changes and drug therapy can reduce both blood pressure and the risk of long-term complications.

Unfortunately, drug therapy does not cure hypertension, it only reduces symptoms. Accordingly, for most patients, treatment must continue lifelong. As a result, noncompliance can be a significant problem.

Many different drugs are used to treat hypertension. All have been introduced in previous chapters. Hence, in this chapter, rather than struggling with a huge array of new drugs, we will simply be discussing the antihypertensive applications of drugs with which we are already familiar.

In approaching our study of antihypertensive therapy, we will begin by discussing the nature of hypertension and nondrug methods of treatment. Following that we will discuss drug therapy of chronic hypertension. We will complete the chapter by discussing drugs used for hypertensive emergencies and for hypertensive disorders of pregnancy.

## Hypertension: Definition, Types, and Consequences

### Definition and Diagnosis

*Hypertension* is defined as systolic blood pressure (SBP) greater than 140 mm Hg or diastolic blood pressure (DBP) greater than 90 mm Hg. If SBP is above 140 mm Hg and DBP is below 90 mm Hg, a diagnosis of *isolated systolic hypertension* applies.

As shown in Table 44–1, hypertension can be classified as stage 1, 2, 3, or 4, based on the degree of blood pressure elevation. This new classification scheme was introduced in the fifth report of the Joint National Committee on Detection, Evaluation, and Treatment of Hypertension (1993). When SBP and DBP fall into different categories, classification is based on the higher category. For example, an individual with a reading of 185/105 mm Hg would be diagnosed as having stage 3 hypertension, and an individual with a reading of 185/85 would be diagnosed as having stage 3 isolated systolic hypertension.

Diagnosis of hypertension should not be based on a single blood pressure determination. Rather, if an initial screening shows that blood pressure is elevated (but does not represent an immediate danger), it should be measured again on two subsequent visits 1 week to several weeks later. At each visit, two measurements should be made and averaged. If these readings confirm that SBP is indeed greater than 140 mm Hg or that DBP is greater than 90 mm Hg, a diagnosis of hypertension can be made.

### Types of Hypertension

There are two broad categories of hypertension: *primary hypertension* and *secondary hypertension*. As indicated in Table 44-2, primary hypertension is by far the most common form of hypertensive disease. Less than 10% of people with hypertension have a secondary form.

## TABLE 44–1. CLASSIFICATION OF BLOOD PRESSURE FOR ADULTS AGE 18 YEARS AND OLDER

| Category* | Systolic (mm Hg) | Diastolic (mm Hg) |
|---|---|---|
| *Normal*[†] | <130 | <85 |
| *High Normal* | 130–139 | 85–89 |
| *Hypertension*[‡] | | |
| STAGE 1 (mild) | 140–159 | 90–99 |
| STAGE 2 (moderate) | 160–179 | 100–109 |
| STAGE 3 (severe) | 180–209 | 110–119 |
| STAGE 4 (very severe) | ≥210 | ≥120 |

*When systolic and diastolic pressure fall into different categories, the *higher* category should be selected to classify the individual's blood pressure status. For instance, 130/80 mm Hg should be classified as high normal, and 180/120 mm Hg should be classified as Stage 4 hypertension.

[†]Optimal blood pressure with respect to cardiovascular risk is SBP <120 mm Hg and DBP <80 mm Hg. However, unusually low readings should be evaluated for clinical significance.

[‡]Based on the average of two or more readings taken at each of two or more visits following an initial screening. Isolated systolic hypertension (ISH) is defined as SBP ≥140 mm Hg and DBP <90 mm Hg and staged appropriately (e.g., 170/85 mm Hg is defined as Stage 2 ISH).

Data from the fifth report of the Joint National Committee on Detection, Evaluation, and Treatment of High Blood Pressure, 1993.

## Primary (Essential) Hypertension

Primary hypertension is defined as hypertension that has no identifiable cause. A diagnosis of primary hypertension is made by ruling out probable specific causes of blood pressure elevation. Primary hypertension is a chronic, progressive disorder. In the absence of treatment, patients will experience a continuous, gradual rise in blood pressure over the remainder of their lives.

In the United States, primary hypertension affects about 20% of adults ages 25 to 74. Some people are more likely to experience hypertension than others: older people experience more hypertension than younger people, African Americans experience more hypertension than white Americans, postmenopausal women experience more hypertension than premenopausal women, and obese people experience more hypertension than people of normal weight.

## TABLE 44–2. TYPES OF HYPERTENSION AND THEIR FREQUENCY

| Type of Hypertension | Frequency (%) |
|---|---|
| *Primary (Essential) Hypertension* | 92 |
| *Secondary Hypertension* | |
| Chronic renal disease | 4 |
| Renovascular disease | 2 |
| Coarctation | 0.3 |
| Primary aldosteronism | 0.2 |
| Cushing's syndrome | 0.1 |
| Pheochromocytoma | 0.1 |
| Oral contraceptive-induced | 1 |

Although the cause of primary hypertension is unknown, the condition *can* be successfully treated. It should be understood, however, that treatment is not curative: drugs can lower blood pressure, but they do not eliminate the underlying pathology. Consequently, treatment must continue lifelong.

Primary hypertension is also referred to as *essential hypertension*. This alternative name preceded the term primary hypertension and reflects our ignorance about the cause of the disease. Historically, it had been noted that as people grew older, their blood pressure rose. Why older people had elevated blood pressure was (and remains) unknown. One hypothesis noted that as people aged, their vascular systems offered greater resistance to blood flow. In order to move blood against this increased resistance, a compensatory increase in blood pressure was required. Therefore, the hypertension that occurred with age was seen as being "essential" for providing adequate perfusion of tissues—hence, the term essential hypertension. Over time, the term essential hypertension came to be applied to all cases of hypertension for which an underlying cause could not be found.

## Secondary Hypertension

Secondary hypertension is defined as an elevation of blood pressure brought on by an identified primary cause. The most common causes are listed in Table 44–2.

Because secondary hypertension is due to an identified cause, it may be possible to treat that cause directly, rather than relying on drugs to provide symptomatic relief. As a result, some individuals with secondary hypertension can actually be cured. For example, if hypertension occurs secondary to pheochromocytoma (a catecholamine-secreting tumor), surgical removal of the tumor may produce permanent cure. When cure is not possible, secondary hypertension can be managed with the same drugs used to lower blood pressure in primary hypertension.

## Consequences of Hypertension

Chronic hypertension is associated with increased morbidity and mortality. Left untreated, chronically elevated blood pressure can lead to *heart disease* (left ventricular hypertrophy, myocardial infarction, angina pectoris), *kidney disease*, *blindness*, and *stroke*. The degree of injury is directly related to the degree of blood pressure elevation: the higher the pressure, the greater the injury. In addition, certain risk factors (e.g., obesity, sedentary lifestyle) can intensify injury. Deaths related to chronic hypertension result largely from cerebral hemorrhage, heart failure, renal failure, and myocardial infarction.

Unfortunately, despite its potential for serious harm, hypertension usually remains asymptomatic until long after injury has begun to develop. That is, hypertension can exist for years before overt pathology is evident. Because injury develops slowly and progressively, and because hypertension rarely causes noticeable discomfort, many people with the disease are unaware of it. Furthermore, many other people, even though diagnosed as hypertensive, forgo therapy because hypertension doesn't make them feel bad. In fact, only 50% of Americans with hypertension undergo treatment, and, of these, only 20% take sufficient medicine to reduce their blood pressure to 140/90 mm Hg.

## Objectives of Antihypertensive Therapy

Treatment of hypertension has two objectives: (1) reduction of blood pressure to 140/90 mm Hg and (2) prevention of long-term complications. These goals should be achieved without decreasing quality of life with the drugs used for treatment. Extensive clinical trials have demonstrated unequivocally that, when the blood pressure of hypertensive individuals is lowered, morbidity is decreased and life is prolonged. Antihypertensive therapy significantly decreases the risk of heart disease, kidney disease, blindness, and stroke.

## Management of Essential Hypertension I: Lifestyle Changes

Lifestyle changes (previously termed nonpharmacologic therapy) can decrease blood pressure in many people with hypertension. These changes are useful by themselves and, when implemented in conjunction with drug therapy, can reduce the number of required drugs and their dosages.

**Weight Reduction.** There is a direct relationship between obesity and elevation of blood pressure. Clinical studies indicate that weight loss can reduce blood pressure in 60% to 80% of overweight hypertensive individuals. Consequently, a restricted-calorie diet is recommended for all patients whose weight exceeds 110% of ideal. The diet should be low in saturated fats, and total dietary fat should not exceed 30% of caloric intake.

**Sodium Restriction.** Reduction of sodium chloride (salt) intake can lower blood pressure in people with hypertension. In addition, salt restriction can enhance the hypotensive effects of drugs. Accordingly, it is recommended that all people with hypertension consume no more than 6 gm of sodium chloride (2.3 gm of sodium) a day. To facilitate salt restriction, patients should be given information on the salt content of foods.

Experts disagree about the relationship between salt intake and blood pressure in *normotensive* patients. In particular, they disagree as to whether a high-salt diet *causes* hypertension. Hence, for people with normal blood pressure, a low-salt diet may be considered healthy or unnecessary, depending on which expert you consult.

**Alcohol Restriction.** Excessive alcohol consumption can raise blood pressure and create resistance to antihypertensive drugs. Accordingly, patients should limit alcohol intake to 1 ounce/day. One ounce of ethanol is equivalent to about two mixed drinks, two glasses of wine, or two cans of beer.

**Exercise.** Regular aerobic exercise (e.g., jogging, walking, swimming, bicycling) can reduce blood pressure by about 10 mm Hg, even in the absence of weight reduction. Patients with a sedentary lifestyle should be encouraged to develop an appropriate exercise program. An activity as simple as brisk walking for 30 to 45 minutes 3 to 5 times a week can be beneficial.

**Smoking Cessation.** Although not directly related to hypertension, smoking is a major risk factor for cardiovascular disease and should be avoided. Furthermore, smoking may impair the ability of antihypertensive drugs to protect against cardiovascular disease. All patients who smoke should be forcefully encouraged to quit.

## Management of Essential Hypertension II: Pharmacologic Therapy

Drug therapy is indicated if blood pressure is still excessive 3 to 6 months after implementation of lifestyle changes. The decision to use drugs should be the result of collaboration between clinician and patient. A wide range of antihypertensive drugs is available, permitting versatility in the regimen. Consequently, for the majority of patients, it should be possible to establish a program that is effective and yet devoid of objectionable side effects. After 12 months of successful therapy, an attempt should

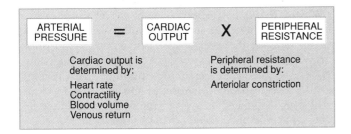

**Figure 44–1. Primary determinants of arterial blood pressure.**

be made to reduce the number of drugs taken and their dosages.

## Review of Blood Pressure Control

Before discussing the antihypertensive drugs, it will be helpful to review the major mechanisms by which blood pressure is controlled. This information will help us understand the mechanisms by which drugs lower blood pressure.

### Principal Determinants of Blood Pressure

The principal determinants of blood pressure are summarized in Figure 44-1. As indicated, arterial pressure is the product of cardiac output and peripheral resistance. An increase in either will increase blood pressure.

As shown in the figure, cardiac output is influenced by four factors: (1) heart rate, (2) myocardial contractility (force of contraction), (3) blood volume, and (4) venous return of blood to the heart. An increase in any of these factors will increase cardiac output, thereby causing blood pressure to rise. Conversely, by reducing these factors, we can make blood pressure fall. Drugs that affect these factors are (1) beta blockers, which decrease heart rate and contractile force; (2) diuretics, which decrease blood volume; and (3) venodilators, which reduce venous return.

Peripheral vascular resistance is regulated by arteriolar constriction. Accordingly, we can reduce blood pressure with drugs that promote arteriolar dilation.

### Systems That Help Regulate Blood Pressure

Having established that blood pressure is determined by heart rate, myocardial contractility, blood volume, venous return, and arteriolar constriction, we will now examine how these factors are regulated. Three regulatory systems are of particular significance: (1) the sympathetic nervous system, (2) the renin-angiotensin system, and (3) the kidney.

*Sympathetic Baroreceptor Reflex.* The sympathetic nervous system employs a reflex circuit—the *baroreceptor reflex*—to keep blood pressure at a preset level. This circuit operates as follows: (1) Baroreceptors in the aortic arch and carotid sinus sense blood pressure and relay this information to the brainstem. (2) When blood pressure is perceived as too low, the brainstem sends impulses along sympathetic nerves to stimulate the heart and blood vessels. (3) Blood pressure is then elevated by (a) stimulation of beta$_1$ receptors in the heart, resulting in increased cardiac output, and (b) stimulation of vascular alpha$_1$ receptors, resulting in vasoconstriction. (4) When blood pressure has been reduced to an acceptable level, sympathetic stimulation of the heart and vascular smooth muscle subsides.

The baroreceptor reflex frequently opposes our attempts to reduce blood pressure with drugs. Opposition occurs because the "set point" of the baroreceptors is high in people with hypertension. That is, the baroreceptors are set to perceive excessively high blood pressure as being "normal" (i.e., appropriate). As a result, the system operates to maintain blood pressure at pathologic levels. Consequently, when we attempt to lower blood pressure using drugs, the reduced (healthier) pressure is interpreted by the baroreceptors as below what it should be, and, in response, signals are sent out along sympathetic nerves to "correct" the reduction. These signals produce reflex tachycardia and vasoconstriction—responses that can counteract the hypotensive effects of drugs. Clearly, if treatment is to succeed, the regimen must compensate for the resistance offered by the baroreceptor reflex. Inclusion of a *beta blocker*, which will block reflex tachycardia, can be an effective method of compensation. Fortunately, when blood pressure has been suppressed with drugs for an extended period, the baroreceptors become reset at a lower level. Consequently, as therapy proceeds, sympathetic reflexes offer progressively less resistance to the hypotensive effects of medication.

*Renin-Angiotensin System.* The renin-angiotensin system (RAS) can elevate blood pressure, thereby negating the hypotensive effects of our drugs. The RAS is discussed at length in Chapter 41 and reviewed briefly here.

How does the RAS elevate blood pressure? The process begins with the release of renin from juxtaglomerular cells of the kidney. These cells release renin in response to reduced renal blood flow, reduced blood volume, reduced blood pressure, and stimulation of beta$_1$-adrenergic receptors on the cell surface. Following its release, renin promotes the conversion of angiotensinogen into angiotensin I, a weak vasoconstrictor. After this, *angiotensin-converting enzyme* (ACE) acts on angiotensin I to form *angiotensin II*, a compound that constricts systemic and renal blood vessels. Constriction of systemic blood vessels elevates blood pressure by increasing peripheral resistance. Constriction of renal blood vessels elevates blood pressure by reducing glomerular filtration, which causes retention of salt and water, which in turn increases blood volume and blood pressure. In addition to causing vasoconstriction, angiotensin II causes release of *aldosterone* from the adrenal cortex. Aldosterone acts on the kidneys to further increase retention of sodium and water.

Since drug-induced reductions in blood pressure can activate the RAS, this system can counteract the effects we are trying to achieve. We have three ways to cope with this problem. First, we can suppress renin release with *beta blockers*. Second, we can prevent the conversion of angiotensin I into angiotensin II with an *ACE inhibitor*. Third, we can block receptors for angiotensin II with an *angiotensin II receptor antagonist.*

***Renal Regulation of Blood Pressure.*** As discussed in Chapter 40, the kidney plays a central role in long-term regulation of blood pressure. When blood pressure falls, glomerular filtration rate (GFR) falls as well, thereby promoting retention of sodium, chloride, and water. The resultant increase in blood volume increases venous return to the heart, causing an increase in cardiac output, which in turn increases arterial pressure. We can negate renal effects on blood pressure with *diuretics*.

## Antihypertensive Mechanisms: Sites of Drug Action and Effects Produced

As discussed above, drugs can lower blood pressure by reducing heart rate, myocardial contractility, blood volume, venous return, and the tone of arteriolar smooth muscle. In this section we survey the principal mechanisms by which drugs produce these effects.

The major mechanisms for lowering blood pressure are summarized in Figure 44–2 and Table 44–3. The figure indicates the nine principal sites at which antihypertensive drugs act. The table summarizes the effects brought about by drug actions exerted at these sites. The sites of drug action and the resultant effects are described briefly below. Sites numbered 1 through 10 below correspond with sites 1 through 10 in the figure and table.

***1. Brainstem.*** Antihypertensive drugs acting in the brainstem suppress sympathetic outflow to the heart and blood vessels, resulting in decreased heart rate, decreased myocardial contractility, and vasodilation. Vasodilation

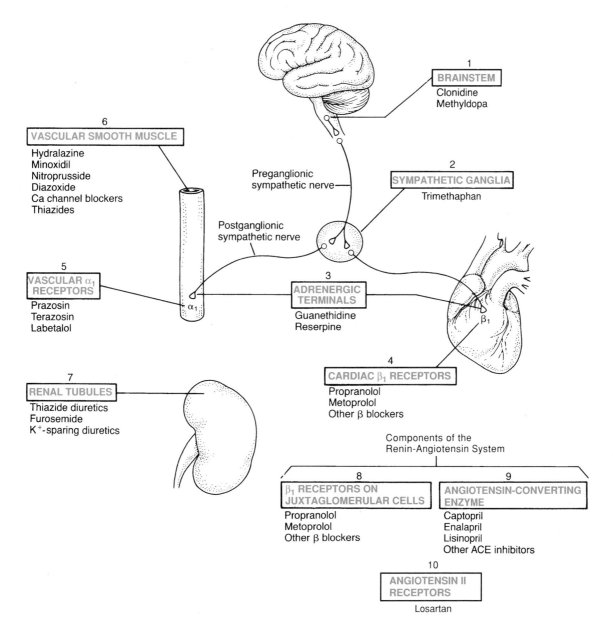

**Figure 44–2. Sites of action of antihypertensive drugs.** Note that some antihypertensive agents act at more than one site: beta blockers act at sites 4 and 8, and thiazides act at sites 6 and 7. The hemodynamic consequences of drug actions at the sites depicted are summarized in Table 44–3.

## TABLE 44–3. SUMMARY OF ANTIHYPERTENSIVE EFFECTS ELICITED BY DRUG ACTIONS AT SPECIFIC SITES

| Site of Drug Action* | Representative Drug | Drug Effects |
|---|---|---|
| 1. Brainstem | Clonidine | Suppression of sympathetic outflow decreases sympathetic stimulation of the heart and blood vessels. |
| 2. Sympathetic ganglia | Trimethaphan | Ganglionic blockade reduces sympathetic stimulation of the heart and blood vessels. |
| 3. Adrenergic nerve terminals | Guanethidine | Reduced norepinephrine release decreases sympathetic stimulation of the heart and blood vessels. |
| 4. Cardiac beta$_1$ receptors | Propranolol | Beta$_1$ blockade decreases heart rate and myocardial contractility. |
| 5. Vascular alpha$_1$ receptors | Prazosin | Alpha$_1$ blockade causes vasodilation. |
| 6. Vascular smooth muscle | Hydralazine | Relaxation of vascular smooth muscle causes vasodilation. |
| 7. Renal tubules | Chlorothiazide | Promotion of diuresis results in decreased blood volume. |
| 8. Beta$_1$ receptors on juxtaglomerular cells | Propranolol | Beta$_1$ blockade suppresses renin release, resulting in (1) vasodilation secondary to reduced production of angiotensin II, and (2) prevention of aldosterone-mediated volume expansion. |
| 9. Angiotensin-converting enzyme (ACE) | Captopril | Inhibition of ACE decreases formation of angiotensin II and thereby prevents (1) vasoconstriction, and (2) aldosterone-mediated volume expansion. |
| 10. Angiotenson II receptors | Losartan | Blockade of angiotensin II receptors prevents angiotensin-mediated vasoconstriction and aldosterone-mediated volume expansion. |

*Sites 1 through 10 in this table correspond to sites 1 through 10 in Figure 44-2.

contributes most to reductions in blood pressure. Dilation of *arterioles* reduces blood pressure by decreasing vascular resistance. Dilation of *veins* decreases blood pressure by decreasing venous return to the heart.

**2. Sympathetic Ganglia.** Ganglionic blockade reduces sympathetic stimulation of the heart and blood vessels. Antihypertensive effects result primarily from dilation of arterioles and veins. Ganglionic blocking agents produce such a profound reduction in blood pressure that they are employed only for hypertensive emergencies.

**3. Terminals of Adrenergic Nerves.** Antihypertensive agents acting at adrenergic nerve terminals decrease the release of norepinephrine, resulting in decreased sympathetic stimulation of the heart and blood vessels.

**4. Beta$_1$-Adrenergic Receptors on the Heart.** Blockade of cardiac beta$_1$ receptors prevents sympathetic stimulation of the heart. As a result, heart rate and myocardial contractility decline.

**5. Alpha$_1$-Adrenergic Receptors on Blood Vessels.** Blockade of vascular alpha$_1$ receptors promotes dilation of arterioles and veins. Arteriolar dilation reduces peripheral resistance. Venous dilation reduces venous return of blood to the heart.

**6. Vascular Smooth Muscle.** Several antihypertensive drugs (Fig. 44-2) act directly on vascular smooth muscle to cause relaxation. Two of these agents—sodium nitroprusside and diazoxide—are used only for hypertensive emergencies. The rest are used for essential hypertension.

**7. Renal Tubules.** Diuretics act on renal tubules to promote salt and water excretion. As a result, blood volume declines, causing blood pressure to fall.

**8. Beta$_1$ Receptors on Juxtaglomerular Cells.** Blockade of beta$_1$ receptors on juxtaglomerular cells suppresses release of renin. The resultant decrease in angiotensin II levels has three effects: peripheral vasodilation, renal vasodilation, and suppression of aldosterone-mediated volume expansion.

**9. Angiotensin-Converting Enzyme.** Inhibitors of angiotensin-converting enzyme suppress formation of angiotensin II. This results in peripheral vasodilation, renal vasodilation, and suppression of aldosterone-mediated volume expansion.

**10. Angiotensin II Receptors.** Blockade of angiotensin II receptors prevents the actions of angiotensin II. Hence blockade results in peripheral vasodilation, renal vasodilation, and suppression of aldosterone-mediated volume expansion.

## The Antihypertensive Drugs

In this section we consider the principal drugs employed to treat *essential hypertension*. Drugs used in *hypertensive emergencies* and *hypertensive disorders of pregnancy* are considered below.

The antihypertensive drugs and their classes are summarized in Table 44-4. All of these drugs have been discussed in previous chapters. Accordingly, discussion here

## TABLE 44-4. DRUGS FOR CHRONIC HYPERTENSION

| Diuretics | Sympatholytics | Others |
|---|---|---|
| **Thiazides and Related Diuretics** | **Beta Blockers** | **ACE Inhibitors** |
| Bendroflumethiazide | Acebutolol | Benazepril |
| Benzthiazide | Atenolol | Captopril |
| Chlorothiazide | Betaxolol | Enalapril |
| Cyclothiazide | Bisoprolol | Fosinopril |
| Hydrochlorothiazide | Metoprolol | Lisinopril |
| Hydroflumethiazide | Nadolol | Moexipril |
| Indapamide | Penbutolol | Quinapril |
| Methyclothiazide | Pindolol | Ramipril |
| Metolazone | Propranolol | Trandolapril |
| Polythiazide | Timolol | **Angiotensin II Receptor Antagonists** |
| Quinethazone | **Alpha₁ Blockers** | Losartan |
| Trichlormethiazide | Doxazosin | Valsartan |
| **Loop Diuretics** | Prazosin | **Calcium Channel Blockers** |
| Furosemide | Terazosin | Amlodipine |
| Ethacrynic acid | **Alpha/Beta Blockers** | Diltiazem |
| Bumetanide | Labetalol | Felodipine |
| Torsemide | Carvedilol | Isradipine |
| **Potassium-Sparing Diuretics** | **Centrally Acting Alpha₂ Agonists** | Nifedipine |
| Spironolactone | Clonidine | Nicardipine |
| Triamterene | Methyldopa | Nimodipine |
| Amiloride | Guanabenz | Nislodipine |
| | Guanfacine | Verapamil |
| | **Adrenergic Neuron Blockers** | **Direct-Acting Vasodilators** |
| | Guanethidine | Hydralazine |
| | Guanadrel | Minoxidil |
| | Reserpine | |

| Combinations with Diuretics | Trade Name |
|---|---|
| **Thiazide Plus Potassium-Sparing Diuretic** | |
| Hydrochlorothiazide + spironolactone | Aldactazide |
| Hydrochlorothiazide + triamterene | Dyazide, Maxide |
| Hydrochlorothiazide + amiloride | Moduretic |
| **Thiazide Plus Beta Blocker** | |
| Hydrochlorothiazide + propranolol | Inderide |
| Hydrochlorothiazide + metoprolol | Lopressor HCT |
| Hydrochlorothiazide + timolol | Timolide |
| Hydrochlorothiazide + bisoprolol | Ziac |
| Chlorthalidone + atenolol | Tenoretic |
| **Thiazide Plus ACE Inhibitor** | |
| Hydrochlorothiazide + captopril | Capozide |
| Hydrochlorothiazide + benazepril | Lotensin HCT |

is limited to their use in hypertension. Of primary interest are mechanisms of antihypertensive action and major adverse effects.

## Diuretics

Diuretics are a mainstay of antihypertensive therapy. These drugs reduce blood pressure when used alone, and they can enhance the effects of other hypotensive drugs. The basic pharmacology of the diuretics is discussed in Chapter 38.

**Thiazide Diuretics.** The thiazide diuretics (e.g., hydrochlorothiazide) are the most commonly used antihypertensive drugs. Thiazides reduce blood pressure by two mechanisms: reduction of blood volume and reduction of arterial resistance. Reduced blood volume is responsible for initial antihypertensive effects. Reduced vascular resistance develops over time and is responsible for long-term antihypertensive effects. The mechanism by which thiazides reduce vascular resistance has not been established.

The principal adverse effect of thiazides is *hypokalemia*. This effect can be minimized by consuming potassium-rich foods (e.g., bananas, citrus fruits) and by using potassium supplements or a potassium-sparing diuretic. Other side effects include *dehydration, hyperglycemia,* and *hyperuricemia.*

***High-Ceiling (Loop) Diuretics.*** High-ceiling diuretics (e.g., furosemide) produce much greater diuresis than the thiazides. For most individuals with essential hypertension, the amount of fluid loss that loop diuretics can produce is greater than needed or desirable. Consequently, loop diuretics are not used routinely. Rather, they are reserved for (1) patients who need greater diuresis than can be achieved with thiazides and (2) patients with a low GFR (since thiazides won't work when GFR is low). Like the thiazides, the loop diuretics lower blood pressure by reducing blood volume and promoting vasodilation.

Most adverse effects are like those of the thiazides: *hypokalemia, dehydration, hyperglycemia,* and *hyperuricemia.* In addition, high-ceiling agents can cause *hearing loss.*

***Potassium-Sparing Diuretics.*** The degree of diuresis induced by the potassium-sparing agents (e.g., spironolactone) is small. Consequently, these drugs are not very effective as hypotensive agents. However, because of their ability to conserve potassium, these drugs can play an important role in an antihypertensive regimen. That role is to balance potassium loss caused by thiazides or loop diuretics. The most significant adverse effect of the potassium-sparing agents is *hyperkalemia.* Because of the risk of hyperkalemia, potassium-sparing diuretics must not be used in combination with one another or with potassium supplements. Also, they should not be used routinely with ACE inhibitors, which also promote hyperkalemia.

## Sympatholytics (Adrenergic Antagonists)

Sympatholytic drugs suppress the influence of the sympathetic nervous system on the heart, blood vessels, and other structures. These drugs are used widely in the treatment of hypertension.

As indicated in Table 44-4, there are five subcategories of sympatholytic drugs: (1) beta-adrenergic blockers, (2) centrally acting alpha$_2$ agonists, (3) adrenergic neuron blockers, (4) alpha$_1$-adrenergic antagonists, and (5) alpha$_1$/beta blockers.

***Beta-Adrenergic Blockers.*** The beta blockers (e.g., propranolol, metoprolol) are among the most widely used antihypertensive drugs. However, despite their efficacy and frequent use, the exact mechanism by which these drugs reduce blood pressure is somewhat uncertain.

The beta blockers have at least four useful actions in hypertension. First, blockade of cardiac beta$_1$ receptors decreases heart rate and contractility, thereby decreasing cardiac output. Second, beta blockers can suppress reflex tachycardia caused by vasodilators in the regimen. Third, blockade of beta$_1$ receptors on juxtaglomerular cells of the kidney reduces release of renin, thereby reducing angiotensin II–mediated vasoconstriction and aldosterone-mediated volume expansion. Fourth, recent studies indicate that long-term use of beta blockers reduces peripheral vascular resistance—by a mechanism that is unknown. This newly discovered action could readily account for most of the antihypertensive effects of these drugs.

Beta blockers can produce a variety of adverse effects. Blockade of cardiac beta$_1$ receptors can produce *bradycardia, decreased atrioventricular (AV) conduction,* and *reduced contractility.* Consequently, beta blockers should not be used by patients with sick sinus syndrome, congestive heart failure, or second- or third-degree AV block. Blockade of beta$_2$ receptors in the lung can promote *bronchoconstriction.* Accordingly, beta blockers should be avoided by patients with asthma. If an asthmatic individual absolutely must use a beta blocker, a beta$_1$-selective agent (e.g., metoprolol) should be employed. Beta blockers can mask signs of hypoglycemia, and therefore must be used with caution in patients with *diabetes.* Through actions exerted in the central nervous system, beta blockers can cause *depression, insomnia, bizarre dreams,* and *sexual dysfunction.*

The basic pharmacology of the beta blockers is discussed in Chapter 19.

***Centrally Acting Alpha$_2$ Agonists.*** As discussed in Chapter 20, these drugs (e.g., clonidine, methyldopa) act within the brainstem to suppress sympathetic outflow to the heart and blood vessels. The result is vasodilation and reduced cardiac output, both of which help lower blood pressure. All central alpha$_2$ agonists can cause *drying of the mouth* and *sedation.* In addition, clonidine can cause severe *rebound hypertension* if treatment is abruptly discontinued. Additional adverse effects of methyldopa are *hemolytic anemia* (accompanied by a positive direct Coombs' test) and *liver disorders.*

***Adrenergic Neuron Blockers.*** This group consists of three drugs: guanethidine, guanadrel, and reserpine. All three decrease blood pressure through actions exerted within the terminals of postganglionic sympathetic neurons. Guanethidine and guanadrel inhibit release of norepinephrine, whereas reserpine causes norepinephrine depletion. Both actions result in decreased sympathetic stimulation of the heart and blood vessels.

The major adverse effect of *guanethidine* and *guanadrel* is *severe orthostatic hypotension* resulting from decreased sympathetic tone to veins. Because of the risk of postural hypotension, these drugs are last-choice agents for chronic hypertension.

The major adverse effect of *reserpine* is *depression.* Accordingly, reserpine is absolutely contraindicated for patients with a history of depressive illness.

The basic pharmacology of reserpine and guanethidine is discussed in Chapter 20.

***Alpha$_1$-Adrenergic Blockers.*** The alpha$_1$ blockers (e.g., prazosin, terazosin) prevent stimulation of alpha$_1$ receptors on arterioles and veins, thereby preventing sympathetically mediated vasoconstriction. The resultant vasodilation reduces both peripheral resistance and venous return to the heart.

The most disturbing side effect of alpha blockers is *orthostatic hypotension*. Hypotension can be especially severe with the initial dose. Significant hypotension continues with subsequent doses but is less profound.

The basic pharmacology of the alpha blockers is discussed in Chapter 19.

***Alpha/Beta-Adrenergic Blockers: Labetalol and Carvedilol.*** Labetalol and carvedilol are unusual in that they can block alpha$_1$ receptors as well as beta receptors. Blood pressure reduction results from a combination of actions: (1) alpha$_1$ blockade promotes dilation of arterioles and veins, (2) blockade of cardiac beta$_1$ receptors reduces heart rate and contractility, and (3) blockade of beta$_1$ receptors on juxtaglomerular cells suppresses release of renin. Presumably, these drugs also share the ability of other beta blockers to reduce peripheral vascular resistance. Like other nonselective beta blockers, labetalol and carvedilol can exacerbate bradycardia, AV heart block, heart failure, and asthma. Blockade of venous alpha$_1$ receptors can produce postural hypotension.

## Direct-Acting Vasodilators: Hydralazine and Minoxidil

Hydralazine and minoxidil reduce blood pressure by promoting dilation of *arterioles*. Neither drug causes significant dilation of veins. Because venous dilation is minimal, these agents produce very little orthostatic hypotension. With both drugs, lowering of blood pressure may be followed by reflex tachycardia, renin release, and fluid retention. Reflex tachycardia and release of renin can be prevented with a beta blocker. Fluid retention can be prevented with a diuretic.

The most disturbing adverse effect of *hydralazine* is a syndrome resembling *systemic lupus erythematosus* (SLE). Fortunately, this reaction is rare when the drug is used at recommended doses. If an SLE-like reaction occurs, hydralazine should be withdrawn. Hydralazine is considered a third-choice drug for chronic hypertension.

*Minoxidil* is substantially more toxic than hydralazine. By causing fluid retention, minoxidil can promote *pericardial effusion* (accumulation of fluid beneath the myocardium) that in some cases progresses to *cardiac tamponade* (compression of the heart). A less serious effect is *hypertrichosis* (excessive hair growth). Because of its capacity for significant harm, minoxidil is not used routinely in chronic hypertension. Instead, the drug is reserved for patients with severe hypertension who have not responded to less dangerous drugs.

The basic pharmacology of hydralazine and minoxidil is discussed in Chapter 43.

## Calcium Channel Blockers

The calcium channel blockers used most frequently are verapamil, diltiazem, and nifedipine. Discussion here is limited to these three drugs. All three reduce blood pressure by causing dilation of *arterioles*.

Like other vasodilators, calcium channel blockers can cause *reflex tachycardia*. This reaction is greatest with nifedipine and minimal with verapamil and diltiazem.

Reflex tachycardia is low with verapamil and diltiazem because these drugs have direct suppressant effects on the heart. Since nifedipine does not block cardiac calcium channels, reflex tachycardia with this drug can be substantial.

Because of their ability to compromise cardiac performance, verapamil and diltiazem must be used cautiously in patients with bradycardia, heart failure, or AV heart block. These precautions do not apply to nifedipine.

The *rapid-acting* formulation of nifedipine has been associated with increased mortality in patients with myocardial infarction and unstable angina. As a result, the National Heart, Lung, and Blood Institute has recommended that rapid-acting nifedipine be used with great caution, if at all.

The basic pharmacology of the calcium channel blockers is discussed in Chapter 42.

## Angiotensin-Converting Enzyme Inhibitors

The ACE inhibitors used most frequently in hypertension are captopril and enalapril. Discussion here is limited to these two drugs. Both agents lower blood pressure by preventing the conversion of angiotensin I into angiotensin II, thereby preventing angiotensin II–mediated vasoconstriction and aldosterone-mediated volume expansion. Principal adverse effects are *persistent cough*, *first-dose hypotension*, and *hyperkalemia* (secondary to suppression of aldosterone release). Because of the risk of hyperkalemia, combined use with potassium supplements or potassium-sparing diuretics should generally be avoided. ACE inhibitors can cause fetal harm during the second and third trimesters of pregnancy, and hence must not be given to pregnant women. These are the only antihypertensive drugs that are specifically contraindicated for use during pregnancy. The basic pharmacology of the ACE inhibitors is discussed in Chapter 41.

## Angiotensin II Receptor Antagonists

Angiotensin II receptor antagonist (AngIIRAs) are new drugs for use in hypertension. At this time, only two AngIIRAs are available: losartan and valsartan. Both drugs lower blood pressure in much the same way as the ACE inhibitors do. That is, like the ACE inhibitors, AngIIRAs prevent angiotensin II–mediated vasoconstriction and release of aldosterone. The only difference is that AngIIRAs do so by blocking angiotensin II receptors, whereas the ACE inhibitors prevent angiotensin II formation. Since AngIIRAs are new drugs, their niche in antihypertensive therapy has not been established. The basic pharmacology of these drugs is discussed in Chapter 41.

# Fundamentals of Antihypertensive Therapy

## The Basic Strategy

The basic approach to treating hypertension is outlined in Figure 44–3. As shown, lifestyle changes should be tried first. If these fail to produce an adequate response, they

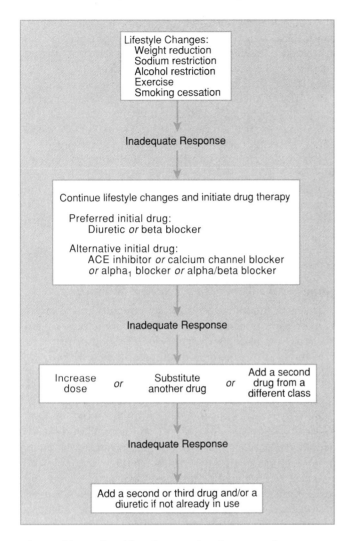

**Figure 44–3. Algorithm for treating hypertension.**

**TABLE 44-5. CHOICE OF ANTIHYPERTENSIVE DRUGS: INITIAL AND SUPPLEMENTAL AGENTS**

| DRUGS FOR INITIAL THERAPY | |
|---|---|
| *Preferred Agents** | *Alternatives†* |
| Beta Blockers | ACE Inhibitors |
| Diuretics | Alpha₁ blockers |
| | Alpha/Beta blockers |
| | Calcium channel blockers |

| SUPPLEMENTAL DRUGS |
|---|
| Centrally acting sympatholytics |
| Adrenergic neuron blockers |
| Direct-acting vasodilators |

*Diuretics and beta blockers are preferred because these drugs have a demonstrated ability to reduce morbidity and mortality.
†Although these drugs can reduce blood pressure, we do not yet know if they can reduce morbidity and mortality.
Based on recommendations in the fifth report of the Joint National Committee on Detection, Evaluation, and Treatment of High Blood Pressure, 1993.

should be continued and drug therapy should be started. Treatment should begin with a single drug, usually a diuretic or a beta blocker. If the initial drug fails to produce an adequate response, another drug may be added or substituted. However, before another drug is considered, possible reasons for failure with the initial drug should be assessed. These include insufficient dosage, poor compliance, excessive salt intake, and the presence of secondary hypertension. If treatment with two drugs is unsuccessful, a third may be added.

## Guidelines for Drug Selection

As indicated in Table 44-5, the antihypertensive drugs can be placed in two major therapeutic groups: (1) drugs for initial therapy and (2) supplemental drugs. For initial therapy, a *diuretic* or a *beta blocker* is generally preferred. This preference is based on long-term controlled trials that show conclusively that beta blockers and diuretics can reduce morbidity and mortality in hypertensive patients. The alternative drugs for initial therapy— *ACE inhibitors, calcium channel blockers, alpha₁-adrenergic blockers,* and *alpha/beta adrenergic*

*blockers*—are equally effective in reducing blood pressure. However, because these drugs have not been used in long-term controlled trials, we do not yet know if they reduce morbidity and mortality. Hence, authorities recommend they be reserved for special indications and for patients who have not responded to beta blockers and diuretics. The drugs classified as supplemental—*centrally acting sympatholytics, adrenergic neuron blockers,* and *direct-acting vasodilators*—are associated with a high incidence of undesirable effects; hence, these drugs are not well suited for initial monotherapy.

An important guideline for drug selection is that each drug in the regimen should belong to a different class. That is, each drug should have a different mechanism of action. In accord with this guideline, it would be appropriate to combine a beta blocker, a diuretic, and a vasodilator, since each lowers blood pressure by a different mechanism. In contrast, it would be inappropriate to combine two thiazide diuretics or two beta blockers or two vasodilators.

To ensure maximum benefits with minimum harm, it is essential that treatment be tailored to the individual patient. This important topic is addressed later under *Individualizing Therapy.*

## Benefits of Multidrug Therapy

Treatment with multiple drugs can offer significant benefits. First, by employing drugs that have different mechanisms of action, we can increase the chance of success: attacking blood pressure control at several sites is more likely to be effective than an attack that centers on just one site. Second, when drugs are used in combination, each can be administered in a lower dosage than would be possible if it were used alone; as a result, both the frequency and the intensity of side effects are reduced. Third, when proper combinations are selected, one agent can offset the adverse effects of another. For example, if a vasodilator is used alone, reflex tachycardia is likely. However, if a vasodilator is combined with a beta blocker, reflex tachycardia will be minimal.

## Dosing

For each drug in the regimen, *dosage should be low initially and then gradually increased*. There are several reasons for this approach. First, for most people with chronic hypertension, the disease poses no immediate threat to well-being. Hence there is no need to lower blood pressure rapidly using large doses. Second, when blood pressure is reduced slowly, baroreceptors gradually reset to the new, lower pressure. As a result, sympathetic reflexes will offer less resistance to the hypotensive effects of therapy. Third, since there is no need to drop blood pressure rapidly, and since higher doses carry a higher risk of adverse effects, use of high initial doses would needlessly increase the risk of unpleasant responses.

## Step-Down Therapy

After blood pressure has been controlled for at least 1 year, an attempt should be made to reduce dosages and the number of drugs in the regimen. Of course, lifestyle modifications should be continued. When reductions are made slowly and progressively, many patients are able to maintain blood pressure control with less medication—and some can be maintained with no medication at all. If drugs are discontinued, regular follow-up is essential, since blood pressure usually returns to hypertensive levels—although it may take years to do so.

## Individualizing Therapy

### Treating Patients with Co-existing Diseases

Antihypertensive drugs that can exacerbate co-existing disorders must be avoided. In our discussion of specific antihypertensive drugs, we noted that certain agents can aggravate certain disease states. We saw, for example, that reserpine can intensify depression and that beta blockers can exacerbate heart failure, AV block, and asthma. Other conditions that can be aggravated by antihypertensive drugs are presented in Table 44–6. To help avoid drug-disease mismatches, the medical history should identify all co-existing pathophysiology. With this information, the prescriber will be able to choose drugs that are least likely to make co-existing disorders worse.

### Treating Patients in Special Populations

*African Americans.* Hypertension is the major health problem of African American adults. Hypertension develops earlier in blacks than in whites, has a much higher incidence, and is likely to be more severe. As a result, African Americans face a greater risk of heart disease, end-stage renal disease, and stroke. Available data indicate that blacks and whites respond equally to treatment—although not always to the same drugs. Controlled trials have shown that *diuretics* can decrease morbidity and mortality in blacks. Accordingly, these agents are drugs of first choice. Monotherapy with calcium channel blockers, alpha$_1$ blockers, and labetalol are equally effective in blacks and whites. In contrast, *beta blockers* and *ACE inhibitors* are less effective in blacks than in whites. Because African Americans have a high incidence of salt sensitivity, obesity, and cigarette use, lifestyle changes are especially important in this group.

*Children.* The incidence of secondary hypertension in children is much higher than in adults. Accordingly, efforts to diagnose and treat an underlying cause should be especially diligent. For children with primary hypertension, treatment is the same as for adults.

*The Elderly.* The incidence of hypertension in people over age 60 is approximately 65%, and the prevalence of isolated systolic hypertension is greater than in younger adults. In clinical trials, treatment has reduced the incidence of stroke by 36% and myocardial infarction by 27%. Although all antihypertensive drugs are effective in older adults, only the *beta blockers* and *diuretics* have been shown in controlled trials to reduce morbidity and mortality. Hence, these drugs are often preferred. Since cardiovascular reflexes are blunted in the elderly, treatment carries a significant risk of orthostatic hypotension. Accordingly, initial doses should be lower than for younger adults. Furthermore, drugs that are especially likely to cause orthostatic hypotension (e.g., guanethidine, alpha blockers, alpha/beta blockers) should be used with caution.

*Diabetics.* ACE inhibitors help protect against diabetic nephropathy. Accordingly, for diabetics who have hypertension, these drugs can serve the dual purpose of preserving kidney function and lowering blood pressure. Beta blockers should be used with caution for two reasons: they suppress glycogenolysis and mask early signs of hypoglycemia. Thiazides and high-ceiling diuretics promote hyperglycemia and should be used with care.

## Minimizing Adverse Effects

Antihypertensive drugs can produce many unwanted effects, including hypotension, sedation, and disruption of sexual function. (Although not stressed previously, practically all antihypertensive drugs can interfere with sexual feelings or performance.)

The fundamental strategy for decreasing side effects is to tailor the regimen to the sensitivities of the patient. Simply put, if one drug causes effects that are objectionable, a more acceptable drug should be substituted. The best way to identify unacceptable responses is to encourage the patient to report them.

Adverse effects caused by exacerbation of co-existing diseases are both predictable and avoidable. By taking a thorough medical history, we can greatly reduce the chances of an inappropriate drug-disease match.

Use of high initial doses and rapid dosage escalation can increase the incidence and severity of adverse effects. Accordingly, doses should be low initially and then gradually increased. Remember, there is usually no need to re-

## TABLE 44–6. PATHOPHYSIOLOGIC CONDITIONS THAT REQUIRE CAUTIOUS USE OR COMPLETE AVOIDANCE OF CERTAIN ANTIHYPERTENSIVE DRUGS

| Pathophysiologic Condition | Drugs to Be Avoided or Used with Caution | Reason for Concern |
|---|---|---|
| *Cardiovascular* | | |
| Congestive heart failure | Beta blockers Labetalol Verapamil Diltiazem | These drugs act on the heart to decrease myocardial contractility and can thereby further reduce cardiac output. |
| AV heart block | Beta blockers Labetalol Verapamil Diltiazem | These drugs act on the heart to suppress AV conduction and can thereby intensify AV block. |
| Coronary artery disease | Guanethidine Hydralazine | Reflex tachycardia induced by these drugs can precipitate an anginal attack. |
| Post-myocardial infarction | Guanethidine Hydralazine | Reflex tachycardia induced by these drugs can increase cardiac work and oxygen demand. |
| *Other* | | |
| Renal insufficiency | $K^+$-sparing diuretics $K^+$-supplements | Use of these agents can lead to dangerous accumulations of potassium. |
| Asthma | Beta blockers Labetalol | $Beta_2$ blockade promotes bronchoconstriction. |
| Depression | Reserpine | Reserpine causes depression. |
| Diabetes mellitus | Thiazides Furosemide Beta blockers | Thiazides and furosemide promote hyperglycemia; beta blockers suppress glycogenolysis and can mask signs of hypoglycemia. |
| Gout | Thiazides Furosemide | These diuretics promote hyperuricemia. |
| Hyperkalemia | $K^+$-sparing diuretics ACE inhibitors | These drugs cause potassium accumulation. |
| Hypokalemia | Thiazides Furosemide | These diuretics promote potassium loss. |
| Collagen diseases | Hydralazine | Hydralazine can precipitate a lupus erythematosus–like syndrome. |
| Liver disease | Methyldopa | Methyldopa is hepatotoxic. |
| Pre-eclampsia | ACE inhibitors | These drugs can injure the fetus. |

duce blood pressure rapidly. Hence, it makes no sense to give large initial doses that can produce a rapid fall in blood pressure but that also produce intense undesired responses.

## Promoting Compliance

The major cause of treatment failure in patients with chronic hypertension is lack of adherence to the therapeutic regimen. In this section we consider the causes of noncompliance and then discuss some solutions.

### Why Compliance Can Be Difficult to Achieve

Much of the difficulty in promoting compliance stems from the nature of hypertension itself. Hypertension is a chronic, slowly progressing disease that, through much of its course, is devoid of overt symptoms. Because symp-toms are absent, it can be difficult to convince patients that they are ill and need treatment. In addition, since there are no symptoms to relieve, drugs cannot produce an obvious therapeutic response. In the absence of such a response, it can be difficult for patients to believe that their medication is doing anything useful.

Because hypertension progresses very slowly, the disease tends to encourage procrastination. For most people, the adverse effects of hypertension will not become manifest for many years. Realizing this, patients may reason (incorrectly) that they can postpone therapy without significantly increasing their risk.

The negative aspects of treatment also contribute to noncompliance. Antihypertensive regimens can be complex and expensive. In addition, treatment must continue lifelong. Lastly, antihypertensive drugs can cause a number of adverse effects, ranging from sedation to hypotension to disruption of sexual function. It is difficult to convince people who are feeling good to take drugs that may make them feel worse. Some people may decide that exposing themselves to the negative effects of therapy today is paying too high a price to avoid the adverse consequences of hypertension at some indefinite time in the future.

### Ways to Promote Compliance

*Patient Education.* Compliance requires motivation; patient education can help provide it. Patients should be taught about the consequences of hypertension and the benefits of treatment. Because hypertension does not cause discomfort, it may not be clear to patients that their condition is indeed serious. Patients must be made to understand that, left untreated, hypertension can cause heart disease, kidney disease, blindness, and stroke. In addition, patients should appreciate that with proper therapy the risks of these long-term complications can be minimized, resulting in a longer and healthier life. Lastly, patients must understand that drugs do not cure hypertension—they only control symptoms. Hence, for treatment to be effective, medication must usually be taken lifelong.

*Self-Monitoring.* Patients should be taught the goal of treatment (reduction of blood pressure to 140/90 mm Hg), and they should be taught to monitor and record their blood pressure daily. This increases patient involvement and provides positive feedback that can help promote compliance.

*Minimize Side Effects.* Common sense dictates that if we expect patients to comply with long-term treatment, we must keep undesired effects to a minimum. As discussed above, adverse effects can be minimized by (1) encouraging patients to report side effects, (2) discontinuing objectionable drugs and substituting more acceptable ones, (3) avoiding drugs that can exacerbate co-existing pathology, and (4) using doses that are low initially and then gradually increased.

*Establish a Collaborative Relationship.* The patient who feels like a collaborative partner in the treatment program is more likely to comply than is the patient who feels that treatment is being imposed. Collaboration allows the patient to help set treatment goals, create the treatment program, and evaluate progress. In addition, a collaborative relationship facilitates communication about side effects. This is especially important with respect to drug-induced sexual dysfunction, which patients may be reluctant to discuss.

*Simplify the Regimen.* Antihypertensive regimens may consist of several drugs taken multiple times a day. Such complex regimens deter compliance. Therefore, in order to promote compliance, steps should be taken to make the dosing schedule as simple as possible. Once an effective regimen has been established, an attempt should be made to switch to once-a-day or twice-a-day dosing. If an appropriate combination product is available (e.g., a fixed-dose combination of a thiazide diuretic plus a potassium-sparing diuretic), the combination product may be substituted for its components.

*Other Measures.* Compliance can be promoted by giving positive reinforcement when therapeutic goals are achieved. Involvement of family members in the program can be helpful. Also, compliance can be promoted by scheduling office visits at convenient times and by following up when appointments are missed. For many patients, antihypertensive therapy represents a significant economic burden; devising a regimen that is effective and yet keeps costs low will certainly encourage compliance.

## Drugs for Hypertensive Emergencies

A hypertensive emergency exists when diastolic blood pressure exceeds 120 mm Hg. The severity of the emergency is determined by the likelihood of organ damage. When excessive blood pressure is associated with papilledema (edema of the retina), intracranial hemorrhage, myocardial infarction, or acute congestive heart failure, a severe emergency exists—and blood pressure must be lowered rapidly (within 1 hour). If severe hypertension is present but does not yet pose an immediate threat of organ damage, it is preferable to reduce blood pressure more slowly (over 24 to 48 hours). (Rapid reductions in blood pressure can cause cerebral ischemia, myocardial infarction, and renal failure. Hence pressure should be reduced gradually whenever possible.)

The major drugs used for hypertensive emergencies are discussed below. All reduce blood pressure by causing vasodilation. With the exception of short-acting nifedipine, all are administered intravenously.

*Sodium Nitroprusside.* When acute, severe hypertension demands a rapid but controlled reduction in pressure, intravenous nitroprusside [Nipride, Nitropress] is usually the drug of first choice. Nitroprusside is a direct-acting vasodilator that relaxes smooth muscle of arterioles and veins. Effects begin in seconds and then fade rapidly when administration ceases. Nitroprusside is administered by continuous IV infusion using a pump to control the infusion rate. The usual rate is 0.5 to 8 µg/kg/min. To avoid overshoot, continuous monitoring of blood pressure is required. Because nitroprusside has an extremely short duration of action, overshoot can be corrected quickly by reducing the rate of the infusion. Prolonged infusion (longer than 72 hours) can produce toxic accumulation of thiocyanate and should be avoided. The basic pharmacology of nitroprusside is discussed in Chapter 43.

*Nifedipine.* Short-acting nifedipine [Adalat, Procardia] has been widely used for hypertensive emergencies. This calcium channel blocker lowers blood pressure by dilating arterioles. In patients with severe hypertension, nifedipine produces a 20% reduction in systolic and diastolic pressure within 20 to 30 minutes. The dosage is 5 to 20 mg repeated every 4 to 6 hours. To ensure a rapid response, patients must bite the nifedipine capsule and swallow its contents.

Until recently, short-acting nifedipine had been the drug of choice for most hypertensive emergencies. However, we now know that short-acting nifedipine can cause serious dysrhythmias and cardiac arrest—even when used for hypertensive emergencies. Hence, the drug can no longer be considered safe for this application. Nonetheless, nifedipine continues to be a common treatment in emergency situations. The basic pharmacology of nifedipine is discussed in Chapter 42.

**Labetalol.** Labetalol [Trandate, Normodyne] blocks alpha- and beta-adrenergic receptors. Blood pressure is reduced by arteriolar dilation secondary to alpha blockade. Beta blockade prevents reflex tachycardia in response to reduced arterial pressure; hence, the drug is probably safe for patients with angina pectoris and myocardial infarction. Beta blockade can aggravate bronchial asthma, heart failure, AV block, cardiogenic shock, and bradycardia. Accordingly, labetalol should not be given to patients with these disorders. Administration is by slow IV injection.

**Diazoxide.** Diazoxide [Hyperstat IV] causes selective dilation of arterioles. Effects begin within minutes and may persist for hours. The drug can be administered by IV bolus or by slow IV infusion (over 15 to 30 minutes). Diazoxide can produce reflex tachycardia and should be avoided in patients with angina. Reflex tachycardia can be reduced with a beta blocker. Fluid retention may occur and can be controlled with a diuretic. Hyperglycemia may be a complication for patients with diabetes. The basic pharmacology of diazoxide is discussed in Chapter 43.

**Trimethaphan.** Trimethaphan [Arfonad] is a ganglionic blocking agent that dilates arterioles and veins. Effects begin and end within minutes. Like nitroprusside, trimethaphan must be administered by continuous IV infusion, using a pump to control the rate of flow. Continuous monitoring of blood pressure is required. Prominent side effects—dry mouth, blurred vision, urinary retention, paresis of the bowel—result from parasympathetic blockade. The basic pharmacology of trimethaphan is discussed in Chapter 17.

# Drugs for Hypertensive Disorders of Pregnancy

Hypertension is the most common complication of pregnancy, with an incidence of about 10%. When hypertension develops, it is essential to distinguish between chronic hypertension and pre-eclampsia, since chronic hypertension is relatively benign, whereas pre-eclampsia can lead to life-threatening complications for the mother and fetus.

## Chronic Hypertension

Chronic hypertension is defined as hypertension that was present prior to pregnancy or that developed before the 20th week of gestation. Since elevated maternal blood pressure is not a direct threat to the fetus, the goal of treatment is to minimize the risk of hypertension to the mother while avoiding drug-induced harm to the fetus. With the exception of the ACE inhibitors, antihypertensive drugs that were being taken before pregnancy can be continued. *ACE inhibitors are contraindicated because of their potential for harm* (fetal growth retardation, congenital malformations, neonatal renal failure, neonatal

death). When drug therapy is initiated during pregnancy, *methyldopa* is the drug of choice. The drug has no effect on uteroplacental hemodynamics or fetal hemodynamics, nor does it affect the fetus or neonate. Regardless of the drug selected, treatment should not be too aggressive, since an excessive drop in blood pressure could compromise uteroplacental blood flow.

## Pre-Eclampsia and Eclampsia

Pre-eclampsia is a hypertensive disorder that develops after the 20th week of pregnancy. The condition is characterized by elevated blood pressure, proteinuria, and generalized edema. Liver dysfunction and coagulation abnormalities may also be present. Pre-eclampsia can rapidly progress to eclampsia, the convulsive phase of the disorder.

Management is based on the severity of the disease, the status of mother and fetus, and the length of gestation. The objective is to preserve the health of the mother and deliver an infant that will not require intensive and prolonged neonatal care. Success requires close maternal and fetal monitoring. Although drugs can help reduce blood pressure, delivery is the only cure.

Management of *mild* pre-eclampsia is controversial and depends on the duration of gestation. If pre-eclampsia develops near term, and if fetal maturity is certain, induction of labor is advised. However, if mild pre-eclampsia develops earlier in gestation, experts disagree as to what should be done. Suggested measures include bed rest, prolonged hospitalization, treatment with antihypertensive drugs, and prophylaxis with anticonvulsants. Studies to evaluate these strategies have generally failed to demonstrate benefits from any of them, including treatment with antihypertensive drugs.

Management of *severe* pre-eclampsia presents a dilemma. Since the condition can deteriorate rapidly, with grave consequences for mother and fetus, immediate delivery is recommended. However, if the fetus is not sufficiently mature, immediate delivery could threaten its life. Hence the dilemma: do we deliver the fetus immediately, which would eliminate risk for the mother but present a serious risk for the fetus—or do we postpone delivery, which would reduce risk for the fetus but greatly increase risk for the mother? If the patient elects to postpone delivery, then blood pressure can be lowered with drugs. Because severe pre-eclampsia can be life threatening, treatment must be done in a tertiary care center to permit close monitoring of mother and fetus. The major objective of treatment is to prevent cerebral complications (e.g., hemorrhage, encephalopathy). The drug of choice for lowering blood pressure is *hydralazine* (5 mg by IV bolus); dosing may be repeated 3 times at 20-minute intervals. If blood pressure is still too high, the patient may be given *nifedipine* (10 mg PO) or *labetalol* (20 mg IV).

Because pre-eclampsia can (rarely) evolve into eclampsia, the patient may be given anticonvulsants, such as magnesium sulfate or phenytoin, for either prophylaxis or treatment. In the United States, it has been common practice to give magnesium sulfate prophylactically during labor and postpartum to all women with pre-eclampsia.

However, since the risk of eclamptic convulsions is very low to begin with, it has been difficult to prove that anticonvulsant prophylaxis actually reduces the risk any further. Nonetheless, if anticonvulsant prophylaxis is to be used, *magnesium sulfate* is the drug of choice. If convulsions *do* develop, *magnesium sulfate* is considered the best agent to treat them.

## KEY POINTS

Key points are limited to information specific to hypertension. Key points for individual drugs and drug families are presented in their own chapters.

- Hypertension is defined as systolic blood pressure greater than 140 mm Hg or diastolic pressure greater than 90 mm Hg.
- Primary hypertension (essential hypertension), which is defined as hypertension that has no identifiable cause, is the most common form of hypertension.
- Untreated hypertension can lead to heart disease, kidney disease, blindness, and stroke.
- Management of hypertension should begin with lifestyle changes. These are weight reduction, smoking cessation, reduction of salt and alcohol intake, and increased exercise.
- The baroreceptor reflex, the kidneys, and the renin-angiotensin system can oppose attempts to lower blood pressure with drugs. We can counteract the baroreceptor reflex with beta blockers, the kidneys with diuretics, and the renin-angiotensin system with ACE inhibitors and AngIIRAs.
- Thiazide diuretics (e.g., hydrochlorothiazide) and loop diuretics (e.g., furosemide) reduce blood pressure in two ways: they reduce blood volume (by promoting diuresis) and they reduce arterial resistance (by an unknown mechanism).
- Loop diuretics should be reserved for patients who need greater diuresis than can be achieved with thiazides and for patients with a low GFR (since thiazides won't work when GFR is low).
- Beta blockers (e.g., propranolol) appear to lower blood pressure primarily by reducing peripheral vascular resistance (by an unknown mechanism). They may also lower blood pressure by decreasing myocardial contractility and by suppressing reflex tachycardia (through

beta$_1$ blockade in the heart), and by decreasing renin release (through beta$_1$ blockade in the kidney).
- Alpha$_1$ blockers (e.g., prazosin) lower blood pressure by preventing sympathetically mediated vasoconstriction.
- Direct-acting vasodilators (e.g., hydralazine) and calcium channel blockers (e.g., diltiazem, nifedipine) reduce blood pressure by promoting dilation of arterioles.
- ACE inhibitors and AngIIRAs lower blood pressure by preventing angiotensin II–mediated vasoconstriction and aldosterone-mediated volume expansion. ACE inhibitors do so by blocking angiotensin II formation; AngIIRAs does so by blocking angiotensin II receptors.
- Beta blockers and diuretics are the preferred drugs for initial therapy of hypertension.
- When a combination of drugs is used for hypertension, each drug should have a different mechanism of action from the others.
- Dosages of antihypertensive drugs should be low initially and then gradually increased. This approach minimizes adverse effects and permits baroreceptors to reset to a lower pressure.
- Lack of patient compliance is the major cause of treatment failure in antihypertensive therapy.
- Compliance is difficult to achieve because (1) hypertension has no symptoms (so drug benefits aren't obvious), (2) hypertension progresses slowly (so patients think they can postpone treatment), and (3) treatment is complex and expensive, continues lifelong, and can cause adverse effects.
- A hypertensive emergency exists when diastolic blood pressure exceeds 120 mm Hg.
- Nitroprusside (IV) is a drug of choice for hypertensive emergencies.
- Although short-acting nifedipine continues to be used for hypertensive emergencies, the drug is not safe for this application.
- Hypertension is the most common complication of pregnancy.
- Methyldopa is the drug of choice for treating chronic hypertension of pregnancy.
- ACE inhibitors are contraindicated for treating hypertension of pregnancy.
- Although antihypertensive drugs may help reduce blood pressure in pre-eclampsia, delivery is the only cure.
- Hydralazine (IV) is the drug of choice for lowering blood pressure in pre-eclampsia.

# Summary of Major Nursing Implications*

## Antihypertensive Drugs

### Preadministration Assessment

#### Therapeutic Goal
The objective of antihypertensive therapy is to reduce blood pressure to 140/90 mm Hg, prevent the long-term

sequelae of hypertension (heart disease, kidney disease, blindness, stroke), and minimize drug effects that can reduce quality of life.

#### Baseline Data
The following tests should be done in all patients: blood pressure; electrocardiogram; complete urinalysis; hemoglobin and hematocrit; and blood levels of sodium, potassium, calcium, creatinine, glucose, uric acid, triglycerides, and cholesterol (total and HDL cholesterol).

*Patient education information is highlighted in color.

## Identifying High-Risk Patients

When taking the patient history, attempt to identify drugs that can raise blood pressure or that can interfere with the effects of antihypertensive drugs. Some drugs of concern are listed below under *Minimizing Adverse Interactions.*

The patient history should identify co-existing pathologies that either contraindicate use of specific agents (e.g., heart failure generally contraindicates use of beta blockers) or require that drugs be used with special caution (e.g., thiazide diuretics must be used with caution in patients with gout or diabetes). For risk factors that pertain to specific antihypertensive drugs, refer to the chapters in which those drugs are discussed.

## Implementation: Administration

### Routes

All drugs for chronic hypertension can be administered orally. None are injected.

### Dosage

To minimize adverse effects, dosages should be low initially and then gradually increased. It is counterproductive to employ high initial dosages that produce a rapid fall in pressure while also producing intense undesired responses that can discourage compliance. After 12 months of successful treatment, an attempt should be made to reduce dosages to their lowest effective level.

### Simplifying the Regimen

An antihypertensive regimen can consist of several drugs taken multiple times a day. Once an effective regimen has been established, attempt to switch to once-a-day or twice-a-day dosing. If an appropriate combination product is available (e.g., a fixed-dose combination of a thiazide diuretic plus a potassium-sparing diuretic), substitute the combination product for its components.

## Implementation: Measures to Enhance Therapeutic Effects

### Lifestyle Changes

Lifestyle changes can lower blood pressure. These should be tried for 3 to 6 months before implementing drug therapy and should continue even if drug therapy is required.

*Weight Reduction.* Help overweight patients develop a restricted-calorie diet. The diet should be low in saturated fats, and total fat should not exceed 30% of caloric intake. Target weight is 110% of ideal weight or less.

*Sodium Restriction.* Encourage patients to consume no more than 6 gm of salt (2.3 gm of sodium) daily and provide them with information on the salt content of foods.

*Alcohol Restriction.* Encourage patients to limit consumption of alcohol to 1 ounce a day. One ounce of ethanol is equivalent to about two mixed drinks, two glasses of wine, or two cans of beer.

*Exercise.* Encourage patients who have a sedentary lifestyle to establish a regular program of aerobic exercise (e.g., walking, jogging, swimming, bicycling).

*Smoking Reduction or Cessation.* Strongly encourage patients to quit smoking.

## Promoting Compliance

Noncompliance is the major cause of treatment failure. Compliance can be difficult to achieve for the following reasons: hypertension is devoid of overt symptoms; drugs do not make people feel better—and may make them feel worse; regimens can be complex and expensive; complications of hypertension take years to develop, thereby providing a misguided rationale for postponing treatment; and treatment is usually lifelong.

*Provide Patient Education.* Educate patients about the long-term consequences of hypertension and the ability of lifestyle changes and drug therapy to decrease morbidity and prolong life. Inform patients that drugs do not cure hypertension, and therefore must usually be taken lifelong.

*Encourage Self-Monitoring.* Make certain that patients know the treatment goal (reduction of blood pressure to 140/90 mm Hg) and teach them to monitor and chart their own pressure. This will increase patient involvement and help them see the benefits of therapy.

*Minimize Side Effects.* Adverse drug effects are an obvious deterrent to compliance. Measures to reduce undesired effects are discussed below, under *Minimizing Adverse Effects.*

*Establish a Collaborative Relationship.* Encourage patients to be active partners in setting treatment goals, creating a treatment program, and evaluating progress.

*Simplify the Regimen.* Simplification measures are discussed above, under *Simplifying the Regimen.*

*Other Measures.* Additional measures to promote compliance include providing positive reinforcement when treatment goals are achieved, involving family members in the treatment program, scheduling office visits at convenient times, following up on patients who miss an appointment, and devising a program that is effective but keeps costs low.

## Ongoing Evaluation and Interventions

### Evaluating Treatment

Monitor blood pressure periodically. The goal is to reduce it 140/90 mm Hg. Teach patients to self-monitor their blood pressure and to maintain a blood pressure record.

### Minimizing Adverse Effects

*General Considerations.* The fundamental strategy for decreasing adverse effects is to tailor the regimen to the sensitivities of the patient. If a drug causes objectionable effects, a more acceptable drug should be substituted.

Inform patients about the potential side effects of treatment and encourage them to report objectionable responses.

Avoid drugs that can exacerbate co-existing pathology. For example, don't give beta blockers to patients who have heart failure, bradycardia, AV block, or asthma. A list of pathologies and drugs to avoid is given in Table 44-6.

Initiate therapy with low doses and increase them gradually.

***Adverse Effects of Specific Drugs.*** For measures to minimize adverse effects of specific antihypertensive drugs (e.g., beta blockers, diuretics, ACE inhibitors), refer to the chapters in which those drugs are discussed.

## Minimizing Adverse Interactions

When taking the patient history, identify drugs that can raise blood pressure or interfere with the effects of antihypertensive drugs. Drugs of concern include oral contraceptives, nasal decongestants and other cold remedies, nonsteroidal anti-inflammatory drugs, glucocorticoids, appetite suppressants, tricyclic antidepressants, monoamine oxidase inhibitors, cyclosporine, erythropoietin, and alcohol (in large quantities).

Antihypertensive regimens frequently contain two or more drugs, thereby posing a potential risk of adverse interactions (e.g., ACE inhibitors can increase the risk of hyperkalemia caused by potassium-sparing diuretics). For interactions that pertain to specific antihypertensive drugs, refer to the chapters in which those drugs are discussed.

# CHAPTER 45

# Drugs for Angina Pectoris

Angina pectoris is defined as sudden pain beneath the sternum, often radiating to the left shoulder and arm. Anginal pain is precipitated when the oxygen supply to the heart is insufficient to meet oxygen demand. Most often, anginal pain occurs secondary to atherosclerosis of the coronary arteries. Hence, angina should be seen as a symptom of a disease and not as a disease in its own right.

Three drug families are used to treat angina. These are *organic nitrates* (e.g., nitroglycerin), *beta blockers* (e.g., propranolol), and *calcium channel blockers* (e.g., verapamil). Most of the chapter focuses on the organic nitrates. Beta blockers and calcium channel blockers are discussed at length in earlier chapters; hence, consideration here is limited to their use in angina.

## Determinants of Cardiac Oxygen Demand and Oxygen Supply

Before discussing angina pectoris, we need to review the major factors that determine cardiac oxygen demand and oxygen supply.

*Oxygen Demand.* The principal determinants of cardiac oxygen demand are heart rate, myocardial contractility, and, most importantly, intramyocardial wall tension. Wall tension is determined by two factors: cardiac preload and cardiac afterload. (Preload and afterload are defined in Chapter 40.) In summary, cardiac oxygen demand is determined by four major factors: (1) heart rate, (2) contractility, (3) preload, and (4) afterload. Drugs that reduce these factors will reduce oxygen demand.

*Oxygen Supply.* Cardiac oxygen supply is determined by myocardial blood flow. Under resting conditions, the heart extracts nearly all of the oxygen delivered to it by the coronary vessels. Hence, the only way to accommodate an increase in oxygen demand is to increase blood flow. When oxygen demand increases, coronary arterioles dilate; the resultant decrease in vascular resistance allows blood flow to increase. During exertion, coronary blood flow increases to 4 to 5 times the flow rate at rest. It is important to note that myocardial perfusion takes place only during diastole (i.e., when the heart relaxes). Perfusion does not take place during systole because the vessels that supply the myocardium are squeezed shut when the heart contracts.

## Angina Pectoris: Pathophysiology and Treatment Strategy

Angina pectoris has three forms: (1) chronic stable angina (exertional angina), (2) variant angina (Prinzmetal's or vasospastic angina), and (3) unstable angina. Our focus is on stable angina and variant angina. Consideration of unstable angina is brief.

### Chronic Stable Angina (Exertional Angina)

*Pathophysiology.* Stable angina is triggered most often by an increase in physical activity. Emotional excitement, large meals, and cold exposure may also precipitate an attack. Because stable angina usually occurs in response to

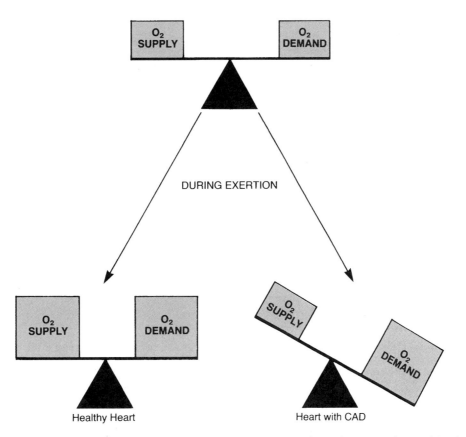

**Figure 45–1. Effect of exertion on the balance between oxygen supply and oxygen demand in the healthy heart and the heart with CAD.** In the healthy heart, $O_2$ supply and $O_2$ demand are always in balance; during exertion, coronary arteries dilate, producing an increase in blood flow to meet the increase in $O_2$ demand. In the heart with CAD, $O_2$ supply and demand are in balance only during rest. During exertion, dilation of coronary arteries cannot compensate for the increase in $O_2$ demand, and an imbalance results.

strain, this condition is known alternatively as *exertional angina* or *angina of effort.*

The underlying cause of exertional angina is *coronary artery disease* (CAD), a condition characterized by deposition of fatty plaque on the arterial wall. If an artery is only partially occluded by plaque, blood flow will be reduced and angina pectoris will result. However, if complete vessel blockage occurs, blood flow will stop and myocardial infarction (heart attack) will result.

The impact of CAD on the balance between myocardial oxygen demand and oxygen supply is illustrated in Figure 45-1. As the figure depicts, in both the healthy heart and the heart with CAD, oxygen supply and oxygen demand are in balance during rest. (In the presence of CAD, resting oxygen demand is met through dilation of arterioles distal to the partial occlusion. This dilation reduces resistance to blood flow and thereby compensates for the increase in resistance created by the plaque.)

The picture is very different during exertion. In the healthy heart, as cardiac oxygen demand rises, coronary arterioles dilate, causing blood flow to increase. This increase keeps oxygen supply in balance with oxygen de-

mand. In people with CAD, arterioles in the affected region are already fully dilated at rest. Hence, when exertion occurs, there is no way to increase blood flow to compensate for the increase in oxygen demand. The resultant imbalance between oxygen supply and oxygen demand is the cause of anginal pain.

***Treatment Strategy.*** The goal of therapy is to reduce the intensity and frequency of anginal attacks. Because anginal pain results from an imbalance between oxygen supply and oxygen demand, logic dictates two possible remedies: (1) we might increase cardiac oxygen supply or (2) we might decrease oxygen demand. Since the underlying cause of stable angina is occlusion of the coronary arteries, there is little we can do to increase cardiac oxygen supply. Hence, the first remedy is not a real option. Consequently, the principal way that we can relieve the pain of stable angina is to *decrease cardiac oxygen demand.* As discussed above, we can reduce oxygen demand with drugs that decrease heart rate, contractility, afterload, and preload.

***Overview of Therapeutic Agents.*** Stable angina can be treated with three types of drugs: *organic nitrates, beta*

## TABLE 45-1. MECHANISMS OF ANTIANGINAL ACTION

| | Mechanism of Pain Relief | |
| --- | --- | --- |
| Drug Class | Stable Angina | Variant Angina |
| *Nitrates* | *Decrease oxygen demand* by dilating veins, which decreases preload | *Increase oxygen supply* by relaxing coronary vasospasm |
| *Beta Blockers* | *Decrease oxygen demand* by decreasing heart rate and contractility | Not used |
| *Calcium Channel Blockers* | *Decrease oxygen demand* by dilating arterioles, which decreases afterload (all calcium blockers), and by decreasing heart rate and contractility (verapamil and diltiazem) | *Increase oxygen supply* by relaxing coronary vasospasm |

*blockers*, and *calcium channel blockers*. All of these agents relieve the pain of stable angina primarily by decreasing cardiac oxygen demand (Table 45-1). It should be noted that drugs only provide symptomatic relief; they do not affect the underlying pathology (CAD). To reduce the risk of myocardial infarction, all patients should receive an *antiplatelet drug* (e.g., aspirin) unless it is contraindicated.

**Nondrug Therapy.** Patients should attempt to avoid factors that can precipitate angina. These include overexertion, heavy meals, emotional stress, and exposure to cold.

Risk factors for stable angina should be corrected. Important among these are smoking, obesity, hypertension, hyperlipidemia, and a sedentary lifestyle. Patients should be strongly encouraged to quit smoking. Overweight patients should be given a restricted-calorie diet; the diet should be low in saturated fats, and total fat content should not exceed 30% of caloric intake. The target weight is 110% of ideal or less. Patients with a sedentary lifestyle should be encouraged to establish a regular program of aerobic exercise (e.g., walking, jogging, swimming, bicycling). Hypertension and hyperlipidemia are major risk factors and should be treated. These disorders are discussed in Chapters 44 and 49, respectively.

## Variant Angina (Prinzmetal's Angina, Vasospastic Angina)

**Pathophysiology.** Variant angina is caused by *coronary artery spasm*, which restricts blood flow to the myocardium. Hence, as in stable angina, pain is secondary to insufficient oxygenation of the heart. In contrast to stable angina, whose symptoms occur primarily at times of exertion, variant angina can produce pain at any time, even during rest and sleep. Frequently, variant angina occurs in conjunction with stable angina. Alternative names for vari-

ant angina are *vasospastic angina* and *Prinzmetal's angina*.

**Treatment Strategy.** The goal of therapy is to reduce the incidence and severity of attacks. In contrast to stable angina, which is treated primarily by reducing oxygen demand, variant angina is treated by *increasing cardiac oxygen supply*. This makes sense since the pain is caused by a reduction in oxygen supply, rather than by an increase in demand. Oxygen supply is increased with vasodilators, which act to prevent or relieve coronary artery spasm.

**Overview of Therapeutic Agents.** Vasospastic angina is treated with two groups of drugs: *calcium channel blockers* and *organic nitrates*. Both drug classes act by relaxing coronary artery spasm. *Beta blockers*, which are effective in stable angina, are not effective against variant angina. As with stable angina, therapy is symptomatic only; drugs do not alter the underlying pathology.

## Unstable Angina

**Pathophysiology.** Unstable angina is a medical emergency. Symptoms result from severe CAD complicated by vasospasm, platelet aggregation, and transient coronary thrombi or emboli. The patient may present with either (1) symptoms of angina at rest, (2) new-onset exertional angina, or (3) intensification of existing angina. Unstable angina poses a greater risk of death than stable angina, and a smaller risk of death than myocardial infarction. The risk of dying is greatest initially and then declines to baseline in about 2 months (unless death occurs first).

**Treatment.** The treatment strategy is to *maintain oxygen supply* and *decrease oxygen demand*. The goal is to reduce pain and prevent progression to myocardial infarction or death. Acute management consists of:

- *Anticoagulants* (heparin and aspirin) to maintain oxygen supply

- *Intravenous nitrates* to increase oxygen supply and decrease oxygen demand
- *Beta blockers* to reduce oxygen demand
- *Calcium channel blockers* if nitrates and beta blockers are inadequate
- *Morphine* if pain persists

# Organic Nitrates

The organic nitrates are the oldest and most frequently used antianginal drugs. These agents relieve angina by causing vasodilation. Nitroglycerin, the most familiar organic nitrate, will serve as our prototype for the family. A complete listing of organic nitrates appears in Table 45-2.

| TABLE 45-2. TRADE NAMES FOR ORGANIC NITRATES | |
| --- | --- |
| **Generic Name** | **Trade Name(s)** |
| *Nitroglycerin* | |
| Sublingual tablets | Nitrostat |
| Translingual spray | Nitrolingual |
| Transmucosal tablets | Nitrogard |
| Oral tablets, SR | Nitrong |
| Oral capsules, SR | Nitro-Bid Plateau Caps, Nitroglyn, Nitrocine Timecaps |
| Transdermal patches | Deponit, Minitran, Nitrodisc Nitro-Dur, Nitrocine, Transderm-Nitro |
| Topical ointment | Nitro-Bid, Nitrol |
| Intravenous | Nitro-Bid IV, Tridil |
| *Isosorbide Mononitrate* | |
| Oral tablets, IR | ISMO, Monoket |
| Oral tablets, SR | Imdur |
| *Isosorbide Dinitrate* | |
| Sublingual tablets | Isordil, Sorbitrate |
| Chewable tablets | Sorbitrate |
| Oral tablets, IR | Isordil Titradose, Sorbitrate |
| Oral tablets, SR | Isordil Tembids, Sorbitrate SA |
| Oral capsules, SR | Dilatrate-SR, Iso-Bid, Isordil Tembids, Isotrate Timecelles |
| *Erythrityl Tetranitrate* | |
| Sublingual tablets | Cardilate |
| Oral tablets | Cardilate |
| *Pentaerythritol Tetranitrate* | |
| Oral tablets, IR | Pentylan, Peritrate |
| Oral tablets, SR | Peritrate SA |
| Oral capsules, SR | Duotrate, Duotrate 45 |
| *Amyl Nitrite* | |
| Inhalant | Generic only |

SR = sustained release, IR = immediate release.

## Nitroglycerin

Nitroglycerin has been used to treat angina since 1879. This drug is effective, fast acting, and inexpensive. Despite the development of newer antianginal agents, nitroglycerin remains the drug of choice for relieving acute anginal attacks.

### Vasodilator Actions

Nitroglycerin acts directly on vascular smooth muscle (VSM) to promote vasodilation. At usual therapeutic doses, the drug acts primarily on *veins*; dilation of arterioles is only modest.

The biochemical events that lead to vasodilation are outlined in Figure 45-2. The process begins with uptake of nitrate by VSM, followed by conversion of nitrate to its active form: *nitric oxide*. As indicated, this conversion requires the presence of *sulfhydryl groups*. Nitric oxide activates guanylate cyclase, an enzyme that catalyzes the formation of cyclic GMP. Through a series of reactions, cyclic GMP decreases intracellular calcium levels. Since calcium is required for VSM contraction, the reduction in calcium results in vasodilation. For our purposes, the most important aspect of this sequence is the conversion of nitrate to its active form—nitric oxide—in the presence of a sulfhydryl source.

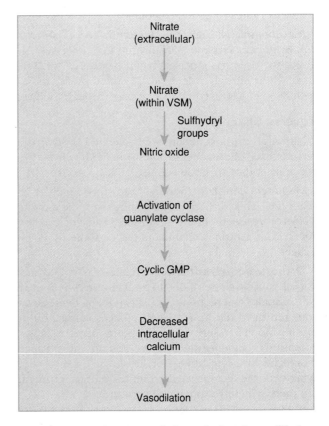

**Figure 45-2. Biochemistry of nitrate-induced vasodilation.** Note that sulfhydryl groups are needed to catalyze the conversion of nitrate to its active form, nitric oxide. If sulfhydryl groups are depleted from VSM, tolerance to nitrates will occur.

## Mechanism of Antianginal Effects

*Stable Angina.* Nitroglycerin decreases the pain of exertional angina primarily by *decreasing cardiac oxygen demand.* Oxygen demand is decreased as follows: by dilating veins, nitroglycerin decreases venous return to the heart, and thereby decreases ventricular filling; the resultant decrease in wall tension (preload) decreases oxygen demand.

In patients with stable angina, nitroglycerin does not appear to increase blood flow to ischemic areas of the heart. This statement is based on two observations. First, nitroglycerin does not dilate atherosclerotic coronary arteries. Second, when nitroglycerin is injected directly into coronary arteries during an anginal attack, the drug does not relieve pain. Both observations suggest that the antianginal effects of nitroglycerin result from effects on peripheral blood vessels—and not from effects on coronary blood flow.

*Variant Angina.* In patients with variant angina, nitroglycerin acts by relaxing or preventing spasm in coronary arteries. Hence, the drug *increases oxygen supply.* It does not reduce oxygen demand.

## Pharmacokinetics

*Absorption.* Nitroglycerin is *highly lipid soluble* and crosses membranes with ease. Because of this property, nitroglycerin can be administered by uncommon routes (sublingual, buccal, transdermal) as well as by more conventional routes (oral, intravenous).

*Metabolism.* Nitroglycerin undergoes *rapid inactivation* by hepatic enzymes (organic nitrate reductases). As a result, the drug has a plasma half-life of only 5 to 7 minutes. When nitroglycerin is administered orally, most of each dose is destroyed on its first pass through the liver.

## Adverse Effects

Nitroglycerin is generally well tolerated. Principal adverse effects—headache, hypotension, and tachycardia—occur secondary to vasodilation.

*Headache.* Initial therapy can produce severe headache. This response diminishes over the first few weeks of treatment. In the meantime, headache can be reduced with aspirin, acetaminophen, or some other mild analgesic.

*Orthostatic Hypotension.* Relaxation of venous smooth muscle causes blood to pool in veins when the patient assumes an erect posture. This pooling decreases venous return to the heart, which reduces cardiac output, causing blood pressure to fall. Symptoms of orthostatic hypotension include lightheadedness and dizziness. Patients should be instructed to sit or lie down if these occur. Lying with the feet elevated promotes venous return, and can thereby help restore blood pressure.

*Reflex Tachycardia.* Nitroglycerin lowers blood pressure—primarily by decreasing venous return, and partly by dilating arterioles. By lowering blood pressure, the drug can activate the baroreceptor reflex, thereby causing sympathetic stimulation of the heart. The resultant increase in heart rate and contractile force increases cardiac oxygen demand, which negates the benefits of therapy. Pretreatment with a beta blocker or verapamil (a calcium channel blocker that directly suppresses the heart) can prevent sympathetic cardiac stimulation.

## Drug Interactions

*Hypotensive Drugs.* Nitroglycerin can intensify the effects of other hypotensive agents. Consequently, care should be exercised when nitroglycerin is used concurrently with beta blockers, calcium channel blockers, diuretics, and all other drugs that can lower blood pressure. Also, patients should be advised to avoid alcohol.

*Beta Blockers, Verapamil, and Diltiazem.* These drugs can suppress nitroglycerin-induced tachycardia. Beta blockers do so by preventing sympathetic activation of beta$_1$-adrenergic receptors on the heart. Verapamil and diltiazem prevent tachycardia through direct suppression of pacemaker activity in the sinoatrial (SA) node.

## Tolerance

Tolerance to nitroglycerin-induced vasodilation can develop rapidly (over the course of a single day). The principal mechanism appears to be depletion of sulfhydryl groups in VSM; in the absence of sulfhydryl groups, nitroglycerin cannot be converted to nitric oxide, its active form. Patients who develop tolerance to nitroglycerin display cross-tolerance to all other nitrates and vice versa. Development of tolerance is most likely with high-dose therapy and with uninterrupted therapy. To prevent tolerance, nitroglycerin and other nitrates should be used in the lowest effective dosages, and long-acting formulations (e.g., patches, sustained-release preparations) should be used on an intermittent schedule that allows at least 8 drug-free hours every day, usually during the night. If pain occurs during the nitrate-free interval, it can be managed with sparing use of a short-acting nitrate (e.g., sublingual nitroglycerin) or by adding a beta blocker or calcium channel blocker to the regimen. Tolerance can be reversed by withholding nitrates for a short time.

## Preparations and Routes of Administration

Nitroglycerin is available in an assortment of formulations for administration by a variety of routes. This proliferation of dosage forms reflects efforts to delay hepatic metabolism, and thereby prolong therapeutic effects.

All nitroglycerin preparations produce qualitatively similar responses; differences relate only to onset and duration of action (Table 45–3). With some preparations, effects begin rapidly (in 1 to 5 minutes) and then fade in less than 1 hour. With others, effects begin slowly but last for several hours. Only three preparations have both a rapid onset *and* long duration.

Applications of specific preparations are based on their time course. Preparations with a *rapid onset* are employed to *terminate an ongoing anginal attack.* When used for this purpose, rapid-acting preparations are administered as soon as pain begins. Rapid-acting preparations can also be used for *acute prophylaxis of angina.* For this purpose, these preparations are taken just prior to

## TABLE 45-3. ORGANIC NITRATES: TIME COURSE OF ACTION

| Drug and Dosage Form | Onset* | Duration† |
|---|---|---|
| *Nitroglycerin* | | |
| Sublingual tablets | Rapid (1-3 min) | Brief (30-60 min) |
| Translingual spray | Rapid (2-3 min) | Brief (30-60 min) |
| Transmucosal tablets | Rapid (1-2 min) | Long (3-5 hr) |
| Oral tablets, SR | Slow (20-45 min) | Long (3-8 hr) |
| Oral capsules, SR | Slow (20-45 min) | Long (3-8 hr) |
| Transdermal patches | Slow (30-60 min) | Long (24 hr)‡ |
| Topical ointment | Slow (30-60 min) | Long (2-12 hr) |
| *Isosorbide Mononitrate* | | |
| Oral tablets, IS | Slow (30-60 min) | Long (6-10 hr) |
| Oral tablets, SR | Slow (30-60 min) | Long (7-12 hr) |
| *Isosorbide Dinitrate* | | |
| Sublingual tablets | Rapid (2-5 min) | Long (1-3 hr) |
| Chewable tablets | Rapid (2-5 min) | Long (1-3 hr) |
| Oral tablets, IR | Slow (20-40 min) | Long (4-6 hr) |
| Oral tablets, SR | Slow (30 min) | Long (6-8 hr) |
| Oral capsules, SR | Slow (30 min) | Long (6-8 hr) |
| *Erythrityl Tetranitrate* | | |
| Sublingual tablets | Rapid (5 min) | Long (3 hr) |
| Oral tablets | Slow (15-30 min) | Long (6-8 hr) |
| *Pentaerythritol Tetranitrate* | | |
| Oral tablets, IR | Slow (20-60 min) | Long (4-5 hr) |
| Oral tablets, SR | Slow (30 min) | Long (<12 hr) |
| Oral capsules, SR | Slow (30 min) | Long (<12 hr) |

*Nitrates with a *rapid* onset have two uses: (1) termination of an ongoing anginal attack and (2) short-term prophylaxis prior to anticipated exertion. Of the rapid-acting nitrates, nitroglycerin (sublingual or spray) is preferred to the others for terminating an ongoing attack.

†*Long-acting* nitrates are used for sustained prophylaxis (prevention) of anginal attacks. All cause tolerance if used without interruption.

‡Although patches can release nitroglycerin for up to 24 hours, they should be removed after 12 to 14 hours to avoid tolerance.

IR = immediate release, SR = sustained release.

anticipated exertion. *Long-acting preparations* are used to provide *sustained protection* against anginal attacks. To provide protection, these preparations are administered on a fixed schedule (but one that permits at least 8 drug-free hours each day).

Dosages for nitroglycerin preparations are summarized in Table 45-4. Trade names are shown in Table 45-2.

**Sublingual Tablets.** When administered sublingually (beneath the tongue), nitroglycerin is absorbed directly through the oral mucosa and into the bloodstream. Hence, unlike orally administered drugs, which must pass through the liver on their way to the systemic circulation, sublingual nitroglycerin bypasses the liver, and thereby temporarily avoids metabolism. Because the liver is bypassed, sublingual doses can be low (between 0.15 and 0.6 mg). These doses are about 10 times lower than those required when nitroglycerin is taken orally.

Effects of sublingual nitroglycerin begin rapidly—in 1 to 3 minutes—and persist for up to 1 hour. Because sublingual administration works fast, this route is ideal for

(1) termination of an ongoing anginal attack and (2) short-term prophylaxis when exertion is anticipated.

To terminate an acute anginal attack, sublingual nitroglycerin should be administered as soon as pain begins. Administration should not be delayed until the pain has become severe. If 1 tablet is insufficient, 1 or 2 additional tablets should be taken at 5-minute intervals. If pain persists, the patient should contact a physician or report to an emergency department, since anginal pain that is unresponsive to nitroglycerin may indicate myocardial infarction.

Sublingual administration is unfamiliar to most patients. Accordingly, education is needed. The patient should be instructed to place the tablet under the tongue and leave it there while it dissolves. Nitroglycerin tablets formulated for sublingual use are ineffective if swallowed.

Nitroglycerin tablets are chemically unstable and can lose effectiveness over time. Shelf life can be prolonged by storing tablets in a tightly closed, dark container. Under these conditions, tablets should remain effective for at

## TABLE 45–4. ORGANIC NITRATE DOSAGES

| Drug and Formulation | Usual Dosage |
|---|---|
| *Nitroglycerin* | |
| Sublingual tablets | 0.15–0.6 mg as needed |
| Translingual spray | 0.4–0.8 mg as needed |
| Transmucosal tablets | 1–2 mg every 3–8 hr |
| Oral tablets and capsules, SR | 2.5–6.5 mg 3 or 4 times daily; to avoid tolerance, administer only once or twice daily; do not crush or chew |
| Transdermal patches | 1 patch a day; to avoid tolerance, remove after 12–14 hr, allowing 10–12 patch-free hr each day |
| Topical ointment | 1–2 inches (12–30 mg) every 4–8 hr |
| Intravenous | 5 µg/min initially, then increased gradually as needed; tolerance develops with prolonged continuous infusion |
| *Isosorbide Mononitrate* | |
| Oral tablets, IR | 20 mg twice daily; to avoid tolerance, take the 1st dose upon awakening and the 2nd dose 7 hr later |
| Oral tablets, SR | 60–120 mg once a day; do not crush or chew |
| *Isosorbide Dinitrate* | |
| Sublingual tablets | 2.5–10 mg every 4–6 hr; do not crush or chew |
| Chewable tablets | 5–10 mg every 2–3 hr |
| Oral tablets, IR | 5–30 mg every 6 hr; to avoid tolerance, take only 2 or 3 times daily, with the last dose no later than 7 PM |
| Oral tablets and capsules, SR | 40 mg every 6–12 hr; to avoid tolerance, take only once or twice daily (at 8 AM and 2 PM) |
| *Erythrityl Tetranitrate* | |
| Sublingual tablets | 5–10 mg as needed |
| Oral tablets | 10 mg 3 times a day |
| *Pentaerythritol Tetranitrate* | |
| Oral tablets, IR | 10–40 mg 4 times a day |
| Oral tablets and capsules, SR | 30–80 mg every 12 hr; do not crush or chew |
| *Amyl Nitrite* | |
| Inhalant | 0.18 or 0.3 ml |

IR = immediate release, SR = sustained release.

least 6 months after the container is first opened. As a rule, nitroglycerin tablets should be discarded after this time. Patients should be instructed to write the date of opening on the container and to discard unused tablets 6 months later.

**Sustained-Release Oral Tablets and Capsules.** Sustained-release oral formulations are intended for long-term prophylaxis only; these formulations cannot act fast enough to terminate an ongoing anginal attack. Sustained-release tablets and capsules contain a large dose of nitroglycerin that is slowly absorbed across the gastrointestinal wall. In theory, doses are large enough so that amounts of nitroglycerin sufficient to produce a therapeutic response will survive passage through the liver. Because they produce sustained blood levels of nitroglycerin, these formulations can cause tolerance. To reduce the risk of tolerance, these products should be taken only once or twice daily. Patients should be instructed to swallow sustained-release formulations intact.

**Transdermal Delivery Systems.** Nitroglycerin patches look like Band-Aids and contain a reservoir from which nitroglycerin is slowly released. Following its release, the drug is absorbed through the skin and then into the blood. The rate of release is constant for any particular transdermal patch and, depending upon the patch used, can range from 0.1 to 0.6 mg/hr. Effects begin within 30 to 60 minutes and persist as long as the patch remains in place (up to 14 hours). Patches are applied once daily to a hairless area of skin. The site should be rotated to avoid local irritation.

Tolerance develops if patches are used continuously (24 hours a day every day). Accordingly, a daily "patch-free" interval of 10 to 12 hours is recommended. This can be accomplished by applying a new patch each morning, leaving it in place for 12 to 14 hours, and then removing it in the evening.

Because of their long duration, patches are well suited for sustained prophylaxis. Since patches have a delayed onset, they cannot be used to abort an ongoing attack.

***Translingual Spray.*** Nitroglycerin can be delivered to the oral mucosa using a metered-dose spray device. Each activation delivers a 0.4-mg dose. Indications for nitroglycerin spray are the same as for sublingual tablets: suppression of an acute anginal attack and prophylaxis of angina when exertion is anticipated. As with sublingual tablets, no more than three doses should be administered within a 15-minute interval. *Patients should be instructed not to inhale the spray.*

***Transmucosal (Buccal) Tablets.*** Administration of transmucosal nitroglycerin tablets consists of placing the tablet between the upper lip and the gum, or in the buccal area between the cheek and the gum. The tablet adheres to the oral mucosa and slowly dissolves over 3 to 5 hours. As the tablet dissolves, nitroglycerin is absorbed directly through the oral mucosa and into the blood, thereby bypassing the liver. Like sublingual nitroglycerin, transmucosal nitroglycerin has a rapid onset of action. Hence, transmucosal administration can be used to terminate an ongoing anginal attack, and to provide short-term prophylaxis prior to exertion. In addition, since the effects of transmucosal nitroglycerin are prolonged, this formulation can be used for sustained prophylaxis. Patients should be instructed not to chew or swallow these tablets.

***Topical Ointment.*** Topical nitroglycerin ointment is used for sustained protection against anginal attacks. The ointment is applied to the skin of the chest, back, abdomen, or anterior thigh. (Since nitroglycerin acts primarily by dilating peripheral veins, there is no mechanistic advantage to applying topical nitroglycerin directly over the heart.) Following topical application, nitroglycerin is absorbed through the skin and then into the blood. Effects begin within 20 to 60 minutes and may persist for up to 12 hours.

Nitroglycerin ointment (2%) is dispensed from a tube, and the length of the ribbon squeezed from the tube determines the dosage. (One inch contains about 15 mg of nitroglycerin.) The usual adult dosage is 1 to 2 inches applied every 4 to 8 hours. The ointment should be spread over a 6-inch by 6-inch area and then covered with a plastic wrap. Sites of application should be rotated to minimize irritation of the skin. As with other long-acting formulations, uninterrupted use can cause tolerance.

***Intravenous Infusion.*** Intravenous nitroglycerin is employed only rarely to treat angina pectoris. When used for angina, IV nitroglycerin is limited to patients who have failed to respond to other medications. Additional uses of IV nitroglycerin include treatment of congestive heart failure associated with acute myocardial infarction, treatment of perioperative hypertension, and production of controlled hypotension for surgery.

Intravenous nitroglycerin has a very short duration of action; hence, continuous infusion is required. The rate is 5 µg/min initially and then increased gradually until an adequate response has been achieved. Heart rate and blood pressure must be monitored continuously.

Stock solutions of nitroglycerin must be diluted for intravenous therapy. Since ampules of nitroglycerin prepared by different manufacturers can differ in both volume and nitroglycerin concentration, the label must be read carefully when dilutions are made.

Administration should be performed using a glass IV bottle and the administration set provided by the manufacturer. Nitroglycerin absorbs into standard polyvinyl chloride tubing; hence this tubing should be avoided.

## Discontinuing Nitroglycerin

Long-acting preparations (transdermal patches, topical ointment, sustained-release oral tablets or capsules) should be discontinued slowly. If these preparations are withdrawn abruptly, vasospasm may result.

## Summary of Therapeutic Uses

***Acute Therapy of Angina.*** For acute treatment of angina pectoris, nitroglycerin is administered in sublingual tablets, transmucosal tablets, and a translingual spray. All three dosage forms can be used to abort an ongoing anginal attack and to provide prophylaxis in anticipation of exertion.

***Sustained Therapy of Angina.*** For sustained prophylaxis against angina, nitroglycerin is administered in the following formulations: transdermal patches, topical ointment, transmucosal tablets, and sustained-release oral tablets or capsules.

***Intravenous Therapy.*** Intravenous nitroglycerin is indicated for perioperative control of blood pressure, production of controlled hypotension during surgery, and treatment of congestive heart failure associated with acute myocardial infarction. In addition, IV nitroglycerin is used to treat unstable angina and angina when symptoms cannot be controlled with preferred medications.

### Other Organic Nitrates

**Isosorbide Dinitrate, Isosorbide Mononitrate, Erythrityl Tetranitrate, Pentaerythritol Tetranitrate**

All of these nitrates have pharmacologic actions identical to those of nitroglycerin. All are used for angina, all are taken orally, and all produce headache, hypotension, and reflex tachycardia. Differences among them relate only to route of administration and time course of action. Time course determines whether a particular drug or dosage form will be used for acute therapy, sustained prophylaxis, or both. As with nitroglycerin, tolerance can develop to long-acting preparations. To avoid tolerance, long-acting preparations should be used on an intermittent schedule that allows at least 8 drug-free hours a day. Trade names, time courses, and dosages are summarized in Tables 45-2, 45-3, and 45-4, respectively.

### Amyl Nitrite

Amyl nitrite is an ultrashort-acting agent used to treat acute episodes of angina pectoris. The drug has the same mechanism as nitroglycerin. Amyl nitrite is a volatile liquid that is dispensed in glass ampules. For administration, an ampul is crushed, allowing the volatile compound to be inhaled. Effects begin within 30 seconds and terminate in 3 to 5 minutes. Amyl nitrite is highly flammable and should not be used near flame. The drug is reputed to intensify sexual orgasm and has been abused for that purpose (see Chapter 37).

# Beta Blockers

Beta blockers (e.g., propranolol, metoprolol) are important drugs for *stable angina*, but are *not* effective against vasospastic angina. When administered on a fixed schedule, beta blockers can provide sustained protection against effort-induced anginal pain. Exercise tolerance is increased and the frequency and intensity of anginal attacks are lowered. All of the beta blockers appear equally effective.

Beta blockers reduce anginal pain by *decreasing cardiac oxygen demand.* This is accomplished primarily through blockade of beta₁ receptors in the heart, which decreases heart rate and contractility. Beta blockers can reduce oxygen demand further by causing a modest reduction in arterial pressure (afterload). In patients taking vasodilators (e.g., nitroglycerin), beta blockers provide the additional benefit of blunting reflex tachycardia.

For treatment of stable angina, dosage should be low initially and then gradually increased. The dosing goal is to lower resting heart rate to 50 to 60 beats/min, and limit exertional heart rate to about 100 beats/min. Beta blockers should not be withdrawn abruptly, since doing so can increase the incidence and intensity of anginal attacks, and may even precipitate myocardial infarction.

Beta blockers can produce a variety of adverse effects. Blockade of cardiac beta₁ receptors can produce *bradycardia, decreased atrioventricular (AV) conduction,* and *reduction of contractility.* Consequently, beta blockers should not be used by patients with sick sinus syndrome, heart failure, or second- or third-degree AV block. Blockade of beta₂ receptors in the lung can promote *bronchoconstriction.* Accordingly, beta blockers should be avoided by patients with asthma. If an asthmatic individual absolutely must use a beta blocker, a beta₁-selective agent (e.g., metoprolol) should be selected. Beta blockers can *mask signs of hypoglycemia,* and therefore must be used with caution in patients with diabetes. Through effects on the central nervous system, these drugs can cause *insomnia, depression, bizarre dreams,* and *sexual dysfunction.*

The basic pharmacology of the beta blockers is discussed in Chapter 19.

## Calcium Channel Blockers

The calcium channel blockers used most frequently are *verapamil, diltiazem,* and *nifedipine.* Accordingly, our discussion focuses on these three drugs. *All three* can block calcium channels in *vascular smooth muscle,* primarily in arterioles. The result is arteriolar dilation and reduction of peripheral resistance (afterload). In addition, all three can relax coronary vasospasm. *Verapamil* and *diltiazem* also block calcium channels in the heart, and can thereby decrease heart rate, AV conduction, and contractility.

Calcium channel blockers are used to treat both stable angina and variant angina. In *variant angina,* these drugs promote relaxation of coronary artery spasm, thereby *increasing cardiac oxygen supply.* In *stable angina,* these drugs promote relaxation of peripheral arterioles; the resultant decrease in afterload *reduces cardiac oxygen demand.* Verapamil and diltiazem can produce modest additional reductions in oxygen demand by suppressing heart rate and contractility.

The major adverse effects of the calcium channel blockers are cardiovascular. Dilation of peripheral arterioles lowers blood pressure, and can thereby induce *reflex tachycardia.* This reaction is greatest with nifedipine and minimal with verapamil and diltiazem. Because of their suppressant effects on the heart, verapamil and diltiazem must be used cautiously in patients taking beta blockers and in patients with bradycardia, heart failure, or AV block. These precautions do not apply to nifedipine.

The basic pharmacology of the calcium channel blockers is discussed in Chapter 42.

# Invasive Treatments for Angina: CABG and PTCA

## Coronary Artery Bypass Graft Surgery

Coronary artery bypass graft (CABG) surgery is used to increase blood flow to ischemic areas of the heart. In this procedure, one end of a segment of healthy blood vessel (internal mammary artery or saphenous vein) is grafted onto the aorta, and the other end is connected to the diseased coronary artery at a point distal to the region of atherosclerotic plaque. Hence, the graft constitutes a shunt whereby blood flow can circumvent the occluded section of a diseased coronary vessel. Following surgery, most patients remain in the hospital for a week, and then recuperate for another 6 weeks at home. Once considered exotic, CABG surgery is now commonplace; more than 300,000 Americans undergo the procedure each year.

Vessel blockage can recur over time, thereby requiring repeat surgery. When an artery is used for the graft, the incidence of reblockage is only 4% after 10 years. In contrast, when a vein is used, the incidence of reblockage at 10 years is nearly 50%.

A new procedure, called *minimally invasive direct coronary artery bypass* (MIDCAB) surgery, is an alternative to CABG surgery for some patients. MIDCAB surgery is much less invasive than CABG surgery, and therefore faster and cheaper. Furthermore, MIDCAB surgery is performed on the beating heart; hence heart-lung bypass machinery is not needed. At this time, MIDCAB surgery is used only to bypass blockage in the left ascending coronary artery.

## Percutaneous Transluminal Coronary Angioplasty

Percutaneous transluminal coronary angioplasty (PTCA) is an alternative to CABG surgery for patients with stable angina. In PTCA, a miniature catheter containing a deflated balloon is inserted into the femoral artery, threaded up into the aorta, and then manipulated into the occluded coronary artery. The balloon is then inflated, thereby flattening the obstruction and allowing blood to flow. Unfortunately, re-occlusion occurs in about one third of patients within 6 to 8 months, necessitating either repeat PCTA or CABG surgery. PCTA is performed on about 400,000 Americans annually.

## Comparison of CABG Surgery with PTCA

CABG surgery and PTCA are equally safe and almost equally effective. The 5-year survival rate after either procedure is about 90%. However, in other respects, the procedures differ substantially. Compared with PTCA, CABG surgery is more traumatic, more expensive, requires a longer hospital stay, and recovery is slower. On the other hand, CABG surgery is more effective: coronary blood flow is better, relief of angina is superior, exercise tolerance is higher, and patients require less antianginal medication. Moreover, the incidence of reblockage after CABG surgery is far less. For example, after 5 years, the rate of reblockage with PTCA is 54%, compared with only 3% following CABG surgery. At this time, CABG surgery is considered the treatment of choice for patients with multivessel disease. For patients with single-vessel disease, either procedure is generally appropriate; the choice between them is based on patient preference.

# Summary of Therapeutic Measures

In the preceding sections, we discussed three drug families and two invasive procedures that can be used to treat angina pectoris. In this section, we consider guidelines for implementing these therapeutic modalities. It should be noted that these guidelines are general and intended only to provide a basic understanding as to when a specific modality might be employed.

## Stable Angina Pectoris

Treatment of stable angina can be approached in a stepwise fashion (Table 45–5). Progression from one step to the next is based on the frequency and intensity of attacks and on the patient's response to therapy. Some patients can be treated with a single drug, some require two or three drugs, and some may require surgical intervention.

***Step 1.*** If anginal attacks are infrequent (no more than one a day), then PRN therapy with sublingual nitroglyc-

---

### TABLE 45–5. STEPWISE THERAPY OF STABLE ANGINA PECTORIS

Step 1: Nitrates

Step 2: Nitrates + beta blocker *or*
Nitrates + calcium channel blocker

Step 3: Nitrates + beta blocker + calcium channel blocker

Step 4: CABG *or* PTCA

At all stages, the treatment program should encourage reduction of angina risk factors: obese patients should lose weight, smokers should quit, sedentary patients should get aerobic exercise, and patients with hypertension or hyperlipidemia should receive appropriate therapy.

---

erin or another fast-acting nitrate is often sufficient. Likewise, if attacks occur predictably with exertion, taking a fast-acting nitrate 5 minutes before the anticipated activity may be all that is needed.

***Step 2.*** When anginal episodes occur more than once a day, a drug that can provide sustained prophylaxis should be added to the regimen. A beta blocker is usually chosen. In fact, in the absence of specific contraindications (asthma, bradycardia, heart failure, AV block), a trial with a beta blocker is recommended for all patients who have frequent anginal attacks. To be effective, the drug must be taken on a fixed schedule. Therapy with a fast-acting nitrate should continue on a PRN basis. In addition to providing prophylaxis, the beta blocker will suppress nitrate-induced reflex tachycardia.

Calcium channel blockers are an alternative to beta blockers for sustained prophylaxis. Since calcium channel blockers do not promote bronchoconstriction, they are preferred to beta blockers for patients with asthma. Nifedipine, which lacks cardiosuppressant effects, is safer than beta blockers for patients with bradycardia, AV block, or heart failure. This is not true of verapamil and diltiazem—calcium channel blockers that, like beta blockers, can suppress cardiac function. When used for prophylaxis of angina, calcium channel blockers must be taken on a regular schedule. A fast-acting nitrate should be used as needed to supplement antianginal effects.

Long-acting nitrate preparations (e.g., transdermal nitroglycerin) can also be used for sustained prophylaxis. However, because tolerance can develop quickly, these preparations would seem less well suited than beta blockers or calcium channel blockers for continuous protection against angina.

***Step 3.*** Patients who do not respond to two drugs (a nitrate plus either a beta blocker or a calcium channel blocker) should receive a trial with three drugs: a nitrate, a beta blocker, and a calcium channel blocker (usually nifedipine). The benefit of taking three drugs is that oxygen demand is reduced by multiple mechanisms: nitrates reduce preload (by dilating veins); calcium channel blockers reduce afterload (by dilating arterioles); and beta blockers reduce heart rate and contractility. It should be noted that when a calcium channel blocker is to be combined with a beta blocker, nifedipine is preferred to verapamil and diltiazem. Nifedipine is preferred because it does not directly affect the heart and, therefore, will not intensify the cardiosuppressant effects of beta blockade.

***Step 4.*** If the combination of a nitrate, a beta blocker, and a calcium channel blocker fails to provide relief from angina, CABG surgery or PTCA may be indicated. Note that invasive procedures should be considered only after more conservative treatment has been attempted.

***Reduction of Risk Factors.*** At all stages, the treatment program should reduce anginal risk factors: obese patients should lose weight, smokers should quit, sedentary patients should get aerobic exercise, and patients with hypertension or hyperlipidemia should receive appropriate therapy.

## Variant Angina Pectoris

Treatment of vasospastic angina can proceed in three steps. For initial therapy, either a calcium channel blocker or a nitrate is selected. If either drug alone is inadequate, then combined therapy with a calcium channel blocker *plus* a nitrate should be tried. If this combination fails to control anginal attacks, CABG surgery may be indicated.

## KEY POINTS

- Anginal pain occurs when cardiac oxygen supply is insufficient to meet oxygen demand.
- Cardiac oxygen demand is determined by heart rate, contractility, preload, and afterload. Drugs that reduce these factors will help relieve anginal pain.
- Cardiac oxygen supply is determined by myocardial blood flow. Drugs that increase oxygen supply will reduce anginal pain.
- Angina pectoris has three forms: chronic stable angina, variant angina, and unstable angina.
- The underlying cause of stable angina is coronary artery atherosclerosis.
- The underlying cause of variant angina is coronary artery spasm.
- Drugs relieve pain of stable angina by decreasing cardiac oxygen demand. They do not increase oxygen supply.
- Drugs relieve pain of variant angina by increasing cardiac oxygen supply. They do not decrease oxygen demand.
- Nitroglycerin and other organic nitrates are vasodilators.
- To cause vasodilation, nitroglycerin must first be converted to nitric oxide, its active form. This reaction requires a sulfhydryl source.
- Nitroglycerin relieves pain of stable angina by dilating veins, which decreases venous return, which decreases preload, which decreases oxygen demand.
- Nitroglycerin relieves pain of variant angina by relaxing coronary vasospasm, which increases oxygen supply.
- Nitroglycerin is highly lipid soluble, and therefore is readily absorbed through the oral mucosa and skin.
- Nitroglycerin undergoes very rapid inactivation in the liver. Hence, when the drug is administered orally, most of each dose is destroyed before reaching the systemic circulation.

- When nitroglycerin is administered sublingually, it is absorbed directly into the systemic circulation, and therefore temporarily bypasses the liver. Hence, to produce equivalent effects, sublingual doses can be much smaller than oral doses.
- Nitroglycerin causes three characteristic side effects: headache, orthostatic hypotension, and reflex tachycardia. All three occur secondary to vasodilation.
- Reflex tachycardia from nitroglycerin can be prevented with beta blockers, verapamil, or diltiazem.
- Continuous use of nitroglycerin can produce tolerance within 24 hours. The probable mechanism is depletion of sulfhydryl groups.
- To prevent tolerance, nitroglycerin should be used in the lowest effective dosage, and long-acting formulations should be used on an intermittent schedule that allows at least 8 drug-free hours every day, usually during the night.
- Nitroglycerin preparations with a rapid onset (e.g., sublingual nitroglycerin) are used to abort ongoing anginal attacks and to provide acute prophylaxis when exertion is expected. Administration is PRN.
- Nitroglycerin preparations with a long duration (e.g., patches, sustained-release oral tablets) are used for extended protection against anginal attacks. Administration is on a fixed schedule (but one that allows at least 8 drug-free hours each day).
- Beta blockers prevent pain of stable angina by decreasing heart rate and contractility, which reduces cardiac oxygen demand.
- Beta blockers are administered on a fixed schedule, not PRN.
- Beta blockers are not used for variant angina.
- Calcium channel blockers relieve pain of stable angina by reducing cardiac oxygen demand. Two mechanisms are involved. First, all calcium channel blockers relax peripheral arterioles, and thereby decrease afterload. Second, verapamil and diltiazem reduce heart rate and contractility (in addition to decreasing afterload).
- Calcium channel blockers relieve pain of variant angina by increasing cardiac oxygen supply. The mechanism is relaxation of coronary artery spasm.
- When a calcium channel blocker is combined with a beta blocker, nifedipine is preferred to verapamil or diltiazem. This is because verapamil and diltiazem will intensify cardiosuppression caused by the beta blocker, whereas nifedipine will not.

# Summary of Major Nursing Implications*

## Nitroglycerin

### Preadministration Assessment

#### Therapeutic Goal
Reduction of the frequency and intensity of anginal attacks.

*Patient education information is highlighted in color.

### Baseline Data
Obtain baseline data on the frequency and intensity of anginal attacks, the location of anginal pain, and the factors that precipitate attacks.

The patient interview and physical examination should identify risk factors for angina pectoris, including treatable contributing pathophysiologic conditions (e.g., hypertension, hyperlipidemia).

## Identifying High-Risk Patients

Use with *caution* in *hypotensive patients* and patients taking *drugs that can lower blood pressure*, including alcohol and antihypertensive medications.

## Implementation: Administration

### Routes and Administration

*Sublingual Tablets.* Use: prophylaxis or termination of an acute anginal attack.

Instruct patients to place the tablet under the tongue and leave it there until fully dissolved; the tablet should not be swallowed.

Inform patients that if 1 tablet fails to relieve pain, 1 or 2 additional tablets should be taken at 5-minute intervals. Instruct patients to seek medical help immediately if pain is not relieved within 15 minutes.

Instruct patients to store tablets in a dark, tightly closed bottle that contains no other medications. Instruct patients to write the date of opening on the bottle and to discard unused medication after 6 months.

*Sustained-Release Oral Tablets and Capsules.* Use: sustained protection against anginal attacks.

To avoid tolerance, administer only once or twice daily. Instruct patients to swallow these preparations intact, without chewing or crushing.

*Transdermal Delivery Systems.* Use: sustained protection against anginal attacks.

Instruct patients to apply transdermal patches to a hairless area of skin, using a new patch and a different site each day.

Instruct patients to remove the patch after 12 to 14 hours, allowing 10 to 12 "patch-free" hours each day. This will prevent tolerance.

*Intravenous.* Uses: (1) angina pectoris refractory to more conventional therapy, (2) perioperative control of blood pressure, (3) production of controlled hypotension during surgery, and (4) heart failure associated with acute myocardial infarction.

Perform IV administration using a glass IV bottle and the administration set provided by the manufacturer; avoid standard IV tubing. Dilute stock solutions before use.

Administer by continuous infusion. The rate is slow initially (5 μg/min) and then gradually increased until an adequate response is achieved.

Monitor cardiovascular status constantly.

*Translingual Spray.* Use: prophylaxis or termination of an acute anginal attack.

Instruct patients to direct the spray against the oral mucosa. Warn patients not to inhale the spray.

*Transmucosal (Buccal) Tablets.* Uses: (1) prophylaxis or termination of an acute anginal attack and (2) sustained prophylaxis.

Instruct patients to place the transmucosal tablet between the upper lip and the gum or in the buccal area between the cheek and the gum. Inform patients that the tablet will adhere to the oral mucosa and slowly dissolve

over 3 to 5 hours. To achieve sustained prophylaxis, a tablet should be administered every 3 to 8 hours.

*Topical Ointment.* Use: sustained protection against anginal attacks.

Before applying a new dose, remove ointment remaining from the previous dose.

Technique of administration: (1) squeeze a ribbon of ointment of prescribed length onto the applicator paper provided; (2) using the applicator paper, spread the ointment over a 6-inch by 6-inch area (application may be made to the chest, back, abdomen, upper arm, or anterior thigh); and (3) cover the ointment with plastic wrap. Avoid touching the ointment.

Rotate the application site to minimize local irritation.

### Terminating Therapy

Warn patients against abrupt withdrawal of long-acting preparations (transdermal systems, topical ointment, sustained-release tablets and capsules).

## Implementation: Measures to Enhance Therapeutic Effects

### Reducing Risk Factors

*Precipitating Factors.* Advise patients to avoid activities that are likely to elicit an anginal attack (e.g., overexertion, heavy meals, emotional stress, cold exposure).

*Weight Reduction.* Help overweight patients develop a restricted-calorie diet. The diet should be low in saturated fats, and total fat should not exceed 30% of caloric intake. Target weight is 110% of ideal or less.

*Exercise.* Encourage patients who have a sedentary lifestyle to establish a regular program of aerobic exercise (e.g., walking, jogging, swimming, bicycling).

*Smoking Cessation.* Strongly encourage patients to quit smoking.

*Contributing Disease States.* Ensure that patients with contributing pathology (especially hypertension or hypercholesterolemia) are receiving appropriate treatment.

## Ongoing Evaluation and Interventions

### Evaluating Therapeutic Effects

Have the patient keep a record of the frequency and intensity of anginal attacks, the location of anginal pain, and the factors that precipitate attacks.

### Minimizing Adverse Effects

*Headache.* Inform patients that headache will diminish with continued drug use. Advise patients that headache can be relieved with aspirin, acetaminophen, or some other mild analgesic.

*Orthostatic Hypotension.* Inform patients about symptoms of hypotension (e.g., dizziness, lightheadedness), and advise them to sit or lie down if these occur. Inform patients that hypotension can be minimized by moving slowly when changing from a sitting or supine position to an upright posture.

**Reflex Tachycardia.** This reaction can be suppressed by concurrent treatment with a beta blocker, verapamil, or diltiazem.

### Minimizing Adverse Interactions

**Hypotensive Agents.** Nitroglycerin can interact with other hypotensive drugs to produce excessive lowering of blood pressure. Advise patients to avoid alcohol. Exercise caution when nitroglycerin is used in combination with beta blockers, calcium channel blockers, diuretics, and all other drugs that can lower blood pressure.

## Isosorbide Mononitrate, Isosorbide Dinitrate, Erythrityl Tetranitrate, Pentaerythritol Tetranitrate

All four drugs have pharmacologic actions identical to those of nitroglycerin. Differences relate only to dosage forms, routes of administration, and time course of action. Hence, the implications presented for nitroglycerin apply to these drugs as well.

# CHAPTER 46

# Drugs for Heart Failure

Heart failure is a serious, progressive disorder characterized by ventricular dysfunction, reduced cardiac output, insufficient tissue perfusion, and signs of volume overload (e.g., peripheral edema, shortness of breath). Of the estimated 2 million Americans who have heart failure, 10 percent are likely to die within 1 year, and 50 percent within 5 years. Heart failure results in 1 million hospitalizations each year, at a cost of $7 billion. With improved evaluation and outpatient care, many hospitalizations could be prevented. The total annual health care cost related to heart failure is $10 billion.

Heart failure is commonly referred to as *congestive heart failure.* This term has been used because heart failure frequently causes fluid accumulation (congestion) in the lungs and peripheral tissues. However, since many patients do not have signs of pulmonary or systemic congestion, the term *heart failure* seems more appropriate.

The principal drugs employed to treat heart failure are *vasodilators*, *diuretics*, and *inotropic agents.* Most of this chapter is dedicated to digoxin, the inotropic drug encountered most frequently. Since vasodilators and diuretics are discussed at length in other chapters, their consideration here is brief.

In order to understand heart failure and the drugs used for treatment, you need a basic understanding of hemodynamics. In particular, you need to understand the contribution of venous pressure, afterload, and the Starling mechanism in determining cardiac output. You also need to understand the role of the baroreceptor reflex, renin-angiotensin system, and kidneys in regulating arterial pressure. If your understanding of these concepts is a little hazy, you can refresh your memory by reading Chapter 40 (Review of Hemodynamics).

## Pathophysiology of Heart Failure

Heart failure is a syndrome in which the heart is unable to pump sufficient blood to meet the metabolic needs of tissues. The syndrome is characterized by signs of *inadequate tissue perfusion* (fatigue, shortness of breath, exercise intolerance) and/or signs of *volume overload* (venous distention, peripheral and pulmonary edema). Heart failure can be precipitated by multiple factors, including hypertension, valvular heart disease, coronary artery disease, myocardial infarction, dysrhythmias, and aging of the myocardium. Early symptoms include fatigue and shortness of breath. As cardiac performance deteriorates further, blood backs up behind the failing ventricles, causing venous distention, peripheral edema, and pulmonary edema. Heart failure is a chronic disorder that requires continuous treatment with drugs.

### Primary Pathology of Heart Failure

The primary defect in heart failure is a reduction in ventricular contractility. This decrease in contractile force is responsible for the reduction in cardiac output that characterizes heart failure. The cellular changes that underlie reduced contractility are unknown.

### Physiologic Adaptations to Reduced Cardiac Output

In response to reductions in the pumping ability of the heart, the body undergoes several adaptive changes. Some of these help improve tissue perfusion, whereas others may compound existing problems.

***Cardiac Dilation.*** Dilation of the heart is characteristic of heart failure. Cardiac dilation results from a combination of increased venous pressure (see below) and reduced contractile force. Reduced contractility lowers the amount of blood ejected during systole, causing end-systolic volume to rise. The increase in venous pressure increases diastolic filling, which causes the heart to expand even further.

Because of the Starling mechanism, the increase in heart size that occurs during heart failure helps improve cardiac output. That is, as the heart fails and its volume expands, contractility increases, causing a corresponding increase in stroke volume. However, it must be noted that the maximal contractile force that can be developed by the failing heart is considerably lower than the maximal force of the healthy heart. This limitation is reflected in the curve for the failing heart shown in Figure 46-1.

If cardiac dilation is insufficient to maintain cardiac output, other factors come into play. As discussed below, these are not always beneficial.

***Increased Sympathetic Tone.*** Heart failure causes arterial pressure to fall. In response, the baroreceptor reflex increases sympathetic output to the heart, veins, and arterioles. At the same time, parasympathetic effects on the heart are reduced. The consequences of increased sympathetic tone are summarized below.

- *Increased heart rate.* Acceleration of heart rate increases cardiac output, thereby helping improve tissue perfusion. However, if heart rate increases too much, there will be insufficient time for ventricular filling, and cardiac output will fall.
- *Increased contractility.* Increased myocardial contractility has the obvious benefit of increasing cardiac output. The only detriment is an increase in cardiac oxygen demand.
- *Increased venous tone.* Elevation of venous tone increases venous pressure, and thereby increases ventricular filling. Because of the Starling mechanism, increased filling increases stroke volume. Unfortunately, if venous pressure is excessive, blood will back up behind the failing ventricles, thereby aggravating pulmonary and peripheral edema. Furthermore, excessive filling pressure can dilate the heart so much that stroke volume will begin to decline (see Fig. 46-1).
- *Increased arteriolar tone.* Elevation of arteriolar tone increases arterial pressure, thereby increasing perfusion of vital organs. Unfortunately, increased arterial pressure also means that the heart must pump against greater resistance. Since cardiac reserve is minimal in heart failure, the heart may be unable to meet this challenge, and cardiac output may decline.

***Water Retention and Increased Blood Volume.*** *Mechanisms.* Water retention results from two mechanisms. First, reduced cardiac output causes a reduction in renal blood flow (RBF), which in turn decreases glomerular filtration rate. As a result, urine production is de-

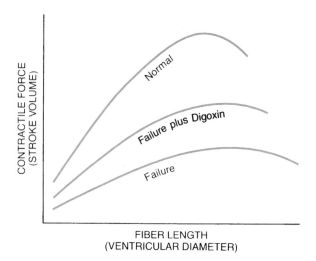

**Figure 46–1. Relationship of ventricular diameter to contractile force.** In the normal heart and the failing heart, increased fiber length produces increased contractile force. However, for any given fiber length, contractile force in the failing heart is much less than in the healthy heart. By increasing cardiac contractility, digoxin shifts the relationship between fiber length and stroke volume in the failing heart toward that in the normal heart.

creased and water is retained. Retention of water increases blood volume.

Second, heart failure activates the *renin-angiotensin system.* Activation occurs in response to reduced blood pressure and reduced RBF. Once activated, the renin-angiotensin system promotes water retention by increasing circulating levels of *aldosterone* and *angiotensin II.* Aldosterone acts directly on the kidneys to promote retention of sodium and water. Angiotensin II causes constriction of renal blood vessels, which decreases renal blood flow, and thereby further decreases urine production. In addition to promoting water retention, angiotensin II causes constriction of systemic arterioles and veins, and thereby increases venous and arterial pressure.

*Consequences.* As with other adaptive responses to heart failure, increased blood volume can be both beneficial and harmful. Increased blood volume increases venous pressure, and thereby increases venous return. As a result, ventricular filling and stroke volume are increased. The resultant increase in cardiac output can improve tissue perfusion. However, as noted above, if venous pressure is too high, edema of the lungs and periphery may result. More importantly, *if the increase in cardiac output is insufficient to maintain adequate kidney function, renal retention of water will continue unabated. The resultant accumulation of fluid will cause severe cardiac, pulmonary, and peripheral edema—and, ultimately, death.*

## The Vicious Cycle of "Compensatory" Physiologic Responses

As discussed above, reduced cardiac output leads to compensatory responses: (1) cardiac dilation, (2) activation of the sympathetic nervous system, (3) activation of the renin-angiotensin system, and (4) retention of water and expansion of blood volume. Although these responses represent the body's attempt to compensate for reduced cardiac output, they can actually make matters worse: excessive heart rate can reduce ventricular filling; excessive arterial pressure can lower cardiac output; and excessive venous pressure can cause pulmonary and peripheral edema. Hence, as depicted in Figure 46–2, the "compensatory" responses can create a self-sustaining cycle of maladaptation that further impairs cardiac output and tissue perfusion. If cardiac output becomes too low to maintain sufficient production of urine, the resultant accumulation of water will eventually cause death. The actual cause is complete cardiac failure secondary to excessive cardiac dilation and cardiac edema.

### Signs and Symptoms of Heart Failure

The prominent signs and symptoms of heart failure are a direct consequence of the pathophysiology described above. Decreased tissue perfusion results in reduced exercise tolerance, fatigue, and shortness of breath; shortness of breath may also stem from pulmonary edema. Increased sympathetic tone produces tachycardia. Increased ventricular filling and reduced systolic ejection result in cardiomegaly (increased heart size). The combination of increased venous tone plus increased blood volume helps cause pulmonary edema, peripheral edema, hepatomegaly (increased liver size), and distention of the jugular veins. Weight gain results from fluid retention.

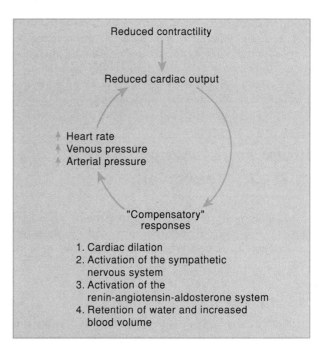

**Figure 46–2. The vicious cycle of maladaptive compensatory responses to a failing heart.**

## Treatment Goals and Strategies

Therapy of heart failure has three major goals: (1) relief of pulmonary and peripheral congestive symptoms, (2) improvement of functional capacity and quality of life, and (3) prolongation of life expectancy. To achieve these goals, three strategies are employed. First, we need to treat correctable underlying causes of heart failure, such as hypertension, dysrhythmias, and aortic stenosis. Second, we need to implement nondrug measures. Third, if the first two strategies prove insufficient, drug therapy should be employed.

## Nondrug Therapy of Heart Failure

Nondrug measures are an essential component of treatment. Salt intake should be limited to 2 gm/day. Excessive fluids must be avoided. Alcohol ingestion should be discouraged. Excessive, chronic consumption of alcohol is a leading cause of cardiomyopathy. In patients with heart failure, acute consumption of alcohol can suppress contractility. Accordingly, patients who drink alcohol should be advised to consume no more than one drink each day. Obese patients should be encouraged to adopt a reduced-calorie diet. In the past, bed rest was recommended. However, regular mild exercise (e.g., walking, cycling) is now advised; being active helps avoid atrophy of skeletal muscle, and there are no data indicating that activity is harmful.

## Evaluating Treatment of Heart Failure

Evaluation is based on symptoms and physical findings. Reductions in dyspnea on exertion, paroxysmal nocturnal dyspnea, and orthopnea (difficulty breathing, except in the upright position) indicate success. The physical examination should assess for reductions in jugular distention, edema, and rales. Success is also indicated by increased capacity for physical activity. Accordingly, patients should be interviewed to determine improvements in the maximal activity they can perform without symptoms, the type of activity that regularly produces symptoms, and the maximal activity that they can tolerate. (Activity is defined as walking, stair climbing, activities of daily living, or any other activity that is appropriate for the patient.) Successful treatment should also improve health-related quality of life in general. Hence the interview should look for improvements in sleep, sexual function, outlook on life, cognitive function (alertness, memory, concentration), and ability to participate in usual social, recreational, and work activities.

Routine measurement of ejection fraction or maximal exercise capacity is not recommended. Although the degree of reduction in ejection fraction measured at the beginning of therapy is predictive of outcome, improvement in the ejection fraction does not necessarily indicate that the prognosis has changed.

# Overview of Drugs Used to Treat Heart Failure

Heart failure is treated with three major classes of drugs: (1) vasodilators, (2) diuretics, and (3) inotropic agents. In addition, beta blockers are being tried in some patients.

## Vasodilators

In recent years, vasodilators have assumed a primary role in treating heart failure. These agents reduce symptoms and can prolong life. Vasodilators differ from one another with respect to route of administration (oral versus intravenous) and site of action (arterioles, veins, or both). Route of administration determines whether a drug is used acutely or long term. Site of action determines the specific hemodynamic benefits the drug offers.

### Principles of Use

*Venodilators.* Drugs that dilate *veins* increase venous capacitance, and thereby decrease venous pressure. As a result, venodilators reduce venous return and cardiac filling, which in turn decreases excessive ventricular stretching and cardiac oxygen demand. In addition to their beneficial effects on the heart, venodilators decrease pulmonary congestion and peripheral edema.

*Arteriolar Dilators.* Drugs that dilate *arterioles* have three beneficial effects: (1) arteriolar dilation reduces cardiac afterload, thereby allowing stroke volume and cardiac output to increase; (2) by increasing cardiac output and dilating arterioles in the kidney, these drugs increase renal perfusion, thereby promoting loss of fluid; and (3) in skeletal muscle, arteriolar dilation increases local perfusion.

### Oral Agents for Long-Term Therapy

*Angiotensin-Converting Enzyme Inhibitors.* Angiotensin-converting enzyme (ACE) inhibitors (e.g., captopril, enalapril) are the most frequently used vasodilators for long-term therapy of heart failure. In the absence of specific contraindications, *all* patients should receive one of these drugs. ACE inhibitors improve functional status and reduce mortality. These drugs can be used as sole therapy if heart failure is moderate and volume overload is absent.

ACE inhibitors suppress production of angiotensin II, and thereby *dilate arterioles and veins* and *decrease release of aldosterone.* Arteriolar dilation improves regional blood flow and, by reducing afterload, increases stroke volume and cardiac output. Venous dilation reduces venous pressure, and thereby reduces pulmonary

congestion, peripheral edema, and cardiac dilation. By dilating renal blood vessels, ACE inhibitors improve renal blood flow, and thereby enhance excretion of sodium and water. Suppression of aldosterone release further enhances excretion of sodium, while causing retention of potassium. From the foregoing, we can see that giving an ACE inhibitor is much like giving three different drugs: an arteriolar dilator, a venodilator, and a diuretic. ACE inhibitors are especially useful for patients with heart failure plus hypertension, angina, or elevated plasma renin activity.

The principal adverse effects of the ACE inhibitors are *hypotension* (secondary to arteriolar dilation), *hyperkalemia* (secondary to decreased aldosterone release), and *cough* (the mechanism of which is unknown). Because of their ability to elevate potassium levels, ACE inhibitors should be used with caution in patients taking potassium supplements or potassium-sparing diuretics. ACE inhibitors can cause *fetal injury* if taken during the second or third trimester. In addition, they can cause *renal failure in patients with bilateral renal artery stenosis.* The basic pharmacology of the ACE inhibitors is discussed in Chapter 41.

*Isosorbide Dinitrate Plus Hydralazine.* For treatment of heart failure, isosorbide dinitrate (ISDN) and hydralazine are usually combined. The combination is an alternative to ACE inhibitors for patients who cannot tolerate those drugs.

Isosorbide dinitrate [Isordil, Sorbitrate] belongs to the same drug family as nitroglycerin. Like nitroglycerin, ISDN causes selective dilation of *veins.* In patients with severe refractory heart failure, the drug can reduce congestive symptoms and improve exercise capacity. Principal adverse effects are orthostatic *hypotension* and *reflex tachycardia.* The basic pharmacology of ISDN and other organic nitrates is discussed in Chapter 45.

Hydralazine [Apresoline] causes selective dilation of *arterioles.* By doing so, the drug can improve cardiac output and renal blood flow. For treatment of heart failure, hydralazine is always used in combination with ISDN, since hydralazine by itself is relatively ineffective. Principal adverse effects are *hypotension*, *tachycardia*, and a syndrome that resembles *systemic lupus erythematosus.* The basic pharmacology of hydralazine is discussed in Chapter 43.

### Intravenous Agents for Acute Care

*Nitroglycerin.* Intravenous nitroglycerin is a powerful *venodilator* that produces a dramatic reduction in venous pressure. The drug's effects have been described as being equivalent to "pharmacologic phlebotomy." In heart failure, nitroglycerin is used to relieve acute severe pulmonary edema. Principal adverse effects are *hypotension* and resultant *reflex tachycardia.* The basic pharmacology of nitroglycerin is discussed in Chapter 45.

*Sodium Nitroprusside.* Sodium nitroprusside [Nipride, Nitropress] acts rapidly to dilate *arterioles* and *veins.* Arteriolar dilation reduces afterload and thereby increases cardiac output. Venodilation reduces venous pressure and thereby decreases pulmonary and peripheral congestion. The drug is indicated for short-term therapy of severe refractory heart failure. The principal adverse effect is *profound hypotension.* Blood pressure must be monitored continuously. The basic pharmacology of nitroprusside is discussed in Chapter 43.

## Diuretics

Diuretics are first-line drugs for all patients with signs of volume overload. By reducing blood volume, these drugs can decrease venous pressure, arterial pressure (afterload), pulmonary edema, peripheral edema, and cardiac dilation. It is important to note, however, that excessive diuresis is hazardous and must be avoided: if blood volume drops too low, cardiac output and blood pressure may fall precipitously, thereby further compromising tissue perfusion. Nonetheless, for most patients, diuretics offer a high benefit/risk ratio. The basic pharmacology of the diuretics is discussed in Chapter 38.

**Thiazide Diuretics.** The thiazide diuretics (e.g., hydrochlorothiazide) produce moderate diuresis. These oral agents are used for long-term therapy of heart failure when edema is not too great. Since thiazides are ineffective when glomerular filtration rate (GFR) is low, these drugs cannot be used if cardiac output is greatly reduced. The principal adverse effect of the thiazides is *hypokalemia*, which increases the risk of *digoxin-induced dysrhythmias* (see below).

**High-Ceiling (Loop) Diuretics.** The loop diuretics (e.g., furosemide) produce profound diuresis. In contrast to the thiazides, these drugs can promote fluid loss even when GFR is low. Hence, loop diuretics are preferred to thiazides when cardiac output is greatly reduced. Administration may be oral or intravenous. Because they can mobilize large volumes of water, and because they work when GFR is low, loop diuretics are drugs of choice for patients with severe heart failure. Like the thiazides, these drugs can cause *hypokalemia*, thereby increasing the risk of *digoxin toxicity*. In addition, loop diuretics can cause severe *hypotension* secondary to excessive volume reduction.

**Potassium-Sparing Diuretics.** In contrast to the thiazides and loop diuretics, the potassium-sparing diuretics (e.g., spironolactone) promote only scant diuresis. In patients with heart failure, these drugs are employed to counteract potassium loss caused by thiazide and loop diuretics, thereby lowering the risk of digoxin-induced dysrhythmias. Not surprisingly, the principal adverse effect of the potassium-sparing drugs is *hyperkalemia*. Because *ACE inhibitors* also carry a risk of hyperkalemia, caution is needed if they are combined with a potassium-sparing diuretic. Accordingly, when therapy with an ACE inhibitor is initiated, the potassium-sparing diuretic should be discontinued. It can be resumed later if needed.

## Inotropic Agents

Inotropic agents are drugs that increase the force of myocardial contraction. These agents are given to improve performance of the failing heart. Three types of inotropic drugs are available: *cardiac glycosides, sympathomimetics,* and *phosphodiesterase (PDE) inhibitors*. The sympathomimetics and PDE inhibitors that are currently available can be administered only by intravenous infusion. Accordingly, use is generally restricted to acute care of the hospitalized patient. At this time, the cardiac glycosides are the only inotropic agents that can be used orally. Hence they are the only inotropics suited for long-term therapy.

### Cardiac Glycosides

The cardiac glycosides (e.g., digoxin) are the oldest and most frequently prescribed inotropic drugs. These agents are used widely for long-term therapy of heart failure. Unfortunately, although these drugs reduce symptoms, they do not prolong life. The pharmacology of the cardiac glycosides is discussed at length later in the chapter.

### Sympathomimetic Drugs: Dopamine and Dobutamine

The basic pharmacology of dopamine and dobutamine is presented in Chapter 18. Discussion here is limited to the use of these drugs in heart failure.

**Dopamine.** Dopamine [Dopastat, Intropin] is a catecholamine that can activate (1) beta$_1$-adrenergic receptors in the heart, (2) dopamine receptors in the kidney, and (3) at high doses, alpha$_1$-adrenergic receptors in blood vessels. Activation of beta$_1$ receptors increases myocardial contractility, thereby improving cardiac performance. Beta$_1$ activation also increases heart rate, creating a risk of tachycardia. Activation of dopamine receptors dilates renal blood vessels, thereby increasing renal blood flow and urine output. Activation of alpha$_1$ receptors increases vascular resistance (afterload), and can thereby reduce cardiac output. Dopamine is administered by continuous infusion. Constant monitoring of blood pressure, the electrocardiogram (EKG), and urine output is required. Dopamine is employed as a short-term rescue measure for patients with severe, acute cardiac failure.

**Dobutamine.** Dobutamine [Dobutrex] is a synthetic catecholamine that causes selective activation of beta$_1$-adrenergic receptors. By doing so, the drug can increase myocardial contractility, thereby improving cardiac performance. Like dopamine, dobutamine can cause tachycardia. In contrast to dopamine, dobutamine does not activate alpha$_1$ receptors, and therefore does not increase vascular resistance. As a result, the drug is generally preferred to dopamine for short-term treatment of acute heart failure. Administration is by continuous infusion.

#### Phosphodiesterase Inhibitors

**Amrinone.** Amrinone [Inocor] has been called an *inodilator*, because it increases myocardial contractility and promotes vasodilation. Increased contractility results from intracellular accumulation of cyclic AMP (cAMP) secondary to inhibition of phosphodiesterase III, the enzyme that normally degrades cAMP. The mechanism underlying vasodilation is unclear. Comparative studies indicate that improvements in cardiac function elicited by amrinone are superior to those elicited by dopamine or dobutamine. Like dopamine and dobutamine, amrinone is administered by intravenous infusion, and therefore is not suitable for outpatient use. Amrinone is indicated for short-term (2- to 3-day) treatment of heart failure in patients who have not responded to vasodilators, diuretics, and digoxin. The drug should be protected from light and should not be mixed with glucose-containing solutions. Constant monitoring is required. The initial dose is 0.75 mg/kg (IV) administered over 2 to 3 minutes. The maintenance infusion is 5 to 10 µg/kg/min.

***Milrinone.*** Like amrinone, milrinone [Primacor] is an inodilator. Increased contractility results from accumulation of cAMP secondary to inhibition of phosphodiesterase III. Milrinone is administered by IV infusion and is indicated only for short-term therapy of severe heart failure. Dosing is complex.

***Vesnarinone.*** Like other phosphodiesterase inhibitors, vesnarinone [Arkin-Z] increases myocardial contractility and promotes vasodilation. In addition, by affecting cardiac sodium and potassium channels, the drug prolongs action potential duration and slows heart rate, thereby decreasing the risk of dysrhythmias.

Clinical effects are dose dependent. When administered in *high* doses (120 mg/day), vesnarinone produces a fivefold *increase* in mortality, which is greater than the increase in mortality reported for any other inotropic drug. In striking contrast, when given in *low* doses (60 mg/day), vesnarinone *decreases* mortality by 62%, which is two to four times greater than the decrease in mortality reported for any other drug used for heart failure. Because the toxic dose (120 mg/day) is only twice the beneficial dose (60 mg/day), vesnarinone clearly has a very narrow margin of safety.

The mechanism underlying reduced mortality is not known. The low doses that are responsible for reduced mortality produce no significant hemodynamic change. Hence, it would appear that reduced mortality cannot be explained by an increase in contractility.

The major adverse effect of vesnarinone is reversible neutropenia, which occurs in 2.5% of patients. Neutrophil counts must be monitored.

## Beta Blockers

Although beta blockers were traditionally contraindicated during heart failure, recent studies indicate these drugs can (paradoxically) improve cardiac performance, at least for some patients. Recall that blockade of cardiac beta$_1$-adrenergic receptors *reduces* contractility—an effect that is clearly detrimental, given that contractility is already compromised by heart failure. Nonetheless, with careful control of dosage, beta blockers can gradually improve patient status. Controlled trials have shown that three beta blockers—metoprolol, bisoprolol, and carvedilol—when added to conventional therapy, can decrease symptoms, improve exercise tolerance, slow progression of heart failure, and reduce the need for hospitalization. The mechanism underlying these benefits is subject to speculation. Because beta blockade has the potential to acutely reduce contractility, dosage must be very low initially and then gradually increased. Full benefits may not be seen for 1 to 3 months. At this time, carvedilol [Coreg] is the only beta blocker approved by the FDA for use in heart failure. The basic pharmacology of the beta blockers is discussed in Chapter 19.

## Drug Selection in Chronic Heart Failure

The choice of drugs for treating chronic heart failure has undergone significant change in recent years. Vasodilators are now considered first-line therapy. In contrast, use of cardiac glycosides has declined. In the past, practically all patients were given a cardiac glycoside. However, it is now clear that not every patient needs one. Patients with mild to moderate heart failure may respond adequately to nondrug measures. If these are insufficient, drugs are indicated. Treatment can begin with just one agent. In the absence of volume overload, initial therapy with an ACE inhibitor is indicated. If volume overload is present, a diuretic should be combined with the ACE inhibitor. If more intensive therapy is needed, we can treat with three drugs: an ACE inhibitor plus a diuretic plus digoxin. For patients with moderate to severe heart failure, this triple therapy is considered standard. Patients who cannot tolerate ACE inhibitors may be given a combination of hydralazine and isosorbide dinitrate instead.

## Pharmacology of the Cardiac (Digitalis) Glycosides

The cardiac glycosides are naturally occurring compounds that have profound effects on the mechanical and electrical properties of the heart. By improving mechanical function of the heart, these drugs can reduce symptoms of heart failure. By altering electrical properties of the heart, these drugs can both suppress dysrhythmias and cause them. Because they are prepared by extraction from *Digitalis purpura* (purple foxglove) and *Digitalis lanata* (white foxglove), the cardiac glycosides are also known as *digitalis glycosides.*

The cardiac glycosides are among the most widely used prescription drugs, and they are also among the most dangerous. The frequent use of these drugs stems from their ability to improve cardiac performance in patients with heart failure. The high incidence of toxicity results from their propensity to cause dysrhythmias—at doses that are close to therapeutic. There is no question that the cardiac glycosides are a mixed blessing, having the potential for life-enhancing benefits as well as life-threatening harm. Accordingly, it is essential that we use these drugs with respect, caution, and skill.

In the United States, only two cardiac glycosides are available: digoxin and digitoxin. Of the two, digoxin is by far the more widely prescribed.

### Digoxin

Digoxin [Lanoxin, Lanoxicaps] is indicated for heart failure and dysrhythmias. Use for heart failure is discussed here; use for dysrhythmias is discussed in Chapter 48. When used for heart failure, digoxin can reduce symptoms, increase exercise tolerance, and decrease hospitalizations. However, the drug does not prolong life. Of all prescription medications employed in the United States, digoxin is among the 10 most frequently prescribed.

#### Chemistry

Digoxin consists of three components: a steroid nucleus, a lactone ring, and three molecules of digitoxose (a sugar). It is because of the sugars that digoxin is known as a glycoside. The region of the molecule composed of the steroid nucleus plus the lactone ring (i.e., the region without the sugar molecules) is responsible for the pharmacologic effects of digoxin. The sugars only increase solubility.

## Mechanical Effects on the Heart

Digoxin exerts a *positive inotropic action* on the heart. That is, the drug *increases the force of ventricular contraction*, and thereby increases cardiac output.

### Mechanism of Inotropic Action.

Digoxin increases myocardial contractility by inhibiting an enzyme known as *sodium, potassium-ATPase* ($Na^+,K^+$-ATPase). By way of an indirect process (see below), inhibition of $Na^+,K^+$-ATPase promotes *calcium accumulation* within cardiac cells. The calcium then augments contractile force by facilitating the interaction of myocardial contractile proteins—actin and myosin.

To understand how inhibition of $Na^+,K^+$-ATPase causes intracellular calcium to rise, we must first understand the normal role of $Na^+,K^+$-ATPase in the cardiac cell. That role is illustrated in Figure 46–3. As indicated, when an action potential passes along the cardiac cell membrane (sarcolemma), $Na^+$ ions and $Ca^{++}$ ions enter the cell, and $K^+$ ions exit. Once the action potential has passed, these ion fluxes must be reversed so that the original ionic composition of the cell can be restored. $Na^+,K^+$-ATPase is critical to this restorative process. As shown in the figure, $Na^+,K^+$-ATPase acts as a "pump" to draw extracellular $K^+$ ions into the cell, while simultaneously extruding intracellular $Na^+$. The energy required for pumping $Na^+$ and $K^+$ is provided by the breakdown of ATP—hence, the name $Na^+,K^+$-ATPase. To complete the normalization of cellular ionic composition, $Ca^{++}$ ions must leave the cell. Extrusion of $Ca^{++}$ is accomplished through an exchange process in which extracellular $Na^+$ ions are taken into the cell while $Ca^{++}$ ions exit. This exchange of $Na^+$ for $Ca^{++}$ is a passive (energy-independent) process.

We can now answer the question, how does the ability of digoxin to inhibit $Na^+,K^+$-ATPase produce an increase in intracellular $Ca^{++}$ levels? By inhibiting $Na^+,K^+$-ATPase, digoxin prevents the cardiac cell from restoring its proper ionic composition following the passage of an action potential. Inhibition of $Na^+,K^+$-ATPase blocks uptake of $K^+$ and extrusion of $Na^+$. Hence, with each successive action potential, intracellular $K^+$ levels decline while levels of $Na^+$ within the cell rise. It is this rise in $Na^+$ that leads to the rise in intracellular $Ca^{++}$. In the presence of excess intracellular $Na^+$, further $Na^+$ entry is suppressed. Since $Na^+$ entry is suppressed, the passive exchange of $Ca^{++}$ for $Na^+$ cannot take place; hence, $Ca^{++}$ accumulates within the cell.

### Relationship of Potassium to Inotropic Action.

Potassium ions compete with digoxin for binding to $Na^+,K^+$-ATPase. This competition is of great clinical significance. Because potassium competes with digoxin, when potassium levels are low, binding of digoxin to $Na^+,K^+$-ATPase increases. This increase can produce excessive inhibition of $Na^+,K^+$-ATPase with resultant toxicity. Conversely, when levels of potassium are high, inhibition of $Na^+,K^+$-ATPase by digoxin is reduced, causing a reduction in the therapeutic response. Because an increase in potassium can impair therapeutic responses, whereas a decrease in potassium can cause toxicity, it is imperative that potassium levels be kept within the normal physiologic range (3.5 to 5 mEq/L).

## Beneficial Effects in Heart Failure

### Increased Cardiac Output.

The primary effect of digoxin is to increase myocardial contractility, which in turn causes an increase in cardiac output. As shown in Figure 46–1, by increasing contractility, digoxin shifts the relationship of fiber length to stroke volume in the failing heart toward that in the healthy heart. Consequently, at any given heart size, the stroke volume of the failing heart increases, causing cardiac output to rise.

### Consequences of Increased Cardiac Output.

As a result of increased cardiac output, three major secondary responses occur: (1) sympathetic tone declines, (2) urine production increases, and (3) renin release declines. These responses can lead to reversal of virtually all signs and symptoms of heart failure.

*Decreased Sympathetic Tone.* By increasing contractile force and cardiac output, digoxin increases arterial pressure. In response, sympathetic nerve traffic to the heart and blood vessels is reduced via the baroreceptor reflex. (Recall that a compensatory *increase* in sympathetic tone had taken place because of heart failure.)

The decrease in sympathetic tone has several beneficial effects. First, heart rate is reduced, thereby allowing more

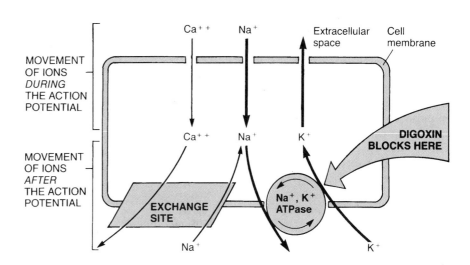

**Figure 46–3. Ion fluxes across the cardiac cell membrane.** During the action potential, $Na^+$ and $Ca^{++}$ enter the cardiac cell and $K^+$ exits. Following the action potential, $Na^+,K^+$-ATPase pumps $Na^+$ out of the cell and takes up $K^+$. $Ca^{++}$ leaves the cell in exchange for the uptake of $Na^+$. By inhibiting $Na^+,K^+$-ATPase, digoxin prevents the extrusion of $Na^+$, causing $Na^+$ to accumulate inside the cell. The resulting buildup of intracellular $Na^+$ suppresses the $Na^+$-$Ca^{++}$ exchange process, thereby causing intracellular levels of $Ca^{++}$ to rise.

complete ventricular filling. Second, afterload is reduced (because of reduced arteriolar constriction), thereby allowing more complete ventricular emptying. Third, venous pressure is reduced (because of reduced venous constriction), thereby reducing cardiac distention, pulmonary congestion, and peripheral edema.

*Increased Urine Production.* The increase in cardiac output increases renal blood flow, and thereby increases production of urine. The resultant loss of water reduces blood volume, which in turn reduces cardiac distention, pulmonary congestion, and peripheral edema.

*Decreased Renin Release.* In response to increased arterial pressure, renin release declines, causing levels of aldosterone and angiotensin II to decline as well. The decrease in angiotensin II decreases vasoconstriction, thereby further reducing afterload and venous pressure. The decrease in aldosterone reduces retention of sodium and water, which reduces blood volume, which in turn further reduces venous pressure.

**Summary of Effects in Heart Failure.** In summary, we can see that, through direct and indirect mechanisms, digoxin has the potential to reverse all of the overt manifestations of heart failure: cardiac output improves, heart rate decreases, heart size declines, constriction of arterioles and veins decreases, water retention reverses, blood volume declines, peripheral and pulmonary edema decrease, and weight is lost (because of water loss). In addition, exercise tolerance improves and fatigue is reduced. Given this impressive spectrum of responses, in combination with the prevalence of heart disease, we can appreciate why digoxin is widely prescribed. There is, however, one important caveat to keep in mind: Although digoxin can produce substantial improvement in symptoms, the drug does not alter the natural course of heart failure, and does not prolong life.

## Electrical Effects on the Heart

The effects of digoxin on the electrical activity of the heart are of therapeutic and toxicologic importance. It is because of its electrical effects that digoxin is useful for treating dysrhythmias (see Chapter 48). Ironically, these same electrical effects are responsible for *causing* dysrhythmias—the most serious toxicity of digoxin.

The electrical effects of digoxin can be bewildering in their complexity. Through a combination of actions, digoxin can alter the electrical activity in noncontractile tissue (sinoatrial node, atrioventricular node, Purkinje fibers) as well as in ventricular muscle. In these various tissues, digoxin can alter automaticity, refractoriness, and impulse conduction. Whether these parameters are increased or decreased depends on cardiac status, digoxin dosage, and the particular tissue examined.

Although the electrical effects of digoxin are many and varied, only a few are clinically significant. These are discussed below.

*Mechanisms for Altering Electrical Activity of the Heart.* Digoxin alters the electrical properties of the heart by *inhibiting* $Na^+,K^+$*-ATPase* and by *enhancing vagal influences on the heart.* By inhibiting $Na^+,K^+$-ATPase, digoxin alters the distribu-

tion of ions ($Na^+$, $K^+$, $Ca^{++}$) across the cardiac cell membrane. This change in ion distribution can alter the electrical responsiveness of the cells involved. Since hypokalemia intensifies inhibition of $Na^+,K^+$-ATPase, hypokalemia intensifies alterations in cardiac electrical properties.

Digoxin acts in two ways to enhance vagal effects on the heart. First, the drug acts in the central nervous system to increase the firing rate of vagal fibers that innervate the heart. Second, digoxin increases the responsiveness of the sinoatrial (SA) node to acetylcholine (the neurotransmitter released by the vagus). The net result of these vagotonic effects is (1) decreased automaticity of the SA node, and (2) decreased conduction through the atrioventricular (AV) node.

**Effects on Specific Regions of the Heart.** In the SA node, digoxin decreases automaticity (by the vagotonic mechanisms just mentioned). In the AV node, digoxin decreases conduction velocity and prolongs the effective refractory period; these effects, which can promote varying degrees of AV block, result primarily from the drug's vagotonic actions. In Purkinje fibers, digoxin-induced inhibition of $Na^+,K^+$-ATPase results in increased automaticity; this increase can generate ectopic foci that, in turn, can cause ventricular dysrhythmias. In the ventricular myocardium, digoxin acts to shorten the effective refractory period and to (possibly) increase automaticity.

## Cardiotoxicity: Generation of Dysrhythmias

Dysrhythmias are the most serious adverse effect of digoxin. The drug causes dysrhythmias by altering the electrical properties of the heart.

Because serious dysrhythmias are a potential consequence of therapy, all patients should be evaluated frequently for changes in heart rate and rhythm. If significant changes occur, digoxin should be withheld and the physician consulted. Outpatients should be taught to monitor their pulses and instructed to report any significant changes in rate or regularity.

**Types of Digoxin-Induced Dysrhythmias.** Digoxin can mimic practically all types of dysrhythmias. AV block with escape beats is among the most common. Ventricular flutter and ventricular fibrillation are the most dangerous.

**Mechanism of Ventricular Dysrhythmia Generation.** Digoxin-induced ventricular dysrhythmias result from a combination of four factors:

- decreased automaticity of the SA node
- decreased conduction of impulses through the AV node
- spontaneous discharge of Purkinje fibers (caused in part by increased automaticity)
- shortening of the effective refractory period in ventricular muscle.

Increased Purkinje fiber discharge and shortening of the ventricular effective refractory period predispose the ventricles to developing ectopic beats. Potential ectopic beats become manifest because the effects of digoxin on the SA and AV nodes decrease the ability of the normal pacemaker to drive the ventricles, thereby allowing ventricular ectopic beats to take over.

**Predisposing Factors.** *Hypokalemia. The most common cause of dysrhythmias in patients receiving digoxin is* *hypokalemia secondary to the use of diuretics.* Less common causes of hypokalemia include vomiting and diarrhea. Hypokalemia promotes dysrhythmias by increasing digoxin-induced inhibition of $Na^+,K^+$-ATPase, which in turn leads to increased automaticity of Purkinje fibers. Because low potassium can precipitate dysrhythmias, *it is imperative that serum potassium levels be kept within a normal range.* If diuretic therapy causes potassium levels to fall, a potassium-sparing diuretic (e.g., spironolactone) can be added to the regimen to correct the problem. Potassium supplements may also be used. Patients should be taught to recognize symptoms of hypokalemia (e.g., muscle weakness) and instructed to notify the physician if these develop.

*Elevated Digoxin Levels. Digoxin has a narrow therapeutic range: drug levels only slightly higher than therapeutic greatly increase the risk of toxicity.* Possible causes of excessive digoxin levels include (1) intentional or accidental overdose, (2) increased digoxin absorption, and (3) decreased digoxin elimination.

If digoxin levels are kept within the therapeutic range, the chances of a dysrhythmia will be reduced. However, it is important to note that careful control over drug levels does not eliminate the risk entirely. As discussed above, there is only a loose relationship between digoxin levels and clinical effects. As a result, some patients may experience dysrhythmias even when drug levels are well within what is normally considered the therapeutic range.

*Heart Disease.* The ability of digoxin to cause dysrhythmias is greatly increased by the presence of heart disease. Doses of digoxin that have no adverse effects on healthy volunteers can precipitate serious dysrhythmias in patients with heart failure. The probability and severity of a dysrhythmia are directly related to the severity of the underlying disease. Since heart disease is the reason for taking digoxin, it should be no surprise that people taking the drug are at risk of dysrhythmias.

*Diagnosis of Cardiotoxicity.* Diagnosis of digoxin-induced dysrhythmias is not a simple matter. Much of the difficulty stems from the fact that the failing heart is prone to developing dysrhythmias spontaneously. Hence, when a dysrhythmia occurs, we cannot simply assume that digoxin is the cause; the possibility that the dysrhythmia is the direct result of heart disease must be considered. Compounding diagnostic difficulties is the poor correlation between plasma digoxin levels and dysrhythmia onset. Because of this loose correspondence, the presence of an apparently excessive digoxin level does not necessarily indicate that digoxin is responsible for the problem. Laboratory data required for diagnosis include digoxin level, serum electrolytes, and an EKG. Ultimately, diagnosis is based on experience and clinical judgment. Resolution of the dysrhythmia following digoxin withdrawal confirms the diagnosis.

*Management of Digoxin-Induced Dysrhythmias.* With proper treatment, digoxin-induced dysrhythmias can almost always be controlled. Basic management measures are as follows:

- *Withdraw digoxin and potassium-wasting diuretics.* For many patients, no additional treatment is needed. To help ensure that medication is stopped, a written order to withhold digoxin should be made.
- *Monitor serum potassium.* If the potassium level is low or nearly normal, potassium (IV or PO) should be administered. Potassium displaces digoxin from $Na^+,K^+$-ATPase and thereby helps reverse toxicity. However, if potassium levels are high or if AV block is present, no more potassium should be given. Under these conditions, more potassium may cause complete AV block.
- Some patients may require an antidysrhythmic drug. *Phenytoin* and *lidocaine* are most effective. Quinidine, another antidysrhythmic drug, can cause plasma levels of digoxin to rise, and therefore should not be used.
- Patients who develop bradycardia or AV block can be treated with atropine. (Atropine helps by blocking the vagal influences that underlie bradycardia and AV block.) Alternatively, electronic pacing may be employed.
- When overdose is especially severe, digoxin levels can be lowered using *Fab antibody fragments* [Digibind]. Following IV administration, these fragments bind digoxin, and thereby prevent it from acting. Treatment is expensive: a full neutralizing dose costs $2000 to $3000. *Cholestyramine* and *activated charcoal*, agents that also bind digoxin, can be administered orally to suppress absorption of digoxin from the gastrointestinal tract.

## Noncardiac Adverse Effects

The principal noncardiac toxicities of digoxin concern the GI system and the central nervous system (CNS). Since adverse effects on these systems frequently precede development of dysrhythmias, symptoms involving the GI tract and CNS can provide advance warning of more serious toxicity. Accordingly, patients should be taught to recognize these effects and instructed to notify the physician if they occur.

*Anorexia, nausea,* and *vomiting* are the most common GI effects of digoxin. These responses result primarily from stimulation of the chemoreceptor trigger zone of the medulla. Digoxin rarely causes diarrhea.

*Fatigue* is the most frequent CNS effect. *Visual disturbances* (e.g., blurred vision, yellow tinge to vision, appearance of halos around dark objects) are also relatively common.

## Reducing the Risk of Toxicity

Patient education can help reduce the incidence of toxicity. Patients should be warned about digoxin-induced dysrhythmias and instructed to take their medication exactly as prescribed. In addition, they should be informed about symptoms of developing toxicity (altered heart rate or rhythm, visual or GI disturbances) and instructed to notify the physician if these develop. If a potassium supple-

## TABLE 46-1. DRUG INTERACTIONS WITH DIGOXIN

| Drug | Effect |
|---|---|
| *Pharmacodynamic Interactions* | |
| Thiazide diuretics | Promote potassium loss |
| Loop diuretics | and thereby increase |
| | the risk of digoxin- |
| | induced dysrhythmias |
| Beta blockers | Decrease contractility |
| Verapamil | and heart rate |
| Diltiazem | |
| Sympathomimetics | Increase contractility |
| | and heart rate |
| *Pharmacokinetic Interactions* | |
| Cholestyramine | *Decrease digoxin levels* |
| Kaolin-pectin | by decreasing digoxin |
| Neomycin | absorption or |
| Sulfasalazine | bioavailability |
| Aminoglycosides | *Increase digoxin levels* |
| Antacids | by increasing digoxin |
| Colestipol | absorption or |
| Erythromycin | bioavailability |
| Omeprazole | |
| Tetracycline | |
| Alprazolam | *Increase digoxin levels* |
| Amiodarone | by decreasing |
| Captopril | excretion of digoxin, |
| Diltiazem | altering distribution |
| Nifedipine | of digoxin, or both |
| Nitrendipine | |
| Propafenone | |
| Quinidine | |
| Verapamil | |

ment or potassium-sparing diuretic is part of the regimen, it should be taken exactly as prescribed.

## Drug Interactions

Digoxin is subject to a large number of significant drug interactions. Some are pharmacodynamic and some are pharmacokinetic. Several important interactions are discussed below. A summary of interactions is presented in Table 46-1.

**Diuretics.** *Thiazide diuretics* and *loop diuretics* promote loss of potassium, and thereby increase the risk of digoxin-induced dysrhythmias. Accordingly, when digoxin and these diuretics are used concurrently, serum potassium levels must be monitored and maintained within a normal range (3.5 to 5 mEq/L). If hypokalemia develops, potassium levels can be restored with potassium supplements, a potassium-sparing diuretic, or both.

**Sympathomimetics.** Sympathomimetic drugs (e.g., dopamine, dobutamine) act on the heart to increase the rate and force of contraction. The increase in contractile force can add to the positive inotropic effects of digoxin. These complementary actions can be beneficial. In con-

trast, the ability of sympathomimetics to increase heart rate may be detrimental in that the risk of a tachydysrhythmia is increased.

**Quinidine.** Quinidine is an antidysrhythmic drug that can cause plasma levels of digoxin to rise. Quinidine increases digoxin levels by (1) displacing digoxin from tissue binding sites and (2) reducing the renal excretion of digoxin. By elevating levels of free digoxin, quinidine can promote digoxin toxicity. Accordingly, concurrent use of quinidine and digoxin should be avoided.

**Verapamil.** Verapamil, a calcium channel blocker, can significantly increase plasma levels of digoxin. If the combination is employed, digoxin dosage must be reduced. In addition, verapamil can suppress myocardial contractility, and can thereby counteract the benefits of digoxin.

## Pharmacokinetics

**Absorption.** Absorption of oral digoxin can be variable. The extent of absorption is lowest and most variable with digoxin *tablets*, ranging between 60% and 80%. Absorption from digoxin capsules [Lanoxicaps] is more complete and less variable, ranging between 90% and 100%. However, although digoxin capsules permit excellent absorption, they do have one drawback: they are much more expensive than the tablets. Hence it may be preferable to reserve the capsules for patients in whom stable drug levels cannot be achieved with tablets.

Several factors can decrease digoxin bioavailability. For example, meals high in bran can decrease absorption significantly. Bioavailability can also be decreased by cholestyramine, kaolin-pectin, and certain other drugs (see Table 46-1). Taking digoxin with meals slows the rate of absorption, but does not decrease the extent of absorption.

Until recently, there was considerable variability in the absorption of digoxin from tablets prepared by different manufacturers. This variability resulted from differences in the rate and extent of tablet dissolution. Because of this variable bioavailability, it had been recommended that patients not switch between different digoxin brands. Today, bioavailability of digoxin in tablets produced by different companies is fairly uniform, making brands of digoxin more interchangeable than in the past. However, given the narrow therapeutic range of the digoxin, some authorities still recommend that patients not switch between brands of digoxin tablets—even when prescriptions are written generically—except with the approval and supervision of the physician.

**Distribution.** Digoxin undergoes wide distribution throughout the body and crosses the placenta. High levels are achieved in cardiac and skeletal muscle, owing largely to binding to $Na^+,K^+$-ATPase. About 23% of digoxin in plasma is bound to proteins (mainly albumin).

**Elimination.** Digoxin is eliminated primarily by *renal excretion*. Hepatic metabolism is minimal. Because digoxin is eliminated by the kidneys, alterations in renal function can have a significant impact on digoxin blood levels: if kidney function declines, digoxin may accumulate to levels that are toxic. Accordingly, dosage must be reduced in patients with renal impairment. Because digoxin is not metabolized to any significant extent, changes in liver function do not affect plasma digoxin levels.

*Half-Life and Time to Plateau.* The half-life of digoxin is about 1.5 days. Hence, in the absence of a loading dose, about 6 days (4 half-lives) are required for plateau levels to be achieved. When use of the drug is discontinued, another 6 days are required for digoxin stores to be eliminated.

*Single-Dose Time Course.* Effects of a single oral dose begin 30 minutes to 2 hours after administration and peak within 4 to 6 hours. Effects of intravenous digoxin begin rapidly (within 5 to 30 minutes) and peak in 1 to 4 hours.

*A Note on Plasma Digoxin Levels.* Most hospitals are equipped to measure plasma levels of digoxin. The therapeutic range is 0.5 to 2.0 ng/ml. Levels above 2.5 ng/ml are toxic. Knowledge of plasma levels can be useful for:

- Establishing dosage
- Monitoring compliance
- Diagnosing toxicity
- Determining the cause of therapeutic failure.

Once a stable blood level has been achieved, routine measurement of digoxin levels is unnecessary; rather, an annual determination is usually sufficient. However, measurements should be made whenever

- Digoxin dosage is changed
- Symptoms of heart failure intensify
- Kidney function deteriorates
- Signs of toxicity appear
- Drugs that can affect digoxin levels are added to or deleted from the regimen.

Although knowledge of digoxin plasma levels can aid the clinician, it must be understood that the extent of this aid is limited. The correlation between plasma levels of digoxin and clinical effects—both therapeutic and adverse—is not very tight: drug levels that are safe and effective for patient A may be subtherapeutic for patient B and toxic for patient C. Because of interpatient variability, knowledge of digoxin levels does not permit precise predictions of therapeutic effects or toxicity. Hence, information regarding drug levels must not be relied upon too heavily. Rather, this information should be seen as but one factor among several to be considered when evaluating clinical responses.

## Preparations, Dosage, and Administration

*Preparations.* Digoxin is available in tablets (0.125, 0.25, and 0.5 mg), a pediatric elixir (0.05 mg/ml), an injection (0.1 and 0.25 mg/ml), and in capsules that contain digoxin in solution (0.05, 0.1, and 0.2 mg). Trade names are Lanoxin (for the tablets and elixir) and Lanoxicaps (for the capsules).

*Administration.* Digoxin can be administered *orally* and *intravenously. Intramuscular* administration causes severe pain and tissue damage and should be avoided. Prior to administration, the rate and regularity of the heart beat should be determined. If heart rate is less than 60 beats/min or if a change in rhythm is detected, digoxin should be withheld and the physician notified. When digoxin is given IV, cardiac status should be monitored continuously for 1 to 2 hours.

*Dosage in Heart Failure.* For several reasons, establishing a safe and effective dosage is difficult. First, since digoxin has a narrow therapeutic range, the dosing target is small, making it difficult to hit. Second, when treating heart failure with digoxin, we lack a clear-cut therapeutic endpoint. Without such an endpoint, we cannot determine with certainty if the dosage is greater or smaller than required. Third, monitoring digoxin plasma levels is only moderately helpful. Because of substantial interpatient variability, drug levels that may be safe and effective in one patient may be ineffective or toxic in another. Hence, we cannot rely heavily on the concept of "standard therapeutic plasma levels" when attempting to establish digoxin dosage. Ultimately, determining the most desirable dosage must be based on careful observation of the patient: signs of beneficial and adverse responses must be monitored and the dosage adjusted accordingly.

*Digitalization.* When maximal effects must be achieved rapidly, a loading dose is required. (As noted above, 6 days are needed for plasma drug levels to reach plateau if no loading dose is employed.) By convention, the process of using a loading dose to achieve high levels of digoxin quickly is termed *digitalization.* Digitalization can be accomplished with an initial oral dose of 0.5 to 0.75 mg followed by doses of 0.25 to 0.5 mg at intervals of 6 to 8 hours until digitalization is complete (usually with a total dose of 0.75 to 1.25 mg). For most patients, digitalization is unnecessary.

*Maintenance Doses.* The dosing objective in maintenance therapy is to establish doses that are high enough to be effective but not so high as to cause toxicity. As discussed above, *dosing is highly individualized and based largely on clinical observation.* Because digoxin is eliminated by the kidneys, *maintenance doses must be reduced if renal function declines.* Maintenance dosages for adults usually range from 0.125 to 0.5 mg daily. A typical adult dose is 0.25 mg/day.

If digoxin therapy is initiated with digitalization, a transition to smaller doses for maintenance is required. When this is done, it is imperative that a new medication order be written. This will help prevent inadvertent continued administration of the large digitalizing doses.

### Digitoxin

Digitoxin [Crystodigin] is similar to digoxin in most respects. These drugs have the same mechanism of action (inhibition of $Na^+,K^+$-ATPase), the same applications (treatment of heart failure and dysrhythmias), and they produce the same major toxicities (dysrhythmias). The principal differences between these drugs are pharmacokinetic. The most outstanding property of digi-

## TABLE 46-2. PHARMACOKINETIC PROPERTIES OF DIGOXIN AND DIGITOXIN

| Property | Digoxin | Digitoxin |
|---|---|---|
| Route | PO, IV | PO |
| Liquid solubility | Moderate | High |
| Oral absorption (%) | | |
| Tablets | 60–80 | 100 |
| Elixir | 70–80 | — |
| Solution in capsules | 90–100 | — |
| Plasma protein binding (%) | 23 | 97 |
| Elimination | Renal | Hepatic |
| Half-life | | |
| Liver and kidney healthy | 1.6 days | 1 week |
| Severe renal dysfunction | 4–5 days | 1 week |
| Liver dysfunction | 1.6 days | Prolonged? |
| Time to plateau* | 6–7 days | 4–5 weeks |
| Plasma levels (ng/ml)† | | |
| Therapeutic | 0.5–2.0 | 10–35 |
| Toxic | >2.5 | >35 |

*In the absence of a loading dose.
†There is significant individual variation in responses to digoxin and digitoxin. Levels that are safe and effective for patient A may be subtherapeutic for patient B and toxic for patient C.

toxin is its prolonged half-life—a characteristic that makes management of toxicity very difficult. Accordingly, digitoxin is used much less frequently than digoxin.

### Contrasts with Digoxin

The major differences between digitoxin and digoxin concern pharmacokinetics, especially absorption, route of elimination, and plasma half-life. Pharmacokinetic contrasts between these drugs are summarized in Table 46-2.

*Absorption.* Digitoxin is highly lipid soluble. As a result, the drug undergoes complete absorption following oral administration. In contrast, absorption of digoxin is both incomplete and variable.

*Elimination.* Unlike digoxin, which is eliminated by the kidneys, digitoxin is eliminated by the *liver.* The capacity of the liver to metabolize digitoxin is large—so large, in fact, that inactivation of digitoxin continues at a high rate even in the presence of liver disease. Hence, a decline in liver function rarely necessitates a reduction in dosage.

*Half-Life and Time to Plateau.* The half-life of digitoxin is about 7 days—considerably longer than the 1.6-day half-life of digoxin. Because of its prolonged half-life, digitoxin requires about 4 weeks to reach plateau in the absence of a loading dose. More importantly, the drug's long half-life dictates that, in the event of toxicity, plasma levels will take a long time to decline to ones that are safe. This slow decline makes management of digitoxin overdose very difficult.

*Plasma Drug Levels.* As indicated in Table 46-2, the usual therapeutic range for *total* plasma digitoxin is 10 to 35 ng/ml. Toxicity occurs at levels above 35 ng/ml. These levels are much higher than those for digoxin. This is because digitoxin is highly bound to plasma proteins. As a result, plasma levels of digitoxin must be higher than those of digoxin in order to produce equivalent concentrations of *free* drug—the form that is responsible for therapeutic and toxic effects.

### Therapeutic Use

For most patients with heart failure, digoxin is preferred to digitoxin. This preference is based on the relatively short half-life of digoxin, a property that allows digoxin levels to be reduced more quickly in the event of toxicity. However, although digoxin is usually preferred, when there is a need for plasma drug levels to be very stable, digitoxin—with its prolonged half-life and reliable absorption—might be superior. Similarly, when compliance is a problem, maintenance of therapeutic drug levels can be achieved best with digitoxin: if a dose is missed, the long half-life of digitoxin will prevent plasma drug levels from declining significantly during the extended interval between doses. If kidney function is poor, elimination of digoxin will be delayed, possibly resulting in drug accumulation; hence, in patients with renal impairment, digitoxin may be preferred.

### Preparations, Dosage, and Administration

Digitoxin [Crystodigin] is dispensed in tablets (0.05, 0.1, 0.15, and 0.2 mg) for oral use. As with digoxin, dosing is highly individualized. If plateau drug levels must be achieved quickly, an initial series of digitalizing doses is required. For rapid digitalization in adults, an initial oral dose of 0.8 mg is followed by two or three doses of 0.2 mg at 6- to 8-hour intervals. Maintenance dosages for adults range from 0.05 to 0.3 mg/day.

## KEY POINTS

- Heart failure is characterized by ventricular dysfunction, reduced cardiac output, signs of inadequate tissue perfusion (fatigue, shortness of breath, exercise intolerance) and signs of volume overload (venous distention, peripheral edema, pulmonary edema).
- The primary defect in heart failure is a reduction in ventricular contractility, which results in reduced cardiac output.
- Reduced cardiac output leads to compensatory responses: (1) cardiac dilation, (2) activation of the sympathetic nervous system, (3) activation of the renin-angiotensin system, and (4) retention of water and expansion of blood volume.
- If the compensatory responses are insufficient to maintain adequate production of urine, water will continue to accumulate, eventually causing death (from complete cardiac failure secondary to excessive cardiac dilation and cardiac edema).
- Therapy of heart failure has three major goals: (1) relief of pulmonary and peripheral congestion, (2) improvement of functional capacity and quality of life, and (3) prolongation of life expectancy.
- Heart failure is treated with three major classes of drugs: vasodilators, diuretics, and inotropic agents.
- Drugs that dilate veins decrease venous pressure, and thereby decrease excessive ventricular stretching and cardiac oxygen demand. The decrease in venous pressure also reduces pulmonary and peripheral edema.
- Drugs that dilate arterioles reduce afterload, and thereby allow stroke volume and cardiac output to increase. By increasing cardiac output and dilating arterioles in the kidney, arteriolar dilators increase renal perfusion, and thereby promote loss of fluid.

- ACE inhibitors block formation of angiotensin II and reduce release of aldosterone. As a result, they cause dilation of veins and arterioles, and promote renal excretion of water.

- In patients with heart failure, ACE inhibitors improve functional status and reduce mortality. In the absence of specific contraindications, all patients should receive one of these drugs.

- ACE inhibitors can cause hypotension, hyperkalemia, and cough.

- The combination of isosorbide dinitrate (which dilates veins) and hydralazine (which dilates arterioles) can be used in place of an ACE inhibitor for patients who cannot tolerate ACE inhibitors.

- Diuretics are first-line drugs for all patients with volume overload. By reducing blood volume, these drugs can decrease venous pressure, arterial pressure, pulmonary edema, peripheral edema, and cardiac dilation.

- Thiazide diuretics are ineffective when GFR is low, and hence cannot be used if cardiac output is greatly reduced.

- Loop diuretics are effective even when GFR is low, and hence are preferred to thiazides if heart failure is severe.

- Thiazide diuretics and loop diuretics can cause hypokalemia, and can thereby increase the risk of digoxin-induced dysrhythmias.

- Potassium-sparing diuretics are used to counteract potassium loss caused by thiazide diuretics and loop diuretics.

- Potassium-sparing diuretics can cause hyperkalemia. By doing so, they can increase the risk of hyperkalemia in patients taking ACE inhibitors.

- Inotropic agents (e.g., cardiac glycosides, sympathomimetics) increase the force of myocardial contraction, and thereby increase cardiac output.

- Of the available inotropic agents, the cardiac glycosides (e.g., digoxin) are the only ones that are effective and safe orally, and hence are the only ones currently suitable for long-term use.

- Digoxin increases contractility by inhibiting myocardial $Na^+,K^+$-ATPase, thereby (indirectly) increasing intracellular calcium content, which in turn facilitates the interaction of actin and myosin.

- Potassium competes with digoxin for binding to $Na^+,K^+$-ATPase. Therefore, if potassium levels are low, excessive inhibition of $Na^+,K^+$-ATPase can occur, resulting in toxicity. Conversely, if potassium levels are high, insufficient inhibition can occur, resulting in loss of therapeutic effects. Accordingly, it is imperative that we keep potassium levels in the normal physiologic range—3.5 to 5 mEq/L.

- By increasing cardiac output, digoxin can reverse all of the overt manifestations of heart failure: cardiac output improves, heart rate decreases, heart size declines, constriction of arterioles and veins decreases, water retention reverses, blood volume declines, peripheral and pulmonary edema decrease, weight is lost (because of water loss), and exercise tolerance improves. Unfortunately, although digoxin can reduce symptoms, it does not alter the natural course of heart failure, and does not prolong life.

- Digoxin causes dysrhythmias by altering the electrical properties of the heart (secondary to inhibition of $Na^+,K^+$-ATPase).

- The most common reason for digoxin-related dysrhythmias is diuretic-induced hypokalemia.

- If a severe overdose is responsible for dysrhythmias, digoxin levels can be lowered using Fab antibody fragments [Digibind].

- In addition to dysrhythmias, digoxin can cause GI effects (anorexia, nausea, vomiting) and CNS effects (fatigue, visual disturbances). GI and CNS effects often precede dysrhythmias, and therefore can provide advance warning of serious toxicity.

- Digoxin has a narrow therapeutic range.

- Because digoxin has a narrow therapeutic range, and because tablets from different manufacturers may vary in bioavailability, some authorities recommend that patients not switch between brands of digoxin tablets unless instructed to do so by the physician.

- Digoxin is eliminated by renal excretion.

- Digoxin has a half-life of 1.5 days. Hence, in the absence of a loading dose, about 6 days (four half-lives) are required to achieve plateau.

- Although routine monitoring of digoxin levels is generally unnecessary (once an effective dosage has been established), monitoring can be helpful when dosage is changed, symptoms of heart failure intensify, kidney function declines, signs of toxicity appear, or drugs that affect digoxin levels are added to or deleted from the regimen.

- Maintenance doses of digoxin are based primarily on observation of the patient: doses should be large enough to minimize symptoms but not so large as to cause adverse effects.

- Maintenance doses must be reduced if renal function declines.

- When maximal effects of digoxin are needed quickly, therapy should be initiated with a loading (digitalizing) dose.

## Summary of Major Nursing Implications*

## Digoxin

### Preadministration Assessment

#### Therapeutic Goal

Digoxin is used to treat heart failure and cardiac dysrhythmias. Be sure to confirm which disorder the drug is being used for.

#### Baseline Data

Assess for signs and symptoms of heart failure, including fatigue, weakness, cough, breathing difficulty (orthopnea, dyspnea on exertion, paroxysmal nocturnal dyspnea), jugular distention, and edema.

Determine baseline values for maximal activity without symptoms, activity that regularly causes symptoms, and maximal tolerated activity.

Laboratory tests should include an EKG, serum electrolytes, measurement of ejection fraction, and evaluation of kidney function.

#### Identifying High-Risk Patients

Digoxin is *contraindicated* for patients experiencing *ventricular fibrillation*, *ventricular tachycardia*, or *digoxin toxicity*. Exercise *caution* in the presence of conditions that can predispose the patient to serious adverse responses to digoxin, such as *hypokalemia*, *partial AV block*, *advanced heart failure*, and *renal impairment*.

### Implementation: Administration

#### Routes

Oral, slow IV injection.

#### Administration

*Oral.* Determine heart rate and regularity prior to administration. If heart rate is less than 60 beats per minute or if a change in rhythm is detected, withhold digoxin and notify the physician.

Dosing may be initiated with small (maintenance) doses or with large (digitalizing) doses. If large doses are used initially, be sure that the switch to maintenance doses is accompanied by a written order, to help ensure that the large doses are not continued inadvertently.

Warn patients not to "double up" on doses in attempts to compensate for missed doses.

*Intravenous.* Monitor cardiac status closely for 1 to 2 hours following IV injection.

#### Promoting Compliance

Since digoxin has a narrow therapeutic range, rigid adherence to the prescribed dosage is essential. Inform patients that failure to take digoxin exactly as prescribed

may lead to toxicity or therapeutic failure. Warn patients against switching between brands or formulations of digoxin, since variations in bioavailability may lead to altered responses. If poor compliance is suspected, serum drug levels may help in assessing the extent of noncompliance.

### Implementation: Measures to Enhance Therapeutic Effects

Advise patients to limit salt intake to 2 gm/day, and to avoid excessive fluids. Advise patients who drink alcohol to consume no more than one drink each day. Advise obese patients to adopt a reduced-calorie diet. Help patients establish an appropriate program of regular, mild exercise (e.g., walking, cycling). Precipitating factors for heart failure (e.g., hypertension, valvular heart disease) should be corrected.

### Ongoing Evaluation and Interventions

#### Evaluating Therapeutic Effects

Evaluation is based on symptoms and physical findings. Assess for reductions in orthopnea, dyspnea on exertion, paroxysmal nocturnal dyspnea, neck vein distention, edema, and rales, and for increased capacity for physical activity. In addition, assess for improvements in sleep, sexual function, outlook on life, cognitive function, and ability to participate in social, recreational, and work activities.

Measurement of plasma drug levels can help determine the cause of therapeutic failure. The therapeutic range for digoxin is 0.5 to 2 ng/ml.

#### Minimizing Adverse Effects

*Cardiotoxicity.* Dysrhythmias are the most serious adverse effect of digoxin.

Monitor hospitalized patients for alterations in heart rate or rhythm, and withhold digoxin if significant changes develop.

Inform outpatients about the danger of dysrhythmias. Teach them to monitor their pulses for rate and rhythm, and instruct them to notify the physician if significant changes occur. Provide the patient with an EKG rhythm strip; this can be used by physicians unfamiliar with the patient (e.g., when the patient is traveling) to verify suspected changes in rhythm.

Hypokalemia, usually diuretic-induced, is the most frequent underlying cause of dysrhythmias. Monitor serum potassium concentrations. If hypokalemia develops, potassium levels can be raised with potassium supplements, with a potassium-sparing diuretic, or both. Teach patients to recognize early signs of hypokalemia (e.g., muscle weakness), and instruct them to notify the physician if these develop. Severe vomiting and diarrhea can in-

---

*Patient education information is highlighted in color.

crease potassium loss; exercise caution if these events occur.

To treat digoxin-induced dysrhythmias: (1) withdraw digoxin and diuretics (make sure that a written order for digoxin withdrawal is made); (2) administer potassium (unless potassium levels are above normal or AV block is present); (3) administer an antidysrhythmic drug (phenytoin or lidocaine, but not quinidine) if indicated; (4) manage bradycardia with atropine or electrical pacing; and (5) treat with Fab fragments if toxicity is life threatening.

***Noncardiac Effects.*** *Nausea*, *vomiting*, *diarrhea*, *fatigue*, and *visual disturbances* (blurred or yellow vision) frequently foreshadow more serious toxicity (dysrhythmias) and should be reported immediately. Inform patients about these early indications of toxicity, and instruct them to notify the physician if they develop.

## Minimizing Adverse Interactions

***Diuretics.*** *Thiazide diuretics* and *loop diuretics* increase the risk of dysrhythmias by promoting potassium loss. Monitor potassium levels. If hypokalemia develops, it should be corrected with potassium supplements, a potassium-sparing diuretic, or both.

***Sympathomimetic Agents.*** Sympathomimetic drugs (e.g., dopamine, dobutamine) stimulate the heart, thereby increasing the risk of tachydysrhythmias and ectopic pacemaker activity. When sympathomimetics are combined with digoxin, monitor closely for dysrhythmias.

***Quinidine.*** Quinidine can elevate plasma levels of digoxin. If quinidine is employed concurrently with digoxin, digoxin dosage must be reduced. Do not use quinidine to treat digoxin-induced dysrhythmias.

# CHAPTER 47

# Management of Myocardial Infarction

Myocardial infarction (MI) is defined as necrosis of the myocardium resulting from acute occlusion of a coronary artery. In the United States, MI strikes about 1.5 million people each year and is the most common cause of death. Risk factors include advanced age, a family history of MI, sedentary lifestyle, obesity, high serum cholesterol, hypertension, smoking, and diabetes. The objectives of this chapter are to describe the pathophysiology of MI and to discuss interventions that can help reduce morbidity and mortality.

## Pathophysiology of Myocardial Infarction

Myocardial infarction occurs when blood flow to a region of the myocardium (heart muscle) is stopped because of platelet plugging and thrombus formation in a coronary artery—almost always at a site of a fissured or ruptured atherosclerotic plaque. Myocardial injury is ultimately the result of an imbalance between oxygen demand and oxygen supply.

In response to local ischemia (insufficient oxygen), a dramatic redistribution of ions takes place. Hydrogen ions accumulate in the myocardium, and calcium ions become sequestered in mitochondria. The resultant acidosis and functional calcium deficiency alter the distensibility of cardiac muscle. Sodium ions accumulate in myocardial cells and promote edema. Potassium ions are lost from myocardial cells, thereby setting the stage for dysrhythmias.

Local metabolic changes begin rapidly following coronary artery occlusion. Within seconds, metabolism shifts from aerobic to anaerobic. High energy stores of ATP and creatine phosphate become depleted. As a result, contraction ceases in the affected region.

If blood flow is not restored, cell death occurs within 2 to 6 hours. Clear indices of cell death—myocyte disruption, coagulative necrosis, elevation of serum enzymes—are present by 24 hours. By 4 days, monocyte infiltration and removal of dead myocytes weaken the infarcted area, making it vulnerable to expansion and rupture. Healing begins in 10 to 12 days with deposition of collagen, and is usually complete with dense scar formation in 4 to 6 weeks.

The degree of residual cardiac dysfunction depends on how much of the myocardium was damaged. With infarction of 10% of left ventricular (LV) mass, the ejection fraction is reduced. With 25% LV infarction, dilatation and congestive heart failure occur. With 40% LV infarction, cardiogenic shock and death are likely.

## Diagnosis of Myocardial Infarction

Myocardial infarction is diagnosed by the presence of chest pain, characteristic electrocardiographic (EKG) changes, and elevated serum levels of myocardial cellular components (creatine kinase, troponin). Other symptoms include sweating, weakness, and a sense of impending doom. About 20% of people with MI experience no symptoms.

***Chest Pain.*** Patients undergoing acute MI typically experience severe substernal pressure that they characterize as unbearable crushing or constricting pain. The pain often radiates down the arms and up to the jaw. Acute MI can be differentiated from angina pectoris in that pain caused by MI lasts longer (20 to 30 minutes) and is not relieved by nitroglycerin. Some patients confuse the pain of MI with indigestion.

***Electrocardiographic Changes.*** Myocardial infarction often produces characteristic changes in the EKG (Fig.

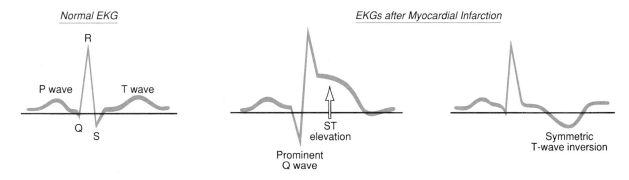

**Figure 47–1. EKG changes associated with myocardial infarction.**

47-1). These changes occur because conduction of electrical impulses through the heart becomes altered in the region of myocardial injury and cell death. Elevation of the ST segment occurs almost immediately in response to acute ischemia. Following a period of ST elevation, a prominent Q wave (>0.04-second duration) develops in the majority of patients. (Q waves are small or absent in the normal EKG.) Over time, the ST segment returns to baseline, after which a symmetrical inverted T wave appears. This T wave inversion may resolve within weeks to months. Q waves may resolve over a period of years.

***Biochemical Markers for MI.*** Components of damaged myocardial cells are released into the blood following an acute MI. Hence elevations in these cellular components can be diagnostic. The component measured most commonly is the *MB isozyme of creatine kinase* (CK-MB). Since CK-MB is found primarily in cardiac muscle rather than in skeletal muscle, an increase in serum CK-MB is highly suggestive of cardiac injury. Following MI, serum levels of CK-MB begin to rise in 4 to 8 hours, peak in 24 hours, and return to baseline in 36 to 72 hours. In some patients, the increase in CB may be too small to allow a definitive diagnosis, even though significant myocardial injury has occurred.

Like CK-MB, *troponin I* and *troponin T* are released by injured myocardial cells. Studies show a good correlation between the degree of troponin elevation and the risk of MI complications. Compared with measurements of CK-MB, measurements of troponin I and troponin T produce fewer false-positive or false-negative results.

# Management of Myocardial Infarction

The acute phase of management refers to the interval between the onset of symptoms and discharge from the hospital (usually in 6 to 10 days). The goal is to bring cardiac oxygen supply back in balance with oxygen demand. This can be accomplished by reperfusion therapy, which restores blood flow to the myocardium, and by reducing my-

ocardial oxygen demand. The first few hours of treatment are the most critical. The major threats to life during acute MI are ventricular dysrhythmias, cardiogenic shock, and congestive heart failure.

## Reperfusion Therapy

The goal of reperfusion therapy is to restore blood flow through the blocked coronary artery. Reperfusion therapy is the most effective way to preserve myocardial function and limit infarct size. Reperfusion can be accomplished with thrombolytic drugs or with angioplasty. Both approaches are equally effective. Authorities disagree about which is superior.

### Thrombolytic Therapy

Thrombolytic drugs dissolve clots. They accomplish this by converting plasminogen into plasmin, a proteolytic enzyme that digests the fibrin meshwork that holds clots together. At this time, five thrombolytic drugs are available: *alteplase* (tissue plasminogen activator, or tPA), *reteplase, streptokinase, urokinase,* and *anistreplase.* The basic pharmacology of these drugs is presented in Chapter 50. Discussion here is limited to their use in MI.

Thrombolytic therapy is now standard treatment for early MI. When thrombolytics are given soon enough, the occluded artery can be opened in 80% of patients. Clinical trials have shown that timely therapy improves ventricular function, limits infarct size, and reduces mortality. Restoration of blood flow reduces or eliminates chest pain, and often reduces ST elevation as well. To be most effective, treatment should be initiated within 4 to 6 hours of the onset of symptoms—and preferably sooner. Current guidelines restrict thrombolytic therapy to patients younger than 75 and to those whose ischemic pain has been present no more than 12 hours. Patients in whom thrombolytic therapy is contraindicated are listed in Table 47-1. Under *typical* conditions, all of the available thrombolytics are equally beneficial. However, under *ideal* conditions (i.e., treatment within 4 to 6 hours of pain onset), alteplase is most effective, especially in patients under the age of 75 (see discussion of the GUSTO trial in Chapter 50). Unfortunately, alteplase is also very

## TABLE 47–1. CONTRAINDICATIONS TO THROMBOLYTIC THERAPY

*Absolute Contraindications*

Active bleeding
Aortic dissection
Acute pericarditis
Cerebral neoplasm
History of intracranial hemorrhage
Cerebral vascular disease (aneurysm, arteriovenous malformation)

*Relative Contraindications*

Either urogenital hemorrhage, cerebral hemorrhage, or ischemic stroke within the prior 6 months
Either major surgery, organ biopsy, puncture of a noncompressible vessel, prolonged cardiopulmonary resuscitation, major trauma, or head trauma within the prior 2 to 4 weeks
Severe uncontrolled hypertension (systolic pressure >200 mm Hg, dias≈tolic pressure >120 mm Hg, or both)
Diabetic proliferative retinopathy
History of bleeding diathesis
History of hepatic dysfunction
History of cancer
Pregnancy

*As recommended by the Fourth American College of Chest Physicians Consensus Conference on Antithrombotic Therapy.

---

expensive. With two drugs—streptokinase and anistreplace—neutralizing antibodies may develop within 5 days of initial use. Since these antibodies prevent anistreplase and streptokinase from acting, a different agent must be used if thrombolytic therapy must be repeated.

The major complication of thrombolytic therapy is bleeding, which occurs in 1% to 5% of patients. Intracranial hemorrhage (ICH) is the greatest concern. ICH has an incidence of 0.5% to 1%, and is most likely in the elderly. Nonetheless, the benefits of thrombolysis generally outweigh the risks. ICH occurs slightly more often with alteplase than with streptokinase.

### Percutaneous Transluminal Coronary Angioplasty (PTCA)

PTCA is a mechanical technique for recanalizing an occluded coronary artery. In this procedure, a catheter containing a deflated balloon is worked into the affected artery, and then the balloon is inflated. This opens the vessel and allows blood to flow. PTCA can be used as primary therapy for acute MI, or as secondary therapy when thrombolysis fails. When PTCA is used as primary therapy, the success rate is equal to that of thrombolysis. Moreover, after 2 days, recurrence of ischemia is much lower with PTCA than with thrombolytic therapy. After 6 to 8 months, the rate of re-occlusion with PTCA is about 30%. At this time, we do not know which procedure—PTCA or thrombolysis—provides the best long-term reduction in morbidity and mortality.

## Adjunctive Drug Therapy

### Morphine

Intravenous morphine controls the pain of MI and improves hemodynamics. By promoting venodilation, the drug reduces cardiac preload. By promoting modest arterial dilation, morphine may cause some reduction in afterload. The combined reductions in preload and afterload lower cardiac oxygen demand, thereby helping preserve the ischemic myocardium.

### Aspirin

Low-dose aspirin (160 to 325 mg/day) suppresses platelet aggregation. In ISIS-2 (Second International Study of Infarct Survival), aspirin produced a substantial reduction in mortality. Moreover, benefits were synergistic with thrombolytic drugs: mortality was 13.2% with thrombolytics alone, and dropped to 8% with the addition of aspirin. Therapy should begin immediately after onset of symptoms, and should continue indefinitely. Prolonged therapy with aspirin reduces the risk of reinfarction, stroke, and death.

### Anticoagulants

*Warfarin.* Warfarin [Coumadin] is an oral anticoagulant with benefits much like those of aspirin. That is, like aspirin, warfarin can reduce the risk of reinfarction, thromboembolism, and early death. However, since aspirin is cheaper, safer (causes less bleeding), and doesn't require monitoring of prothrombin time, aspirin is preferred. Among patients with acute MI, the principal indications for warfarin are (1) a large anterior infarction and (2) a left ventricular thrombus. In both cases, warfarin can decrease the risk of thrombotic embolization. Treatment should begin immediately and continue for 3 to 6 months.

*Heparin.* Heparin is a parenteral anticoagulant agent that was used widely to treat MI before thrombolytics became available. The drug was shown to decrease mortality, reinfarction, stroke, pulmonary embolism, and deep vein thrombosis. However, among patients who receive thrombolytic therapy, indications for heparin are limited. Heparin offers no additional benefits to patients treated with *streptokinase* or *anistreplase*; hence, the drug is not recommended following these antithrombotics. In contrast, heparin does reduce the risk of coronary artery re-occlusion following therapy with *alteplase*, a thrombolytic drug with a short half-life. Accordingly, follow-up therapy with intravenous heparin is strongly recommended. Heparin is also recommended after reperfusion therapy with PTCA, since PTCA causes vascular trauma that can encourage thrombus formation. For all patients, the main complication of heparin therapy is bleeding. The basic pharmacology of heparin is discussed in Chapter 50.

### Nitroglycerin

Nitroglycerin reduces preload, and thereby reduces oxygen demand. The drug may also increase collateral blood flow in the ischemic region of the heart. When given IV during acute MI, nitroglycerin limits infarct size and improves left ventricular function. However, combining nitroglycerin with thrombolytics does not offer any mortality advantage over thrombolytic therapy alone. Nonetheless, since nitroglycerin is easily administered, offers hemodynamic benefits, and helps relieve ischemic chest pain, it continues to be used.

## Beta-Adrenergic Blocking Agents

When given to patients undergoing acute MI, beta blockers (e.g., atenolol, metoprolol) reduce cardiac pain, infarct size, and short-term mortality. Recurrent ischemia and reinfarction are also decreased. Reduction in myocardial wall tension may decrease the risk of myocardial rupture. Continued use increases long-term survival.

Benefits result from several mechanisms. As an MI evolves, traffic along sympathetic nerves to the heart increases greatly, as does the number of beta receptors on the heart. As a result, heart rate and force of contraction rise substantially, thereby increasing cardiac oxygen demand. By preventing beta receptor activation, beta blockers lower heart rate and contractility, and thereby reduce oxygen demand. They reduce oxygen demand further by lowering blood pressure. By prolonging diastolic filling time, beta blockers increase coronary blood flow and oxygen supply. Additional benefits derive from antidysrhythmic actions.

Beta blockers should be used routinely in the absence of specific contraindications. For patients who reach the hospital within 24 hours of symptom onset, administration should be IV. Otherwise, oral therapy is recommended. Treatment should continue for at least 2 to 3 years, and perhaps longer. Beta blockers are especially good for patients with reflex tachycardia, systolic hypertension, atrial fibrillation, and atrioventricular conduction abnormalities. Contraindications include overt heart failure, pronounced bradycardia, hypotension, and advanced heart block. The basic pharmacology of the beta blockers is presented in Chapter 19.

## Angiotensin-Converting Enzyme Inhibitors

In patients with acute MI, angiotensin-converting enzyme (ACE) inhibitors (e.g., captopril, enalapril, lisinopril) decrease mortality, severe heart failure, and recurrent MI. As discussed in Chapter 46, ACE inhibitors are standard therapy for patients with heart failure. Benefits derive from reducing preload and afterload, and from promoting water loss. In MI patients who develop left ventricular dysfunction, ACE inhibitors slow progression of heart failure and decrease mortality. Mortality is also reduced in patients who do not have left ventricular dysfunction. Because of their benefits, ACE inhibitors should be given to all MI patients in the absence of specific contraindications. Treatment should start within 24 hours of symptom onset and should continue 4 to 6 weeks; in patients with signs of left ventricular dysfunction, treatment should continue for at least 3 years, and perhaps indefinitely. The possibility that long-term therapy may also benefit patients who do not have left ventricular dysfunction is

being evaluated in large-scale trials. The major adverse effects of ACE inhibitors are hypotension and cough. Contraindications to ACE inhibitors are hypotension, bilateral renal artery stenosis, renal failure, and a history of ACE inhibitor–induced cough or angioedema. The basic pharmacology of the ACE inhibitors is presented in Chapter 41.

## Lidocaine

Lidocaine, a class I antidysrhythmic agent (see Chapter 48), is a drug of choice for treating ischemic ventricular dysrhythmias. Among patients with acute MI, 4% to 8% experience potentially fatal ventricular fibrillation within the first 24 to 48 hours of symptom onset. In the past, lidocaine was given *prophylactically* to prevent dysrhythmias from occurring. However, prophylactic treatment has been abandoned. Why? Because even though lidocaine does indeed reduce the incidence of serious ventricular dysrhythmias, prophylactic use actually *increases* mortality, probably because of the drug's prodysrhythmic actions (see Chapter 48). Accordingly, lidocaine is now reserved for *treating* serious ventricular dysrhythmias once they occur. Specific indications include ventricular fibrillation, ventricular tachycardia (sustained or nonsustained), and ventricular premature beats (more than 6 per minute). Small clinical studies suggest that prophylaxis with *amiodarone*, an antidysrhythmic drug with complex actions, can prevent dysrhythmias without increasing mortality. Larger trials are needed to confirm this possibility.

### Magnesium

Magnesium has several potential cardioprotective effects. The drug decreases platelet aggregation, increases coronary blood flow, reduces cardiac afterload, and lowers the risk of serious ventricular dysrhythmias. In several small trials, magnesium infusion decreased mortality from MI. However, in ISIS-4, a trial involving over 58,000 patients, adding magnesium to thrombolytic therapy failed to reduce mortality—and actually *increased* the incidence of bradycardia, congestive heart failure, and death from cardiogenic shock. Accordingly, magnesium is not recommended for routine use. In patients who are not candidates for reperfusion therapy, magnesium may offer some benefit.

### Calcium Channel Blockers

Because of their antianginal, vasodilatory, and antihypertensive actions, calcium channel blockers were presumed beneficial for patients with acute MI, and hence have been used widely. However, in large-scale controlled trials, these drugs have failed to decrease mortality either during or after an acute MI. Accordingly, calcium channel blockers are not recommended for treatment.

## Complications of Myocardial Infarction

Myocardial infarction predisposes the heart and vascular system to serious complications. Among the most severe are ventricular dysrhythmias, cardiogenic shock, and congestive heart failure.

***Ventricular Dysrhythmias.*** These develop frequently and are the major cause of death following MI. Sudden death from dysrhythmias occurs in 15% of patients during the first hour. Ultimately, ventricular dysrhythmias cause 60% of infarction-related deaths. Acute management of ventricular fibrillation consists of defibrillation followed by intravenous lidocaine for 24 to 48 hours. Programmed ventricular stimulation with guided antidysrhythmic therapy may be lifesaving for some patients.

Attempts to prevent dysrhythmias by giving antidysrhythmic drugs *prophylactically* have failed to reduce mortality. Worse yet, attempted prophylaxis of ventricular dysrhythmias with two drugs—encainide and flecainide—actually increased mortality. Similarly, when quinidine was employed to prevent supraventricular dysrhythmias, it too increased mortality. Therefore, since prophylaxis with antidysrhythmic drugs does not reduce mortality—and may in fact increase mortality—antidysrhythmic drugs should be withheld until a dysrhythmia actually occurs.

***Cardiogenic Shock.*** Shock results from greatly reduced tissue perfusion secondary to impaired cardiac function. Shock develops in 7% to 15% of patients during the first few days after MI and has a mortality rate of up to 90%. Patients at highest risk are those with large infarcts, a previous infarct, a low ejection fraction (less than 35%), diabetes, and advanced age. Drug therapy includes inotropic agents (e.g., dopamine, dobutamine) to increase cardiac output and vasodilators (nitroglycerin, nitroprusside) to improve tissue perfusion and reduce cardiac work and oxygen demand. Unfortunately, although these drugs can improve hemodynamic status, they do not seem to reduce mortality. Restoration of cardiac perfusion with PTCA or coronary artery bypass grafting (CABG) may be of value.

***Congestive Heart Failure.*** Congestive heart failure (CHF) secondary to acute MI can be treated with a combination of drugs. A diuretic (e.g., furosemide) is given to decrease preload and pulmonary congestion. Inotropic agents (e.g., digoxin) increase cardiac output by enhancing contractility. Vasodilators (e.g., nitroglycerin, nitroprusside) improve hemodynamic status by reducing preload, afterload, or both. ACE inhibitors, which reduce both preload and afterload, can be especially helpful.

***Cardiac Rupture.*** Weakening of the myocardium predisposes the heart wall to rupture. Following rupture, shock and circulatory collapse develop rapidly. Death is often immediate. Fortunately, cardiac rupture is relatively rare (less than 2% incidence). Patients at highest risk are those with a large anterior infarction. Cardiac rupture is most likely within the first days after MI. Early treatment with vasodilators and beta blockers may reduce the risk of wall rupture.

***Arterial Embolism and Deep Venous Thrombosis.*** Arterial embolism occurs when a thrombus in the heart breaks free and becomes lodged in a systemic artery. The incidence of embolism is 2% to 6%. Deep venous thrombosis of the legs develops in 17% to 38% of patients, usually within a few days of the MI. The incidence of embolism and thrombosis can be reduced with heparin (IV or SC). Treatment should begin soon (within 12 to 18 hours) after the onset of MI symptoms and should continue for 10 days.

***Pericarditis.*** About 10% of patients with acute MI develop pericarditis, usually within 2 to 4 days. Inflammation develops in response to transmural necrosis. Symptoms can be reduced with anti-inflammatory doses of aspirin.

## Risk Reduction

As a rule, patients who survive the acute phase of MI can be discharged from the hospital after 6 to 10 days. However, these patients are still at risk of reinfarction (5% to 15% incidence within the first year) and other complications (e.g., dysrhythmias, heart failure). Lifestyle changes and reduction of risk factors can improve outcome.

Reduction of risk factors for MI can increase long-term survival. Patients who smoke must be discouraged from doing so. Patients with high serum cholesterol should be given an appropriate dietary plan and, if necessary, treated with lipid-lowering drugs. Diabetes and hypertension increase the risk of mortality and must be controlled.

Exercise training can be valuable for two reasons: (1) it reduces complications associated with prolonged bed rest and (2) it accelerates return to an optimal level of functioning. Although exercise is safe for most patients, there is concern about cardiac risk and impairment of infarct healing in patients whose infarct is large.

## KEY POINTS

- MI is defined as necrosis of the myocardium secondary to acute occlusion of a coronary artery. The usual cause is platelet plugging and thrombus formation at the site of a ruptured atherosclerotic plaque.
- Myocardial infarction is diagnosed by the presence of chest pain, characteristic EKG changes, and elevated serum levels of myocardial cellular components: CK-MB, troponin I, or troponin T.
- Reperfusion therapy, which restores blood flow through blocked coronary arteries, is the most beneficial treatment for MI.
- Reperfusion can be accomplished with thrombolytic drugs or PTCA. Experts disagree as to which is superior.
- Thrombolytic drugs dissolve clots by converting plasminogen into plasmin, an enzyme that digests the fibrin meshwork that holds clots together.
- Under *typical* conditions, all thrombolytic drugs are equally effective. However, when treatment is initiated within 4 to 6 hours of pain onset, alteplase is most effective (but also very expensive).

- The major complication of thrombolytic therapy is bleeding. Intracranial hemorrhage is the greatest concern.
- PTCA can be used as primary reperfusion therapy, or as secondary therapy when thrombolysis fails.
- Aspirin suppresses platelet aggregation, and thereby decreases mortality, reinfarction, and stroke. Low-dose therapy (160 to 325 mg/day) should be initiated immediately after symptom onset and continued indefinitely.
- Aspirin and warfarin offer similar benefits, but aspirin is cheaper, safer, and easier to use. Accordingly, aspirin is preferred.
- Heparin offers no additional benefits to patients treated with streptokinase or anistreplase, but does reduce the risk of coronary artery re-occlusion following PTCA or treatment with alteplase.

- In patients undergoing acute MI, beta blockers reduce cardiac pain, infarct size, short-term mortality, recurrent ischemia, and reinfarction. Continued use increases long-term survival. All patients should receive a beta blocker in the absence of specific contraindications.
- In patients with acute MI, ACE inhibitors decrease mortality, severe heart failure, and recurrent MI. All patients should receive an ACE inhibitor in the absence of specific contraindications.
- Lidocaine is a drug of choice for treating severe ischemic ventricular dysrhythmias (e.g., ventricular fibrillation). However, neither lidocaine nor any other drug is currently recommended for prophylaxis of ischemic dysrhythmias.

# CHAPTER 48

# Antidysrhythmic Drugs

A dysrhythmia is defined as an abnormality in the rhythm of the heart beat. In their mildest forms, dysrhythmias have only modest effects on cardiac output. However, in their most severe forms, dysrhythmias can so disable the heart that no blood is pumped at all. Because of their ability to compromise cardiac function, dysrhythmias are associated with a high degree of morbidity and mortality.

There are two basic types of dysrhythmias: *tachydysrhythmias* (dysrhythmias in which heart rate is increased) and *bradydysrhythmias* (dysrhythmias in which heart rate is slowed). In this chapter, we will only consider the tachydysrhythmias. This is by far the largest group of dysrhythmias and the group that responds best to drugs. We will not discuss the bradydysrhythmias because they are few in number and are commonly treated with electronic pacing. When drugs are indicated, atropine (see Chapter 15) and isoproterenol (see Chapter 18) are usually the agents of choice.

It is important to appreciate that virtually all of the drugs used to treat dysrhythmias can also cause dysrhythmias. These drugs can create new dysrhythmias and worsen existing ones. Accordingly, antidysrhythmic drugs should be employed only when the benefits of treatment clearly outweigh the risks.

A note on terminology: dysrhythmias are also known as *arrhythmias*. Since the term *arrhythmia* denotes an absence of cardiac rhythm whereas *dysrhythmia* denotes an *abnormal* rhythm, dysrhythmia would seem to be the more appropriate term.

## Electrical Properties of the Heart

Dysrhythmias result from alteration of the electrical impulses that regulate cardiac rhythm—and antidysrhythmic drugs produce rhythm control by correcting or compensating for these alterations. Accordingly, if we want to understand the generation of dysrhythmias as well as the drugs used to treat them, we must first understand the electrical properties of the heart. To establish that understanding, we will review the following: (1) timing and pathways of impulse conduction, (2) cardiac action potentials, and (3) basic elements of the electrocardiogram.

### Impulse Conduction: Pathways and Timing

For the heart to pump effectively, contraction of the atria and ventricles must be coordinated. Coordination is achieved through precise timing and routing of impulse conduction. In the healthy heart, impulses originate in the sinoatrial (SA) node, spread rapidly through the atria, pass slowly through the atrioventricular (AV) node, and then

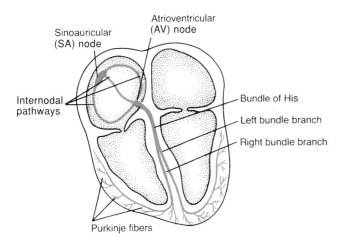

**Figure 48–1. Cardiac conduction pathways.**

spread rapidly through the ventricles via the His-Purkinje system (Fig. 48-1). Details of conduction are discussed below.

**Sinoatrial Node.** Under normal circumstances, the SA node serves as the pacemaker for the heart. Pacemaker activity results from spontaneous phase 4 depolarization (see below). Since sinus node cells usually discharge at a rate higher than that of other cells that display automaticity, the SA node normally dominates all other potential pacemakers.

After the SA node discharges, impulses spread rapidly through the atria along the *internodal pathways.* This rapid conduction allows the atria to contract in unison.

**Atrioventricular Node.** Impulses originating in the atria must travel through the AV node in order to reach the ventricles. In the healthy heart, impulses arriving at the AV node are delayed before going on to produce ventricular excitation. This delay at the AV node provides time for blood to fill the ventricles prior to ventricular contraction.

**His-Purkinje System.** The fibers of the His-Purkinje system consist of specialized conducting tissue. The function of these fibers is to conduct electrical excitation very rapidly to all parts of the ventricles. Stimulation of the His-Purkinje system is caused by impulses leaving the AV node. These impulses are conducted rapidly down the bundle of His, enter the right and left bundle branches, and then distribute to the many fine branches of the Purkinje fibers (see Fig. 48-1). Because impulses travel quickly through this system, all regions of the ventricles are stimulated almost simultaneously, producing synchronized ventricular contraction with resultant forceful ejection of blood.

## Cardiac Action Potentials

Cardiac cells can initiate and conduct action potentials—self-propagating waves of depolarization followed by repolarization. As in neurons, cardiac action potentials are generated by the movement of ions into and out of cells. These ion fluxes take place by way of specific channels in the cell membrane. In the resting cardiac cell, negatively

charged ions cover the inner surface of the cell membrane while positively charged ions cover the external surface. Because of this separation of charge, the cell membrane is said to be *polarized.* Under proper conditions, channels in the cell membrane open, allowing positively charged ions to rush in. This influx eliminates the charge difference across the cell membrane; hence, the cell is said to *depolarize.* Following depolarization, positively charged ions are extruded from the cell, causing the cell to return to its original polarized state.

In the heart, two kinds of action potentials occur: *fast potentials* and *slow potentials.* These potentials differ from each other with respect to the mechanisms by which they are generated, the kinds of cells in which they occur, and the drugs to which they respond.

Profiles of fast and slow potentials are depicted in Figure 48-2. Please note that action potentials in this figure represent the electrical activity of *single cardiac cells.* Such single-cell recordings, which are made using experimental preparations, should not be confused with the electrocardiogram, which is made using surface electrodes, and reflects the electrical activity of the entire *heart.*

### Fast Potentials

Fast potentials occur in fibers of the *His-Purkinje system* and in *atrial* and *ventricular muscle.* These responses serve to conduct electrical impulses rapidly throughout the heart.

As indicated in panel A of Figure 48-2, fast potentials have five distinct phases, labeled 0, 1, 2, 3, and 4. As we discuss each phase, we will focus on its ionic basis and its relationship to the actions of antidysrhythmic drugs.

**Phase 0.** In phase 0, the cell undergoes *rapid depolarization* in response to *influx of sodium ions.* Phase 0 is important in that the speed of phase 0 depolarization determines the velocity of impulse conduction. Drugs that decrease the rate of phase 0 depolarization (by blocking sodium channels) slow impulse conduction though the His-Purkinje system and myocardium.

**Phase 1.** During phase 1, rapid (but partial) repolarization takes place. Phase 1 has no relevance to antidysrhythmic drugs.

**Phase 2.** Phase 2 consists of a prolonged plateau in which the membrane potential remains relatively stable. During this phase, *calcium* enters the cell and promotes contraction of atrial and ventricular muscle. Drugs that reduce calcium entry during phase 2 do *not* influence *cardiac rhythm.* However, since calcium influx is required for contraction, these drugs can reduce myocardial contractility.

**Phase 3.** In phase 3, rapid repolarization takes place. This repolarization is caused by *extrusion of potassium* from the cell. Phase 3 is relevant in that delay of repolarization prolongs the action potential duration, and thereby prolongs the effective refractory period (ERP). (The ERP is the time during which a cell is unable to respond to excitation and initiate a new action potential. Hence, extending the ERP prolongs the minimum inter-

### A  Myocardium and His-Purkinje System

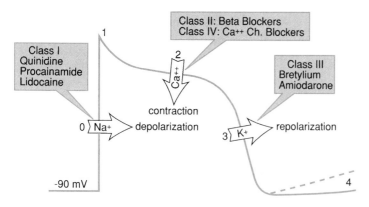

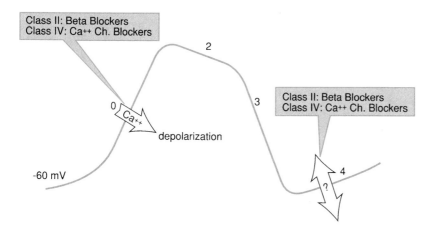

**Figure 48–2. Ion fluxes during cardiac action potentials and effects of antidysrhythmic drugs.** *A*, Fast potential of the His-Purkinje system and atrial and ventricular myo-cardium. Blockade of sodium influx by class I drugs slows conduction in the His-Purkinje system. Blockade of calcium influx by beta blockers and calcium channel blockers decreases contractility. Blockade of potassium efflux by class III drugs delays repolarization and thereby prolongs the effective refractory period. *B*, Slow potential of the sinoatrial (SA) node and atrioventricular (AV) node. Blockade of calcium influx by beta blockers and calcium channel blockers slows AV conduction. These same drugs decrease SA nodal automaticity (phase 4 depolarization); the ionic basis of this effect is not understood.

val between two propagating responses.) Phase 3 repolarization can be delayed by drugs that block potassium channels.

***Phase 4.*** During phase 4, two types of electrical activity are possible: (1) the membrane potential may remain *stable* (solid line in Fig. 48-2A), or (2) the membrane may undergo *spontaneous depolarization* (dotted line). In cells undergoing spontaneous depolarization, the membrane potential gradually rises until a threshold potential is reached. At this point, rapid phase 0 depolarization takes place, setting off a new action potential. Hence, it is phase 4 depolarization that gives cardiac cells *automaticity* (the ability to initiate an action potential through self-excitation). The capacity for self-excitation makes potential pacemakers of all cells that have it.

Under normal conditions, His-Purkinje cells undergo very slow spontaneous depolarization, and myocardial cells do not undergo any. However, under pathologic conditions, significant phase 4 depolarization may occur in all of these cells, and especially in Purkinje fibers. When this happens, a dysrhythmia can result.

### Slow Potentials

Slow potentials occur in cells in the *SA node* and *AV node.* The profile of a slow potential is depicted in Figure

48-2B. Like fast potentials, slow potentials are generated by ion fluxes. However, the specific ions involved are not the same for every phase.

From a physiologic and pharmacologic perspective, slow potentials have three features of special significance: (1) phase 0 depolarization is slow and mediated by calcium influx, (2) these potentials conduct slowly, and (3) spontaneous phase 4 depolarization in the SA node normally determines heart rate.

***Phase 0.*** Phase 0 (depolarization phase) of slow potentials differs significantly from phase 0 of fast potentials. As we can see from Figure 48-2, whereas phase 0 of fast potentials is caused by an *inward rush of sodium*, phase 0 of slow potentials is caused by *slow influx of calcium.* Because calcium influx is slow, the rate of depolarization is slow; and because depolarization is slow, these potentials conduct slowly. This explains why impulse conduction through the AV node is delayed. Phase 0 of the slow potential is of therapeutic significance in that drugs that suppress calcium influx during phase 0 can suppress AV conduction.

***Phases 1, 2, and 3.*** Slow potentials lack a phase 1 (see Fig. 48-2B). Phases 2 and 3 of the slow potential are not significant with respect to the actions of antidysrhythmic drugs.

**Phase 4.** Cells of the SA node and AV node undergo spontaneous phase 4 depolarization. The ionic basis of this phenomenon is complex and incompletely understood.

Under normal conditions, the rate of phase 4 depolarization in cells of the SA node is faster than in all other cells of the heart. As a result, the SA discharges first and determines heart rate. Hence, the SA node is referred to as the cardiac *pacemaker.*

As indicated in Figure 48–2B, two classes of drugs (beta blockers and calcium channel blockers) can suppress phase 4 depolarization. By doing so, these agents can decrease automaticity in the SA node.

### The Electrocardiogram

The electrocardiogram (EKG) provides a graphic representation of cardiac electrical activity. The EKG can be used to identify dysrhythmias and to monitor responses to therapy. (*Note:* In referring to the electrocardiogram, two abbreviations may be used: EKG and ECG. Many people prefer EKG over ECG, since ECG sounds much like EEG [electroencephalogram] when spoken aloud.)

The major components of an EKG are illustrated in Figure 48–3. As we can see, three features are especially prominent: the P wave, the QRS complex, and the T wave. The P wave is caused by *depolarization in the atria.* Hence, the P wave corresponds to atrial contraction. The QRS complex is caused by *depolarization of the ventricles.* Hence, the QRS complex corresponds to ventricular contraction. If conduction through the ventricles is slowed, the QRS complex will widen. The T wave is caused by *repolarization of the ventricles.* Hence, this wave is not associated with overt physical activity of the heart.

In addition to the features just described, the EKG has three other components of interest: the PR interval, the QT interval, and the ST segment. The PR interval is defined as the time between the onset of the P wave and the onset of the QRS complex. Lengthening of this interval indicates a delay in conduction through the AV node.

Several drugs increase the PR interval. The QT interval is defined as the time between the onset of the QRS complex and the completion of the T wave. This interval is prolonged by drugs that delay ventricular repolarization. The ST segment is the portion of the EKG that lies between the end of the QRS complex and the beginning of the T wave. Digoxin depresses the ST segment.

## Generation of Dysrhythmias

Dysrhythmias arise from two fundamental causes: *disturbances of impulse formation* (automaticity) and *disturbances of impulse conduction.* One or both of these disturbances underlie all dysrhythmias. Factors that may lead to altered automaticity or conduction include hypoxia, electrolyte imbalance, cardiac surgery, reduced coronary blood flow, myocardial infarction, and all of the antidysrhythmic drugs.

### Disturbances of Automaticity

Disturbances of automaticity can occur in any area of the heart. Cells normally capable of automaticity (cells of the SA node, AV node, and His-Purkinje system) can produce dysrhythmias if their normal rate of discharge changes. In addition, dysrhythmias may be produced if tissues that do not normally express automaticity (atrial and ventricular muscle) develop spontaneous phase 4 depolarization.

Altered automaticity in the SA node can produce tachycardia or bradycardia. Excessive discharge of sympathetic neurons that innervate the SA node can augment automaticity to such a degree that *sinus tachycardia* results. Excessive vagal (parasympathetic) discharge can suppress automaticity to such a degree that sinus bradycardia results.

Increased automaticity of Purkinje fibers is a common cause of dysrhythmias. The increase can be brought on by injury and by excessive stimulation of Purkinje fibers by the sympathetic nervous system. If Purkinje fibers begin to discharge faster than the SA node, they will escape control by the SA node and potentially serious dysrhythmias may result.

Under special conditions, automaticity may develop in cells of atrial and ventricular muscle. Dysrhythmias will result if these cells begin to fire faster than the SA node.

### Disturbances of Conduction

*Atrioventricular Block.* Impaired conduction through the AV node produces varying degrees of AV block. If impulse conduction is delayed (but not prevented entirely), the block is termed *first degree.* If some impulses pass through the node but others do not, the block is termed *second degree.* If all traffic through the AV node stops, the block is termed *third degree.*

*Reentry (Recirculating Activation).* Reentry, also referred to as recirculating activation, is a generalized mechanism by which dysrhythmias can be produced. Reentry causes dysrhythmias by establishing a localized, self-

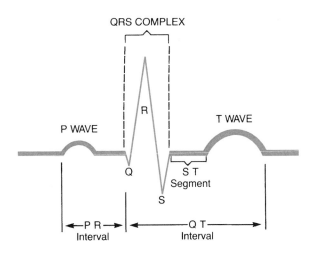

**Figure 48–3. The electrocardiogram.**

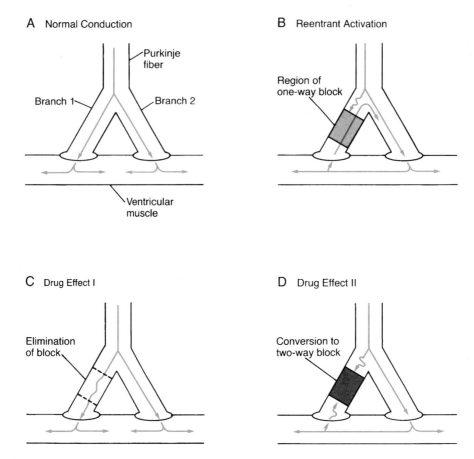

**Figure 48–4. Reentrant activation: mechanism and drug effects.** *A*, In normal conduction, impulses from the branched Purkinje fiber stimulate the strip of ventricular muscle in two places. Within the muscle, waves of excitation spread from both points of excitation, meet between the Purkinje fibers, and cease further travel. *B*, In the presence of one-way block, the strip of muscle is excited at only one location. Impulses spreading from this area meet no impulses coming from the left and can therefore travel far enough to stimulate branch 1 of the Purkinje fiber. This stimulation passes back up the fiber, past the region of one-way block, and then stimulates branch 2, causing reentrant activation. *C*, Elimination of reentry by a drug that improves conduction in the sick branch of the Purkinje fiber. *D*, Elimination of reentry by a drug that further suppresses conduction in the sick branch, thereby converting one-way block into two-way block.

sustaining circuit capable of repetitive cardiac stimulation. Reentry results from a unique form of conduction disturbance. The mechanism of reentrant activation and the effects of drugs on this process are described below.

The mechanism for establishing a reentrant circuit is depicted in Figure 48-4, panels A and B. In the figure, the inverted Y-shaped structure represents a branched Purkinje fiber terminating on a strip of ventricular muscle; the muscle appears as a horizontal bar. Normal impulse conduction is shown in Figure 48-4A. As indicated by the arrows, impulses travel down both branches of the Purkinje fiber to cause excitation of the muscle at two separate locations. Impulses created within the muscle travel in both directions (to the right and to the left) away from their sites of origin. Those impulses that are moving toward each other meet at a point midway between the two branches of the Purkinje fiber. Since the muscle in the wake of both impulses is in a refractory state, neither impulse can proceed further, and both impulses come to a stop.

Figure 48-4B depicts a reentrant circuit. The shaded area in branch 1 of the Purkinje fiber represents a region of one-way conduction block. This region prevents conduction of impulses

downward (toward the muscle) but does not prevent impulses from traveling upward. (Impulses can travel back up the block because impulses in muscle are very strong and, therefore, are able to pass the block, whereas impulses in the Purkinje fiber are weaker and unable to pass.) A region of one-way block is essential for reentrant activation.

How does one-way block lead to reentrant activation? As an impulse travels down the Purkinje fiber, it is stopped in branch 1 but continues unimpeded in branch 2. Upon reaching the tip of branch 2, the impulse stimulates the muscle. As described above, the impulse in the muscle travels to the right and to the left away from its site of origin. However, in this new situation, as the impulse travels toward the impaired branch of the Purkinje fiber, it meets no impulse coming from the other direction; hence, the impulse continues on, resulting in the stimulation of the terminal end of branch 1. This stimulation causes an impulse to travel backward up the Purkinje fiber. Since blockade of conduction is unidirectional, the impulse passes through the region of block and then back down into branch 2, causing reentrant activation of this branch. Under proper conditions, the impulse will continue to cycle indefinitely, resulting in repetitive ectopic beats.

## TABLE 48-1. VAUGHAN WILLIAMS CLASSIFICATION OF ANTIDYSRHYTHMIC DRUGS

**Class I: Sodium Channel Blockers**

**Class IA**
Quinidine [Quinidex, others]
Procainamide [Pronestyl, others]
Disopyramide [Norpace]

**Class IB**
Lidocaine [Xylocaine]
Phenytoin [Dilantin]
Mexiletine [Mexitil]
Tocainide [Tonocard]

**Class IC**
Flecainide [Tambocor]
Propafenone [Rythmol]

**Other Class I**
Moricizine [Ethmozine]

**Class II: Beta Blockers**

Propranolol [Inderal]
Acebutolol [Sectral]
Esmolol [Brevibloc]

**Class III: Potassium Channel Blockers (Drugs That Delay Repolarization)**

Amiodarone [Cordarone]
Bretylium [Bretylol]
Sotalol [Betapace]

**Class IV: Calcium Channel Blockers**

Diltiazem [Cardizem, others]
Verapamil [Isoptin, Calan, Verelan]

**Other Antidysrhythmic Drugs**

Adenosine [Adenocard]
Digoxin [Lanoxin, Lanoxicaps]
Ibutilide [Corvert]

There are two mechanisms by which drugs can abolish a reentrant dysrhythmia. First, drugs can improve conduction in the sick branch of the Purkinje fiber, and can thereby eliminate the one-way block (Fig. 48-4C). Alternatively, drugs can suppress conduction in the sick branch, and thereby convert unidirectional block into two-way block (Fig. 48-4D).

## Classification of Antidysrhythmic Drugs

According to the Vaughan Williams classification scheme, the antidysrhythmic drugs fall into five groups (Table 48-1). As indicated in the table, there are four major classes of antidysrhythmic drugs (classes I, II, III, and IV) and a fifth group that includes adenosine, digoxin, and magnesium. Membership in classes I through IV is determined by effects on ion movements during slow and fast potentials (see Fig. 48-2).

**Class I: Sodium Channel Blockers.** Class I drugs produce blockade of cardiac sodium channels (see Fig. 48-2). By doing so, these drugs slow the rate of impulse conduc-

tion in the atria, ventricles, and His-Purkinje system. Class I constitutes the largest group of antidysrhythmic drugs.

**Class II: Beta Blockers.** Class II consists of beta-adrenergic blocking agents. As suggested by Figure 48-2, these drugs reduce calcium entry (during fast and slow potentials) and they depress phase 4 depolarization (in slow potentials only). Beta blockers have three prominent effects on the heart: (1) in the SA node they reduce automaticity; (2) in the AV node they slow conduction velocity; and (3) in the atria and ventricles they reduce contractility. Cardiac effects of the beta blockers are nearly identical to those of the calcium channel blockers.

**Class III: Potassium Channel Blockers (Drugs That Delay Repolarization).** Class III drugs block potassium channels (Fig. 48-2A), and thereby delay repolarization of fast potentials. By delaying repolarization, these drugs prolong both the action potential duration and the effective refractory period.

**Class IV: Calcium Channel Blockers.** Only two calcium channel blockers—verapamil and diltiazem—are employed as antidysrhythmics. As indicated in Figure 48-2, calcium channel blockade has the same impact on cardiac action potentials as beta blockade. Accordingly, verapamil, diltiazem, and beta blockers have nearly identical effects on cardiac function—namely, reduction of automaticity in the SA node, delay of conduction through the AV node, and reduction of myocardial contractility. Antidysrhythmic effects derive from suppressing AV nodal conduction.

**Other Antidysrhythmic Drugs.** Digoxin, adenosine, and ibutilide do not fit into the four major classes of antidysrhythmic drugs. Digoxin and adenosine decrease conduction through the AV node and reduce automaticity in the SA node. Ibutilide prolongs the action potential duration, but, unlike class III drugs, does not block potassium channels.

## Prodysrhythmic Effects of Antidysrhythmic Drugs

Virtually all of the drugs used to treat dysrhythmias have prodysrhythmic (proarrhythmic) effects. That is, *all of these drugs can worsen existing dysrhythmias and generate new ones.* This ability was documented dramatically in the CAST study (Cardiac Arrhythmia Suppression Trial), in which use of class IC drugs (encainide and flecainide) to prevent dysrhythmias after myocardial infarction actually *doubled the mortality rate.* Because of their prodysrhythmic actions, antidysrhythmic drugs should be used only when dysrhythmias are symptomatically significant, and only when the potential benefits of treatment clearly outweigh the risks. Applying this guideline, it would be inappropriate to give antidysrhythmic drugs to a patient with nonsustained ventricular tachycardia, since this dysrhythmia does not significantly reduce cardiac output.

Conversely, when a patient is facing death from ventricular fibrillation, any therapy that might work must be tried; in this case, the risk of prodysrhythmic effects is clearly outweighed by the potential benefits of stopping the fibrillation. Regardless of the particular circumstances of drug use, all patients must be followed closely.

# Overview of Common Dysrhythmias and Their Treatment

The common dysrhythmias can be divided into two major groups: *supraventricular dysrhythmias* and *ventricular dysrhythmias*. In general, ventricular dysrhythmias are more dangerous than supraventricular dysrhythmias. With either type, intervention is required only if the dysrhythmia interferes with effective ventricular pumping.

Treatment usually proceeds in two phases: (1) *termination* of the dysrhythmia (with electrical countershock, drugs, or both), followed by (2) *long-term suppression* with drugs.

Therapy of the common dysrhythmias is summarized in Table 48–2. As indicated, drugs are not always the preferred treatment. In fact, drugs constitute the first line of treatment for only two of the common dysrhythmias: ventricular premature beats and digoxin-induced ventricular dysrhythmias. For several dysrhythmias, direct current (DC) cardioversion (electrical countershock) is the preferred therapy. In one case (supraventricular tachycardia), maneuvers that increase vagal tone are the treatment of choice.

It is important to appreciate that drug therapy of dysrhythmias is highly empirical (i.e., based largely on the response of the patient and not on scientific principles). In practice, this means that even after a dysrhythmia has been identified, we cannot predict with certainty just which drugs will be effective. Frequently, trials with several drugs are required before control of rhythm is

## TABLE 48-2. TREATMENT OF COMMON DYSRHYTHMIAS

| Type of Dysrhythmia | Acute Treatment | | Long-Term Suppression |
|---|---|---|---|
| | Preferred | Alternatives | |
| *Supraventricular* | | | |
| Supraventricular tachycardia | Vagotonic maneuvers | To terminate:<br>Beta blocker (II)<br>Verapamil (IV)<br>Diltiazem (IV)<br>Digoxin<br>Adenosine | Quinidine (IA)<br>Procainamide (IA)<br>Other drugs |
| Atrial flutter and atrial fibrillation | DC cardioversion | To slow ventricular response:<br>Beta-blocker (II)<br>Verapamil (IV)<br>Diltiazem (IV)<br>Digoxin | Quinidine (IA)*<br>Procainamide (IA)<br>Other drugs |
| *Ventricular* | | | |
| Sustained ventricular tachycardia | DC cardioversion | Lidocaine (IB)<br>Procainamide (IA)<br>Amiodarone (III)<br>Bretylium (III) | Quinidine (IA)<br>Procainamide (IA)<br>Sotalol (III)<br>Other Drugs |
| Ventricular fibrillation | Defibrillation | Lidocaine (IB)[†]<br>Procainamide (IA)[†]<br>Amiodarone (III)<br>Bretylium (III)[†] | Amiodarone (III) |
| Ventricular premature beats | Asymptomatic patients need no treatment | Beta-blocker (II)[‡] | |
| Digoxin-induced ventricular dysrhythmias | Digoxin-immune Fab (digoxin antibody fragments) | Lidocaine (IB)<br>Phenytoin (IB) | |

*Quinidine may *increase* mortality in these patients.
[†]Defibrillation is the treatment of choice. Drugs are given to prevent recurrence.
[‡]Beta blockers are used only if the dysrhythmia is symptomatic.

achieved. In the discussion below, only first-choice drugs are considered.

## Supraventricular Dysrhythmias

Supraventricular dysrhythmias are dysrhythmias that arise in areas of the heart above the ventricles (atria, SA node, AV node). Supraventricular dysrhythmias per se are not especially harmful. This is because dysrhythmic activity within the atria does not significantly reduce cardiac output (except in patients with valvular disorders and heart failure). Supraventricular tachydysrhythmias *can* be dangerous, however, in that atrial impulses are likely to traverse the AV node, resulting in excitation of the ventricles. If the atria drive the ventricles at an excessive rate, diastolic filling will be incomplete and cardiac output will decline. Hence, when treating supraventricular tachydysrhythmias, the objective is frequently one of *blocking impulse conduction through the AV node* and not elimination of the dysrhythmia itself. Of course, if treatment did abolish the dysrhythmia, this outcome would not be undesirable. As indicated in Table 48–2, acute treatment of supraventricular dysrhythmias is accomplished with vagotonic maneuvers, DC cardioversion, and certain drugs: class II agents, class IV agents, adenosine, and digoxin.

***Sustained Supraventricular Tachycardia.*** Supraventricular tachycardia (SVT) is usually caused by an AV nodal reentrant circuit. Heart rate is increased to 150 to 250 beats/min. SVT is best treated by maneuvers that increase vagal tone, such as carotid sinus massage or the Valsalva maneuver. If vagal maneuvers are ineffective, intravenous adenosine or verapamil should be given. If these drugs fail, others may be tried (see Table 48–2). Once the dysrhythmia has been controlled, long-term prophylaxis with quinidine may prevent its recurrence.

***Atrial Flutter.*** Atrial flutter is caused by an ectopic atrial focus discharging at a rate of 250 to 350 times a minute. Ventricular rate is considerably slower than this, however, because the AV node is unable to transmit impulses at such a high rate. Typically, one atrial impulse out of three manages to reach the ventricles. The treatment of choice is DC cardioversion, which almost always converts atrial flutter to normal sinus rhythm. If cardioversion is ineffective, drugs may be employed; the objective is to decrease the number of atrial impulses that pass to the ventricles. The drug of choice for atrial flutter is digoxin. Verapamil, diltiazem, or a beta blocker may also be effective. Long-term therapy with quinidine has been used to prevent the dysrhythmia from recurring. However, recent analysis of older data indicates that quinidine can actually increase mortality in these patients. It is not known whether other drugs used for prophylaxis pose a similar danger.

***Atrial Fibrillation.*** Atrial fibrillation is caused by multiple atrial ectopic foci firing in random order; each focus stimulates only a small area of atrial muscle. This chaotic excitation produces a highly irregular atrial rhythm. Depending upon the extent of impulse transmission through the AV node, ventricular rate may be rapid or nearly normal.

Treatment is the same as for atrial flutter. DC cardioversion is the preferred therapy. If DC cardioversion is ineffective, ventricular rate can be controlled with a beta blocker, calcium channel blocker, or digoxin. Long-term quinidine therapy may prevent the dysrhythmia from recurring, but may also increase the risk of mortality.

Atrial fibrillation carries a high risk of intracardiac thrombus formation. This occurs because some blood can become trapped in the atria, rather than flowing straight through to the ventricles. When normal sinus rhythm is restored, intracardiac thrombi may become dislodged, creating a risk of embolism. To reduce this risk, patients are given an anticoagulant drug (warfarin) for 3 to 4 weeks prior to treating the dysrhythmia, and for another 4 weeks after normal rhythm has been restored.

## Ventricular Dysrhythmias

In contrast to atrial dysrhythmias, which are generally benign, ventricular dysrhythmias can cause significant disruption of cardiac pumping. Accordingly, the usual objective is to abolish the dysrhythmia. Cardioversion is often the treatment of choice. When antidysrhythmic drugs are indicated, agents in class I or class III are usually employed.

***Sustained Ventricular Tachycardia.*** Ventricular tachycardia arises from a single, rapidly firing ventricular ectopic focus, typically located at the border of an old infarction. The focus drives the ventricles at a rate of 150 to 250 beats/min. Since the ventricles cannot pump effectively at these rates, immediate treatment is required. Cardioversion is the treatment of choice. If cardioversion fails to normalize rhythm, lidocaine should be administered. If lidocaine is also ineffective, bretylium, procainamide, or amiodarone should be tried. For long-term management, drugs (e.g., sotalol) or an implantable cardioverter/defibrillator may be employed.

***Ventricular Fibrillation.*** Ventricular fibrillation is a life-threatening emergency that requires immediate treatment. This dysrhythmia results from the asynchronous discharge of multiple ventricular ectopic foci. Because many different foci are firing, and because each focus initiates contraction in its immediate vicinity, localized twitching takes place all over the ventricles, making coordinated ventricular contraction impossible. As a result, the pumping action of the heart stops. In the absence of blood flow, the patient becomes unconscious and cyanotic. If heartbeat is not restored rapidly, death soon follows. Electrical countershock (defibrillation) is applied to eliminate fibrillation and restore cardiac function. If necessary, lidocaine can be used to enhance the effects of defibrillation. Procainamide and bretylium may also be helpful. Amiodarone can be used for long-term suppression. As an alternative, an implantable cardioverter/defibrillator may be employed.

***Ventricular Premature Beats.*** Ventricular premature beats (VPBs) are beats that occur before they should in the cardiac cycle. These beats are caused by ectopic ventricular foci. VPBs may arise from a single ectopic focus or from several foci. In the absence of additional signs of heart disease, VPBs are benign and not usually treated. However, in the presence of acute myocardial infarction, VPBs may predispose the patient to ventricular fibrillation. In this case, therapy is required. A beta blocker is the agent of choice. Because VPBs are associated with a premature QRS complex on the EKG, this dysrhythmia is also known as *premature ventricular complexes.*

**Digoxin-Induced Ventricular Dysrhythmias.** Digoxin toxicity can mimic practically all types of dysrhythmias. Varying degrees of AV block are among the most common. Ventricular flutter and ventricular fibrillation are the most dangerous. Digoxin causes dysrhythmias by increasing automaticity in the atria, ventricles, and His-Purkinje system, and by decreasing conduction through the AV node.

With proper treatment, digoxin-induced dysrhythmias can almost always be controlled. Treatment is discussed at length in Chapter 46. If antidysrhythmic drugs are required, lidocaine and phenytoin are the agents of choice. In patients with digoxin toxicity, DC cardioversion may bring on ventricular fibrillation. Accordingly, this procedure should be used only when absolutely required.

# Class I: Sodium Channel Blockers

Class I antidysrhythmic drugs block cardiac sodium channels. By doing so, these drugs decrease conduction velocity in the atria, ventricles, and His-Purkinje system.

There are three subgroups of class I agents. Drugs in all three groups block sodium channels. In addition, class IA agents delay repolarization, whereas class IB agents accelerate repolarization. Class IC agents have pronounced prodysrhythmic actions.

The class I drugs are similar in action and structure to the local anesthetics. In fact, one of these drugs—lidocaine—has both local anesthetic and antidysrhythmic applications. Because of their relationship to the local anesthetics, class I agents are sometimes referred to as *local anesthetic antidysrhythmic agents.*

Some important properties of the class I drugs (and other antidysrhythmics) are summarized in Table 48–3.

## Class IA Agents

### Quinidine

Quinidine is the oldest and most thoroughly studied of the class IA drugs. Accordingly, quinidine will serve as our prototype for the group. Quinidine is the most frequently used oral antidysrhythmic agent. Like other antidysrhythmic drugs, quinidine has prodysrhythmic actions.

**Chemistry and Source.** Quinidine is similar to quinine in structure and actions. The natural source of both drugs

is the bark of the South American cinchona tree. Accordingly, these agents are referred to as *cinchona alkaloids.* Like quinine, quinidine has antimalarial and antipyretic properties.

**Effects on the Heart.** By blocking sodium channels, quinidine *slows impulse conduction* in the atria, ventricles, and His-Purkinje system. In addition, the drug *delays repolarization* at these sites. Both actions contribute to suppression of dysrhythmias.

Quinidine is strongly *anticholinergic* (atropine-like) and blocks vagal input to the heart. The resultant *increase* in SA nodal automaticity and AV conduction can drive the ventricles at an excessive rate. To prevent excessive ventricular stimulation, patients are usually pretreated with digoxin, verapamil, or a beta blocker, all of which suppress AV conduction.

**Effects on the EKG.** Quinidine has two pronounced effects on the EKG. The drug *widens the QRS complex* (by slowing depolarization of the ventricles) and *prolongs the QT interval* (by delaying ventricular repolarization).

**Therapeutic Uses.** Quinidine is a broad-spectrum drug that is active against *supraventricular* and *ventricular dysrhythmias.* The drug's principal indication is long-term suppression of dysrhythmias, including supraventricular tachycardia, atrial flutter, atrial fibrillation, and sustained ventricular tachycardia. To prevent quinidine from increasing ventricular rate, patients are usually pretreated with an AV nodal blocking agent (digoxin, verapamil, beta blocker). A recent analysis of older studies indicates that quinidine may actually *increase* mortality in patients with *atrial flutter* and *atrial fibrillation.*

**Pharmacokinetics.** Quinidine is rapidly absorbed following oral administration. Peak responses to *quinidine sulfate* develop in 30 to 90 minutes; responses to *quinidine gluconate* develop more slowly, peaking after 3 to 4 hours. Elimination is by hepatic metabolism, and patients with liver dysfunction may require a reduction in dosage. Therapeutic plasma levels are 2 to 5 µg/ml.

**Adverse Effects.** *Diarrhea.* Diarrhea and other GI symptoms develop in about 33% of patients. These reactions can be immediate and intense, and frequently force discontinuation of treatment. Gastric upset can be reduced by administering quinidine with food.

*Cinchonism.* Cinchonism is characterized by tinnitus (ringing in the ears), headache, nausea, vertigo, and disturbed vision. These symptoms can develop with just one quinidine dose.

*Cardiotoxicity.* At high concentrations, quinidine can cause severe cardiotoxicity (sinus arrest, AV block, ventricular tachydysrhythmias, asystole). These reactions occur secondary to increased automaticity of Purkinje fibers and reduced conduction throughout all regions of the heart.

As cardiotoxicity develops, the EKG will change. Important danger signals are *widening of the QRS complex* (by 50% or more) and *excessive prolongation of the QT interval.* The physician should be notified immediately if these changes occur.

*Arterial Embolism.* Embolism is a potential complication of treating *atrial fibrillation.* During atrial fibrillation, thrombi may

## TABLE 48-3. PROPERTIES OF ANTIDYSRHYTHMIC DRUGS

| Drug | Usual Route | Effects on the EKG | Antidysrhythmic Applications |
|---|---|---|---|
| *Class IA* | | | |
| Quinidine | PO | Widens QRS, prolongs QT | Broad spectrum: used for long-term suppression of ventricular and supraventricular dysrhythmias |
| Procainamide | PO | Widens QRS, prolongs QT | Broad spectrum: similar to quinidine, but toxicity makes it less desirable for long-term use |
| Disopyramide | PO | Widens QRS, prolongs QT | Ventricular dysrhythmias |
| *Class IB* | | | |
| Lidocaine | IV | No significant change | Ventricular dysrhythmias |
| Mexiletine | PO | No significant change | Ventricular dysrhythmias |
| Tocainide | PO | No significant change | Life-threatening ventricular dysrhythmias |
| Phenytoin | PO | No significant change | Digoxin-induced ventricular dysrhythmias |
| *Class IC* | | | |
| Flecainide | PO | Widens QRS, prolongs PR | Life-threatening ventricular dysrhythmias |
| Propafenone | PO | Widens QRS, prolongs PR | Life-threatening ventricular dysrhythmias |
| *Other Class I* | | | |
| Moricizine | PO | Widens QRS, prolongs PR | Life-threatening ventricular dysrhythmias |
| *Class II* | | | |
| Propranolol | PO | Prolongs PR, bradycardia | Dysrhythmias caused by excessive sympathetic activity; control of ventricular rate in patients with supraventricular tachydysrhythmias |
| Acebutolol | PO | Prolongs PR, bradycardia | Premature ventricular beats |
| Esmolol | IV | Prolongs PR, bradycardia | Control of ventricular rate in patients with supraventricular tachydysrhythmias |
| *Class III* | | | |
| Amiodarone | PO | Widens QRS, prolongs PR and QT | Life-threatening ventricular dysrhythmias |
| Bretylium | IV | Prolongs QT | Life-threatening ventricular dysrhythmias |
| Sotalol | IV | Prolongs PR and QT, bradycardia | Life-threatening ventricular dysrhythmias |
| *Class IV* | | | |
| Verapamil | PO | Prolongs PR, bradycardia | Control of ventricular rate in patients with supraventricular tachydysrhythmias |
| Diltiazem | IV | Prolongs PR, bradycardia | Same as verapamil |
| *Others* | | | |
| Adenosine | IV | Prolongs PR | Termination of paroxysmal supraventricular tachycardia |
| Digoxin | PO | Prolongs PR, depresses ST | Control of ventricular rate in patients with supraventricular tachydysrhythmias |
| Ibutilide | IV | Prolongs QT | Atrial flutter, atrial fibrillation |

form in the atria. When sinus rhythm is restored, these thrombi may be dislodged and cause embolism. To reduce the risk of embolism, warfarin (an anticoagulant) is given for 3 to 4 weeks prior to quinidine, and is maintained for an additional 4 weeks. Signs of embolism (e.g., sudden chest pain, dyspnea) should be reported immediately.

*Other Adverse Effects.* Quinidine can cause alpha-adrenergic blockade, resulting in vasodilation and subsequent *hypotension*. This reaction is much more serious with intravenous therapy than with oral therapy. Rarely, quinidine has caused *hypersensitivity reactions*, including fever, anaphylactic reactions, and thrombocytopenia.

**Drug Interactions.** *Digoxin.* Quinidine can double digoxin levels. The increase is caused by displacing digoxin from plasma albumin and by decreasing digoxin elimina-

tion. When these drugs are used concurrently, digoxin dosage must be reduced. Also, patients should be monitored closely for digoxin toxicity (dysrhythmias). Because of its interaction with digoxin, quinidine is a last-choice drug for treating digoxin-induced dysrhythmias.

*Other Interactions.* Because of its anticholinergic actions, quinidine can intensify the effects of other atropine-like drugs; one possible result is excessive tachycardia. Phenobarbital, phenytoin, and other drugs that induce hepatic drug metabolism can shorten the half-life of quinidine by as much as 50%. Quinidine can intensify the effects of warfarin by a mechanism that is not known.

**Preparations, Dosage, and Administration.** *Preparations.* Quinidine is available as three salts: *quinidine sulfate*, *quinidine gluconate*, and *quinidine polygalacturonate*. Because these salts have different molecular weights, equal doses of these preparations (on a milligram basis) do not provide equal amounts of quinidine. A 200-mg dose of quinidine sulfate is equivalent to 275 mg of either quinidine gluconate or quinidine polygalacturonate. *Quinidine sulfate* [Quinora, Quinidex Extentabs] is dispensed in standard tablets (200 and 300 mg) and sustained-release tablets (300 mg). *Quinidine gluconate* [Quinalan, Quinaglute Dura-Tabs] is available in sustained-release tablets (324 mg) and as an injection (80 mg/ml). *Quinidine polygalacturonate* [Cardioquin] is available in 275-mg tablets.

*Dosage.* The usual dosage of *quinidine sulfate* is 200 to 400 mg every 4 to 6 hours. The usual dosage of *quinidine gluconate* is 324 to 648 mg every 8 to 12 hours. Dosage is adjusted to produce plasma quinidine levels between 2 and 5 μg/ml.

*Administration.* Quinidine is almost always administered by mouth. If time permits, a small test dose (200 mg PO or IM) should be given prior to the full therapeutic dose in order to assess for hypersensitivity. Intramuscular administration is painful and produces erratic absorption. Intravenous injection carries a great risk of adverse cardiovascular reactions; hence continuous cardiovascular monitoring is required.

## Procainamide

Procainamide [Pronestyl, Procan SR] is similar to quinidine in actions and applications. Like quinidine, procainamide is active against a broad spectrum of dysrhythmias. Unfortunately, serious side effects frequently limit the drug's use.

***Effects on the Heart and EKG.*** Like quinidine, procainamide blocks cardiac sodium channels, thereby decreasing conduction velocity in the atria, ventricles, and His-Purkinje system. Also, the drug delays repolarization. In contrast to quinidine, procainamide is only weakly anticholinergic. Hence, procainamide is not likely to increase ventricular rate. Effects on the EKG are the same as those of quinidine: widening of the QRS complex and prolongation of the QT interval.

***Therapeutic Uses.*** Procainamide is effective against a broad spectrum of atrial and ventricular dysrhythmias. Like quinidine, the drug can be used for long-term suppression. However, since prolonged therapy is often associated with serious adverse effects (see below), procainamide is less desirable than quinidine for long-term use. In contrast to quinidine, procainamide can be used to terminate ventricular tachycardia and ventricular fibrillation.

***Pharmacokinetics.*** Routes are oral, IV, and IM. Peak plasma levels develop 1 hour after oral administration. Procainamide has a short half-life and requires more frequent dosing than quinidine.

Elimination is by hepatic metabolism and renal excretion. The major metabolite—*N*-acetylprocainamide (NAPA)—has antidysrhythmic properties of its own. NAPA is excreted by the kidneys and can accumulate to toxic levels in patients with renal dysfunction.

***Adverse Effects.*** *Systemic Lupus Erythematosus-like Syndrome.* Prolonged treatment with procainamide is associated with severe immunologic reactions. Within a year, about 70% of patients develop antinuclear antibodies (ANA)—antibodies directed against the patient's own nucleic acids. If procainamide is continued, between 20% and 30% of patients with ANA go on to develop symptoms resembling those of systemic lupus erythematosus (SLE). These symptoms include pain and inflammation of the joints, pericarditis, fever, and hepatomegaly. When procainamide is withdrawn, symptoms usually slowly subside. If the patient has a life-threatening dysrhythmia for which no alternative drug is available, procainamide can be continued and the symptoms of SLE can be controlled with a nonsteroidal anti-inflammatory agent (e.g., aspirin) or a glucocorticoid. All patients taking procainamide chronically should be tested for ANA.

If the ANA titer rises, discontinuation of treatment should be considered.

*Blood Dyscrasias.* About 0.5% of patients develop blood dyscrasias, including neutropenia, thrombocytopenia, and agranulocytosis. Fatalities have occurred. These reactions usually develop during the first 12 weeks of treatment. Complete blood counts should be obtained weekly during this time and periodically thereafter. Also, complete blood counts should be obtained promptly at the first sign of infection, bruising, or bleeding. If blood counts indicate bone marrow suppression, procainamide should be withdrawn. Hematologic status usually returns to baseline within 1 month.

*Cardiotoxicity.* Procainamide has cardiotoxic actions like those of quinidine. Danger signs are QRS widening (>50%) and excessive prolongation of the QT interval. If these develop, the drug should be withheld and the physician informed.

*Other Adverse Effects.* Like quinidine, procainamide can cause *GI symptoms* and *hypotension.* However, these are much less prominent than with quinidine. Procainamide is a derivative of procaine (a local anesthetic) and patients with a history of procaine allergy are at high risk of having an *allergic response* to procainamide. As with quinidine, *arterial embolism* may occur during treatment of atrial fibrillation.

***Preparations, Dosage, and Administration.*** *Oral.* Procainamide [Pronestyl, Procan SR] is available in tablets and capsules (250, 375, and 500 mg) and sustained-release tablets (250, 500, 750, and 1000 mg). The usual maintenance dosage is 50 mg/kg/day in divided doses. Standard tablets and capsules are administered every 3 to 4 hours and sustained-release tablets every 6 hours. Dosage is adjusted to maintain plasma drug levels between 4 and 10 μg/ml.

*Parenteral.* Procainamide injection (100 and 500 mg/ml) is available for IM and IV administration. Intramuscular injection is made deep into the gluteal muscle; dosage is 0.5 to 1.0 gm repeated every 4 to 8 hours.

Intravenous infusion may be performed at an initial rate of 20 mg/min (maximal loading dose is 500 to 600 mg). After the loading period, an infusion rate of 2 to 6 mg/min should be employed. Once the dysrhythmia has been controlled, the patient should be switched to oral procainamide. Three hours should elapse between terminating the infusion and the first oral dose.

## Disopyramide

Disopyramide is a class I drug with actions like those of quinidine. However, because of prominent side effects, indications for disopyramide are limited.

***Effects on the Heart and EKG.*** Cardiac effects are similar to those of quinidine. By blocking sodium channels, disopyramide decreases conduction velocity in the atria, ventricles, and His-Purkinje system. In addition, the drug delays repolarization. Anticholinergic actions are greater than those of quinidine. In contrast to quinidine, disopyramide causes a pronounced reduction in contractility. Like quinidine, disopyramide causes widening of the QRS complex and prolongation of the QT interval.

***Adverse Effects.*** Anticholinergic responses are most common. These include dry mouth, blurred vision, constipation, and urinary hesitancy or retention. Urinary retention frequently requires discontinuation of treatment.

Because of its negative inotropic effects, disopyramide can cause severe hypotension (secondary to reduced cardiac output) and can exacerbate congestive heart failure (CHF). The drug should not be administered to patients with CHF or to patients taking beta blockers. Whenever disopyramide is used, pressor drugs should be immediately available.

***Therapeutic Uses.*** Disopyramide is indicated only for ventricular dysrhythmias (VPBs, ventricular tachycardia, ventricular fibrillation). The drug is reserved for patients who cannot tolerate safer medications (e.g., quinidine, procainamide).

***Preparations, Dosage, and Administration.*** Disopyramide [Norpace] is available in standard and extended-release capsules (100 and 150 mg). An initial loading dose (200 to 300 mg) is followed by maintenance doses (100 to 200 mg) every 6 hours.

## Class IB Agents

As a group, class IB agents differ from quinidine and the other class IA agents in two respects: (1) whereas class IA agents *delay* repolarization, class IB agents *accelerate* repolarization, and (2) class IB agents have little or no effect on the EKG.

### Lidocaine

Lidocaine [Xylocaine], an intravenous agent, is used only against ventricular dysrhythmias. In addition to its antidysrhythmic applications, lidocaine is employed as a local anesthetic (see Chapter 26).

***Effects on the Heart and EKG.*** Lidocaine has three significant effects on the heart: (1) like other class I drugs, lidocaine blocks cardiac sodium channels and thereby *slows conduction* in the atria, ventricles, and His-Purkinje system; (2) the drug *reduces automaticity* in the ventricles and His-Purkinje system by a mechanism that is not understood; and (3) lidocaine *accelerates repolarization* (shortens action potential duration and the ERP). In contrast to quinidine and procainamide, lidocaine is devoid of anticholinergic properties. Also, lidocaine has no significant impact on the EKG: a small reduction in the QT interval may occur, but there is no widening of the QRS complex.

***Pharmacokinetics.*** Lidocaine undergoes rapid metabolism by the liver. If the drug were administered orally, most of each dose would be inactivated on its first pass through the liver. For this reason, administration is by intravenous infusion.

Because lidocaine is rapidly degraded, plasma drug levels can be easily controlled: if drug levels climb too high, the infusion can be slowed and the liver will quickly remove excess drug from the circulation. The therapeutic range for lidocaine is 1.5 to 5 µg/ml.

***Antidysrhythmic Use.*** Antidysrhythmic use of lidocaine is limited to short-term therapy of *ventricular* dysrhythmias. Because its levels can be easily controlled, lidocaine is the drug of choice for several ventricular dysrhythmias, including those associated with myocardial infarction, cardiac surgery, and digoxin toxicity. Lidocaine is not active against supraventricular dysrhythmias.

***Adverse Effects.*** Lidocaine is generally well tolerated. However, adverse central nervous system (CNS) effects can occur. High therapeutic doses can cause *drowsiness, confusion,* and *paresthesias.* Toxic doses may produce *convulsions* and *respiratory arrest.* Consequently, whenever lidocaine is used, equipment for resuscitation must be available. Convulsions can be managed with diazepam or phenytoin.

***Preparations, Dosage, and Administration.*** Administration is parenteral only. The usual route is intravenous. Intramuscular injection can be used in emergencies. Blood pressure and the EKG should be monitored for signs of toxicity.

*Intravenous Use.* Lidocaine [Xylocaine] preparations intended for intravenous administration are clearly labeled as such. These contain no preservatives or catecholamines. (Lidocaine used for local anesthesia frequently contains epinephrine.) *Preparations that contain epinephrine or another catecholamine must never be administered intravenously, since doing so can cause severe hypertension and life-threatening dysrhythmias.*

Intravenous therapy is initiated with a loading dose followed by continuous infusion for maintenance. The usual loading dose is 50 to 100 mg (1 mg/kg) administered at a rate of 25 to 50 mg/min. An infusion rate of 1 to 4 mg/min is used for maintenance; the rate is adjusted on the basis of cardiac response. Intravenous lidocaine should be discontinued as soon as possible, usually within 24 hours. Lidocaine for IV administration is dispensed in concentrated and dilute formulations. The concentrated forms must be diluted with 5% dextrose in water.

To avoid toxicity, the dosage should be reduced in patients with impaired hepatic function or impaired hepatic blood flow (e.g., elderly patients; patients with cirrhosis, shock, or CHF).

*Intramuscular Use.* Lidocaine is dispensed in an automatic injection device [Lido-Pen Auto-Injector] for IM administration. A dose of 300 mg is injected into the deltoid muscle. This dose can be repeated in 60 to 90 minutes if necessary. The patient should be switched to IV lidocaine as soon as possible.

### Phenytoin

Phenytoin [Dilantin] is an antiseizure drug that is also used to treat digoxin-induced dysrhythmias. The basic pharmacology of phenytoin is presented in Chapter 23 (Drugs for Epilepsy). Discussion here is limited to antidysrhythmic applications.

***Effects on the Heart and EKG.*** Like lidocaine, phenytoin reduces automaticity (especially in the ventricles), and has little or no effect on the EKG. In contrast to lidocaine (and practically all other antidysrhythmic agents), phenytoin increases AV nodal conduction.

***Pharmacokinetics.*** Phenytoin has two unfortunate kinetic properties. First, metabolism of the drug is subject to wide interpatient variation. Second, doses only slightly greater than therapeutic are likely to cause toxicity. Because of these characteristics, maintenance of therapeutic plasma levels (5 to 20 µg/ml) is difficult.

***Adverse Effects and Interactions.*** The most common adverse reactions are sedation, ataxia, and nystagmus. With too rapid intravenous administration, phenytoin can cause hypotension, dysrhythmias, and cardiac arrest. Gingival hyperplasia is a frequent complication of long-term treatment. Phenytoin is subject to a large number of undesirable drug interactions (see Chapter 23).

***Antidysrhythmic Applications.*** Phenytoin is a second-choice drug after lidocaine for treating digoxin-induced dysrhythmias. The ability of phenytoin to increase AV nodal conduction can help counteract the reduction in AV conduction caused by digoxin intoxication. Phenytoin should not be used to treat atrial fibrillation or atrial flutter, since enhanced AV conduction could increase the number of atrial impulses reaching the ventricles, thereby driving the ventricles at an excessive rate.

***Dosage and Administration.*** Phenytoin [Dilantin] is administered orally and intravenously. For oral therapy, a loading dose (14 mg/kg) is followed by daily maintenance doses (200 to 400 mg).

Intravenous administration is reserved for severe, acute dysrhythmias. Blood pressure and the EKG must be monitored continuously. Phenytoin is not soluble in water and must be diluted in the medium supplied by the manufacturer. This medium is highly alkaline (pH 12) and will cause phlebitis if given by continuous infusion. Consequently, administration is by intermittent injections. Intravenous injections must be performed slowly (50 mg/min or less), since rapid injection can cause cardiovascular collapse. Treatment is begun with a series of loading doses (50 to 100 mg every 5 minutes until the dysrhythmia has been controlled or until toxicity appears). Maintenance dosages range from 200 to 400 mg/day.

### Mexiletine

Mexiletine [Mexitil] is an oral congener of lidocaine used to treat symptomatic ventricular dysrhythmias. Principal indications are VPBs and sustained ventricular tachycardia. Like lidocaine, mexiletine does not alter the EKG. The drug is eliminated by hepatic metabolism; hence, effects may be prolonged in patients with liver disease or reduced hepatic blood flow. The most common adverse effects are gastrointestinal disturbances (nausea, vomiting, diarrhea, constipation) and neurologic disorders (tremor, dizziness, sleep disturbances, psychosis, convulsions). About 40% of patients find these intolerable. The initial dosage is 100 to 200 mg every 8 hours. The maintenance dosage is 100 to 300 mg every 6 to 12 hours. All doses should be taken with food.

### Tocainide

Like mexiletine, tocainide [Tonocard] is an oral analog of lidocaine used to treat ventricular dysrhythmias. Effects on the EKG are minimal. Elimination is by hepatic metabolism and renal excretion. As with mexiletine, the most common side effects are gastrointestinal disturbances (especially nausea) and neurologic disorders (especially tremor). In addition, tocainide can cause serious blood dyscrasias, including a 2% incidence of agranulocytosis; hence, blood counts should be monitored. The drug can also cause pulmonary fibrosis and pneumonitis. Because of its serious adverse effects, tocainide should be reserved for patients with severe ventricular dysrhythmias that have not responded to safer drugs. The initial dosage is 200 to 400 mg every 8 hours. The maintenance dosage is 200 to 600 mg every 8 hours.

### Class IC Agents

Class IC antidysrhythmics block cardiac sodium channels and thereby reduce conduction velocity in the atria, ventricles, and His-Purkinje system. In addition, these drugs delay ventricular repolarization, causing a small increase in the effective refractory period. All class IC agents can exacerbate existing dysrhythmias and create new ones. Currently, only two class IC agents are available: flecainide and propafenone. A third agent—encainide [Enkaid]—was voluntarily withdrawn from the market.

### Flecainide

Flecainide [Tambocor] is employed for oral therapy of severe ventricular dysrhythmias. Like other class IC agents, the drug decreases cardiac conduction and increases the effective refractory period. Prominent effects on the EKG are prolongation of the PR interval and widening of the QRS complex. Excessive QRS widening indicates a need for dosage reduction. Flecainide has prodysrhythmic effects. As a result, the drug can intensify existing dysrhythmias and can provoke new ones. In patients with asymptomatic ventricular tachycardia associated with acute myocardial infarction, flecainide caused a twofold increase in mortality. Flecainide decreases myocardial contractility and can thereby exacerbate or precipitate heart failure. Accordingly, the drug should not be combined with others that can decrease contractile force (e.g., beta blockers, verapamil). Elimination is by hepatic metabolism and renal excretion. Dosage is low initially (100 mg every 12 hours) and then gradually increased to a maximum of 400 mg/day. Because of its potential for serious side ef-

fects, flecainide should be reserved for severe ventricular dysrhythmias that have not responded to safer drugs. Patients should be monitored closely.

### Propafenone

Propafenone [Rythmol] is similar to flecainide in actions and uses. By blocking cardiac sodium channels, the drug decreases conduction velocity in the atria, ventricles, and His-Purkinje system. In addition, it causes a small increase in the ventricular effective refractory period. Prominent effects on the EKG are QRS widening and PR prolongation. Like flecainide, propafenone has prodysrhythmic actions that can exacerbate existing dysrhythmias and create new ones. It is not known if propafenone, like flecainide, increases mortality in patients with asymptomatic ventricular dysrhythmias following myocardial infarction. Propafenone has beta-adrenergic blocking properties and can thereby decrease myocardial contractility and promote bronchospasm. Accordingly, the drug should be used with caution in patients with congestive heart failure, AV block, or asthma. Noncardiac adverse effects are generally mild and include dizziness, altered taste, blurred vision, and gastrointestinal symptoms (abdominal discomfort, anorexia, nausea, vomiting). Because of its prodysrhythmic actions, propafenone should be reserved for patients with life-threatening ventricular dysrhythmias that have not responded to safer drugs. Propafenone is dispensed in tablets (150 and 300 mg) for oral use. The dosage is 150 mg every 8 hours initially, and can be gradually increased to 300 mg every 8 hours.

### Other Class I: Moricizine

Moricizine [Ethmozine] is a class I antidysrhythmic drug approved for oral therapy of life-threatening ventricular dysrhythmias. This agent shares properties with other class I drugs but doesn't quite fit any of the existing subclasses (IA, IB, and IC). Like other class I agents, moricizine blocks cardiac sodium channels and thereby decreases conduction velocity in the atria, ventricles, and His-Purkinje system. Prominent effects on the EKG are QRS widening and PR prolongation. The most common adverse effects are dizziness, nausea, and headache. Like other antidysrhythmic drugs, moricizine is prodysrhythmic. In addition, moricizine can cause bradycardia, heart block, and congestive failure. Interactions with digoxin, diuretics, beta blockers, calcium channel blockers, angiotensin-converting enzyme inhibitors, and warfarin have not been reported. Because of its potential for adverse cardiac effects, moricizine should be reserved for life-threatening ventricular dysrhythmias that have not responded to safer drugs. The dosage is 200 mg every 8 hours initially, and may be gradually increased to a maximum of 300 mg every 8 hours.

## Class II: Beta Blockers

Class II consists of beta-adrenergic blocking agents. At this time only four beta blockers—propranolol, acebutolol, esmolol, and sotalol—are approved for treating dysrhythmias. One of these drugs—sotalol—also blocks potassium channels; this agent is discussed under class III. The basic pharmacology of these drugs is discussed in Chapter 19. Discussion here is limited to treatment of dysrhythmias.

### Propranolol

Propranolol [Inderal] is considered a nonselective beta-adrenergic antagonist, since it blocks both beta₁- and beta$_2$-adrenergic receptors. As discussed in Chapter 19, beta$_1$ blockade affects the heart, and beta$_2$ blockade affects the bronchi.

**Effects on the Heart and EKG.** Blockade of cardiac beta$_1$ receptors attenuates sympathetic stimulation of the heart. The result is (1) decreased automaticity of the SA node, (2) decreased velocity of conduction through the AV node, and (3) decreased myocardial contractility. The reduction in AV conduction velocity translates to a prolonged PR interval on the EKG.

It is worth noting that cardiac beta$_1$ receptors are functionally coupled to calcium channels, and that beta$_1$ blockade causes these channels to close. Hence, the effects of beta blockers on heart rate, AV conduction, and contractility all result from decreased calcium influx. Because beta blockers and calcium channel blockers both decrease calcium entry, the effects of these drugs on the heart are very similar.

**Therapeutic Use.** Propranolol is especially useful for treating dysrhythmias caused by excessive sympathetic stimulation of the heart. Among these are sinus tachycardia, severe recurrent ventricular tachycardia, exercise-induced tachydysrhythmias, and paroxysmal atrial tachycardia provoked by emotion or exercise. In patients with supraventricular tachydysrhythmias, propranolol has two beneficial effects: (1) suppression of excessive discharge of the SA node, and (2) slowing of ventricular rate by decreasing transmission of atrial impulses through the AV node.

**Adverse Effects.** Beta blockers are generally well tolerated. Principal adverse effects concern the heart and bronchi. By blocking cardiac beta$_1$ receptors, propranolol can cause *heart failure*, *AV block*, and *sinus arrest*. *Hypotension* can occur secondary to reduced cardiac output. In patients with asthma, blockade of beta$_2$ receptors in the lung can cause *bronchospasm*. Because of its cardiac and pulmonary effects, propranolol is contraindicated for patients with asthma, sinus bradycardia, high-degree heart block, and heart failure.

**Dosage and Administration.** Propranolol can be administered orally and, in life-threatening emergencies, by IV injection. Dosages with either route show wide individual variation. Oral dosages range from 10 to 80 mg every 6 to 8 hours. The usual intravenous dose is 1 to 3 mg injected at a rate of 1 mg/min.

### Acebutolol

Acebutolol [Sectral] is a cardioselective beta blocker approved for oral therapy of ventricular premature beats (VPBs). Adverse effects are like those of propranolol: bradycardia, congestive heart failure, heart block, and—despite cardioselectivity—bronchospasm. Accordingly, acebutolol is contraindicated for patients with congestive heart failure, severe bradycardia, AV heart block, and asthma. Acebutolol can also cause adverse immunologic reactions; titers of antinuclear antibodies may rise, resulting in myalgia, arthralgia, and arthritis. For suppression of VPBs, the initial dosage is 200 mg twice daily. Usual maintenance dosages range from 600 to 1200 mg/day.

### Esmolol

Esmolol [Brevibloc] is a cardioselective beta blocker with a very short half-life (9 minutes). Administration is by IV infusion.

The drug is employed for immediate control of ventricular rate in patients with atrial flutter and atrial fibrillation. Use is short term only (e.g., in patients with dysrhythmias associated with surgery). The most common adverse reaction is hypotension. However, like other beta blockers, esmolol can also cause bradycardia, heart block, congestive heart failure, and bronchospasm (at higher doses). In addition, pain can occur at the infusion site. Esmolol is available in two concentrations: 10 mg/ml and 250 mg/ml; the concentrated formulation must be diluted prior to use. Treatment is begun with a loading dose of 500 µg/kg infused over 1 minute. The usual maintenance infusion rate is 100 µg/kg/min.

## Class III: Potassium Channel Blockers (Drugs That Delay Repolarization)

Three class III antidysrhythmics are available: bretylium, amiodarone, and sotalol (which is also a beta blocker). All three drugs delay repolarization of fast potentials. Hence all three prolong action potential duration and the effective refractory period and, by doing so, prolong the QT interval. In addition, each drug can affect the heart in other ways. Hence, these agents are not interchangeable.

### Bretylium

Bretylium [Bretylol] is used only for short-term therapy of severe ventricular dysrhythmias. The drug's principal adverse effect is profound hypotension.

**Effects on the Heart and EKG.** Therapeutic effects result from blockade of potassium channels in Purkinje fibers and ventricular muscle (see Fig. 48-2A). By doing so, bretylium delays repolarization and thereby prolongs both the action potential duration and the effective refractory period. Because ventricular repolarization is delayed, the QT interval on the EKG is prolonged.

When first administered, bretylium is taken up by sympathetic neurons, where it causes a transient increase in catecholamine release followed by blockade of further release. In the heart, the initial increase in release can briefly exacerbate dysrhythmias. In blood vessels, the extended blockade of release produces hypotension.

**Adverse Effects.** Profound and persistent hypotension is the most troubling side effect of therapy. This reaction is common, occurring in up to 66% of those treated. Blood pressure may fall in subjects who are supine as well as standing. Hypotension results from blockade of norepinephrine release in sympathetic neurons that promote contraction of vascular smooth muscle. Patients should undergo continuous monitoring of blood pressure. If hypotension develops, blood pressure may be raised with dopamine or norepinephrine.

**Therapeutic Use.** Bretylium is indicated for short-term therapy of ventricular fibrillation and recurrent ventricular tachycardia in patients who have been refractory to more conventional therapy (cardioversion, lidocaine). For these patients, bretylium may be life saving.

*Preparations, Dosage, and Administration.* Bretylium tosylate [Bretylol] is dispensed in solution (50 mg/ml). The drug must be diluted for certain applications. In all cases, the EKG and blood pressure should be monitored continuously.

*Intravenous.* For nonemergency treatment, bretylium is administered by slow IV infusion. Rapid injection is reserved for emergencies. To manage ventricular fibrillation, the following protocol may be employed: (1) rapid IV injection of a 5-mg/kg dose, (2) rapid IV injection of additional doses (10 mg/kg) until the dysrhythmia has been controlled, and (3) slow IV infusion of maintenance doses (5 to 10 mg/kg) every 6 hours. (Maintenance doses are infused slowly because rapid administration results in nausea and vomiting. Initial doses are injected rapidly, despite the risk of nausea and vomiting, because of the need for rapid rhythm control.)

*Intramuscular.* Bretylium is used undiluted for IM injection. The initial dose is 5 to 10 mg/kg. Dosing may be repeated every 6 to 8 hours. Injection sites should be rotated.

## Amiodarone

Amiodarone [Cordarone, Cordarone IV] is a class III antidysrhythmic drug that has complex effects on the heart. Serious side effects are common, and may persist for months after therapy has stopped. In the United States, the drug is approved only for life-threatening ventricular dysrhythmias that have been refractory to other therapy.

Amiodarone is available for oral and IV use. Indications, electrophysiologic effects, time course of action, and adverse effects are different for each use. Accordingly, we will consider oral and IV therapy separately.

*Oral Therapy. Therapeutic Use.* Although amiodarone is very effective, toxicity limits its use. In the United States, oral amiodarone is approved only for long-term therapy of two life-threatening ventricular dysrhythmias: *recurrent ventricular fibrillation* and *recurrent hemodynamically unstable ventricular tachycardia.* Treatment should be reserved for patients who have not responded to safer drugs. Outside the United States, amiodarone is also used to treat atrial dysrhythmias.

*Effects on the Heart and EKG.* Amiodarone has complex effects on the heart. Like bretylium, amiodarone delays repolarization, and thereby prolongs the action potential duration and the ERP. The underlying cause of these effects may be blockade of potassium channels. Additional cardiac effects include reduced automaticity in the SA node, reduced contractility, and reduced conduction velocity in the AV node, ventricles, and His-Purkinje system. These effects occur secondary to blockade of sodium channels, calcium channels, and beta receptors. Prominent effects on the EKG are QRS widening and prolongation of the PR and QT intervals. Amiodarone also acts on coronary and peripheral blood vessels to promote dilation.

*Pharmacokinetics.* Amiodarone is highly lipid soluble and accumulates in many tissues, especially the liver and lungs. Elimination is by hepatic metabolism and excretion in the bile. Amiodarone has an extremely long half-life, ranging from 25 to 110 days. Because of its slow elimination, amiodarone continues to act long after administration has ceased.

*Adverse Effects.* Amiodarone produces many serious adverse effects. Since the drug's half-life is protracted, toxicity can continue for weeks or months after drug withdrawal.

*Pulmonary toxicity* (pneumonitis, alveolitis, pulmonary fibrosis) is the most serious adverse effect. Symptoms (dyspnea, cough, chest pain) resemble those of congestive heart failure and pneumonia. Pulmonary toxicity develops in 2% to 17% of patients and carries a 10% risk of mortality. Patients at highest risk

are those receiving long-term, high-dose therapy. A baseline chest x-ray and pulmonary function test are required. Pulmonary function should be monitored throughout treatment.

Amiodarone may cause a paradoxical *increase in dysrhythmic activity.* In addition, by suppressing the SA and AV nodes, the drug can cause *sinus bradycardia* and *AV heart block.* By reducing contractility, amiodarone can precipitate *heart failure.*

Virtually all patients develop *corneal microdeposits,* which may cause *photophobia* or *blurred vision.* Between 2% and 5% of patients experience *blue-gray discoloration of the skin. Gastrointestinal reactions* (anorexia, nausea, vomiting) are common. Possible *CNS reactions* include ataxia, dizziness, tremor, mood alteration, and hallucinations. *Hepatitis* and *thyroid dysfunction* (hypothyroidism, hyperthyroidism) have occurred; hence, all patients should undergo periodic liver and thyroid tests.

*Drug Interactions.* Amiodarone can increase plasma levels of several drugs, including quinidine, procainamide, phenytoin, digoxin, diltiazem, and warfarin. Dosages of these agents may require reduction.

*Dosage.* Amiodarone for oral use is available in 200-mg tablets. Treatment should be initiated in a hospital setting. The following schedule is used for loading: 800 to 1600 mg daily for 1 to 3 weeks followed by 600 to 800 mg daily for 4 weeks. The daily maintenance dosage is 100 to 400 mg.

*Intravenous Therapy.* Intravenous amiodarone is indicated for initiation of treatment and prophylaxis of *recurrent ventricular fibrillation* and *hemodynamically unstable ventricular tachycardia* in patients refractory to safer drugs. For these indications, the drug may be more effective than IV bretylium.

In contrast to oral amiodarone, which affects multiple aspects of cardiac function, IV amiodarone affects primarily the AV node. Specifically, the drug slows AV conduction and prolongs AV refractoriness. Both effects probably result from antiadrenergic actions. The mechanism underlying antidysrhythmic effects is unknown.

The most common adverse effects are hypotension and bradydysrhythmias. Hypotension develops in 15% to 20% of patients, and may require discontinuation of treatment. Bradycardia or AV block occur in 5% of patients; discontinuation of treatment or insertion of a pacemaker may be needed. Concentrations above 3 mg/ml (in 5% dextrose-in-water) produce a high incidence of phlebitis, and hence should be administered through a central venous catheter. Torsades de pointes in association with QT prolongation occurs rarely.

Dosing is complex. During the first 24 hours, a total dose of 1050 mg is infused. After that, a maintenance infusion (0.5 mg/min) is given around the clock. The usual duration of treatment is 2 to 4 days. However, maintenance infusions may be continued for up to 3 weeks before switching to oral amiodarone.

## Sotalol

*Actions and Uses.* Sotalol [Betapace] is a beta blocker that also delays repolarization. Hence, the drug has combined class II and class III properties. Prodysrhythmic properties are pronounced. Sotalol is approved only for ventricular dysrhythmias, such as sustained ventricular tachycardia, that are considered life threatening. The drug is not approved for hypertension or angina pectoris (the primary indications for other beta-adrenergic blockers).

*Pharmacokinetics.* Sotalol is administered orally and undergoes nearly complete absorption. The drug is excreted unchanged in the urine. Its half-life is 12 hours.

*Adverse Effects.* The major adverse effect is torsades de pointes, a serious dysrhythmia that develops in about 5% of patients. The risk of this dysrhythmia is increased by hypokalemia and by other drugs that prolong the QT interval.

At therapeutic doses, sotalol produces substantial beta blockade. Hence, the drug can cause bradycardia, AV block, congestive heart failure, and bronchospasm. Accordingly, the usual contraindications to beta blockers apply.

***Preparations, Dosage, and Administration.*** Sotalol is dispensed in tablets (80, 160, and 240 mg) for oral use. Treatment should start in a hospital. The initial dosage is 80 mg twice daily. The usual maintenance dosage is 160 to 320 mg/day in two or three divided doses. The dosing interval should be increased in patients with renal impairment.

# Class IV: Calcium Channel Blockers

Only two calcium channel blockers—verapamil [Calan, others] and diltiazem [Cardizem, others]—are able to block calcium channels in the heart. Hence, these are the only calcium channel blockers used to treat dysrhythmias. The basic pharmacology of these drugs is discussed in Chapter 42. Consideration here is limited to their use against dysrhythmias.

***Effects on the Heart and EKG.*** Blockade of cardiac calcium channels has three effects: (1) reduction of SA nodal automaticity, (2) delay of AV nodal conduction, and (3) reduction of myocardial contractility. Note that these effects are identical to those of the beta blockers (which makes sense in that beta blockers promote calcium channel closure in the heart). The principal effect on the EKG is prolongation of the PR interval, reflecting delay of AV conduction.

***Therapeutic Uses.*** Verapamil and diltiazem have two antidysrhythmic uses. First, they can slow ventricular rate in patients with atrial fibrillation or atrial flutter. Second, they can terminate supraventricular tachycardia caused by an AV nodal reentrant circuit. In both cases, benefits derive from suppressing AV nodal conduction. With intravenous administration, effects can be seen in 2 to 3 minutes. Verapamil and diltiazem are not active against ventricular dysrhythmias.

***Adverse Effects.*** Although generally safe, these drugs can cause undesired effects. Blockade of cardiac calcium channels can cause *bradycardia*, *AV block*, and *heart failure*. Blockade of calcium channels in vascular smooth muscle can cause vasodilation, resulting in *hypotension* and *edema*. Blockade of calcium channels in intestinal smooth muscle can produce *constipation*.

***Drug Interactions.*** Both verapamil and diltiazem can elevate levels of *digoxin*, thereby increasing the risk of digoxin toxicity. Also, since digoxin shares with verapamil and diltiazem the ability to decrease AV conduction, combining digoxin with either drug increases the risk of AV block

Since verapamil, diltiazem, and *beta blockers* have nearly identical suppressant effects on the heart, combining verapamil or diltiazem with a beta blocker increases the risk of bradycardia, AV block, and heart failure.

***Preparations, Dosage, and Administration.*** *Verapamil.* Administration may be intravenous or oral. Intravenous therapy is preferred for initial treatment. Oral therapy is used for maintenance.

Verapamil for *intravenous* use is dispensed in solution (5 mg/2 ml). The initial dose is 5 to 10 mg injected slowly (over 2 to 3 minutes). If the dysrhythmia persists, an additional 10 mg may be administered in 30 minutes. An IV infusion (0.375 mg/min) can be used for maintenance. Intravenous verapamil can cause serious adverse cardiovascular effects. Accordingly, blood pressure and the EKG should be monitored, and equipment for resuscitation should be immediately available.

Verapamil for *oral* use is available in standard and sustained-release tablets. The maintenance dosage is 40 to 120 mg 3 or 4 times a day.

*Diltiazem.* For treatment of dysrhythmias, diltiazem is administered IV. Therapy is initiated with an IV bolus (0.25 mg/kg); if the response is inadequate, a second bolus (0.35 mg/kg) may be administered 15 minutes later. If appropriate, initial therapy may be followed with a continuous IV infusion (up to 24 hours' duration) at a rate of 5 to 15 mg/hr.

## Other Antidysrhythmic Drugs

### Digoxin

Although its primary indication is heart failure, digoxin [Lanoxin] is also used to treat supraventricular dysrhythmias. The basic pharmacology of digoxin is discussed in Chapter 46. Consideration here is limited to treatment of dysrhythmias.

***Effects on the Heart.*** Digoxin suppresses dysrhythmias by decreasing conduction through the AV node and by decreasing automaticity in the SA node. The drug decreases AV conduction by (1) a direct depressant effect on the AV node, and (2) acting in the CNS to increase vagal (parasympathetic) impulses to the AV node. Digoxin decreases automaticity of the SA node by increasing vagal traffic to the node and by decreasing sympathetic traffic. It should be noted that, although digoxin decreases automaticity in the SA node, this drug can *increase* automaticity in *Purkinje* fibers. The latter effect contributes to the dysrhythmias that are *caused* by digoxin.

***Effects on the EKG.*** By slowing AV conduction, digoxin prolongs the PR interval. The QT interval may be shortened, reflecting accelerated repolarization of the ventricles. Depression of the ST segment is common. The T wave may be depressed or even inverted. There is little or no change in the QRS complex.

***Adverse Effects and Interactions.*** The major adverse effect is *cardiotoxicity* (dysrhythmias). The risk of dysrhythmias is increased by hypokalemia, which can result from concurrent therapy with diuretics (thiazides and high-ceiling agents). Accordingly, it is essential that potassium levels be kept within the normal range (3.5 to 5 mEq/L). The most common adverse effects are gastrointestinal disturbances (anorexia, nausea, vomiting, abdominal discomfort). CNS responses (fatigue, visual disturbances) are also relatively common.

***Antidysrhythmic Uses.*** Digoxin is used only for supraventricular dysrhythmias. The drug is inactive against ventricular dysrhythmias.

*Atrial Fibrillation and Atrial Flutter.* Digoxin is used to slow ventricular rate in patients with atrial fibrillation and atrial flutter.

Ventricular rate is decreased by reducing the number of atrial impulses that pass through the AV node. It should be noted that although atrial fibrillation and flutter respond to digoxin and other drugs, cardioversion is the treatment of choice.

*Supraventricular Tachycardia.* Digoxin may be employed acutely and chronically to treat supraventricular tachycardia (SVT). Acute therapy is used to abolish the dysrhythmia. Chronic therapy is used to prevent its return. Digoxin suppresses SVT by increasing cardiac vagal tone and by decreasing sympathetic tone.

**Dosage and Administration.** Oral therapy is generally preferred. The initial dosage is 1 to 1.5 mg administered in three or four doses over 24 hours. The maintenance dosage is 0.125 to 0.5 mg/day.

### Adenosine

Adenosine [Adenocard] is an expensive intravenous drug used to terminate paroxysmal supraventricular tachycardia. Adverse effects are minimal because the drug is rapidly cleared from the blood.

**Effects on the Heart and EKG.** Adenosine decreases automaticity in the SA node and greatly slows conduction through the AV node. The most prominent EKG change is prolongation of the PR interval, which occurs because of delayed AV conduction.

**Therapeutic Use.** Adenosine is approved only for termination of paroxysmal supraventricular tachycardia, including Wolff-Parkinson-White syndrome. The drug is not active against atrial fibrillation, atrial flutter, or ventricular dysrhythmias.

**Pharmacokinetics.** Adenosine has an extremely short plasma half-life (several seconds) owing to rapid uptake by cells and deactivation by circulating adenosine deaminase. Because of its rapid clearance from the blood, adenosine must be administered by IV bolus, as close to the heart as possible.

**Adverse Effects.** Adverse effects are short lived, lasting for less than 1 minute. The most common effects are sinus bradycardia, dyspnea (from bronchoconstriction), hypotension and facial flushing (from vasodilation), and chest discomfort (perhaps from stimulation of pain receptors in the heart).

**Drug Interactions.** Methylxanthines (aminophylline, caffeine) block receptors for adenosine. Hence, asthma patients taking aminophylline or theophylline need larger doses of adenosine, and even then adenosine may not work.

**Preparations, Dosage, and Administration.** Adenosine [Adenocard] is dispensed in solution (6 mg/2-ml vial) for bolus IV administration. The injection should be made as close to the heart as possible, and should be followed by a saline flush. The initial dose is 6 mg. If there is no response in 1 or 2 minutes, 12 mg may be tried and repeated once. If a response is going to occur, it should happen as soon as the drug reaches the AV node.

### Ibutilide

Ibutilide [Corvert] is a new intravenous agent for terminating atrial flutter and atrial fibrillation of recent onset (i.e., that has been present no longer than 90 days). Conversion to sinus rhythm occurs during the infusion or within 90 minutes of its termination. Ibutilide is more effective against atrial flutter (48% to 70% success) than atrial fibrillation (22% to 43% success). Like class III agents, ibutilide prolongs the action potential duration; however, the mechanism does not involve blockade of potassium channels. Because it prolongs action potential duration, ibutilide prolongs the QT interval. Up to 8% of patients develop torsades de pointes, frequently in association with QT prolongation. Oral doses are teratogenic and embryocidal in rats. For patients who weigh over 60 kg, the dosage is 1 mg infused over 10 minutes. If the dysrhythmia does not convert within 10 minutes of terminating the infusion, a second 1-mg infusion may be made.

## Principles of Antidysrhythmic Drug Therapy

### Balancing Risks and Benefits

Therapy with antidysrhythmic drugs is based on a simple but important concept: treat only if there is a clear benefit—and then only if the benefit outweighs the risks. As a rule, this means that intervention is needed only when the dysrhythmia interferes with ventricular pumping.

Treatment offers two potential benefits: reduction of symptoms and reduction of mortality. Symptoms that can be reduced include palpitations, angina, dyspnea, and faintness. For most antidysrhythmic drugs, there is little or no evidence of reduced mortality; in fact, mortality may actually increase.

Antidysrhythmic therapy carries considerable risk. Because of their *prodysrhythmic actions*, antidysrhythmic drugs can exacerbate existing dysrhythmias and generate new ones. Examples abound: toxic doses of digoxin can generate a wide variety of dysrhythmias; drugs that prolong the QT interval can cause torsades de pointes; many drugs can cause ventricular ectopic beats; several drugs (quinidine, encainide, flecainide, propafenone) can cause atrial flutter; and two drugs—encainide and flecainide—can produce incessant ventricular tachycardia. Because of their prodysrhythmic actions, antidysrhythmic drugs can *increase mortality*. Other risks associated with these agents include heart failure and third-degree AV block (caused by calcium channel blockers and beta blockers), as well as many noncardiac effects, including severe diarrhea (quinidine), a lupus-like syndrome (procainamide), and pulmonary toxicity (amiodarone).

### Properties of the Dysrhythmia to Be Considered

- *Sustained versus Nonsustained Dysrhythmias.* As a rule, nonsustained dysrhythmias require intervention only when they are symptomatic; in the absence of symptoms, treatment is usually unnecessary. In contrast, sustained dysrhythmias can be dangerous; hence the benefits of treatment generally outweigh the risks.
- *Asymptomatic versus Symptomatic Dysrhythmias.* No study has demonstrated a benefit to treating dysrhythmias that are asymptomatic or minimally symptomatic. In contrast, therapy may be beneficial for dysrhythmias that produce symptoms (palpitations, angina, dyspnea, faintness).
- *Supraventricular versus Ventricular Dysrhythmias.* Supraventricular dysrhythmias are generally benign. The primary harm comes from driving the ventricles too rapidly to allow adequate filling. The goal of treatment is to either (1) terminate the dysrhythmia

or (2) prevent excessive atrial beats from reaching the ventricles (using a beta blocker, calcium channel blocker, or digoxin). In contrast to supraventricular dysrhythmias, ventricular dysrhythmias frequently interfere with pumping. Accordingly, the goal of treatment is to terminate the dysrhythmia and prevent its recurrence.

### Phases of Treatment

Treatment has two phases: acute and long term. The goal of acute treatment is to terminate the dysrhythmia. For many dysrhythmias, termination is accomplished with DC cardioversion (electrical countershock) or vagotonic maneuvers (e.g., carotid sinus massage), rather than with drugs. The goal of long-term therapy is to prevent dysrhythmias from recurring. Quite often, the risks of long-term prophylactic therapy outweigh the benefits.

### Long-Term Treatment: Drug Selection and Evaluation

Selecting a drug for long-term therapy is largely an empiric process. There are many drugs that might be employed, and we usually can't predict which one is going to work. Hence, finding an effective drug is done by trial and error.

Drug selection can be aided with electrophysiologic testing. In this testing, a dysrhythmia is generated artificially by programmed electrical stimulation of the heart. If a candidate drug is able to suppress the electrophysiologically induced dysrhythmia, it may also work against the real thing.

Holter monitoring can be used to evaluate treatment. A Holter monitor is a portable EKG device that is worn by the patient around the clock. If Holter monitoring indicates that dysrhythmias are still occurring with the present drug, a different drug should be tried.

### Minimizing Risks

Several measures can help minimize risk. These include:

* Starting with low doses and increasing them gradually
* Using a Holter monitor during initial therapy to detect danger signs—especially QT prolongation, which can precede torsades de pointes
* Monitoring plasma drug levels. Unfortunately, although drug levels can be good predictors of noncardiac toxicity (e.g., quinidine-induced nausea), they are less helpful for predicting adverse cardiac effects.

## Nonpharmacologic Treatment of Dysrhythmias

### Implantable Cardioverter/Defibrillators

Implantable cardioverter/defibrillators (ICDs) are surgically implanted devices that monitor and analyze cardiac rhythm, and, by delivering electrical shocks to the heart, terminate any dysrhythmias that develop. Termination is accomplished with either a series of pacing stimuli, which are usually imperceptible, or with a defibrillating shock, which can be painful. It is important to note that ICDs do not prevent dysrhythmias; rather, they neutralize the ones that occur. ICDs are indicated for patients with recurrent ventricular fibrillation or sustained ventricular tachycardia. For these patients, ICDs significantly reduce the risk of sudden death. The major complication associated with ICDs is mortality during surgical implantation. The mortality rate had been as high as 8%, but is declining due to use of newer techniques. ICDs cost about $20,000 to $25,000. The cost for implantation, including hospitalization, adds another $30,000 to 50,000.

### Radiofrequency Catheter Ablation

Radiofrequency (RF) catheter ablation is a technique in which cardiac tissue responsible for causing a dysrhythmia is identified and destroyed; the result is often permanent cure. Prior to RF ablation, the patient undergoes electrophysiologic cardiac testing to identify the small region of the heart that is generating the dysrhythmia. Next, an RF catheter is placed at the site. Activation of the catheter generates RF energy, which heats (and thereby destroys) all tissue within 5 to 8 mm of the catheter tip. Destruction of the offending tissue eliminates the dysrhythmia. Success rates depend on the dysrhythmia being treated. In patients with atrial tachycardia, AV nodal reentrant tachycardia, or dysrhythmias associated with Wolf-Parkinson-White syndrome, the rate of permanent cure is between 90% and 100%. In patients with atrial flutter, initial responses are generally good, but recurrence is common. Complications develop in less than 5% of procedures. The most common complications are AV block and myocardial perforation. Complications that require intervention or that result in long-term injury occur in only 1% of patients. When RF catheter ablation is done on an outpatient basis, the cost is about $10,000.

## KEY POINTS

* Dysrhythmias result from alteration of the electrical impulses that regulate cardiac rhythm. Antidysrhythmic drugs control rhythm by correcting or compensating for these alterations.
* In the healthy heart, the SA node is the pacemaker.
* Impulses originating in the SA node must travel through the AV node to reach the ventricles. Impulses arriving at the AV node are delayed before going on to excite the ventricles.
* The His-Purkinje system conducts impulses rapidly throughout the ventricles, thereby causing all parts of the ventricles to contract in near-synchrony.
* The heart employs two kinds of action potentials: fast potentials and slow potentials.
* Fast potentials occur in the His-Purkinje system, atrial muscle, and ventricular muscle.

- Slow potentials occur in the SA node and AV node.
- Phase 0 of fast potentials (depolarization) is generated by rapid influx of sodium. Because depolarization is fast, these potentials conduct rapidly.
- During phase 2 of fast potentials, calcium enters myocardial cells, thereby promoting contraction.
- Phase 3 of fast potentials (repolarization) is generated by rapid extrusion of potassium.
- Phase 0 of slow potentials (depolarization) is caused by slow influx of calcium. Because depolarization is slow, these potentials conduct slowly.
- Spontaneous phase 4 depolarization (of fast or slow potentials) confers automaticity upon cells. Spontaneous phase 4 depolarization of cells in the SA node normally determines heart rate.
- The P wave (of an EKG) is caused by depolarization of the atria.
- The QRS complex is caused by depolarization of the ventricles. Widening of the QRS complex indicates slowed conduction through the ventricles.
- The T wave is caused by repolarization of the ventricles.
- The PR interval represents the time between onset of the P wave and onset of the QRS complex. PR prolongation indicates delayed AV conduction.
- The QT interval represents the time between onset of the QRS complex and completion of the T wave. QT prolongation indicates delayed ventricular repolarization.
- Dysrhythmias arise from disturbances of impulse formation (automaticity) or impulse conduction.
- Reentrant dysrhythmias result from a localized, self-sustaining circuit capable of repetitive cardiac stimulation.
- Dysrhythmias can be divided into two major groups: supraventricular dysrhythmias and ventricular dysrhythmias. In general, ventricular dysrhythmias disrupt cardiac pumping more than supraventricular dysrhythmias do.
- Treatment of supraventricular tachydysrhythmias is often directed at blocking impulse conduction through the AV node, rather than eliminating the dysrhythmia.
- Treatment of ventricular dysrhythmias is usually directed at eliminating the dysrhythmia.
- All antidysrhythmic drugs are also prodysrhythmic (proarrhythmic). That is, they all can worsen existing dysrhythmias and generate new ones.
- Class I antidysrhythmic drugs block cardiac sodium channels, and thereby slow impulse conduction through the atria, ventricles, and His-Purkinje system.
- Slowing ventricular conduction widens the QRS complex.
- Quinidine (a class IA drug) blocks sodium channels and delays ventricular repolarization. Delaying ventricular repolarization prolongs the QT interval.
- Quinidine causes diarrhea and other GI symptoms in 33% of patients. These effects frequently force drug withdrawal.

- Quinidine can cause dysrhythmias. Widening of the QRS complex (by 50% or more) and excessive prolongation of the QT interval are warning signs.
- Quinidine elevates digoxin levels. If the drugs are used together, digoxin dosage must be reduced.
- Class IB agents differ from class IA agents in two ways: they accelerate repolarization and have little or no effect on the EKG.
- Lidocaine (a class IB agent) is used only for ventricular dysrhythmias. The drug is not active against supraventricular dysrhythmias.
- Lidocaine undergoes rapid inactivation by the liver. As a result, the drug must be administered by continuous IV infusion.
- Propranolol and other class II drugs block cardiac beta$_1$ receptors.
- By blocking cardiac beta$_1$ receptors, propranolol attenuates sympathetic stimulation of the heart, and thereby decreases SA nodal automaticity, AV conduction velocity, and myocardial contractility.
- By decreasing AV conduction velocity, propranolol prolongs the PR interval.
- The effects of propranolol on the heart result (ultimately) from suppressing calcium entry. Hence the effects of propranolol and the effects of calcium channel blockers are nearly identical.
- Propranolol is especially useful for treating dysrhythmias caused by excessive sympathetic stimulation of the heart.
- In patients with supraventricular tachydysrhythmias, propranolol helps by (1) slowing discharge of the SA node and (2) decreasing conduction through the AV node, which prevents the atria from driving the ventricles at an excessive rate.
- Class III antidysrhythmics block potassium channels, and thereby delay repolarization of fast potentials. As a result, they prolong the action potential duration and the effective refractory period. By delaying ventricular repolarization, they prolong the QT interval.
- Bretylium (a class III agent) is used only for short-term therapy of severe ventricular dysrhythmias that have been refractory to safer treatments.
- Bretylium blocks release of norepinephrine from sympathetic nerves, and thereby causes profound and persistent hypotension in up to 66% of patients.
- Verapamil and diltiazem (class IV antidysrhythmics) block cardiac calcium channels, and thereby reduce automaticity of the SA node, conduction through the AV node, and myocardial contractility. These effects are identical to those of the beta blockers.
- By suppressing AV conduction, verapamil and diltiazem prolong the PR interval.
- Verapamil and diltiazem are used to slow ventricular rate in patients with atrial fibrillation or atrial flutter and to terminate supraventricular tachycardia caused by an AV nodal reentrant circuit. In both cases, benefits derive from suppressing AV nodal conduction.

# Summary of Major Nursing Implications*

Summaries are limited to the major antidysrhythmic drugs. Summaries for beta blockers, calcium channel blockers, phenytoin, and digoxin appear in other chapters.

## Quinidine

### Preadministration Assessment

#### Therapeutic Goal
The usual goal is long-term suppression of atrial and ventricular dysrhythmias.

#### Baseline Data
Obtain a baseline EKG and laboratory evaluation of liver function. Determine blood pressure.

#### Identifying High-Risk Patients
Quinidine is *contraindicated* for patients with a history of *hypersensitivity to quinidine or other cinchona alkaloids* and for patients with *complete heart block, digoxin intoxication*, or *conduction disturbances associated with marked QRS widening and QT prolongation*. Exercise *caution* in patients with *partial AV block, heart failure, hypotensive states*, and *hepatic dysfunction*.

### Implementation: Administration

#### Routes
*Usual Route.* Oral.
*Rare Routes.* IM and IV.

#### Administration
Before giving full therapeutic doses, assess for hypersensitivity by giving a small test dose (200 mg PO or IM). Advise patients to take quinidine with meals. Warn patients not to crush or chew sustained-release formulations.

Dosing must account for the particular quinidine salt being used: 200 mg of quinidine sulfate is equivalent to 275 mg of quinidine gluconate or quinidine polygalacturonate.

### Ongoing Evaluation and Interventions

#### Evaluating Therapeutic Effects
Monitor for beneficial changes in the EKG. Plasma drug levels should be kept between 2 and 5 μg/ml.

#### Minimizing Adverse Effects
*Diarrhea.* Diarrhea and other gastrointestinal disturbances occur in one third of patients and frequently force

drug withdrawal. These effects can be reduced by administering quinidine with meals.

*Cinchonism.* Inform patients about symptoms of cinchonism (tinnitus, headache, nausea, vertigo, disturbed vision), and instruct them to notify the physician if these develop.

*Cardiotoxicity.* Monitor the EKG for signs of cardiotoxicity, especially widening of QRS complex (by 50% or more) and excessive prolongation of the QT interval. Monitor pulses for significant changes in rate or regularity. If cardiotoxicity develops, withhold quinidine and notify the physician.

*Arterial Embolism.* Embolism may occur during therapy of atrial fibrillation. The risk can be reduced with warfarin (an anticoagulant). Observe for signs of thromboembolism (e.g., sudden chest pain, dyspnea) and report these immediately.

### Minimizing Adverse Interactions
*Digoxin.* Quinidine can double digoxin levels. When these drugs are combined, digoxin dosage should be reduced. Monitor patients for digoxin toxicity (dysrhythmias).

## Procainamide

### Preadministration Assessment

#### Therapeutic Goal
Procainamide is indicated for acute and long-term management of ventricular and supraventricular dysrhythmias. Because of toxicity with long-term use, quinidine is preferred to procainamide for chronic suppression.

#### Baseline Data
Obtain a baseline EKG, complete blood counts, and laboratory evaluations of liver and kidney function. Determine blood pressure.

#### Identifying High-Risk Patients
Procainamide is *contraindicated* for patients with *systemic lupus erythematosus, complete AV block*, and *second- or third-degree AV block in the absence of an electronic pacemaker*. Exercise *caution* in patients with *hepatic or renal dysfunction or a history of procaine allergy*.

### Implementation: Administration

#### Routes
Oral, IM, IV.

## Administration

Instruct patients to administer procainamide at evenly spaced intervals around the clock. Warn patients not to crush or chew sustained-release preparations.

When switching from IV procainamide to oral procainamide, allow 3 hours to elapse between stopping the infusion and giving the first oral dose.

Give IM injections deep into the gluteal muscle.

## Ongoing Evaluation and Interventions

### Evaluating Therapeutic Effects

Monitor the EKG for beneficial changes. Plasma drug levels should be kept between 3 and 10 μg/ml.

### Minimizing Adverse Effects

*Systemic Lupus Erythematosus-like Syndrome.* Prolonged therapy can produce a syndrome resembling SLE. Inform patients about manifestations of SLE (joint pain and inflammation; hepatomegaly; unexplained fever; soreness of the mouth, throat, or gums), and instruct them to notify the physician if these develop. If SLE is diagnosed, procainamide should be discontinued. If discontinuation is impossible, signs and symptoms can be controlled with a nonsteroidal anti-inflammatory drug (e.g., aspirin) or with a glucocorticoid. The ANA titer should be measured periodically; if it rises, withdrawal of procainamide should be considered.

*Blood Dyscrasias.* Procainamide can cause agranulocytosis, thrombocytopenia, and neutropenia. Death has occurred. Obtain complete blood counts weekly during the first 3 months of treatment and periodically thereafter. Instruct patients to inform the physician at the first sign of infection (fever, chills, sore throat), bruising, or bleeding. If subsequent blood counts indicate hematologic disturbance, discontinue procainamide immediately.

*Cardiotoxicity.* Procainamide can cause dysrhythmias. Monitor pulses for changes in rate or regularity. Monitor the EKG for excessive QRS widening (greater than 50%) and for PR prolongation. If these occur, withhold procainamide and notify the physician.

*Arterial Embolism.* Embolism may occur during therapy of atrial fibrillation. The risk can be reduced with warfarin. Observe for signs of thromboembolism (e.g., sudden chest pain, dyspnea) and report these immediately.

## Lidocaine

## Preadministration: Assessment

### Therapeutic Goal

Management of ventricular dysrhythmias.

### Baseline Data

Obtain a baseline EKG and determine blood pressure.

### Identifying High-Risk Patients

Lidocaine is *contraindicated* for patients with *Stokes-Adams syndrome, Wolff-Parkinson-White syndrome,* and *severe degrees of SA, AV, or intraventricular block in the absence of electronic pacing.* Exercise *caution* in patients with *hepatic dysfunction* or *impaired hepatic blood flow.*

## Implementation: Administration

### Routes

*Usual.* IV.

*Emergencies.* IM.

### Administration

*Intravenous.* Make certain the lidocaine preparation is labeled for IV use (i.e., is devoid of preservatives and catecholamines). Dilute concentrated preparations with 5% dextrose in water.

The initial dose is 50 to 100 mg (1 mg/kg) infused at a rate of 25 to 50 mg/min. For maintenance, monitor the EKG and adjust the infusion rate on the basis of cardiac response. The usual rate is 1 to 4 mg/min.

*Intramuscular.* Reserve for emergencies. The usual dose is 300 mg injected into the deltoid muscle. Switch to IV lidocaine as soon as possible.

## Ongoing Evaluation and Interventions

### Evaluating Therapeutic Effects

Continuous EKG monitoring is required. Plasma drug levels should be kept between 1.5 and 5 μg/ml.

### Minimizing Adverse Effects

Excessive doses can cause convulsions and respiratory arrest. Equipment for resuscitation should be available. Convulsions can be managed with diazepam or phenytoin.

## Drugs Summarized in Other Chapters

# CHAPTER 49

# Prophylaxis of Coronary Artery Disease: Drugs that Lower LDL-Cholesterol Levels

Our topic in this chapter is cholesterol and its impact on atherosclerosis, especially of the coronary arteries. Coronary artery disease (CAD) begins with deposition of fatty plaque on the arterial wall. As atherosclerotic plaque grows, it impedes coronary blood flow, causing anginal pain. Worse yet, coronary atherosclerosis encourages formation of thrombi, which can block flow entirely, thereby causing myocardial infarction (heart attack).

The risk of developing CAD is directly related to increased levels of blood cholesterol in the form of low-density lipoproteins (LDLs). By reducing levels of LDL-cholesterol, we can slow progression of atherosclerosis, reduce the risk of serious CAD, and prolong life. The primary method for lowering LDL-cholesterol is modification of diet. Drugs are employed only when diet modification is insufficient.

In approaching the topic of cholesterol and its impact on CAD, we will begin by discussing (1) cholesterol itself, (2) plasma lipoproteins (structures that transport cholesterol in blood), and (3) the process of atherogenesis. Next we will consider guidelines for cholesterol screening and management of high cholesterol. After that we will discuss the pharmacology of the cholesterol-lowering drugs.

## Cholesterol

Cholesterol has multiple physiologic roles. Of greatest importance, cholesterol is a component of all cell membranes, as well as the membranes of intracellular organelles. In addition to these structural roles, cholesterol is required for synthesis of certain hormones (estrogen, progesterone, testosterone, adrenal corticosteroids) and for synthesis of bile salts, which are needed for digestion and absorption of fats. Also, cholesterol is deposited in stratum corneum of the skin, where it reduces evaporation of water and blocks transdermal absorption of water-soluble compounds.

Some of our cholesterol comes from dietary sources (exogenous cholesterol) and some is manufactured by cells (endogenous cholesterol), primarily in the liver. More cholesterol comes from endogenous production than from the diet. A critical step in hepatic synthesis of cholesterol is catalyzed by an enzyme named hydroxymethylglutaryl coenzyme A (HMG CoA) reductase. Drugs that inhibit this enzyme constitute our most widely used class of cholesterol-lowering agents. During the night, endogenous synthesis of cholesterol increases. Hence HMG CoA reductase inhibitors are more effective when given in the evening than in the morning.

An increase in dietary cholesterol produces only a small increase in cholesterol in the blood, primarily because increased ingestion of cholesterol inhibits endogenous cholesterol synthesis. Interestingly, an increase in dietary saturated fats produces a substantial (15% to 25%) increase in circulating cholesterol. The reason is that saturated fats are a substrate for cholesterol production by the liver. Accordingly, when we want to reduce cholesterol levels, it is more important to reduce intake of saturated fats than to reduce intake of cholesterol itself, although cholesterol intake should definitely be lowered.

# Plasma Lipoproteins

## Structure and Function of Lipoproteins

*Function.* Lipoproteins serve as carriers for transporting lipids—cholesterol and triglycerides—in blood. Like all other nutrients and metabolites, lipids use the bloodstream to move throughout the body. However, since cholesterol and triglycerides are not water soluble, these substances cannot dissolve directly in plasma. Lipoproteins represent a means of solubilizing these lipids, thereby allowing their transport.

*Basic Structure.* The basic structure of lipoproteins is depicted in Figure 49–1. As indicated, lipoproteins are tiny, spherical structures that consist of a *hydrophobic core*, composed of cholesterol and triglycerides, surrounded by a *hydrophilic shell*, composed primarily of phospholipids arranged in a monolayer. Since the hydrophilic (water-soluble) shell completely covers the lipid core, the entire structure is soluble in plasma.

*Apolipoproteins.* All lipoproteins have one or more *apolipoprotein* molecules embedded in their shells (Fig 49–1). Apolipoproteins, which constitute the protein component of lipoproteins, have three functions:

- They serve as recognition sites for cell-surface receptors, and thereby allow cells to bind and ingest lipoproteins.
- They activate enzymes that metabolize lipoproteins.
- They increase the structural stability of lipoproteins.

The apolipoproteins of greatest clinical interest are labeled A-I, A-II, and B-100. All lipoproteins that deliver cholesterol and triglycerides to nonhepatic tissues contain *apolipoprotein B-100.* Conversely, all lipoproteins that transport lipids from nonhepatic tissues back to the liver (i.e., that remove lipids from tissues) contain *apolipoprotein A-I.*

## Classes of Lipoproteins

There are six major classes of plasma lipoproteins. Distinctions among classes are based on size, density, apolipoprotein content, transport function, and primary core lipids (cholesterol or triglycerides). From a pharmacologic perspective, the features of greatest interest are *lipid content, apolipoprotein content,* and *transport function.*

The topic of lipoprotein *density* deserves comment for two reasons. First, naming of lipoproteins is based on their density. Second, differences in density provide the basis for the physical isolation and subsequent measurement of plasma lipoproteins. The various classes of lipoproteins differ in density as a result of dissimilarities in their percent composition of lipid and protein. Because protein is more dense than lipid, lipoproteins that have a high percentage of protein (and a low percentage of lipid) have a relatively high density. Conversely, lipoproteins with a lower percentage of protein have a lower density.

Of the six major classes of lipoproteins, three are of particular relevance to coronary atherosclerosis. These classes are named (1) very-low-density lipoproteins (VLDLs), (2) low-density lipoproteins (LDLs), and (3) high-density lipoproteins (HDLs). Properties of these three classes are summarized in Table 49–1.

### Very-Low-Density Lipoproteins

VLDLs contain *triglycerides* (and some cholesterol) as their core lipids, and account for nearly all of the triglycerides in blood. The physiologic role of VLDLs is *delivery of triglycerides* from the liver to adipose tissue and muscle. Each VLDL particle contains one molecule of *apolipoprotein B-100,* which allows VLDLs to bind cell-surface receptors and thereby transfer their lipid content to cells.

The role of VLDLs in atherosclerosis is unclear. Although several studies suggest a link between elevated levels of VLDLs and development of atherosclerosis, this link has not been firmly established. However, we do know that elevation of triglyceride levels (>500 mg/dl) increases the risk of *pancreatitis.*

### Low-Density Lipoproteins

LDLs contain *cholesterol* as their primary core lipid, and account for the majority (60% to 70%) of all cholesterol in blood. The physiologic role of LDLs is *delivery of cholesterol to nonhepatic tissues.* Each LDL particle contains one molecule of *apolipoprotein B-100,* which is needed for binding of LDL particles to LDL receptors on cells. LDLs can be looked on as by-products of VLDL metabolism, in that the lipids and apolipoproteins that compose LDLs are remnants of VLDL degradation.

Cells that require cholesterol meet their needs through endocytosis (engulfment) of LDLs, a process that begins with binding of LDL particles to LDL receptors on the cell surface. When cellular demand for cholesterol increases,

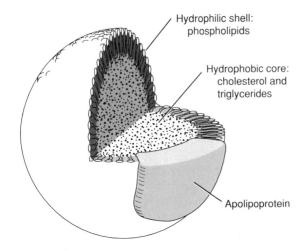

**Figure 49–1. Basic structure of plasma lipoproteins.**

Hydrophilic shell: phospholipids

Hydrophobic core: cholesterol and triglycerides

Apolipoprotein

**TABLE 49–1. PROPERTIES OF THE PLASMA LIPOPROTEINS THAT AFFECT ATHEROSCLEROSIS**

| Lipoprotein Class* | Major Core Lipids | Apolipoproteins | Transport Function | Influence on Atherosclerosis |
|---|---|---|---|---|
| VLDL | Triglycerides | B-100, E, others | Delivery of triglycerides to nonhepatic tissues | *Probably contribute* to atherosclerosis |
| LDL | Cholesterol | B-100 | Delivery of cholesterol to nonhepatic tissues | *Definitely contribute* to atherosclerosis |
| HDL | Cholesterol | A-I, A-II, A-IV | Transport of cholesterol from nonhepatic tissues back to the liver | *Protect* against atherosclerosis |

*VLDL = very-low-density lipoproteins; LDL = low-density lipoproteins; HDL = high-density lipoproteins.

cells synthesize more LDL receptors, and thereby increase their capacity for LDL uptake. Cells that are unable to make more LDL receptors are unable to increase cholesterol absorption. An important mechanism by which drugs reduce LDL levels is to increase the number of LDL receptors on cells.

*Of all lipoproteins, LDLs make the greatest contribution to coronary atherosclerosis.* The probability of developing CAD is directly related to the level of LDLs in blood. Conversely, by reducing LDL levels, we decrease the risk of CAD. Accordingly, when cholesterol-lowering drugs are used, the primary goal is to reduce LDL levels. Multiple studies have shown that, by reducing LDL levels, we can arrest or reverse atherosclerosis, and can thereby reduce mortality from CAD. For individuals with elevated levels of LDLs, a 25% reduction may reduce the risk of serious coronary events by 50%.

**High-Density Lipoproteins**

Like LDLs, HDLs contain *cholesterol* as their primary core lipid, and account for 20% to 30% of all cholesterol in blood. In contrast to LDLs, whose function is delivery of cholesterol to peripheral tissues, HDLs carry cholesterol from peripheral tissues back to the liver. That is, *HDLs promote cholesterol removal.*

The influence of HDLs on CAD is dramatically different from that of LDLs. Whereas elevation of LDLs *increases* the risk of CAD, elevation of HDLs *reduces* the risk of CAD. That is, elevation of HDL levels actively *protects* against CAD.

Not all HDL particles are the same. Some contain only apolipoprotein A-I, whereas others contain apolipoproteins A-I *and* A-II. Available data suggest that cardioprotection is conferred by the HDLs that contain only *apolipoprotein A-I.*

## LDL-Cholesterol versus HDL-Cholesterol

From the foregoing, it is clear that not all cholesterol in plasma has the same impact on CAD. As discussed, a rise in cholesterol associated with LDLs increases the risk of

CAD. In contrast, a rise in cholesterol associated with HDLs lowers the risk of CAD. Consequently, when speaking of plasma cholesterol levels, we need to distinguish between cholesterol that is associated with HDLs and cholesterol that is associated with LDLs. To make this distinction, we will use the terms *HDL-cholesterol* and *LDL-cholesterol.*

## LDL-Cholesterol and Atherosclerosis

LDLs initiate and fuel development of atherosclerosis. The process begins with transport of LDLs from the arterial lumen into endothelial cells and from there into the space that underlies the arterial epithelium. Once in the subendothelial space, components of LDLs undergo *oxidation.* This step is critical in that oxidized LDLs

- Attract monocytes from the circulation into the subendothelial space, after which the monocytes undergo conversion to macrophages
- Inhibit macrophage mobility, thereby keeping macrophages at the site of atherogenesis
- Undergo uptake by macrophages (macrophages do not take up LDLs that have not been oxidized)
- Are cytotoxic, and hence can damage the endothelium directly

As macrophages engulf more and more cholesterol, they become large and vacuolated. When macrophages assume this form, they are referred to as *foam cells.* Accumulation of foam cells beneath the arterial epithelium produces a fatty streak, which makes the surface of the arterial wall lumpy. Continued accumulation of foam cells can eventually cause rupture of the endothelium, thereby exposing the underlying tissue to the blood. This results in platelet adhesion and formation of microthrombi. As the process continues, smooth muscle cells migrate to the site, synthesis of collagen increases, and there can be repeated rupturing and healing of the endothelium. The end result is a mature atherosclerotic lesion, characterized by a large lipid core and a tough fibrous cap. In less mature lesions, the fibrous cap is not strong, and hence the lesions are unstable. As a result, arterial pressure and shear forces from moving blood can cause the cap to rupture; accumulation of platelets at the site can rapidly cause thrombosis, and can thereby cause infarction. Infarction is less likely at sites of mature atherosclerotic lesions.

# Cholesterol Testing and Follow-up

Given the clear relationship between high LDL-cholesterol and CAD, it is recommended that all adults undergo periodic cholesterol evaluation. For individuals with existing CAD, the guidelines for cholesterol testing and follow-up differ from the guidelines for individuals without CAD. The guidelines presented here reflect recommendations in the Second Report of the National Cholesterol Education Program (NCEP) Expert Panel on Detection, Evaluation, and Treatment of High Blood Cholesterol in Adults.

## Individuals Without Coronary Artery Disease

**Total Cholesterol and HDL-Cholesterol.** All adults over the age of 20 should be tested for *total blood cholesterol* at least every 5 years; when possible, *HDL-cholesterol* should be determined at the same time. Measurements can be made without prior fasting. Classification of *total blood cholesterol* in individuals without CAD is as follows:

- <200 mg/dl = desirable blood cholesterol
- 200 to 239 mg/dl = borderline high-risk blood cholesterol
- >240 mg/dl = high-risk blood cholesterol

An *HDL-cholesterol* level of less than 35 mg/dl is classified as *low HDL-cholesterol* (which is undesirable). As indicated in the top half of Table 49–2, follow-up to this initial screen is based on (1) the total cholesterol level, (2) the presence of low HDL-cholesterol (<35 mg/dl is a risk factor for CAD), and (3) the presence of additional risk factors for CAD. If these considerations suggest a risk of CAD, the individual should then be evaluated for *LDL-cholesterol*.

**LDL-Cholesterol.** Management decisions for lowering blood cholesterol are based on LDL-cholesterol levels, not on levels of total cholesterol or HDL-cholesterol. Hence, if screening for total cholesterol and HDL-cholesterol suggests that the patient may be at risk, an LDL-cholesterol determination is required. Blood for the determination should be drawn after fasting for 9 to 12 hours. An LDL-cholesterol level below 130 mg/dl is classified as desirable, and no treatment is needed. Conversely, levels above 130 mg/dl require intervention. Management guidelines

are summarized in the bottom half of Table 49–2. Note that the recommended follow-up depends on (1) the LDL-cholesterol level and (2) the presence or absence of other CAD risk factors (e.g., hypertension, smoking, diabetes mellitus, suboptimal levels of HDL-cholesterol).

## Individuals with Existing Coronary Artery Disease

Individuals with evidence of CAD are at highest risk. Accordingly, guidelines for cholesterol testing and follow-up are more stringent than for individuals without CAD. Patients with existing CAD should be evaluated *annually*. An *LDL-cholesterol* determination is required. As indicated in Table 49–3, an LDL-cholesterol level below 100 mg/dl is considered *optimal*, and no treatment is needed. Conversely, levels above 100 mg/dl are classified as *higher than optimal* and require intervention; the goal is to reduce LDL-cholesterol to 100 mg/dl or less. Note that, in patients with existing CAD, the acceptable level of LDL-cholesterol (100 mg/dl) is not as high as the acceptable level in individuals without CAD (130 mg/dl).

# Management of High LDL-Cholesterol

## Nondrug Therapy

**Diet Modification.** Diet modification is the cornerstone of treatment for reducing LDL-cholesterol. Depending on the severity of LDL-cholesterol elevation, diet modification may be the only treatment needed.

Diet modification has two objectives: (1) reduction of LDL-cholesterol and (2) reduction of body weight (for individuals who are obese). To achieve these objectives, the patient should

- Limit *total fat* to 30% or less of caloric intake
- Limit *saturated fats* (animal fats and some vegetable oils) to 10% or less of caloric intake
- Limit *cholesterol* to 300 mg/day or less

If these measures fail to reduce LDL-cholesterol to an acceptable level, consumption of saturated fat and cholesterol should be restricted further: saturated fat should be limited to 7% of caloric intake, and cholesterol should not exceed 200 mg/day. Patients should be given instructions on diet modification and encouraged to follow them. Consultation with a dietitian may be appropriate. A list of specific foods to choose or avoid is shown in Table 49–4.

**Reduction of Risk Factors.** Major risk factors for CAD are summarized in Table 49–5. These should be identified, and then corrected when possible. *Cigarette smoking* raises LDL-cholesterol and lowers HDL-cholesterol, thereby increasing the risk of CAD; patients should be forcefully encouraged to quit smoking. *Diabetes mellitus*, *hypertension*, and *obesity* all carry an increased risk of CAD; these conditions should be treated.

**TABLE 49–2. CHOLESTEROL TESTING AND FOLLOW-UP FOR INDIVIDUALS WITHOUT CAD**

### Total Cholesterol

| mg/dl | Classification | Recommended Follow-up |
|---|---|---|
| <200 | Desirable blood cholesterol | For patients with HDL-cholesterol ≥35 mg/dl: repeat tests of total and HDL-cholesterol within 5 years<br>For patients with HDL-cholesterol <35 mg/dl: obtain lipoprotein analysis; further management based on LDL-cholesterol level |
| 200–239 | Borderline high-risk blood cholesterol | For patients with HDL-cholesterol ≥35 mg/dl and less than two CAD risk factors*: provide dietary information and recheck total and HDL-cholesterol within 1 to 2 years<br>For patients with HDL-cholesterol <35 mg/dl or two or more CAD risk factors: obtain lipoprotein analysis; further management based on LDL-cholesterol level |
| >240 | High-risk blood cholesterol | Obtain lipoprotein analysis; further management based on LDL-cholesterol level |

### LDL-Cholesterol

| mg/dl | Classification | Recommended Follow-up |
|---|---|---|
| <130 | Desirable LDL-cholesterol | Retest total and HDL-cholesterol within 5 years |
| 130–159 | Borderline high-risk LDL-cholesterol | For patients with less than two CAD risk factors*: recheck LDL-cholesterol annually<br>For patients with two or more CAD risk factors: institute dietary therapy to bring LDL-cholesterol below 130 mg/dl |
| 160–189 | High-risk LDL-cholesterol | For patients with less than two CAD risk factors: institute dietary therapy to bring LDL-cholesterol below 160 mg/dl<br>For patients with two or more risk factors; institute dietary therapy, followed by drug therapy if needed, to bring LDL-cholesterol below 130 mg/dl |
| >190 | High-risk LDL-cholesterol | For patients with less than two CAD risk factors: institute dietary therapy, followed by drug therapy if needed, to bring LDL-cholesterol below 160 mg/dl<br>For patients with two or more risk factors: institute dietary therapy followed by drug therapy to bring LDL-cholesterol below 130 mg/dl |

*CAD risk factors: see Table 49–5.
Based on recommendation in the Summary of the Second Report of the National Cholesterol Education Program Adult Treatment Panel, published in JAMA 269:3015, 1993.

A *sedentary lifestyle* carries an increased risk of CAD. Conversely, regular exercise lowers the risk of CAD. Running and swimming, for example, can decrease LDL-cholesterol and elevate HDL-cholesterol, thereby reducing CAD risk. When appropriate, an exercise program should be instituted.

Risk factors that cannot be corrected, but nonetheless should be identified, include *a family history of premature CAD*, *a history of cerebrovascular or peripheral vascular disease*, and *advancing age* (>45 for men, >55 for women).

*Low HDL-cholesterol* (<35 mg/dl) is an independent risk factor for CAD. Unfortunately, we have no specific method for raising HDL-cholesterol at this time (although some of the drugs given to lower LDL-cholesterol also pro-

duce a modest increase in HDL-cholesterol). As indicated in Table 49–5, *high* HDL-cholesterol (>60 mg/dl) is a *negative* risk factor. That is, high HDL-cholesterol protects against CAD.

## Drug Therapy

*Drugs are not the first-line therapy for lowering LDL-cholesterol. Rather, drugs should be employed only if diet modification and an exercise program fail to reduce LDL-cholesterol to an acceptable level—and then only if the combination of elevated LDL-cholesterol and other risk factors justifies drug use.* Specific NCEP guidelines for implementing drug therapy are presented in Tables 49–2 and 49–3. When drugs are employed, it is es-

**TABLE 49-3. LDL-CHOLESTEROL TESTING AND FOLLOW-UP FOR PATIENTS WITH EVIDENCE OF CAD***

| LDL-Cholesterol[†] (mg/dl) | Classification | Recommended Follow-up |
|---|---|---|
| <100 | Optimal | Provide instruction on diet and exercise; repeat LDL-cholesterol measurement annually |
| 100–129 | Higher than optimal | Institute dietary therapy, followed by drug therapy if needed, to bring LDL-cholesterol to 100 mg/dl or less |
| ≥130 | Higher than optimal | Institute drug therapy to bring LDL-cholesterol to 100 mg/dl or less |

*Based on recommendations in the Summary of the Second Report of the National Cholesterol Education Program Adult Treatment Panel, published in JAMA 269:3015, 1993.
[†]Average of two measurements made 1 to 8 weeks apart; measurements are made following an 8- to 12-hour fast.

sential that dietary therapy continue; beneficial effects of diet and drugs are additive—and drugs alone may be unable to produce adequate LDL-cholesterol reduction.

The objective of drug therapy is to lower LDL-cholesterol without also lowering HDL-cholesterol. At this time, the preferred drugs for reducing LDL-cholesterol are the *HMG CoA reductase inhibitors*. Alternatives include *cholestyramine, colestipol,* and *nicotinic acid* (niacin). For some patients, single-drug therapy is effective. Others may require a combination of drugs. Since LDL-cholesterol levels will return to pretreatment values if drugs are withdrawn, *treatment must continue lifelong*; patients must be made aware of this requirement. It is important to note that the principal benefit of drug therapy is *prophylaxis*: drugs are much more effective at preventing or retarding CAD than they are at promoting regression of coronary atherosclerosis that has already occurred.

Periodic monitoring of cholesterol is required. Levels should be measured monthly early in treatment and at longer intervals thereafter.

# Pharmacology of the Lipid-Lowering Drugs

Drugs that lower LDL-cholesterol levels include HMG CoA reductase inhibitors, bile acid–binding resins, and nicotinic acid. All are effective to varying degrees. The HMG CoA reductase inhibitors cause the fewest adverse effects and are tolerated best.

## HMG CoA Reductase Inhibitors (Statins)

HMG CoA reductase inhibitors are the most effective drugs for lowering LDL-cholesterol levels and cause few adverse effects. As a result, they are the most widely used cholesterol-lowering drugs.

At this time, five HMG CoA reductase inhibitors are available: lovastatin, fluvastatin, pravastatin, simvastatin, and atorvastatin. Because all of these drugs have *statin* in their names, an alternative name for the family is *statins*. Dosages are summarized in Table 49-6.

### Mechanism of Action

The mechanism by which statins decrease LDL-cholesterol levels is complex, and depends ultimately on reducing the number of LDL receptors on hepatocytes (liver cells). The process begins with inhibition of hepatic HMG CoA reductase, the rate-limiting enzyme in cholesterol biosynthesis. In response to decreased cholesterol production, hepatocytes synthesize more HMG CoA reductase. As a result, cholesterol synthesis is largely restored to pretreatment levels. However, for reasons that are not fully understood, inhibition of cholesterol synthesis causes hepatocytes to synthesize more LDL receptors. As a result, hepatocytes are able to remove more LDLs from the blood. In patients who are genetically unable to synthesize LDL receptors, statins fail to reduce LDL levels, indicating that (1) inhibition of cholesterol synthesis, by itself, is not sufficient to explain cholesterol-lowering effects; and (2) in order for statins to be effective, production of LDL receptors must increase.

In addition to inhibiting HMG CoA reductase, statins decrease production of apolipoprotein B-100. As a result, hepatocytes decrease production of VLDLs. This lowers VLDL levels along with LDL levels. Statins also *raise* HDL levels by 8%.

### Therapeutic Use

Statins are given to lower elevated levels of LDL-cholesterol. Responses are dose dependent: low doses decrease LDL-cholesterol by about 25%; large doses decrease levels by as much as 45%. Reductions are significant within 2 weeks and maximal within 4 to 6 weeks. Because cholesterol synthesis normally increases during the night, statins are more effective when given in the evening than in the morning. Concurrent use of a *bile*

## TABLE 49-4. RECOMMENDED DIETARY MODIFICATIONS TO LOWER SERUM CHOLESTEROL

| | Recommendation | |
| --- | --- | --- |
| **Food Type** | Choose | Decrease |
| Fish, chicken, turkey, and lean meats | Fish; poultry without skin; lean cuts of beef, lamb, pork, or veal; shellfish | Fatty cuts of beef, lamb, or pork; spare-ribs; organ meats; regular cold cuts; sausage; hot dogs |
| Skim and low-fat milk, cheese, yogurt, and dairy products | Skim and 1% fat milk (liquid, powdered, evaporated), buttermilk | 4% fat milk (regular, evaporated, condensed), 2% fat milk, cream, half and half, imitation milk products, most nondairy creamers, whipped toppings |
| | Nonfat (%) or low-fat yogurt | Whole-milk yogurt |
| | Low-fat cottage cheese (1% or 2% fat) | Whole-milk cottage cheese (4%) |
| | Low-fat cheeses, farmer or pot cheeses (all of these cheeses should be no more than 2 to 6 gm of fat per ounce) | All natural cheeses (e.g., blue, Roquefort, Camembert, cheddar, Swiss) |
| | | Cream cheese (including low-fat and "light" types), sour cream (including low-fat and "light" types) |
| | Sherbet, sorbet | Ice cream |
| Eggs | Egg whites (2 whites = 1 whole egg in recipes), cholesterol-free egg substitutes | Egg yolks |
| Fruits and vegetables | Fresh, frozen, canned, and dried fruits and vegetables | Vegetables prepared in butter, cream, and other sauces |
| Breads and cereals | Homemade baked goods using unsaturated oils sparingly, angel food cake, low-fat crackers, low-fat cookies | Commercial baked goods: pies, cakes, muffins, doughnuts, croissants, biscuits, high-fat crackers, high-fat cookies |
| | Rice, pasta | Egg noodles |
| | Whole-grain breads and cereals (oatmeal, whole wheat, rye, bran, multigrain, etc) | Breads in which eggs are a major ingredient |
| Fats and oils | Unsaturated vegetable oils: corn, olive, rapeseed (canola oil), safflower, sesame, soybean, sunflower | Butter, coconut oil, palm oil, palm kernel oil, lard, bacon fat |
| | Margarine (regular or diet), shortening made from one of the unsaturated oils listed above | |
| | Mayonnaise, salad dressings made with one of the unsaturated oils listed above, low-fat dressings | Dressings made with egg yolk |
| | Seeds and nuts | Coconut |
| | Baking cocoa | Chocolate |

From the National Cholesterol Education Program Adult Treatment Panel report. Arch. Intern. Med. 148:36, 1988.

*acid-binding resin* (cholestyramine or colestipol) can decrease LDL levels by an additional 20% to 25%. Adding nicotinic acid to the regimen can decrease LDL levels 15% to 20% more. If statins are withdrawn, serum cholesterol will return to pretreatment levels. Hence, treatment must continue lifelong.

Statins slow progression of CAD, decrease the number of cardiac events, and reduce mortality. In patients with evidence of existing CAD (angina or previous myocardial infarction), statins reduce the risk of death from cardiac causes. This was demonstrated conclusively in the landmark Scandinavian Simvastatin Survival Study. In this trial,

the death rate was 12% among patients taking placebo and 8% in patients taking simvastatin—a 30% decrease in overall mortality. Benefits were due to a decrease in cardiac-related mortality; deaths from noncardiac causes were the same in both groups.

### Pharmacokinetics

Statins are administered orally. The amount absorbed ranges between 30% and 90%, depending on the drug in question. Regardless of how much is absorbed, most of an absorbed dose is extracted from the blood on its first pass through the liver, the principal site at which statins act. In general, statins undergo rapid hepatic metabolism followed by excretion in the bile. Only

## TABLE 49-5. RISK FACTORS FOR CAD (OTHER THAN HIGH LDL-CHOLESTEROL)*

*Positive Risk Factors*[†]

Age (years)
    Male ≥45
    Female ≥55
Family history of premature CAD
Cigarette smoking
Hypertension
Diabetes mellitus
Low HDL-cholesterol (<35 mg/dl)

*Negative Risk Factors*

High HDL-cholesterol (≥60 mg/dl)

---

*Net risk status is determined by adding the number of positive risk factors and then subtracting one risk factor if HDL-cholesterol is ≥60 mg/dl (since high HDL-cholesterol protects against CAD).

[†]*Obesity* and *physical inactivity* are not listed as separate risk factors. *Obesity* is not listed because it operates through other risk factors that are included (hypertension, hyperlipidemia, low HDL-cholesterol, and diabetes mellitus); however, obesity is nonetheless a target for intervention. Although *physical inactivity* is not listed, it too is a target for intervention.

Adapted from the Summary of the Second Report of the National Cholesterol Education Program Adult Treatment Panel. JAMA 269:3015, 1993.

---

a small fraction of each dose reaches the general circulation. Statins cross the blood-brain barrier and placenta.

## Adverse Effects

Statins are generally well tolerated. Side effects are uncommon. Some patients develop headache, rash, or GI disturbances (dyspepsia, cramps, flatulence, constipation, abdominal pain). However, these effects are usually mild and transient. Serious adverse effects—hepatotoxicity and myopathy—are rare.

**Hepatotoxicity.** Liver injury, as evidenced by elevations in serum transaminase levels, develops in 1% to 2% of patients treated 1 year or longer. However, jaundice and other clinical signs are rare. Because of the risk of liver injury, hepatic function should be assessed before treatment, every 4 to 6 weeks during the first 3 months of treatment, every 6 to 8 weeks for the next 12 months, and periodically thereafter. If serum transaminase levels rise to three times normal and remain there, statins should be discontinued. Transaminase levels decline to pretreatment levels following drug withdrawal. Caution should be exercised in patients with liver disease and in those who consume alcohol in excess.

**Myopathy.** Muscle injury coupled with elevation of creatine phosphokinase (CPK) develops in about 0.5% of patients. If statins are not withdrawn, the condition may progress to severe *myositis* (muscle inflammation) and *rhabdomyolysis* (muscle disintegration or dissolution), possibly associated with acute renal failure. The risk of myopathy is highest with lovastatin, especially when the drug is combined with gemfibrozil, nicotinic acid, cyclosporine (an immunosuppressant), or erythromycin. Patients should be instructed to notify the physician if unexplained muscle pain or tenderness is noted. Statins should be withdrawn if myositis is diagnosed or if CPK levels become excessive (10 times normal).

## Use in Pregnancy

*Statins are classified in FDA Pregnancy Category X: the risks to the fetus outweigh any potential benefits of treatment.* When administered to pregnant rats in doses 500 times greater than the maximal recommended dosage for humans, lovastatin produced fetal skeletal malformations. Teratogenic effects in humans have not been reported. However, because statins inhibit synthesis of cholesterol, and since cholesterol is required for synthesis of cell membranes and several hormones, concern regarding human fetal injury remains. Moreover, there is no compelling reason to continue lipid-lowering drugs during pregnancy. Women of child-bearing age should be informed about the potential for fetal harm and warned against becoming pregnant. If pregnancy occurs, statins should be withdrawn.

## Bile Acid-Binding Resins: Cholestyramine and Colestipol

Bile acid–binding resins lower LDL-cholesterol levels. Two resins are available: *cholestyramine* [Questran, Prevalite] and *colestipol* [Colestid]. Since these drugs are alike in practically all respects, we will discuss them jointly. Both

## TABLE 49-6. DOSAGES FOR HMG CoA REDUCTASE INHIBITORS

| Drug | Initial Dose | Usual Dose | Maximal Dosage | Comments |
|------|-------------|-----------|----------------|----------|
| Atorvastatin [Lipitor] | 10 mg at bedtime | | 80 mg at bedtime | May be taken with or without food |
| Fluvastatin [Lescol] | 20 mg at bedtime | 20 mg at bedtime | 40 mg at bedtime or 20 mg bid | May be taken with or without food |
| Lovastatin [Mevacor] | 20 mg at dinner | 20 mg with dinner | 40 mg bid | Take with food to increase bioavailability |
| Pravastatin [Pravachol] | 10 mg at bedtime | 20 mg at bedtime | 40 mg at bedtime | Take with food to reduce dyspepsia |
| Simvastatin [Zocor] | 5 mg at bedtime | 10 mg at bedtime | 40 mg bid | Take with food to reduce dyspepsia |

agents are unusually safe, although constipation, abdominal discomfort, and bloating are common.

***Effect on Plasma Lipoproteins.*** The principal response to bile acid-binding resins is a reduction in LDL-cholesterol levels. LDL levels begin to fall during the first week of therapy, and maximum reductions (about a 20% drop) develop within 1 month. When these drugs are discontinued, LDL-cholesterol returns to pretreatment levels in 3 to 4 weeks.

Bile acid-binding resins may *increase* VLDL levels in some patients. In most cases, the elevation is brief and mild. However, if VLDL levels are elevated prior to treatment, the increment induced by bile acid-binding resins may be sustained and substantial. Accordingly, bile acid-binding resins are not drugs of choice for lowering LDL-cholesterol in patients whose VLDL levels are elevated.

***Pharmacokinetics.*** Bile acid-binding resins are biologically inert. These drugs are insoluble in water, cannot be absorbed from the GI tract, and are impervious to digestive enzymes. Following oral administration, they simply pass through the intestine and become excreted in the feces.

***Mechanism of Action.*** The bile acid-binding resins lower LDL-cholesterol through a mechanism that ultimately depends on increasing LDL receptors on hepatocytes. Following ingestion, these resins form an insoluble complex with bile acids present in the intestine; this complex prevents the reabsorption of bile acids, and thereby accelerates their excretion. Since bile acids are normally reabsorbed, the increase in excretion creates a demand for increased synthesis, which takes place in the liver. Since bile acids are made from cholesterol, liver cells must have an increased cholesterol supply in order to increase bile acid production. The required cholesterol is provided by LDL. To avail themselves of more LDL-cholesterol, liver cells increase their number of LDL receptors, thereby increasing their capacity for LDL uptake. The resultant increase in LDL absorption from plasma decreases LDL levels in blood. Individuals who are genetically incapable of increasing LDL receptor synthesis are unable to benefit from these drugs.

***Therapeutic Use.*** The bile acid-binding resins are preferred drugs for lowering elevated levels of LDL-cholesterol. When used in conjunction with a low-cholesterol diet, these agents can produce a 15% to 20% reduction in LDL-cholesterol levels. LDL levels can be reduced even further (up to a total of 50%) by adding nicotinic acid. Combining a statin with one of the resins can decrease LDL-cholesterol by an additional 20% to 25%.

***Adverse Effects.*** The bile acid-binding resins are not absorbed from the GI tract, and hence are devoid of systemic effects. Accordingly, these agents are safer than all other lipid-lowering drugs.

Adverse effects are limited to the GI tract. *Constipation* is the principal undesired response. This can be minimized by increasing dietary fiber and fluids. If necessary, a mild laxative may be used. Other GI effects include *bloating*, *indigestion*, and *nausea*. Rarely, these resins de-

crease fat absorption, and may thereby *decrease uptake of fat-soluble vitamins* (vitamins A, D, E, and K). Vitamin supplements may be required.

***Drug Interactions.*** The bile acid-binding resins can form complexes with drugs. Medications that undergo binding cannot be absorbed, and hence are not available for systemic effects. Drugs known to form complexes with these resins include *thiazide diuretics*, *digoxin*, *warfarin*, and *some antibiotics*. To reduce formation of complexes, oral medications should be administered either 1 hour before the resin or 4 hours after.

***Preparations, Dosage, and Administration.*** *Cholestyramine.* Cholestyramine [Questran, Questran Light, Prevalite] is dispensed in powdered form. Patients should be instructed to mix the powder with fluid, since swallowing it dry can cause esophageal irritation and impaction. Appropriate liquids for mixing include water, fruit juices, and soups. Pulpy fruits with a high fluid content (e.g., applesauce, crushed pineapple) may also be used. The usual dosage is 4 to 12 gm twice a day.

*Colestipol.* Colestipol hydrochloride [Colestid] is dispensed in granular form (5 gm) and 1-gm tablets. The dosage for the *granules* is 5 to 30 gm/day administered in one or more doses. Patients should be instructed to mix the granules with fluids or pulpy fruits before ingestion. The dosage for the tablets is 2 to 16 gm/day administered in one or more doses. Tablets should be swallowed whole and taken with fluid.

## Nicotinic Acid (Niacin)

Nicotinic acid reduces LDL and VLDL levels, and increases HDL levels. Prior to recent trials with statins, nicotinic acid was the only drug proved to reduce coronary mortality and recurrence of myocardial infarction in patients with high LDL-cholesterol. Unfortunately, although nicotinic acid is effective, the drug causes a variety of side effects. For example, nearly all patients experience flushing. Because of its side-effect profile, nicotinic acid has limited clinical utility.

***Mechanism of Action.*** The primary effect of nicotinic acid is to decrease production of VLDLs. Since LDLs are by-products of VLDL degradation, the fall in VLDL levels causes LDL levels to fall as well. There appear to be several mechanisms by which nicotinic acid decreases VLDL production. Notable among these is inhibition of lipolysis in adipose tissue.

***Effect on Plasma Lipoproteins.*** Nicotinic acid reduces LDL-cholesterol by 15% to 25% and triglycerides by 30% to 60%. In addition, it raises HDL-cholesterol by 25% to 35%. VLDL levels begin to fall within the first 4 days of therapy. LDL levels decline more slowly, taking 3 to 5 weeks to reach maximum reductions. If a bile acid-binding resin is added to the regimen, a 40% to 60% decrease in LDL may be achieved. Triple therapy (nicotinic acid plus a bile acid-binding resin plus a statin) can decrease LDL-cholesterol by 70% or more.

***Therapeutic Use.*** Although nicotinic acid is effective, side effects limit its use. Nicotinic acid is a drug of choice for lowering VLDL levels in patients at risk of pancreatitis. Additional indications include mixed elevation of LDLs and triglycerides (VLDLs), and elevation of triglycerides in combination with low levels of HDLs.

Nicotinic acid (niacin) also has a role as a vitamin. The doses employed to correct niacin deficiency are much smaller than those employed to lower lipoprotein levels. The role of nicotinic acid as a vitamin is discussed in Chapter 74.

**Adverse Effects.** The most frequent adverse reactions involve the skin (flushing, itching) and GI tract (gastric upset, nausea, vomiting, diarrhea). *Intense flushing* of the face, neck, and ears occurs in practically all patients receiving nicotinic acid in pharmacologic doses. This reaction diminishes in several weeks, and can be attenuated by taking 325 mg of aspirin 30 minutes before each dose. (Aspirin reduces flushing by preventing synthesis of prostaglandins, which mediate the flushing response.)

In addition to its common side effects, nicotinic acid may induce more serious reactions. The most troubling is *hepatotoxicity*, which occurs almost exclusively with the *sustained-release* formulation. Accordingly, sustained-release nicotinic acid should not be used routinely. If this formulation *must* be used, the dosage should not exceed 1500 mg/day. Because of the risk of hepatotoxicity, liver function should be assessed before treatment and periodically thereafter. Other serious adverse effects include *hyperglycemia* and *gouty arthritis*.

**Preparations, Dosage, and Administration.** Nicotinic acid (niacin) is marketed generically and under multiple trade names. Three formulations are available: tablets, sustained-release capsules, and an elixir. Because of the risk of hepatotoxicity, sustained-release capsules should not be used routinely. The usual maintenance dosage is 1000 to 2000 mg 3 times a day, administered with or after meals. (*Note:* When nicotinic acid is taken as a vitamin, the dosage is only about 25 mg/day—much lower than the dosages employed to lower plasma lipoproteins.)

### Gemfibrozil

Gemfibrozil [Lopid] decreases triglyceride (VLDL) levels and raises HDL-cholesterol levels. The drug does not reduce LDL-cholesterol. Its principal indication is hypertriglyceridemia.

**Effects on Plasma Lipoproteins.** Gemfibrozil decreases plasma triglyceride content by lowering VLDL levels. Maximum reductions in VLDLs range from 40% to 55%, and are achieved within 3 to 4 weeks of treatment. Gemfibrozil can raise HDL-cholesterol by about 25%. The drug has little effect on LDL-cholesterol levels.

**Mechanism of Action.** The mechanism by which gemfibrozil lowers VLDL levels is not known. Gemfibrozil decreases lipolysis in adipose tissue and reduces uptake of fatty acids by the liver. Both actions can decrease hepatic synthesis of triglycerides. Since triglycerides are the primary core lipids in VLDLs, there is speculation that reducing triglyceride production may underlie the decrease in LDL levels. There is no explanation why gemfibrozil increases levels of HDL.

**Therapeutic Use.** The principal indication for gemfibrozil is elevation of plasma triglycerides (VLDLs). Treatment is limited to patients who have not responded adequately to weight loss and diet modification. Although gemfibrozil can reduce LDL-cholesterol, other drugs (statins, cholestyramine, colestipol) are more effective.

**Adverse Effects.** Gemfibrozil is generally well tolerated. The most common reactions are rashes and GI disturbances (nausea, abdominal pain, diarrhea).

Gemfibrozil increases biliary cholesterol saturation, thereby increasing the risk of *gallstones*. Patients should be informed about manifestations of gallbladder disease (e.g., upper abdominal discomfort, intolerance of fried foods, bloating) and instructed to notify the physician if these develop. Patients with pre-existing gallbladder disease should not take the drug.

Gemfibrozil is *hepatotoxic*. The drug can disrupt liver function and may also present a risk of liver cancer. Periodic tests of liver function are required.

**Drug Interactions.** *Gemfibrozil displaces warfarin from plasma albumin*, thereby increasing anticoagulant effects. Prothrombin time should be measured frequently to assess coagulation status. Warfarin dosage may need to be reduced.

Gemfibrozil increases the risk of *statin-induced myopathy*. The combination of a statin with gemfibrozil should be used with caution.

**Preparations, Dosage, and Administration.** Gemfibrozil [Lopid] is dispensed in 300-mg capsules and 600-mg tablets. The usual adult dosage is 600 mg twice daily, administered 30 minutes before the morning and evening meals.

### Clofibrate

After years of use, clofibrate [Atromid-S] has failed to display a convincing ability to reduce mortality from myocardial infarction. Moreover, long-term therapy may actually *increase* mortality. Consequently, the drug should be employed only when clearly indicated, and then only if the perceived benefits outweigh the risks. In the United States, clofibrate use has essentially stopped. An extended discussion of clofibrate can be found in the previous edition of this book.

## Estrogen

In postmenopausal women, estrogen replacement therapy (0.625 mg/day) reduces LDL-cholesterol by 15% to 25% and increases HDL-cholesterol by 10% to 15%. As a result, the risk of CAD is reduced by about 45% (compared with the risk in postmenopausal women who do not take estrogen). Accordingly, estrogen replacement is considered a treatment of choice for postmenopausal women with elevated LDL-cholesterol levels. The basic pharmacology of estrogen as well as its use for replacement therapy is discussed at length in Chapter 57.

## KEY POINTS

- Lipoproteins are structures that transport lipids (cholesterol and triglycerides) in blood.
- Lipoproteins consist of a hydrophobic core, a hydrophilic shell, plus at least one apolipoprotein, which serves as a recognition site for receptors on cells.
- Lipoproteins that contain apolipoprotein B-100 transport cholesterol and/or triglycerides from the liver to peripheral tissues.
- Lipoproteins that contain apolipoproteins A-I or A-II transport cholesterol from peripheral tissues back to the liver.
- VLDLs transport triglycerides to peripheral tissues.
- The contribution of VLDLs to CAD is unclear.

- LDLs transport cholesterol to peripheral tissues.
- Elevation of LDL-cholesterol greatly increases the risk of CAD.
- By reducing LDL-cholesterol levels, we can arrest or reverse atherosclerosis, and can thereby reduce morbidity and mortality from CAD.
- HDLs transport cholesterol back to the liver.
- HDLs protect against CAD.
- Atherogenesis begins with accumulation of LDLs beneath the arterial endothelium, followed by oxidation of LDLs.
- NCEP guidelines recommend that all adults over the age of 20 be tested for total blood cholesterol (and HDL-cholesterol when possible) at least every 5 years. If these tests indicate a risk for CAD, then LDL-cholesterol should be measured. LDL-cholesterol measurement is needed because management of high cholesterol is based on LDL-cholesterol levels, not on total cholesterol.
- Diet modification is the primary method for reducing LDL-cholesterol. Drugs are employed only if diet modification and exercise fail to reduce LDL-cholesterol to acceptable levels.
- Therapy with cholesterol-lowering drugs must continue lifelong. If these drugs are withdrawn, cholesterol levels will return to pretreatment values.
- Statins (HMG CoA reductase inhibitors) are the most effective drugs for lowering LDL-cholesterol and cause minimal adverse effects.
- Statins can slow progression of CAD, decrease the number of adverse cardiac events, and reduce mortality.

- Statins reduce LDL-cholesterol levels by increasing the number of LDL receptors on hepatocytes, thereby enabling hepatocytes to remove more LDLs from blood. The process by which LDL receptor number is increased begins with inhibition of HMG CoA reductase, the rate-limiting enzyme in cholesterol synthesis.
- Statins should not be used during pregnancy.
- Bile acid-binding resins—cholestyramine and colestipol—reduce LDL-cholesterol levels by increasing the number of LDL receptors on hepatocytes. The mechanism is complex and begins with preventing reabsorption of bile acids in the intestine.
- Bile acid–binding resins are not absorbed from the GI tract, and hence do not cause systemic adverse effects. However, they do cause constipation and other GI effects.
- Bile acid–binding resins can form complexes with other drugs, and thereby prevent their absorption. Accordingly, oral medications should be administered 1 hour before these resins or 4 hours after.
- Nicotinic acid reduces LDL and VLDL levels and raises HDL levels, but also causes adverse effects in nearly all patients. As a result, its clinical utility is limited.
- Nicotinic acid causes intense flushing of the face, neck, and ears in most patients.
- The sustained-release formulation of nicotinic acid causes liver injury, and therefore should not be used routinely.
- Estrogen replacement therapy in postmenopausal women reduces LDL-cholesterol and increases HDL-cholesterol, and thereby reduces the risk of CAD by about 45%.

# Summary of Major Nursing Implications*

## Implications That Apply to All Drugs That Lower LDL-Cholesterol

### Preadministration Assessment

#### Baseline Data

Obtain laboratory values for total cholesterol, LDL-cholesterol, HDL-cholesterol, and triglycerides (VLDLs).

#### Identifying CAD Risk Factors

The patient history and physical examination should identify CAD risk factors. These include smoking, obesity, age (men >45 yr, women >55 yr), family history of premature CAD, a personal history of cerebrovascular or peripheral vascular disease, reduced levels of HDL-cholesterol (<35 mg/dl), diabetes mellitus, and hypertension.

*Patient education information is highlighted in color.

## Measures to Enhance Therapeutic Effects

### Diet Modification

Diet modification should precede and accompany drug therapy for elevated LDL-cholesterol. Inform patients about the importance of diet in controlling cholesterol levels and arrange for diet counseling. Provide patients with the following dietary guidelines:

- Restrict total dietary fat to 30% (or less) of caloric intake
- Restrict saturated fats to 10% (or less) of caloric intake
- Restrict cholesterol to 300 mg/day

If these restrictions fail to reduce cholesterol to a desirable level, saturated fats should be reduced further (to 7% of caloric intake) and cholesterol should be restricted to 200 mg/day.

### Exercise

Regular exercise can reduce LDL-cholesterol and elevate HDL-cholesterol, thereby reducing the risk of CAD.

Help the patient establish an appropriate exercise program.

### Reduction of CAD Risk Factors

Correctable CAD risk factors should be addressed. Encourage cigarette smokers to quit. Encourage obese patients to lose weight. Disease states that promote CAD—diabetes mellitus and hypertension—must be treated.

### Promoting Compliance

Drug therapy for elevated LDL-cholesterol must continue lifelong; if drugs are withdrawn, cholesterol levels will return to pretreatment values. Inform patients about the need for continuous therapy, and encourage them to adhere to the prescribed regimen.

## HMG CoA Reductase Inhibitors (Statins)

| | |
|---|---|
| Atorvastatin | Pravastatin |
| Fluvastatin | Simvastatin |
| Lovastatin | |

In addition to the implications discussed below, *see above* for implications that apply to all drugs that lower LDL-cholesterol.

### Preadministration Assessment

#### Therapeutic Goal

Statins, in combination with diet modification and exercise, are used to lower elevated levels of LDL-cholesterol.

#### Baseline Data

Obtain baseline values for total cholesterol, LDL-cholesterol, HDL-cholesterol, and triglycerides (VLDLs).

#### Identifying High-Risk Patients

Statins are *contraindicated* for patients with *active liver disease* and during *pregnancy*. Exercise *caution* in patients taking *cyclosporine, gemfibrozil, nicotinic acid,* or *erythromycin.*

### Implementation: Administration

#### Route

Oral.

#### Administration

Instruct patients to take statins with the evening meal or at bedtime, and to take *lovastatin, pravastatin,* and *simvastatin* with food.

### Ongoing Evaluation and Interventions

#### Evaluating Therapeutic Effects

Cholesterol levels should be monitored monthly early in treatment and at longer intervals thereafter.

#### Minimizing Adverse Effects

Statins are very well tolerated. Side effects are uncommon, and serious adverse effects—hepatotoxicity and myopathy—are rare.

*Hepatotoxicity.* Statins can injure the liver, but jaundice and other clinical signs are rare. Liver function should be assessed every 4 to 6 weeks during the first 3 months of treatment and periodically thereafter. If serum transaminase becomes persistently excessive (more than three times normal), statins should be discontinued.

*Myopathy.* Statins can cause muscle injury. If statins are not withdrawn, the condition may progress to severe myositis or rhabdomyolysis. Inform patients about the risk of myopathy, and instruct them to notify the physician if unexplained muscle pain or tenderness develops. If CPK levels are excessive (more than 10 times normal), statins should be withdrawn. Concurrent use of *gemfibrozil, nicotinic acid, cyclosporine,* and *erythromycin* increases the risk of myopathy.

#### Use in Pregnancy

Statins are contraindicated during pregnancy. Inform women of child-bearing age about the potential for fetal harm and warn them against becoming pregnant. If pregnancy occurs, statins should be withdrawn.

#### Minimizing Adverse Interactions

The risk of muscle injury is increased by concurrent use of *cyclosporine, gemfibrozil, nicotinic acid,* and *erythromycin.* The combinations should be used with caution.

## Bile Acid-Binding Resins

| |
|---|
| Cholestyramine |
| Colestipol |

In addition to the implications discussed below, *see above* for implications that apply to all drugs that lower LDL-cholesterol.

### Preadministration Assessment

#### Therapeutic Goal

Bile acid–binding resins, in conjunction with diet modification and exercise, are used to reduce elevated levels of LDL-cholesterol.

#### Baseline Data

Obtain laboratory values for total cholesterol, LDL-cholesterol, HDL-cholesterol, and triglycerides (VLDLs).

### Implementation: Administration

#### Route

Oral.

#### Administration

Instruct patients to mix cholestyramine powder and colestipol granules with water, fruit juice, soup, or pulpy fruit (e.g., applesauce, pineapple) to reduce the risk of esophageal irritation and impaction. Inform patients that these resins are not water soluble, and therefore mixtures will be cloudy suspensions, not clear solutions.

## Ongoing Evaluation and Interventions

### Evaluating Therapeutic Effects

Cholesterol levels should be monitored monthly early in treatment and at longer intervals thereafter.

### Minimizing Adverse Effects

*Constipation.* Inform patients that constipation can be minimized by increasing dietary fiber and fluids. A mild laxative may be used if needed. Instruct patients to notify the physician if constipation becomes bothersome.

*Vitamin Deficiency.* Absorption of fat-soluble vitamins (A, D, E, and K) may be impaired. Vitamin supplements may be required.

### Minimizing Adverse Interactions

Bile acid–binding resins can bind to other drugs and prevent their absorption. Administer other medications 1 hour before the resin or 4 hours after.

## Nicotinic Acid (Niacin)

In addition to the implications discussed below, *see above* for implications that apply to all drugs that lower LDL-cholesterol.

## Preadministration Assessment

### Therapeutic Goal

Nicotinic acid, in conjunction with diet modification and exercise, is used to reduce elevated levels of LDL-cholesterol, VLDLs, and triglycerides.

### Baseline Data

Obtain laboratory values for total cholesterol, LDL-cholesterol, HDL-cholesterol, and triglycerides (VLDLs). Obtain a baseline test of liver function.

### Identifying High-Risk Patients

Nicotinic acid is *contraindicated* for patients with *active liver disease*. Exercise *caution* in patients with *diabetes mellitus* and *gout.*

## Implementation: Administration

### Route

Oral.

### Administration

Instruct patients to take nicotinic acid with meals to reduce GI upset.

## Measures to Enhance Therapeutic Effects

### Dietary Therapy

Diet modification should precede and accompany drug therapy for elevated triglycerides and VLDLs. Inform patients about the importance of diet in controlling lipid levels and arrange for dietary counseling. In addition to the guidelines presented above for all drugs that reduce LDL-cholesterol, patients with hypertriglyceridemia should restrict consumption of alcohol and other sources of triglycerides.

## Ongoing Evaluation and Interventions

### Evaluating Therapeutic Effects

Blood lipid levels should be monitored monthly early in treatment and at longer intervals thereafter.

### Minimizing Adverse Effects

*Flushing.* Nicotinic acid causes flushing of the face, neck, and ears in most patients. Advise patients that flushing can be reduced by taking 325 mg of aspirin 30 minutes before each dose.

*Hepatotoxicity.* Nicotinic acid (primarily the sustained-release formulation) may injure the liver, causing jaundice or other symptoms. Liver function should be assessed before treatment and periodically thereafter.

*Hyperglycemia.* Nicotinic acid may cause hyperglycemia and reduced glucose tolerance. Blood glucose should be monitored frequently. Exercise caution in patients with diabetes.

*Hyperuricemia.* Nicotinic acid can elevate blood levels of uric acid. Exercise caution in patients with gout.

## Gemfibrozil

## Preadministration Assessment

### Therapeutic Goal

Gemfibrozil, in conjunction with diet modification, is used to reduce elevated levels of VLDLs. The drug is not very effective at lowering LDL-cholesterol.

### Baseline Data

Obtain laboratory values for total cholesterol, LDL-cholesterol, HDL-cholesterol, and triglycerides (VLDLs).

### Identifying High-Risk Patients

Gemfibrozil is *contraindicated* for patients with *liver disease, severe renal dysfunction*, and *gallbladder disease.* Use with *caution* in patients taking *statins.*

## Implementation: Administration

### Route

Oral.

## Administration

Instruct patients to administer gemfibrozil 30 minutes before the morning and evening meals.

## Ongoing Evaluation and Interventions

### Evaluating Therapeutic Effects

Obtain periodic tests of blood lipids.

### Minimizing Adverse Effects

*Gallstones.* Gemfibrozil increases gallstone development. Inform patients about symptoms of gallbladder disease (e.g., upper abdominal discomfort, intolerance of fried foods, bloating), and instruct them to notify the physician if these develop.

*Liver Disease.* Gemfibrozil may disrupt liver function. Cancer of the liver may also be a risk. Obtain periodic tests of liver function.

### Minimizing Adverse Interactions

*Warfarin.* Gemfibrozil enhances the effects of warfarin, thereby increasing the risk of bleeding. Obtain frequent measurements of prothrombin time and observe the patient for signs of bleeding. Reduction of warfarin dosage may be required.

*Lovastatin.* Gemfibrozil increases the risk of statin-induced myopathy. Use the combination with caution.

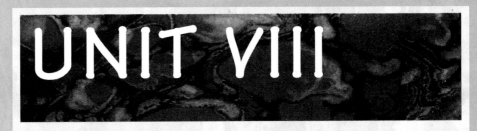

# UNIT VIII

## Drugs That Affect the Blood

**Anticoagulants, Antiplatelet Drugs, and Thrombolytics**

**Drugs for Deficiency Anemias**

**Hematopoietic Growth Factors**

# CHAPTER 50

# Anticoagulants, Antiplatelet Drugs, and Thrombolytics

The drugs discussed in this chapter are used to prevent formation of thrombi (intravascular blood clots) and to dissolve thrombi that have already formed. These drugs act in several ways: some suppress coagulation, some inhibit platelet aggregation, and some promote clot dissolution. All of these drugs interfere with normal hemostasis. As a result, all carry a significant risk of hemorrhage.

## Physiology and Pathophysiology of Coagulation

### Hemostasis

Hemostasis is the physiologic process by which bleeding is stopped. Hemostasis occurs in two stages: (1) formation of a platelet plug, followed by (2) reinforcement of the platelet plug with fibrin. Both processes are set in motion by injury to a blood vessel.

*Stage One: Formation of a Platelet Plug.* Platelet aggregation is initiated when platelets come in contact with collagen on the exposed surface of a damaged blood vessel. In response to contact with collagen, platelets adhere to the site of vessel injury. Following adhesion to the vessel wall, platelets release *adenosine diphosphate* (ADP), a substance that causes more platelets to stick to the developing aggregate. In addition to ADP, platelets release *thromboxane $A_2$* ($TXA_2$), an inducer of platelet aggrega-

tion that is more powerful than ADP. Under the influence of $TXA_2$ and ADP, a platelet plug quickly forms and bleeding is stopped. This plug is unstable, however, and must be reinforced with fibrin if protection is to last.

*Stage Two: Coagulation.* Coagulation is defined as production of fibrin, a protein that reinforces the platelet plug. Fibrin is produced by way of two convergent pathways (Fig. 50-1). Both consist of a series of cascading reactions. These pathways are referred to as the *intrinsic system* and the *extrinsic system*. The intrinsic system is so named because all necessary clotting factors are present within the vascular system. The extrinsic system is so named because tissue thromboplastin, a factor from outside the vascular system, is required for the extrinsic system to work. As Figure 50-1 indicates, the two systems converge at factor Xa, after which they employ the same final series of reactions. Both systems are required for optimal production of fibrin.

Characteristic of both the intrinsic and extrinsic systems is the fact that each reaction in these sequences serves to enhance the reaction that follows (see Fig. 50-1). Looking at the intrinsic system, we can see that the reaction cascade begins with the conversion of clotting factor XII into its active form, XIIa. The active form of factor XII then stimulates the conversion of factor XI into its active form (XIa), and so on. Hence, once the sequence is initiated, it becomes self-sustaining and self-reinforcing.

Important to our understanding of anticoagulant drugs is the fact that *four coagulation factors—factors VII, IX, X, and prothrombin—require vitamin K for their synthesis.* These factors appear in colored boxes in Figure

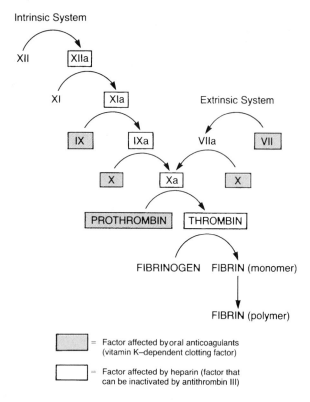

**Figure 50–1. Outline of the coagulation cascade showing factors affected by anticoagulant drugs.** Common names for factors shown: VII = proconvertin, IX = Christmas factor, X = Stuart factor, XI = plasma thromboplastin antecedent, and XII = Hageman factor.

50-1. The significance of the vitamin K-dependent factors will become apparent when we discuss warfarin, an oral anticoagulant.

***Keeping Hemostasis Under Control.*** To protect against widespread coagulation, the body must inactivate any clotting factors that stray from the site of vessel injury. This inactivation is accomplished with *antithrombin III*, a protein that forms a complex with clotting factors, and thereby inhibits their activity. The clotting factors that can be neutralized by antithrombin III appear in uncolored boxes in Figure 50-1. As we shall see, antithrombin III is intimately involved in the action of *heparin*, an injectable anticoagulant drug.

***Physiologic Removal of Clots.*** As healing of an injured vessel proceeds, removal of the clot is eventually necessary. The body accomplishes this with *plasmin*, an enzyme that digests the fibrin meshwork of the clot. Plasmin is produced through the activation of its precursor, *plasminogen*. The *thrombolytic drugs*—streptokinase, urokinase, alteplase, and anistreplase—act by promoting conversion of plasminogen into plasmin.

## Thrombosis

A thrombus is a blood clot formed within a blood vessel or within the heart. Thrombosis (thrombus formation) reflects pathologic functioning of hemostatic mechanisms.

***Arterial Thrombosis.*** Formation of an arterial thrombus begins with adhesion of platelets to the arterial wall. Following adhesion, platelets release ADP and $TXA_2$, and thereby attract additional platelets to the evolving thrombus. With continued platelet aggregation, occlusion of the artery takes place. As blood flow comes to a stop, the coagulation cascade is initiated, causing the original plug to undergo reinforcement with fibrin. The consequence of an arterial thrombus is localized tissue injury owing to lack of perfusion.

***Venous Thrombosis.*** Venous thrombi develop at sites where blood flow is slow. Stagnation of blood initiates the coagulation cascade, resulting in the production of fibrin, which enmeshes red blood cells and platelets to form the thrombus. The typical venous thrombus has a long tail that can break off to produce an *embolus*. Such emboli travel within the vascular system and become lodged at faraway sites, frequently the pulmonary arteries. Hence, unlike an arterial thrombus, whose harmful effects are localized, injury from a venous thrombus occurs secondary to embolization at a site distant from the original thrombus.

## Overview of Drugs Used to Treat Thromboembolic Disorders

The drugs considered in this chapter fall into three major categories: (1) anticoagulants, (2) antiplatelet drugs, and (3) thrombolytic drugs. *Anticoagulants* (heparin, warfarin) are drugs that disrupt the coagulation cascade, and thereby suppress production of fibrin. *Antiplatelet* drugs (primarily aspirin) inhibit platelet aggregation. *Thrombolytic drugs* (e.g., alteplase, streptokinase) promote lysis of fibrin, and thereby cause dissolution of thrombi. Characteristic features of these drug classes are summarized in Table 50-1.

Although the anticoagulants and the antiplatelet drugs both suppress thrombosis, they do so by different mechanisms. As a result, these drugs differ in their effects and applications. The *antiplatelet drugs* are most effective at preventing *arterial* thrombosis. In contrast, *anticoagulants* (heparin and warfarin) act to prevent *venous* thrombosis.

## Parenteral Anticoagulants

### Heparin

Heparin is a rapid-acting anticoagulant administered only by injection. Heparin differs from the oral anticoagulants in several respects, including mechanism of action, time course of effects, indications, and management of overdose.

## TABLE 50-1. OVERVIEW OF DRUGS USED TO TREAT THROMBOEMBOLIC DISORDERS

| Drug Class | Prototype | Drug Action | Therapeutic Effect |
|---|---|---|---|
| *Anticoagulants: parenteral* | Heparin | ↓ Fibrin formation (by promoting inactivation of clotting factors) | Prevention of venous thrombosis |
| *Anticoagulants: oral* | Warfarin | ↓ Fibrin formation (by decreasing synthesis of clotting factors) | Prevention of venous thrombosis |
| *Antiplatelet drugs* | Aspirin | ↓ Platelet aggregation | Prevention of arterial thrombosis |
| *Thrombolytic drugs* | Streptokinase | Promotion of fibrin digestion | Removal of newly formed thrombi |

## Source

Heparin is present in a variety of mammalian tissues. The heparin employed clinically is prepared from two sources: lungs of cattle and intestines of pigs. The anticoagulant activity of heparin from either source is equivalent. Although heparin occurs naturally, its physiologic role is unknown.

## Chemistry

Heparin is not a single molecule, but rather a mixture of long polysaccharide chains, with molecular weights that range from 3000 to 30,000. The active site is a unique pentasaccharide (five-sugar) sequence found randomly along the chain. An important feature of heparin's structure is the presence of many negatively charged groups. Because of these negative charges, heparin is highly polar, and hence cannot readily cross membranes.

## Mechanism of Anticoagulant Action

Heparin suppresses coagulation by helping antithrombin III inactivate thrombin, factor Xa, and other clotting factors. As depicted in Figure 50-2, heparin helps inactivate *thrombin* in *two* ways. First, heparin binds antithrombin III, thereby causing a configurational change in antithrombin III that greatly increases its ability to interact with and inactivate thrombin. Second, heparin serves as a template to which both antithrombin III and thrombin can bind, thereby facilitating interaction between these compounds. It is important to remember that, in addition to helping antithrombin III inactivate thrombin, heparin helps antithrombin III inactivate factor Xa and most other active clotting factors (see Fig. 50-1). By promoting the inactivation of clotting factors, heparin ultimately suppresses formation of fibrin. Since fibrin forms the framework of thrombi in *veins*, heparin is especially useful for prophylaxis of *venous thrombosis*. Because heparin, in combination with antithrombin III, acts directly to inhibit clotting factor activity, the anticoagulant effects of heparin develop *quickly* (within minutes of IV administration). This contrasts with the oral anticoagulants, whose full effects take *days* to develop.

## Pharmacokinetics

***Absorption and Distribution.*** Because of its polarity and large size, heparin is unable to cross membranes, including those of the GI tract. Consequently, heparin cannot be absorbed if given orally, and therefore must be given by injection (IV or SC). Since it cannot cross membranes, heparin does not traverse the placenta and does not enter breast milk.

***Protein and Tissue Binding.*** Heparin chains bind nonspecifically to plasma proteins, mononuclear cells, and endothelial cells. As a result, plasma levels of free heparin can be highly variable following IV or SC administration. Because of this variability, intensive monitoring is required (see below).

***Metabolism and Excretion.*** Heparin undergoes hepatic metabolism followed by renal excretion. Under normal conditions, the half-life of heparin is short (about 1.5 hours). However, in patients with hepatic or renal disease, the half-life is prolonged.

***Time Course of Effects.*** Therapy is initiated with a bolus IV injection and effects begin immediately. Duration of action is brief (hours) and varies with dosage. Effects are prolonged in patients with hepatic or renal impairment.

## Therapeutic Uses

Heparin is the preferred anticoagulant for use during *pregnancy* and in situations that require rapid onset of anticoagulant effects, including *pulmonary embolism*, *evolving stroke*, and *massive deep vein thrombosis* (DVT). In addition, heparin is required for patients undergoing *open heart surgery* and *renal dialysis*; during these procedures, heparin serves to prevent coagulation in devices of extracorporeal circulation (heart-lung machines, dialyzers). Low-dose therapy is used to *prevent postoperative venous thrombosis*. Heparin may also be useful for treating *disseminated intravascular coagulation* (DIC), a complex disorder in which fibrin clots form throughout the vascular system and in which bleeding tendencies may be present; bleeding can occur because massive fibrin

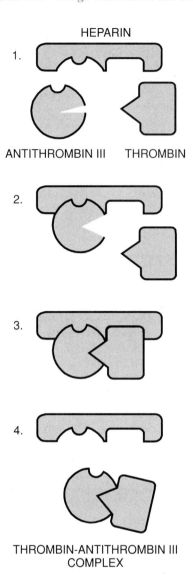

HEPARIN

1.

ANTITHROMBIN III    THROMBIN

2.

3.

4.

THROMBIN-ANTITHROMBIN III
COMPLEX

**Figure 50–2. Inactivation of thrombin by heparin and antithrombin III.** (1) Heparin, thrombin, and antithrombin III are free in the blood. (2) Binding of heparin to antithrombin III causes a configurational change in antithrombin III that increases its ability to interact with thrombin. (3) Thrombin forms a complex with heparin and antithrombin III, after which thrombin and antithrombin III react, causing permanent inactivation of thrombin. (4) The thrombin–antithrombin III complex dissociates from heparin, freeing heparin to act again. *IMPORTANT NOTE:* Thrombin is not the only clotting factor that is inactivated by the heparin–antithrombin III complex. Heparin–antithrombin III also inactivates factor Xa and several other clotting factors.

production consumes available supplies of clotting factors. Heparin is also used as an adjunct to thrombolytic therapy of *acute myocardial infarction.*

## Adverse Effects

*Hemorrhage.* Bleeding develops in about 10% of patients and is the principal complication of treatment. Hemorrhage can occur at any site and may be fatal.

Patients should be monitored closely for signs of blood loss. These include reduced blood pressure, increased heart rate, bruises, petechiae, hematomas, red or black stools, cloudy or discolored urine, pelvic pain (suggestive of ovarian hemorrhage), headache or faintness (suggestive of cerebral hemorrhage), and lumbar pain (suggestive of adrenal hemorrhage). If bleeding develops, heparin should be withdrawn. Severe overdose can be treated with *protamine sulfate* (see below).

The risk of hemorrhage can be decreased in several ways. First, dosage should be carefully controlled so that the activated partial thromboplastin time (see below) does not exceed two times the control value. In addition, candidates for heparin therapy should be screened for risk factors (see *Warnings and Contraindications*). Finally, antiplatelet drugs (e.g., aspirin) should be avoided.

*Thrombocytopenia.* Heparin may decrease platelet counts. Moderate reductions in platelet counts are common and result from heparin-induced platelet aggregation. Severe reductions are rare and result from development of antiplatelet antibodies. If severe thrombocytopenia develops (platelet count <100,000/mm$^3$), heparin should be discontinued. If anticoagulant therapy must be maintained, an oral anticoagulant (warfarin) may be substituted for heparin. Platelet counts should be obtained before treatment and frequently thereafter.

Heparin-induced thrombocytopenia is associated with a seemingly paradoxical *increase* in thrombotic events. These include deep vein thrombosis, pulmonary embolism, cerebral thrombosis, myocardial infarction, and ischemic injury to the arms or legs. The potential for severe morbidity or even mortality is obvious. Hence, even though thrombocytopenia itself is rarely a threat, the increase in thrombosis definitely is.

*Hypersensitivity Reactions.* Since commercial heparin is extracted from animal tissues, these preparations may be contaminated with antigens that can promote allergy. Possible allergic responses include chills, fever, and urticaria. Anaphylactic reactions are rare. To minimize the risk of severe reactions, patients should receive a small test dose of heparin prior to the full therapeutic dose.

*Other Adverse Effects.* Subcutaneous administration may produce *local irritation* and *hematoma. Vasospastic reactions* that persist for several hours may develop after 1 or more weeks of treatment. Long-term, high-dose therapy may cause *osteoporosis.*

## Warnings and Contraindications

*Contraindications.* Heparin is contraindicated for patients with *thrombocytopenia* and *uncontrollable bleeding.* In addition, heparin should be avoided both *during and immediately after surgery of the eye, brain,* or *spinal cord. Lumbar puncture* and *regional anesthesia* are additional contraindications.

*Warnings.* Heparin must be used with extreme caution in all patients for whom there is a high likelihood of bleeding. Included are individuals with *hemophilia, increased capillary permeability, dissecting aneurysm, peptic ulcer disease, severe hypertension,* or *threatened abor-*

*tion.* Heparin must also be used cautiously in patients with *severe disease of the liver or kidneys.*

## Drug Interactions

In heparin-treated patients, platelet aggregation is the major remaining defense against hemorrhage. Drugs that depress platelet function (e.g., aspirin, ibuprofen, indomethacin) will weaken this defense and must be employed with caution.

## Protamine Sulfate for Heparin Overdose

Protamine sulfate is an antidote to severe heparin overdose. Protamine is a small protein that has multiple positively charged groups. These charged groups bond ionically with the negatively charged groups on heparin, thereby forming a heparin-protamine complex that is devoid of anticoagulant activity. Neutralization of heparin occurs immediately and lasts for 2 hours, after which additional protamine may be needed. Protamine is administered by slow intravenous injection (no faster than 20 mg/min or 50 mg in 10 min). Dosage can be estimated by employing the knowledge that 1 mg of protamine will inactivate 100 units of heparin. Hence, for each 100 units of heparin in the body, 1 mg of protamine should be injected.

## Laboratory Monitoring

The objective of anticoagulant therapy is to reduce blood coagulability to a level that is low enough to prevent thrombosis, but not so low as to promote spontaneous bleeding. Because heparin levels can be highly variable, achieving this goal is difficult, and requires careful control of dosage based on frequent tests of coagulation. The laboratory test employed most commonly to monitor heparin therapy is the *activated partial thromboplastin time* (APTT). The normal value for APTT is 40 seconds. At therapeutic levels, heparin increases the APTT by a factor of 1.5 to 2, making the APTT 60 to 80 seconds. Since heparin has a rapid onset and brief duration, if an APTT value should fall outside the therapeutic range, coagulability can be quickly corrected through an adjustment in dosage: if the APTT is too long (>80 seconds), the dosage should be lowered; conversely, if the APTT is too short (<60 seconds), the dosage should be increased. Measurements of APTT should be made frequently (every 4 to 6 hours) during the initial phase of therapy. Once an effective dosage has been established, one APTT measurement a day will suffice.

## Unitage and Preparations

*Unitage.* Heparin is prescribed in units, not in milligrams. The heparin unit is an index of anticoagulant activity, and is defined as the amount of heparin that will prevent 1.0 ml of sheep plasma from coagulating for 1 hour. Heparin is prescribed in units because heparin preparations tend to differ from one another in anticoagulant activity when compared on a milligram basis.

*Preparations.* Two salts of heparin are available: heparin sodium and heparin calcium. *Heparin sodium* [Liquaemin

Sodium] is dispensed in single-dose vials; multiple-dose vials; and unit-dose, preloaded syringes that have their own needles. Concentrations range from 1000 to 40,000 units/ml. Heparin sodium for use in heparin locks [Hep-Lock] is dispensed in dilute solutions (10 and 100 units/ml) that are too weak to produce systemic anticoagulant effects.

*Heparin calcium* [Calciparine] is dispensed in single-dose (5000 units) prefilled syringes. Heparin calcium may carry a lower risk of local hematoma than heparin sodium.

## Dosage and Administration

*General Considerations.* Heparin is administered by injection only. Two routes are employed: (1) intravenous (either intermittent or continuous) and (2) subcutaneous. Intramuscular injection causes hematoma and must not be used. Heparin is not administered orally because heparin is too large and too polar for intestinal absorption.

Dosage varies with the specific application. Postoperative prophylaxis of thrombosis, for example, requires relatively small doses. In other situations, such as open heart surgery, much larger doses are required. The dosages given below are for "general anticoagulant therapy." As a rule, the APTT should be employed as a guideline for dosage determination; increases in APTT of 1.5- to 2-fold are therapeutic. Since heparin is dispensed in widely varying concentrations, the label must be read carefully to ensure that dosing is correct.

*Intermittent Intravenous Therapy.* Intermittent intravenous heparin is administered via an indwelling rubber-capped needle (heparin lock). Therapy is initiated with a dose of 10,000 units. Subsequent doses of 5000 to 10,000 units are given every 4 to 6 hours. The APTT should be taken 1 hour before each injection until dosage is stabilized. To avoid venous injury, the site of the heparin lock should be moved every 2 or 3 days. When heparin is administered intermittently, plasma levels of the drug will fluctuate. These fluctuations may result in alternating periods of excessive and insufficient anticoagulation.

*Continuous Intravenous Infusion.* Intravenous infusion provides steady levels of heparin, and therefore is preferred to intermittent injections. Dosing is begun with a bolus of 5000 to 10,000 units; this loading dose is followed by infusion at a rate of 1000 units/hr. During the initial phase of treatment, the APTT should be measured once every 4 hours and the infusion rate adjusted accordingly. To decrease the risk of overdose, when heparin solutions are prepared, the amount made up should be sufficient for no more than a 6-hour infusion. Heparin should be infused using an electric pump, and the rate should be checked every 30 to 60 minutes.

*Deep Subcutaneous Injection.* Subcutaneous injections are made deep into the fatty layer of the abdomen (but not within 2 inches of the umbilicus). The heparin solution should be withdrawn using a 20- to 22-gauge needle. This needle is then discarded and replaced with a small needle (1/2 to 5/8 inch, 25- or 26-gauge) to make the injection. Following administration, firm but gentle pressure should be applied to the injection site for 1 to 2 minutes. The initial SC dose is 10,000 to 20,000 units (preceded immediately by an IV loading dose of 5000 units). The initial SC dose is followed by either (1) 8000 to 10,000 units every 8 hours or (2) 15,000 to 20,000 units every 12 hours. Dosage is adjusted on the basis of APTT taken 4 to 6 hours after each injection. Injection sites should be rotated.

*Low-Dose Therapy.* Heparin in low doses is given for prophylaxis against postoperative thromboembolism. The initial dose (5000 units SC) is given 2 hours prior to surgery. Additional doses of 5000 units are given every 8 to 12 hours for 7 days (or until the patient is ambulatory). Low-dose heparin is also employed as adjunctive therapy for patients with myocardial infarction. During low-dose therapy, monitoring of APTT is not usually required.

## Low-Molecular-Weight Heparins

### Group Properties

Low-molecular-weight (LMW) heparins are simply heparin preparations composed of molecules that are shorter than those found in standard heparin. LMW heparins are as effective as standard heparin, and offer several advantages. Most importantly, LMW heparins can be given on a fixed-dose schedule and don't require APTT monitoring. As a result, LMW heparins can be used at home, whereas standard heparin must be given in a hospital. At this time, only two LMW heparins are available in the United States. Their names are enoxaparin [Lovenox] and dalteparin [Fragmin]. Differences between LMW heparins and standard heparin are summarized in Table 50-2.

**Production.** LMW heparins are produced by depolymerizing standard heparin (i.e., breaking standard heparin into smaller pieces). Molecular weights in LMW preparations range between 1000 and 9000, with a mean of 4000 to 5000. In comparison, molecular weights in standard heparin preparations range between 3000 and 30,000, with a mean of 12,000 to 15,000.

**Mechanism of Action.** Anticoagulant activity of LMW heparin is mediated by the same active pentasaccharide sequence that mediates anticoagulant action of standard heparin. However, because LMW heparin molecules are short, they do not have quite the same effect as standard heparin. In particular, whereas standard heparin is equally good at inactivating factor Xa *and* thrombin, *LMW heparin preferentially inactivates factor Xa*, being much less able to inactivate thrombin. Why the difference? In order to inactivate thrombin, a heparin chain must contain not only the pentasaccharide sequence that activates antithrombin III, it must also be long enough to provide a binding site for thrombin. This binding site is necessary because inactivation of thrombin requires simultaneous binding of thrombin with heparin and antithrombin III (see Fig. 50-2). In contrast to standard heparin chains, most LMW heparin chains are too short to allow thrombin binding, and hence are unable to inactivate this clotting factor.

Inactivation of factor Xa differs from inactivation of thrombin. Specifically, unlike thrombin, factor Xa need only bind with antithrombin III (that has been activated by heparin) to undergo inactivation; simultaneous binding of factor Xa with heparin and antithrombin III is unnecessary. Accordingly, since LMW heparin can activate antithrombin III just as well as standard heparin can, LMW heparin is fully able to inactivate factor Xa—even though LMW heparin molecules are generally too short to facilitate inactivation of thrombin.

**Therapeutic Use.** In the United States, LMW heparins are approved only for prophylaxis of deep vein thrombosis (DVT) following hip replacement surgery or high-risk abdominal surgery. Although lacking approval, LMW heparins have also been employed to treat existing DVT. When used for prophylaxis or treatment of DVT, LMW heparins are at least as effective as standard heparin, and possibly more effective.

**Pharmacokinetics.** LMW heparin differs from standard heparin with respect to nonspecific binding and half-life.

## TABLE 50-2. COMPARISON OF STANDARD (UNFRACTIONATED) HEPARIN WITH LOW-MOLECULAR-WEIGHT HEPARIN

| Property | Type of Heparin | |
| --- | --- | --- |
| | Standard | LMW |
| Molecular weight range | 3000–30,000 | 1000–9000 |
| Mean molecular weight | 12,000–15,000 | 4000–5000 |
| Mechanism of action | Inactivation of factor Xa and thrombin | Preferential inactivation of factor Xa |
| Routes | IV, SC | SC only |
| Nonspecific binding | Widespread | Minimal |
| Laboratory monitoring | APTT monitoring is essential | No APTT monitoring required |
| Dosage | Dosage must be adjusted on basis of APTT | Dosage is fixed |
| Setting for use | Hospital | Hospital or home |
| Cost | $3/day for heparin itself, but hospitalization and APTT monitoring greatly increase the real cost | $14/day for LMW heparin, but home use and absence of APTT monitoring greatly reduce the real cost |

In contrast to standard heparin, LMW heparin does not undergo nonspecific binding to proteins and tissues. As a result, plasma levels of LMW heparin are highly predictable. The elimination half-life of LMW heparin is two to four times longer than that of standard heparin.

***Administration, Dosing, and Monitoring.*** LMW heparins are administered SC. Dosage is based on body weight. Because plasma levels of LMW heparin are predictable for any given dose, these preparations can be administered on a fixed schedule without the need for laboratory monitoring. This contrasts with standard heparin therapy, which requires adjustment of dosage on the basis of APTT measurements. Because LMW heparin has an extended half-life, dosing can be done once or twice daily. For prophylaxis of DVT, dosing is begun in the perioperative period and continued for 5 to 10 days.

***Adverse Effects and Interactions.*** *Bleeding* is the major adverse effect of LMW heparin. However, the incidence of bleeding complications is less than with standard heparin. Despite the potential for bleeding, LMW heparin is considered safe for outpatient use. Like standard heparin, LMW heparin can cause *thrombocytopenia*, but the incidence may be lower than with standard heparin. Moreover, when thrombocytopenia does occur, it is not associated with an increase in thrombotic events. As with standard heparin, overdosage with LMW heparin can be treated with protamine sulfate. Like standard heparin, LMW heparin should be used with caution in patients taking antiplatelet drugs (e.g., aspirin) or warfarin.

***Cost.*** LMW heparins cost more than standard heparin (e.g., about $13/day for dalteparin vs. $3/day for standard heparin). However, since LMW heparins can be used at home and don't require monitoring of APTT, the overall cost of treatment is far less than with standard heparin.

### Individual Preparations

In the United States, two LMW heparin preparations are available: enoxaparin and dalteparin. Other LMW heparins are available outside this country. Each LMW preparation is unique. Hence clinical experience with one LMW heparin may not apply fully to the others and vice versa.

***Enoxaparin.*** Enoxaparin [Lovenox] was the first LMW heparin available in the United States. The drug is prepared by depolymerization of unfractionated porcine heparin. Molecular weights range between 2000 and 8000. The drug is approved for prevention of DVT following hip and knee replacement surgery. For these indications, the recommended dosage is 30 mg twice daily administered by deep SC injection. Dosing should begin as soon after surgery as possible, and no longer than 24 hours after. The average duration of treatment is 7 to 10 days. In the event of overdose, hemorrhage can be controlled with protamine sulfate; the dosage is 1 mg of protamine sulfate for each milligram of enoxaparin administered.

***Dalteparin.*** Dalteparin [Fragmin] was the second LMW heparin to be marketed in the United States. The drug is prepared by depolymerization of porcine heparin. Molecular weights range between 2000 and 9000, the average being about 5000. The only approved indication for dalteparin is prevention of DVT after abdominal surgery in patients considered at risk for thrombotic complications. Included are obese patients, those over 40, and those with malignancy or a history of DVT or pulmonary em-

bolism. For prophylaxis of DVT, the recommended dosage is 2500 anti–factor Xa IU injected SC once daily, beginning 1 or 2 hours before surgery and continuing for 5 to 10 days postoperatively. Overdose is treated with 1 mg of protamine sulfate for every 100 anti–factor Xa IU of dalteparin administered.

# Oral Anticoagulants

Oral anticoagulants are similar to heparin in some respects and quite different in others. Like heparin, oral anticoagulants are used to prevent thrombosis. In contrast to heparin, oral agents have a delayed onset of action, which makes them inappropriate for emergency use. However, because they don't require injection, these drugs are well suited for long-term prophylaxis. As with heparin, oral anticoagulants carry a significant risk of hemorrhage. This risk is amplified by the many drug interactions to which the oral agents are subject. In the United States, only two oral anticoagulants are available: warfarin and anisindione. Of these, warfarin is by far the most frequently prescribed.

## Warfarin

Warfarin [Coumadin, Panwarfin, Sofarin] is the oldest member of the oral anticoagulant family and will serve as our prototype for the group.

### History

The history of warfarin underscores the potential hazards of the oral anticoagulants. The story of warfarin began with the observation that ingestion of spoiled clover silage could induce bleeding in cattle; the causative agent was identified as bishydroxycoumarin (dicumarol). Research into derivatives of dicumarol resulted in the synthesis of warfarin. When warfarin was first developed, clinical use was ruled out because of concerns about hemorrhage. Instead of becoming a medicine, warfarin was used to kill rats. The drug proved especially effective in this application and remains one of our most widely used rodenticides. Clinical interest in warfarin was renewed following the report of a failed suicide attempt using huge doses of a warfarin-based rat poison. The clinical trials triggered by that event soon demonstrated that warfarin could be employed safely in humans.

### Mechanism of Action

Warfarin suppresses coagulation by acting as an *antagonist of vitamin K*. Four clotting factors (factors VII, IX, X, and prothrombin) require vitamin K for their synthesis. By antagonizing vitamin K, warfarin blocks the biosynthesis of these vitamin K–dependent factors.

### Pharmacokinetics

***Absorption, Distribution, and Elimination.*** Warfarin is readily absorbed following oral administration. Once in the bloodstream, about 99% of warfarin becomes bound to albumin. This binding provides the basis of several drug interactions. Those warfarin molecules that remain free (unbound) can readily cross membranes, including those of the placenta and milk-producing glands. Warfarin undergoes hepatic metabolism followed by excretion in the urine and feces.

***Time Course of Effects.*** Although warfarin acts quickly to inhibit clotting factor synthesis, noticeable anticoagulant effects are delayed. The delay occurs because warfarin has no effect on clotting factors that already exist at the time of drug administration. Until these clotting factors decay, coagulation remains unaffected. Since decay of clotting factors occurs with a half-life of 6 hours to 2.5 days (depending on the clotting factor under consideration), initial responses to warfarin may not be evident until 8 to 12 hours after administration. Peak effects do not develop for several days.

After warfarin is discontinued, coagulation remains inhibited for 2 to 5 days. This residual effect is due to the long half-life of warfarin (1.5 to 2 days). Because warfarin leaves the body slowly, synthesis of new clotting factors remains suppressed, despite cessation of drug administration.

### Therapeutic Uses

Warfarin is employed most frequently for long-term prophylaxis of thrombosis. Specific indications are (1) prevention of venous thrombosis and associated pulmonary embolism, (2) prevention of thromboembolism in patients with prosthetic heart valves, and (3) prevention of thrombosis during atrial fibrillation. For all of these indications, warfarin is the oral anticoagulant of choice. Because onset of effects is delayed, warfarin is not useful in emergencies. When rapid action is needed, therapy can be initiated with heparin.

### Monitoring Treatment

The anticoagulant effects of warfarin are evaluated by monitoring *prothrombin time* (PT)—a coagulation test that is especially sensitive to alterations in vitamin K-dependent factors. The average pretreatment value for PT is 12 seconds. Treatment with warfarin prolongs PT.

Traditionally, PT test results have been reported as a *PT ratio*, which is simply the ratio of the patient's PT to a control PT. However, there is a serious problem with this form of reporting: test results can vary widely among laboratories. The underlying cause of variability is thromboplastin, a critical reagent employed in the PT test. To ensure that test results from different laboratories are comparable, results are now reported in terms of an *international normalized ratio* (INR). The INR is determined by multiplying the observed PT ratio by a correction factor specific to the particular thromboplastin preparation employed in the test.

The objective of treatment is to raise the INR to an appropriate value. Recommended INR ranges are summarized in Table 50–3. As indicated, an INR of 2 to 3 is appropriate for most patients—although for some patients the target INR is 3 to 4.5. If the INR is below the recommended range, warfarin dosage should be increased. Conversely, if the INR is above the recommended range,

### TABLE 50–3. MONITORING ORAL ANTICOAGULANT THERAPY: RECOMMENDED RANGES OF PROTHROMBIN TIME-DERIVED VALUES

| Condition Being Treated | Recommended Ranges | |
| --- | --- | --- |
| | Observed PT Ratio* | INR[†] |
| Acute myocardial infarction[‡] | 1.3–1.5 | 2.0–3.0 |
| Atrial fibrillation[‡] | 1.3–1.5 | 2.0–3.0 |
| Valvular heart disease[‡] | 1.3–1.5 | 2.0–3.0 |
| Pulmonary embolism | 1.3–1.5 | 2.0–3.0 |
| Venous thrombosis[§] | 1.3–1.5 | 2.0–3.0 |
| Tissue heart valves[‡] | 1.3–1.5 | 2.0–3.0 |
| Mechanical heart valves | 1.5–2.0 | 3.0–4.5 |
| Systemic embolism | | |
| Prevention | 1.3–1.5 | 2.0–3.0 |
| Recurrent | 1.5–2.0 | 3.0–4.5 |

*Observed PT ratio = ratio of patient's prothrombin time (PT) to a control PT value. In this particular case, the reagent used to determine the control PT value is one of the preparations of rabbit brain thromboplastin employed in the United States. Had a different preparation of thromboplastin been used, the observed PT ratio could be very different.

[†]INR = international normalized ratio. This value is calculated from the observed PT ratio. The INR is equivalent to the PT ratio that would have been obtained if the patient's PT has been compared to a PT value obtained using the International Reference Preparation, a standardized human brain thromboplastin prepared by the World Health Organization. In contrast to PT ratios, INR values are comparable from one laboratory to the next throughout the United States and the rest of the world.

[‡]For prevention of systemic embolism.

[§]Prophylaxis in high-risk surgery; treatment.

the dosage should be reduced. Unfortunately, since warfarin has a delayed onset and prolonged duration of action, the INR cannot be altered quickly: once the dosage has been changed, the desired INR may take a week or more to be reached.

PT must be determined frequently during warfarin therapy. PT should be measured daily during the first 5 days of treatment, twice a week for the next 1 to 2 weeks, once a week for the next 1 to 2 months, and every 2 to 4 weeks thereafter. In addition, PT should be determined whenever a drug that interacts with warfarin is added to or deleted from the regimen.

Concurrent therapy with heparin can influence PT values. To minimize this influence, blood for PT determinations should be drawn no sooner than 5 hours after an intravenous injection of heparin, and no sooner than 24 hours after a subcutaneous injection.

### Adverse Effects

***Hemorrhage.*** Bleeding is the major complication of warfarin therapy. Hemorrhage can occur at any site. Patients should be monitored closely for signs of bleeding. For specific signs, refer to the discussion of heparin-induced hemorrhage. If bleeding develops, warfarin should be discontinued. Severe overdose can be treated with *vitamin K* (see below). Patients should be encouraged to carry identification (e.g., Medic Alert bracelet) to inform emergency personnel of warfarin use.

Several measures can reduce the risk of bleeding. Candidates for treatment must be carefully screened for risk factors (see *Warnings and Contraindications*). Prothrombin time must be measured frequently. A variety of drugs can potentiate warfarin's effects (see below); these must be used with extreme care. Patients should be given detailed verbal and written instructions regarding signs of bleeding, dosage size and timing, and scheduling of PT tests. When a patient is incapable of accurate self-medication, a responsible individual must supervise therapy. Patients should be advised to record administration of each dose, rather than relying on memory. A soft toothbrush can reduce gingival bleeding. An electric razor can reduce cuts from shaving.

Warfarin intensifies bleeding during surgery and dental procedures. Surgeons and dentists must be informed of warfarin use. Patients anticipating elective procedures should discontinue warfarin several days prior to the appointment. If an emergency procedure must be performed, injection of vitamin K will help suppress bleeding.

**Fetal Hemorrhage and Teratogenesis from Use During Pregnancy.** Warfarin can cross the placenta and affect the developing fetus. Fetal hemorrhage and death have occurred. In addition, the drug can cause gross malformation, central nervous system (CNS) defects, and optic atrophy. Accordingly, *warfarin is classified in FDA Pregnancy Category X: the risks to the developing fetus outweigh any possible benefits of treatment.* Women of child-bearing age should be informed about the potential for teratogenesis and advised to postpone pregnancy. If pregnancy occurs, the possibility of termination should be discussed. If an anticoagulant is needed during pregnancy, heparin, which does not cross the placenta, should be employed.

**Use During Lactation.** Warfarin enters breast milk. Women should be advised against breast-feeding.

**Other Adverse Effects.** Adverse effects other than hemorrhage are uncommon. Possible undesired responses include skin necrosis, alopecia, urticaria, dermatitis, fever, GI disturbances, and red-orange discoloration of urine, which must not be confused with hematuria.

## Drug Interactions

**General Considerations.** Warfarin is subject to a large number of clinically significant adverse interactions—perhaps more than any other drug. As a result of drug interactions, anticoagulant effects may be reduced to the point of permitting thrombosis, or they may be increased to the point of causing hemorrhage. Patients must be informed about the potential for hazardous interactions and instructed to avoid all drugs not specifically approved by the physician. This prohibition includes prescription drugs and over-the-counter preparations.

Interactions between warfarin and other drugs are summarized in Table 50-4. As indicated, the interactants fall into three major categories: (1) *drugs that increase anticoagulant effects*, (2) *drugs that promote bleeding*, and (3) *drugs that decrease anticoagulant effects*. The major mechanisms by which anticoagulant effects can be *increased* are (1) displacement of warfarin from plasma albumin and (2) inhibition of the hepatic enzymes that degrade warfarin. The major mechanisms for *decreasing* anticoagulant effects are (1) acceleration of warfarin degradation through induction of hepatic drug-metabolizing enzymes, (2) increased synthesis of clotting factors, and (3) inhibition of warfarin absorption. Mechanisms by which drugs can *promote bleeding*, and thereby complicate anticoagulant therapy, include (1) inhibition of platelet aggregation, (2) inhibition of the coagulation cascade, and (3) generation of gastrointestinal ulcers.

The existence of an interaction between warfarin and another drug does not absolutely preclude using the combination. Such an interaction does mean, however, that the combination must be used with due caution. The potential for harm is greatest when an interacting drug is being added to or deleted from the regimen. At these times, prothrombin time must be monitored, and the dosage of warfarin must be adjusted to compensate for the impact of removing or adding an interacting drug.

**Specific Interacting Drugs.** Of the many drugs listed in Table 50-4, a few are especially likely to produce interactions of clinical significance. Three of these agents are discussed below.

*Heparin.* The interaction of heparin with warfarin is obvious: being an anticoagulant itself, heparin directly increases the bleeding tendencies brought on by warfarin. Combined therapy with heparin plus warfarin must be performed with care.

*Aspirin.* Aspirin inhibits platelet aggregation. By blocking aggregation, aspirin can suppress formation of the platelet plug that initiates hemostasis. To make matters worse, aspirin can act directly on the GI tract to cause ulcers, thereby initiating bleeding. Hence, when the antifibrin effects of warfarin are coupled with the antiplatelet and ulcerogenic effects of aspirin, the potential for hemorrhagic disaster is substantial. Accordingly, patients should be warned specifically against using any product that contains aspirin, unless the physician has prescribed aspirin therapy. Drugs similar to aspirin (e.g., indomethacin, ibuprofen) should be avoided as well.

*Barbiturates.* Barbiturates (e.g., phenobarbital) are powerful inducers of hepatic drug-metabolizing enzymes. Hence barbiturates can accelerate warfarin degradation, thereby decreasing anticoagulant effects. Accordingly, if a barbiturate is added to the regimen, warfarin dosage must be increased. Of equal importance, when barbiturates are withdrawn, causing rates of drug metabolism to decline, a compensatory decrease in warfarin dosage must be made.

*Other Notable Interactions.* *Vitamin K* increases clotting factor synthesis, and can thereby decrease anticoagulant effects. *Rifampin* (a drug for tuberculosis) and *glutethimide* (a CNS depressant) can stimulate drug metabolism, and can thereby reduce anticoagulant effects. Conversely, *cimetidine* (a drug for ulcers) and *disulfiram* (a drug for treating alcoholism) can inhibit warfarin metabolism, and can thereby increase anticoagulant ef-

## TABLE 50-4. INTERACTIONS BETWEEN HEPARIN AND OTHER DRUGS

| Drug Category | Mechanism of Interaction | Representative Interacting Drugs |
|---|---|---|
| Drugs that *increase* the effects of warfarin | Displacement of warfarin from albumin | Aspirin and other salicylates Phenylbutazone Sulfonamides Chloral hydrate |
| | Inhibition of warfarin degradation | Cimetidine Disulfiram Phenylbutazone Sulfonamides |
| | Decreased synthesis of clotting factors | Oral antibiotics |
| Drugs that *promote* bleeding | Inhibition of platelet aggregation | Aspirin and other salicylates Dipyridamole Phenylbutazone Indomethacin |
| | Inhibition of clotting factors | Heparin Antimetabolites |
| | Promotion of ulcer formation | Aspirin Indomethacin Phenylbutazone Glucocorticoids |
| Drugs that *decrease* the effects of warfarin | Induction of drug-metabolizing enzymes | Barbiturates Carbamazepine Glutethimide Phenytoin |
| | Promotion of clotting factor synthesis | Vitamin $K_1$ Oral contraceptives |
| | Reduction of warfarin absorption | Cholestyramine Colestipol |

fects. *Sulfonamides* (antibacterial drugs) and *chloral hydrate* (a CNS depressant) can increase the effects of warfarin by displacing it from albumin.

## Warnings and Contraindications

Like heparin, warfarin is *contraindicated* for patients with *severe thrombocytopenia* or *uncontrollable bleeding* and for patients undergoing *lumbar puncture, regional anesthesia*, or *surgery of the eye, brain, or spinal cord*. Also like heparin, warfarin must be used with extreme *caution* in patients at high risk of bleeding, including those with *hemophilia, increased capillary permeability, dissecting aneurysm, GI ulcers*, and *severe hypertension*, and in women anticipating *abortion*. In addition, warfarin is contraindicated in the presence of *vitamin K deficiency, liver disease*, and *alcoholism*—conditions that can disrupt hepatic synthesis of clotting factors. Also, warfarin is contraindicated during *pregnancy* and *lactation*.

## Vitamin K₁ for Warfarin Overdose

The effects of warfarin overdose can be overcome with vitamin $K_1$ (phytonadione). Vitamin $K_1$ is an antagonist of warfarin action that can reverse warfarin-induced inhibition of clotting factor synthesis. (Vitamin $K_3$—mena-

dione—has no effect on warfarin action.) For mild bleeding, vitamin $K_1$ should be administered orally; a dose of 10 to 20 mg will cause prothrombin levels to normalize within 24 hours. If bleeding is severe, parenteral vitamin $K_1$ (5 to 50 mg) is indicated. If vitamin K fails to control bleeding, levels of clotting factors can be raised quickly by infusing fresh whole blood, fresh-frozen plasma, or plasma concentrates of vitamin K–dependent clotting factors.

Therapy with vitamin K is not without problems. The residual effects of vitamin K will hamper restoration of anticoagulant therapy once bleeding has stopped. This problem can be minimized by keeping vitamin K dosage low. Intravenous vitamin K has been associated with severe anaphylactoid reactions. Accordingly, IV administration should be employed only if other routes are not feasible, and only if the potential benefits outweigh the risks. The pharmacology of vitamin K is discussed in Chapter 74.

## Contrasts Between Warfarin and Heparin

Although heparin and warfarin are both anticoagulants, these drugs have several important differences. Whereas administration of warfarin is oral, heparin must be given by injection. Although both drugs decrease fibrin formation, they do so by different mechanisms: heparin works through antithrombin III, whereas warfarin inhibits syn-

## TABLE 50–5. SUMMARY OF CONTRASTS BETWEEN HEPARIN AND WARFARIN

|  | Heparin | Warfarin |
|---|---|---|
| *Mechanism of action* | Promotes action of antithrombin III | Inhibits synthesis of vitamin K-dependent clotting factors |
| *Route* | Intravenous or subcutaneous | Oral |
| *Onset* | Rapid (minutes) | Slow (hours) |
| *Duration* | Brief (hours) | Prolonged (days) |
| *Monitoring* | APTT* | PT† |
| *Antidote for overdose* | Protamine | Vitamin K₁ |

*Activated partial thromboplastin time.
†Prothrombin time. Test results are reported in terms of a PT ratio or in terms of an INR (international normalized ratio).

thesis of vitamin K-dependent clotting factors. Heparin and warfarin differ markedly with respect to time course of action: effects of heparin begin and fade rapidly, whereas effects of warfarin begin slowly but then persist for several days. Different tests are used to monitor therapy: changes in APTT are used to monitor heparin treatment, whereas changes in PT are used to monitor warfarin. Finally, these drugs differ with respect to management of overdose: protamine is given to counteract heparin; vitamin K₁ is given to counteract warfarin. These differences are summarized in Table 50–5.

### Preparations, Dosage, and Administration

Warfarin sodium [Coumadin, Panwarfin, Sofarin] is dispensed in tablets (1, 2, 2.5, 5, 7.5, and 10 mg) for oral use. The initial dosage is 10 mg/day. Maintenance dosages range from 2 to 10 mg/day and are determined by the target INR value: for most patients, dosage should be adjusted to produce an INR between 2 and 3.

## Anisindione

Anisindione [Miradon] has actions and uses like those of warfarin. However, since the incidence of severe side effects with this drug is much greater than with warfarin, use of anisindione is rare. The drug is dispensed in 50-mg tablets for oral administration. The initial dose is 300 mg. Maintenance dosages range from 25 to 250 mg/day.

# Antiplatelet Drugs

Antiplatelet drugs are agents that suppress platelet aggregation. Since a platelet core constitutes the bulk of an *arterial thrombus*, the principal indication for the antiplatelet drugs is prevention of thrombosis in *arteries*. In contrast, the principal indication for heparin and warfarin is prevention of thrombosis in veins. The antiplatelet drug employed most frequently is aspirin.

## Aspirin

The basic pharmacology of aspirin is discussed in Chapter 64. Consideration here is limited to the use of aspirin to prevent arterial thrombosis.

***Mechanism of Antiplatelet Action.*** Aspirin suppresses platelet aggregation by causing *irreversible inhibition of cyclooxygenase*, an enzyme required by platelets to synthesize thromboxane A₂ (TXA₂). As noted earlier, TXA₂ acts on platelets to promote aggregation. In addition, TXA₂ acts on vascular smooth muscle to promote vasoconstriction. Both actions promote hemostasis. By inhibiting cyclooxygenase, aspirin suppresses TXA₂-mediated vasoconstriction and platelet aggregation, thereby reducing the risk of arterial thrombosis. Since inhibition of cyclooxygenase by aspirin is irreversible, and since platelets lack the machinery to synthesize new cyclooxygenase, the effects of a single dose of aspirin persist for the life of the platelet (7 to 10 days).

In addition to inhibiting the synthesis of TXA₂, aspirin can inhibit synthesis of *prostacyclin* by the blood vessel wall. Since prostacyclin has effects that are exactly opposite to those of TXA₂—namely, suppression of platelet aggregation and promotion of vasodilation—suppression of prostacyclin synthesis can partially counteract the beneficial effects of aspirin therapy. Fortunately, aspirin is able to inhibit synthesis of TXA₂ at doses that are lower than those needed to inhibit synthesis of prostacyclin. Accordingly, if we keep the dosage of aspirin *low* (325 mg/day or less), we can minimize inhibition of prostacyclin production, while maintaining inhibition of TXA₂ production.

***Indications for Antiplatelet Therapy.*** Antiplatelet therapy with aspirin has three applications of proven efficacy: (1) primary prophylaxis of myocardial infarction (MI), (2) prevention of reinfarction in patients who have experienced an acute MI, and (3) prevention of stroke in patients with a history of transient ischemic attacks (TIAs). In all three situations, prophylactic therapy with aspirin can reduce morbidity and mortality.

***Dosing.*** Dosages for antiplatelet therapy should be low—325 mg/day or less. Higher doses offer no therapeutic advantage, but do increase the risk of adverse effects, especially bleeding. In patients who have experienced an MI, dosages of 160 to 325 mg/day can be used to help prevent reinfarction. To reduce the incidence of TIAs, doses of 30 to 325 mg/day have been employed.

## Other Antiplatelet Drugs

### Ticlopidine

***Actions and Uses.*** Ticlopidine [Ticlid] is an oral antiplatelet drug approved only for prevention of thrombotic stroke. The drug is at least as effective as aspirin, but is much more expensive and carries a risk of neutropenia and agranulocytosis. In contrast to aspirin, ticlopidine acts by inhibiting ADP-mediated platelet aggregation, and not by inhibiting synthesis of thromboxane A₂. Suppression of aggregation persists for the life of the platelet.

***Pharmacokinetics.*** Ticlopidine is well absorbed following oral administration. Antiplatelet effects begin within 48 hours and become maximal in about a week. The drug undergoes extensive hepatic metabolism followed by renal excretion. Ticlopidine has a long half-life (4 to 5 days), and effects persist for a week or more after drug withdrawal.

*Adverse Effects.* The most common effects are *GI disturbances* (diarrhea, abdominal pain, flatulence, nausea, dyspepsia) and *dermatologic reactions* (rash, purpura, pruritus).

The most serious effects are hematologic. *Neutropenia* develops in 2.4% of those treated, and is sometimes severe. *Agranulocytosis* has occurred rarely. Both effects reverse within 1 to 3 weeks after drug withdrawal. Complete blood counts and a white cell differential should be obtained every 2 weeks through the first 3 months of treatment and at any sign of infection. Ticlopidine should be withdrawn if neutropenia or agranulocytosis develop.

*Preparations and Dosage.* Ticlopidine [Ticlid] is dispensed in 250-mg tablets for oral administration. The recommended dosage is 250 mg twice a day, administered with food.

### Dipyridamole

Dipyridamole [Persantine] suppresses platelet aggregation, perhaps by increasing plasma levels of adenosine. The drug is approved only for prevention of thromboembolism following heart valve replacement surgery. For this application, the drug is always employed in combination with warfarin. The recommended dosage is 75 to 100 mg 4 times a day.

### Abciximab

*Use and Dosage.* Abciximab [ReoPro] is an expensive drug used to prevent reocclusion of coronary blood vessels following percutaneous transluminal coronary angioplasty (PTCA). Reocclusion is a common problem because PTCA damages the blood vessel wall, and thereby encourages platelet aggregation. Abciximab treatment consists of an IV bolus (25 mg/kg) administered 10 to 60 minutes prior to PTCA, followed by an infusion (10 µg/min) for 12 hours. The cost of bolus plus infusion is about $1200. Abciximab is intended for use in combination with aspirin and heparin.

*Mechanism of Action.* Abciximab is a purified Fab fragment of a monoclonal antibody. The drug acts by blocking glycoprotein IIb/IIIa receptors on the platelet surface. As a result, fibrinogen and other adhesive glycoproteins are unable to attach to activated platelets, and hence aggregation is prevented.

*Adverse Effects.* Abciximab doubles the risk of major bleeding, especially at the PTCA access site in the femoral artery. The drug may also cause gastrointestinal, urogenital, and retroperitoneal bleeds. However, it does not increase the risk of fatal hemorrhage or hemorrhagic stroke. In the event of severe bleeding, infusion of abciximab and heparin should be discontinued.

# Thrombolytic Drugs

As their name implies, thrombolytic drugs act to remove thrombi that have already formed. This contrasts with the anticoagulants, which act to prevent thrombus formation. Five thrombolytic drugs are available: streptokinase, alteplase, reteplase, urokinase, and anistreplase. All five carry a risk of serious bleeding, and hence should be administered only by clinicians skilled in their use. Thrombolytic agents are employed acutely and only for severe thrombotic disease. Because of their mechanism of action, these agents are also known as *fibrinolytics.*

Properties of individual agents are summarized in Table 50-6.

## Streptokinase

Streptokinase [Kabikinase, Streptase] was the first thrombolytic drug available and will serve as our prototype for the group.

### Mechanism of Action

Streptokinase acts by an indirect mechanism. The drug first binds to *plasminogen* to form a complex. This complex then acts on other molecules of plasminogen (a proenzyme present in blood) to cause their conversion into plasmin, an enzyme that digests the fibrin meshwork of clots. In addition to digesting clots, plasmin degrades fibrinogen and other clotting factors; these actions do not contribute to lysis of thrombi, but they do increase the risk of hemorrhage.

### Therapeutic Uses

Streptokinase has three major indications: (1) acute coronary thrombosis (acute MI), (2) deep vein thrombosis, and (3) massive pulmonary emboli. In all three situations, timely intervention is essential. For example, in patients with acute MI, results are best when thrombolytic therapy is started within 4 to 6 hours of the onset of symptoms. Thrombolytic therapy of acute MI is discussed further in Chapter 47 (Management of Myocardial Infarction).

### Pharmacokinetics

Streptokinase may be administered by IV infusion or by infusion directly into an occluded coronary artery. Because of rapid inactivation, the drug has a plasma half-life of only 40 to 80 minutes.

### Adverse Effects

*Bleeding.* Bleeding is the major complication of treatment. Intracranial hemorrhage (ICH), which occurs in 1% of patients, is by far the most serious concern. Bleeding occurs for two reasons: (1) plasmin can destroy pre-existing clots, and can thereby promote recurrence of bleeding at sites of recently healed injury; and (2) by degrading clotting factors, plasmin can disrupt the coagulation cascade, and can thereby interfere with new clot formation in response to vascular injury. Likely sites of bleeding include recent wounds, sites of needle puncture, and sites at which invasive procedures have been performed. Anticoagulants (heparin, warfarin) and antiplatelet drugs (e.g., aspirin) further increase the risk of hemorrhage. Accordingly, high-dose therapy with these drugs must be avoided until thrombolytic effects of streptokinase have abated.

Management of bleeding depends on the severity. Oozing at sites of cutaneous puncture can be controlled with a pressure dressing. If severe bleeding occurs, streptokinase should be discontinued. Patients who require blood replacement can be given whole blood or blood

## TABLE 50-6. PROPERTIES OF THROMBOLYTIC DRUGS

| Property | Drug | | | | |
|---|---|---|---|---|---|
| | Streptokinase | Alteplase (tPA) | Reteplase | Anistreplase | Urokinase |
| *Trade name* | Kabikinase, Streptase | Activase | Retavase | Eminase | Abbokinase |
| *Description* | A compound that forms an active complex with plasminogen | A compound identical to human tissue plasminogen activator (tPA) | A compound that contains the active sequence of amino acids present in tPA | An equimolar complex of acetylated streptokinase and human plasminogen | An enzyme that converts plasminogen to plasmin |
| *Source* | Streptococcal culture | Recombinant DNA technology | Recombinant DNA technology | Streptococcal culture and human plasma | Cultured human fetal kidney cells |
| *Mechanism* | All five drugs act directly or indirectly to convert plasminogen to plasmin, an enzyme that degrades the fibrin matrix of thrombi | | | | |
| *Adverse effects* | | | | | |
| Bleeding | Yes | Yes | Yes | Yes | Yes |
| Allergic reactions | Yes | No | No | Yes | No |
| *Half-life (min)* | 40–80 | 5–10 | 13–16 | 40–60 | 15–20 |
| *Dosage and administration for acute MI* | *Intravenous:* 1.5 million IU infused over 30–60 min *Intracoronary:* 20,000 IU bolus, then 2000 IU/min for 60 min | *Intravenous:* 15 mg bolus, then 50 mg infused over 30 min, then 35 mg infused over 60 min | *Intravenous:* 10 IU bolus 2 times, separated by 30 min | *Intravenous:* 30 IU injected over 2-5 min | *Intracoronary:* 6000 IU/min for 2 hr or less |
| *Cost* | $300 | $2300 | $2200 | $2000 | $3800 |

products (packed red blood cells, fresh-frozen plasma). As a rule, blood replacement restores hemostasis. However, if this approach fails, excessive fibrinolysis can be reversed with IV *aminocaproic acid* [Amicar], a compound that prevents activation of plasminogen and directly inhibits plasmin.

The risk of bleeding can be lowered by:

• Minimizing physical manipulation of the patient
• Avoiding subcutaneous and intramuscular injections
• Minimizing invasive procedures
• Minimizing concurrent use of anticoagulants (heparin, warfarin)
• Minimizing concurrent use of antiplatelet drugs (e.g., aspirin)

Because of the risk of hemorrhage, streptokinase and other thrombolytic drugs must be avoided by patients at high risk for bleeding complications, and must be used with great caution in patients at lower risk of bleeding. A list of absolute and relative contraindications to thrombolytic therapy is presented in Table 50-7.

**Antibody Production.** Streptokinase is a foreign protein extracted from cultures of streptococci. As a result, antibodies may form. Two consequences are possible: *allergic reactions* and *neutralization of streptokinase*. The most common allergic reactions are urticaria, itching, flushing, and headache. These can be treated with antihistamines. Severe anaphylaxis is rare. Because neutralizing antibodies may develop within a few days of streptokinase administration, repeat courses of streptokinase may be ineffective. Hence, if a repeat course is needed, a different thrombolytic (e.g., alteplase) should be chosen.

**Hypotension.** Streptokinase may cause significant hypotension soon after administration. The incidence is 1% to 10%. Hypotension is not related to bleeding or allergic reactions. Blood pressure should be monitored. If hypotension develops, it may be necessary to slow the streptokinase infusion.

**Fever.** Temperature elevation of 1.5°F or more occurs in one third of those treated. Only 3.5% of patients develop temperatures above 104°F. Acetaminophen—not aspirin—should be used to lower temperature.

### Preparations, Dosage, and Administration

Streptokinase [Kabikinase, Streptase] is dispensed as a powder and must be reconstituted for use. Solutions are prepared with either 0.9% saline or 5% dextrose. Dosage is prescribed in International Units.

For treatment of *pulmonary embolism, DVT*, and *arterial thrombosis or embolism*, streptokinase is administered by IV infusion. Therapy is usually initiated with an IV loading dose of 250,000 IU infused over 30 minutes. After the loading dose, infusion is continued for 1 to 3 days at a rate of 100,000 IU/hr.

For treatment of an evolving *myocardial infarction*, streptokinase may be infused through a catheter placed in the oc-

## TABLE 50–7. CONTRAINDICATIONS OF THROMBOLYTIC THERAPY*

*Absolute Contraindications*

  Active bleeding
  Aortic dissection
  Acute pericarditis
  Cerebral neoplasm
  History of intracranial hemorrhage
  Cerebral vascular disease (aneurysm, arteriovenous
    malformation)

*Relative Contraindications*

  Either urogenital hemorrhage, cerebral hemorrhage,
    or ischemic stroke within the prior 6 months
  Either major surgery, organ biopsy, puncture of a
    noncompressible vessel, prolonged cardiopulmonary
    resuscitation, major trauma, or head trauma within
    the prior 2 to 4 weeks
  Severe uncontrolled hypertension (systolic pressure
    >200 mm Hg, diastolic pressure >120 mm Hg, or both)
  Diabetic proliferative retinopathy
  History of bleeding diathesis
  History of hepatic dysfunction
  History of cancer
  Pregnancy

* As recommended by the Fourth American College of Chest
  Physicians Consensus Conference on Antithrombotic Therapy.

cluded coronary artery. This technique offers two benefits: first, high levels of streptokinase are achieved at the site where the drug is needed; and second, high levels are avoided at other sites, thereby minimizing generalized bleeding. Timing of therapy is critical: streptokinase is most effective when therapy is initiated within 6 hours of the onset of symptoms.

## Alteplase (tPA)

Alteplase [Activase], also known as tissue plasminogen activator (tPA), is produced commercially by recombinant DNA technology. The commercial preparation is identical to naturally occurring human tPA, an enzyme that promotes conversion of plasminogen to plasmin, which then acts to digest the fibrin matrix of clots. Low therapeutic doses produce selective activation of plasminogen that is bound to fibrin in thrombi. As a result, activation of plasminogen in the general circulation is minimal. However, despite selective activation of fibrin-bound plasminogen, bleeding tendencies with alteplase are equivalent to those seen with the other thrombolytic drugs. Furthermore, the risk of intracranial bleeding is higher with alteplase than with streptokinase. Since alteplase is devoid of foreign proteins, the drug does not cause allergic reactions. In contrast to streptokinase, alteplase does not induce hypotension. Alteplase has a short half-life (5 to 10 minutes) owing to rapid hepatic inactivation.

Like streptokinase, alteplase is indicated for acute MI and pulmonary embolism. In addition, alteplase was recently approved for treating ischemic stroke. As discussed below, the GUSTO trial has shown that alteplase is slightly better than streptokinase for treating acute MI. Unfortunately, alteplase is also much more expensive: a single course of treatment costs about $2300, compared with $300 for treatment with streptokinase.

Alteplase is now given by an "accelerated" or "front-loaded" schedule. In this schedule, the infusion time is only 90 minutes, compared with the 2 hours that had been used previously. For patients who weigh over 67 kg, the total dose for treating acute MI is 100 mg. Administration is divided into three phases: a 15-mg IV bolus, followed by 50 mg infused over 30 minutes, followed in turn by 35 mg infused over 60 minutes. Total doses in excess of 100 mg are associated with an increased risk of intracranial bleeding and should be avoided.

## Other Thrombolytic Drugs

Urokinase, anistreplase, and reteplase are similar to streptokinase and alteplase with regard to mechanism of action, indications, and ability to promote bleeding. Principal differences among these drugs relate to half-life, source, antigenicity, cost, and specific indications.

### Urokinase

Urokinase [Abbokinase] is an enzyme that occurs naturally in human urine. Commercial urokinase is prepared by extraction from cultures of human fetal kidney cells. Like streptokinase, urokinase promotes the conversion of plasminogen into plasmin, its active form. As with other thrombolytics, bleeding is the principal adverse effect. Since urokinase is human derived, it is not antigenic; hence allergic reactions do not occur. Urokinase has a short half-life (15 to 20 minutes) owing to rapid inactivation by the liver. The drug is approved for acute MI, DVT, and clearance of IV catheters. For treatment of acute MI, urokinase is infused for 2 hours or less at a rate of 6000 IU/hr. Because of its high cost (see Table 50–6), urokinase is used much less frequently than streptokinase.

### Anistreplase (APSAC)

Anistreplase [Eminase] is an acylated complex of streptokinase plus human plasminogen. The streptokinase is obtained from streptococcal culture; the human plasminogen is obtained by extraction from human plasma. Because it is acylated, the plasminogen in anistreplase is inactive. Once in the body, the drug undergoes gradual deacylation followed by conversion to plasmin, which then acts to digest fibrin in clots. In addition to degrading fibrin in thrombi, anistreplase can degrade circulating fibrinogen. Both actions (digestion of fibrin and degradation of fibrinogen) promote bleeding. The risk of bleeding complications with anistreplase is the same as with the other thrombolytic drugs. Since anistreplase contains streptokinase (a foreign protein), the drug can cause allergic reactions. Like streptokinase, anistreplase may cause hypotension. Anistreplase differs from the other thrombolytics in that it can be administered by slow IV injection instead of by infusion. This makes anistreplase more convenient to use. The recommended dosage for acute MI is 30 units injected over 2 to 5 minutes. Like urokinase and alteplase, anistreplase is expensive, costing over $2000 for one course of treatment. An alternative name for anistreplase is anisoylated plasminogen-streptokinase activator complex, or APSAC.

### Reteplase

Reteplase [Retavase] is a derivative of tPA produced by recombinant DNA technology. In contrast to tPA, which contains 527 amino acids, reteplase is composed of only 355 amino acids. Like tPA, reteplase converts plasminogen to plasmin, which in turn digests the fibrin matrix of the thrombus. Reteplase has a short half-life (13 to 16 minutes) because of rapid clearance by the liver and kidneys. As with other thrombolytic drugs, bleeding is the major adverse effect. The risk of bleeding is increased by concurrent use of heparin and aspirin. Allergic reactions have not been reported.

Reteplase was compared with front-loaded alteplase in RAPID II (Reteplase vs. Alteplase Patency Investigation During Myocardial Infarction Study). The results indicate that reteplase produces higher rates of early reperfusion than alteplase without increasing the risk of hemorrhagic stroke or other complications.

Reteplase is approved only for acute MI. Treatment consists of two 10-unit doses separated by 30 minutes. Each dose is given by IV bolus injected over a 2-minute interval. Reteplase should not be administered through a line that contains heparin. If a heparin-containing line must be used, it should be flushed prior to giving reteplase.

## Streptokinase versus Alteplase: The GUSTO Trial

The GUSTO trial (Global Utilization of Streptokinase and tPA for Occluded Coronary Arteries) is the largest study ever conducted on the treatment of acute MI. Over 41,000 patients from 15 countries participated. The results indicate that *mortality* from MI in patients receiving alteplase (tPA) is somewhat lower than in patients receiving streptokinase (SK)—although the risk of *hemorrhagic stroke* with tPA is higher. However, as discussed below, the apparent superiority of tPA as seen in GUSTO may not be relevant to everyday clinical practice.

In GUSTO, each participant received one of the following treatments (30-day mortality rates are in parentheses):

- tPA + IV heparin (6.3%)
- SK + IV heparin (7.4%)
- SK + SC heparin (7.2%)
- SK + tPA + IV heparin (7.0%)

As the mortality figures indicate, 7.4 of each 100 patients who received SK (plus IV heparin) died within 30 days. In contrast, only 6.3 of each 100 patients who received tPA (plus IV heparin) died within 30 days. Hence, by using tPA instead of SK, we might expect to save 1 additional life for each 100 patients.

What the above figures don't indicate is the timing of tPA administration with respect to onset of MI symptoms. In GUSTO, nearly 90% of patients received treatment within 2 to 4 hours of symptom onset. Among patients who received tPA within 2 hours of symptom onset, the death rate was only 5.4%; among those treated 2 to 4 hours after symptom onset, the rate increased to 6.6%; and among those treated 4 to 6 hours after symptom onset, the rate jumped to 9.4%. Not only do these figures underscore the importance of early treatment of MI, they also bring into question the relevance to GUSTO to ordinary clinical practice—since, in usual practice, very few patients are treated as early as those in GUSTO. Furthermore, among patients who are treated *after* 4 hours, GUSTO showed no significant difference in mortal-

ity between treatment with tPA and treatment with SK. Hence, although tPA may be superior to SK when these drugs are employed under *ideal* conditions, tPA may not be superior in everyday practice. When this observation is coupled with two others—the much higher cost of tPA and the greater incidence of hemorrhagic stroke with tPA—the desirability of tPA over SK is not entirely obvious. Regardless of whether tPA is significantly better than SK, there is no question that treatment with either drug is much better than no treatment at all. Put another way, selecting some thrombolytic drug is much more important than which one is selected.

## KEY POINTS

- Hemostasis occurs in two stages: formation of a platelet plug, followed by coagulation (i.e., production of fibrin, a protein that reinforces the platelet plug).
- Fibrin is produced by two pathways, known as the intrinsic and extrinsic systems. These converge with production of factor Xa, which catalyzes formation of thrombin, which in turn catalyzes formation of fibrin.
- Four factors in the coagulation pathways require vitamin K for synthesis.
- Plasmin, the active form of plasminogen, serves to dissolve the fibrin meshwork of clots.
- A thrombus is a blood clot formed within a blood vessel or within the heart.
- Arterial thrombi begin with formation of a platelet plug, which is then reinforced with fibrin.
- Venous thrombi begin with formation of fibrin, which then enmeshes red blood cells and platelets.
- Arterial thrombi are best prevented with antiplatelet drugs (e.g., aspirin), whereas venous thrombi are best prevented with anticoagulants (warfarin, heparin).
- Heparin is a large polymer (MW range = 3000 to 30,000) that carries many negative charges.
- Heparin suppresses coagulation by helping antithrombin III inactivate thrombin, factor Xa, and other clotting factors.
- Heparin is administered IV or SC. Because of its large size and negative charges, heparin is unable to cross membranes, and hence cannot be administered PO.
- Anticoagulant effects of heparin develop within minutes of IV administration.
- The major adverse effect of heparin is bleeding.
- Severe heparin-induced bleeding can be treated with protamine sulfate, a drug that binds heparin and thereby stops it from working.
- Heparin can cause thrombocytopenia. Two mechanisms are involved: promotion of platelet aggregation (common) and production of antiplatelet antibodies (rare).
- Heparin is contraindicated for patients with thrombocytopenia or uncontrollable bleeding, and must be used with extreme caution in all patients for whom there is a high likelihood of bleeding.
- Heparin therapy is monitored by measuring APTT (activated partial thromboplastin time). The target APTT is

60 to 80 seconds (i.e., 1.5 to 2 times the normal value of 40 seconds).

- Low-molecular-weight (LMW) heparin is produced by breaking molecules of standard heparin into smaller pieces.
- In contrast to standard heparin, which inactivates factor Xa and thrombin equally, LMW heparin preferentially inactivates factor Xa.
- In contrast to standard heparin, LMW heparin does not bind nonspecifically to plasma proteins and tissues. As a result, plasma levels of LMW heparin are highly predictable.
- Because plasma levels of LMW heparin are predictable, LMW heparin can be administered on a fixed schedule with no need for laboratory monitoring. As a result, LMW heparin can be used at home.
- Warfarin is the prototype of the oral anticoagulants.
- Warfarin antagonizes vitamin K, and thereby blocks the biosynthesis of vitamin K–dependent clotting factors.
- Anticoagulant responses to warfarin develop slowly and persist for several days after warfarin is discontinued.
- Warfarin therapy is monitored by measuring prothrombin time (PT). Results are expressed as an international normalized ratio (INR). An INR of 2 to 3 is the target for most patients.
- Bleeding is the major complication of warfarin therapy.
- Warfarin overdose is treated with vitamin K.
- Warfarin must not be used during pregnancy. The drug can cause fetal malformation, central nervous system defects, and optic atrophy.
- Warfarin is subject to a large number of clinically significant drug interactions. Drugs can increase anticoagulant effects by displacing warfarin from plasma albumin and by inhibiting hepatic enzymes that degrade warfarin. Drugs can decrease anticoagulant effect by inducing hepatic drug-metabolizing enzymes, increasing synthesis of clotting factors, and inhibiting warfarin absorption. Drugs that promote bleeding, such as heparin and aspirin, will obviously increase the risk of bleeding in patients taking warfarin. Instruct patients to avoid all drugs—prescription and nonprescription—that have not been specifically approved by the physician.
- Aspirin and other antiplatelet drugs suppress thrombus formation in arteries.
- Aspirin inhibits platelet aggregation by causing irreversible inhibition of cyclooxygenase. Since platelets are unable to synthesize new cyclooxygenase, inhibition persists for the life of the platelet (7 to 10 days).
- In its role as an antiplatelet drug, aspirin is given for primary prophylaxis of MI, prevention of MI recurrence, and prevention of stroke in patients with a history of TIAs.
- When used to suppress platelet aggregation, aspirin is administered in low doses—typically 160 to 325 mg/day.
- Thrombolytic drugs (e.g., streptokinase, alteplase [tPA]) are used to dissolve existing thrombi (rather than prevent thrombi from forming).
- Thrombolytic drugs work by converting plasminogen to plasmin, an enzyme that degrades the fibrin matrix of thrombi.
- Thrombolytic therapy is most effective when started early (i.e., within 4 to 6 hours of symptom onset).
- Thrombolytic drugs carry a significant risk of bleeding. Intracranial hemorrhage is the greatest concern.
- For patients with acute MI, tPA is slightly more effective than streptokinase, but costs much more and causes more intracranial bleeding.

# Summary of Major Nursing Implications*

## Heparin

### Preadministration Assessment

#### Therapeutic Goal

The objective of treatment is to prevent thrombosis without inducing spontaneous bleeding.

Heparin is the preferred anticoagulant for use during *pregnancy* and in situations that require rapid onset of effects, including *pulmonary embolism, evolving stroke,* and *massive deep vein thrombosis.* Other indications include *open heart surgery, renal dialysis,* and *disseminated intravascular coagulation.* Low doses are used to prevent *postoperative venous thrombosis* and to enhance thrombolytic therapy of *myocardial infarction.*

#### Baseline Data

Obtain baseline values for blood pressure, heart rate, complete blood cell counts, platelet counts, hematocrit, and activated partial thromboplastin time (APTT).

#### Identifying High-Risk Patients

Heparin is *contraindicated* for patients with *severe thrombocytopenia* or *uncontrollable bleeding* and for patients undergoing *lumbar puncture, regional anesthesia,* or *surgery of the eye, brain, or spinal cord.*

Use with *extreme caution* in *patients at high risk of bleeding,* including those with *hemophilia, increased capillary permeability, dissecting aneurysm, gastrointestinal ulcers,* or *severe hypertension. Caution* is also needed in patients with *severe hepatic or renal dysfunction.*

### Implementation: Administration

#### Routes

Intravenous (continuous infusion or intermittent) and subcutaneous. Avoid IM injections!

## Administration

***General Considerations.*** Dosage is prescribed in units, not milligrams. Heparin preparations vary widely in concentration; read the label carefully to ensure correct dosing.

***Intermittent Intravenous Administration.*** Administer through a heparin lock every 4 to 6 hours. APTT should be determined before each dose during the early phase of treatment, and daily thereafter. Rotate the injection site every 2 to 3 days.

***Continuous Intravenous Infusion.*** Administer with a constant infusion pump or some other approved volume control unit. Policy may require that dosage be double-checked by a second person. Check the infusion rate every 30 to 60 minutes. During the early phase of treatment, APTT should be determined every 4 hours. Check the site of needle insertion periodically for extravasation.

***Deep Subcutaneous Injection.*** Perform SC injections into the fatty layer of the abdomen (but not within 2 inches of the umbilicus). Withdraw heparin solution using a 20- to 22-gauge needle, and then discard that needle and replace it with a small needle (1/2 to 5/8 inch, 25- or 26-gauge) to make the injection. Apply firm but gentle pressure to the injection site for 1 to 2 minutes following administration. Rotate and record injection sites.

## Ongoing Evaluation and Interventions

### Evaluating Treatment

Periodic determinations of APTT are used to evaluate treatment. Heparin should increase the APTT by 1.5- to 2-fold above baseline.

### Minimizing Adverse Effects

***Hemorrhage.*** Heparin overdose may cause hemorrhage. Monitor closely for signs of bleeding. These include lowering of blood pressure, elevation of heart rate, discoloration of urine or stool, bruises, petechiae, hematomas, persistent headache or faintness (suggestive of cerebral hemorrhage), pelvic pain (suggestive of ovarian hemorrhage), and lumbar pain (suggestive of adrenal hemorrhage). Laboratory data suggesting hemorrhage include reductions in the hematocrit and blood cell counts. If bleeding occurs, heparin should be discontinued. Severe overdose can be treated with *protamine sulfate* administered by slow IV injection. The risk of bleeding can be reduced by ensuring that the APTT does not exceed two times the baseline value.

***Thrombocytopenia.*** Heparin can decrease platelet counts, thereby increasing the risk of bleeding. Platelet counts should be monitored. If they drop below 100,000/mm$^3$, heparin should be discontinued.

***Hypersensitivity Reactions.*** Allergy may develop to antigens in heparin preparations. To minimize the risk of severe reactions, administer a small test dose prior to the full therapeutic dose.

### Minimizing Adverse Interactions

***Antiplatelet Drugs.*** Concurrent use of antiplatelet drugs (e.g., aspirin) increases the risk of bleeding. Use these agents with caution.

# Warfarin

## Preadministration Assessment

### Therapeutic Goal

The goal of therapy is to prevent thrombosis without inducing spontaneous bleeding. Specific indications include prevention of venous thrombosis and associated pulmonary embolism, prevention of thromboembolism in patients with prosthetic heart valves, and prevention of thrombosis during atrial fibrillation.

### Baseline Data

Obtain a thorough medical history, making sure to identify use of any medications that might interact adversely with warfarin. Obtain baseline values of vital signs and prothrombin time.

### Identifying High-Risk Patients

Warfarin is *contraindicated* in the presence of *vitamin K deficiency*, *liver disease*, *alcoholism*, *thrombocytopenia*, *uncontrollable bleeding*, *pregnancy*, and *lactation*, and for patients undergoing *lumbar puncture*, *regional anesthesia*, or *surgery of the eye, brain, or spinal cord*.

Use with *extreme caution* in patients at high risk of bleeding, including those with *hemophilia*, *increased capillary permeability*, *dissecting aneurysm*, *GI ulcers*, and *severe hypertension*.

## Implementation: Administration

### Route

Oral.

### Administration

For most patients, dosage is adjusted to maintain an international normalized ratio (INR) value of 2 to 3. Maintain a flow chart for hospitalized patients indicating INR values and dosage size and timing.

## Implementation: Measures to Enhance Therapeutic Effects

### Promoting Compliance

Safe and effective therapy requires rigid adherence to the dosing schedule. Achieving adherence requires active and informed participation by the patient. Provide the patient with detailed written and verbal instructions regarding the purpose of treatment, dosage size and timing, and the importance of strict adherence to the dosing schedule. Also, provide the patient with a chart on which to keep an ongoing record of warfarin use. If the patient is incompetent (e.g., mentally ill, alcoholic, senile), ensure that a responsible individual supervises treatment.

### Nondrug Measures

Advise the patient to (1) avoid prolonged immobility, (2) elevate the legs when sitting, (3) avoid garments that can restrict blood flow in the legs, (4) participate in exercise activities, and (5) wear support hose. These measures will reduce venous stasis, and will thereby reduce the risk of thrombosis.

## Ongoing Evaluation and Interventions

### Evaluating Therapeutic Effects

*Monitoring Prothrombin Time.* Evaluate therapy by monitoring prothrombin time (PT). Test results are reported as an INR. For most patients, the target INR is 2 to 3. If the INR is below this range, dosage should be increased. Conversely, if the INR is above this range, dosage should be reduced.

Prothrombin time should be measured frequently: daily during the first 5 days, twice a week for the next 1 to 2 weeks, once a week for the next 1 to 2 months, and every 2 to 4 weeks thereafter. In addition, PT should be determined whenever a drug that interacts with warfarin is added to or deleted from the regimen.

If heparin is being employed concurrently, blood for PT determinations should be drawn no sooner than 5 hours after IV administration of heparin, and no sooner than 24 hours after SC administration.

### Minimizing Adverse Effects

*Hemorrhage.* Hemorrhage is the major complication of warfarin therapy. Warn patients about the danger of hemorrhage, and inform them about signs of bleeding. These signs include lowering of blood pressure, elevation of heart rate, discoloration of urine or stools, bruises, petechiae, hematomas, persistent headache or faintness (suggestive of cerebral hemorrhage), pelvic pain (suggestive of ovarian hemorrhage), and lumbar pain (suggestive of adrenal hemorrhage). Laboratory data suggesting hemorrhage include reductions in the hematocrit and blood cell counts.

Instruct the patient to withhold warfarin and notify the physician if signs of bleeding are noted. Advise the patient to wear some form of identification (e.g., Medic Alert bracelet) indicating warfarin use.

To reduce the incidence of bleeding, advise the patient to avoid excessive consumption of alcohol. Suggest use of a soft toothbrush to prevent bleeding from the gums. Advise patients to shave with an electric razor.

Warfarin intensifies bleeding during surgical or dental procedures. Instruct the patient to make certain that the surgeon or dentist is aware that warfarin is being used. Warfarin should be discontinued several days prior to elective procedures. If emergency surgery must be performed, vitamin K$_1$ can help reduce bleeding.

Warfarin-induced bleeding can be controlled with vitamin K$_1$. If bleeding is minor, oral vitamin K will suffice. For severe bleeding, vitamin K is given by injection. The physician may advise the patient to keep a supply of vitamin K on hand for use in emergencies, but only after consultation with a physician.

*Use in Pregnancy and Lactation.* Warfarin can cross the placenta, causing fetal hemorrhage and malformation. Inform women of child-bearing age about potential risks to the fetus, and warn them against becoming pregnant. If pregnancy develops, termination should be considered.

Warfarin enters breast milk and may harm the nursing infant. Warn women against breast-feeding.

### Minimizing Adverse Interactions

Inform patients that warfarin is subject to a large number of potentially dangerous drug interactions. Instruct patients to avoid all drugs—prescription and nonprescription—that have not been specifically approved by the physician. Prior to treatment, take a complete medication history to identify any drugs that might interact adversely with warfarin.

# Thrombolytic Drugs

| | |
|---|---|
| Streptokinase | Urokinase |
| Alteplase (tPA) | Anistreplase |
| Reteplase | |

## Preadministration Assessment

### Therapeutic Goal

Thrombolytic drugs are used to treat acute MI, massive pulmonary emboli, ischemic stroke, and deep vein thrombosis.

### Baseline Data

Obtain baseline values for blood pressure, heart rate, platelet counts, hematocrit, APTT, PT, and fibrinogen level.

### Identifying High-Risk Patients

Thrombolytic drugs are *contraindicated* for patients with *active bleeding*, *aortic dissection*, *acute pericarditis*, *cerebral neoplasm*, *cerebral vascular disease*, or a *history of intracranial bleeding*. Use with *great caution* in patients with relative contraindications, including *pregnancy*, *severe hypertension*, *ischemic stroke within the prior 6 months*, and *major surgery within the prior 2 to 4 weeks*. See Table 50-7 for a complete list of absolute and relative contraindications.

## Implementation: Administration

### Routes

Intracoronary, intravenous (see Table 50-6)

### Administration

Depending on the drug employed and the specific application, administration may be by IV infusion, slow IV injection, IV bolus, intracoronary infusion, or intracoronary bolus. (See Table 50-6 for administration during acute MI.)

Do not administer heparin and streptokinase through the same IV line.

## Ongoing Evaluation and Interventions

### Minimizing Adverse Effects

*Hemorrhage.* Thrombolytics may cause bleeding; intracranial hemorrhage (ICH), is the greatest concern. To reduce the risk of major bleeding, minimize manipulation of the patient, avoid SC and IM injections, minimize invasive procedures, and minimize concurrent use of anticoagulants (heparin, warfarin) and antiplatelet drugs (e.g., aspirin). Manage oozing at cutaneous puncture sites with a pressure dressing.

For severe bleeding, discontinue streptokinase and give whole blood or blood products (packed red blood cells, fresh-frozen plasma). If bleeding continues, give IV aminocaproic acid.

### Minimizing Adverse Interactions

*Anticoagulants and Antiplatelet Drugs.* Anticoagulants (heparin, warfarin) and antiplatelet drugs (e.g., aspirin) increase the risk of bleeding from antithrombotics. Avoid high-dose therapy with these drugs until thrombolytic effects have subsided.

# CHAPTER 51

# Drugs for Deficiency Anemias

Anemia is defined as a decrease in erythrocyte number, size, or hemoglobin content. Causes include blood loss, hemolysis, bone marrow dysfunction, and deficiencies of substances essential for red blood cell formation and maturation. The majority of deficiency anemias result from a deficiency in iron, vitamin B$_{12}$, or folic acid—and of these, iron deficiency anemia is by far the most common.

In discussing the deficiency anemias, we will limit our scope to deficiencies of iron, vitamin B$_{12}$, and folic acid. Iron is considered first, followed by vitamin B$_{12}$ and folic acid. To facilitate discussion, we will begin with a review of red blood cell development.

## Red Blood Cell Development

Red blood cells begin developing in the bone marrow and reach maturity in the blood. As developing red cells grow and divide, they evolve through four principal stages (Fig. 51-1). In their earliest stage, red cells lack hemoglobin and are known as *proerythroblasts*. In the next stage, they gain hemoglobin and are called *erythroblasts*. Both the erythroblasts and the proerythroblasts reside in the bone marrow. After the erythroblast stage, red cells evolve into *reticulocytes* (immature erythrocytes) and enter the systemic circulation. Following the reticulocyte stage, circulating red cells reach full maturity and are referred to as *erythrocytes*.

Development of red blood cells requires the cooperative interaction of several factors: the bone marrow must be healthy; erythropoietin (a stimulant of red cell maturation) must be present; iron must be available for hemoglobin synthesis; and other factors, including vitamin B$_{12}$ and folic acid, must be available to support synthesis of deoxyribonucleic acid (DNA). If any of these factors is absent or amiss, anemia will result.

## Iron Deficiency

Iron deficiency is the most common cause of nutrition-related anemia. Worldwide, people with iron deficiency number in the hundreds of millions. In the United States, between 5% and 10% of the population is iron deficient.

### Biochemistry and Physiology of Iron

In order to understand the consequences of iron deficiency as well as the rationale behind iron therapy, we must first understand the biochemistry and physiology of iron. This information is reviewed below.

#### Metabolic Functions

Iron is essential to the function of hemoglobin, myoglobin (the oxygen-storing molecule of muscle), and a variety of iron-containing enzymes. From a quantitative perspective, the most significant use of iron is in hemoglobin: between 70% and 80% of all iron in the body is dedicated to hemoglobin production. Although the iron in myoglobin and certain enzymes is clearly important, the amount involved is small.

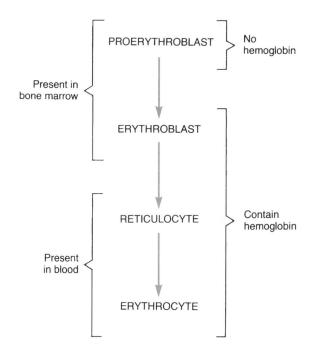

**Figure 51-1. Stages of red blood cell development..**

## Fate in the Body

The major pathways for iron movement and utilization are shown in Figure 51-2. In the discussion below, the numbers in parentheses refer to the circled numbers in the figure.

*Uptake and Distribution.* The life cycle of iron begins with (1) the uptake of iron into mucosal cells of the small intestine. These cells absorb between 5% and 20% of dietary iron; the maximum absorptive capacity is 3 to 4 mg of iron a day. Iron in the ferrous form ($Fe^{++}$) is absorbed more readily than iron in the ferric form ($Fe^{+++}$). Food greatly reduces absorption.

Following uptake, iron can either (2a) undergo storage within mucosal cells in the form of *ferritin* (a complex consisting of iron plus a protein used for iron storage) or (2b) undergo binding to *transferrin* (the iron transport protein) for distribution throughout the body.

*Utilization and Storage.* Iron that is bound to transferrin can undergo one of three fates. The majority of transferrin-bound iron is (3a) taken up by cells of the bone marrow for incorporation into hemoglobin. Small amounts are (3b) taken up by the liver and other tissues for storage as ferritin; these stores make up about 18% of the iron in the body. Lastly (3c), some of the iron in plasma is taken up by muscle (for production of myoglobin) and some is taken up by all tissues (for production of iron-containing enzymes). These last two uses account for about 10% of the iron in the body.

*Recycling.* As Figure 51-2 depicts, iron associated with hemoglobin undergoes continuous recycling. After hemoglobin is made in bone marrow, iron re-enters the circulation (4) as a component of hemoglobin in erythrocytes. (The iron in circulating erythrocytes accounts for

about 70% of total body iron.) After 120 days of useful life, red cells are catabolized (5). Iron released by this process re-enters the plasma bound to transferrin (6)—and then the cycle begins anew.

*Elimination.* Excretion of iron is minimal. Under normal circumstances, only 1 mg of iron is excreted each day. At this rate, if none of the lost iron were replaced, body stores would decline by only 10% a year.

Iron leaves the body by several routes. Most excretion occurs via the bowel: iron in ferritin is lost as mucosal cells slough; iron also enters the bowel in the bile. Small amounts of iron are excreted in the urine and sweat.

It should be noted that although very little iron leaves the body as a result of excretion (i.e., normal physiologic loss), substantial amounts can leave because of blood loss. Hence, menorrhagia (excessive menstrual flow), hemorrhage, and blood donations can all cause iron deficiency.

*Regulation of Body Iron Content.* The amount of iron in the body is regulated through control of intestinal absorption. As noted, most of the iron that enters the body stays in the body. Hence, if all dietary iron were readily absorbed, body iron content could rapidly build to toxic levels. Such *excessive buildup is prevented through control of iron uptake*: as body stores rise, *uptake of iron declines*; conversely, as body stores become depleted, *uptake increases*. For example, when body stores of iron are high, only 2% to 3% of dietary iron is absorbed. In contrast, when body stores are depleted, iron absorption may climb to 20%. Although it is clear that iron absorption adjusts to meet needs, the mechanisms underlying these adjustments are unknown.

## Daily Requirements

Requirements for iron are determined largely by the rate of erythrocyte production. When red cell production is low, iron needs are small; conversely, when red cell production is high, iron needs are high as well. Accordingly, infants and children—individuals whose rapid growth rate requires massive red cell synthesis—have iron requirements that are high (relative to body weight). In contrast, the daily iron needs of adults are relatively low. Adult males need only 10 mg of dietary iron per day. Adult females need somewhat more—to compensate for iron loss during menstruation.

During pregnancy, requirements for iron increase dramatically. This increase results from (1) expansion of maternal blood volume and (2) production of red blood cells by the fetus. In most cases, the iron needs of pregnant women are too great to be met by diet alone. Consequently, iron supplements (about 30 mg/day) are recommended during pregnancy and for 2 to 3 months after parturition.

Table 51-1 summarizes the recommended dietary allowances (RDAs) of iron as a function of age. For each age, the table presents two iron values. The first is the actual physiologic need for iron. The second is the RDA. Note that RDA values are about 10 times greater than the values for physiologic need. This disparity reflects the fact

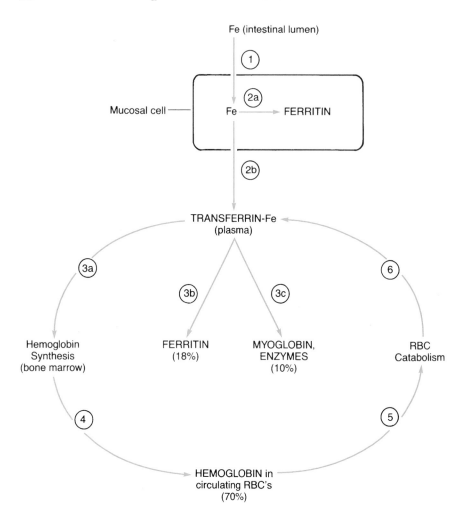

**Figure 51–2. Fate of iron in the body.** Pathways labeled with circled numbers are explained in the text. Values in parentheses indicate percentage of total body stores. Elimination of iron is not shown since most iron is rigidly conserved. (Fe = iron, RBC = red blood cell.)

that, on average, only 10% of dietary iron is absorbed. Hence, if physiologic requirements are to be met, the diet must contain 10 times more iron than the body actually needs.

### Dietary Sources

Iron is available in foods of plant and animal origin. Foods that are especially rich in iron include liver, egg yolk, brewer's yeast, and wheat germ. Other foods with a high iron content include muscle meats, fish, fowl, cereal grains, beans, and green leafy vegetables. Foods that do not provide much iron include milk and most nongreen vegetables. Since iron can be extracted from cooking utensils, the use of iron pots and pans can augment dietary iron. Except for individuals who have very high iron requirements (infants, pregnant women, those undergoing chronic blood loss), the average diet is sufficient to meet iron needs.

## Iron Deficiency: Causes, Consequences, and Diagnosis

### Causes

Iron deficiency results when there is an imbalance between iron uptake and iron demand. Most commonly, this imbalance results from increased demand and not from reduced uptake. The most common causes of increased iron demand (and resulting iron deficiency) are (1) blood volume expansion during pregnancy coupled with red blood cell synthesis by the developing fetus, (2) blood volume expansion during infancy and early childhood, and (3) chronic blood loss, which is usually of GI or uterine origin. Rarely, iron deficiency results from reduced iron uptake; potential causes include gastrectomy and sprue.

### Consequences

Iron deficiency has multiple effects, the most conspicuous being *iron deficiency anemia*. In the absence of iron for hemoglobin synthesis, red blood cells become *microcytic* (small) and *hypochromic* (pale). The reduced oxygen-carrying capacity of blood results in listlessness, fatigue, and pallor of the skin and mucous membranes. If tissue oxygenation is severely compromised, tachycardia, dyspnea, and angina may result. In addition to causing anemia, iron deficiency impairs myoglobin production and reduces synthesis of iron-containing enzymes.

### Diagnosis

The hallmarks of iron deficiency anemia are (1) the presence of microcytic, hypochromic erythrocytes, and (2) the absence of hemosiderin (aggregated ferritin) in bone marrow. Additional laboratory data that can help

## TABLE 51-1. RECOMMENDED DIETARY ALLOWANCES FOR IRON

| | Age (years) | Physiologic Requirement for Iron (mg/day) | RDA* for Iron (mg/day) |
|---|---|---|---|
| Infants | 0-0.5 | 0.6 | 6 |
| | 0.5-1 | 1.0 | 10 |
| Children | 1-10 | 1.0 | 10 |
| Males | 11-18 | 1.2 | 12 |
| | 18+ | 1.0 | 10 |
| Females | 11-50 | 1.5 | 15 |
| | 50+ | 1.0 | 10 |
| Pregnant and 2-3 months postpartum | — | 5 | 30† |

*Since only a small fraction of dietary iron is absorbed, the RDA is higher than the actual physiologic need.
†Iron requirements during pregnancy cannot be met through dietary sources alone; supplements are recommended.

confirm a diagnosis of iron deficiency anemia include reduced red cell count, reduced hemoglobin and hematocrit values, reduced serum iron content, and increased serum iron-binding capacity (IBC).*

When a diagnosis of iron deficiency anemia is made, it is imperative that the underlying cause be determined. This is especially true when the suspected cause is blood loss of GI origin. Such blood loss may be indicative of peptic ulcer disease or GI cancer, conditions that demand immediate treatment.

## Oral Iron Preparations I: Ferrous Sulfate

Ferrous sulfate is the least expensive of the oral iron preparations and is the standard against which other oral preparations are measured. Ferrous sulfate will serve as our prototype for the group.

### Indications

Ferrous sulfate is the drug of choice for treating iron deficiency anemia. This compound is also employed for prophylaxis of iron deficiency in people whose need for iron cannot be met by diet alone (e.g., pregnant women, individuals experiencing chronic blood loss).

### Adverse Effects

**Gastrointestinal Disturbances.** The most significant adverse effects of oral iron preparations involve the GI tract. These effects, which are dose dependent, include nausea, pyrosis (heartburn), bloating, constipation, and di-

*Serum IBC measures iron binding by transferrin. An increase in IBC indicates an increase in the amount of transferrin that is not carrying any iron, and hence signals reduced iron availability.

arrhea. Gastrointestinal reactions are most intense during the initial phase of therapy, and become less disturbing with continued drug use. Because of their effects on the GI tract, oral iron preparations can aggravate peptic ulcers, regional enteritis, and ulcerative colitis. Accordingly, patients with these disorders should not take iron orally. In addition to its other GI effects, oral iron may impart a dark green or black coloration to stools. This effect is harmless and should not be interpreted as a sign of bleeding.

**Staining of Teeth.** Liquid iron preparations can stain the teeth. This effect can be prevented by (1) diluting liquid preparations with juice or water, (2) administering the iron through a straw or with a dropper, and (3) rinsing the mouth after administration.

### Toxicity

Iron in large amounts is toxic. Poisoning is almost always the result of accidental or intentional overdose; poisoning from proper therapeutic use of iron is rare. Death from iron poisoning is most likely in the very young. Death in adults is uncommon. For children, the lethal dose of elemental iron is 2 to 10 gm. To reduce the chances of pediatric poisoning, iron should be stored in child-proof containers and kept out of reach.

**Symptoms.** The effects of iron poisoning are complex. Early reactions include nausea, vomiting, diarrhea, and shock. These are followed by acidosis, gastric necrosis, hepatic failure, pulmonary edema, and vasomotor collapse.

**Diagnosis and Treatment.** With rapid diagnosis and treatment, mortality from iron poisoning is low (about 1%). Serum iron should be measured and the intestine x-rayed to determine if unabsorbed tablets are present. Induction of vomiting will remove iron from the stomach. Acidosis and shock should be treated as required.

If the plasma level of iron is high (above 500 µg/dl) it should be lowered using *deferoxamine*. Deferoxamine absorbs iron and

## TABLE 51-2. ORAL IRON PREPARATIONS

| Iron Salt | Dosage Forms | % Iron (by weight) | Dose Providing 100 mg Iron |
|---|---|---|---|
| Ferrous sulfate | C, E, L, Sy, T, T-TR | 20 | 500 mg |
| Ferrous sulfate (dried) | C, C-TR, T, T-SR | ~30 | 330 mg |
| Ferrous fumarate | Su, T, T-Ch, T-TR, L | 33 | 300 mg |
| Ferrous gluconate | C, E, T, T-SR | 11.6 | 860 mg |

C = capsule; C-TR = capsule, timed-release; E = elixir; L = liquid; Su = suspension; Sy = syrup; T = tablet; T-Ch = tablet, chewable; T-SR = tablet, sustained-release; T-TR = tablet, timed-release.

thereby prevents toxic effects. The pharmacology of deferoxamine is discussed in Chapter 100 (Management of Poisoning).

### Drug Interactions

Interaction of iron with other drugs can alter the absorption of iron, the other agent, or both. *Antacids* reduce the absorption of iron. Coadministration of iron with tetracyclines decreases the absorption of both agents. *Ascorbic acid* (vitamin C) promotes iron absorption but also increases its adverse effects. Accordingly, attempts to promote iron uptake by combining iron with ascorbic acid offer no advantage over a simple increase in iron dosage.

### Formulations

Oral iron is available in several dosage forms (Table 51-2). Some of these formulations (timed- or sustained-release capsules and tablets) are intended to reduce gastric disturbances. Unfortunately, although side effects may be lowered, these dosage forms have disadvantages: iron may be released at inconstant rates, causing variable, unpredictable absorption; in addition, these preparations are expensive. Ordinary tablets do not have these drawbacks.

### Dosage and Administration

*General Considerations.* Dosing with oral iron is complicated by the fact that the oral iron salts differ from one another with regard to percentage of elemental iron (see Table 51-2). Ferrous *sulfate*, for example, contains 20% iron by weight. In contrast, ferrous *gluconate* contains only 11.6% iron. Consequently, in order to provide equivalent amounts of elemental iron, we must use different doses of these iron preparations. For example, if we wished to provide 100 mg of elemental iron, we would need to administer a 500-mg dose of ferrous *sulfate*. To provide this same amount of elemental iron using ferrous *fumarate*, the dose would be only 300 mg. In the discussion below, dosage values refer to milligrams of *elemental* iron, and not to milligrams of any particular iron salt needed to provide that amount of elemental iron.

Food affects therapy with oral iron in two ways. First, food helps protect against iron-induced GI distress. Second, food decreases absorption of iron by 50% to 70%. Hence, we have a dilemma: *absorption is best* when iron is taken *between* meals, but *side effects are lowest* when iron is taken *with* meals. As a rule, it is recommended that

iron be administered between meals, thereby maximizing absorption; if necessary, the dosage can be lowered to render GI effects more acceptable.

For two reasons, it may be desirable to take iron *with* food during *initial* therapy. First, since the GI effects of iron are most intense as treatment commences, the salving effects of food can be especially beneficial at this time. Second, by reducing GI discomfort during the early phase of therapy, administering iron with food can help promote compliance.

*Use in Iron Deficiency Anemia.* Dosing with oral iron represents a compromise between a desire to replenish lost iron rapidly and a desire to keep adverse GI effects to a minimum. For most adults, this compromise can best be achieved with doses of 65 mg administered 3 times a day, yielding a total daily dose of approximately 200 mg. Since there is a ceiling to intestinal absorption of iron, doses above this level provide only a modest increase in therapeutic effect. On the other hand, at dosages greater than 200 mg/day, GI disturbances become disproportionately high. Hence, elevation of the daily dosage above 200 mg would augment adverse effects without offering a significant increase in benefits. When treating iron deficiency in infants and children, a typical dosage is 5 mg/kg/day administered in three or four divided doses.

Timing of iron administration is important: doses should be spaced evenly throughout the day. This schedule provides the bone marrow with a continuous iron supply, thereby maximizing red cell production.

Duration of therapy is determined by the therapeutic objective. If correction of anemia is the sole objective of treatment, a few months of therapy is sufficient. However, if the objective also includes replenishment of ferritin, treatment must continue for an additional 4 to 6 months. It should be noted, however, that drugs are usually unnecessary for ferritin replenishment; in most cases, diet alone can do the job. Accordingly, once anemia has been corrected, pharmaceutical iron can usually be discontinued.

*Prophylactic Use of Iron.* Pregnancy is the principal indication for prophylactic iron therapy. A daily dose of 30 mg taken between meals is recommended. Other candidates for iron prophylaxis include infants, children, and women experiencing menorrhagia.

$$\text{mg iron} = 0.66 \times \text{kg body weight} \times \left(100 - \frac{\text{hemoglobin value in g/dl}}{14.8}\right)$$

**Figure 51–3. Formula for estimating total dosage of parenteral iron dextran.**

### Oral Iron Preparations II: Ferrous Gluconate and Ferrous Fumarate

In addition to ferrous sulfate, two other iron salts—ferrous gluconate and ferrous fumarate—are available for oral use. Except for differences in percentage of iron content (see Table 51–2), all of these preparations are equivalent. Hence, when dosage is adjusted to provide equal amounts of elemental iron, ferrous gluconate and ferrous fumarate produce pharmacologic effects identical to those of ferrous sulfate: all three agents produce equivalent therapeutic responses, and all three cause the same degree of GI distress. Patients who fail to respond to one of these agents will not respond to the others. Patients who cannot tolerate the GI effects of one agent will find the others intolerable too.

## Parenteral Iron: Iron Dextran

Iron dextran is the only parenteral iron preparation available in the United States. This preparation is a complex consisting of ferric hydroxide and dextrans (polymers of glucose). The rate of response to parenteral iron is equal to that seen with oral iron. Iron dextran is dangerous—fatal anaphylactic reactions have occurred—and should be used only when circumstances demand.

### Indications

Iron dextran is reserved for patients with a clear diagnosis of iron deficiency and for whom oral iron is either ineffective or intolerable. Primary candidates for parenteral iron are patients who, because of intestinal disease, are unable to absorb iron administered orally. Iron dextran is also indicated when blood loss is so great (500 to 1000 ml/week) that oral iron cannot be absorbed rapidly enough to meet hematopoietic needs. Parenteral iron may also be employed when there is concern that oral iron might exacerbate pre-existing disease of the stomach or bowel. Lastly, parenteral iron can be employed for the rare patient for whom the GI effects of oral iron are intolerable.

### Adverse Effects

*Anaphylactic Reactions.* Potentially fatal anaphylaxis is the most serious adverse effect of iron dextran. Although these reactions are rare, the possibility of their occurrence demands that iron dextran be used only when clearly required. Whenever iron dextran is administered, injectable epinephrine and facilities for resuscitation should be at hand.

*Other Adverse Effects.* Iron dextran can cause headache, fever, urticaria, and arthralgia. More serious reactions—circulatory failure and cardiac arrest—have also occurred. When administered IM, iron dextran can cause persistent pain and prolonged, localized discoloration. Very rarely, tumors have developed at sites of IM injection. Intravenous administration may result in lymphadenopathy and phlebitis.

### Preparations, Dosage, and Administration

*Preparations.* Iron dextran [InFeD] is dispensed in 10-ml vials and 2-ml ampules, all containing 50 mg/ml of elemental iron.

*Dosage.* Dosage determination is complex. Dosage will vary depending on the degree of anemia, the weight of the patient, and the presence of persistent bleeding. For the patient with iron deficiency anemia who is not losing blood, the equation in Figure 51–3 provides a guideline for estimating total iron dosage.

*Administration.* Iron dextran may be administered IM or IV. Intravenous administration is preferred. This route is just as effective as IM administration but causes fewer anaphylactic reactions and other adverse effects.

*Intravenous.* To minimize anaphylactic reactions, intravenous iron dextran should be administered by the following protocol: (1) administer a tiny test dose (25 mg over 5 minutes) and observe the patient for at least 15 minutes; (2) if the test dose appears safe, slowly administer a larger dose (500 mg over a 10- to 15-minute interval); and (3) if the 500-mg dose is uneventful, additional doses may be given as needed.

*Intramuscular.* Intramuscular iron dextran has significant drawbacks and should be avoided. Disadvantages include persistent pain and discoloration at the injection site, possible development of tumors, and a greater risk of anaphylaxis than with IV administration. When IM administration must be performed, iron dextran should be injected deep into each buttock using the Z-track technique. (Z-track injection keeps the iron dextran deep in the muscle, thereby minimizing leakage and surface discoloration.) As with IV iron dextran, a small test dose should precede the full therapeutic dose.

## Guidelines for Treating Iron Deficiency

*Assessment.* Prior to initiation of therapy, the cause of iron deficiency must be determined. This information is required if treatment is to be appropriate. Potential causes of deficiency include pregnancy, bleeding, inadequate diet, and, rarely, reduced intestinal absorption.

The objective of therapy is to increase the production of hemoglobin and erythrocytes. When therapy is successful, reticulocytes will increase within 4 to 7 days; within 1 week, increases in hemoglobin and the hematocrit will be apparent; and within 1 month, hemoglobin levels will rise by at least 2 gm/dl. If these responses fail to occur, the patient should be evaluated for (1) compliance, (2) continued bleeding, (3) inflammatory disease (which can interfere with hemoglobin production), and (4) malabsorption of oral iron.

*Routes of Administration.* Iron preparations are available for oral, intravenous, and intramuscular administration. Oral iron (e.g., ferrous sulfate) is preferred to parenteral iron (iron dextran). Oral administration is safer than parenteral administration while being just as effective. Parenteral iron should be used only when oral iron is ineffective or intolerable. Of the two parenteral routes, IV is safer and preferred.

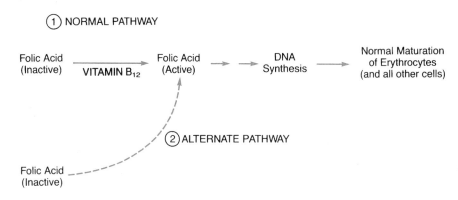

**Figure 51–4. Relationship of folic acid and vitamin B$_{12}$ to DNA synthesis and cell maturation.** Folic acid requires activation to be of use. Normally, activation occurs via a vitamin B$_{12}$-dependent pathway. However, when folic acid is present in large amounts, activation can occur via an alternative pathway, thereby bypassing the requirement for vitamin B$_{12}$.

***Duration of Therapy.*** Therapy with oral iron should be continued until hemoglobin levels become normal (about 15 gm/dl). This phase of treatment may require 1 to 2 months. After this time, continued treatment can help to replenish stores of ferritin. However, for most patients, diet alone is sufficient to replenish these stores.

***Therapeutic Combinations.*** As a rule, combinations of antianemic agents should be avoided. Combining oral iron with parenteral iron can lead to iron toxicity. Accordingly, use of oral iron should cease prior to giving iron injections. Combinations of iron with vitamin B$_{12}$ or folic acid should be avoided; as discussed in the following sections, these combinations can confuse interpretation of hematologic responses.

# Vitamin B$_{12}$ Deficiency

The term *vitamin B$_{12}$* refers not to a single compound but rather to a group of compounds that have very similar structures. These compounds are large molecules that contain an atom of cobalt. Because of the cobalt atom, members of the vitamin B$_{12}$ family are known as *cobalamins*.

The most prominent consequences of vitamin B$_{12}$ deficiency are *anemia* and *injury to the nervous system*. Anemia reverses rapidly following vitamin B$_{12}$ administration. Neurologic damage takes longer for repair and, in some cases, may never fully recover. Additional effects of B$_{12}$ deficiency include GI disturbances and impaired production of white blood cells and platelets.

## Biochemistry and Physiology of Vitamin B$_{12}$

In order to understand the consequences of vitamin B$_{12}$ deficiency and the rationale behind therapy, we must first understand the normal biochemistry and physiology of B$_{12}$. This background information is reviewed below.

## Metabolic Function

Vitamin B$_{12}$ is essential for synthesis of DNA, and hence is required for the growth and division of virtually all of our cells. The mechanism by which this vitamin influences DNA synthesis is depicted in Figure 51–4. As indicated, vitamin B$_{12}$ helps catalyze the conversion of folic acid to its active form. Active folic acid then participates in several reactions essential for DNA synthesis. Hence, *it is by permitting utilization of folic acid that vitamin B$_{12}$ influences cell growth and division*—and it is the absence of usable folic acid that underlies the blood cell abnormalities seen during vitamin B$_{12}$ deficiency.

## Fate in the Body

***Absorption.*** Absorption of vitamin B$_{12}$ requires *intrinsic factor*, a compound secreted by parietal cells of the stomach. Following ingestion, vitamin B$_{12}$ forms a complex with intrinsic factor. Upon reaching the ileum, the B$_{12}$-intrinsic factor complex interacts with specific receptors on the intestinal wall, causing the complex to be absorbed. In the absence of intrinsic factor, absorption of vitamin B$_{12}$ is nearly impossible.

***Distribution and Storage.*** Following absorption, the vitamin B$_{12}$-intrinsic factor complex dissociates. Free B$_{12}$ then binds to *transcobalamin II* for transport to tissues. Most vitamin B$_{12}$ goes to the liver and is stored. Total body stores of B$_{12}$ are minute, ranging from 1 to 10 mg.

***Elimination.*** Excretion of vitamin B$_{12}$ takes place very slowly; daily losses are about 0.05% of total body stores. Because B$_{12}$ is excreted so slowly, years are required for B$_{12}$ deficiency to develop—even when virtually no replenishment of lost B$_{12}$ has been taking place.

### Daily Requirements

Because very little vitamin B$_{12}$ is excreted, and because body stores are small to begin with, daily requirements for this vitamin are minuscule. The average adult needs only 3 μg of B$_{12}$ per day. Children need even less.

### Dietary Sources

The ability to biosynthesize vitamin B$_{12}$ is limited to microorganisms; higher plants and animals are unable to synthesize this compound. The microorganisms that make $B_{12}$ reside in the soil, sewage, and the intestines of humans and other animals. Unfortunately, vitamin $B_{12}$ produced in the human GI tract is unavailable for absorption. Consequently, humans must obtain the majority of their $B_{12}$ by consuming animal products. Liver and dairy products are especially good sources.

## Vitamin $B_{12}$ Deficiency: Causes, Consequences, and Diagnosis

### Causes

In the majority of cases, vitamin $B_{12}$ deficiency is the result of impaired absorption. Insufficient $B_{12}$ in the diet is rarely a cause of deficiency. Potential causes of poor absorption include (1) regional enteritis, (2) celiac disease (a malabsorption syndrome involving abnormalities in the intestinal villi), and (3) development of antibodies directed against the vitamin $B_{12}$–intrinsic factor complex.

Most frequently, impaired absorption of vitamin $B_{12}$ occurs secondary to a lack of intrinsic factor. The principal causes of intrinsic factor deficiency are atrophy of gastric parietal cells and surgery of the stomach (total gastric resection).

When vitamin $B_{12}$ deficiency is caused by an absence of intrinsic factor, the resulting syndrome is called *pernicious anemia*—a term suggesting a highly destructive or fatal condition. Pernicious anemia is an old term that refers back to the days when, for most patients, vitamin $B_{12}$ deficiency had no effective therapy. Hence, the condition was uniformly fatal. Today, vitamin $B_{12}$ deficiency secondary to lack of intrinsic factor can be managed successfully. Hence, the label pernicious no longer bears its original ominous connotation.

### Consequences

Many of the consequences of vitamin $B_{12}$ deficiency result from disruption of DNA synthesis. Tissues that are affected most are those that have a high proportion of cells undergoing growth and division. Accordingly, vitamin $B_{12}$ deficiency has profound effects on the bone marrow (the site where blood cells are produced) and the epithelial cells lining the mouth and GI tract.

*Megaloblastic Anemia.* The most conspicuous consequence of vitamin $B_{12}$ deficiency is an anemia in which large numbers of *megaloblasts* (oversized erythroblasts) appear in the bone marrow, and in which *macrocytes* (oversized erythrocytes) appear in the blood. These strange cells are produced because of impaired DNA synthesis: lacking sufficient DNA, growing cells are unable to divide; hence, as erythroblasts mature and their division is prevented, oversized cells result. Most megaloblasts die within the bone marrow; only a few evolve into the macrocytes that can be seen in the blood. Because of these unusual cells, the anemia associated with vitamin $B_{12}$ deficiency is often referred to as either *megaloblastic* or *macrocytic* anemia.

Severe anemia is the principal cause of mortality from $B_{12}$ deficiency. Anemia produces peripheral and cerebral hypoxia. Heart failure and dysrhythmias are the most frequent causes of death.

It is important to note that the hematologic effects of vitamin $B_{12}$ deficiency can be reversed with large doses of folic acid. As indicated in Figure 51–4, when folic acid is present in large amounts, some of it can be activated by an alternative pathway that is independent of vitamin $B_{12}$. This pathway bypasses the metabolic block caused by vitamin $B_{12}$ deficiency, thereby permitting DNA synthesis to proceed.

*Neurologic Damage.* Deficiency of vitamin $B_{12}$ causes demyelination of neurons, primarily in the spinal cord and brain. A variety of signs and symptoms can result. Early manifestations include paresthesias (tingling, numbness) of the hands and feet and a reduction in deep tendon reflexes. Late-developing responses include loss of memory, mood changes, hallucinations, and psychosis. If vitamin $B_{12}$ deficiency is prolonged, neurologic damage can be permanent.

The precise mechanism by which vitamin $B_{12}$ deficiency results in neuronal damage is unknown. We do know, however, that *neurologic damage is not related to effects on folic acid or DNA*. That is, the mechanism that underlies neuronal damage is different from the mechanism that underlies disruption of hematopoiesis. Consequently, although administration of large doses of folic acid can correct the hematologic consequences of vitamin $B_{12}$ deficiency, folic acid will not affect the neurologic picture.

*Other Effects.* As noted, vitamin $B_{12}$ deficiency can adversely affect virtually all tissues in which a high proportion of cells are undergoing growth and division. Hence, in addition to disrupting the production of erythrocytes, lack of vitamin $B_{12}$ also prevents the bone marrow from making leukocytes (white blood cells) and thrombocytes (platelets). Loss of these blood cells can lead to infection and spontaneous bleeding. Disruption of DNA synthesis can also suppress division of the cells that form the epithelial lining of the mouth, stomach, and intestine, thereby causing oral ulceration and a variety of gastrointestinal disturbances.

### Diagnosis

When megaloblastic anemia occurs, it may be due to vitamin $B_{12}$ deficiency or other causes, especially a lack of folic acid. Hence, if therapy is to be appropriate, a definitive diagnosis must be made. Two tests are particularly helpful. The first is obvious: measurement of plasma $B_{12}$ content. The second procedure, known as the Schilling test[†], measures vitamin $B_{12}$ absorption. The combination of megaloblastic anemia plus low plasma vitamin $B_{12}$ plus evidence of $B_{12}$ malabsorption permits a clear diagnosis of vitamin $B_{12}$ deficiency.

[†]The Schilling test is performed by administering a small dose of radiolabeled vitamin $B_{12}$, after which the urine is monitored for radioactivity. If the urine remains free of radioactivity, we can conclude that vitamin $B_{12}$ absorption is impaired.

## Vitamin B$_{12}$ Preparations I: Cyanocobalamin

Cyanocobalamin is a purified, crystalline form of vitamin B$_{12}$. This compound is the drug of choice for all forms of vitamin B$_{12}$ deficiency.

### Adverse Effects

Cyanocobalamin is generally devoid of serious adverse effects. One potential response, *hypokalemia*, may occur as a natural consequence of increased erythrocyte production. Erythrocytes incorporate significant amounts of potassium. Hence, as large numbers of new red cells are produced, levels of free potassium may fall.

### Dosage and Administration

*Parenteral.* Parenteral forms of cyanocobalamin can be administered by *intramuscular or deep subcutaneous* injection. *Cyanocobalamin must NOT be given intravenously.* Intramuscular and SC injections rarely cause pain or other local reactions.

Parenteral administration is required for all patients who are unable to absorb oral vitamin B$_{12}$. If the cause of malabsorption is irreversible (e.g., parietal cell atrophy, total gastrectomy), parenteral therapy must continue lifelong. A typical dosing schedule for megaloblastic anemia is 30 µg/day for 5 to 10 days followed by 100 to 200 µg monthly until remission is complete. After anemia has been corrected, doses of 100 µg are administered monthly for life.

*Oral.* Oral cyanocobalamin is employed almost exclusively as a dietary supplement. The usual supplemental dose is 6 µg/day. Oral preparations are not useful for treating B$_{12}$ deficiency caused by malabsorption.

### Vitamin B$_{12}$ Preparations II: Miscellaneous Preparations

*Hydroxocobalamin.* Hydroxocobalamin is very similar to cyanocobalamin. Both drugs are alike in structure and therapeutic effects. Hydroxocobalamin differs from cyanocobalamin in that hydroxocobalamin can be administered only by IM injection. Of greater importance, hydroxocobalamin can stimulate production of antibodies directed against the vitamin B$_{12}$-transcobalamin II complex. Accordingly, hydroxocobalamin is not recommended.

*Liver Extracts.* Liver extracts have large amounts of vitamin B$_{12}$. Although liver extracts can be used to treat vitamin B$_{12}$ deficiency, purified cyanocobalamin is by far the treatment of choice. Liver extracts are administered by IM injection.

## Guidelines for Treating Vitamin B$_{12}$ Deficiency

*Route of B$_{12}$ Administration.* *Parenteral* administration is required for all patients who cannot absorb vitamin B$_{12}$ given orally. In this group are patients with pernicious anemia (i.e., lack of intrinsic factor) and those with ileal disease. *Oral* administration is used only when intestinal absorption is unimpaired.

*Treatment of Moderate B$_{12}$ Deficiency.* The primary manifestations of moderate B$_{12}$ deficiency are megaloblasts in the bone marrow and macrocytes in peripheral blood. Moderate deficiency does not cause leukopenia, thrombocytopenia, or neurologic complications. Moderate deficiency can be managed with vitamin B$_{12}$ alone; no other measures are required.

*Treatment of Severe B$_{12}$ Deficiency.* Severe deficiency produces multiple effects, all of which must be attended to. Unlike mild B$_{12}$ deficiency, in which erythrocytes are the only blood cells affected, severe deficiency disrupts production of all blood cells. Loss of erythrocytes leads to hypoxia, cerebrovascular insufficiency, and congestive heart failure; loss of leukocytes encourages infection; and loss of thrombocytes promotes bleeding. In addition to causing serious hematologic deficits, severe B$_{12}$ deficiency has adverse effects on the nervous system and GI tract.

Treatment of severe deficiency involves the following: (1) IM injection of vitamin B$_{12}$ and folic acid (the folic acid accelerates recovery of hematologic deficits); (2) administration of 2 to 3 units of packed red blood cells (to correct anemia quickly); (3) transfusion of platelets (to suppress bleeding); and (4) therapy with antibiotics if infection has developed.

Following treatment with vitamin B$_{12}$ plus folic acid, recovery from anemia occurs quickly. Within 1 to 2 days, megaloblasts disappear from the bone marrow; within 3 to 5 days, reticulocyte counts become elevated; by the 10th day, the hematocrit begins to rise; and within 2 to 3 weeks, the hematocrit becomes normal.

Recovery from neurologic damage is slow and depends on how long the damage had been present. Patients with deficits that have been present for only 2 to 3 months tend to recover with relative haste. Patients with deficits that have been present for many months or for years recover more slowly: months may pass before any improvement is apparent, and complete recovery may never occur.

*Long-Term Treatment.* For patients who lack intrinsic factor, or who suffer from some other permanent cause of vitamin B$_{12}$ malabsorption, *lifelong treatment with parenteral vitamin B$_{12}$ is required.* These people must be made aware of their condition, and arrangements should be made to ensure monthly receipt of an injection. During prolonged therapy, the effectiveness of treatment should be periodically assessed: plasma levels of vitamin B$_{12}$ should be measured every 3 to 6 months, blood samples should be examined for the return of macrocytes, and blood counts should be performed.

*Potential Hazard of Folic Acid.* If care is not exercised, use of folic acid in patients with vitamin B$_{12}$ deficiency can result in exacerbation of the neurologic consequences of vitamin B$_{12}$ deficiency. Recall that folic acid, by itself, can reverse the hematologic effects of B$_{12}$ deficiency—but will not alleviate neurologic deficits. By correcting the most obvious manifestation of B$_{12}$ deficiency (anemia), folic acid can obscure the fact that a deficiency of B$_{12}$ still exists. *By masking B$_{12}$ deficiency, use of folic acid can lead to undertreatment with B$_{12}$ itself, and can thereby permit neurologic damage to progress.* Clearly, folic acid is not a substitute for vitamin B$_{12}$, and vitamin B$_{12}$ deficiency should never be treated with folic acid alone. Whenever folic acid is employed during treatment of vitamin B$_{12}$ de-

## TABLE 51-3. VITAMIN B₁₂ DEFICIENCY VERSUS FOLIC ACID DEFICIENCY

|  | Vitamin B$_{12}$ Deficiency | Folic Acid Deficiency |
| --- | --- | --- |
| *Usual Cause* | Vitamin B$_{12}$ malabsorption from lack of intrinsic factor | Low dietary folic acid |
| *Primary Hematologic Effect* | Megaloblastic anemia | Megaloblastic anemia |
| *Neurologic Effect* | Damage to brain and spinal cord | None |
| *Diagnosis* | Low plasma vitamin B$_{12}$; low vitamin B$_{12}$ absorption (Schilling test) | Low plasma folic acid |
| *Treatment (Usual Route)* | Cyanocobalamin (IM) | Folic acid (PO) |
| *Usual Duration of Therapy* | Lifelong | Short-term |

ficiency, extra care must be taken to ensure that vitamin B$_{12}$ dosage is adequate.

## Folic Acid Deficiency

In one respect, folic acid deficiency is identical to a vitamin B$_{12}$ deficiency: in both states, *megaloblastic anemia* is the most conspicuous pathology. However, in other important ways, folic acid deficiency and vitamin B$_{12}$ deficiency are dissimilar (Table 51-3 provides a summary). Consequently, when a patient presents with megaloblastic anemia, it is essential to determine whether the cause is a deficiency of folic acid, vitamin B$_{12}$, or both.

### Physiology and Biochemistry of Folic Acid

#### Metabolic Function

As we noted when discussing vitamin B$_{12}$, folic acid (also known as *folate*) is an essential factor for DNA synthesis; without folic acid, DNA replication and cell division become disrupted.

In order to be usable, dietary folic acid must first be converted into an active form. Under normal conditions, activation occurs via a pathway employing vitamin B$_{12}$ (see Fig. 51-4). However, when large amounts of folate are ingested, some can be activated via an alternative pathway—one that does not employ vitamin B$_{12}$. Hence, even in the absence of vitamin B$_{12}$, if sufficient amounts of folic acid are consumed, active folate will be available for DNA synthesis.

#### Fate in the Body

Folic acid is absorbed in the early segment of the small intestine. Following absorption, folic acid is transported to the liver and other tissues, where it is either used or stored.

Folic acid in the liver undergoes extensive enterohepatic recirculation. That is, folate from the liver is excreted into the intestine, after which it is reabsorbed and then returned to the liver through the hepatic-portal circulation. This enterohepatic recirculation helps salvage up to 200 µg of folate/day. Accordingly, this process is an important means of maintaining folic acid stores.

In contrast to vitamin B$_{12}$, folic acid is not conserved rigidly: every day, significant amounts are excreted. As a result, if intake of folic acid were to cease, signs of deficiency would develop rapidly (within weeks if body stores were already low when intake stopped).

#### Daily Requirements

The RDA of folic acid is 200 µg/day for adult males, 180 µg/day for adult females who do not plan on becoming pregnant soon, and 400 µg/day if they do plan on becoming pregnant soon. The RDA increases to 400 µg/day during pregnancy and is 280 µg/day for nursing mothers. Individuals with malabsorption syndromes (e.g., tropical sprue) may require as much as 2000 µg (2 mg) per day; at these high doses, folate will be taken up in sufficient quantity despite impaired absorption.

#### Dietary Sources

Folic acid is present in all foods. Green vegetables, liver, and yeast are especially rich sources. It should be noted, however, that with prolonged cooking, folic acid is destroyed.

### Folic Acid Deficiency: Causes, Consequences, and Diagnosis

#### Causes

Folic acid deficiency has two principal causes: (1) poor diet (especially as seen in alcoholics), and (2) malabsorption secondary to intestinal disease. Rarely, certain drugs may cause folate deficiency.

*Alcoholism.* Alcoholism, either acute or chronic, may be the most common cause of folate deficiency. Deficiency results for two reasons: (1) insufficient folic acid in the diet and (2) derangement of enterohepatic recirculation because of alcohol-induced injury to the liver. Fortunately, with improved diet and reduced alcohol consumption, alcohol-related folate deficiency can often be reversed.

*Sprue.* Sprue is an intestinal malabsorption syndrome that decreases folic acid uptake. Since sprue does not block folate absorption entirely, deficiency can be corrected by giving large doses of folic acid orally.

### Consequences

With the important exception that folic acid deficiency does not injure the nervous system, the effects of folate deficiency are identical to those of vitamin $B_{12}$ deficiency. Hence, as with $B_{12}$ deficiency, the most prominent consequence of folate deficiency is *megaloblastic anemia*. In addition, like $B_{12}$ deficiency, lack of folic acid may result in leukopenia, thrombocytopenia, and injury to the oral and gastrointestinal mucosa. Since we have already observed that many of the consequences of vitamin $B_{12}$ deficiency result from depriving cells of active folic acid, the similarities between folate deficiency and vitamin $B_{12}$ deficiency should come as no surprise.

### Diagnosis

When patients present with megaloblastic anemia, it is essential to distinguish between folic acid deficiency and vitamin $B_{12}$ deficiency as the cause. We can make this distinction by comparing plasma levels of folate and vitamin $B_{12}$. If folic acid levels are low and vitamin $B_{12}$ levels are normal, a diagnosis of folic acid deficiency is suggested. Conversely, if folate levels are normal and $B_{12}$ is low, $B_{12}$ deficiency would be the likely diagnosis. A decision against folic acid deficiency would be strengthened if neurologic deficits were observed.

## Folic Acid Preparations

### Nomenclature

Nomenclature regarding folic acid preparations can be confusing and deserves comment. Two forms of folic acid are available. One form is inactive as administered (but undergoes activation once it has been absorbed). The second form is active to start with. Both forms of folic acid have several generic names: the *inactive form* is referred to as *folacin, folate, pteroylglutamic acid,* and *folic acid;* the *active form* is referred to as *leucovorin calcium, folinic acid,* and *citrovorum factor.* The inactive form is by far the most commonly used preparation.

### Folic Acid (Pteroylglutamic Acid)

*Chemistry.* Folic acid is inactive as administered and cannot support DNA synthesis. Activation takes place rapidly following absorption.

*Indications.* Folic acid has three uses: (1) treatment of megaloblastic anemia resulting from folic acid deficiency, (2) prophylaxis of folate deficiency, especially during pregnancy and lactation, and (3) initial treatment of severe megaloblastic anemia resulting from vitamin $B_{12}$ deficiency.

*Adverse Effects.* Oral folic acid is nontoxic. Massive dosages (e.g., as much as 15 mg/day) have been taken with no ill effects.

*Warning.* If taken in sufficiently large doses, folic acid can correct the hematologic consequences of vitamin $B_{12}$ deficiency, thereby masking the fact that a deficiency in vitamin $B_{12}$ still exists. Since folic acid will not prevent the neurologic consequences of vitamin $B_{12}$ deficiency (despite correcting the hematologic picture), this masking effect may allow irreversible damage to the nervous system. To reduce the chances of this problem, folate should not be used indiscriminately: unless specifically indicated, consumption of folic acid should not exceed 0.1 mg/day. Furthermore, whenever folic acid is given to patients known to have a deficiency in vitamin $B_{12}$, special care must be taken to ensure that the vitamin $B_{12}$ dosage is adequate.

*Formulations and Routes of Administration.* Folic acid is available in tablets (0.4, 0.8, and 1.0 mg) and as a 0.5-mg/ml injection [Folvite]. The injection may be administered IM, IV, or SC. As a rule, oral therapy is preferred to parenteral. Injections are reserved for patients with severely impaired absorption.

*Dosage.* For treatment of folate-deficient megaloblastic anemia in adults, the usual oral dosage is 1 to 2 mg/day. Once symptoms have resolved, a maintenance dosage of 0.4 mg/day is given. For prophylaxis during pregnancy and lactation, doses of 1.0 mg/day may be used.

### Leucovorin Calcium (Folinic Acid)

Leucovorin calcium is an active form of folic acid used primarily as an adjunct to cancer chemotherapy (see Chapter 96). Leucovorin is not used routinely to correct folic acid deficiency. This is because folic acid is just as effective and less expensive.

## Guidelines for Treating Folic Acid Deficiency

*Choice of Treatment Modality.* The modality for treating folic acid deficiency should be matched with the cause. If folic acid deficiency is due to poor diet, the deficiency should be corrected by dietary measures—not with drugs. Ingestion of one fresh vegetable or one glass of fruit juice a day will usually suffice. In contrast, when folate deficiency is the result of malabsorption, diet alone cannot correct the deficiency, and a pharmaceutical preparation of folate will be needed.

*Route of Administration.* Oral administration is preferred for most patients. Unlike vitamin $B_{12}$, folic acid is rarely administered by injection. Even in the presence of intestinal disease, oral folic acid can be effective, providing the dosage is big enough.

*Prophylactic Use of Folic Acid.* Folic acid should be taken prophylactically only when clearly appropriate. The principal indications are pregnancy and lactation. Since folic acid may mask vitamin $B_{12}$ deficiency, indiscriminate use of folate should be avoided.

***Treatment of Severe Deficiency.*** Folic acid deficiency can produce severe megaloblastic anemia. To ensure a rapid response, therapy should be initiated with an IM injection of folic acid and vitamin $B_{12}$. (Because of the metabolic interrelationship between folic acid and vitamin $B_{12}$, the combination of these agents helps accelerate recovery.) After the initial injection, treatment should be continued with folic acid alone. Folic acid should be given orally in a dosage of 1 to 2 mg/day for 1 to 2 weeks. After this, maintenance doses of 0.4 mg/day may be required.

Therapy is evaluated by monitoring the hematologic picture. When treatment has been effective, megaloblasts will disappear from the bone marrow within 48 hours; the reticulocyte count will increase measurably within 2 to 3 days; and the hematocrit will begin to rise in the second week.

## KEY POINTS

- The principal cause of iron deficiency is increased iron demand secondary to (1) maternal and fetal blood volume expansion during pregnancy, (2) blood volume expansion during infancy and early childhood, or (3) chronic blood loss, usually of GI or uterine origin.
- The major consequence of iron deficiency is microcytic, hypochromic anemia.
- Ferrous sulfate, given PO, is the drug of choice for iron deficiency.

- Iron-deficient patients who cannot tolerate or absorb oral ferrous salts are treated with parenteral iron dextran, preferably administered IV.
- The major adverse effects of ferrous sulfate are gastrointestinal disturbances. These are best managed by reducing the dosage (rather than by administering the drug with food, which would greatly reduce its absorption).
- The principal cause of vitamin $B_{12}$ deficiency is impaired absorption secondary to lack of intrinsic factor.
- The principal consequences of vitamin $B_{12}$ deficiency are megaloblastic (macrocytic) anemia and neurologic injury.
- Vitamin $B_{12}$ deficiency is treated with lifelong injections (IM or SC) of cyanocobalamin.
- For initial therapy of *severe* vitamin $B_{12}$ deficiency, folic acid is injected along with cyanocobalamin.
- When folic acid is combined with $B_{12}$ to treat $B_{12}$ deficiency, it is essential that the dosage of $B_{12}$ be adequate. This is because folic acid can mask continued $B_{12}$ deficiency (by improving the hematologic picture), while allowing the neurologic consequences of $B_{12}$ deficiency to progress.
- The principal causes of folic acid deficiency are poor diet (usually in alcoholics) and malabsorption secondary to intestinal disease.
- The principal consequence of folic acid deficiency is megaloblastic anemia.
- Folic acid deficiency is treated by improving the diet (when poor diet is the cause) or with oral pharmaceutical folic acid (when malabsorption is the cause).

## Summary of Major Nursing Implications[‡]

## Iron Preparations

|  |  |
|---|---|
| Ferrous Fumarate | Ferrous Sulfate |
| Ferrous Gluconate | Iron Dextran |

Except where indicated, the implications summarized below apply to all of the iron preparations.

## Preadministration Assessment

### Therapeutic Goal
Prevention or treatment of iron deficiency anemias.

### Baseline Data
Prior to treatment, assess the degree of anemia. Fatigue, listlessness, and pallor indicate mild anemia; dyspnea, tachycardia, and angina suggest severe anemia. Laboratory findings indicative of anemia are subnormal hemoglobin levels, subnormal hematocrit, subnormal hemosiderin in bone marrow, and the presence of microcytic, hypochromic erythrocytes.

The cause of iron deficiency (e.g., pregnancy, occult bleeding, menorrhagia, inadequate diet, malabsorption) must be determined.

### Identifying High-Risk Patients
All iron preparations are *contraindicated* for patients with *anemias other than iron-deficiency anemia.*

*Iron dextran* is *contraindicated* for patients who have had a *severe allergic reaction to this preparation in the past.*

Use *oral* preparations with *caution* in patients with *peptic ulcer disease, regional enteritis,* and *ulcerative colitis.*

## Implementation: Administration

### Routes
*Oral.* Ferrous sulfate, ferrous fumarate, ferrous gluconate.

*Parenteral.* Iron dextran.

### Oral Administration
Food reduces GI distress from oral iron but also greatly reduces absorption. Instruct the patient to administer oral iron between meals to maximize uptake. If GI distress is

intolerable, the dosage may be reduced. If absolutely necessary, oral iron may be administered with meals.

Liquid preparations can stain the teeth. Instruct the patient to dilute liquid preparations with juice or water, administer them through a straw, and rinse the mouth after.

Warn the patient not to crush or chew sustained-release preparations.

Warn the patient against ingesting iron salts together with antacids or tetracyclines.

Inform the patient that oral iron salts are not identical and warn him or her against changing from one salt to another.

### Parenteral Administration

Iron dextran may be given IV or IM. Intravenous administration is safer and preferred.

*Intravenous.* To minimize anaphylactic reactions, follow this protocol: (1) Inject 1 or 2 drops as a test dose and observe the patient for at least 15 minutes. (2) If the test dose appears safe, infuse 500 mg over 10 to 15 minutes. (3) If the 500-mg dose proves uneventful, give additional doses as needed.

*Intramuscular.* Intramuscular injection can cause significant adverse reactions (anaphylaxis, persistent pain, localized discoloration, promotion of tumors) and is generally avoided. Make injections deep into each buttock using the Z-track technique. Give a small test dose before giving the full therapeutic dose.

## Implementation: Measures to Enhance Therapeutic Effects

If diet is poor in iron, advise the patient to increase consumption of iron-rich foods (e.g., liver, egg yolks, brewer's yeast, wheat germ, muscle meats, fish, fowl).

## Ongoing Evaluation and Interventions

### Evaluating Therapeutic Responses

Evaluate treatment by monitoring the blood. Reticulocyte number should increase within 4 to 7 days, hemoglobin content and the hematocrit should begin to rise within 1 week, and hemoglobin levels should rise by at least 2 gm/dl within 1 month. If these responses do not occur, evaluate the patient for compliance, persistent bleeding, inflammatory disease, and malabsorption.

### Minimizing Adverse Effects

*Gastrointestinal Disturbances.* Forewarn patients about possible GI reactions (nausea, vomiting, constipation, diarrhea) and inform them that these will diminish over time. If GI distress is severe, the dosage may be reduced, or, if absolutely necessary, iron may be administered with food.

Forewarn patients that iron will impart a harmless dark green or black color to stools.

*Anaphylactic Reactions.* Parenteral iron dextran can cause potentially fatal anaphylaxis. Before giving the drug, ensure that injectable epinephrine and facilities for resuscitation are immediately available. After administration, observe the patient for 60 minutes. Follow the administration protocol described above.

### Management of Acute Toxicity

Iron poisoning can be fatal to young children. Instruct parents to store iron out of reach and in child-proof containers. If poisoning occurs, rapid treatment is imperative. Induce vomiting to remove iron from the stomach. Administer deferoxamine if plasma levels of iron exceed 500 µg/ml. Manage acidosis and shock as required.

# Cyanocobalamin (Vitamin B$_{12}$)

## Preadministration Assessment

### Therapeutic Goal

Correction of megaloblastic anemia and other sequelae of vitamin B$_{12}$ deficiency.

### Baseline Data

Assess the extent of vitamin B$_{12}$ deficiency. Record signs and symptoms of anemia (e.g., pallor, dyspnea, palpitations, fatigue). Determine the extent of neurologic damage. Assess GI involvement.

Baseline laboratory data include plasma vitamin B$_{12}$ levels, erythrocyte and reticulocyte counts, and hemoglobin and hematocrit values. Bone marrow may be examined for megaloblasts. A Schilling test may be ordered to assess vitamin B$_{12}$ absorption.

### Identifying High-Risk Patients

Use with *caution* in patients receiving *folic acid*.

## Implementation: Administration

### Routes

Oral, IM, SC.

Parenteral administration is required for most patients. Oral administration is effective only for patients with modest dietary deficiency.

### Administration

Most patients require monthly injections for life.

## Implementation: Measures to Enhance Therapeutic Effects

### Promoting Compliance

Patients with permanent impairment of vitamin B$_{12}$ absorption require lifelong vitamin B$_{12}$ therapy. To promote compliance, educate patients about the nature of their condition and impress upon them the need for regular monthly injections. Schedule appointments conveniently.

### Improving Diet

When vitamin $B_{12}$ deficiency is not due to impaired absorption, a change in diet may accelerate recovery. Advise the patient to increase consumption of vitamin $B_{12}$-rich foods (e.g., muscle meats, dairy products).

## Ongoing Evaluation and Interventions

### Evaluating Therapeutic Effects

Assess for improvements in hematologic and neurologic status. Over a period of 2 to 3 weeks, megaloblasts should disappear, reticulocyte counts should rise, and the hematocrit should normalize. Neurologic damage may take months to improve; in some cases, full recovery may never occur.

For patients receiving long-term therapy, vitamin $B_{12}$ levels should be measured every 3 to 6 months, and blood counts should be performed.

### Minimizing Adverse Effects

*Hypokalemia* may develop during the first days of therapy. Monitor serum potassium levels and observe the patient for signs of potassium insufficiency (e.g., muscle weakness, dysrhythmias).

### Minimizing Adverse Interactions

*Folic acid* can mask hematologic symptoms of vitamin $B_{12}$ deficiency, resulting in undertreatment and progression of neurologic injury from $B_{12}$ insufficiency. When folic acid and cyanocobalamin are used concurrently, special care must be taken to ensure that the cyanocobalamin dosage is adequate.

## Folic Acid (Folacin, Folate, Pteroylglutamic Acid)

## Preadministration Assessment

### Therapeutic Goal

Folic acid is used for (1) treatment of megaloblastic anemia resulting from folic acid deficiency, (2) initial treatment of severe megaloblastic anemia resulting from vitamin $B_{12}$ deficiency, and (3) prevention of folic acid deficiency (especially during pregnancy).

### Baseline Data

Assess the extent of folate deficiency. Record signs and symptoms of anemia (e.g., pallor, dyspnea, palpitations, fatigue). Determine the extent of gastrointestinal damage.

Baseline laboratory data include serum folate levels, erythrocyte and reticulocyte counts, and hemoglobin and hematocrit values. In addition, bone marrow may be evaluated for megaloblasts. To rule out vitamin $B_{12}$ deficiency, vitamin $B_{12}$ determinations and a Schilling test may be ordered.

### Identifying High-Risk Patients

Folic acid is *contraindicated* for patients with *pernicious anemia* (except during the acute phase of treatment). Inappropriate use of folic acid by these patients can mask signs of vitamin $B_{12}$ deficiency, thereby allowing further neurologic deterioration.

## Implementation: Administration

### Routes

Oral, SC, IV, and IM. Oral administration is most common and preferred. Injections are employed only when intestinal absorption is severely impaired.

## Implementation: Measures to Enhance Therapeutic Effects

### Improving Diet

If the diet is deficient in folic acid, advise the patient to increase consumption of folate-rich foods (e.g., green vegetables, liver, yeast). Warn the patient that prolonged cooking destroys folic acid. If alcoholism underlies dietary deficiency, counseling should be offered.

## Ongoing Evaluation and Interventions

### Evaluating Therapeutic Effects

Monitor hematologic status. Within 2 weeks, megaloblasts should disappear, reticulocyte counts should increase, and the hematocrit should begin to rise.

# CHAPTER 52

# Hematopoietic Growth Factors

**Epoetin Alfa (Erythropoietin)**
**Filgrastim (Granulocyte Colony-Stimulating Factor)**
**Sargramostim (Granulocyte-Macrophage**
 **Colony-Stimulating Factor)**

Hematopoiesis is the process by which new blood cells are produced. This process is regulated in part by hematopoietic growth factors—naturally occurring hormones that (1) stimulate the proliferation and differentiation of hematopoietic stem cells, and (2) enhance function in the mature forms of those cells (neutrophils, monocytes, macrophages, and erythrocytes). In a laboratory setting, hematopoietic growth factors can cause stem cells to form colonies of mature blood cells. Because of this action, hematopoietic growth factors are also known as *colony-stimulating factors*. Therapeutic applications of hematopoietic growth factors include (1) acceleration of neutrophil repopulation after cancer chemotherapy, (2) acceleration of bone marrow recovery after autologous bone marrow transplantation, and (3) stimulation of erythrocyte production in patients with chronic renal failure.

The names used for the hematopoietic growth factors are a potential source of confusion. At this time, three hematopoietic growth factors are available for clinical use. The *biologic* names of these three hormones are *erythropoietin, granulocyte colony-stimulating factor,* and *granulocyte-macrophage colony-stimulating factor*. In addition to their biologic name, each compound has two types of *pharmacologic* names: a *generic* name and one or more *proprietary* (trade) names. The generic and proprietary names for the three growth factors are listed in Table 52-1. Keep in mind that the biologic, generic, and trade names for each compound all refer to the identical chemical.

## Epoetin Alfa (Erythropoietin)

Epoetin alfa [Epogen, Procrit] is a drug produced by recombinant DNA technology. Chemically, the compound is a glycoprotein containing 165 amino acids. The protein portion of epoetin alfa is identical to that of human erythropoietin, a naturally occurring hormone. Epoetin alfa is used to maintain erythrocyte counts in (1) patients with chronic renal failure, (2) HIV-infected patients taking zi-

dovudine, and (3) patients with nonmyeloid malignancies who have anemia secondary to chemotherapy.

### Physiology

Erythropoietin is a glycoprotein hormone that stimulates production of red blood cells (erythrocytes). The hormone is produced by peritubular cells in the proximal tubules of the kidney. In response to anemia or hypoxia, circulating levels of erythropoietin rise dramatically, triggering an increase in erythrocyte synthesis. However, since production of erythrocytes requires iron, folic acid, and vitamin $B_{12}$, the response to erythropoietin will be minimal if any of these factors is deficient.

### Therapeutic Uses

*Anemia of Chronic Renal Failure.* Epoetin alfa can reverse anemia associated with chronic renal failure (CRF). The drug is effective in patients on dialysis and in patients who do not yet require dialysis. Effective treatment virtually eliminates the need for transfusions. Initial effects can be seen within 1 to 2 weeks. The hematocrit reaches normal levels (30% to 33%) in 2 to 3 months. Patients experience an improved quality of life and increased energy levels. Unfortunately, treatment does not prevent progressive renal deterioration.

For therapy to be effective, iron stores must be adequate. Transferrin saturation should be at least 20%, and ferritin concentration should be at least 100 ng/ml. If pretreatment assessment shows these values to be low, they must be restored with iron supplements.

*HIV-Infected Patients Taking Zidovudine.* Epoetin alfa is approved for treating anemia caused by therapy with zidovudine (AZT) in patients with AIDS. For these patients, treatment can maintain or elevate erythrocyte counts and reduce the need for transfusions. However, if endogenous levels of erythropoietin are at or above 500 mU/ml, raising them further with epoetin is not likely to help.

*Chemotherapy-Induced Anemia.* Epoetin alfa is used to treat chemotherapy-induced anemia in patients with *nonmyeloid malignancies*, thereby reducing or eliminat-

## TABLE 52-1. NOMENCLATURE FOR HEMATOPOIETIC GROWTH FACTORS

| Biologic Name | Pharmacologic Names | |
| --- | --- | --- |
| | Generic Name | Trade Name |
| Granulocyte colony-stimulating factor (G-CSF) | Filgrastim | Neupogen |
| Granulocyte-macrophage-colony-stimulating factor (GM-CSF) | Sargramostim | Leukine |
| Erythropoietin (EPO) | Epoetin alfa | Epogen, Procrit |

ing the need for periodic transfusions. Since transfusions require hospitalization, whereas epoetin can be self-administered at home, epoetin therapy can spare patients considerable inconvenience. Because epoetin works slowly (the hematocrit may take 2 to 4 weeks to recover), transfusions are still indicated when rapid replenishment of red blood cells is required. Please note that epoetin is not approved for patients with *leukemias* and *other myeloid malignancies* because it may stimulate proliferation of these cancers.

*Investigational Use.* Epoetin has been used with success to increase the harvest of red blood cells for autologous transfusion in patients anticipating elective surgery.

### Pharmacokinetics

Epoetin alfa is administered parenterally (IV or SC). The drug cannot be given orally because, being a glycoprotein, it would be degraded in the gastrointestinal tract. The plasma half-life of the drug is highly variable and is not changed by dialysis.

### Adverse Effects and Interactions

Epoetin alfa is generally well tolerated. Although the drug is a protein, no serious allergic reactions have been reported. The most significant adverse effect is hypertension. There are no significant drug interactions.

*Hypertension.* In patients with CRF, epoetin is frequently associated with an increase in blood pressure. The extent of hypertension is directly related to the rate of rise in the hematocrit. To minimize the risk of hypertension, blood pressure should be monitored and, if necessary, controlled with antihypertensive drugs. If hypertension cannot be controlled, the dosage of epoetin should be reduced. In patients with pre-existing hypertension (a common complication of CRF), it is imperative that blood pressure be under control prior to epoetin use. About 30% of dialysis patients receiving epoetin require an adjustment in their antihypertensive therapy once the hematocrit has been normalized.

### Monitoring

The hematocrit should be determined prior to treatment and twice weekly thereafter until the target level has been reached and a maintenance dose established.

Complete blood counts with a differential should be done routinely. Blood chemistry—blood urea nitrogen (BUN), uric acid, creatinine, phosphorus, and potassium—should be monitored. Iron should be measured periodically and maintained at an adequate level.

### Preparations, Dosage, and Administration

Epoetin alfa [Epogen, Procrit] is dispensed in 1-ml vials (2000, 3000, 4000, and 10,000 units) for SC and IV injection. Vials should not be shaken since epoetin is a protein that can be denatured by agitation. Use only one dose per vial and discard the unused portion. Don't mix epoetin with other drugs. Store at 2°C to 8°C; don't freeze.

*Patients with Chronic Renal Failure.* The initial dosage is 50 to 100 U/kg 3 times a week. Administration is by IV bolus for dialysis patients and by IV bolus or SC injection for nondialysis patients. The dosage should be reduced when the therapeutic endpoint is reached (hematocrit of 30% to 33%) or if the rate of rise in the hematocrit exceeds 4 units in 2 weeks. Once the target hematocrit has been achieved, an individualized maintenance dosage should be established: for dialysis patients, the median maintenance dosage is 75 U/kg 3 times a week; for nondialysis patients, the median maintenance dosage is 75 to 100 U/kg once a week. If the hematocrit rises above 36%, epoetin should be temporarily withheld.

*HIV-Infected Patients Taking Zidovudine.* Prior to treatment, measure the endogenous erythropoietin level. If this level is already at or above 500 mU/ml, epoetin alfa is unlikely to be helpful.

Therapy is begun at 100 U/kg (IV or SC injection) 3 times a week. If the response is insufficient, the dosage may be increased by increments of 50 to 100 U/kg until a maximum of 300 U/kg 3 times a week has been reached. When the hematocrit has been restored to the desired level, an individualized maintenance dosage should be established.

*Patients Receiving Cancer Chemotherapy.* The initial dosage is 150 U/kg SC 3 times a week. If the response is inadequate by 8 weeks, the dosage may be increased to 300 U/kg 3 times a week.

## Filgrastim (Granulocyte Colony-Stimulating Factor)

Filgrastim [Neupogen] is produced by recombinant DNA technology. This agent is essentially identical in structure and actions to human granulocyte colony-stimulating factor (G-CSF), a naturally occurring hormone. Filgrastim has two principal uses: elevation of neutrophil counts in cancer patients and treatment of severe chronic neutropenia.

## Physiology

G-CSF acts on cells in bone marrow to increase production of neutrophils (granulocytes). In addition, it enhances phagocytic and cytotoxic actions of mature neutrophils. The hormone is produced by monocytes, fibroblasts, and endothelial cells in response to inflammation and allergic challenge. This suggests that the hormone's natural role is to help fight infections and cancer.

## Therapeutic Uses

*Cancer.* *Patients Undergoing Myelosuppressive Chemotherapy.* Filgrastim is given to reduce the risk of infection in patients undergoing cancer chemotherapy. Many anticancer drugs act on the bone marrow to suppress production of neutrophils, thereby greatly increasing the risk of infection. By stimulating production of neutrophils, filgrastim can decrease the risk of infection. Clinical trials have shown that the drug (1) reduces the incidence of severe neutropenia, (2) produces a dose-dependent increase in circulating neutrophils, (3) reduces the incidence of infection, (4) reduces the need for hospitalization, and (5) reduces the need for intravenous antibiotics. Unfortunately, this useful drug is very expensive: the cost to the pharmacist for a single course of treatment is $1800 to $2800. Because filgrastim stimulates proliferation of bone marrow cells, it should be used with great caution in patients with cancers that originated in the marrow.

*Patients Undergoing Bone Marrow Transplant.* Filgrastim is given to shorten the duration of neutropenia in patients who have undergone high-dose chemotherapy followed by a bone marrow transplant. As noted above, the drug is not used when the cancer is of myeloid origin.

*Severe Chronic Neutropenia.* Filgrastim provides effective treatment for *congenital neutropenia* (Kostmann's syndrome), a condition characterized by pronounced neutropenia and frequent, severe infections. Therapy causes resolution of existing infections and decreases the incidence of subsequent infections. Because treatment is chronic, the cost is extremely high. In addition to congenital neutropenia, filgrastim is used in patients with *idiopathic neutropenia* and *cyclic neutropenia*.

*Investigational Uses.* Filgrastim can reverse *zidovudine-induced neutropenia* in HIV-infected patients. However, the drug does not reduce the incidence of opportunistic infections in these people. In patients with *acute myelogenous leukemia*, filgrastim has been given to stimulate division of cancer cells, thereby making them more sensitive to chemotherapeutic agents. Filgrastim has also been employed in patients with *aplastic anemia* and *myelodysplasia*.

## Pharmacokinetics

Administration is parenteral (IV or SC). Filgrastim cannot be used orally because, being a protein, it would be destroyed in the gastrointestinal tract. Other aspects of the drug's kinetics are unremarkable.

## Adverse Effects and Interactions

When used on a short-term basis, filgrastim is generally devoid of serious adverse effects. There are no drug interactions of note.

*Bone Pain.* Filgrastim causes bone pain in about 25% of those treated. Pain is dose-related and usually of mild to moderate intensity. In most cases, relief can be achieved with a nonopioid analgesic (e.g., acetaminophen). If not, an opioid may be tried.

*Leukocytosis.* When administered in doses greater than 5 μg/kg/day, filgrastim has caused white cell counts to rise above 100,000/mm$^3$ in 2% of patients. Although no adverse effects were associated with this degree of leukocytosis, avoidance of leukocytosis would nonetheless be prudent. Excessive white cell counts can be avoided by obtaining complete blood counts twice weekly during treatment and by reducing filgrastim dosage if leukocytosis develops.

*Other Adverse Effects.* Treatment frequently causes elevation of plasma uric acid, lactate dehydrogenase, and alkaline phosphatase. These increases are usually moderate and reverse spontaneously. Long-term therapy has caused splenomegaly in some patients.

## Preparations, Dosage, and Administration

*Preparations and Storage.* Filgrastim [Neupogen] is dispensed in solution (300 μg/ml) in 1- and 1.6-ml single-dose vials. The drug is stored at 2°C to 8°C—not frozen.

*Dosage and Administration.* *General Considerations.* Prior to administration, filgrastim can be kept at room temperature for up to 6 hours. It should not be agitated. Only 1 dose per vial should be used, and the vial should not be re-entered.

*Cancer Chemotherapy.* The usual dosage is 5 μg/kg once daily, administered IV or SC. Therapy should start no sooner than 24 hours after termination of chemotherapy, and should continue for up to 2 weeks after the expected chemotherapy-induced nadir, or until the absolute neutrophil count has reached 10,000/mm$^3$. Administer by SC bolus, short IV infusion, or continuous IV or SC infusion. A complete blood count and platelet count should be obtained prior to treatment and twice weekly during treatment.

*Bone Marrow Transplant.* The initial dosage is 10 μg/kg/day administered by slow IV or SC infusion. During the period of neutrophil recovery, the dosage is titrated against the neutrophil count.

*Severe Chronic Neutropenia.* The dosage is 6 μg/kg SC administered twice a day every day.

# Sargramostim (Granulocyte-Macrophage Colony-Stimulating Factor)

Sargramostim [Leukine], like filgrastim and epoetin, is produced by recombinant DNA technology. This drug is nearly identical in structure and actions to human granulocyte-macrophage colony-stimulating factor (GM-CSF), a naturally occurring hormone. Sargramostim is given to accelerate bone marrow recovery following a bone marrow transplant.

## Physiology

GM-CSF acts on cells in bone marrow to increase production of neutrophils, monocytes, macrophages, and eosinophils. In addition, the hormone acts on the mature forms of these cells to enhance their function. For example, GM-CSF acts on neutrophils and macrophages to increase their chemotactic, antifungal, and antiparasitic actions. Also, the hormone acts on monocytes and polymorphonuclear leukocytes to enhance their actions against cancer cells. GM-CSF is synthesized by T lymphocytes, monocytes, fibroblasts, and endothelial cells. Like G-CSF, GM-CSF is produced in response to inflammation and allergic challenge, suggesting that its natural role is to help fight infections and cancers.

## Therapeutic Uses

### Adjunct to Autologous Bone Marrow Transplantation.
Sargramostim can accelerate myeloid recovery in cancer patients who have undergone an autologous bone marrow transplant (BMT) following high-dose chemotherapy (with or without concurrent irradiation). The drug is approved for promoting myeloid recovery following BMT in patients with acute lymphoblastic leukemia, non-Hodgkin's lymphoma, and Hodgkin's disease. In these patients, sargramostim can (1) accelerate neutrophil engraftment, (2) reduce the duration of antibiotic use, (3) reduce the duration of infectious episodes, and (4) reduce the duration of hospitalization. Therapy is expensive: the cost to the pharmacist for a 21-day course of sargramostim is more than $4000.

### Treatment of Failed Bone Marrow Transplants.
Sargramostim is approved for patients in whom an autologous or allogenic BMT has failed to take. For these patients, the drug can produce a significant increase in survival time.

*Investigational Uses.* In *HIV-infected patients*, sargramostim can reverse neutropenia caused by zidovudine (a drug that inhibits HIV replication) and by ganciclovir (a drug for cytomegalovirus retinitis).

In patients with *aplastic anemia* (a syndrome characterized by pancytopenia and high mortality from infection and bleeding), sargramostim can increase neutrophil counts and reduce the incidence and severity of infections.

Sargramostim is beneficial for patients with *myelodysplastic syndrome* (MDS), a chronic disorder characterized by greatly reduced hematopoiesis. Patients with MDS are neutropenic, thrombocytopenic, and anemic, putting them at high risk for serious infections and bleeding. The syndrome has a mortality rate of 66%—and those who survive often develop leukemia. Treatment with sargramostim can increase counts of neutrophils, eosinophils, and monocytes. However, the premalignant clone still exists and may eventually cause leukemia.

## Pharmacokinetics

Sargramostim is administered by IV infusion. Since the drug is a protein and would be degraded in the digestive tract, it cannot be administered by mouth. Other aspects of the drug's kinetics are unremarkable.

## Adverse Effects and Interactions

Sargramostim is generally well tolerated. A variety of acute reactions have been observed, including *diarrhea*, *weakness*, *rash*, *malaise*, and *bone pain* that can be managed with nonopioid analgesics (e.g., acetaminophen). *Pleural and pericardial effusions* have occurred, but only when sargramostim dosage was massive (16 times the recommended dosage). There are no drug interactions of note.

### Leukocytosis and Thrombocytosis.
Stimulation of the bone marrow can produce excessive elevations in white blood cells and platelets. Complete blood counts should be done twice weekly during therapy. If the white cell count rises above 50,000/mm$^3$, if the absolute neutrophil count rises above 20,000/mm$^3$, or if the platelet count rises above 500,000/mm$^3$, sargramostim should be interrupted or the dosage reduced.

### Preparations, Dosage, and Administration

*Preparations.* Sargramostim [Leukine] is dispensed as a powder (250 and 500 µg) in single-use vials to be reconstituted for IV infusion.

*Reconstitution and Storage.* To reconstitute the powder, add 1 ml of sterile water and swirl gently; don't shake. To prepare the final solution for infusion, dilute the reconstituted concentrate in either (1) 0.9% sodium chloride (if the final concentration of sargramostim is to be 10 µg/ml or more) or in (2) 0.9% sodium chloride plus 0.1% albumin (if the final concentration is to be less than 10 µg/ml). Since the solution contains no antibacterial preservatives, it should be used as soon as possible—and no later than 6 hours after preparation. Sargramostim (powder, reconstituted concentrate, final IV solution) should be kept at 2°C to 8°C (never frozen) until used.

*Dosage and Administration.* For acceleration of myeloid recovery after an autologous bone marrow transplant, the recommended dosage is 250 µg/m$^2$ (as a 2-hour IV infusion) administered once daily for 21 days beginning 2 to 4 hours after the bone marrow infusion.

For patients in whom an autologous or allogenic bone marrow transplant has failed or in whom engraftment has been delayed, the recommended dosage is 250 µg/m$^2$ (as a 2-hour IV infusion) administered once daily for 14 days. After a 7-day hiatus, the 14-day series of infusions can be repeated if needed. After another 7-day hiatus, the 14-day series can be repeated once more if needed. If the graft still has not taken, further treatment is unlikely to be of benefit.

## KEY POINTS

- Epoetin alfa is given to increase red blood cell counts. Specific indications are anemia associated with (1) chronic renal failure, (2) zidovudine therapy in AIDS patients, and (3) cancer chemotherapy.
- By increasing the hematocrit, epoetin alfa can cause or exacerbate hypertension.
- Filgrastim is given to elevate neutrophil counts, and thereby reduce the risk of infection. Specific indications are chronic severe neutropenia and neutropenia associated with cancer chemotherapy or a bone marrow transplant.
- The principal adverse effects of filgrastim are bone pain and leukocytosis.
- Sargramostim is used to accelerate recovery from a bone marrow transplant and to treat patients in whom a bone marrow transplant has failed.
- The principal adverse effect of sargramostim is leukocytosis.
- Since epoetin alfa, filgrastim, and sargramostim stimulate proliferation of bone marrow cells, these drugs should be used with great caution, if at all, in patients with cancers of bone marrow origin.

# Summary of Major Nursing Implications

## Epoetin Alfa (Erythropoietin)

### Preadministration Assessment

#### Therapeutic Goal
Restoration and maintenance of erythrocyte counts in (1) patients with chronic renal failure, (2) HIV-infected patients receiving zidovudine, and (3) patients receiving cancer chemotherapy.

#### Baseline Data
*All Patients.* Obtain blood pressure; blood chemistry (BUN, uric acid, creatinine, phosphorus, potassium); complete blood counts with differential and platelet count; hematocrit; degree of transferrin saturation (should be at least 20%); and ferritin concentration (should be at least 100 ng/ml).

*HIV-Infected Patients.* Obtain an erythropoietin level. (If the level is above 500 mU/ml, epoetin is unlikely to help.)

#### Identifying High-Risk Patients
Epoetin alfa is *contraindicated* for patients with *uncontrolled hypertension* or *hypersensitivity to mammalian cell-derived products or albumin.* Use with *caution* in patients with *cancers of myeloid origin.*

### Implementation: Administration

#### Routes
Subcutaneous, intravenous.

#### Handling and Storage
Epoetin alfa is dispensed in single-use vials; don't re-enter the vial, and discard the unused portion. Don't agitate. Don't mix with other drugs. Store at 2°C to 8°C; don't freeze.

#### Administration
*Chronic Renal Failure.* For dialysis patients, administer by IV bolus. For nondialysis patients, administer by IV bolus or SC injection.

*Zidovudine-Induced Anemia.* Administer by IV or SC injection.

*Chemotherapy-Induced Anemia.* Administer by SC injection.

### Ongoing Evaluation and Interventions

#### Monitoring Summary
Determine the hematocrit twice weekly until the target level has been reached and a maintenance dosage established. Obtain complete blood counts with a differential and platelet counts routinely. Monitor blood chemistry, including BUN, uric acid, creatinine, phosphorus, and potas-

sium. Monitor iron stores and maintain at an adequate level. Monitor blood pressure.

#### Minimizing Adverse Effects
*Hypertension.* Monitor blood pressure and, if necessary, control with antihypertensive drugs. If hypertension cannot be controlled, reduce epoetin dosage. In patients with pre-existing hypertension (a common complication of CRF), make certain that blood pressure is controlled prior to epoetin use.

## Filgrastim (Granulocyte Colony-Stimulating Factor)

### Preadministration Assessment

#### Therapeutic Goal
Filgrastim is given to promote neutrophil recovery in cancer patients following myelosuppressive chemotherapy or a bone marrow transplant. The drug is also used to treat severe chronic neutropenia.

#### Baseline Data
Obtain complete blood counts and platelet counts.

#### Identifying High-Risk Patients
Filgrastim is *contraindicated* for patients with *hypersensitivity to E. coli-derived proteins.* Use with *caution* in patients with *cancers of bone marrow origin.*

### Implementation: Administration

#### Routes
Subcutaneous, intravenous.

#### Handling and Storage
Filgrastim is dispensed in single-use vials; don't re-enter the vial, and discard the unused portion. Don't agitate. Store at 2°C to 8°C; don't freeze. Prior to administration, filgrastim may be kept at room temperature for up to 6 hours.

#### Administration
*Cancer Chemotherapy.* Administer by SC bolus, short IV infusion, or continuous IV or SC infusion.

*Bone Marrow Transplant.* Administer by slow IV or SC infusion.

*Chronic Severe Neutropenia.* Inject SC twice daily every day.

### Ongoing Evaluation and Interventions

#### Evaluating Therapeutic Effects
Obtain complete blood counts twice weekly. Discontinue treatment when the absolute neutrophil count reaches 10,000/mm$^3$.

## Minimizing Adverse Effects

***Bone Pain.*** Evaluate for bone pain and treat with a nonopioid analgesic (e.g., acetaminophen). Consider a more powerful (opioid) analgesic if the nonopioid is insufficient.

***Leukocytosis.*** Massive doses of filgrastim can cause leukocytosis (white blood cell counts above 100,000/mm³). If leukocytosis develops, reduce filgrastim dosage.

# Sargramostim (Granulocyte-Macrophage Colony-Stimulating Factor)

## Preadministration Assessment

### Therapeutic Goal

Acceleration of myeloid recovery in cancer patients who have undergone an autologous bone marrow transplant following high-dose chemotherapy (with or without concurrent irradiation).

Treatment of patients for whom an autologous or allogenic bone marrow transplant has failed to take.

### Baseline Data

Obtain complete blood counts with differential and platelet count.

### Identifying High-Risk Patients

Sargramostim is *contraindicated* in the presence of *hypersensitivity to yeast-derived products* and *excessive leukemic myeloid blasts in bone marrow or peripheral blood*. Exercise *caution* in patients with *cardiac disease, hypoxia, peripheral edema, pleural or pericardial effusion*, or *cancers of bone marrow origin*.

## Implementation: Administration

### Route

Intravenous (by infusion).

### Handling and Storage

Sargramostim is dispensed in single-use vials; don't re-enter the vial, and discard the unused portion. Don't agitate. Don't mix with other drugs. Administer as soon as possible—and no later than 6 hours after reconstitution. Store sargramostim (powder, reconstituted concentrate, final IV solution) at 2°C to 8°C until used.

### Administration

Administer by 2-hour IV infusion.

## Ongoing Evaluation and Interventions

### Minimizing Adverse Effects

***Leukocytosis and Thrombocytosis.*** Obtain complete blood counts with a differential and platelet counts twice weekly. If the white blood cell count rises above 50,000/mm³, if the absolute neutrophil count rises above 20,000/mm³, or if the platelet count rises above 500,000/mm³, temporarily interrupt sargramostim or reduce its dosage.

# UNIT IX

# Endocrine Drugs

# CHAPTER 53

# Drugs for Diabetes Mellitus

## Diabetes Mellitus: Overview of the Disease and Its Treatment

The term *diabetes mellitus* is derived from the Greek word for *fountain* and the Latin word for *honey*. Hence, the name *diabetes mellitus* describes one of the prominent symptoms of untreated diabetes: production of large volumes of glucose-rich urine. In this chapter we will use the terms *diabetes mellitus* and *diabetes* interchangeably.

Diabetes is primarily a disorder of carbohydrate metabolism. Symptoms result from a deficiency of insulin or from resistance to insulin's actions. The principal sign of diabetes is sustained hyperglycemia, which rapidly causes polyuria, polydipsia, ketonuria, and weight loss. Over time, hyperglycemia can lead to hypertension, heart disease, blindness, renal failure, neuropathy, amputations, impotence, and stroke.

Diabetes is a major public health concern. In the United States, diabetes is the most common endocrine disorder, and the fourth leading cause of death. About 16 million Americans have diabetes, although only half are diagnosed. In 1992, the direct medical cost of diabetes was $45 billion. Put another way, one of every seven health care dollars was spent on this disease.

## Types of Diabetes Mellitus

There are two principal forms of diabetes: (1) insulin-dependent diabetes mellitus (IDDM) and (2) noninsulin-dependent diabetes mellitus (NIDDM). Several less common forms (e.g., gestational diabetes) have also been identified. The distinguishing characteristics of IDDM and NIDDM are summarized in Table 53-1 and discussed below.

### Insulin-Dependent Diabetes Mellitus

IDDM accounts for 5% to 10% of all cases of diabetes. Approximately 700,000 Americans have this disorder. IDDM is known by three alternative names: *type 1 diabetes mellitus*, *juvenile-onset diabetes mellitus*, and *ketosis-prone diabetes mellitus*. As a rule, IDDM develops during childhood or adolescence. Onset of symptoms is usually abrupt.

The primary defect in IDDM is *destruction of pancreatic beta cells*—the cells responsible for insulin synthesis. Insulin levels are reduced early in the disease and *completely absent* later. Beta cell destruction is the result of an autoimmune process (i.e., development of antibodies against the patient's own beta cells). Although the trigger for this immune response is unknown, infection with Coxsackie virus is a leading candidate.

### Noninsulin-Dependent Diabetes Mellitus

NIDDM is the most prevalent form of diabetes. Approximately 15 million Americans have this disease. NIDDM has two alternative names: *type 2 diabetes mellitus* and *adult-onset diabetes mellitus*. The disease usually begins in middle age and progresses gradually. Obesity is almost always present. In contrast to IDDM, NIDDM carries little risk of ketoacidosis. However, NIDDM does carry the same long-term risks as IDDM (see below).

## TABLE 53–1. CHARACTERISTICS OF THE MAJOR FORMS OF DIABETES MELLITUS

| | Types of Diabetes Mellitus | |
|---|---|---|
| **Characteristics** | Insulin-Dependent (IDDM) | Noninsulin-Dependent (NIDDM) |
| Alternative names | Type 1 diabetes mellitus, juvenile-onset diabetes mellitus, ketosis-prone diabetes mellitus | Type 2 diabetes mellitus, adult-onset diabetes mellitus |
| Age of onset | Usually childhood or adolescence | Usually over 40 |
| Speed of onset | Abrupt | Gradual |
| Family history | Usually negative | Frequently positive |
| Prevalence | 5% to 10% of diabetics have IDDM | 90% to 95% of diabetics have NIDDM |
| Etiology | Autoimmune process | Unknown—but there is a strong familial association, suggesting heredity as the underlying cause |
| Primary defect | Loss of pancreatic beta cells | Insulin resistance and inappropriate insulin secretion |
| Insulin levels | Reduced early in the disease and completely absent later | Levels may be low (indicating deficiency), normal, or high (indicating resistance) |
| Treatment | Insulin replacement is mandatory, along with strict dietary control; oral hypoglycemic drugs are not effective | Exercise and a reduced-calorie diet may be sufficient; if not, an oral hypoglycemic agent and/or insulin is required |
| Blood glucose | Levels fluctuate widely in response to infection, exercise, and changes in caloric intake and insulin dose | Levels are more stable than in IDDM |
| Symptoms | Polyuria, polydipsia, polyphagia, weight loss | May be asymptomatic |
| Body composition | Usually thin and undernourished | Frequently obese |
| Ketosis | Common, especially if insulin dosage is insufficient | Uncommon |

Symptoms result from a combination of insulin resistance and altered insulin secretion. In contrast to patients with IDDM, patients with NIDDM are capable of insulin synthesis. In fact, insulin levels tend to be normal or slightly elevated. However, although insulin is still produced, its secretion is no longer tightly coupled to plasma glucose content: release of insulin is delayed and peak output is subnormal. Furthermore, the target tissues of insulin (liver, muscle, adipose tissue) exhibit insulin resistance. Resistance appears to result from two causes: reduced binding of insulin to its receptors and reduced receptor responsiveness. Although the underlying cause of NIDDM is not known, there is a strong familial association, suggesting that heredity may be a major factor.

## Short-Term Complications of Diabetes

Acute complications are seen primarily in patients with IDDM. Principal concerns are *hyperglycemia* and *hypoglycemia*. Hyperglycemia results when insulin dosage is insufficient. Conversely, hypoglycemia results when insulin dosage is excessive. Ketoacidosis, a potentially fatal acute complication, develops when hyperglycemia is allowed to persist. All three complications are discussed further below.

## Long-Term Complications of Diabetes

The long-term sequelae of IDDM and NIDDM take years to develop. More than 90% of diabetic deaths result from long-term complications, not from hypoglycemia or ketoacidosis. Most complications occur secondary to disruption of blood flow—because of either macrovascular or microvascular damage. Ironically, insulin can be viewed as having made long-term complications possible: prior to the discovery of insulin, diabetics died long before chronic disorders could arise.

The landmark Diabetes Complications and Control Trial (DCCT) demonstrated that, with rigorous control of blood glucose, development of long-term complications can be greatly reduced. For example, compared with patients whose glucose was only moderately controlled, patients whose glucose was tightly controlled experienced 76% less retinopathy, 60% less neuropathy, and 35% to 56% less nephropathy. Although all participants in the DCCT had IDDM, the benefits of tight glucose control are believed to apply equally to patients with NIDDM.

**Macrovascular Disease.** Cardiovascular complications are the leading cause of death among diabetics. Diabetes carries an increased risk of *hypertension*, *heart disease*, and *stroke*. Much of this pathology is due to atherosclerosis, which develops earlier in diabetics than in nondiabetics and progresses at an accelerated rate. Macrovascular complications result from a combination of hyperglycemia and altered lipid metabolism.

**Microvascular Disease.** Microangiopathy is common. The basement membrane of capillaries thickens, causing blood flow in the microvasculature to decline. Destruction of small blood vessels leads to kidney damage and blindness. Microvascular complications are directly related to the degree and duration of hyperglycemia.

**Retinopathy.** Diabetes is the major cause of blindness among American adults. Every year, 12,000 to 24,000 diabetics lose their sight. Visual losses result most commonly from damage to retinal capillaries. Microaneurysms may occur, followed by scarring and proliferation of new vessels; the overgrowth of new retinal capillaries reduces visual acuity. Capillary damage may also impair vision by causing local ischemia, with resultant death of retinal cells. Retinopathy is accelerated by hyperglycemia, hypertension, and smoking. Accordingly, these risk factors should be controlled or eliminated.

**Nephropathy.** Diabetic nephropathy is characterized by proteinuria, reduced glomerular filtration, and increased arterial blood pressure. Diabetic nephropathy is the most common cause of end-stage renal disease, a condition that requires dialysis or a kidney transplant for survival. Between 10% and 21% of people with diabetes have kidney disease. The risk of nephropathy among patients with IDDM is 12 times higher than among patients with NIDDM. Nephropathy is the primary cause of morbidity and mortality in patients with IDDM. If the injured kidney is replaced with a transplant, the new kidney is likely to fail within a few years unless tight control of diabetes is established.

Onset of diabetic nephropathy can be delayed and the extent of injury can be reduced. The DCCT revealed that tight glucose control decreases the risk of nephropathy by 35% to 56%. As discussed in Chapter 41, treatment with an angiotensin-converting enzyme (ACE) inhibitor can delay the onset of overt nephropathy and retard progression of nephropathy that is already present. It must be noted, however, that ACE inhibitors increase the risk of hypoglycemia, and hence must be used with care.

**Neuropathy.** Nerve degeneration often begins early in the course of diabetes, but symptoms are usually absent for years. Sensory and motor nerves may be affected. Symptoms of diabetic neuropathy include tingling sensations in the fingers and toes, pain, suppression of reflexes, and loss of sensation (especially vibratory sensation). Nerve damage is directly related to sustained hyperglycemia. In the DCCT, tight glycemic control reduced the incidence of neuropathy by 60%.

**Amputations.** Diabetes is responsible for more than 50% of lower limb amputations in the United States. Each year, 54,000 diabetics lose a foot or leg because of their disease. Amputations result in part because of severe nerve damage.

**Impotence.** The combination of blood vessel injury and neuropathy can cause impotence. About 13% of men with IDDM and 8% of men with NIDDM suffer diabetes-related impotence.

**Gastroparesis.** Diabetic gastroparesis affects 20% to 30% of patients with longstanding diabetes. Manifestations include nausea, vomiting, delayed gastric emptying, and abdominal distention secondary to atony of the GI tract. Injury to the autonomic nerves that control GI motility may be the underlying cause. Symptoms can be reduced with metoclopramide [Reglan], a drug that promotes gastric emptying.

## Diabetes and Pregnancy

Before the discovery of insulin, virtually all babies born to diabetic mothers died during infancy. Although insulin therapy has greatly improved this picture, successful management of the diabetic pregnancy remains a challenge. Three factors contribute to the problem. First, the placenta produces hormones that can antagonize insulin's actions. Second, production of cortisol, a hormone that promotes hyperglycemia, increases threefold during pregnancy. Both of these factors increase the need for insulin. Third, since glucose can pass freely from the maternal circulation to the fetal circulation, hyperglycemia in the mother will stimulate secretion of fetal insulin; the resultant hyperinsulinemia can have multiple adverse effects on the developing fetus.

Successful management of the diabetic pregnancy demands that proper glucose levels be maintained in *both* the fetus and the mother; failure to do so may be teratogenic or otherwise detrimental to the fetus. Achieving glucose control requires diligence on the part of the mother and her physician. Blood glucose levels must be monitored six to seven times a day. Insulin dosage and food intake must be adjusted accordingly.

Since fetal death frequently occurs near term, it is desirable that delivery take place as soon as development of the fetus will permit. Hence, when tests indicate sufficient fetal maturation, it is common practice to deliver the infant early—either by cesarean section or by induction of labor with drugs.

*Gestational diabetes* is defined as diabetes that appears during pregnancy and then subsides rapidly after delivery. Gestational diabetes is managed in much the same manner as any other diabetic pregnancy: blood glucose should be monitored and then controlled with insulin and diet. In most cases, the diabetic state disappears almost immediately after delivery. In these cases, insulin should be discontinued. However, if the diabetic condition persists beyond parturition, it is no longer considered gestational and should be re-diagnosed and treated accordingly.

## Diagnosis of Diabetes

Excessive blood glucose is diagnostic of diabetes. Three tests are employed to determine if blood glucose is too high.

**Fasting Blood Glucose Test.** To determine fasting glucose levels, blood is drawn 8 to 10 hours after the last meal. In nondiabetics, fasting glucose levels are less than 115 mg/dL. If fasting glucose levels exceed 140 mg/dL, diabetes is indicated. As a rule, the physician will make a diagnosis of diabetes if fasting glucose exceeds 140 mg/dL on two tests.

**Random Blood Glucose Test.** For this test, blood can be drawn at any time. Fasting is not required. If blood glucose exceeds 200 mg/mL, and if the patient has classic signs and symptoms (polyuria, polydipsia, ketonuria, rapid weight loss), diabetes is diagnosed.

**Oral Glucose Tolerance Test.** This test is used when diabetes is suspected but could not be definitively diagnosed by measuring fasting or nonfasting blood glucose. The glucose tolerance test is performed by giving an oral glucose load (75 gm to adults) and measuring plasma glucose levels 1 and 2 hours later. In nondiabetic individuals, glucose levels will be less than 200 mg/dL 1 hour after the glucose challenge and below 140 mg/dL at 2 hours. A diagnosis of diabetes is made if plasma glucose levels exceed 200 mg/dL for both the 1-hour and 2-hour determinations.

## Overview of Treatment

### Insulin-Dependent Diabetes Mellitus

The goal of therapy is to maintain glucose levels within an acceptable range. This prevents acute complications and reduces or prevents long-term complications. Glycemic control is accomplished with an integrated program of *diet, blood glucose monitoring, exercise,* and *insulin replacement.*

*Proper diet, balanced by insulin replacement, is the cornerstone of treatment.* Since patients with IDDM are usually thin, the dietary goal is to maintain weight—not lose weight. The recommended diet consists of 55% to 60% carbohydrates (unrefined or fiber-containing refined), 15% protein, and no more than 30% fat (primarily unsaturated and monosaturated). Cholesterol should be limited to 300 mg/day. Total caloric intake should be spread evenly throughout the day, with meals spaced 4 to 5 hours apart.

Unless specifically contraindicated, regular exercise should be part of the treatment program. Exercise increases cellular responsiveness to insulin, and may also increase glucose tolerance. Since strenuous exercise can produce hypoglycemia, close oversight is needed to establish a safe balance between exercise, glucose intake, and insulin dosage. Exercise should be avoided if glycemic control is unstable.

*Survival requires daily administration of insulin.* Before insulin replacement therapy became available, people with IDDM invariably died within a few years of the onset of their disease; the cause of death was ketoacidosis. It is essential to coordinate insulin dosage with caloric intake. If caloric intake is too great or too small with respect to insulin dosage, hyperglycemia or hypoglycemia will result.

It should be noted that *oral hypoglycemic* agents, which can be helpful for patients with NIDDM, are *not* effective for patients with IDDM.

### Noninsulin-Dependent Diabetes Mellitus

As with IDDM, the goal of therapy with NIDDM is to maintain blood glucose levels within an acceptable range. However, for patients with NIDDM, the core of treatment is *diet and exercise alone*; insulin or oral hypoglycemics are employed only as adjuncts. Since patients are often obese, the usual dietary goal is to promote weight loss and establish a more lean body composition. Clinical experience has shown that dietary measures, by themselves, often normalize insulin release and decrease insulin resistance. Frequently, these beneficial responses precede loss of weight. Exercise provides the additional benefit of promoting glucose uptake by muscle, even when insulin is low or absent.

If diet and exercise fail to produce adequate glycemic control, pharmacotherapy will be needed. An *oral hypoglycemic agent* and/or *insulin* is employed. It must be stressed, however, that drugs should be used only as a *supplement* to caloric restriction and exercise; drugs are not a substitute for nondrug measures.

## Monitoring Treatment

The goal of monitoring is to determine whether glucose levels are being maintained in a safe range. Home measurement of blood glucose levels is now the standard method for routine monitoring. Measurement of urinary glucose is reserved for patients who cannot or will not monitor their blood glucose. Glycosylated hemoglobin is measured to assess long-term success.

**Home Blood Glucose Monitoring.** Home blood glucose monitoring (HBGM) is now standard for self-monitoring. The test is performed by placing a drop of blood on a chemically treated strip, which is then read by a small machine. The test is rapid, relatively inexpensive, and can be performed in almost any setting. Information on blood glucose content provides a basis for "fine tuning" insulin dosage. Target values for blood glucose are 80 to 120 mg/dL before meals and 100 to 140 mg/dL at bedtime.

HBGM does have certain drawbacks. These tests are more expensive than urine tests and are more difficult to perform. Also, the machines employed require periodic calibration and patients require education on how to apply test results. Because of these disadvantages, HBGM may not be practical for patients with limited economic resources or for patients who are unable or unwilling to learn how to use the device and apply the results.

HBGM is far superior to measuring glucose in urine: with HBGM, hyperglycemia can be detected long before blood glucose levels are high enough to cause spilling of glucose into urine. Furthermore, HBGM can detect *hypoglycemia*, something that urinary measurements simply can't do.

**Urine Glucose Monitoring.** In the past, this procedure was the mainstay for assessing glycemic control. Urine testing is inexpensive and easy to perform. Unfortunately, urine testing has limited utility. There is a poor correlation between urine glucose concentration and blood glucose levels. Furthermore, a negative urine glucose test tells us only that blood glucose is below 180 mg/dL, the usual threshold for spilling glucose from blood to urine. What a negative test does not tell us is how much below the threshold the glucose level is. Hence, a patient with a negative urine glucose test could be hypoglycemic, normoglycemic, or even slightly hyperglycemic; without some other means of evaluation, we cannot distinguish among these possibilities. Accordingly, although urine testing is superior to no testing at all, it is clearly inferior to blood glucose monitoring.

**Glycosylated Hemoglobin.** Glucose interacts with hemoglobin to form glycosylated derivatives; the most prevalent is named *hemoglobin A$_{1c}$*. With *prolonged hyperglycemia*, levels of hemoglobin A$_{1c}$ gradually increase. Since red blood cells have a long life span (120 days), levels of hemoglobin A$_{1c}$ reflect *average* glucose levels over an extended time. Hence, by measuring hemoglobin A$_{1c}$ every 3 to 4 months, we can get a picture of *long-term* glycemic control. These measurements are a useful adjunct to daily blood glucose monitoring, but are definitely not a substitute. For patients with diabetes, the target value for hemoglobin A$_{1c}$ is 7% or less.

# Insulin

## Physiology

**Structure.** The structure of insulin is depicted in Figure 53–1. As indicated, insulin consists of two amino acid chains: the "A" (acidic) chain and the "B" (basic) chain. The A and B chains are linked to each other by two disulfide bridges.

**Biosynthesis.** Insulin is synthesized in the pancreas by beta cells located in the islets of Langerhans. The immediate precursor of insulin is called proinsulin (see Fig. 53–1). Proinsulin consists of insulin itself plus a peptide loop that runs from the A chain to the B chain. This loop is referred to as *connecting peptide* or *C-peptide*. In the final step of insulin synthesis, C-peptide is enzymatically clipped from the proinsulin molecule.

Measurement of plasma C-peptide levels offers a way to assess residual capacity for insulin synthesis. Since commercial insulin preparations are devoid of C-peptide, and since endogenous C-peptide is only present as a by-product of in-

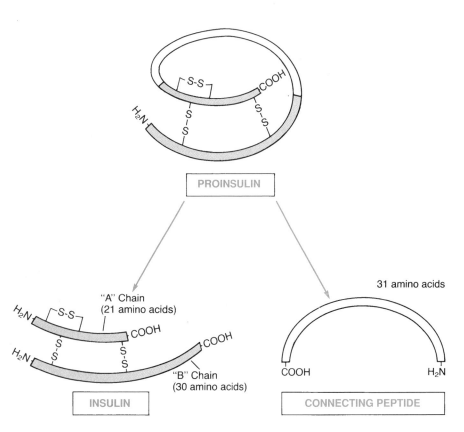

**Figure 53–1. Conversion of proinsulin to insulin and connecting peptide.**

sulin biosynthesis, the presence of C-peptide in the blood of a diabetic indicates the pancreas is still producing some insulin of its own.

**Secretion.** The principal stimulus for insulin release is glucose. Under normal conditions, there is tight coupling between elevations in blood glucose content and increased secretion of insulin. Insulin release may also be triggered by amino acids, fatty acids, and ketone bodies.

The sympathetic nervous system provides additional control of insulin release. Activation of beta$_2$-adrenergic receptors in the pancreas *promotes* secretion of insulin. Conversely, activation of pancreatic alpha-adrenergic receptors *inhibits* insulin release.

**Metabolic Actions.** The metabolic actions of insulin are primarily *anabolic* (i.e., conservative or constructive). Insulin promotes conservation of energy and buildup of energy stores. The hormone also promotes cell growth and division.

Insulin acts in two ways to promote anabolic effects. First, insulin stimulates cellular transport (uptake) of glucose, amino acids, nucleotides, and potassium. Second, insulin promotes synthesis of complex organic molecules. Under the influence of insulin and other factors, glucose is converted into glycogen, amino acids are assembled into proteins, and fatty acids are incorporated into triglycerides. The principal metabolic actions of insulin are summarized in Table 53-2.

## Metabolic Consequences of Insulin Deficiency

Insulin deficiency puts the body into a *catabolic* mode (i.e., a metabolic state that favors the breakdown of complex molecules into their simple constituents). Hence, in the absence of insulin, glycogen is converted into glucose, proteins are degraded into amino acids, and fats are converted to glycerol (glycerin) and free fatty acids. These catabolic effects contribute to the signs and symptoms of diabetes. Note that the catabolic effects produced by insulin deficiency are opposite to the anabolic effects seen when insulin levels are normal.

Insulin deficiency promotes *hyperglycemia* by three mechanisms: (1) increased glycogenolysis, (2) increased gluconeogenesis, and (3) reduced glucose utilization. *Glycogenolysis*, by definition, generates free glucose by breaking down glycogen. The raw materials that allow increased *gluconeogenesis* are the amino acids and fatty acids produced by degradation of proteins and fats. *Reduced glucose utilization* occurs because insulin deficiency decreases cellular uptake of glucose, and decreases conversion of glucose to glycogen.

*Diabetic ketoacidosis* occurs secondary to disruption of glucose and fat metabolism. This potentially fatal syndrome is discussed separately later in the chapter.

## Therapeutic Uses

The principal indication for insulin is *diabetes mellitus*; the drug is required by *all* patients with IDDM and by some with NIDDM. Intravenous insulin is used to treat *diabetic ketoacidosis*. Because of its ability to promote cellular uptake of potassium and thereby lower plasma potassium levels, insulin infusion is employed to treat *hyperkalemia*. The use of insulin in diabetes is discussed further below.

## Preparations

Insulin is available in several forms. These differ with respect to time course of action, route of administration, and source.

### Types of Insulin

There are five types of insulin: "natural" insulin and four modified insulins. One of the modified insulins (lispro insulin) acts more rapidly than natural insulin but has a shorter duration of action. The other modified insulins act more slowly than natural insulin but have longer durations

### TABLE 53-2. METABOLIC ACTIONS OF INSULIN

| Substances Affected | Insulin Action | Site of Action |
|---|---|---|
| *Carbohydrates* | ↑ Glucose uptake | Muscle, adipose tissue |
| | ↑ Glucose oxidation | Muscle |
| | ↑ Glucose storage | Muscle, liver |
| | ↑ Glycogen synthesis | |
| | ↓ Glycogenolysis | |
| | ↓ Gluconeogenesis* | Liver |
| *Amino acids and proteins* | ↑ Amino acid uptake | Muscle |
| | ↓ Amino acid release | Muscle |
| | ↑ Protein synthesis | Muscle |
| *Lipids* | ↑Triglyceride synthesis | Adipose tissue |
| | ↓ Release of FFA[†] and glycerol | Adipose tissue |
| | ↑ Oxidation of FFA to ketoacids[‡] | Liver |

*Because of decreased delivery of substrate (fatty acids and amino acids) to the liver.
[†]Free fatty acids.
[‡]Because of decreased delivery of FFA to the liver.

### TABLE 53-3. INSULIN PREPARATIONS: TIME COURSE OF ACTION

| Insulin Type | Onset (hr) | Peak (hr) | Duration (hr) |
|---|---|---|---|
| *Short Acting* | | | |
| Lispro insulin | 5 min | 0.5–1 | 2–4 |
| Regular insulin | 0.5–1 | 2–4 | 5–7 |
| *Intermediate Acting* | | | |
| NPH insulin | 1–2 | 6–12 | 18–24 |
| Lente insulin | 1–2 | 6–12 | 18–24 |
| *Long Acting* | | | |
| Ultralente insulin | 4–6 | 16–18 | 20–36 |

of action. Two processes have been used to prolong insulin effects: (1) complexing natural insulin with a protein and (2) altering the physical state of natural insulin by mixing it with zinc. When classified according to time course, insulin preparations fall into three groups: short acting, intermediate acting, and long acting (Table 53–3). Trade names for insulin preparations are presented in Table 53–4.

**Regular (Natural) Insulin.** Regular insulin is unmodified crystalline insulin. As shown in Table 53–3, regular insulin has a rapid onset and short duration. Regular insulin is dispensed as a *clear solution* and is the only form of insulin that can be administered *intravenously*. The usual route, however, is *subcutaneous*. Following SC injection, molecules of regular insulin forms small aggregates (dimers and hexamers). As a result, absorption is slightly delayed.

In the past, preparations of regular insulin were unstable at room temperature, and therefore required constant refrigeration. The stability of formulations available today is greatly improved. As a result, the insulin bottle in current use (usually a 2- to 4-week supply) does not have to be kept cold, although exposure to sunlight and extreme heat must be avoided.

**Lispro Insulin.** Lispro insulin [Humalog] is a new, rapid-acting form of insulin. Effects begin within 5 minutes of SC injection and persist for 2 to 4 hours. Lispro insulin acts more rapidly than regular insulin but has a shorter duration of action. Because of its rapid onset, lispro insulin can be administered immediately before eating. In contrast, regular insulin is generally administered 30 to 60 minutes before meals. Unlike other insulins, which are available over the counter, lispro insulin is available only by prescription.

The structure of lispro insulin is nearly identical to that of natural insulin. The only difference is that the position of two amino acids has been switched. In lispro insulin, lysine occupies position 28 in the B chain and proline occupies position 29—the reverse of their natural order.

## TABLE 53–4. INSULIN PREPARATIONS

| Insulin Type and Trade Names | Insulin Type* | Manfacturer† |
|---|---|---|
| *Lispro Insulin* | | |
| Humalog | Modified human | Lilly |
| *Regular Insulin* | | |
| Regular Iletin I | Beef/Pork | Lilly |
| Regular Iletin II | Pork | Lilly |
| Regular Purified Pork Insulin | Pork | Novo Nordisk |
| Humulin R | Human | Lilly |
| Novolin R | Human | Novo Nordisk |
| Velosulin BR‡ | Human | Novo Nordisk |
| *NPH (Isophane) Insulin* | | |
| NPH Iletin I | Beef/Pork | Lilly |
| Pork NPH Iletin II | Pork | Lilly |
| NPH Purified (N) | Pork | Novo Nordisk |
| Humulin N | Human | Lilly |
| Novolin N | Human | Novo Nordisk |
| *Lente Insulin* | | |
| Lente Iletin I | Beef/Pork | Lilly |
| Lente Iletin II (Pork) | Pork | Lilly |
| Lente (L) Purified Pork Insulin | Pork | Novo Nordisk |
| Humulin L | Human | Lilly |
| Novolin L | Human | Novo Nordisk |
| *Ultralente Insulin* | | |
| Humulin U Ultralente | Human | Lilly |
| *NPH/Regular Mixture (70%/30%)* | | |
| Humulin 70/30 | Human | Lilly |
| Novolin 70/30 | Human | Novo Nordisk |
| *NPH/Regular Mixture (50%/50%)* | | |
| Humulin 50/50 | Human | Lilly |

*Insulins listed as *human* or *modified human* are produced by recombinant DNA technology.
†Lilly = Eli Lilly and Company.
‡Phosphate buffered; preferred for use in insulin pumps.

Because of this change, molecules of lispro insulin aggregate less than molecules of regular insulin, which explains why lispro insulin acts more rapidly. Lispro insulin is produced by recombinant DNA technology.

**Neutral Protamine Hagedorn (NPH) Insulin.** NPH insulin is prepared by conjugating regular insulin with protamine (a large protein). The presence of protamine decreases the solubility of NPH insulin and thereby retards its absorption. As a result, onset of action is delayed and duration of action is extended. NPH insulin is classified as intermediate acting. Since protamine is a foreign protein, allergic reactions are possible.

**Lente Insulin and Ultralente Insulin.** The lente series of insulins consists of *semilente insulin*, *lente insulin*, and *ultralente insulin*. These are produced by complexing regular insulin with zinc, which changes the physical state of insulin and thereby reduces its solubility. Semilente insulin is the most rapid acting member of the series. Insulin in this preparation is amorphous (noncrystalline) and present as particles of small size. Semilente insulin is no longer available by itself. In *ultralente insulin*, insulin is present as large crystals; these dissolve slowly and thereby give ultralente insulin a long duration of action. *Lente insulin* is a stable mixture composed of 70% ultralente insulin and 30% semilente insulin. This preparation has an intermediate duration of action. Because no proteins are added, the lente insulins are less allergenic than NPH insulin.

### Sources of Insulin

Insulins are prepared from animal sources or by recombinant DNA technology. Table 53–4 indicates the source of insulins used in the United States.

**Beef or Pork Pancreas.** Much of commercial insulin is prepared by extraction from beef pancreas or pork pancreas. Insulin from both sources is similar in structure to human insulin. Pork insulin is identical to human insulin with the exception of one amino acid. Beef insulin contains three amino acids that differ from those of human insulin. Because beef and pork insulins are not identical to human insulin, antibodies against these foreign insulins may develop.

**Recombinant DNA Technology.** In this process, the genetic code for human proinsulin is inserted into *Escherichia coli* or yeast, which then produce large amounts of proinsulin. The proinsulin is converted to insulin by enzymatic cleavage of C-peptide from proinsulin. The insulins made by recombinant DNA technology are identical to insulin produced by the human pancreas. Insulins listed as "human" in Table 53–4 are produced by recombinant DNA technology.

### Concentration

In the United States, insulin is available in two concentrations: 100 U/ml (U-100) and 500 U/ml (U-500). Preparations containing 40 U/ml are available in other countries but are no longer used here. U-100 insulins are employed for routine replacement therapy. U-500 insulin, which is available from the manufacturer by special request, is reserved for emergencies and for patients with severe insulin resistance (i.e., patients who need doses in excess of 200 U/day).

## Administration and Storage

### Usual Routes of Administration

Insulin is given by injection. Because of its peptide structure, insulin would be inactivated by the digestive system if it were given by mouth. All insulins may be injected *subcutaneously*. Only *regular insulin* may also be administered *intravenously* and *intramuscularly*.

In emergencies, *regular* insulin (and only regular insulin) may be administered *intravenously*. Since regular insulin forms a true *solution*, it is safe for intravenous use. In contrast, all other insulin preparations (except lispro insulin) consist of particles in suspension; introduction of these particles into the bloodstream could produce serious adverse effects. When administered by IV infusion, insulin can adsorb to the infusion set, thereby reducing the dosage received. Since the extent of adsorption is not predictable, monitoring the therapeutic response is essential. If emergency treatment by the intravenous route is impossible, regular insulin may be administered IM instead.

### Preparation for Injection

With the exception of regular insulin and lispro insulin, all insulin preparations consist of particles in suspension. Hence, to ensure correct dosing, these particles must be evenly dispersed prior to loading the syringe. Dispersion is accomplished by rolling the insulin vial between the palms of the hands. Mixing must be gentle, since vigorous agitation will cause frothing and render accurate dosing impossible. If granules or clumps remain after gentle agitation, the vial should be discarded.

Unlike insulin suspensions, which are cloudy, regular insulin and lispro insulin are dispensed as clear, colorless solutions. Because they are in solution, these preparations can be administered without prior agitation. If a preparation of regular or lispro insulin becomes cloudy or discolored, or if a precipitate develops, it should be discarded.

Before loading the syringe, the bottle cap should be swabbed with alcohol. Air bubbles should be eliminated from the syringe and needle after loading. The skin should be cleaned with alcohol prior to injection.

### Sites of Injection

The most common sites of SC injection are the upper arms, thighs, and abdomen. Since rates of absorption vary among these sites, it is recommended that injections be made using only one general locale (e.g., thigh or abdomen). Regardless of whether one general locale or several are used, specific sites of injection within the locale should be rotated. This practice will reduce the incidence of lipohypertrophy (see below). About 1 inch should be allowed between sites of injection. Ideally, each site should be used only once every month.

## Mixing Insulins

When the treatment plan calls for the use of two different insulin preparations (e.g., regular insulin plus NPH insulin), it is usually desirable to mix the preparations rather than inject them separately since this eliminates the need for an additional injection. However, although mixing insulins offers convenience, it can alter the time course of the response. Therefore, to ensure a consistent response, insulins should be mixed according to established guidelines (see below). Also, only those insulins that are compatible with each other should be mixed.

*Regular Insulin.* Regular insulin is compatible with all other insulin preparations except lispro insulin. When preparing a mixture of regular insulin with another insulin preparation, the regular insulin should be drawn into the syringe first. This sequence will avoid contaminating the stock vial of regular insulin with insulin of another type.

*Lispro Insulin.* Information on mixing lispro insulin is limited. In clinical trials, the drug was mixed with NPH insulin, lente insulin, and ultralente insulin. All mixtures were administered immediately after preparation. Lispro insulin is produced by Eli Lilly and Company (Lilly), and all mixtures employed during clinical trials were made with Lilly products. Until more information is available, mixtures should be made only with other insulins made by Lilly (see Table 53-4) and should be injected immediately after they are prepared.

*NPH Insulin.* This preparation is compatible with regular insulin and lispro insulin. Mixtures of NPH and regular insulin may be prepared by the patient or may be purchased premixed (70% NPH/30% regular or 50%NPH/50% regular). Mixtures of regular and NPH insulin are stable and do not alter the kinetics of either component. Mixtures with lispro insulin should be injected immediately.

*Lente Insulins.* Lente, semilente, and ultralente insulin may be mixed with one another or with regular insulin. When the lente insulins are mixed with one another, no change in time course occurs. In contrast, when lente insulins are mixed with regular insulin, zinc present in the lente-type insulin can complex with the regular insulin, thereby delaying and prolonging its actions. Since this reaction begins soon after mixing, these mixtures should be injected immediately to avoid altering the regular insulin.

## Storage

Insulin in *unopened vials* should be stored *under refrigeration* until needed. Vials should not be frozen. When stored unopened under refrigeration, insulin can be used up to the expiration date on the vial.

*The vial in current use can be kept at room temperature for up to 1 month without significant loss of activity.* Direct sunlight and extreme heat must be avoided. Partially filled vials should be discarded after several weeks if left unused. Injection of insulin stored at room temperature causes less pain than cold insulin.

*Mixtures* of insulin prepared in *vials* are stable for 1 month at room temperature and for 3 months under refrigeration.

*Mixtures* of insulin in *prefilled syringes* (plastic or glass) should be stored in a refrigerator, where they will be stable for at least 1 week and perhaps 2. The syringe should be stored vertically with the needle pointing up to avoid clogging the needle. Prior to administration, the syringe should be agitated gently to re-suspend the insulin.

### Alternative Methods of Insulin Delivery

Insulin is usually administered subcutaneously using a syringe and needle. The devices discussed below represent alternatives to the traditional method of insulin administration.

*Jet Injectors.* These devices shoot insulin directly through the skin into subcutaneous tissue. No needle is used. Hence, for patients who dislike needles, a jet injector may be attractive. However, these devices do have a downside. They are expensive ($500 to $900) and can be difficult to use. Moreover, because insulin is delivered under high pressure, they can cause stinging, burning, and pain. In addition, bruising can occur in people with reduced subcutaneous fat (children, the elderly, thin people).

*Pen Injectors.* These devices are similar to a syringe and needle but more convenient. Pen injectors look like a fountain pen but have a disposable needle where the writing tip would be and a disposable insulin-filled cartridge inside. Administration is accomplished by sticking the needle under the skin and injecting the insulin manually. Dosage can be adjusted in 2-unit increments.

*Portable Insulin Pumps.* These computerized devices deliver a basal infusion of regular insulin plus bolus doses before each meal. The basal infusion is usually about 1 U/hr and can be programmed to match the patients metabolism. Mealtime boluses are calculated to match caloric intake. The pumps are about the size of a call-pager, weigh only 4 ounces, and are worn on the belt or in a pocket. An infusion set delivers insulin from the pump to a subcutaneous needle, usually located on the abdomen. The infusion set should be replaced every 1 to 3 days, at which time the needle should be moved to a new site (at least 1 inch away from the old site). Since the pump delivers regular (short-acting) insulin, insulin levels will drop quickly if the pump is removed. Accordingly, the pump should remain in place most of the day. However, it can be removed for an hour or two on special occasions. External insulin pumps cost between $3000 and $5000. Infusion sets, insulin, and glucose monitoring materials add another $300/month to the bill. Aside from expense, the main drawback of the pumps is underdelivery of insulin owing to formation of insulin microdeposits.

*Implantable Insulin Pumps.* These devices are surgically implanted in the abdomen and deliver insulin either intraperitoneally or intravenously. Like external pumps, internal pumps deliver a basal insulin infusion plus bolus doses with meals. Insulin delivery is adjusted by an external telemetry device. Compared with multiple daily injections, implantable pumps produce superior glycemic control, cause less hypoglycemia and weight gain, and improve quality of life. As with external pumps, delivery of insulin can be impeded by formation of insulin microprecipitates. Implantable pumps are experimental and not yet available for general use.

*Intranasal Insulin.* Intranasal administration of insulin is experimental. When insulin is administered by this route, effects have a rapid onset and brief duration. Hence, intranasal administration is suitable for delivery of mealtime insulin supplements, but cannot meet basal insulin needs. Therefore, long-acting SC insulin is still required. Additional problems are discomfort and expense. In order for absorption to occur, insulin must be administered with surfactants, which irritate the nasal mucosa; intranasal insulin is expensive because only 10% of each dose is absorbed, which means the dose must be 10 times greater than an SC dose to produce equivalent effects.

## Insulin Therapy of Diabetes Mellitus

Insulin is given to all patients who have IDDM and to many who have NIDDM. In addition, insulin is employed

**TABLE 53-5. TARGETS FOR GLYCEMIC CONTROL IN DIABETES**

| Monitoring Parameter | Target Value for Diabetics | Normal Value for Nondiabetics |
|---|---|---|
| Premeal blood glucose | 80-120 mg/dL | <115 mg/dL |
| Bedtime blood glucose | 100-140 mg/dL | <120 mg/dL |
| Hemoglobin $A_{1c}$ | <7% | <6% |

to manage gestational diabetes. In treating these disorders, the objective is to maintain levels of blood glucose within an acceptable range (see Table 53-5). When therapy is successful, both hyperglycemia and hypoglycemia will be avoided, and the long-term complications of diabetes will be minimized.

### Tight Glucose Control: Benefits and Drawbacks

The process of maintaining glucose levels within a normal range is referred to as tight glucose control. The *Diabetes Control and Complications Trial* (DCCT), a 9-year study whose results were announced in the summer of 1993, has shown conclusively that tight glucose control can greatly reduce the long-term complications of diabetes. In this study, patients with IDDM received either *conventional insulin therapy* (i.e., one or two injections/day) or *intensive insulin therapy* (four injections/day). The patients who received intensive therapy experienced a 50% decrease in clinically significant kidney disease, a 35% to 56% decrease in neuropathy, and a 76% decrease in serious ophthalmic complications. Moreover, onset of ophthalmic problems was delayed and progression of existing problems was slowed. All of these benefits were correlated with improved glycemic control. Hence, with rigorous control of blood glucose, the high degree of morbidity traditionally associated with diabetes can be markedly reduced. Although the participants in this study had IDDM, we can assume that tight glucose control would be of similar benefit to patients with NIDDM, who are at risk for the same long-term complications experienced by patients with IDDM.

Unfortunately, intensive insulin therapy has its drawbacks. The greatest concern is hypoglycemia. Since glucose levels are kept relatively low, the possibility of hypoglycemia secondary to a modest insulin overdose is significantly increased. Compared with patients using conventional insulin therapy, those using intensive insulin therapy experienced three times as many hypoglycemic events requiring the assistance of another person, and three times as many episodes of hypoglycemia-induced coma or seizures. In addition, patients on intensive insulin therapy gain more weight (about 10 pounds, on average). Other disadvantages are greater inconvenience, increased complexity, and a need for greater patient motivation. Finally, the annual expense per patient is much higher: whereas traditional therapy costs about $1700, intensive therapy costs about $4000 (for multiple daily injections) or $5800 (for continuous infusion with a pump).

### Dosage

To achieve tight glucose control, insulin dosage must be closely matched with insulin needs. If caloric intake is increased, insulin dosage must be increased as well. When a meal is missed or is low in calories, the dosage of insulin must be decreased. Dosage must undergo additional adjustments to meet specialized needs. For example, insulin needs are *increased* by infection, stress, obesity, the adolescent growth spurt, and pregnancy (after the first trimester). Conversely, insulin needs are *decreased* by exercise and pregnancy (during the first trimester). To ensure that insulin dosage is coordinated with insulin requirements, the patient and physician must work together to establish an integrated program of nutrition, exercise, blood glucose monitoring, and insulin replacement therapy.

Total daily dosages may range from 0.1 U/kg body weight to more than 2.5 U/kg. For patients with IDDM, initial dosages typically range from 0.5 to 0.6 U/kg/day. For patients with NIDDM, initial dosages typically range from 0.2 to 0.6 U/kg/day.

### Dosing Schedules

The schedule of insulin administration helps determine the extent to which tight glucose control is achieved. Three dosing schedules are compared below. These modes are referred to as (1) conventional therapy, (2) intensified conventional therapy, and (3) continuous subcutaneous insulin infusion.

***Conventional Therapy.*** Several dosing schedules fall under the heading of conventional therapy. A representative schedule is summarized in Table 53-6. In this schedule, a combination of regular insulin (a fast-acting preparation) plus lente insulin (an intermediate-acting preparation) is administered 15 to 30 minutes before breakfast and again before the evening meal. No insulin is administered with the noon meal. Typically, two thirds of the total daily dose is given in the morning and the remainder is given late in the day. Dosage remains rigidly fixed from one day to the next.

*Conventional therapy does not provide tight glucose control.* The weak point of this schedule is that there is no provision for adjusting insulin dosage in response to ongoing changes in insulin needs. Hence, if a meal is abnormally large, insulin levels will be insufficient and hyperglycemia will result. Conversely, if a meal is delayed, reduced in size, or missed entirely, hypoglycemia will follow.

***Intensified Conventional Therapy.*** This form of therapy is designed to provide tight glucose control. A representative regimen is presented in Table 53-6. In this regimen, the patient injects ultralente insulin (a long-acting preparation) in the evening and also injects regular insulin (a rapid-acting preparation) 15 to 30 minutes before each meal.* The *ultralente* preparation provides a *basal* level

---

*Lispro insulin can be used instead of regular insulin. The advantage of lispro insulin is that it can be administered just a few minutes before eating.

## TABLE 53–6. INSULIN THERAPY OF DIABETES MELLITUS: CONVENTIONAL VERSUS INTENSIFIED CONVENTIONAL THERAPY

| Regimen | Insulin Type and Dosing Schedule | | | |
|---|---|---|---|---|
| | Breakfast | Lunch | Supper | Bedtime |
| Conventional therapy* | Regular + lente | None | Regular + lente | None |
| Intensified conventional therapy† | Regular | Regular | Regular | Ultralente |

*Dosage is *fixed* (2/3 daily total in AM, 1/3 daily total in PM). As a result, flexibility of timing and composition of meals is not possible.
†Dosage of regular insulin is *adjusted for each meal*; hence, timing and composition of meals can be varied.

of insulin throughout the night and the following day. The mealtime doses of *regular* insulin accommodate the *acute* needs that occur at times of caloric loading. Note that insulin is injected *four times each day*, rather than just twice as in conventional therapy.

The most significant feature of intensified conventional therapy (ICT) is *adaptability*. Unlike conventional therapy, in which doses never change, the preprandial doses given in ICT are adjusted to match the caloric content of each meal: if no meal is eaten, no insulin is administered; if a meal is delayed, so is the dose of regular insulin; if a meal is larger than usual, the insulin dose is increased proportionately. Since insulin dosage is determined by the timing and size of each meal, ICT offers patients a degree of glycemic control and dietary flexibility that is not possible with conventional therapy.

Home blood glucose monitoring (HBGM) is an essential component of ICT. Blood glucose should be measured three to five times a day. HBGM is discussed above under *Monitoring Treatment*.

***Continuous Subcutaneous Insulin Infusion.*** Continuous subcutaneous insulin infusion (CSII) is accomplished using a portable infusion pump connected to an indwelling subcutaneous catheter. The only form of insulin employed for CSII is regular insulin. To provide a basal level of insulin, the pump is set to infuse the hormone continuously at a slow but steady rate. To accommodate insulin needs created by eating, the pump is triggered manually to provide a bolus dose of insulin matched in size to the caloric content of each meal. Hence, like ICT, CSII can adapt to changes in insulin needs. As with ICT, home monitoring of blood glucose is an essential. CSII is equivalent to ICT for achieving tight glucose control. Portable infusion pumps are discussed above under *Alternative Methods of Insulin Delivery*.

### Achieving Tight Glucose Control

As we have seen, the primary requirement for achieving tight glucose control is a method of insulin delivery that permits adjustments in dosage to accommodate ongoing variations in insulin needs. ICT and CSII meet this criterion. In addition to an adaptable method of insulin de-

livery, achieving tight glucose control requires the following:

- Careful attention to all elements of the treatment program (diet, exercise, insulin replacement therapy)
- A defined glycemia target (see Table 53-5)
- Home monitoring of blood glucose three to five times daily
- A high degree of patient motivation
- Extensive patient education

Tight glucose control cannot be achieved without the informed participation of the patient. Accordingly, patients must receive thorough instruction on the following:

- The nature of diabetes
- The importance of tight glucose control
- The major components of the treatment routine (insulin replacement, HBGM, diet, exercise)
- Procedures for purchasing insulin, syringes, and needles
- The importance of avoiding arbitrary changes between human, pork, and beef/pork insulins
- The importance of avoiding arbitrary changes between insulins from different manufacturers
- Methods of insulin storage
- Procedures for mixing insulins
- Calculation of dosage adjustments
- Techniques of insulin administration
- Methods for monitoring blood glucose

In the final analysis, responsibility for managing diabetes rests with the patient. The health care team can design a treatment program and can provide education and guidance. However, tight glucose control will be achieved only if the patient is actively involved in his or her own therapy.

## Complications of Insulin Treatment

### Hypoglycemia

Hypoglycemia (blood glucose <50 mg/dL) occurs when insulin levels exceed insulin needs. A major cause of insulin excess is overdose. Imbalance between insulin levels and insulin needs can also result from reduced intake of food, vomiting and diarrhea (which reduce absorption of nutrients), excessive consumption of alcohol (which promotes hypoglycemia), unaccustomed exercise (which promotes glucose uptake and utilization), and parturition (which reduces insulin requirements).

Diabetic patients and their families should be familiar with the signs and symptoms of hypoglycemia. Some symptoms result from activation of the sympathetic nervous system, whereas others arise from the central nervous system (CNS). When glucose levels fall *rapidly*, activation of the sympathetic nervous system occurs, resulting in tachycardia, palpitations, sweating, and nervousness. However, if the decline in glucose is *gradual*, symptoms may be limited to those of CNS origin. Mild CNS symptoms include headache, confusion, drowsiness, and fatigue. If hypoglycemia is severe, convulsions, coma, and death may follow.

Rapid treatment of hypoglycemia is mandatory; if hypoglycemia is allowed to persist, irreversible brain damage or death may result. In conscious patients, glucose levels can be restored with a fast-acting oral sugar (e.g., glucose tablets, orange juice, sugar cubes, honey, corn syrup, nondiet soda). However, if the swallowing reflex or the gag reflex is suppressed, nothing should be administered by mouth. In cases of severe hypoglycemia, intravenous glucose is the preferred therapy. Parenteral *glucagon* is an alternative method of treatment. (The pharmacology of glucagon is discussed separately at the end of the chapter.)

In anticipation of hypoglycemic episodes, diabetics should always have an oral carbohydrate available (e.g., Life Savers, candy, glucose tablets, sugar cubes). Many physicians recommend that patients keep glucagon on hand as well. Patients should carry some sort of identification (e.g., Medic Alert bracelet) to inform emergency personnel of their condition.

In some patients, hypoglycemia occurs without producing the symptoms noted above. As a result, the patient is unaware of hypoglycemia until blood sugar has become dangerously low. Hypoglycemia unawareness is a particular problem among patients practicing tight glucose control. The risk of dangerous hypoglycemia can be minimized by frequently monitoring blood glucose.

Severe hypoglycemia and diabetic ketoacidosis (see below) can both produce coma. Of these two causes of diabetic coma, hypoglycemia is the more common. Since treatment of these two conditions is very different (hypoglycemia involves withholding insulin, whereas ketoacidosis requires insulin administration), it is essential that coma from these causes be differentiated. The most definitive diagnosis is made by measuring plasma or urinary glucose levels: in hypoglycemic coma, glucose levels are very low; in ketoacidosis, glucose levels are very high.

### Other Complications

*Lipodystrophies.* Altered deposition of subcutaneous fat (lipodystrophy) can occur at sites of insulin injection. Two types of change may be seen: (1) *lipoatrophy* (loss of subcutaneous fat), and (2) *lipohypertrophy* (accumulation of subcutaneous fat).

*Lipoatrophy* produces a depression in the skin at the site of insulin injection. The cause of atrophy appears to be immunologic. Accordingly, fat atrophy is most likely with use of insulin preparations that have a high concentration of antigenic contaminants. Because the insulin preparations in use today are much purer than those used in the past, lipoatrophy is now rare. When lipoatrophy occurs, subcutaneous fat can often be restored by injecting a highly purified insulin preparation (e.g., purified pork insulin or human insulin) directly into the site of fat loss. Some improvement can be seen in 4 weeks, but full recovery takes 3 to 6 months.

*Lipohypertrophy* occurs at sites of frequent insulin injection. Fat accumulates because insulin stimulates fat synthesis. When use of the site is discontinued, excess fat will eventually be lost. Lipohypertrophy can be minimized through systematic rotation of injection sites.

**Allergic Reactions.** Insulin injection can produce local and systemic allergic responses. Fortunately, allergic reactions are rare.

With local reactions, the injection site becomes red and hardened. These reactions are usually delayed, taking several hours to develop. Local reactions occur in response to a contaminant in the insulin preparation, and not to the insulin itself. Because insulins in use today are highly purified, local reactions are uncommon.

Systemic reactions take place rapidly, and are characterized by the widespread appearance of red and intensely itchy welts. Breathing difficulty may develop. Systemic reactions occur in response to insulin itself, not to a contaminant. Beef insulin, which differs from human insulin by three amino acids, is the most frequent cause of systemic allergy. Generalized reactions are least likely with pork and human insulins. If severe allergy develops in a patient who nonetheless must continue insulin use, a desensitization procedure can be performed. This process entails giving small initial doses of purified pork or human insulin, followed by a series of progressively larger doses.

## Drug Interactions

*Hypoglycemic Agents.* Drugs with the ability to lower blood glucose levels can intensify hypoglycemia induced by insulin. Drugs that promote hypoglycemia include *sulfonylureas*, *troglitazone*, *alcohol* (used acutely), and *beta-adrenergic blocking agents*. When these drugs are combined with insulin, special care must be taken to ensure that blood glucose content does not fall too low.

*Hyperglycemic Agents.* Drugs with the ability to increase blood glucose, such as *thiazide diuretics*, *glucocorticoids*, and *sympathomimetics*, can counteract the therapeutic effects of insulin. When these agents are combined with insulin, an increase in insulin dosage may be required.

*Beta-Adrenergic Blocking Agents.* Beta blockers can delay awareness of insulin-induced hypoglycemia by masking signs that are associated with stimulation of the sympathetic nervous system (e.g., tachycardia, palpitations). Furthermore, since beta blockade impairs glycogenolysis, and since glycogenolysis is one means by which the diabetic can counteract a fall in blood glucose, beta blockers can make insulin-induced hypoglycemia even worse.

# Oral Hypoglycemics

There are four families of oral hypoglycemic drugs: sulfonylureas, biguanides, alpha-glucosidase inhibitors, and thiazolidinediones. These agents are indicated only for treatment of NIDDM; they are not used to treat IDDM. Oral hypoglycemics should be used only after a program of diet modification and exercise has failed to produce glycemic control. Actions and adverse effects of the oral hypoglycemics are summarized in Table 53-7.

## Sulfonylureas

The sulfonylureas were the first oral hypoglycemics available. These drugs are derivatives of the sulfonamide antibiotics, but lack antimicrobial activity. All of the sulfonylureas may be used alone or in combination with insulin. Dosages are summarized in Table 53-8.

The sulfonylureas fall into two groups: *first-generation agents* and *second-generation agents*. Both generations reduce glucose levels to the same extent. The principal difference between the generations is that the second-generation agents are more potent. That is, second-generation agents produce their effects at much lower doses than the first-generation agents do. However, although the differences in potency are large, these differences are of minimal clinical significance. More important than differences in potency are differences in duration of action (see Table 53-8), since agents with longer durations can be given once daily.

## Tolbutamide

Tolbutamide [Orinase], a first-generation agent, will serve as our prototype for the sulfonylurea family. As with the other oral hypoglycemics, use of tolbutamide is restricted to patients with NIDDM.

***Mechanism of Action.*** Tolbutamide acts primarily by stimulating the release of insulin from pancreatic islets. If the pancreas is incapable of insulin synthesis, tolbutamide will be ineffective. It is for this reason that tolbutamide is of no value to insulin-dependent diabetics. With prolonged use, tolbutamide may increase cellular sensitivity to insulin.

***Pharmacokinetics.*** Tolbutamide is readily absorbed following oral administration. Plasma levels peak within 3 to 5 hours. The drug undergoes extensive hepatic metabolism followed by urinary excretion. Because of its mode of elimination, tolbutamide must be used with caution in patients with hepatic or renal impairment. Tolbutamide has a relatively short half-life (about 6 hours), and hence must be administered two to three times a day.

***Therapeutic Use.*** Sulfonylureas are employed only in the treatment of NIDDM. These drugs are of no help to patients with IDDM. Sulfonylureas should be employed only if blood glucose cannot be lowered by a program of caloric restriction and exercise. When these agents are to be used, they should be employed as an *adjunct* to nondrug therapy—not as a substitute. Tolbutamide and other sulfonylureas may be used alone or together with insulin.

***Adverse Effects.*** *Hypoglycemia.* Tolbutamide and all other sulfonylureas can cause excessive lowering of blood

---

## TABLE 53-7. ORAL HYPOGLYCEMICS FOR NIDDM

| Class and Specific Agents | Actions | Major Adverse Effects |
|---|---|---|
| *Sulfonylureas* | | |
| Tolbutamide [Orinase] Glipizide [Glucotrol] Glyburide [Micronase] (See Table 53-8 for other sulfonylureas) | Promote insulin secretion by the pancreas; may also increase tissue response to insulin | Hypoglycemia |
| *Biguanides* | | |
| Metformin [Glucophage] | Decrease glucose production by liver and increase glucose uptake by muscle | GI symptoms: decreased appetite, nausea, diarrhea Lactic acidosis (rarely) |
| *Alpha-Glucosidase Inhibitors* | | |
| Acarbose [Precose] Miglitol [Glyset] | Inhibit carbohydrate digestion and absorption, thereby decreasing the postprandial rise in blood glucose | GI symptoms: flatulence, cramps, abdominal distention, borborygmus |
| *Thiazolidinediones* | | |
| Troglitazone [Rezulin] | Decreases insulin resistance, and thereby increases glucose uptake by muscle and decreases glucose production by the liver | Hypoglycemia, but only in the presence of excessive insulin |

## TABLE 53–8. SULFONYLUREAS: TIME COURSE AND DOSAGE

| Generic Name [Trade Name] | Duration (hr) | Dosage* |
|---|---|---|
| *First-Generation Agents* | | |
| Tolbutamide [Orinase] | 6–12 | Initial: 1–2 gm/day in 1 to 3 doses<br>Maximum: 2–3 gm/day in 1 to 3 doses |
| Acetohexamide [Dymelor] | 12–24 | Initial: 0.25–1.5 gm/day in 1 or 2 doses<br>Maximum: 1.5 gm/day in 1 or 2 doses |
| Tolazamide [Tolinase] | 12–24 | Initial: 100–200 mg/day with breakfast<br>Maximum: 0.75–1 gm in 2 divided doses |
| Chlorpropamide [Diabinese] | 24–72 | Initial: 250 mg once a day<br>Maximum: 750 mg once a day |
| *Second-Generation Agents* | | |
| Glipizide | | |
| Standard [Glucotrol] | 12–24 | Initial: 5 mg once a day with breakfast<br>Maximum: 40 mg/day in 2 divided doses |
| Sustained release [Glucotrol XL] | 24 | Initial: 5 mg/day with breakfast<br>Maximum: 20 mg/day with breakfast |
| Glyburide | | |
| Nonmicronized [DiaBeta, Micronase] | 12–24 | Initial: 2.5–5 mg/day with breakfast<br>Maximum: 20 mg/day in 1 or 2 doses |
| Micronized [Glynase PresTab] | 24 | Initial: 1.5–3 mg/day with breakfast<br>Maximum: 12 mg/day in 1 or 2 doses |
| Glimepiride [Amaryl] | 24 | Initial: 1–2 mg with breakfast<br>Maximum: 8 mg with breakfast |

*The dosages listed are for nonelderly patients. Elderly patients should use a smaller dose.

glucose. Although hypoglycemia is usually mild, fatalities have occurred. Hypoglycemia is sometimes persistent, requiring infusion of dextrose for several days. Hypoglycemic reactions are most likely in patients with kidney or liver dysfunction, because accumulation of tolbutamide may occur. If signs of hypoglycemia develop (fatigue, excessive hunger, profuse sweating, palpitations), the physician should be notified.

*Use in Pregnancy and Lactation.* Oral hypoglycemics should be avoided during pregnancy. Although adequate studies in humans are lacking, sulfonylureas are teratogenic in animals. Furthermore, since sulfonylurea therapy during pregnancy often fails to provide good glycemic control, and since even mild hyperglycemia may be hazardous to the fetus, insulin is generally preferred to sulfonylureas for managing the diabetic pregnancy.

It is especially important to avoid tolbutamide near term. Newborns exposed to sulfonylureas at the time of delivery have experienced severe hypoglycemia lasting as long as 4 to 10 days. Hence, if an oral hypoglycemic has been taken during pregnancy, it should be discontinued at least 48 hours prior to the anticipated time of delivery.

Tolbutamide should not be taken by women who are nursing. The drug is excreted into breast milk, posing a risk of hypoglycemia to the infant. If a woman wishes to breast-feed, she should substitute insulin for the sulfonylurea.

*Cardiovascular Toxicity.* There has been controversy regarding the possibility of adverse cardiovascular reactions to oral hypoglycemics. In 1970, the University Group Diabetes Program

(UGDP) published results indicating that sulfonylureas carried an increased risk of mortality from cardiovascular causes. In the UGDP study, cardiovascular mortality was 2.5 times greater among subjects treated with a combination of diet plus tolbutamide than among control subjects who received dietary therapy alone. The UGDP study has been criticized on several grounds, including design, patient selection, dosing, and compliance. Subsequent clinical trials by other groups have failed to confirm the conclusions of the UGDP report. The American Diabetes Association, which initially endorsed the UGDP study, has since withdrawn its support.

**Drug Interactions.** *Alcohol.* When alcohol is combined with tolbutamide, a disulfiram-like reaction may occur. This syndrome includes flushing, palpitations, and nausea. Disulfiram reactions are discussed fully in Chapter 36. As noted above, alcohol can also potentiate the hypoglycemic effects of tolbutamide. Patients taking tolbutamide must be warned against alcohol consumption.

*Drugs That Can Intensify Hypoglycemia.* A variety of drugs, acting by diverse mechanisms, can intensify hypoglycemic responses to sulfonylureas. Included are *nonsteroidal anti-inflammatory drugs*, *sulfonamide antibiotics*, *ethanol* (used acutely), *ranitidine*, and *cimetidine*. Caution must be exercised when a sulfonylurea is used in combination with these drugs.

*Beta-Adrenergic Blocking Agents.* Beta blockers can interfere with tolbutamide's action by suppressing insulin release. (Recall that activation of beta receptors is one way to promote insulin release.) Since beta blockers can also mask sympathetic responses (e.g., tachycardia, tremors) to declining blood glucose, use of beta blockers can delay awareness of tolbutamide-induced hypoglycemia.

### Other Sulfonylureas

In addition to tolbutamide, six other sulfonylureas are available (see Table 53-8). All of these drugs have similar actions and side effects, and they all share the same application: treatment of noninsulin-dependent diabetes. All sulfonylureas can cause hypoglycemia.

The oral hypoglycemics differ significantly from one another with respect to duration of action. For example, the shortest acting sulfonylurea (tolbutamide) has effects that last 6 to 12 hours. In contrast, chlorpropamide, the longest acting oral hypoglycemic, has effects that last as long as 3 days. Time courses and dosages are summarized in Table 53-8.

## Biguanides: Metformin

Metformin [Glucophage] was approved for treatment of NIDDM in the United States in 1994. The drug has been available in Canada and Europe since 1959. Phenformin, a chemical relative of metformin, was withdrawn from the U.S. market in 1977 because of a high incidence of lactic acidosis. Both metformin and phenformin are classified chemically as biguanides. Metformin frequently causes GI disturbances; lactic acidosis occurs rarely.

*Mechanism of Action.* Metformin lowers blood glucose primarily by decreasing production of glucose by the liver. The underlying mechanism is suppression of gluconeogenesis. In addition to reducing hepatic glucose output, the drug enhances glucose utilization by muscle. In contrast to sulfonylureas, metformin does not does promote insulin release from the pancreas and does not cause hypoglycemia.

*Pharmacokinetics.* Metformin is administered by mouth and absorbed slowly from the small intestine. Of particular interest, the drug is excreted unchanged by the kidneys. In the event of renal insufficiency, metformin will accumulate to toxic levels.

*Therapeutic Use.* Metformin is used to lower blood sugar in patients who have not responded adequately to a program of diet modification and exercise. The drug may be used alone or in combination with a sulfonylurea. When used alone, metformin lowers basal and postprandial blood glucose levels. When metformin is combined with a sulfonylurea, the combination lowers blood sugar more effectively than either drug used alone—which is to be expected since metformin and sulfonylureas act by different mechanisms. Since metformin does not act by causing insulin release, the drug is able to reduce blood sugar in patients who can no longer produce insulin. This contrasts with the sulfonylureas, which require pancreatic production of insulin to work.

*Side Effects.* The most common side effects are decreased appetite, nausea, and diarrhea. These generally subside over time. However, in 3% to 5% of patients, GI effects lead to discontinuation of treatment. Metformin decreases absorption of vitamin $B_{12}$ and folic acid, which can result in deficiency. In contrast to sulfonylureas, metformin does not cause weight gain; in fact, patients *lose* an average of 7 to 8 pounds—probably because metformin causes nausea and decreases appetite.

*Toxicity: Lactic Acidosis.* Metformin and other biguanides inhibit mitochondrial oxidation of lactic acid, and can thereby cause lactic acidosis. This condition is a medical emergency and has a mortality rate of about 50%. Fortunately, lactic acidosis is rare (about 3 cases/100,000 patient years) when metformin is used at recommended doses in patients with good renal function. However, in the event of renal insufficiency, metformin can rapidly accumulate to toxic levels. Accordingly, the drug must never be used in patients with kidney disease. In addition, metformin must be avoided in patients who are prone to increased lactic acid production. This includes patients with liver disease, severe infection, or a history of lactic acidosis; patients who consume alcohol to excess; and patients with heart failure, shock, and other conditions that can result in hypoxemia. All patients should be informed about early signs of lactic acidosis—hyperventilation, myalgia, malaise, unusual somnolence—and instructed to report these to the physician. Metformin should be withdrawn until lactic acidosis has been ruled out. If lactic acidosis is present, hemodialysis can correct the acidosis and remove accumulated metformin.

*Preparations, Dosage, and Administration.* Metformin [Glucophage] is available in 500- and 850-mg tablets for oral administration. The recommended initial dosage is 500 mg twice daily, taken with the morning and evening meals. The usual maintenance dosage is 850 mg twice daily. The maximum dosage is 850 mg 3 times a day.

## Alpha-Glucosidase Inhibitors

### Acarbose

*Mechanism of Action.* Acarbose [Precose] delays absorption of dietary carbohydrates, and thereby reduces the rise in blood glucose that occurs after meals. In order to be absorbed, oligosaccharides and complex carbohydrates must be broken down to monosaccharides by alpha-glucosidase, an enzyme located on the brush border of intestinal cells. Acarbose inhibits this enzyme. As a result, the drug slows digestion of carbohydrates, and hence reduces the postprandial rise in blood glucose.

*Therapeutic Use.* Acarbose is indicated for patients with NIDDM whose hyperglycemia is not controlled by diet modification and exercise. The drug may be used alone or in combination with insulin, metformin, or a sulfonylurea. In clinical trials, 24 weeks of therapy with acarbose alone reduced mean peak postprandial glucose levels by 56 mg/dL, compared with 71 mg/dL for tolbutamide alone, and 85 mg/dL for acarbose plus tolbutamide. In addition to lowering glucose levels after meals, acarbose lowers glycosylated hemoglobin levels, indicating an overall improvement in glycemic control.

*Adverse Effects and Interactions.* Acarbose frequently causes *flatulence, cramps, abdominal distention, borborygmus* (rumbling bowel sounds), and *diarrhea.* These result from bacterial fermentation of unabsorbed carbohydrates in the colon. In addition to causing GI effects, acarbose can decrease absorption of iron, thereby posing a risk of anemia.

*Hypoglycemia* does not occur with acarbose alone, but may develop when acarbose is combined with *insulin* or a *sulfonylurea.* When hypoglycemia develops, sucrose cannot be used for oral therapy, since acarbose will impede its hydrolysis and thereby delay its absorption. Accordingly, in patients taking acarbose, oral therapy of hypoglycemia must be accomplished with glucose.

The combination of *metformin* and acarbose should probably be avoided. Both drugs cause significant GI side effects, hence the combination could be very unpleasant. Furthermore, acarbose decreases metformin absorption.

***Preparations, Dosage, and Administration.*** Acarbose [Precose] is available in 50- and 100-mg tablets. The drug is taken at the beginning of each meal. The initial dosage is 25 mg 3 times a day. Depending on tolerability and postprandial blood glucose levels, the dosage may be increased at 4- to 8-week intervals. The maximum dosage is 50 mg 3 times a day (for patients under 60 kg) and 100 mg 3 times a day (for patients over 60 kg).

### Miglitol

Miglitol [Glyset] is the second alpha-glucosidase inhibitor to be approved for use in the United States. Like acarbose, miglitol delays conversion of oligosaccharides and complex carbohydrates to glucose and other monosaccharides, and thereby reduces the postprandial rise in blood glucose. In clinical trials, the drug was especially effective among Hispanics and African-Americans. Like acarbose, miglitol causes flatulence, abdominal discomfort, and other GI effects. The drug is administered three times daily with meals. A dose of 50 mg or 100 mg has been employed.

## Thiazolidinediones: Troglitazone

Troglitazone [Rezulin] belongs to a new class of antihyperglycemic agents known as thiazolidinediones. The drug is not related chemically or functionally to sulfonylureas, biguanides, or alpha-glucosidase inhibitors.

***Actions and Use.*** Troglitazone acts primarily by decreasing insulin resistance. That is, the drug increases the ability of target cells to respond to insulin. Accordingly, insulin must be present for troglitazone to work. In animal models of diabetes, the drug increases uptake of glucose by muscle and decreases glucose production by the liver. In insulin-resistant patients, the drug decreases postprandial and fasting plasma glucose, improves glucose tolerance, and reduces plasma insulin content to near-normal levels.

Troglitazone is approved for patients with NIDDM who are currently using insulin but remain hyperglycemic despite injecting at least 30 units of insulin a day. In clinical trials, troglitazone significantly reduced insulin requirements, allowing some patients to stop taking insulin. At this time, there is little or no information regarding concurrent use of troglitazone with sulfonylureas, biguanides, or alpha-glucosidase inhibitors.

***Pharmacokinetics.*** Troglitazone is rapidly absorbed following oral administration. Food increases absorption;

hence troglitazone should be administered with food to improve bioavailability. Troglitazone undergoes extensive hepatic metabolism followed by excretion in the feces. Only 3% of the drug is eliminated in the urine.

***Adverse Effects.*** Troglitazone is generally well tolerated. Side effects are usually mild or absent. In clinical trials, the incidence of adverse effects was essentially the same as in patients taking placebo. Hypoglycemia has not been observed in patients using troglitazone as monotherapy, but can occur in the presence of too much insulin. Safety for use in pregnancy and lactation has not been determined.

***Drug Interactions.*** *Cholestyramine* (a drug for lowering cholesterol) greatly reduces troglitazone absorption. Accordingly, troglitazone and cholestyramine should not be administered at the same time. Troglitazone reduces levels of *oral contraceptives* and *terfenadine* (an antihistamine), perhaps by inducing synthesis of drug-metabolizing enzymes.

***Preparations, Dosage, and Administration.*** Troglitazone [Rezulin] is available in 200- and 400-mg tablets. The initial dosage is 200 mg once daily with breakfast. If, after 2 to 4 weeks, the response is inadequate, the dosage should be increased to 400 mg once daily. The maximum daily dosage is 600 mg. When fasting plasma glucose falls below 120 mg/dL, insulin dosage should be reduced by 10% to 25%.

## Diabetic Ketoacidosis

Ketoacidosis is the most severe manifestation of insulin deficiency. This syndrome is characterized by hyperglycemia, production of ketoacids, hemoconcentration, acidosis, and coma. Before insulin became available, practically all insulin-dependent diabetics died from ketoacidosis.

### Pathogenesis

Diabetic ketoacidosis is brought on by derangements of glucose and fat metabolism. Altered glucose metabolism causes hyperglycemia, water loss, and hemoconcentration. Altered fat metabolism causes production of ketoacids. Figure 53–2 outlines the sequence of metabolic events by which ketoacidosis develops. Note that, in its final stages, the syndrome consists of hemoconcentration and shock in addition to ketoacidosis itself. The alterations in fat and glucose metabolism that lead to ketoacidosis are described in detail below.

***Altered Fat Metabolism.*** Alterations in fat metabolism lead to production of ketoacids. As indicated in Figure 53–2, insulin deficiency promotes lipolysis (breakdown of fats) in adipose tissue. The products of lipolysis are glycerol and free fatty acids (FFA). Both of these metabolites are transported to the liver. In the liver, oxidation of FFA results in the production of two ketoacids (beta-hydroxybutyric acid and acetoacetic acid), which are also referred to as ketone bodies. Accumulation of ketoacids puts the body in a state of ketosis. Ketosis can be detected by an odor of decaying apples that ketones impart to the urine. As buildup of ketoacids increases, frank acidosis develops. At this point, the patient's condition changes from ketosis to ketoacidosis.

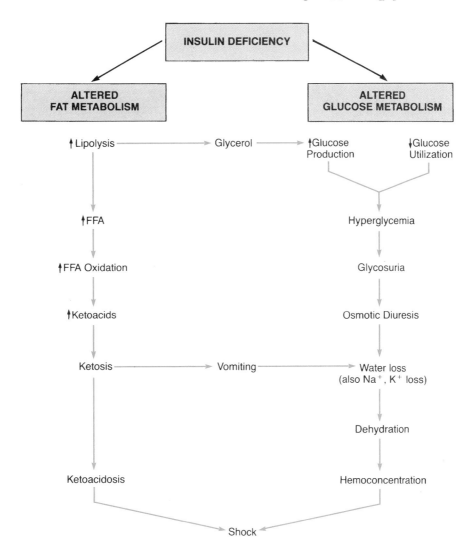

**Figure 53–2. Pathogenesis of diabetic ketoacidosis.** The syndrome of ketoacidosis is caused by derangements of fat and glucose metabolism that occur in response to lack of insulin. (FFA = free fatty acids.)

(Ketoacidosis can be distinguished from ketosis by the presence of hyperventilation.) Acidosis contributes to the development of shock.

***Alterations in Glucose Metabolism.*** Deranged glucose metabolism leads to hyperglycemia, water loss, and hemoconcentration. As shown in Figure 53–2, insulin deficiency has two direct effects on the metabolism of glucose: (1) an increase in glucose production and (2) a decrease in glucose utilization. (The glycerol released by lipolysis is a substrate for glucose synthesis, and therefore helps increase glucose production.) Since more glucose is being made, and less is being used, plasma levels of glucose rise, causing hyperglycemia. Glycosuria develops when plasma glucose content becomes so high that the amount of glucose filtered by the glomeruli exceeds the capacity of the renal tubules for glucose reuptake. As the concentration of glucose in the urine increases, osmotic diuresis develops, resulting in the loss of large volumes of water. Dehydration is worsened because of vomiting brought on by ketosis. Vomiting is a direct source of fluid loss and, more importantly, is an impediment to rehydration with oral fluids. (It should be noted that, along with loss of water, sodium and potassium are also lost. These positive ions are excreted in conjunction with ketone bodies, compounds that carry a negative charge.) As dehydration becomes more severe, hemoconcentration develops. Hemoconcentration

causes cerebral dehydration, which, together with acidosis, leads to shock.

## Treatment

Diabetic ketoacidosis is a life-threatening emergency. Treatment is directed at the following: restoration of insulin levels, correction of acidosis, replacement of lost water and sodium, and normalization of potassium and glucose levels. Details of therapy are presented below.

***Insulin Replacement.*** Insulin levels are restored with an initial 10-U IV bolus of regular insulin followed by continuous infusion at 0.1 U/kg/hr. The total dose should range from 35 to 40 units. The dosing objective is to achieve an optimum blood level of insulin (about 100 to 150 μU/ml). Dosage is not determined by the degree of glycemia or ketonemia.

Intravenous infusion of insulin is preferred to subcutaneous injection. When insulin is administered SC, insulin levels cannot be lowered quickly in response to excessive dosing; hence, avoiding hypoglycemia may be difficult. In contrast, since insulin levels will drop quickly when an infusion is terminated, infusion permits better regulation of blood glucose content.

***Bicarbonate for Acidosis.*** Acidosis is a serious problem with a straightforward solution. Severe acidosis (pH less than 7.1 and plasma bicarbonate less than 10 mEq/L) is corrected by administering sodium bicarbonate IV. pH will equilibrate about 30 minutes after bicarbonate administration. When acidosis is moderate, no specific treatment is needed.

**Water and Sodium Replacement.** Dehydration and sodium loss are both corrected with intravenous saline. Depending on the specific needs of the patient, either 0.9% or 0.45% saline is employed. Adults usually require between 8 and 10 L of fluid during the first 12 hours of treatment. In elderly patients and patients with heart disease, central venous pressure should be monitored.

**Potassium Replacement.** Loss of potassium is a serious problem and must be corrected. Potassium can be replenished through oral or IV administration. Since hypokalemia predisposes the patient to dysrhythmias, EKG monitoring is essential.

Treatment of potassium loss is tricky. This is because plasma potassium levels may be normal even though intracellular potassium is very low. When insulin is administered, causing cellular uptake of potassium to increase, severe hypokalemia can develop as plasma potassium rushes into potassium-depleted cells. Because of this relationship between insulin administration and plasma potassium levels, the following guidelines apply: (1) if plasma potassium is normal, no potassium should be administered until plasma levels decline in response to insulin; (2) if plasma potassium is low, potassium should be given immediately (and then re-administered if potassium levels fall following insulin administration).

**Normalization of Glucose Levels.** Treatment of ketoacidosis with insulin may convert hyperglycemia into hypoglycemia. Because cellular uptake of glucose is impaired by insulin deficiency, ketoacidosis is likely to be associated with a reduction in intracellular glucose—despite elevations in plasma glucose content. Under these conditions, insulin administration will cause plasma glucose to rush into the glucose-depleted cells, thereby causing plasma levels of glucose to drop precipitously. If insulin therapy induces hypoglycemia, plasma glucose can be restored by administering either glucagon or glucose itself.

## Glucagon for Insulin Overdose

Glucagon is a polypeptide hormone produced by alpha cells of the pancreatic islets. The hormone increases plasma levels of glucose and relaxes smooth muscle of the GI tract. The drug can be used to elevate blood glucose levels following insulin overdose.

Glucagon has effects on carbohydrate metabolism that are exactly opposite to those of insulin. Specifically, glucagon promotes the breakdown of glycogen, reduces glycogen synthesis, and stimulates biosynthesis of glucose. Hence, whereas insulin acts to lower plasma glucose content, glucagon causes glucose levels to rise. In addition, glucagon acts on gastrointestinal smooth muscle to promote relaxation.

Glucagon is used to treat hypoglycemia resulting from insulin overdose. In unconscious patients, arousal usually occurs within 20 minutes of glucagon injection. If no response occurs by this time, intravenous dextrose (glucose) must be administered. Once consciousness has been produced, oral carbohydrates should be given; these will help prevent recurrence of hypoglycemia and will help restore hepatic glycogen content.

Glucagon cannot correct hypoglycemia resulting from starvation. Since glucagon acts in large part by promoting glycogen breakdown, and since starvation depletes glycogen stores, glucagon cannot elevate glucose levels in individuals who are starved.

Glucagon is administered parenterally (IM, SC, and IV). The drug is dispensed in powder form and must be reconstituted to a concentration of 1 mg/ml using the diluent supplied by the manufacturer. A dose of 0.5 to 1 mg is usually effective.

## KEY POINTS

- Diabetes mellitus (diabetes) is characterized by sustained hyperglycemia.
- Diabetes has two major forms: insulin-dependent diabetes mellitus (IDDM; type 1 diabetes) and noninsulin-dependent diabetes mellitus (NIDDM; type 2 diabetes).
- Symptoms of IDDM result from a complete absence of insulin. The underlying cause is autoimmune destruction of pancreatic beta cells.
- Symptoms of NIDDM result primarily from cellular resistance to insulin's actions, and not from an absence of insulin.
- IDDM and NIDDM share the same long-term complications: hypertension, heart disease, stroke, blindness, renal failure, neuropathy, lower limb amputations, impotence, and gastroparesis.
- Diabetes is diagnosed if (1) fasting blood glucose exceeds 140 mg/dL, (2) random blood glucose exceeds 200 mg/dL, or (3) blood glucose exceeds 200 mg/dL 1 and 2 hours after an oral glucose challenge.
- IDDM is treated with insulin replacement. Oral hypoglycemics are not used.
- NIDDM is treated with oral hypoglycemics and/or insulin—but only in conjunction with a program of diet modification and exercise, and only if glycemic control cannot be maintained by diet and exercise alone.
- Home blood glucose monitoring (HBGM) is the standard method for day-to-day monitoring of diabetes therapy. Target values are 80 to 120 mg/dL before meals and 100 to 140 mg/dL at bedtime.
- Glycosylated hemoglobin (hemoglobin $A_{1c}$) can be measured every few months to assess long-term glycemic control. The target value is 7% or less.
- Insulin is anabolic. That is, the hormone promotes conservation of energy and buildup of energy stores.
- Insulin has two basic effects: (1) it stimulates uptake of glucose, amino acids, nucleotides, and potassium; and (2) it promotes synthesis of complex organic molecules (glycogen, proteins, triglycerides).
- Insulin deficiency puts the body into a catabolic mode. As a result, glycogen is converted into glucose, proteins are degraded into amino acids, and fats are converted to glycerol (glycerin) and free fatty acids.
- Insulin deficiency promotes hyperglycemia by increasing glycogenolysis and gluconeogenesis and decreasing glucose utilization.
- Five forms of insulin are used in the United States: regular insulin, lispro insulin, NPH insulin, lente insulin, and ultralente insulin.
- Lispro insulin has a very rapid onset and short duration.
- Regular insulin has a rapid onset and short duration.
- NPH insulin and lente insulin have intermediate durations.
- Ultralente insulin has a prolonged duration.
- All insulins can be injected SC. Regular insulin can be administered IV and IM in addition to SC.

- Insulin suspensions (NPH insulin, lente insulin, ultralente insulin) should be gently agitated before use. Insulin solutions (regular insulin, lispro insulin) do not need agitation.
- Insulin is used to treat all patients with IDDM and some patients with NIDDM.
- When insulin therapy produces tight glucose control, it can markedly reduce the long-term complications of diabetes, as demonstrated in the Diabetes Complications and Control Trial (DCCT).
- To achieve tight glucose control, patients must practice intensive insulin therapy, consisting of either (1) an evening injection of ultralente insulin supplemented with mealtime injections of regular insulin or lispro insulin, or (2) continuous SC infusion of regular insulin supplemented with mealtime bolus doses. With both approaches, the mealtime dose is adjusted to match caloric intake. Tight glucose control cannot be achieved with conventional insulin therapy (i.e., one or two injections a day).
- HBGM is an essential component of intensive therapy. Blood glucose should be measured three to five times a day.
- Compared with conventional therapy, intensive insulin therapy carries a greater risk of hypoglycemia. Other drawbacks are an increase in cost, inconvenience, complexity, and weight gain.
- The principal adverse effect of insulin therapy is hypoglycemia (blood glucose <50 mg/dL), which occurs whenever insulin levels exceed insulin needs. Symptoms include tachycardia, palpitations, sweating, headache, confusion, drowsiness, and fatigue. If hypoglycemia is severe, convulsions, coma, and death may follow.
- Beta blockers can delay awareness of hypoglycemia by masking signs that are caused by activation of the sympathetic nervous system (e.g., tachycardia, palpitations).
- Insulin-induced hypoglycemia can be treated with a fast-acting oral sugar (e.g., glucose tablets, orange juice, sugar cubes), intravenous glucose, or parenteral glucagon.
- Oral hypoglycemic drugs—sulfonylureas, metformin, alpha-glucosidase inhibitors, troglitazone—are indicated only for treatment of NIDDM. They are not used for IDDM.
- Sulfonylureas stimulate release of insulin from the pancreas. They may also increase cellular sensitivity to insulin.
- The major adverse effect of sulfonylureas is hypoglycemia.
- Metformin (a biguanide) decreases glucose production by the liver and increases glucose uptake by muscle.
- The major adverse effects of metformin are gastrointestinal: decreased appetite, nausea, and diarrhea.
- Rarely, metformin causes lactic acidosis, which can be fatal. The risk of lactic acidosis is greatly increased by renal impairment, which decreases metformin excretion and thereby causes drug levels to rise rapidly.
- Acarbose (an alpha-glucosidase inhibitor) inhibits digestion and absorption of carbohydrates, and thereby reduces the postprandial rise in blood glucose. To be effective, the drug must be taken with every meal.
- The major adverse effects of acarbose are gastrointestinal: flatulence, cramps, and abdominal distention.
- Troglitazone decreases insulin resistance, and thereby increases glucose uptake by muscle and decreases glucose production by the liver. The drug is approved only for patients who are already taking insulin.
- Troglitazone can cause hypoglycemia, but only in the presence of excessive insulin.

# Summary of Major Nursing Implications†

## Insulin

### Preadministration Assessment

#### Therapeutic Goal
Insulin is required by all patients with IDDM and by some with NIDDM. The goal of therapy is to maintain plasma glucose levels within an acceptable range (see Table 53-5).

#### Baseline Data
Assess for clinical manifestations of diabetes (e.g., polyuria, polydipsia, polyphagia, weight loss) and for indications of hyperglycemia. Baseline laboratory tests may include random blood glucose, fasting blood glucose, a glucose tolerance test, hemoglobin $A_{1c}$, urinary glucose and ketones, and serum electrolytes.

#### Identifying High-Risk Patients
Special care is needed in patients taking drugs that can raise or lower blood glucose levels, such as *sympathomimetics, beta blockers, glucocorticoids, sulfonylureas,* and *troglitazone.*

Patients with a history of severe allergic reactions to insulin derived from beef or pork pancreas should be treated with lispro insulin or one of the human insulins.

### Implementation: Administration

#### Routes
All insulins may be administered SC. None are given PO. Regular insulin may be administered IM and IV in addition to SC.

---

†Patient education information is highlighted in color.

## Preparation for Subcutaneous Injection

Teach the patient to prepare for SC injections as follows:

- Before loading the syringe, disperse insulin suspensions (i.e., all forms of insulin except lispro insulin and regular insulin) by rolling the vial gently between the palms. Vigorous agitation causes frothing and must be avoided. If granules or clumps remain after mixing, discard the vial.
- Regular insulin and lispro insulin are clear solutions, and hence can be administered without mixing. If a preparation becomes cloudy or discolored, or if a precipitate develops, discard the vial.
- Before loading the syringe, swab the bottle cap with alcohol.
- Eliminate air bubbles from the syringe and needle after loading.
- Cleanse the skin with alcohol prior to injection.

## Sites of Injection

Provide the patient with the following instruction regarding sites of SC injection:

- Usual sites of injection are the upper arms, thighs, and abdomen. To minimize variability in responses, it is preferable to make all injections in just one of these areas.
- Rotate the injection site within the general area employed (i.e., abdomen, thigh, or upper arm). Allow about 1 inch between sites. If possible, use each site just once every month.

## Insulin Storage

Teach the patient the following about insulin storage:

- Store unopened vials of insulin in the refrigerator, but do not freeze. When stored under these conditions, insulin can be used up to the expiration date on the vial.
- The vial in current use can be stored at room temperature for up to 1 month, but must be kept out of direct sunlight and extreme heat. Discard partially filled vials after several weeks if left unused.
- Mixtures of insulin prepared in vials may be stored for 1 month at room temperature, and for 3 months under refrigeration.
- Mixtures of insulin in prefilled syringes (plastic or glass) should be stored in a refrigerator, where they will be stable for at least 1 week, and perhaps 2. Store the syringe vertically (needle pointing up) to avoid clogging the needle. Gently agitate the syringe prior to administration to resuspend the insulin.

## Dosage Adjustment

The dosing goal is to maintain blood glucose levels within an acceptable range. Dosage must be adjusted to balance changes in caloric intake and other factors that can decrease insulin needs (strenuous exercise, pregnancy during the first trimester) or increase insulin needs (illness, trauma, stress, adolescent growth spurt, pregnancy after the first trimester).

Regular insulin can adsorb in varying amounts onto IV infusion sets. Dosage adjustments made to compensate for losses are based on the therapeutic response.

## Patient and Family Education

Patient and family education is an absolute requirement for safe and successful glycemic control. Provide patients and their families with thorough instruction on

- The nature of diabetes
- The importance of tight glucose control
- The major components of the treatment routine (insulin, blood glucose monitoring, diet, exercise)
- Procedures for purchasing insulin, syringes, and needles
- Methods of insulin storage
- Procedures for mixing insulins
- Calculation of dosage adjustments
- Techniques of insulin injection
- Rotation of injection sites
- Measurement of blood glucose content
- Signs and management of hypoglycemia
- Signs and management of hyperglycemia
- Special problems of diabetic pregnancy
- The procedure for obtaining Medic Alert registration
- The importance of not making arbitrary changes between insulins made by different manufacturers and between human, pork, or beef/pork insulins.

# Ongoing Evaluation and Interventions

## Evaluating Therapeutic Effects

Whenever practical, HBGM should be employed to evaluate treatment. Teach patients how to use the HBGM measuring device, and encourage them to monitor blood glucose daily. Urinary glucose may be monitored as an alternative, but these measurements are much less useful than HBGM. The physician may request periodic hemoglobin $A_{1c}$ tests to assess long-term glycemic control.

## Minimizing Adverse Effects

*Hypoglycemia.* Hypoglycemia occurs whenever insulin levels exceed insulin needs. Inform the patient about potential causes of hypoglycemia (e.g., reduced food intake, vomiting, diarrhea, excessive consumption of alcohol, unaccustomed exercise, termination of pregnancy), and teach the patient and family members to recognize the early signs and symptoms of hypoglycemia (tachycardia, palpitations, sweating, nervousness, headache, confusion, drowsiness, fatigue).

Rapid treatment is mandatory. If the patient is conscious, oral carbohydrates are indicated (e.g., glucose tablets, orange juice, sugar cubes, honey, corn syrup, nondiet soda). However, if the swallowing or gag reflex is suppressed, nothing should be administered PO. For unconscious patients, IV glucose is the treatment of choice. Parenteral glucagon is an alternative.

Hypoglycemic coma must be differentiated from coma of diabetic ketoacidosis (DKA). The differential diagnosis is made by measuring plasma or urinary glucose content: hypoglycemic coma is associated with very low levels of glucose, whereas high levels signify DKA.

***Lipohypertrophy.*** Accumulation of subcutaneous fat can occur at sites of frequent insulin injection. Inform the patient that lipohypertrophy can be minimized by systematic rotation of the injection site.

***Systemic Allergic Reactions.*** Systemic reactions (widespread urticaria, impairment of breathing) are rare. Systemic allergy is most common with beef insulin and is less likely with pork or human insulin. If systemic allergy develops, it can be reduced through desensitization (i.e., administration of small initial doses of purified pork or human insulin followed by a series of progressively larger doses).

### Minimizing Adverse Interactions

***Hypoglycemic Agents.*** Several drugs, including sulfonylureas, troglitazone, alcohol (used acutely), and beta-adrenergic blocking agents, can intensify hypoglycemia induced by insulin. When any of these drugs is combined with insulin, special care must be taken to ensure that blood glucose content does not fall too low.

***Hyperglycemic Agents.*** Several drugs, including thiazide diuretics, glucocorticoids, and sympathomimetics, can elevate blood glucose, and can thereby counteract the beneficial effects of insulin. When these agents are combined with insulin, increased insulin dosage may be required.

***Beta-Adrenergic Blocking Agents.*** Beta blockade can mask sympathetic responses (e.g., tachycardia, palpitations, tremors) to declining blood glucose, and can thereby delay awareness of insulin-induced hypoglycemia. Also, since beta blockade impairs glycogenolysis, beta blockers can make insulin-induced hypoglycemia even worse.

## Sulfonylureas

| | |
|---|---|
| Acetohexamide | Glyburide |
| Chlorpropamide | Tolazamide |
| Glimepiride | Tolbutamide |
| Glipizide | |

### Preadministration: Assessment

#### Therapeutic Goal

Sulfonylureas are used as an adjunct to caloric restriction and exercise to maintain glycemic control in patients with NIDDM. These drugs are not useful for patients with IDDM.

#### Identifying High-Risk Patients

These drugs are contraindicated for during *pregnancy* and *breast-feeding*. Use with *caution* in patients with *kidney or liver dysfunction*. Sulfonylureas should not be used in conjunction with *alcohol*.

### Implementation: Administration

#### Route

Oral.

#### Administration

Advise patients to administer with food if GI upset occurs.

Note that dosages for the second-generation agents are much lower than dosages for first-generation agents (Table 53–8).

Sulfonylureas are intended only as supplemental therapy of NIDDM. Encourage patients to maintain their established program of exercise and caloric restriction.

### Ongoing Evaluation and Interventions

#### Minimizing Adverse Effects

***Hypoglycemia.*** Inform patients about signs of hypoglycemia (palpitations, tachycardia, sweating, fatigue, excessive hunger), and instruct them to notify the physician if these occur. Treat severe hypoglycemia with IV glucose.

#### Use in Pregnancy and Lactation

***Pregnancy.*** Discontinue sulfonylureas during pregnancy. If a hypoglycemic agent is needed, insulin is the drug to use.

***Lactation.*** Sulfonylureas are excreted into breast milk, posing a risk of hypoglycemia to the nursing infant. Women who choose to breast-feed should substitute insulin for the sulfonylurea.

# CHAPTER 54

# Drugs for Thyroid Disorders

hyroid hormones have profound effects on metabolism, cardiac function, growth, and development. These hormones stimulate the metabolic rate of most cells, and increase the force and rate of cardiac contraction. During infancy and childhood, thyroid hormones promote maturation; an absence of these hormones can produce dwarfism and permanent mental impairment. Fortunately, most abnormalities of thyroid function can be effectively treated.

We will begin our study of thyroid drugs by reviewing thyroid physiology. Next we will review the pathophysiology of hypothyroid and hyperthyroid states. With this background, we will then discuss the agents used to treat thyroid disorders.

## Thyroid Physiology

### Chemistry and Nomenclature

The thyroid gland produces two active hormones: *triiodothyronine* (T$_3$) and *thyroxine* (T$_4$, tetraiodothyronine). As Figure 54-1 shows, the structures of these hormones are nearly identical, the only difference being that T$_4$ contains four atoms of iodine, whereas T$_3$ contains only three. The biologic effects of T$_3$ and T$_4$ are qualitatively similar. However, when compared on a molar basis, T$_3$ is more potent than T$_4$.

The preparations of T$_3$ and T$_4$ employed clinically are manmade. These synthetic compounds have structures identical to those of the naturally occurring hormones. Synthetic T$_3$ has the generic name *liothyronine*; synthetic T$_4$ is called *levothyroxine*. A fixed-ratio mixture of T$_3$ plus T$_4$, known as *liotrix*, is also available.

### Thyroid Hormone Actions

Thyroid hormones have three principal actions: (1) stimulation of energy use, (2) stimulation of the heart, and (3) promotion of growth and development. Stimulation of energy use elevates the basal metabolic rate, resulting in increased oxygen consumption and increased heat production. Stimulation of the heart increases both the rate and force of contraction, resulting in increased cardiac output and increased oxygen demand. Thyroid effects on growth and development are profound: thyroid hormones are essential for normal development of the brain and other components of the nervous system; these hormones also have a significant impact on maturation of skeletal muscle.

### Synthesis and Fate of Thyroid Hormones

*Synthesis.* Synthesis of thyroid hormones takes place in four basic steps (Fig. 54–2). The circled numbers in the figure correspond with the steps below.

*Step 1.* Formation of thyroid hormone begins with the active transport of *iodide* into the thyroid. Under normal conditions, this uptake process produces concentrations of iodide within the thyroid that are 20 to 50 times greater than the concentration of iodide in plasma. When plasma iodide levels are extremely low, intrathyroid iodide content may reach levels that are more than 100 times greater than those in plasma.

*Step 2.* Following uptake, iodide undergoes oxidation to *iodine*, the active form of iodide. Oxidation of iodide is catalyzed by an enzyme called *peroxidase*.

*Step 3.* In this step, activated iodine becomes incorporated into tyrosine residues that are bound to *thyroglobulin*, a large glycoprotein molecule. As indicated in Figure 54–2, one tyrosine molecule may receive either one or

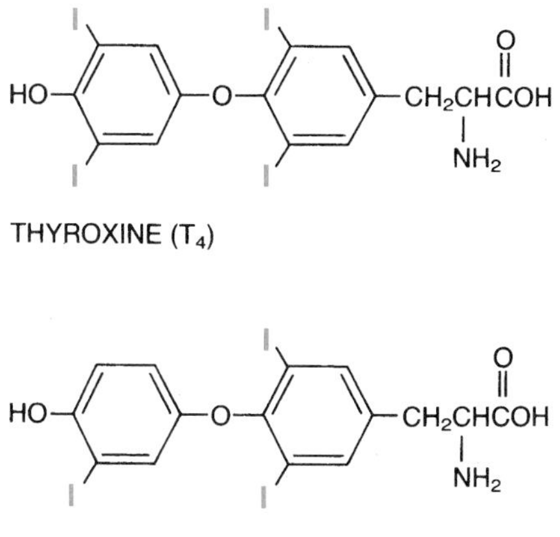

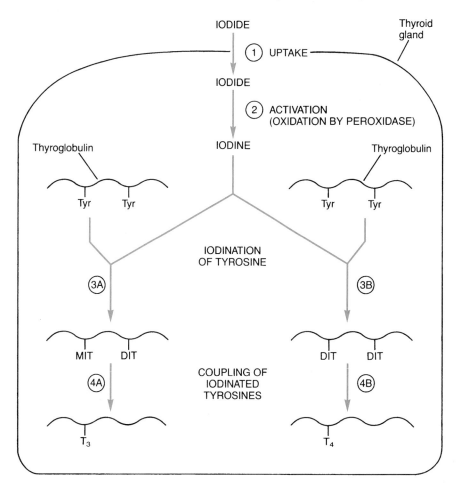

THYROXINE (T₄)

TRIIODOTHYRONINE (T₃)

**Figure 54–1. Structural formulas of the thyroid hormones.**

two iodine atoms, resulting in the production of mono-iodotyrosine (MIT) and diiodotyrosine (DIT), respectively.

*Step 4.* In the final step of thyroid hormone synthesis, iodinated tyrosine molecules are coupled. Coupling of one DIT with one MIT forms $T_3$ (Step 4A); coupling of one DIT with another DIT forms $T_4$ (Step 4B).

**Fate.** Thyroid hormones are released from the thyroid gland by a proteolytic process. The amount of $T_4$ released is substantially greater than the amount of $T_3$. However, much of the $T_4$ that is released undergoes conversion to $T_3$ by enzymes in peripheral tissues. In fact, conversion of $T_4$ to $T_3$ accounts for the majority (about 80%) of the $T_3$ found in plasma.

More than 99.5% of the $T_3$ and $T_4$ in plasma is bound to plasma proteins. Consequently, only a tiny fraction of circulating thyroid hormone is free to produce biologic effects.

Thyroid hormones are eliminated primarily by hepatic metabolism. Because $T_3$ and $T_4$ are extensively bound to plasma proteins, metabolism takes place slowly. As a result, the half-lives of these hormones are prolonged. $T_3$ has a half-life of 1.5 days and $T_4$ has a half-life of 1 week.

## Regulation of Thyroid Function by the Hypothalamus and Anterior Pituitary

The functional relationship between the hypothalamus, anterior pituitary, and thyroid is depicted in Figure 54–3. As indicated, thyrotropin-releasing hormone (TRH), secreted by the hypothalamus, acts on the pituitary to cause secretion of thyrotropin (thyroid-stimulating hormone; TSH). TSH then acts on the thyroid to stimulate all aspects of thyroid function: thyroid size is enlarged, iodine uptake is augmented, and synthesis and release of thyroid hormones are increased. In response to rising plasma levels of

**Figure 54–2. Steps in thyroid hormone synthesis.** The reactions at each step (circled numbers) are explained in the text. (Tyr = tyrosine, MIT = monoiodotyrosine, DIT = diiodotyrosine, $T_3$ = triiodothyronine, $T_4$ = thyroxine.)

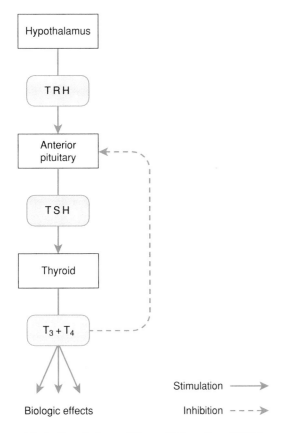

**Figure 54–3. Regulation of thyroid function.** TRH from the hypothalamus stimulates release of TSH from the pituitary. TSH stimulates all aspects of thyroid function, including release of $T_3$ and $T_4$. $T_3$ and $T_4$ act on the pituitary to suppress further TSH release. (TRH = thyrotropin-releasing hormone, TSH = thyrotropin [thyroid-stimulating hormone], $T_3$ = triiodothyronine, $T_4$ = thyroxine.)

$T_3$ and $T_4$, further release of TSH is suppressed. The stimulatory effect of TSH on the thyroid followed by the inhibitory effect of thyroid hormones on the pituitary constitutes a negative feedback loop.

### Influence of Iodine Levels on Thyroid Function

*Low Iodine.* When iodine availability is diminished, production of thyroid hormones decreases. The ensuing drop in thyroid hormone levels promotes release of TSH. In response to increased levels of TSH, thyroid size increases (causing goiter), and the ability of the thyroid to concentrate iodine increases as well. If the iodine deficiency is not too severe, the increased capacity for iodine uptake will permit production of thyroid hormones in amounts sufficient to return plasma levels of $T_3$ and $T_4$ to normal.

*High Iodine.* The effect of extremely high iodine levels on thyroid function is opposite to that of low iodine: uptake of iodide is suppressed, and synthesis and release of thyroid hormones decline. The mechanisms underlying these effects are not understood.

# Thyroid Pathophysiology

## Hypothyroidism

Hypothyroidism can occur at any age. In the adult, mild deficiency of thyroid hormone is referred to simply as *hypothyroidism*; severe deficiency in adults is called *myxedema*. When hypothyroidism occurs in infancy, the resulting condition is called *cretinism*.

### Hypothyroidism in Adults

*Clinical Presentation.* Hypothyroidism in adults produces a characteristic set of signs and symptoms. The face is pale, puffy, and expressionless. The skin is cold and dry. The hair is brittle. Heart rate and temperature are lowered. The patient may complain of lethargy, fatigue, and intolerance to cold. Mentality may be impaired. Thyroid enlargement (goiter) may occur if reduced levels of $T_3$ and $T_4$ promote excessive release of TSH.

*Causes.* Hypothyroidism in the adult is usually due to malfunction of the thyroid itself. In iodine-sufficient countries, the principal cause of thyroid malfunction is *chronic autoimmune thyroiditis (Hashimoto's disease)*. Other causes are insufficient iodine in the diet, surgical removal of the thyroid, and destruction of the thyroid by radioactive iodine. Adult hypothyroidism may also result from insufficient secretion of TSH and TRH.

*Therapeutic Strategy.* Hypothyroidism in adults requires replacement therapy with thyroid hormones. In almost all cases, treatment must continue lifelong. For mild deficiency, oral hormones are employed; levothyroxine ($T_4$) is the preferred preparation. For severe deficiency, IV therapy is required; either liothyronine ($T_3$) or $T_4$ may be used. When replacement doses are adequate, they eliminate all signs and symptoms of thyroid deficiency.

### Hypothyroidism in Infants

*Clinical Presentation.* Thyroid deficiency in infants (cretinism) causes mental retardation and derangement of growth. In the absence of thyroid hormones, the child develops a large and protruding tongue, potbelly, and dwarfish stature. Development of the nervous system, bones, teeth, and muscles is impaired.

*Causes.* Cretinism usually results from a failure in thyroid development. Other causes include autoimmune disease, severe iodine deficiency, TSH deficiency, and exposure to radioactive iodine *in utero*.

*Therapeutic Strategy.* Hypothyroidism in newborns requires replacement therapy with thyroid hormones. If treatment is initiated within a few days of birth, physical and mental development will be normal. However, if therapy is delayed for several months, some permanent retardation will be evident, although the physical effects of thyroid deficiency will reverse. Replacement therapy must continue for life.

# Hyperthyroidism

There are two major forms of hyperthyroidism: *Graves' disease* and *toxic nodular goiter* (also known as *Plummer's disease*). Of the two, Graves' disease is the more common. Signs and symptoms of both disorders are similar; the principal difference is that Graves' disease may cause exophthalmos, whereas toxic nodular goiter does not. If levels of thyroid hormone rise extremely high, patients with either form of hyperthyroidism may experience *thyrotoxic crisis*.

## Graves' Disease

Graves' disease is the most common cause of excessive thyroid hormone secretion. This disorder occurs most frequently in women 20 to 40 years of age. The incidence in females is 6 times greater than in males.

**Clinical Presentation.** Most clinical manifestations of Graves' disease result from elevated levels of thyroid hormone. Heart beat is rapid and strong, and dysrhythmias and angina may develop. The central nervous system is stimulated, resulting in rapid thought flow and rapid speech, nervousness, and insomnia. Skeletal muscles may weaken and atrophy. Metabolic rate is raised, resulting in increased heat production, increased body temperature, intolerance to heat, and skin that is warm and moist. Appetite is increased; however, despite increased food consumption, weight loss occurs if caloric intake fails to match the increase in metabolic rate. Collectively, the above signs and symptoms are referred to as *thyrotoxicosis*.

In addition to thyrotoxicosis, patients with Graves' disease often present with *exophthalmos* (protrusion of the eyeballs). The cause is obscure. However, we do know this condition is not caused by increased levels of thyroid hormones.

**Cause.** Thyroid stimulation in Graves' disease is caused by thyroid-stimulating immunoglobulins (TSIs). These immunoglobulins are antibodies produced by an autoimmune process. TSIs increase thyroid activity by stimulating receptors for TSH on the thyroid gland. That is, TSIs mimic the effects of TSH on thyroid function. TSIs are not responsible for exophthalmos.

**Treatment.** Treatment for Graves' disease is directed at decreasing the production of thyroid hormones. Three modalities are employed: (1) surgical removal of thyroid tissue, (2) destruction of thyroid tissue with radioactive iodine, and (3) suppression of thyroid hormone synthesis with antithyroid drugs (e.g., propylthiouracil). Of the three, radiation and surgery are most definitive.

Propranolol and nonradioactive iodine may be used as adjunctive therapy. Propranolol suppresses tachycardia by blocking beta-adrenergic receptors on the heart. Nonradioactive iodine inhibits synthesis and release of thyroid hormones.

Since exophthalmos is not the result of hyperthyroidism per se, this condition is not improved by lowering thyroid hormone production. If exophthalmos is severe, it can be treated with high doses of oral glucocorticoids.

## Toxic Nodular Goiter (Plummer's Disease)

Toxic nodular goiter is the result of thyroid adenoma. Clinical manifestations are much like those of Graves' disease, except exophthalmos is absent. Toxic nodular goiter is a persistent condition that rarely undergoes spontaneous remission. Treatment modalities are the same as for Graves' disease. However, if antithyroid drugs are used, symptoms return rapidly upon their discontinuation. Accordingly, surgery and radiation, which provide long-term control, are often preferred.

## Thyrotoxic Crisis (Thyroid Storm)

Thyrotoxic crisis occurs when levels of thyroid hormone become extremely high. The syndrome is characterized by hyperthermia, severe tachycardia, and profound weakness. Unconsciousness, coma, and heart failure may ensue. Thyrotoxic crisis can be caused by excessive production of endogenous thyroid hormones or by overdose with thyroid hormones during replacement therapy.

Thyrotoxic crisis can be life threatening and requires immediate treatment. High doses of potassium iodide or strong iodine solution are given to suppress thyroid hormone release; propylthiouracil is given to suppress thyroid hormone synthesis and conversion of $T_4$ to $T_3$ in the periphery; and propranolol is given to reduce heart rate. Additional measures include sedation, cooling, and giving glucocorticoids and IV fluids.

# Thyroid Function Tests

Several laboratory tests can be used to evaluate thyroid function. Three are described below.

**Serum $T_4$ Test.** The serum $T_4$ test measures total (bound plus free) *thyroxine*. Since serum $T_4$ levels reflect overall thyroid activity, this test is useful for initial screening of thyroid function: levels of $T_4$ will be low in hypothyroid patients and high in hyperthyroid patients. The test can also be used to monitor thyroid-hormone replacement therapy; all thyroid preparations, except liothyronine, should cause $T_4$ levels to rise.

**Serum $T_3$ Test.** The $T_3$ test measures total (bound plus free) *triiodothyronine*. This test is useful for diagnosing hyperthyroidism, since in this disorder levels of $T_3$ often rise sooner and to a greater extent than levels of $T_4$. $T_3$ determinations can also be employed to monitor thyroid-hormone replacement therapy; all thyroid preparations should increase levels of $T_3$.

**Serum TSH.** Measurement of serum TSH is the most sensitive method for diagnosing hypothyroidism. This is because very small reductions in serum $T_3$ and $T_4$ cause a

## TABLE 54–1.  THYROID HORMONE PREPARATIONS

| Generic Name | Trade Names | Dosage Forms | Equivalent Dosage | Description |
|---|---|---|---|---|
| Levothyroxine | Levothroid, Synthroid, Eltroxin, Levoxyl, Levo-T | Tablets, injection | 50–60 μg | Synthetic preparation of $T_4$ identical to the naturally occurring hormone |
| Liothyronine | Cytomel, Triostat | Tablets, injection | 15–37 μg | Synthetic preparation of $T_3$ identical to the naturally occurring hormone |
| Liotrix | Euthroid, Thyrolar | Tablets | 60 μg | Synthetic $T_4$ plus synthetic $T_3$ in a 4:1 fixed ratio |
| Thyroglobulin | Proloid | Tablets | 60 mg | Purified extract of hog thyroid |
| Thyroid | Armour Thyroid, S-P-T, Thyrar, Thyroid USP, Thyroid Strong | Tablets, capsules | 60 mg | Desiccated animal thyroid glands |

dramatic rise in serum TSH. Hence, even when the degree of hypothyroidism is minimal, it will be reflected by an abnormally high level of TSH. When replacement therapy is instituted, TSH levels should return to normal.

Serum TSH determinations can also be used to distinguish primary hypothyroidism from secondary hypothyroidism. In primary (thyroidal) hypothyroidism, TSH levels are high, whereas in secondary hypothyroidism (hypothyroidism resulting from anterior pituitary dysfunction), TSH levels are low.

# Thyroid Hormone Preparations for Hypothyroidism

Thyroid hormones are available as pure, synthetic compounds and as extracts of animal thyroid glands. All of these preparations have qualitatively similar effects. The synthetic preparations are more stable and better standardized than the animal gland extracts. As a result, the synthetics are preferred to the natural products. Properties of the thyroid hormone preparations are summarized in Table 54–1.

## Levothyroxine ($T_4$)

Levothyroxine [Levothroid, Synthroid, others] is a synthetic preparation of thyroxine ($T_4$), a naturally occurring thyroid hormone. The structure of levothyroxine is identical to that of the natural hormone. Levothyroxine is the drug of choice for most patients who require thyroid hormone replacement. Consequently, levothyroxine will serve as our prototype for the thyroid hormone preparations.

### Pharmacokinetics

*Absorption.* Absorption of oral levothyroxine is variable. Depending upon the preparation, absorption may range from 42% to 74%.

*Conversion to $T_3$.* Much of an administered dose of levothyroxine is converted to $T_3$ in the body. As a result, levothyroxine can produce nearly normal levels of both $T_3$ and $T_4$. Hence, for most patients, there is no need to give $T_3$ along with levothyroxine.

*Half-Life and Plasma Levels.* Because levothyroxine is highly protein bound (about 99.97%), the hormone has a prolonged half-life (about 7 days). From a clinical perspective, this long half-life has advantages as well as disadvantages. On the negative side, about 1 month (four half-lives) is required for plasma levels of levothyroxine to reach plateau. As a result, onset of full effects is delayed. On the positive side, a long half-life causes hormone levels to remain steady between doses. This property permits once-a-day dosing, which makes levothyroxine desirable for lifelong therapy.

### Therapeutic Uses

Levothyroxine is indicated for all forms of hypothyroidism, regardless of cause. The drug is used for cretinism, myxedema coma, ordinary hypothyroidism in adults and children, and simple goiter. Levothyroxine is also used to treat hypothyroidism resulting from insufficient TSH (secondary to pituitary malfunction) and from insufficient TRH (secondary to hypothalamic malfunction). In addition, levothyroxine is used to maintain proper levels of thyroid hormones following thyroid surgery, irradiation, and treatment with antithyroid drugs.

*Levothyroxine and other thyroid hormones should not be taken to treat obesity.* These hormones will accelerate metabolism and promote weight reduction only if the dosage is high enough to establish a pathologic (hyperthyroid) state.

### Adverse Effects

When administered in appropriate dosage, levothyroxine rarely causes adverse effects. If the dosage is excessive, *thyrotoxicosis* may be produced. Signs and symptoms include tachycardia, angina, tremor, nervousness, insomnia, hyperthermia, heat intolerance, and sweating. The patient should be informed about these signs and instructed to notify the physician if they develop. If the dosage is especially large, *thyrotoxic crisis* may occur.

## Drug Interactions

***Drugs That Reduce Levothyroxine Absorption.*** Cholestyramine [Questran] and colestipol [Colestid], which are used to treat high cholesterol, can bind levothyroxine and thereby significantly reduce its absorption. To minimize this interaction, several hours should separate administration of levothyroxine and administration of these two drugs. Other drugs that may reduce levothyroxine absorption include sucralfate [Carafate], aluminum hydroxide, and ferrous sulfate.

***Warfarin.*** Levothyroxine accelerates the degradation of vitamin K–dependent clotting factors. As a result, effects of warfarin, an oral anticoagulant, are enhanced. If thyroid hormone replacement therapy is instituted in a patient who has been taking warfarin, the dosage of warfarin should be reduced.

***Catecholamines.*** Thyroid hormones increase cardiac responsiveness to catecholamines (epinephrine, dopamine, dobutamine), thereby increasing the risk of catecholamine-induced dysrhythmias. Caution must be exercised when administering catecholamines to patients receiving levothyroxine and other thyroid preparations.

***Other Interactions.*** Levothyroxine can increase requirements for insulin and digitalis. Hence, when converting patients from a hypothyroid to a euthyroid state, dosages of *insulin* and *digitalis* may need to be increased.

## Dosage and Administration I: General Considerations

***Routes of Administration.*** Levothyroxine is almost always administered by mouth. Oral doses should be taken on an empty stomach to enhance absorption. Dosing is usually done in the morning before breakfast.

Intravenous administration is used for myxedema coma and for patients who cannot take levothyroxine orally. Intravenous doses are about one half the size of oral doses.

***Evaluation.*** The goal of thyroid hormone replacement therapy is to provide a dosage that will compensate precisely for the existing thyroid deficit. This dosage is determined using a combination of clinical judgment and laboratory tests. When therapy is successful in adults, clinical evaluation should reveal a reversal of the signs and symptoms of thyroid deficiency—and an absence of signs of thyroid excess. Successful therapy of infants is reflected in normalization of intellectual function and normalization of growth and development. Monthly determinations of height provide a good index of success.

Laboratory determinations of serum TSH are an important means of evaluation. Successful therapy will cause elevated TSH levels to fall. These levels will begin their decline within hours of the onset of therapy and will continue to drop as plasma levels of thyroid hormone build up. If an adequate dosage is established, TSH levels will remain suppressed for the duration of treatment. For some patients, serum $T_4$ must be used to evaluate levothyroxine therapy. In young children, TSH secretion

may remain high even though levels of thyroid hormone have been restored. In such patients, TSH determinations are not helpful. For these patients, serum $T_4$ levels can be employed to evaluate dosage; when the dosage is appropriate, $T_4$ levels will be in the normal to high-normal range.

***Duration of Therapy.*** For most hypothyroid patients, replacement therapy must be continued for life. Treatment provides symptomatic relief but does not produce cure. The patient must be made fully aware of the chronic nature of the condition. In addition, the patient should be forewarned that, although therapy will cause symptoms to improve, these improvements do not constitute a reason to interrupt or discontinue drug use.

### Dosage and Administration II: Specific Applications

***Hypothyroidism in Adults.*** The dosage should be low initially and then increased gradually until full replacement doses have been achieved. A typical dosing schedule consists of 50 µg daily (PO) for 2 weeks followed by 100 µg daily for 2 additional weeks. Thereafter, daily doses of 150 µg are taken for life.

***Myxedema Coma.*** Myxedema coma is a rare but serious condition and requires rapid treatment. Levothyroxine is administered intravenously in a dose of 200 to 500 µg. If required, an additional dose of 100 to 300 µg can be given 1 day later. Adrenal corticosteroids (e.g., hydrocortisone) are also required.

***Cretinism.*** In cretinism, thyroid hormone dosage decreases with age. For infants less than 6 months old, the dosage is 10 µg/kg/day; for children age 6 to 8 months, 8 µg/kg/day; for children age 1 to 5 years, 6 µg/kg/day; and for children age 5 to 10 years, 4 µg/kg/day.

***Simple Goiter.*** In simple goiter, the thyroid is enlarged and levels of thyroid hormones are reduced. Thyroid enlargement is caused by TSH that has been released in response to low levels of thyroid hormone. When treating simple goiter, the goal is to provide full replacement doses of thyroid hormone so as to suppress further TSH release. This can usually be achieved with 100 to 200 µg of levothyroxine per day.

## Liothyronine (T₃)

Liothyronine [Cytomel, Triostat] is a synthetic preparation of triiodothyronine ($T_3$), a naturally occurring thyroid hormone. The structure of liothyronine is identical to that of thyroid-derived $T_3$. The effects of liothyronine are qualitatively similar to those of levothyroxine.

***Contrasts with Levothyroxine.*** Liothyronine differs from levothyroxine in three important ways: (1) liothyronine has a shorter half-life and shorter duration of action, (2) liothyronine has a more rapid onset of action, and (3) liothyronine is more expensive. Because of its high price and relatively brief duration of action, liothyronine is less desirable than levothyroxine for long-term use. However, because its effects develop quickly, liothyronine may be superior to levothyroxine in situations that require speedy results, especially myxedema coma.

***Evaluation.*** As with levothyroxine, the dosage of liothyronine is adjusted on the basis of clinical evaluation and laboratory data. Two laboratory tests are useful: serum $T_3$ and serum TSH. Since liothyronine is not converted into $T_4$, plasma levels of $T_4$ remain low. Hence, $T_4$ levels cannot be used to assess treatment.

***Dosage and Administration.*** Liothyronine is usually administered by mouth, although IV administration may also be employed. Dosage of liothyronine is about one half the dosage of levothyroxine.

## Other Thyroid Preparations

### Liotrix

Liotrix is a mixture of synthetic $T_4$ plus synthetic $T_3$ in a 4:1 fixed ratio. (This ratio is similar to the ratio of these hormones in plasma.) The rationale for use of liotrix is that the mixture can produce plasma levels of $T_4$ and $T_3$ similar to those that occur naturally. However, since levothyroxine alone produces the same ratio of $T_4$ to $T_3$, liotrix offers no advantage over levothyroxine for most indications.

Dosing with liotrix can be confusing. Two brands of liotrix are available—Euthroid and Thyrolar—and both use the same designations for tablet strength (1/2, 1, 2, 3). However, although the designations are the same, tablets with a particular designation (e.g., 1/2) produced by one manufacturer do not contain the same amount of hormone as tablets with the same designation produced by the other manufacturer. Because of these differences, care should be taken if patients are switched from one brand of liotrix to the other, or from liotrix to a different thyroid preparation.

### Natural Thyroid Products

*Thyroid.* Thyroid consists of desiccated animal thyroid glands. Standardization of this preparation is based on content of iodine, levothyroxine, and liothyronine; the ratio of levothyroxine to liothyronine is not less than 5:1. Thyroid is dispensed in tablets ranging from 16 to 325 mg. Capsules are also available. For practical purposes, thyroid is obsolete: use is limited to those patients who have been taking the preparation for years. Thyroid is rarely prescribed for patients starting therapy today.

*Thyroglobulin.* Thyroglobulin [Proloid] is a purified extract of hog thyroid glands. Like thyroid, thyroglobulin is standardized on the basis of its content of iodine, levothyroxine, and liothyronine; the ratio of levothyroxine to liothyronine is at least 2.8:1. Thyroglobulin is available in tablets ranging from 32 to 200 mg.

---

# Drugs for Hyperthyroidism

---

## Propylthiouracil

Propylthiouracil (PTU) inhibits thyroid hormone synthesis. The drug is a member of the thionamide category of antithyroid drugs and will serve as prototype for the group. Only one other thionamide—methimazole—is currently employed.

## Mechanism of Action

Therapeutic responses to PTU result primarily from blockade of thyroid hormone synthesis, which occurs in two ways: (1) PTU prevents the oxidation of iodide, thereby inhibiting incorporation of iodine into tyrosine, and (2) PTU prevents iodinated tyrosines from coupling. Both effects result from inhibiting peroxidase, the enzyme that catalyzes both reactions. In addition to blocking thyroid hormone synthesis, PTU acts in the periphery to suppress conversion of $T_4$ to $T_3$, the more active form of thyroid hormone.

It should be noted that although PTU prevents thyroid hormone synthesis, PTU does not destroy existing stores of thyroid hormone. Hence, once therapy has begun, it may take 1 to 2 weeks for existing stores to become de-

pleted. Until depletion occurs, therapeutic effects will not be evident.

## Pharmacokinetics

Propylthiouracil is rapidly absorbed following oral administration. Therapeutic effects begin within 30 minutes. The plasma half-life of PTU is short (about 2 hours). As a result, PTU must be administered several times each day. The drug can cross the placenta and can enter breast milk.

## Therapeutic Uses

Propylthiouracil has four applications in hyperthyroidism. First, PTU can be used alone as the sole form of therapy for Graves' disease. Second, PTU can be employed as an adjunct to radiation therapy; PTU is administered to control hyperthyroidism until the effects of radiation become manifest. Third, PTU can be given to suppress thyroid hormone synthesis in preparation for thyroid gland surgery (subtotal thyroidectomy). Fourth, PTU is given to patients experiencing thyrotoxic crisis; benefits derive from suppressing thyroid hormone synthesis and from preventing conversion of $T_4$ to $T_3$.

## Adverse Effects

Adverse responses to PTU are relatively rare. However, severe adverse effects can occur.

*Agranulocytosis.* Agranulocytosis is the most serious toxicity of PTU. This reaction is rare and usually occurs during the first 2 months of therapy. Sore throat and fever may be the earliest indications; patients should be instructed to report these immediately. Since agranulocytosis often develops rapidly, periodic blood counts cannot guarantee early detection. If agranulocytosis occurs, PTU should be discontinued; agranulocytosis will then reverse. Treatment with granulocyte colony-stimulating factor [Neupogen] may accelerate recovery.

*Hypothyroidism.* Excessive dosing with PTU may convert the patient from a hyperthyroid state to a hypothyroid state. If this occurs, the dosage should be reduced. Temporary administration of thyroid hormone may be required.

*Pregnancy and Lactation.* Propylthiouracil crosses the placenta and has caused neonatal hypothyroidism and goiter. Accordingly, the drug must be used judiciously during pregnancy. To minimize effects on the fetus, the dosage should be kept as low as possible. As an alternative, some physicians recommend treatment with full doses of PTU combined with thyroid hormone replacement therapy. However, this practice is controversial. Propylthiouracil enters breast milk and is contraindicated for nursing mothers.

*Other Adverse Effects.* The most common undesired effect of PTU is rash. The drug may also cause nausea, arthralgia, headache, dizziness, and paresthesias.

### Preparations, Dosage, and Administration

Propylthiouracil is available in 50-mg tablets for oral administration. Because of its short half-life, PTU is usually administered in multiple daily doses. A typical adult *maintenance* dosage is 50 mg every 8 hours. *Initial* doses may total up to 900 mg daily.

## Methimazole

Methimazole [Tapazole] is similar to PTU in most respects. Like PTU, methimazole suppresses thyroid hormone synthesis. However, in contrast to PTU, methimazole does not block conversion of $T_4$ to $T_3$ in the periphery. Like PTU, methimazole can cause agranulocytosis, but the risk may be lower. Methimazole crosses the placenta more readily than PTU; hence, if a thionamide must be used in pregnancy, PTU is preferred. Like PTU, methimazole is contraindicated for nursing mothers. Methimazole is dispensed in 5- and 10-mg tablets. The usual adult maintenance dosage is 5 to 15 mg/day administered in three divided doses.

## Radioactive Iodine ($^{131}$I)

### Physical Properties

$^{131}$I, a radioactive isotope of stable iodine, emits a combination of beta particles and gamma rays. Radioactive decay of $^{131}$I takes place with a half-life of 8 days. Hence, after 56 days (7 half-lives), less than 1% of the radioactivity in a dose of $^{131}$I remains.

### Use in Graves' Disease

$^{131}$I can be used to destroy thyroid tissue in patients with hyperthyroidism. The objective is to produce clinical remission without causing complete destruction of the gland. Unfortunately, delayed hypothyroidism, due to excessive thyroid damage, is a frequent complication.

***Effect on the Thyroid.*** Like stable iodine, $^{131}$I is concentrated in the thyroid gland. Destruction of thyroid tissue is produced primarily by emission of beta particles. (The gamma rays from $^{131}$I are relatively harmless.) Since beta particles have a very limited ability to penetrate any type of physical barrier, these particles do not travel outside the thyroid; hence damage to surrounding tissue is minimal.

Reduction of thyroid function is gradual. Initial effects take days or weeks to become apparent. Full effects require 2 to 3 months to develop.

Not all patients respond satisfactorily to a single $^{131}$I treatment. About 66% of patients with Graves' disease are cured with a single exposure to $^{131}$I; others require two or more treatments.

***Advantages and Disadvantages of $^{131}$I Therapy.*** The advantages of $^{131}$I treatment are considerable: (1) cost is low; (2) patients are spared the risks, discomfort, and expense of thyroid surgery; (3) death from $^{131}$I treatment has never occurred, nor is it ever likely to; and (4) no tissue other than the thyroid is injured (patients should be reassured of this fact).

Treatment with $^{131}$I is not without drawbacks. First, the effect of treatment is delayed, taking several months to become maximal. Second, and more important, treatment is associated with a significant incidence of *delayed hypothyroidism*. Hypothyroidism results from excessive dosage and occurs in 10% of patients within the first year following $^{131}$I exposure. An additional 2% to 3% develop hypothyroidism each year thereafter.

***Who Should Be Treated and Who Should Not.*** Patients over the age of 30 may be candidates for $^{131}$I ther-

apy. $^{131}$I also is indicated for patients who have not responded adequately to antithyroid drugs or to subtotal thyroidectomy.

Children are considered inappropriate candidates. The likelihood of delayed hypothyroidism is higher in children than in adults. Also, there is concern that administration of $^{131}$I to young patients may carry a slight risk of cancer. It should be noted, however, that there is no evidence that the use of $^{131}$I in Graves' disease has ever caused cancer of the thyroid or any other tissue.

*$^{131}$I is contraindicated in pregnancy and lactation.* Exposure of the fetus to $^{131}$I after the first trimester may damage the immature thyroid, and exposure to radiation at any point in fetal life carries a risk of generalized developmental harm. Since $^{131}$I enters breast milk, women receiving this agent should not breast-feed.

***Dosage.*** Dosage of $^{131}$I is determined by thyroid size and by the rate of thyroidal iodine uptake. For Graves' disease, the dosage usually ranges between 4 and 10 mCi.

### Use in Thyroid Cancer

$^{131}$I can be used to destroy malignant thyroid cells. However, since most forms of thyroid cancer do not accumulate iodine, only a small percentage of patients are candidates for $^{131}$I therapy.

The doses of $^{131}$I used to treat cancer are large, ranging from 50 to 150 mCi. These doses are much higher than those used in Graves' disease. Because high amounts of radioactivity are involved, body wastes must be disposed of properly. In addition, adverse effects from large doses of $^{131}$I can be severe: radiation sickness may occur; leukemia may be produced; and bone marrow function may be depressed, resulting in leukopenia, thrombocytopenia, and anemia.

### Diagnostic Use

$^{131}$I is employed to diagnose a variety of thyroid disorders, including hyperthyroidism, hypothyroidism, and goiter. Following $^{131}$I administration, the thyroid is scanned for uptake of radioactivity; the amount and location of $^{131}$I uptake reveals the extent of thyroid activity. Doses used for diagnosis are minuscule (less than 1 μCi for children and less than 10 μCi for adults). These tracer doses pose virtually no threat to health.

### Preparations

$^{131}$I is dispensed in capsules and solution for oral administration. Both preparations are odorless and tasteless. Capsules contain between 0.8 and 100 mCi of $^{131}$I. Vials of oral solution contain between 3.5 and 150 mCi of $^{131}$I. Capsules and oral solutions are available generically (as sodium iodide $^{131}$I) and under the trade name Iodotope.

## Iodide Products (Nonradioactive)

Three iodide preparations are available. All three have the same mechanism of action and similar pharmacologic effects, although their specific applications may differ.

### Strong Iodine Solution (Lugol's Solution)

***Description.*** Lugol's solution is a mixture containing 5% elemental iodine and 10% potassium iodide. The iodine undergoes reduction to iodide within the gastrointestinal tract prior to absorption.

***Mechanism of Action.*** When present in high concentrations, iodide has a paradoxical suppressant effect on the thyroid. This suppression is brought about in three ways. First, high concentrations of iodide decrease iodine uptake by the thyroid. Second, high concentrations of iodide inhibit thyroid hormone synthesis by suppressing both the iodination of tyrosine and the coupling of iodinated tyrosine residues. Third, high concentrations of iodine inhibit release of thyroid hormone into the bloodstream. All three actions combine to decrease circulating levels of $T_3$ and $T_4$.

Unfortunately, the effects of iodide on thyroid function cannot be sustained indefinitely; with long-term iodide administration, suppressant effects become weaker. Accordingly, iodide is rarely used alone to produce thyroid suppression.

***Therapeutic Use.*** Strong iodine solution is given to hyperthyroid individuals to suppress thyroid function in preparation for thyroidectomy. Initial effects develop within 24 hours; peak effects develop in 10 to 15 days. In most cases, plasma levels of thyroid hormone are reduced with PTU before initiating strong iodine solution. Then iodine solution (along with more PTU) is administered for the last 10 days prior to surgery. In addition to its use prior to thyroidectomy, strong iodine solution is employed in thyrotoxic crisis and also as an antiseptic (see Chapter 90).

***Adverse Effects.*** Chronic ingestion of iodine can produce *iodism.* Signs and symptoms include a brassy taste, a burning sensation in the mouth and throat, soreness of the teeth and gums, frontal headache, coryza (nasal inflammation and sneezing), salivation, and various skin eruptions. All of these fade rapidly upon discontinuation of iodine use.

***Overdose.*** Iodine is corrosive, and overdose will injure the gastrointestinal tract. Symptoms include abdominal pain, vomiting, and diarrhea. Swelling of the glottis may result in asphyxiation. Treatment consists of gastric lavage (to remove iodine from the stomach) and administration of sodium thiosulfate (to reduce iodine to iodide).

***Dosage and Administration.*** When used to prepare hyperthyroid patients for thyroidectomy, strong iodine solution is administered in a dosage of 2 to 6 drops 3 times daily for 10 days immediately preceding surgery. Iodine solution should be mixed with juice or some other beverage to disguise its unpleasant taste. The dosage for thyrotoxic crisis is 5 to 8 drops every 6 hours.

### Sodium Iodide (IV)

Intravenous sodium iodide is employed for the acute management of *thyrotoxic crisis.* Benefits derive from the ability of high concentrations of iodide to rapidly suppress thyroid hormone release. In the treatment of thyrotoxic crisis, sodium iodide is used in combination with propylthiouracil and propranolol. Sodium iodide for IV use is dispensed as a 10% solution in 10-ml ampules. The dosage is 0.5 to 1 g every 12 hours.

Although intravenous sodium iodide rarely causes adverse effects, *severe hypersensitivity reactions* have occurred. These may develop immediately or may be delayed by several hours. The most characteristic feature is angioedema. Skin eruptions, serum sickness, and edema of the larynx may also develop. Death has occurred. There is no specific antidote to these hypersensitivity reactions; hence, treatment is purely supportive.

### Potassium Iodide

***Use in Radiation Emergencies.*** Potassium iodide [Thyro-Block] taken orally can be used to protect the thyroid gland in the event of a radiation emergency. If a nuclear accident should release radioactive iodine into the environment, thyroidal uptake of this radioactive iodide would damage the gland. By administering large doses of nonradioactive iodide, uptake of radioactive material can be blocked. The dosage of potassium iodide is 130 mg/day for all people over the age of 1 year; children less than 1 year old should receive 65 mg daily. Duration of use is likely to last from 3 to 10 days. Potassium iodide tablets for blocking radioactive iodine uptake are available only through state and federal agencies.

***Use in Thyroid Disease.*** A concentrated solution of potassium iodide, containing 1 g of potassium iodide per milliliter, can be used to treat Graves' disease and thyrotoxic crisis.

In Graves' disease, potassium iodide has the same effect as Lugol's solution: suppression of iodine uptake by the thyroid, inhibition of thyroid hormone synthesis, and inhibition of thyroid hormone release. All three actions reduce circulating levels of $T_3$ and $T_4$. The dosage is 1 to 3 drops of concentrated potassium iodide solution PO 3 times a day.

In patients experiencing thyrotoxic crisis, potassium iodide is given to suppress thyroid hormone release. The dosage is 5 to 8 drops PO every 6 hours.

### Propranolol

Propranolol can suppress tachycardia and other symptoms of *Graves' disease.* Benefits derive from beta-adrenergic blockade, not from reducing levels of $T_3$ or $T_4$. One advantage of propranolol is that its effects occur rapidly, unlike those of propylthiouracil and $^{131}$I. The dosage for hyperthyroidism is highly individualized, ranging from 40 to 240 mg/day in divided doses.

Propranolol is also beneficial in *thyrotoxic crisis.* In the absence of contraindications (e.g., asthma, congestive heart failure), all patients should receive propranolol immediately. Administration may be oral or intravenous. The dosage is 80 to 120 mg PO every 6 hours or 2 to 4 mg IV every 4 hours.

The basic pharmacology of propranolol is discussed in Chapter 19.

## KEY POINTS

- The thyroid gland produces two active hormones: triiodothyronine ($T_3$), which is highly active; and thyroxine ($T_4$; tetraiodothyronine), which is less active.
- Thyroid hormones have three principal actions: stimulation of energy use, stimulation of the heart, and promotion of growth and development.
- Hormonal regulation of thyroid function occurs as follows: TRH from the hypothalamus causes the pituitary to release TSH, which causes the thyroid to make and release $T_3$ and $T_4$, which then act on the pituitary to suppress further release of TSH.
- The four steps in thyroid hormone synthesis are (1) uptake of iodide by the thyroid, (2) conversion of iodide to iodine, (3) linking of iodine to tyrosine, and (4) coupling of two iodinated tyrosines to form $T_3$ or $T_4$.
- Much of the $T_4$ released by the thyroid is converted to $T_3$ in the periphery.
- Low levels of iodine stimulate synthesis of $T_3$ and $T_4$; high levels of iodine suppress synthesis of $T_3$ and $T_4$.
- In iodine-sufficient areas, the major cause of hypothyroidism is chronic autoimmune thyroiditis (Hashimoto's disease).
- A goiter is an enlargement of the thyroid.

- Testing serum for elevated levels of TSH is the most sensitive way to diagnose hypothyroidism.
- Most patients with hypothyroidism require lifelong replacement therapy with thyroid hormones.
- Levothyroxine (synthetic $T_4$), sold as Levothroid and Synthroid, is the drug of choice for most patients who require thyroid hormone replacement.
- Cholestyramine [Questran], colestipol [Colestid], sucralfate [Carafate], aluminum hydroxide, and ferrous sulfate can significantly reduce levothyroxine absorption.
- Levothyroxine can intensify the anticoagulant effects of warfarin.
- The most common form of hyperthyroidism is Graves' disease.
- Thyrotoxic crisis (thyroid storm) occurs if levels of thyroid hormone rise exceptionally high.

- Graves' disease can be treated by surgical removal of thyroid tissue, destruction of thyroid tissue with radioactive iodine ($^{131}I$), or treatment with antithyroid drugs.
- Propylthiouracil, an antithyroid drug, benefits patients with hyperthyroidism by suppressing thyroid hormone synthesis and by inhibiting conversion of $T_4$ to $T_3$ in the periphery.
- The most serious adverse effect of propylthiouracil is agranulocytosis.
- Propylthiouracil is contraindicated for nursing mothers and must be used with caution during pregnancy.
- Full effects of $^{131}I$ require 2 to 3 months to develop.
- $^{131}I$ is contraindicated during pregnancy and lactation.
- Strong iodine solution (Lugol's solution) can be used to suppress thyroid hormone synthesis.

## Summary of Major Nursing Implications*

## Levothyroxine

### Preadministration Assessment

#### Therapeutic Goal
Resolution of signs and symptoms of hypothyroidism and restoration of normal laboratory values for serum TSH and thyroid hormones.

#### Baseline Data
Obtain plasma levels of TSH and $T_4$.

### Implementation: Administration

#### Routes
Oral, IV.

#### Administration
*Oral.* Instruct the patient to take levothyroxine on an empty stomach, preferably in the morning before breakfast. Not all products have equal bioavailability; warn the patient against switching from one brand to another.

Make certain the patient understands that replacement therapy must continue for life. Caution the patient against discontinuing treatment without consulting the physician.

*Intravenous.* Intravenous administration is reserved for treating myxedema coma and for patients who cannot take levothyroxine orally.

### Ongoing Evaluation and Interventions

#### Evaluating Therapeutic Effects
*Adults.* Clinical evaluation should reveal reversal of signs of thyroid deficiency and an absence of signs of thyroid excess (e.g., tachycardia). Laboratory tests should indicate normal plasma levels of TSH and $T_4$.

*Infants.* Clinical evaluation should reveal normalization of intellectual function, growth, and development. Monthly measurements of height provide a good index of thyroid sufficiency. Laboratory tests should show normal plasma levels of TSH and $T_4$. (*Note:* TSH levels may remain abnormal in some children, despite adequate dosing.)

#### Minimizing Adverse Effects
*Thyrotoxicosis.* Overdosage may cause thyrotoxicosis. Inform patients about symptoms of thyrotoxicosis (tachycardia, angina, tremor, nervousness, insomnia, hyperthermia, heat intolerance, sweating) and instruct them to notify the physician if these develop.

#### Minimizing Adverse Interactions
*Drugs That Reduce Levothyroxine Absorption.* Absorption of levothyroxine can be reduced by cholestyramine, colestipol, sucralfate, aluminum hydroxide, and ferrous sulfate. Allow several hours to separate administration of levothyroxine and these drugs.

*Warfarin.* Levothyroxine can intensify the effects of warfarin. The dosage of warfarin should be reduced.

*Catecholamines.* Thyroid hormones sensitize the heart to catecholamines (epinephrine, dopamine, dobutamine) and may thereby promote dysrhythmias. Exercise caution when catecholamines and levothyroxine are used concomitantly.

## Liothyronine ($T_3$)

With the exceptions noted below, the nursing implications for liothyronine are the same as those for levothyroxine.

---

*Patient education information is highlighted in color.

## Evaluation of Therapeutic Effects

Success is indicated by resolution of the signs and symptoms of hypothyroidism and by normalization of plasma $T_3$ and TSH levels. $T_4$ levels cannot be used to evaluate therapy.

# Propylthiouracil

## Preadministration Assessment

### Therapeutic Goals

PTU has four indications: (1) reduction of thyroid hormone production in Graves' disease, (2) control of hyperthyroidism until the effects of radiation on the thyroid become manifest, (3) suppression of thyroid hormone production prior to subtotal thyroidectomy, and (4) treatment of thyrotoxic crisis.

### Baseline Data

Obtain plasma levels of $T_3$ and $T_4$.

### Identifying High-Risk Patients

PTU is *contraindicated* for *nursing mothers*. Use with *caution* during *pregnancy*.

## Implementation: Administration

### Route

Oral.

### Administration

Instruct the patient to take PTU at regular intervals around the clock (usually every 8 hours).

## Ongoing Evaluation and Interventions

### Summary of Monitoring

Evaluate treatment by monitoring for weight gain, decreased heart rate, and other indications that levels of thyroid hormone have declined. Laboratory tests should indicate a decrease in plasma content of $T_3$ and $T_4$.

### Minimizing Adverse Effects

*Agranulocytosis.* Inform patients about early signs of agranulocytosis (fever, sore throat) and instruct them to notify the physician if these develop. If follow-up blood tests reveal leukopenia, PTU should be withdrawn. Administration of granulocyte colony-stimulating factor may accelerate recovery.

*Hypothyroidism.* PTU may cause excessive reductions in thyroid hormone synthesis. If signs of hypothyroidism develop or if plasma levels of $T_3$ and $T_4$ become subnormal, PTU dosage should be reduced. Supplemental thyroid hormone may be needed.

*Use in Pregnancy and Lactation.* PTU can cause fetal hypothyroidism and goiter; use with caution during pregnancy. PTU is contraindicated for nursing mothers.

# Radioactive Iodine ($^{131}$I)

## Use in Graves' Disease

*Therapeutic Goal.* Suppression of thyroid hormone production.

*Identifying High-Risk Patients.* $^{131}$I is *contraindicated* during *pregnancy and lactation*.

*Dosage and Administration.* $^{131}$I is administered in capsules or an oral liquid. The dosing objective is to reduce thyroid hormone production without causing complete thyroid destruction. The dosage for Graves' disease is 4 to 10 mCi.

*Promoting Therapeutic Effects.* Responses take 2 to 3 months to develop fully. Propylthiouracil may be required during this interval.

*Minimizing Adverse Effects.* Excessive thyroid destruction can cause *hypothyroidism*. Patients who develop thyroid insufficiency need thyroid hormone supplements.

## Use in Thyroid Cancer

High doses (50 to 150 mCi) are required. These doses can cause radiation sickness, leukemia, and bone marrow depression. Monitor for these effects. Body wastes will be contaminated with radioactivity and must be disposed of appropriately.

## Diagnostic Use

$^{131}$I is used to diagnose hyperthyroidism, hypothyroidism, and goiter. Diagnostic doses are so small (less than 10 μCi) as to be virtually harmless.

# Strong Iodine Solution (Lugol's Solution)

## Preadministration Assessment

### Therapeutic Goal

Suppression of thyroid hormone production in preparation for subtotal thyroidectomy. Also used to suppress thyroid hormone release in patients experiencing thyroid storm.

### Baseline Data

Obtain tests of thyroid function.

## Implementation: Administration

### Route

Oral.

## Administration

Advise the patient to dilute strong iodine solution with fruit juice or some other beverage to increase palatability.

## Ongoing Evaluation and Interventions

### Minimizing Adverse Effects

*Mild Toxicity.* Inform patients about symptoms of iodism (brassy taste, burning sensations in the mouth, soreness of gums and teeth) and instruct them to discontinue treatment and notify the physician if these occur. Symptoms fade upon drug withdrawal.

*Severe Toxicity.* Iodine solution can cause corrosive injury to the gastrointestinal tract. Instruct the patient to discontinue drug use and notify the physician immediately if severe abdominal distress develops. Treatment includes gastric lavage and administration of sodium thiosulfate.

# CHAPTER 55

# Drugs Related to Hypothalamic and Pituitary Function

The hypothalamus and pituitary are intimately related both anatomically and functionally. Working together, these structures help regulate practically all bodily processes. To achieve their widespread effects, the hypothalamus and pituitary employ at least 15 hormones and regulatory factors (Fig. 55-1). The endocrinology of these two structures is exceedingly complex. Fortunately, from the perspective of therapeutics, the picture is much less imposing. This is because the clinical applications of the hypothalamic and pituitary hormones are limited. In this chapter, we emphasize three agents: growth hormone, antidiuretic hormone, and prolactin. Additional hypothalamic and pituitary hormones of therapeutic interest are considered briefly and discussed at greater length in other chapters.

## Overview of Hypothalamic and Pituitary Endocrinology

### Anatomic Considerations

The pituitary sits in a depression in the skull located just below the third ventricle of the brain; the hypothalamus is located immediately above (see Fig. 55-1). The pituitary has two divisions: the *anterior pituitary* (or *adenohypophysis*) and the *posterior pituitary* (or *neurohypophysis*). Both divisions are under hypothalamic control. As indicated in Figure 55-1, the hypothalamus communicates with the *anterior* pituitary by way of release-regulating factors delivered through a system of portal blood vessels. In contrast, communication with the *posterior* pituitary is neuronal.

### Hormones of the Anterior Pituitary

The anterior pituitary produces six major hormones. Production and release of these hormones is controlled largely by the hypothalamus. Functions of the anterior pituitary hormones are summarized briefly as follows:

- *Growth hormone* (GH) stimulates growth in practically all tissues and organs.
- *Adrenocorticotropic hormone* (ACTH) acts on the adrenal cortex to promote synthesis and release of adrenocortical hormones.
- *Thyrotropin* (thyroid-stimulating hormone; TSH) acts on the thyroid gland to promote synthesis and release of thyroid hormones.
- *Follicle-stimulating hormone* (FSH) acts on the ovary to promote follicular growth and development. In the testes, FSH promotes spermatogenesis.
- *Luteinizing hormone* (LH) acts in women to promote ovulation and development of the corpus luteum. In men, LH, which is also known as *interstitial cell–stimulating hormone*, acts on the testes to promote androgen production.
- *Prolactin* stimulates milk production after parturition.

### Hormones of the Posterior Pituitary

The posterior pituitary has only two hormones: *oxytocin* and *antidiuretic hormone* (ADH). The principal function of oxytocin is to facilitate uterine contractions at term. Antidiuretic hormone promotes renal conservation of water.

Although oxytocin and ADH are considered hormones of the posterior pituitary, these agents are actually synthesized in the hypothalamus. The cells that make oxytocin and ADH are called neurosecretory cells. As indicated in

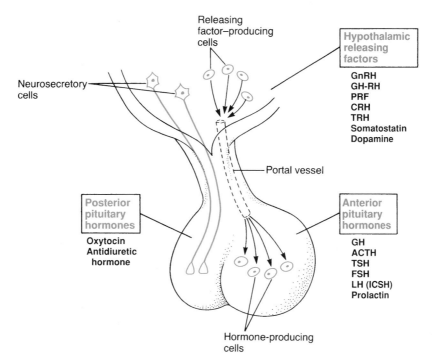

**Figure 55–1. Hormones and releasing factors of the hypothalamus and pituitary.** *Hypothalamic releasing factors:* GnRH = gonadotropin-releasing hormone, GH-RH = growth hormone–releasing hormone, PRF = prolactin-releasing factor, CRH = corticotropin-releasing hormone, TRH = thyrotropin-releasing hormone.
  *Anterior pituitary hormones:* GH = growth hormone, ACTH = adrenocorticotropic hormone, TSH = thyroid-stimulating hormone, FSH = follicle-stimulating hormone, LH (ICSH) = luteinizing hormone (interstitial cell–stimulating hormone).

Figure 55–1, these cells originate in the hypothalamus and project their axons to the posterior pituitary. Oxytocin and ADH are produced within the bodies of these cells and then transported down the axons to the cell terminals for storage. When appropriate stimuli impinge upon the bodies of the neurosecretory cells, impulses are sent down the axon, causing the hormones to be released.

## Hypothalamic Release-Regulating Factors

The hypothalamus has the primary responsibility for regulating the release of hormones from the *anterior* pituitary. To accomplish this, the hypothalamus employs eight different release-regulating factors (see Fig. 55–1). Most of these factors *stimulate* the release of anterior pituitary hormones. However, two of these factors regulate release by exerting an *inhibitory* influence. As indicated in Figure 55–1, the hypothalamic release-regulating factors are delivered to the anterior pituitary via portal blood vessels. Although the hypothalamic releasing factors are of extreme *physiologic* importance, only two of these factors (thyrotropin-releasing hormone and gonadotropin-releasing hormone) have *clinical applications*. These are the only hypothalamic release-regulating factors that we will discuss.

## Feedback Regulation of Hypothalamus and Anterior Pituitary

With few exceptions, the release of hypothalamic and anterior pituitary hormones is regulated by a *negative feedback loop*. Such a loop is illustrated in Figure 55–2. In this example, the loop begins with the secretion of releasing-factor X from the hypothalamus. Factor X then acts on the anterior pituitary to stimulate the release of hormone A. Hormone A then acts on its target gland to promote the release of hormone B. Hormone B has two actions: (1) it produces its designated biologic effects and (2) it acts on the hypothalamus and pituitary to inhibit further release of factor X and hormone A. This feedback inhibition of the hypothalamus and pituitary suppresses further release of hormone B itself, thereby keeping levels of hormone B within an appropriate range.

# Growth Hormone

Growth hormone is a large polypeptide hormone (191 amino acids) produced by the anterior pituitary. As its name suggests, this hormone helps regulate growth. An absence of growth hormone during childhood results in *dwarfism*. Excessive growth hormone results in *acromegaly*.

## Physiology
### Regulation of Release

The factors regulating growth hormone release are summarized in Figure 55–3. As indicated, the hypothala-

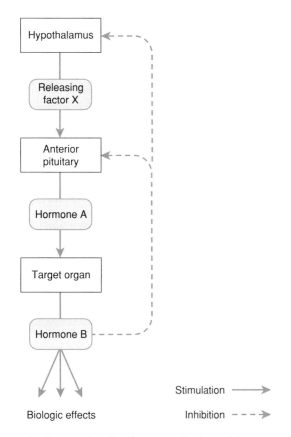

**Figure 55–2. Negative feedback regulation of the hypothalamus and anterior pituitary.** The feedback loop works as follows: Factor X stimulates the pituitary to release hormone A, which stimulates its target organ, causing release of hormone B. Hormone B then acts on the hypothalamus and pituitary to suppress further release of factor X and hormone A, thereby suppressing further release of hormone B itself.

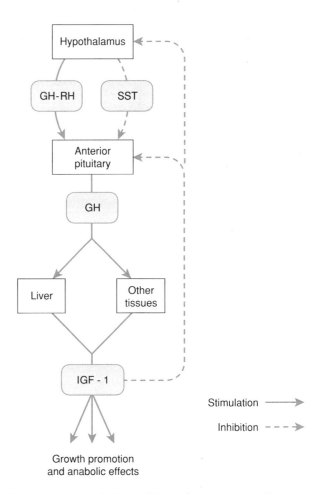

**Figure 55–3. Regulation of Growth Hormone Release.** GH-RH = growth hormone–releasing hormone, GH = growth hormone, SST = somatostatin, IGF-1 = insulin-like growth factor-1.

mus first releases growth hormone–releasing hormone (GH-RH), which stimulates release of growth hormone (GH) from the pituitary. Growth hormone then acts on the liver and other tissues to cause release of insulin-like growth factor-1 (IGF-1). IGF-1 has two actions: (1) it is the hormone that actually mediates increases in growth, and (2) it acts on the hypothalamus and pituitary to suppress release of GH-RH and GH, thereby completing a negative feedback loop. One additional hormone—somatostatin—helps regulate GH release; as shown in Figure 55–3, somatostatin is produced in the hypothalamus and acts on the pituitary to inhibit release of GH.

## Biologic Effects

*Promotion of Growth.* Growth hormone, acting through IGF-1, stimulates the growth of practically all organs and tissues. If administered to a GH-deficient subject prior to epiphyseal closure, GH will increase bone length, producing a corresponding increase in height. The size and number of muscle cells is increased, resulting in enlargement of muscle mass, and the internal organs are stimulated to grow in proportion to overall body growth. The only organs that do not respond noticeably to growth hormone are the brain and eyes.

*Promotion of Protein Synthesis.* For growth to occur, cells must increase their production of protein. Growth hormone facilitates this process by increasing amino acid uptake and utilization. Since amino acids have substantial nitrogen content, increased protein synthesis results in net nitrogen retention. This retention is reflected in reduced urinary nitrogen excretion. Increased amino acid utilization also causes blood urea nitrogen (BUN) to fall.

*Effect on Carbohydrate Metabolism.* Administration of growth hormone reduces glucose utilization. Hence, plasma levels of glucose tend to rise. When growth hormone is administered to nondiabetics, elevation of blood glucose stimulates release of insulin, thereby maintaining plasma levels of glucose within a normal range. In contrast, when growth hormone is administered to diabetics, insulin cannot be released; hence, the hyperglycemic action of growth hormone is unopposed, and plasma glucose levels may climb dramatically.

## Growth Hormone Deficiency
### Consequences of Deficiency

Growth hormone is essential for normal growth of children; hormone deficiency results in *dwarfism*. In children who are growth hormone deficient, growth is retarded to an equal extent in all parts of the body. Hence, the dwarf, although small, has normal proportions. Dwarfism is not associated with mental impairment. In contrast to normal individuals, whose growth ceases at puberty, the dwarf continues to grow throughout life. The only treatment for growth hormone deficiency is replacement therapy with human growth hormone.

## Growth Hormone Replacement Therapy

***Who Should Be Treated?*** The only approved indication for growth hormone is treatment of children whose growth has been retarded because of proven growth hormone deficiency. Except in experimental protocols, growth hormone should not be given to promote growth in children who are short for reasons unrelated to lack of growth hormone. In addition, this agent should not be given during or after epiphyseal closure; to avoid this misuse, epiphyseal status should be assessed annually.

***Expected Response.*** Treatment is prolonged, and responses are usually satisfactory. When treatment is started early, adult height may be increased by as much as 6 inches. To monitor treatment, height and weight should be measured monthly. Therapy should continue until a satisfactory adult height has been achieved, until epiphyseal closure occurs, or until a response can no longer be elicited. Efficacy of therapy declines as the patient grows older and is usually lost entirely by age 20 to 24 years. If treatment fails to promote growth, growth hormone should be discontinued and the diagnosis of growth hormone deficiency re-evaluated.

***Adverse Effects.*** *Hyperglycemia.* Growth hormone is diabetogenic. When used in patients with pre-existing diabetes, significant hyperglycemia may result. Glucose levels should be monitored and insulin dosage should be adjusted accordingly.

*Hypothyroidism.* Growth hormone therapy is associated with a decline in thyroid function. Function of the thyroid should be assessed periodically. If thyroid hormone levels are subnormal, replacement therapy should be instituted.

*Antibodies to Growth Hormone.* Two forms of growth hormone are used clinically: somatropin and somatrem. Although antibodies may develop to either form, they are much more common with somatrem. Fortunately, these antibodies rarely decrease the effectiveness of treatment.

*Poverty.* Growth hormone is expensive. One year of treatment costs about $20,000.

***Interaction with Glucocorticoids.*** Glucocorticoids can oppose the growth-stimulating effects of growth hormone. Patients receiving growth hormone should not be given glucocorticoids in doses that exceed the equivalent of 10 to 15 mg/m$^2$ of hydrocortisone.

***Preparations.*** *Somatrem.* Somatrem [Protropin] is a form of growth hormone produced by recombinant DNA technology. With the exception of one amino acid, the structure of somatrem is identical to that of growth hormone produced by the human pituitary. The biologic activity of somatrem is indistinguishable from that of the naturally occurring hormone.

*Somatropin.* Like somatrem, somatropin [Humatrope, Nutropin], is produced by recombinant DNA technology. The structure and actions of somatropin are identical to those of growth hormone produced by the human pituitary.

***Dosage and Administration.*** Growth hormone is administered parenterally (IM and SC). It cannot be used orally because of rapid inactivation by the digestive system. Intramuscular administration has been traditional. However, studies indicate that SC administration is less painful than IM while being just as safe and effective.

Growth hormone is dispensed as a lyophilized powder for reconstitution with 1 to 5 ml of diluent. *Mix gently; do not shake.* Do not inject the drug if the preparation is cloudy or contains particulate matter.

Dosage is individualized. For *somatrem* [Protropin], the maximum recommended dosage is 0.26 IU/kg (0.1 mg/kg) 3 times a week. For *somatropin*, the dosage depends on the brand: for Humatrope, the maximum recommended dosage is 0.16 IU/kg (0.06 mg/kg) 3 times a week; for Nutropin, the recommended dosage is 0.043 mg/kg (0.11 IU/kg) once a day.

### Growth Hormone Excess

#### Consequences of Growth Hormone Excess

Growth hormone excess causes *acromegaly*, a syndrome characterized by enlargement of many parts of the skeleton, especially the extremities. Facial features are coarse and the hands and feet are wide. Arthralgias, headaches, and excessive sweating are common. Levels of IGF-1 are elevated in all patients; elevation of GH levels may or may not be detected. Since manifestations of acromegaly develop very slowly, the disease may be present for years prior to diagnosis. The cause of GH excess is almost always a pituitary adenoma. Acromegaly is a rare disorder, with only 250 new cases reported each year in the United States.

#### Treatment

Acromegaly may be treated with surgery, radiation, or drugs. Surgical excision of the pituitary adenoma is the preferred initial treatment for most patients. Radiation therapy may be used as primary treatment or as an adjunct to surgery. When used as primary treatment, radiation takes 10 to 20 years to produce a full response.

***Octreotide.*** Octreotide [Sandostatin], a synthetic analog of somatostatin, is our most effective drug for suppressing GH release. The drug works by mimicking the suppressant actions of somatostatin on the pituitary (see Fig. 55–3). Octreotide can be used as primary therapy for acromegaly or as an adjunct to surgery or radiation. The usual dosage is 100 µg SC 3 times a day. Unfortunately, although octreotide is effective, it is also very expensive: for a dosage of 300 µg/day, the annual cost is $7800. Gastrointestinal side effects (nausea, cramps, diarrhea, flatulence) are common initially but subside in 1 to 2 weeks. Within a year, cholesterol gallstones develop in about 25% of patients; however, the stones are usually asymptomatic.

## Prolactin

Prolactin is a polypeptide hormone produced by the anterior pituitary. The principal function of prolactin is stimulation of milk production after parturition. Prolactin deficiency is generally without symptoms, except for disturbance of lactation. In contrast, overproduction of prolactin causes multiple adverse effects.

## Regulation of Release

Regulation of prolactin release is predominantly *inhibitory*. Under the influence of dopamine released from the hypothalamus, release of prolactin by the pituitary is suppressed. When release of dopamine declines, release of prolactin is allowed to increase. Another hypothalamic factor, known as prolactin-releasing factor (PRF), acts to promote prolactin release. However, the stimulatory influence of PRF is usually dominated by dopamine-mediated inhibition. The most powerful stimulus to prolactin release is suckling, an action that presumably suppresses release of dopamine from the hypothalamus.

## Prolactin Hypersecretion

Excessive secretion of prolactin produces adverse effects in males and females. Women may experience amenorrhea, galactorrhea (excessive milk flow), and infertility. In men, libido and potency are reduced, and occasionally galactorrhea occurs. Puberty may be delayed in boys and in girls. Causes of prolactin hypersecretion include pituitary adenoma, injury to the hypothalamus, and certain drugs (e.g., antipsychotics, estrogens).

## Bromocriptine for Suppression of Prolactin Release

Excessive secretion of prolactin can be reduced with bromocriptine, a dopaminergic agonist. By binding to dopaminergic receptors in the pituitary, bromocriptine exerts the same inhibitory influence on prolactin release as does dopamine released from the hypothalamus. Bromocriptine is used to inhibit prolactin release in postpartum women and to decrease the release of prolactin by pituitary adenomas. The usual dosage is 2.5 mg administered 2 to 3 times daily. Adverse effects are common early in therapy and include nausea, vomiting, dizziness, and hypotension. Other uses of bromocriptine include management of infertility (see Chapter 59) and treatment of Parkinson's disease (see Chapter 22).

## Thyrotropin

Thyrotropin (thyroid-stimulating hormone; TSH) is a hormone produced by the anterior pituitary. The physiologic role of thyrotropin is stimulation of thyroid gland function. In promoting thyroid function, thyrotropin causes (1) increased thyroidal uptake of iodine, (2) increased synthesis of thyroid hormones, (3) increased release of thyroid hormones, and (4) thyroid growth.

Thyrotropin is employed clinically to diagnose thyroid failure. Specifically, thyrotropin is used to differentiate primary hypothyroidism (failure of the thyroid gland itself) from secondary hypothyroidism (hypothyroidism resulting from insufficient production of thyrotropin by the pituitary). Testing is performed as follows: thyrotropin is administered (IM or SC) in a dose of 10 IU for 1 to 3 days; 24 hours after the last dose, radioactive iodine is administered, and thyroidal uptake of the radioactive iodine is then measured. In patients with primary hypothyroidism, the thyroid is unable to respond to thyrotropin; hence, uptake of radioactive iodine is low. In contrast, if lack of endogenous thyrotropin is the cause of hypothyroidism, administration of thy-

rotropin will promote substantial iodine uptake. Thyrotropin used for diagnosis of thyroid failure is marketed under the trade name Thytropar. Thyroid diseases and their treatment are discussed in Chapter 54.

## Corticotropin

Corticotropin (adrenocorticotropic hormone; ACTH) is a polypeptide hormone produced by the anterior pituitary. This hormone acts on the adrenal cortex to stimulate the production and release of adrenocortical hormones (e.g., cortisol, aldosterone). The principal use of corticotropin is diagnosis of adrenocortical dysfunction. A synthetic analog of corticotropin, called cosyntropin, is available. Corticotropin and cosyntropin, along with the hormones of the adrenal cortex, are discussed in Chapter 56.

## Gonadotropins

The anterior pituitary produces two gonadotropic hormones: *follicle-stimulating hormone* (FSH) and *luteinizing hormone* (LH). (Note: LH is also known as *interstitial cell-stimulating hormone* or ICSH.) LH and FSH are produced by the pituitaries of males and females and serve to regulate gonadal function in both sexes. In women, FSH acts on the ovary to promote follicular growth and development. In men, FSH supports sperm production. The role of LH in women is to promote ovulation and formation of the corpus luteum. In men, LH stimulates testosterone synthesis by Leydig cells of the testicular interstitium. Plasma levels of LH and FSH are relatively stable in males. In females, levels of both hormones vary with the phase of the menstrual cycle. The physiology of LH and FSH in females is discussed further in Chapter 57.

LH and FSH are employed clinically to treat infertility in men and women. In women, fertility is increased by promoting follicular development and ovulation. In men, increased fertility results from enhancement of spermatogenesis.

Two preparations of gonadotropins are used clinically: menotropins and urofollitropin. Menotropins [Pergonal, Humegon] is a 50:50 mixture of LH and FSH. Urofollitropin [Metrodin] is primarily FSH. The use of gonadotropins to treat infertility is discussed further in Chapter 59.

# Antidiuretic Hormone

Antidiuretic hormone (ADH) is a tripeptide hormone that acts on the kidney to cause reabsorption (conservation) of water. Deficiency of ADH produces *hypothalamic diabetes insipidus*, a condition in which large volumes of dilute urine are produced.

## Physiology

*Actions.* Antidiuretic hormone promotes renal conservation of water. The hormone accomplishes this by acting on the collecting ducts of the kidney to increase their permeability to water, which results in increased water reabsorption. Because water is withdrawn from the tubular urine (back into the extracellular space), urine that entered the collecting ducts in a relatively dilute state becomes highly concentrated by the time it leaves.

In addition to its renal actions, ADH can stimulate contraction of vascular smooth muscle and the smooth muscle of the GI tract. Because of its ability to cause vasoconstriction, ADH is known alternatively as *vasopressin*. It should be noted that the plasma levels of ADH required to cause smooth muscle contraction are higher than those that occur physiologically.

**Production and Storage.** Antidiuretic hormone is produced within the cell bodies of neurosecretory cells of the hypothalamus, and is then transported down the axons of those cells to their terminals in the posterior pituitary. ADH is stored in these terminals until released.

**Regulation of Release.** Release of ADH is regulated by the hypothalamus, the brain center responsible for maintaining body fluids at their proper osmolality. When the hypothalamus senses that osmolality has risen too high, it instructs the posterior pituitary to release ADH. The resultant increase in water reabsorption dilutes body fluids, causing osmolality to decline. Release of ADH can also be stimulated by hypotension and by reduced plasma volume.

## Hypothalamic Diabetes Insipidus

**Causes, Signs, and Symptoms.** Hypothalamic diabetes insipidus is a syndrome caused by partial or complete deficiency of ADH. The syndrome is characterized by polydipsia (excessive thirst) and excretion of large volumes of dilute urine. The deficiency of ADH may be inherited or it may result from head trauma, neurosurgery, cancer, and other causes. (In contrast to hypothalamic diabetes insipidus, *nephrogenic diabetes insipidus* results from a failure of the kidney to produce concentrated urine despite adequate levels of ADH.)

**Treatment.** The best treatment for hypothalamic diabetes insipidus is replacement therapy with ADH. (Although two other drugs—chlorpropamide and clofibrate—are effective, they are not recommended because of their side effects.) Of the ADH preparations available, *desmopressin* is the agent of choice. Desmopressin is preferred over other ADH preparations because of its prolonged duration of action, ease of administration, and lack of significant side effects, especially vasoconstriction. The response to treatment is rapid, and urine volume quickly drops to normal amounts. Desmopressin is administered by nasal spray, usually twice daily. Because desmopressin is expensive, and because excessive dosing can result in water intoxication (see below), the smallest effective dosage should be employed.

## Antidiuretic Hormone Preparations

Three preparations with ADH activity are available: *vasopressin*, *desmopressin*, and *lypressin*. Vasopressin is identical in structure to naturally occurring ADH; desmopressin and lypressin are structural analogs of natural ADH. These three preparations differ from one another with respect to routes of administration, duration of action, and therapeutic applications (Table 55-1). They also differ in their ability to cause vasoconstriction (see *Cardiovascular Effects*). All three agents may be employed to treat diabetes insipidus. However, because of its prolonged effects, convenient route (intranasal), and freedom from significant side effects, desmopressin is the drug of choice.

## Adverse Effects

**Water Intoxication.** Excessive water retention can cause water intoxication. Early signs include drowsiness, listlessness, and headache. Severe intoxication progresses to convulsions and terminal coma. Patients experiencing early symptoms of intoxication should notify the physician. Treatment of water intoxication includes restriction of fluid intake and diuretic therapy.

A major cause of water intoxication is failure to reduce water intake once ADH therapy has begun. Since treatment prevents continued fluid loss, failure to decrease fluid intake will result in water buildup and intoxication. Hence, at the onset of treatment, patients should be instructed to reduce their accustomed fluid intake.

## TABLE 55-1. ADH PREPARATIONS: ROUTES, DURATION, DOSAGE, AND USES

| Generic Name [Trade Name] | Routes | Duration of Antidiuretic Action (hr) | Therapeutic Uses | Usual Adult Dosage |
|---|---|---|---|---|
| Desmopressin [DDAVP, Stimate] | Intranasal, SC, IV, PO | 8–20 | Diabetes insipidus | 0.1 ml (10 µg) intranasally 2 times/day **or** 0.25–0.5 ml SC or IV twice daily |
| | | | Hemophilia* | 0.3 µg/kg IV over 15–30 min |
| Lypressin [Diapid] | Intranasal | 3–8 | Diabetes insipidus | 1–2 sprays (about 2–4 pressor units) into each nostril 4 times/day |
| Vasopressin [Pitressin Synthetic] | IM, SC† | 2–8 | Diabetes insipidus | 5–10 units IM or SC 3–4 times/day |
| | | | Postoperative abdominal distention | 5 units IM initially; then 10 units IM every 3–4 hours |
| | | | Abdominal radiography (to dispel gas shadows) | 10 units 2 hr before and again 30 min before the procedure |

*Desmopressin controls bleeding by increasing levels of clotting factor VIII.
†Sometimes administered intranasally or IV.

***Cardiovascular Effects.*** Because of its powerful vasoconstrictor actions, *vasopressin* can cause severe adverse cardiovascular effects. Desmopressin and lypressin, which possess only weak pressor activity, do not adversely affect hemodynamics. By constricting arteries of the heart, vasopressin can cause angina pectoris and even myocardial infarction—especially if given to patients with coronary insufficiency. In addition, vasopressin may cause gangrene by decreasing blood flow in the periphery. Because it can reduce cardiac perfusion, vasopressin must be used with extreme caution in patients with coronary artery disease. This warning does not apply to desmopressin and lypressin.

## Oxytocin

Oxytocin is produced by neurosecretory cells of the hypothalamus, and is then transported down the axons of these cells for storage in the posterior pituitary. Oxytocin has two physiologic roles: (1) promotion of uterine contraction during labor and (2) stimulation of milk ejection during breast-feeding. The principal therapeutic application of oxytocin is induction of labor near term. In addition, the hormone can be used by nursing mothers to promote milk ejection. The physiology, pharmacology, and applications of oxytocin are discussed in Chapter 60.

## Drugs Related to Hypothalamic Function

Of the seven regulatory factors found in the hypothalamus, only three—gonadotropin-releasing hormone (GnRH), thyrotropin-releasing hormone (TRH), and somatostatin—have clinical applications. GnRH and its synthetic analogs are used to treat prostatic cancer and endometriosis, and to induce ovulation. TRH is used to diagnose thyroid disorders. As discussed above, somatostatin is used to treat acromegaly.

### Gonadotropin-Releasing Hormone

Gonadotropin-releasing hormone is produced by the hypothalamus and promotes release of gonadotropins (LH and FSH) from the pituitary. Four preparations of GnRH are available: *leuprolide, goserelin, nafarelin,* and *gonadorelin*. The actions and uses of gonadorelin and nafarelin are discussed in Chapter 59 (Drugs for Infertility). Leuprolide and goserelin are discussed in Chapter 96 (Anticancer Drugs).

### Thyrotropin-Releasing Hormone

Thyrotropin-releasing hormone is produced by the hypothalamus and acts on the pituitary to stimulate release of thyrotropin (thyroid-stimulating hormone; TSH). A synthetic preparation of TRH, called *protirelin*, is used clinically. Protirelin is thought to be identical to TRH made by the hypothalamus. Protirelin is employed in the diagnosis of thyroid, pituitary, and hypothalamic disorders. Testing is performed by injecting protirelin (IV) and then sampling the blood for increases in TSH content. Interpretation of test findings can be difficult and will not be discussed here. Protirelin is marketed under the trade names Thypinone and Relefact-TRH. For a general discussion of thyroid physiology and pharmacology, refer to Chapter 54.

## KEY POINTS

- Release of hormones from the anterior pituitary is stimulated by releasing factors from the hypothalamus and inhibited by negative feedback loops.
- The growth-promoting actions of growth hormone (GH) are mediated by insulin-like growth factor-1 (IGF-1).
- Growth hormone deficiency causes dwarfism.
- Growth hormone replacement is indicated only for children who are GH deficient; GH is not indicated for children who are short simply because of their genetic heritage.
- Exogenous glucocorticoids can inhibit responses to GH.
- Growth hormone can elevate glucose levels in children with diabetes.
- Prolactin stimulates milk production after delivery.
- Excessive production of prolactin can be suppressed with bromocriptine, a drug that mimics the inhibitory action of hypothalamic dopamine on the pituitary.
- Antidiuretic hormone (ADH) acts on the kidney to cause reabsorption (conservation) of water.
- ADH deficiency results in hypothalamic diabetes insipidus.
- Hypothalamic diabetes insipidus can be treated by replacement therapy with desmopressin, a synthetic form of ADH.
- When initiating ADH replacement therapy, warn the patient to decrease water intake, since failure to do so can cause water intoxication.
- Vasopressin, a drug identical to natural ADH, can cause profound vasoconstriction.

# Summary of Major Nursing Implications*

## Growth Hormone: Somatrem and Somatropin

### Preadministration Assessment

#### Therapeutic Goal
Normalization of growth and development in children with proven growth hormone deficiency.

#### Baseline Data
Assess developmental status (height, weight, etc.). Obtain thyroid function tests.

#### Identifying High-Risk Patients
Growth hormone is *contraindicated during and after epiphyseal closure*. Use with *caution* in patients with *diabetes mellitus* and *hypothyroidism*.

### Implementation: Administration

#### Routes
IM, SC.

*Patient education information is highlighted in color.

## Administration

Reconstitute the lyophilized powder with 1 to 5 ml of diluent. *Mix gently; do not shake.* Do not inject if the preparation is cloudy or contains particulate matter.

## Ongoing Evaluation and Interventions

### Evaluating Treatment

Monitor height and weight monthly. Continue therapy until a satisfactory adult height has been achieved, until epiphyseal closure occurs, or until a response can no longer be elicited (usually by age 20 to 24).

If no stimulation of growth occurs, discontinue treatment and re-evaluate the diagnosis of growth hormone deficiency.

### Minimizing Adverse Effects and Interactions

*Hyperglycemia.* Growth hormone can elevate plasma glucose levels in diabetics. Increase insulin dosage as needed.

*Hypothyroidism.* Growth hormone may suppress thyroid function. Assess thyroid function before treatment and periodically thereafter. If levels of thyroid hormone fall, institute replacement therapy.

*Interaction with Glucocorticoids.* Glucocorticoids can oppose the growth-stimulating effects of growth hormone. Dosage of glucocorticoids should not exceed the equivalent of 10 to 15 mg/m² of hydrocortisone.

## Antidiuretic Hormone

Desmopressin
Lypressin
Vasopressin

The nursing implications summarized here apply only to the use of ADH preparations for *hypothalamic diabetes insipidus.*

## Preadministration Assessment

### Therapeutic Goal

Normalization of urinary water excretion in patients with hypothalamic diabetes insipidus.

### Baseline Data

Determine fluid and electrolyte status.

### Identifying High-Risk Patients

Use *vasopressin* with *caution* in patients with *coronary artery disease* and *other vascular diseases.*

## Implementation: Administration

### Routes

IM, IV, SC, intranasal. The route depends upon the preparation (see Table 55-1).

### Administration

Teach the patient the technique for intranasal administration. To promote compliance, make certain the patient understands that treatment is lifelong.

## Ongoing Evaluation and Interventions

### Evaluating Therapeutic Effects

Teach the patient to monitor and record daily intake and output of fluid. If ADH dosage is correct, urine volume should rapidly drop to normal.

### Minimizing Adverse Effects

*Water Intoxication.* Excessive retention of water can produce water intoxication; this is most likely at the beginning of therapy. Instruct patients to decrease their accustomed fluid intake at the start of treatment. Inform patients about early signs of water intoxication (drowsiness, listlessness, and headache) and instruct them to notify the physician if these occur. Treatment includes fluid restriction and diuretic therapy.

*Cardiovascular Effects.* *Vasopressin*, but not desmopressin or lypressin, is a powerful vasoconstrictor. Excessive vasoconstriction can produce angina pectoris, myocardial infarction, and gangrene (from extravasation of IV vasopressin). Use vasopressin with caution, especially in patients with coronary insufficiency.

# CHAPTER 56

# Drugs for Disorders of the Adrenal Cortex

The hormones of the adrenal cortex affect multiple physiologic processes, including maintenance of glucose availability, regulation of water and electrolyte balance, development of sexual characteristics, and life-preserving responses to stress. As one might guess, when production of adrenal hormones goes awry, the consequences can be profound. The two most familiar forms of adrenocortical dysfunction are *Cushing's syndrome*, caused by adrenal hormone excess, and *Addison's disease*, caused by adrenal hormone deficiency.

In approaching the drugs used for disorders of the adrenal cortex, we will begin by reviewing adrenocortical endocrinology. After that, we will discuss the disease states associated with adrenal hormone excess and adrenal hormone insufficiency. Having established this background, we will discuss the agents used for diagnosis and treatment of adrenocortical disorders.

## Physiology of the Adrenocortical Hormones

The adrenal cortex produces three classes of steroid hormones: *glucocorticoids*, *mineralocorticoids*, and *androgens*. Glucocorticoids influence carbohydrate metabolism and other processes; mineralocorticoids modulate salt and water balance; and adrenal androgens contribute to expression of sexual characteristics. When referring to either the glucocorticoids or the mineralocorticoids, the terms *corticosteroids*, *adrenocorticoids*, or *corticoids*

may be used. These terms are not used in reference to adrenal androgens.

## Glucocorticoids

Glucocorticoids are so named because of their ability to increase the availability of glucose. Of the several glucocorticoids produced by the adrenal cortex, *cortisol* is the most important. The structural formula of cortisol is shown in Figure 56–1.

When considering the glucocorticoids, it is important to distinguish between *physiologic effects* and *pharmacologic effects*. *Physiologic* effects occur at *low* levels of glucocorticoids (i.e., the levels produced by release of glucocorticoids from healthy adrenals or by administration of exogenous glucocorticoids in low doses). *Pharmacologic* effects occur at *high* levels of glucocorticoids. These are the levels achieved when exogenous glucocorticoids are administered in the large doses required to treat disorders unrelated to adrenocortical function (e.g., allergic reactions, asthma, inflammation). In this chapter, we will limit discussion to the *physiologic* role of glucocorticoids. The use of glucocorticoids for nonendocrine purposes (which is the major application of these agents) is discussed in Chapter 65.

### Physiologic Effects

*Carbohydrate Metabolism.* Supplying the brain with glucose is essential for survival. Glucocorticoids help meet this need. Glucocorticoids promote glucose availability in three ways: (1) stimulation of gluconeogenesis, (2) reduction of peripheral glucose utilization, and (3) promotion of glucose storage (in the form of glycogen). All three actions

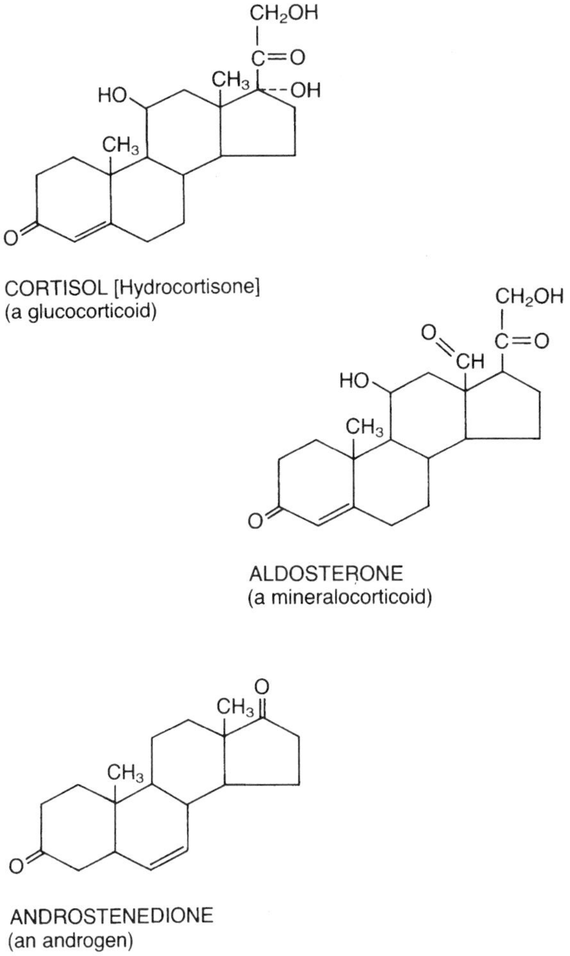

**Figure 56–1. Structural formulas of representative adrenocortical hormones.**

increase glucose availability during fasting, and thereby help ensure that the brain will not be deprived of its primary source of energy.

The effects of glucocorticoids on carbohydrate metabolism are opposite to those of insulin: whereas insulin lowers plasma levels of glucose, glucocorticoids raise them. When present chronically in high concentrations, glucocorticoids produce symptoms much like those of diabetes.

*Protein Metabolism.* Glucocorticoids promote protein catabolism (breakdown). This action, which is opposite to that of insulin, provides amino acids for glucose synthesis. If present at high levels for a prolonged time, glucocorticoids will cause thinning of the skin, muscle wasting, and negative nitrogen balance.

*Fat Metabolism.* Glucocorticoids promote lipolysis (fat breakdown). When present at high levels for an extended period, as occurs in Cushing's syndrome, glucocorticoids cause fat redistribution, giving the patient a potbelly, "moon face," and "buffalo hump" on the back.

*Cardiovascular System.* Glucocorticoids are required to maintain the functional integrity of the vascular system.

When levels of glucocorticoids are depressed, capillary permeability is increased, the ability of vessels to constrict is reduced, and blood pressure falls.

Glucocorticoids have multiple effects on blood cells. These hormones increase red blood cell counts and levels of hemoglobin. Of the white blood cells, only the polymorphonuclear leukocytes increase; in contrast, lymphocytes, eosinophils, basophils, and monocytes decrease.

*Skeletal Muscle.* Glucocorticoids support function of striated muscle, primarily by maintaining circulatory competence. In the absence of sufficient levels of glucocorticoids, muscle perfusion decreases, causing work capacity to decrease as well.

*Central Nervous System.* Glucocorticoids affect mood, central nervous system (CNS) excitability, and the electroencephalogram. Glucocorticoid insufficiency is associated with depression, lethargy, and irritability. Rarely, outright psychosis occurs. In contrast, when present in excess, glucocorticoids can produce generalized excitation and euphoria.

*Stress.* In response to stress (e.g., anxiety, exercise, trauma, infection, surgery), the adrenal cortex secretes increased amounts of glucocorticoids, and the adrenal medulla secretes increased amounts of epinephrine. Working together, glucocorticoids and epinephrine serve to maintain blood pressure and plasma glucose content. If glucocorticoid levels are insufficient, hypotension and hypoglycemia can occur. If the stress is extreme (e.g., trauma, surgery, severe infection), glucocorticoid deficiency can result in circulatory collapse and death. Accordingly, it is essential that patients with adrenal insufficiency be given glucocorticoid supplements when severe stress occurs.

*Respiratory System in Neonates.* During labor and delivery, the adrenals of the full-term fetus release a burst of glucocorticoids. Within hours, these steroids act on the lungs to accelerate their maturation. In the premature infant, the adrenals only produce small amounts of glucocorticoids. As a result, preterm infants experience a high incidence of respiratory distress syndrome.

## Regulation of Synthesis and Secretion

Adrenal storage of glucocorticoids is minimal; hence, glucocorticoids must be synthesized as they are needed. Accordingly, the amount of glucocorticoid released from the adrenals per unit time closely approximates the amount being made.

Synthesis and release of glucocorticoids are regulated by a negative feedback loop (Fig. 56–2). The loop begins with the release of corticotropin-releasing factor (CRF) from the hypothalamus. CRF acts on the anterior pituitary to cause release of adrenocorticotropic hormone (ACTH), which stimulates the adrenal cortex, causing synthesis and release of cortisol and other glucocorticoids. Following release, cortisol acts in two ways: (1) it promotes its designated biologic effects and (2) it acts on the hypothalamus and pituitary to suppress further release of CRF and ACTH. Hence, as cortisol levels rise, they act to

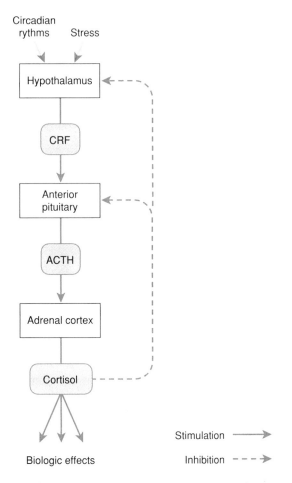

**Figure 56–2. Negative feedback regulation of glucocorticoid synthesis and secretion.** (CRF = corticotropin-releasing factor, ACTH = adrenocorticotropic hormone.)

suppress further stimulation of glucocorticoid production, thereby keeping plasma levels of glucocorticoids within an appropriate range.

The hypothalamic-pituitary-adrenal system is activated by signals from the CNS. These signals turn the system on by causing the hypothalamus to release CRF. As indicated in Figure 56-2, two modes of activation are involved. One mode provides a basal level of stimulation. Basal stimulation follows a circadian rhythm, peaking in the early morning and reaching a nadir late in the evening. The second mode of activation is stress. Stressful events that can activate the loop include injury, infection, and surgery. The signals generated by stress produce intense stimulation of the hypothalamus. The resultant release of CRF and ACTH can cause plasma levels of cortisol to increase by a factor of 10. Because stress is such a powerful stimulus, it overrides feedback inhibition by cortisol.

## Mineralocorticoids

The mineralocorticoids influence renal processing of sodium, potassium, and hydrogen. Of the mineralocorticoids made by the adrenal cortex, *aldosterone* is the most important.

***Physiologic Effects.*** Aldosterone acts on the collecting ducts of the nephron to promote sodium reabsorption in exchange for secretion of potassium and hydrogen. The total amount of hydrogen and potassium lost equals the amount of sodium reabsorbed. It should be noted that, as sodium is reabsorbed, water is reabsorbed along with it. In the absence of aldosterone, renal excretion of sodium and water is greatly increased, whereas excretion of potassium and hydrogen is reduced. As a result, aldosterone insufficiency causes hyponatremia, hyperkalemia, acidosis, cellular dehydration, and reduction of extracellular fluid volume. Left uncorrected, the condition can lead to renal failure, circulatory collapse, and death.

***Control of Secretion.*** Secretion of aldosterone is regulated by the renin-angiotensin system—not by ACTH. The mechanisms by which the renin-angiotensin system regulates aldosterone are discussed in Chapter 41. It is important to note that, since aldosterone is not regulated by ACTH, conditions in which secretion of ACTH is altered do not affect the release of aldosterone.

## Adrenal Androgens

The adrenal cortex produces several steroids that have androgenic properties. *Androstenedione* is representative of these compounds. Under normal conditions, the effects of the adrenal androgens are minimal. In adult males, the influence of adrenal androgens is overshadowed by the effects of testosterone produced by the testes. In adult females, a metabolite of the adrenal androgens (testosterone) contributes to development of sexual hair and maintenance of normal libido. Although adrenal androgens normally have very little effect, when secretion of these hormones is excessive, as occurs in congenital adrenal hyperplasia, virilizing actions can be pronounced.

# Pathophysiology of the Adrenocortical Hormones

## Adrenal Hormone Excess

### Cushing's Syndrome

***Causes.*** Signs and symptoms of Cushing's syndrome result from excess levels of circulating glucocorticoids. Principal causes of excess are (1) hypersecretion of ACTH by pituitary adenomas (Cushing's disease), (2) hypersecretion of glucocorticoids by adrenal adenomas and carcinomas, and (3) administration of exogenous glucocorticoids in the large doses used to treat arthritis and other nonendocrine disorders.

***Clinical Presentation.*** Cushing's syndrome is characterized by obesity, hyperglycemia, glycosuria, hypertension, fluid and electrolyte disturbances, osteoporosis, muscle weakness, myopathy, hirsutism, menstrual irregularities, and decreased resistance to infection. The skin is weakened, resulting in striae (stretch marks) and increased susceptibility to injury. Fat undergoes redistribution to the abdomen, face, and upper back, giving the patient a characteristic potbelly, "moon face," and "buffalo hump." Psychiatric changes are common.

**Treatment.** Treatment of Cushing's syndrome is directed at the cause. The treatment of choice for adrenal adenoma and carcinoma is surgical removal of the diseased adrenal gland. If bilateral adrenalectomy is performed, replacement therapy with glucocorticoids and mineralocorticoids will be needed. For patients with inoperable adrenal carcinoma, treatment with *mitotane* is indicated. Mitotane is an anticancer drug that produces selective destruction of adrenocortical cells. The pharmacology of mitotane is discussed in Chapter 96.

When Cushing's syndrome is caused by pituitary adenoma, surgery is the preferred form of treatment. Partial removal of the pituitary often lowers ACTH secretion to safe levels, while leaving other pituitary functions intact. If partial adenectomy is unsuccessful, the remainder of the pituitary may be removed. As an alternative, pituitary irradiation may be employed.

The role of drugs in treating Cushing's syndrome is limited. Most commonly, drugs are employed as adjuncts to radiation and surgery; drugs are rarely the primary therapeutic modality. Drugs can relieve symptoms by inhibiting corticosteroid synthesis. Two drugs that act by this mechanism—*aminoglutethimide* and *ketoconazole*—are discussed below.

### Primary Hyperaldosteronism

**Clinical Presentation and Causes.** Hyperaldosteronism (excessive secretion of aldosterone) causes hypokalemia, metabolic alkalosis, and hypertension. Muscle weakness and changes in the electrocardiogram develop secondary to hypokalemia. Hyperaldosteronism is frequently caused by an aldosterone-producing adrenal adenoma. The condition may also result from bilateral adrenal hyperplasia.

**Treatment.** Management of hyperaldosteronism is dependent on the cause. When an adrenal adenoma is responsible, surgical resection of the adrenal is usually curative. When bilateral adrenal hyperplasia underlies hyperaldosteronism, an aldosterone antagonist is the preferred treatment. The antagonist employed most frequently is *spironolactone*, a drug we normally think of as a potassium-sparing diuretic. Under the influence of spironolactone, potassium levels may normalize in 2 weeks. To achieve full control of hypertension, an additional diuretic may be required. The basic pharmacology of spironolactone is discussed in Chapter 38 (Diuretics). Pharmacologic alternatives to spironolactone are *amiloride* (another potassium-sparing diuretic) or an *angiotensin-converting enzyme inhibitor* (e.g., captopril).

## Adrenal Hormone Insufficiency
### General Therapeutic Considerations

Adrenal hormone insufficiency can result from multiple causes, including destruction of the adrenals, inborn deficiencies of the enzymes required for corticosteroid syn-

thesis, and reduced secretion of ACTH and CRF. Regardless of the cause, adrenal insufficiency requires lifelong replacement therapy with appropriate corticosteroids. All patients require a *glucocorticoid*. Some may require a *mineralocorticoid* as well. Of the glucocorticoids available, *cortisone* and *hydrocortisone* are drugs of first choice. When a mineralocorticoid is indicated, *fludrocortisone* is the drug of choice.

Replacement therapy should mimic normal patterns of corticosteroid secretion. For glucocorticoids, this can be accomplished by dividing the daily dosage, giving two thirds in the morning and one third in the evening. Mineralocorticoids can be administered once a day. Doses of glucocorticoids and mineralocorticoids should approximate the amounts normally secreted by the adrenals. It is important to note that, when glucocorticoids are employed for replacement therapy, doses are much smaller than the doses employed to treat nonendocrine disorders.

*At times of stress, patients must increase their glucocorticoid dosage.* The importance of doing so cannot be overemphasized: *failure to increase the dosage can be fatal.* Recall that healthy adrenals increase their output of glucocorticoids in response to stress. For patients with adrenal insufficiency, the extra glucocorticoids that would normally be supplied by the adrenals must instead be supplied through supplemental dosing. For mild stress (e.g., upper respiratory infection), doubling the normal dosage should suffice. For severe stress (e.g., surgery), the dosage should be increased fivefold. To ensure availability of glucocorticoids in emergencies, the patient should carry an adequate supply at all times. This supply should include an injectable preparation plus an oral preparation. Furthermore, the patient should wear some form of identification (e.g., Medic Alert bracelet) to inform emergency health care personnel about glucocorticoid requirements.

### Addison's Disease (Primary Adrenocortical Insufficiency)

**Clinical Presentation and Causes.** Addison's disease is characterized by weakness, emaciation, hypoglycemia, and increased pigmentation of the skin and mucous membranes. Hyperkalemia, hyponatremia, and hypotension are present as well. These symptoms result from a deficiency of glucocorticoids and mineralocorticoids occurring secondary to adrenal atrophy. Potential causes of adrenal atrophy include carcinoma, infection, and autoimmune disease.

**Treatment.** Replacement therapy with adrenocorticoids is required. *Hydrocortisone* and *cortisone* are the drugs of choice. Both agents exert a combination of mineralocorticoid and glucocorticoid activity. Hence, therapy with either agent alone may be sufficient. If additional mineralocorticoid activity is needed, *fludrocortisone*, the only mineralocorticoid available, can be added to the regimen.

### Secondary and Tertiary Adrenocortical Insufficiency

Secondary adrenocortical insufficiency results from decreased secretion of ACTH, and tertiary insufficiency results from decreased secretion of CRF. In both cases, adrenal secretion of glucocorticoids is diminished, whereas secretion of mineralocorticoids is usually not affected. Glucocorticoid insufficiency produces a characteristic set of symptoms: hypoglycemia, malaise, loss of appetite, and reduced capacity to respond to stress. For secondary and tertiary insufficiency, treatment consists of replacement therapy with a glucocorticoid (e.g., hydrocortisone, cortisone). A mineralocorticoid is needed only rarely.

### Acute Adrenal Insufficiency (Adrenal Crisis)

*Clinical Presentation.* Acute adrenal insufficiency is characterized by hypotension, dehydration, weakness, lethargy, and gastrointestinal symptoms (e.g., vomiting, diarrhea). Left untreated, the syndrome progresses to shock and then death.

*Causes.* Adrenal crisis may be brought on by adrenal failure, pituitary failure, and failure to provide patients receiving replacement therapy with adequate doses of corticosteroids. Adrenal crisis may also be triggered by abrupt withdrawal from chronic, high-dose glucocorticoid therapy.

*Treatment.* Patients require rapid replacement of fluid, salt, and glucocorticoids. They also need glucose for energy. These needs are met by injecting 100 mg of hydrocortisone (as an IV bolus) followed by IV infusion of normal saline with dextrose. Additional hydrocortisone is given by infusion at a rate of 100 mg every 8 hours.

### Congenital Adrenal Hyperplasia

*Clinical Presentation and Causes.* Congenital adrenal hyperplasia results from an inborn deficiency of enzymes needed for glucocorticoid synthesis. The capacity to make glucocorticoids is decreased, but not eliminated. In an attempt to enhance glucocorticoid synthesis, the pituitary releases amounts of ACTH that are much greater than normal. The resultant high levels of ACTH produce powerful stimulation of the adrenals, causing growth of the adrenals (hyperplasia) and increased synthesis of glucocorticoids and androgens. (Synthesis of mineralocorticoids is relatively unaffected.) Frequently, stimulation of glucocorticoid synthesis may be sufficient to bring levels of cortisol up to normal. Unfortunately, the amounts of ACTH required to normalize glucocorticoid production are so large that synthesis of adrenal androgens becomes excessive. In girls, increased androgen levels cause masculinization of the external genitalia. The ovaries, uterus, and fallopian tubes are not affected. Increased androgen levels in boys may cause precocious penile enlargement. In children of both sexes, linear growth is accelerated. However, because androgens cause premature closure of the epiphyses, adult height is usually diminished.

*Treatment.* The therapeutic objective is to ensure adequate levels of glucocorticoids while preventing excessive production of adrenal androgens. This goal is achieved through lifelong administration of glucocorticoids. *Hydrocortisone* and *cortisone* are the drugs of choice. By supplying glucocorticoids exogenously, we can suppress secretion of ACTH; since ACTH release is diminished, the adrenals are no longer stimulated to produce excessive quantities of androgens. As a rule, suppression of ACTH secretion can be achieved with daily doses of hydrocortisone equivalent to twice the amount secreted each day by normal adrenals. To assess the efficacy of therapy, children should be monitored every 3 months for growth rate and signs of virilization.

# Agents for Replacement Therapy in Adrenocortical Insufficiency

Patients with adrenocortical insufficiency require replacement therapy with corticosteroids. A glucocorticoid is always required, and some patients require a mineralocorticoid as well. The principal glucocorticoids employed are *hydrocortisone* and *cortisone*. *Fludrocortisone* is the only mineralocorticoid available.

It should be noted that classification of a drug as a "glucocorticoid" or "mineralocorticoid" may be an oversimplification. That is, a drug that we classify as a glucocorticoid may also exhibit salt-retaining (mineralocorticoid) activity. Conversely, a drug that we classify as a mineralocorticoid may also display typical glucocorticoid activity.

## Hydrocortisone

Hydrocortisone is a synthetic steroid whose structure is identical to that of cortisol, the principal glucocorticoid produced by the adrenal cortex (see Fig. 56–1). Hydrocortisone is a drug of choice for adrenocortical insufficiency and will serve as our prototype of the glucocorticoids employed clinically. It should be noted that, despite its classification as a glucocorticoid, hydrocortisone also has mineralocorticoid properties.

### Therapeutic Uses

*Replacement Therapy.* Hydrocortisone is a preferred drug for all forms of adrenocortical insufficiency. *Oral* hydrocortisone is ideal for chronic replacement therapy. *Parenteral* administration is used for acute adrenal insufficiency and to supplement oral doses at times of stress. Because of its mineralocorticoid actions, hydrocortisone can sometimes suffice as sole therapy for adrenal insufficiency, even when salt loss is a symptom.

*Nonendocrine Applications.* Hydrocortisone and other glucocorticoids are used to treat a broad spectrum of nonendocrine disorders, ranging from allergic reactions to inflammation to cancer. The doses required in these disorders are considerably higher than the doses employed in replacement therapy. The use of glucocorticoids for nonendocrine diseases is discussed in Chapter 65.

## Adverse Effects

When given in the low doses required for replacement therapy, hydrocortisone and other glucocorticoids are devoid of adverse effects. In contrast, when taken chronically in the large doses employed to treat nonendocrine disorders, glucocorticoids are highly toxic. The adverse effects of chronic, high-dose therapy include adrenal suppression and production of Cushing's syndrome. These and other adverse effects are discussed in Chapter 65.

### Preparations, Dosage, and Administration

**Preparations.** For replacement therapy, four hydrocortisone preparations are used: *hydrocortisone base*, *hydrocortisone cypionate*, *hydrocortisone sodium phosphate*, and *hydrocortisone sodium succinate*. The base and the cypionate salt can be administered orally. Because they are insoluble, these preparations must not be administered IV. The sodium phosphate and sodium succinate salts are water soluble and can be used IV and IM.

**Dosage and Administration.** The oral route is employed for chronic treatment. Intravenous and IM administration are reserved for emergencies. For oral therapy of chronic adrenal insufficiency, the total daily dose ranges from 12 to 15 mg/m². This dose may be divided, giving two thirds in the morning and one third in the afternoon. For emergency treatment, IV doses of 50 to 100 mg are employed. When IV injections can't be used, IM doses of 100 to 250 mg may be given instead. Doses for nonendocrine disorders are given in Chapter 65.

## Cortisone

Cortisone is a prodrug that undergoes conversion to its active form—hydrocortisone (cortisol)—within the body. Like hydrocortisone itself, cortisone has both glucocorticoid and mineralocorticoid actions, and is a drug of choice for chronic adrenal insufficiency. In contrast to hydrocortisone, which can be administered orally, IV, and IM, cortisone can only be used orally and IM. Cortisone is insoluble in water and must never be administered IV. Absorption of intramuscular cortisone is unpredictable, hence cortisone injections are not recommended for acute adrenal insufficiency. For management of chronic adrenal insufficiency, the usual oral dosage is 12 to 15 mg/m²/day.

## Fludrocortisone

Fludrocortisone [Florinef] is a potent mineralocorticoid that also possesses significant glucocorticoid activity. Fludrocortisone is the only mineralocorticoid available and is the drug of choice for chronic mineralocorticoid replacement.

**Therapeutic Uses.** Fludrocortisone is a preferred drug for treating Addison's disease, primary hypoaldosteronism, and congenital adrenal hyperplasia (when salt wasting is a feature of the syndrome). In most cases, fludrocortisone must be used in combination with a glucocorticoid (e.g., hydrocortisone, cortisone).

**Adverse Effects.** Adverse effects are a direct consequence of fludrocortisone's mineralocorticoid actions. When the dosage is too high, salt and water are retained in excess, while excessive amounts of potassium are lost. These effects on salt and water can result in expansion of blood volume, hypertension, edema, cardiac enlargement, and hypokalemia. Patients should be monitored for weight gain and elevation of blood pressure. If these changes occur, fludrocortisone should be temporarily withdrawn. Fluid and electrolyte imbalance should resolve spontaneously within days.

**Preparations, Dosage, and Administration.** Fludrocortisone acetate [Florinef Acetate] is available in 0.1-mg tablets for oral administration. The usual daily dose is 0.1 mg. If excessive salt retention occurs, the daily dose should be decreased to 0.05 mg.

# Agents for Diagnostic Testing of Adrenocortical Function

## Corticotropin and Cosyntropin

Corticotropin and cosyntropin mimic the effects of human ACTH. That is, both compounds act on the adrenal cortex to stimulate synthesis and secretion of cortisol and other adrenal corticosteroids. Corticotropin is prepared from animal pituitary glands and is nearly identical in structure to human ACTH. Cosyntropin is a synthetic polypeptide whose structure corresponds to the first 24 amino acids of ACTH. Since corticotropin, cosyntropin, and ACTH all produce equivalent stimulation of the adrenal cortex, we will use the term ACTH in reference to all three compounds.

### Clinical Applications

ACTH is used primarily for diagnostic tests. For reasons discussed below, ACTH has only limited utility as a medication.

**Diagnosis of Adrenal Insufficiency.** Suspected adrenal insufficiency can be assessed by administering ACTH and then measuring plasma cortisol content. In patients with primary adrenocortical insufficiency, ACTH is unable to promote cortisol synthesis. Hence, plasma levels of the hormone will not be raised. If ACTH succeeds in elevating cortisol levels, primary adrenal insufficiency can be ruled out.

**Therapeutic Uses.** Because of its ability to stimulate glucocorticoid production, ACTH can, in theory, be used to treat a variety of conditions responsive to glucocorticoids. In practice, however, ACTH is rarely used for therapeutics. There are several reasons for this: (1) responses to ACTH are highly variable; (2) ACTH cannot be given orally, whereas glucocorticoids can; (3) ACTH can produce undesired side effects by stimulating production of adrenal androgens, and possibly aldosterone as well; (4) since the therapeutic effects of ACTH derive from enhanced glucocorticoid production, ACTH is only useful in patients with functioning adrenal glands; and (5) there is no evidence that treatment with ACTH offers any benefits over treatment with glucocorticoids themselves. Consequently, in most cases where ACTH might be employed, it is preferable to treat with glucocorticoids directly.

## Preparations

There are three preparations of corticotropin and one of cosyntropin. *Corticotropin injection* [Acthar, ACTH] is dispensed in 25- and 40-unit vials; routes are IM, SC, and IV. *Repository corticotropin* injection [H.P. Acthar Gel, ACTH-40, ACTH-80] is dispensed in 40- and 80-unit vials; routes are IM and SC. *Corticotropin zinc hydroxide* [Cortrophin-Zinc] is dispensed in 40-unit vials; administration is IM. *Cosyntropin* [Cortrosyn] is dispensed in 0.25-mg vials; routes are IM and IV.

## Dexamethasone

Dexamethasone is a synthetic steroid that has pronounced glucocorticoid properties and very little mineralocorticoid activity. The drug is used primarily to treat nonendocrine disorders. Dexamethasone is also employed in the diagnostic tests described below.

### Overnight Dexamethasone Suppression Test

The overnight dexamethasone suppression test is used to diagnose Cushing's syndrome. This test is performed by administering 1 mg of dexamethasone at 11 PM followed by measurement of plasma cortisol levels at 8 o'clock the following morning. In normal individuals, dexamethasone acts on the pituitary to suppress release of ACTH, thereby suppressing synthesis and release of cortisol. If the patient has Cushing's syndrome, little or no suppression of cortisol production will occur.

### Prolonged Dexamethasone Suppression Test

Once Cushing's syndrome has been diagnosed, the prolonged dexamethasone suppression test can be used to distinguish between excessive ACTH release as the cause versus dysfunction of the adrenal cortex itself. This test is performed as follows: (1) baseline measurement of *urinary* 17-hydroxycorticosteroids is made (these compounds provide an index of adrenal corticosteroid production); (2) dexamethasone is administered in 2-mg doses every 6 hours for 48 hours; and (3) 24-hour urine is collected for determination of 17-hydroxycorticosteroids. If primary adrenal dysfunction is responsible for the symptoms of Cushing's syndrome, no suppression of 17-hydroxycorticosteroid production will occur. In contrast, if excessive ACTH release underlies Cushing's syndrome, prolonged administration of dexamethasone should produce some suppression of ACTH secretion, and therefore should cause a small but measurable reduction in urinary 17-hydroxycorticosteroids.

It should be noted that the dexamethasone suppression test is not the best method for determining the underlying cause of Cushing's syndrome. The preferred procedure is to measure plasma ACTH and cortisol content directly. If plasma cortisol levels are high and ACTH levels are normal, adrenal dysfunction is responsible for the observed signs. If levels of both ACTH and cortisol are high, excessive ACTH secretion is likely to be the underlying problem.

# Inhibitors of Corticosteroid Synthesis

Several drugs have been employed to inhibit excessive corticosteroid synthesis in patients with Cushing's disease. Two of these drugs—ketoconazole and aminoglutethimide—are discussed below. Although these agents can help relieve hypercortisolism, they are not a preferred form of therapy. Instead, they are used primarily as adjuncts to radiation therapy during the time required for irradiation of the pituitary to produce its effects (usually several months).

## Ketoconazole

Ketoconazole [Nizoral] is an antifungal drug that also inhibits glucocorticoid synthesis. In fact, ketoconazole is the most effective inhibitor of glucocorticoid synthesis available. In patients with Cushing's syndrome, the drug may be used as an adjunct to surgery or radiation, but not as primary treatment. The dosage for suppression of steroid synthesis is 600 to 800 mg/day—much higher than doses employed for antifungal therapy. At these high doses, ketoconazole can cause significant liver dysfunction. In addition, if combined with a nonsedating antihistamine (e.g., terfenadine, astemizole), the drug can induce fatal ventricular dysrhythmias. The basic pharmacology of ketoconazole is discussed in Chapter 86 (Antifungal Agents).

### Aminoglutethimide

*Actions.* Aminoglutethimide [Cytadren] blocks the conversion of cholesterol to pregnenolone, the first step in the synthesis of all adrenal steroids. As a result, production of glucocorticoids, mineralocorticoids, and androgens declines.

*Therapeutic Use.* Aminoglutethimide has been employed as a temporary means of decreasing excessive corticosteroid production in patients awaiting more definitive therapy (e.g., surgery). Duration of treatment is seldom greater than 3 months. In patients with adrenal adenoma, adrenal carcinoma, and ectopic ACTH-secreting tumors, morning plasma levels of cortisol are reduced by about 50%. Aminoglutethimide does not affect the underlying disease process; hence, if therapy is stopped, excessive production of adrenal corticoids will resume.

*Adverse Effects.* Untoward effects are common. The most frequent are drowsiness, nausea, anorexia, and morbilliform rash. Additional effects include headache, dizziness, hematologic abnormalities, hypothyroidism, muscle pain, and fever. Masculinization may occur in females. Precocious sexual development may occur in males.

*Preparations, Dosage, and Administration.* Aminoglutethimide [Cytadren] is available in 250-mg tablets for oral use. The initial dosage is 250 mg every 6 hours. If steroid synthesis remains excessive, the dosage may be gradually increased, but should not exceed 2 gm/day.

# KEY POINTS

- The adrenal cortex produces three classes of steroid hormones: glucocorticoids, mineralocorticoids, and androgens.
- Glucocorticoids influence the metabolism of carbohydrates, proteins, and fats; in addition, they affect skeletal muscle, the cardiovascular system, and the CNS. At times of stress, glucocorticoids are essential for survival.

- Synthesis and release of glucocorticoids is regulated by a negative feedback loop involving CRF from the hypothalamus, ACTH from the pituitary, and cortisol from the adrenal cortex.
- Aldosterone, the major mineralocorticoid, acts on the kidney to promote the retention of sodium and water and the excretion of potassium and hydrogen.
- Glucocorticoid excess causes Cushing's syndrome.
- The principal treatment for Cushing's syndrome is surgical removal of the adrenals (if adrenal cancer is the cause) or part of the pituitary (if pituitary cancer is the cause).
- Ketoconazole can be used to suppress synthesis of adrenal steroids in patients with Cushing's syndrome. However, this drug is only employed as an adjunct to surgery or radiation.
- Adrenal insufficiency causes Addison's disease.
- Adrenal insufficiency is treated by replacement therapy with glucocorticoids, usually cortisone or hydrocortisone. Fludrocortisone, a pure mineralocorticoid, may be added if the mineralocorticoid actions of cortisone or hydrocortisone are inadequate.
- In patients with adrenal insufficiency, it is absolutely essential to increase glucocorticoid doses at times of stress (e.g., surgery, trauma). Failure to do so may be fatal.
- When used in the low (physiologic) doses needed for replacement therapy, glucocorticoids have no adverse effects. In contrast, when used chronically in the high (pharmacologic) doses needed for nonendocrine diseases (e.g., arthritis), glucocorticoids can cause severe adverse effects (see Chapter 65).
- Corticotropin and cosyntropin are drugs that act like ACTH (i.e., they stimulate the synthesis and release of corticosteroids).
- Corticotropin and cosyntropin are used only for diagnosis of adrenal insufficiency—not for treatment.

# Summary of Major Nursing Implications*

## Glucocorticoids: Hydrocortisone and Cortisone

The nursing implications summarized here apply only to the use of glucocorticoids for *replacement therapy*. Nursing implications that apply to use of glucocorticoids for *nonendocrine disorders* are summarized in Chapter 65.

### Use in Addison's Disease

*Administration.* Instruct the patient to take two thirds of the daily dose in the morning and one third in the afternoon. Make certain the patient understands that replacement therapy must continue lifelong.

*Emergency Preparedness.* Warn the patient that the dosage must be increased at times of stress (e.g., infection, surgery, trauma). Advise the patient to carry an emergency supply of glucocorticoids at all times. This supply should include an injectable glucocorticoid plus an oral preparation. Advise the patient to wear identification (e.g., Medic Alert bracelet) to inform emergency medical personnel of glucocorticoid requirements.

### Use in Congenital Adrenal Hyperplasia

To assess therapy, monitor the child at 3-month intervals for signs of excess androgen production (e.g., excessive growth rate, virilization in girls, precocious penile enlargement in boys). Suppression of these effects indicates success.

### Minimizing Adverse Effects

Excessive doses can produce symptoms of Cushing's syndrome. Observe the patient for signs of Cushing's syndrome and notify the physician if these develop.

## Fludrocortisone (a Mineralocorticoid)

### Route

Oral.

### Minimizing Adverse Effects

Excessive doses cause retention of sodium and water and excessive excretion of potassium, resulting in expansion of blood volume, hypertension, cardiac enlargement, edema, and hypokalemia. Inform patients about signs of salt and water retention (e.g., unusual weight gain, swelling of the feet or lower legs), and instruct them to notify the physician if these occur. Treatment consists of temporary withdrawal of fludrocortisone; fluid and electrolyte balance should normalize within days.

---

*Patient education information is highlighted in color.

# CHAPTER 57

# Estrogens and Progestins

**The Menstrual Cycle**
**Estrogens**
    Biosynthesis
    Physiologic and Pharmacologic Effects
    Clinical Pharmacology

**Progestins**
    Biosynthesis
    Physiologic and Pharmacologic Effects
    Clinical Pharmacology
**Hormone Replacement Therapy after Menopause**
**Premenstrual Syndrome**

Estrogens and progestins are hormones that promote the maturation and ongoing activity of female reproductive organs. These hormones also promote development of secondary sex characteristics in females. In addition, estrogen protects against coronary heart disease and osteoporosis. The principal endogenous estrogen is estradiol. The principal endogenous progestational hormone is progesterone. Both hormones are produced by the ovaries. During pregnancy, large amounts are also produced by the placenta.

Clinical applications of the female sex hormones fall into two major categories: contraception and noncontraceptive applications. In this chapter, our focus is on noncontraceptive uses; contraception is discussed in Chapter 58. The principal noncontraceptive application of estrogens and progestins is in hormone replacement therapy: estrogens are given to replace estrogens lost following menopause; progestins are given to prevent adverse effects of estrogens on the endometrium.

## The Menstrual Cycle

Since much of the clinical pharmacology of the estrogens and progestins is related to their actions during the menstrual cycle, understanding the menstrual cycle is essential to understanding these hormones. Accordingly, we will begin our discussion with a review of the menstrual cycle. The anatomic and hormonal changes that take place during the cycle are summarized in Figure 57-1. As indicated in the figure, the first half of the cycle (days 1 through 14) is referred to as the *follicular phase*; the second half is referred to as the *luteal phase*. The whole cycle typically takes 28 days.

***Ovarian and Uterine Events.*** The menstrual cycle consists of a coordinated series of ovarian and uterine events. In the ovary, the following sequence occurs: (1) several ovarian follicles ripen; (2) one of the ripe follicles ruptures, causing ovulation; (3) the ruptured follicle evolves into a corpus luteum; and (4) if fertilization of the ovum does not occur, the corpus luteum dissolves. As these ovarian events are taking place, parallel events take place in the uterus: (1) while ovarian follicles ripen, the endometrium prepares for nidation (implantation of a fertilized ovum) by increasing in thickness and vascularity; (2) following ovulation, the uterus continues its preparation by increasing its secretory activity; and (3) if nidation fails to occur, the thickened endometrium breaks down, causing menstruation, and the cycle begins anew.

***The Roles of Estrogens and Progesterone.*** The uterine changes that take place during the menstrual cycle are brought about under the influence of estrogens and progesterone produced by the ovaries. During the first half of the cycle, estrogens are secreted by the maturing ovarian follicles. As suggested by Figure 57-1, these estrogens act on the uterus to cause proliferation of the endometrium. At midcycle, one of the ovarian follicles ruptures and then evolves into a corpus luteum. For most of the second half of the cycle, estrogens and progesterone are produced by the newly formed corpus luteum. These hormones maintain the endometrium in its hypertrophied state. At the end of the cycle, the corpus luteum atrophies, causing production of estrogens and progesterone to decline. In response to the diminished supply of ovarian hormones, the endometrium breaks down.

***The Role of Pituitary Hormones.*** Two anterior pituitary hormones—follicle-stimulating hormone (FSH) and luteinizing hormone (LH)—play central roles in regulating the menstrual cycle. During the first half of the cycle, FSH acts on the developing ovarian follicles, causing the follicles to grow and secrete estrogens. The resultant rise in estrogen levels exerts a negative feedback influence on the pituitary, thereby suppressing further FSH release. At midcycle, LH levels rise abruptly (see Fig. 57-1). This LH surge, which is triggered by rising estrogen levels, causes

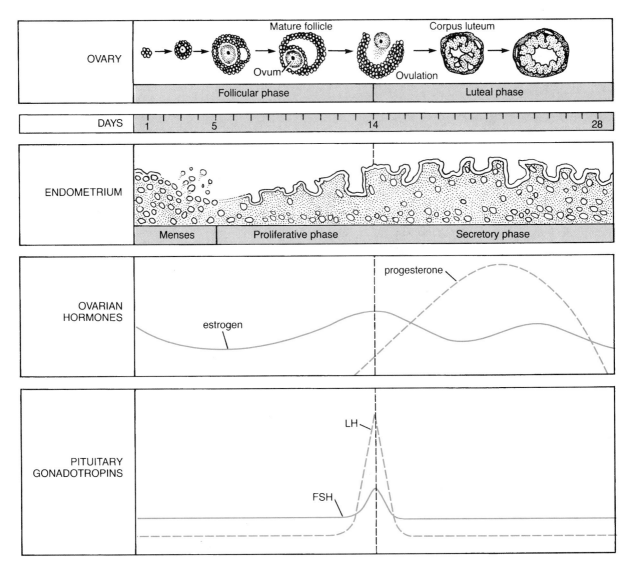

**Figure 57–1. The menstrual cycle: anatomic and hormonal changes.** (LH = luteinizing hormone, FSH = follicle-stimulating hormone.)

one of the mature follicles to swell rapidly, burst, and release its ovum. (Why only one follicle undergoes ovulation remains a mystery.) Following ovulation, LH acts on the newly formed corpus luteum to promote secretion of estrogens and progesterone.

From the foregoing, it is clear that precisely timed alterations in the secretion of FSH and LH are responsible for coordinating the structural and secretory changes that occur throughout the menstrual cycle. The mechanisms that regulate secretion of FSH and LH are complex and incompletely understood.

## Estrogens

### Biosynthesis

***Females.*** In premenopausal women, the ovary is the principle organ of estrogen production. During the follic-

ular phase of the menstrual cycle, estrogens are synthesized by ovarian follicles under the direction of FSH; during the luteal phase, estrogens are synthesized by the corpus luteum under the direction of LH. The major estrogen produced by the ovaries is *estradiol*. In the periphery, some of the estradiol secreted by the ovaries is converted into *estrone* and *estriol*; these estrogens are less potent than estradiol itself. Estrogens are eliminated by a combination of hepatic metabolism and urinary excretion.

During pregnancy, large quantities of estrogens are produced by the placenta. Excretion of these hormones results in high levels of estrogens in the urine. (The urine of pregnant mares is extremely rich in estrogens and serves as a commercial source of these hormones.)

***Males.*** Estrogen production is not limited to females. In the human male, small amounts of testosterone are converted into estradiol and estrone by the testes. Enzymatic conversion of testosterone in peripheral tissues (e.g., liver, fat, skeletal muscle) results in additional estrogen production. Underscoring the capacity of males to produce estrogen is the curious fact that stallions, despite their reputation for virility, excrete even greater quantities of urinary estrogens than do pregnant mares.

## Physiologic and Pharmacologic Effects

### Effects on Primary and Secondary Sex Characteristics of Females

Estrogens support the development and maintenance of the female reproductive tract and secondary sex characteristics. These hormones are required for the growth and maturation of the uterus, vagina, fallopian tubes, and breasts. In addition, estrogens direct development of pubic and axillary hair as well as pigmentation of the nipples and genitalia.

Estrogens have a profound influence on physiologic processes related to reproduction. During the follicular phase of the menstrual cycle, estrogens cause proliferation of the vaginal and uterine epithelium; secretions by the cervical glands are increased; and breast enlargement is induced. Estrogens increase vaginal acidity by promoting deposition of glycogen in the vaginal epithelium. At the end of the menstrual cycle, a decline in estrogen levels can bring on menstruation; however, it is the fall in progesterone levels at the end of the cycle that normally causes breakdown of the endometrium and resultant menstrual bleeding. Following menstruation, estrogens promote endometrial restoration. Although the effects of estrogens on the release of pituitary gonadotropins are not completely understood, it is clear that high levels of estrogen can suppress release of FSH. During pregnancy, estrogens stimulate uterine growth and blood flow. In addition, estrogens (along with progestins) act on the breasts to promote development of the acini.

### Metabolic Actions

Estrogens can affect various nonreproductive tissues. Important among these are bone, blood vessels, the heart, liver, and central nervous system.

**Bone.** Estrogens have a positive effect on bone mass. Under normal circumstances, bone undergoes a continuous process of remodeling, in which bone mineral is resorbed and deposited in equal amounts. The principal effect of estrogens on the process is to block bone resorption, although estrogens may also promote mineral deposition. In young girls, estrogens promote the rapid growth of the long bones that occurs during puberty; in addition, they direct epiphyseal closure, thereby bringing linear growth to a halt. In post menopausal women, estrogen replacement therapy can help maintain bone mass.

**Cholesterol.** Estrogens have favorable effects on cholesterol levels: levels of low-density lipoprotein (LDL) cholesterol are reduced, while levels of high-density lipoprotein (HDL) cholesterol are elevated. These beneficial effects on cholesterol metabolism result at least in part from actions of estrogens in the liver. There is specu-

lation, but no proof, that effects on cholesterol metabolism may explain the low incidence of myocardial infarction observed in premenopausal women.

Estrogens alter cholesterol excretion. Specifically, they increase the cholesterol content of bile and decrease the content of bile acids, which are needed to keep cholesterol soluble. These effects may explain why some women taking estrogens develop cholesterol gallstones.

## Clinical Pharmacology

### Adverse Effects

The principal concerns with estrogen therapy are the potential for endometrial hyperplasia, endometrial cancer, and breast cancer. Other adverse effects are more of a nuisance than a concern.

***Endometrial Hyperplasia and Carcinoma.*** Prolonged use of estrogens *alone* by postmenopausal women is associated with an increased risk of endometrial carcinoma. However, when estrogens are used in combination with a progestin, there is little or no risk of uterine cancer. Why? When used alone, estrogens act on the endometrium to cause proliferation and hyperplasia; in a few cases, hyperplasia progresses to carcinoma. Progestins eliminate (or at least greatly reduce) the risk of cancer by antagonizing estrogen-mediated endometrial proliferation and by reversing hyperplasia. Accordingly, whenever estrogens are given to postmenopausal women who have an intact uterus, progestins should be given as well. If persistent or recurrent vaginal bleeding develops during the course of estrogen use, the possibility of endometrial carcinoma should be evaluated. In addition, the patient should receive an endometrial biopsy every 2 to 3 years.

***Breast Cancer.*** The question of whether estrogens cause breast cancer has been investigated intensively—yet remains unresolved. More than 30 studies have been published. Two important studies reported in 1995 illustrate the confusion. The first study, published in the *New England Journal of Medicine*, reported a definitive link between long-term (greater than 5 years) estrogen therapy and breast cancer. The second study, published 1 month later in *JAMA* (Journal of the American Medical Association), found no such connection. Altogether, the available data suggest that estrogens pose a possible, albeit small, risk of breast cancer. A definitive answer should come from the Women's Health Initiative—a large, randomized, prospective trial whose initial results should be available in 2005. For now, however, the bottom line is we just don't know. Because all women are at potential risk for breast cancer, and because estrogens may increase that risk, women taking estrogens should be especially diligent about doing monthly breast self-exams and having a yearly mammogram.

Regardless of whether estrogens *cause* breast cancer, there is no question that these compounds promote the growth of certain cancers that have estrogen receptors. Accordingly, estrogen-dependent breast cancer must be ruled out before initiating estrogen treatment.

***Adverse Effects Associated with Use during Pregnancy.***
Use of estrogens during pregnancy can cause cancer and developmental abnormalities. Accordingly, women who become pregnant while taking estrogens should be apprised of the risks to the fetus. *Estrogens are classified in FDA Pregnancy Category X: the risks of use during pregnancy clearly outweigh any potential benefit.*

Diethylstilbestrol (DES), a nonsteroidal estrogen, has caused vaginal and cervical cancer in women who were exposed to this drug during fetal life (i.e., in women whose mothers took DES during pregnancy). Estimates of the incidence of vaginal and cervical cancer resulting from *in utero* exposure to DES range from 0.01% to 0.1%. These cancers appear most commonly when women who were exposed to DES reach 19 years of age; after the age of 30, the chance of developing these malignancies is very low. Although DES is the only estrogen clearly linked to induction of vaginal and cervical cancers, there is no reason to believe that other estrogens do not present a similar risk.

Use of DES during pregnancy has produced genital abnormalities (e.g., testicular hypoplasia) in the male fetus. Abnormal semen production has also occurred. There have been no reports of cancer in males following *in utero* exposure to DES.

***Nausea and Other Gastrointestinal Disturbances.***
*Nausea* is the most frequent undesired response to the estrogens. Fortunately, this reaction diminishes with continued use, and is rarely so severe as to necessitate cessation of therapy. Nausea can be minimized by administering estrogens with food and by initiating therapy with low doses. If taken in large doses, estrogens may cause anorexia, vomiting, and diarrhea.

***Other Adverse Effects.*** Use of estrogens during menopause produces a small increase in the risk of *gallbladder disease*. Treatment of breast cancer and bone metastases can result in severe *hypercalcemia*. Estrogens may cause *jaundice* in patients with pre-existing liver dysfunction. *Central nervous system (CNS) reactions* include headache, dizziness, and depression.

## Therapeutic Uses

In this chapter, discussion is limited to the noncontraceptive uses of estrogens. Use of estrogens for contraception is discussed in Chapter 58.

***Hormone Replacement Therapy after Menopause.***
Replacement therapy in postmenopausal women is the most common noncontraceptive use of estrogens. This use is discussed separately below.

***Female Hypogonadism.*** In the absence of estrogens, pubertal transformation will not take place. Causes of estrogen deficiency include primary ovarian failure, hypopituitarism, and bilateral oophorectomy (i.e., removal of both ovaries). In girls with estrogen insufficiency, puberty can be induced by administering exogenous estrogens. This treatment promotes breast development, maturation of the reproductive organs, and development of pubic and axillary hair. To simulate normal patterns of estrogen secretion, the regimen should consist of continuous low-dose therapy (for about a year) followed by cyclic administration of higher estrogen doses.

***Prostate Cancer.*** Growth of prostate cancer is dependent upon the presence of androgens (e.g., testosterone). Estrogens can help patients by suppressing androgen production. Estrogens reduce androgen synthesis by suppressing secretion of LH (also known as interstitial cell-stimulating hormone), the hormone required by the testes to support androgen production. Since gonadotropin-releasing hormone analogs (e.g., leuprolide) are also able to suppress LH secretion, but do not cause the feminizing side effects seen with estrogens, these agents have largely replaced estrogens for treatment of prostate cancer.

### Routes of Administration

***Oral, Intramuscular, Intravenous.*** The principal routes of administration are *oral* and *intramuscular*. With only one exception (conjugated estrogens), preparations that are used orally are not administered IM, and vice versa. As a rule, the oral preparations, because of their convenience, are preferred to parenteral estrogens. In addition to oral and IM use, some estrogens may be applied *intravaginally*. One preparation—conjugated estrogens—may be administered *intravenously*.

***Transdermal.*** Estradiol is available in transdermal patch formulations. Patches are applied to the skin of the trunk (but not the breasts), allowing estrogen to be absorbed through the skin and then directly into the bloodstream. When compared with oral administration, the patches have two significant advantages: (1) the total dosage of estrogen is greatly reduced (because the liver is bypassed) and (2) serum levels of estrogen produced by patches more closely resemble premenopausal estrogen levels than do the serum levels produced by oral estrogens. Rates of estrogen absorption range from 37.5 to 100 μg/hr, depending on the patch employed. Trade names are Estraderm, Climara, and Vivelle.

# Progestins

Progestins are compounds that have actions like those of progesterone, the principal endogenous progestational hormone. As their name implies, the progestins act prior to gestation to prepare the uterus for implantation of a fertilized ovum. In addition, progestins help maintain the uterus throughout pregnancy.

## Biosynthesis

Progesterone is produced by the ovaries and placenta. Ovarian production occurs during the second half of the menstrual cycle. During this period, progesterone is synthesized by the corpus luteum. Production of progesterone by the corpus luteum is regulated by LH secreted by the anterior pituitary. If implantation of a fertilized ovum fails to occur, progesterone production by the corpus luteum ceases, and menstrual flow begins. However, if implantation does take place, the developing trophoblast will produce its own luteotropic hormone (chorionic gonadotropin) that will act on the corpus luteum to promote continued progesterone secretion. By the second or third month of pregnancy, the placenta begins to produce progesterone of its own (along with estrogens). After this time, ovarian progesterone is no longer needed to support gestation. Placental synthesis of progesterone and estrogens continues throughout the remainder of pregnancy.

## Physiologic and Pharmacologic Effects

*Effects on the Endometrium and Endocervical Glands.* Progesterone secreted during the second half of the menstrual cycle converts the endometrium from a proliferative state into a secretory state. At the end of the menstrual cycle, progesterone production ceases. The resultant abrupt fall in progesterone levels is the principal stimulus for the onset of menstruation. In addition to affecting the endometrium, progesterone acts on the endocervical glands, causing their secretions to become scant and viscous. This action is opposite to that of estrogen, which promotes the flow of profuse, watery secretions.

*Effects during Pregnancy.* As noted above, progesterone levels increase during pregnancy. These high levels of progesterone are thought to have two actions that help to sustain pregnancy. First, progesterone inhibits uterine contraction. Second, progesterone may suppress the maternal immune response, thereby preventing immune rejection of the fetus.

*Other Effects.* Pharmacologic doses of progesterone can suppress release of pituitary gonadotropins (LH and FSH). This prevents maturation of follicles and ovulation. Also, individual progestin preparations display varying degrees of estrogenic, androgenic, and anabolic activity.

## Clinical Pharmacology

### Adverse Effects

*Teratogenic Effects.* Administration of progestins in high doses during the first 4 months of pregnancy has been associated with an increased incidence of birth defects (limb reductions, heart defects, masculinization of the female fetus). Accordingly, use of progestins during early pregnancy is not recommended. Women who become pregnant while taking progestins should be apprised of the potential risk to the fetus.

*Gynecologic Effects.* Because of their actions on the endometrium, progestins can cause breakthrough bleeding, spotting, and amenorrhea. Other effects include breast tenderness and alteration of cervical secretions. To facilitate evaluation of potential adverse drug responses, the patient should undergo examination of the breasts and pelvic organs prior to therapy. In addition, a Papanicolaou smear should be obtained and evaluated. Patients should be instructed to report any episodes of abnormal vaginal bleeding.

*Other Adverse Effects.* Progestins have been associated with depression, jaundice, edema, lethargy, photosensitivity, nausea, bloating, breast tenderness, and exacerbation of acute intermittent porphyria.

### Therapeutic Uses

Discussion in this chapter is limited to the noncontraceptive uses of progestins. Use of progestins for contraception is considered in Chapter 58.

*Hormone Replacement Therapy after Menopause.* The primary noncontraceptive use of progestins is to counteract the adverse effects of estrogen on the endometrium in women undergoing hormone replacement therapy. This application is discussed below.

*Dysfunctional Uterine Bleeding.* This condition occurs when progesterone levels are insufficient to balance the stimulatory influence of estrogen on the endometrium. In the absence of sufficient progesterone, estrogen puts the endometrium in a state of continuous proliferation. Since progesterone is unavailable to induce monthly endometrial breakdown, the excessively proliferative endometrium undergoes spontaneous sloughing at irregular intervals. Irregular breakdown of the endometrium can result in periodic episodes of severe menstrual bleeding. Alternatively, chronic spotting may be produced. Dysfunctional uterine bleeding is often associated with anovulatory cycles. The disorder occurs most commonly in adolescents and in women approaching menopause.

Treatment has two objectives: the initial goal is cessation of hemorrhage; the long-term goal is to establish a regular monthly cycle. Excessive bleeding can be stopped by administering a progestin for several days. Dosing may be continued for 2 weeks for sustained suppression. When progestin administration is stopped, withdrawal bleeding will take place. This bleeding is likely to be profuse and associated with cramping.

Cyclic therapy is employed to establish a regular monthly cycle. In this regimen, administration of an oral progestin is initiated 5 days after the onset of each menstrual period and continued for the next 20 days. This form of therapy promotes a repeating pattern of endometrial proliferation followed by endometrial breakdown and menstruation.

*Amenorrhea.* Progestins can induce menstrual flow in selected women who are experiencing amenorrhea. If endogenous estrogen levels are adequate, treatment with a progestin for 5 to 10 days will be followed by withdrawal bleeding when the progestin is discontinued. If estrogen levels are low, it may be necessary to induce endometrial proliferation with an estrogen prior to giving the progestin. Cyclic therapy can be used to promote regular monthly flow. This form of treatment consists of estrogen administration for 25 days coupled with progestin administration on days 15 through 25. The regimen is repeated beginning on the first day of each month.

*Endometriosis.* Endometriosis is a disorder in which endometrial tissue has become implanted in an abnormal location (e.g., uterine wall, ovary, extragenital sites). This condition is painful and a frequent cause of infertility and spontaneous abortion. Endometriosis can be treated surgically, or growth of the implants can be suppressed with drugs. When drug therapy is indicated, the medication most commonly employed is danazol. This agent inhibits synthesis of estrogens and progesterone, thereby depriving the implant of the hormones required to support its growth.

Before danazol became available, progestins (alone or in combination with an estrogen) were the preferred pharmacologic therapy of endometriosis. Continuous (noncyclic) treatment for 6 to 9 months can often produce symptomatic relief as well as regression of ectopic endometrial growths. Progestins that have been used against endometriosis include medroxyprogesterone acetate (MPA) and norethindrone.

*Endometrial Carcinoma.* Progestins can induce beneficial responses (palliation, regression of tumor size, remission) in women with metastatic endometrial carcinoma. Several months of treatment may be required before a response is observed. The progestins employed for this indication are *medroxyprogesterone acetate* (MPA) and *megestrol acetate*. MPA is given once weekly by IM injection; megestrol acetate is administered daily by mouth. In addition to its use against endometrial carcinoma, megestrol acetate may provide palliation for women with breast cancer.

***Premenstrual Syndrome.*** Progesterone has been widely prescribed for premenstrual syndrome (PMS). However, it is now clear that the practice should cease. In controlled studies, progesterone was shown to be no more effective than placebo. Furthermore, there is evidence that progesterone may actually cause PMS symptoms. PMS is discussed further below.

### Preparations and Routes

Progestins may be administered orally or parenterally (IM). Oral progestins include *medroxyprogesterone acetate* [Provera], *norethindrone* [Micronor, Nor-Q.D.], *norethindrone acetate* [Aygestin], and *megestrol acetate* [Megace]. Intramuscular progestins are *medroxyprogesterone acetate* [Depo-Provera], *hydroxyprogesterone caproate* [Hylutin, Hypògest 250], and *progesterone* (in oil).

# Hormone Replacement Therapy after Menopause

Menopause results from a decline in ovarian follicles. Onset usually occurs at about 50 years of age. During the initial phase, the menstrual cycle is irregular; anovulatory cycles may occur, and periods of amenorrhea may alternate with menses. Eventually, ovulation and menstruation cease entirely. Production of ovarian estrogens decreases gradually, coming to a complete stop several years after menstruation has ceased.

Loss of estrogen has multiple physiologic consequences. Prominent among these are vasomotor symptoms (hot flushes), accelerated bone loss, and increased risk of coronary heart disease.

Hormone replacement therapy (HRT) typically consists of an estrogen combined with a progestin. The purpose of the estrogen is to replace the estrogen that was lost at menopause. The purpose of the progestin is to counteract adverse effects that unopposed estrogen has on the endometrium. In women who no longer have a uterus, the progestin is omitted.

### Benefits of Hormone Replacement Therapy

Replacement of estrogen offers three primary benefits: suppression of vasomotor symptoms, prevention of osteoporosis, and prevention of coronary heart disease. For suppression of vasomotor symptoms, HRT is employed short term. For prevention of osteoporosis and heart disease, HRT should continue lifelong.

***Suppression of Vasomotor Symptoms.*** In most women, estrogen decline causes vasomotor symptoms, characterized by hot flushes (flashes) that may alternate with sweating or chilliness. Vasomotor symptoms generally respond well to HRT. *Clonidine* [Catapres], a centrally acting alpha$_2$ agonist, can help as well. Since vasomotor symptoms gradually subside over time, the need for continued HRT should be periodically reassessed (unless, of course, the objective of therapy includes prevention of the long-term sequelae of estrogen loss).

***Prevention of Osteoporosis.*** Osteoporosis is characterized by demineralization and weakening of the bones.

Compression fractures of the vertebrae are common. Fractures of the hip and wrist can be caused by minimal trauma. Osteoporosis occurs in a majority (about 70%) of elderly white females; males and black females rarely experience this disorder. The condition develops following surgical removal of the ovaries as well as after menopause. Estrogen deficiency is the principal cause.

In postmenopausal women, HRT decreases bone loss and reduces the incidence of fractures. However, it must be stressed that HRT is primarily prophylactic: estrogens do little to reverse bone loss that has already occurred. Exercise and calcium supplements are important adjuncts to estrogen therapy. To prevent osteoporosis, HRT must continue lifelong. Osteoporosis and its treatment are discussed at length in Chapter 75.

***Protection against Coronary Heart Disease.*** In the United States, cardiovascular disease is the leading killer of women over age 65. The underlying cause appears to be loss of the protective effects of estrogen. This conclusion is based on three observations: (1) the incidence of cardiovascular disease increases after menopause; (2) the incidence of angina pectoris and myocardial infarction is lower in postmenopausal women who use HRT than in those who do not; and (3) the incidence of myocardial infarction is lower in premenopausal women than in men of the same age. Estrogens protect against cardiovascular disease at least in part by elevating HDL cholesterol and lowering LDL cholesterol.

***Maintenance of Estrogen-Dependent Tissues.*** Estrogen loss is also associated with degenerative changes in estrogen-dependent tissues: the endometrium atrophies, uterine muscle mass declines, and the vaginal epithelium becomes reduced in thickness and glycogen content. Changes in the vaginal epithelium may lead to atrophic vaginitis. To prevent these changes, estrogens must be taken long term. Administration may be oral or transdermal. For atrophic vaginitis, estrogens may be administered orally or in a vaginal cream.

### Risks of Hormone Replacement Therapy

Minor adverse effects can be common; serious problems are rare. Nausea occurs in up to 20% of women during the first 2 to 3 months of HRT. Fluid retention may result in weight gain and breast tenderness. With cyclic regimens, menstrual bleeding occurs. Because estrogens are now combined with a progestin in HRT, the risk of endometrial cancer is low or nonexistent. The biggest concern with HRT is the possibility of an increased risk of breast cancer.

### Making a Decision about Hormone Replacement Therapy

Women going through menopause must make a decision about HRT. With short-term therapy, the choice is relatively easy. Estrogens can be taken for a few years to relieve vasomotor symptoms and vaginal dryness, while causing only minor side effects (e.g., initial nausea, breast tenderness, vaginal bleeding). There is general agreement that HRT poses no risk of breast cancer when used for less than 5 years.

Deciding on long-term HRT is much more difficult. Lifelong therapy has important benefits—protection against osteoporosis and heart disease—but, as discussed earlier, may (or may not) increase the risk of breast cancer. Given the uncertainty about breast cancer, how can a decision be made? One argument regarding the dilemma goes like this: since many more women die early from heart disease than from breast cancer, more lives will be prolonged by reducing the risk of heart disease with HRT than will be shortened by (possibly) increasing the risk of breast cancer. Looking at the issue from a more personal perspective, if a woman has high LDL cholesterol, low HDL cholesterol, and hypertension, if she smokes a lot, and if her mother suffered a hip fracture, she may well be a good candidate for HRT. Conversely, if a woman is not at increased risk for coronary heart disease, has good bone mass, and has a long family history of cancer, prolonged HRT may be a bad choice. Ultimately, each woman must make her own decision. Factors to consider are family history of cancer, heart disease, and osteoporosis; personal risk factors; and fears. Unfortunately, until questions regarding breast cancer have been answered, the choice will remain difficult.

### Regimens for Hormone Replacement Therapy

Every women undergoing HRT receives an estrogen, and every woman with an intact uterus also receives a progestin (to counteract the adverse effects of estrogen on the endometrium). Although several schedules of administration may be employed, in the protocol recommended most, estrogen is administered *continuously* (i.e., every day of the month), whereas the progestin is administered *cyclically* (i.e., on calendar days 1 through 12). Cyclic pro-

gestin administration has the disadvantage of promoting monthly menstrual bleeding, but has the advantage of being the only schedule thus far proved both safe and effective.

Some drug preparations for HRT are listed in Table 57-1. The estrogens employed most often are conjugated estrogens [Premarin], estradiol [Estrace], and transdermal estrogen [Estraderm, others]. The progestins employed most often are medroxyprogesterone acetate [Provera, Cycrin, others] and norethindrone acetate [Aygestin, Micronor, Nor-Q.D.].

## Premenstrual Syndrome

Premenstrual syndrome consists of a constellation of psychologic and physical symptoms that develop in the luteal phase of the menstrual cycle and then resolve a few days after the onset of menses. Common psychologic symptoms include irritability, depression, mood lability, crying spells, and social withdrawal. Common physical symptoms include acne, breast tenderness, abdominal bloating, and appetite disturbance. Additional symptoms are listed in Table 57-2. Psychologic symptoms are much more disabling than physical symptoms. Other names for PMS are *premenstrual dysphoric disorder* and *late luteal phase dysphoric disorder*. Premenstrual syndrome is among the most common disorders in women of reproductive age.

### Diagnosis

To make a diagnosis of PMS, symptoms must be *intense* and they must be *intermittent* (i.e., there must be a symptom-free interval between days 4 and 12 of the men-

**TABLE 57-1. ESTROGENS AND PROGESTINS USED FOR HRT**

| Drug | Trade Names | Dosage* |
|---|---|---|
| *Estrogens, oral* | | |
| Conjugated estrogens | Premarin | 0.625 mg/day |
| Estropipate | Ogen, Otho-Est | 0.625 mg/day |
| Estradiol | Estrace | 0.5 mg/day |
| Ethinyl estradiol | Estinyl | 0.02 mg/day |
| *Estrogens, transdermal* | | |
| Estradiol | Estraderm, Climara, Vivelle | 0.5 mg over 24 hr |
| *Progestins (oral)* | | |
| Medroxyprogesterone acetate | Provera, Cycrin, others | 5 or 10 mg on days 1–12 |
| Norethindrone acetate | Aygestin | 0.35–2.5 mg on days 1–12 |
| Norethindrone | Micronor, Nor-Q.D. | 0.35–2.5 mg on days 1–12 |

*For estrogens: minimum daily dosage to prevent bone loss.

## TABLE 57-2. COMMON SYMPTOMS OF PMS

| Psychologic and Behavioral Symptoms | Physical Symptoms |
| --- | --- |
| Irritability | Acne |
| Depression, sadness, or hopelessness | Breast tenderness |
| Mood lability: alternating sadness and anger | Abdominal bloating |
| Hypersensitivity to trivial events | Ankle edema |
| Loneliness and social withdrawal | Fatigue |
| Crying spells | Headache |
| Anxiety | Backache |
| Difficulty concentrating | Constipation or diarrhea |
| Decreased sense of well-being | Nausea, vomiting |
| Reduced efficiency or work performance | Food craving (especially carbohydrates) |
| Restlessness, agitation | Weight gain |
| Tension | Joint and muscle pain |

strual cycle). Practically all women experience some PMS-like symptoms in the late luteal phase of the menstrual cycle. However, in the vast majority of women, symptoms are of low intensity, and are therefore considered physiologic—not pathologic. These normal physiologic symptoms are referred to as *molimina*. In contrast to women who experience molimina, about 3% to 5% of women have luteal phase symptoms that are severe enough to be considered pathologic. Timing of symptoms is critical to a diagnosis. On days 4 through 12 of the cycle, symptoms should be absent, or at least no greater than would be expected in the population at large. Symptoms should begin in the third week of the cycle, and become most intense in the fourth week (i.e., late in the luteal phase). To make a diagnosis, total symptom severity in the fourth week must be at least twice the intensity of any symptoms present in the second week. Daily charting of symptoms for at least two menstrual cycles is needed to establish whether symptoms occur in the appropriate pattern and are of sufficient intensity to permit a diagnosis of PMS.

### Etiology

Although PMS is clearly of neuroendocrine origin, the exact cause is unknown. At one time, hormonal abnormality was suspected. However, we now know that hormone levels in women who experience PMS are identical to those in women who do not. Hence, hormonal abnormality cannot be the cause. Nonetheless, since symptoms are synchronized with the menstrual cycle, it would seem that hormones are in some way involved—even if they are normal. One reasonable hypothesis is that women who experience PMS are sensitive to hormonal changes in a way that other women are not; because of this special sensitivity, normal hormonal changes are able to trigger PMS. The ability of serotonin reuptake inhibitors to relieve dysphoric symptoms (see below) suggests that susceptibility to mood changes, which are the principal complaint in PMS, may result from altered serotonergic transmission in the CNS.

### Drug Therapy

Over the years, many different drugs have been tried. Unfortunately, none has proved consistently effective. Selective serotonin uptake inhibitors are currently considered drugs of first choice.

***Selective Serotonin Reuptake Inhibitors (SSRIs).*** Fluoxetine [Prozac] and other SSRIs are the most effective therapy known for PMS. These agents can significantly reduce depression, anger, irritability, tension, fatigue, and confusion in many women. Success rates range from 50% to 75%. Since symptoms of PMS are much like the symptoms of depression states that have been linked to serotonergic dysregulation, the efficacy of SSRIs in PMS is not surprising. SSRIs do not relieve the physical symptoms of PMS.

The dosage used most frequently is 20 mg/day administered on a continuous schedule. However, intermittent therapy appears equally effective. For intermittent therapy, dosing is begun on day 14 of the menstrual cycle, stopped on day 2 of the following cycle, resumed on day 14, and so forth. Because SSRIs cause CNS stimulation, they are usually taken in the morning.

In clinical trials, about 15% of women discontinued treatment because of side effects. These include insomnia, agitation, gastrointestinal disturbances, headache, and sexual dysfunction. Contrary to reports in the popular press, fluoxetine does not increase suicidal tendencies. If side effects are intolerable, initial doses as low as 5 mg/day can be tried.

The basic pharmacology of the SSRIs is discussed in Chapter 30 (Antidepressants).

***Alprazolam.*** Alprazolam [Xanax], a member of the benzodiazepine family, is superior to placebo for reducing irritability, anxiety, severe tension, and the feeling of being out of control. Unfortunately, daytime sedation is significant at the doses needed to suppress these symptoms. Alprazolam is administered only during the luteal phase. Doses should be tapered to minimize withdrawal symptoms.

**Gonadotropin-Releasing Hormone Agonists.** Leuprolide and other gonadotropin-releasing hormone (Gn-RH) agonists can reduce physical and psychologic symptoms of PMS. Treatment has relieved breast tenderness, bloating, depression, nervous tension, anxiety, and loss of control. These agents act by suppressing release of LH and FSH from the pituitary, which in turn causes levels of estrogen and progesterone to fall to postmenopausal levels. Unfortunately, loss of estrogen increases the risk of osteoporosis and cardiovascular disease. Hence, even though Gn-RH agonists may help reduce symptoms of PMS, serious adverse effects preclude their use for more than 6 months. The pharmacology of Gn-RH agonists is discussed further in Chapter 59.

**Danazol and Bromocriptine.** Both of these drugs can reduce cyclical breast tenderness and pain. Side effects of danazol include virilization, edema, and liver dysfunction. Side effects of bromocriptine include nausea, headache, dizziness, fatigue, and abdominal cramps. Both drugs are discussed further in Chapter 59.

**Spironolactone.** Spironolactone [Aldactone], a potassium-sparing diuretic, can counteract water retention, and thereby relieve bloating. Treatment should be reserved for women with documented weight gain, and should be limited to the luteal phase.

**Analgesics.** *Aspirin*, *acetaminophen*, and *ibuprofen* have no effect on mood, but can reduce headache, dysmenorrhea, cramps, muscle pain, and joint pain.

**Drugs That Offer Little or No Benefit.** *Progesterone* has been used for years on the theory that it may produce a favorable hormonal balance. However, we now know that progesterone is no more effective than placebo, and in fact may exacerbate some symptoms (bloating, breast tenderness, emotional lability). *Pyridoxine* (vitamin B$_6$) offers no benefits in PMS, and using it can cause sensory neuropathies. Other drugs that have no proven benefits include *tamoxifen*, *lithium*, *atenolol*, *magnesium*, and *calcium*.

# KEY POINTS

- Estradiol is the principal endogenous estrogen.
- Progesterone is the principal endogenous progestational hormone.
- The first half of the 28-day menstrual cycle is called the follicular phase; the second half is called the luteal phase.
- During the follicular phase, estrogens produced by maturing ovarian follicles cause proliferation of the endometrium.
- During the luteal phase, estrogens and progesterone produced by the corpus luteum maintain the endometrium in its hypertrophied state.
- Toward the end of the menstrual cycle, progesterone levels decline, causing the hypertrophied endometrium to break down, which results in bleeding.
- In addition to their role in the menstrual cycle, estrogens are required for the growth and maturation of the uterus, vagina, fallopian tubes, and breasts. Estrogens also control development of pubic and axillary hair as well as pigmentation of the nipples and genitalia.
- Estrogens suppress bone mineral resorption, and thereby have a positive effect on bone mass.
- Estrogens raise levels of HDL cholesterol and reduce levels of LDL cholesterol. These actions may explain the low incidence of coronary heart disease in premenopausal women.
- Nausea is the most common adverse effect of exogenous estrogens.
- Prolonged use of estrogens *alone* is associated with an increased risk of endometrial carcinoma. However, when estrogens are used in combination with a progestin, there is little or no risk of uterine cancer.
- When taken less than 5 years, estrogens pose no risk of breast cancer. When taken longer than 5 years, estrogens may (or may not) pose a risk of breast cancer.
- Use of estrogens during pregnancy can cause vaginal and cervical cancer in female offspring and genital malformation in male fetuses. Accordingly, estrogens are contraindicated during pregnancy.
- Progestins may cause birth defects during the first 4 months of pregnancy; hence their use during pregnancy is not recommended.
- Because of their actions on the endometrium, exogenous progestins can cause breakthrough bleeding, spotting, and amenorrhea.
- The principal consequences of estrogen loss after menopause are vasomotor symptoms (hot flushes), accelerated bone loss, and increased risk of coronary heart disease.
- HRT in postmenopausal women typically consists of an estrogen combined with a progestin. The estrogen replaces the estrogen that was lost at menopause. The progestin counteracts adverse effects that unopposed estrogen has on the endometrium. In women who no longer have a uterus, the progestin is omitted.
- Replacement of estrogen offers three primary benefits: suppression of vasomotor symptoms, prevention of osteoporosis, and prevention of coronary heart disease.
- Short-term HRT (i.e., 5 years or less) poses no risk of breast cancer or any other cancer. Long-term HRT may (or may not) increase the risk of breast cancer.
- Premenstrual syndrome (PMS) consists of a constellation of psychologic and physical symptoms that develop in the luteal phase of the menstrual cycle and then resolve a few days after the onset of menses.
- Psychologic symptoms of PMS (e.g., irritability, depression, mood lability, crying spells, social withdrawal) are more disabling that physical symptoms (e.g., acne, breast tenderness, abdominal bloating, appetite disturbance).
- To make a diagnosis of PMS, symptoms must be sufficiently intense, and must be *absent* between days 4 and 12 of the menstrual cycle.
- Fluoxetine [Prozac] and other SSRIs are the most effective drugs known for PMS. These agents relieve psychologic symptoms, which are the principal complaint in PMS, but do not relieve physical symptoms.

## Summary of Major Nursing Implications*

# Estrogens

| | |
|---|---|
| Conjugated estrogens | Estrone |
| Diethylstilbestrol | Estropipate |
| Estradiol | Ethinyl estradiol |

## Preadministration Assessment

### Therapeutic Goal

Estrogens are used primarily for contraception (see Chapter 58) and for hormone replacement therapy in postmenopausal women. Additional indications are female hypogonadism, breast cancer, prostatic cancer, and dysfunctional uterine bleeding.

### Baseline Data

Assessment should include a breast examination, pelvic examination, Papanicolaou smear, lipid profile, mammography, and blood pressure measurement. If the objective is hormone replacement therapy, menopause should be verified.

### Identifying High-Risk Patients

Estrogens are *contraindicated* during *pregnancy* and for patients with *estrogen-dependent cancer, undiagnosed abnormal vaginal bleeding, active thrombophlebitis or thromboembolic disorders,* or a *history of estrogen-associated thrombophlebitis, thrombosis, or thromboembolic disorders.*

## Implementation: Administration

### Routes

Oral, IM, IV, transdermal, and intravaginal.

### Administration

**Transdermal.** Give the patient the following instructions for using the estradiol transdermal system: (1) apply the transdermal patch to an area of clean, dry, intact skin on the abdomen or some other region of the trunk (but not the breasts or waistline) by pressing the patch firmly in place and holding for 10 seconds; (2) if the patch falls off, reapply the same patch or, if necessary, apply a new patch; (3) remove the old patch and apply a new one twice weekly; and (4) rotate the application site such that the same site is not used more than once each week.

**Intravaginal.** Instruct the patient to apply the estrogen preparation high into the vagina using the applicator provided.

### Dosing Schedule for Hormone Replacement Therapy

In the schedule recommended most, estrogen is administered every day of the month, and, for women with an intact uterus, a progestin is administered on the first 12 days of the month. The progestin is eliminated if the woman has no uterus. *Note:* many other dosing schedules are possible.

## Ongoing Evaluation and Interventions

### Monitoring Summary

The patient should receive a yearly follow-up breast and pelvic exam. An endometrial biopsy should be performed every 2 to 3 years.

### Minimizing Adverse Effects

**Nausea.** Nausea is common early in treatment but diminishes with time. Inform the patient that nausea can be reduced by taking estrogens with food.

**Endometrial Hyperplasia and Cancer.** Therapy with estrogen alone during menopause increases the risk of endometrial carcinoma. Adding a progestin to the regimen eliminates (or at least greatly reduces) this risk. Instruct the patient to notify the physician if persistent or recurrent vaginal bleeding develops so that the possibility of endometrial carcinoma can be evaluated. Also, the patient should receive an endometrial biopsy every 2 to 3 years.

**Breast Cancer.** Estrogens may (or may not) produce a small increase in the risk of breast cancer. Either way, educate the patient about the importance of doing monthly breast self-exams and having a yearly mammogram.

**Use during Pregnancy.** *In utero* exposure to estrogens can cause genital abnormalities in males and vaginal cancer in females. Accordingly, estrogens are *contraindicated during pregnancy.* Inform women of child-bearing age about the potential risks to the fetus. Instruct the patient to discontinue estrogens immediately if pregnancy is suspected.

**Effects Resembling Those Caused by Oral Contraceptives.** Use of estrogens for noncontraceptive purposes can produce adverse effects similar to those caused by oral contraceptives (e.g., abnormal vaginal bleeding, hypertension, benign hepatic adenoma, reduced glucose tolerance). Nursing implications regarding these effects are summarized in Chapter 58.

### Minimizing Adverse Interactions

The interactions of estrogens are probably similar to those seen with the oral contraceptives. Implications regarding these interactions are summarized in Chapter 58.

# Progestins

| | |
|---|---|
| Hydroxyprogesterone acetate | Megestrol |
| Levonorgestrel | Norethindrone |
| Medroxyprogesterone acetate | Norgestrel |
| | Progesterone |

## Preadministration Assessment

### Therapeutic Goal

Progestins are used primarily for contraception (see Chapter 58) and to counteract the adverse endometrial effects of estrogens during HRT. Other uses include dysfunctional uterine bleeding, amenorrhea, and endometriosis.

### Baseline Data

The physical examination should include breast and pelvic examinations. A Papanicolaou smear should be obtained.

### Identifying High-Risk Patients

Progestins are *contraindicated* in the presence of *undiagnosed abnormal vaginal bleeding, thrombophlebitis, thromboembolic disorders, severe liver disease*, and *carcinoma of the breast and reproductive organs*. Progestins should be *avoided* during *pregnancy*.

## Implementation: Administration

### Routes

Oral, IM.

### Administration

Advise the patient to take oral progestins with food if gastrointestinal upset occurs.

## Ongoing Evaluation and Interventions

### Minimizing Adverse Effects

***Teratogenic Effects.*** Progestins can cause birth defects (limb reductions, heart defects, masculinization of the female fetus) if taken during the first 4 months of pregnancy. Inform women of child-bearing age about the potential risks to the fetus. Instruct the patient to discontinue progestins immediately if pregnancy is suspected.

***Gynecologic Effects.*** Inform the patient about potential side effects (breakthrough bleeding, spotting, amenorrhea, alteration of cervical secretions, breast tenderness). Instruct the patient to notify the physician if abnormal vaginal bleeding occurs.

# CHAPTER 58

# Birth Control

Birth control can be accomplished by interfering with the reproductive process at any step from gametogenesis to nidation (implantation of a fertilized ovum). Pharmacologic methods of contraception include oral contraceptives, levonorgestrel implants, depot medroxyprogesterone acetate, a progesterone-containing intrauterine device, and gossypol (an investigational agent that suppresses sperm production). Nonpharmacologic methods include surgical sterilization (tubal ligation, vasectomy), mechanical devices (condom, diaphragm, cervical cap), and avoiding intercourse during periods of fertility (calendar method, temperature method, cervical mucus method).

Although we have birth control methods that are safe and effective, statistics show that unwanted pregnancy is common—suggesting that available methods are not used as widely or effectively as they could be, and that alternatives to current methods are needed. In the United States, nearly 6 of every 10 pregnancies is unplanned or unwanted. Among girls ages 15 to 17, the pregnancy rate is 1 in 10. However, although much attention is focused on teenage pregnancy, fully 80% of unplanned pregnancies occur in woman age 20 or older. Of the 3.6 million unplanned pregnancies that occur annually, about 2 million are carried to term; the other 1.6 million end in abortion.

Our principal focus in this chapter is on oral contraceptives. These agents are the second most widely used form of birth control (sterilization is first), and are among the most effective methods available. In preparing to study these agents and other forms of contraception, you should review Chapter 57, paying special attention to information on the menstrual cycle and the physiologic and pharmacologic effects of estrogens and progestins.

## Effectiveness and Safety of Birth Control Methods

### Effectiveness

The effectiveness of a birth control method can be expressed in terms of the percentage of accidental pregnancies that occur during use of that particular technique. Employing this criterion, Table 58-1 compares the effectiveness of the major birth control methods. As we can see, the most effective methods are Norplant, Depo-Provera, IUDs, and sterilization. Oral contraceptives are close behind. The least reliable methods include periodic abstinence, spermicides, and the cervical cap.

Note that Table 58-1 contains two columns of figures, one labeled *optimal* and the other *typical*. The *optimal* figures are the pregnancy rates that are likely when a method of birth control is employed exactly as it should be (i.e., consistently and with proper technique). The *typical* figures represent pregnancy rates observed in actual practice. The higher pregnancy rates reported in the typical column are largely an indication that methods of birth control are not always used when and as they should be.

### Safety

The issue of the relative safety of birth control measures is complex. Contributing to this complexity is the fact that much of our information on the adverse effects of oral contraceptives (OCs) was gathered when these agents were employed in doses higher than those employed today. Newer data show that OCs, as currently prescribed, are considerably safer than older studies indicate. An additional complication regarding the safety of birth control measures stems from the fact that the risk of mortality associated with pregnancy and delivery is greater than the risk associated with any form of birth control. Hence, a birth control measure that is inherently more safe than others, but is also less effective, may become relatively less safe when the dangers associated with a greater pregnancy rate are factored into the equation.

Keeping the above provisos in mind, we can make the following observations on birth control safety. Of the contraceptive methods available, OCs produce the broadest spectrum of adverse effects, ranging from nausea to menstrual irregularity to rare thromboembolic disorders. However, despite their wide variety of undesired actions, when used by nonsmoking women with normal cardiovascular function, OCs produce no greater mortality than other active forms of birth control. The lowest mortality rate is seen when barrier methods (diaphragm, condom, cervical cap) are used together with abortion (if contraceptive failure should occur). As discussed below, women who are at risk for sexually transmitted disease should not use an intrauterine device (IUD).

## Selecting a Birth Control Method

Figure 58-1 indicates the percentage of users who select particular forms of birth control. Perhaps surprisingly, the method chosen most often is sterilization: female sterilization (tubal ligation) plus male sterilization (vasectomy) are selected by over 42% of birth control users. Oral contraceptives or condoms are chosen by most of the remaining birth control users. Diaphragms, periodic abstinence, and IUDs account for only a small fraction of birth control use.

Several factors should be considered when choosing a method of birth control. Chief among these are *effectiveness, safety,* and *personal preference*. As indicated in Table 58-1, the most effective methods are levonorgestrel subdermal implants [Norplant], intramuscular medroxyprogesterone acetate [Depo-Provera], sterilization, and IUDs. Oral contraceptives are close behind. The remaining methods—condoms, diaphragm, cervical cap, spermicides, and periodic abstinence—must be used in a near-perfect fashion to provide any reasonable level of protection.

When factoring safety into the choice of a birth control method, several guidelines apply. Oral contraceptives should be avoided by women with certain cardiovascular disorders (see below) and should be used with caution by women who smoke heavily. For women in these categories, a barrier method or an IUD would be preferable to OCs. Although OCs are both effective and relatively convenient, they can also cause many side effects; women who consider the benefit-to-risk ratio unfavorable should be advised about alternative contraceptive techniques. Women who are at risk for a sexually transmitted disease (i.e., women who are not in a mutually monogamous relationship) should not use an IUD.

Personal preference is a major factor in providing the motivation needed for consistent implementation of a birth control method. Since even the best form of contraception will be ineffective if improperly practiced, the importance of personal preference cannot be stressed too strongly. Practitioners should take pains to educate clients about the various contraceptive methods available so that expressions of preference can be based on understanding.

Additional factors that bear on selection of a birth control method include family planning goals, age, frequency of sexual intercourse, and the individual's capacity for compliance. If family planning goals have already been met, sterilization of either the male or female partner may be desirable. For women who engage in coitus frequently, OCs or a long-term method (Norplant, Depo-Provera, IUD) are reasonable choices. Conversely, when sexual activity is limited, use of a spermicide, condom, or diaphragm may be most appropriate. Since barrier methods combined with spermicides can offer some protection against venereal disease (as well as providing contraception), these combinations may be of special benefit to individuals who have multiple partners. If compliance is a problem (as it can be with OCs, condoms, and diaphragms), use of a long-term method (IUD, Norplant, Depo-Provera) would confer reliable protection.

## Oral Contraceptives

### Classification

There are two main categories of OCs: (1) those that contain both an estrogen and a progestin, known as *combination OCs,* and (2) those that contain only a progestin, known as "minipills" or *progestin-only OCs*. Of the two groups, combination OCs are by far the more widely used.

The combination OCs have four subgroups: *monophasic, biphasic, triphasic* and *estrophasic*. In a monophasic regimen, the daily estrogen and progestin dosage remains constant throughout the monthly cycle of use. In a biphasic regimen, the estrogen dosage remains constant, but the progestin dosage is increased during the second half of the cycle. In triphasic regimens, the monthly cycle is divided into three phases. In all triphasic regimens, the progestin dosage changes for each phase of the cycle; in one regimen, the estrogen dosage also varies. In the estrophasic regimen, the progestin dose remains constant and the estrogen dose gradually increases through the monthly cycle.

### Combination Oral Contraceptives

Since their introduction in the late 1950s, combination OCs have become one of our most widely prescribed families of drugs. As indicated in Table 58-1, these agents are nearly 100% effective, making them one of the most efficacious forms of birth control available. Not only are these drugs highly effective, they are also very safe, although minor side effects are relatively common.

## TABLE 58-1. EFFECTIVENESS OF BIRTH CONTROL METHODS

| Birth Control Method | Failure Rate* (%) | |
| --- | --- | --- |
| | Typical[†] | Optimal[‡] |
| Levonorgestrel subdermal implant [Norplant] | 0.09% | 0.09% |
| Surgical sterilization | | |
| *Female: tubal ligation* | 0.4% | 0.2% |
| *Male: vasectomy* | 0.15% | 0.1% |
| Intramuscular medroxyprogesterone acetate [Depo-Provera] | 0.3% | 0.3% |
| Intrauterine devices | | |
| *Copper T 380A* [ParaGard] | 0.8% | 0.6% |
| *Progesterone T* [Progestasert] | 2% | 1.5% |
| Oral contraceptives | | |
| *Combination pills* | 3% | 0.1% |
| *Progestin-only pills* | 2% | 0.5% |
| Condoms | | |
| *Male* | 12% | 3% |
| *Female* | 21% | 5% |
| Diaphragm with spermicide | 18% | 6% |
| Cervical cap with spermicide | 18% | 11.5% |
| Spermicide alone | 21% | 6% |
| Periodic abstinence | 20% | 2–10% |
| No birth control | Pregnancy rate would be 80%–85% | |

*Failure rate = percentage of women who have an accidental pregnancy during first year of use.
[†]Typical = failure rate usually observed in actual practice.
[‡]Optimal = failure rate that would be expected if the birth control method were practiced exactly as it should be.

## Chemistry

Combination OCs consist of an *estrogen* plus a *progestin*. Only two estrogens are employed: *ethinyl estradiol* and *mestranol* (see Table 58-3). In contrast, several progestins are used, *norethindrone* being employed most often.

## Mechanism of Action

Combination OCs decrease fertility in several ways. The principal effect of these agents is *inhibition of ovulation*. The precise mechanism by which inhibition occurs is not known. In addition, OCs can promote thickening of the cervical mucus, thereby creating a barrier to the passage of sperm. Also, OCs can modify the endometrium, making it less favorable for nidation.

## Adverse Effects

Combination OCs can cause a wide variety of adverse effects. However, although many types of effects may be produced, severe effects are rare. Hence, when compared with the serious risks associated with pregnancy and childbirth, the risks of OCs are low.

Since OCs are taken by women who are healthy, and since OCs represent a potential health hazard (albeit small), it is important that steps be taken to minimize any risks associated with OC use. Accordingly, a thorough physical examination should be performed. This examination should include blood pressure determination, examination of the breasts and pelvic organs, and a Papanicolaou smear. These tests should be repeated at least once a year.

***Thromboembolic Disorders.*** Combination OCs have been associated with venous and arterial thromboembolism, pulmonary embolism, myocardial infarction, and thrombotic stroke. These thrombotic disorders are caused by the *estrogen* component of combination OCs—not by the progestin. Thrombosis results at least in part from an increase in circulating levels of clotting factors. Thrombosis is not due to atherosclerosis.

In contrast to older OCs, the OCs available today carry a low risk of thrombosis. When combination OCs first became available, they contained *high* doses of estrogens (e.g., 100 µg ethinyl estradiol). As a result, these preparations carried a significant risk of thrombotic disorders. Because today's OCs contain *low* doses of estrogens—no more than 50 µg ethinyl estradiol, and usually less—the risk of thrombosis among users is only slightly greater than among nonusers.

The risk of thromboembolic phenomena from OCs is increased in the presence of other risk factors, espe-

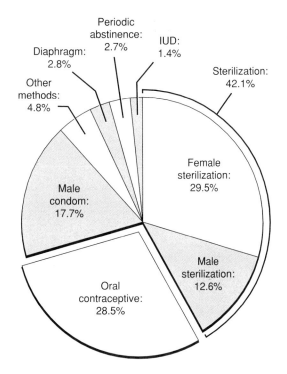

**Figure 58–1. Percentage use for birth control methods.**
*Note:* the segment labeled "other methods" refers to douching, withdrawal, contraceptives sponges, spermicides, and other techniques.

cially *heavy smoking* and a *history of thromboembolism*. Additional risk factors include cerebrovascular disease, coronary artery disease, myocardial infarction, and surgery in which postoperative thrombosis might be expected.

Until recently, OCs were not recommended for women over the age of 35. This was because earlier studies indicated a dramatic increase in the risk of thrombosis for this group. However, newer data show that today's low-estrogen OCs may be used up to menopause with no greater risk of thrombosis than among younger women.

Several measures can help minimize thromboembolic phenomena. First, the estrogen dose in OCs should be no greater than required for contraceptive efficacy. Second, OCs should not be prescribed for women who are heavy smokers, for women with a history of thromboembolism, or for women with other risk factors for thrombosis. Third, OCs should be discontinued at least 4 weeks prior to surgery in which postoperative thrombosis might be expected. Lastly, women should be informed about the symptoms of thrombosis and thromboembolism (e.g., leg tenderness or pain, sudden chest pain, shortness of breath, severe headache, sudden visual disturbance) and instructed to cease OC use and notify the physician if these occur.

**Hypertension.** The incidence of hypertension among OC users is 3 to 6 times greater than among nonusers. Oral contraceptives elevate blood pressure by increasing blood levels of both angiotensin (a potent vasoconstrictor) and aldosterone (a hormone that promotes salt and water retention). The risk of hypertension increases with age and duration of OC use. Women taking OCs should undergo periodic determination of blood pressure. If hypertension develops, OCs should be discontinued. Blood pressure usually declines to pretreatment levels within a few months after OCs have been withdrawn.

**Cancer.** The risk of cancer from OCs is extremely low. Although estrogen use by postmenopausal women is associated with an increased incidence of endometrial carcinoma (see Chapter 57), OCs appear to *protect* against this form of cancer. In addition, OCs protect against ovarian cancer. The question of whether OCs increase the risk of breast cancer remains unresolved: some studies show a small increase in risk; others show no increase in risk. Regardless, since estrogens can promote the growth of existing breast carcinoma, women with this disease should not use OCs. As discussed in Chapter 57, women who had been exposed to diethylstilbestrol (DES), a nonsteroidal estrogen, during fetal life are at increased risk of developing cervical and vaginal cancer upon maturing. To minimize this risk to the fetus, OCs should be discontinued if contraceptive failure occurs.

**Teratogenic Effects.** Birth defects can be produced by estrogens and progestins. Exposure of the male fetus to DES can cause testicular hypoplasia and abnormal semen production. Progestin use during early pregnancy has been associated with a variety of teratogenic defects (e.g., limb reductions, heart abnormalities, masculinization of the female fetus). Accordingly, if pregnancy should occur, OCs should be discontinued immediately.

**Abnormal Uterine Bleeding.** By inducing endometrial regression, OCs may decrease or eliminate menstrual flow during the initial months of use. Breakthrough bleeding and spotting may occur, especially when OCs with low estrogen and progestin content are employed. If bleeding irregularities persist, the possibility of malignancy should be investigated. If two consecutive periods are missed, the client should be evaluated for pregnancy. Following discontinuation of OC use, a period of 1 to 3 months may be required before normal menstruation resumes. In extreme cases, cyclic menses may not return for up to 1 year.

**Effects Related to Estrogen or Progestin Imbalance.** Many of the mild side effects of OCs result from an excess or deficiency of estrogen or progestin. Effects that can result from an excess of estrogen include nausea, breast tenderness, and edema. Progestin excess can produce increased appetite, fatigue, and depression. A deficiency in either class of hormone can cause menstrual irregularities. Side effects related to hormonal imbalance are summarized in Table 58–2. By making appropriate adjustments in the estrogen and progestin content of an OC regimen, many of these effects can be minimized.

**Use in Pregnancy and Lactation.** Because OCs are teratogenic and can cause cancer in females exposed to them *in utero, OCs are contraindicated for use during pregnancy* (FDA Pregnancy Category X). Pregnancy should be ruled out prior to initiation of OC therapy. If pregnancy occurs during OC use, the OC should be discontinued immediately. OCs enter breast milk and reduce milk produc-

## TABLE 58-2. SIDE EFFECTS CAUSED BY AN EXCESS OR DEFICIENCY IN THE ESTROGEN OR PROGESTIN CONTENT OF AN ORAL CONTRACEPTIVE REGIMEN

| Estrogen | | Progestin | |
|---|---|---|---|
| Excess | Deficiency | Excess | Deficiency |
| Nausea | Early or midcycle | Increased appetite | Late breakthrough |
| Breast tenderness | breakthrough | Weight gain | bleeding |
| Edema | bleeding | Depression | Amenorrhea |
| Bloating | Increased spotting | Tiredness | Hypermenorrhea |
| Hypertension | Hypomenorrhea | Fatigue | |
| Migraine headache | | Hypomenorrhea | |
| Cervical mucorrhea | | Breast regression | |
| Polyposis | | Monilial vaginitis | |
| | | Acne, oily scalp* | |
| | | Hair loss* | |
| | | Hirsutism* | |

*Caused by progestins that have androgenic activity.

tion. Accordingly, OCs should not be taken by women who are breast-feeding.

***Benign Hepatic Adenoma.*** Hepatic adenoma is a rare complication of OC use. Although nonmalignant, these tumors are highly vascular, and hence can be the source of severe hemorrhage if they rupture. Women using OCs should undergo periodic palpation of the liver. If a mass is detected, further tests should be performed to establish a definitive diagnosis. If hepatic adenoma is diagnosed, OCs must be discontinued; spontaneous regression of the tumor usually follows.

***Multiple Births.*** The incidence of twin births is increased in women who become pregnant shortly after discontinuing OCs. Women who desire pregnancy, but wish to reduce the chances of multiple births, should employ an alternative form of birth control for approximately 3 months after stopping OCs.

***Glucose Intolerance.*** Oral contraceptives can elevate plasma glucose levels. This diabetogenic effect is caused by the *progestin* in OCs. Glucose intolerance is most likely in patients who are already diabetic or have experienced gestational diabetes. Since hypoglycemic agents (e.g., insulin) can control glucose elevations induced by OCs, the presence of diabetes does not preclude OC use. Prediabetic women should be monitored for development of hyperglycemia. Glucose intolerance may occur less with OCs that contain *desogestrel* or *norgestimate* as their progestin component.

***Other Adverse Effects.*** Rarely, OCs cause *gallbladder disease* accompanied by jaundice. This condition reverses following termination of treatment. OCs can cause a variety of *ocular lesions* (e.g., retinal vascular occlusion, retinal edema, optic neuropathy). Accordingly, OCs should be withdrawn in the event of unexplained visual disturbance. *Melanoderma* (darkening of the skin) may occur during OC use; a reduction in dosage may cause pigmentation to decrease. Progestins with androgenic actions may cause *acne, hirsutism,* and *hair loss*; these may occur less with OCs that contain desogestrel or norgestimate, rather than older progestins.

### Summary of Contraindications and Precautions

Combination OCs are *contraindicated* during pregnancy and for women with the following disorders (or a history thereof): thrombophlebitis, thromboembolic disorders, cerebrovascular accident, coronary artery disease, known or suspected breast carcinoma, known or suspected estrogen-dependent neoplasm, benign or malignant liver tumors, and undiagnosed abnormal genital bleeding.

Combination OCs should be used with *caution* by women with diabetes, women who are heavy smokers (more than 15 cigarettes a day), women who have risk factors for cardiovascular disease (e.g., hypertension, obesity, hypercholesterolemia), and women anticipating elective surgery in which postoperative thrombosis might be expected.

### Noncontraceptive Benefits of Oral Contraceptives

Oral contraceptives decrease the risk of several diseases, including ovarian cancer, endometrial cancer, ovarian cysts, pelvic inflammatory disease, premenstrual syndrome, fibrocystic breast disease, toxic shock syndrome, and anemia. In addition, OCs favorably affect menstrual symptoms: cramps are reduced, menstrual flow is smaller and of shorter duration, and menses are more predictable.

### Drug Interactions

***Drugs That Reduce the Effects of Oral Contraceptives.*** The effectiveness of OCs can be decreased by a variety of drugs. *Rifampin* (used for tuberculosis) and several *anticonvulsants* (phenobarbital, phenytoin, primidone) can induce synthesis of hepatic drug-metabolizing enzymes, and can thereby accelerate OC degradation. A number of antibiotics, including *tetracyclines* and *ampicillin*, can also lower OC efficacy: by killing gut flora, these agents reduce enterohepatic recirculation of OCs, and thereby accelerate OC elimination. Women taking OCs in combination with any of the above agents should be alert for indications of reduced OC blood levels (e.g., breakthrough bleeding, spotting). If these signs appear, it may be necessary to increase OC dosage or use an alternative form of birth control.

***Drugs Whose Effects Are Reduced by Oral Contraceptives.*** Oral contraceptives can reduce the effects of several drugs. By increasing levels of clotting factors, OCs can decrease the effectiveness of *warfarin*, an anticoagulant. OCs can also reduce the effects of *insulin and other hypoglycemic agents*. Hence, when combined with OCs, warfarin and hypoglycemic agents may require increased dosage.

***Drugs Whose Effects Are Increased by Oral Contraceptives.*** Oral contraceptives can impair the hepatic metabolism of several agents, including *theophylline* (used for asthma) and *imipramine* (an antidepressant). Because of reduced metabolic breakdown, these drugs may accumulate to toxic levels. Accordingly, women taking these drugs in combination with OCs should be alert for signs of toxicity; a reduction in the dosage of theophylline or imipramine may be required.

### Preparations

The combination OCs currently available are listed in Table 58–3. As shown, the principal estrogen in OCs is *ethinyl estradiol*. The principal progestin is *norethindrone*. The preparations in Table 58–3 are listed in order of increasing estrogen content. OCs with lower amounts of estrogen are less likely to produce serious side effects. The table also indicates which preparations belong to each of the four subgroups of combination OCs: monophasic, biphasic, triphasic and progressive. The biphasic and triphasic preparations reflect efforts to more closely simulate ovarian production of estrogens and progestins. However, these preparations offer little if any advantage over monophasic OCs.

### Dosage and Administration

***Dosing Schedules.*** Most OCs are taken in a sequence that consists of 21 days of OC use followed by 7 days on which either (1) no pill is taken, (2) an inert pill is taken, or (3) an iron-containing pill is taken. The sequence is begun on the fifth day of the menstrual cycle (i.e., 5 days after the onset of menses) and is repeated for as long as appropriate. Successive cycles should commence every 28 days, regardless of whether breakthrough bleeding or spotting has occurred. Pills should be taken at the same hour every day (e.g., with a meal, at bedtime). During the first week of OC use, an additional form of birth control (e.g., condom, diaphragm) is recommended. Postpartum use of OCs can be initiated immediately after delivery, as long as breast-feeding is not intended.

***Adjustments to Estrogen and Progestin Dosage.*** In most cases, therapy is initiated with an OC whose estrogen content is equivalent to 35 µg of estrogen or less. If this low-estrogen preparation results in signs of estrogen deficiency (e.g., spotting, breakthrough bleeding), an OC with higher estrogen content may be substituted. Conversely, if signs of estrogen excess become apparent (e.g., nausea, edema, breast discomfort), a preparation with

lower estrogen content may be selected. In a similar fashion, the progestin content of the regimen can be adjusted so as to alleviate symptoms of progestin excess or deficiency. When substituting one combination OC for another, the change can be made at the beginning of any new cycle; the change will not affect contraceptive efficacy.

***What to Do in the Event of Missed Dosage.*** The chances of ovulation (and hence pregnancy) from missing one OC dose are small. However, the risk of pregnancy becomes progressively larger with each consecutive omission. If only one dose is missed, that dose should be taken together with the next scheduled dose. If two doses are missed, two doses should be taken per day on the following 2 days. If three doses are missed, a new cycle should be initiated, starting 7 days after the last pill was taken. An additional form of birth control should be used during the first 2 weeks of the new cycle.

## Progestin-Only Oral Contraceptives

Progestin-only OCs, also known as "minipills," contain a progestin (norethindrone or norgestrel) but no estrogen. Because they lack estrogen, minipills do not cause thromboembolic disorders and most of the other adverse effects associated with combination OCs. Unfortunately, although somewhat safer than combination OCs, the progestin-only preparations are less effective and cause more menstrual irregularity (breakthrough bleeding, spotting, amenorrhea, inconsistent cycle length, variations in the volume and duration of monthly flow). Because of these drawbacks, minipills are considerably less popular than combination OCs. Three progestin-only preparations are currently available (see Table 58–3).

Contraceptive effects of the minipill result largely from alteration of cervical secretions. Under the influence of progestin, cervical glands produce a thick, sticky mucus that acts as a barrier to penetration by sperm. Progestins also modify the endometrium, making it less favorable for nidation. In comparison to combination OCs, minipills are relatively ineffective as inhibitors of ovulation; hence suppression of ovulation is not a major mechanism by which minipills prevent conception.

Unlike combination OCs, whose administration is cyclic, progestin-only OCs are taken continuously. Use is initiated on day 1 of the menstrual cycle and a pill is taken every day thereafter. Each pill should be taken at the same time of day.

The following guidelines apply in the event of missed dosage. If one pill is missed, it should be taken as soon as remembered; the next pill should be taken as scheduled. If two pills are missed, one should be taken as soon as remembered and the other should be discarded; the next pill should be taken as originally scheduled. If three pills are missed, administration should be discontinued, and use should not be resumed until menstruation occurs or until pregnancy has been ruled out. (Progestins are teratogenic, and therefore must not be taken if there is any suspicion of conception.)

## TABLE 58–3. COMPOSITION OF ORAL CONTRACEPTIVES

| Trade Name | µg | Estrogen | mg | Progestin |
|---|---|---|---|---|
| *Combination OCs: Monophasic* | | | | |
| Loestrin 21 1/20 | 20 | Ethinyl estradiol | 1 | Norethindrone |
| Loestrin Fe 1/20 | 20 | Ethinyl estradiol | 1 | Norethindrone |
| Alesse | 20 | Ethinyl estradiol | 0.1 | Levonorgestrel |
| Levlen | 30 | Ethinyl estradiol | 0.15 | Levonorgestrel |
| Nordette | 30 | Ethinyl estradiol | 0.15 | Levonorgestrel |
| Lo/Ovral | 30 | Ethinyl estradiol | 0.3 | Norgestrel |
| Loestrin 21 1.5/30 | 30 | Ethinyl estradiol | 1.5 | Norethindrone |
| Loestrin Fe 1.5/30 | 30 | Ethinyl estradiol | 1.5 | Norethindrone |
| Desogen | 30 | Ethinyl estradiol | 0.15 | Desogestrel |
| Ortho-Cept | 30 | Ethinyl estradiol | 0.15 | Desogestrel |
| Levora | 30 | Ethinyl estradiol | 0.15 | Norgestimate |
| Demulen 1/35 | 35 | Ethinyl estradiol | 1 | Ethynodiol diacetate |
| Ovocon-35 | 35 | Ethinyl estradiol | 0.4 | Norethindrone |
| Brevicon | 35 | Ethinyl estradiol | 0.5 | Norethindrone |
| Genora 0.5/35 | 35 | Ethinyl estradiol | 0.5 | Norethindrone |
| Modicon | 35 | Ethinyl estradiol | 0.5 | Norethindrone |
| Nelova 0.5/35 | 35 | Ethinyl estradiol | 0.5 | Norethindrone |
| Genora 1/35 | 35 | Ethinyl estradiol | 1 | Norethindrone |
| N.E.E. 1/35 | 35 | Ethinyl estradiol | 1 | Norethindrone |
| Nelova 1/35E | 35 | Ethinyl estradiol | 1 | Norethindrone |
| Norethin 1/35E | 35 | Ethinyl estradiol | 1 | Norethindrone |
| Norinyl 1 + 35 | 35 | Ethinyl estradiol | 1 | Norethindrone |
| Ortho-Novum 1/35 | 35 | Ethinyl estradiol | 1 | Norethindrone |
| Ortho-Cyclen | 35 | Ethinyl estradiol | 0.250 | Norgestimate |
| Ovral | 50 | Ethinyl estradiol | 0.5 | Norgestrel |
| Demulin 1/50 | 50 | Ethinyl estradiol | 1 | Ethynodiol diacetate |
| Ovocon-50 | 50 | Ethinyl estradiol | 1 | Norethindrone |
| Genora 1/50 | 50 | Mestranol | 1 | Norethindrone |
| Nelova 1/50M | 50 | Mestranol | 1 | Norethindrone |
| Norethin 1/50M | 50 | Mestranol | 1 | Norethindrone |
| Ortho-Novum 1/50 | 50 | Mestranol | 1 | Norethindrone |
| Norinyl 1 + 50 | 50 | Mestranol | 1 | Norethindrone |
| *Combination OC: Biphasic* | | | | |
| Ortho-Novum 10/11, | 35 | Ethinyl estradiol | 0.5 | Norethindrone (phase 1) |
| Nelova 10/11, | 35 | Ethinyl estradiol | 1.0 | Norethindrone (phase 2) |
| Janest 28 | | | | |
| *Combination OCs: Triphasic* | | | | |
| Tri-Norinyl | 35 | Ethinyl estradiol | 0.5 | Norethindrone (phase 1) |
| | 35 | Ethinyl estradiol | 1.0 | Norethindrone (phase 2) |
| | 35 | Ethinyl estradiol | 0.5 | Norethindrone (phase 3) |
| Ortho-Novum 7/7/7 | 35 | Ethinyl estradiol | 0.5 | Norethindrone (phase 1) |
| | 35 | Ethinyl estradiol | 0.75 | Norethindrone (phase 2) |
| | 35 | Ethinyl estradiol | 1.0 | Norethindrone (phase 3) |
| Tri-Levlen, Triphasil | 30 | Ethinyl estradiol | 0.05 | Levonorgestrel (phase 1) |
| | 40 | Ethinyl estradiol | 0.075 | Levonorgestrel (phase 2) |
| | 30 | Ethinyl estradiol | 0.125 | Levonorgestrel (phase 3) |
| Ortho Tri-Cyclen | 35 | Ethinyl estradiol | 0.18 | Norgestimate (phase 1) |
| | 35 | Ethinyl estradiol | 0.215 | Norgestimate (phase 2) |
| | 35 | Ethinyl estradiol | 0.25 | Norgestimate (phase 3) |
| *Combination OC: Estrophasic* | | | | |
| Estrostep | 20 | Ethinyl estradiol | 1.0 | Norethindrone (phase 1) |
| | 30 | Ethinyl estradiol | 1.0 | Norethindrone (phase 2) |
| | 35 | Ethinyl estradiol | 1.0 | Norethindrone (phase 3) |
| *Progestin-Only OCs:* | | | | |
| Micronor | | | 0.35 | Norethindrone |
| Nor-Q.D. | | | 0.35 | Norethindrone |
| Orvette | | | 0.075 | Norgestrel |

# Long-Acting Contraceptives

## Subdermal Levonorgestrel Implants

A subdermal system [Norplant System] for delivery of levonorgestrel is available for long-term, reversible contraception. As indicated in Table 58-1, subdermal implants are the most effective contraceptives available. Unfortunately, implants also have a high incidence of side effects.

**Description.** The Norplant System consists of 6 tiny Silastic rubber capsules (2.4 mm × 34 mm), each containing 36 mg of levonorgestrel, a synthetic progestin. Under local anesthesia, the capsules are surgically implanted on the inside of the upper arm through a small incision. Levonorgestrel then diffuses slowly and continuously from the capsules, providing blood levels sufficient for contraception for up to 5 years. The capsules are removed after 5 years, and then replaced if continued contraception is desired.

**Mechanism of Action.** Subdermal levonorgestrel implants act much like progestin-only OCs. Cervical mucous is made thick and sticky, creating a barrier to migration of sperm. Endometrial growth is suppressed, thereby discouraging nidation. In some women, ovulation is suppressed.

**Pharmacokinetics.** The daily release of levonorgestrel is about 80 µg initially and declines over time. Plasma drug levels vary widely among users. The drug is slowly metabolized by the liver. Following removal of the capsules, blood levels become undetectable within 10 to 14 days.

**Adverse Effects.** Menstrual irregularities are common. Their incidence is as follows: prolonged bleeding or many bleeding days (28%), spotting (17%), amenorrhea (9.4%), irregular onset of bleeding (7.6%), and frequent bleeding (7%). Other common reactions include breast discharge, cervicitis, musculoskeletal pain, abdominal discomfort, leukorrhea, and vaginitis—all of which have an incidence of 5% or more. In about 6% of users, removal of the implants has been difficult: some implants break during removal, some are displaced and hard to find, and some are too embedded to remove easily on the initial attempt.

## Depot Medroxyprogesterone Acetate

Following a single IM injection, medroxyprogesterone acetate (MPA) [Depo-Provera] provides safe and effective contraception for 3 months or more. Injections of 150 mg are repeated every 3 months to provide continuous protection. MPA prevents pregnancy in three ways: (1) suppression of ovulation, (2) thickening of the cervical mucus, and (3) alteration of the endometrium such that nidation is discouraged. When injections are discontinued, an average of 12 months is required for fertility to return; however, some women remain infertile as long as 2.5 years.

Adverse effects of MPA are typical of those seen with other progestins. Menstrual disturbances are common; cycles become irregular at first and, after 6 to 12 months, menstruation may cease entirely. Because the drug is used on a long-term basis, osteoporosis may be a concern: in one study, bone density was lower following 5 years of MPA; however, in another study, bone density increased after MPA was discontinued. Other adverse effects include weight gain, abdominal bloating, headache, depression, and decreased libido. Although MPA has produced uterine and mammary cancers in animals, a large-scale study has shown no increase in the risk of cervical, ovarian, or breast cancer in women—and the risk of endometrial cancer is actually reduced.

Although used worldwide for contraception for many years, MPA did not receive approval for contraceptive use in the United States until 1992. Approval had been withheld in large part because (1) MPA has caused cancer in laboratory animals and (2) when undesired effects occur with MPA, they are prolonged. These drawbacks are not seen with other forms of contraception (e.g., oral contraceptives). Furthermore, it had been argued that, with the advanced health care system that exists in the United States, the need for a long-acting, injectable contraceptive was much smaller than in many other parts of the world. Despite these arguments, it is clear that MPA does have attractive features, most notably high contraceptive efficacy (see Table 58-1) and infrequent administration. With these qualities, MPA would seem to be a desirable form of birth control for women who are incapable of using other methods reliably or for whom other forms of contraception are contraindicated.

### Intrauterine Devices

Intrauterine devices (IUDs) are among the most reliable forms of reversible birth control (see Table 58-1). In addition, the IUDs available today are very safe for the right clients (see below). However, despite their safety and efficacy, IUDs are not used widely in the United States: only 1.4% of American women who use birth control choose an IUD.

Nonuse of IUDs is largely the legacy of the Dalcon Shield, an IUD that caused miscarriages, pelvic infections, and infertility—as well as 18 deaths. The cause of these problems was a tiny string, composed of hundreds of nylon filaments and encased in a sheath. Once in the body, the sheath rotted and thereby exposed the string, which then acted as a wick, drawing bacteria into the uterus.

With proper client selection, today's IUDs are very safe. The principal problem is pelvic inflammatory disease (PID) secondary to a sexually transmitted disease (STD). If PID occurs during the course of IUD use, the risk of infertility is about 7%. Accordingly, IUDs should be used only by women with a low risk for STDs—that is, women who are monogamous, and who are confident that their partners are monogamous too. The major side effects of IUDs are cramps and increased menstrual bleeding. Pain and cramping are likely immediately following insertion, but are less intense in women who have had one or more children. If pregnancy occurs while an IUD is in place, there is an increased risk of ectopic pregnancy.

Two IUDs are available: (1) the *copper T 380A* [ParaGard] and (2) an *intrauterine progesterone contraceptive system* [Progestasert]. Both are T-shaped. ParaGard, which can remain in place for 8 years, is by far the more widely used. Progestasert, which must be replaced annually, is generally prescribed only for specific health reasons, such as allergy to the copper in ParaGard. As indicated in Table 58-1, the failure rate with ParaGard is less than 1%, compared with 1.5% to 2% for Progestasert.

How IUDs prevent conception is uncertain. ParaGard, whose active ingredient is copper, was initially thought to prevent implantation. However, more recent studies suggest that the device causes a harmless inflammation of the endometrium, and thereby interferes with sperm motility and fertilization.

The mechanism for Progestasert—but is also uncertain. This IUD contains a 38-mg reservoir of progesterone. The device releases progesterone at a rate of 65 µg/day, an amount too small to elevate systemic progesterone levels. We do know that Progestasert does not inhibit ovulation. Furthermore, since models of this IUD that lack progesterone are not effective, it is clear that localized actions of progesterone are required for contraceptive effects. It has been hypothesized that the device may work by altering the endometrium to prevent nidation or by reducing the viability of sperm. To ensure that progesterone release remains adequate, a new device must be inserted annually.

## Spermicides

Spermicides are dispensed in the form of foams, gels, creams, and suppositories; until recently, a spermicide-impregnated sponge was also available. All of these preparations can be purchased without a prescription. When used alone, and especially when used in combination with a diaphragm or condom, spermicides can provide effective contraception (see Table 58-1). As indicated in Table 58-4, spermicidal preparations employ either *nonoxynol 9* or *octoxynol 9* as their active ingredient. These agents are chemical surfactants that kill sperm by destroying

their cell membrane. Adverse effects are minimal. Most studies show no relationship between spermicide use and birth defects.

Correct use of spermicides is required for contraceptive efficacy. The spermicide must be applied prior to coitus, but no more than 1 hour in advance (when used alone). Containers for foam preparations must be shaken thoroughly before each use to ensure dispersal of the spermicide. Suppositories or tablets should be inserted a minimum of 10 to 15 minutes before intercourse to allow time for dissolution. Spermicides should be reapplied each time intercourse is anticipated. Douching should be postponed for at least 6 hours following coitus.

The contraceptive sponge differs somewhat from other spermicidal preparations. The sponge acts in three ways to prevent conception: it (1) releases nonoxynol 9, (2) provides a barrier to sperm, and (3) absorbs seminal fluid. Unlike other spermicides, which must be reapplied every time intercourse takes place, a single sponge provides contraception for repeated coitus over a 24-hour period. The sponge should remain in place no longer than 1 day. The most common adverse effects are vaginal irritation and dryness. The only manufacturer of spermicidal sponges in the United States discontinued production in 1995.

## Barrier Devices

Barrier devices—male and female condoms, diaphragms, and the cervical cap—are nonpharmacologic options for birth control. Of the barrier devices available, condoms for men are by far the most commonly employed.

***Condoms for Men.*** Condoms are made from three materials: latex, polyurethane, and lamb intestine. In the United States, most condoms are made of latex, which is impermeable to bacteria and viruses. Hence, in addition to protecting against pregnancy, latex condoms protect against sexually transmitted diseases. Lubricants that contain mineral oil can very rapidly

---

### TABLE 58-4. SPERMICIDES

| Formulation | Active Ingredient | Trade Name |
|---|---|---|
| *Foam* | Nonoxynol 9 (12.5%) | Delfen Contraceptive, Koromex |
| | Nonoxynol 9 (8%) | Because, Emko, Emko Pre-Fil |
| *Jelly* | Nonoxynol 9 (5%) | Ramses |
| | Nonoxynol 9 (3%) | Koromex, Gynol II Extra Strength Contraceptive |
| *Gel* | Nonoxynol 9 (4%) | Conceptrol Disposable Contraceptive |
| | Nonoxynol 9 (3.5%) | Advantage 24* |
| | Nonoxynol 9 (2.2%) | K-Y Plus* |
| | Nonoxynol 9 (2%) | Gynol II Contraceptive,* Koromex Crystal Clear,* Shur Seal* |
| | Octoxynol 9 (1%) | Ortho Gynol Contraceptive* |
| *Cream* | Nonoxynol 9 (5%) | Conceptrol Birth Control |
| | Nonoxynol 9 (2%) | Ortho Creme Contraceptive* |
| | Octoxynol 9 (3%) | Koromex* |
| *Suppository* | Nonoxynol 9 (2.27%) | Encare |
| | Nonoxynol 9 (100 mg) | Semicid |
| | Nonoxynol 9 (150 mg) | Conceptrol Contraceptive Inserts |
| *Sponge* | Nonoxynol 9 (1 g) | Today† |
| *Vaginal Film* | Nonoxynol 9 (28%) | VCF |

*Intended for use only in combination with a diaphragm.
†No longer manufactured in the United States.

decrease the barrier strength of latex—by as much as 90%—and therefore should be avoided. Allergy to latex can develop in men and women, especially with repeated exposure. Like latex condoms, polyurethane condoms protect against STDs. In addition, they are thinner than latex condoms, possibly stronger, and don't cause allergies. In contrast to latex and polyurethane condoms, condoms made from lamb intestine are permeable to viruses, and hence do not protect against viral STDs. As indicated in Figure 58-1, condoms are the fourth most common form of birth control. The typical-use failure rate is 12%.

**Condom for Women.** The *Reality* female condom is a loose-fitting, tubular polyurethane pouch that has flexible rings at both ends. The ring at the closed end anchors the pouch over the cervix. The ring at the open end, which is larger than the ring at the closed end, is placed over the labia and serves as an external anchor. The Reality condom is prelubricated, available without prescription, cannot be combined with a male condom, and should be used just once and then discarded. Like male condoms, the female condom provides protection against STDs. The failure rate with typical use is 21%.

**Diaphragm.** The diaphragm is a soft rubber cap with a metal spring that reinforces its rim. The device must be fitted by a health care provider, and the user must be taught how to insert it. When in place over the cervical os, the diaphragm blocks access of sperm to the cervix. Because the device does not fit tightly enough to completely block penetration of sperm, it must be filled with spermicidal jelly or cream before insertion. Spermicide must be reapplied with repeated intercourse. The diaphragm can be inserted as long as 6 hours prior to intercourse, and must remain in place for at least 6 hours after. Because of the risk of toxic shock syndrome, the diaphragm should not remain in place for more than 24 hours. With typical use, the failure rate is about 18%.

**Cervical Cap.** The *Prentif Cavity-Rim Cervical Cap* is a small, pliant, cup-shaped device that fits snugly over the cervix. Suction holds it in place. The device must be fitted by a health care provider, and the user must be taught how to insert it. Because only four sizes are available, some women cannot be fitted. Like the diaphragm, the cap is filled with spermicidal cream or jelly prior to use, and can be inserted up to 6 hours before intercourse. There is no need to apply additional spermicide with repeated intercourse. The cap should remain in place for at least 8 hours after intercourse, and probably no longer than 24 hours (although the manufacturer says it can stay in place for 48 hours). The typical-use failure rate is about 18%.

## Emergency Postcoital Contraception

Postcoital contraceptives, also known as "morning-after" pills, can prevent pregnancy when taken following intercourse. To be effective, these drugs should be taken no later than 72 hours after coitus. Because their side effects can be intense, postcoital contraceptives are not considered substitutes for traditional methods of birth control. Rather, these drugs should be reserved for isolated instances of unprotected intercourse. Hence, they might be used to prevent an unplanned and unwanted pregnancy resulting from sexual assault, contraceptive failure (e.g., torn condom), or occasional lack of forethought.

### Combination Oral Contraceptives

Table 58-5 lists seven combination OCs that have proven ability to prevent pregnancy following unprotected intercourse. Ovral, which has a success rate of about 99%, might be considered the preparation of choice. For postcoital contraception, 2 Ovral tablets are taken within 72 hours of coitus, and 2 more are

### TABLE 58-5. DRUGS FOR EMERGENCY POSTCOITAL CONTRACEPTION

#### I. Combination Oral Contraceptives

| Trade Name | Composition* | Dosage |
|---|---|---|
| Ovral | 50 µg EE, 500 mg NG | 2 tablets immediately, 2 tablets 12 hr later |
| Lo/Ovral | 30 µg EE, 300 mg NG | 4 tablets immediately, 4 tablets 12 hr later |
| Levlen Levora Nordette | 30 µg EE, 150 mg NG | 4 tablets immediately, 4 tablets 12 hr later |
| Tri-Levlen† Triphasil† | 30 µg EE, 125 mg LNG | 4 tablets immediately, 4 tablets 12 hr later |

#### II. High-Dose Estrogens

| Drug | Dosage |
|---|---|
| Diethylstilbestrol | 25 mg bid for 5 days |
| Ethinyl estradiol | 2.5 mg bid for 5 days |
| Conjugated estrogens | 10 mg tid for 5 days |
| Estrone | 5 mg tid for 5 days |

*EE = ethinyl estradiol, NG = norgestrel, LNG = levonorgestrel.
†Yellow (phase 3) pills only.

taken 12 hours later. Pregnancy is prevented because the hormones in Ovral impede migration of the ovum through the fallopian tubes and also discourage nidation. The high estrogen content of the regimen produces a high incidence of side effects: nausea (60%), vomiting (17%), headache (70%), and breast tenderness (46%). Since estrogens and progestins can harm a developing fetus, pre-existing pregnancy should be ruled out before Ovral is given. Furthermore, if Ovral fails to prevent pregnancy, abortion should be considered. Dosages for emergency contraception using Ovral and other combination oral contraceptives are listed in Table 58–5.

### High-Dose Estrogens

High doses of estrogens taken within 72 hours of intercourse will block nidation, and thereby prevent pregnancy. The success rate is 97.6% to 100%. Dosages for four estrogens are given in Table 58–5. All are taken for 5 days. The most common side effects are nausea (70%) and vomiting (33%). If a dose is not retained because of vomiting, it should be repeated. Because of the high risk of teratogenicity, abortion should be considered if pregnancy is not prevented. Also, pre-existing pregnancy should be ruled out before giving high-dose estrogens.

### Mifepristone (RU-486)

Mifepristone is effective both for emergency postcoital contraception and early abortion. Both uses are discussed immediately below.

## Drugs for Medical Abortion

### Mifepristone (RU 486) with Misoprostol

Mifepristone (RU 486) is a synthetic steroid that blocks receptors for progesterone. The drug is used for "morning-after" contraception and for termination of early pregnancy (abortion). In addition, mifepristone is under investigation for treatment of recurrent breast cancer, certain meningiomas, Cushing's syndrome, and glaucoma. The drug has been used in France, the United Kingdom, and Sweden for years, and should be available in the United States soon.

***Abortion Early in Pregnancy.*** Mifepristone, followed by misoprostol, is a safe and effective alternative to surgery for termination of early pregnancy. The combination stimulates uterine contractions, causing the conceptus to undergo detachment and expulsion. In contrast to surgical abortion, which is generally unavailable before 8 weeks of gestation, abortion with mifepristone is performed early—within 7 weeks of conception.

In a study conducted in France, the abortion success rate with mifepristone-misoprostol was nearly 99%. (Success was defined as termination of pregnancy with complete expulsion of the conceptus.) All women in the study had amenorrhea for less than 50 days prior to receiving mifepristone. Dosing was done as follows: each patient received a 600-mg oral dose of mifepristone and, if abortion had not occurred within 48 hours, each was given a 400-μg dose of oral misoprostol; a second dose of misoprostol (200 μg) was offered if abortion had not occurred by 4 hours after the first dose. Only 5.5% of the pregnancies terminated prior to dosing with misoprostol; with the addition of misoprostol (1 or 2 doses), the cumulative success rate was 98.7%. In the majority of patients (69%), abortion occurred within 4 hours of the first misoprostol dose.

The principal adverse effect of mifepristone-misoprostol is prolonged bleeding, which may persist for 1 to 2 weeks. Rarely, a transfusion is required. About 80% of patients experience transient cramping, beginning 1 hour after taking misoprostol; about 15% require a nonopioid analgesic for relief. Other common side effects are nausea (40%), vomiting (15%), and diarrhea (10%).

A recent study demonstrated that *intravaginal* misoprostol is more effective and better tolerated than oral misoprostol. In this study, all women received 600 mg of oral mifepristone, followed by 800 μg of misoprostol, either PO or intravaginally. Following intravaginal misoprostol, 95% of conceptuses were expelled without the need for surgery, compared with only 87% following oral misoprostol. With intravaginal administration, abortion occurred within 4 hours in 93% of patients, compared with 78% of patients receiving oral misoprostol. The incidence of nausea and vomiting with intravaginal administration was significantly lower than with oral administration.

***Emergency Postcoital Contraception.*** For postcoital contraception, mifepristone is given in a single, 600-mg oral dose no later than 72 hours after unprotected intercourse. Misoprostol is not employed. Like Ovral and other combination oral contraceptives, mifepristone prevents pregnancy by blocking nidation. Mifepristone would seem preferable to combination oral contraceptives for two reasons. First, only one dose is required. Second, side effects are less frequent: headache occurs in 49% of patients, nausea in 40%, breast tenderness in 27%, and vomiting in 3%. The major disadvantage of mifepristone is that onset of menstruation may be delayed, which can be very stressful to a woman concerned about possibly being pregnant.

***The Status of Mifepristone in the United States.*** Mifepristone has been a battleground in the abortion controversy. The drug is strongly opposed by antiabortion groups. In support are many women's organizations and some major physicians' groups, including the American Medical Association. Mifepristone is of special importance to both camps in that it represents a medical alternative to surgical termination of pregnancy—and as such would decentralize abortion availability. That is, whereas surgical abortions are performed almost exclusively at specialized clinics, virtually any physician can facilitate abortion with mifepristone. Not only does this make abortion much more accessible and discreet, it makes the task of anti-abortion activists much more difficult. (It's relatively easy to focus opposition on a few abortion clinics and their doctors—but clearly impossible to picket every doctor's office in the country.)

Because of political and ideologic opposition, availability of mifepristone in the United States has been slow in coming. Hoechst-Roussel, the European company that holds the patent to mifepristone, wanted no part of our abortion debate—and hence made no attempt to market the drug in the United States, despite potentially huge profits. In 1994, in an arrangement brokered by the FDA, Hoechst-Roussel agreed to license mifepristone to the Population Council, a not-for-profit research group in the United States. In the summer of 1996, following research conducted by the Population Council, the FDA declared mifepristone (in combination with misoprostol) safe and effective for abortion, provided it is given within 7 weeks of conception. The approved regimen is 600 mg of mifepristone followed in 2 days by 400 μg of misoprostol. Marketing and distribution of mifepristone are to be arranged by Advances in Health Technology, a not-for-profit company created by the Population Council. Mifepristone should be available in 1997 or 1998.

### Other Drugs for Medical Abortion
#### Methotrexate with Misoprostol

Methotrexate, followed by misoprostol, is a safe and effective alternative to surgical termination of early pregnancy. Methotrexate induces abortion because of its toxicity to trophoblastic tissue; misoprostol contributes by promoting uterine contraction. Abortion is accomplished by giving an intramuscular injection of methotrexate (50 mg/m$^2$) followed in 5 days by 800 μg of intravaginal misoprostol; if abortion does not occur in 24 hours, dosing with misoprostol is repeated. In one study, 14%

of patients required the second dose of misoprostol, but 96% eventually aborted. The procedure is more effective at 49 days of gestation (or less) than between 50 and 56 days of gestation. Side effects include nausea, vomiting, diarrhea, headache, dizziness, and hot flushes. Acetaminophen plus codeine is sufficient to relieve pain in most cases. The vast majority of women who have undergone the procedure said they would recommend it.

### Carboprost Tromethamine and Dinoprostone

Carboprost tromethamine [Hemabate] and dinoprostone [Prostin E2] are prostaglandins used for second-trimester abortion. These agents cause abortion by inducing uterine contraction. The pharmacology of these prostaglandins and their use for abortion is discussed in Chapter 60 (Uterine Stimulants and Relaxants).

## KEY POINTS

- The most effective methods of birth control are levonorgestrel subdermal implants [Norplant], intramuscular medroxyprogesterone acetate [Depo-Provera], IUDs, and sterilization. Oral contraceptives are a close second.
- Sterilization is the most common form of birth control. Oral contraceptives and condoms come next.
- A long-term method of birth control—Norplant, Depo-Provera, IUD—is a good choice when compliance is a problem.
- There are two main categories of OCs: (1) combination OCs, which contain an estrogen plus a progestin, and (2) progestin-only OCs (minipills).
- The principal estrogen in combination OCs is ethinyl estradiol; the principal progestin is norethindrone.
- Combination OCs act primarily by inhibiting ovulation.
- Although combination OCs can cause a wide variety of adverse effects, serious effects are rare.
- The low-estrogen combination OCs used today pose only a minimal risk of thromboembolism—except in heavy smokers and women with a history of thromboembolic disorders.

- When used by nonsmoking women with normal cardiovascular function, OCs produce no greater mortality than other active forms of birth control.
- Combination OCs protect against ovarian and endometrial cancer. Whether these drugs carry a small risk of causing breast cancer is unresolved.
- Many of the mild side effects of OCs result from an excess or deficiency of estrogen or progestin, and hence can be minimized by adjusting the estrogen and/or progestin content of the OC regimen.
- Because OCs are teratogenic and can cause cancer in female offspring, they are contraindicated during pregnancy, and should be discontinued immediately if accidental pregnancy occurs.
- Oral contraceptive efficacy can be reduced by drugs that induce hepatic drug-metabolizing enzymes (e.g., rifampin, phenobarbital) and by certain antibiotics (e.g., ampicillin, tetracyclines) that kill gut flora and thereby decrease enterohepatic recirculation of OCs, which in turn accelerates their excretion.
- Because they lack estrogen, progestin-only OCs are slightly safer than combination OCs—but are less effective and cause more menstrual irregularity.
- Progestin-only OCs prevent pregnancy by promoting production of thick, sticky mucus (which creates a barrier to migration of sperm) and by suppressing endometrial growth (which discourages nidation).
- Subdermal levonorgestrel implants [Norplant] are active for 5 years, and are the most effective contraceptives available.
- Norplant has the same mechanism as progestin-only pills: production of thick, sticky mucus and alteration of the endometrium.
- Intramuscular medroxyprogesterone acetate [Depo-Provera] is active for 3 months, and is one of the most effective contraceptives available.
- Depo-Provera prevents pregnancy in three ways: (1) it suppresses ovulation, (2) it thickens the cervical mucus, and (3) it alters the endometrium such that nidation is discouraged.

## Summary of Major Nursing Implications*

### Combination Oral Contraceptives

### Preadministration Assessment

#### Therapeutic Goal
Prevention of unwanted pregnancy.

#### Baseline Data
Assess for a history of hypertension, diabetes, thrombophlebitis, thromboembolic disorders, cerebrovascular disease, coronary artery disease, breast carcinoma, estrogen-dependent neoplasm, and benign or malignant liver tumors.

#### Identifying High-Risk Patients
Combination OCs are *contraindicated* during *pregnancy* and for women with the following disorders (or a history thereof): *thrombophlebitis, thromboembolic disorders, cerebrovascular disease, coronary artery disease, myocardial infarction, known or suspected breast carcinoma, known or suspected estrogen-dependent neoplasm, benign or malignant liver tumors,* and *undiagnosed abnormal genital bleeding.*

Combination OCs should be used with *caution* in women with *diabetes,* women who *smoke heavily* (more

---

*Patient education information is highlighted in color.

than 15 cigarettes a day), *women who have risk factors for cardiovascular disease* (e.g., hypertension, obesity, hypercholesterolemia), and women *anticipating elective surgery in which postoperative thrombosis might be expected.*

## Implementation: Administration

### Dosing Schedule

Provide the client with the following instructions on administration: (1) initiate administration 5 days after the onset of menstruation; (2) the administration sequence consists of 21 days of drug use followed by 7 days off (for the 7 "off" days, the manufacturer may provide inert tablets, iron-containing tablets, or no tablets); and (3) take pills at the same time each day (e.g., with a meal, at bedtime).

### Responding to Missed Doses

Provide the client with the following instructions regarding missed doses: (1) if only one dose is missed, take the omitted dose together with the next scheduled dose; (2) if two doses are missed, take two doses per day on the following 2 days; and (3) if three doses are missed, initiate a new cycle (starting 7 days after the last pill was taken) and use an additional form of contraception (e.g., condom, diaphragm) during the first 2 weeks of the new cycle.

### Postpartum Use

Inform the client that OCs can be initiated immediately after delivery if breast-feeding is not intended.

### Promoting Compliance

Counsel the client about the importance of taking OCs as prescribed. Encourage the client to read the package insert provided with combination OCs.

## Ongoing Evaluation and Interventions

### Monitoring Summary

Periodic evaluations should include pelvic and breast examinations, palpation of the liver, blood pressure determination, and a Papanicolaou smear.

### Minimizing Adverse Effects

*Thrombotic Disorders.* Because of their estrogen content, combination OCs slightly increase the risk of thrombosis and thromboembolism. To minimize thrombosis and thromboembolism, (1) use OCs of low estrogen content, (2) avoid use of OCs by women with known risk factors for thrombotic disorders, and (3) discontinue OCs at least 4 weeks prior to elective surgeries in which postoperative thrombosis might be expected. Inform the client about symptoms of thrombosis and thromboembolism (e.g., leg tenderness or pain, sudden chest pain, shortness of breath, severe headache, sudden visual disturbance), and instruct her to notify the physician if these develop.

*Hypertension.* Perform periodic determinations of blood pressure. If hypertension is detected, discontinue OCs. Blood pressure usually normalizes within a few months.

*Abnormal Uterine Bleeding.* During initial use, combination OCs may reduce or eliminate menstrual flow; breakthrough bleeding or spotting may also occur. Menstrual irregularities may be greater with low-estrogen preparations.

Instruct the client to notify the physician if two consecutive periods are missed; the possibility of pregnancy must be evaluated.

Instruct the client to notify the physician if bleeding irregularities persist; the possibility of malignancy must be investigated.

Inform the client that menstruation may take several months to normalize following OC withdrawal.

*Effects Related to Estrogen or Progestin Imbalance.* An excess or deficiency of estrogen or progestin can cause specific side effects (see Table 58–2). By adjusting the estrogen or progestin content of the OC regimen, these effects can be reduced or eliminated. Substitution of one combination OC for another can be made at the beginning of any new cycle.

*Use in Pregnancy and Lactation.* OCs are teratogenic and may cause cancer in female offspring, and are therefore contraindicated during pregnancy. Pregnancy should be ruled out prior to OC use. Instruct the client to cease OC use immediately if pregnancy should occur.

Inform the client that oral contraceptives enter breast milk and can reduce milk production. Instruct her not to breast-feed while taking OCs.

*Benign Hepatic Adenoma.* Women taking OCs should undergo periodic palpation of the liver; if a mass is detected, further tests are required for definitive diagnosis. If benign hepatoma is present, OC use must cease; regression of the tumor usually follows.

*Glucose Intolerance.* Oral contraceptives can elevate plasma glucose levels. Advise the diabetic client to monitor blood glucose content closely; an increase in dosage of insulin or oral hypoglycemic medication may be needed. Monitor the prediabetic client for hyperglycemia.

*Multiple Births.* The incidence of twin births is increased when conception takes place shortly after termination of OC use. Advise the client to employ another form of birth control for 3 months after termination of OC use if she wishes to reduce the chances of multiple births.

### Minimizing Adverse Interactions

*Drugs That Reduce Oral Contraceptive Levels.* Several *anticonvulsants* (phenobarbital, phenytoin, primidone) and certain *antibiotics* (e.g., rifampin, tetracycline, ampicillin) can accelerate OC elimination. Advise the client who is taking OCs in combination with these agents to be alert for indications of reduced OC levels (e.g., breakthrough bleeding, spotting), and to notify the physician if these occur. An increase in OC dosage or use of an alternative method of birth control may be required.

*Drugs Whose Effects Are Reduced by Oral Contraceptives.* Oral contraceptives can reduce the effects of some drugs, including *warfarin*, *insulin*, and *oral hypoglycemic agents*. When combined with OCs, these drugs may require greater than normal dosages.

*Drugs Whose Effects Are Increased by Oral Contraceptives.* Oral contraceptives can increase blood levels of several drugs, including *theophylline* and *imipramine*. Women using these drugs in combination with OCs should be alert for signs of toxicity; dosage reduction for theophylline or imipramine may be required.

# Progestin-Only Oral Contraceptives

## Preadministration Assessment

### Therapeutic Goal
Prevention of unwanted pregnancy.

### Identifying High-Risk Patients
Progestin-only pills are *contraindicated* during *pregnancy*.

## Implementation: Administration

### Dosing Schedule
Instruct the client to initiate OC use on day 1 of the menstrual cycle and to take one pill every day thereafter. Pills should be taken at the same time each day (e.g., with a meal or at bedtime).

### Responding to Missed Doses
Provide the client with the following instructions regarding missed doses: (1) if one pill is missed, take it as soon as the omission is noticed; (2) if two pills are missed, take one pill as soon as the omission is noticed, discard the second pill, and take the next scheduled pill at its normal time; and (3) if three pills are missed, terminate OC use. Do not resume use until menstruation occurs or until pregnancy has been ruled out.

## Ongoing Evaluation and Interventions

### Minimizing Adverse Effects
*Menstrual Irregularities.* Breakthrough bleeding, spotting, amenorrhea, inconsistent cycle length, and variations in the amount and duration of monthly flow are common and unavoidable. Forewarn the client of these effects.

# CHAPTER 59

# Drug Therapy of Infertility

*nfertility* (subfertility) is defined as a decrease in the ability to reproduce. This contrasts with *sterility*, which is the complete absence of reproductive ability. About 15% of couples attempting to have children experience infertility. Failure to conceive may be due to reproductive dysfunction of the male partner, the female partner, or both. When medical treatment is implemented, approximately one half of infertile couples achieve pregnancy. To date, drug therapy of female infertility has been considerably more successful than drug therapy of male infertility.

In treating infertility, the chances of success are greatly enhanced by accurate diagnosis. A variety of diagnostic procedures may be employed, including semen analysis, determination of basal body temperature patterns, measurement of estrogen and progesterone levels, endometrial biopsy, and evaluation of fallopian tube patency. A complete medical history of both partners is essential. This history should include information on frequency and timing of coitus and use of drugs that might lower fertility.

In approaching the drugs employed to increase fertility, we will begin with a discussion of causes of reproductive dysfunction. Following this we will discuss the fertility-promoting drugs. In preparation for the study of these agents, you should review the following from Chapter 57: information on the menstrual cycle and information on the biosynthesis and physiologic and pharmacologic effects of the female hormones (estrogens and progestins). In addition, you should review the section on testosterone in Chapter 61. In both chapters, pay special attention to the roles of pituitary gonadotropins (luteinizing hormone [LH], follicle-stimulating hormone [FSH]) in male and female reproduction.

## Infertility: Causes and Treatment Strategies

### Female Infertility

Female infertility can result from disruption of any phase of the reproductive process. The most critical phases are follicular maturation, ovulation, transport of the ovum through the fallopian tubes, fertilization of the ovum, nidation, and growth and development of the conceptus. These events cannot take place unless the ovaries, uterus, hypothalamus, and pituitary are functioning properly. If the activity of any of these structures is disturbed, fertility can be impaired. The causes of female infertility that respond to drug therapy are discussed below.

#### Anovulation and Failure of Follicular Maturation

In the absence of adequate hormonal stimulation, ovarian follicles will not ripen and ovulation will not take place. Frequently, these causes of infertility can be corrected with drugs. The agents used to promote follicular maturation and/or ovulation are *clomiphene, gonadorelin, menotropins, urofollitropin,* and *human chorionic gonadotropin* (HCG). Clomiphene and gonadorelin induce follicular maturation and ovulation by promoting release of FSH and LH from the pituitary; in some cases, induction of ovulation requires co-treatment with HCG. Menotropins and urofollitropin are used in conjunction with HCG: menotropins and urofollitropin act directly on the ovary to promote follicular development; after the follicle has matured, HCG is given to induce ovulation. Since HCG acts on the mature follicle to cause ovulation, the drug is used only after follicular maturation has been induced with another agent (menotropins, urofollitropin, or clomiphene). The pharmacology of clomiphene, gonadorelin, menotropins, urofollitropin, and HCG is discussed later.

### Unfavorable Cervical Mucus

In the periovulatory period, the cervical glands normally secrete large volumes of thin, watery mucus. These secretions, which are produced under the influence of estrogen, facilitate passage of sperm through the cervical canal. If the cervical mucus is scant or of inappropriate consistency (thick, sticky), sperm will be unable to pass through to the uterus. Production of unfavorable mucus may occur spontaneously or as a side effect of clomiphene (see below).

Cervical mucus can be restored to its proper volume and consistency by administering *estrogens*. Two regimens have been employed. In one regimen, ethinyl estradiol is given beginning early in the menstrual cycle (on day 6, 7, or 8) and continued through day 12 or 13; dosages range from 20 to 80 µg/day. In the second regimen, conjugated estrogens are administered from day 5 through day 15 of the cycle; dosages range from 2.5 to 5 mg/day. When used to counteract the effects of clomiphene on the cervical mucus, estrogens are administered for 10 days beginning 1 day after the last clomiphene dose.

### Hyperprolactinemia

Elevation of prolactin levels may be caused by a pituitary adenoma or by disturbed regulation of the healthy pituitary. Amenorrhea, galactorrhea, and infertility may all occur in association with excessive prolactin secretion. The mechanism by which hyperprolactinemia impairs fertility is not known. Hyperprolactinemia can be treated with *bromocriptine*.

### Luteal Phase Defect

The term *luteal phase defect* refers to a group of disorders in which secretion of progesterone by the corpus luteum is insufficient to maintain endometrial integrity. Dysfunction of the corpus luteum may be spontaneous or may occur secondary to hyperprolactinemia or to use of clomiphene. Luteal phase defect can be diagnosed by making serial determinations of plasma progesterone levels or by taking a biopsy of the endometrium.

*Progesterone* is the preferred therapy for luteal phase defect. This hormone will correct the defect regardless of its etiology. Only progesterone itself should be used; synthetic progestins are teratogenic and may also induce degeneration of the corpus luteum. Progesterone treatment should commence after ovulation has occurred, and should continue through the first 8 to 10 weeks of pregnancy (i.e., until the placenta has developed the capacity to make its own progestins).

Progesterone may be administered by IM injection (12.5 mg/day) or by a vaginal suppository (25 mg twice daily). Because progesterone injections are both painful and inconvenient, the suppositories are preferred.

### Endometriosis

Endometriosis is a condition in which endometrial tissue has become implanted in an abnormal location (e.g., uterine wall, ovary, extragenital sites). These implants respond to hormonal stimulation in much the same fashion as the normally situated endometrium. Endometriosis is a common cause of infertility and, when pregnancies do occur, the rate of spontaneous abortion is high (about 50%).

The mechanism by which endometriosis reduces fertility is not always clear. In some cases, infertility results from ovarian or tubal adhesions that impede transport of the ovum. However, when endometriosis is mild, visible causes of infertility are frequently absent.

Endometriosis can be treated surgically, with drugs, or with a combination of both. Surgery reduces symptoms of endometriosis and increases fertility. In contrast, although drugs can reduce symptoms, there is no conclusive proof that they enhance fertility. In recent years, the drug employed most frequently has been *danazol*. Before danazol became available, progestins (alone and in combination with an estrogen) were the preferred pharmacologic therapy. Most recently, *nafarelin* and *leuprolide* (synthetic analogs of gonadotropin-releasing hormone) have been used. Oral contraceptives can reduce symptoms of endometriosis, but obviously won't promote fertility.

### Androgen Excess

Overproduction of androgens can decrease fertility. Excess androgens may be of ovarian or adrenal origin. The most common condition associated with androgen excess is polycystic ovary (PCO). This condition is characterized by the presence of multiple polycystic follicles within a thickened capsule; ovulation is absent. *Clomiphene* is the treatment of choice for PCO. If clomiphene alone fails to induce ovulation, addition of HCG to the regimen may improve results. If the androgen excess is of adrenal origin, a combination of *clomiphene plus dexamethasone* (a glucocorticoid) may prove effective; dexamethasone decreases adrenal androgen synthesis by suppressing release of adrenocorticotropic hormone from the pituitary.

## Male Infertility

For about 30% of couples who experience infertility, failure to conceive is due entirely to reproductive dysfunction in the male. Male infertility is due most often to decreased density or motility of sperm, or to semen of abnormal volume or quality. The most obvious manifestation of male infertility is impotence (inability to achieve erection). In most cases, infertility in males is not associated with an identifiable endocrine disorder. Unfortunately, male infertility is generally unresponsive to drugs.

### Hypogonadotropic Hypogonadism

A few males may be incapable of spermatogenesis because of insufficient gonadotropin secretion. In these rare cases, drug therapy may be helpful. If the gonadotropin deficiency is only partial, sperm counts can be increased using HCG (alone or in combination with menotropins). If the deficiency is severe, treatment with androgens is required (see Chapter 61). If therapy with HCG and menotropins is intended, the patient should be informed that treatment will be prolonged (3 to 4 years) and very expensive.

## Impotence

Inability to achieve erection is the most conspicuous cause of male infertility. In recent years, vasoactive drugs (phentolamine, papaverine, alprostadil) have been given to produce erection. Use of these agents is discussed below.

## Idiopathic Male Infertility

Idiopathic infertility is defined as infertility for which no cause can be identified. It is estimated that 25% to 40% of male infertility is idiopathic. Since the cause is unknown, specific drug therapy is impossible. Accordingly, treatment is empiric (trial and error). Several drugs, including androgens, clomiphene, and HCG, have been administered in hopes of improving idiopathic infertility in males. Unfortunately, none of these agents has been especially successful.

# Drugs Used to Treat Infertility

The majority of drugs used to increase fertility are directed at improving reproductive function in females. Drugs can increase female fertility by helping promote the following: (1) maturation of ovarian follicles, (2) ovulation, (3) production of favorable cervical mucus, (4) control of endometriosis, and (5) reduction of excessive prolactin levels. The ability of drugs to increase fertility in males is limited. In some cases, therapy may improve semen and sperm production. Recently, drugs have been employed to facilitate erection.

## Clomiphene

**Therapeutic Use.** Clomiphene [Clomid, Milophene, Serophene] is used to promote follicular maturation and ovulation in selected infertile women.

**Mechanism of Fertility Promotion.** Clomiphene blocks receptors for estrogen. By blocking these receptors in the hypothalamus and the pituitary, clomiphene makes it appear to these structures that estrogen levels are low. In response, the pituitary increases secretion of gonadotropins (LH and FSH) and these hormones then stimulate the ovary, promoting follicular maturation and ovulation. In properly selected patients, the ovulation rate is about 90%. Because of its mechanism of action, clomiphene can induce ovulation only if the pituitary is capable of producing LH and FSH, and only if the ovaries are capable of responding to these hormones. Success is impossible in women with primary failure of either the pituitary

or ovaries. Accordingly, pituitary and ovarian function should be verified prior to clomiphene therapy. If treatment produces follicular maturation but ovulation fails to occur, it may be possible to induce ovulation by adding HCG to the regimen (see below). The occurrence of ovulation can be determined by three methods: (1) monitoring for an increase in basal body temperature, (2) monitoring for an increase in progesterone levels, and (3) examining a biopsy of the endometrium for evidence of secretory transformation.

**Adverse Effects.** Common side effects include hot flushes (similar to the vasomotor responses of menopause), nausea, abdominal discomfort, bloating, and breast engorgement. Some patients experience visual disturbances (blurred vision, visual flashes), which usually reverse following clomiphene withdrawal. Multiple births (usually twins) occur in 8% to 10% of clomiphene-facilitated pregnancies. Patients should be informed of this possibility.

Excessive stimulation of the ovaries can produce *ovarian enlargement*. This reaction is most likely in women with polycystic ovaries. Hyperstimulation of the ovaries can be minimized by avoiding unnecessarily large clomiphene doses. If undue ovarian enlargement occurs, administration of clomiphene should cease. The ovaries will regress to normal size following drug withdrawal.

Some actions of clomiphene may *interfere* with conception. Luteal phase defect may be induced. This response can be corrected by administering progesterone. Because of its antiestrogenic actions, clomiphene may force the production of scant and viscous cervical mucus; estrogen therapy will render cervical secretions more hospitable to sperm.

It is recommended that clomiphene be avoided during pregnancy. Although no human fetal defects have been reported, clomiphene has produced developmental abnormalities in animals.

**Preparations, Dosage, and Administration.** Clomiphene [Clomid, Milophene, Serophene] is dispensed in 50-mg tablets for oral use. The initial course of treatment consists of 50 mg once daily for 5 days. If cyclic menstrual bleeding has been occurring, therapy should begin on the fifth day after the onset of menses. If menstruation has been absent, therapy can commence at any time (assuming that pregnancy has been ruled out). If the first course of treatment fails to induce ovulation, a second 5-day course (using 100 mg/day) may be tried. The second course may begin as early as 30 days after the previous course. Doses may be increased in subsequent courses. However, doses above 100 mg/day are rarely needed. Once a dose that induces ovulation has been established, that dose should be used for a maximum of three cycles. If pregnancy has not occurred, further treatment is unlikely to succeed. When ovulation does occur, it is usually within 5 to 10 days after the last clomiphene dose; patients should be instructed to have coitus at least every other day during this time.

## Menotropins

Menotropins [Pergonal, Humegon] (also known as human menopausal gonadotropin, or HMG) is a hormonal preparation having equal amounts of LH and FSH activity.

Commercial menotropins is prepared by extraction from the urine of postmenopausal women.

**Therapeutic Actions and Use.** Menotropins is employed in conjunction with HCG to promote follicular maturation and ovulation. Menotropins acts directly on the ovaries to cause maturation of follicles. Once follicles have ripened, HCG is administered to induce ovulation.

Menotropins is employed when gonadotropin secretion by the pituitary is insufficient to provide adequate ovarian stimulation. Candidates for menotropins therapy must have ovaries capable of responding to FSH and LH; menotropins is of no help in women with primary ovarian failure. Among properly selected patients, the rate of ovulation approaches 100%. It should be noted that therapy with menotropins is not cheap: a single cycle of treatment can cost between $500 and $1500 (in addition to physicians' fees and laboratory costs). Menotropins has also been used to treat infertility in males (hypogonadotropic hypogonadism, idiopathic male infertility).

**Adverse Effects.** The most serious adverse response is *ovarian hyperstimulation syndrome*, a condition characterized by sudden enlargement of the ovaries. Mild to moderate ovarian enlargement is common, occurring in about 20% of patients. This condition is benign and resolves spontaneously upon discontinuation of drug use. Of greater concern is ovarian enlargement that occurs rapidly and that may be accompanied by ascites, pleural effusion, and considerable pain. If this manifestation of ovarian stimulation occurs, menotropins should be withdrawn and the patient hospitalized. Treatment is usually supportive (bed rest, analgesics, fluid and electrolyte replacement). If rupture of ovarian cysts occurs, surgery may be required to stop bleeding. Enlargement of the ovaries is most likely during the first 2 weeks of treatment. To ensure early detection, the patient should be examined at least every other day while taking menotropins, and for 2 weeks after termination of treatment. Ovarian stimulation can be minimized by keeping the dosage as low as possible.

In addition to causing excessive ovarian stimulation, menotropins may produce *spontaneous abortion* (in about 25% of menotropins-facilitated pregnancies) and *multiple births* (15% of pregnancies result in twins; 5% of pregnancies have three or more conceptuses).

**Monitoring Therapy.** Ovarian responses to menotropins must be monitored to determine timing of HCG administration and to minimize the risk of ovarian enlargement. Responses can be followed by measuring serum estrogen levels and by ultrasonography of the developing follicles. When estrogen levels rise to twice the pretreatment baseline, or when ultrasonography indicates that follicles have enlarged to 16 to 20 mm, administration of menotropins should cease and HCG should be injected. However, if estrogen production is excessive (serum levels 3 to 4 times the pretreatment baseline), HCG should be withheld, since there is a risk of ovarian hyperstimulation under these conditions. In addition, HCG should be withheld if ultrasonography indicates the presence of four or more mature follicles.

**Preparations, Dosage, and Administration.** Menotropins [Pergonal, Humegon] is dispensed as a powder to be reconstituted with sterile saline immediately prior to use. Each Pergonal ampule contains 75 international units (IU) of FSH activity and 75 IU of LH activity. Each Humegon ampule contains 150 IU of FSH activity and 150 IU of LH activity. Administration is by IM injection.

Menotropins is used sequentially with HCG: after follicular maturation has been induced with menotropins, HCG is injected to promote ovulation. For the initial cycle, the contents of one menotropins ampule is injected daily for 9 to 12 days. When estrogen measurements indicate follicular maturation has occurred, menotropins is discontinued; HCG (5000 to 10,000 USP units) is injected 24 hours after the last menotropins dose. Ovulation occurs 2 to 3 days after injection of HCG. Accordingly, patients should be instructed to have intercourse on the eve of HCG injection and on the following 2 to 3 days. If there is evidence of ovulation but conception does not take place, treatment should be repeated for two more courses using the same menotropins dosage. If treatment remains ineffective, two additional courses may be tried, using twice as much menotropins as previously. If there is still no conception, further treatment is unlikely to help.

## Urofollitropin

Urofollitropin [Metrodin] is a preparation of FSH made from the urine of postmenopausal women. Its actions, uses, and adverse effects are like those of menotropins (a 50:50 mixture of FSH and LH). Like menotropins, urofollitropin acts directly on the ovary to stimulate follicle maturation. For treatment of infertility, urofollitropin is used sequentially with HCG: urofollitropin is given first to promote follicle maturation; then HCG is given to stimulate ovulation. As with menotropins, the principal adverse effect of urofollitropin is ovarian hyperstimulation syndrome.

## Gonadorelin

**Therapeutic Use and Mechanism of Action.** Gonadorelin [Lutrepulse] is a synthetic polypeptide identical in structure to human gonadotropin-releasing hormone (Gn-RH). The drug is given to treat infertility resulting from hypothalamic failure to secrete Gn-RH.

Under physiologic conditions, Gn-RH is secreted from the hypothalamus in a *pulsatile* pattern; following secretion, the hormone acts on the pituitary to promote release of LH and FSH, which in turn act on the ovary to promote follicular maturation and ovulation. To be effective, gonadorelin must be administered in "pulses" that mimic physiologic secretion of Gn-RH. When administered in this pattern, the drug is able to promote follicular maturation and ovulation.

**Adverse Effects.** Because administration is via an indwelling intravenous catheter, there is a risk of inflammation, infection, phlebitis, and hematoma at the site of infusion. Like menotropins, gonadorelin can cause hyperstimulation of the ovaries, but the risk is much lower with gonadorelin. There is a 12% incidence of multiple births, twins being most common.

**Preparations, Dosage, and Administration.** Gonadorelin acetate [Lutrepulse] is dispensed as a lyophilized powder to be reconstituted for IV use. The drug is administered through an indwelling catheter, usually in a forearm vein, using a portable infusion pump (Lutrepulse pump) supplied by the manufacturer.

The initial dosing schedule is 5 μg every 90 minutes for 21 days or until ovulation occurs. If pregnancy occurs, administration may be continued for an additional 2 weeks to support the corpus luteum. Throughout the procedure, the catheter should be moved every 24 hours. Treatment is expensive, costing $750 to $1000 per cycle.

## Human Chorionic Gonadotropin

Human chorionic gonadotropin is a polypeptide hormone produced by the placenta. HCG is similar in structure and identical in action to luteinizing hormone.

*Therapeutic Use.* HCG is used to induce ovulation in women who are infertile because of ovulatory failure. The drug causes ovulation by simulating the midcycle LH surge. When HCG is used to promote ovulation, follicular maturation must first be induced with another agent, usually menotropins. HCG can also be used in conjunction with clomiphene when treatment with clomiphene alone has failed to promote ovulation.

*Adverse Effects.* The most severe adverse response to HCG is *ovarian hyperstimulation syndrome*. If this reaction occurs, hospitalization and discontinuation of HCG are indicated. HCG may also provoke *rupture of ovarian cysts* with resultant bleeding into the peritoneal cavity. *Multiple births* may be induced; the patient should be informed of this possibility. Additional adverse effects include *edema*, *pain at the site of injection*, and *central nervous system disturbances* (headache, irritability, restlessness, fatigue).

*Preparations, Dosage, and Administration.* Commercial HCG is prepared by extraction from the urine of pregnant women. HCG is dispensed as a powder and must be reconstituted for use. Administration is by IM injection. The usual dose for induction of ovulation is 5000 to 10,000 USP units. Trade names are A.P.L., Chorex, Choron, Gonic, Pregnyl, and Profasi.

Prior to giving HCG, follicular maturation must be induced with another agent (menotropins, urofollitropin, or clomiphene). When used in conjunction with menotropins or urofollitropin, HCG is injected 1 day after the last menotropins/urofollitropin dose. When used as an adjunct to clomiphene, HCG is administered 7 to 9 days after the last clomiphene dose.

## Bromocriptine

*Therapeutic Uses.* Bromocriptine [Parlodel] is used to correct amenorrhea and infertility associated with excessive prolactin secretion. If galactorrhea is present, this consequence of hyperprolactinemia may also be corrected. When the source of excessive prolactin is a pituitary adenoma, bromocriptine can induce regression of the tumor, in addition to reducing prolactin secretion. Continuous treatment can suppress tumor growth for years. Bromocriptine is also used in Parkinson's disease (see Chapter 22).

*Mechanism of Fertility Promotion.* Bromocriptine stimulates receptors for dopamine. By stimulating dopamine receptors in the anterior pituitary, bromocriptine inhibits prolactin secretion. Reductions in prolactin levels are accompanied by normalization of the menstrual cycle and a return of fertility. The mechanism by which lowering of prolactin levels leads to a return of ovulation is not known.

*Adverse Effects.* When bromocriptine is given to treat infertility, adverse effects are frequent but usually mild. Nausea occurs in 50% of patients. Headache, dizziness, fatigue, and abdominal cramps are also common. Orthostatic hypotension may occur, but is rare at the doses employed to decrease prolactin secretion. Teratogenic effects have not been reported. Adverse effects can be minimized by taking bromocriptine with meals and by initiating treatment at low doses.

*Preparations, Dosage, and Administration.* Bromocriptine mesylate [Parlodel] is dispensed in 2.5-mg tablets and 5-mg capsules. Dosing is begun at 2.5 mg once a day and then gradually increased to 2.5 mg 2 or 3 times a day. All doses should be administered with food. Normalization of the menstrual cycle may occur rapidly (within a few days) or may require up to 2 months of treatment. As soon as pregnancy is achieved, use of bromocriptine should cease. As a rule, administration should not resume until after delivery. If treatment is not reinstated, hypersecretion of prolactin is almost certain to recur within a year.

## Drugs for Endometriosis

### Danazol

*Therapeutic Use.* Danazol [Danocrine] is used to treat *endometriosis and associated infertility*. Treatment leads to complete resolution of endometrial implants in the majority of patients. In most cases, ovulation is restored within 1 to 3 months after danazol has been discontinued. Since danazol may temporarily impair the ability of the endometrium to support pregnancy, attempts at conception should be postponed for about 3 months following danazol withdrawal. It should be noted that, when endometriosis is mild, danazol may *reduce* fertility rather than increase it. In addition to the therapy of endometriosis, danazol has been used to treat *angioneurotic edema* and *fibrocystic breast disease*.

*Mechanism of Action.* Danazol acts by multiple mechanisms to induce regression of endometrial implants. First, danazol inhibits several of the enzymes required for synthesis of ovarian hormones, thereby depriving the implant of the hormonal environment needed for its maintenance. Second, danazol suppresses secretion of pituitary gonadotropins (FSH and LH), thereby further decreasing the availability of ovarian hormones. Lastly, danazol may act directly on the implant to block ovarian hormone receptors. All of these actions result in atrophy of ectopic endometrial tissue. The normal endometrium atrophies as well.

*Adverse Effects and Interactions.* Danazol is weakly androgenic and may induce virilization. Potential manifestations include acne, deepening of the voice, and growth of facial hair. These effects are usually reversible upon cessation of treatment. If taken during pregnancy, danazol may cause masculinization of the female fetus. Danazol may also cause edema, and therefore should be used with caution in patients with cardiac and renal disorders. Liver dysfunction has been reported; liver function should be assessed before therapy and periodically thereafter. Danazol may intensify the effects of oral anticoagulants (e.g., warfarin).

***Preparations, Dosage, and Administration.*** Danazol [Danocrine] is dispensed in capsules (50, 100, and 200 mg) for oral administration. A dosage of 200 to 300 mg twice daily is usually effective. To ensure that danazol is not taken during pregnancy, therapy should be initiated at the time of menstruation. The usual course of treatment is 3 to 9 months.

## Gonadotropin-Releasing Hormone Analogs

Nafarelin [Synarel] and leuprolide [Lupron] are synthetic analogs of gonadotropin-releasing hormone used to treat endometriosis. Although both drugs reduce symptoms of endometriosis, there is no proof that they increase fertility.

***Nafarelin.*** *Mechanism of Action.* Ectopic endometrial implants, like the normal endometrium, are dependent on ovarian hormones. Nafarelin suppresses endometriosis by indirectly suppressing ovarian hormone production.

How does nafarelin suppress production of ovarian hormones? *Initial* doses of nafarelin actually *increase* hormone production. This increase occurs because nafarelin, like endogenous Gn-RH, acts on the pituitary to promote release of FSH and LH, which in turn act on the ovary to stimulate hormone production. However, in contrast to endogenous Gn-RH, which has a short half-life and is released in a *pulsatile* fashion, nafarelin has a long half-life and is administered on a continuing basis. As a result, nafarelin causes *continuous* stimulation of pituitary Gn-RH receptors. This continuous stimulation has the paradoxical effect of *suppressing* FSH and LH release, thereby depriving the ovary of the stimulation needed for hormone production.

*Therapeutic Use.* Nafarelin is approved for treatment of *endometriosis*. The drug is about as effective as danazol for this application. Nafarelin reduces the area of endometriosis and improves symptoms. The drug's ability to promote pregnancy is not clear. Because of concern about bone loss (see below), nafarelin should not be used for more than 6 months.

It must be stressed that nafarelin, like danazol, does not produce cure. Within 6 months after discontinuation of treatment, symptoms return in up to 50% of women who had previously been rendered symptom free.

*Adverse Effects.* Most undesired effects are secondary to estrogen deficiency. Common responses include hot flushes, vaginal dryness, decreased libido, mood changes, and headache. Nasal irritation also occurs (administration is by nasal spray). Nafarelin is teratogenic and must not be used during pregnancy.

The adverse effect of greatest concern is bone loss. After 3 to 6 months of treatment, bone mass and mineral content have decreased in some patients. To minimize the risk of osteoporosis, the manufacturer recommends that treatment last no longer than 6 months.

*Preparations, Dosage, and Administration.* Nafarelin [Synarel] is dispensed in a spray for intranasal administration. (The drug cannot be given orally because of rapid degradation by gastrointestinal enzymes.) For treatment of endometriosis, the initial dosage is 200 µg (one spray) in the morning and another 200 µg in the evening. Doses should alternate between nostrils. Treatment should begin between days 2 and 4 of the menstrual cycle.

***Leuprolide.*** Like nafarelin, leuprolide [Lupron Depot] is a Gn-RH analog that can reduce symptoms of endometriosis. However, proof of its ability to enhance fertility is lacking. Leuprolide has the same mechanism as nafarelin (suppression of LH and RH release with continued use) as well as the same adverse effects (hot flushes, vaginal dryness, amenorrhea, headache, depression, osteoporosis). For treatment of endometriosis, a depot formulation of leuprolide is used; the dosage is 3.75 mg IM once a month. In addition to endometriosis, leuprolide is indicated for advanced cancer of the prostate.

## Drugs for Impotence

### Papaverine Plus Phentolamine

***Therapeutic Use.*** The combination of papaverine (a smooth muscle relaxant) plus phentolamine (an alpha-adrenergic blocking agent) can counteract impotence when injected directly into the corpus cavernosum of the penis. Erection develops within minutes and lasts for 2 to 4 hours. In clinical trials, erection suitable for coitus was produced in 65% to 100% of males whose impotence was of neurologic or vascular origin. For patients who do not respond to papaverine plus phentolamine, addition of alprostadil may help (see below).

***Mechanism of Action.*** Papaverine and phentolamine produce erection by increasing arterial inflow to the penis and decreasing venous outflow. Arterial inflow is augmented by alpha-adrenergic blockade (causing arterial dilation) and by the direct relaxant action of papaverine on arterial smooth muscle. Venous outflow is reduced, probably because relaxation of corporal smooth muscle results in occlusion of the venules that drain the corporal spaces.

***Adverse Effects.*** *Priapism* (persistent erection lasting more than 6 hours) occurs in about 10% of patients. Persistent erection can be relieved by aspiration of blood from the corpus followed by irrigation with a solution containing a vasoconstrictor (e.g., epinephrine, phenylephrine, metaraminol). Development of painless *fibrotic nodules* in the corpus is common. Other adverse effects include *orthostatic hypotension with dizziness, transient paresthesias, ecchymosis* (extravasation of blood into subcutaneous tissue), and *difficulty in achieving orgasm or ejaculation.*

***Dosage and Administration.*** For males with psychogenic or neurogenic impotence, erection can be achieved by injecting as little as 0.1 ml of a solution containing 30 mg of papaverine/ml and 1.0 mg of phentolamine/ml. A 1-ml syringe with a 27-gauge or 28-gauge, 3/8-inch needle is used. Injections are made directly into the corpus cavernosum through the lateral aspect of the shaft of the penis. These injections are nearly painless and can be administered by the patient.

### Alprostadil (Prostaglandin E₁)

***Intracavernous.*** Like the combination of phentolamine plus papaverine, alprostadil [Caverject] can produce erection in impotent males when injected directly into the corpus cavernosum. Erection results from increased inflow of arterial blood and reduced outflow of venous blood. Dosages may range from 5 to 40 µg and should be determined in the physician's office. The dosing endpoint is an erection that is sufficient for intercourse, but that does not last for more than 1 hour. Alprostadil should be used no more than 3 times a week and not more than once in 24 hours. Acute adverse effects are penile pain (37%), prolonged erection (4%), and priapism (erection lasting more than 6 hours; 0.4%). Penile fibrosis may develop with continued use.

*Transurethral.* Alprostadil pellets [Muse], inserted into the urethra, are an alternative to intracavernous injection of the drug. Administration is accomplished by loading a pellet into a small plastic applicator, which is then inserted an inch and a half into the penis. The procedure is painless. Erection develops 5 to 10 minutes after drug insertion and lasts 30 to 60 minutes. Alprostadil pellets are available in 4 sizes: 125, 250, 500, and 1000 µg. Dosage should be determined in the physician's office; the objective is to employ the smallest dose required to produce an erection sufficient for intercourse. Alprostadil pellets should be used no more than twice every 24 hours. The most common adverse effect, dull ache in the penis, has an incidence of 11%. Priapism and penile fibrosis, which have occurred with alprostadil injections, have not been reported with the pellets.

## KEY POINTS

- Infertility (subfertility) is defined as a decrease in reproductive ability, whereas sterility is a complete absence of reproductive ability.
- Infertility in a couple may result from infertility in the male partner, the female partner, or both.
- Clomiphene is used to promote follicular maturation and ovulation.
- Clomiphene acts by blocking estrogen receptors in the hypothalamus and pituitary, causing a compensatory increase in the release of LH and FSH, which then act on the ovary to promote follicular maturation and ovulation.
- Menotropins is a 50:50 mixture of LH and FSH.
- Menotropins is used sequentially with HCG: menotropins is given to promote follicular maturation, then HCG is given to promote ovulation.
- The most serious adverse effect of menotropins is ovarian hyperstimulation syndrome, which is characterized by *sudden* enlargement of the ovaries.
- Gonadorelin is a synthetic polypeptide identical to human Gn-RH.
- When administered in a pulsatile fashion, gonadorelin acts on the pituitary to cause release of LH and FSH, which then act on the ovary to promote follicular maturation and ovulation.
- HCG is given to stimulate ovulation (after another drug, such as menotropins, has been given to promote follicular maturation).
- Like menotropins, HCG can cause ovarian hyperstimulation syndrome.
- Bromocriptine is given to suppress excessive prolactin release.
- Danazol is used to treat endometriosis.
- Danazol acts by multiple mechanisms: it reduces synthesis of ovarian hormones, it suppresses release of FSH and LH, and it blocks hormone receptors on endometrial implants.
- Nafarelin and leuprolide are Gn-RH analogs used to treat endometriosis.
- Nafarelin and leuprolide act by (indirectly) suppressing production of the ovarian hormones needed to support endometrial implants.
- Papaverine plus phentolamine is injected directly into the corpus cavernosum of the penis to promote erection in impotent males. Priapism (erection lasting more than 6 hours) may occur.
- Alprostadil (prostaglandin $E_1$), administered by intracavernous injection or transurethral pellet, is an alternative to papaverine plus phentolamine for treating impotence.

## Summary of Major Nursing Implications*

## Clomiphene

The implications summarized here apply only to the use of clomiphene for promoting maturation of ovarian follicles and ovulation. (Clomiphene has also been used investigationally to increase fertility in males.)

### Preadministration Assessment

#### Therapeutic Goal
Promotion of follicular maturation and ovulation in carefully selected patients.

#### Baseline Data
Take a complete health and gynecologic history; a pelvic examination and an endometrial biopsy are also required. Ovarian and pituitary function must be confirmed. Pregnancy must be ruled out.

#### Identifying High-Risk Patients
Clomiphene is *contraindicated* during *pregnancy* and in women with *liver disease* and *abnormal uterine bleeding of undetermined origin*.

### Implementation: Administration

#### Route
Oral.

*Patient education information is highlighted in color.

## Administration Schedule

If cyclic menstrual bleeding has been occurring, begin therapy 5 days after the onset of menses. If menstruation has been absent, begin treatment at any time.

The initial course consists of 50-mg doses once daily for 5 days. If ovulation fails to occur, additional courses may be tried, each beginning no sooner than 30 days after the previous course.

## Implementation: Measures to Enhance Therapeutic Effects

### Timing of Coitus

Advise the patient to have coitus at least every other day during the 5- to 10-day period that follows the last clomiphene dose.

### Adjunctive Use of Human Chorionic Gonadotropin

If ovulation fails to occur under the influence of clomiphene alone, injection of HCG 7 to 9 days after the last clomiphene dose may yield success.

## Ongoing Evaluation and Interventions

### Evaluating Therapeutic Effects

Successful induction of ovulation is evaluated by monitoring for an increase in basal body temperature or plasma progesterone levels, or by examining an endometrial biopsy for evidence of secretory transformation.

### Minimizing Adverse Effects

*Ovarian Enlargement.* Instruct the patient to notify the physician if pelvic pain occurs (an indication of ovarian enlargement). If ovarian enlargement is diagnosed, clomiphene should be withdrawn, after which ovarian size usually regresses spontaneously.

*Reduced Fertility.* Clomiphene may cause luteal phase defect; this response can be corrected with progesterone. Alteration of cervical mucus may occur; estrogens can be used to restore the volume and fluidity of cervical secretions.

*Multiple Births.* Inform the patient that multiple births (usually twins) are not uncommon in clomiphene-facilitated pregnancies.

*Visual Disturbances.* Forewarn the patient about possible visual disturbances (blurred vision, visual flashes), and instruct her to notify the physician if these occur. Visual aberrations usually cease following drug withdrawal.

*Other Adverse Effects.* Common side effects include hot flushes (similar to the vasomotor responses of menopause), nausea, abdominal discomfort, bloating, and breast engorgement. Forewarn the patient about these effects and instruct her to notify the physician if they are especially disturbing.

# Menotropins

The implications summarized here refer only to the use of menotropins (together with HCG) for induction of follicular maturation and ovulation. (Menotropins is also used to treat certain forms of infertility in males.)

## Preadministration Assessment

### Therapeutic Goal

Induction of follicular maturation and ovulation (in conjunction with HCG) in carefully selected patients.

### Baseline Data

A thorough gynecologic and endocrinologic evaluation should precede treatment. Ovarian function must be verified. Obtain a baseline value for serum estrogen.

### Identifying High-Risk Patients

Menotropins is *contraindicated* in the presence of *pregnancy*, *primary ovarian failure*, *thyroid dysfunction*, *adrenal dysfunction*, *ovarian cysts*, and *ovarian enlargement* (other than that caused by polycystic ovary syndrome).

## Implementation: Administration

### Route

Intramuscular.

### Administration

Reconstitute powdered menotropins with sterile saline immediately prior to injection.

Menotropins is employed sequentially with HCG. Administer menotropins for 9 to 12 days (to promote follicular maturation). Twenty-four hours after the last dose, inject HCG. Ovulation follows in 2 to 3 days.

Serum estrogen content and ultrasonography are used to assess follicular maturation; upon follicular maturation, menotropins is discontinued and HCG is injected. If estrogen production is excessive (3 to 4 times the pretreatment baseline) or if ultrasonography indicates the presence of four or more mature follicles, withhold HCG.

## Implementation: Measures to Enhance Therapeutic Effects

### Timing of Coitus

Advise the patient to have intercourse on the eve of HCG injection and on the following 2 to 3 days (i.e., during the probable period of ovulation).

## Ongoing Evaluation and Interventions

### Minimizing Adverse Effects

*Ovarian Hyperstimulation Syndrome.* Rapid ovarian enlargement can occur, sometimes associated with ascites, pleural effusion, and pain. If ovarian enlargement is excessive, discontinue menotropins and hospitalize the patient. Treatment is supportive (bed rest, analgesics, fluid and electrolyte replacement). If ovarian cysts rupture, surgery may be required to stop bleeding. To ensure early detection of ovarian enlargement, the patient should be examined at least every other day during menotropins use, and for 2 weeks following drug withdrawal. Since HCG can intensify ovarian stimulation, if serum estrogen levels rise to 3 to 4 times the pretreatment baseline (suggesting existing hyperstimulation of the ovaries), HCG should not be given.

***Other Adverse Effects.*** Forewarn the patient that treatment may result in *spontaneous abortion*. Inform the patient that *multiple births* are relatively common in menotropins-facilitated pregnancies.

# Human Chorionic Gonadotropin

The implications summarized here apply only to the use of HCG in the treatment of female infertility.

## Preadministration Assessment

### Therapeutic Goal
Induction of ovulation in women who are infertile because of anovulation. Pretreatment with menotropins, urofollitropin, or clomiphene is required.

## Implementation: Administration

### Route
Intramuscular.

### Administration
HCG must be used in conjunction with menotropins, urofollitropin, or clomiphene. When used with menotropins or urofollitropin, HCG is injected 1 day after the last menotropins dose. When used with clomiphene, HCG is administered 7 to 9 days after the last clomiphene dose.

## Ongoing Evaluation and Interventions

### Minimizing Adverse Effects
***Ovarian Hyperstimulation Syndrome.*** See implications for menotropins.

***Multiple Births.*** Inform the patient that multiple births are common in HCG-facilitated pregnancies.

# Bromocriptine

The implications summarized here refer only to the use of bromocriptine for hyperprolactinemia. They do not apply to treatment of Parkinson's disease.

## Preadministration Assessment

### Therapeutic Goal
Treatment of female infertility occurring secondary to hyperprolactinemia.

### Identifying High-Risk Patients
Bromocriptine is *contraindicated* during *pregnancy* and in patients with *severe ischemic heart disease* or *peripheral vascular disease*.

## Implementation: Administration

### Route
Oral.

### Administration
Instruct the patient to take bromocriptine with food.

Normalization of the menstrual cycle may occur within a few days or may require up to 2 months of treatment.

Bromocriptine should be withdrawn when pregnancy is achieved, and administration should not resume until after delivery.

## Ongoing Evaluation and Interventions

### Minimizing Adverse Effects
***Nausea.*** Inform the patient that nausea can be reduced by taking bromocriptine with meals.

***Other Adverse Effects.*** Headache, dizziness, fatigue, and abdominal cramps can be reduced by initiating therapy at low doses.

# Danazol

The implications summarized here refer only to the use of danazol in the treatment of endometriosis. (Danazol may also be used to treat angioneurotic edema and fibrocystic breast disease.)

## Preadministration Assessment

### Therapeutic Goal
Regression of ectopic endometrial implants (endometriosis) and reversal of infertility occurring secondary to endometriosis.

### Baseline Data
Obtain tests of liver function.

### Identifying High-Risk Patients
Danazol is *contraindicated* during *pregnancy* and for women with *undiagnosed genital bleeding* or *severe impairment of cardiac, renal, or hepatic function*.

## Implementation: Administration

### Route

Oral.

### Administration

Initiate therapy during menstruation. Treatment typically lasts 3 to 9 months. Ovulation and fertility are usually restored 1 to 3 months after danazol withdrawal.

## Ongoing Evaluation and Interventions

### Minimizing Adverse Effects

*Impairment of Pregnancy.* Danazol may temporarily impair the ability of the endometrium to support pregnancy. Caution the patient to avoid conception for about 3 months following danazol withdrawal.

*Virilization.* Danazol is weakly androgenic. Inform the patient about signs of masculinization (acne, deepening of the voice, growth of facial hair), and instruct her to notify the physician if these occur. Virilization usually reverses following danazol withdrawal.

*Use in Pregnancy.* If taken during pregnancy, danazol may cause masculinization of the female fetus. Warn the patient against becoming pregnant prior to danazol withdrawal.

*Edema.* Danazol may cause edema. Use with caution in the presence of cardiac and renal disease.

*Liver Dysfunction.* Liver dysfunction has been reported. Liver function should be assessed prior to danazol use and periodically throughout the course of treatment.

# CHAPTER 60

# Uterine Stimulants and Relaxants

**Uterine Stimulants (Oxytocics)**
 Oxytocin
 Ergot Alkaloids: Ergonovine and Methylergonovine
 Prostaglandins: Carboprost and Dinoprostone

**Uterine Relaxants (Tocolytics)**
 Beta$_2$-Adrenergic Agonists: Ritodrine and Terbutaline
 Other Uterine Relaxants

Uterine contraction can be intensified or diminished with drugs. Drugs that stimulate contraction are known as *oxytocics*. Drugs that suppress contraction are known as *tocolytics*. Oxytocic agents have three applications: (1) induction or augmentation of labor, (2) control of postpartum bleeding, and (3) induction of abortion. The tocolytic drugs have only one major use: suppression of preterm labor.

## Uterine Stimulants (Oxytocics)

There are three groups of uterine stimulants: (1) *oxytocin* (in a group by itself), (2) *ergot alkaloids*, and (3) *prostaglandins*. The principal use for oxytocin is induction of labor; the principal use of ergot alkaloids is control of postpartum bleeding; and the principal use of prostaglandins is abortion.

### Oxytocin

Oxytocin [Pitocin, Syntocinon] is a peptide hormone produced by the posterior pituitary. This hormone promotes uterine contraction during parturition and stimulates the milk-ejection reflex. The primary therapeutic use of oxytocin is induction of labor near term, a procedure for which oxytocin is the agent of choice.

#### Physiologic and Pharmacologic Effects

*Uterine Stimulation.* Oxytocin can increase the force, frequency, and duration of uterine contractions. The ability of the uterus to respond to oxytocin depends on the stage of gestation: early in pregnancy, uterine sensitivity to oxytocin is low; as pregnancy proceeds, the uterus becomes progressively more responsive; and just prior to term, a large and abrupt increase in responsiveness develops. These increases in sensitivity occur because the number of oxytocin receptors on uterine smooth muscle in-

creases throughout pregnancy. Although uterine sensitivity to oxytocin is low early in pregnancy, oxytocin can still initiate and enhance contractions at this stage; however, the doses required are much larger than those needed to stimulate the uterus at term.

Despite the profound effects of oxytocin on uterine contractility, the precise role of oxytocin in spontaneous labor and delivery has not been established. We do know that administration of exogenous oxytocin can elicit contractions identical to those seen during spontaneous labor. However, we also know that parturition can take place with virtually no oxytocin present, although labor will be prolonged. Furthermore, during normal labor or during labor induced artificially (through rupture of the membranes), only modest increases in plasma oxytocin levels occur. From these observations we can conclude that, although oxytocin is not absolutely required for parturition, it is very likely that oxytocin serves to facilitate contractions. However, it is not certain that oxytocin is responsible for actually *initiating* the process of labor.

*Milk Ejection.* Milk is produced by glandular tissue of the breast and is later transferred, via small channels, into large sinuses within the breast. Once in these sinuses, milk is readily accessible to the suckling infant. Transfer of milk to the sinuses is brought about by the milk-ejection reflex: when the infant sucks on the breast, neuronal stimuli are sent to the posterior pituitary, causing release of oxytocin; oxytocin then causes contraction of the smooth muscle surrounding the small milk channels, thereby forcing milk into the large sinuses. In the absence of oxytocin, milk ejection does not occur.

*Water Retention.* Oxytocin is similar in structure to antidiuretic hormone (ADH), which acts on the kidney to decrease excretion of water. Although less potent than ADH, oxytocin can nonetheless promote renal retention of water.

#### Pharmacokinetics

Oxytocin is usually administered IV or IM. To promote milk ejection, intranasal administration is employed. The plasma half-life of oxytocin is short, ranging from 12 to 17 minutes. Elimination is by a combination of hepatic metabolism and renal excretion.

## Use for Induction of Labor

*Rationale.* Induction of labor is reserved for those pregnancies in which early vaginal delivery is likely to decrease morbidity and mortality for either the mother or the infant. The most common reason for induction is premature rupture of the membranes. Other acceptable indications include severe maternal infection, diabetes mellitus, placental insufficiency, renal insufficiency, anemia, and pre-eclampsia (at or near term). Labor should be induced only when continued pregnancy constitutes a greater risk to the mother and fetus than the risk of induction itself. Induction for elective purposes (e.g., convenience of the obstetrician) is controversial.

*Precautions and Contraindications.* Improper use of oxytocin can be hazardous. Uterine rupture may occur, which may result in death of the mother, the infant, or both. The likelihood of trauma is especially high in the presence of cephalopelvic disproportion, fetal malpresentation, placental abnormalities, previous uterine surgery, and fetal distress. Oxytocin is contraindicated in pregnancies with any of these characteristics. Induction of labor in women of high parity (five or more pregnancies) carries a high risk of uterine rupture; oxytocin must be used with special caution in these patients.

*Adverse Effect: Water Intoxication.* When administered in large doses, oxytocin exerts an antidiuretic effect. If large volumes of fluid have been administered along with oxytocin, retention of water may produce intoxication. However, at the doses employed to induce labor, water intoxication is rare.

*Dosage and Administration.* For induction of labor, oxytocin is administered by intravenous infusion. The flow rate must be carefully controlled with an infusion pump. Solutions should be dilute (e.g., 10 mU/ml) and infused at an initial rate of no more than 1 to 2 mU/min. The infusion rate is then gradually increased (by increments of 1 to 2 mU/min every 30 to 60 minutes) until uterine contractions resembling those of spontaneous labor have been produced (i.e., contractions every 2 to 3 minutes and lasting 45 to 60 seconds). The infusion rate should rarely exceed 10 mU/min.

During oxytocin infusion, constant monitoring is required. The mother should be monitored for uterine contractility (frequency, duration, intensity), blood pressure, and pulse rate. The fetus should be monitored for heart rate and rhythm. In the event of significant maternal or fetal distress, the infusion should be stopped; this will cause contractions to diminish rapidly. Complications that usually require interruption of the infusion are (1) elevation of resting uterine pressure above 15 to 20 mm $H_2O$, (2) contractions that persist for more than 90 seconds, (3) contractions that occur more often than every 2 to 3 minutes, and (4) pronounced alteration in fetal heart rate or rhythm.

### Additional Therapeutic Uses

*Augmentation of Labor.* Oxytocin may be employed if labor is *dysfunctional*. However, patients must be judiciously selected, and oxytocin dosage must be regulated with special care. As a rule, oxytocic agents should not be used to promote labor that is already in progress, even if that labor is proceeding slowly: by intensifying the force of contractions, oxytocin may cause uterine damage (laceration or rupture) or trauma to the infant.

*Postpartum Use.* Oxytocin can be administered after placental delivery to control bleeding or hemorrhage and to increase uterine tone. Administration may be IM or IV.

*Milk Ejection.* Oxytocin has been used to promote milk ejection in nursing mothers. When employed for this purpose, the drug is administered by nasal spray 2 to 3 minutes prior to breastfeeding. Unfortunately, this treatment frequently fails. In addition, since oxytocin acts only to cause milk ejection, this agent will be of no help in cases of insufficient milk production.

*Abortion.* Oxytocin has been employed during the second trimester for management of incomplete abortion. Intravenous infusion of 10 units at a rate of 10 to 20 mU/min is often effective in emptying the uterus. However, oxytocin is not a method of choice.

### Preparations

Oxytocin [Pitocin, Syntocinon] is available as an injection (10 U/ml) for IV and IM administration. The drug is also dispensed as a spray (40 U/ml) for intranasal application.

## Ergot Alkaloids: Ergonovine and Methylergonovine

Ergot is a dried preparation of *Claviceps purpurea*, a fungus that grows on rye plants. The ergot alkaloids are compounds present in ergot. Ergot is capable of inducing powerful uterine contractions, a fact known to midwifes for centuries. Analysis of ergot has revealed the presence of several pharmacologically active constituents. Of these, *ergonovine* has proved the most effective uterine stimulant. A derivative of ergonovine—*methylergonovine*—has been synthesized and produces effects very much like those of ergonovine. Because the actions of ergonovine and methylergonovine are so similar, we will consider these agents jointly.

### Pharmacologic Effects

The ergot alkaloids produce their effects by stimulating a variety of receptors (adrenergic, dopaminergic, serotonergic). These drugs exert their most profound effects on uterine and vascular smooth muscle.

*Effects on the Uterus.* Ergot alkaloids stimulate uterine contraction. In small doses, these agents produce contractions of moderate strength that alternate with uterine relaxation of a normal degree and duration. With large doses, the force and frequency of contractions are greatly increased, and the extent of uterine relaxation is reduced; sustained contraction is not uncommon. Because contractions may be prolonged, *ergot alkaloids are not employed for induction of labor.*

*Vascular Effects.* Ergot alkaloids can cause constriction of arterioles and veins. This ability is the basis for using certain ergot alkaloids—ergotamine and dihydroergota-mine—to treat migraine headache (see Chapter 28).

## Pharmacokinetics

Regardless of route of administration, ergonovine and methylergonovine act rapidly. Uterine contractions begin within 60 seconds of IV injection, and within 10 minutes of oral and IM administration. Effects persist for several hours.

## Therapeutic Uses

*Postpartum Use.* The ergot alkaloids are given post-partum and postabortion to increase uterine tone and de-crease bleeding. The ability of these drugs to induce sus-tained uterine contraction makes them especially well suited for these purposes. Administration is usually de-layed until after delivery of the placenta. The patient should be monitored for blood pressure, pulse rate, and uterine contractility. Cramping occurs as part of the ther-apeutic response, but may also indicate overdose.

*Augmentation of Labor.* Because contractions may be both intense and prolonged, ergot alkaloids are not recommended for use during labor. If these drugs are given during labor, excessive uterine tone can cause trauma to the mother and fetus. Placental blood flow may be reduced, resulting in fetal hypoxia and uter-ine rupture. In addition, cervical laceration may occur.

*Migraine.* Ergot alkaloids relieve migraine in part by con-stricting dilated cerebral blood vessels. The two ergot prepara-tions employed in migraine are ergotamine and dihydroergot-amine. The pharmacology of these drugs and the treatment of migraine are discussed in Chapter 28 (Drugs for Headache).

## Adverse Effects

When ergot alkaloids are given orally or IM, significant adverse effects are rare. In contrast, IV administration fre-quently results in *hypertension*. This reaction can be se-vere and may be associated with nausea, vomiting, and headache; convulsions and even death have occurred. Accordingly, IV injection should be reserved for emergen-cies. Furthermore, patients with pre-existing hypertension should not be given these drugs. Caution should be exer-cised in patients with cardiovascular, renal, or hepatic dis-orders.

## Contraindications

Ergot alkaloids are contraindicated for women who are pregnant, hypertensive, or hypersensitive to these drugs. These drugs are also contraindicated for induction of labor and for use in the presence of threatened or ongo-ing spontaneous abortion.

### Preparations, Dosage, and Administration

*Preparations.* Ergonovine maleate [Ergotrate Maleate] and methylergonovine maleate [Methergine] are both dispensed in solution (0.2 mg/ml) for IV and IM administration. Methyl-ergonovine is also available in 0.2 mg tablets.

*Dosage and Administration.* For *parenteral* therapy, er-gonovine and methylergonovine are usually administered IM; in-travenous administration is hazardous and should be reserved for emergency control of postpartum hemorrhage. Treatment is usually initiated only after passage of the placenta. Dosages for both drugs are as follows: *intramuscular* (for control of post-

partum bleeding), 0.2 mg initially, repeated in 2 to 4 hours if needed; *intravenous* (for control of uterine hemorrhage), 0.2 mg infused over 60 seconds or more.

The *oral* dosage for methylergonovine (to minimize postpar-tum bleeding) is 0.2 to 0.4 mg every 6 to 8 hours (for no more than 1 week).

## Prostaglandins: Carboprost and Dinoprostone

Prostaglandins are synthesized in all tissues of the body, where they act as local hormones. Unlike true hormones, which travel to distant sites to produce their effects, prostaglandins act on the very tissues in which they are made; degradation of prostaglandins is so rapid that these agents rarely escape their tissue of origin intact. Although the prostaglandins produce a broad spectrum of physio-logic effects, clinical use of these compounds is limited. In obstetrics, prostaglandins are indicated for induction of abortion, induction of cervical ripening, and control of postpartum hemorrhage.

Nomenclature of the prostaglandins can be confusing and deserves comment. Each prostaglandin has three names: a traditional name, an official generic name, and a trade name. Carboprost and dinoprostone are generic names for the two drugs considered below. For *carbo-prost*, the traditional name is *15-methyl-prostaglandin F$_2$ alpha*; the trade name is *Hemabate*. For *dinoprostone*, the traditional name is *prostaglandin E$_2$*; trade names are *Prostin E$_2$* and *Prepidil*.

## Physiologic and Pharmacologic Effects

*Uterine Stimulation.* Prostaglandins, like oxytocin, can increase the force, frequency, and duration of uterine con-tractions. In the early months of pregnancy, the uterus is more responsive to prostaglandins than to oxytocin. During the second and third trimesters, prostaglandins can induce contractions of sufficient strength to cause complete evacuation of the uterus.

Like oxytocin, prostaglandins appear to have a physio-logic role as promoters of uterine contraction, sponta-neous labor, and delivery. Observations supporting this statement include: (1) exogenous prostaglandins can in-duce uterine contractions that are very similar in fre-quency and duration to those that occur spontaneously; (2) the ability of the uterus to synthesize prostaglandins in-creases at term; (3) the prostaglandin content of amniotic fluid, umbilical blood, and maternal blood increases at term and during labor; and (4) labor is delayed and pro-longed by agents that inhibit prostaglandin synthesis.

*Cervical Softening.* Local application of prostaglandins produces cervical softening. This softening results from breakdown of collagen, and hence mimics the process by which natural cervical ripening occurs. Softening of the cervix is not dependent on uterine stimulation.

## Therapeutic Uses

*Abortion.* Prostaglandins are used to induce second-trimester abortion. Uterine contractions develop slowly.

As a result, about 18 hours must pass before expulsion of the fetus takes place. Unlike other abortifacients, prostaglandins are not feticidal; hence, the aborted fetus may show transient signs of life. Prostaglandins have been proved teratogenic in animals. Therefore, if abortion fails, it is important that pregnancy be terminated by an alternative procedure (e.g., administration of oxytocin or hypertonic saline). Following passage of the fetus and placenta, the patient should be examined for possible cervical or uterine laceration.

**Other Applications.** One prostaglandin—carboprost—is indicated for control of *postpartum hemorrhage*. This drug is reserved for bleeding that has been refractory to more conventional agents (oxytocin, ergot alkaloids). In these situations, carboprost may be lifesaving. Another prostaglandin—dinoprostone—is used to *initiate ripening of the cervix* (prior to induction of labor); also, the drug has been used investigationally for *induction of labor*.

### Adverse Effects

**Gastrointestinal Disturbances.** Gastrointestinal reactions are extremely common and result from the ability of prostaglandins to stimulate smooth muscle of the alimentary canal. Vomiting and diarrhea occur in up to 60% of those treated. Nausea also occurs frequently. These responses can be reduced by pretreatment with antiemetic and antidiarrheal medications.

**Cervical or Uterine Laceration.** Intense uterine contractions can result in cervical or uterine laceration. The patient should be examined thoroughly for trauma following expulsion of the fetus and placenta.

**Other Adverse Effects.** *Fever* is common. When hyperthermia develops, it is important to distinguish between drug-induced fever and pyrexia resulting from endometritis. With *dinoprostone*, there is a 10% incidence of *headache*, *shivering*, and *chills*.

### Precautions and Contraindications

Prostaglandins are contraindicated for women with acute pelvic inflammatory disease and active disease of the heart, lungs, kidneys, or liver. These drugs should be used with caution in women with a history of asthma, hypotension, hypertension, diabetes, or uterine scarring.

#### Preparations, Dosage, and Administration

**Carboprost Tromethamine.** Carboprost tromethamine [Hemabate] is dispensed as an injection containing 250 μg of carboprost per milliliter. Administration is IM. For *induction of abortion* (weeks 13 to 20), the dosage is 250 μg initially followed by 250 μg every 1.5 to 3.5 hours as needed. For *control of postpartum bleeding*, a single 250 μg dose is injected.

**Dinoprostone.** Dinoprostone is available in two formulations: (1) 20-mg vaginal suppositories and (2) a gel (0.5 mg dinoprostone/2.5 ml gel) in prefilled syringes with shielded endocervical catheters (10- and 20-mm tip). Dinoprostone suppositories [Prostin E2] are used for abortion. Dinoprostone gel [Prepidil] is used for cervical ripening.

For *induction of abortion* (weeks 12 to 20), one 20-mg vaginal suppository is inserted initially, followed by one suppository every 3 to 5 hours as needed.

For *cervical ripening*, 0.5 mg of dinoprostone gel is introduced into the cervical canal just below the level of the internal os. The drug is administered using the prefilled syringe supplied by the manufacturer and fitted with the appropriate endocervical catheter. If the desired response has not occurred within 6 hours, an additional 0.5-mg dose can be given. If necessary, a third 0.5-mg dose can be given 6 hours later.

# Uterine Relaxants (Tocolytics)

Uterine relaxants (tocolytics) are given to prevent premature delivery (i.e., delivery prior to the 37th week of gestation). The drugs employed most frequently are beta$_2$-adrenergic agonists.

## Beta$_2$-Adrenergic Agonists: Ritodrine and Terbutaline

Two beta$_2$-adrenergic agonists—ritodrine and terbutaline—are used to delay preterm labor. Although both drugs are effective, only ritodrine has received FDA approval for this application.

### Ritodrine

Ritodrine [Yutopar] is classified as a beta$_2$-selective adrenergic agonist. Despite this classification, ritodrine also stimulates beta$_1$-adrenergic receptors, although less readily than beta$_2$ receptors. By causing beta$_1$ and beta$_2$ stimulation, ritodrine can elicit all of the effects characteristic of other beta-adrenergic agonists. These effects are described fully in Chapter 19.

**Effect on the Uterus.** Stimulation of uterine beta$_2$ receptors relaxes uterine smooth muscle. Following oral or IV administration, ritodrine decreases both the intensity and frequency of uterine contractions. Ritodrine-induced relaxation can be prevented with a beta-adrenergic blocker (e.g., propranolol).

**Therapeutic Use.** The only indication for ritodrine is suppression of preterm labor. Delivery may be delayed for weeks (to permit full-term intrauterine development) or labor may be suppressed for just a few *days* (while glucocorticoids are given to promote maturation of the fetal lungs). Ritodrine is not given if gestation has been less than 20 weeks, and use of ritodrine beyond the 34th week of gestation is rare. Therapy is most effective early in pregnancy and early in labor. Efficacy in advanced labor is uncertain. Treatment is begun with an intravenous infusion (for about 12 hours). Thereafter, oral therapy is instituted to maintain suppression of labor.

**Adverse Effects.** Significant adverse effects with *oral* ritodrine are rare. The adverse effects described below are associated with *intravenous* administration.

**Pulmonary Edema.** Intravenous ritodrine has caused pulmonary edema. The risk appears higher when glucocorticoids are given concurrently and when the infusion fluid is isotonic saline. Accordingly, 5% dextrose may be the preferred fluid. Some physicians recommend limiting total fluid intake to 2.5 L over 24 hours. The patient should be monitored for fluid overload. If pulmonary edema develops, the infusion should be discontinued and standard treatment implemented.

*Tachycardia.* Intravenous ritodrine almost always elevates maternal and fetal heart rate. Tachycardia results from stimulation of beta$_1$ receptors in the heart. Maternal and fetal heart rate should be monitored. Excessive tachycardia can usually be corrected by reducing the rate of infusion.

*Hypotension.* Blood pressure may be reduced because of vasodilation brought about by stimulation of beta$_2$ receptors on blood vessels. Hypotension can be minimized by keeping the patient in a left-lateral recumbent position.

*Hyperglycemia.* Intravenous ritodrine elevates blood glucose levels by stimulating beta$_2$ receptors in the liver. For most patients, hyperglycemia is transient. However, hyperglycemia is likely to persist in insulin-dependent diabetics. Insulin infusion is usually required to prevent ketoacidosis in these patients.

*Precautions and Contraindications.* Ritodrine should be employed only if the benefits of continued pregnancy outweigh the risks associated with drug-induced delay of delivery. Conditions for which the risks are considered too high include eclampsia, severe pre-eclampsia, hemorrhage, chorioamnionitis, maternal heart disease, and gestation of less than 20 weeks' duration. In these cases ritodrine is contraindicated. In addition, ritodrine must be used with caution in women with hyperthyroidism (because of heightened cardiac sensitivity to beta$_1$ stimulants) and in women with insulin-dependent diabetes.

*Preparations, Dosage, and Administration.* Ritodrine hydrochloride [Yutopar] is dispensed as an injection (10 and 15 mg/ml) for intravenous administration and in tablets (10 mg) for oral administration.

Intravenous therapy is used initially to arrest labor rapidly; later, the patient is switched to oral ritodrine for long-term suppression. Infusion is begun at a rate of 0.1 mg/min. This rate may be increased gradually until contractions have ceased or until the maximum acceptable rate (0.35 mg/min) has been reached. Infusion is continued for 12 hours after labor has stopped. Oral therapy is begun 30 minutes prior to terminating the infusion. The initial oral dosage is 10 mg every 2 hours for 24 hours. After this, the dosage is 10 to 20 mg every 4 to 6 hours (to a maximum of 120 mg daily). Oral therapy is continued for as long as suppression of labor is considered desirable. If contractions recur, IV treatment can be reinstated.

### Terbutaline

Terbutaline [Brethine, Bricanyl], is a beta$_2$-selective adrenergic agonist that is much like ritodrine in its actions, adverse effects, and potential uses. The principal indication for terbutaline is asthma (see Chapter 69). In addition, the drug is used widely to delay preterm labor, although it is not FDA approved for this application. Therapy is initiated with an IV infusion at a rate of 10 μg/min; the rate is then gradually increased to a maximum of 80 μg/min. After contractions have been suppressed with IV therapy, oral therapy (2.5 mg every 4 to 6 hours) is used for maintenance. For delay of labor, terbutaline appears superior to ritodrine in two ways: (1) recurrence of labor during oral therapy with terbutaline is less common than during oral therapy with ritodrine, and (2) terbutaline is much less expensive than ritodrine.

## Other Uterine Relaxants

*Magnesium Sulfate (Intravenous).* The primary obstetric use of magnesium sulfate is control of seizures associated with eclampsia and severe pre-eclampsia. However, magnesium may also be given to suppress preterm labor. Magnesium sulfate causes uterine relaxation through a direct effect on uterine smooth muscle; both the force and frequency of contractions are reduced. Arrest of labor is achieved at plasma levels of magnesium ranging from 4 to 7 mEq/L. At levels greater than these, substantial inhibition of cardiac conduction and neuromuscular transmission may occur, resulting in cardiac arrest and respiratory depression. Because it does not sensitize the heart to catecholamines or promote hyperglycemia, magnesium sulfate may be preferred to beta$_2$ agonists for suppressing preterm labor in women with hyperthyroidism or diabetes.

*Indomethacin.* Indomethacin is a third-line agent for suppressing preterm labor. The drug acts by inhibiting synthesis of prostaglandins, which are needed for uterine contraction (see discussion of prostaglandins above). Indomethacin is an effective tocolytic, but has been associated with significant neonatal complications, including bronchopulmonary dysplasia, respiratory distress syndrome, necrotizing enterocolitis, and intracranial hemorrhage. Furthermore, by inhibiting fetal synthesis of prostaglandins, the drug may promote premature closure of the ductus arteriosus. To suppress preterm labor, treatment is initiated with a 50-mg loading dose (usually rectal), followed by 25-mg doses every 6 hours for 2 to 3 days.

*Nifedipine.* Nifedipine [Procardia, Adalat] is a calcium channel blocker that has been used to suppress preterm labor. The drug is at least as effective as ritodrine. Presumably, nifedipine suppresses contractions by blocking calcium entry into uterine smooth muscle. Maternal side effects include transient tachycardia, facial flushing, and headache. In animal studies, calcium channel blockers have caused acidosis, hypoxemia, and hypercapnia in the newborn. To suppress preterm labor, an initial 10-mg dose (sublingual) is followed at 20-minute intervals by two or three additional 10-mg doses, after which 10- or 20-mg maintenance doses are given every 4 to 6 hours. The basic pharmacology of the calcium channel blockers is discussed in Chapter 42.

## KEY POINTS

- Oxytocic agents stimulate contraction of uterine smooth muscle.
- Oxytocics have three major applications: induction or augmentation of labor, induction of abortion, and control of postpartum bleeding.
- The principal indication for oxytocin is induction of labor, primarily for pregnancies in which early vaginal delivery is likely to decrease morbidity or mortality for the mother or infant. Induction of labor for convenience is controversial.
- Used improperly (e.g., in pregnancies with cephalopelvic disproportion), oxytocin can cause uterine rupture.
- Ergonovine and methylergonovine are powerful oxytocics used primarily to control postpartum bleeding.
- Because they produce very strong uterine contractions, ergonovine and methylergonovine are contraindicated for use in pregnancy.
- When administered IV, ergonovine and methylergonovine can cause severe hypertension. Oral or IM administration is much safer.

- Carboprost (15-methyl-prostaglandin $F_2$ alpha) and dinoprostone (prostaglandin $E_2$) are oxytocic agents employed primarily for second-trimester abortion.
- In addition to stimulating the uterus, carboprost and dinoprostone stimulate gastrointestinal smooth muscle, causing vomiting and diarrhea in about 60% of patients. Pretreatment with antiemetic and antidiarrheal agents reduces these responses.

- Tocolytic drugs suppress uterine contractions.
- The only indication for tocolytics is delay of preterm labor.
- Two beta$_2$-adrenergic agonists—ritodrine and terbutaline—are the principal tocolytics in use.
- *Intravenous* ritodrine and terbutaline can cause pulmonary hypertension, tachycardia, hypotension, and hyperglycemia. In contrast, oral therapy is very safe.

# Summary of Major Nursing Implications*

## Oxytocin

The implications summarized here apply only to the use of oxytocin for induction of labor, the principal use of this drug.

### Preadministration Assessment

#### Therapeutic Goal
Give oxytocin to initiate or improve uterine contractions so as to achieve early vaginal delivery. Reserve treatment for pregnancies in which induction is likely to decrease morbidity and mortality for the mother or the infant.

#### Baseline Data
The history should determine parity, previous obstetric problems, stillbirths, and abortions. Full maternal and fetal status should be assessed.

#### Identifying High-Risk Patients
Induction of labor is *contraindicated* in the presence of *cephalopelvic disproportion, fetal malpresentation, placental abnormality, previous major surgery to the uterus or cervix,* and *fetal distress.*
Use with *caution* in *women of high parity* (five or more pregnancies).

### Implementation: Administration

#### Route
Intravenous.

#### Administration
Administer by carefully controlled infusion, using an infusion pump.

### Ongoing Evaluation and Interventions

#### Minimizing Adverse Effects
Uterine contractions of excessive intensity, frequency, and duration can cause maternal and fetal harm. Monitor uterine contractility (frequency, duration, intensity), maternal blood pressure, and fetal and maternal heart rate. Interrupt the infusion if any of the following occur: (1)

resting intrauterine pressure rises above 15 to 20 mm $H_2O$, (2) individual contractions persist longer than 1 minute, (3) contractions occur more often than every 2 to 3 minutes, and (4) fetal heart rate or rhythm changes significantly.

## Ergot Alkaloids: Ergonovine and Methylergonovine

### Preadministration Assessment

#### Therapeutic Goal
Prevention and treatment of postpartum and postabortion hemorrhage.

#### Identifying High-Risk Patients
Ergot alkaloids are *contraindicated during pregnancy, for induction of labor, in women with hypertension or allergy to ergot alkaloids,* and *in the presence of threatened or ongoing spontaneous abortion.*

### Implementation: Administration

#### Routes
*Oral and IM.* Usual routes.
*Intravenous.* Hazardous; reserve for hemorrhagic emergencies.

#### Administration
As a rule, administer after passage of the placenta.
Perform IV injections slowly (over 60 seconds or more).

### Ongoing Evaluation and Interventions

#### Evaluating Therapeutic Effects
Monitor blood pressure, pulse rate, and uterine activity. Report sudden increases in blood pressure, excessive uterine bleeding, and insufficient uterine tone. Cramping is normal but may also indicate overdose.

#### Minimizing Adverse Effects
Significant adverse effects—*hypertension, nausea, vomiting, headache, convulsions, death*—usually occur only with IV administration. To minimize risk, infuse slowly (over 60 seconds or more) and reserve IV administration for emergencies.

---

*Patient education information is highlighted in color.

# Prostaglandins: Carboprost and Dinoprostone

## Preadministration Assessment

### Therapeutic Goal
Prostaglandins are used for induction of abortion (carboprost, dinoprostone), control of postpartum hemorrhage (carboprost), induction of labor (dinoprostone), and initiation of cervical ripening (dinoprostone).

### Identifying High-Risk Patients
Prostaglandins are *contraindicated* for women with *acute pelvic inflammatory disease* and *active disease of the heart, lungs, kidneys,* or *liver.* Use with *caution* in women with a *history of asthma, hypotension, hypertension, diabetes,* or *uterine scarring.*

## Implementation: Administration

### Routes
*Carboprost.* Intramuscular.

*Dinoprostone.* Vaginal suppository, gel for intracervical instillation.

## Ongoing Evaluation and Interventions

### Evaluation of Therapeutic Effects
*Termination of Pregnancy.* Monitor and record intensity, frequency, and duration of contractions. If treatment fails to terminate pregnancy, implement an alternative procedure (e.g., use of oxytocin or hypertonic saline).

### Minimizing Adverse Effects
*Gastrointestinal Disturbances.* Nausea, vomiting, and diarrhea can be reduced by pretreatment with antiemetic and antidiarrheal drugs.

*Fever.* Fever may be prostaglandin induced or it may indicate endometritis. If fever develops, a differential diagnosis must be made.

*Cervical or Uterine Laceration.* Use for abortion may result in cervical or uterine laceration. Examine the patient thoroughly for trauma following expulsion of the fetus and placenta.

# Ritodrine and Terbutaline: Beta₂-Adrenergic Agonists Used to Delay Preterm Labor

## Preadministration Assessment

### Therapeutic Goal
Delay of preterm labor in pregnancies between 20 and 34 weeks' duration. An accurate determination of gestational age is required.

### Baseline Data
Determine maternal heart rate, blood pressure, blood glucose, and fluid status. Determine fetal heart rate.

### Identifying High-Risk Patients
Ritodrine is *contraindicated* in women with *eclampsia, severe pre-eclampsia, hemorrhage, chorioamnionitis, heart disease,* and *gestation of less than 20 weeks' duration.* Exercise *caution* in women with *hyperthyroidism* and *insulin-dependent diabetes.*

## Implementation: Administration

### Routes
Oral, IV.

### Administration
Begin therapy with an IV infusion and continue the infusion for 12 hours after contractions cease. Begin oral maintenance therapy 30 minutes before terminating the infusion. Continue oral therapy for as long as suppression of labor is considered desirable. If contractions recur, reinstitute IV administration.

## Ongoing Evaluation and Interventions

### Monitoring Summary
Monitor maternal blood pressure, heart rate, blood glucose, and fluid status. Monitor fetal heart rate.

### Evaluating Therapeutic Effects
Warn the outpatient on oral therapy that contractions may resume. Instruct her to return to the hospital for intravenous therapy if oral therapy becomes ineffective.

### Minimizing Adverse Effects
Significant adverse effects occur primarily with IV administration; side effects of oral therapy are usually minor.

*Pulmonary Edema.* Intravenous ritodrine may cause pulmonary edema. Monitor the patient for fluid overload. If pulmonary edema develops, discontinue the infusion.

Concurrent therapy with glucocorticoids increases the risk of edema, as does the use of isotonic saline for the infusion fluid. The risk may be reduced by using 5% dextrose for the infusion fluid and by limiting total fluid intake to 2.5 L over 24 hours.

*Tachycardia.* Intravenous treatment almost always causes maternal and fetal tachycardia. Monitor maternal and fetal heart rate and reduce the dosage if tachycardia is excessive.

*Hypotension.* Ritodrine- and terbutaline-induced vasodilation can cause hypotension. Monitor blood pressure. Minimize hypotension by having the patient assume a left-lateral recumbent position.

*Hyperglycemia.* Intravenous beta₂ agonists elevate blood glucose. Monitor blood glucose levels. Insulin-dependent diabetics are likely to require insulin infusion.

# CHAPTER 61

# Androgens

### Testosterone
Biosynthesis and Secretion
Mechanism of Action
Physiologic and Pharmacologic Effects

### Clinical Pharmacology of the Androgens
Classification
Therapeutic Uses
Adverse Effects
Preparations, Dosage, and Administration
### Androgen (Anabolic Steroid) Abuse by Athletes

The androgen hormones are produced by the testes, ovaries, and adrenal cortex. The major endogenous androgen is testosterone. Androgens are noted most for their ability to promote expression of male sex characteristics. However, androgens can also influence sexuality in females. In addition, androgens have significant physiologic and pharmacologic effects unrelated to sex. The primary clinical application of the androgens is management of androgen deficiency in males. Principal adverse effects are virilization and hepatotoxicity.

## Testosterone

Testosterone is the prototype of the androgen hormones. This compound is the principal endogenous androgen in both males and females. In addition to its physiologic role, testosterone is representative of the androgens employed clinically. The structural formula of testosterone is shown in Figure 61-1.

### Biosynthesis and Secretion

*Males.* Testosterone is made by Leydig cells of the testes. Daily production in men ranges from 2.5 to 10 mg. Synthesis of testosterone is promoted by two hormones of the anterior pituitary: follicle-stimulating hormone (FSH) and luteinizing hormone (LH), which is also known as interstitial cell–stimulating hormone. Production of testosterone is under negative feedback control: rising plasma levels of testosterone act on the pituitary to suppress further release of FSH and LH, thereby reducing the stimulus for further testosterone formation.

Some of the testosterone present in plasma is produced by the adrenals. However, androgenic activity of adrenal origin is much less than that of testicular origin. Hence, in

men, adrenal androgens have minimal functional significance.

*Females.* In women, preandrogens (precursors of testosterone) are secreted by the adrenal cortex and the ovaries. Conversion of these precursors into testosterone takes place in peripheral tissues. Synthesis of preandrogens by the adrenals is regulated by adrenocorticotropic hormone (ACTH), whereas ovarian production of preandrogens is under the control of LH. Total daily secretion of testosterone is about 0.25 mg—that is, 10 to 40 times less than the amount produced in men. In the event of ovarian or adrenocortical pathology (e.g., adenoma, carcinoma, hyperplasia), secretion of androgens can be greatly increased, and may be sufficient to produce virilization.

### Mechanism of Action

The effects of testosterone on its target tissues are mediated by specific receptors located in the cell cytoplasm. Following binding of testosterone to its receptor, the hormone-receptor complex migrates to the cell nucleus, and then acts on DNA to promote synthesis of specific messenger RNA molecules. These, in turn, serve as templates for production of specific proteins. It is through these proteins that the effects of testosterone become manifest. It should be noted that in some tissues—prostate, seminal vesicles, and hair follicles—androgen receptors do not interact with testosterone itself; rather, they interact with dihydrotestosterone, which is a metabolite of testosterone.

### Physiologic and Pharmacologic Effects
#### Effects on Sex Characteristics in Males

*Pubertal Transformation.* Increased production of testosterone brings on the transformations that signal puberty in males. Under the influence of testosterone, the testes enlarge, followed by growth of the penis and scro-

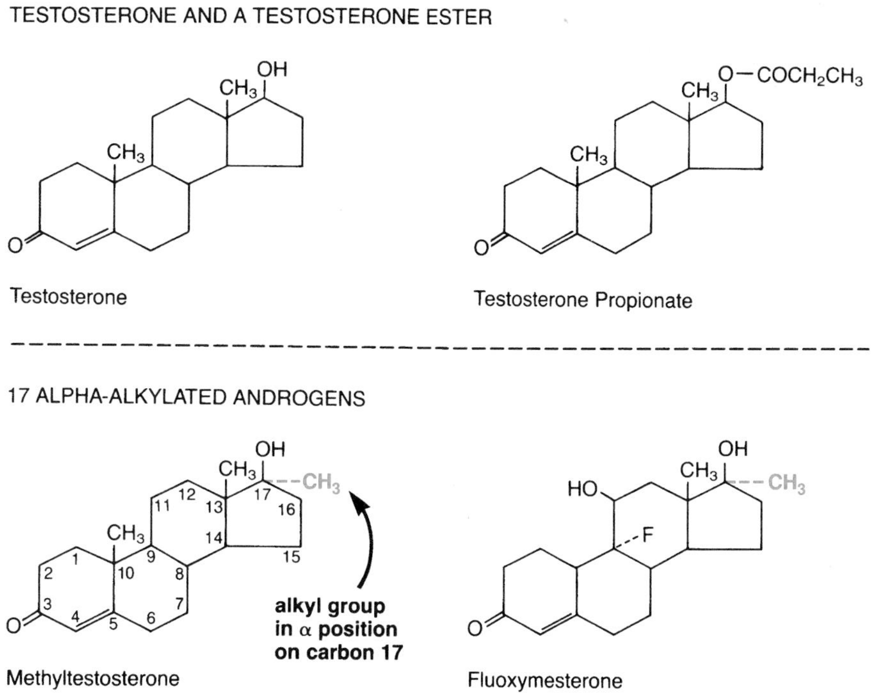

TESTOSTERONE AND A TESTOSTERONE ESTER

Testosterone

Testosterone Propionate

17 ALPHA-ALKYLATED ANDROGENS

alkyl group
in α position
on carbon 17

**Figure 61–1. Structural formulas of representative androgens.**

Methyltestosterone

Fluoxymesterone

tum. Pubic and axillary hair appear, and hair on the trunk, arms, and legs assumes adult male patterns. Testosterone stimulates bone growth and growth of skeletal muscle, causing height and weight to increase rapidly. Testosterone also accelerates epiphyseal closure, causing bone growth to cease within a few years. The larynx enlarges, thereby deepening the voice. Sebaceous glands increase in number, causing the skin to become oily; acne results if the glands become clogged and infected. The final pubertal change is beard development. Several years are required for all of these transformations to take place.

*Spermatogenesis.* Androgens are necessary for production of sperm by the seminiferous tubules, and for maturation of sperm as they pass through the epididymis and vas deferens. Androgen deficiency causes sterility.

### Effects on Sex Characteristics in Females

Under physiologic conditions, endogenous androgens have only moderate effects in females. Principal effects are promotion of clitoral growth and, perhaps, maintenance of normal libido. However, when production of androgens becomes excessive (e.g., in girls with congenital adrenal hyperplasia), virilization can take place. Virilization can also occur in response to therapeutic use of androgens (see below).

### Anabolic Effects

Testosterone promotes growth of skeletal muscle. This anabolic effect results from the binding of androgens to the same type of receptor that mediates androgen actions in other tissues. Effects in young males and in females of any age can be dramatic. In contrast, effects in healthy adult males are more modest. This is because the testes of

the adult male produce enough testosterone to cause near-maximal stimulation of the musculature. Hence, the increment in muscle mass that can be achieved with exogenous androgens is relatively small.

### Erythropoietic Effects

Testosterone promotes synthesis of erythropoietin, a hormone that acts on bone marrow to increase production of erythrocytes. This action of testosterone, together with the high levels of testosterone present in males, explains why men have a greater hematocrit than women. When women are given testosterone, the hematocrit rises and hemoglobin levels increase by an average of 4.3 gm/dl. In contrast, since men have high testosterone levels to begin with, the increase in plasma hemoglobin content that can be elicited with exogenous androgens is only 1 gm/dl.

## Clinical Pharmacology of the Androgens

In addition to testosterone, a number of other androgens are employed clinically. All of these agents can bind to androgen receptors, and therefore all can elicit similar responses. Major differences among individual androgens pertain to route of administration, pharmacokinetics, adverse effects, and specific applications.

### Classification

The androgens fall into three basic categories: (1) testosterone and testosterone esters, (2) 17-alpha-alkylated com-

668  Unit IX  Endocrine Drugs

## TABLE 61-1. APPLICATIONS OF INDIVIDUAL ANDROGENS

| Androgens | Androgens | | | | | | | |
|---|---|---|---|---|---|---|---|---|
| | Hypogonadism (male) | Delayed puberty (male) | Breast cancer (female) | Anemias | Hereditary angioedema | Catabolic states | Breast engorgement | Osteoporosis |
| *Testosterone and Testosterone Esters* | | | | | | | | |
| Testosterone | ✔ | ✔ | ✔ | | | | | |
| Testosterone cypionate | ✔ | ✔ | ✔ | | | | | |
| Testosterone enanthate | ✔ | ✔ | ✔ | | | | | |
| Testosterone propionate | ✔ | ✔ | ✔ | | | | ✔ | |
| *17-Alpha-Alkylated Androgens* | | | | | | | | |
| Fluoxymesterone | ✔ | | ✔ | | | | ✔ | |
| Methyltestosterone | ✔ | | ✔ | | | | ✔ | |
| Oxandrolone | | | | | | ✔ | | ✔ |
| Oxymetholone | | | | ✔ | | | | |
| Stanozolol | | | | | ✔ | | | |
| *Other Androgens* | | | | | | | | |
| Danazol | | | | | ✔ | | | |
| Nandrolone decanoate | | | | ✔ | | | | |
| Nandrolone phenpropionate | | | ✔ | | | | | |
| Testolactone | | | ✔ | | | | | |

pounds (noted for their hepatotoxicity), and (3) miscellaneous androgens. The androgens that belong to each of these classes are indicated in Table 61-1.

When speaking of testosterone-like compounds, it is traditional to distinguish between "androgens" and "anabolic steroids." However, we will not make this distinction. It is now clear that the receptor type that mediates the anabolic actions of the androgens is the same receptor type that mediates the androgenic actions of these hormones. Consequently, it has not been possible to separate anabolic activity from androgenic activity: virtually all anabolic hormones are also androgenic. Accordingly, rather than creating two categories—androgens versus anabolic steroids—and assigning some agents to one category and some to the other, we will simply refer to all of the testosterone-like drugs as androgens.

### Therapeutic Uses

Individual androgens differ from one another in their applications. No single androgen is employed for all of the uses discussed below. Specific applications of individual androgens are summarized in Table 61-1.

***Male Hypogonadism.*** Hypogonadism in males is the principal indication for androgens. In this condition, the testes fail to produce adequate amounts of testosterone, hence replacement therapy is required. Male hypogonadism may be hereditary or may result from other causes, including pituitary failure, hypothalamic failure, and primary dysfunction of the testes.

When complete hypogonadism occurs in boys, puberty will not take place unless exogenous androgens are supplied. To induce puberty, a long-acting parenteral preparation (usually *testosterone enanthate* or *testosterone cypionate*) is chosen; injections are given IM every 2 to 4 weeks for 3 to 4 years. Under the influence of this therapy, the normal sequence of pubertal changes occurs: growth is accelerated, the penis enlarges, the voice deepens, and other secondary sex characteristics are expressed. As in normal males, these changes take place over several years.

Androgen replacement therapy is also beneficial when testicular failure occurs in adult males. Treatment restores libido, increases ejaculate volume, and supports expression of secondary sex characteristics. However, treatment will not restore fertility. Therapy can be accomplished with a long-acting testosterone ester (usually *testosterone enanthate* or *testosterone cypionate*) injected IM every 2 weeks, or with a *transdermal formulation* of testosterone itself. Two transdermal formulations are now available: (1) *Testoderm*, which is applied daily to the scrotum, and (2) *Androderm*, which is applied daily to the upper arm, thigh, back, or abdomen—but *not* the scrotum.

**Delayed Puberty.** In some boys, puberty fails to occur at the usual age (i.e., prior to 15). Most often, this failure reflects a familial pattern of delayed puberty and is not indicative of pathology. Puberty can be expected to occur spontaneously, but at an age somewhat older than normal. Hence, although androgen therapy can be employed, treatment is not an absolute necessity. However, although therapy is not required, the psychologic pressures of delayed sexual maturation are sometimes greater than a boy (or his parents) can tolerate. In these cases, a limited course of androgen therapy is indicated. If delayed puberty is the result of true hypogonadism, long-term replacement therapy should be instituted.

**Breast Cancer.** Testosterone and other androgens have been used to provide palliation in women with advanced and metastatic breast carcinoma. The mechanism of palliation is unknown. For treatment of breast cancer, high doses of androgens are required. As a result, some virilization is inevitable; the patient should be forewarned of this likelihood. (In contrast to their beneficial effects in women, androgens exacerbate breast cancer in males. Accordingly, androgens are contraindicated for this use in men.)

**Hereditary Angioedema.** Hereditary angioedema is a disorder in which an inhibitor of the complement system is deficient. Lack of the inhibitor allows uncontrolled activation of the complement cascade, resulting in increased vascular permeability and angioedema (localized swelling of the subcutaneous tissue of the face, hands, feet, and genitalia). Androgens provide prophylaxis against this response by elevating plasma levels of the deficient inhibitor. For treatment of hereditary angioedema, *stanozolol* and *danazol* are the androgens of choice.

**Anemias.** Androgens may be used in men and women to treat anemias that have been refractory to other therapy. Anemias that may respond include aplastic anemia, anemia associated with renal failure, Fanconi's anemia, and anemia caused by cancer chemotherapy. Androgens help relieve anemia by promoting synthesis of erythropoietin, the renal hormone that stimulates production of red blood cells. In addition to increasing erythrocyte count, androgens may stimulate production of white blood cells and platelets.

## Adverse Effects

**Virilization.** This is the most common complication of androgen therapy. When taken in high doses by women, androgens can cause acne, deepening of the voice, proliferation of facial and body hair, male-pattern baldness, increased libido, clitoral enlargement, and menstrual irregu-larities. Clitoral growth, hair loss, and lowering of the voice may be irreversible. Masculinization can also occur in children: boys may experience growth of pubic hair, phallic enlargement, increased frequency of erections, and even priapism (persistent erection). In girls, growth of pubic hair and clitoral enlargement may occur. To prevent irreversible masculinization, androgens must be discontinued when virilizing effects first appear. In the treatment of breast carcinoma, some virilization should be tolerated.

**Premature Epiphyseal Closure.** When given to children, androgens can accelerate epiphyseal closure, thereby decreasing adult height. To evaluate androgen effects on the epiphyses, x-ray examination of the hand and wrist should be performed every 6 months.

**Hepatotoxicity.** Androgens can cause *cholestatic hepatitis* and other disorders of the liver. Clinical *jaundice* may occur, but this is rare. Patients receiving androgens should undergo periodic tests of liver function. If jaundice develops, it will reverse following discontinuation of androgen use. Androgens may also be carcinogenic: *hepatocellular carcinoma* has developed in some patients following prolonged use of these drugs.

It must be emphasized that not all androgens are hepatotoxic: liver damage is associated primarily with the *17-alpha-alkylated androgens*. As indicated in Figure 61–1 (see methyltestosterone), these androgens all share a structural feature in common—an alkyl group substituted on carbon 17 of the steroid nucleus. Because of their capacity to cause liver damage, *the 17-alpha-alkylated compounds should not be used chronically.* In contrast to the 17-alpha-alkylated androgens, the testosterone esters (testosterone propionate, testosterone cypionate, testosterone enanthate) have never been associated with liver disease.

**Effects on Cholesterol Levels.** Androgens can lower plasma levels of HDL-cholesterol ("good cholesterol") and elevate plasma levels of LDL-cholesterol ("bad cholesterol"). These actions may increase the risk of atherosclerosis.

**Use in Pregnancy.** *Because of their ability to induce masculinization of the female fetus, androgens are contraindicated during pregnancy.* Potential fetal changes include vaginal malformation, clitoral enlargement, and formation of a structure resembling the male scrotum. Virilization is most likely when androgens are taken during the first trimester. Women who become pregnant while using androgens should be informed about the possible consequences to the fetus. Androgens are classified in FDA Pregnancy Category X.

**Edema.** Edema can result from androgen-induced retention of salt and water. This complication is of concern for patients with heart failure and for those with a predisposition to developing edema from other causes. Treatment consists of discontinuing the androgen; a diuretic may also be needed.

**Gynecomastia.** Breast enlargement may occur in males receiving androgen replacement therapy. This effect results from conversion of certain androgens into estrogen.

## TABLE 61-2. ANDROGENS IN CLINICAL USE

| Class | Generic Name | Trade Name | Route | Usual Dosage |
|---|---|---|---|---|
| *Testosterone and Testosterone Esters* | Testosterone, intramuscular | Histerone, Tesamone, Testandro | IM | 10–25 mg 2–3 times weekly (for androgen deficiency) |
| | Testosterone, transdermal | Androderm | TD* | Two 12.2-mg patches release 4.4 mg in 24 hr |
| | | Testoderm | TD* | 10-mg patch releases 4 mg in 24 hr; 15-mg patch releases 6 mg in 24 hr |
| | Testosterone cypionate | Depo-Testosterone, others | IM | 50–400 mg every 2–4 weeks (for androgen deficiency) |
| | Testosterone enanthate | Delatestryl, others | IM | 50–400 mg every 2–4 weeks (for androgen deficiency) |
| | Testosterone propionate | | IM | 10–25 mg 2–4 times weekly (for androgen deficiency) |
| *17-Alpha-Alkylated Androgens* | Fluoxymesterone | Halotestin | PO | 5–20 mg daily (for androgen deficiency) 5–40 mg daily (for breast carcinoma) |
| | Methyltestosterone | Oreton Methyl, others | PO | *Oral:* 10–40 mg daily (for male hypogonadism) *Buccal:* 5–25 mg daily (for androgen deficiency) |
| | Oxandrolone | Oxandrin | PO | 5–10 mg daily (for anabolic effects) |
| | Oxymetholone | Anadrol-50 | PO | 1–5 mg/kg daily (for anemia) |
| | Stanozolol | Winstrol | PO | 6 mg daily (for hereditary angioedema) |
| *Other Androgens* | Danazol | Danocrine | PO | 400–600 mg daily (for hereditary angioedema) |
| | Nandrolone decanoate | Deca-Durabolin, Androlone-D, others | IM | 50–200 mg weekly (for anemia of renal disease in adults) |
| | Nandrolone phenpropionate | Durabolin, Hybolin, Nandrobolic | IM | 50–100 mg weekly (for breast carcinoma) |
| | Testolactone | Teslac | PO | 250 mg 4 times daily (for breast carcinoma) |

*TD = transdermal.

***Abuse Potential.*** As discussed below, androgens are frequently misused (abused) to enhance athletic performance. Because of their abuse potential, most androgens are now regulated under the Controlled Substances Act. Of the androgens listed in Table 61-1, all but danazol are classified as Schedule III drugs; danazol remains unregulated.

## Preparations, Dosage, and Administration

Preparations, dosages, and routes are summarized in Table 61-2. As indicated, three routes are employed: oral, intramuscular, and transdermal. With the exception of testosterone, individual androgens are administered by only one route: oral or intramuscular. Testosterone differs in that it may be administered by two routes: oral and transdermal.

*Transdermal formulations* of testosterone are new and require comment. Two formulations are available: Testoderm and Androderm. *Testoderm* is applied once daily to the scrotum, which must first be shaved. Despite

shaving, the patch may fall off during exercise. In men with primary hypogonadism, the scrotum may be too small to accept the patch. The principal adverse effect is scrotal rash.

*Androderm* can be applied to the upper arm, thigh, back, or abdomen—but not the scrotum. Two patches are applied each evening. The principal adverse effect—rash at the site of application—is more intense than the rash caused by Testoderm.

## Androgen (Anabolic Steroid) Abuse by Athletes

Many athletes take androgens (anabolic steroids) to enhance athletic performance. The potential benefits of this practice, although substantial, are accompanied by substantial risks. The drugs taken most commonly by athletes are nandrolone [Durabolin], stanozolol [Winstrol], and methenolone (not available in the United States). Of

## TABLE 61-3. IMPACT OF TESTOSTERONE ON MUSCLE MASS AND STRENGTH IN NORMAL MEN*

| Regimen | Increase in Muscle Mass (pounds) | Increase in Bench Press (pounds) |
|---|---|---|
| Testosterone[†] alone | 7 | 20 |
| Exercise alone | 4 | 20 |
| Testosterone[†] + exercise | 13 | 48 |

*Data adapted from Bhasin, S., Storer, T.W., Berman, N. The effects of supraphysiologic doses of testosterone on muscle size and strength in normal men. N. Engl. J. Med., 335:1, 1996.
[†]Testosterone dosage = 600 mg testosterone enanthate, IM, daily for 10 weeks.

course, all of these drugs are regulated by the Controlled Substances Act, making their use by athletes illegal.

Who takes steroids? Steroid use is especially prevalent among football players, weight lifters, discus throwers, shot putters, and body builders. The drugs are also used by sprinters and by athletes in endurance sports (e.g., cycling, Nordic skiing). Steroids are used by athletes of all ages (professionals as well as athletes in college, high school, and junior high). Use is not limited to males: some females also take these drugs, despite masculinizing effects.

What can anabolic steroids do for the athlete? The answer to this question depends partly on the age and gender of the athlete, and partly on whether an athlete or a scientist is answering the question. Scientists and athletes have agreed for years that steroids can increase muscle mass in *young males* and in *females of all ages*. However, it was not until 1996 that scientists finally demonstrated what athletes have claimed for years: exogenous androgens can significantly increase muscle mass and strength in *sexually mature males*. In order to demonstrate these effects, scientists gave normal men *large* daily injections of testosterone enanthate for 10 weeks. Some subjects did regular strength training along with drug treatment; some only took the drug. As indicated in Table 61–3, testosterone treatment produced a 7-pound increase in muscle mass in the subjects who did not exercise, and a 13-pound increase in the subjects who exercised along with taking the drug. In contrast, exercise in the absence of exogenous testosterone produced only a 4-pound increase in muscle mass. Similar increases were shown in the subjects' ability to bench press weights (Table 61–3). Why has it taken so long for scientists to agree with the athletes? The principal reason is that, in studies performed prior to 1996, the doses of androgens employed were too small to elicit a clear response. When sufficiently large doses were finally given, the results were unequivocal. (In the 1996 study, the testosterone dosage was equivalent to 6 to 8 times the amount produced by the testes.)

The potential for adverse effects of androgens is significant. Salt and water retention can lead to hypertension. When administered in the high doses used by athletes, androgens suppress release of LH and FSH, resulting in testicular shrinkage and sterility. Acne is common. Reduction of HDL-cholesterol and elevation of LDL-

cholesterol may accelerate development of atherosclerosis (although no effect was seen on lipids in the study discussed above). Because most of the androgens that athletes take are 17-alpha-alkylated compounds, hepatotoxicity (cholestatic hepatitis, jaundice, hepatocellular carcinoma) is an ever-present danger. In females, androgens can cause menstrual irregularities and virilization (growth of facial hair, deepening of the voice, decreased breast size, uterine atrophy, clitoral enlargement, and male-pattern baldness); hair loss, growth of facial hair, and voice change may be irreversible. In boys and girls, androgens promote premature epiphyseal closure, thereby reducing attainable adult height. In boys, androgens can induce premature puberty.

What about psychologic effects? Interestingly, although androgens are reputed to cause manic episodes, depression, and excessive aggressiveness ('roid rage), none of these effects was observed in the 1996 study discussed above. The authors suggested that, if an athlete is mentally healthy, testosterone will not make him into a beast. On the other hand, if an athlete is already psychologically unbalanced, it is possible that steroids could intensify aberrant behavior.

Long-term androgen use can lead to an "abuse" or "addiction" syndrome. Characteristics of the syndrome include preoccupation with androgen use and difficulty in stopping use. When androgens finally are discontinued, an abstinence syndrome can develop similar to that produced by withdrawal of alcohol, opioids, and cocaine. Because of their abuse potential, most androgens are now classified under Schedule III of the Controlled Substances Act.

## KEY POINTS

- Testosterone is the principal endogenous androgen.
- Important physiologic effects of androgens are pubertal transformation in males, maintenance of adult male sexual characteristics, promotion of muscle growth, and stimulation of erythropoiesis.
- The major indication for androgens is male hypogonadism.
- The major side effects of androgens are edema, virilization in females, premature epiphyseal closure in chil-

dren, and liver toxicity (with the 17-alpha-alkylated androgens).

- Androgens are contraindicated during pregnancy.
- Two transdermal formulations of testosterone are available: Testoderm is applied to the scrotum; Androderm is applied to the upper arm, thigh, back, or abdomen, but not the scrotum.
- Large doses of androgens can increase muscle mass and strength in athletes. However, athletic use of androgens is illegal and carries significant risks.

# Summary of Major Nursing Implications*

## Androgens

| | |
|---|---|
| Testosterone | Methyltestosterone |
| Testosterone cypionate | Nandrolone phenpropionate |
| Testosterone enanthate | Nandrolone decanoate |
| Testosterone propionate | Oxandrolone Oxymetholone |
| Danazol | Stanozolol |
| Fluoxymesterone | Testolactone |

## Preadministration Assessment

### Therapeutic Goals

*Males.* Treatment of hypogonadism and delayed puberty.

*Females.* Treatment of breast cancer and breast engorgement.

*Males and Females.* Treatment of anemias, hereditary angioedema, catabolic states, and osteoporosis.

### Identifying High-Risk Patients

Androgens are *contraindicated during pregnancy* and for *males who have breast cancer.* Also, androgens are *contraindicated for enhancing athletic performance.*

## Implementation: Administration

### Routes

PO, IM, transdermal.

### Administration

*Oral.* Advise patients to take oral androgens with food if gastrointestinal upset occurs.

*Transdermal.* Advise patients using *Testoderm* to shave the scrotum before application.

## Ongoing Evaluation and Interventions

### Minimizing Adverse Effects

*Virilization.* Virilization may occur in women, girls, and boys. Inform female patients about signs of virilization (deepening of the voice, acne, changes in body and facial hair, menstrual irregularities), and instruct them to notify the physician if these occur. Irreversible changes may be avoided if androgens are withdrawn early. In the treatment of breast carcinoma, some virilization should be tolerated.

*Premature Epiphyseal Closure.* Accelerated bone maturation can decrease attainable adult height. Monitor effects on epiphyses with x-rays of the hand and wrist twice yearly.

*Hepatotoxicity.* The *17-alpha-alkylated androgens* can cause cholestatic hepatitis, jaundice, and other liver disorders. Rarely, liver cancer develops. Obtain periodic tests of liver function. Inform patients about signs of liver dysfunction (jaundice, malaise, anorexia, fatigue, nausea), and instruct them to notify the physician if these occur. Liver function normalizes following cessation of drug use. Avoid long-term use of 17-alpha-alkylated preparations.

*Edema.* Salt and water retention may result in edema. Inform patients about signs of salt and water retention (swelling of the extremities, unusual weight gain), and instruct them to notify the physician if these occur. Treatment consists of androgen withdrawal and, if necessary, use of a diuretic.

*Teratogenesis.* Androgens can cause masculinization of the female fetus. Rule out pregnancy prior to androgen use. Warn women against becoming pregnant while taking androgens.

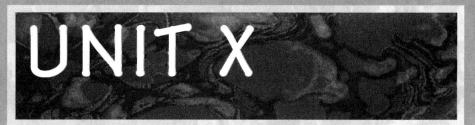

# UNIT X

# Anti-inflammatory, Antiallergic, and Immunologic Drugs

# CHAPTER 62

# Review of the Immune System

**Introduction to the Immune System**
**Antibody-Mediated (Humoral) Immunity**
   Production of Antibodies
   Antibody Effector Mechanisms

**Cell-Mediated Immunity**
   Delayed-Type Hypersensitivity
   Cytolytic T Lymphocytes

L ife is a constant battle—and the immune system is the army that helps us prevail. This system protects us from invading organisms (viruses, bacteria, fungi, parasites) and can destroy cancer cells before they destroy us. Unfortunately, the army does not always act in our best interest: it can attack transplanted organs and tissues and, when it runs amok, can turn on the very cells it was intended to protect.

In approaching the immune system, we will begin by establishing an overview of the system, after which we will discuss the two major types of specific immune responses: antibody-mediated immunity (humoral immunity) and cell-mediated immunity.

## Introduction to the Immune System

Our objective in this section is to establish an overview of immune system components and how they function. Much of the information introduced here is amplified later.

### Natural Immunity versus Specific Acquired Immunity

Our bodies can mount two types of immune responses, referred to as *natural immunity* (innate or native immunity) and *specific acquired immunity*. Factors that confer natural immunity include physical barriers (e.g., skin), phagocytic cells, and natural killer (NK) cells. All of these factors are present prior to exposure to a particular infectious agent and all respond nonspecifically. In contrast, specific acquired immune responses occur only after exposure to a foreign substance. The foreign substances that induce specific responses are called *antigens*, and the objective of the immune response is to destroy the antigen. With each succeeding re-exposure to a particular antigen, the specific immune response to that antigen becomes more rapid and more intense. Specific immune responses

are possible because certain cells of the immune system (T lymphocytes and B lymphocytes) possess receptors that can recognize individual antigens. In this chapter, our focus is on specific acquired immunity and not on natural immunity.

### Cell-Mediated Immunity versus Antibody-Mediated (Humoral) Immunity

Specific acquired immune responses can be classified as either *cell mediated* or *humoral*. *Cell-mediated immunity* refers to immune responses in which targets are attacked directly by immune system cells—specifically, cytolytic T cells and macrophages. *Humoral immunity* refers to immune responses that are mediated by *antibodies*. (The term *humoral*—defined as "pertaining to elements dissolved in blood or body fluids"—simply connotes that antibodies are present dissolved in the blood.)

### Introduction to Cells of the Immune System

Immune responses are mediated by several types of cells, some of which play more central roles than others. The major actors are the *lymphocytes* (B cells, cytolytic T cells, helper T cells), dendritic cells, and *macrophages*. Accessory cells include neutrophils and basophils. With the exception of some dendritic cells, all of the cells involved in the immune response arise from pluripotent stem cells in the bone marrow (Figure 62-1) and, for at least part of their life cycle, circulate in the blood. Defining characteristics of individual immune system cells are summarized in Table 62-1.

*B Lymphocytes (B Cells).* B lymphocytes have the job of making *antibodies*. Hence, B cells mediate humoral immunity. As discussed below, antibody specificity is determined by the structure of highly specific receptors present on the surface of B cells. Like all other lymphocytes, B cells circulate in both the blood and the lymph. B cells are so named because in chickens, where B cells were discovered, these cells are produced in the *bursa of Fabricius*, a structure not found in mammals. In humans and other mammals, B cells are produced in the bone marrow.

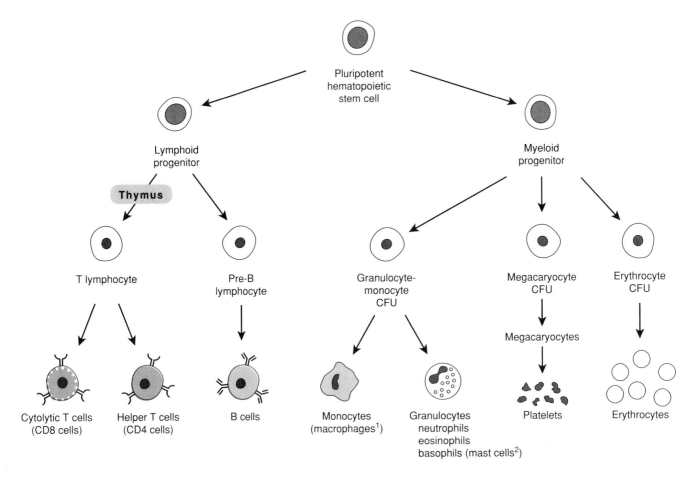

**Figure 62–1. Maturation of blood cells.** With the exception of platelets and erythrocytes, all of the mature blood cells shown participate in immune responses. However, only cells of lymphoid origin (cytolytic T cells, helper T cells, B cells) possess receptors that can recognize specific antigens. CFU = colony forming unit.

[1]Monocytes that move into tissues are called macrophages.

[2] Basophils that move into tissues are called mast cells.

***Cytolytic T Lymphocytes (Cytolytic T Cells, CD8 Cells).*** Cytolytic T cells are key players in cellular immunity. These cells do not produce antibodies. Rather, they attack and kill target cells directly. Specificity of attack is determined by the presence of antigen molecules on the surface of the target and specific receptors for that antigen on the surface of the T cell. Cytolytic T cells are also known as *CD8 cells* and *cytotoxic T cells.* The designation "CD8" refers to the presence of cell-surface marker molecules known as *cell differentiation complex 8.* The "T" in T cell stands for thymus, the organ in which cytolytic T cells and helper T cells mature. Like B cells, cytolytic T cells circulate in the blood and the lymph.

***Helper T Lymphocytes (Helper T Cells, CD4 Cells).*** Helper T cells contribute to the immune response in three ways: (1) they have an essential role in antibody production by B cells, (2) they release factors that promote delayed-type hypersensitivity (DTH), and (3) they participate in the activation of cytolytic T cells. Specificity of B cells is achieved through highly specific cell-surface receptors that recognize individual antigens. Like other lymphocytes, helper T cells circulate in the blood

and the lymph. Helper T cells carry CD4 marker molecules on their surface and, hence, are referred to as CD4 cells.

The term *helper* is somewhat misleading, in that it connotes a useful but dispensable role. Nothing could be further from reality. Helper T cells are not simply nice to have around, they are absolutely required for an effective immune response. The critical nature of their contribution—and the grim consequences of their absence—are manifested in people with AIDS: helper T cells are the immune cells that the HIV virus attacks; because of helper T cell loss, AIDS patients are at high risk of death from opportunistic infections.

***Macrophages.*** Macrophages begin their existence in bone marrow, enter the blood as monocytes, and then infiltrate tissues where they evolve into macrophages. Macrophages are present in all organs and tissues.

The primary function of macrophages is *phagocytosis* (i.e., ingestion of microbes, other foreign material, and cellular debris). In their role as phagocytes, macrophages are the principal scavengers of the body. Although their major job is phagocytosis, macrophages also have an im-

## TABLE 62-1. CELLS OF THE IMMUNE SYSTEM

| Cell Type | Synonyms | Primary Immune-Related Actions |
|---|---|---|
| *Major Cell Types* | | |
| B lymphocytes | B cells | • Produce antibodies |
| Cytolytic T lymphocytes (CTLs) | Cytolytic T cells, cytotoxic T cells, CD8 cells | • Lyse target cells |
| Helper T lymphocytes | Helper T cells, CD4 cells | • Promote proliferation and differentiation of B cells and CTLs<br>• Initiate delayed-type hypersensitivity |
| Macrophages | | • Promote proliferation and differentiation of helper T cells and CTLs by serving as antigen-presenting cells<br>• Participate in delayed-type hypersensitivity<br>• Phagocytize cells tagged with antibodies<br>• Phagocytize cells in the effector stage of DTH |
| Dendritic cells | | • Promote proliferation of cytolytic T cells and helper T cells by serving as antigen-presenting cells |
| *Accessory Cells* | | |
| Mast cells | | • Mediate immediate hypersensitivity reactions |
| Basophils | | • Mediate immediate hypersensitivity reactions |
| Neutrophils | Polymorphonuclear leukocytes | • Phagocytize foreign particles (e.g., bacteria), especially those tagged with IgG<br>• Mediate inflammation |
| Eosinophils | | • Attack helminths and other foreign particles that have been coated with IgE<br>• Contribute to immediate hypersensitivity reactions |

portant role in specific immunity, natural immunity, and inflammation.

In specific acquired immunity, macrophages have three functions: (1) they are required for activation of T cells (both helper Ts and cytolytic Ts), (2) they are the final mediators of delayed-type hypersensitivity, and (3) they phagocytize cells that have been tagged with antibodies. Of these three immune-related roles, activation of T cells is perhaps the most critical. When performing this function, macrophages are referred to as *antigen-presenting cells*. Since antigen presentation is an absolute requirement for a specific immune response to occur (see below), we can appreciate how important macrophages are to immunity.

**Dendritic Cells.** Dendritic cells perform the same antigen-presenting task as do macrophages. However, unlike macrophages, dendritic cells do not also serve as scavengers. Dendritic cells are found in lymph nodes and other lymphoid tissues.

**Mast Cells and Basophils.** These cells mediate immediate hypersensitivity reactions. Mast cells, which are derived from basophils, are concentrated in the skin and other soft tissues; basophils circulate in the blood. Both cell types release histamine, heparin, and other compounds that cause the symptoms of immediate hypersensitivity. Release of these mediators is triggered when an

antigen binds to antibodies on the cell surface. The role of mast cells and basophils in allergic reactions is discussed further in Chapter 63 (Antihistamines).

**Neutrophils.** Neutrophils, also known as *polymorphonuclear leukocytes*, phagocytize bacteria and other foreign particles. As discussed below, neutrophils avidly devour cells that have been tagged with antibodies of the IgG class. Accordingly, neutrophils can be viewed as important effectors in humoral immunity. Neutrophils are also major contributors to inflammation.

**Eosinophils.** Eosinophils attack and destroy foreign particles that have been coated with antibodies of the IgE class. Their usual target is helminths (parasitic worms). Eosinophils also contribute to tissue injury and inflammation associated with immediate hypersensitivity reactions.

## Antibodies

Antibodies are a family of structurally related glycoproteins that mediate humoral immunity. The most characteristic feature of antibodies is their ability to recognize and bind specific antigens. Alternative names for antibodies are *immunoglobulins* and *gamma globulins.*

All antibodies are produced by B lymphocytes. Some of the antibodies that B cells produce are retained on the surface of the B cell, where they serve as the receptors whereby B cells recognize specific antigens. However,

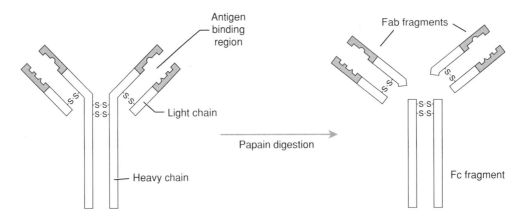

**Figure 62–2. Antibody structure.** The basic antibody structure depicting heavy and light chains is shown on the left. Variable regions of the heavy and light chains, which form the antigen-binding site, appear in color. As shown on the right, papain digestion of antibodies produces two types of fragments: Fab fragments, which retain the ability to bind antigen, and Fc fragments, which do not bind antigen and tend to crystallize in the test tube.

most of the antibodies that B cells produce are secreted from the cell, after which they bind their specific antigen, thereby initiating the effector phase of humoral immunity. The process of antibody production is discussed in detail below.

All antibodies are composed of units that have the same basic structure. As shown in Figure 62-2, antibodies have four chains: two heavy chains and two light chains. Disulfide bridges connect the four chains to form a unit. Each heavy chain and each light chain has two regions, one in which the sequence of amino acids is *constant* and one in which the sequence is highly *variable*. The variable regions form the antigen-binding site.

There are five classes of antibodies, known as immunoglobulin A (IgA), immunoglobulin D (IgD), immunoglobulin E (IgE), immunoglobulin G (IgG), and immunoglobulin M (IgM). All are constructed from the same basic unit described above. However, the heavy chains differ for each class. Primary functions of the five classes are summarized in Table 62-2.

When antibodies are subjected to digestion by papain in the laboratory, they break down into three pieces (Fig. 62-2). Two of the pieces retain the ability to bind antigen, and hence are called *Fab fragments* (fragment, antigen binding). The third piece does not bind antigen and tends to form crystals in the test tube, and hence is called the *Fc fragment* (fragment, crystalline).

### Antigens

Antigens are molecules that induce specific immune responses and, as a result, become the targets of those responses. By way of analogy, an antigen is like the child who pokes a stick in a hornet's nest, at once triggering a response and becoming its target. An antigen may trigger production of antibodies, cytotoxic T cells, or both—all of which can then attack the antigen.

Most antigens are large molecules. Because antigens are big, the antigen-binding region of the resultant antibodies cannot recognize and bind the entire antigen molecule.

Rather, the antibodies recognize and bind selected small portions of the antigen, referred to as *epitopes* or *antigenic determinants*. All antigens have multiple epitopes. As a result, more than one antibody can bind the antigen.

In research and in clinical practice, we may want to generate antibodies to molecules that are too small to induce an immune response. To overcome this obstacle, we can link the small molecule to a larger molecule, usually a protein. When this is done, the small molecule is referred to as a *hapten*, and the large molecule is referred to as a *carrier*. At least some of the resultant antibodies will be selective for the hapten.

### Characteristic Features of Immune Responses

Cell-mediated immunity and humoral immunity share five characteristic features: specificity, diversity, memory, time limitation, and selectivity for antigens of nonself origin (i.e., the ability to discriminate between self and nonself).

*Specificity.* Cell-mediated and humoral immune responses are triggered by specific antigens, and their purpose is to destroy the antigen that triggered the response. The ability to respond to a specific antigen (i.e., the ability to make subtle distinctions among related molecules) is conferred by highly specific receptors on B cells and T cells.

*Diversity.* Our immune systems can respond to millions of different antigenic determinants. This is possible because our immune systems have millions of clones of B and T lymphocytes—each of which is programmed to recognize a different antigenic determinant. As noted above, this ability to discriminate between antigens is the result of having unique cell-surface receptors.

*Memory.* Exposure to an antigen affects the immune system such that re-exposure produces a faster, larger, and more prolonged response than the initial exposure (Fig. 62-3). Why does this happen? Because during the initial response, B and T lymphocytes that recognize the anti-

## TABLE 62-2. FUNCTIONS OF ANTIBODY CLASSES

| Class | Function |
|-------|----------|
| IgA | • Located in mucous membranes of the GI tract and lungs and in many secretions, where it serves as the first line of defense against microbes entering the body via these routes<br>• Transferred to infants via breast milk; is not absorbed from the GI tract but does protect the infant against microbes *in* the GI tract |
| IgD | • Found only on the surface of mature B cells, where it serves as a receptor for antigen recognition (along with IgM) |
| IgE | • Binds to surface of mast cells; subsequent binding of antigen to IgE stimulates release of histamine, heparin, and other mediators from the mast cells, thereby causing symptoms of allergy (e.g., hives, hay fever)<br>• Binds to parasitic worms, after which eosinophils bind to IgE and release compounds that lyse the worms |
| IgG | • Produced in copious amounts in response to antigenic stimulation, and hence is the major antibody in blood<br>• Fixes complement and thereby promotes target-cell lysis<br>• Binds target cells and thereby enhances phagocytosis<br>• Transferred across the placenta to the fetal circulation, thereby providing neonatal immunity |
| IgM | • First class of antibody produced in response to antigen<br>• Fixes complement and thereby promotes target-cell lysis<br>• Present on surface of mature B cells, where it serves as a receptor for antigen recognition (along with IgD) |

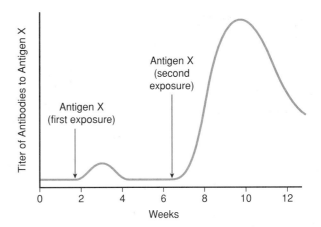

**Figure 62–3. Memory and time limitation of immune responses.** After the initial exposure to antigen X, antibody levels rise slowly, peak at a low level, and then decline rapidly. After the secondary exposure to antigen X, antibody levels rise more rapidly, reach a higher peak, persist longer, and then slowly decline.

gen undergo proliferation. Most of the new cells participate in the attack against the antigen. However, some of the new cells become *memory cells*, thereby increasing the pool of antigen-specific cells available to respond in the future. Hence, when the antigen is encountered again, the memory cells mobilize, and thereby accelerate and intensify the response.

***Time Limitation.*** As indicated in Figure 62–3, immune responses don't persist indefinitely. Rather they are time limited. The reasons are twofold. First, as the immune response proceeds, it greatly decreases the level of antigen that initiated the response, thereby attenuating the stimulus for continuing. Second, activated B cells and T cells only function for a short time, after which they become quiescent or die. Hence, in the absence of a continuing stimulus to generate more active B and T cells, the immune response fades.

***Selectivity for Antigens of Nonself Origin.*** Under normal conditions, our immune systems only target foreign antigens, leaving potentially antigenic molecules on our

own cells untouched. Sparing of self is possible because, as T cells develop in the thymus, cells that are able to react with antigens of self origin are eliminated. As discussed below, this discrimination between self and nonself is made possible by *major histocompatibility complex* (MHC) molecules. When the ability to discriminate between self and nonself fails, our immune systems can attack our own cells. The result is an autoimmune disease. Diseases that result from autoimmune attack include rheumatoid arthritis, myasthenia gravis, and type I diabetes (insulin-dependent diabetes).

### Phases of the Immune Response

Specific immune responses can be viewed as having three main phases, named the recognition phase, the activation phase, and the effector phase.

***Recognition Phase.*** The recognition phase occurs when a mature lymphocyte encounters its matching antigen. All specific immune responses begin with antigen recognition by B cells and T cells. Antigen recognition is possible because of antigen-specific receptors on the lymphocyte surface.

***Activation Phase.*** Antigen recognition causes the lymphocyte involved to become activated. The activated lymphocyte then undergoes proliferation and differentiation. Some of the daughter cells differentiate into cells that actively participate in the immune response, attacking the source of the antigen. Other daughter cells differentiate into memory cells, thereby preparing the host for a more intense and rapid response in the event of antigen exposure in the future.

***Effector Phase.*** In this stage, the immune system attempts to eliminate the specific antigen that initiated the response. With both cell-mediated and antibody-mediated immunity, several effector mechanisms can be involved. In cell-mediated immunity, antigen-bearing cells can be lysed by cytolytic T cells or they can be ingested by macrophages. In antibody-mediated immunity, target cells may be primed for attack by phagocytes or for destruction by the complement system.

## Major Histocompatibility Complex Molecules

The *major histocompatibility complex* (MHC) is a group of *genes* that code for *MHC molecules*, which become expressed on the surface of all cells. MHC molecules are critical to immune system function. They play a key role in the activation of helper and cytotoxic T lymphocytes; they guide cytotoxic T lymphocytes toward target cells; and they provide the basis for distinguishing between self and nonself.

There are two classes of MHC gene products, referred to as *class I MHC molecules* and *class II MHC molecules.* Class I MHC molecules are found on virtually all cells except erythrocytes; class II MHC molecules are found pri-marily on B cells and antigen-presenting cells (i.e., dendritic cells and macrophages). As discussed below, *class I MHC molecules* on the surface of antigen-presenting cells (APCs) help initiate immune responses by "presenting" antigen to *cytotoxic T cells.* In contrast, *class II MHC molecules* on the surface of APCs help initiate immune responses by presenting antigen to *helper T cells.*

As a rule, the sequence of amino acids in the MHC molecules produced by one individual differs from the sequence of amino acids in the MHC molecules produced by everyone else. That is, it is rare for two individuals to have MHC molecules that are identical. As a result, MHC molecules from one individual are recognized as foreign (nonself) by the immune systems of nearly everyone else. Hence, when we attempt to transplant organs between individuals who are not identical twins, immune rejection of the transplant is likely. To reduce the risk of rejection, we can treat patients with immunosuppressant drugs (see Chapter 67).

## Cytokines, Lymphokines, and Monokines

The terms *cytokine*, *lymphokine*, and *monokine* are encountered frequently when discussing the immune system and can be a source of confusion. Accordingly, clarification is in order. The term *cytokine* refers to any mediator molecule (other than an antibody) released by *any* immune-system cell. A *lymphokine* is simply a cytokine released by a *lymphocyte*, and a *monokine* is simply a cytokine released by a *mononuclear phagocyte* (*monocyte* or *macrophage*). Put another way, *cytokine* is a generic term for the whole class of nonantibody mediators released by immune cells, whereas the terms *lymphokine* and *monokine* are more restrictive, referring only to nonantibody mediators released by lymphocytes and mononuclear phagocytes, respectively. Examples of cytokines and their functions are listed in Table 62–3.

### TABLE 62-3. FUNCTIONS OF SELECTED CYTOKINES

| Cytokine | Function |
| --- | --- |
| Interleukin-1 | Stimulation of lymphocyte progenitor cells |
| Interleukin-2 | Stimulates proliferation and differentiation of helper T cells and cytolytic T cells |
| Interleukin-3 | Stimulates proliferation of bone marrow lineage cells, B cells, and T cells |
| Interleukin-4 | Activates B cells, T cells, and macrophages |
| Interleukin-5 | Stimulates generation of eosinophils |
| Interleukin-6 | Stimulates proliferation of bone marrow cells and plasma cells |
| Interleukin-7 | Stimulates B cells and T cells |
| Interleukin-8 | Attracts neutrophils, B cells, and T cells |
| Interleukin-9 | Stimulates proliferation of mast cells |
| Interleukin-10 | Inhibits some T cells |
| Interleukin-11 | Enhances actions of inteleukin-3 |
| Interleukin-12 | Enhances actions of interleukin-2 |
| Interferon alpha | Activates macrophages, cytotoxic T cells, and NK cells |
| Interferon gamma | Activates macrophages and T cells and enhances expression of MHC molecules |
| Tumor necrosis factor | Kills tumor cells; promotes inflammation |
| Granulocyte-macrophage colony-stimulating factor | Stimulates proliferation of monocytes, macrophages, and granulocytes (neutrophils, eosinophils, basophils) |

# Antibody-Mediated (Humoral) Immunity

As noted above, there are two types of immune responses: humoral immunity and cell-mediated immunity. Our objective in this section is to review humoral immunity, focusing on (1) how antibodies are produced and (2) the mechanisms by which antibodies protect us. Cell-mediated immunity is discussed in the section that follows.

## Production of Antibodies

Antibody production requires the cooperative interaction of three types of cells: *B cells*, which actually make the antibodies; *helper T cells* (CD4 cells), which stimulate the B cells; and an *antigen-presenting cell* (either a macrophage or dendritic cell), which activates the CD4 cells so that they can then help the B cells. The major steps in the process are depicted in Figure 62–4.

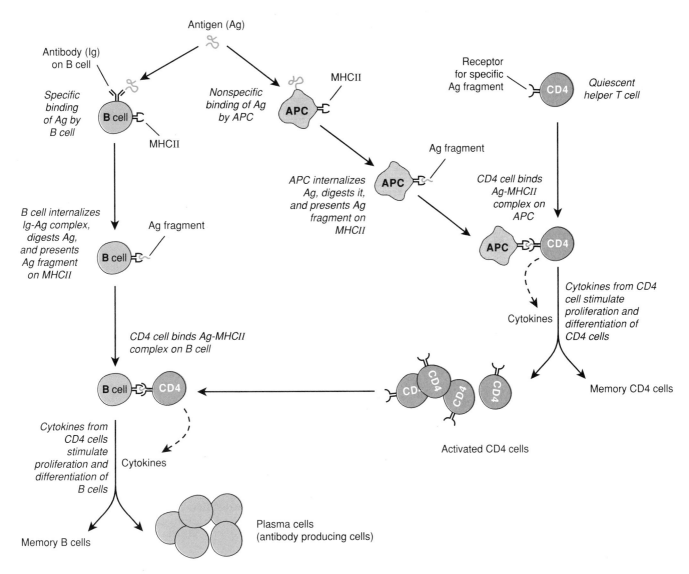

**Figure 62–4. Major events in antibody-mediated (humoral) immunity.** Humoral immunity requires three types of cells: B cells, APCs, and helper T cells (CD4 cells). Binding of a CD4 cell to an APC activates the CD4, which then binds to a B cell and releases cytokines, which then stimulate the B cell. MHC II = class II MHC molecule; APC = antigen-presenting cell (macrophage or dendritic cell); Ig = immunoglobulin (antibody).

## Overview of Antibody Production

As indicated in Figure 62–4, production of antibodies begins with binding of a specific antigen (Ag) to two types of cells: a virgin B cell and an antigen-presenting cell (APC). The APC may be either a macrophage or dendritic cell. After processing the Ag, the APC is able to bind with a specific CD4 cell, thereby causing the CD4 cell to proliferate and differentiate into active CD4 cells and memory CD4 cells. The active CD4 cells then bind with processed Ag on B cells, thereby causing the B cells to proliferate and differentiate into plasma cells, which manufacture the antibodies, and memory B cells, which await the next antigen exposure.

## Specific Cellular Events in Antibody Production

*B Cells.*  Participation of B cells in the immune response begins with recognition and binding of a *specific* Ag. The receptor that B cells employ for Ag recognition is actually an antibody (IgD or IgM). For any given B cell, this antibody (receptor) is highly specific for just one antigenic determinant. After the Ag binds the B-cell receptor, the receptor-Ag complex is internalized and the Ag is broken down into small peptide fragments. Each fragment is then complexed with a *class II MHC molecule*, after which the *MHC II–Ag complexes* are transported to the cell surface. (In Fig. 62–4, only one such complex is shown. However, in a real cell, many such complexes, each with a different piece of the antigen, would appear on the cell surface.) The final step of B-cell activation occurs when a CD4 helper T cell recognizes and binds to an MHC II–Ag complex on the B cell. This binding causes the CD4 cell to secrete cytokines, which then stimulate the B cell to proliferate and differentiate into two types of cells: plasma cells and memory B cells. The plasma cells are the cells that make the antibodies; the memory cells serve to hasten and intensify the immune response if antigen exposure should occur again.

***Antigen-Presenting Cells.*** APCs are essential for activation of CD4 helper T cells. The reason is that CD4 cells cannot recognize antigen that is free in solution. Rather, they can only recognize antigen that has been complexed with an MHC II molecule.

Participation of APCs in the immune response begins with nonspecific binding of Ag to the APC (Fig. 62-4). Next, as in B cells, the Ag is internalized and broken into fragments, which are then complexed with MHC II molecules and transported to the cell surface, where they are available for interaction with CD4 cells.

***Helper T Cells (CD4 Cells).*** The role of CD4 cells in humoral immunity is to activate B cells. In the absence of stimulation by CD4 cells, B cells are unable to proliferate and produce antibodies.

Participation of CD4 cells in the immune response begins when these cells bind with an MHC II–Ag complex on the surface of an APC. Binding is mediated by a receptor on the CD4 cell that is specific for the particular antigen in the MHC II–Ag complex. (As noted above, in order for the CD4 cell to recognize the Ag, the Ag must be complexed with an MHC II molecule, which is why the APC is essential for CD4 cell activation.) Upon binding to the MHC II–Ag complex, the CD4 cell releases cytokines, which then cause the CD4 cell itself to proliferate and differentiate into memory CD4 cells and activated CD4 cells. The activated CD4 cells then bind to their corresponding MHC II–Ag complexes on B cells, release cytokines, and thereby cause proliferation and differentiation of the B cells.

## Antibody Effector Mechanisms

Antibodies are simply molecules with the ability to bind to other molecules. Antibodies have no special destructive powers. Hence, in order to rid the body of antigens, which is what antibodies are for, antibodies usually work in conjunction with other factors, namely, *phagocytic cells* and the *complement system.* The only antigens that antibodies can neutralize without help are bacterial toxins and viruses.

### Opsonization of Bacteria

One mechanism for ridding the body of pathogenic bacteria is phagocytosis by macrophages and neutrophils. However, because of their structures, some bacteria are difficult for phagocytes to grab hold of, and hence are resistant to ingestion. Antibodies help promote phagocytosis of these bacteria by acting as *opsonins.* (An opsonin is a molecule that binds to a bacterium or other target particle and thereby promotes phagocytosis by providing a handle for phagocytes to grab on to.)

Bacterial opsonization by antibodies occurs in two steps. First, the antigen-binding region of the antibody binds to antigen on the bacterial surface, which leaves the Fc portion of the antibody projecting away from the surface. Second, phagocytes link up with the Fc portion of the antibody, which brings them in close contact with the bacterium and hence enables them to commence phagocytosis. Phagocytes are able to bind the Fc fragment because they have high-affinity receptors for Fc on their surface. Most of the antibodies that act as opsonins belong to the IgG class.

### Activation of the Complement System

The complement cascade is a complex system consisting of at least 20 serum proteins, which, when activated, can cause multiple effects, including cell lysis, opsonization, degranulation of mast cells, and infiltration of phagocytes. The system may be activated in two ways, known as the *classical pathway* and the *alternative pathway.* The classical pathway is activated by *antibodies*; the alternative pathway is not. However, with both pathways, the end results are essentially the same. Consideration here is limited to the classical pathway.

The classical pathway is turned on when C1 (the first component of the complement system) encounters an antigen-antibody complex and then binds to the Fc region of the antibody. C1 will not bind with antibody that is free in solution; hence, free antibodies cannot activate the system. Activation of the complement system triggers a cascade of reactions that amplify the response at each stage. The result is production of compounds that can injure target cells.

Lysis of target cells that have been tagged with antibodies is the most dramatic effect of the complement system. Lysis is caused by cylindrical *membrane attack complexes*, which are formed by the complement cascade. Following their insertion into the target cell membrane, the attack complexes act as pores through which fluid can enter the cell. As a result of fluid influx, the cell swells and eventually bursts.

### Neutralization of Viruses and Bacterial Toxins

Neutralization of toxins and viruses is the only protective action that antibodies can perform unassisted. In order to hurt us, bacterial toxins must first bind to receptors on our cells. Similarly, in order to infect us, viruses must first bind to cell-surface receptors. By binding to antigenic determinants on toxins and viruses, antibodies make it impossible for toxins and viruses to bind to cellular receptors. As a result, these agents can no longer harm us.

## Cell-Mediated Immunity

Cell-mediated immunity has two branches, one mediated by *helper T lymphocytes* (CD4 cells) and *macrophages*, and one mediated primarily by *cytolytic T lymphocytes* (CD8 cells). In the branch mediated by CD4 cells and macrophages, the result is called *delayed-type hypersensitivity.* In the branch mediated by CD8 cells, the result is *target-cell lysis.*

## Delayed-Type Hypersensitivity

The object of delayed-type hypersensitivity (DTH) is to rid the body of bacteria that replicate primarily within macrophages (e.g., *Listeria monocytogenes, Mycobac-terium tuberculosis*). For DTH to occur, two cells are needed: an *infected macrophage* and a *CD4 helper T cell*. The macrophage serves to activate the CD4 cell, which in turn activates the macrophage, thereby enabling the macrophage to kill the bacteria residing within it. Hence, the same cell (i.e., the macrophage) is both the activator of the CD4 cell and the recipient of the activated CD4 cell's help.

***Activation of Helper T Cells.*** Activation of CD4 cells in DTH is essentially identical to the activation of CD4 cells in humoral immunity. As shown in Figure 62–5, the process begins when a macrophage becomes infected with intracellular bacteria. As in humoral immunity, the macrophage breaks down the antigen to small peptides, complexes each peptide with a class II MHC molecule, and then presents the antigen–MHC II complexes on its surface. In the next step, a CD4 cell binds to an antigen–MHC II complex on the macrophage. As discussed above, selectivity of binding is determined by receptors on the CD4 cell that recognize a specific antigen fragment, but only when the fragment is bound to a class II MHC molecule. Binding of the CD4 cell to the APC causes the CD4 cell to release (1) cytokines that cause the CD4 cell itself to proliferate and differentiate into memory cells and (2) mediators of DTH, including interferon gamma and tumor necrosis factor.

***Activation of Macrophages.*** *Interferon gamma*, released from the activated CD4 cell, is the major stimulus for macrophage activation. In response to interferon gamma, macrophages increase production of lysosomes and reactive oxygen. The reactive oxygen is ultimately responsible for killing bacteria inside the macrophage. In addition to ridding macrophages of bacteria, DTH produces local inflammation.

## Cytolytic T Lymphocytes

Cytolytic lymphocytes (CTLs, CD8 cells) kill other cells. Their principal job is to kill self cells that are infected with viruses, thereby halting viral replication. In addition, CTLs participate in rejection of transplants. In this chapter, we will limit discussion to killing of virally infected cells.

The process by which CTLs kill other cells has two stages: activation of CTLs, followed by recognition and killing of the target cell. The overall process is depicted in Figure 62–6.

***Activation of Cytolytic T Cells.*** Activation of CTLs requires the participation of an *antigen-presenting cell* and a *helper T cell* (CD4 cell). The process is very similar to the activation of CD4 cells discussed above. However, there is one important difference: whereas CD4 cells specifically recognize antigen that is bound to a *class II* MHC molecule on an APC, CTLs specifically recognize antigen that is bound to a *class I* MHC molecule on an APC.

In viral infections, activation of CTLs begins with processing of viral antigens by an APC. As shown in Figure 62–6, the APC combines the antigen with a class I MCH molecule and then presents the antigen–MHC I complex on its surface. Next, a pre-CTL binds to the antigen–MHC I complex. (Like CD4 cells, each pre-CTL has receptors that are specific for a particular antigen–MHC complex.)

**Figure 62–5. Cell-mediated immunity: delayed-type hypersensitivity.** DTH requires two cells: an infected macrophage and a CD4 cell. Binding of the CD4 cell to the macrophage activates the CD4 cell, which then releases interferon gamma and several cytokines. Interferon gamma activates the macrophage. The cytokines cause the CD4 cell to proliferate and differentiate into memory cells. Ag = antigen; MHC II = class II MHC molecule.

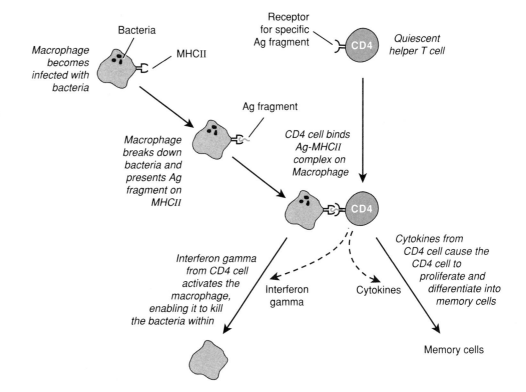

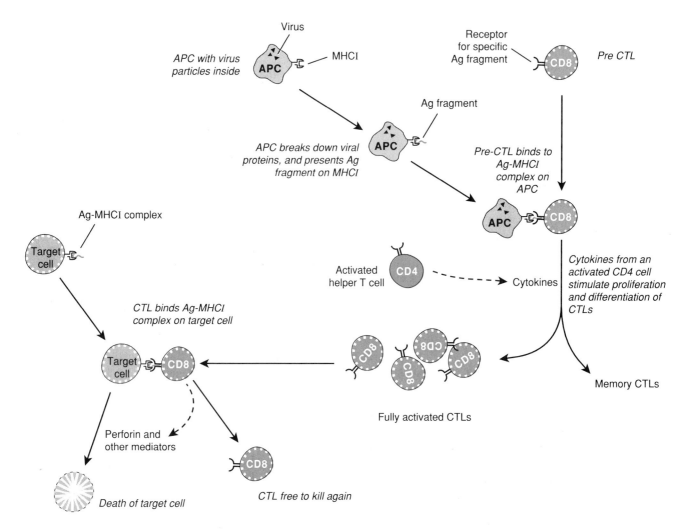

**Figure 62–6. Cell-mediated immunity: cytolytic T cells.** This branch of cell-mediated immunity requires three types of cells: CTLs, APCs, and CD4 cells. Binding of the CTL to the APC begins the activation of the CTL. Stimulation of the CTL by cytokines from the CD4 cell completes the activation of the CTL, which then binds with and kills its target. Activation of the CD4 cells, which is not shown, takes place essentially as depicted in Figures 62–4 and 62–5. CTL = cytolytic T lymphocyte; Ag = antigen;  MHC I = class I MHC molecule; APC = antigen-presenting cell.

Linking of the pre-CTL to the APC primes the pre-CTL for the next stage of activation: stimulation by cytokines (interleukin-2, interferon gamma, and probably others) provided by an activated CD4 cell. (Activation of the CD4 cell, which is not shown in Figure 62–6, occurs when the CD4 cell encounters an APC with a viral antigen–MHC II complex.) In response to the cytokines released by the CD4 cell, the pre-CTL undergoes proliferation and differentiation into memory CTLs and activated CTLs.

***Recognition of Virally Infected Target Cells.*** CTLs recognize their targets by the presence of an antigen–MHC I complex. This is the same process by which CTLs recognize APCs. As noted earlier, virtually all cells in the body carry class I MHC molecules. (Class II molecules are limited to APCs and B cells). Hence, when a cell is infected with a virus, viral antigens form intracellular complexes with MHC I molecules, after which the antigen–MHC I complexes are presented on the cell surface. As shown in Figure 62–6, activated CTLs recognize the antigen–MHC I complex, and hence bind to the target cell. Since only

cells that are infected with the virus will bear viral antigens on their class I MHC molecules, attack by CTLs is limited to infected cells; all other cells are spared.

***Mechanisms of Cell Kill.*** Binding of a CTL to its target cell causes the CTL to release mediators that kill the target. Two mechanisms of cell kill are involved: *lysis* and *apoptosis* (programmed cell death). The mediator of lysis is called *perforin*, a molecule that forms pores in the target cell membrane; the resultant influx of fluid causes the cell to swell and then burst. (This mechanism is very similar to one by which the complement system causes cell lysis.) The mediators of apoptosis have not been identified with certainty. However, their effects are very clear. The initial effect is activation of intracellular enzymes that digest the cell's own DNA. This is followed by fragmentation of the nucleus and cell death. Only the target cell is harmed; bystander cells and the CTL itself are not touched. In fact, after releasing its mediators, the CTL disconnects from the doomed target and goes on to seek other victims.

# KEY POINTS

- The immune system helps us by attacking invading organisms (viruses, bacteria, fungi, parasites) and cancer cells. The immune system can hurt us by attacking transplants and our own healthy cells.
- There are two basic types of immune responses: natural immunity (native or innate immunity) and specific acquired immunity.
- There are two types of specific acquired immunity: cell-mediated immunity and humoral (antibody-mediated) immunity.
- The immune system has five major types of cells: B lymphocytes (B cells), helper T lymphocytes (CD4 cells), cytolytic T lymphocytes (CD8 cells, CTLs), macrophages, and dendritic cells.
- Only lymphocytes have receptors that can recognize specific antigens.
- B cells make antibodies.
- CTLs kill target cells directly.
- Helper T cells are essential for the activation of B cells, CTLs, and the macrophages involved in delayed type hypersensitivity (DTH).
- Macrophages have three functions in specific immunity: (1) they serve as antigen-presenting cells (APCs) in the activation of helper T cells and CTLs, (2) they are involved in DTH, and (3) they phagocytize opsonized cells in humoral immunity.
- Like macrophages, dendritic cells serve as APCs.
- An antigen is a molecule that triggers a specific immune response (and then becomes the target of that response).
- Most antigens are large molecules.
- Antibodies bind to specific, small regions of an antigen, referred to as epitopes or antigenic determinants.
- The major histocompatibility complex (MHC) is a group of genes that codes for MHC molecules, which are found on the cell surface.
- MHC molecules have three major functions: they play a key role in the activation of helper T cells and CTLs, they guide CTLs toward target cells, and they provide the basis for distinguishing between self and nonself.
- Class II MHC molecules are found only on B cells and APCs, whereas class I MHC molecules are found on virtually all cells (including B cells and APCs).
- It is rare for two individuals to have MHC molecules that are precisely the same. As a result, MHC molecules from one individual are usually recognized as foreign (nonself) by the immune systems of everyone else.
- A cytokine is defined as any mediator molecule (other than an antibody) released by any immune-system cell.
- The most characteristic feature of antibodies is their ability to recognize specific antigens.

- Antibody production requires the cooperative interaction of three types of cells: B cells, which make the antibodies; helper T cells (CD4 cells), which stimulate the B cells; and APCs, which activate the CD4 cells so that they can then activate B cells.
- B cells have antibodies on their surface that serve as receptors for recognizing specific antigens. Binding of antigen to the receptor is the first step in B-cell activation.
- Activation of B cells is completed when a CD4 cell binds to an antigen–MHC II complex on the B cell and then releases cytokines, which then stimulate the B cell.
- In order to activate a B cell, a CD4 cell must first become activated itself. CD4 activation is initiated by binding of the CD4 cell to an antigen–MHC II complex on an APC.
- Antibodies eliminate antigens by three mechanisms: (1) direct neutralization of toxins and viruses, (2) opsonization of bacteria, and (3) activation of the complement system.
- Opsonization (coating bacteria with antibodies) helps macrophages and neutrophils hold on to bacteria, and thereby facilitates phagocytosis.
- The complement system forms pores in the bacterial cell membrane, thereby promoting death by lysis.
- Cell-mediated immunity can result in delayed-type hypersensitivity (DTH) and lysis of target cells by CTLs.
- DTH involves two types of cells: an infected macrophage and a CD4 cell. The macrophage activates the CD4 cell, which then releases interferon gamma, which in turn stimulates the macrophage, thereby enabling the macrophage to kill the bacteria within it.
- The major role of CTLs is to kill self cells that have become infected with viruses.
- Activation of CTLs proceeds in two steps: first, the CTL binds to an APC; second, the CTL is stimulated by cytokines provided by a CD4 cell.
- Binding of CTLs to APCs differs from binding of CD4 cells to APCs in that CTLs specifically recognize antigen that is bound to a class I MHC molecule on the APC, whereas CD4 cells specifically recognize antigen that is bound to a class II MHC molecule.
- CTLs kill target cells in two ways: (1) they release perforin, which creates pores in the cell, thereby causing death by lysis; and (2) they release compounds that cause apoptosis (programmed cell death).
- Activated CTLs only attack self cells that have antigen–MHC I complexes; all other self cells, including the CTLs, are spared.
- Specific immune responses result in production of memory T cells and memory B cells. As a result, the next time an antigen is encountered, the immune response occurs faster and with greater intensity.

# Antihistamines

H istamine is an endogenous compound found in specialized cells throughout the body. This substance plays an important role in allergic reactions and regulation of gastric acid secretion. The antihistamines, one of our most widely used families of drugs, are agents that block histamine's actions.

In order to understand the antihistamines, we must first understand histamine itself. Accordingly, we will begin the chapter with a discussion of histamine, emphasizing its contribution to allergic responses. Having established this background, we will discuss the antihistamines.

## Histamine

Histamine is a locally acting substance with prominent and varied effects. In the vascular system, histamine dilates small blood vessels and increases capillary permeability. In the bronchi, histamine produces constriction. In the stomach, histamine stimulates secretion of acid. In the central nervous system (CNS), histamine acts as a neurotransmitter. Despite this impressive spectrum of effects, clinical applications for histamine itself are limited. Currently, use of histamine is restricted to diagnostic procedures. However, although its clinical utility is minimal, histamine is still of great medical interest because of its involvement in two common pathologic states: allergies and peptic ulcer disease.

### Distribution, Synthesis, Storage, and Release

**Distribution.** Histamine is present in practically all tissues of the body. Levels of histamine are especially high in the skin, lungs, and GI tract. The histamine content of plasma is relatively low.

**Synthesis and Storage.** Histamine is synthesized and stored in two types of cells: *mast cells* and *basophils*. Mast cells are present in the skin and other soft tissues; basophils are present in the blood. In both mast cells and basophils, histamine is stored in structures called secretory granules. (In addition to histamine, secretory granules contain other substances that, like histamine, are mediators of allergic reactions.)

**Release.** Release of histamine from mast cells and basophils is produced by allergic and nonallergic mechanisms.

*Allergic Release.* The initial requirement for allergic release of histamine is the production of antibodies of the immunoglobulin E class. These antibodies are generated in response to exposure to specific allergens (e.g., pollens, insect venoms, certain drugs). Following synthesis, the antibodies become attached to the outer surface of mast cells and basophils (Fig. 63–1). When the subject is re-exposed to the allergen, the allergen becomes bound by the antibodies. As indicated in Figure 63–1, binding of allergen to *adjacent* antibodies creates a bridge between those antibodies. By a mechanism that is not fully understood, this bridging process mobilizes intracellular calcium. The calcium, in turn, causes the histamine-containing storage granules to fuse with the cell membrane and disgorge their contents into the extracellular space. Note that allergic release of histamine requires *prior exposure* to the allergen; an allergic reaction cannot occur during initial contact with an allergen.

*Nonallergic Release.* A number of agents (certain drugs, radiocontrast media, plasma expanders) can act directly on mast cells to cause histamine release. With these agents, no prior sensitization is needed. Cell injury can also cause direct release of histamine.

### Physiologic and Pharmacologic Effects

Histamine acts through two types of receptors, named $H_1$ and $H_2$. Responses to stimulation of these receptors are discussed below.

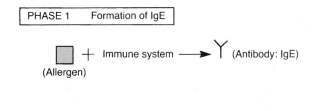

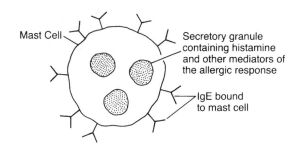

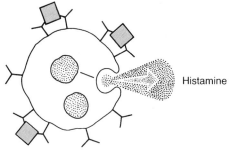

**Figure 63–1. Release of histamine by allergen-antibody interaction.**

### Effects of H₁ Stimulation

**Vasodilation.** Stimulation of H₁ receptors causes dilation of small blood vessels (arterioles and venules). Vasodilation is prominent in the skin of the face and upper body. In these areas, release of histamine causes the skin to become warm and flushed. If vasodilation is extensive, total peripheral resistance will be reduced and blood pressure will fall.

**Increased Capillary Permeability.** H₁ stimulation increases capillary permeability by causing contraction of capillary endothelial cells. This contraction produces openings between endothelial cells through which fluid, protein, and platelets can flow. Escape of fluid and protein into the interstitial space produces edema. If loss of intravascular fluid is substantial, blood pressure may fall.

**Bronchoconstriction.** H₁ stimulation causes constriction of the bronchi. If histamine is administered to an individual with asthma, severe bronchoconstriction will follow. However, although *exogenous* histamine is clearly capable of inducing bronchial constriction, histamine is not the cause of bronchoconstriction during a spontaneous asthma attack. Consequently, antihistamines are of no use for treating asthma.

**Other Effects.** Stimulation of H₁ receptors located on sensory nerves produces *itching and pain*. H₁ stimulation also promotes *secretion of mucus*. In the CNS, histamine acts as a neurotransmitter, causing *sedation* and other effects.

### Effects of H₂ Stimulation

The principal response to H₂-receptor stimulation is *secretion of gastric acid*. Histamine acts directly on parietal cells of the stomach to promote acid release. Histamine is the dominant regulator of gastric acidity. Acetylcholine and gastrin, two modulators of acid production, play a subordinate role: in the presence of H₂ blockade, acetylcholine and gastrin are unable to elicit acid secretion.

## Histamine in Allergic Responses

Allergic reactions are mediated by histamine and other compounds (e.g., prostaglandins, leukotrienes). The intensity of an allergic reaction is determined by which of these substances is mediating the reaction.

**Mild Allergy.** The symptoms of mild allergy (e.g., rhinitis, itching, localized edema) are caused largely by histamine (acting at H₁ receptors). As a result, mild allergic conditions (e.g., hay fever, acute urticaria, mild transfusion reactions) are generally responsive to antihistamine therapy.

**Severe Allergic Reactions (Anaphylaxis).** Severe allergic reactions manifest as anaphylactic shock, a syndrome characterized by bronchoconstriction, hypotension, and edema of the glottis. Although histamine is involved in these responses, it is only a minor contributor; other substances (e.g., leukotrienes) are the principal causative agents. Since histamine has little to do with producing anaphylaxis, it follows that antihistamines will be of little help as treatment. The drug of choice for management of anaphylaxis is *epinephrine*. The rationale for using epinephrine is discussed in Chapter 19.

## The Two Types of Antihistamines: H₁ Antagonists and H₂ Antagonists

Antihistamines fall into two basic categories: H₁-receptor antagonists and H₂-receptor antagonists. The H₁ antagonists produce selective blockade at H₁ receptors. The H₂ antagonists produce selective blockade at H₂ receptors. The principal application of the H₁ blockers is management of mild allergic disorders. The H₂ antagonists are used to treat gastric and duodenal ulcers. Since the H₂ antagonists do not block $H_1$ receptors, these drugs are of no use for allergies. In this chapter, our focus is on the $H_1$ antagonists. The $H_2$ blockers, which are important and widely used, are discussed in Chapter 71 (Drugs for Peptic Ulcer Disease).

# $H_1$ Antagonists I: Basic Pharmacology

The $H_1$ antagonists are the classic antihistamines. These agents were in use long before the $H_2$ blockers were developed. In fact, before $H_2$ blockers became available, the term *$H_1$ antagonist* did not exist; the drugs that we now call $H_1$ antagonists or $H_1$ blockers were simply referred to as *antihistamines*. Because of its historical use, the term *antihistamines* is still employed as a synonym for the subgroup of histamine antagonists that produce selective $H_1$ blockade. In this chapter, we will respect tradition and continue to use the term *antihistamine* interchangeably with *$H_1$ blocker* and *$H_1$ antagonist*.

Although the many $H_1$ antagonists available have similar antihistaminic actions, these drugs differ significantly in their side effects. Because of these differences, selection of a prototype to represent the group is not feasible. Hence, rather than structuring discussion around one prototypic drug, we will discuss the $H_1$ antagonists collectively. Differences between individual antihistamines are addressed where appropriate.

## Classification of $H_1$ Antagonists

The $H_1$ antagonists fall into two major groups: *first-generation $H_1$ antagonists* and *second-generation $H_1$ antagonists*. The principal difference between these groups is that the first-generation agents are highly *sedating*, whereas the second-generation agents are essentially *nonsedating*. In the prior edition of this text, the second-generation agents were referred to simply as nonsedating antihistamines.

## Mechanism of Action

$H_1$ blockers bind selectively to $H_1$-histaminic receptors, thereby preventing the actions of histamine at these sites. The $H_1$ antagonists have no effect at $H_2$ receptors. Antihistamines do not act by preventing the release of histamine from mast cells or basophils.

It should be noted that, although interaction of the classic antihistamines with *histaminic* receptors is limited to the $H_1$-receptor subtype, these drugs can also bind to *nonhistaminic* receptors. Of particular significance is the ability of certain antihistamines to bind to and block muscarinic receptors. Blockade of muscarinic receptors underlies several important side effects of these drugs.

## Pharmacologic Effects

***Peripheral Effects.*** The major effects of the $H_1$ antagonists can be attributed to preventing the actions of histamine at $H_1$ receptors. In arterioles and venules, $H_1$ block-

ers inhibit the dilator actions of histamine, and thereby reduce localized flushing. In capillary beds, the antihistamines prevent histamine-induced increases in permeability, and thereby reduce edema. By blocking the actions of histamine at sensory nerves, $H_1$ antagonists reduce itching and pain. Blockade of $H_1$ receptors in mucous membranes suppresses secretion of mucus.

***Effects on the Central Nervous System.*** Antihistamines can cause both excitation and depression of the CNS. At *therapeutic doses*, antihistamines usually produce CNS *depression*: reaction time is slowed, alertness is diminished, and drowsiness is likely. These effects are more pronounced with some antihistamines than with others; with the second-generation antihistamines (e.g., terfenadine, astemizole) CNS depression is negligible.

*Stimulation* of the CNS is most common following antihistamine overdose. Convulsions frequently result. Very young children are especially sensitive to CNS stimulation by these drugs.

***Other Pharmacologic Effects.*** Blockade of muscarinic cholinergic receptors by antihistamines can produce typical *anticholinergic* responses. These are discussed below under *Adverse Effects*. Several antihistamines can suppress nausea and vomiting (see below under *Motion Sickness*).

## Therapeutic Uses

All of the $H_1$ antagonists are useful in treating allergic disorders. Some of these drugs are also indicated for other conditions (e.g., motion sickness, insomnia).

***Mild Allergy.*** Antihistamines can reduce symptoms of mild allergies. In people with *seasonal allergic rhinitis* (hay fever), $H_1$ blockers can reduce sneezing, rhinorrhea, and itching of the eyes, nose, and throat. In patients with *acute urticaria*, these drugs can reduce redness, itching, and edema. The antihistamines can also reduce symptoms of *allergic conjunctivitis* and urticaria associated with *mild transfusion reactions*. In all of these conditions, benefits result from $H_1$-receptor blockade—and not from preventing allergen-induced release of histamine from mast cells and basophils. Since mild allergic reactions may be mediated by other substances in addition to histamine, relief of symptoms with antihistamines may not be complete.

***Severe Allergy.*** As noted above, the major symptoms of anaphylaxis (hypotension, laryngeal edema, bronchospasm) are caused by mediators other than histamine. Hence, although antihistamines may be employed as adjuncts to epinephrine in the treatment of anaphylaxis, the benefits of antihistamines are minimal.

***Motion Sickness.*** Some antihistamines, such as promethazine [Phenergan] and dimenhydrinate [Dramamine], are labeled for use in motion sickness. Benefits derive from blockade of $H_1$ receptors and muscarinic receptors in the pathway leading from the vestibular apparatus of the inner ear to the vomiting center of the medulla. Motion sickness and its treatment are discussed in Chapter 73. The antihistamines employed for motion sickness, along with their dosages, are listed in Table 73-1.

## TABLE 63-1. PHARMACOLOGIC EFFECTS OF H₁ ANTAGONISTS

| Drug | H₁-Blocking Activity | Sedative Effects | Anticholinergic Effects |
|---|---|---|---|
| **FIRST-GENERATION AGENTS** | | | |
| *Alkylamines* | | | |
| Brompheniramine | +++ | + | ++ |
| Chlorpheniramine | ++ | + | ++ |
| Dexchlorpheniramine | +++ | + | ++ |
| Triprolidine | ++ to +++ | + | ++ |
| *Ethanolamines* | | | |
| Carbinoxamine | + to ++ | ++ | +++ |
| Clemastine | + to ++ | ++ | +++ |
| Diphenhydramine | + to ++ | +++ | +++ |
| *Ethylenediamines* | | | |
| Pyrilamine | + to ++ | + | ± |
| Tripelennamine | + to ++ | ++ | ± |
| *Phenothiazines* | | | |
| Methdilazine | +++ | + | +++ |
| Promethazine | +++ | +++ | +++ |
| Trimeprazine | +++ | ++ | +++ |
| *Piperidines* | | | |
| Azatadine | ++ | ++ | ++ |
| Cyproheptadine | ++ | + | ++ |
| Phenindamine | ++ | * | ++ |
| **SECOND-GENERATION (NONSEDATING) AGENTS** | | | |
| Astemizole | ++ to +++ | ± | ± |
| Cetirizine | +++ | ± | ± |
| Fexofenadine | +++ | ± | ± |
| Loratadine | ++ to +++ | ± | ± |
| Terfenadine | ++ to +++ | ± | ± |

± = low to none; + = low; ++ = moderate; +++ = high.
*May cause excitation.

**Insomnia.** The ability of antihistamines to cause CNS depression has been exploited in the treatment of insomnia. Practically every over-the-counter (OTC) sleep aid contains an H₁ antagonist (diphenhydramine or pyrilamine) as its active ingredient. However, although antihistamines can induce sleep when used in sufficient dosage, the doses recommended for OTC preparations are usually too small to be effective.

**Common Cold.** Despite their widespread presence in cold remedies, antihistamines are of practically no value as treatment for the common cold. These drugs neither prevent colds nor shorten their duration. Moreover, since histamine does not mediate symptoms of colds, H₁ blockade cannot even provide symptomatic relief. The only benefit that these drugs may offer is a moderate reduction in rhinorrhea, an effect that derives from the *anticholinergic* properties of the H₁ antagonists.

## Adverse Effects

All of the H₁ blockers can produce undesired effects. As a rule, these responses are more of a nuisance than a source of serious discomfort or danger. Frequently, side effects subside with continued drug use. Since individual antihistamines differ in their abilities to produce particular side effects (Table 63-1), adverse responses can be minimized by judicious drug selection.

**Sedation.** Sedation is the most common undesired effect of the antihistamines. Fortunately, tolerance to this effect often develops within a few days or weeks. If a preparation with a long half-life is being used, daytime sedation can be minimized by administering the entire daily dose at night. Patients should be advised to avoid driving and other hazardous activities if alertness is impaired. Also, patients should be warned against using alcohol and other CNS depressants since these agents will intensify the depressant effects of the H₁ antagonist.

The second-generation antihistamines exert little or no sedative effect. These agents—astemizole, loratadine, terfenadine, and cetirizine—are unable to cross the blood-brain barrier, and therefore do not alter CNS function. For patients experiencing disabling sedation with a first-generation H₁ antagonist, therapy with a second-generation (nonsedating) antihistamine may be helpful. Unfortunately, the nonsedating agents are considerably more expensive than the first-generation agents. The sedative properties of individual antihistamines are indicated in Table 63–1.

**Cardiac Dysrhythmias.** Potentially fatal cardiac dysrhythmias (torsades de pointes, ventricular fibrillation, others) have occurred rarely in patients taking *astemizole* or *terfenadine*, two of the second-generation antihistamines. These drugs predispose the patient to dysrhythmias by prolonging the QT interval, but only when drug levels are excessive. The major causes of excessive levels are *overdose* and *reduced metabolism*. The causes of reduced metabolism are *liver dysfunction* and inhibition of metabolism by another drug. Currently, only four drugs have been proved to inhibit antihistamine metabolism; these are *erythromycin, clarithromycin, ketoconazole,* and *itraconazole*. Three related drugs—azithromycin, dirithromycin, and fluconazole—do *not* inhibit metabolism of terfenadine and astemizole.

The relationship of metabolism to therapeutic effects and dysrhythmias requires explanation. Under normal conditions, both terfenadine and astemizole are rapidly converted to metabolites. It is these metabolites, and not the parent drug, that mediate therapeutic effects. Conversely, it is the parent drug that causes dysrhythmias. Because rapid metabolism normally keeps levels of parent drug low, dysrhythmias are rare.

Since terfenadine and astemizole promote dysrhythmias by prolonging the QT interval, it is possible that other drugs that prolong the QT interval will increase the risk. However, this potential interaction has not yet been proved. Nonetheless, it would seem prudent to avoid such agents in patients taking terfenadine and astemizole. Some drugs that prolong the QT interval are listed in Table 63-2.

Several measures can reduce the risk of dysrhythmias. To avoid overdose, patients should be cautioned against exceeding the prescribed dosage, even if the prescribed dosage has failed to relieve allergic symptoms. To avoid excessive drug levels at normal doses, terfenadine and astemizole should not be given to patients with significant liver dysfunction or to patients taking erythromycin, clarithromycin, ketoconazole, or itraconazole. Avoiding terfenadine and astemizole in patients receiving other drugs that prolong the QT interval may also help. In some patients, syncope (fainting) has preceded development of dysrhythmias; patients who experience syncope should discontinue terfenadine and astemizole and undergo evaluation for potential dysrhythmias.

**Nonsedative CNS Effects.** In addition to sedation, antihistamines can cause dizziness, incoordination, confusional states, and fatigue. The elderly are especially sensitive to these actions. In some patients, paradoxical excitation occurs, resulting in insomnia, nervousness, tremors, and even convulsions. CNS stimulation is most common in children and following overdose.

**Gastrointestinal Effects.** Gastrointestinal disturbances are common. Responses include nausea, vomiting, loss of appetite, and diarrhea or constipation. These reactions can be minimized by administering antihistamines with meals.

**Anticholinergic Effects.** The $H_1$ antagonists possess weak atropine-like properties. These antimuscarinic actions can produce drying of mucous membranes in the mouth, nasal passages, and throat. Cholinergic blockade may also result in urinary hesitancy, constipation, and palpitations. If dry mouth becomes distressing, discomfort can be minimized by sucking on hard (sugarless) candy and by taking frequent sips of fluid. Antihistamines should be used with caution in patients with asthma, since thickening of bronchial secretions may impair breathing. Care should also be exercised in patients with other conditions that may be exacerbated by muscarinic blockade (e.g., urinary retention, prostatic hypertrophy, hypertension). The antimuscarinic efficacy of individual $H_1$ blockers is

**TABLE 63-2. AGENTS THAT DO (OR DON'T) INCREASE THE RISK OF DYSRHYTHMIAS FROM TERFENADINE AND ASTEMIZOLE**

| Definitely Increase Risk | Possibly Increase Risk | Do NOT Increase Risk |
|---|---|---|
| *By raising antihistamine level* | *By raising antihistamine level* | *Do NOT raise antihistamine level* |
| Erythromycin | Grapefruit juice | Azithromycin |
| Clarithromycin | *By prolonging QT interval* | Fluconazole |
| Ketoconazole | | Dirithromycin |
| Itraconazole | Disopyramide | |
| Nefazodone | Haloperidol | |
| | Probucol | |
| | Procainamide | |
| | Quinidine | |
| | Quinine | |
| | Sotalol | |
| | Thioridazine | |

indicated in Table 63-1. As can be seen, the second-generation antihistamines are also the least anticholinergic.

## Drug Interactions

***CNS Depressants.*** *Alcohol and other CNS depressants* (e.g., barbiturates, benzodiazepines, opioids) can intensify the depressant effects of the $H_1$ antagonists. Patients should be advised against consumption of alcoholic beverages. If medications with CNS-depressant properties are combined with $H_1$ blockers, dosage of the depressant may need to be lowered.

***Drugs That Increase the Risk of Dysrhythmias.*** *Erythromycin*, *clarithromycin*, *itraconazole*, and *ketoconazole* inhibit the metabolism of terfenadine and astemizole, and thereby increase the risk of dysrhythmias. Accordingly, concurrent use of terfenadine or astemizole with these antimicrobial drugs is contraindicated. Drugs that prolong the QT interval (e.g., quinidine) and grapefruit juice, which inhibits metabolism of terfenadine and astemizole, may also increase the risk of toxicity.

## Use in Pregnancy and Lactation

***Pregnancy.*** The margin of safety of antihistamines in pregnancy is not known. There have been reports of fetal malformation, but direct involvement of $H_1$ antagonists has not been proved. Given the uncertainty over the safety of these drugs, it is recommended that antihistamines be used only when clearly necessary, and only when the benefits of treatment outweigh the potential risks to the fetus. Antihistamines should be avoided late in the third trimester, since newborns are particularly sensitive to the adverse actions of these drugs.

***Lactation.*** The $H_1$ antagonists can be excreted in breast milk, thereby posing a risk to the nursing infant. Since infants, and especially newborns, are unusually sensitive to antihistamines, these drugs should not be used by women who are breast-feeding.

## Acute Toxicity

Although the antihistamines have a large margin of safety, acute poisoning is nonetheless common, owing to the widespread use of these drugs. CNS effects are prominent, especially anticholinergic reactions. Specific symptoms and treatment are described below.

***Symptoms.*** The anticholinergic actions of $H_1$ blockers produce symptoms resembling those of atropine poisoning (dilated pupils, flushed face, hyperpyrexia, tachycardia, dry mouth, urinary retention). In children, CNS excitation is prominent, manifesting as hallucinations, incoordination, ataxia, and convulsions. In extreme cases, intoxication progresses to coma, cardiovascular collapse, and death.

***Treatment.*** There is no specific antidote to antihistamine poisoning. Hence, treatment is directed at drug removal and management of symptoms. Emesis should be induced to expel the drug from the stomach. Following this, activated charcoal plus a cathartic is given to minimize absorption of any drug that remains in the GI tract. Convulsions should be treated with IV phenytoin. Anticonvulsants that have CNS-depressant properties must be avoided. Hyperthermia can be reduced by application of ice packs or by sponge baths.

# $H_1$ Antagonists II: Preparations

## First-Generation $H_1$ Antagonists

The first-generation (sedating) $H_1$ antagonists can be grouped in five major categories: alkylamines, ethanolamines, ethylenediamines, phenothiazines, and piperidines. As indicated in Table 63-1, these groups differ in antihistaminic efficacy and the ability to cause sedation and muscarinic blockade. Given these differences, it is often possible, through judicious drug selection, to produce effective $H_1$ blockade while minimizing undesired side effects.

Sedation can be a significant problem. Among the first-generation agents, CNS depression is most prominent with the ethanolamines (e.g., diphenhydramine) and phenothiazines (e.g., promethazine), and least prominent with the alkylamines (e.g., chlorpheniramine). For most patients, the alkylamines can provide effective $H_1$ blockade while causing only a modest reduction in alertness. If sedation remains excessive with an alkylamine, a second-generation agent may be tried.

All of the $H_1$ blockers can be administered by mouth. In addition, some can be given parenterally or by rectal suppository. Routes and dosages for individual $H_1$ antagonists are summarized in Table 63-3.

## Second-Generation (Nonsedating) $H_1$ Antagonists

Five second-generation antihistamines are available: terfenadine, astemizole, loratadine, fexofenadine, and cetirizine. Sedation does not occur because these drugs are unable to cross the blood-brain barrier. Unfortunately, these agents are much more expensive than first-generation antihistamines; they cost, for example, about 20 times more than chlorpheniramine, a representative traditional agent. Accordingly, it would seem prudent to reserve the newer antihistamines for patients who experience too much sedation with the older drugs. Although the nonsedative antihistamines are generally well tolerated, two of them—terfenadine and astemizole—have caused fatal cardiac dysrhythmias.

### Terfenadine

Terfenadine [Seldane] was the first nonsedating antihistamine to become available and will serve as our prototype for the group. As noted above, sedation is minimal because the drug does not cross the blood-brain barrier. No synergism has been seen with alcohol and other CNS depressants. In addition to being nonsedating, terfenadine is essentially devoid of anticholinergic actions.

Although generally well tolerated, terfenadine can cause *fatal dysrhythmias* when drug levels are excessive. Accordingly, patients should be warned not to exceed the prescribed dosage. Also, the drug should be avoided in patients with significant severe liver dysfunction and in those taking nefazodone, erythromycin, clarithromycin,

## TABLE 63-3. H₁ ANTAGONISTS: TRADE NAMES, ROUTES, AND DOSAGE

| Generic Name | Trade Names | Routes | Usual Adult Oral Dosage |
|---|---|---|---|
| **FIRST-GENERATION AGENTS** | | | |
| *Alkylamines* | | | |
| Brompheniramine | Dimetane, others | PO, IV, IM, SC | 4 mg q 4-6 h |
| Chlorpheniramine | Chlor-Trimeton, others | PO, IV, IM, SC | 4 mg q 4-6 h |
| Dexchlorpheniramine | Polaramine, others | PO | 2 mg q 4-6 h |
| Triprolidine | Actidil, Myidil | PO | 2.5 mg q 4-6 h |
| *Ethanolamines* | | | |
| Carbinoxamine | Clistin | PO | 4-8 mg q 6-8 h |
| Clemastine | Tavist | PO | 1.34 mg q 12 h |
| Diphenhydramine | Benadryl, others | PO, IV, IM | 25-50 mg q 6-8 h |
| *Ethylenediamines* | | | |
| Pyrilamine | Nisaval | PO | 25-50 mg q 6-8 h |
| Tripelennamine | PBZ, Pelamine | PO | 25-50 mg q 4-6 h |
| *Phenothiazines* | | | |
| Methdilazine | Tacaryl | PO | 8 mg q 6-12 h |
| Promethazine | Phenergan, others | PO, IV, IM, R* | 12.5-25 mg q 6-24 h |
| Trimeprazine | Temaril | PO | 2.5 mg q 6 h |
| *Piperidines* | | | |
| Azatadine | Optimine | PO | 1-2 mg q 12 h |
| Cyproheptadine | Periactin | PO | 4 mg q 6-8 h |
| Phenindamine | Nolahist | PO | 25 mg q 4-6 h |
| **SECOND-GENERATION (NONSEDATING) AGENTS** | | | |
| Astemizole | Hismanal | PO | 10 mg q 24 h |
| Cetirizine† | Zyrtec | PO | 5 or 10 mg q 24 h |
| Fexofenadine | Allegra | PO | 60 mg q 12 h |
| Loratadine | Claritin | PO | 10 mg q 24 h |
| Terfenadine | Seldane | PO | 60 mg q 12 h |

*R = Rectal suppository
†Cetirizine has mild sedating effects.

itraconazole, or ketoconazole. Caution should be exercised in patients with pre-existing cardiac disease. Because of the risk of serious adverse effects, the Food and Drug Administration (FDA) has recommended that terfenidine be withdrawn from the market.

Terfenadine is dispensed in 60-mg tablets for oral administration. The usual adult dosage is 60 mg twice daily.

### Astemizole

Astemizole [Hismanal] is much like terfenadine. The drug does not cross the blood-brain barrier, does not produce significant sedation, and does not intensify the effects of alcohol and other CNS depressants. Also, astemizole has minimal anticholinergic actions.

Like terfenadine, astemizole has been associated with fatal cardiac dysrhythmias. Patients should be warned not to exceed the prescribed dosage. As with terfenadine, the drug should be avoided in patients with severe liver disease and in those taking nefazodone, erythromycin, clarithromycin, itraconazole, or ketoconazole.

Astemizole is available in 10-mg tablets for oral administration. Absorption is reduced greatly (by 60%) in the presence of food;

hence, the drug should be administered 1 hour before meals or 2 hours after. Astemizole has a long half-life (9 days)—much longer than that of terfenadine. As a result, astemizole is effective when given just once a day. Because of its long half-life, astemizole can take several days to reach effective plasma concentrations. To achieve therapeutic levels more quickly, a loading schedule is used. This schedule consists of 30 mg once on day 1, 20 mg once on day 2, and 10 mg once daily thereafter.

### Loratadine

Loratadine [Claritin] is much like terfenadine and astemizole, but does not cause dysrhythmias. Like terfenadine and astemizole, loratadine is nonsedating and does not intensify sedation from alcohol and other CNS depressants. Loratadine is available in 10-mg tablets for oral administration. The drug should be taken on an empty stomach. The usual adult dosage is 10 mg once daily.

### Cetirizine

Cetirizine [Zyrtec] is new second-generation antihistamine approved for allergic rhinitis and chronic urticaria. The drug is highly effective, poses no risk of dysrhythmias, and is devoid of anticholinergic actions. Cetirizine crosses the blood-brain barrier poorly and sedation appears to be minimal (mild sedation was reported in some clinical trials, but not in others.) Dosages range from 5 to 20 mg/day.

### Fexofenadine

Fexofenadine [Allegra] is a new nonsedating antihistamine approved for treatment of seasonal allergic rhinitis. The drug is manufactured by Hoechst Marion Roussel, which also produces terfenadine. The company is marketing fexofenadine as a replacement for terfenadine [Seldane], which the FDA recommended be withdrawn because of the risk of fatal dysrhythmias. (Fexofenadine does not affect the heart and does not pose a risk of dysrhythmias.) The recommended dosage is 60 mg twice daily.

## KEY POINTS

- Histamine is synthesized and stored in mast cells and basophils. Release may be triggered by allergic and non-allergic mechanisms.
- There are two classes of histamine receptors: $H_1$ receptors and $H_2$ receptors.
- Stimulation of $H_1$ receptors causes vasodilation, increased capillary permeability, pain, itching, bronchoconstriction, and sedation.
- Stimulation of $H_2$ receptor causes release of gastric acid from parietal cells of the stomach.
- Histamine is an important mediator of *mild* allergic reactions, but only a minor contributor to severe (anaphylactic) allergic reactions.
- There are two major classes of histamine receptor antagonists: $H_1$-receptor antagonists, which are used to treat mild allergic reactions, and $H_2$-receptor antagonists, which are used to treat gastric and duodenal ulcers (see Chapter 71).
- $H_1$-receptor antagonists relieve allergic symptoms by blocking histamine receptors on small blood vessels, capillaries, and sensory nerves. These drugs do *not* block release of histamine from mast cells and basophils.
- There are two major classes of $H_1$-receptor antagonists, known as first-generation $H_1$-receptor antagonists and second-generation $H_1$-receptor antagonists.
- First-generation $H_1$-receptor antagonists frequently cause sedation; second-generation agents do not.
- CNS depression from first-generation $H_1$-receptor antagonists can be intensified by alcohol and other drugs with CNS-depressant actions.
- When present at high levels, *terfenadine* and *astemizole* can cause potentially fatal dysrhythmias.
- Blood levels of terfenadine and astemizole, and hence the risk of dysrhythmias, can be increased by overdose, significant liver dysfunction, and concurrent use of nefazodone, erythromycin, clarithromycin, ketoconazole, or itraconazole.

## Summary of Major Nursing Implications*

## $H_1$-Receptor Antagonists

### Preadministration Assessment

#### Therapeutic Goal

*Oral Therapy.* Relief of symptoms of mild to moderate allergic disorders (e.g., seasonal rhinitis, allergic conjunctivitis, uncomplicated urticaria and angioedema).

*Parenteral Therapy.* Treatment of allergic reactions to blood or plasma; adjunctive therapy of anaphylaxis.

#### Identifying High-Risk Patients

Antihistamines are *contraindicated* during the *third trimester of pregnancy* and for *nursing mothers* and *newborns*. *Terfenadine* and *astemizole* are *contraindicated* for patients with *severe liver disease* and for patients taking *nefazodone, erythromycin, clarithromycin, itraconazole,* or *ketoconazole.*

Exercise *caution* when treating *young children, the elderly,* and *patients with conditions that may be aggravated by muscarinic blockade,* including *asthma, urinary retention, open-angle glaucoma, hypertension,* and *prostatic hypertrophy.*

Use *astemizole* and *terfenadine* with *caution* in patients with *cardiac disease*.

### Implementation: Administration

#### Routes

All $H_1$ blockers can be administered orally. Some can also be administered parenterally or by rectal suppository (see Table 63-3).

#### Administration

Advise the patient to take all antihistamines (except astemizole) with food if GI upset occurs.

Instruct the patient to take *astemizole* at least 1 hour before eating or 2 hours after.

Warn the patient not to crush or chew enteric-coated preparations.

### Ongoing Evaluation and Interventions

#### Minimizing Adverse Effects

*Sedation.* For most patients, an antihistamine in the alkylamine group (see Table 63-1) can provide effective $H_1$ blockade with minimal sedation. If sedation is unacceptable with these agents, a nonsedating antihistamine—

*Patient education information is highlighted in color.

*astemizole, cetirizine, fexofenadine, loratadine,* or *terfenadine*—can be used. With long-acting antihistamines, daytime sedation can be minimized by administering the entire daily dose in the evening. Caution the patient to avoid hazardous activities if sedation is significant.

**Anticholinergic Effects.** Advise the patient that dryness of the mouth and throat can be reduced by sucking on hard (sugarless) candy and by taking frequent sips of liquids. Other atropine-like responses (urinary hesitancy, tachycardia, constipation) are not usually problems. Second-generation antihistamines have minimal anticholinergic effects.

**Gastrointestinal Distress.** Advise the patient that GI disturbances (nausea, vomiting) can be minimized by taking antihistamines with meals.

**Cardiac Dysrhythmias.** *Astemizole* and *terfenadine* can cause potentially fatal cardiac dysrhythmias. Warn the patient not to exceed the prescribed dosage. Use with caution in patients with cardiac disease. Syncope has preceded dysrhythmias in some patients; if syncope occurs, discontinue astemizole and terfenadine and evaluate for potential dysrhythmias. The risk of dysrhythmias is increased by concurrent use of nefazodone, erythromycin, clarithromycin, itraconazole, or ketoconazole; accordingly, concurrent use of these agents is contraindicated. The risk of dysrhythmias is also increased by severe liver disease; do not give astemizole or terfenadine to these patients.

## Minimizing Adverse Interactions

**CNS Depressants.** *Alcohol* and *other CNS depressants* can intensify the depressant actions of the $H_1$ antagonists. Warn the patient against consumption of alcohol. Dosages of CNS depressants (e.g., barbiturates, benzodiazepines, opioids) may need to be reduced. Second-generation antihistamines have no CNS depressant effects and do not potentiate the actions of CNS depressants.

**Drugs That Increase the Risk of Dysrhythmias.** *Nefazodone, erythromycin, clarithromycin, itraconazole,* and *ketoconazole* increase the risk of serious dysrhythmias from astemizole or terfenadine. Concurrent use of these agents is contraindicated.

Drugs that prolong the QT interval (e.g., quinidine) and grapefruit juice, which inhibits metabolism of terfenadine and astemizole, may also increase the risk of toxicity.

## Management of Toxicity

There is no specific antidote for antihistamine overdose; treatment is directed at removing the drug and managing symptoms. To remove the drug, give an emetic and, after vomiting has occurred, give activated charcoal and a cathartic. Treat hyperthermia with ice packs or cooling sponge baths. Control convulsions with IV phenytoin.

# CHAPTER 64

# Aspirin-Like Drugs: Nonsteroidal Anti-inflammatory Drugs and Acetaminophen

**Nonsteroidal Anti-inflammatory Drugs**
    Aspirin
    Other NSAIDs That Inhibit Cyclooxygenase-1 and
       Cyclooxygenase-2
    NSAIDs That Selectively Inhibit Cyclooxygenase-2
**Acetaminophen**

The family of aspirin-like drugs consists of aspirin itself and a large number of related agents. Most of these drugs can produce three clinically useful effects: (1) suppression of inflammation, (2) relief of pain, and (3) reduction of fever. As discussed below, all three responses are produced through one central mechanism: inhibition of cyclooxygenase, the enzyme responsible for synthesis of prostaglandins. This same mechanism underlies the principal adverse effects of these drugs: (1) gastric ulceration, (2) suppression of platelet aggregation, and (3) induction of acute renal failure. Because of their pronounced anti-inflammatory actions, the aspirin-like drugs are commonly referred to as *nonsteroidal anti-inflammatory drugs* (NSAIDs) to distinguish them from cortisone and other steroids used to treat inflammatory disorders. Because of their ability to relieve pain, these drugs are also known as *nonopioid analgesics* (to distinguish them from morphine and other opioid analgesics).

The aspirin-like drugs fall into two major categories: (1) agents that possess anti-inflammatory properties (NSAIDs) and (2) agents that lack anti-inflammatory properties. With the exception of acetaminophen, all of the aspirin-like drugs suppress inflammation, and hence belong to the NSAID category.

## Nonsteroidal Anti-inflammatory Drugs

The NSAIDs are a large and commonly prescribed family of drugs. These agents are a mainstay of treatment for inflammatory disorders (e.g., rheumatoid arthritis) and are used widely to relieve mild to moderate pain, suppress fever, and relieve symptoms of primary dysmenorrhea. All of the NSAIDs in current use pose a risk of gastric ulceration, bleeding, and acute renal failure. However, new drugs that can suppress inflammation without causing these serious adverse effects will soon be available. Aspirin, the oldest member of the NSAID family, will serve as our prototype for the group.

### Aspirin

Aspirin is an important drug whose effectiveness is frequently underappreciated. Given that aspirin is available without prescription, widely advertised in the media, and used somewhat casually by the general public, you may be surprised to hear that aspirin is a highly valuable and effective medication. The drug provides excellent relief of mild to moderate pain, reduces fever, and has been the initial drug of choice for rheumatoid arthritis and other inflammatory disorders. You may also be surprised to hear that aspirin can cause serious toxicity (e.g., gastric ulceration). Despite the introduction of many new NSAIDs, aspirin remains the most widely prescribed member of the group, and is the standard against which the others must be compared.

#### Chemistry

Aspirin belongs to a chemical family known as *salicylates*. All members of this group are derivatives of salicylic acid (Fig. 64–1). Aspirin is produced by substituting an acetyl group onto salicylic acid. Because of this acetyl group, aspirin is commonly known as *acetylsalicylic acid*, or simply ASA.

#### Mechanism of Action

Although aspirin has been in use since 1899, it was not until 1970 that its mechanism of action began to be revealed. It is now clear that most of the therapeutic and

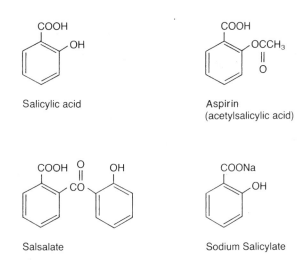

**Figure 64–1. Structural formulas of aspirin and related salicylates.**

adverse effects of aspirin result from *inhibition of cyclooxygenase*, an enzyme required for biosynthesis of *prostaglandins* and related metabolites of arachidonic acid (i.e., prostacyclin and thromboxane $A_2$).

Prostaglandins and other metabolites of arachidonic acid produce a wide variety of biologic effects. These agents mediate inflammatory responses, increase the responsiveness of pain receptors, and cause fever. In the stomach, prostaglandins serve three functions: they suppress output of gastric acid, promote secretion of cytoprotective mucus and bicarbonate, and support normal submucosal blood flow. In platelets, thromboxane $A_2$ stimulates aggregation. In the kidney, prostaglandins promote vasodilation, thereby increasing renal blood flow. In the uterus, prostaglandins promote contraction at term.

By inhibiting synthesis of prostaglandins and thromboxane $A_2$, aspirin can produce beneficial effects and undesired effects. The principal benefits that derive from inhibiting cyclooxygenase are (1) suppression of inflammation, (2) relief of pain, and (3) reduction of fever. By decreasing prostaglandin synthesis in the stomach, aspirin increases gastric acidity, reduces secretion of cytoprotective mucus and bicarbonate, and reduces submucosal blood flow; this combination of effects can lead to gastric ulceration. Inhibition of thromboxane $A_2$ synthesis suppresses platelet aggregation, an effect that can be both beneficial and harmful: reduced platelet aggregation can help prevent myocardial infarction but can also promote bleeding. By decreasing prostaglandin synthesis in the kidney, aspirin can reduce renal blood flow, which in turn can lead to acute renal failure. By decreasing uterine production of prostaglandins, aspirin can prolong gestation and suppress contractions during labor.

Recently, researchers have discovered that cyclooxygenase has two forms, which they named *cyclooxygenase-1* (COX-1) and *cyclooxygenase-2* (COX-2). COX-1 is found in practically all cells. In contrast, COX-2 is found only in cells that promote inflammatory and immune responses.

Aspirin and all other NSAIDs currently available inhibit both COX-1 and COX-2. Inhibition of COX-1 is responsible for the major adverse effects of these drugs—namely, gastric ulceration, bleeding tendencies, and disruption of kidney function. Inhibition of COX-1 may also underlie two beneficial effects: reduction of pain and fever. Inhibition of COX-2, on the other hand, is responsible for decreasing inflammation, the principal beneficial effect of the NSAIDs. Because traditional NSAIDs cannot inhibit COX-2 without also inhibiting COX-1, these drugs cannot suppress inflammation without posing a risk of serious adverse effects.

It is important to note that aspirin is an *irreversible* inhibitor of cyclooxygenase. This contrasts with all other NSAIDs, which are reversible (competitive) inhibitors. Because inhibition of cyclooxygenase by aspirin is irreversible, the drug's duration of action depends on how quickly tissues synthesize new enzyme. With other NSAIDs, effects decline as soon as drug levels fall.

## Pharmacokinetics

*Absorption.* Aspirin is absorbed rapidly and completely following oral administration. The principal site of absorption is the small intestine. When administered by rectal suppository, aspirin is absorbed slowly and blood levels are lower than with oral therapy.

*Metabolism.* Aspirin has a very short half-life (15 to 20 minutes) because of rapid conversion to salicylic acid, an active metabolite. The rate of salicylic acid inactivation depends on the amount present: at *low* therapeutic levels, salicylic acid has a half-life of approximately 2 hours; at *high* therapeutic levels, the half-life may exceed 20 hours.

*Distribution.* Salicylic acid is extensively bound to plasma albumin. At therapeutic levels, binding is between 80% and 90%. Aspirin undergoes distribution to all body tissues and fluids, including breast milk, fetal tissues, and the central nervous system (CNS).

*Excretion.* Salicylic acid and its metabolites are excreted by the kidneys. Excretion of salicylic acid is highly dependent on urinary pH. Accordingly, by raising the pH of urine from 6 to 8, we can increase the excretion of salicylic acid by a factor of 4.

*Plasma Drug Levels.* Low therapeutic doses of aspirin produce plasma salicylate levels in the range of 100 μg/ml. Anti-inflammatory doses produce salicylate levels of about 400 μg/ml. Signs of salicylism (toxicity) begin to appear when plasma salicylate levels exceed 200 μg/ml. Severe toxicity occurs at levels above 400 μg/ml.

## Therapeutic Uses

*Suppression of Inflammation.* Aspirin is an initial drug of choice for rheumatoid arthritis, osteoarthritis, and juvenile arthritis. Aspirin is also indicated for other inflammatory disorders (e.g., rheumatic fever, tendinitis, bursitis). The dosages employed to suppress inflammation are considerably larger than those employed for analgesia or reduction of fever. The use of aspirin and other NSAIDs to treat arthritis is discussed further in Chapter 66.

The precise mechanisms by which aspirin decreases inflammation have not been established. We do know that prostaglandins contribute to several (but not all) components of the inflammatory process. Hence, inhibition of prostaglandin synthesis provides a partial explanation of aspirin's anti-inflammatory effects. Other possible mechanisms include modulation of T-cell function, suppression of inflammatory cell infiltration, and stabilization of lysosomes.

**Analgesia.** Aspirin is our most widely used medication for relieving mild to moderate pain. Just how much analgesia is produced depends on the type of pain. Aspirin is most active against joint pain, muscle pain, and headache. For some forms of postoperative pain, aspirin can be more effective than opioids. However, aspirin is relatively inactive against severe pain of visceral origin. In contrast to the opioid analgesics, aspirin produces neither tolerance nor physical dependence. In addition, aspirin is safer than the opioids.

Aspirin relieves pain primarily by actions in the periphery. At sites of injury, prostaglandins act to sensitize pain receptors to mechanical and chemical stimulation. Aspirin reduces pain by inhibiting synthesis of these prostaglandins. In addition to this peripheral mechanism, aspirin has actions in the CNS that contribute to pain relief.

**Reduction of Fever.** Aspirin is the drug of choice for reducing temperature in febrile individuals. However, because of the risk of Reye's syndrome (see below), *aspirin should not be used to treat fever in children suspected of having chickenpox or influenza*. Although aspirin readily reduces fever, the drug will not lower normal body temperature, nor will it lower temperature that has become elevated in response to physical activity or a rise in external temperature.

How does aspirin reduce fever? Body temperature is regulated by the hypothalamus, which maintains a balance between heat production and heat loss. Fever occurs when the set point of the hypothalamus becomes elevated, causing the hypothalamus to increase heat production and decrease in heat loss. Set-point elevation is triggered by local synthesis of prostaglandins in response to endogenous pyrogens (fever-promoting substances). Aspirin lowers the set point by inhibiting pyrogen-induced synthesis of prostaglandins.

**Dysmenorrhea.** Aspirin can provide relief from primary dysmenorrhea. Benefits derive from inhibiting prostaglandin synthesis in uterine smooth muscle. (Prostaglandins promote uterine contraction; hence, suppression of prostaglandin synthesis relieves cramping.) Some of the newer aspirin-like drugs (e.g., ibuprofen, naproxen) are superior to aspirin for relieving dysmenorrhea. The efficacy of the newer drugs is attributed to a greater ability to inhibit uterine cyclooxygenase.

**Suppression of Platelet Aggregation.** As noted above, synthesis of thromboxane $A_2$ by platelets promotes aggregation. Aspirin suppresses platelet aggregation by causing *irreversible* inhibition of platelet cyclooxygenase, the enzyme required for production of thromboxane $A_2$. Since platelets lack the machinery to synthesize new cyclooxygenase, the effects of a single dose of aspirin persist for the life of the platelet (about 8 days). When administered in low doses (e.g., 160 mg/day) following myocardial infarction (MI), aspirin decreases the risk of reinfarction and death. Aspirin also decreases the risk of acute MI in patients with unstable angina pectoris. In addition, it can decrease the risk of thrombotic stroke in patients with a history of transient ischemic attacks. Antiplatelet effects of aspirin are discussed further in Chapter 50.

**Prevention of Colorectal Cancer.** There is a growing body of evidence that regular use of aspirin decreases the risk of colorectal cancer. This disease kills 55,000 Americans each year and is second only to lung cancer as the leading cause of cancer deaths. Although the protective dosage of aspirin has not been determined, the minimum appears to be 2 or 3 tablets a week. Benefits are not apparent until years of use. The mechanism underlying protection is unknown. One theory is that aspirin stops the growth of precancerous polyps.

Who should take aspirin for prophylaxis? One authority recommends that people at risk for colorectal cancer take 1 aspirin tablet (325 mg) every other day (assuming there is no contraindication to using the drug). Individuals at risk include patients with inflammatory bowel disease; those with previous large-bowel cancer; those with breast, ovarian, or endometrial cancer; and those with a family history of colorectal cancer.

## Adverse Effects

When administered in analgesic or antipyretic (fever-reducing) doses, aspirin rarely causes serious adverse effects. However, significant toxicity is common at the higher doses required to treat inflammatory disorders.

**Gastrointestinal Effects.** The most common side effects of aspirin are gastric distress, heartburn, and nausea. These reactions can be reduced by taking aspirin with food or with a full glass of water.

*Occult gastrointestinal bleeding* occurs frequently. In most cases, the amount of blood lost each day is insignificant. However, with chronic aspirin use, cumulative blood loss can result in anemia.

Long-term high-dose therapy causes *gastric ulceration* in 25% of patients. The FDA estimates that aspirin-induced ulcers and their complications are responsible for 10,000 to 20,000 deaths annually. Ulcers result from (1) increased secretion of acid and pepsin, (2) decreased production of cytoprotective mucus and bicarbonate, (3) decreased submucosal blood flow, and (4) the direct irritant action of aspirin on the gastric mucosa. The first three effects occur secondary to inhibition of prostaglandin synthesis. Injury to the stomach is most likely with aspirin preparations that dissolve slowly: because of slow dissolution, particulate aspirin becomes entrapped in folds of the stomach wall, causing prolonged exposure to high concentrations of the drug. Because aspirin-induced ulcers are often asymptomatic, perforation and upper GI hemorrhage can occur without premonitory signs. (Hemorrhage is due in part to erosion of the stomach wall and in part to suppression of platelet aggregation.) Factors that increase the risk of ulceration include (1) advanced age, (2) a history of peptic ulcer disease, (3) previous intolerance to aspirin or other NSAIDs, (4) cigarette smoking, and (5) a history of alcoholism. Because alcohol intensifies the irritant effects of aspirin, alcohol should not be consumed during aspirin therapy.

Aspirin-induced ulcers can be managed by discontinuing aspirin and giving an antiulcer medication—usually an *H₂-receptor antagonist* (e.g., cimetidine, famotidine) or *sucralfate*. In some cases, it may be possible to continue aspirin therapy while treating the ulcer with *omeprazole*, a powerful suppressant of acid production. The pharmacology of sucralfate, omeprazole, and the $H_2$-receptor blockers is discussed in Chapter 71 (Drugs for Peptic Ulcer Disease).

The only drug approved for *prophylaxis* against aspirin-induced ulcers is *misoprostol*, a synthetic prostaglandin. Misoprostol helps prevent ulcers by (1) suppressing secretion of gastric acid, (2) promoting secretion of cytoprotective mucus and bicarbonate, and (3) maintaining normal submucosal blood flow. Because misoprostol can stimulate uterine contractions, the drug is absolutely contraindicated during pregnancy. The pharmacology of misoprostol is discussed in Chapter 71.

**Bleeding.** Aspirin can promote bleeding by suppressing platelet aggregation. After ingestion of just 2 aspirin tablets, bleeding time is doubled for approximately 1 week. (Recall that platelets are unable to replace aspirin-inactivated cyclooxygenase. Hence bleeding time is prolonged for the life of the platelet.) Because of its effects on platelets, *aspirin is contraindicated for patients with bleeding disorders* (e.g., hemophilia, vitamin K deficiency, hypoprothrombinemia). In order to minimize blood loss during elective surgery and parturition, aspirin should be discontinued at least 1 week prior to these procedures. Care must be exercised when aspirin is used in conjunction with anticoagulants.

**Renal Effects.** For most patients, the risk of aspirin-induced renal dysfunction is very low. However, among patients with predisposing risk factors—advanced age, pre-existing renal dysfunction, hypovolemia, hepatic cirrhosis, or congestive heart failure—the incidence of aspirin-induced renal failure may be as high as 20%, although a recent study suggests the risk may be much lower.

Aspirin impairs kidney function by inhibiting the synthesis of prostaglandins that cause renal vasodilation. The resultant vasoconstriction decreases renal blood flow, decreases glomerular filtration rate, and promotes renal ischemia. These effects can combine to cause acute renal failure. Fortunately, aspirin does not affect renal function in most patients. Why? Because under normal conditions prostaglandins do not participate in the regulation of renal blood flow. Rather, prostaglandins serve to maintain renal blood flow primarily in patients with the risk factors noted above.

Development of renal impairment is signaled by reduced urine output, weight gain despite use of diuretics, and a rapid rise in serum creatinine and blood urea nitrogen. If any of these signs is observed, aspirin should be withdrawn immediately. In most cases, kidney function then returns to baseline level.

The risk of renal impairment can be reduced by identifying high-risk patients and treating them with the smallest aspirin dosages possible.

**Salicylism.** Salicylism is a syndrome that begins to develop when aspirin levels climb just slightly above therapeutic. Overt signs include *tinnitus* (ringing in the ears), *sweating*, *headache*, and *dizziness*. Acid-base disturbance may occur also (see below). If salicylism develops, aspirin should be withheld until symptoms subside; therapy should then resume, but with a small reduction in dosage. In some cases, development of tinnitus can be used to adjust aspirin dosage: when tinnitus occurs, the maximum acceptable dose has been achieved. However, this guideline may be inappropriate for older patients, since they may fail to develop tinnitus even when aspirin levels become toxic.

Acid-base disturbance results from the effects of aspirin on respiration. When administered in high therapeutic doses, aspirin acts on the CNS to stimulate breathing. The resultant increased loss of $CO_2$ produces *respiratory alkalosis*. In response to alkalosis, the kidneys excrete increased amounts of bicarbonate. As a result, plasma pH returns to normal and a state of *compensated respiratory alkalosis* is produced.

**Reye's Syndrome.** This syndrome is a rare but serious illness of childhood that has a mortality rate of 20% to 30%. Epidemiologic data suggest a relationship between Reye's syndrome and use of aspirin by children who have influenza or chickenpox. However, a direct causal link has not been established. Because of the possible relationship between aspirin and development of Reye's syndrome, *it is recommended that aspirin (and other NSAIDs) be avoided by children and teenagers suspected of having influenza or chickenpox.*

### Adverse Effects Associated with Use during Pregnancy.
Aspirin poses risks to the pregnant patient and the developing fetus. Accordingly, the drug is classified in *FDA Pregnancy Category D: there is evidence of human fetal risk, but the potential benefits from use of the drug during pregnancy may outweigh the potential for harm.* The principal risks to pregnant women are (1) anemia (from GI blood loss), and (2) postpartum hemorrhage. In addition, by inhibiting prostaglandin synthesis, aspirin may suppress spontaneous uterine contractions, and may thereby prolong gestation and labor.

Aspirin crosses the placenta and may adversely affect the fetus. Since prostaglandins help keep the ductus arteriosus patent, inhibition of prostaglandin synthesis by aspirin may induce premature closure of the ductus arteriosus. Aspirin therapy has also been associated with low birth weight, stillbirth, intracranial hemorrhage in premature infants, and neonatal death.

**Hypersensitivity Reactions.** Hypersensitivity develops in about 0.3% of aspirin recipients. Reactions are most likely in adults who have certain predisposing conditions: asthma, hay fever, chronic urticaria, or nasal polyps. Hypersensitivity reactions are uncommon in children. The aspirin hypersensitivity reaction begins with profuse, watery rhinorrhea and may progress to generalized urticaria, bronchospasm, laryngeal edema, and shock. Despite its resemblance to severe anaphylaxis, this reaction is not allergic and is not mediated by the immune system. Since individuals who react to aspirin are also sensitive to most other NSAIDs, it is thought that hypersensitivity reactions are in some way related to inhibition of cyclooxygenase. However, it is not clear why the reaction is limited to those adults who have the predisposing conditions noted. As with severe anaphylactic reactions, *epinephrine* is the treatment of choice. Hypersensitivity to aspirin is a contraindication to using other drugs with aspirin-like properties.

## Summary of Precautions and Contraindications

Aspirin is contraindicated in patients with *peptic ulcer disease*, *bleeding disorders* (e.g., hemophilia, vitamin K deficiency, hypoprothrombinemia), and *hypersensitivity to aspirin itself or other NSAIDs*. In addition, the drug should be used with extreme caution by *pregnant women* and by *children who have chickenpox or influenza*. Caution should also be exercised when treating *elderly patients*, *patients who smoke cigarettes*, and *patients with congestive heart failure*, *hepatic cirrhosis*, *hypovolemia*, *renal dysfunction*, *asthma*, *hay fever*, *chronic urticaria*, *nasal polyps*, or a *history of alcoholism*. Aspirin should be withdrawn 1 week prior to elective surgery or the anticipated date of parturition.

## Drug Interactions

Because of its widespread use, aspirin has been reported to interact with many other medications. However, most of these interactions have little clinical significance. Significant interactions are discussed below.

*Warfarin.* The most important interactions of aspirin occur with warfarin, an oral anticoagulant. Because aspirin suppresses platelet function and can decrease prothrombin production, aspirin will intensify the anticoagulant effects of warfarin. Furthermore, since aspirin can initiate gastric bleeding, augmentation of anticoagulant effects can increase the risk of gastric hemorrhage. Accordingly, the combination of aspirin with warfarin must be used with great care.

*Glucocorticoids.* Like aspirin, glucocorticoids promote gastric ulceration. Accordingly, the risk of ulcers is greatly increased when these drugs are combined—as may happen when treating arthritis. To reduce the risk of gastric ulceration, patients can be given *misoprostol* for prophylaxis.

## Acute Poisoning

Aspirin overdosage is a common cause of poisoning. Although rarely fatal in adults, aspirin poisoning may prove lethal in children. The lethal dose for adults is 20 to 25 gm. In contrast, as little as 4 gm may be sufficient to kill a child.

*Signs and Symptoms.* Initially, aspirin overdosage produces a state of compensated respiratory alkalosis—the same state seen in mild salicylism. As poisoning progresses, respiratory excitation is replaced by respiratory depression. Acidosis, hyperthermia, sweating, and dehydration are prominent, and electrolyte imbalance is likely. Stupor and coma result from effects in the CNS. Death usually results from respiratory failure. The mechanisms that underlie these clinical manifestations are described below.

Many symptoms of aspirin overdosage occur secondary to uncoupling of oxidative phosphorylation, the process by which the energy released during the oxidation of carbohydrates, fats, and proteins is used to form ATP from ADP. When oxidative phosphorylation becomes uncoupled, energy from metabolism of carbohydrates and other nutrients can no longer be transferred to ATP and stored. The consequences of this uncoupling are threefold: (1) Production of $CO_2$ is increased (secondary to the increased rates of metabolism that take place in futile attempts to form needed ATP). (2) There is increased production of lactic and pyruvic acids (as by-products of increased metabolism). (3) Production of heat is increased because the energy that would normally be used to make ATP is released in the form of heat. Increased heat production is responsible for hyperthermia and dehydration, two of the more serious consequences of aspirin overdosage.

The acidosis that characterizes aspirin poisoning results from multiple causes. Respiratory acidosis occurs because $CO_2$ production is increased and because toxic levels of salicylate act on the CNS to decrease respiration, thereby allowing even more $CO_2$ to accumulate. Respiratory acidosis remains uncompensated because bicarbonate stores become depleted during the initial phase of poisoning. Superimposed on respiratory acidosis is true metabolic acidosis. Metabolic acidosis results from (1) the acidity of aspirin and its metabolites, (2) increased production of lactic and pyruvic acids, and (3) accumulation of acidic products of metabolism (e.g., sulfuric and phosphoric acids) because of aspirin-induced impairment of renal excretion.

Acidosis is intensified by the following cycle: (1) Because of the pH partitioning effect, acidosis promotes penetration of salicylate into the CNS. (2) Increased entry of salicylate deepens respiratory depression. (3) Deepening of respiratory depression increases accumulation of $CO_2$, thereby increasing acidosis. (4) Increasing acidosis causes even more salicylate to enter the CNS, producing even further deepening of respiratory depression. This cycle continues until respiration ceases.

*Treatment.* Aspirin poisoning is an acute medical emergency that requires hospitalization. The immediate threats to life are respiratory depression, hyperthermia, dehydration, and acidosis. Treatment is largely symptomatic. If respiration is inadequate, mechanical ventilation should be instituted. External cooling (e.g., sponging with tepid water) can help reduce hyperthermia. Intravenous fluids are administered to correct dehydration; the composition of these fluids is determined by electrolyte and acid-base status. Slow infusion of bicarbonate is given to reverse acidosis. Several measures (induction of emesis, gastric lavage, administration of activated charcoal) can reduce further gastrointestinal absorption of aspirin. Alkalinization of the urine with bicarbonate accelerates excretion of aspirin and salicylate. If necessary, hemodialysis or peritoneal dialysis can be used to remove salicylates from the body.

## Formulations

Aspirin is available in several formulations, including plain and buffered tablets, enteric-coated preparations, and tablets used to produce a buffered solution. These different formulations reflect efforts to increase rates of absorption and decrease gastric irritation. For the most part, the clinical utility of the more complex formulations is no greater than that of plain aspirin tablets.

**Aspirin Tablets (Plain).** All brands are essentially the same with respect to analgesic efficacy, time of onset, and duration of action. Some of the less expensive tablets have greater particle size, which results in slower dissolution and prolonged contact with the gastric mucosa. These effects can augment gastric irritation. Over time, aspirin in tablets decomposes and emits an odor of vinegar (acetic acid); these tablets should be discarded.

**Aspirin Tablets (Buffered).** The amount of buffer in buffered aspirin tablets is too small to produce significant elevation of gastric pH. An equivalent effect on pH can be achieved by taking plain aspirin tablets with a glass of water or with food. Buffered aspirin tablets are no different from plain tablets with respect to analgesic effects and incidence of gastric distress. Buffered tablets may dissolve faster than plain tablets, resulting in a somewhat faster onset of action.

**Buffered Aspirin Solution.** A buffered aspirin solution is produced by dissolving effervescent aspirin tablets [Alka-Seltzer] in a glass of water. This solution has considerable buffering capacity due to its high content of sodium bicarbonate. Effects on gastric pH are sufficient to decrease the incidence of gastric irritation and bleeding. In addition, absorption is accelerated and peak blood levels are increased. Unfortunately, these benefits do not come without a price. The sodium content of buffered aspirin solution can be detrimental to individuals on a sodium-restricted diet. Also, absorption of bicarbonate can result in elevation of urinary pH, an effect that will accelerate aspirin excretion. Lastly, this highly buffered preparation is expensive. Because of this combination of benefits and drawbacks, the buffered aspirin solution is well suited for occasional use but is generally inappropriate for long-term therapy.

**Enteric-Coated Preparations.** Enteric-coated preparations dissolve in the intestine rather than the stomach, thereby reducing gastric irritation. Unfortunately, absorption from these formulations can be delayed and erratic. Patients should be advised not to crush or chew them.

**Timed-Release Tablets.** Timed-release tablets offer no advantage over plain aspirin tablets. Since the half-life of salicylic acid is long to begin with, and since aspirin produces irreversible inhibition of cyclooxygenase, timed-release tablets cannot increase duration of action.

**Rectal Suppositories.** Rectal suppositories have been employed for patients who cannot take aspirin orally. Absorption can be variable, resulting in plasma drug levels that are insufficient in some patients and excessive in others. Also, rectal irritation can occur. Because of these undesirable properties, aspirin suppositories are not generally recommended.

### Dosage and Administration

Aspirin is almost always administered by mouth. Gastric irritation can be minimized by administering aspirin with a glass of water or with food. Dosage depends on the age of the patient and the condition being treated. Adult and pediatric dosages for major indications are summarized in Table 64-1.

## Other NSAIDs That Inhibit Cyclooxygenase-1 and Cyclooxygenase-2

In attempts to produce an aspirin-like drug with fewer gastrointestinal and hemorrhagic effects than aspirin, the pharmaceutical industry has produced a large number of drugs with actions very similar to those of aspirin. In the United States, over 20 NSAIDs are now available (Table 64-2). Like aspirin, all of the traditional NSAIDs are nonselective inhibitors of cyclooxygenase. That is, they inhibit both COX-1 and COX-2. However, in contrast to aspirin, which cause *irreversible* inhibition of cyclooxygenase, other NSAIDs cause *reversible* inhibition. All of these drugs display anti-inflammatory, analgesic, and antipyretic properties. In addition, they all can promote gastric ulceration, bleeding, and renal failure—although the intensity of these effects may be less with some NSAIDs than with others. Patients who are hypersensitive to aspirin are likely to experience cross-hypersensitivity with the newer aspirin-like drugs. For most of the NSAIDs, safety during pregnancy has not been established; hence their use by pregnant women is not recommended.

The principal indications for the nonaspirin NSAIDs are rheumatoid arthritis and other inflammatory disorders. In addition, certain NSAIDs are used to treat fever, bursitis,

| TABLE 64-1. ASPIRIN DOSAGE | | |
|---|---|---|
| **Indication** | **Adult Dosage** | **Pediatric Dosage** |
| Aches and pains; fever | 325-650 mg every 4 hr | 2-3 years old: 160 mg<br>4-5 years old: 240 mg<br>6-8 years old: 325 mg<br>9-10 years old: 405 mg<br>11 years old: 485 mg<br>Over 11 years old: 650 mg<br>*All of the above doses are administered every 4 hr* |
| Acute rheumatic fever | 5-8 gm/day in divided doses | 100 mg/kg/day (initially) then 75 mg/kg/day for 4 to 6 wk |
| Rheumatoid arthritis | 3.6-5.4 gm/day in divided doses | 90-130 mg/kg/day in divided doses at 4- to 6-hr intervals |
| Postmyocardial infarction | 160 mg/day | |
| Prevention of transient ischemic attacks (in men) | 650 mg 2 times a day or 325 mg 4 times a day | |

tendinitis, mild to moderate pain, and primary dysmenorrhea (see Table 64–2).

Although individual NSAIDs differ from one another chemically, pharmacokinetically, and to some extent pharmacodynamically, all of these drugs are very similar clinically: they all produce essentially equivalent antirheumatic effects and they all present an essentially equal risk of serious adverse effects (gastric ulceration and renal failure). However, for reasons that are not understood, individual patients may respond better to one

## TABLE 64–2. CLINICAL PHARMACOLOGY OF THE NONSTEROIDAL ANTI-INFLAMMATORY DRUGS

| Generic Name [Trade Name] | Maximum Daily Dosage (mg) | Plasma Half-Life (hr) | Major Indications | | | | |
|---|---|---|---|---|---|---|---|
| | | | Rheumatoid Arthritis | Moderate Pain | Fever | Primary Dysmenorrhea | Bursitis/ Tendinitis |
| *Salicylates* | | | | | | | |
| Aspirin (many trade names) | 8000 | 0.2–0.3 | A | A | A | | |
| Choline salicylate [Arthropan] | 5200 | 2–30* | A | A | A | | |
| Magnesium salicylate [Magan] | 4800 | 2–30* | A | A | A | | |
| Sodium salicylate (generic) | 3900 | 2–30* | A | A | A | | |
| Salsalate [Disalcid, Mono-Gesic] | 3000 | 2–30* | A | A | A | | |
| *Propionic Acid Derivatives* | | | | | | | |
| Fenoprofen [Nalfon] | 3200 | 2–3 | A | A | | | |
| Flurbiprofen [Ansaid] | 300 | 2.6–5 | A | I | I | I | I |
| Ibuprofen [Motrin, Advil, others] | 3200 | 1.8–2.5 | A | A | A | A | |
| Ketoprofen [Orudis, others] | 300 | 1.4–2.2 | A | A | A | A | |
| Naproxen [Naprosyn] | 1500 | 12–16 | A | A | A | A | A |
| Naproxen sodium [Anaprox, Aleve] | 1375 | 12–13 | A | A | A | A | A |
| Oxaprozin [Daypro] | 1800 | 50–60 | A | | | | |
| *Other NSAIDs* | | | | | | | |
| Diclofenac [Voltaren, Cataflam] | 200 | 0.9–1.3 | A | I | | | |
| Diflunisal [Dolobid] | 1500 | 11–15 | A | A | | | |
| Etodolac [Lodine] | 1200 | 3–6 | I | A | | | I |
| Indomethacin [Indocin] | 200 | 3.9–5.3 | A | | | | A |
| Ketorolac [Toradol] | 40 | 2.4–8.6 | | A | | | |
| Meclofenamate [Meclomen] | 400 | 2–3 | A | A | | | |
| Mefenamic acid [Ponstel] | 1000 | 2–4 | | A | | A | |
| Nabumetone [Relafen] | 2000 | 21–31 | A | | | | |
| Piroxicam [Feldene] | 20 | 35–79 | A | | | I | |
| Sulindac [Clinoril] | 400 | 6–22 | A | | | | A |
| Tolmetin [Tolectin] | 2000 | 0.7–1.3 | A | | | | |

A = FDA approved indication; I = investigational use.
*Half-life increases with increasing dosage.

NSAID than to another. Furthermore, individual patients may tolerate one NSAID better than another. Therefore, in order to optimize therapy for the individual patient, therapeutic trials with more than one NSAID may be needed.

### Nonacetylated Salicylates: Choline Salicylate, Magnesium Salicylate, Sodium Salicylate, and Salsalate

***Similarities to Aspirin.*** The nonacetylated salicylates are similar to aspirin (an acetylated salicylate) in most respects. Like aspirin, these drugs inhibit prostaglandin synthesis and are employed to treat arthritis, moderate pain, and fever. The most common adverse effects are gastrointestinal disturbances. As with aspirin, these drugs should not be given to children with chickenpox or influenza, because of the possibility of precipitating Reye's syndrome.

***Contrasts with Aspirin.*** In contrast to aspirin, the nonacetylated salicylates cause little or no suppression of platelet aggregation. Accordingly, these drugs are preferred to aspirin for use by surgical patients and by patients with bleeding disorders.

Because of its sodium content, *sodium salicylate* should be avoided by patients on a sodium-restricted diet (e.g., patients with hypertension or congestive heart failure).

*Magnesium salicylate* may accumulate to toxic levels in patients with chronic renal insufficiency. Accordingly, magnesium salicylate should be avoided by these people.

*Salsalate* is a prodrug that breaks down to release two molecules of salicylate in the alkaline environment of the small intestine. Because the stomach is not exposed to salicylate, salsalate produces less gastric irritation than aspirin.

Like salsalate, *choline salicylate* causes less gastric irritation than aspirin.

***Preparations, Dosage, and Administration.*** *Choline salicylate* [Arthropan] is dispensed in solution (870 mg/5 ml) for oral use. The usual dosage is 870 mg every 3 to 4 hours.

*Magnesium salicylate* [Magan, others] is dispensed in caplets (325 and 500 mg) and tablets (545 and 600 mg) for oral administration. The usual dosage is 650 mg every 4 hours or 1090 mg every 8 hours. The maximum dosage is 4800 mg/day administered in three or four doses.

*Sodium salicylate* (generic) is dispensed in enteric-coated tablets (325 and 650 mg) for oral use. The usual dosage is 325 to 650 mg every 4 hours.

*Salsalate* [Disalcid, Mono-Gesic, others] is dispensed in capsules (500 mg) and tablets (500 and 750 mg) for oral use. The usual dosage is 3000 mg/day in divided doses.

### Ibuprofen

Ibuprofen [Advil, Motrin, others] is the prototype of the propionic acid derivatives. Other members of the family are listed in Table 64–2, and discussed individually below. Like aspirin, ibuprofen inhibits prostaglandin synthesis and has anti-inflammatory, analgesic, and antipyretic actions. The drug is used to treat fever, mild to moderate pain, and arthritis. In addition, ibuprofen appears superior to most other NSAIDs for relief of primary dysmenorrhea. This property has been attributed to unusually effective inhibition of prostaglandin synthesis in uterine smooth muscle.

The incidence of adverse effects is low, and ibuprofen is generally well tolerated. The drug produces less gastric bleeding than aspirin and causes less inhibition of platelet aggregation. Consequently, ibuprofen is one of the safer NSAIDs for use with anticoagulants.

Ibuprofen is available in four formulations: (1) standard tablets (100 to 800 mg), (2) chewable tablets (50 and 100 mg), (2) a 20-mg/ml oral suspension [Children's Advil, Children's Motrin], and (4) 40-mg/ml oral drops [Children's Motrin]. The dosage for

arthritis ranges from 1.2 to 3.2 gm/day administered in three or four divided doses. The dosage for primary dysmenorrhea is 400 mg every 4 hours. Administration with meals or milk can reduce gastric distress.

### Fenoprofen

Fenoprofen [Nalfon] belongs to the propionic acid family of NSAIDs. Like other NSAIDs, the drug inhibits synthesis of prostaglandins, thereby causing anti-inflammatory, analgesic, and antipyretic effects. Fenoprofen is indicated for arthritis and mild to moderate pain. The most common adverse effects are gastrointestinal disturbances. Fenoprofen is dispensed in capsules (200 and 300 mg) and tablets (600 mg) for oral use. The usual dosage for rheumatoid arthritis is 300 to 600 mg 3 or 4 times a day. The maximum daily dosage is 3.2 gm.

### Flurbiprofen

Flurbiprofen [Ansaid] is chemically related to ibuprofen and the other derivatives of propionic acid. The drug is approved for treating arthritis and has been used on an investigational basis to treat bursitis, tendinitis, moderate pain, fever, and primary dysmenorrhea. The most common adverse effects are gastrointestinal disturbances (dyspepsia, nausea, diarrhea, abdominal pain). The risk of serious gastrointestinal effects (ulceration, perforation, hemorrhage) may be greater than with ibuprofen. Like other NSAIDs, flurbiprofen can exacerbate renal impairment. The drug is dispensed in tablets (50 and 100 mg) for oral administration. The usual dosage for rheumatoid arthritis is 200 to 300 mg/day administered in two to four divided doses.

### Ketoprofen

Ketoprofen [Orudis, Oruvail, Actron Caplets] belongs to the propionic acid family of NSAIDs. The drug inhibits synthesis of prostaglandins and has anti-inflammatory, analgesic, and antipyretic effects. Indications are rheumatoid arthritis, mild to moderate pain, and primary dysmenorrhea. The most common adverse effects are dyspepsia (11.5%), nausea, vomiting, and abdominal pain. Ketoprofen is dispensed in standard capsules (12.5, 25, 50, and 75 mg) and extended-release capsules (100, 150, and 200 mg). The usual dosage for rheumatoid arthritis is 150 to 300 mg/day administered in three or four divided doses. The dosage for moderate pain or primary dysmenorrhea is 25 to 50 mg every 6 to 8 hours.

### Naproxen and Naproxen Sodium

***Actions and Uses.*** Naproxen [Naprosyn, others] and naproxen sodium [Aleve, Anaprox, others] belong to the propionic acid family of NSAIDs. Because these drugs have prolonged half-lives (see Table 64–2), they needn't be administered as frequently as the other propionic acid derivatives (e.g., ibuprofen). Naproxen and naproxen sodium are approved for treating arthritis, bursitis, tendinitis, primary dysmenorrhea, and mild to moderate pain. In addition, they are used investigationally to reduce fever. Like other NSAIDs, they act primarily by inhibiting synthesis of prostaglandins.

***Adverse Effects.*** Naproxen and naproxen sodium are among the better tolerated NSAIDs. The most common adverse effects are gastrointestinal disturbances. Like other NSAIDs, these drugs can compromise renal function by decreasing renal blood flow. Bleeding time can be prolonged secondary to reversible inhibition of platelet aggregation.

***Preparations, Dosage, and Administration.*** *Naproxen* is dispensed in standard tablets (250, 375, and 500 mg), 375- and 500-mg delayed release enteric-coated tablets [EC Naprosyn], 375- and 500-mg controlled-release tablets [Naprelan], and as an oral suspension (25 mg/ml). The usual dosage for rheumatoid arthritis is 250 to 500 mg twice daily. The dosage for mild to moderate pain is 500 mg initially followed by 250 mg every 6 to 8 hours.

*Naproxen sodium* is dispensed in tablets (220, 275, and 550 mg) for oral use. The usual dosage for rheumatoid arthritis is 275 to 550 mg twice daily. The dosage for mild to moderate pain is 550 mg initially followed by 275 mg every 6 to 8 hours.

### Diclofenac

Diclofenac [Voltaren, Cataflam] is approved for rheumatoid arthritis, osteoarthritis, ankylosing spondylitis, and primary dysmenorrhea. Like other NSAIDs, diclofenac produces its anti-inflammatory, analgesic, and antipyretic effects by inhibiting the synthesis of prostaglandins.

Diclofenac is well absorbed following oral administration, but undergoes extensive (40% to 50%) metabolism on its first pass through the liver. In blood, about 99.5% of the drug is protein bound, primarily to albumin. Diclofenac is metabolized by the liver and excreted in the urine.

The most common adverse effects are abdominal pain, dyspepsia, and nausea. Diclofenac can cause fluid retention, and this can exacerbate hypertension and congestive heart failure. The risk of liver dysfunction is greater than with other NSAIDs. Accordingly, patients should receive periodic tests of liver function, and should be instructed to report manifestations of liver injury (e.g., jaundice, fatigue, nausea).

Diclofenac is dispensed in standard tablets (50 mg) and enteric-coated delayed-release tablets (25, 50, and 75 mg) for oral administration. The dosage for rheumatoid arthritis is 150 to 200 mg/day administered in two or three divided doses. The dosage for osteoarthritis is 100 to 150 mg/day administered in two or three divided doses.

### Diflunisal

Diflunisal [Dolobid] is a derivative of salicylic acid. However, unlike the salicylates, diflunisal is not converted to salicylic acid in the body. The drug is indicated for mild to moderate pain and rheumatoid arthritis. Like other NSAIDs, the drug inhibits prostaglandin synthesis and can cause gastrointestinal disturbances, suppression of platelet aggregation, and impairment of kidney function. Diflunisal has a prolonged half-life (11 to 15 hours), which allows the drug to be administered only 2 or 3 times a day. Diflunisal is dispensed in tablets (250 and 500 mg) for oral use. For treatment of arthritis and mild to moderate pain, the initial dose is 500 to 1000 mg. Maintenance doses of 250 to 500 mg are administered every 8 to 12 hours.

### Etodolac

Etodolac [Lodine] is indicated for osteoarthritis and moderate pain. The drug has been used on an investigational basis to treat rheumatoid arthritis, bursitis, and tendinitis. Like other NSAIDs, etodolac produces many of its effects by suppressing the synthesis of prostaglandins. The drug's most common adverse effects are dyspepsia (10%), nausea, vomiting, diarrhea, and abdominal pain. Etodolac may cause less gastric ulceration and bleeding than other NSAIDs. The drug is dispensed in capsules (200 and 300 mg) for oral use. The recommended dosage for osteoarthritis is 800 to 1200 mg/day in divided doses. The dosage for moderate pain is 200 to 400 mg every 6 to 8 hours.

### Indomethacin

***Actions and Uses.*** Indomethacin [Indocin] is an effective anti-inflammatory agent approved for arthritis, bursitis, tendinitis, and, as discussed in Chapter 66, acute gouty arthritis. The drug can reduce pain and fever but is not routinely used for these effects (because of its potential for toxicity).

***Adverse Effects.*** Untoward effects are seen in 35% to 50% of those treated. About 20% of patients discontinue the drug. The most common adverse effect is severe frontal headache, which

occurs in 25% to 50% of recipients. Other CNS effects (dizziness, vertigo, confusion) are also common. Seizures and psychiatric changes (e.g., depression, psychosis) have occurred. Mild gastrointestinal reactions (nausea, vomiting, indigestion) are experienced by 3% to 9% of users. More severe GI effects (ulceration with perforation, hemorrhage) may also develop. Hematologic reactions (neutropenia, thrombocytopenia, aplastic anemia) have occurred but are rare. Indomethacin suppresses platelet aggregation.

***Precautions and Contraindications.*** Because of its adverse effects, indomethacin is contraindicated for infants and children under the age of 14, patients with peptic ulcer disease, and women who are pregnant or breast-feeding. Caution is required in patients with epilepsy and psychiatric disorders, in patients involved in hazardous activities, and in patients receiving anticoagulant therapy.

***Pharmacokinetics.*** Indomethacin is well absorbed following oral administration and distributes to all body fluids and tissues. The drug is metabolized in the liver. Metabolites and parent drug are excreted in the urine and feces.

***Preparations, Dosage, and Administration.*** Indomethacin [Indocin] is dispensed in standard capsules (25 and 50 mg), sustained-release capsules (75 mg), an oral suspension (5 mg/ml), and rectal suppositories (50 mg). For treatment of rheumatoid arthritis, the initial dosage is 25 mg 2 or 3 times a day. The maximum daily dosage is 200 mg. Gastrointestinal reactions can be reduced by administering indomethacin with meals. Dosages for gout are presented in Chapter 66.

### Ketorolac

***Actions and Uses.*** Ketorolac [Toradol] is a powerful analgesic with minimum anti-inflammatory actions. Pain relief is equivalent to that produced with morphine and other opioids. Although ketorolac lacks the serious adverse effects associated with opioids (respiratory depression, tolerance, dependence, abuse potential), it nonetheless has serious adverse effects of its own. Accordingly, use should be short term and restricted to managing acute pain of moderate to severe intensity. Ketorolac is not indicated for chronic therapy use or for treatment of minor aches and pains. The usual indication is postoperative pain, for which ketorolac is as effective as morphine. Therapy should begin with parenteral administration, followed by oral ketorolac if needed. Because of the risks associated with prolonged use, treatment (parenteral plus oral) should not exceed 5 days. Like other NSAIDs, ketorolac suppresses prostaglandin synthesis. This action is thought to underlie the drug's analgesic effects.

***Pharmacokinetics.*** Ketorolac is administered orally and parenterally (IM or IV). With parenteral administration, analgesia begins within 30 minutes, peaks in 1 to 2 hours, and persists 4 to 6 hours. The drug is eliminated by a combination of hepatic metabolism and urinary excretion. In young adults, ketorolac has a half-life of 4 to 6 hours. The half-life may be prolonged in the elderly and in patients with renal impairment.

***Adverse Effects and Contraindications.*** Ketorolac can cause all of the adverse effects associated with other NSAIDs, including peptic ulcers, GI bleeding or perforation, prolonged bleeding time, renal failure, hypersensitivity reactions, suppression of uterine contractions, and premature closure of the ductus arteriosus. Concurrent use with other NSAIDs increases the risk of these effects and is therefore contraindicated. Other contraindications include active peptic ulcer disease, history of peptic ulcer disease or recent GI bleeding, advanced renal impairment, confirmed or suspected intracranial bleeding, use prior to major surgery, history of NSAID hypersensitivity reactions, and use during labor and delivery.

***Preparations, Dosage, and Administration.*** Ketorolac [Toradol] is available in 10-mg tablets for oral administration and in preloaded syringes (15 and 30 mg/ml) for parenteral administration.

*Parenteral therapy* can be accomplished with a single injection or with multiple injections. When a single injection is used, the IM dose is 30 or 60 mg, and the IV dose is 15 or 30 mg. When multiple injections are given, the dosage (IM or IV) is 15 or 30 mg every 6 hours. In all cases, the smaller dosage option is employed for patients over 65 years old, patients with impaired kidney function, and patients who weigh less than 50 kg (110 pounds). Intravenous doses should be administered over 15 seconds or longer. Intramuscular injections should be done slowly and deep in the muscle. Treatment should not exceed 5 days.

*Oral ketorolac* is indicated only as a continuation of therapy with parenteral ketorolac. Initial oral doses are based on preceding parenteral doses. The usual oral maintenance dosage is 10 mg every 4 to 6 hours. Combined oral and parenteral treatment should not exceed 5 days.

## Mefenamic Acid

Mefenamic acid [Ponstel] is indicated for relief of primary dysmenorrhea and moderate pain. The principal adverse effect is diarrhea, which is sometimes severe. Mefenamic acid is dispensed in 250-mg capsules for oral administration. The dosage for primary dysmenorrhea is 500 mg initially followed by 250 mg every 6 hours. The drug should be administered with food or milk to reduce gastric distress. Duration of treatment is usually 2 to 3 days.

## Nabumetone

Nabumetone [Relafen] is a prodrug that undergoes conversion to its active form (6-MNA) in the liver. In contrast to other currently available NSAIDs, which are nonselective inhibitors of cyclooxygenase, 6-MNA inhibits COX-2 more than COX-1. Although nabumetone has antipyretic, analgesic, and anti-inflammatory properties, the drug is approved only for treatment of arthritis. Principal adverse effects are diarrhea (14%), abdominal cramps (13%), dyspepsia (12%), and nausea (3% to 9%). Nabumetone causes much less gastrointestinal ulceration than other NSAIDs, probably because it preferentially inhibits COX-2. Nabumetone is dispensed in 500- and 750-mg tablets for oral use. Treatment of rheumatoid arthritis is begun with a single dose of 1000 mg. After this, the daily dosage is 1500 to 2000 mg administered in one or two doses. Administration with food increases the rate of absorption.

## Piroxicam

Piroxicam [Feldene] has anti-inflammatory, analgesic, and antipyretic properties. However, the drug is approved only for treatment of arthritis. The most outstanding feature of piroxicam is its long half-life (about 50 hours). Because the drug is eliminated so slowly, therapeutic effects can be maintained with once-a-day dosing. In general, piroxicam is better tolerated than aspirin. Undesired effects are seen in 11% to 46% of those treated, and between 4% and 12% discontinue therapy. Gastrointestinal reactions are most common, occurring in about 20% of recipients. The incidence of gastric ulceration is about 1%. Like aspirin, piroxicam inhibits platelet aggregation and prolongs bleeding time. The drug is dispensed in 10- and 20-mg capsules for oral administration. The usual dosage is 20 mg once a day.

## Sulindac

Sulindac [Clinoril] is a prodrug that undergoes conversion to its active form within the body. The drug is approved for rheumatoid arthritis, tendinitis, bursitis, and acute gouty arthri-

tis. Principal adverse effects are abdominal distress, dyspepsia, nausea, vomiting, and diarrhea. Gastric ulceration is less common than with some other NSAIDs, perhaps because sulindac is not active as administered. Like other NSAIDs, sulindac causes reversible inhibition of platelet aggregation, prolongs bleeding time, and causes acute renal failure. The drug is dispensed in 150- and 200-mg tablets for oral administration. The usual dosage is 150 mg administered twice daily with meals. The maximum daily dosage is 400 mg.

## Tolmetin

Tolmetin [Tolectin] is used to treat arthritis and related inflammatory disorders. The drug has analgesic and antipyretic properties but is not employed for relief of fever or pain unrelated to inflammation. Adverse effects occur in 25% to 40% of those treated. Between 5% and 10% of patients discontinue the drug. Gastrointestinal effects (nausea, vomiting, indigestion) are most common. Gastric ulceration has occurred, but this reaction is less frequent than with aspirin. Nonetheless, caution should be exercised in patients with a history of peptic ulcer disease. Hypersensitivity reactions occur more frequently than with aspirin. Effects on the CNS (headache, dizziness, anxiety, drowsiness) are less severe and less frequent than with indomethacin. Unlike most other NSAIDs, tolmetin does not augment the effects of warfarin, an oral anticoagulant. The drug is dispensed in tablets (200 and 600 mg) and capsules (400 mg) for oral administration. For rheumatoid arthritis, the initial dosage is 400 mg 3 times a day. The maximum daily dosage is 2 gm. Gastrointestinal distress can be minimized by administering tolmetin with food.

# NSAIDs That Selectively Inhibit Cyclooxygenase-2

NSAIDs that produce selective inhibition of COX-2 are in clinical trials and should be available in a few years. The importance of these agents cannot be stated too strongly. Recall that NSAIDS reduce inflammation by inhibiting COX-2, and produce serious side effects (gastrointestinal ulceration, bleeding tendencies, kidney failure) by inhibiting COX-1. Because of their selectivity, the COX-2 inhibitors are able to suppress inflammation without causing gastrointestinal ulceration and the other dangerous side effects associated with inhibition of COX-1. For people with rheumatoid arthritis and other chronic inflammatory conditions, the COX-2 inhibitors represent a near-miraculous therapeutic advance. When drugs in this new generation of NSAIDs become available, they are certain to replace older NSAIDs for long-term therapy of inflammation.

***Celecoxib.*** Celecoxib, an investigational COX-2 inhibitor, is 300 times more selective for COX-2 than for COX-1. As a result, the drug can suppress inflammation while causing minimal side effects. Furthermore, because it does not decrease synthesis of protective prostaglandins, it can be given in higher doses than traditional NSAIDs, and can thereby produce more intense anti-inflammatory effects.

Celecoxib demonstrated the clinical potential of the COX-2 inhibitors in recently completed phase II trials. In patients with rheumatoid arthritis and osteoarthritis, celecoxib reduced pain and inflammation while producing

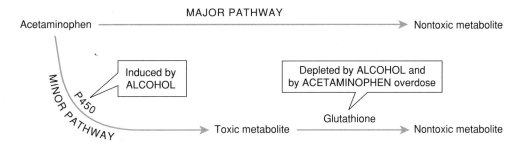

**Figure 64–2. Metabolism of acetaminophen.**

side effects similar to those of placebo. In healthy volunteers, gastrointestinal effects were like those of placebo and significantly less than those of naproxen, a nonselective cyclooxygenase inhibitor. Studies have also demonstrated that celecoxib does not inhibit platelet aggregation. From the foregoing, we can see that this selective COX-2 inhibitor offers all the anti-inflammatory benefits of traditional NSAIDs while being devoid of major side effects.

# Acetaminophen

Acetaminophen [Tylenol, others] is similar to aspirin in some respects but quite different in others. Acetaminophen has *analgesic* and *antipyretic* properties equivalent to those of aspirin. However, in contrast to aspirin and the other NSAIDs, *acetaminophen is devoid of clinically useful anti-inflammatory and antirheumatic actions*. In addition, acetaminophen does not suppress platelet aggregation, does not cause gastric ulceration, and does not decrease renal blood flow or cause renal failure. Furthermore, acetaminophen overdosage differs from overdosage with aspirin both in manifestations and treatment.

## Mechanism of Action

Differences between the effects of acetaminophen and aspirin are thought to result from selective inhibition of prostaglandin synthesis. Whereas aspirin can inhibit synthesis of prostaglandins in both the CNS and the periphery, inhibition by acetaminophen is limited to the CNS; acetaminophen has only minimal effects on prostaglandin synthesis at peripheral sites. By decreasing prostaglandin synthesis in the CNS, acetaminophen is able to reduce fever and pain. The inability of acetaminophen to inhibit prostaglandin synthesis outside the CNS may explain the absence of anti-inflammatory effects, gastric ulceration, and adverse effects on the kidneys and platelets.

## Pharmacokinetics

Acetaminophen is readily absorbed following oral administration and undergoes wide distribution. Most of an administered dose is metabolized by the liver, and the re-

sultant metabolites are excreted in the urine. The plasma half-life of the drug is approximately 2 hours.

Acetaminophen can be metabolized by two pathways; one is major and the other is minor (Fig. 64-2). In the major pathway, acetaminophen undergoes conjugation with glucuronic acid and other compounds to form nontoxic metabolites. In the minor pathway, acetaminophen is oxidized by a P-450–containing enzyme into a highly reactive and toxic compound. At therapeutic doses, practically all of the drug is converted to nontoxic compounds via the major pathway. Only a small fraction is converted into the toxic metabolite via the minor pathway. Under normal conditions, the toxic metabolite undergoes rapid conversion to a nontoxic form; glutathione is required for the conversion. When an overdose of acetaminophen is taken, a larger than normal amount is processed via the minor pathway; hence, a large quantity of the toxic metabolite is produced. As the liver attempts to detoxify the metabolite, glutathione is rapidly depleted, and further detoxification stops. As a result, the toxic metabolite accumulates, causing damage to the liver (see below).

## Adverse Effects

Adverse effects are rare at therapeutic doses. As noted above, acetaminophen does not cause gastric ulceration, does not inhibit platelet aggregation, and does not decrease renal blood flow or cause renal failure. In addition, there is no evidence linking acetaminophen with Reye's syndrome. Individuals who are hypersensitive to aspirin only rarely experience cross-hypersensitivity to acetaminophen. Overdosage can cause severe liver injury.

## Drug Interactions

***Alcohol.*** Regular alcohol consumption increases the risk of liver injury from acetaminophen. Three mechanisms are involved. First, alcohol induces synthesis of the P-450–containing enzyme in the minor pathway, thereby increasing production of the toxic metabolite (Fig. 64-2). Second, stores of glutathione are depleted in chronic alcoholics; as a result, the liver is unable to convert the toxic metabolite to a nontoxic form (Fig. 64-2). Third, chronic alcoholics often have pre-existing liver damage, which renders them less able to tolerate injury caused by acetaminophen.

There is some evidence that even moderate consumption of alcohol (2 to 4 drinks a day) can increase the risk of serious liver injury from *therapeutic* doses of acetaminophen. Accordingly, some authorities recommend that people who consume alcohol routinely take no more than 2 gm of acetaminophen a day (i.e., half the normally recommended maximum). To date, no liver damage has been reported at this reduced acetaminophen dosage.

## Therapeutic Uses

Acetaminophen is indicated for relief of pain and fever in patients who cannot tolerate the side effects of aspirin (e.g., patients with bleeding disorders or peptic ulcer disease). Because of its lack of association with Reye's syndrome, acetaminophen is preferred to aspirin for use by children suspected of having chickenpox or influenza. In addition, acetaminophen may be a safe alternative to aspirin for patients who have experienced aspirin hypersensitivity reactions. Because of its weak anti-inflammatory actions, acetaminophen is *not* useful for treating arthritis or rheumatic fever.

## Acute Toxicity

Overdose with acetaminophen causes liver damage. The risk of liver injury is increased by fasting and by chronic consumption of alcohol.

***Signs and Symptoms.*** The principal feature of acetaminophen overdose is *hepatic necrosis*. Severe poisoning can progress to hepatic failure, coma, and death. Early symptoms of poisoning (nausea, vomiting, diarrhea, sweating, abdominal discomfort) belie the severity of intoxication. It is not until 48 to 72 hours after drug ingestion that overt indications of hepatic injury appear.

***Treatment.*** Liver damage can be minimized by administering *acetylcysteine* [Mucomyst], a specific antidote to acetaminophen toxicity. Acetylcysteine reduces injury by substituting for depleted glutathione in the reaction that converts the toxic metabolite of acetaminophen to its nontoxic form. Although acetylcysteine is most effective when given shortly after acetaminophen ingestion, the drug can still provide significant protection when administered as long as 24 hours after poisoning has occurred. Acetylcysteine is dispensed in 10% and 20% solutions, and should be diluted to 5% with water, fruit juice, or a cola beverage. The initial dose is 140 mg/kg. Additional doses of 70 mg/kg are administered at 4-hour intervals for the next 72 hours. Acetylcysteine has an extremely unpleasant odor and may induce vomiting. If vomiting interferes with oral treatment, the drug can be administered through an oroduodenal tube.

### Preparations, Dosage, and Administration

Acetaminophen is dispensed in a variety of oral formulations (standard tablets, chewable tablets, effervescent granules, capsules, liquids, elixirs, solutions) and in rectal suppositories. The dosage for adults and children over 12 years is 325 to 650 mg every 4 to 6 hours. Doses for younger children vary with age, progressing from 40 mg (for children aged 3 months or younger) up to 480 mg (for children age 11 years); these doses may be administered up to 5 times a day.

## KEY POINTS

- Aspirin is the prototype of the traditional nonsteroidal anti-inflammatory drugs (NSAIDs).
- NSAIDs have four beneficial actions: suppression of inflammation, relief of mild to moderate pain, reduction of fever, and reduction of thrombus formation (secondary to suppression of platelet aggregation).
- NSAIDs have three major adverse effects: gastric ulceration, acute renal failure, and increased bleeding tendencies (secondary to suppression of platelet aggregation).
- NSAIDs produce their beneficial and adverse effects by inhibiting cyclooxygenase, an enzyme needed to form prostaglandins and related compounds from arachidonic acid.
- Cyclooxygenase has two forms: COX-1 and COX-2.
- Inhibition of COX-2 reduces inflammation.
- Inhibition of COX-1 causes gastric ulceration and the other major adverse effects of NSAIDs.
- Traditional NSAIDs inhibit both COX-1 and COX-2.
- A new generation of NSAIDs causes selective inhibition of COX-2, and therefore suppresses inflammation without causing the serious adverse effects associated with inhibition of COX-1.
- Aspirin causes irreversible inhibition of cyclooxygenase. In contrast, all other NSAIDs produce reversible (competitive) inhibition.
- The effects of aspirin persist until cells can make more cyclooxygenase. The effects of all other NSAIDs decline as soon as drug levels decline.
- Because platelets are unable to synthesize new cyclooxygenase, the effects of a single dose of aspirin persist for the life of the platelet (about 8 days).
- Anti-inflammatory doses of aspirin are much higher than analgesic or antipyretic doses.
- Aspirin and other NSAIDs are drugs of first choice for rheumatoid arthritis and other chronic inflammatory conditions.
- Aspirin is a very effective analgesic. It can be as effective as opioids for some types of postoperative pain.
- The risk of NSAID-induced gastric ulcers can be reduced by prophylactic treatment with misoprostol, a synthetic prostaglandin.
- Because of its antiplatelet actions, aspirin should be discontinued 1 week prior to elective surgery or parturition.
- Because of its antiplatelet actions, aspirin intensifies the anticoagulant response to warfarin.
- The risk of acute renal failure from aspirin is limited to patients in whom renal blood flow is supported by production of prostaglandins. These patients include the elderly and those with hypovolemia, hepatic cirrhosis, heart failure, and pre-existing renal dysfunction.
- Because of the risk of Reye's syndrome, aspirin and other NSAIDs should be avoided by children and teenagers with influenza or chickenpox.
- Use of aspirin and other NSAIDs during labor and delivery can suppress spontaneous uterine contractions, induce premature closure of the ductus arteriosus, and intensify bleeding.

- Although rarely fatal in adults, aspirin poisoning may prove lethal in children.
- Acetaminophen inhibits prostaglandin synthesis in the CNS, but not in the periphery. As a result, acetaminophen differs from the NSAIDs in four ways: it lacks anti-inflammatory actions, does not cause gastric ulceration, does not suppress platelet aggregation, and does not cause renal failure.
- Hepatic necrosis from acetaminophen overdose results from accumulation of a toxic metabolite.

- Chronic alcohol consumption promotes acetaminophen-induced liver damage primarily by inducing P-450 (which increases production of the toxic metabolite of acetaminophen) and depleting stores of glutathione (which reduces detoxification of the metabolite).
- Acetaminophen poisoning is treated with acetylcysteine, a drug that substitutes for depleted glutathione in the reaction that removes the toxic metabolite of acetaminophen.

# Summary of Major Nursing Implications*

## Nonsteroidal Anti-inflammatory Drugs

Except where noted, the nursing implications summarized below apply to aspirin and all other NSAIDs.

### Preadministration Assessment

#### Therapeutic Goal

Major indications for the NSAIDs are inflammatory disorders (e.g., rheumatoid arthritis), mild to moderate pain, fever, primary dysmenorrhea, tendinitis, bursitis, and prevention of cardiovascular disease. Applications of individual NSAIDs are summarized in Table 64–2.

#### Identifying High-Risk Patients

NSAIDs are *contraindicated* for patients with a *history of severe NSAID hypersensitivity*.

NSAIDs should be used with *extreme caution* by *pregnant women* and by patients with *peptic ulcer disease* and *bleeding disorders* (e.g., hemophilia, vitamin K deficiency, hypoprothrombinemia) and by patients taking *warfarin* or *glucocorticoids*. *Caution* is also needed when treating *elderly* patients and patients with *heart failure, hypovolemia, hepatic cirrhosis, renal dysfunction, asthma, hay fever, chronic urticaria, nasal polyps*, or a *history of alcoholism or heavy cigarette smoking*.

NSAIDs (especially aspirin) should be avoided by children with chickenpox or influenza.

NSAIDs should be discontinued 1 week prior to elective surgery or the anticipated date of parturition.

### Implementation: Administration

#### Routes

*Oral.* All NSAIDs.

*Intramuscular.* Ketorolac.

*Rectal (by suppository).* Aspirin and indomethacin.

### Administration

Advise patients to take NSAIDs with food, milk, or a glass of water to reduce gastric upset.

Instruct patients not to crush or chew enteric-coated or sustained-release formulations.

Advise patients to discard aspirin preparations that smell of vinegar.

### Ongoing Evaluation and Interventions

#### Minimizing Adverse Effects

*Gastrointestinal Effects.* NSAIDs frequently cause mild GI reactions (dyspepsia, abdominal pain, nausea). To minimize these effects, advise patients to take NSAIDs with food, milk, or a glass of water.

Long-term, high-dose therapy can cause gastric ulceration, perforation, and hemorrhage. To reduce the risk of these reactions, avoid NSAIDs in patients with a recent history of peptic ulcer disease and use NSAIDs with caution in patients with other risk factors (advanced age, previous intolerance to NSAIDs, heavy cigarette smoking, history of alcoholism). Warn patients not to consume alcohol.

Instruct patients to notify the physician if gastric irritation is severe or persistent. Switching to a different NSAID (e.g., ibuprofen) may be helpful.

Manage GI ulcers by discontinuing the NSAID and giving an antiulcer medication (usually an $H_2$-receptor antagonist or sucralfate). Alternatively, it may be possible to continue the NSAID while treating the ulcer with omeprazole.

Misoprostol can be given for prophylaxis of NSAID-induced ulcers in high-risk patients. Because misoprostol can stimulate uterine contractions, the drug is absolutely contraindicated during pregnancy.

*Bleeding.* Aspirin promotes bleeding by causing irreversible suppression of platelet aggregation. Aspirin should be discontinued 1 week prior to elective surgery or anticipated date of parturition. Exercise caution when using aspirin in conjunction with warfarin. Avoid aspirin in patients with bleeding disorders (e.g., hemophilia, vitamin K deficiency, hypoprothrombinemia).

The nonacetylated salicylates—sodium salicylate, choline salicylate, and magnesium salicylate—have mini-

*Patient education information is highlighted in color.

mal effects on platelet aggregation. Accordingly, these drugs are preferred for use in surgical patients and patients with bleeding disorders.

**Renal Impairment.** NSAIDs can cause acute renal insufficiency in elderly patients and in patients with heart failure, hypovolemia, hepatic cirrhosis, or pre-existing renal dysfunction. Keep NSAID dosages as low as possible in these patients. Monitor high-risk patients for indications of renal impairment (reduced urine output, weight gain despite diuretic therapy, rapid elevation of serum creatinine and blood urea nitrogen). Discontinue NSAIDs if these signs occur.

**Hypersensitivity Reactions.** These reactions are most likely in patients with asthma, hay fever, chronic urticaria, or nasal polyps. NSAIDs should be used with caution by these patients. If a severe hypersensitivity reaction occurs, parenteral epinephrine is the treatment of choice. Avoid NSAIDs in patients with a history of NSAID hypersensitivity.

**Salicylism.** Aspirin and other salicylates can cause salicylism. Educate patients about manifestations of salicylism (tinnitus, sweating, headache, dizziness), and advise them to notify the physician if these occur. Aspirin should be withheld until symptoms subside, after which therapy can resume but at a slightly reduced dosage.

**Reye's Syndrome.** Use of NSAIDs (especially aspirin) by children with chickenpox or influenza may precipitate Reye's syndrome. Advise parents to consult a physician before administering NSAIDs to children suspected of having these viral infections.

**Use in Pregnancy.** NSAIDs can cause maternal anemia and prolongation of labor and gestation. In addition, they can promote premature closure of the ductus arteriosus. NSAIDs should be avoided by expectant mothers unless the potential benefits outweigh the risks. If NSAIDs are employed during pregnancy, they should be discontinued at least 1 week before the anticipated day of delivery.

### Minimizing Adverse Interactions

**Warfarin.** NSAIDs can increase the risk of spontaneous bleeding in patients taking warfarin. Monitor patients for signs of bleeding.

**Glucocorticoids.** Glucocorticoids increase the risk of gastric ulceration in patients taking NSAIDs. Prophylactic therapy with misoprostol can decrease the risk.

### Managing Aspirin Toxicity

Aspirin poisoning is an acute medical emergency that requires hospitalization. Treatment is largely supportive and consists of external cooling (e.g., sponging with tepid water), infusion of fluids (to correct dehydration and elec-

trolyte loss), infusion of bicarbonate (to reverse acidosis and promote renal excretion of salicylates), and mechanical ventilation (if respiration is severely depressed). Absorption of aspirin can be reduced by gastric lavage, induction of emesis, and administration of activated charcoal. If necessary, hemodialysis or peritoneal dialysis can accelerate salicylate removal.

## Acetaminophen

### Preadministration Assessment

#### Therapeutic Goal

Acetaminophen is indicated for relief of pain and suppression of fever in patients who are intolerant to aspirin and other NSAIDs. Acetaminophen is preferred to NSAIDs for use in children with chickenpox or influenza.

#### Identifying High-Risk Patients

Use with *caution* in *chronic alcoholics* and in patients who *consume moderate amounts of alcohol daily*.

### Implementation: Administration

#### Routes

Oral, rectal.

#### Administration

Do not exceed recommended doses.

### Ongoing Evaluation and Interventions

#### Minimizing Adverse Effects

Acetaminophen is devoid of significant adverse effects at usual therapeutic doses, except perhaps in people who consume alcohol on a regular basis.

#### Minimizing Adverse Interactions

**Alcohol.** Moderate daily consumption of alcohol may increase the risk of liver injury from therapeutic doses of acetaminophen. Accordingly, some authorities recommend giving no more than half the normal maximum daily dose of acetaminophen to alcohol drinkers.

#### Managing Toxicity

Overdose can cause hepatic necrosis. *Acetylcysteine* is a specific antidote. Acetylcysteine has an extremely unpleasant odor and may induce vomiting. If vomiting interferes with oral administration, acetylcysteine can be administered through an oroduodenal tube.

# CHAPTER 65

# Glucocorticoids in Nonendocrine Diseases

The glucocorticoid drugs (e.g., cortisone, prednisone), which are also known as *corticosteroids*, are nearly identical to the glucose-regulating steroids produced by the adrenal cortex. Accordingly, we can look on the glucocorticoids as having two kinds of effects: physiologic and pharmacologic. *Physiologic* effects, such as modulation of glucose metabolism, are elicited by *low* doses of glucocorticoids. In contrast, *pharmacologic* effects (e.g., suppression of inflammation) require *high* doses.

As implied by the chapter title, glucocorticoids have both endocrine and nonendocrine applications. In low (physiologic) doses, glucocorticoids are used to treat endocrine disorders (e.g., adrenocortical insufficiency). In high (pharmacologic) doses, these agents are used to treat inflammatory disorders (e.g., rheumatoid arthritis, asthma) and certain cancers and to suppress immune responses in patients receiving organ transplants. The endocrine applications of the glucocorticoids are discussed in Chapter 56. Nonendocrine uses, which are the most common applications of these drugs, are the subject of this chapter.

Toxicity of the glucocorticoids can be severe and is determined by the pattern of drug use. Glucocorticoids are devoid of toxicity when used in physiologic doses. However, when taken in pharmacologic doses, especially for extended periods, glucocorticoids can produce multiple, severe adverse effects.

All of the glucocorticoid drugs can elicit the same spectrum of therapeutic effects. Differences among individual agents pertain to time course of action and side effects. Since the similarities among these drugs are much more striking than the differences, we will forego our practice of focusing on a prototypic agent and discuss the glucocorticoids as a group. In approaching the glucocorticoids, we will begin with a review of their physiology, after which we will discuss their pharmacology.

# Review of Glucocorticoid Physiology

## Physiologic Effects

Physiologic responses can be elicited with low doses of glucocorticoids. When the dosage is high, these effects will simply be more intense. When glucocorticoids are used to treat nonendocrine disorders, physiologic responses will occur as side effects. Physiologic effects of the glucocorticoids are discussed in depth in Chapter 56. The discussion below is a review.

*Metabolic Effects.* Glucocorticoids influence the metabolism of carbohydrates, proteins, and fats. The principal effect on carbohydrate metabolism is elevation of blood glucose content. This is accomplished by promoting synthesis of glucose from amino acids and by reducing peripheral glucose utilization. Glucocorticoids also promote storage of glucose in the form of glycogen.

Glucocorticoids have an unfavorable impact on protein metabolism. These agents suppress synthesis of proteins from amino acids and divert amino acids for production of glucose. These actions can cause a reduction in muscle mass, thinning of the skin, and a decrease in the protein matrix of bone. Nitrogen balance becomes negative.

The most consistent effect of glucocorticoids on fat metabolism is stimulation of lipolysis (fat breakdown). Long-term, high-dose therapy can cause fat redistribution, resulting in the potbelly, "moon face," and "buffalo hump" that characterize Cushing's disease.

*Cardiovascular Effects.* Glucocorticoids are required to maintain the functional integrity of the vascular system. When levels of endogenous glucocorticoids are low, capillaries become more permeable, vasoconstriction is sup-

**TABLE 65–1. GLUCOCORTICOIDS: HALF-LIVES, RELATIVE POTENCIES AND EQUIVALENT DOSES**

| Drug | Biologic Half-Life (hr) | Relative Mineralocorticoid Potency* | Relative Glucocorticoid (Anti-Inflammatory) Potency | Equivalent Anti-Inflammatory Dose (mg)[†] |
|---|---|---|---|---|
| *Short-Acting* | | | | |
| Cortisone | 8–12 | 2 | 0.8 | 25 |
| Hydrocortisone | 8–12 | 2 | 1.0 | 20 |
| *Intermediate-Acting* | | | | |
| Prednisone | 18–36 | 1 | 4 | 5 |
| Prednisolone | 18–36 | 1 | 4 | 5 |
| Methylprednisolone | 18–36 | 0 | 5 | 4 |
| Triamcinolone | 18–36 | 0 | 5 | 4 |
| *Long-Acting* | | | | |
| Betamethasone | 36–54 | 0 | 20–30 | 0.75 |
| Dexamethasone | 36–54 | 0 | 20–30 | 0.75 |

*Relative mineralocorticoid activity (sodium and water retention; potassium depletion): 0 = very low; 1 = moderate; 2 = high.
[†]Approximate *oral* or *intravenous* dose needed to produce equivalent anti-inflammatory effects.

pressed, and blood pressure falls. Glucocorticoids increase the number of circulating red blood cells and polymorphonuclear leukocytes. Counts of lymphocytes, eosinophils, basophils, and monocytes are reduced.

**Effects during Stress.** At times of stress (e.g., anxiety, surgery, infection, trauma), the adrenals secrete large quantities of glucocorticoids and epinephrine. Working together, these compounds help maintain blood pressure and plasma levels of glucose. In the absence of sufficient amounts of glucocorticoids, hypotension and hypoglycemia will occur. If the stress is especially severe, glucocorticoid insufficiency can result in circulatory failure and death.

**Effects on Water and Electrolytes.** To varying degrees, individual glucocorticoids can exert actions like those of aldosterone, the major mineralocorticoid released by the adrenals. Accordingly, glucocorticoids can act on the kidney to promote retention of sodium and water while increasing urinary excretion of potassium. The net result of these effects is hypernatremia, hypokalemia, and edema. Fortunately, most of the glucocorticoids employed as drugs have very low mineralocorticoid activity (see Table 65–1).

**Respiratory System in Neonates.** During labor and delivery, the adrenals of the full-term fetus release a burst of glucocorticoids, which act to hasten maturation of the lungs. In the premature infant, production of glucocorticoids is low, resulting in a high incidence of respiratory distress syndrome.

## Control of Synthesis and Secretion

Synthesis and release of glucocorticoids are regulated by a negative feedback loop. The principal components of this

loop are the hypothalamus, the anterior pituitary, and the adrenal cortex (Fig. 65–1). The loop is turned on when stress or some other stimulus from the central nervous system (CNS) acts on the hypothalamus to cause release of corticotropin-releasing factor (CRF). CRF then stimulates the pituitary to release adrenocorticotropic hormone (ACTH), which in turn acts on the adrenal cortex to promote synthesis and release of cortisol (the principal endogenous glucocorticoid). Cortisol then exerts two kinds of effects: (1) it promotes physiologic responses and (2) it acts on the hypothalamus and pituitary to suppress further release of CRF and ACTH. By inhibiting release of these factors, cortisol suppresses its own production. Hence, this negative feedback system serves to keep glucocorticoid levels within an appropriate range. As discussed later, when glucocorticoids are administered chronically in large doses, the feedback loop remains continuously suppressed. This persistent inhibition can be very detrimental.

## Pharmacology of the Glucocorticoids

## Pharmacologic Actions

When administered in the high doses employed to treat nonendocrine disorders, the glucocorticoids have powerful anti-inflammatory and immunosuppressive actions. These actions do not occur when glucocorticoid doses are physiologic. In addition to these pharmacologic effects, high-dose therapy intensifies the type of responses seen at physiologic doses.

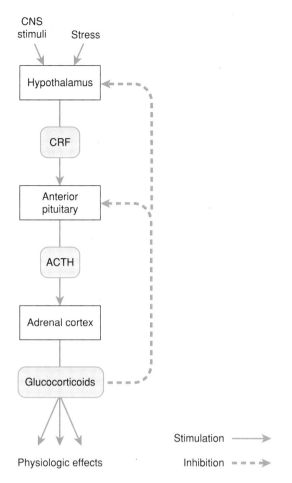

**Figure 65–1. Feedback regulation of glucocorticoid synthesis and secretion.** (CRF = corticotropin-releasing factor, ACTH = adrenocorticotropic hormone.)

## Effects on Metabolism and Electrolytes

Qualitatively, the effects of high-dose therapy on metabolism and electrolytes are the same as those that occur at physiologic doses; these responses are simply more intense when the dosage is high. Hence, with pharmacologic doses, glucose levels rise, protein synthesis is suppressed, and fat deposits are mobilized. As noted above, most glucocorticoids have very little mineralocorticoid activity. Accordingly, these drugs do not usually induce significant sodium retention or potassium loss. However, these effects do occur in some patients and can be hazardous. In addition, high-dose therapy can inhibit intestinal absorption of calcium. This effect is not seen when doses are physiologic.

## Anti-inflammatory and Immunosuppressant Effects

The major clinical applications of the glucocorticoids stem from the ability of these drugs to suppress immune responses and inflammation. Since effects on the immune system and inflammation are interrelated, we will consider these effects together.

Before discussing the actions of glucocorticoids, it will be helpful to review the process of inflammation. The characteristic symptoms of inflammation are pain, swelling, redness, and warmth. These effects are initiated by chemical mediators (prostaglandins, histamine, leukotrienes) and are amplified by the actions of lymphocytes and phagocytic cells (neutrophils and macrophages). Prostaglandins and histamine promote several symptoms of inflammation—swelling, redness, and warmth—by causing vasodilation and by increasing capillary permeability. Prostaglandins and histamine also help cause pain: histamine acts by stimulating pain receptors directly; prostaglandins act by sensitizing pain receptors to histamine and other stimuli. Neutrophils and macrophages heighten inflammation by releasing lysosomal enzymes (enzymes that cause direct tissue injury). Lymphocytes, which are important elements of the immune system, intensify inflammation by (1) causing direct cell injury and (2) promoting formation of antibodies that serve to perpetuate the inflammatory response.

Glucocorticoids act through several mechanisms to interrupt the inflammatory processes. These drugs can inhibit synthesis of chemical mediators (prostaglandins, leukotrienes, histamine) and thereby reduce swelling, warmth, redness, and pain. In addition, these agents suppress infiltration of phagocytes. Hence, damage from release of lysosomal enzymes is averted. Lastly, glucocorticoids suppress proliferation of lymphocytes, and thereby reduce the immune component of inflammation.

On a molecular level, most effects of glucocorticoids can be attributed to promoting the synthesis of specific regulatory proteins. Stimulation of protein synthesis is accomplished as follows: (1) glucocorticoids penetrate the cell membrane and then bind to intracellular receptors; (2) the receptor-steroid complex migrates to the cell nucleus, where it binds to chromatin in DNA; and (3) the interaction with chromatin triggers transcription of messenger RNA molecules that code for regulatory proteins, thereby increasing synthesis of these regulatory molecules.

It is important to note that the mechanisms by which glucocorticoids suppress inflammation are broader in scope than the mechanisms by which nonsteroidal anti-inflammatory drugs (NSAIDs) act. As discussed in Chapter 64, the anti-inflammatory effects of the NSAIDs can be attributed largely to inhibition of prostaglandin biosynthesis. The glucocorticoids share this mechanism and, as indicated above, act in several other ways as well. It is because of this multiplicity of mechanisms that the anti-inflammatory effects of glucocorticoids are much greater than those of the NSAIDs.

### Pharmacokinetics

***Absorption.*** The rate of glucocorticoid absorption depends on route of administration and the particular glucocorticoid derivative being administered. With oral administration, absorption of all glucocorticoids is rapid and nearly complete. Following IM injection, absorption is rapid with two types of glucocorticoid esters (sodium phosphates and sodium succinates) and relatively slow with other derivatives (e.g., acetates, acetonides, tebutates). Absorption from local sites of injection (e.g., intra-articular, intrasynovial) is slower than from IM sites.

*Duration of Action.* Duration of action is a function of dosage, route of administration, and solubility. For glucocorticoids administered orally or IV, duration of action is determined largely by biologic half-life (see Table 65–1). With IM administration, duration of action is a function of water solubility: highly soluble preparations have a shorter duration than less soluble preparations. For locally administered glucocorticoids, duration is determined by solubility and by the specific site of administration.

*Metabolism and Excretion.* Glucocorticoids are metabolized primarily by the liver. As a rule, metabolites are inactive. Excretion of glucocorticoid metabolites is renal.

## Therapeutic Uses in Nonendocrine Disorders

Glucocorticoids are used to treat endocrine disorders and nonendocrine disorders. Endocrine disorders (e.g., Addison's disease, acute adrenal insufficiency) can be managed with low-dose therapy and are considered in Chapter 56. Nonendocrine applications, which require much higher doses, are discussed below. Because prolonged, high-dose therapy can produce serious adverse effects, the potential benefits of treatment must be weighed carefully against the very real risks.

*Rheumatoid Arthritis.* Glucocorticoids are indicated for adjunctive treatment of acute exacerbations of rheumatoid arthritis. These drugs can reduce inflammation and pain, but do not alter the course of the disease. Because of the risk of serious complications, prolonged systemic use should be avoided.

When arthritis is limited to just a few joints, intra-articular injections should be employed. Local injections can be highly effective, and cause less toxicity than systemic therapy. Frequently, reductions in pain and inflammation may be so dramatic as to prompt vigorous use of joints that were previously immobile. Since excessive use of diseased joints can cause injury, patients should be warned against overactivity, even though their symptoms may have abated.

The use of glucocorticoids in rheumatoid arthritis is discussed further in Chapter 66.

*Systemic Lupus Erythematosus.* Systemic lupus erythematosus (SLE) is a chronic disease similar in many ways to rheumatoid arthritis. However, in SLE, inflammation is not limited to joints; rather, inflammation occurs throughout the body. Symptoms frequently include pleuritis, pericarditis, and nephritis. A severe episode of SLE can be fatal. Fortunately, manifestations of SLE can usually be controlled with prompt and aggressive glucocorticoid therapy.

*Inflammatory Bowel Disease.* Glucocorticoids are used to treat severe cases of ulcerative colitis and Crohn's disease, the two most common forms of inflammatory bowel disease. Administration may be oral, by injection, or by enema. Glucocorticoid therapy of these disorders is considered further in Chapter 73.

*Miscellaneous Inflammatory Disorders.* Glucocorticoids are useful in treating a variety of inflammatory disorders in addition to those discussed above. Conditions that re-

spond to glucocorticoid therapy include *bursitis, tendonitis, synovitis, osteoarthritis, gouty arthritis,* and *inflammatory disorders of the eye.*

*Allergic Conditions.* Glucocorticoids can control symptoms of allergic reactions. Responsive conditions include bee stings, hay fever (see Chapter 65), and drug-induced allergies. Since responses to glucocorticoids are delayed, these agents have little value as acute therapy for severe allergic reactions (e.g., anaphylaxis). For life-threatening allergic reactions, epinephrine is the treatment of choice.

*Asthma.* Glucocorticoids are the most effective antiasthmatic agents available. For treatment of asthma, these drugs may be administered orally or by inhalation. Because oral therapy can be associated with serious toxicity, oral glucocorticoids should be reserved for patients who have failed to respond to safer medications (beta$_2$-adrenergic agonists, theophylline, cromolyn sodium). Fortunately, adverse effects are minimal when glucocorticoids are administered by inhalation. The use of glucocorticoids in asthma is discussed further in Chapter 69.

*Dermatologic Disorders.* Glucocorticoids are beneficial in a wide variety of skin diseases, including pemphigus, psoriasis, mycosis fungoides, seborrheic dermatitis, contact dermatitis, and exfoliative dermatitis. For mild disease, topical administration is usually adequate. Systemic steroids are generally reserved for severe disorders. It should be noted that absorption of topically applied glucocorticoids can be sufficient to produce systemic toxicity. Topical therapy is discussed further in Chapter 98.

*Neoplasms.* Glucocorticoids are used in conjunction with other anticancer agents to treat acute lymphocytic leukemia, Hodgkin's disease, and non-Hodgkin's lymphomas. Benefits derive from the direct toxicity of glucocorticoids to malignant lymphocytes. Treatment kills lymphoid cells and causes regression of lymphatic tissue. The use of glucocorticoids to treat cancers is discussed further in Chapter 96.

*Suppression of Allograft Rejection.* Glucocorticoids, together with other immunosuppressant agents, are used to prevent rejection of organ transplants. Treatment with glucocorticoids is initiated at the time of surgery and continued indefinitely. The use of glucocorticoids for immunosuppression is discussed further in Chapter 67.

*Preterm Labor and Delivery.* Preterm infants are at high risk of respiratory distress syndrome because their adrenals cannot produce the glucocorticoids needed for lung maturation. When preterm delivery is imminent, injection of the mother with glucocorticoids (dexamethasone or betamethasone) reduces the risk of respiratory distress syndrome by 50% and mortality by 40%. Steroids may also reduce the incidence of intraventricular hemorrhage and necrotizing enterocolitis (inflammation of the small intestine and colon).

## Adverse Effects

The adverse effects discussed below occur in response to *pharmacologic* doses of glucocorticoids. The intensity of these effects increases with dosage size and duration of treatment. These toxicities are not seen when dosage is physiologic. Furthermore, most are not seen when treatment is brief (a few days or less), even when doses are high.

**Adrenal Insufficiency.** Pharmacologic doses of glucocorticoids can suppress production of glucocorticoids by the adrenals, resulting in adrenal insufficiency. The mechanism, consequences, and management of adrenal insufficiency are discussed in depth below.

**Osteoporosis.** Osteoporosis is a frequent and serious complication of chronic glucocorticoid therapy. The ribs and vertebrae are affected most, and vertebral compression fractures are common, sometimes occurring only weeks after beginning glucocorticoid use. Patients should be observed for signs of compression fractures (back and neck pain) and for indications of fractures in other bones. If the technology is available, bone status should be evaluated periodically by employing bone densitometry.

Osteoporosis results from a combination of decreased formation of bone and increased bone resorption. Glucocorticoids inhibit the activity of osteoblasts, the cells responsible for formation of bone and increase the activity of osteoclasts, the cells responsible for resorption of bone. Also, glucocorticoids decrease intestinal absorption of calcium, and thereby promote hypocalcemia. In response to hypocalcemia, release of parathyroid hormone is increased, promoting mobilization of calcium from bone.

Development of osteoporosis can be reduced by taking calcium supplements along with calcitriol (the most active form of vitamin D). Recent evidence suggests that adding calcitonin or a bisphosphonate to the regimen can be of further benefit. The roles of calcium, calcitriol, calcitonin, and bisphosphonates in the prophylaxis and treatment of osteoporosis are discussed fully in Chapter 75.

**Infection.** By suppressing host defenses (immune responses and phagocytic activity of neutrophils and macrophages), glucocorticoids can increase susceptibility to infection. The risk of acquiring a new infection is increased, as is the risk of reactivating a latent infection (e.g., tuberculosis). In addition, since suppression of the immune system and neutrophils reduces inflammation and other manifestations of infection, a fulminant infection may develop without detection. Hence, not only do glucocorticoids increase susceptibility to infection, they can mask the presence of an infection as it progresses. To minimize acquisition of infection, patients should avoid close contact with individuals who have communicable diseases. If a significant infection occurs, glucocorticoids should be continued only if absolutely necessary, and then only in combination with appropriate antimicrobial or antifungal therapy.

One infection, *Pneumocystis carinii* pneumonia (PCP), occurs with alarming frequency in people receiving high doses of glucocorticoids (and not just in people with AIDS, among whom PCP is the most common opportunistic infection). Accordingly, it has been suggested that PCP prophylaxis be considered for all people taking glucocorticoids in high doses.

**Glucose Intolerance.** Because of their effects on glucose production and utilization, glucocorticoids can increase plasma glucose levels, causing hyperglycemia and glycosuria. For patients with diabetes, these effects may necessitate an increase in insulin dosage or a reduction in caloric intake. For patients with normal pancreatic function, significant elevations of blood glucose are unlikely. However, since use of glucocorticoids can unmask latent diabetes, nondiabetics should undergo periodic evaluation of blood glucose levels.

**Myopathy.** High-dose glucocorticoid therapy can cause myopathy, manifested as muscle weakness. The proximal muscles of the arms and legs are affected most. Damage to muscle may be sufficient to prevent ambulation. If myopathy develops, glucocorticoid dosage should be reduced. Myopathy then gradually resolves over several months.

**Fluid and Electrolyte Disturbance.** Because of their mineralocorticoid activity, glucocorticoids can cause sodium and water retention and potassium loss. Retention of water and sodium can cause hypertension and edema. Hypokalemia can predispose the patient to dysrhythmias and toxicity from digitalis. Fortunately, most of the glucocorticoids in current use have minimal mineralocorticoid activity (see Table 65–1). Hence, serious fluid and electrolyte disturbance is rare. The risk of fluid and electrolyte disturbance can be reduced by (1) using glucocorticoids that have low mineralocorticoid activity, (2) restricting sodium intake, and (3) taking potassium supplements or consuming potassium-rich foods (e.g., bananas, citrus fruits). Patients should be informed about signs of fluid retention (e.g., weight gain, swelling of the lower extremities) and advised to contact the physician if these develop. Patients should also be alert for signs of hypokalemia (e.g., muscle weakness or fatigue, irregular pulses).

**Growth Retardation.** Glucocorticoids can suppress growth in children. Growth retardation is probably the result of reduced DNA synthesis and decreased cell division. To assess effects on growth, height and weight should be measured at regular intervals. Growth suppression can be minimized with alternate-day therapy. This dosing schedule is discussed below.

**Psychologic Disturbances.** Rarely, glucocorticoids have caused hallucinations, mood changes (depression, euphoria, mania), and other psychologic disturbances. These effects are related more to dosage size than to duration of treatment, and can occur within the first few days of drug use. Previous psychiatric illness does not appear to predispose patients to adverse psychologic effects of glucocorticoids. Conversely, a history of good mental health does not guarantee immunity from psychologic disturbance.

**Cataracts.** Cataracts are a common complication of long-term glucocorticoid therapy. Risk factors are in dispute; cataract development may be related to age, dosage, or individual susceptibility. To facilitate early detection, patients should receive an ophthalmologic examination every 6 months. Also, patients should be advised to contact the physician if vision becomes cloudy or blurred.

**Peptic Ulcer Disease.** Although glucocorticoids have actions that could lead to peptic ulcer disease, whether they actually cause gastrointestinal ulceration is controversial. By inhibiting prostaglandin synthesis, glucocorticoids can augment secretion of gastric acid and pepsin, inhibit production of cytoprotective mucus, and reduce gastric mucosal blood flow. These actions predispose the patient to gastrointestinal ulceration. Making matters worse, glucocorticoids can decrease gastric pain, thereby masking ulcer development. As a result, perforation and hemorrhage can occur without warning. The risk of ulceration is increased by concurrent use of other ulcerogenic drugs, such as aspirin and other NSAIDs. To provide early detection of ulcer formation, stools should be periodically checked for occult blood. Patients should be instructed to notify the physician if feces become black and tarry. If gastrointestinal ulceration occurs, glucocorticoids should be slowly withdrawn (unless their continued use is considered essential to support life). Treatment with antiulcer medication is indicated.

**Iatrogenic Cushing's Syndrome.** Long-term glucocorticoid therapy can induce a cushingoid syndrome whose symptoms are identical to those of naturally occurring Cushing's disease. Prominent symptoms are hyperglycemia, glycosuria, fluid and electrolyte disturbances, osteoporosis, muscle weakness, cutaneous striations, and lowered resistance to infection. Redistribution of fat produces a potbelly, "moon face," and "buffalo hump."

## Use in Pregnancy and Lactation

**Pregnancy.** Glucocorticoids can cross the placenta and affect the developing fetus. Animal studies indicate an increased incidence of cleft palate, spontaneous abortion, and low birth weight. No adequate studies of these effects have been done in humans. Prolonged therapy with very large doses can cause fetal adrenal hypoplasia. Hence, when large doses have been employed, the infant should be assessed for adrenal insufficiency and given replacement therapy if indicated. Whenever glucocorticoids are to be used during pregnancy, the benefits must be carefully weighed against the potential risk to the fetus.

**Lactation.** Glucocorticoids enter breast milk. When physiologic doses or low pharmacologic doses are used, the concentration achieved in milk is probably too low to affect the nursing infant. However, when large pharmacologic doses are employed (e.g., doses greater than 5 mg/day of prednisone or its equivalent) the amount ingested by the infant may be sufficient to cause growth retardation and other adverse effects. Consequently, women receiving high-dose glucocorticoid therapy should be warned against breast-feeding.

## Drug Interactions

**Interactions Related to Potassium Loss.** As discussed above, glucocorticoids can increase urinary loss of potas-

sium, and can thereby induce hypokalemia. Consequently, glucocorticoids must be used with caution when combined with *digoxin* (because hypokalemia increases the risk of digoxin-induced dysrhythmias) and when combined with *thiazide diuretics* or *loop diuretics* (because these potassium-depleting diuretics will increase the risk of hypokalemia). When glucocorticoids are given together with any of the above drugs, it is advisable to monitor plasma potassium levels and be alert for signs of cardiac toxicity.

**Nonsteroidal Anti-inflammatory Drugs.** NSAIDs have the same effects on the gastrointestinal tract as do glucocorticoids. Accordingly, concurrent use of these agents increases the risk of ulceration.

**Insulin and Oral Hypoglycemics.** As noted, glucocorticoids promote hyperglycemia. To maintain glycemic control, diabetic patients may require increased doses of a glucose-lowering drug (insulin or an oral hypoglycemic agent).

**Vaccines.** Because of their immunosuppressant actions, glucocorticoids can decrease antibody responses to vaccines. Furthermore, if a live-virus vaccine is employed, there is an increased risk of developing viral disease. Accordingly, attempts at immunization should not be made while glucocorticoids are being used.

## Summary of Precautions and Contraindications

**Contraindications.** Glucocorticoids are contraindicated for patients with *systemic fungal infections* and for patients receiving *live-virus vaccines.*

**Precautions.** Glucocorticoids must be used with caution in *pediatric patients* and in *women who are pregnant or breast-feeding.* Caution is also required in patients with *hypertension*, *heart failure*, *renal impairment*, *esophagitis*, *gastritis*, *peptic ulcer disease*, *myasthenia gravis*, *diabetes mellitus*, *osteoporosis*, and *infections that are resistant to treatment.* In addition, caution is required during concurrent therapy with *potassium-depleting diuretics*, *digoxin*, *insulin*, *oral hypoglycemics*, and *NSAIDs.*

## Adrenal Suppression

**Development of Adrenal Suppression.** Like the naturally occurring glucocorticoids (e.g., cortisol), the glucocorticoids that we administer as drugs suppress the release of both CRF from the hypothalamus and ACTH from the anterior pituitary. By doing so, glucocorticoid drugs inhibit the synthesis and release of endogenous glucocorticoids by the adrenals. During long-term therapy, the pituitary loses much of its ability to manufacture ACTH and, in response to the prolonged absence of ACTH, the adrenals atrophy and lose their ability to synthesize cortisol and other glucocorticoids. As a result, when prolonged therapy with glucocorticoids is discontinued, there is a period during which the adrenals are unable to produce glucocorticoids. Recovery of adrenal function may take from a few weeks to more than a year. The extent of adrenal suppression and the time required for recovery are determined primarily by the duration of glucocorticoid use; dosage size is of secondary importance. Development of adrenal suppression can be minimized through alternate-day dosing. This procedure is discussed below.

***Adrenal Suppression and Stress.*** As noted above, the adrenals normally secrete large amounts of glucocorticoids at times of stress. When stress is severe (e.g., trauma, surgery) these glucocorticoids are essential for supporting life. Accordingly, *it is imperative that patients receiving long-term glucocorticoid therapy be given increased doses at times of stress* (unless the dosage is already very high). Furthermore, *once glucocorticoid use has ceased, supplemental doses are required whenever stress occurs until recovery of adrenal function is complete.* Patients should carry an identification card or bracelet informing emergency health care personnel of their glucocorticoid needs. In addition, patients should always have an emergency supply of glucocorticoids on hand.

***Glucocorticoid Withdrawal.*** Withdrawal of glucocorticoids should be done slowly. The withdrawal schedule is determined by the degree of adrenal suppression. A representative schedule is as follows: (1) taper the dosage to a physiologic range over 7 days; (2) switch from multiple daily doses to single doses administered each morning; (3) taper the dosage to 50% of physiologic values over the next month; and (4) monitor for production of endogenous cortisol and, when basal levels have returned to normal, cease routine steroid administration (but be prepared to give supplemental glucocorticoids at times of stress).

In addition to unmasking adrenal insufficiency, cessation of glucocorticoid use may produce a withdrawal syndrome. Symptoms include hypotension, hypoglycemia, myalgia, arthralgia, and fatigue. In patients being treated for arthritis and certain other disorders, these symptoms may be confused with return of the underlying disease. Discomfort of withdrawal can be minimized by gradual dosage reduction and by concurrent treatment with NSAIDs.

## Preparations and Routes of Administration

### Preparations

The glucocorticoids employed clinically include hydrocortisone (cortisol) and synthetic derivatives of this compound. Individual glucocorticoids differ from one another with respect to (1) biologic half-life, (2) mineralocorticoid potency, and (3) glucocorticoid (anti-inflammatory) potency (see Table 65-1).

The term *biologic half-life* refers to the time required for glucocorticoids to leave body tissues. In most cases, these drugs are cleared from tissues more slowly than from the blood. Hence, the biologic half-life is usually longer than the plasma half-life. When glucocorticoids are administered by mouth or by IV injection, it is the biologic

half-life, not the plasma half-life, that determines duration of action. Because of differences in their biologic half-lives, individual glucocorticoids can be classified as short-acting, intermediate-acting, or long-acting (Table 65-1).

Glucocorticoids with high *mineralocorticoid potency* (cortisone, hydrocortisone) can cause significant retention of sodium and water, coupled with depletion of potassium. These mineralocorticoid effects can be especially hazardous for patients with hypertension or heart failure and for patients taking digoxin. Because of the potential dangers of sodium retention and potassium loss, glucocorticoids with high mineralocorticoid activity should not be administered systemically for long periods.

The differences in *glucocorticoid potency* summarized in Table 65-1 are reflected in the doses required to produce anti-inflammatory effects (and not mineralocorticoid effects). As with other drugs, potency is a relatively unimportant characteristic. However, it *is* important to appreciate that, in order to produce equivalent therapeutic effects, dosages for some glucocorticoids must be much larger than for others.

### Routes of Administration

Glucocorticoids can be administered *orally*, *parenterally* (IV, IM, SC), *topically*, by *local injection* (e.g., intra-articular, intralesional), and by *inhalation*. Topical application is reserved for dermatologic disorders (see Chapter 98), and inhalational therapy is reserved primarily for asthma (see Chapter 69). Since local therapy (topical application, inhalation, local injection) minimizes systemic toxicity, this form of treatment is preferred to systemic therapy (oral, parenteral). When systemic effects are needed, oral administration is preferred to parenteral. It is important to note that, even when glucocorticoids are administered for local effects, absorption can be sufficient to produce systemic effects. That is, local administration does not eliminate the risk of systemic toxicity.

Individual glucocorticoids are available as various esters (e.g., acetate, sodium phosphate, tebutate). When glucocorticoids are administered by routes other than oral or intravenous, the particular ester being used is a major determinant of duration of action. As indicated in Table 65-2, not all esters can be employed by all routes. Hence, when preparing to administer a glucocorticoid, you should verify that the particular ester to be used is appropriate for the intended route.

### Dosage

#### General Guidelines for Dosing

For most patients, the objective of glucocorticoid therapy is to reduce symptoms to an acceptable level. Complete relief of symptoms is usually not an appropriate goal.

Dosages are highly individualized; for any patient with any disease, the dosage must be determined empirically (by trial and error). For patients whose disease is not an immediate threat to life, the dosage should be low initially

## TABLE 65-2. GLUCOCORTICOID ROUTES OF ADMINISTRATION*

| Drug | Systemic | | | | Local | | | | |
|---|---|---|---|---|---|---|---|---|---|
| | PO | IM | IV | SC | IA | IB | IL | IS | ST |
| Betamethasone | ✔ | | | | | | | | |
| Betamethasone sodium phosphate | | ✔ | ✔ | | ✔ | | ✔ | | ✔ |
| Betamethasone acetate/sodium phosphate | | ✔ | | | ✔ | | ✔ | ✔ | ✔ |
| Cortisone acetate | ✔ | ✔ | | | | | | | |
| Dexamethasone | ✔ | | | | | | | | |
| Dexamethasone acetate | | ✔ | | | ✔ | | ✔ | | ✔ |
| Dexamethasone sodium phosphate | | ✔ | ✔ | | ✔ | | ✔ | ✔ | ✔ |
| Hydrocortisone | ✔ | | | | | | | | |
| Hydrocortisone acetate | | | | | ✔ | ✔ | ✔ | ✔ | ✔ |
| Hydrocortisone cypionate | ✔ | | | | | | | | |
| Hydrocortisone sodium phosphate | | ✔ | ✔ | ✔ | | | | | |
| Hydrocortisone sodium succinate | | ✔ | ✔ | | | | | | |
| Methylprednisolone | ✔ | | | | | | | | |
| Methylprednisolone acetate | | ✔ | | | ✔ | | ✔ | | ✔ |
| Methylprednisolone sodium succinate | | ✔ | ✔ | | | | | | |
| Prednisolone | ✔ | | | | | | | | |
| Prednisolone acetate | | ✔ | | | | | | | |
| Prednisolone acetate/sodium phosphate | | ✔ | | | ✔ | ✔ | | ✔ | ✔ |
| Prednisolone sodium phosphate | | ✔ | ✔ | | ✔ | | ✔ | | ✔ |
| Prednisolone tebutate | | | | | ✔ | | ✔ | | ✔ |
| Prednisone | ✔ | | | | | | | | |
| Triamcinolone | ✔ | | | | | | | | |
| Triamcinolone acetonide | | ✔ | | | ✔ | ✔ | ✔ | | |
| Triamcinolone diacetate | | ✔ | | | ✔ | | ✔ | ✔ | ✔ |
| Triamcinolone hexacetonide | | | | | ✔ | | ✔ | | |

*Topical preparations are listed in Table 98–1.
†PO = oral; IM = intramuscular; IV = intravenous; SC = subcutaneous; IA = intra-articular; IB = intrabursal; IL = intralesional; IS = intrasynovial; ST = soft tissue.

and then increased gradually until symptoms are under control. In the event of life-threatening disease, a large initial dose should be used, and, if a response does not occur rapidly, the dose should be doubled or tripled. When glucocorticoids are used for a prolonged period, the dosage should be reduced until the smallest effective amount has been established. Prolonged treatment with high doses should be done only if the disorder (1) is life threatening or (2) has the potential to cause permanent disability. During long-term treatment, an increase in dosage will be needed at times of stress (unless the dosage is very high to begin with). If disease status changes, appropriate adjustment of dosage must be made.

As noted above, abrupt termination of long-term therapy may unmask adrenal insufficiency. To minimize the impact of adrenal insufficiency, withdrawal of glucocorticoids should be gradual. Patients must be warned against abrupt discontinuation of treatment.

### Alternate-Day Therapy

In alternate-day therapy, a large dose (of an intermediate-acting agent) is given every other morning. This dosing schedule contrasts with traditional therapy, in which multiple smaller doses are administered daily. Benefits of alternate-day therapy are (1) reduced adrenal suppression, (2) reduced risk of growth retardation, and (3) reduced toxicity overall. Adrenal insufficiency is decreased because, over the extended interval between doses, plasma glucocorticoids decline to a level that is low enough to permit some production of ACTH, thereby promoting some synthesis of cortisol by the adrenals. To allow maximal recovery of endocrine function, doses should be administered prior to 9 in the morning, and long-acting agents should be avoided. Early morning administration is also helpful in that it mimics the burst of glucocorticoids normally released by the adrenals each dawn.

Unfortunately, alternate-day therapy does have one drawback: in the long interval between doses, drug levels may fall to a subtherapeutic value, thus permitting a flare-up of symptoms. Symptoms are likely to be most intense late on the second day after a dose is given. If symptoms become intolerable, switching to a single daily dose may be sufficient to provide control. As with alternate-day treatment, patients taking single daily doses should administer their medicine before 9 AM.

## KEY POINTS

- Glucocorticoids are used in low (physiologic) doses to treat endocrine disorders (see Chapter 56) and in high (pharmacologic) doses to treat nonendocrine disorders (e.g., arthritis, asthma).
- Glucocorticoids are beneficial in nonendocrine disorders primarily because of their ability to suppress inflammatory and immune responses.
- Glucocorticoids reduce inflammation by multiple mechanisms, including suppression of (1) the synthesis of inflammatory mediators (prostaglandins, leukotrienes, histamine), (2) infiltration of phagocytes, (3) release of lysosomal enzymes, and (4) proliferation of lymphocytes.

- Important nonendocrine indications for glucocorticoids include arthritis, allergic disorders, asthma, cancer, and suppression of allograft rejection.
- When used in pharmacologic doses, especially for prolonged times, glucocorticoids can cause severe adverse effects. These are not seen at physiologic doses.
- Adverse effects of the glucocorticoids include adrenal insufficiency, osteoporosis, increased vulnerability to infection, muscle wasting, thinning of the skin, fluid and electrolyte imbalance, glucose intolerance, and possibly peptic ulcer disease.
- By causing potassium loss, glucocorticoids can increase the risk of toxicity from digoxin, and they can exacerbate potassium loss caused by thiazide and loop diuretics.
- Concurrent use of NSAIDs with glucocorticoids increases the risk of peptic ulcer disease.
- Prolonged glucocorticoid use causes adrenal insufficiency.
- Patients with adrenal insufficiency must be given supplemental doses of glucocorticoids at times of stress (e.g., surgery, trauma). Failure to do so may be fatal!
- To minimize expression of adrenal insufficiency when glucocorticoids are discontinued, doses should be tapered very gradually.
- Following glucocorticoid withdrawal, supplemental glucocorticoids are needed at times of stress until adrenal function has fully recovered.
- Alternate-day dosing can help minimize development of adrenal insufficiency.
- Glucocorticoids should be administered before 9 AM. This helps minimize adrenal insufficiency and mimics the burst of glucocorticoids released naturally by the adrenals each morning.

## Summary of Major Nursing Implications*

## Glucocorticoids

The nursing implications summarized here apply to all glucocorticoids, but only to their use for *nonendocrine diseases*. Implications that apply specifically to use of glucocorticoids for *replacement therapy* are summarized in Chapter 56.

### Preadministration Assessment

#### Therapeutic Goal
Glucocorticoids are used to suppress rejection of organ transplants, and to treat a variety of inflammatory, allergic, and neoplastic disorders. When treating inflammatory and allergic disorders, the goal is to suppress signs and symptoms to an acceptable level, not to eliminate them entirely.

#### Baseline Data
Make a full assessment of the specific disorder (e.g., rheumatoid arthritis, asthma, psoriasis) to be treated.

These data are used to determine the initial dosage as well as dosage adjustments as treatment proceeds.

#### Identifying High-Risk Patients
Glucocorticoids are *contraindicated* for patients with *systemic fungal infections* and for *individuals receiving live-virus vaccines.* Use glucocorticoids with *caution* in *pediatric patients* and in *women who are pregnant or breast-feeding.* In addition, exercise *caution* in patients with *hypertension, heart failure, renal impairment, esophagitis, gastritis, peptic ulcer disease, myasthenia gravis, diabetes mellitus, osteoporosis,* and *infections that are resistant to treatment,* and in *patients receiving potassium-depleting diuretics, digoxin, insulin, oral hypoglycemics,* or *NSAIDs.*

### Implementation: Administration and Dosage

#### Routes and Administration
Glucocorticoids are administered orally, parenterally (IV, IM, SC), topically (to skin and mucous membranes), by inhalation, and by local injection (e.g., intra-articular,

---

*Patient education information is highlighted in color.

intralesional). Routes for specific preparations are summarized in Table 65-2. When preparing to administer a glucocorticoid, verify that the preparation is appropriate for the intended route.

## Dosage

Dosage is determined empirically. For patients whose disease does not threaten life, the dosage should be low initially and then gradually increased until the desired response is achieved. For life-threatening disease, initial doses should be as large as needed to control symptoms. During prolonged therapy, the dosage should be reduced to the smallest effective amount. Supplemental doses are needed at times of stress (unless the dosage is very high to begin with).

## Alternate-Day Therapy

Alternate-day dosing reduces adrenal suppression and other toxicities. Instruct patients to take their medicine before 9 AM.

## Drug Withdrawal

Glucocorticoids must be withdrawn gradually. Warn the patient against abrupt discontinuation of treatment. Following termination, supplemental doses are needed during times of stress until adrenal function has recovered fully.

## Ongoing Evaluation and Interventions

### Evaluating Therapeutic Effects

Evaluate therapy by making periodic comparisons of current signs and symptoms with the pretreatment assessment. Dosage is adjusted on the basis of these evaluations.

### Minimizing Adverse Effects

*General Measures.* (1) Keep the dosage as low as possible and the duration of treatment as short as possible. (2) Use alternate-day therapy if possible. (3) When appropriate, administer glucocorticoids topically, by inhalation, or by local injection, rather than systemically.

*Adrenal Insufficiency.* Long-term therapy suppresses the adrenal's ability to make glucocorticoids. Increase the dosage when stress occurs (e.g., surgery, trauma, infection) unless the dosage is very high to begin with. Following termination of therapy, supplemental doses are required at times of stress until recovery of adrenal function is complete. Advise the patient to carry some sort of identification (e.g., Medic Alert bracelet) to ensure proper dosing in emergencies. Advise the patient to have an emergency supply of glucocorticoids on hand at all times. Expression of adrenal insufficiency will be reduced by withdrawing glucocorticoids gradually. Adrenal insufficiency can be minimized through alternate-day dosing and use of glucocorticoids that have an intermediate duration of action.

*Osteoporosis.* Glucocorticoid-induced osteoporosis can predispose the patient to fractures, especially of the ribs and vertebrae. Monitor patients for signs of compression fractures (neck or back pain) and for indications of

other fractures. Ideally, bone status should be evaluated periodically by bone densitometry. Development of osteoporosis can be reduced with calcium supplements, calcitriol (vitamin D), and edtidronate.

*Infection.* Glucocorticoids increase the risk of morbidity from infection. Warn patients against contact with persons who have communicable diseases. Inform patients about early signs of infection (e.g., fever, sore throat), and instruct them to notify the physician if these occur. Treat established infections with appropriate antimicrobial drugs, and withdraw glucocorticoids unless they are absolutely required.

*Glucose Intolerance.* Glucocorticoids can cause hyperglycemia and glycosuria. Diabetic patients may need to decrease their caloric intake and increase their dosage of hypoglycemic medication (insulin or oral hypoglycemic).

*Fluid and Electrolyte Disturbance.* Glucocorticoids can cause sodium and water retention and loss of potassium. These effects can be minimized by (1) using glucocorticoids that have low mineralocorticoid activity, (2) restricting sodium intake, and (3) taking potassium supplements or consuming potassium-rich foods (e.g., bananas, citrus fruits). Educate patients about signs and symptoms of fluid retention (e.g., weight gain, swelling of the lower extremities) and instruct them to notify the physician if these develop.

*Growth Retardation.* Glucocorticoids can suppress growth in children. Evaluate growth retardation by making periodic measurements of height and weight. Alternate-day therapy minimizes growth suppression.

*Cataracts.* Cataracts are a common complication of long-term therapy. The patient should receive an ophthalmologic examination every 6 months. Instruct the patient to notify the physician if vision becomes cloudy or blurred.

*Peptic Ulcer Disease.* Glucocorticoids may increase the risk of ulcer formation and can mask ulcer symptoms. Instruct the patient to notify the physician if feces become black and tarry. Have stools checked periodically for occult blood. If ulcers develop, glucocorticoids should be slowly withdrawn (unless their continued use is considered essential for life), and antiulcer therapy should be instituted.

*Use in Pregnancy and Lactation.* Glucocorticoids can induce adrenal hypoplasia in the developing fetus. When large doses have been employed, the newborn should be assessed for adrenal insufficiency, and given replacement therapy if indicated.

During high-dose therapy, the glucocorticoid content of breast milk may become high enough to affect the nursing infant. Warn women who are receiving high-dose therapy not to breast-feed.

*Other Adverse Effects. Psychologic disturbances, myopathy,* and *Cushing's syndrome* can be minimized by implementing the general measures noted at the beginning of this section. There are no specific measures to prevent these complications.

## Minimizing Adverse Interactions

*Interactions Related to Potassium Loss.* Glucocorticoid-induced potassium loss can be augmented by *potassium-depleting diuretics* (thiazides, loop diuretics) and can increase the risk of toxicity from *digoxin*. If digoxin and glucocorticoids are used concurrently, potassium levels should be monitored. Also, be alert for indications of cardiotoxicity.

*Nonsteroidal Anti-inflammatory Drugs.* NSAIDs can increase the risk of gastric ulceration during glucocorticoid therapy. Exercise caution when this combination is employed.

*Insulin and Oral Hypoglycemics.* Glucocorticoids can elevate blood levels of glucose. Diabetic patients may need to increase their dosage of insulin or oral hypoglycemic drug.

*Vaccines.* Glucocorticoids can decrease antibody responses to vaccines and can increase the risk of infection from live-virus vaccines. Attempts at immunization should not be made while glucocorticoids are being used.

# CHAPTER 66

# Drug Therapy of Rheumatoid Arthritis and Gout

In this chapter we will focus on the drug therapy of two inflammatory disorders: rheumatoid arthritis and gout. Some of the agents used to treat arthritis have been discussed in the preceding two chapters. Several additional agents are introduced here.

## Drug Therapy of Rheumatoid Arthritis

Rheumatoid arthritis is the most common systemic inflammatory disease, affecting between 5 and 8 million Americans. Although the disease can develop at any age, initial symptoms usually appear during the third and fourth decades. In younger patients, the incidence of arthritis is about 2.5 times greater in females than in males. However, in patients over 60, the incidence in men and women is equal. Rheumatoid arthritis follows a progressive course and can eventually cripple its victim. For some patients, drug therapy can halt the advance of the disease. However, for many patients benefits may be limited to symptomatic relief.

### Pathophysiology of Arthritis

Rheumatoid arthritis is an inflammatory disorder whose onset is heralded by symmetric joint stiffness and pain. Symptoms are most intense in the morning and abate as the day advances. Joints become swollen, tender, and warm. For some patients, periods of spontaneous remission occur. For others, injury progresses steadily. In addition to joint injury, rheumatoid arthritis is associated with weakness, fatigue, anorexia, and weight loss. An especially severe manifestation is vasculitis.

The progression of joint deterioration is depicted in Figure 66–1. Inflammation begins in the synovium—the membrane that encloses the joint cavity. The inflammatory process is self-reinforcing and complex; mediators include prostaglandins, immune factors, and other endogenous compounds. As inflammation intensifies, the synovial membrane thickens and begins to envelop the articular cartilage. This overgrowth is referred to as *pannus*. Damage to the cartilage is caused by enzymes released from the pannus and by chemicals and enzymes produced by the inflammatory process raging within the synovial space. Ultimately, the articular cartilage undergoes total destruction, resulting in direct contact between bones of the joint, followed by eventual bone fusion. After this, inflammation subsides. Although it is clear that an autoimmune process is central to the events described, the pathogenesis of rheumatoid arthritis remains incompletely understood.

### Overview of Therapy

Treatment has three major objectives: (1) relief of symptoms (pain, inflammation, stiffness), (2) maintenance of joint function and range of motion, and (3) prevention of deformity. To achieve these goals, a combination of pharmacologic and nonpharmacologic measures is employed.

#### Nondrug Measures

Nondrug measures for management of arthritis include physical therapy, exercise, and surgery. Physical therapy may consist of massage, warm baths, and application of heat to the affected regions. These procedures can enhance mobility and reduce inflammation. A balanced program of rest and exercise can decrease joint stiffness and improve function. However, excessive rest or exercise should be avoided: too much rest will foster stiffness, and too much activity can intensify inflammation.

Orthopedic surgery has made marked advances. For patients with severe disease of the hip or knee, total joint replacement can be performed. When joints of the hands or

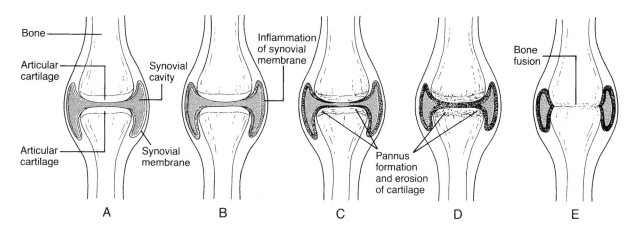

**Figure 66–1. Progressive joint degeneration in rheumatoid arthritis.** *A,* Healthy joint. *B,* Inflammation of synovial membrane. *C,* Onset of pannus formation and cartilage erosion. *D,* Pannus formation progresses and cartilage deteriorates further. *E,* Complete destruction of joint cavity together with fusion of articulating bones.

wrists have been damaged severely, function can be improved through removal of the diseased synovium and repair of ruptured tendons. Plastic implants can help correct deformities.

A complete program of treatment should include patient education and counseling. The patient should be informed about the nature of rheumatoid arthritis, the possible consequences of joint degeneration, management measures, and the benefits and limitations of drug therapy. If loss of mobility limits function at home, on the job, or in school, consultation with a social worker, occupational therapist, or specialist in vocational rehabilitation may be appropriate.

## Drug Therapy

Antiarthritic drugs can produce symptomatic relief, and, in some cases, may induce protracted remission. However, remission is rarely complete, and the disease usually advances steadily. As a result, drug therapy is chronic. Accordingly, successful treatment requires both motivation and cooperation on the part of the patient.

***Classification of Antiarthritic Drugs.*** As indicated in Table 66–1, the antiarthritic drugs fall into three major categories: (1) *nonsteroidal anti-inflammatory drugs* (NSAIDs), (2) *disease-modifying antirheumatic drugs* (DMARDs), and (3) *glucocorticoids* (adrenal corticosteroids). The NSAIDs can be subdivided into *salicylates* (e.g., aspirin, choline salicylate) and *nonsalicylates* (e.g., ibuprofen, naproxen). The DMARDs can be subdivided into (1) first-choice DMARDs (e.g., methotrexate, hydroxychloroquine), and (2) other DMARDs (e.g., gold salts, azathioprine).

The three major groups of antiarthritic drugs differ from one another with respect to (1) time course of action, (2) toxicity, and (3) ability to alter the progression of rheumatoid arthritis. The NSAIDs provide rapid relief of symptoms but do not alter disease progression. These drugs are safer than the DMARDs and the glucocorticoids; hence, treatment requires less vigorous monitoring. Like the NSAIDs, glucocorticoids provide rapid relief of symptoms

but do not retard disease progression. Since glucocorticoids can cause serious toxicity with long-term use, treatment is usually restricted to short courses. In contrast to the NSAIDs and glucocorticoids, DMARDs often retard the progression of rheumatoid arthritis. However, the onset of therapeutic effects is delayed, typically for 3 to 5 months. The DMARDs are more toxic than NSAIDs, and therefore vigorous monitoring is required.

***Drug Selection.*** Drug therapy of arthritis is based on severity of symptoms, the patient's response to treatment, and the patient's ability to tolerate a drug's side effects. A scheme for drug selection is depicted in Figure 66–2. As indicated, NSAIDs are the initial drugs of choice. Because of cost considerations, aspirin or another salicylate is usually chosen first. If side effects of the salicylates are intolerable, one of the newer (nonsalicylate) NSAIDs may be tried. If symptoms cannot be controlled with an NSAID, a DMARD is indicated. Unfortunately, the DMARDs are more toxic than the NSAIDs, and take several months to produce their effects. Since therapeutic effects are delayed, therapy with an NSAID should be continued until the DMARD has produced an adequate response. Of the DMARDs in use, the preferred agents are methotrexate, hydroxychloroquine, and sulfasalazine. (Rheumatologists have different opinions as to which of these three is best.) The other DMARDs—gold salts, azathioprine, penicillamine, and cyclosporine—should be employed only if the preferred (safer) DMARDs have been ineffective. Glucocorticoids are generally used on a short-term basis to provide symptomatic relief while responses to DMARDs are developing, and to supplement the effects of other drugs if symptoms "flare."

Until recently, patients with mild symptoms were treated with NSAIDs alone; DMARDs were employed only when NSAIDs were ineffective or produced intolerable side effects. Today, many rheumatologists initiate therapy with a DMARD together with an NSAID. This approach is employed in an effort to delay joint degeneration. Recall that NSAIDs only provide symptomatic relief; they do not retard the progression of rheumatoid arthritis. In contrast,

DMARDs may be able to arrest the disease process. Accordingly, by instituting DMARD therapy early (rather than waiting until joint degeneration has progressed to the point where NSAIDs can no longer control symptoms), it may be possible to delay or prevent serious joint injury. Since the effects of DMARDs take several months to develop, whereas responses to NSAIDs are immediate,

treatment is initiated with an NSAID along with the DMARD; once the DMARD has had time to act, the NSAID can be withdrawn.

Recently, combination therapy with two or more DMARDs has been tried. Available data indicate that these combinations can be more effective than therapy with just one DMARD.

## TABLE 66–1. DRUGS FOR RHEUMATOID ARTHRITIS

**NONSTEROIDAL ANTI-INFLAMMATORY DRUGS (NSAIDs)***

*Salicylates*

Aspirin
Choline salicylate [Arthropan]
Choline magnesium salicylate [Trilisate]
Magnesium salicylate [Magan, Mobidin]
Salsalate [Disalcid, Mono-Gesic]
Sodium salicylate

*Nonsalicylate NSAIDs*

Diclofenac [Voltaren]
Diflunisal [Dolobid]
Etodolac [Lodine]
Fenoprofen [Nalfon]
Flurbiprofen [Ansaid]
Ibuprofen [Motrin, Rufen]
Indomethacin [Indocin]
Ketoprofen [Orudis]
Meclofenamate [Meclomen]
Nabumetone [Relafen]
Naproxen [Naprosyn]
Naproxen sodium [Anaprox]
Oxaprozin [Daypro]
Piroxicam [Feldene]
Sulindac [Clinoril]
Tolmetin [Tolectin]

**DISEASE-MODIFYING ANTIRHEUMATIC DRUGS (DMARDs)†**

*First-Choice DMARDs*

Hydroxychloroquine [Plaquenil]
Methotrexate [Rheumatrex]
Sulfasalazine [Azulfidine]

*Other DMARDs*

Azathioprine [Imuran]
Cyclosporine [Sandimmune]
Gold Salts
  Auranofin [Ridaura]
  Aurothioglucose [Solganal]
  Gold sodium thiomalate [Myochrysine]
Penicillamine [Cuprimine, Depen]

**GLUCOCORTICOIDS‡**

Prednisolone
Prednisone

---

*NSAIDs relieve symptoms rapidly but do not retard the progression of rheumatoid arthritis. NSAIDs are safer than DMARDs and glucocorticoids and require less vigorous monitoring.
†DMARDs have a delayed onset of action (typically 3 to 5 months), and hence are also known as *slow-acting antirheumatic drugs* (SAARDs). DMARDs may retard the progression of arthritis. DMARDs are more toxic than NSAIDs and require more vigorous monitoring.
‡Glucocorticoids relieve symptoms rapidly but do not retard the progression of rheumatoid arthritis. Because of their toxicity, glucocorticoids are generally reserved for short-term therapy.

## Pharmacology of the Antiarthritic Drugs

### Salicylates

The basic pharmacology of the salicylates is discussed in Chapter 64. Consideration here is limited to the use of these drugs in arthritis.

*Role in Arthritis Therapy.* For most patients with rheumatoid arthritis, therapy is initiated with aspirin or another salicylate. These drugs are effective, fast acting, and inexpensive. Relief of symptoms is due primarily to anti-inflammatory actions, although analgesic effects are also beneficial. Salicylates only provide symptomatic relief; they do not slow progression of the disease.

*Adverse Effects.* Primary adverse effects are *gastrointestinal disturbances* (nausea, gastric distress, ulceration) and *suppression of platelet aggregation*. Use of enteric-coated tablets decreases the risk of gastrointestinal bleeding. Tinnitus and other signs of salicylism usually indicate toxicity. Accordingly, if these signs develop, salicylates should be temporarily withdrawn. Once symptoms have subsided, treatment should resume, but at a slightly reduced dosage. About 0.2% of patients experience hypersensitivity reactions. These reactions are most likely in patients who have nasal polyps, asthma, and hay fever.

*Dosage.* The dosages employed for anti-inflammatory effects are considerably higher than those required for analgesia or reduction of fever. Patients may need as much as 5.2 gm (16 standard tablets) of aspirin a day. Although there is no precise relationship between plasma salicylate levels and therapeutic responses, levels in the range of 15 to 30 mg/dl are usually effective. Dosages for the salicylates are summarized in Table 66–2.

*Achieving Compliance.* Because aspirin is such a commonplace drug—advertised on television and available over the counter—many patients do not believe in its efficacy. Consequently, if compliance is to be achieved, an effort must be made to convince patients that aspirin really works. In some cases, use of a prescription formulation may help persuade the patient that aspirin is indeed a legitimate and effective medication.

### Nonsalicylate NSAIDs

Like the salicylates, the nonsalicylate NSAIDs (e.g., ibuprofen, naproxen) are effective anti-inflammatory drugs and analgesics. Antirheumatic actions are equivalent to those of aspirin. However, for reasons that are not clear, some patients who fail to respond adequately to salicylates may respond more favorably to one of the nonsalicylates. Moreover, a particular patient may respond

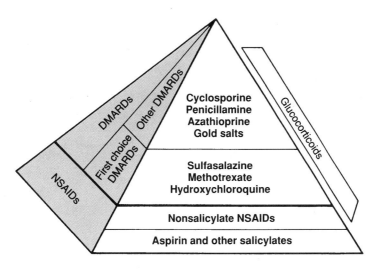

**Figure 66–2. Drug-selection pyramid for antiarthritic drugs.** Treatment is initiated with agents at the base of the pyramid. As the disease progresses, agents higher up the pyramid are indicated. Glucocorticoids may be used on a short-term basis at any stage of treatment. Drugs high on the pyramid are considerably more toxic than those near the base. (NSAIDs = nonsteroidal anti-inflammatory drugs, DMARDs = disease-modifying antirheumatic drugs.)

better to one nonsalicylate NSAID than to another. Consequently, trials with several different nonsalicylates may be needed before an optimal response is achieved. The nonsalicylate NSAIDs differ from the salicylate NSAIDs in two significant ways: (1) nonsalicylate NSAIDs are *more expensive* than the salicylates and (2) they tend to cause *less gastrointestinal bleeding* and *tinnitus.* Because of these differences, the nonsalicylates are usually

reserved for patients who began therapy with a salicylate but were unable to tolerate its side effects. However, if cost were not a factor, the nonsalicylate NSAIDs would probably replace the salicylates as the drugs of first choice for arthritis therapy. Antiarthritic dosages for the nonsalicylate NSAIDs are summarized in Table 66-2. A more complete discussion of these drugs is presented in Chapter 64.

## TABLE 66-2. ANTIARTHRITIC DOSAGES FOR NONSTEROIDAL ANTI-INFLAMMATORY DRUGS

| Generic Name | Trade Name | Daily Dosage |
| --- | --- | --- |
| *Salicylates* | | |
| Aspirin (extended release) | | 1.6 gm bid |
| Choline magnesium salicylate | Trisalate | 3 gm/day (in 1 to 3 doses) |
| Choline salicylate | Arthropan | 4.8-7.2 gm/day (in divided doses) |
| Magnesium salicylate | Magan | 1090 mg tid or qid |
| Salsalate | Disalcid, Mono-Gesic | 3.0-4.0 gm/day (in divided doses) |
| Sodium salicylate | | 3.6-5.4 gm/day (in divided doses) |
| *Nonsalicylate NSAIDs* | | |
| Diclofenac | Voltaren | 150-200 mg/day (in 3 or 4 doses) |
| Diflunisal | Dolobid | 250-500 mg bid |
| Etodolac | Lodine | 600-1200 mg/day (in 2 to 4 doses) |
| Fenoprofen | Nalfon | 300-600 mg tid or qid |
| Flurbiprofen | Ansaid | 200-300 mg/day (in 2 to 4 doses) |
| Ibuprofen | Motrin, Rufen | 600-800 mg tid or qid |
| Indomethacin | Indocin | 25-50 mg tid |
| Ketoprofen | Orudis | 150-300 mg (in 3 or 4 doses) |
| Meclofenamate | Meclomen | 200-400 mg/day (in 3 or 4 doses) |
| Nabumetone | Relafen | 1.5-2 gm/day (in 1 or 2 doses) |
| Naproxen | Naprosyn | 250-500 mg bid |
| Naproxen sodium | Anaprox | 250-500 mg bid |
| Oxaprozin | Daypro | 1.2 gm qd |
| Piroxicam | Feldene | 5 mg qid |
| Sulindac | Clinoril | 150-200 mg bid |
| Tolmetin | Tolectin | 200-400 mg tid |

## Glucocorticoids

The glucocorticoids are powerful anti-inflammatory drugs that can *relieve symptoms* of severe rheumatoid arthritis. These drugs do not induce remission and they do not halt the progression of the disease. For patients with generalized symptoms, *oral* glucocorticoids are indicated. However, if only one or two joints are affected, *intra-articular injections* may be employed. Because long-term oral therapy can cause serious toxicity (e.g., osteoporosis, gastric ulceration, adrenal suppression), oral glucocorticoids should be restricted to short-term use whenever possible. Most often, these drugs are given to provide temporary relief until drugs with a slower onset of action (e.g., methotrexate, hydroxychloroquine) can provide control. Long-term therapy should be limited to patients who have failed to respond adequately to all other forms of treatment. The most commonly employed oral glucocorticoids are prednisone and prednisolone. The usual dosage for either drug is 5 to 7.5 mg a day. The pharmacology of the glucocorticoids is discussed at length in Chapter 65 (Glucocorticoids in Nonendocrine Diseases).

## Methotrexate

Methotrexate [Rheumatrex] is the fastest acting of the disease-modifying antiarthritic drugs; therapeutic effects may be seen as early as 3 to 6 weeks. Many rheumatologists consider methotrexate the first-choice drug among the DMARDs. Major toxicities are *hepatic fibrosis*, *bone marrow suppression*, *gastrointestinal ulceration*, and *pneumonitis*. Periodic tests of liver and kidney function are mandatory, as are complete blood counts and platelet counts. Methotrexate can cause fetal death and congenital abnormalities, and hence is contraindicated during pregnancy. Methotrexate may be administered once weekly, beginning with a 5-mg dose. The weekly dose is then gradually increased to a maximum of 15 to 20 mg. The pharmacology of methotrexate is discussed at length in Chapter 96 (Anticancer Drugs).

## Hydroxychloroquine

*Actions and Uses.* Hydroxychloroquine [Plaquenil], a drug with antimalarial actions, can produce remission in patients with rheumatoid arthritis. Traditionally, the drug was reserved for patients who had not responded to NSAIDs. Today, the drug may be prescribed earlier in the course of the disease in an effort to delay joint degeneration. Hydroxychloroquine has a delayed onset of action; full therapeutic effects take 3 to 6 months to develop. Concurrent therapy with anti-inflammatory agents (NSAIDs or glucocorticoids) is indicated during the latency period. The mechanism by which hydroxychloroquine acts is not known.

*Toxicity.* The most serious toxicity is *retinal damage*. Retinopathy may be irreversible and can produce blindness. Visual loss is directly related to hydroxychloroquine dosage. Low doses may be used in long-term treatment with little risk. When dosage has been excessive, retinal damage may appear after treatment has ceased and may progress in the absence of continued drug use. Patients should receive a thorough ophthalmologic examination prior to treatment and every 6 months thereafter. Hydroxychloroquine should be discontinued at the first sign of retinal injury. Patients should be advised to contact the physician if any visual disturbance is noted.

*Preparations, Dosage, and Administration.* Hydroxychloroquine [Plaquenil] is dispensed in 200-mg tablets for oral administration. The initial dosage is 200 mg twice daily. Maintenance dosages range from 200 to 400 mg/day. The daily dosage should not exceed 6.4 mg/kg of body weight.

## Sulfasalazine

Sulfasalazine [Azulfidine], a drug used for years to treat inflammatory bowel disease (see Chapter 73), is now used to treat rheumatoid arthritis (although it is not approved by the FDA for this indication). Sulfasalazine can retard progression of joint deterioration and may be superior to hydroxychloroquine in this regard. In one clinical trial, sulfasalazine was as effective as intramuscular gold and caused less toxicity. Gastrointestinal reactions (nausea, vomiting, diarrhea, anorexia, abdominal pain) are the most common reason for discontinuing treatment. These reactions can be minimized by using enteric-coated formulations and by dividing the daily dosage. Dermatologic reactions (pruritus, rash, urticaria) are also common. Fortunately, serious adverse effects—hepatitis and bone marrow suppression—are relatively rare. To ensure early detection of these reactions, periodic monitoring for hepatitis and bone marrow function (complete blood counts, platelet counts) should be performed. The initial dosage for arthritis is 500 mg/day. This can be gradually increased to a maximum of 2 gm/day, administered in divided doses.

## Gold Salts

*Actions and Uses.* The beneficial effects of gold in rheumatoid arthritis have been known since the 1930s. Gold can relieve pain and stiffness and, for some patients, may arrest the progression of joint degeneration. Symptomatic improvement is seen in 60% to 70% of patients. About 15% experience remission. Because the toxicity of gold can be severe, therapy is often reserved for patients who have not responded adequately to salicylates or other NSAIDs. However, since gold salts may prevent joint degeneration, but cannot reverse damage that has already occurred, many rheumatologists begin treatment with gold early in the course of the disease.

Therapeutic effects take 4 to 6 months to develop. So that expectations can be realistic, patients should be made aware of this latency. Until a response has occurred, concurrent treatment with anti-inflammatory agents is indicated. If remission is less than complete, continued use of NSAIDs is needed.

Gold preparations are available for intramuscular and oral use. Patients receiving IM therapy require repeated injections over a prolonged period. The oral preparation is more convenient and less toxic than the IM preparations. Unfortunately, the oral preparation is also less effective.

The exact mechanism by which gold induces remission and relieves symptoms has not been determined. Likely contributory mechanisms are suppression of lysozyme release and suppression of the immune response.

*Toxicity.* Gold has a number of toxicities that can limit its use; about 15% to 20% of patients discontinue treatment because of adverse effects. Among the most common reactions are *intense pruritus*, *rashes*, and *stomatitis* (lesions of the oral mucosa). *Renal toxicity*, manifested as proteinuria, occurs frequently. *Severe blood dyscrasias* (thrombocytopenia, leukopenia, agranulocytosis, aplastic anemia) have developed, but these are rare. Other serious toxicities include encephalitis, hepatitis, peripheral neuritis, pulmonary infiltrates, and profound hypotension. *Oral* gold causes less mucocutaneous and renal toxicity than the intramuscular preparations, but *gastrointestinal reactions* (diarrhea, nausea, abdominal pain) with oral gold are common.

***Monitoring.*** Frequent laboratory tests and clinical evaluations are required to monitor toxicity. At each office visit the patient should be examined for dermatologic reactions and stomatitis. In addition, kidney and liver function must be monitored, and complete blood counts should be performed. The urine should be analyzed for protein. If signs of toxicity are detected, gold should be discontinued immediately. If the adverse reactions are mild, therapy may be resumed 2 to 3 weeks after symptoms have subsided. However, many rheumatologists believe that once *any* toxicity has occurred, further use of gold should be avoided. The chances of severe toxicity can be reduced by initiating treatment at low doses.

***Preparation, Dosage, and Administration.*** *Preparations.* Three gold preparations are available. Two of these—*aurothioglucose* [Solganal] and *gold sodium thiomalate* [Myochrysine]—are administered IM. The third preparation—*auranofin* [Ridaura]—is taken orally.

*Intramuscular Dosing.* On the first day of treatment, a 10-mg test dose is administered. This is followed on days 7 and 14 by doses of 25 mg. After this, 50-mg doses are injected weekly until a cumulative dose of 1 gm has been administered. If beneficial effects occur, therapy is continued but the dosing interval is gradually lengthened, first to 2 weeks, then to 3 weeks, and then to 1 month. In the absence of toxicity, monthly maintenance injections can be continued indefinitely.

*Oral Dosing.* The usual adult dosage is 6 mg/day (administered in one or two doses). If, after 6 months, the response is inadequate, the dosage may be increased to 3 mg 3 times a day for an additional 3 months. If the response is still insufficient, therapy should be discontinued.

## Penicillamine

Penicillamine [Cuprimine, Depen] can induce remission in patients with rheumatoid arthritis. However, treatment may be associated with serious toxicity, especially *bone marrow depression* and *autoimmune disorders*. Consequently, the drug is reserved for patients with severe disease who have failed to respond to more conventional therapy. Therapeutic effects take 2 to 3 months to develop. Arthritic symptoms can be suppressed with NSAIDs or glucocorticoids during this latency period. The initial dosage is 125 mg/day. The daily dosage can be increased by 125-mg increments every 2 to 3 months. Usual maintenance dosages range from 750 to 1000 mg daily. The pharmacology of penicillamine is discussed further in Chapter 100.

## Azathioprine

The antiarthritic effects of azathioprine [Imuran] are equivalent to those of gold salts and penicillamine. Benefits derive from immunosuppressive and anti-inflammatory actions. Serious toxicities include *hepatitis* and *blood dyscrasias* (leukopenia, thrombocytopenia, anemia). To monitor for these effects, complete blood counts, platelet counts, and tests of liver function are required. Azathioprine is teratogenic in animals and should not be used during pregnancy. The drug may also pose a small risk of malignancy. For treatment of arthritis, the initial dosage is 1 mg/kg/day. The dosage may be gradually increased to a maximum of 2.5 mg/kg/day. In addition to its use in arthritis, azathioprine is employed to prevent organ rejection in patients receiving kidney transplants. This application is discussed in Chapter 67.

### Investigational Agents

***Cyclosporine.*** Cyclosporine [Sandimmune], an immunosuppressive drug used to prevent rejection of transplanted organs, can reduce symptoms of arthritis. Because it can cause kidney damage and other serious adverse effects, cyclosporine is reserved for severe, progressive arthritis that has not responded to safer agents. In patients with an inadequate response to methotrexate, addition of cyclosporine has produced significant improvement. For treatment of arthritis, the dosage is 3 mg/kg/day. Cyclosporine is discussed at length in Chapter 67.

***Minocycline.*** There has long been speculation that *Mycoplasma* or *Chlamydia* may cause some cases of rheumatoid arthritis. Supporting this theory is the observation that minocycline [Minocin], an antibiotic in the tetracycline family, can improve arthritis symptoms.

***Antibodies to Tumor Necrosis Factor.*** When symptoms of rheumatoid arthritis flare, levels of tumor necrosis factor (TNF) in synovial fluid rise dramatically, suggesting that TNF may be an important causative factor. To test this possibility, researchers developed a monoclonal antibody that selectively binds TNF, thereby rendering TNF inactive. In early clinical trials, treatment with these anti-TNF antibodies has reduced joint swelling and pain.

## Drug Therapy of Gout

### Pathophysiology of Gout

Gout is a recurrent inflammatory disorder characterized by *hyperuricemia* (high blood levels of uric acid) and episodes of severe joint pain, typically in the large toe. Hyperuricemia can occur through two mechanisms: (1) excessive uric acid production and (2) impaired renal excretion of uric acid. Acute attacks are precipitated by crystallization of sodium urate (the sodium salt of uric acid) in the synovial space. Deposition of urate crystals promotes inflammation by triggering a complex series of events. A key feature of the inflammatory process is infiltration of leukocytes; once inside the synovial cavity, these cells phagocytize urate crystals and then break down, causing release of destructive lysosomal enzymes. When hyperuricemia is chronic, large and gritty deposits, known as *tophi*, may form in the affected joint. Also, renal damage may result from deposition of urate crystals in the kidney. Fortunately, when gout is detected and treated early, the disease can be arrested and these chronic sequelae avoided.

In the absence of treatment, gout progresses through four stages. Stage one consists of *asymptomatic hyperuricemia*. Stage two is characterized by attacks of *acute gouty arthritis*. In stage three, symptoms subside; hence, this phase is known as the *asymptomatic intercritical period*. Stage four—*tophaceous gout*—is distinguished by development of tophi in joints.

### Overview of Therapy

Five principal drugs are employed to treat gout. Two of these agents—*colchicine* and *indomethacin*—relieve inflammation. The other three—*allopurinol, probenecid,* and *sulfinpyrazone*—reduce hyperuricemia. Allopurinol reduces hyperuricemia by inhibiting uric acid formation. In contrast, probenecid and sulfinpyrazone reduce hyperuricemia by promoting uric acid excretion. Because they facilitate urate excretion, probenecid and sulfinpyrazone are called *uricosuric drugs*. In addition to the above agents, *glucocorticoids* and several *nonsteroidal anti-inflammatory drugs* may be employed.

Drug selection is determined by the stage of gout being treated. During stage one—asymptomatic hyperuricemia—drugs are rarely employed; treatment is indicated only if symptoms de-

## TABLE 66–3. DRUG THERAPY OF GOUT

| Stage of Gout | Drug Therapy | Comments |
|---|---|---|
| Asymptomatic hyperuricemia | Drugs rarely indicated | |
| Acute gouty arthritis | Colchicine, indomethacin, and other nonsteroidal anti-inflammatory agents Glucocorticoids | Colchicine is the drug of choice for the first episode. Indomethacin, which has fewer gastrointestinal side effects, is preferred for subsequent attacks. Glucocorticoids are reserved for patients who fail to respond to other agents. |
| Asymptomatic intercritical period | Colchicine Antihyperuricemics: Allopurinol Probenecid Sulfinpyrazone | Allopurinol is indicated if 24-hr urate excretion is high (>800 mg), indicating urate overproduction. A uricosuric agent (sulfinpyrazone, probenecid) is indicated if 24-hour urate excretion is <800 mg, indicating impaired urate excretion. |
| Chronic tophaceous gout | Allopurinol | The treatment objective is to decrease plasma urate below 7 mg/dl in males and 6 mg/dl in females. |

velop or if blood levels of uric acid rise exceptionally high. Stage two—acute gouty arthritis—is treated with colchicine (for the initial episode) and indomethacin (for subsequent attacks). Stage two may also be treated with nonsteroidal anti-inflammatory drugs and, in extreme cases, with glucocorticoids. Allopurinol and the uricosuric drugs should be avoided during stage two. Treatment during stage three—the intercritical period—is variable. Some patients do well on small doses of colchicine, others respond well to antihyperuricemic agents, and still others require no treatment at all. The objective in treating stage four—chronic tophaceous gout—is to promote dissolution of tophi by lowering plasma levels of urate. Allopurinol is the preferred agent for this stage. Drug therapy of gout is summarized in Table 66–3.

### Pharmacology of the Drugs Used to Treat Gout

#### Colchicine

Colchicine is an anti-inflammatory agent whose effects are specific for gout; the drug is ineffective for other inflammatory disorders. Colchicine is not an analgesic and does not relieve pain in conditions other than gout. The drug's principal adverse effect is gastrointestinal toxicity.

**Therapeutic Use.** Colchicine has three distinct applications in gout. The drug can be used to (1) treat acute gouty attacks, (2) reduce the incidence of attacks in chronic gout, and (3) abort an impending attack.

*Acute Gouty Arthritis.* When taken in large doses, colchicine produces dramatic relief of acute gouty attacks. Within hours, patients whose pain had made movement impossible are able to walk. Inflammation disappears completely within 2 to 3 days. Administration may be either intravenous or oral. With intravenous administration, symptoms resolve sooner than with oral administration, and gastrointestinal reactions are minimal. However, if extravasation occurs, intravenous colchicine can cause severe local necrosis.

*Prophylaxis of Gouty Attacks.* When taken during the asymptomatic intercritical period, small doses of colchicine (e.g., 0.5 to 1.0 mg/day) can decrease the frequency and intensity of acute attacks. Colchicine is also given for prophylaxis when therapy

with antihyperuricemic agents is initiated, since there is a tendency for gouty episodes to increase at this time.

*Abortion of an Impending Attack.* During prophylactic therapy with colchicine, patients may experience prodromal signs of a developing gouty attack. If large amounts of colchicine (e.g., 0.5 mg every 2 hours) are taken immediately, the attack may be prevented. Consequently, it is recommended that patients with chronic gout always have colchicine tablets on hand.

**Mechanism of Action.** We do not fully understand the mechanisms by which colchicine relieves or prevents episodes of gout. It is clear that the drug does not influence either the production or excretion of uric acid. An important contributory action is inhibition of leukocyte infiltration; in the absence of leukocytes, there is no phagocytosis of uric acid and no subsequent release of lysosomal enzymes. Leukocyte migration is inhibited by disruption of microtubules, the structures required for cellular motility. Since microtubules are also required for cell division, colchicine is toxic to any tissue that has a large percentage of proliferating cells. Disruption of cell division underlies the gastrointestinal toxicity of colchicine.

**Pharmacokinetics.** Colchicine is readily absorbed following oral administration. At therapeutic doses, large amounts re-enter the intestine via the bile and intestinal secretions. The drug is excreted primarily in the feces.

**Adverse Effects.** The most characteristic signs of colchicine toxicity are *nausea, vomiting, diarrhea,* and *abdominal pain.* These responses, which occur during treatment of acute gouty attacks, result from injury to the rapidly proliferating cells of the gastrointestinal epithelium. If gastrointestinal symptoms develop, colchicine should be discontinued immediately, regardless of the status of joint pain. As noted above, intravenous administration avoids most gastrointestinal toxicity. Diarrhea from colchicine can be managed with opioids.

**Precautions.** Colchicine should be used with care in elderly and debilitated patients, and in patients with cardiac, renal, and gastrointestinal diseases. Colchicine is classified in FDA Pregnancy Category C (for oral use) and Category D (for IV use). Since the drug can cause fetal harm, it should be avoided during pregnancy unless the perceived benefits outweigh the potential risks to the fetus.

***Preparations, Dosage, and Administration.*** Colchicine is dispensed in tablets (0.5 and 0.6 mg) for oral administration and in solution (1 mg/2 ml ampule) for intravenous administration.

*Oral.* For an acute gouty attack, the dosage is 0.5 to 1.2 mg initially followed by doses of 0.5 to 1.2 mg every 1 to 2 hours. Administration is repeated until pain is relieved or until signs of gastrointestinal toxicity appear. The total dose should not exceed 8 mg. The dosage for prophylaxis is 0.5 to 1.0 mg/day. The dosage for aborting an impending attack is 0.5 mg every 2 hours.

*Intravenous.* Intravenous administration can be used to treat an acute gouty attack. In many cases, relief can be achieved with a single 2-mg injection. To minimize vascular injury, the contents of 1 ampule (1 mg) should be diluted in 20 ml of sterile 0.9% sodium chloride and then injected slowly (over 5 minutes or more). Extravasation can result in local necrosis with sloughing of skin and subcutaneous tissue. Accordingly, care must be taken to ensure that the IV line remains in place.

### Indomethacin

Indomethacin [Indocin] is a nonsteroidal anti-inflammatory drug (NSAID) used to treat acute gouty arthritis. For treatment of gout, the drug's efficacy is equivalent to that of colchicine. Like colchicine, indomethacin does not reduce hyperuricemia. Rather, benefits derive from suppressing inflammation. In contrast to colchicine, indomethacin is devoid of severe gastrointestinal effects. Consequently, indomethacin is the drug of choice for treating acute gouty attacks once a diagnosis has been firmly established. The most characteristic side effect of indomethacin is *severe frontal headache*. Like other NSAIDs, indomethacin can promote *gastric ulceration* and should be avoided by patients with a history of peptic ulcer disease. *Probenecid* delays excretion of indomethacin. Accordingly, if probenecid and indomethacin are used together, a reduction in indomethacin dosage may be required. For relief of acute gouty arthritis, the adult dosage is 50 mg initially followed by 25-mg doses 3 to 4 times a day. Pain is relieved rapidly (within 2 to 4 hours); swelling subsides in 3 to 5 days. After this time, the dosage should be rapidly reduced, and then treatment should cease entirely. The pharmacology of indomethacin is discussed further in Chapter 64.

### Allopurinol

Allopurinol [Zyloprim] is used to reduce blood levels of uric acid. The drug is indicated for primary hyperuricemia of gout and for hyperuricemia occurring secondary to certain blood dyscrasias (e.g., polycythemia vera, leukemia) and to therapy with anticancer drugs.

***Mechanism of Action.*** Allopurinol and its major metabolite—alloxanthine—reduce uric acid levels by inhibiting uric acid production. Allopurinol and alloxanthine are *inhibitors of xanthine oxidase*, an enzyme required for uric acid formation. As indicated in Figure 66–3, xanthine oxidase catalyzes the final two reactions that lead to formation of uric acid from breakdown of DNA. By inhibiting xanthine oxidase, these compounds can reduce uric acid formation.

***Pharmacokinetics.*** Allopurinol is well absorbed following oral administration. Once absorbed, the drug undergoes rapid conversion to alloxanthine, an active metabolite. Since alloxanthine has a prolonged half-life (about 25 hours), therapeutic effects are long lasting. Consequently, allopurinol requires only once-a-day dosing.

***Use in Chronic Tophaceous Gout.*** Allopurinol is the drug of choice for chronic tophaceous gout. By reducing uric acid production and blood levels, the drug prevents tophus formation and promotes regression of tophi that have already formed, allowing joint function to improve. In addition, reversal of hyperuricemia decreases the risk of nephropathy that can occur from deposition of urate crystals in the kidney. During the initial months of treatment, allopurinol may *increase* the incidence of acute gouty arthritis; chances of an attack can be reduced by concurrent treatment with colchicine or indomethacin.

***Use in Secondary Hyperuricemia.*** Hyperuricemia may occur secondary to treatment with anticancer drugs. Uric acid levels are elevated because of the breakdown of DNA that occurs following cell death. To minimize elevations in plasma urate levels, allopurinol should be administered prior to initiation of cancer chemotherapy. Allopurinol is also useful for treating hyperuricemia that may occur secondary to certain blood dyscrasias (e.g., polycythemia vera, myeloid metaplasia, leukemia).

***Adverse Effects.*** Allopurinol is generally well tolerated. The most serious toxicity is a rare but potentially fatal *hypersensitivity syndrome*, characterized by rash, fever, eosinophilia, and dysfunction of the liver and kidneys. If rash or fever develops, allopurinol should be discontinued immediately. Many patients recover spontaneously; others may require hemodialysis or treatment with glucocorticoids.

Mild side effects seen occasionally include *gastrointestinal reactions* (nausea, vomiting, diarrhea, abdominal discomfort) and *neurologic effects* (drowsiness, headache, metallic taste). A few patients using allopurinol for a long time have developed *cataracts*; periodic ophthalmic examinations are recommended.

***Drug Interactions.*** Allopurinol can inhibit hepatic drug-metabolizing enzymes, thereby delaying the inactivation of other

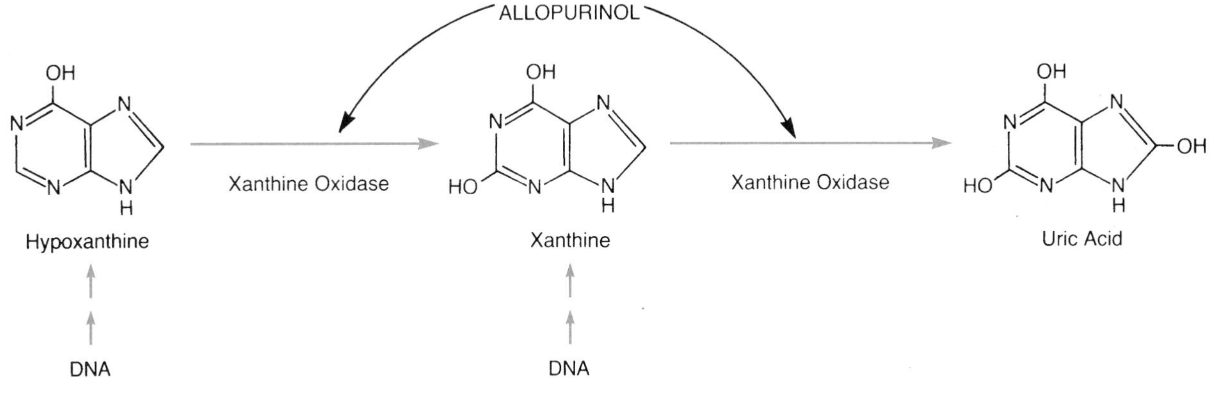

**Figure 66–3. Reduction of uric acid formation by allopurinol.**

drugs. This interaction is of particular concern for patients taking *oral anticoagulants* (e.g., warfarin), whose dosage should be reduced. Similarly, if allopurinol is combined with *mercaptopurine* or *azathioprine* in the treatment of cancer, dosages of mercaptopurine and azathioprine should be lowered by as much as 75%. The combination of allopurinol plus *ampicillin* is associated with a high incidence of rash; if rash develops, allopurinol should be discontinued immediately.

**Preparations, Dosage, and Administration.** Allopurinol [Zyloprim] is dispensed in 100- and 300-mg tablets for oral use.

For *treatment of chronic tophaceous gout*, the objective is to decrease plasma urate content to 7 mg/dl (or less) in males and 6 mg/dl (or less) in females. Dosages should be individualized to achieve this goal. The usual initial dosage is 100 mg once daily. The dosage is then increased by 100-mg increments at intervals of 1 week until urate has been reduced to an acceptable level, usually at doses of 200 to 300 mg/day. To prevent renal injury, fluid intake should be sufficient to maintain a urine flow of at least 2 L/day.

For *secondary hyperuricemias in adults*, dosages range from 100 to 800 mg/day. For *children* ages 6 to 10 years who are undergoing cancer chemotherapy, the recommended dosage is 300 mg daily. The dosage for children under 6 years is 150 mg/day.

### Probenecid

**Actions and Uses.** Probenecid [Benemid, Probalan] acts on renal tubules to inhibit reabsorption of uric acid. As a result, excretion of uric acid is increased and hyperuricemia is reduced. By lowering plasma urate levels, probenecid prevents formation of new tophi and facilitates regression of tophi that have already formed. The drug may exacerbate acute episodes of gout, and therefore treatment should be delayed until the acute attack has been controlled. During the initial months of therapy, probenecid may induce acute attacks of gout. If an attack occurs, colchicine or indomethacin should be added to the regimen. In addition to its use in gout, probenecid may be employed to prolong the effects of penicillins and cephalosporins (by delaying their excretion by the kidneys).

**Adverse Effects.** Probenecid is well tolerated by most patients. Mild gastrointestinal effects (nausea, vomiting, anorexia) occur occasionally. These responses can be reduced by administering the drug with food. Hypersensitivity reactions, usually manifested as rash, develop in about 4% of patients. Renal injury may occur from deposition of urate in the kidney. The risk of kidney damage can be minimized by alkalinizing the urine and consuming 2.5 to 3 L of fluid daily during the first few days of treatment.

**Drug Interactions.** Aspirin and other salicylates interfere with the uricosuric action of probenecid. Accordingly, probenecid should not be used concurrently with these drugs. Probenecid inhibits the renal excretion of several drugs, including indomethacin and sulfonamides; dosages of these agents may require reduction.

**Preparations, Dosage, and Administration.** Probenecid [Benemid, Probalan] is dispensed in 500-mg tablets. The initial dosage for adults is 250 mg twice daily for 1 week. The maintenance dosage is 500 mg twice daily. Administration with food decreases gastrointestinal upset. Therapy should not be initiated during an acute gouty attack.

### Sulfinpyrazone

**Actions and Uses.** Like probenecid, sulfinpyrazone [Anturane] is a uricosuric agent and is employed to reduce hyperuricemia in patients with *chronic* gout. The drug lacks antiinflammatory and analgesic actions and is of no benefit during an *acute* gouty attack. During the first few months of therapy, sulfinpyrazone may precipitate an acute gouty attack. The risk of an attack can be decreased by concurrent use of colchicine or indomethacin.

**Adverse Effects.** Gastrointestinal effects (nausea, abdominal pain) are common but rarely necessitate cessation of treatment. These reactions can be reduced by administering sulfinpyrazone with meals. Sulfinpyrazone can exacerbate gastrointestinal ulcers. The drug should be used cautiously in patients with a history of gastric ulcers and is contraindicated in patients with active ulcers. As with probenecid, there is a risk of uric acid deposition in the kidney. This risk can be reduced by alkalinizing the urine and ingesting large volumes of fluids.

**Drug Interactions.** *Salicylates* will counteract the uricosuric action of sulfinpyrazone; these drugs should not be taken concurrently. Sulfinpyrazone can inhibit hepatic metabolism of *tolbutamide* (causing hypoglycemia) and *warfarin* (causing bleeding tendencies). If combined with sulfinpyrazone, these drugs may require a reduction in dosage.

**Preparations, Dosage, and Administration.** Sulfinpyrazone [Anturane] is dispensed in 100-mg tablets and 200-mg capsules. Administration with meals decreases gastrointestinal side effects. The initial adult dosage is 100 to 200 mg twice daily. Maintenance dosages range from 200 to 800 mg/day in divided doses.

## KEY POINTS

- Therapy of rheumatoid arthritis has three objectives: reduction of symptoms (pain, inflammation, stiffness), maintenance of joint function and range of motion, and prevention of deformity.
- Arthritis is treated with three classes of drugs: nonsteroidal antiinflammatory drugs (NSAIDs), glucocorticoids, and disease-modifying antirheumatic drugs (DMARDs), which are also known as slow-acting antirheumatic drugs (SAARDs).
- NSAIDs and glucocorticoids act quickly to relieve symptoms of arthritis, but do not slow the progression of the disease.
- DMARDs slow the progression of rheumatoid arthritis, but their onset is delayed for weeks to months.
- NSAIDs are much safer than glucocorticoids or DMARDs.
- Traditionally, treatment of arthritis was initiated with NSAIDs alone; DMARDs were added only after NSAIDs could no longer control symptoms. Today, many rheumatologists begin therapy with NSAIDs *plus* a DMARD in an effort to delay joint degeneration.
- Because glucocorticoids cause serious toxicity when used long term, they are generally used short term to (1) control symptoms while responses to DMARDs are developing or (2) supplement other drugs when symptoms flare.
- The doses of NSAIDs used for rheumatoid arthritis are much higher than the doses used for pain or fever.
- Nonsalicylate NSAIDs (e.g., ibuprofen) are more expensive than salicylates (e.g., aspirin), but may cause less gastrointestinal bleeding.
- Methotrexate has a much faster onset than other DMARDs and is considered the DMARD of choice by many rheumatologists.
- Hydroxychloroquine can cause blindness secondary to retinal damage.

# CHAPTER 67

# Immunosuppressants

**Cyclosporine and Tacrolimus**
  Cyclosporine
  Tacrolimus

**Glucocorticoids**
**Cytotoxic Drugs**
**Antibodies**

mmunosuppressive drugs inhibit immune responses. These agents have two principal applications: (1) prevention of organ rejection in transplant patients, and (2) treatment of autoimmune disorders (e.g., rheumatoid arthritis, systemic lupus erythematosus). At the doses required to suppress allograft rejection, all of these drugs are toxic. Two toxicities are of particular concern: (1) increased risk of infection and (2) increased risk of neoplasms. Sites of action of immunosuppressants are summarized in Figure 67–1.

## Cyclosporine and Tacrolimus

Cyclosporine and tacrolimus are the most effective immunosuppressants available. Although these drugs are structurally dissimilar, they act by similar mechanisms. The principal application of these agents is prevention of organ rejection following transplantation. Cyclosporine was developed before tacrolimus and is used more frequently.

### Cyclosporine

Cyclosporine [Sandimmune, Neoral] is a powerful immunosuppressant and the drug of choice for preventing organ rejection following allogenic transplants. Major adverse effects are nephrotoxicity and increased risk of infection.

#### Mechanism of Action

Cyclosporine acts on T lymphocytes to suppress production of interleukin-2, gamma interferon, and other cytokines. The drug's primary molecular target is a protein known as *cyclophilin*. After binding to cyclophilin, cyclosporine inhibits *calcineurin*, a key enzyme in the pathway that leads to cytokine synthesis. In contrast to cytotoxic immunosuppressants (e.g., methotrexate), cyclosporine does not depress the bone marrow.

#### Therapeutic Uses

Cyclosporine is used primarily to prevent rejection of allogenic kidney, liver, and heart transplants. A glucocorticoid (prednisone) is usually given concurrently. Azathioprine may be given as well. In addition to its use in transplant patients, cyclosporine has been employed on an investigational basis to treat autoimmune diseases, including rheumatoid arthritis, psoriasis, myasthenia gravis, and early stages of insulin-dependent diabetes.

#### Pharmacokinetics

Oral administration is preferred; intravenous administration is reserved for patients who cannot take the drug orally. Absorption from the GI tract is incomplete (about 30%) and erratic. Accordingly, to avoid toxicity (from high drug levels) and organ rejection (from low drug levels), blood levels of cyclosporine should be measured periodically during long-term use.

Most cyclosporine in the body is bound. In the blood, the drug is bound to red cells (60% to 70%), leukocytes (10% to 20%), and plasma lipoproteins. Outside the vascular system, the drug is bound to tissues.

Cyclosporine undergoes extensive metabolism by hepatic microsomal enzymes. Hence, drugs that increase or decrease the activity of microsomal enzymes can have a significant impact on cyclosporine levels. Excretion of cyclosporine and its metabolites is via the bile. Practically none of the drug appears in the urine.

#### Adverse Effects

The most common adverse effects are nephrotoxicity, infection, hypertension, tremor, and hirsutism. Of these, nephrotoxicity and infection are the most serious.

*Nephrotoxicity.* Renal damage occurs in as many as 75% of patients. Injury manifests as reduced renal blood flow and reduced glomerular filtration rate. These effects are dose dependent and usually reverse following a decrease in cyclosporine dosage.

Nephrotoxicity is evaluated by monitoring for elevated blood urea nitrogen (BUN) and serum creatinine. However, be aware that a rise in these values could also indicate rejection of a kidney transplant. Patients should be informed about the possibility of kidney damage and the importance of periodic tests for BUN and creatinine.

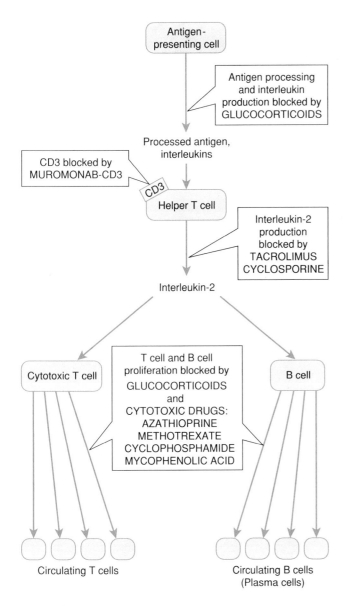

**Figure 67–1.** Sites of action of immunosuppressant drugs.

**Infection.** Cyclosporine increases the risk of infection, although less so than the cytotoxic immunosuppressants. Infectious complications occur in 74% of those treated. Patients should be warned about early signs of infection (fever, sore throat) and instructed to report these immediately.

**Hepatotoxicity.** Liver damage occurs in 4% to 7% of patients. Injury is evaluated by monitoring for serum bilirubin and liver transaminases. Signs of liver injury reverse rapidly with a reduction in dosage. Inform the patient about the need for periodic tests of liver function.

**Lymphomas.** Cyclosporine and other immunosuppressants can cause lymphoproliferative diseases. The incidence with cyclosporine alone is low. However, when cyclosporine is combined with other immunosuppressants, the risk of malignant lymphomas increases.

**Other Common Adverse Effects.** *Hypertension*, indicated by a 10% to 15% increase in blood pressure, develops in 13% to 53%

of patients. *Tremor* (21% to 55%) and *hirsutism* (21% to 45%) are also common. Less frequently, patients experience *leukopenia* (6%), *gingival hyperplasia* (4%), *gynecomastia* (4%), *sinusitis* (3% to 7%), and *hyperkalemia*.

**Anaphylactic Reactions.** These reactions are rare, occurring in 1 patient per 1000 treated. Signs of anaphylaxis are flushing, respiratory distress, hypotension, and tachycardia. Anaphylaxis occurs only with IV therapy—not with oral cyclosporine. Patients should be monitored for 30 minutes after the onset of IV treatment. If anaphylaxis develops, discontinue the infusion and treat with epinephrine and oxygen.

**Use in Pregnancy and Lactation.** At doses two to five times those used clinically, cyclosporine is embryotoxic and fetotoxic to rats and rabbits. However, experience to date shows minimal fetal risk in humans. Nonetheless, prudence dictates avoiding the drug during pregnancy if possible. Patients taking cyclosporine should be advised to use a mechanical form of contraception (condom, diaphragm); oral contraceptives should not be used. Cyclosporine is classified in FDA Pregnancy Category C. The drug is excreted in breast milk and nursing should be avoided.

## Drug and Food Interactions

Many interactions have been reported. However, only a few appear to be of clinical significance. Important interactions are considered below.

**Drugs That Can Decrease Cyclosporine Levels.** Drugs that induce hepatic microsomal enzymes can accelerate metabolism of cyclosporine, causing cyclosporine levels to fall. This can result in organ rejection. Drugs known to lower cyclosporine levels include *phenytoin*, *phenobarbital*, *rifampin*, and *trimethoprim-sulfamethoxazole*. Cyclosporine levels should be monitored and the dosage adjusted in patients taking these drugs.

**Drugs That Can Increase Cyclosporine Levels.** *Ketoconazole*, *erythromycin*, and *amphotericin B* can elevate cyclosporine levels (by inhibiting hepatic microsomal enzymes). When either of these drugs is combined with cyclosporine, the dosage of cyclosporine must be reduced to prevent accumulation to toxic levels.

Some physicians administer ketoconazole concurrently with cyclosporine for the express purpose of permitting a reduction in cyclosporine dosage. By slowing metabolism of cyclosporine, ketoconazole permits cyclosporine dosage to be reduced by up to 88%, while continuing to maintain cyclosporine levels within the therapeutic range. The lowered dosage greatly reduces the cost of treatment—from about $7000 per year to about $3000 per year.

**Nephrotoxic Drugs.** Renal damage may be intensified by concurrent use of other nephrotoxic drugs. These include *amphotericin B*, *aminoglycosides*, and *nonsteroidal anti-inflammatory drugs* (NSAIDs).

**Grapefruit Juice.** A compound present in grapefruit juice inhibits metabolism of cyclosporine. As a result, consuming grapefruit juice can raise cyclosporine levels by 50% to 200%, thereby greatly increasing the risk of toxicity.

### Preparations, Dosage, and Administration

**Preparations and Storage.** Cyclosporine is available under two trade names: Sandimmune and Neoral. Neoral differs from

Sandimmune in that cyclosporine is present as a microemulsion. As a result, absorption of Neoral is greater than absorption of Sandimmune. As Sandimmune, cyclosporine is available in capsules (25, 50, and 100 mg), an oral solution (100 mg/ml), and an IV solution (50 mg/ml). As Neoral, cyclosporine is available in capsules (25 and 100 mg) and an oral solution (100 mg/ml).

**Oral Therapy.** To improve palatability, the oral solution can be mixed with milk, chocolate milk, or orange juice just before administration. The initial dose is 15 mg/kg given 4 to 24 hours prior to surgery. This dose is continued once daily for 1 to 2 weeks. Dosage is then gradually reduced to a maintenance level of 3 to 10 mg/kg/day.

**Intravenous Therapy.** One milliliter of concentrate is diluted in 20 to 100 ml of 0.9% sodium chloride or 5% dextrose. The initial dose is 5 to 6 mg/kg (one-third the oral dose) administered over 2 to 6 hours. The solution should be protected from light. Because of the risk of anaphylaxis, epinephrine and oxygen must be immediately available. The patient should be switched to oral therapy as soon as possible.

**Monitoring.** Dosage is adjusted on the basis of nephrotoxicity and cyclosporine levels. Blood for drug levels is drawn just prior to the next dose. Target levels are generally 50 to 100 ng/ml in plasma or 250 to 800 ng/ml in whole blood.

## Tacrolimus

Tacrolimus [Prograf], formerly known as FK506, is an alternative to cyclosporine for prevention of organ rejection in patients receiving transplants. The drug is somewhat more effective than cyclosporine, but also more toxic.

**Therapeutic Use.** At this time, tacrolimus is approved only for prophylaxis of organ rejection in patients receiving liver transplants. Concurrent use of glucocorticoids is recommended. Compared with patients receiving cyclosporine, those receiving tacrolimus experienced fewer episodes of acute transplant rejection, but twice as many discontinued the drug because of toxicity. Tacrolimus is under investigation for use in patients receiving kidney, bone marrow, heart, pancreas, and small bowel transplants.

**Mechanism of Action.** Tacrolimus acts much like cyclosporine, although the two drugs are structurally dissimilar. Like cyclosporine, tacrolimus inhibits calcineurin, and thereby prevents T cells from producing interleukin-2, gamma interferon, and other cytokines. Tacrolimus and cyclosporine differ only in that cyclosporin must first bind to cyclophilin in order to act, whereas tacrolimus must first bind to a molecule named FK506-binding protein.

**Pharmacokinetics.** Tacrolimus may be administered orally or IV. Following oral administration, absorption is slow and incomplete; bioavailability is less than 25%. The drug is metabolized in the liver by an isozyme of cytochrome P-450. Excretion is via the bile. Less than 1% is excreted unchanged in the urine. The mean plasma half-life is 8 to 9 hours.

**Adverse Effects.** Adverse effects of tacrolimus are much like those of cyclosporine. As with cyclosporine, *nephrotoxicity* is the major concern; the incidence is 33% to 40%. Other common reactions include *neurotoxicity* (headache, tremor, insomnia), *GI effects* (diarrhea, nausea, vomiting), *hypertension*, *hyperkalemia*, and *hyperglycemia*. *Anaphylaxis* can occur with IV administration. Like other immunosuppressants, tacrolimus increases the risk of *infection* and *lymphomas*.

**Drug and Food Interactions.** Since tacrolimus is metabolized by an isozyme of cytochrome P-450, agents that inhibit the isozyme—erythromycin, ketoconazole, fluconazole, grapefruit juice—can increase tacrolimus levels. Like tacrolimus, NSAIDs can injure the kidneys. Accordingly, NSAIDs should be avoided.

**Preparations, Dosage, and Administration.** *Preparations.* Tacrolimus [Prograf] is dispensed in capsules (1 and 5 mg) for oral use and in solution (5 mg/ml) for IV use. For initial therapy, administration may be oral (if tolerated) or IV. For maintenance therapy, administration is oral.

*Intravenous.* The dosage range is 50 to 100 µg/kg/day. Administration is by continuous infusion. Treatment should begin no sooner than 6 hours after transplantation. Patients should switch to oral tacrolimus as soon as possible (usually 2 to 3 days after surgery).

*Oral.* The dosage range is 75 to 150 µg/kg every 12 hours. Oral therapy should begin 8 to 12 hours after the last IV dose. If treatment is initiated with oral therapy, the first dose should be given no sooner than 6 hours after surgery.

## Glucocorticoids

Glucocorticoids (e.g., prednisone) are used widely to suppress immune responses. Immunosuppressant applications range from suppression of transplant rejection to treatment of asthma to treatment of autoimmune disorders, such as rheumatoid arthritis and systemic lupus erythematosus.

Glucocorticoids have multiple effects on elements of the immune system. They cause lysis of antigen-activated lymphocytes, suppression of lymphocyte proliferation, and sequestration of lymphocytes at extravascular locations. In addition, they reduce production of interleukin-2 by monocytes and lymphocytes, and they reduce the responsiveness of T lymphocytes to interleukin-1.

Immunosuppressive doses are large. For example, to prevent organ rejection, an initial dose of 0.5 to 2 mg/kg of prednisone is employed. To treat episodes of acute organ rejection, 500 to 1500 mg of IV methylprednisolone is given.

Because large doses are employed, the full range of glucocorticoid adverse effects can be expected. These include increased risk of infection, thinning of the skin, bone dissolution with resultant fractures, impaired growth in children, and suppression of the hypothalamic-pituitary-adrenal axis.

The pharmacology of glucocorticoids is discussed at length in Chapter 65 (Glucocorticoids in Nonendocrine Diseases).

## Cytotoxic Drugs

Cytotoxic drugs suppress immune responses by killing B and T lymphocytes that are undergoing proliferation. With the exception of mycophenolate mofetil, these drugs are also toxic to all other proliferating cells. As a result, they can cause bone marrow depression, gastrointestinal disturbances, reduced fertility, and alopecia. Neutropenia and thrombocytopenia from bone marrow suppression are of particular concern. Because of their serious adverse effects, the cytotoxic drugs are usually reserved for patients who do not respond to safer immunosuppressants (cyclosporine and glucocorticoids).

### Azathioprine

*Mechanism of Action.* Azathioprine [Imuran] suppresses cell-mediated and humoral immune responses by inhibiting the proliferation of B and T lymphocytes. Azathioprine is a prodrug and must be converted to its active form—mercaptopurine—in the body. Mercaptopurine suppresses cell proliferation by inhibiting DNA synthesis. Hence, the drug acts selectively during the S phase of the cell cycle. As discussed in Chapter 96, mercaptopurine itself is used to treat cancer.

*Therapeutic Uses.* Prior to the advent of cyclosporine, azathioprine (combined with prednisone) was the principal drug employed to suppress rejection of renal transplants. Today, the drug is generally used as an adjunct to cyclosporine and glucocorticoids to help suppress transplant rejection. In addition, azathioprine is approved for severe refractory rheumatoid arthritis in nonpregnant adults (see Chapter 66). Azathioprine has been used on an investigational basis to treat various autoimmune diseases, including myasthenia gravis, systemic lupus erythematosus, Crohn's disease, ulcerative colitis, and insulin-dependent diabetes.

*Adverse Effects and Interactions.* Although uncommon at usual therapeutic doses, *neutropenia* and *thrombocytopenia* from bone marrow suppression can be serious concerns. Accordingly, patients should receive complete blood counts at regular intervals. Azathioprine is *mutagenic and teratogenic* in animals, and should be avoided during pregnancy. Long-term therapy is associated with an increased incidence of *neoplasms*.

*Allopurinol* delays conversion of mercaptopurine to inactive products, increasing the risk of toxicity. If allopurinol and azathioprine are used concurrently, the dose of azathioprine must be reduced by about 70%.

*Preparations, Dosage, and Administration.* Azathioprine [Imuran] is available in 50-mg tablets for oral administration, and as a powder to be reconstituted with sterile water for IV administration. Immunosuppressive therapy is initiated with a single daily dose of 3 to 5 mg/kg, usually beginning on the day of renal transplantation. Daily maintenance doses range from 1 to 3 mg/kg. Oral administration is preferred to intravenous.

### Cyclophosphamide

Cyclophosphamide [Cytoxan], an anticancer drug, is discussed at length in Chapter 96. Discussion here is limited to its immunosuppressant actions. Cyclophosphamide is a prodrug that is converted to its active form by the liver. The active form is an alkylating agent that cross-links DNA, leading to cell injury and death. Immunosuppressant effects result from a decrease in the number and activity of B and T lymphocytes. Toxicity to other cells produces adverse effects. These include neutropenia (from bone marrow suppression), hemorrhagic cystitis, and sterility in males and females. Cyclophosphamide has been used for its immunosuppressant actions to treat rheumatoid arthritis, systemic lupus erythematosus, and multiple sclerosis. The drug is as effective as azathioprine for suppressing rejection of renal transplants.

### Methotrexate

Methotrexate [Folex, Mexate, others] is an anticancer drug (see Chapter 96) that is also employed for immunosuppression.

As an immunosuppressant, the drug is approved for severe, refractory rheumatoid arthritis (see Chapter 66) and psoriasis. Methotrexate has also been used to suppress graft-versus-host disease in bone marrow recipients. These beneficial effects result from suppression of B and T lymphocytes secondary to interference with folate metabolism. The doses employed for immunosuppression are lower than those employed to treat cancers. As a result, toxicities differ with the two applications: in cancer chemotherapy, bone marrow suppression, ulcerative stomatitis, and renal damage are primary concerns, whereas in immunosuppressive therapy, hepatic fibrosis and cirrhosis are primary concerns.

### Mycophenolate Mofentil

*Therapeutic Use.* Mycophenolate mofentil [CellCept] is approved for prophylaxis of organ rejection in patients with allogenic renal transplants. The drug should be combined with cyclosporine and glucocorticoids.

*Mechanism of Action.* Following oral administration, mycophenolate mofentil is rapidly converted to mycophenolic acid (MPA), its active form. MPA then acts on B and T lymphocytes to inhibit inosine monophosphate dehydrogenase, an enzyme required for *de novo* synthesis of purines. Since these cells are uniquely dependent on *de novo* synthesis for proliferation (other cells acquire needed purines via salvage pathways), MPA causes selective inhibition of B and T lymphocyte proliferation.

*Pharmacokinetics.* Mycophenolate mofentil is administered orally, and undergoes nearly complete absorption, followed by rapid and nearly complete hydrolysis to MPA. MPA is converted in the liver to an inactive metabolite, which is then excreted in the urine. The half-life of MPA is about 18 hours.

*Adverse Effects.* Major adverse effects include *diarrhea, severe neutropenia, vomiting*, and *sepsis* (primarily cytomegalovirus viremia). As with other immunosuppressive drugs, there is an *increased risk of infection and malignancies*, especially lymphomas.

*Drug Interactions.* Absorption of mycophenolate can be decreased by *antacids* that contain magnesium and aluminum hydroxides and by *cholestyramine*, a drug used to lower cholesterol levels. Accordingly, mycophenolate should not be given simultaneously with antacids or cholestyramine.

*Use in Pregnancy.* When given to pregnant rats in doses at or below those used clinically, mycophenolate caused fetal malformations and fetal resorption. Controlled studies in women have not been performed. Because of the serious risk of fetal toxicity, the drug should be avoided during pregnancy. Before initiating treatment, pregnancy should be ruled out. During therapy, women of child-bearing age should use *two* reliable forms of contraception.

*Preparations, Dosage, and Administration.* Mycophenolate mofentil [CellCept] is dispensed in 250-mg capsules for oral administration. Treatment should begin no later than 72 hours after transplantation. For patients with renal transplants, the dosage is 1 mg twice daily. The regimen should also include cyclosporine and glucocorticoids.

## Antibodies

Antibodies directed against components of the immune system can suppress immune responses. Three preparations are considered here. Two of these—muromonab-CD3 and lymphocyte immune globulin—are used to manage allograft rejection in renal transplant recipients. The third—Rh₀(D) immune globulin—is used to prevent reactions to Rh-positive blood in Rh-negative women.

## Muromonab-CD3

***Actions and Uses.*** Muromonab-CD3 is a monoclonal antibody developed in mice and directed against the CD3 site on human T lymphocytes. Upon binding to the CD3 site, the antibody blocks all T cell functions. All T cells—both those in the circulation and those in tissues—are affected. Muromonab-CD3 is used primarily to prevent acute allograft rejection of kidney, heart, and liver transplants. In addition, the drug is given to deplete T cells from bone marrow prior to bone marrow transplantation.

***Adverse Effects.*** Relatively mild reactions are common. These include *fever* (73%), *chills* (59%), *dyspnea* (21%), *chest pain* (14%), and *nausea and vomiting* (12%). These effects are most intense on the first day of treatment and then rapidly subside.

In some patients, potentially fatal *anaphylactoid reactions* have occurred. Manifestations include pulmonary edema, cardiovascular collapse, and cardiac or respiratory arrest. Accordingly, patients should be monitored closely. Also, the drug should be used only in facilities with equipment and staffing for cardiopulmonary resuscitation.

***Preparations, Dosage, and Administration.*** Muromonab-CD3 [Orthoclone OKT3] is dispensed in solution (5 mg/5 ml) for IV administration. The usual dosage is 5 mg/day for 10 to 14 days. Administration is by IV bolus. The preparation should be drawn through a filter before injection. Treatment is begun following diagnosis of acute transplant rejection. To minimize first-dose adverse reactions, the patient should be pretreated with IV glucocorticoids.

## Lymphocyte Immune Globulin, Antithymocyte Globulin (Equine)

***Basic Pharmacology.*** Lymphocyte immune globulin [Atgam] is prepared by immunizing horses with human T lymphocytes. Therapeutic effects result from a decrease in the number and activity of thymus-derived lymphocytes. Lymphocyte immune globulin is approved for preventing rejection of renal transplants. Although not approved, it is also given to suppress organ rejection following liver, bone marrow, and heart transplants. Investigational uses include myasthenia gravis and multiple sclerosis. Lymphocyte immune globulin is usually employed in combination with glucocorticoids and azathioprine. Because these other immunosuppressants are present, immune reactions to this horse-derived drug are generally mild (chills, fever, leukopenia, skin reactions). However, anaphylactic reactions can occur. Accordingly, epinephrine and facilities for respiratory support should be immediately available.

***Preparations, Dosage, and Administration.*** Lymphocyte immune globulin is dispensed in solution (50 mg/ml) for IV administration. The concentrate should be diluted in saline according to the manufacturer's instructions, and the infusion apparatus should have an in-line filter. The usual adult dosage is 10 to 30 mg/kg/day administered over 4 hours or more. To minimize phlebitis, a high-flow vein should be employed. The patient must be monitored for anaphylaxis.

## Rh₀(D) Immune Globulin

***Actions and Uses.*** Rh₀(D) immune globulin (RhIG) is a concentrated preparation of immune globulin that contains antibodies to Rh₀(D). RhIG is given to prevent development of antibodies to Rh₀(D) in Rh₀(D)-negative women following exposure to Rh₀(D)-positive blood. Such exposure can occur in association with a Rh₀(D)-positive pregnancy (as a result of the pregnancy itself, full-term delivery, spontaneous or induced abortion, or amniocentesis). RhIG acts by suppressing the immune response of

Rh-negative women to Rh-positive blood cells. In many medical centers, RhIG is administered routinely at 28 weeks of gestation to all Rh₀(D)-negative women.

***Adverse Effects, Precautions, and Contraindications.*** Undesired reactions are uncommon and mild. Temperature may rise slightly. RhIG is contraindicated for Rh-positive women and must not be administered to newborns.

***Preparations, Dosage, and Administration.*** Rh₀(D) immune globulin [Gamulin, RhoGAM, others] is dispensed in vials and prefilled syringes for IM injection. Prevention of anti-Rh₀(D) antibody formation is most successful if the drug is administered twice: at 28 weeks of gestation and again within 72 hours after delivery.

## KEY POINTS

- Immunosuppressants are used to prevent organ rejection in transplant recipients and treat autoimmune disorders (e.g., rheumatoid arthritis).
- Immunosuppressants increase the risk of infection and lymphomas.
- Cyclosporine and tacrolimus are the most effective immunosuppressants available.
- Cyclosporine and tacrolimus are used primarily in transplant recipients.
- Cyclosporine causes kidney injury in up to 75% of patients.
- Renal damage from cyclosporine can be intensified by other nephrotoxic drugs, including amphotericin B, aminoglycosides, and NSAIDs.
- Drugs that inhibit hepatic microsomal enzymes can increase cyclosporine levels, and drugs that induce these enzymes can decrease cyclosporine levels.
- Grapefruit juice inhibits cyclosporine metabolism, and can thereby greatly increase cyclosporine levels.
- Like cyclosporine, tacrolimus causes renal damage, and hence should not be combined with other nephrotoxic drugs.
- Ketoconazole, fluconazole, grapefruit juice, and other agents that inhibit metabolism of tacrolimus can elevate its levels.
- Immunosuppressant applications of glucocorticoids include suppression of transplant rejection and treatment of rheumatoid arthritis and other autoimmune disorders.
- Prolonged use of glucocorticoids can result in osteoporosis, thinning of the skin, increased risk of infection, impaired growth in children, and adrenal insufficiency (secondary to suppression of the hypothalamic-pituitary-adrenal axis).
- Azathioprine and other cytotoxic drugs suppress immune responses by killing B and T lymphocytes.
- Cytotoxic immunosuppressants (except mycophenolate mofentil) injure all proliferating cells. As a result, they can cause bone marrow depression (neutropenia, thrombocytopenia), gastrointestinal disturbances, reduced fertility, and alopecia.
- Immune responses can be suppressed with muromonab-CD3 and other antibodies directed against components of the immune system.

# Summary of Major Nursing Implications*

## Cyclosporine

## Preadministration Assessment

### Therapeutic Goal
Prevention of allograft rejection.

### Baseline Data
Obtain baseline data on kidney function (serum creatinine, BUN), liver function (aspartate aminotransferase, alanine aminotransferase, serum amylase, bilirubin, alkaline phosphatase), and serum potassium levels.

### Identifying High-Risk Patients
Cyclosporine is *contraindicated* in the presence of *hypersensitivity to cyclosporine or to its intravenous vehicle* (polyoxyethylated castor oil), *pregnancy, recent inoculation with live-virus vaccines*, and *recent contact with or active infection with chickenpox or herpes zoster*.

Use with *caution* in patients using *potassium-sparing diuretics* and in those with *intestinal malabsorption, hypertension, hyperkalemia, active infection*, and *renal or hepatic dysfunction*.

## Implementation: Administration

### Routes
Oral, intravenous.

### Patient Education for Oral Administration
Dispense the oral liquid into a glass container using the specially calibrated pipette. Mix well and drink immediately. Rinse the container with diluent and drink to ensure ingestion of the complete dose. Dry the outside of the pipette and return to its cover for storage.

To improve palatability, mix the concentrated drug solution with milk, chocolate milk, or orange juice just before administration.

### Intravenous Dosage and Administration
Dilute 1 ml of concentrate in 20 to 100 ml of 0.9% sodium chloride or 5% dextrose. Protect from light. Administer the initial dose (5 to 6 mg/kg) slowly—over 2 to 6 hours. Because of the risk of anaphylactic reactions, monitor the patient closely for 30 minutes after beginning administration; have epinephrine and oxygen available. Switch to oral therapy as soon as possible.

### Dosage Adjustment
Adjust dosage on the basis of nephrotoxicity and cyclosporine levels. Draw blood for drug levels just prior to the next dose. Target levels are 50 to 100 ng/ml in plasma or 250 to 800 ng/ml in whole blood.

## Ongoing Evaluation and Interventions

### Evaluating Therapeutic Effects
Graft tenderness or fever may indicate rejection. In renal transplant patients, elevated BUN and elevated serum creatinine in conjunction with low cyclosporine may indicate rejection. Therapeutic failure can be confirmed with ultrasound, a biopsy, or renal flow scan.

### Minimizing Adverse Effects
***Nephrotoxicity.*** Cyclosporine can cause a dose-dependent reduction in kidney function. Monitor for elevation of serum creatinine and BUN. Inform outpatients about the importance of receiving periodic tests of kidney function.

***Infection.*** Cyclosporine increases the risk of infection. Inform patients about early signs of infection (fever, sore throat), and instruct them to report these immediately.

***Hepatotoxicity.*** Cyclosporine causes reversible liver damage. Monitor for elevation of serum bilirubin and liver transaminases. Inform patients about the need for periodic tests of liver function.

***Hirsutism.*** Cyclosporine promotes hair growth. Assure the patient that this effect is reversible.

***Use in Pregnancy and Lactation.*** Cyclosporine is embryotoxic. Advise women of child-bearing age to use a mechanical form of contraception (diaphragm, condom) and avoid oral contraceptives. Cyclosporine is excreted in breast milk; warn the patient against breast-feeding.

***Anaphylactic Reactions.*** See *Intravenous Dosage and Administration* above.

### Minimizing Adverse Interactions
***Drugs That Can Decrease Cyclosporine Levels.*** *Phenytoin, phenobarbital, rifampin*, and *trimethoprim-sulfamethoxazole* can reduce cyclosporine levels, leading to organ rejection. Monitor cyclosporine levels and increase the dosage as needed.

***Drugs That Can Increase Cyclosporine Levels.*** *Ketoconazole, erythromycin*, and *amphotericin B* can elevate cyclosporine levels, increasing the risk of toxicity. Monitor cyclosporine levels and reduce the dosage as needed.

***Nephrotoxic Drugs.*** *Amphotericin B, aminoglycosides*, and *nonsteroidal anti-inflammatory drugs* increase the risk of cyclosporine-induced kidney damage. Monitor renal function.

***Grapefruit Juice.*** Grapefruit juice inhibits cyclosporine metabolism, and can thereby increase cyclosporine levels. Toxicity may result.

---

*Patient education information is highlighted in color.

# Pediatric Immunization

The purpose of immunization is to protect against infectious diseases. Because of widespread immunization, the incidence of several infectious diseases has been dramatically reduced, and one disease—polio—has been eliminated entirely. Experience has shown that the most effective way to reduce vaccine-preventable disease is to have a highly immune population. Accordingly, universal vaccination is a national goal. Although immunization carries some risk, the risk from failing to vaccinate is much greater.

## General Considerations

### Definitions

In order to discuss immunization, we need to use some special terminology. Accordingly, we will begin the chapter by defining some important terms.

**Vaccine.** A vaccine is a preparation containing whole or fractionated microorganisms. Administration causes the recipient's immune system to manufacture antibodies directed against the microbe from which the vaccine was made. Most of the preparations discussed in this chapter are vaccines.

**Killed Vaccines versus Live Vaccines.** There are two major classes of vaccines: killed and live (albeit attenuated). Killed vaccines are composed of whole, killed microbes or isolated microbial components (e.g., the polysaccharide of *Haemophilus influenzae* type b or the surface antigen of hepatitis B). In contrast, live, attenuated vaccines are composed of live microbes that have been weakened or rendered completely avirulent. Live vaccines can be dangerous in recipients who are immunocompro-

mised, since these people are unable to mount an effective immune response, even against avirulent organisms.

**Toxoid.** A toxoid is a bacterial toxin that has been changed to a nontoxic form. Administration causes the recipient's immune system to manufacture antitoxins (i.e., antibodies directed against the natural bacterial toxin). Antitoxins protect against injury from toxins, but do not kill the bacteria that produce them. In this chapter, only two toxoids are considered: tetanus toxoid and diphtheria toxoid.

**Vaccination.** The terms *vaccination* and *vaccine* derive from *vaccinia*, a virus whose name in turn derives from *vacca* (Latin for cow). At one time, vaccinia virus was used as a vaccine against smallpox. (Vaccinia itself causes cowpox, a mild sickness, and in the process induces synthesis of smallpox antibodies.) Hence, when the term *vaccination* was originally coined, it had the limited meaning of giving vaccinia to generate immunity against smallpox. Today, vaccination refers broadly to administration of any vaccine or toxoid.

**Immunization: Active versus Passive.** *Immunization* is a more inclusive term than *vaccination*, in that immunization refers to production of both active immunity and passive immunity, whereas vaccination refers only to production of active immunity.

*Active immunity* develops in response to infection or to administration of a vaccine or toxoid. In either case, the result is endogenous production of antibodies. Active immunity takes weeks or months to develop but is long lasting. Discussion in this chapter is limited almost exclusively to active immunization.

*Passive immunity* is conferred by giving a patient *preformed* antibodies (immune globulins). Unlike active immunity, passive immunity protects immediately, but persists only as long as the antibodies remain in the body.

**TABLE 68-1. IMPACT OF VACCINATION ON INCIDENCE OF VACCINE-PREVENTABLE DISEASES**

| | Prevaccine Era: Maximum Number of Reported Cases (Year the Maximum Occurred) | Postvaccine Era: Number of Reported Cases in 1995 | Percentage Change in Reported Cases |
|---|---|---|---|
| Diphtheria | 206,939 (1921) | 0 | -99.99 |
| Pertussis | 265,269 (1934) | 4315 | -98.37 |
| Tetanus | 601 (1948) | 34 | -97.82 |
| Measles | 894,134 (1941) | 309 | -99.97 |
| Mumps | 152,209 (1968) | 840 | -99.45 |
| Rubella | 57,686 (1969) | 146 | -99.75 |
| Poliomyelitis (wild) | 21,269 (1952) | 0 | -99.99 |
| Invasive *Haemophilus influenzae* | 20,000* (1984) | 1164 | -94.18 |

* Estimated because national reporting did not exist in prevaccine era.

***Specific Immune Globulins.*** These preparations contain a high concentration of antibodies directed against a specific antigen (e.g., hepatitis B virus). Administration provides immediate passive immunity. These preparations are made from donated blood and do not transmit infectious diseases.

## Public Health Impact of Immunization

Widespread vaccination has made a profound impact on public health. As shown in Table 68-1, vaccination has greatly reduced the incidence of several infectious diseases (e.g., diphtheria, pertussis, tetanus). With two other diseases—polio and smallpox—results have been even more dramatic: polio has been eliminated from the Western hemisphere, and smallpox has been eliminated from the planet.

Despite these successes, we still have a long way to go. Nationally, more than one child in every three falls behind on his or her immunizations by the age of 2 years. In some parts of the country, more than 50% of the children are not current. The consequences of failing to vaccinate can be enormous. For example, between 1989 and 1991, a measles epidemic occurred; 55,000 cases were reported, 11,000 people were hospitalized, and more than 130 people died, half of them young children.

The Childhood Immunization Initiative, begun in 1993, is directed at preventing such epidemics in the future. The goal of the program is to eliminate all indigenous cases of diphtheria, measles, rubella, tetanus, and *Haemophilus influenzae* b infection from the United States. The program aims to achieve these goals by improving vaccine delivery systems, increasing community participation, reducing vaccine costs to parents, developing safer and simpler vaccines, and involving more federal agencies in providing vaccines to populations who otherwise might not have access to them.

From a strictly economic viewpoint, vaccination is a wonderful investment. On average, we save $14 in future health care costs for each dollar spent on vaccination.

## Adverse Effects of Immunization

Vaccines are generally very safe. Although mild reactions are common, serious events are rare. Many children experience local reactions (discomfort, swelling, and erythema at the injection site). Fever is also common. Potential severe effects include anaphylaxis (e.g., in response to measles, mumps, and rubella virus vaccine); acute encephalopathy (caused by diphtheria, tetanus, and pertussis vaccine); and vaccine-associated paralytic poliomyelitis (caused by *oral* poliovirus vaccine).

*Immunocompromised children* are at special risk from *live* vaccines. The reason is that, in the absence of an adequate immune response, the viruses or bacteria in these normally safe vaccines are able to multiply in profusion, thereby causing serious infection. Accordingly, live vaccines should generally be avoided in children who are severely immunosuppressed. Causes of immunosuppression include congenital immunodeficiency, HIV infection, leukemia, lymphoma, generalized malignancy, and therapy with cytotoxic anticancer drugs, radiation, and high-dose glucocorticoids.

The risk of serious adverse reactions can be minimized by observing appropriate *precautions* and *contraindications*. Table 68-2 lists contraindications that apply to all vaccines. Precautions and contraindications that apply to specific vaccines are discussed in the context of those preparations. Certain conditions, such as diarrhea and mild illness, may be inappropriately regarded as contraindications by some practitioners. As a result, vaccination may be needlessly postponed. Conditions that are often considered contraindications, although they are not, are also listed in Table 68-2.

Practitioners are required to report certain adverse events to the *Vaccine Adverse Events Reporting System* (VAERS). The information is used to help determine whether (1) a particular event that occurs after vaccination is actually caused by the vaccine, and (2) what the risk factors might be. In addition to reporting events that they are required to report on, practitioners should

## TABLE 68-2. CONTRAINDICATIONS THAT APPLY TO ALL VACCINES AND CONDITIONS OFTEN INCORRECTLY REGARDED AS CONTRAINDICATIONS

| True Contraindications (Vaccine Should Not Be Administered) | Not Contraindications (Vaccine May be Administered) |
| --- | --- |
| Anaphylactic reaction to a vaccine contraindicates further doses of that vaccine | Mild to moderate local reaction (soreness, erythema, swelling) following a dose of an injectable vaccine |
| Anaphylactic reaction to a vaccine component contraindicates use of all vaccines that contain that substance | Mild acute illness with or without low-grade fever |
| Moderate or severe illnesses with or without a fever | Diarrhea |
|  | Current antimicrobial therapy |
|  | Convalescent phase of illnesses |
|  | Prematurity (same dosage and indications as for normal, full-term infants) |
|  | Recent exposure to an infectious disease |
|  | Personal or family history of either penicillin allergy or nonspecific allergies |

report all other serious or unusual adverse events, regardless of whether they believe the event was caused by the vaccine. Forms for reporting adverse events can be obtained by calling the VAERS automated recording at 800-822-7967.

The *National Vaccine Injury Compensation Program* (NVCIP), established by the Childhood Vaccine Injury Act of 1986, was created to provide compensation for injury or death resulting from vaccination. The program is intended as an alternative to civil litigation in that negligence need not be proved. As a provision of the law, a table was created listing the vaccines covered by the program and the injuries, disabilities, illness, and conditions (including death) for which compensation may be paid. Compensation may also be paid for injuries not listed in the table, provided that (1) a listed vaccine is involved and (2) causality can be demonstrated. Injuries related to vaccines not listed in the table are not covered under the program. Additional information can be obtained by calling the NVCIP automated recording at 800-338-2382.

### Immunization Records

The National Childhood Vaccine Act of 1986 requires a permanent record of each mandated vaccination a child receives. The information should be recorded in either (1) the permanent medical record of the recipient or (2) a permanent office log or file. The following data are required:

- Date of vaccination
- Route and site of vaccination
- Vaccine type, manufacturer, lot number, and expiration date
- Name, address, and title of the person administering the vaccine

The purpose of these records is twofold. First, they help ensure the child receives appropriate vaccinations. Second, they help avoid overvaccination, and thereby reduce the risk of possible hypersensitivity reactions. To promote uniformity in record keeping, an official immunization card has been adopted by every state and the District of Columbia.

### Reporting Vaccine-Preventable Diseases

Public health officials rely on health care providers to report cases of vaccine-preventable disease. Nearly all vaccine-preventable diseases that occur in the United States are notifiable. Health care providers should report individual cases to their local or state health department. Each week, the state health departments make a report to the Centers for Disease Control and Prevention (CDC). The information gathered is used to (1) determine if an outbreak is occurring, (2) evaluate prevention and control strategies, and (3) evaluate the impact of national immunization policies and practices.

## Target Diseases

Routine childhood vaccination is currently recommended for protection against 10 infectious diseases: diphtheria, tetanus (lockjaw), pertussis (whooping cough), measles, mumps, rubella, invasive *Haemophilus influenzae* type b, hepatitis B, poliomyelitis, and varicella (chickenpox). In the discussion below, some diseases are considered in a group (e.g., measles, mumps, rubella). The reason is that vaccination against these diseases is usually done simultaneously.

## Measles, Mumps, and Rubella

**Measles.** Measles is a highly contagious viral disease characterized by rash and high fever (103°F to 105°F). Infection is spread by inhalation of aerosolized sputum or by direct contact with nasal or throat secretions. Initial symptoms include fever, cough, headache, sore throat, and conjunctivitis. Three days later, rash develops. Rash begins at the hairline, spreads to the rest of the body in 36 hours, and then fades in a few days. Secondary infections can result in pneumonia and otitis media (inner ear infection). However, of the potential complications of measles, *encephalitis* is by far the most serious concern. Sequelae of encephalitis include blindness, deafness, and convulsions. Although encephalitis is rare (0.1% incidence), it carries a 10% risk of death.

**Mumps.** Mumps is a viral disease that primarily affects the parotid glands (the largest of the three pairs of salivary glands). Although mumps can occur in adults, it usually occurs in children ages 5 to 15. As a rule, the first symptom is swelling in one of the parotid glands. Swelling is often associated with pain and tenderness. The patients may also experience fever (100°F to 104°F). Swelling increases for 2 to 3 days and then fades entirely by day 6 or 7. Swelling in the second parotid gland often develops after swelling in the first, but may also occur simultaneously or not at all. Painful *orchitis* (inflammation of the testes) develops in about one-third of adult and adolescent males. Acute aseptic *meningitis* develops in about 10% of all patients; symptoms, which resolve completely, include dizziness, headache, and vomiting. In the United States, the incidence of reported mumps cases has declined from a high of 152,209 in 1968 to only 840 in 1995.

**Rubella.** Rubella, also known as German measles, is a generally mild viral infection. However, if it occurs during pregnancy, the consequences can be severe. Initial symptoms include sore throat, mild fever, and swelling in lymph nodes located behind the ears and the back of the neck. Shortly after, a rash develops on the face and scalp, spreads rapidly to the torso and arms, and then fades in 2 or 3 days. Arthritis may also develop, mainly in women. In pregnant women, rubella can cause miscarriage, stillbirth, and congenital defects, especially if the disease occurs during the first trimester. Possible birth defects include cataracts, heart disease, mental retardation, and deafness. In the United States, the incidence of reported rubella cases peaked at 57,686 in 1969, but was only 146 in 1996.

## Diphtheria, Tetanus, and Pertussis

**Diphtheria.** Diphtheria is a potentially fatal infection caused by *Corynebacterium diphtheriae*, a gram-positive bacillus. The bacterium colonizes the throat and nasal passages, and produces a toxin that spreads throughout the body. Initial symptoms include sore throat, fever, headache, and nausea. Colonization of the airway begins as patches of gray or dirty-yellow membrane that eventually grow together, forming a thick coating. This coating, combined with swelling, can impede swallowing and breathing; in severe cases, a tracheostomy is needed. The toxin produced by *C. diphtheriae* can damage the heart and nerves, resulting in heart failure and paralysis. Treatment of diphtheria includes administration of diphtheria antitoxin and antibiotics (e.g., erythromycin, penicillin G). In the United States, only 37 cases were reported between 1980 and 1992. However, of those infected, about 10% died, mainly children and the elderly. No cases were reported in 1995.

**Tetanus (Lockjaw).** Tetanus, also known as lockjaw, is a frequently fatal disease characterized by painful spasm of all skeletal muscles. The cause is a potent endotoxin elaborated by *Clostridium tetani*, a gram-positive bacillus. Infection with *C. tetani* typically results from puncturing the skin with a nail, splinter, or other object that is contaminated with soil, street dust, or animal or human feces. The first symptom is often stiffness of the jaw, hence the name lockjaw. As infection progresses, the patient may experience stiff neck, difficulty swallowing, restlessness, irritability, headache, chills, fever, and convulsions. Eventually, spasm develops in muscles of the abdomen, back, neck, and face. The case fatality rate is 21%. The yearly incidence of tetanus peaked at 601 cases in 1948, but was only 34 cases in 1995. Treatment options include tetanus antitoxin, a booster dose of tetanus toxoid, and antibiotics (e.g., penicillin G, a tetracycline).

**Pertussis (Whooping Cough).** Pertussis, also known as whooping cough, occurs primarily in infants and young children. The cause is *Bordetella pertussis*, a gram-negative bacillus. Initial symptoms include rhinorrhea, mild fever, and persistent cough. As infection worsens, coughing becomes more intense. The acute phase of the disease can last 4 to 6 weeks. During this time, infants experience difficulty eating, drinking, and breathing. Deaths have occurred. Complications of pertussis include pneumonia, seizures, ear infections, and, rarely, permanent neurologic injury. In the United States, reported cases dropped from a high of 265,269 in 1934 to 4315 in 1995. Worldwide, the disease afflicts about 60 million people, and kills 700,000 each year, mainly infants and young children. The drug of choice for treating pertussis is erythromycin.

## Poliomyelitis

Poliomyelitis, also known as polio or infantile paralysis, is a serious disease in which the poliovirus attacks neurons of the central nervous system that control muscle movement. The result is skeletal muscle paralysis, usually in the legs; however, muscles of respiration and muscles of the arms may also be affected. In about 10% of cases, polio is fatal. The disease is caused by three different polioviruses. Paralytic polio is usually caused by type 1 poliovirus. Polio has no cure. However, proper symptomatic treatment can improve comfort and reduce or prevent some crippling effects. Vaccination against polio has eliminated the disease from the Western hemisphere, except for eight to nine cases annually that are caused by the vaccine itself.

### Haemophilus Influenzae, Type b

*Haemophilus influenzae*, type b, is a gram-negative bacterium that can cause meningitis, pneumonia, and serious throat and ear infections. The bacterium is the leading cause of serious illness in children under the age of 5 years, and the most common cause of bacterial meningitis, which has a mortality rate of 5%. Among children who survive meningitis, between 25% and 35% suffer lasting neurologic sequelae. As a result of childhood vaccination, the annual incidence of infection dropped from an estimated 20,000 cases in 1991 to less than 1200 in 1995. Of the cases that occurred, almost all were in children who were not vaccinated. Infection with *H. influenzae* can be treated successfully with antibiotics.

### Varicella (Chickenpox)

Varicella (chickenpox) is a common, highly contagious, and potentially serious disease of childhood. The causative organism is varicella-zoster virus, a member of the herpesvirus group. Patients typically develop 250 to 500 maculopapular or vesicular lesions, usually on the face, scalp, or trunk. Other symptoms include fever, malaise, and loss of appetite. Among children, the most common complications are bacterial suprainfection and acute cerebellar ataxia; Reye's syndrome and encephalitis develop rarely. Among adults, the most serious common complication is varicella pneumonia. As a rule, symptoms in adults are more severe than in children: hospitalization is 10 times more likely in adults, and death is 20 times more likely. (Although adults account for only 2% of varicella cases, they account for 50% of varicella-induced deaths). Prior to the availability of varicella vaccine, 90% to 95% of children in the United States got chickenpox by age 11, which corresponds to 4 million cases a year.

*Herpes zoster*, also known as *shingles* or simply *zoster*, develops in 15% of cases years after childhood chickenpox has resolved. The cause of zoster is reactivation of varicella-zoster viruses that had been dormant within sensory nerve roots. Episodes of zoster begin with neurologic pain in the area of skin supplied by the affected nerve roots. Blister-like lesions develop within 3 to 4 days, and usually disappear 2 to 3 weeks later. However, in about 14% of patients, neurologic pain persists for a month or more—and in a few cases, pain lasts for years.

### Hepatitis B

Hepatitis B is a serious liver infection caused by the hepatitis B virus. *Acute* infection can cause anorexia, malaise, diarrhea, vomiting, jaundice, pain (in muscles, joints, and stomach), and death. *Chronic* infection can result in cirrhosis, liver cancer, and death. Each year in the United States, hepatitis B infects 150,000 people, puts 11,000 in the hospital, and kills 4000 to 5000. Worldwide, 170 million people have chronic hepatitis B, and 250,000 die from it annually.

Although hepatitis B is found in virtually all body fluids, only blood, serum-derived fluids, saliva, semen, and vaginal fluids are infectious. The most common modes of transmission are needle-stick accidents, sexual contact with an infected partner, maternal-child transmission during birth, and use of contaminated IV equipment or solutions.

## Specific Vaccines and Toxoids

The discussion below is limited to the vaccines and toxoids used most often for childhood immunization. Also, the discussion focuses almost exclusively on immunization of children; vaccination of adults is mentioned only occasionally. The major preparations used for childhood immunization are listed in Table 68–3. Their adverse effects are summarized in Table 68–4. Childhood immunization schedules for 1997, as recommended by the Advisory Committee on Immunization Practices (ACIP) of the Centers for Disease Control and Prevention, the American Academy of Pediatrics (AAP), and the American Academy of Family Physicians (AAFP) are summarized in Figure 68–1.

### Measles, Mumps, and Rubella Virus Vaccine (MMR)

**Description.** Measles, mumps, and rubella vaccine (MMR), marketed under the trade name M-M-R II, is a combination product composed of three live-virus vaccines. Administration induces synthesis of antibodies directed against measles, mumps, and rubella viruses. Immunization with MMR is preferred to immunization with the three vaccines separately.

**Efficacy.** Following a single dose of MMR, an effective response develops in 97% of vaccinees within 2 to 6 weeks.

**Adverse Effects.** *Mild.* Local soreness, erythema, and swelling may develop soon after vaccination. Within 1 to 2 weeks, some children experience glandular swelling in the cheeks and neck and under the jaw. Transient rash develops in 5% to 15% of vaccinees. Fever (103°F or higher) that persists for several days occurs in 5% to 15% of vaccinees 5 to 12 days after vaccination. MMR-induced fever poses a small risk of febrile seizures, but there is no evidence of residual seizure disorders. Within 1 to 3 weeks of the first dose, about 1% of vaccinees experience pain, stiffness, and swelling in one or more joints; these symptoms usually subside in a few days, but on rare occasions persist for a month or more. Fever, soreness, and pain can be reduced with acetaminophen or a nonaspirin nonsteroidal anti-inflammatory drug, such as ibuprofen.

*Severe.* Transient *thrombocytopenia* occurs rarely (0.0025% incidence). MMR-induced thrombocytopenia is generally benign, but hemorrhage has developed in a few vaccinees.

MMR may induce *anaphylactic reactions*. However, the incidence is extremely low: only 11 certain cases have occurred in over 70 million vaccinations. Until recently, MMR-induced anaphylaxis was thought to result from al-

### TABLE 68-3. SOME VACCINES AND TOXOIDS AVAILABLE IN THE UNITED STATES

| Preparation Name (Synonym) | Trade Names | Type of Preparation | Route and Site |
|---|---|---|---|
| Measles, Mumps, and Rubella Virus Vaccine (MMR) | M-M-R II | Live virus | SC, in outer aspect of upper arm |
| Diphtheria and Tetanus Toxoids and Whole-Cell Pertussis Vaccine (DTwP) | Tri-Immunol | Toxoids (diphtheria and tetanus) plus inactivated whole bacteria (pertussis) | IM, in deltoid or medio-lateral thigh |
| Diphtheria and Tetanus Toxoids and Acellular Pertussis Vaccine (DTaP) | Tripedia, Acel-Immune, Infanrix | Toxoids (diphtheria and tetanus) plus inactivated bacterial components (pertussis) | IM, in deltoid or medio-lateral thigh |
| Tetanus and Diphtheria Toxoids (DT [pediatric], Td [adult]) | Generic only | Toxoids | IM, in deltoid or medio-lateral thigh |
| *Haemophilus influenzae* type b (Hib) Conjugate Vaccine | HibTITER, OmniHIB, PedvaxHIB | Bacterial polysaccharide conjugated to protein | IM, in midthigh or outer aspect of upper arm |
| Poliovirus Vaccine, inactivated (IPV, Salk vaccine) | IPOL | Inactivated viruses of all three polio serotypes | SC, in anterolateral thigh |
| Poliovirus Vaccine, oral (OPV, Sabin vaccine) | Orimune | Live viruses of all three of polio serotypes | PO |
| Varicella Virus Vaccine | Varivax | Live virus | SC, in deltoid or antero-lateral thigh |
| Hepatitis B Vaccine (HBV) | Recombivax HB, Energix-B | Inactive viral antigen | IM, in deltoid or antero-lateral thigh |

lergy to eggs (the measles component of the vaccine is produced in chick embryo fibroblasts). However, new studies suggest that egg allergy is not involved. Currently, the leading suspect is a hydrolysis product of gelatin. Until more is known, authorities now recommend that MMR be used with extreme caution in children with a known al-

lergy to gelatin. The ACIP is reconsidering whether caution is still required for children with an allergy to eggs.

***Precautions and Contraindications.*** MMR is *contraindicated* during *pregnancy* and should be used with *caution* in children with a history of (1) *thrombocytopenia* or *thrombocytopenic purpura* or (2) *anaphylactic-*

### TABLE 68-4. ADVERSE EFFECTS OF SOME VACCINES AND TOXOIDS

| Preparation | Mild Effects | Serious Effects |
|---|---|---|
| Measles, Mumps, and Rubella Virus Vaccine | Local reactions; rash; fever; swollen glands in cheeks and neck and under the jaw; pain, stiffness, and swelling in joints | Anaphylaxis, thrombo-cytopenia |
| Diphtheria and Tetanus Toxoids and Pertussis Vaccine, whole-cell or acellular* | Local reactions, fever, fretfulness, drowsiness, anorexia, persistent crying | Acute encephalopathy, convulsions, shock-like state |
| *Haemophilus influenzae* type b conjugate vaccine | Local reactions, fever, crying, diarrhea, vomiting | None |
| Poliovirus Vaccine (IPV and OPV) | Local reactions (only from IPV) | Vaccine-associated paralytic poliomyelitis (only from OPV) |
| Varicella Virus Vaccine | Local reactions, fever, mild varicella-like rash (local or generalized) | None |
| Hepatitis B Vaccine | Local discomfort, fever | Anaphylaxis |

*Acellular DTP causes fever and milder effects than whole-cell DTP.

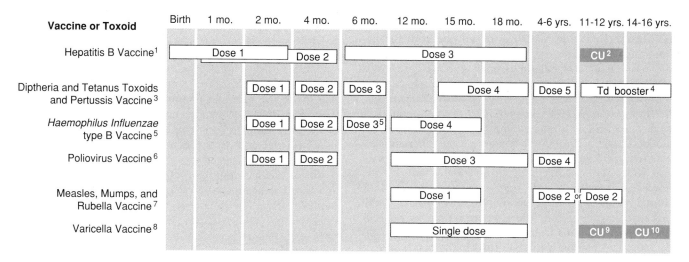

**Figure 68–1. Recommended Childhood Immunization Schedule: United States, 1997.** Based on joint recommendations by the Advisory Committee on Immunization Practices (ACIP) of the Centers for Disease Control and Prevention, the American Academy of Pediatrics (AAP), and the American Academy of Family Physicians (AAFP). *Unshaded boxes* indicate recommended ages for each dose; a box that spans more than one age bracket indicates an acceptable range of ages for that dose. *Shaded boxes* indicate "catch-up" (CU) vaccination.

[1]The immunization schedule for infants is based on whether the mother is *hepatitis B surface antigen (HBsAg)-positive or HBsAg-negative* (i.e., on whether the mother has laboratory evidence of hepatitis B infection). The unshaded boxes indicate the immunization schedule for infants born to HBsAg-negative mothers. The schedule for infants born to HBsAg-positive mothers is discussed in the text under *Hepatitis B Vaccine.*

Children and adolescents who were not vaccinated against hepatitis B during infancy may begin the series at any time. Once the first dose is given, the second dose is given 1 month (or more) later, and the third dose is given 4 months (or more) after the first dose and no less than 2 months after the second dose.

[2]Children who have not been vaccinated with HBV yet should initiate the series at age 11 to 12 years.

[3]*Diphtheria and tetanus toxoids and acellular pertussis vaccine* (DTaP) is the preferred vaccine for all doses in the series, including completion of the series in children who started with one or more doses of *diphtheria and tetanus toxoids plus whole-cell pertussis vaccine* (DPwT). However, although DTaP is preferred, DPwT is an acceptable alternative. The fourth dose of DTaP may be administered to children as young as 12 months, provided 6 months have elapsed since the third dose and the child is considered unlikely to return at age 15 to 18 months.

[4]*Tetanus toxoid plus diphtheria toxoid for adult use* (Td) is recommended at age 11 to 12 years if at least 5 years have elapsed since the last dose of DTwP, DTaP, or diphtheria toxoid plus tetanus toxoid for children. Subsequent routine Td boosters are recommended every 10 years.

[5]Three *Haemophilus influenzae* type b (Hib) conjugate vaccines are licensed in the United States for infant use. If PRP-OMP [PedvaxHIB] is administered at 2 and 4 months, a dose at age 6 months is not required; otherwise, it must be given. After completing the primary series, any Hib conjugate vaccine may be used as a booster.

[6]Two poliovirus vaccines are currently licensed in the United States: *inactivated poliovirus vaccine* (IPV) and *oral poliovirus vaccine* (OPV). Three vaccination schedules are acceptable to the ACIP, AAP, and AAFP. Parents and providers may choose among them:

• IPV at 2 and 4 months and OPV at 12 to 18 months and 4 to 6 years
• IPV at 2, 4, and 12 to 18 months and 4 to 6 years
• OPV at 2, 4, and 6 to 18 months and 4 to 6 years

The ACIP routinely recommends the first schedule. IPV is the only poliovirus vaccine recommended for immunocompromised children and their household contacts.

[7]The second dose of measles-mumps-rubella vaccine is routinely recommended at either 4 to 6 years or 11 to 12 years, but may be administered during any visit provided that (1) at least 1 month has elapsed since the first dose and (2) both doses are administered at or after age 12 months.

[8]Susceptible children may receive varicella vaccine during any visit after the first birthday.

[9]Unvaccinated children who lack a reliable history of chickenpox should be vaccinated at age 11 to 12 years.

[10]Susceptible children ages 13 years and older should receive two doses at least 1 month apart.

*like reactions to gelatin, eggs,* or *neomycin* (MMR contains a small amount of this antibiotic).

MMR can be administered to children with *mild febrile illness* (e.g., upper respiratory infection with or without low-grade fever). However, for children with *moderate or severe febrile illness*, administration should be postponed until the illness has resolved.

Products that contain *immune globulins* (e.g., whole blood, serum, specific immune globulins) contain antibodies against the viruses in MMR, and therefor can inhibit the immune response to the vaccine. Accordingly, in children who have received immune globulins, vaccination with MMR should be postponed for at least 3 to 6 months.

In vaccinees who are *immunocompromised*, replication of the viruses in MMR can be enhanced. If the immunodeficiency is severe, death may occur. However, of the more than 200 million people who have received MMR in the United States, only 5 such deaths have been reported. Nonetheless, *children with severe immunodeficiency should NOT be given MMR*. Severe immunodeficiency may result from immunosuppressive drugs (e.g., glucocorticoids, cytotoxic anticancer drugs), certain cancers (e.g., leukemia, lymphoma, generalized malignancy), and from *advanced* HIV infection. It is important to note, however, that if HIV infection is *asymptomatic*, MMR should be given. In these people, there is no risk of serious adverse events from MMR, whereas there *is* a risk of severe complications from measles if this disease should develop. Vaccination with MMR early in the course of HIV infection is preferred, since the immune response to vaccination diminishes as HIV infection progresses.

**Route, Site, and Immunization Schedule.** MMR is administered SC into the outer aspect of the upper arm. Each child should receive two vaccinations, the first between 12 and 15 months of age, and the second between 4 and 6 years or 11 and 12 years.

## Diphtheria and Tetanus Toxoids and Pertussis Vaccine (DPT)

**Preparations.** Vaccination against diphtheria, tetanus, and pertussis is usually done simultaneously using a combination product. Two types of products are available; one type contains *whole-cell* pertussis and one contains *acellular* pertussis. The whole-cell preparation (DTwP) is composed of diphtheria toxoid, tetanus toxoid, and a whole-cell pertussis vaccine, consisting of *Bordetella pertussis* that has been inactivated or partially detoxified. The acellular preparation (DTaP) also contains diphtheria and tetanus toxoids; however, instead of whole-cell pertussis vaccine, it contains acellular pertussis vaccine. *DTaP is more effective than DTwP and causes fewer and milder side effects.* Vaccination with DTwP or DTaP produces antibodies directed against diphtheria and tetanus toxins and against *Bordetella pertussis*. DTwP is marketed under the trade name Tri-Immunol. DTaP is available under three trade names: Tripedia, Acel-Imune, and Infanrix.

**Efficacy.** Immunization with DTP reduces the risk of disease by 80% to 90%. Protection begins after the third dose and persists 4 to 6 years (against pertussis) and 10 years (against diphtheria and tetanus). Protection against pertussis is better with DTaP than with DTwP.

**Adverse Effects.** *Mild.* Mild reactions are common. The reactions seen most often are *low fever* (50%), *fretfulness* (50%), *drowsiness* (30%), *anorexia* (20%), and *local reactions* (pain [50%], swelling [40%], and redness [30%]). Mild reactions usually develop a few hours to 48 hours after vaccination and then resolve in 1 to 2 days. Acetaminophen or ibuprofen can be used to decrease fever and pain. Mild reactions are much more likely with DTwP than with DTaP.

*Moderate.* Moderate reactions occur less often than mild reactions. *Persistent, inconsolable crying*, lasting 3 hours or longer, occurs in 1% of vaccinees. Crying is most likely with the first dose of DTP and is not associated with long-term sequelae. *Fever* (105°F or higher) occurs in 0.3% of vaccinees; the pertussis component appears responsible. Approximately 0.06% of vaccinees develop *convulsions* (with or without fever). These seizures have no permanent sequelae and do not increase the risk of subsequent febrile or afebrile seizures. A *shock-like state* develops in 0.06% of vaccines and has no lasting sequelae.

*Severe: Encephalopathy.* Very rarely, DTP causes acute encephalopathy. The incidence is between zero and 10.5 episodes per million doses. Most cases occur within 3 days of vaccination. Some of the children who experience acute encephalopathy develop chronic neurologic dysfunction later in life. However, the contribution of acute encephalopathy to long-term neurologic deficits is unclear.

**Precautions and Contraindications.** DTP can be administered to children with *mild febrile illness* (e.g., upper respiratory infection with or without low-grade fever). However, for children with *moderate or severe febrile illness*, administration should be postponed until the illness has resolved.

DPT is *contraindicated* if a prior vaccination with DPT produced (1) an immediate anaphylactic reaction or (2) encephalopathy within 7 days of vaccination.

DPT should be administered with *caution* (if at all) if a prior vaccination with DPT produced any of the following:

- A shock-like state
- Fever (105°F or higher) occurring within 48 hours of vaccination and not attributable to another identifiable cause
- Persistent, inconsolable crying lasting 3 or more hours and occurring within 48 hours of vaccination
- Convulsions (with or without fever) occurring within 3 days of vaccination.

**Route, Site, and Immunization Schedule.** DTP is injected IM into the deltoid or thigh. Most children should receive 5 injections, the first at 2 months, the second at 4 months, the third at 6 months, the fourth between 15 and 18 months, and the fifth between 4 and 6 yours. DTaP is preferred to DTwP for all vaccinations in the series, even for children who began the series with DTwP. Children 11 to 12 years old who completed the DPT series at least 5 years previously should receive a booster shot of tetanus plus diphtheria toxoids for adults (Td). Subsequent Td boosters are recommended every 10 years.

## Poliovirus Vaccine

**Preparations.** We have two vaccines against polioviruses: *oral poliovirus vaccine* (OPV, Sabin vaccine) and *inactivated poliovirus vaccine* (IPV, Salk vaccine). OPV is composed of live, attenuated viruses. In contrast, IPV is composed of *inactivated* polioviruses. As discussed below, OPV has *caused* polio in a few children, whereas IPV has not and cannot. Accordingly, IPV is now recommended by the ACIP for initial immunization. Unfortunately, although IPV is safer than OPV, it is also 50% more expensive. Trade names are IPOL (for IPV) and Orimune (for OPV).

***Efficacy.*** Between 97.5% and 100% of children receiving IPV or OPV develop antibodies to poliovirus types 1, 2, and 3. Antibodies develop after two or more doses and persist for many years.

***Adverse Effects of IPV.*** IPV is devoid of serious adverse effects. As with other injected drugs, local soreness may occur. IPV contains trace amounts of streptomycin, neomycin, and bacitracin. Accordingly, children with an allergy to these drugs should use OPV rather than IPV.

***Adverse Effects of OPV.*** Very rarely, OPV causes *vaccine-associated paralytic poliomyelitis* (VAPP). The severity of VAPP is similar to that of paralytic poliomyelitis caused by the wild-type virus; in immunocompromised children, VAPP can prove fatal. The incidence of VAPP is one case for each 2.4 million doses of OPV administered, which corresponds to 1 case for each 750,000 children starting the vaccination series. In the United States, eight to nine cases of VAPP occur each year. Since wild-type poliovirus has been eliminated from the Western hemisphere, the risk for Americans of acquiring polio from OPV now greatly exceeds the risk of acquiring the disease from the environment. In response to this change in risk/benefit ratio, the ACIP recently changed its recommendations on polio immunization: whereas OCP had been the preferred vaccine for many years, the ACIP now recommends a transition to IVP.

Because of the risk of VAPP, OPV should not be given to individuals who are immunocompromised. This includes those with congenital immunodeficiency or HIV infection, and those taking immunosuppressive drugs (e.g., glucocorticoids, cytotoxic anticancer drugs).

Immunocompetent persons receiving OPV represent a risk for persons who are immunocompromised. This is because the viruses in OPV multiply within the vaccinee's GI tract, and can then be transmitted in saliva and feces. The risk of transmission can be reduced by avoiding contact with saliva (e.g., by not sharing food or utensils) and with feces (e.g., by having someone else change the baby's diapers) and by practicing rigorous hygiene, especially hand washing.

***Route, Site, and Immunization Schedule.*** IPV is administered SC in the anterolateral thigh. OPV is given by mouth (obviously). Three vaccination schedules may be used:

- *Sequential IPV/OPV*—give IPV for the first two doses (at ages 2 and 4 months) and then OPV for the third and fourth doses (at ages 12 to 18 months and 4 to 6 years)
- *All IPV*—give IPV at ages 2 months, 4 months, 12 to 18 months, and 4 to 6 years
- *All OPV*—give OPV at ages 2 months, 4 months, 6 to 18 months, and 4 to 6 years

Because of the risk of acquiring polio from OPV, the ACIP now recommends the sequential IPV/OPV schedule for most children. However, *immunocompromised children* should use the *all IPV* schedule because they are at increased risk of acquiring polio from OPV.

## *Haemophilus influenzae* Type b Conjugate Vaccine

***Preparations.*** Vaccines directed against *Haemophilus influenzae* type b (Hib) vaccines are prepared by conjugating (covalently binding) a purified capsular polysaccharide (PRP) from *H. influenzae* to either (1) diphtheria toxoid, (2) tetanus toxoid, or (3) an outer membrane protein (OMP) isolated from *Neisseria meningitidis*. The reason for conjugating PRP to these compounds is to enhance its antigenicity. The vaccine made with OMP, marketed as PedvaxHIB and abbreviated PRP-OMP, elicits a stronger immune response than the vaccines made with diphtheria toxoid [HibTITER] or tetanus toxoid [OmniHIB].

***Efficacy.*** Immunization with Hib vaccine decreases the risk of disease by 88% to 98%. When PedvaxHIB is used, protection begins 1 week after the first dose. However, when HibTITER or OmniHIB is used, protection is delayed, beginning 1 to 2 weeks after the fourth dose. With all three vaccines, protection persists for several years.

***Adverse Effects.*** Hib vaccine is among the safest of all vaccines. Serious adverse effects have not been reported. The few adverse effects that do occur are generally transient and mild. Between 2% and 5% of vaccinees develop local reactions (swelling, erythema, warmth, tenderness). About 1% experience fever (>101°F), crying, diarrhea, or vomiting.

***Route, Site, and Immunization Schedule.*** Hib vaccines are administered IM into the midthigh or the outer aspect of the upper arm. Most children should receive four doses, the first at 2 months of age, the second at 4 months, the third at 6 months, and the fourth between 12 and 15 months. If PRP-OMP [PedvaxHIB] is used for the first two doses, the third dose (6-month dose) can be omitted.

## Varicella Virus Vaccine

***Preparations.*** Varicella virus vaccine [Varivax] is composed of live, attenuated varicella viruses. Administration induces synthesis of antibodies against the virus. Varicella vaccine was developed in Japan in 1973, but was not available in the United States until March of 1995.

***Efficacy.*** In children less than 12 years old, a single dose of varicella produces antibodies in 97% of recipients; however, in children 13 to 17 years old, only 79% develop antibodies after one dose. In Japan, testing of people who were vaccinated 20 years earlier revealed that antibodies were still present.

Even though most vaccinees develop antibodies to varicella viruses, not everyone with antibodies is fully protected. Immunization *completely* prevents chickenpox in 85% to 96% of vaccinees. Among the 4% to 15% who get chickenpox despite vaccination, symptoms are *always* mild: these children develop fewer lesions (<35, compared with 250 to 500 for unvaccinated children), experience less fever, and recover more quickly. In Japan, herpes zoster (shingles) has not been observed in any adult who received varicella vaccine as a child, even if breakthrough chickenpox occurred. As use of the vaccine in the United States increases, children who remain unvaccinated will be less likely to get chickenpox during childhood, and hence more likely to remain susceptible into adulthood, when the infection is much more severe.

**Adverse Effects.** Varicella vaccine is very safe; no serious adverse events have been reported. About 25% of vaccinees experience erythema, soreness, and swelling at the injection site; 15% develop fever (>102°F); and 3% develop a mild, local varicella-like rash, consisting of just a few lesions. About 5% of healthy children develop a sparse, generalized varicella-like rash within a month of the injection; in children with leukemia, the incidence of generalized rash is much higher—about 50%.

In theory, children receiving the vaccine can transmit vaccine-virus to others. However, among otherwise healthy vaccinees, such transmission has not been reported. In contrast, among leukemic children who developed a rash after vaccination, a few cases of viral transmission have occurred. To reduce the risk of transmission, vaccine recipients should temporarily avoid close contact with susceptible, high-risk individuals (e.g., neonates, pregnant women, immunocompromised people).

**Precautions and Contraindications.** Varicella vaccine is contraindicated during *pregnancy*, for individuals with certain *cancers* (e.g., leukemia, lymphomas), and for those with *hypersensitivity to neomycin or gelatin*, which are in the vaccine. In addition, the vaccine should be avoided by individuals who are *immunocompromised*. This includes those with HIV infection or congenital immunodeficiency and those taking immunosuppressive drugs.

Children receiving the vaccine should avoid *aspirin and other salicylates* for 6 weeks. This precaution is based on the theoretical risk of developing Reye's syndrome: if the child develops chickenpox (albeit a mild case) in response to the vaccine, the very small risk of developing Reye's syndrome is made slightly larger by concurrent use of salicylates.

**Route, Site, and Immunization Schedule.** Varicella vaccine is administered SC into the outer aspect of the upper arm or the anterolateral thigh. Since the vaccine wasn't available in the United States before the spring of 1995, many children missed being vaccinated at the preferred age: 12 to 18 months. Accordingly, the vaccination schedule for older children necessarily differs from that for younger children. Current recommendations are as follows:

- *Children 12 to 18 months old.* Most children in this age group should receive a single dose of vaccine. No additional doses are needed.
- *Children 19 months through 12 years old.* Children in this age group who have not been vaccinated yet and have not had chickenpox can be vaccinated now. A single dose is all that is needed. Many physicians wait until these children are 11 to 12 years old to administer this catch-up dose. However, a single vaccination can be administered at any time prior to the 13th birthday.
- *Children 13 or more years old.* Children in this age group who have not been vaccinated yet and have not had chickenpox can be given a catch-up vaccination now. Since these older children have a reduced response to the vaccine, they need two doses, administered 4 to 8 weeks apart.

## Hepatitis B Vaccine

**Preparations.** Hepatitis B vaccine (HBV) contains *hepatitis B surface antigen* (HBsAg), the primary antigenic protein in the viral envelope. Administration of HBV promotes synthesis of specific antibodies directed against hepatitis B virus. HBV is marketed under two trade names: Recombivax HB and Energix-B. Recombivax is available in formulations that contain 5, 10, and 20 μg of HBsAg/ml. Two formulations of Energix-B are available, both containing 10 μg of HBsAg/ml. The HBsAg in Recombivax HB and Energix-B is produced in yeast using recombinant DNA technology. Because these vaccines are made from a viral component, rather than from a live virus, they cannot cause disease.

**Efficacy.** Greater than 85% of vaccinees are protected after the second dose of HBV, and more than 90% are protected after the third dose. Although the duration of protection has not been determined with precision, it appears to be at least 5 to 7 years.

**Adverse Effects and Contraindications.** HBV is one of our safest vaccines. The most common reactions are soreness at the injection site and mild to moderate fever. Acetaminophen or ibuprofen may be used to relieve discomfort, but aspirin should be avoided. The only contraindication to HBV is a prior anaphylactic reaction to either HBV itself or to baker's yeast.

**Route, Site, and Immunization Schedule.** HBV is injected IM. In neonates and infants, the injection is made into the anterolateral thigh. In adolescents and adults, the injection is made into the deltoid. All vaccinees should receive three doses.

The immunization schedule for *infants* is based on whether the mother is *HBsAg-positive* or *HBsAg-negative* (i.e., on whether the mother has laboratory evidence of hepatitis B infection). The following schedules for infants are recommended:

- Infants whose mothers are *HBsAg-negative*—give 2.5 mg of Recombivax HB or 10 mg of Energix-B sometime between birth and 2 months of age. Give the second dose between 1 and 4 months of age (and at least 1 month after the first dose), and the third dose between 6 and 18 months of age.

- Infants whose mothers are *HBsAg-positive*—give 5 mg of Recombivax HB or 10 mg of Energix-B within 12 hours of birth, and give 0.5 ml of *hepatitis B immune globulin* (HBIG) at the same time but at a separate site. (The purpose of the HBIG is to provide immediate protection against hepatitis B acquired from the mother.) Give the second dose of HBV between 1 and 2 months of age, and the third dose at 6 months of age.

- Infants whose mother's *HBsAg status is unknown*—give 5 mg of Recombivax HB or 10 mg of Energix-B within 12 hours of birth. Subsequent dose are based on the mother's HBsAg status, which is determined by analyzing a maternal blood sample obtained during delivery. If the mother is HBsAg-positive, the infant should be given HBIG as soon as possible—and no later than 1 week after birth.

Children and adolescents who were not vaccinated against hepatitis B during infancy may begin the series at any time. Once the first dose is given, the second is given 1 month (or more) later, and the third is given 4 months (or more) after the first dose and no less than 2 months after the second dose. Children who reach age 11 without being vaccinated should begin a catch-up series at that time.

## KEY POINTS

- Vaccines promote synthesis of antibodies directed against bacteria and viruses, whereas toxoids promote synthesis of antibodies directed against bacterial toxins, but not the bacteria themselves.
- Killed vaccines are composed of whole, killed microbes or isolated microbial components, whereas live vaccines are composed of live microbes that have been weakened or rendered completely avirulent.
- Vaccination is defined as the administration of any vaccine or toxoid.
- Vaccination produces active immunity. Antibodies develop over weeks to months and then persist for years.
- Passive immunity is conferred by administering preformed antibodies (immune globulins). Protection is immediate but persists only as long as the antibodies remain in the body.
- Widespread vaccination has greatly reduced the incidence of several infectious diseases, eliminated polio from the Western hemisphere, and eliminated smallpox from the earth.
- Although vaccines are very safe, mild reactions are common, and serious reactions can occur rarely.

- Immunocompromised children are at special risk from live vaccines and should not receive them.
- Measles, mumps, and rubella vaccine (MMR) is a combination product composed of three live-virus vaccines.
- Rarely, MMR causes thrombocytopenia and anaphylactic reactions. Until recently, anaphylactic reactions were thought to result from allergy to eggs, but we now think they result from allergy to gelatin.
- MMR is contraindicated during pregnancy and should be used with caution in children with a history of thrombocytopenia or of anaphylactic reactions to gelatin, eggs, or neomycin.
- We have two vaccines for protection against diphtheria, tetanus, and pertussis. One (DTwP) contains whole-cell pertussis and the other (DTaP) contains acellular pertussis. DTaP is more effective than DTwP and causes fewer and milder side effects. Accordingly, DTaP is preferred.
- Rarely, DTP causes acute encephalopathy.
- We have two vaccines against polioviruses: oral poliovirus vaccine (OPV, Sabin vaccine) and inactivated poliovirus vaccine (IPV, Salk vaccine). OPV contains live, attenuated viruses, whereas IPV contains inactivated polioviruses.
- Very rarely, vaccination with OPV causes vaccine-associated paralytic poliomyelitis (VAPP). IPV does not cause VAPP. Accordingly, IPV is now recommended for initial immunization.
- *Haemophilus influenzae* type b vaccine is one of our safest vaccines. No serious adverse events have been reported.
- Varicella virus vaccine is composed of live, attenuated varicella viruses.
- Most children receiving varicella vaccine are fully protected against varicella (chickenpox), although some are not. However, among the children who get the disease despite vaccination, symptoms are always mild: vaccinated children develop far fewer lesions than unvaccinated children, experience less fever, and recover more quickly.
- Varicella vaccine is very safe; no serious adverse events have been reported.
- Varicella vaccine is contraindicated for pregnant women, individuals hypersensitive to neomycin or gelatin, and for immunocompromised people.
- Hepatitis B vaccine (HBV) contains hepatitis B surface antigen (HBsAg), the primary antigenic protein in the viral envelope. Administration of HBV promotes synthesis of specific antibodies directed against hepatitis B virus.
- HBV is one of our safest vaccines. The only contraindication is a prior anaphylactic reaction either to HBV itself or to baker's yeast.
- Within 12 hours of birth, infants whose mothers are HBsAg-positive should be injected with hepatis B vaccine and hepatitis B immune globulin.

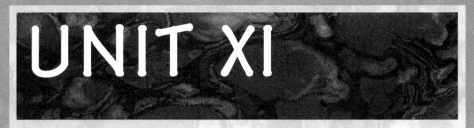

# UNIT XI

## Respiratory Tract Drugs

Drugs for Asthma

Drugs for Rhinitis, Cough, and Colds

# CHAPTER 69

# Drugs for Asthma

Asthma is a common disorder that occurs in children and adults. Characteristic signs and symptoms are a sense of breathlessness and tightness in the chest, together with wheezing, dyspnea, and cough. In the United States, asthma affects about 14 to 15 million people and costs about $6 billion a year to treat. More than 5000 people die each year. However, with proper treatment, most patients can lead full lives with no limitations.

## Pathophysiology of Asthma

Asthma is a *chronic inflammatory disorder* of the airway. In about 50% of children with asthma and in some adults, airway inflammation results from a reaction to known allergens. In the remaining children and in most adults, the cause of airway inflammation is unknown—although as-yet unidentified allergens are suspected.

Figure 69–1 depicts the events that lead to inflammation and bronchoconstriction in patients whose asthma is caused by specific allergens. Although this model may not apply completely to all asthma patients, it nonetheless provides a basis for understanding the drugs used for treatment. The inflammatory process begins with binding of allergen molecules (e.g., house dust mite feces) to antibodies on mast cells. This causes mast cells to release an assortment of mediators, including histamine, leukotrienes, prostaglandins, and interleukins. These mediators have two effects. They act immediately to cause *bronchoconstriction*. In addition, they promote infiltration and activation of inflammatory cells (eosinophils, leukocytes, macrophages). These inflammatory cells then release mediators of their own. The end result is *airway inflamma-*

*tion*, characterized by edema, mucous plugging, and smooth muscle hypertrophy, all of which obstruct airflow. In addition, inflammation produces a state of *bronchial hyperreactivity*. Because of this state, mild trigger factors (e.g., cold air, exercise, tobacco smoke) are able to cause intense bronchoconstriction.

From a therapeutic perspective, the important message here is that symptoms of asthma result from a combination of inflammation and bronchoconstriction; hence, treatment must address both components.

## Overview of Drugs for Asthma

The major drugs for asthma are listed in Table 69–1. As indicated, these fall into two main pharmacologic classes: (1) anti-inflammatory agents and (2) bronchodilators. The principal anti-inflammatory drugs are the *glucocorticoids* and *cromolyn*. The principal bronchodilators are the *beta$_2$ agonists*. For chronic asthma, glucocorticoids are administered on a fixed schedule, usually by inhalation. Beta$_2$ agonists may be administered on a fixed schedule or PRN; the usual route is inhalation. Drug therapy is discussed in detail later.

## Administration of Drugs by Inhalation

Most antiasthmatic drugs can be administered by inhalation, a route with three obvious advantages: (1) therapeutic effects are enhanced (by delivering drugs directly to their site of action), (2) systemic effects are minimized,

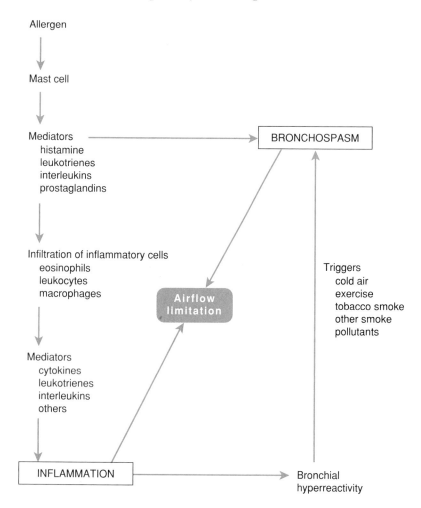

**Figure 69–1. Allergen-induced inflammation and bronchospasm in asthma.**

and (3) relief of acute attacks is rapid. Three types of inhalation devices are employed: metered-dose inhalers, nebulizers, and dry-powder inhalers.

### Metered-Dose Inhalers

Metered-dose inhalers (MDIs) are small, hand-held, pressurized devices that deliver a measured dose of drug with each activation. Dosing is usually accomplished with 1 or 2 puffs. When 2 puffs are needed, an interval of at least 1 minute should separate the first puff from the second. When using an MDI, the patient must begin to inhale prior to activating the device. Hence, hand-lung coordination is required. MDIs can be difficult to use correctly and patients will need a demonstration as well as written and verbal instruction. Even with optimal use, only about 10% of the dose reaches the lungs. About 80% impacts the oropharynx and is swallowed, and the remaining 10% is left in the device or exhaled.

Several kinds of *spacers* are available for use with MDIs. All of these devices, which attach directly to the MDI, serve to increase delivery of drug to the lungs and decrease deposition of drug on the oropharyngeal mucosa (Figure 69–2). Some spacers contain a one-way valve that activates upon inhalation, thereby obviating the need for good hand-lung coordination. Some spacers also contain

an alarm whistle that sounds off when inhalation is too rapid. The ability of spacers to reduce drug deposition in the oropharynx is especially important for inhaled glucocorticoids.

### Dry-Powder Inhalers

Dry-powder inhalers (DPIs) are used to deliver drugs in the form of a dry, micronized powder directly to the lungs. Currently, only two antiasthmatic drugs—cromolyn and albuterol—are available for administration by DPI. Both drugs are dispensed in single-dose capsules that must be inserted into the DPI before each administration. Unlike MDIs, DPIs are breath activated. Hence DPIs don't require the hand-lung coordination needed when using an MDI. When drugs are administered by DPI, up to 20% of the dose can reach the lungs.

### Nebulizers

A nebulizer is a small machine used to convert a drug solution into a mist. The droplets in the mist are much finer than those produced by inhalers. Inhalation of the nebulized mist can be done through a face mask or a mouthpiece held between the teeth. Nebulizers take several minutes to deliver the same amount of drug contained in 1 puff from an inhaler. For some patients, a nebulizer

## TABLE 69-1. OVERVIEW OF MAJOR DRUGS FOR ASTHMA

### ANTI-INFLAMMATORY DRUGS

**Glucocorticoids**
*Inhaled*
  Beclomethasone dipropionate [Beclovent, Vanceril]
  Budesonide [Pulmicort]
  Dexamethasone [Decadron]
  Flunisolide [Aerobid]
  Flucticasone propionate [Flovent]
  Triamcinolone acetonide [Azmacort]
*Oral*
  Prednisone
  Prednisolone

**Cromolyn and Nedocromil**
  Cromolyn, inhaled [Intal]
  Nedocromil, inhaled [Tilade]

**Leukotriene Antagonists**
  Zafirlukast, oral [Accolate]
  Zileuton, oral [Zyflo]

### BRONCHODILATORS

**Beta$_2$-Adrenergic Agonists**
*Inhaled: Short Acting*
  Albuterol [Proventil, Ventolin]
  Bitolterol [Tornalate]
  Pirbuterol [Maxair]
  Terbutaline [Brethaire]
*Inhaled: Long Acting*
  Salmeterol [Serevent]
*Oral*
  Albuterol [Proventil, Ventolin]
  Terbutaline [Brethine, Bricanyl]

**Methylxanthines**
  Theophylline, oral [Slo-Bid Gyrocaps, Theo-Dur, others]

**Anticholinergics**
  Ipratropium, inhaled [Atrovent]

may be more effective than an inhaler. Although nebulizers are usually used at home or in a hospital, these devices, which weigh under 10 pounds, are sufficiently portable for use in other locations.

# Beta$_2$-Adrenergic Agonists

Inhaled beta$_2$ agonists (e.g., albuterol, salmeterol) are the most effective drugs available for relieving acute bronchospasm and preventing exercise-induced bronchospasm. Accordingly, virtually all patients with asthma use these agents. The basic pharmacology of the adrenergic agonists is discussed in Chapter 18. Discussion here is limited to their use in asthma.

## Mechanism of Antiasthmatic Action

The beta$_2$ agonists are sympathomimetic drugs that produce "selective" activation of beta$_2$-adrenergic receptors. By stimulating beta$_2$ receptors in smooth muscle of the lung, these drugs promote *bronchodilation*, and thereby relieve bronchospasm. In addition, beta$_2$ agonists suppress histamine release in the lung and increase ciliary motility. The beta$_2$-selective agents have largely replaced older, less selective sympathomimetics (e.g., epinephrine, isoproterenol) for asthma therapy.

## Antiasthmatic Uses

Beta$_2$ agonists are employed to relieve ongoing attacks and to prevent attacks from occurring. All asthma patients inhale short-acting beta$_2$ agonists on a PRN basis to relieve breakthrough symptoms. Patients who experience frequent attacks may also take these drugs on a fixed schedule; an oral preparation or a long-acting inhaled preparation (e.g., salmeterol) is employed. Patients prone to exercise-induced bronchospasm may inhale a short-acting beta$_2$ agonist immediately prior to exercise as prophylaxis against an attack. For patients undergoing an acute severe attack, a nebulized beta$_2$ agonist is the treatment of choice.

Inhaled beta$_2$ agonists fall into two groups: *short-acting agents* and *long-acting agents* (see Table 69–1). With the short-acting preparations, effects begin almost immediately, peak in 30 to 60 minutes, and persist for 3 to 5 hours. In contrast, with *salmeterol*, the only long-acting preparation available, effects begin slowly but persist for 12 hours or more. As a result, inhaled salmeterol is well suited for prolonged prophylaxis, but is not useful for aborting an ongoing attack.

## Adverse Effects

***Inhaled Preparations.*** Side effects with inhaled beta$_2$ agonists are generally minimal. There have been reports of increased mortality associated with overuse of these drugs. However, it isn't clear whether overuse was the cause of death, or whether severe asthma, which led to increased use, was the actual cause. Although systemic effects—tachycardia, angina, tremor—are usually minimal when beta$_2$ agonists are inhaled, these effects can nonetheless occur.

***Oral and Parenteral Preparations.*** The selectivity of the beta$_2$-adrenergic agonists is only relative—not absolute. Accordingly, when these drugs are administered orally and parenterally, they are likely to produce some activation of beta$_1$ receptors in the heart. If the dosage is excessive, stimulation of cardiac beta$_1$ receptors can cause *angina pectoris* and *tachydysrhythmias*. Patients should be instructed to report chest pain or changes in heart rate or rhythm. When beta$_2$ agonists are inhaled, cardiac stimulation can occur but is minimal.

Systemic beta$_2$ agonists often cause *tremor* by stimulating beta$_2$ receptors on skeletal muscle. Tremor can be reduced by lowering the dosage. With continued drug use, tremor declines spontaneously.

## Preparations, Dosage, and Administration

Five beta$_2$ agonists are available (Table 69–2). All may be administered by inhalation. Albuterol and terbutaline may also be given orally, and terbutaline may be given by injection. Dosages are summarized in Table 69–2.

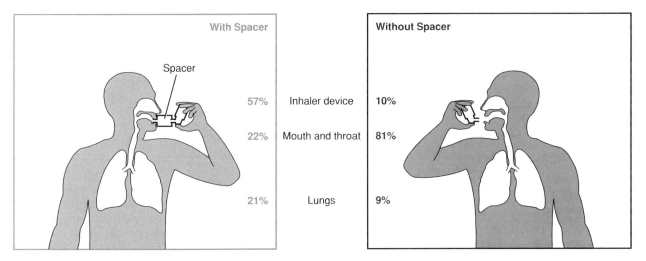

**Figure 69–2. Impact of a spacer device on the distribution of inhaled medication.** Note that in the the presence of a spacer more medication reaches its site of action in the lungs—and less is deposited in the mouth and throat.

*Metered-Dose Inhalers.* All of the beta$_2$ agonists are available in MDIs. With the short-acting agents, the usual dosage is 1 or 2 puffs 3 or 4 times a day. With salmeterol, the only long-acting agent, the usual dosage is 2 puffs every 12 hours. When 2 puffs are needed, an interval of 1 minute or longer should separate puffs. During this interval, some bronchodilation develops, thereby facilitating penetration of the second puff.

*Nebulization.* For certain patients, nebulizers can be superior to inhalers. Experience has shown that some patients who have become unresponsive to a beta$_2$ agonist delivered with an inhaler may respond when the same drug is administered by nebulization. This differential ef-

fect occurs because the nebulizer delivers the dose slowly (over several minutes); as the bronchi gradually dilate, the drug gains deeper and deeper access to the lungs. Nebulization is the preferred method of administration for treating an acute severe attack.

## Glucocorticoids

Glucocorticoids (e.g., beclomethasone, prednisone) are the most effective antiasthma drugs available. Administration is usually by inhalation, but may also be oral or IV.

## TABLE 69-2. BETA₂-ADRENERGIC AGONISTS USED IN ASTHMA

| Generic Name | Trade Name | Daily Dosage | Initial Dosage | |
|---|---|---|---|---|
| | | | Adults | Children |
| Albuterol | Proventil, Ventolin | MDI (90 µg/puff) | 2 puffs q 4-6 h PRN | 2 puffs q 4-6 h PRN |
| | | DPI (200 µg) [Ventol in Rotocaps] | 1-2 caps q 4-6 h PRN | 1-2 caps q 4-6 h PRN |
| | | Nebulized solution (5 mg/ml) | 2.5 mg tid or qid | 0.1-0.15 mg/kg q 4-6 h PRN |
| | | Syrup or tablets | 2 or 4 mg PO tid or qid PRN | 0.1 mg/kg PO q 6-8 h PRN |
| | | Extended-release tablets [Proventil Repetabs] | 4-8 mg PO q 12 h | 0.1-0.2 mg/kg PO q 12 h |
| Bitolterol | Tornalate | MDI (370 µg/puff) | 2-3 puffs q 4-6 h PRN | 2 puffs q 4-6 h PRN |
| Pirbuterol | Maxair | MDI (200 µg/puff) | 2 puffs q 4-6 h PRN | 2 puffs q 4-6 h PRN |
| Salmeterol | Serevent | MDI (21 µg/puff) | 2 puffs q 12 h | 2 puffs q 12 h |
| Terbutaline | Brethaire Brethine, Bricanyl | MDI (200 µg/puff) Tablets Subcutaneous | 2-3 puffs q 4-6 h PRN 2.5-5 mg tid 0.25 mg (repeat after 15-30 min if needed) | 2-3 puffs q 4-6 h PRN 1.25-2.5 mg tid 0.01 mg/kg (repeat after 15-30 min if needed) |

MDI = metered-dose inhaler; DPI = dry-powder inhaler.

Adverse reactions to inhaled glucocorticoids are minor, as are reactions to systemic glucocorticoids taken *acutely*. However, when *systemic* glucocorticoids are used *long term*, severe adverse effects are likely. The basic pharmacology of the glucocorticoids is discussed in Chapter 65. Discussion here is limited to their use in asthma.

## Mechanism of Antiasthmatic Action

Glucocorticoids reduce symptoms of asthma by *suppressing inflammation*. Specific anti-inflammatory effects include (1) decreased synthesis and release of inflammatory mediators (e.g., prostaglandins, leukotrienes, histamine); (2) decreased infiltration and activity of inflammatory cells (e.g., eosinophils, leukocytes); and (3) decreased edema of the airway mucosa (secondary to a decrease in vascular permeability). As a result of suppressing inflammation, glucocorticoids reduce bronchial hyperreactivity. In addition to reducing inflammation, glucocorticoids decrease airway mucus production and increase the number of bronchial beta$_2$ receptors as well as their responsiveness to beta$_2$ agonists.

## Use in Asthma

Glucocorticoids are used for *prophylaxis* of chronic asthma. Accordingly, administration must be done on a fixed schedule—not PRN. Since beneficial effects develop slowly, these drugs are not used to abort ongoing attacks.

*Inhalation Use.* Inhaled glucocorticoids have become first-line therapy for asthma. All patients with moderate to severe asthma should take these drugs daily. In addition to being highly effective, inhaled glucocorticoids are very safe.

*Oral Use.* Oral glucocorticoids are reserved for patients with severe asthma. Because of their potential for toxicity, these drugs are prescribed only when symptoms cannot be controlled with safer medications (inhaled glucocorticoids, cromolyn, beta$_2$ agonists, theophylline). Because the risk of toxicity increases with duration of use, treatment should be as brief as possible.

## Adverse Effects

*Inhaled Glucocorticoids.* These preparations are generally devoid of serious toxicity, even when used in high doses. The most common adverse effects are *oropharyngeal candidiasis* and *dysphonia* (hoarseness, speaking difficulty). Both effects result from local deposition of inhaled glucocorticoids. To minimize these effects, patients should (1) gargle after each administration and (2) employ a spacer device during administration, which will greatly reduce drug deposition in the oropharynx. If candidiasis develops, it can be treated with an antifungal drug. With long-term, high-dose therapy, some adrenal suppression may develop. However, this is rarely clinically significant.

*Oral Glucocorticoids.* When used *acutely* (less than 10 days), even in very high doses, oral glucocorticoids do not cause significant adverse effects. However, prolonged therapy, even in moderate doses, can be hazardous. Potential adverse effects include *adrenal suppression, osteoporosis, hyperglycemia, peptic ulcer disease*, and, in young patients, *suppression of growth.*

Adrenal suppression is of particular concern. As discussed in Chapter 65, prolonged use of glucocorticoids can decrease the ability of the adrenal cortex to produce glucocorticoids of its own. Since high levels of glucocorticoids are required to survive severe stress (e.g., surgery, trauma), and since adrenal suppression prevents production of endogenous glucocorticoids, *patients must be given increased doses of oral or parenteral glucocorticoids at times of stress. Failure to do so may prove fatal!* It should be noted that inhaled glucocorticoids are inadequate as supplements at times of stress. Following withdrawal of oral glucocorticoids, several months are required for recovery of adrenocortical function. Throughout this period, supplemental steroids are required if severe stress occurs.

A complete list of contraindications to oral glucocorticoids is presented in the *Summary of Major Nursing Implications* at the end of this chapter.

## Preparations, Dosage, and Administration

*Inhaled Glucocorticoids.* Five glucocorticoids are available for administration by inhalation (Table 69-3). All are dispensed in metered-dose inhalers (MDIs). Patients should be instructed to employ a *spacer device* (holding chamber) with the MDI, since this will (1) increase the amount of glucocorticoid delivered to the lungs (thereby increasing therapeutic effects), and (2) reduce the amount deposited in the oropharynx (thereby reducing the risk of candidiasis and dysphonia). Penetration of inhaled glucocorticoids to the lungs can be increased by inhaling a beta$_2$ agonist 5 minutes prior to inhaling the glucocorticoid.

Inhaled glucocorticoids are administered on a regular schedule—not PRN. Pediatric and adult dosages are summarized in Table 69-3.

*Oral Glucocorticoids. Prednisone* and *prednisolone* are preferred glucocorticoids for oral therapy of asthma. For acute therapy, the usual adult dosage for either drug is 30 to 40 mg twice daily for 5 to 7 days.

For *long-term* treatment, *alternate-day dosing* is recommended (to minimize adrenal suppression). The *initial adult* dosage is 40 to 60 mg (of prednisone or prednisolone) administered every other morning. The *initial pediatric* dosage is 20 to 40 mg every other morning. After symptoms have been controlled for a month, *adult* and *pediatric* dosages should be reduced by 5 to 10 mg every 2 weeks to the lowest dosage that keeps the patient free of symptoms. As discussed above, supplemental doses are required at times of stress.

# Cromolyn

Cromolyn [Intal] is a very safe and effective drug for *prophylaxis* of asthma, but is not useful for aborting an ongoing attack. Administration is by inhalation.

## Effects on the Lung

Cromolyn suppresses inflammation; it is not a bronchodilator. The drug acts in part by stabilizing the cytoplasmic membrane of mast cells, thereby preventing re-

## TABLE 69-3. DOSAGES FOR INHALED GLUCOCORTICOIDS*

| Generic Name | Trade Name | Dose per Puff (µg) | Initial Dosage | |
| --- | --- | --- | --- | --- |
| | | | Adults | Children |
| Beclomethasone dipropionate | Beclovent, Vanceril | 42 | 2 puffs tid or qid *or* 4 puffs bid | 1 or 2 puffs tid or qid *or* 2-4 puffs bid |
| Dexamethasone sodium phosphate | Decadron Phosphate Respihaler | 84[†] | 3 puffs tid or qid | 2 puffs tid or qid |
| Flunisolide | Aerobid | 250 | 2-4 puffs bid | 2 puffs bid |
| Fluticasone propionate | Flovent | 44, 110, 220 | 2-4 puffs bid | Not approved for children under 12 years |
| Triamcinolone acetonide | Azmacort | 100 | 2 puffs tid or qid | 1 or 2 puffs tid or qid |

*All of these drugs are dispensed in metered-dose inhalers. Use of a spacer device with the inhaler can increase therapeutic effects and reduce local adverse effects (dysphonia and candidiasis).
[†]Each puff releases a dose of dexamethasone phosphate equivalent to 84 µg of dexamethasone.

lease of histamine and other mediators. In addition, cromolyn inhibits eosinophils, macrophages, and other inflammatory cells.

### Pharmacokinetics

Cromolyn is administered by inhalation. The fraction absorbed from the lungs is small (about 8%) and produces no systemic effects. Absorbed cromolyn is excreted unchanged in the urine.

### Therapeutic Uses

*Chronic Asthma.* Cromolyn is a first-line agent for prophylactic therapy of moderate asthma. The drug produces adequate control in 60% to 70% of patients. When administered on a fixed schedule, cromolyn reduces both the frequency and intensity of attacks. No tolerance to the drug is seen with long-term use. To be of benefit, cromolyn must be administered *prior* to the onset of an attack; the drug is without effect if taken after an episode has begun. In patients with chronic asthma, maximal effects may take several weeks to develop. Cromolyn is especially effective for prophylaxis of seasonal allergic attacks and for acute prophylaxis immediately prior to allergen exposure (e.g., when anticipating mowing the lawn). Because of cromolyn's safety and efficacy, many clinicians feel that cromolyn is the anti-inflammatory drug of first choice for childhood asthma.

*Exercise-Induced Bronchospasm.* Cromolyn can prevent bronchospasm in patients subject to exercise-induced asthma. For this use, cromolyn should be administered 15 minutes prior to anticipated exertion.

*Allergic Rhinitis.* *Intranasal* cromolyn [Nasalcrom] can relieve symptoms of allergic rhinitis. This use is discussed in Chapter 70.

### Adverse Effects

Cromolyn is the safest of all antiasthmatic medications. Significant adverse effects occur in fewer than 1 of every 10,000 patients. The most common reactions are wheezing and coughing in response to inhalation of powdered cromolyn.

### Preparations, Dosage, and Administration

Cromolyn for inhalation [Intal] can be administered with three devices: (1) a dry-powder inhaler [Spinhaler], (2) a power-driven nebulizer, and (3) a metered-dose inhaler. Patients will need instruction on how to use these devices. With either the Spinhaler or a nebulizer, the *initial* dosage for adults and children is 20 mg 4 times a day. With the metered-dose inhaler, the *initial* dosage for adults and children is 2 to 4 puffs (1.6 to 3.2 mg) 4 times a day. For *maintenance* therapy with any device, the lowest effective dosage should be established. For therapy of chronic asthma, cromolyn must be administered on a fixed schedule.

## Nedocromil

Nedocromil [Tilade] has actions and uses like those of cromolyn. Like cromolyn, nedocromil has anti-inflammatory and antiallergic actions that derive in part from suppressing the release of histamine and other substances from mast cells. Nedocromil is administered with a metered-dose inhaler. The drug is indicated for prophylactic therapy only; it is not able to abort an ongoing asthma attack. Like cromolyn, nedocromil decreases the incidence and severity of attacks. The most common adverse effect is an unpleasant taste, which about 5% of patients find intolerable. Otherwise, nedocromil is generally well tolerated. The usual dosage is 2 puffs (3.5 mg) 4 times a day. Once symptoms are controlled, 2 puffs a day may suffice. Maximal effects may take several weeks to develop.

## Methylxanthines

We first encountered the methylxanthines (theophylline, caffeine, others) in Chapter 33 (Central Nervous System Stimulants). As discussed in that chapter, the most prominent actions of these drugs are (1) CNS excitation and (2) bronchodilation. Other actions include cardiac stimulation, vasodilation, and diuresis.

## Theophylline

Theophylline is the principal methylxanthine employed to treat asthma. Benefits derive primarily from bronchodilation. Theophylline has a narrow therapeutic range, and hence dosage must be carefully controlled. The drug is usually administered by mouth. Theophylline is not administered by inhalation because it is not active by this route.

At one time, theophylline was a first-line drug for asthma, and nearly all patients with chronic asthma took it. However, use of theophylline has declined sharply, largely because we now have safer and more effective medications (inhaled beta$_2$ agonists, inhaled glucocorticoids, cromolyn).

### Mechanism of Action

Theophylline produces bronchodilation by relaxing smooth muscle of the bronchi. The mechanism of this effect has not been determined. Of the mechanisms that have been proposed, the most probable is blockade of receptors for adenosine.

One frequently discussed mechanism suggests that methylxanthines act by inhibiting an enzyme called phosphodiesterase, and thereby elevate intracellular levels of cyclic AMP. This mechanism was proposed based on the ability of methylxanthines, in high concentrations, to inhibit phosphodiesterase in the test tube. However, since these high concentrations are not achieved in the body, it seems unlikely that inhibition of phosphodiesterase underlies the effects of methylxanthines in humans.

### Use in Asthma

*Oral* theophylline is used for maintenance therapy of chronic stable asthma. Although less effective than beta$_2$ agonists, theophylline has a longer duration of action (when administered in a sustained-release formulation). With regular use, theophylline can decrease the frequency and severity of asthma attacks. Because its effects are prolonged, theophylline may be most appropriate for patients who experience nocturnal attacks.

*Intravenous* theophylline has been employed in emergencies. However, the drug is no more effective than beta$_2$ agonists and glucocorticoids, and is clearly more dangerous.

### Pharmacokinetics

***Absorption.*** Oral theophylline is available in standard and sustained-release formulations. The standard formulations are rapidly absorbed, but produce wide fluctuations in plasma drug levels. The sustained-release preparations are absorbed more slowly and produce plasma levels that are acceptably stable. Absorption from some sustained-release preparations can be affected by food.

***Metabolism.*** Theophylline is metabolized in the liver. Rates of metabolism are affected by multiple factors—age, disease, drugs—and show wide individual variation. As a result, the plasma half-life of theophylline varies considerably among patients. For example, while the *average* half-life in nonsmoking adults is about 8 hours, the half-life can be as short as 2 hours in some adults and as long as 15 hours in others. Smoking cigarettes (one to two packs a day) accelerates metabolism and decreases the half-life of theophylline by about 50%. The average half-life in children is 4 hours. Metabolism is slowed in patients with certain pathologies (e.g., heart disease, liver disease, prolonged fever). Some drugs (e.g., cimetidine, fluoroquinolone antibiotics) decrease theophylline metabolism. Other drugs (e.g., phenobarbi-

tal) accelerate metabolism. Because of these variations in metabolism, individualization of theophylline dosage is essential.

***Plasma Drug Levels.*** Safe and effective therapy requires periodic measurement of theophylline blood levels. Traditionally, dosage has been adjusted to produce theophylline levels between 10 and 20 μg/ml. However, many patients respond well at 5 μg/ml, and as a rule there is little benefit to increasing levels above 15 μg/ml. Hence, levels between 5 and 15 μg/ml are appropriate for most patients. At levels above 20 μg/ml, the risk of significant adverse effects is high.

### Toxicity

***Symptoms.*** Toxicity is related to theophylline levels. Adverse effects are uncommon at plasma levels below 20 μg/ml. At 20 to 25 μg/ml, relatively mild reactions occur (e.g., nausea, vomiting, diarrhea, insomnia, restlessness). Serious adverse effects are most likely at levels above 30 μg/ml. These reactions include severe dysrhythmias (e.g., ventricular fibrillation) and convulsions that can be highly resistant to treatment. Death may result from cardiorespiratory collapse.

***Treatment.*** At the first indication of toxicity, administration of theophylline should cease. If a large amount of the drug has been ingested, ipecac should be given to induce vomiting. After this, absorption can be decreased by administering activated charcoal together with a cathartic. Ventricular dysrhythmias respond to lidocaine. Intravenous diazepam may help control seizures.

### Drug Interactions

***Caffeine.*** Caffeine is a methylxanthine with pharmacologic properties like those of theophylline (see Chapter 33). Accordingly, caffeine can intensify the adverse effects of theophylline on the CNS and heart. In addition, caffeine can compete with theophylline for drug-metabolizing enzymes, thereby causing theophylline levels to rise. Because of these interactions, individuals taking theophylline should avoid caffeine-containing beverages (e.g., coffee, many soft drinks) and other sources of caffeine.

***Drugs That Reduce Theophylline Levels.*** Several agents—including *phenobarbital*, *phenytoin*, and *rifampin*—can lower theophylline levels by causing induction of hepatic drug-metabolizing enzymes. Concurrent use of these agents may necessitate an increase in theophylline dosage.

***Drugs That Increase Theophylline Levels.*** Several drugs—including *cimetidine* and the *fluoroquinolone antibiotics* (e.g., ciprofloxacin)—can elevate plasma levels of theophylline, primarily by inhibiting hepatic metabolism. To avoid theophylline toxicity, the dosage of theophylline should be reduced when the drug is combined with these other agents.

### Oral Formulations

Oral theophylline is available in standard and sustained-release formulations. The standard formulations are rapidly absorbed, require frequent administration, and produce substantial fluctuations in plasma theophylline levels. Sustained-release formulations are more convenient and can produce drug levels that are relatively stable. Accordingly, the sustained-release formulations are preferred for routine therapy. Sustained-release preparations are available in 8-, 12-, and 24-hour forms.

Absorption from sustained-release formulations can be affected markedly by food. For example, absorption from one preparation—Theo-24—is accelerated in the presence of a fatty meal. In contrast, food reduces absorption from a product named Theo-Dur Sprinkle.

Because theophylline has a narrow therapeutic range, and because sustained-release formulations contain large amounts of the drug, accelerated absorption from sustained-release formulations can produce dangerous elevations in theophylline blood levels. Because of this potential hazard, some clinicians avoid the formulations intended for once-a-day administration. These preparations pose the greatest threat because they contain the largest amount of theophylline.

### Dosage and Administration

*Oral.* Dosage must be individualized. Traditionally, dosage has been adjusted to maintain plasma theophylline levels between 10 and 20 µg/ml. However, levels between 5 and 15 µg/ml are appropriate for most patients. To minimize chances of toxicity, doses should be low initially and then gradually increased. If a dose is missed, the following dose should *not* be doubled, since doing so could produce toxicity. Smokers require higher than average doses; conversely, patients with heart disease, liver dysfunction, or prolonged fever are likely to require relatively low doses. Patients should be instructed not to chew the sustained-release formulations. Product information should be consulted for compatibility with food.

Maintenance dosages vary with the age of the patient. A typical maintenance dosage for *adults* is 200 to 300 mg 2 or 3 times a day. Guidelines for *pediatric* dosing are as follows: for children 1 to 9 years old, 22 mg/kg/day; for children 9 to 12 years old, 20 mg/kg/day; and for children 12 to 16 years old, 18 mg/kg/day. The number of daily doses depends upon the duration of action of the preparation employed.

*Intravenous.* Intravenous theophylline is reserved for emergencies. Administration must be done slowly, since rapid injection can cause fatal cardiovascular reactions. Intravenous theophylline is incompatible with many other drugs. Accordingly, compatibility should be verified prior to mixing theophylline with other IV agents. For specific IV dosages, refer to the discussion of *aminophylline* below.

### Other Methylxanthines

#### Aminophylline

Aminophylline [Truphylline] is a theophylline salt that is considerably more soluble than theophylline itself. In solution, each molecule of aminophylline dissociates to yield two molecules of theophylline. Hence the pharmacologic properties of aminophylline and theophylline are identical. Aminophylline is available in formulations for oral, intravenous, and rectal administration. Intravenous administration is employed most frequently.

*Administration and Dosage. Intravenous.* Because of its relatively high solubility, aminophylline is the preferred form of theophylline for intravenous use. Infusions should be done *slowly* (no faster than 25 mg/min), since rapid injection can produce severe hypotension and death. The usual loading dose is 6 mg/kg. The maintenance infusion rate should be adjusted to provide plasma levels of theophylline that are within the therapeutic range (10 to 20 µg/ml). Aminophylline solutions are incompatible with a number of other drugs. Accordingly, compatibility must be verified before mixing aminophylline with other IV agents.

*Oral.* Aminophylline is available in tablets and solution for oral administration. Dosing guidelines are the same as for theophylline.

*Rectal.* Aminophylline is available in *suppositories* and *solution for rectal administration.* Absorption from the suppositories is erratic, and these preparations are not recommended. Rectal solutions provide fast and reliable dosing and are safe for occasional use. Dosages for adults and children are the same as presented above for oral theophylline.

#### Oxtriphylline

Oxtriphylline [Choledyl] is a salt of theophylline that contains 69% theophylline by weight. The drug is administered by mouth and produces the same effects as pure theophylline. Oxtriphyl-

line offers no therapeutic advantage over theophylline itself. The dose of oxtriphylline equivalent to 100 mg of theophylline is 156 mg.

#### Dyphylline

Although structurally similar to theophylline, dyphylline [Dilor, Lufyllin] is nonetheless a completely distinct compound, and is not converted to theophylline in the body. Dyphylline may be administered orally or IM. The drug has a half-life of 2 hours and is eliminated unchanged in the urine. The maximum adult oral dosage is 15 mg/kg 4 times a day. The adult IM dosage is 250 to 500 mg every 6 hours.

## Additional Drugs for Asthma

### Anticholinergic Drug: Ipratropium

Ipratropium [Atrovent] is an atropine derivative administered by inhalation to treat chronic asthma. Like atropine itself, ipratropium is a muscarinic antagonist. By blocking muscarinic cholinergic receptors in the bronchi, ipratropium promotes *bronchodilation.* Therapeutic effects begin within 30 seconds, reach 50% of their maximum in 3 minutes, and persist for about 6 hours. Ipratropium is effective against allergen-induced asthma and exercise-induced asthma, but is less effective than the beta₂ agonists. Because ipratropium and the beta₂-adrenergic agonists promote bronchodilation by different mechanisms, the beneficial effects of these drugs are additive. Ipratropium is a quaternary ammonium compound, and therefore always carries a positive charge. As a result, the drug is not readily absorbed from the lungs or from the digestive tract. Accordingly, systemic effects are minimal. The most common adverse reactions are dryness of the oropharynx (5%) and cough or exacerbation of asthma symptoms (3%). Ipratropium is dispensed in a metered-dose inhaler that delivers 18 µg per activation. The recommended adult dosage is 2 to 4 puffs 4 times a day. The pediatric dosage is 2 puffs 4 times a day.

### Leukotriene Antagonists

Leukotrienes are important contributors to inflammation in asthma; hence, drugs that prevent their effects can reduce symptoms. At this time, two leukotriene antagonists are available. One—zafirlukast—blocks leukotriene receptors. The other—zileuton—blocks leukotriene synthesis. In patients with asthma, these drugs can decrease inflammation, bronchoconstriction, edema, mucous secretion, and recruitment of eosinophils and other inflammatory cells.

*Zafirlukast.* Zafirlukast [Accolate] is the first representative of a new class of anti-inflammatory agents, the *leukotriene receptor antagonists.* The drug is approved for maintenance therapy of chronic asthma in adults and children over 12. Benefits derive in part from reduced infiltration of inflammatory cells and decreased bronchoconstriction. In clinical trials, the drug produced modest symptomatic relief in patients with mild to moderate asthma. Direct comparisons with glucocorticoids are unavailable. Because the drug is new, its therapeutic niche has not been established.

Zafirlukast is administered orally and absorption is rapid. Food reduces absorption by 40%; hence, the drug should be administered at least 1 hour before meals or 2 hours after. Zafirlukast undergoes hepatic metabolism followed by fecal excretion. The half-life is 10 hours, but may be as long as 20 hours in the elderly. The recommended dosage is 20 mg twice a day.

Zafirlukast causes few adverse effects, but has the potential for multiple drug interactions. The most common side effects are headache and gastrointestinal disturbances. Zafirlukast inhibits two isozymes of cytochrome P-450, and therefore can suppress the metabolism of a variety of drugs. Among these are warfarin, glucocorticoids, phenytoin, cyclosporine, and astemizole.

**Zileuton.** Zileuton [Zyflo], an inhibitor of leukotriene synthesis, is approved for prophylaxis and maintenance therapy of asthma in adults and children over 12 years old. Benefits derive from inhibiting 5-lipoxygenase, the enzyme that converts arachidonic acid into leukotrienes. Symptomatic improvement can be seen within 1 to 2 hours of dosing. Since effects are not immediate, zileuton cannot be used to abort an ongoing attack. Because zileuton is a new drug, its therapeutic niche has not been established.

Zileuton is given orally and undergoes rapid absorption, both in the presence and absence of food. Plasma levels peak 2 to 3 hours after dosing. Zileuton is rapidly metabolized in the liver, and the metabolites are excreted in the urine. The drug's plasma half-life is 2.5 hours. The recommended dosage is 600 mg 4 times a day.

Zileuton can injure the liver, as evidenced by increased plasma levels of alanine aminotransferase activity (ALT). A few patients have developed symptomatic hepatitis, which reversed following drug withdrawal. To reduce the risk of serious liver injury, ALT activity should be monitored. The recommended schedule is once a month for 3 months, then every 2 to 3 months for the remainder of the first year, and periodically thereafter. In addition to causing liver injury, zileuton can cause dyspepsia. In mice taking 4 times the human dose, the drug increased the incidence of liver, kidney, and vascular tumors.

Zileuton is metabolized by cytochrome P-450, and hence can compete with other drugs for metabolism, thereby increasing their levels in plasma. In clinical trials, plasma levels of theophylline were increased markedly. Levels of warfarin and propranolol were also increased.

# Management of Asthma

On February 24, 1997, the National Asthma Education and Prevention Program of the National Heart, Lung, and Blood Institute introduced updated guidelines for treatment of asthma in a document titled *Expert Panel Report II: Guidelines for the Diagnosis and Management of Asthma (EPR-II).* The discussion below is based on recommendations in that report.

## Chronic Asthma

Therapy of chronic asthma has undergone significant change in recent years. Use of inhaled glucocorticoids and cromolyn has greatly increased, owing to increased appreciation of the role of inflammation in asthma. Conversely, use of theophylline has sharply declined: once employed as a first-line drug for most patients, theophylline is now considered a second- or third-line agent. Short-acting, inhaled beta$_2$ agonists have been and remain a mainstay of treatment. When asthma medications are used appropriately, most patients can live normal lives, with little or no limitation of activities and few or no side effects.

### Measuring Lung Function

Before considering asthma therapy, we need to address tests of lung function. Two of these are described below.

*Forced expiratory volume* (FEV) is the single most useful test of lung function. Unfortunately, the instrument required—a *spirometer*—is both expensive and cumbersome, and therefore not suited for use at home. To determine FEV, the patient inhales completely, and then exhales as completely and forcefully as possible into the spirometer. The spirometer measures how much air was expelled. Results are then compared to a "predicted normal value" for a healthy person of similar age, sex, height, and weight. Hence, for a patient with asthma, the FEV might be 75% of the predicted value.

*Peak expiratory flow rate* (PEFR) is defined as the maximal rate of air flow during expiration. To determine PEFR, the patient exhales as forcefully as possible into a *peak flow meter*, a relatively inexpensive, hand-held device. Patients should measure their peak flow every morning. If the peak flow is less than 80% of their personal best, more frequent monitoring should be done.

### Classification of Chronic Asthma

As described in EPR-II, chronic asthma has four classes of increasing severity: (1) mild intermittent, (2) mild persistent, (3) moderate persistent, and (4) severe persistent. Diagnostic criteria for these classes are summarized in Table 69-4. As shown in the table, as we progress from mild intermittent asthma to severe persistent asthma, symptoms occur more often and last longer, exacerbations become more frequent, PEF (or FEV) decreases to less than 60% of the predicted value, PEF becomes more variable, and limitations on physical activity become substantial.

### Drug Therapy

Drugs are employed in two ways in chronic asthma: some agents are taken to establish *long-term control* and some are taken for *quick relief* (Table 69-5). Long-term control drugs are administered daily to achieve and maintain control of persistent asthma. Anti-inflammatory drugs—especially inhaled glucocorticoids and cromolyn—provide the foundation for long-term control. Long-acting beta$_2$ agonists—especially inhaled salmeterol—are also valuable for long-term control. Quick-relief medications are taken to promptly reverse bronchoconstriction, and thereby provide rapid relief from cough, chest tightness, and wheezing. By far the most important drugs for quick relief are the short-acting, inhaled beta$_2$ agonists. With all of the drugs used for asthma, the treatment goal is to:

- Prevent chronic and troublesome symptoms (e.g., coughing or breathlessness after exertion or in the night or early morning)
- Maintain normal (or near normal) pulmonary function
- Maintain normal activity levels (including exercise)
- Prevent recurrent exacerbations
- Minimize the need for emergency department visits or hospitalizations
- Provide maximum benefits with minimum adverse effects

## TABLE 69-4. CLASSIFICATION OF ASTHMA SEVERITY*

| Classification | Frequency and Duration of Symptoms[†] | Nighttime Symptoms | Lung Function |
|---|---|---|---|
| STEP 1: Mild intermittent | • Symptoms <2 times a week<br>• Asymptomatic and normal PEF between exacerbations<br>• Exacerbations last a few hours to a few days; intensity may vary | <2 times a month | • PEF or $FEV_1$ ≥80% predicted<br>• PEF variability <20% |
| STEP 2: Mild Persistent | • Symptoms >2 times a week but <1 time a day<br>• Exacerbations may affect activity | >2 times a month | • PEF or $FEV_1$ ≥80% predicted<br>• PEF variability 20%–30% |
| STEP 3: Moderate Persistent | • Daily symptoms<br>• Daily use of inhaled short-acting beta$_2$ agonist<br>• Exacerbations affect activity<br>• Exacerbations >2 times a week and may last days | >1 time a week | • PEF or $FEV_1$ >60% and <80% of predicted<br>• PEF variability >30% |
| STEP 4: Severe Persistent | • Continual symptoms<br>• Limited physical activity<br>• Frequent exacerbations | Frequent | • PEF or $FEV_1$ ≤60% predicted<br>• PEF variability >30% |

*Adapted from National Asthma Education and Prevention Program. Expert Panel Report II: Guidelines for the Diagnosis and Management of Asthma. Bethesda, MD, National Heart, Lung, and Blood Institute, 1997.
[†]Patients at any level of severity can have mild, moderate, or severe exacerbations. Some patients with intermittent asthma experience severe, life-threatening exacerbations separated by long periods of normal lung function and no symptoms.

• Meet patient and family expectations regarding asthma care

The EPR-II recommends *stepwise* therapy of chronic asthma (Table 69–6). The four steps of this approach correspond to the four classes of asthma severity discussed above. For patients with *persistent* asthma (steps 2, 3, and 4), long-term control medications provide the cornerstone of treatment; as the severity of symptoms increases, dosages are increased and additional drugs are added. For *all* patients, a quick-relief drug is taken as needed.

Stepwise therapy may be implemented in two ways. One option is to initiate treatment at the step that corresponds to the patient's asthma severity, and then gradually step up as needed. The second option, which is recommended by the Expert Panel, is to initiate treatment at a step *higher* than the patient's asthma classification, and then step down after control has been achieved. The benefit of this more aggressive approach is faster control of the underlying inflammatory process. As a result, permanent injury to the lungs may be reduced, thereby allowing treatment in the future with lower doses of anti-inflammatory drugs than might otherwise be required. Specific recommendations for stepwise therapy are discussed below and summarized in Table 69–6.

**Step 1: Mild Intermittent Asthma.** Mild intermittent asthma is treated on a PRN basis; long-term control medication is not needed. The occasional acute attack is managed by inhaling a short-acting beta$_2$ agonist. If the patient needs the beta$_2$ agonist more than twice a week, moving to step 2 may be indicated.

**Step 2: Mild Persistent Asthma.** Mild persistent asthma requires a combination of long-term control medication

plus quick-relief medication. The foundation of treatment is daily inhalation of an anti-inflammatory drug. Adults usually begin with an inhaled glucocorticoid (low dose); children usually begin by trying cromolyn or nedocromil. Second-line drugs for long-term control are theophylline and the leukotriene antagonists (zafirlukast and zileuton).

## TABLE 69-5. DRUGS FOR ASTHMA: AGENTS FOR LONG-TERM CONTROL VERSUS QUICK RELIEF

### LONG-TERM CONTROL MEDICATIONS

*Anti-inflammatory Drugs*
  Glucocorticoids (inhaled or oral)
  Cromolyn and nedocromil
  Leukotriene antagonists

*Bronchodilators*
  Long-acting beta$_2$ agonists
    Inhaled (salmeterol)
    Oral (albuterol, SR*)
  Theophylline

### QUICK-RELIEF MEDICATIONS

*Bronchodilators*
  Short-acting inhaled beta$_2$ agonists
  Ipratropium

*Anti-inflammatory Drugs*
  Glucocorticoids, systemic[†]

*SR = sustained release.
[†]Considered quick-relief drugs when used in a short burst (3–10 days) at the start of therapy or during a period of gradual deterioration. Glucocorticoids are not used for immediate relief of an ongoing attack.

### TABLE 69-6. STEPWISE APPROACH FOR MANAGING ASTHMA IN ADULTS AND CHILDREN OVER 5 YEARS OLD

| Classification | Long-Term Control Drugs (Taken Daily) | Quick-Relief Drugs (PRN) |
|---|---|---|
| STEP 1:<br>Mild Intermittent | • No daily medication needed | • Short-acting, inhaled beta$_2$ agonist |
| STEP 2:<br>Mild Persistent | • Inhaled glucocorticoid (low dose),<br>    cromolyn, or nedocromil | • Same as step 1 |
| STEP 3:<br>Moderate Persistent | • Inhaled glucocorticoid (medium dose) **or**<br>• Inhaled glucocorticoid (low-medium dose) *plus*<br>    inhaled salmeterol | • Same as step 1 |
| STEP 4:<br>Severe Persistent | • Inhaled glucocorticoid (high dose) *plus*<br>    inhaled salmeterol<br>• Oral glucocorticoid  (if needed) | • Same as step 1 |

Adapted from National Asthma Education and Prevention Program. Expert Panel Report II: Guidelines for the Diagnosis and Management of Asthma. Bethesda, MD, National Heart, Lung, and Blood Institute, 1997. This table summarizes major treatment options; additional options are discussed in the text.

As in step 1, a short-acting beta$_2$ agonist is inhaled PRN to suppress breakthrough attacks. Inhaling the beta$_2$ agonist every day, or increasing its use, suggests that advancing to step 3 may be needed.

***Step 3: Moderate Persistent Asthma.*** Moderate persistent asthma requires more intensive long-term control than mild persistent asthma. This can be achieved by either (1) inhaling a glucocorticoid in a *moderate* dosage (as compared with the low dosage used in step 1) or (2) inhaling a glucocorticoid in a *low to moderate* dosage and *adding* inhaled salmeterol (a long-acting beta$_2$ agonist). The second option is generally preferred because control is often better and the risk of systemic effects from the glucocorticoid is lower. Alternatives to adding inhaled salmeterol include (1) adding sustained-release theophylline or (2) adding a long-acting, oral beta$_2$ agonist (e.g., sustained-release albuterol). As in steps 1 and 2, breakthrough episodes are managed with a short-acting inhaled beta$_2$ agonist. If the patient inhales the beta$_2$ agonist every day or increases its use, advancing to step 4 may be indicated.

***Step 4: Severe Persistent Asthma.*** Severe chronic asthma is managed with daily inhalation of a glucocorticoid (high dose) plus salmeterol. Alternatives to inhaled salmeterol include sustained-release theophylline or a long-acting, oral beta$_2$ agonist. If symptoms are especially severe, an *oral* glucocorticoid should be *added* to the regimen; administration may be once daily or once every other day. Breakthrough attacks are managed with a short-acting, inhaled beta$_2$ agonist.

***Step-Down.*** Once the treatment goal has been achieved and then sustained, a reduction in drug use may be attempted. The purpose is to identify the minimal therapy required. A step-down attempt is especially important for patients who stepped up because of a seasonal allergy, but may no longer need intensified therapy after the allergy season is over.

## Zone System for Monitoring Treatment

Patients can monitor their treatment using a scheme based on green, yellow, and red "zones," which are analogous to green, yellow, and red traffic lights. By using this system, patients can position themselves for early implementation of corrective measures when control begins to slip or has become dangerously inadequate. To determine which zone they are in, patients must monitor their symptoms and PEFR.

***Green Zone.*** In this zone, patients have no symptoms and their PEFR is greater than 80% of their personal best. The green zone indicates that control is good.

***Yellow Zone.*** In this zone, patients have some symptoms and their PEFR is 50% to 80% of their personal best. The yellow zone indicates that control is insufficient. To regain control, patients should inhale a short-acting beta$_2$ agonist. If this fails to return them to the green zone, a short course (4 days) of oral glucocorticoids may be indicated. Alternatively, the patient may need to advance to a higher step.

***Red Zone.*** In this zone, symptoms occur at rest or interfere with activities, and the PEFR is less than 50% of the patient's personal best. The red zone indicates a medical alert. A beta$_2$ agonist should be inhaled immediately. If the PEFR remains below 50%, the patient should seek medical attention for acute severe asthma (see below).

## Reducing Exposure to Allergens and Triggers

The treatment plan should include measures to control allergens and other factors that can cause airway inflammation and exacerbate symptoms. When successful, these measures can significantly reduce symptoms. Important sources of asthma-associated allergens include the house dust mite, warm-blooded pets, cockroaches, and molds. Factors that can exacerbate asthma include tobacco smoke, wood smoke, and household sprays. To the extent possible, exposure to these factors should be reduced or eliminated. For those who are reluctant to part with Fluffy (the family cat) or Ralph (the family dog), weekly washing of the critter may help. More importantly, the pet should be banned from the patient's bedroom.

The house dust mite is the most notorious cause of asthma. Allergy develops not to the microscopic mite itself, but rather to its even more microscopic feces. Measures to control or avoid dust mites and their feces include:

- Encasing the patient's pillow, mattress, and box spring with covers that are impermeable to allergens
- Washing all bedding and stuffed animals weekly on the hot cycle (130°F)
- Removing carpeting or rugs from the bedroom
- Avoiding sleeping or lying on upholstered furniture
- Keeping indoor humidity below 50%

Routine use of chemicals to kill dust mites is no longer recommended.

## Acute Severe Exacerbations

Acute severe exacerbations of asthma require immediate attention. Hospitalization may be required. The goal is to relieve airway obstruction and hypoxemia, and normalize lung function as soon as possible. The foundation of treatment is repetitive inhalation of a nebulized $beta_2$ agonist. (If the patient is unconscious or unable to generate PEFR, subcutaneous epinephrine should be given.) If there is no response to the first nebulized dose of a $beta_2$ agonist, an intravenous glucocorticoid (e.g., methylprednisolone) should be administered. Oxygen is given to maintain oxygen saturation above 95%. Oral glucocorticoids may be taken for 1 to 2 weeks after discharge. Full recovery of lung function may take weeks.

## Exercise-Induced Bronchospasm

Exercise increases airway obstruction in practically all people with chronic asthma. The cause of obstruction is bronchospasm secondary to loss of heat and/or water from the lung. Exercise-induced bronchospasm usually starts either during or immediately after exercise, peaks in 5 to 10 minutes, and resolves 20 to 30 minutes after that.

With proper medication, most asthmatics can be as active as they wish. Indeed, many world-class athletes have asthma, among them Jackie Joyner-Kersee and other Olympic gold medalists. To prevent symptoms related to exercise, patients should inhale a $beta_2$ agonist or cromolyn prophylactically. $Beta_2$ agonists should be inhaled immediately before exercise; cromolyn should be inhaled 15 minutes before exercise.

## KEY POINTS

- Asthma is a chronic inflammatory disease characterized by inflammation of the airways, bronchial hyperreactivity, and bronchospasm. Allergy is often the underlying cause.

- Asthma is treated with anti-inflammatory drugs and bronchodilators.
- Most drugs for asthma are administered by inhalation, a route that increases therapeutic effects (by delivering drugs directly to their site of action); reduces systemic effects (by minimizing drug levels in blood); and facilitates rapid relief of acute attacks.
- Three devices are used to administer drugs by inhalation: metered-dose inhalers, dry-powder inhalers, and nebulizers. Patients will need instruction on their use.
- Inhaled $beta_2$ agonists are the most effective drugs available for relieving acute bronchospasm and preventing exercise-induced bronchospasm.
- $Beta_2$ agonists promote bronchodilation by stimulating $beta_2$ receptors in bronchial smooth muscle.
- Most inhaled $beta_2$ agonists have a rapid onset and short duration, which makes them useful for short-term prophylaxis and relief of acute attacks.
- Inhaled salmeterol has a delayed onset and extended duration, which makes it useful for prolonged prophylaxis but not for treating acute attacks.
- Inhaled $beta_2$ agonists rarely cause systemic side effects.
- Excessive dosing with oral $beta_2$ agonists can cause tachycardia and angina by stimulating $beta_1$ receptors on the heart. (Selectivity is lost at high doses.)
- Glucocorticoids are the most effective antiasthma drugs available.
- Glucocorticoids reduce symptoms of asthma by suppressing inflammation. As an added bonus, glucocorticoids promote synthesis of bronchial $beta_2$ receptors, and increase their responsiveness to $beta_2$ agonists.
- Inhaled and systemic glucocorticoids are used for long-term prophylaxis of asthma—not to abort ongoing attacks. Accordingly, they are administered on a fixed schedule—not PRN.
- Unless asthma is severe, glucocorticoids should be administered by inhalation.
- Inhaled glucocorticoids are very safe. Their principal side effects are oropharyngeal candidiasis and dysphonia, which can be minimized by employing a spacer device during administration and by gargling after.
- Prolonged therapy with oral glucocorticoids can cause serious adverse effects, including adrenal suppression, osteoporosis, hyperglycemia, peptic ulcer disease, and growth suppression.
- Cromolyn is an inhaled anti-inflammatory drug used for prophylaxis of asthma.
- Cromolyn reduces inflammation primarily by preventing release of mediators from mast cells.
- For long-term prophylaxis, cromolyn is taken daily on a fixed schedule. For prophylaxis of exercise-induced bronchospasm, cromolyn is taken 15 minutes before anticipated exertion.
- Cromolyn is the safest drug for asthma. Serious adverse effects are extremely rare.
- Theophylline, a member of the methylxanthine family, relieves asthma by causing bronchodilation.

- Although theophylline was used widely in the past, it has been largely replaced by safer and more effective medications.
- There are four classes of chronic asthma: mild intermittent, mild persistent, moderate persistent, and severe persistent.
- For therapeutic purposes, asthma drugs can be classified as long-term control medications (e.g., inhaled glucocorticoids, cromolyn) and quick-relief medications (e.g., inhaled, short-acting beta$_2$ agonists).
- In the stepwise approach to asthma therapy, treatment becomes more aggressive as symptoms become more frequent and intense.
- The goals of stepwise therapy are to prevent symptoms, maintain near-normal pulmonary function, maintain normal activity, prevent recurrent exacerbations, minimize emergency room visits, minimize drug side effects, and meet patient and family expectations about treatment.
- Mild intermittent asthma is treated on a PRN basis; a short-acting beta$_2$ agonist is inhaled to abort the few acute episodes that occur.
- For mild persistent asthma, the foundation of therapy is daily inhalation of an anti-inflammatory drug—usually a glucocorticoid or cromolyn. A short-acting beta$_2$ agonist is inhaled PRN to suppress breakthrough attacks.

- For moderate persistent asthma, long-term control is established with either (1) an inhaled glucocorticoid (medium dose) or (2) an inhaled glucocorticoid (low-medium dose) plus inhaled salmeterol.
- For severe persistent asthma, the foundation of therapy is an inhaled glucocorticoid (high dose) plus inhaled salmeterol. An oral glucocorticoid is *added* if required.
- For acute severe exacerbations of asthma, the foundation of treatment is repetitive inhalation of a nebulized beta$_2$ agonist. A systemic glucocorticoid may also be needed.
- Exercise-induced bronchospasm can be avoided by inhaling either cromolyn or a short-acting, inhaled beta$_2$ agonist prior to strenuous activity.
- By daily monitoring of symptoms and peak expiratory flow rate (PEFR), patients can poise themselves for early implementation of corrective measures when asthma control begins to slip or has become dangerously inadequate.
- Patients should avoid allergens that can cause airway inflammation and triggers that can provoke exacerbations. Important sources of allergens are the house dust mite, warm-blooded pets, cockroaches, and molds. Important triggers are tobacco smoke, wood smoke, and household sprays

## Summary of Major Nursing Implications*

## Beta$_2$-Adrenergic Agonists

### Inhaled

| | |
|---|---|
| Albuterol | Salmeterol |
| Bitolterol | Terbutaline |
| Pirbuterol | |

### Oral

| | |
|---|---|
| Albuterol | Terbutaline |

## Preadministration Assessment

### Therapeutic Goal

Short-acting inhaled beta$_2$ agonists are used PRN for prophylaxis of exercise-induced bronchospasm and to relieve ongoing asthma attacks. Oral beta$_2$ agonists and long-acting inhaled agents may be used for maintenance therapy.

### Baseline Data

Determine PEFR (or FEV), the frequency and severity of attacks, and attempt to identify trigger factors.

### Identifying High-Risk Patients

Systemic (oral, parenteral) beta$_2$ agonists are *contraindicated* for patients with *tachydysrhythmias* or *tachycardia associated with digitalis toxicity*. Use systemic beta$_2$ agonists with *caution* in patients with *diabetes, hyperthyroidism, organic heart disease, hypertension*, or *angina pectoris*.

## Implementation: Administration

### Routes

*Usual.* Inhalation.

*Occasional.* Oral, subcutaneous.

### Administration

*Inhalation.* Inhaled beta$_2$ agonists are administered with either a metered-dose inhaler, dry-powder inhaler, or nebulizer. Teach patients how to use these devices. For patients who have difficulty with hand-lung coordination, use of a spacer with a one-way valve may improve results.

Inform patients who are using metered-dose inhalers or dry-powder inhalers that, when 2 puffs are needed, an interval of at least 1 minute should elapse between puffs.

Warn patients against exceeding recommended dosages.

Inform patients that long-acting beta$_2$ agonists should be taken on a fixed schedule—not PRN.

*Oral.* Instruct patients to take oral beta$_2$ agonists on a fixed schedule—not PRN.

Instruct patients to swallow sustained-release preparations intact, without crushing or chewing.

---

*Patient education information is highlighted in color.

## Ongoing Evaluation and Interventions

### Evaluating Therapeutic Effects

Teach patients with chronic asthma to monitor and record PEFR, symptom frequency, and symptom intensity. Teach patients to evaluate whether they are in the green, yellow, or red zone, and what the proper response to being in these zones is.

### Minimizing Adverse Effects

When administered by *inhalation* at recommended doses, beta$_2$ agonists are generally devoid of adverse effects. Cardiac stimulation and tremors are most likely with *systemic* therapy.

*Cardiac Stimulation.* Excessive dosing with systemic beta$_2$ agonists can cause stimulation of beta$_1$ receptors on the heart, resulting in anginal pain and tachydysrhythmias. Instruct the patient to report chest pain and changes in heart rate or rhythm.

*Tremor.* Tremor is common with systemic beta$_2$ agonists, and usually subsides with continued drug use. If necessary, tremor can be reduced by lowering the dosage.

## Glucocorticoids

### Inhaled

| | |
|---|---|
| Beclomethasone dipropionate | Fluticasone propionate |
| Budesonide | Triamcinolone acetonide |
| Dexamethasone | |
| Flunisolide | |

### Oral

| | |
|---|---|
| Prednisone | Prednisolone |

The nursing implications summarized below refer specifically to the use of glucocorticoids in asthma. A full summary of nursing implications for glucocorticoids is presented in Chapter 65.

## Preadministration Assessment

### Therapeutic Goal

Glucocorticoids are used on a fixed schedule to suppress inflammation in chronic asthma. They are not used to abort an ongoing attack.

### Baseline Data

Determine PEFR (or FEV), the frequency and severity of attacks, and attempt to identify trigger factors.

### Identifying High-Risk Patients

*Inhaled Glucocorticoids.* These preparations are *contraindicated* for patients with *persistently positive sputum cultures for Candida albicans.*

*Oral Glucocorticoids.* These preparations are *contraindicated* for patients with *systemic fungal infections* and for individuals receiving *live-virus vaccines.* Use with *caution* in *pediatric patients* and in *women who are pregnant or breast-feeding.* In addition, exercise *caution* in patients with *hypertension, heart failure, renal impairment, esophagitis, gastritis, peptic ulcer disease, myasthenia gravis, diabetes mellitus, osteoporosis,* or *infections that are resistant to treatment* and in patients receiving *potassium-depleting diuretics, digitalis glycosides, insulin, oral hypoglycemics,* or *nonsteroidal anti-inflammatory drugs.*

## Implementation: Administration

### Routes

Inhalation, oral.

### Administration

Inform patients that glucocorticoids are intended for preventive therapy (not for aborting ongoing attacks), and instruct them to administer glucocorticoids on a regular schedule—not on a PRN basis.

*Inhalation.* Advise patients to employ a *spacer device* with the glucocorticoid metered-dose inhaler, and teach them how to use this device. Inform patients that delivery of glucocorticoids to the bronchial tree can be enhanced by inhaling a short-acting beta$_2$ agonist 5 minutes prior to administering the glucocorticoid.

*Oral.* Alternate-day therapy is recommended to minimize adrenal suppression; instruct the patient to take one dose every other day in the morning. During long-term treatment, supplemental doses must be given at times of severe stress.

## Ongoing Evaluation and Interventions

### Evaluating Therapeutic Effects

Teach patients with chronic asthma to monitor and record PEFR, symptom frequency, and symptom intensity. Teach patients to evaluate whether they are in the green, yellow, or red zone, and what the proper response to being in these zones is.

### Minimizing Adverse Effects

*Inhaled Glucocorticoids.* Advise patients to gargle after each administration and to use a spacer with the metered-dose inhaler. These measures will minimize *dysphonia* and *oropharyngeal candidiasis.* If candidiasis develops, it can be treated with antifungal medication.

*Oral Glucocorticoids.* Prolonged therapy can cause *adrenal suppression* and other serious adverse effects, including *osteoporosis, hyperglycemia, peptic ulcer disease,* and *growth suppression.* These effects can be reduced with alternate-day dosing. To compensate for adrenal suppression, patients taking glucocorticoids on a chronic basis must be given supplemental oral or IV glucocorticoids at times of stress (e.g., trauma, surgery, infection). Additional nursing implications that apply to adverse effects of long-term glucocorticoid therapy are summarized in Chapter 65.

# Cromolyn

## Preadministration Assessment

### Therapeutic Goal
Cromolyn is used for acute and long-term *prophylaxis* of asthma. The drug will not abort an ongoing asthma attack.

### Baseline Data
Determine PEFR (or FEV), the frequency and severity of attacks, and attempt to identify trigger factors.

### Identifying High-Risk Patients
Cromolyn is *contraindicated* for the rare patient who *has experienced an allergic response to cromolyn in the past.*

## Implementation: Administration

### Route
Inhalation.

### Administration
*Administration Devices.* Cromolyn is administered with a dry-powder inhaler [Spinhaler], a nebulizer, or a metered-dose inhaler. Instruct patients on the proper use of these devices.

*Acute Prophylaxis.* Instruct patients to administer cromolyn 15 minutes prior to exercise and other precipitating factors (e.g., cold, environmental agents).

*Long-Term Prophylaxis.* Instruct patients to administer cromolyn on a regular schedule, and inform them that full therapeutic effects may take several weeks to develop.

## Ongoing Evaluation and Interventions

### Evaluating Therapeutic Effects
Teach patients with chronic asthma to monitor and record PEFR, symptom frequency, and symptom intensity. Teach patients to evaluate whether they are in the green, yellow, or red zone, and what the proper response to being in these zones is.

### Minimizing Adverse Effects and Interactions
Cromolyn is devoid of significant adverse effects and drug interactions.

# Theophylline

## Preadministration Assessment

### Therapeutic Goal
Theophylline is a bronchodilator taken on a regular schedule to decrease the intensity and frequency of moderate-to-severe asthma attacks.

### Baseline Data
Determine PEFR (or FEV) and the frequency and severity of attacks.

### Identifying High-Risk Patients
Theophylline is *contraindicated* for patients with *untreated seizure disorders* or *peptic ulcer disease.* Use with *caution* in patients with *heart disease, liver or kidney dysfunction,* or *severe hypertension.*

## Implementation: Administration

### Routes
Oral, intravenous.

### Administration
*Oral.* Dosage must be individualized. Doses are low initially and then increased gradually. The dosing objective is to produce plasma theophylline levels in the therapeutic range, which for most patients is 5 to 15 μg/ml. Warn patients that if a dose is missed, the following dose should *not* be doubled.

Instruct patients to swallow enteric-coated and sustained-release formulations intact, without crushing or chewing.

Warn patients not to switch from one sustained-release formulation to another without consulting the physician.

Consult product information regarding compatibility with food, and advise the patient accordingly.

*Intravenous.* Administration must be done slowly. Verify compatibility with other IV drugs prior to mixing.

## Ongoing Evaluation and Interventions

### Evaluating Therapeutic Effects
Monitor drug levels to ensure that they are in the therapeutic range, which for most patients is 5 to 15 μg/ml.

Teach patients with chronic asthma to monitor and record PEFR, symptom frequency, and symptom intensity. Teach patients to evaluate whether they are in the green, yellow, or red zone, and what the proper response to being in these zones is.

### Minimizing Adverse Effects
Mild adverse effects (e.g., nausea, vomiting, diarrhea, insomnia, restlessness) develop as plasma drug levels rise above 20 μg/ml. Severe effects (convulsions, ventricular

fibrillation) can occur at drug levels above 30 μg/ml. Dosage should be adjusted to keep theophylline levels below 20 μg/ml.

## Minimizing Adverse Interactions

*Caffeine.* Caffeine can intensify the adverse effects of theophylline on the heart and CNS and can decrease theophylline metabolism. Caution patients against consuming caffeine-containing beverages (e.g., coffee, many soft drinks) and other sources of caffeine.

*Drugs That Reduce Theophylline Levels.* Phenobarbital, phenytoin, rifampin, and other drugs can lower theophylline levels. In the presence of these drugs, the dosage of theophylline may need to be increased.

*Drugs That Increase Theophylline Levels.* Cimetidine, fluoroquinolone antibiotics, and other drugs can elevate theophylline levels. When combined with these drugs, theophylline should be used in reduced dosage.

## Managing Toxicity

Theophylline overdose can cause severe dysrhythmias and convulsions. Death from cardiorespiratory collapse may occur. Manage toxicity by (1) discontinuing theophylline, (2) administering ipecac (to induce vomiting), and (3) administering activated charcoal (to decrease theophylline absorption) plus a cathartic (to accelerate fecal excretion). Give lidocaine to control ventricular dysrhythmias and IV diazepam to control seizures.

# CHAPTER 70

# Drugs for Rhinitis, Cough, and Colds

**Drugs Used to Treat Rhinitis**
Nasal Decongestants
Antihistamines
Antihistamine-Decongestant Combinations
Intranasal Cromolyn Sodium
Intranasal Glucocorticoids

**Drugs Used to Treat Cough**
Antitussives
Expectorants and Mucolytics
**Cold Remedies: Combination Preparations**

The drugs addressed in this chapter are given to alleviate symptoms of common respiratory disorders. Our principal focus will be on rhinitis. We will also consider cough and the common cold.

## Drugs Used to Treat Rhinitis

Rhinitis is defined as an inflammation of the nasal mucous membranes. Major symptoms are sneezing, rhinorrhea (runny nose), pruritus (itching), and nasal congestion. (Congestion is caused by dilation and engorgement of nasal blood vessels.)

Rhinitis may be allergic or nonallergic. Allergic rhinitis results from release of histamine in response to specific allergens. Nonallergic rhinitis is a frequent symptom of the common cold.

Allergic rhinitis has two forms: seasonal and perennial. Seasonal rhinitis (hay fever) occurs in the spring and fall in reaction to pollens from weeds, grasses, and trees. Perennial (nonseasonal) rhinitis is triggered by allergens present year round, especially the house dust mite and animal hair. Allergic rhinitis is the most common of all allergic disorders, affecting up to 15% of people in the United States.

Several classes of drugs are used to treat rhinitis. Principal among these are (1) nasal decongestants, (2) antihistamines, (3) intranasal cromolyn, and (4) intranasal glucocorticoids. All of these drugs are used to treat allergic rhinitis. In contrast, only the decongestants are used routinely to treat nonallergic rhinitis.

## Nasal Decongestants
### Actions and Uses

Nasal decongestants (e.g., phenylephrine, phenylpropanolamine) act by stimulating alpha$_1$-adrenergic re-

ceptors on smooth muscle of nasal blood vessels. Stimulation of these receptors causes vasoconstriction, resulting in shrinkage of swollen membranes followed by nasal drainage. With *topical* administration, vasoconstriction is both rapid and intense. In contrast, responses to *oral* decongestants are moderate, delayed, and prolonged. Nasal decongestants can relieve stuffiness associated with allergic rhinitis, sinusitis, and colds.

### Adverse Effects

**Rebound Congestion.** Rebound congestion develops when *topical* decongestants are administered on a regular basis for an extended time. With this pattern of use, as the effects of each application wear off, congestion becomes progressively more severe. To overcome this rebound congestion, the patient must use progressively larger and more frequent doses. Hence, once established, rebound congestion can lead to a cycle of escalating congestion and increased drug use. This cycle can be broken by abrupt decongestant withdrawal. However, this tactic can be extremely uncomfortable. A less drastic approach is to discontinue drug use in one nostril at a time. Rebound congestion can be minimized by limiting use of topical agents to no more than 3 to 5 days. Accordingly, topical decongestants are inappropriate for individuals with chronic rhinitis.

**Central Nervous System Stimulation.** Central nervous system (CNS) excitation is the most common adverse effect of the *oral* decongestants. Symptoms include restlessness, irritability, anxiety, and insomnia. These responses are unlikely with topical agents.

**Cardiovascular Effects.** By stimulating alpha$_1$-adrenergic receptors on systemic blood vessels, nasal decongestants can cause widespread vasoconstriction. For most patients, effects on systemic vessels are inconsequential. However, for individuals with hypertension or coronary artery disease, decongestant-induced vasoconstriction can be hazardous. Generalized vasoconstriction is most likely with the orally administered decongestants. However, if taken in excess, even the topical agents can cause significant systemic vasoconstriction.

### Topical Administration

*General Considerations.* Because of the risk of rebound congestion, topical decongestants should be used for no more than 5 consecutive days. To avoid systemic effects, doses should not exceed those recommended by the manufacturer. The applicator should be cleansed after each use to prevent contamination.

*Drops.* Drops should be administered with the patient in a lateral, head-low position. This positioning causes the drops to spread slowly over the nasal mucosa, thereby promoting beneficial effects while reducing the amount that is swallowed. Because the number of drops can be precisely controlled, drops allow better control over dosage than sprays. Accordingly, since young children are particularly susceptible to toxicity, drops are preferred to sprays for these patients.

*Sprays.* Sprays deliver the decongestant in a fine mist. Although convenient, sprays are less effective than an equal volume of properly instilled drops.

### Summary of Contrasts Between Oral and Topical Agents

Oral and topical decongestants differ in several important respects. (1) Topical decongestants act faster than the oral agents and are usually more effective. (2) Oral decongestants are longer acting than topical preparations. (3) Systemic effects (e.g., vasoconstriction, CNS stimulation) are more likely with oral decongestants; topical drugs induce these responses only when dosage is excessive. (4) Whereas rebound congestion is common with prolonged use of topical agents, this reaction is rare with the oral agents.

#### Preparations and Dosage

*Properties of Individual Decongestants. Phenylephrine* is one of the most widely used nasal decongestants. The drug is administered topically (by itself) and orally (as a component of combination preparations). *Phenylpropanolamine* is among the most frequently used oral decongestants; however, there is concern that exceeding the recommended dosage may cause hemorrhagic stroke. *Ephedrine* causes a high incidence of CNS stimulation. CNS effects are much lower with *pseudoephedrine*, a stereoisomer of ephedrine. *Naphazoline*, one of the newer topical agents, can cause severe rebound congestion.

*Dosage and Administration.* Dosages and routes of administration for the nasal decongestants are summarized in Table 70-1.

## Antihistamines

The antihistamines are discussed at length in Chapter 63. Consideration here is limited to the use of these agents for allergic rhinitis.

Antihistamines ($H_1$-receptor antagonists) are the drugs prescribed most frequently to treat *allergic* rhinitis. These agents can relieve sneezing, rhinorrhea, and nasal itching.

However, antihistamines do not decrease nasal congestion. Since histamine does not contribute to symptoms of *infectious* rhinitis, antihistamines are of no value in the treatment of colds.

For therapy of allergic rhinitis, antihistamines are most effective when taken *prophylactically*; these drugs are less helpful when taken after symptoms have appeared. Accordingly, antihistamines should be administered on a regular basis throughout the allergy season, even when symptoms are absent.

Adverse effects are usually mild. The most prominent side effect is *sedation*, which occurs often with first-generation antihistamines (e.g., diphenhydramine), but not with the second-generation agents (e.g., terfenadine). Anticholinergic effects (e.g., dry mouth, constipation, urinary hesitancy) may also occur.

Doses for some commonly used $H_1$ antagonists are presented in Table 70-2. A more complete listing appears in Table 63-3.

## Antihistamine-Decongestant Combinations

Combination therapy with an antihistamine and a decongestant may be used for *allergic rhinitis*. Although antihistamines alone are the first-line treatment for this disorder, they do not relieve nasal congestion, and hence may be inadequate for some patients. In these cases, addition of a decongestant to the regimen may be indicated. This can be accomplished in two ways: by giving the antihistamine and decongestant separately, or by using a combination product. Several popular antihistamine-decongestant combination products are listed in Table 70-2.

## Intranasal Cromolyn Sodium

The basic pharmacology of cromolyn sodium is discussed in Chapter 69 (Drugs for Asthma). Consideration here is limited to the use of cromolyn for allergic rhinitis.

*Actions and Uses.* Intranasal cromolyn sodium is a safe and effective medication for relieving symptoms of *allergic* rhinitis. The drug is of no benefit in the treatment of *nonallergic* rhinitis. Cromolyn reduces symptoms of allergic rhinitis by acting on mast cells to suppress release of histamine and other mediators of the allergic response. Cromolyn is more beneficial to people with seasonal rhinitis than to those with perennial rhinitis. For treatment of seasonal allergic rhinitis, cromolyn is equal in efficacy to the antihistamines but is less effective than intranasal steroids (see below). Like the antihistamines, cromolyn is most effective when taken prior to the onset of symptoms. Beneficial effects may take a week or so to develop, and patients should be informed about this delay. Adverse reactions to intranasal cromolyn are minimal.

*Dosage and Administration.* Intranasal cromolyn sodium [Nasalcrom] is administered with a metered spray device. The usual dosage for adults and children over the age of 6 years is one spray (5.2 mg) per nostril administered 3 to 6 times a day. If nasal congestion is present, a topical decongestant should be used prior to administering cromolyn. Like the antihistamines, cromolyn should be administered on a regular schedule throughout the allergy season.

## Intranasal Glucocorticoids

The basic pharmacology of the glucocorticoids is discussed in Chapter 65. Consideration here is limited to the use of these drugs to treat allergic rhinitis.

*Actions and Uses.* Intranasal glucocorticoids are the most effective drugs for treating both seasonal and perennial rhinitis. Six preparations are available: *beclomethasone, budesonide, dexamethasone, flunisolide, fluticasone,* and *triamcinolone.* All six are equally effective. Because of their anti-inflammatory actions, these drugs can prevent or suppress all of the major symptoms of al-

lergic rhinitis: congestion, rhinorrhea, sneezing, nasal itching, and erythema. As a rule, intranasal steroids are reserved for patients whose symptoms cannot be controlled with more conventional drugs (decongestants, antihistamines, intranasal cromolyn). However, given their safety and superior efficacy, it is possible they may join or replace the $H_1$ antagonists as first-line therapy for allergic rhinitis.

*Adverse Effects.* Adverse effects are mild. The most common effects are drying of the nasal mucosa and sensations of burning or itching. These effects are caused by the vehicle employed for administration and not by the steroids themselves. Preparations that employ an aqueous vehicle (see Table 70–3) are much less irritating than those that use a nonaqueous vehicle (Freon, alcohol, polyethylene glycol).

Systemic effects, including adrenocortical suppression, may occur. However, these responses are rare at recommended doses. Systemic effects are most likely with *dex-*

## TABLE 70–1. NASAL DECONGESTANTS: ROUTES AND DRUGS

| Decongestant | Mode of Administration | Frequency of Dosing | Dosage Size† |
|---|---|---|---|
| Ephedrine | Drops | q 8–12 h | *Adults and children over 6 years:* 2–3 drops (0.5%)<br>*Children under 6 years:* Consult physician |
| Epinephrine | Drops | q 4–6 h | *Adults and children over 6 years:* 1–2 drops (0.1%)<br>*Children under 6 years:* Consult physician |
| Naphazoline | Drops | q 3 h | *Adults and children over 6 years:* 2 drops (0.05%)<br>*Children under 6 years:* Consult physician |
| Oxymetazoline | Drops | q 12 h | *Adults and children over 6 years:* 2–4 drops (0.05%)<br>*Children 2–5 years:* 2–3 drops (0.025%) |
| | Spray | q 12 h | *Adults and children over 6 years:* 2–3 sprays (0.05%) |
| Phenylephrine | Drops | q 2–4 h | *Adults:* Several drops (0.25 to 1%)<br>*Infants:* 1 drop (0.125 to 0.2%) |
| | Spray | q 3–4 h | *Adults:* 1–2 sprays (0.25 to 1%)<br>*Children over 6 years:* 1–2 sprays (0.25%) |
| Phenylpropanolamine | Oral | q 4 h | *Adults:* 25 mg<br>*Children 6–12 years:* 12.5 mg |
| | Oral SR* | q 12 h | Adults: 75 mg |
| Propylhexedrine | Inhaler | PRN | Two inhalations: 0.6–0.8 mg |
| Pseudoephedrine | Oral | q 6–8 h | *Adults:* 60 mg<br>*Children:* 1 mg/kg |
| | Oral SR* | q 12 h | *Adults:* 120 mg |
| Tetrahydrozoline | Drops | q 3 or more h | *Adults and children over 6 years:* 2–4 drops (0.1%)<br>*Children 2–6 years:* 2–3 drops (0.05%) |
| Xylometazoline | Drops | q 8–10 h | *Adults:* 2–3 drops (0.1%)<br>*Children 2–12 years:* 2–3 drops (0.05%) |
| | Spray | q 8–10 h | *Adults:* 2–3 sprays (0.1%) |

*Oral SR = sustained release
†For drops and sprays, dosage listed is applied to *each* nostril; numbers in parentheses indicate concentration of solution employed.

## TABLE 70–2. SOME ORAL DRUGS FOR ALLERGIC RHINITIS

| Drug Class and Generic Name | Trade Name | Adult Dosage |
|---|---|---|
| *Antihistamines: First-Generation (Sedating)* | | |
| Brompheniramine | Dimetane | 4 mg q 4–6 h |
| Chlorpheniramine | Chlor-Trimeton | 4 mg q 4–6 h |
| Diphenhydramine | Benadryl | 25–50 mg q 4–6 h |
| *Antihistamines: Second-Generation (Nonsedating)* | | |
| Astemizole | Hismanal | 10 mg q 24 h |
| Fexofenadine | Allegra | 60 mg bid |
| Loratadine | Claritin | 10 mg q 24 h |
| Terfenadine | Seldane | 60 mg bid |
| Cetirizine | Zyrtec | 5 or 10 mg q 24 h |
| *Decongestants* | | |
| Phenylpropanolamine | Propagest | 20–25 mg q 4–6 h |
| Pseudoephedrine | Sudafed | 60 mg q 4–6 h |
| *Antihistamine-Decongestant Combinations* | | |
| Acravistine-pseudoephedrine | Semprex-D | 8/60* mg qid |
| Chlorpheniramine-pseudoephedrine | Sudafed Plus | 4/60* mg q 4–6 h |
| Chlorpheniramine-phenylpropanolamine | Allerest, Contac | 12/75* mg q 12 h |
| Clemastine-phenylpropanolamine | Tavist-D | 1.34/75* mg q 12 h |
| Terfenadine-pseudoephedrine | Seldane-D | 60/120* mg bid |
| Triprolidine-pseudoephedrine | Actifed | 2.5/60* mg q 4–6 h |

*The first number refers to milligrams of the antihistamine in the combination; the second number refers to milligrams of the decongestant in the combination.

*amethasone*; reactions can be minimized by limiting use of dexamethasone to no more than 30 days. Since the other intranasal glucocorticoids undergo rapid deactivation following absorption, they do not achieve significant blood levels. Hence, systemic effects are minimal. Accordingly, these agents are preferred to dexamethasone for intranasal use.

**Dosage and Administration.** Intranasal glucocorticoids are administered using a metered spray device. Full doses are given initially (Table 70–2). Once symptoms have been controlled, the dosage should be reduced to the lowest effective amount. For patients with seasonal allergic rhinitis, maximal effects may require a week or more to develop. For patients with perennial rhinitis, maximal responses may not be seen for 2 to 3 weeks. If nasal passages are blocked, they should be cleared with a topical decongestant prior to glucocorticoid administration.

# Drugs Used to Treat Cough

Cough is a complex reflex involving the central nervous system, the peripheral nervous system, and the muscles of respiration. The cough reflex can be initiated by irritation of the bronchial mucosa as well as by stimuli arising at sites distant from the respiratory tract. Cough is often beneficial, serving to remove foreign matter and excess secretions from the bronchial tree. Productive cough is

characteristic of chronic lung disease (e.g., emphysema, asthma, bronchitis) and should not be suppressed. Not all cough, however, is useful; cough frequently serves only to deprive us of comfort or sleep. Under these conditions, antitussive medication is appropriate. The most common use of cough medicines is suppression of nonproductive cough associated with the common cold and other upper respiratory infections.

## Antitussives

Antitussives are drugs that suppress cough. Some of these agents act within the CNS, whereas others act peripherally. The antitussives fall into two major groups: (1) opioid antitussives and (2) nonopioid antitussives.

### Opioid Antitussives

All of the opioid analgesics have the ability to suppress cough. The two opioids used most frequently for cough suppression are *codeine* and *hydrocodone*. Both agents act within the CNS to elevate cough threshold. Hydrocodone is somewhat more potent than codeine and carries a greater liability for abuse. The basic pharmacology of the opioids is discussed in Chapter 25.

**Codeine.** Codeine is the most effective cough suppressant available. The drug is active orally and decreases both the frequency and intensity of cough. Doses are low, about one-tenth those needed to relieve pain. At these doses, the risk of physical dependence is small.

| TABLE 70-3. INTRANASAL GLUCOCORTICOIDS | | |
| --- | --- | --- |
| **Generic and Trade Names** | **Vehicle** | **Dosage (Puffs/Nostril)** |
| Beclomethasone | | |
| [Beconase, Vancenase] | Nonaqueous | *Adults:* 1 puff bid-qid |
| [Beconase AQ, Vancenase AQ] | Aqueous | *Children 6-12 years:* 1 puff tid |
| Budesonide | | |
| [Rhinocort] | Nonaqueous | *Adults and Children >6 years:* 2 puffs bid *or* 4 puffs q AM |
| Dexamethasone | | |
| [Decadron Phosphate Turbinaire] | Nonaqueous | *Adults:* 2 puffs bid or tid |
| | | *Children 6-12 years:* 1-2 puffs bid |
| Flunisolide | | |
| [Nasalide] | Nonaqueous | *Adults:* 2 puffs bid |
| | | *Children 6-14 years:* 1 puff tid *or* 2 puffs bid |
| Fluticasone | | |
| [Flonase] | Aqueous | *Adults:* 2 puffs qd *or* 1 puff bid |
| | | *Children 12 or older:* 1 puff qd |
| Triamcinolone | | |
| [Nasocort] | Nonaqueous | *Adults:* 2-4 puffs qd |

Like all opioids, codeine can suppress respiration. Accordingly, the drug should be employed with caution in patients with reduced respiratory reserve. In the event of overdose, respiratory depression may prove fatal; an opioid antagonist (e.g., naloxone) should be used to reverse toxicity.

When dispensed by itself, codeine has a significant potential for abuse, and is classified under Schedule II of the Controlled Substances Act. However, the abuse potential of the antitussive mixtures that contain codeine is low. Accordingly, these mixtures are classified under Schedule V.

For treatment of cough, the adult dosage is 10 to 20 mg orally, 4 to 6 times a day. Codeine is rarely recommended for children.

## Nonopioid Antitussives

**Dextromethorphan.** Dextromethorphan is the most effective of the nonopioid cough medicines. Except when used for severe acute cough, this drug is just as effective as codeine. Like the opioids, dextromethorphan acts within the CNS. Dextromethorphan is a derivative of the opioids but only shares the ability to suppress cough; dextromethorphan does not produce analgesia, euphoria, or physical dependence, and lacks any potential for abuse. At therapeutic doses, dextromethorphan does not depress respiration. Adverse effects are mild and rare. Dextromethorphan is the active ingredient in most nonprescription antitussive preparations. The usual adult dosage is 10 to 30 mg every 4 to 8 hours.

**Other Nonopioid Antitussives.** *Diphenhydramine* is an antihistamine with the ability to suppress cough. The mechanism of antitussive action is unclear. Like other antihistamines, diphenhydramine has sedative and anticholinergic properties. Cough suppression is achieved only at doses that produce prominent sedation. The usual adult dosage is 25 mg every 4 hours.

*Benzonatate* [Tessalon] is a structural analog of tetracaine, a local anesthetic. The drug is believed to suppress cough by decreasing the sensitivity of respiratory tract stretch receptors (components of the cough-reflex pathway); CNS mechanisms may also be involved. Adverse effects are usually mild (e.g., sedation, dizziness, constipation). Benzonatate is dispensed in capsules for oral administration. The capsules should be swallowed intact, since chewing produces anesthesia of the mouth and pharynx. The usual adult dosage is 100 mg 3 times a day. The drug should not be given to infants because anesthesia of the mouth may impair swallowing.

### Expectorants and Mucolytics

**Expectorants.** An expectorant is a drug that renders cough more productive by stimulating the flow of respiratory tract secretions. A variety of compounds (e.g., terpin hydrate, ammonium chloride, iodide products) have been promoted for their supposed expectorant actions. However, in almost all cases, efficacy is doubtful. One agent, *guaifenesin* (glyceryl guaiacolate), may be an exception to this rule. However, for this drug to be effective, doses higher than those normally employed may be needed.

**Mucolytics.** A mucolytic is a drug that reacts directly with mucus to make it more watery. This action should help make cough more productive. Two preparations—*hypertonic saline* and *acetylcysteine*—are employed for their mucolytic actions. Both are administered by inhalation. Unfortunately, both drugs can trigger bronchospasm. Because of its sulfur content, acetylcysteine [Mucomyst] has the additional disadvantage of smelling like rotten eggs.

## Cold Remedies: Combination Preparations

The common cold is an acute upper respiratory infection of viral origin. Symptoms include rhinorrhea, sneezing, cough, sore throat, headache, malaise, and myalgia; fever is common in children but rare in adults. The cold is a self-limited disorder and is usually benign. Persistence or worsening of symptoms suggests development of a secondary bacterial infection.

There is no cure for the cold; hence treatment is purely symptomatic. Since colds are caused by viruses, there is no justification for the routine use of antibacterial drugs. Antibiotics are appropriate only if a bacterial infection arises. There is no evidence that vitamin C can prevent or cure colds.

Because no single drug can relieve all of the symptoms of a cold, the pharmaceutical industry has formulated a vast number of cold remedies that contain a mixture of ingredients. These combination cold remedies should be reserved for patients with multiple symptoms. In addition, the combination chosen should contain only those agents that are appropriate for the symptoms to be treated. Patients who require relief from just a single symptom (e.g., rhinitis, cough, or headache) are best treated with a single-entity preparation.

Combination cold remedies frequently contain two or more of the following: (1) a nasal decongestant, (2) an antitussive, (3) an analgesic, (4) an antihistamine, and (5) caffeine. The purpose of the first three agents is self-evident. In contrast, the roles of antihistamines and caffeine require explanation. Since histamine has nothing to do with the symptoms of a cold, antihistamines are not present to counteract the actions of histamine. Rather, because of their anticholinergic actions, antihistamines are included to suppress secretion of mucus. Caffeine is added to offset the sedative effects of the antihistamine.

Although they can be convenient, combination cold remedies do have disadvantages. As with all fixed-dose combinations, there is the chance that a dosage (e.g., one capsule or one tablet) that produces therapeutic levels of one ingredient may produce levels of other ingredients that are either excessive or subtherapeutic. In addition, the combination may contain ingredients for which the patient has no need. Furthermore, under FDA regulations, a brand-name product can be reformulated and then sold under the same name. Hence, without carefully reading the label, the consumer has no assurance that the brand name product purchased this year contains the same amounts of the same drugs that were present in last year's version of that combination product.

## KEY POINTS

- Allergic rhinitis is the most common of all allergic disorders.
- Allergic rhinitis is treated with antihistamines, decongestants, intranasal cromolyn sodium, and intranasal glucocorticoids.
- Nasal decongestants act by stimulating alpha$_1$-adrenergic receptors on blood vessels, which causes vasoconstriction and thereby shrinks swollen nasal membranes.
- *Topical* decongestants act rapidly and produce minimal systemic effects, but cause rebound congestion when used for more than a few days.
- *Oral* decongestants act slowly and produce CNS stimulation, but do not cause rebound congestion, and hence are suited for long-term use.
- Antihistamines (H$_1$-receptor antagonists) are first-line drugs for treating allergic rhinitis. They relieve rhinorrhea, sneezing, and itching, but *not* congestion.
- Sedation is a common side effect of the first-generation antihistamines but not of the second-generation agents.
- Intranasal cromolyn sodium provides effective treatment of allergic rhinitis, but only when taken prophylactically. Effects take a week or so to develop.
- Intranasal steroids (glucocorticoids) are the most effective drugs for allergic rhinitis. They relieve rhinorrhea, congestion, itching, and sneezing.
- Of the intranasal steroids in use today, only *dexamethasone* presents a significant risk of systemic toxicity.
- Codeine, a member of the opioid family of drugs, is the most effective cough suppressant available. Doses are only one-tenth those used for analgesia.
- Dextromethorphan is the most effective nonopioid cough suppressant available.

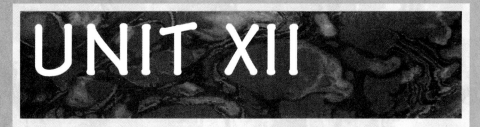

# UNIT XII

# Gastrointestinal Drugs

Drugs for Peptic Ulcer Disease

Laxatives

Other Gastrointestinal Drugs

# Drugs for Peptic Ulcer Disease

The term *peptic ulcer disease* (PUD) refers to a group of upper gastrointestinal disorders characterized by varying degrees of erosion of the gut wall. Severe ulcers can be complicated by hemorrhage and perforation. Although peptic ulcers can develop in any region exposed to acid and pepsin, ulceration is most common in the lesser curvature of the stomach and in the duodenum. PUD is a very common disorder that affects about 10% of Americans at some time in their lives. About 4.5 million Americans get ulcers each year. Until recently, PUD was considered a chronic, relapsing disorder of unknown cause and with no known cure; therapy promoted healing but did not prevent ulcer recurrence. However, we now know that most cases of PUD are caused by infection with *Helicobacter pylori*, and that eradication of this bacterium not only promotes healing, but greatly reduces the chance of ulcer recurrence.

## Pathogenesis of Peptic Ulcers

Peptic ulcers develop when there is an imbalance between mucosal defensive factors and aggressive factors (Fig. 71–1). The major defensive factors are mucus and bicarbonate. The major aggressive factors are *H. pylori*, nonsteroidal anti-inflammatory drugs (NSAIDs), gastric acid, and pepsin.

## Defensive Factors

Defensive factors serve the physiologic role of protecting the stomach and duodenum from self-digestion. When de-

fenses are intact, generation of ulcers is unlikely. Conversely, when defenses are compromised, aggressive factors are able to cause injury. Two important agents that can weaken defenses are *H. pylori* and NSAIDs.

***Mucus.*** Mucus is secreted continuously by cells of the gastrointestinal mucosa, forming a barrier that protects underlying cells from attack by acid and pepsin.

***Bicarbonate.*** Bicarbonate is secreted by epithelial cells of the stomach and duodenum. Most bicarbonate remains trapped in the mucus layer, where it serves to neutralize any hydrogen ions that penetrate the mucus. Bicarbonate produced by the pancreas is secreted into the lumen of the duodenum, where it neutralizes acid delivered from the stomach.

***Blood Flow.*** Blood flow to cells of the gastrointestinal mucosa is essential for maintaining mucosal integrity. If submucosal blood flow is reduced, the resultant local ischemia can lead to cell injury, thereby increasing vulnerability to attack by acid and pepsin.

***Prostaglandins.*** Prostaglandins play an important role in maintaining defenses. These compounds stimulate secretion of mucus and bicarbonate, and they promote vasodilation, which helps maintain submucosal blood flow. Prostaglandins provide additional protection by suppressing secretion of gastric acid.

## Aggressive Factors

***Helicobacter pylori.*** *Helicobacter pylori* is a gram-negative bacillus that can colonize the stomach and duodenum. By taking up residence in the space between epithelial cells and the mucus barrier that protects them, this

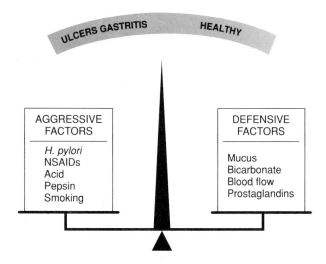

**Figure 71–1. The relationship of mucosal defenses and aggressive factors to health and peptic ulcer disease.** When aggressive factors outweigh mucosal defenses, gastritis and peptic ulcers result. (NSAIDs = nonsteroidal anti-inflammatory drugs.)

organism manages to escape destruction by acid and pepsin. Once established, *H. pylori* can remain in the gastrointestinal tract for decades. Although a vast number of people are infected with *H. pylori*, only a minority develop symptomatic PUD.

Why do we think *H. pylori* causes PUD? First, over 90% of patients with duodenal ulcers and up to 80% of patients with gastric ulcers have *H. pylori* infection. Second, duodenal ulcers are much more common among people with *H. pylori* infection than among people who are not infected. Third, eradication of the bacterium promotes ulcer healing. Fourth, eradication of the bacterium minimizes ulcer recurrence. (Recurrence rates approach 100% when *H. pylori* is not eliminated, and have been as low as 1% when the organism was eradicated.)

Although the mechanism by which *H. pylori* promotes ulcers has not been firmly established, likely possibilities are enzymatic degradation of the protective mucus layer, elaboration of a cytotoxin that injures mucosal cells, and infiltration of neutrophils and other inflammatory cells in response to the organism's presence. Also, *H. pylori* produces urease, an enzyme that forms carbon dioxide and ammonia from urea in gastric juice; the carbon dioxide and ammonia are potentially toxic to the gastric mucosa. In addition to its role in PUD, *H. pylori* is strongly associated with development of gastric adenocarcinoma.

***Nonsteroidal Anti-inflammatory Drugs.*** NSAIDs are the underlying cause of many gastric ulcers and some duodenal ulcers. As discussed in Chapter 64, aspirin and other NSAIDs inhibit the biosynthesis of prostaglandins. By doing so, these drugs can decrease submucosal blood flow, suppress secretion of mucus and bicarbonate, and promote secretion of gastric acid. Furthermore, NSAIDs can irritate the mucosa directly. NSAID-induced ulcers are most likely with long-term, high-dose therapy.

***Gastric Acid.*** Gastric acid is an absolute requirement for peptic ulcer formation: in the absence of acid no ulcer will form. Acid causes ulcers by (1) injuring cells of the gastrointestinal mucosa and (2) activating pepsin, a proteolytic enzyme. In most cases, acid hypersecretion, by itself, is insufficient to generate ulcers. In fact, in most patients with gastric ulcers, acid secretion is normal or reduced, and among patients with duodenal ulcers, only one third produce excessive amounts of acid. From these observations, we can conclude that in the majority of patients with peptic ulcers, factors in addition to acid must be involved.

*Zollinger-Ellison syndrome* is the primary disorder in which hypersecretion of acid alone appears to be the sole cause of ulcer formation. The underlying cause of this syndrome is a tumor that secretes gastrin, a hormone that stimulates gastric acid release. In response to high levels of gastrin, gastric acid is produced in huge quantities—quantities that are sufficient to overwhelm mucosal defenses. Zollinger-Ellison syndrome is a rare disorder that accounts for about 0.1% of duodenal ulcers.

***Pepsin.*** Pepsin is a proteolytic enzyme present in gastric juice. Like gastric acid, pepsin can injure unprotected cells of the gastric and duodenal mucosa.

***Smoking.*** Smoking delays ulcer healing and increases the risk of recurrence. Possible mechanisms for these effects include reduction of the beneficial effects of antiulcer medications, reduced secretion of bicarbonate, and accelerated gastric emptying, which would deliver more acid to the duodenum.

## Summary

Infection with *H. pylori* is now recognized as the most common cause of gastric and duodenal ulcers. However, among people whose PUD can be ascribed to *H. pylori*, additional factors must be involved. We know this because more than 50% of the population harbors *H. pylori*, but only 10% develop ulcers. Factors that may increase the risk of PUD in people infected with *H. pylori* include smoking, increased acid secretion, and reduced bicarbonate production. Following infection with *H. pylori*, the second most common cause of gastric ulcers is use of NSAIDs. Hypersecretion of acid underlies a few cases of PUD that are not caused by *H. pylori* or NSAIDs.

## Overview of Treatment

### Drug Therapy

The goal of drug therapy is to (1) alleviate symptoms; (2) promote healing; (3) prevent complications (hemorrhage, perforation, obstruction); and (4) prevent recurrences. With the exception of antibiotics, antiulcer drugs do not alter the disease process; rather, they simply create conditions conducive to healing. Since nonantibiotic thera-

## TABLE 71-1. CLASSIFICATION OF ANTIULCER DRUGS

| Class | Drugs | Mechanism of Action |
|---|---|---|
| *Antibiotics* | Bismuth [Pepto-Bismol] Metronidazole [Flagyl] Tetracycline [Achromycin V] Amoxicillin [Amoxil] Clarithromycin [Biaxin] | Eradication of *H. pylori* infection |
| *Antisecretory Agents* | | |
| H₂-receptor antagonists | Cimetidine [Tagamet] Famotidine [Pepcid] Nizatidine [Axid] Ranitidine [Zantac] | Suppression of acid secretion by blocking $H_2$ receptors on parietal cells |
| Proton pump inhibitors | Omeprazole [Prilosec] Lansoprazole [Prevacid] | Suppression of acid secretion by inhibiting $H^+$, $K^+$-ATPase, the enzyme that makes gastric acid |
| Muscarinic antagonists | Pirenzepine [Gastrozepine] | Suppression of acid secretion by blocking muscarinic cholinergic receptors (on parietal cells?) |
| *Mucosal Protectant* | Sucralfate [Carafate] | Forms a barrier over the ulcer crater that protects against acid and pepsin |
| *Antisecretory Agent That Enhances Mucosal Defenses* | Misoprostol [Cytotec] | Protects against NSAID-induced ulcers by stimulating secretion of mucus and bicarbonate, maintaining submucosal blood flow, and suppressing secretion of gastric acid |
| *Antacids* | Aluminum hydroxide Magnesium hydroxide Calcium carbonate | Conversion of gastric acid to neutral salts |

pies do not cure ulcers, the relapse rate following their discontinuation is high. In contrast, the relapse rate is low following use of antibiotics.

### Classes of Antiulcer Drugs

As shown in Table 71-1, the antiulcer drugs fall into five major classes: (1) antibiotics, (2) antisecretory agents, (3) mucosal protectants, (4) antisecretory agents that enhance mucosal defenses, and (5) antacids. From this classification, we can see that drugs act in three basic ways to promote ulcer healing. First, drugs can eradicate *H. pylori*; antibiotics do this. Second, drugs can reduce gastric acidity; antisecretory agents, misoprostol, and antacids do this. Third, drugs can enhance mucosal defenses; sucralfate and misoprostol do this.

### Drug Selection

In the past, drugs were given short term to relieve symptoms and promote healing, and then often given long term to prevent ulcer recurrence. In the United States, the drugs employed most frequently for short-term therapy are the H₂-receptor antagonists (H₂RAs) (e.g., ranitidine [Zantac]). These agents are very safe, and, for many patients, effective with once-a-day dosing. Sucralfate [Carafate] and omeprazole [Prilosec] are alternatives.

Sucralfate is just as effective as the H₂RAs but less convenient. The drug must be taken 4 times a day and the tablets are large, making them difficult for some patients to swallow. With omeprazole, rates of healing are faster than with the H₂RAs, but omeprazole is more expensive. In addition, there is some concern about the long-term safety of omeprazole. Antacids are no longer employed as sole therapy of PUD. Although these drugs are as effective as the H₂-receptor antagonists, they are unpleasant to ingest and must be administered 7 times a day. Today, antacids are employed as adjuncts to other antiulcer medications to provide rapid relief of dyspepsia and pain.

Therapy of PUD has changed dramatically in recent years. The reason is *H. pylori*. In 1994, an NIH Consensus Development Conference recommended that all patients with gastric or duodenal ulcers and documented *H. pylori* infection be treated with antibiotics. This recommendation applies to patients with newly diagnosed PUD, recurrent PUD, and PUD in which use of NSAIDs is a contributing factor. To hasten healing and relief of symptoms, an antisecretory agent (usually omeprazole) is given along with the antibiotics. By eliminating *H. pylori*, antibiotics can cure PUD, and thereby prevent recurrence. Diagnosis of *H. pylori* infection and specific antibiotic regimens are discussed below.

Therapy with aspirin and other NSAIDs can cause PUD, especially in elderly patients. Only one drug—*misoprostol*—is approved for prophylaxis of NSAID-induced ulcers. This drug, which is taken along with the NSAID, should be reserved for patients considered at high risk of ulcer development. Since misoprostol stimulates uterine contractions, the drug must never be given to pregnant women. If an ulcer develops despite prophylaxis with misoprostol, the NSAID should be discontinued, or at least given in reduced dosage. The ulcer can be treated with conventional antiulcer drugs (e.g., an $H_2$-receptor antagonist, omeprazole).

### Evaluation

We can evaluate ulcer healing by monitoring for relief of pain and by performing radiologic or endoscopic examination of the ulcer site. Unfortunately, evaluation is seldom straightforward. This is because cessation of pain and disappearance of the ulcer rarely coincide: in most cases, pain subsides prior to complete healing. However, the converse may also be true: pain may persist even though endoscopic or radiologic examination reveals healing is complete.

Eradication of *H. pylori* can be determined with several methods, including a breath test, serologic tests, and microscopic observation of a stained biopsy sample. These methods are discussed below under *Tests for H. pylori*.

#### A Note about the Effects of Drugs on Pepsin

Pepsin is a proteolytic enzyme that can contribute to ulcer formation. This enzyme promotes ulcers by breaking down protein in the gut wall.

Like most enzymes, pepsin is sensitive to alterations in pH. As pH rises from 1.3 (the usual pH of the stomach) to 2, peptic activity increases by a factor of 4. As pH goes even higher, peptic activity begins to decline. At a pH of 5, peptic activity drops below baseline rates. When pH exceeds 6 to 7, pepsin undergoes irreversible inactivation.

Because the activity of pepsin is pH dependent, drugs that elevate gastric pH (e.g., antacids, histamine$_2$ antagonists) can cause peptic activity to increase, thereby enhancing pepsin's destructive effects. For example, treatment that produces a 99% reduction in gastric acidity will cause pH to rise from a base level of 1.3 up to 3.3. At pH 3.3, peptic activity will be significantly increased. To avoid activation of pepsin, drugs that reduce acidity should be administered in doses sufficient to raise gastric pH above 5.

### Nondrug Therapy

Optimal antiulcer therapy requires implementation of nondrug measures in addition to drug therapy.

**Diet.** Despite commonly held beliefs, diet plays a minor role in ulcer management. The traditional "ulcer diet," consisting of bland foods together with milk or cream, does not accelerate healing. Furthermore, there is no convincing evidence that caffeine-containing beverages (coffee, tea, colas) promote ulcer formation or interfere with recovery. A change in *eating pattern* may be beneficial: consumption of five or six small meals a day, rather than three larger ones, can reduce fluctuations in intragastric pH, and may thereby facilitate healing.

**Other Nondrug Measures.** *Smoking* is associated with an increased incidence of ulcers and also retards recovery. Accordingly, cigarettes should be avoided. Because of their ulcerogenic actions, *aspirin and other NSAIDs* should be avoided by patients with PUD. The exception to this rule is use of aspirin to prevent cardiovascular disease; in the low doses employed, aspirin is not a significant factor in PUD. There are no hard data indicating that *alcohol* contributes to PUD. However, if the patient notes a temporal relationship between alcohol consumption and exacerbation of symptoms, then alcohol use should stop. Many people feel that reduction of *stress and anxiety* may encourage ulcer healing; however, there is no good evidence that this is true.

## Antibacterial Drugs

As noted above, antibacterial drugs should be given to all patients with gastric or duodenal ulcers and confirmed infection with *H. pylori*. At this time, antibiotics are not recommended for asymptomatic individuals who test positive for *H. pylori*.

### Tests for *H. pylori*

Several tests for *H. pylori* are available. Some are invasive; some are not. The invasive tests require an endoscopically obtained biopsy sample, which can be evaluated in three ways: (1) staining and viewing under a microscope to see if *H. pylori* is present; (2) assaying for the presence of urease (a marker enzyme for *H. pylori*), and (3) culturing and then assaying for the presence of *H. pylori*. Two types of noninvasive tests are available: breath tests and serologic tests. In the breath tests, patients are given radiolabeled urea. If *H. pylori* is present, the urea is converted to carbon dioxide and ammonia; radiolabeled carbon dioxide can then be detected in the breath. In the serologic tests, blood samples are evaluated for antibodies to *H. pylori*.

### Antibiotics Employed

The antibiotics employed most often are bismuth, metronidazole, tetracycline, amoxicillin, and clarithromycin. None is effective alone. Furthermore, if metronidazole or clarithromycin is used alone, resistance may develop. Resistance has not been reported with bismuth, tetracycline, or amoxicillin.

**Bismuth.** Bismuth compounds act topically to disrupt the cell wall of *H. pylori*, thereby causing lysis and death. Bismuth may also inhibit urease activity and prevent *H. pylori* from adhering to the gastric surface.

Bismuth can impart a harmless black coloration to the tongue and the stool. Patients should be forewarned of these effects. Stool discoloration may confound interpretation of gastric bleeding. Long-term therapy may carry a risk of neurologic injury.

In the United States, bismuth is available (1) by itself as bismuth subsalicylate [Pepto-Bismol, others], and (2) in a complex with ranitidine (ranitidine bismuth citrate), marketed under the trade name Tritec. In Europe the drug is available as bismuth subcitrate [De-Nol].

***Metronidazole.*** Metronidazole is a cornerstone of triple antibiotic therapy (see below). *H. pylori* is highly sensitive to this drug, unless resistance develops. Emergence of resistance can be minimized by combining metronidazole with other antibiotics. The most common side effects are nausea and headache. A disulfiram-like reaction can occur if metronidazole is used with alcohol. Accordingly, alcohol should be avoided. Metronidazole should not be taken during pregnancy. The basic pharmacology of metronidazole is discussed in Chapter 93.

***Tetracycline.*** Tetracycline, an inhibitor of bacterial protein synthesis, is highly active against *H. pylori*. Resistance has not been reported. Because tetracycline can stain developing teeth, it should not be used by pregnant women or young children. The pharmacology of tetracycline is discussed in Chapter 80.

***Amoxicillin.*** *H. pylori* is highly sensitive to amoxicillin. Resistance has not been reported. Amoxicillin kills bacteria by disrupting the cell wall. Antibacterial activity is highest at neutral pH, and hence can be enhanced by reducing gastric acidity with an antisecretory agent (e.g., omeprazole). The most common side effect is diarrhea. The basic pharmacology of amoxicillin and other penicillins is discussed in Chapter 78.

***Clarithromycin.*** Clarithromycin suppresses growth of *H. pylori* by inhibiting protein synthesis. Resistance can develop if the drug is used alone. The combination of clarithromycin with either omeprazole or ranitidine has been approved by the FDA as a regimen for eradicating *H. pylori*. However, the American College of Gastroenterology recommends that either tetracycline or amoxicillin be added as second antibiotics. The most common side effects are nausea, diarrhea, and distortion of taste. The basic pharmacology of clarithromycin is presented in Chapter 80.

## Antibiotic Regimens

Various combinations of antibiotics have been employed to eradicate *H. pylori*. The most effective are summarized in Table 71-2. Because emergence of resistance can be a problem, regimens employ at least two antibiotics, and often three. As a rule, an antisecretory agent (e.g., omeprazole) is given as well. As shown in Table 71-2, the highest eradication rate (94% to 98%) has been achieved by combining triple antibiotic therapy (bismuth

---

**TABLE 71-2. SOME REGIMENS FOR ERADICATING *H. PYLORI***

| Regimen | Dosage | Duration | Eradication |
|---|---|---|---|
| *Three Antibiotics* | | | |
| Bismuth subsalicylate* | 525 mg qid | 14 days | 88-90% |
| Metronidazole | 250 mg qid | 7 days | 86-90% |
| Tetracycline | 500 mg qid | | |
| Bismuth subsalicylate | 525 mg qid | 14 days | 80-86% |
| Metronidazole | 250 mg qid | 7 days | 75-81% |
| Amoxicillin | 500 mg qid | | |
| *Three Antibiotics Plus an Antisecretory Agent* | | | |
| Bismuth subsalicylate | 525 mg qid | 7 days | 94-98% |
| Metronidazole | 250 mg qid | | |
| Tetracycline | 500 mg qid | | |
| Omeprazole | 20 mg bid | | |
| *Two Antibiotics Plus an Antisecretory Agent* | | | |
| Metronidazole | 500 mg bid | 7 days | 87-91% |
| Clarithromycin | 500 mg bid | | |
| Omeprazole | 20 mg bid | | |
| Amoxicillin | 1000 mg bid | 7-14 days | 77-83% |
| Clarithromycin | 500 mg bid | | |
| Omeprazole | 20 mg bid | | |
| Metronidazole | 400 mg tid | 14 days | 90% |
| Amoxicillin | 500 mg tid | | |
| Omeprazole | 40 mg/day | | |

*This three-antibiotic regimen is available in a kit under the trade name Helidac.

subsalicylate, metronidazole, and tetracycline) with omeprazole, an antisecretory drug. However, the eradication rate was only slightly lower (about 90%) when the regimen included either three antibiotics (with no antisecretory agent), or just two antibiotics plus omeprazole. Therapy with a single antibiotic is not recommended.

For several reasons, compliance with antibiotic therapy can be difficult. First, antibiotic regimens are complex, requiring the patient to ingest as many as 12 pills a day. Second, side effects are common. The ones seen most often are nausea and diarrhea. Third, treatment is somewhat expensive (about $200). However, its costs much less to eradicate *H. pylori* with antibiotics than it does to treat ulcers over and over again with traditional antiulcer drugs, which merely promote healing without eliminating the cause.

# Histamine₂-Receptor Antagonists

The histamine₂-receptor antagonists (H₂RAs) are drugs of first choice for treating gastric and duodenal ulcers. These agents promote ulcer healing by suppressing secretion of gastric acid. Four H₂RAs are available: cimetidine, ranitidine, famotidine, and nizatidine. All four are equally effec-

tive, and with all four the incidence of serious side effects is low.

## Cimetidine

Cimetidine [Tagamet] was the first H₂RA available and will serve as our prototype for the family. At one time, cimetidine was the most frequently prescribed drug in the United States.

### Mechanism of Action

As discussed in Chapter 63, histamine acts through two types of receptors, named H₁ and H₂. Activation of H₁ receptors produces symptoms of allergy. In contrast, activation of H₂ receptors, which are located on parietal cells of the stomach (Fig. 71–2), promotes secretion of gastric acid. By blocking H₂ receptors, cimetidine reduces both the volume of gastric juice and its hydrogen ion concentration. Cimetidine suppresses basal acid secretion and reduces stimulation of acid secretion by gastrin and acetylcholine. Since cimetidine produces selective blockade of H₂ receptors, the drug does not reduce symptoms of allergy.

### Pharmacokinetics

Cimetidine is administered orally, intramuscularly, and intravenously. Comparable blood levels are achieved with all three routes. When the drug is taken orally, food de-

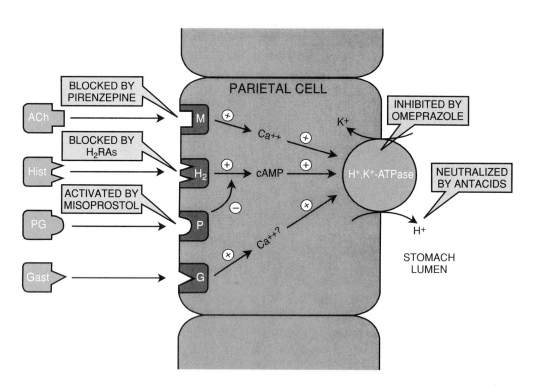

**Figure 71–2. A model of the regulation of gastric acid secretion showing the actions of antisecretory drugs and antacids.** Production of gastric acid is stimulated by three endogenous compounds: (1) acetylcholine (ACh) acting at muscarinic (M) receptors; (2) histamine (hist) acting at histamine₂ (H₂) receptors; and (3) gastrin (gast) acting at gastrin (G) receptors. As indicated, all three compounds act through intracellular messengers—either calcium (Ca⁺⁺) or cyclic AMP (cAMP)—to increase the activity of H⁺, K⁺-ATPase, the enzyme that actually produces gastric acid. Prostaglandins (PG) decrease acid production, perhaps by suppressing production of intracellular cAMP. The actions of histamine₂-receptor antagonists (H₂RAs), other antisecretory drugs, and antacids are indicated. (P = prostaglandin receptor.)

creases the rate of absorption but not the extent. Hence, if cimetidine is taken with meals, absorption will be slowed and beneficial effects prolonged. Cimetidine crosses the blood-brain barrier—albeit with difficulty—and central nervous system (CNS) side effects can occur. Although some hepatic metabolism takes place, most of each dose is eliminated intact in the urine. The half-life of cimetidine is relatively short (about 2 hours), but increases in patients with renal impairment. Dosage should be reduced in these patients.

## Therapeutic Uses

*Gastric and Duodenal Ulcers.* Cimetidine promotes healing of gastric and duodenal ulcers. To heal duodenal ulcers, 4 to 6 weeks of therapy are generally required. To heal gastric ulcers, 8 to 12 weeks may be needed. Long-term therapy with low doses may be given as prophylaxis against recurrence of gastric and duodenal ulcers.

*Gastroesophageal Reflux Disease.* Reflux esophagitis is an inflammatory condition caused by reflux of gastric contents back into the esophagus. Cimetidine is a drug of choice for relieving symptoms. However, cimetidine does little to hasten healing.

*Zollinger-Ellison Syndrome.* This syndrome is characterized by hypersecretion of gastric acid and development of peptic ulcers. The underlying cause is secretion of gastrin from a gastrin-producing tumor. Cimetidine can promote healing of ulcers in patients with Zollinger-Ellison syndrome, but only if high doses are employed. These high doses may cause significant adverse effects.

*Aspiration Pneumonitis.* Anesthesia suppresses the glottal reflex, permitting aspiration of gastric acid. When acid is aspirated, pulmonary injury develops in seconds and can be fatal. Surgical patients at high risk for this disorder include obese patients and women undergoing obstetric procedures. Cimetidine is a drug of choice for preventing aspiration pneumonitis. Gastric acidity can be reduced substantially by administering the drug 60 to 90 minutes prior to anesthesia.

*Heartburn, Acid Indigestion, and Sour Stomach.* Cimetidine is now available over the counter for treatment of these common acid-related symptoms.

## Adverse Effects

The incidence of side effects with cimetidine is low. Furthermore, the effects that do occur are usually benign.

*Antiandrogenic Effects.* Cimetidine binds to androgen receptors, producing receptor blockade. This action may result in *gynecomastia*, *reduced libido*, and *impotence*. These effects reverse following termination of treatment.

*CNS Effects.* Effects on the CNS are most likely in elderly patients who have renal or hepatic impairment. Possible reactions include *confusion*, *hallucinations*, *CNS depression* (lethargy, somnolence), and *CNS excitation* (restlessness, seizures).

*Other Adverse Effects.* When administered as an IV bolus, cimetidine can cause *hypotension* and *dysrhythmias*. These reactions are rare and do not occur with oral therapy. By reducing gastric acidity, cimetidine *may permit growth of Candida within the stomach. Hematologic effects* (neutropenia, leukopenia, thrombocytopenia) occur rarely. *Minor side effects* include headache, dizziness, myalgia, nausea, diarrhea, constipation, rash, and pruritus.

## Drug Interactions

*Interactions Related to Inhibition of Drug Metabolism.* Cimetidine inhibits hepatic drug-metabolizing enzymes. By reducing drug metabolism, cimetidine can cause levels of many other drugs to rise. Agents of particular concern are *warfarin*, *phenytoin*, *theophylline*, and *lidocaine*, all of which have a narrow margin of safety. If these agents are used concurrently with cimetidine, their dosages should be reduced.

*Antacids.* Antacids can decrease the absorption of cimetidine. Accordingly, cimetidine and antacids should be administered at least 1 hour apart from each other.

### Preparations, Dosage, and Administration

*Oral.* Cimetidine [Tagamet] is available in tablets (200, 300, 400, and 800 mg) and solution (300 mg/5 ml) for oral administration. For treatment of duodenal and gastric ulcers, the drug may be given once daily (800 mg at bedtime), twice daily (400 mg each dose), or 4 times a day (300 mg with meals and at bedtime). In patients with renal impairment, the dosage should be lowered to 300 mg every 12 hours. For prophylaxis against recurrence of ulcers, a single 400-mg dose at bedtime may be employed. Patients with Zollinger-Ellison syndrome require high doses, but not more than 2.4 gm/day.

*Parenteral.* Parenteral cimetidine is reserved for patients with hypersecretory conditions (e.g., Zollinger-Ellison syndrome) and ulcers that have failed to respond to oral therapy. The usual dosage (IM or IV) is 300 mg every 6 to 8 hours. Intramuscular injections are made with a concentrated solution (300 mg/2 ml). For IV administration, two concentrations may be employed: (1) the dose may be diluted in a total volume of 20 ml and injected slowly (over 2 minutes), or (2) it may be diluted in 100 ml and infused over 15 minutes.

## Ranitidine

Ranitidine [Zantac] shares many of the properties of cimetidine. However, although similar to cimetidine, ranitidine does differ in three important respects: ranitidine is more potent than cimetidine, produces fewer adverse effects, and causes fewer drug interactions.

*Actions.* Like cimetidine, ranitidine suppresses secretion of gastric acid by blocking $H_2$ receptors on parietal cells. The drug does not block $H_1$ receptors, and hence does not reduce symptoms of allergy.

*Pharmacokinetics.* Ranitidine can be administered orally, IM, and IV. Oral bioavailability is about 50%. In contrast to cimetidine, ranitidine is absorbed at the same rate in the presence or absence of food. The ability of ranitidine to enter the CNS is even less than that of cimetidine. Elimination is by a combination of hepatic metabolism and renal excretion. Accumulation will occur in patients with renal impairment unless the dosage is reduced. The half-life of ranitidine is 2 to 3 hours.

*Adverse Effects.* Significant side effects are uncommon. Because ranitidine penetrates the blood-brain barrier poorly, CNS effects are rare. In contrast to cimetidine, ranitidine does not bind to androgen receptors and, hence, does not cause antiandrogenic effects (e.g., gynecomastia, impotence).

*Drug Interactions.* Ranitidine has few drug interactions. In contrast to cimetidine, ranitidine is only a weak inhibitor of hepatic drug-metabolizing enzymes, and therefore does not greatly depress metabolism of other drugs. Antacids have only a small effect on ranitidine absorption.

***Therapeutic Uses.*** Ranitidine has the same indications as cimetidine. The drug is approved for (1) short-term treatment of gastric and duodenal ulcers, (2) prophylaxis of recurrent duodenal ulcers, (3) treatment of Zollinger-Ellison syndrome and other hypersecretory states, and (4) treatment of gastroesophageal reflux disease. Because it produces fewer side effects than cimetidine, and because of its greater potency, ranitidine is preferred to cimetidine for treating hypersecretory states (e.g., Zollinger-Ellison syndrome).

***Preparations, Dosage, and Administration.*** Ranitidine [Zantac, Zantac EFFERdose] is available in standard tablets (150 and 300 mg), effervescent tablets or granules (150 mg), a syrup (15 mg/ml), and as an injection (0.5 and 25 mg/ml).

***Oral.*** The usual adult dosage for therapy of gastric and duodenal ulcers is 150 mg twice a day. (Note that this dosage is considerably lower than that for cimetidine.) Alternatively, a 300-mg dose can be given once daily at bedtime. For patients with Zollinger-Ellison syndrome, higher doses may be required. The dosage for preventing recurrence of duodenal ulcers is 150 mg once daily at bedtime. Since its absorption is not affected by food, ranitidine can be administered without regard to meals.

***Parenteral.*** The usual parenteral dosage (IM or IV) is 50 mg every 6 to 8 hours. Intramuscular doses can be injected without dilution. For IV injection, the preparation should be diluted to a volume of 20 ml and administered slowly (over 5 or more minutes). For IV infusion, the drug should be diluted in 100 ml and administered over 15 to 20 minutes.

### Famotidine and Nizatidine

***Contrasts with Ranitidine.*** Famotidine [Pepcid] and nizatidine [Axid Pulvules] are very similar to ranitidine. Both agents are approved for (1) treatment of duodenal ulcers and preventing recurrence, (2) treatment of gastric ulcers, and (3) treatment of gastroesophageal reflux. In addition, famotidine is approved for treatment of hypersecretory states (e.g., Zollinger-Ellison syndrome), and the over-the-counter formulation [Pepcid AC Acid Controller] is approved for heartburn, acid indigestion, and sour stomach. Like ranitidine, famotidine and nizatidine do not bind to androgen receptors, and hence do not have antiandrogenic effects. Neither drug inhibits hepatic drug-metabolizing enzymes, and hence neither suppresses the metabolism of other drugs.

***Dosage.*** For treatment of duodenal and gastric ulcers, the dosage for famotidine is 20 mg twice daily or 40 mg once daily at bedtime; the dosage for nizatidine is 150 mg twice daily or 300 mg once daily at bedtime. For preventing the recurrence of duodenal ulcers, the dosage for famotidine is 20 mg once daily at bedtime and the dosage for nizatidine is 150 mg once daily at bedtime. For treatment of gastroesophageal reflux disease, the dosage of famotidine is 20 to 40 mg twice daily and the dosage of nizatidine is 150 mg twice daily.

# Proton Pump Inhibitors

## Omeprazole

Omeprazole [Prilosec] is the prototype of the proton pump inhibitors, the most effective agent available for suppressing secretion of gastric acid. Side effects from short-term therapy are minimal. With long-term therapy there is some concern about possible carcinogenesis.

***Mechanism of Action.*** Omeprazole is a prodrug that undergoes conversion to its active form within parietal cells of the stomach. The active form causes irreversible inhibition of $H^+,K^+$-ATPase—the enzyme that generates gastric acid (see Fig. 71-2). Because it blocks the final common pathway of gastric acid production, omeprazole can inhibit basal and stimulated acid release. A single 30-mg oral dose reduces production of gastric acid by 97% within 2 hours. Because inhibition of the ATPase is irreversible, effects persist until new enzyme is synthesized. Partial recovery of acid production occurs 3 to 5 days after termination of treatment. Full recovery may take weeks.

***Pharmacokinetics.*** Administration is oral. Since the drug is acid labile, it is dispensed in capsules that contain protective enteric-coated granules; the capsule dissolves in the stomach, but the granules do not dissolve until they reach the relatively alkaline environment of the duodenum, thereby protecting the drug from destruction by stomach acid. About 50% of each dose reaches the systemic circulation. The drug undergoes hepatic metabolism followed by renal excretion. The plasma half-life of omeprazole is short (about 1 hour). However, since omeprazole acts by irreversible enzyme inhibition, its effects persist long after the drug has been cleared from the blood.

***Therapeutic Use.*** Omeprazole is approved for short-term therapy of duodenal ulcers, gastric ulcers, and gastroesophageal reflux disease, and for long-term therapy of hypersecretory conditions (e.g., Zollinger-Ellison syndrome). Except for therapy of hypersecretory states, treatment should be limited to 4 to 8 weeks.

In clinical trials, duodenal ulcers healed faster with omeprazole (40 mg/day) than with conventional doses of $H_2RAs$. However, by the end of 8 weeks, the success rate was equivalent with both treatments. Patients who fail to respond to $H_2RAs$ can often benefit from omeprazole. The 6-month relapse rate following discontinuation of omeprazole is equivalent to that seen with $H_2RAs$.

***Adverse Effects.*** Effects seen with short-term therapy are generally inconsequential. Like the $H_2RAs$, omeprazole can cause headache, diarrhea, nausea, and vomiting. The incidence of these effects is less than 1%.

With long-term therapy, there is concern about the risk of cancer. Gastric carcinoid tumors have developed in rats given omeprazole daily for 2 years. These tumors are related to hypersecretion of gastrin, which occurs in response to omeprazole-induced suppression of gastric acidity. Gastrin has a trophic effect on cells of the gastric epithelium; hyperplasia of these cells may precede development of gastric carcinoid tumors. To date, no gastric tumors have been attributed to omeprazole therapy. However, experience with long-term use of the drug is limited. Accordingly, until more is understood about the consequences of prolonged therapy, use of omeprazole should be limited to 4 to 8 weeks by most patients.

***Preparations, Dosage, and Administration.*** Omeprazole [Prilosec] is dispensed in 20-mg sustained-release capsules for oral administration. For treatment of active duodenal ulcer and gastroesophageal reflux, the usual dosage is 20 mg once a day for 4 to 8 weeks. For treatment of Zollinger-Ellison syndrome and other hypersecretory states, doses up to 120 mg 3 times a day may be needed.

## Lansoprazole

Lansoprazole [Prevacid] is the second proton pump inhibitor to become available. Its mechanism of action, indications, and adverse effects are the same as those of omeprazole. Like omeprazole, lansoprazole is acid labile, and therefore is administered in an enteric-coated formulation. The dosage recommended by the manufacturer is 15 mg/day for active duodenal ulcer, 30 mg/day for erosive gastritis, and 60 mg/day for Zollinger-Ellison syndrome. All doses are taken before breakfast.

# Other Antiulcer Drugs

## Sucralfate

Sucralfate [Carafate] is an effective antiulcer medication notable for its minimal side effects and lack of significant drug interactions. The drug promotes ulcer healing by creating a protective barrier against acid and pepsin. Sucralfate has no acid-neutralizing capacity and does not decrease acid secretion.

***Mechanism of Antiulcer Action.*** Sucralfate is a complex substance composed of sulfated sucrose and aluminum hydroxide. Under mildly acidic conditions (pH less than 4), sucralfate undergoes polymerization and cross-linking reactions. The resultant product is a viscid and very sticky gel that adheres to the ulcer crater, creating a barrier to back diffusion of hydrogen ions, pepsin, and bile salts. Attachment to the ulcer appears to last for up to 6 hours.

***Pharmacokinetics.*** Sucralfate is administered orally, and systemic absorption is minimal (3% to 5%). About 90% of each dose is eliminated in the feces.

***Therapeutic Uses.*** Sucralfate is approved for acute therapy and maintenance therapy of duodenal ulcers. Rates of healing are comparable to those achieved with cimetidine. Controlled trials indicate that sucralfate can also promote healing of gastric ulcers.

***Adverse Effects.*** Sucralfate has no known serious adverse effects. The most significant side effect is constipation, and this occurs in only 2% of patients. Since sucralfate is not absorbed, systemic effects are absent.

***Drug Interactions.*** Interactions with other drugs are minimal. By raising gastric pH above 4, antacids may interfere with sucralfate's effects. This interaction can be minimized by administering these drugs at least 30 minutes apart from each other.

Sucralfate may impede the absorption of some drugs, including phenytoin, theophylline, digoxin, warfarin, and the fluoroquinolone antibiotics (e.g., ciprofloxacin, nor-floxacin). These interactions can be minimized by administering sucralfate at least 2 hours apart from these other drugs.

***Preparations, Dosage, and Administration.*** Sucralfate [Carafate] is dispensed in 1-gm tablets and a suspension (1 gm/10 ml) for oral administration. The drug should be taken on an empty stomach. The recommended adult dosage is 1 gm 4 times a day, administered 1 hour before meals and at bedtime. However, a dosing schedule of 2 gm twice a day appears to be equally effective. Treatment should continue for 4 to 8 weeks.

Sucralfate tablets are large and can be difficult to swallow, especially by the elderly. The oral suspension is much easier to ingest.

## Misoprostol

***Therapeutic Use.*** Misoprostol [Cytotec] is an analog of prostaglandin $E_1$. In the United States, the drug is approved only for *preventing gastric ulcers caused by long-term therapy with nonsteroidal anti-inflammatory drugs (NSAIDs).* In other countries, misoprostol is also used to treat peptic ulcers unrelated to NSAIDs. In addition to its use in PUD, misoprostol, in combination with mifepristone (RU-486), can be used for abortion (see Chapter 58).

***Mechanism of Action.*** In normal individuals, prostaglandins help protect the stomach by (1) suppressing secretion of gastric acid, (2) promoting secretion of bicarbonate and cytoprotective mucus, and (3) maintaining submucosal blood flow (by promoting vasodilation). As discussed in Chapter 64, aspirin and other NSAIDs cause gastric ulcers in part by inhibiting prostaglandin biosynthesis. Misoprostol prevents NSAID-induced ulcers by serving as a replacement for endogenous prostaglandins.

***Adverse Effects.*** The most common reactions are dose-related *diarrhea* (13% to 40%) and abdominal pain (7% to 20%). Some women experience spotting and dysmenorrhea.

*Misoprostol is contraindicated for use during pregnancy. The drug is classified in FDA Pregnancy Category X: the risk of use by pregnant women clearly outweighs any possible benefits.* Prostaglandins stimulate uterine contractions. Administration during pregnancy has caused partial or complete expulsion of the developing fetus. If women of child-bearing age are to use misoprostol, they must (1) be able to comply with birth control measures, (2) be given oral and written warnings about the dangers of misoprostol, (3) have a negative serum pregnancy test result within 2 weeks prior to beginning therapy, and (4) begin therapy only on the second or third day of the next normal menstrual cycle.

***Preparations, Dosage, and Administration.*** Misoprostol [Cytotec] is dispensed in 100- and 200-μg tablets for oral administration. The usual dosage is 200 μg 4 times a day administered with meals and at bedtime. Patients who cannot tolerate this dosage may try 100 μg 4 times a day.

## Antacids

Antacids are alkaline compounds that neutralize stomach acid. The principal indications for these drugs are peptic ulcer disease and gastroesophageal reflux disease.

## Beneficial Actions

Antacids react with gastric acid to produce neutral salts or salts of low acidity. By neutralizing acid, these drugs decrease destruction of the gut wall. In addition, if acid neutralization is sufficient to elevate gastric pH above 5, activity of pepsin declines as well. In addition to neutralizing acid and inactivating pepsin, antacids may be able to enhance mucosal protection by stimulating production of prostaglandins. Antacids do not coat the ulcer crater to protect it from acid and pepsin. With the exception of sodium bicarbonate, antacids are poorly absorbed, and therefore do not alter systemic pH.

## Therapeutic Uses

*Peptic Ulcer Disease.* The primary indication for antacids is peptic ulcer disease. Rates of healing are equivalent to those achieved with H$_2$RAs. At one time, antacids were the mainstay of antiulcer therapy. However, these drugs have been largely replaced by newer medications (H$_2$RAs, proton pump inhibitors, sucralfate) that are equally effective, more convenient to administer, and cause fewer side effects.

*Other Uses.* Antacids are administered prior to anesthesia to prevent aspiration pneumonitis. In addition, these drugs can provide prophylaxis against stress-induced ulcers. For patients with gastroesophageal reflux disease, antacids can produce symptomatic relief, but they do not accelerate healing. Although these drugs are used widely by the general public to relieve functional symptoms (dyspepsia, heartburn, acid indigestion), there are no controlled studies that demonstrate efficacy in these conditions.

## Potency, Dosage, and Formulations

*Potency.* Antacid potency is expressed in terms of acid-neutralizing capacity (ANC). ANC is defined as the number of milliequivalents of hydrochloric acid that can be neutralized by a given weight or volume of antacid. Individual antacids differ widely in ANC. The ANC of commonly used proprietary preparations is listed in Table 71-3.

*Dosage.* The objective of peptic ulcer therapy is to promote healing, and not simply to relieve pain. Consequently, antacids should be taken on a regular schedule, not just in response to discomfort. In the usual dosing schedule, antacids are administered 7 times a day: 1 and 3 hours after each meal and at bedtime.

Dosage recommendations should be based on ANC and not on weight or volume of antacid. The ANC of a single dose usually ranges from 20 to 80 mEq. Single doses for gastric ulcers are relatively low (20 to 40 mEq), whereas single doses for duodenal ulcers are higher (40 to 80 mEq). Frequent administration of even larger doses (120 mEq) may be required if ulceration is especially severe.

To provide maximum benefits, treatment should elevate gastric pH above 5. At this pH there is inhibition of pepsin's activity in addition to nearly complete (greater than 99.9%) neutralization of acid.

Antacids are inconvenient and unpleasant to ingest, making compliance difficult to achieve—especially in the absence of pain. Patients should be encouraged to take their medication as prescribed, even after symptoms have subsided.

*Formulations.* Antacids are available in solid (tablet) and liquid formulations. Antacid tablets should be chewed thoroughly

### TABLE 71-3. COMPOSITION AND ACID-NEUTRALIZING CAPACITY OF COMMONLY USED OVER-THE-COUNTER ANTACID SUSPENSIONS

| Product | Acid Neutralizing Capacity (mEq/5 ml) | Active Ingredients (mg/5 ml) | | | | Sodium (mg/5 ml) |
|---|---|---|---|---|---|---|
| | | Al(OH)$_3$ | Mg(OH)$_2$ | Simethicone | Other | |
| AlternaGEL | 16 | 600 | | | | <2.5 |
| Aludrox | 12 | 307 | 103 | | | 2.3 |
| Amphojel | 10 | 320 | | | | 2.3 |
| Basaljel | 12 | | | | Al(OH)CO$_3$* | 2.9 |
| DiGel | — | 200 | 200 | 20 | | <5 |
| Gelusil-II | 24 | 400 | 400 | 30 | | 1.3 |
| Kudrox DS† | 25 | 565 | 180 | | | <15 |
| Maalox | 15 | 225 | 200 | | | 1.4 |
| Maalox TC† | 27 | 600 | 300 | | | 0.8 |
| Milk of Magnesia | 14 | | 390 | | | 0.1 |
| Mylanta-II | 25 | 400 | 400 | 40 | | 1.1 |
| Riopan | 15 | | | | Magaldrate 540 | <0.1 |
| Riopan Plus | 15 | | | 20 | Magaldrate 540 | <0.1 |
| Riopan Plus 2 | 30 | | | 30 | Magaldrate 1080 | 0.3 |

*Equivalent to 400 mg Al(OH)$_3$.
†DS = double strength, TC = therapeutic concentrate.

## TABLE 71-4. CLASSIFICATION OF ANTACIDS

*Aluminum Compounds*

Aluminum hydroxide
Aluminum carbonate
Aluminum phosphate
Dihydroxyaluminum sodium carbonate

*Magnesium Compounds*

Magnesium hydroxide (milk of magnesia)
Magnesium oxide

*Calcium Compounds*

Calcium carbonate

*Sodium Compounds*

Sodium bicarbonate

*Other*

Magaldrate (a complex of magnesium and aluminum compounds)

and followed with a glass of water or milk. Liquid preparations should be shaken before dispensing. As a rule, liquids (suspensions) are more effective than tablets.

### Adverse Effects

***Constipation and Diarrhea.*** Most antacids affect the bowel. Some (e.g., aluminum hydroxide) promote constipation, whereas others (e.g., magnesium hydroxide) promote diarrhea. Effects on the bowel can be minimized by combining an antacid that promotes constipation with one that promotes diarrhea. Patients should be taught to adjust the dosage of one agent or the other to normalize bowel function.

***Sodium Loading.*** Some antacid preparations contain substantial amounts of sodium (see Table 71-3). Since sodium excess can exacerbate hypertension and heart failure, patients with these disorders should avoid preparations that have a high sodium content.

### Drug Interactions

By raising gastric pH, antacids can influence the dissolution and absorption of many other drugs, including *cimetidine* and *ranitidine*. These interactions can be minimized by allowing 1 hour between antacid administration and administration of other drugs.

Antacids can interfere with the actions of *sucralfate*, a locally acting antiulcer medication. To minimize this interaction, these drugs should be administered 1 hour apart from each other.

If absorbed in substantial amounts, antacids can alkalinize the urine. This elevation of urinary pH can accelerate excretion of acidic drugs and delay excretion of basic drugs.

### Antacid Families

There are four major groups of antacids: (1) aluminum compounds, (2) magnesium compounds, (3) calcium compounds, and (4) sodium compounds. Individual agents that belong to these groups are listed in Table 71-4. Representative members of these groups are discussed below.

### Representative Antacids

Antacids differ from one another with respect to ANC, onset and duration of action, effects on the bowel, systemic effects, and special applications. In this section, we discuss the two most commonly used antacids—magnesium hydroxide and aluminum hydroxide—and two less commonly used drugs—calcium carbonate and sodium bicarbonate. The distinguishing properties of these agents are summarized in Table 71-5.

***Magnesium Hydroxide.*** This antacid is rapid acting, has high ANC, and produces effects of long duration. These properties make magnesium hydroxide an antacid of choice. The liquid formulation of magnesium hydroxide is often referred to as milk of magnesia.

The most prominent adverse effect is diarrhea, which results from retention of water in the intestinal lumen. To compensate for this effect, magnesium hydroxide is usually administered in combination with aluminum hydroxide, an antacid that promotes constipation. However, if the dose of magnesium hydroxide is sufficiently high, no amount of aluminum hydroxide will prevent diarrhea. Since stimulation of the bowel can be hazardous for patients with intestinal obstruction or appendicitis, magnesium hydroxide should be avoided in patients with undiagnosed abdominal pain. Because of its effect on the bowel, magnesium hydroxide is frequently employed as a laxative (see Chapter 72). In patients with renal impairment, magnesium may accumulate to high levels, causing signs of toxicity (e.g., CNS depression).

## TABLE 71-5. REPRESENTATIVE ANTACIDS: SUMMARY OF DISTINGUISHING PROPERTIES

| Antacid | Effect on the Bowel | | Raises Systemic pH | Comments |
|---|---|---|---|---|
| | Constipation | Diarrhea | | |
| Aluminum hydroxide | + | − | − | Can cause hypophosphatemia; can treat hyperphosphatemia. |
| Magnesium hydroxide | − | + | − | Can cause Mg toxicity (CNS depression) in patients with renal impairment. |
| Calcium carbonate | + | − | − | May cause acid rebound or milk-alkali syndrome; releases $CO_2$. |
| Sodium bicarbonate | − | − | + | Not used routinely to treat ulcers; used to treat acidosis and to alkalanize urine; high risk of sodium loading; releases $CO_2$. |

**Aluminum Hydroxide.** This drug has relatively low ANC and is slow acting, but produces effects of long duration. Although rarely used alone, this preparation is widely used in combination with magnesium hydroxide (see Table 71-3). Aluminum hydroxide preparations contain significant amounts of sodium, and appropriate caution should be exercised. The most common adverse effect is constipation.

Aluminum hydroxide adsorbs a variety of compounds. Binding of certain drugs (e.g., tetracyclines, warfarin, digoxin) may reduce their therapeutic effects. Aluminum hydroxide has a high affinity for phosphate. By binding phosphate, the drug can reduce phosphate absorption, and can thereby cause hypophosphatemia. Aluminum hydroxide can also bind to pepsin, which may facilitate ulcer healing.

**Calcium Carbonate.** Calcium carbonate, like magnesium hydroxide, is rapid acting, has high ANC, and produces effects of long duration. Because of these properties, calcium carbonate was once considered the ideal antacid. However, because of concerns about acid rebound (stimulation of acid secretion), use of calcium carbonate has declined. The principal adverse effect is constipation. This can be overcome by using the drug in combination with a magnesium-containing antacid (e.g., magnesium hydroxide). Calcium carbonate releases carbon dioxide in the stomach, and can thereby cause eructation (belching) and flatulence. Rarely, systemic absorption is sufficient to produce the milk-alkali syndrome, a condition characterized by hypercalcemia, metabolic alkalosis, soft tissue calcification, and impaired renal function. The palatability of calcium carbonate is low and this can detract from compliance.

**Sodium Bicarbonate.** Although capable of neutralizing gastric acid, sodium bicarbonate is unfit for treating ulcers. This agent has a rapid onset but its effects are short lasting. Like calcium carbonate, sodium bicarbonate liberates carbon dioxide, thereby increasing intra-abdominal pressure and promoting eructation and flatulence. Absorption of sodium can exacerbate hypertension and heart failure. In patients with renal impairment, sodium bicarbonate can cause systemic alkalosis. (Other antacids rarely alter systemic pH.) Because of its brief duration, high sodium content, and capacity for causing alkalosis, sodium bicarbonate is inappropriate for treating PUD. The drug *is* useful, however, for treating acidosis and elevating urinary pH to promote excretion of acidic drugs following overdosage.

### Anticholinergics

Atropine and other classic muscarinic antagonists have a very limited role in treating PUD. This is because the doses required to inhibit acid secretion are so high that they produce muscarinic blockade throughout the body. Hence, when used to treat ulcers, these drugs cause a high incidence of anticholinergic side effects, such as dry mouth, constipation, urinary retention, and disturbance of vision.

**Pirenzepine.** Pirenzepine [Gastrozepine] is a unique muscarinic antagonist available for treatment of PUD. In contrast to the classic anticholinergic drugs, pirenzepine produces "selective" blockade of the muscarinic receptors that regulate gastric acid secretion (see Fig. 71-2). As a result, the drug can inhibit acid secretion without causing pronounced anticholinergic side effects. For treatment of duodenal ulcers, pirenzepine (50 mg 2 to 3 times/day) is about equal to cimetidine (1 gm/day).

Following oral administration, about 20% to 30% of the drug is absorbed. Very little crosses the blood-brain barrier. About 80% is excreted unchanged in the urine. The drug has a half-life of approximately 10 hours.

The most common side effect is dry mouth. In addition, pirenzepine can cause constipation, visual disturbances, nausea, vomiting, and diarrhea.

## KEY POINTS

- The term *peptic ulcer disease* (PUD) refers to a group of upper gastrointestinal disorders characterized by varying degrees of erosion of the gut wall.
- PUD develops when aggressive factors (*H. pylori*, NSAIDs, acid, pepsin) outweigh defensive factors (mucus, bicarbonate, submucosal blood flow, prostaglandins).
- Gastric acid is an absolute requirement for ulcer formation. In the absence of acid, no ulcer will form.
- The major underlying cause of PUD is infection with *H. pylori*. The second most common cause is use of NSAIDs.
- The goal of PUD therapy is to alleviate symptoms, promote healing, prevent complications (hemorrhage, perforation, obstruction), and prevent recurrences.
- The major drugs for treating ulcers are antibiotics, antisecretory agents (H2RAs, proton pump inhibitors), and sucralfate, a mucosal protectant.
- With the exception of antibiotics, antiulcer drugs do not alter the disease process; rather, they simply create conditions conducive to healing. Since nonantibiotic therapies do not cure ulcers, the relapse rate following their discontinuation is high. In contrast, the relapse rate following successful antibiotic therapy is very low.
- All patients with gastric or duodenal ulcers and confirmed infection with *H. pylori* should be treated with antibiotics. (An antisecretory agent may be given as well.)
- The antibiotics employed most often are bismuth, metronidazole, tetracycline, amoxicillin, and clarithromycin.
- To avoid resistance and increase efficacy, at least two antibiotics should be used.
- To date, the most effective regimen for eradicating *H. pylori* has been triple antibiotic therapy (bismuth, metronidazole, and tetracycline) combined with omeprazole.
- Cimetidine and other H2RAs suppress secretion of gastric acid by blocking histamine2 receptors on parietal cells of the stomach.
- Cimetidine inhibits hepatic drug-metabolizing enzymes, and can thereby cause levels of other drugs to rise.
- In contrast to cimetidine, ranitidine [Zantac] has little effect on drug metabolism.
- The proton pump inhibitors—omeprazole and lansoprazole—act by inhibiting gastric $H^+,K^+$-ATPase, the enzyme that actually generates gastric acid. These agents are the most effective inhibitors of acid secretion.
- Sucralfate promotes ulcer healing by creating a protective barrier against acid and pepsin.
- Misoprostol, an analog of prostaglandin $E_1$, is used to prevent gastric ulcers caused by NSAIDs.
- Misoprostol stimulates uterine contraction and is therefore contraindicated during pregnancy.

# Summary of Major Nursing Implications*

## H₂-Receptor Antagonists

> Cimetidine
> Ranitidine
> Famotidine
> Nizatidine

## Preadministration Assessment

### Therapeutic Goal
The objective in treating PUD is to relieve pain, promote healing, prevent ulcer recurrence, and prevent complications.

### Baseline Data
Diagnosis requires radiographic or endoscopic visualization of the ulcer and testing for *H. pylori* infection.

### Identifying High-Risk Patients
Use H₂RAs with *caution* in patients with *renal or hepatic dysfunction.*

## Implementation: Administration

### Routes
**Cimetidine and ranitidine.** Oral, IM, and IV.
**Famotidine.** Oral and IV.
**Nizatidine.** Oral only.

### Administration
**Oral.** Inform patients that H₂RAs may be taken without regard to meals.

Dosing may be done once daily at bedtime, twice daily, or 4 times a day. Make sure the patient knows which dosing schedule has been prescribed.

**Intramuscular.** *Cimetidine and ranitidine*: use concentrated solutions for IM injections.

**Intravenous.** *Cimetidine, famotidine, and ranitidine*: for IV injection, dilute in a small volume (e.g., 20 ml) and inject slowly (over 5 or more minutes). For IV infusion, dilute in a large volume (100 ml) and infuse over 15 to 20 minutes.

## Implementation: Measures to Enhance Therapeutic Effects

Advise patients to avoid cigarettes and ulcerogenic over-the-counter drugs (aspirin and other NSAIDs). Advise patients to stop drinking alcohol if drinking exacerbates ulcer symptoms. Inform patients that five or six small meals per day may be preferable to three larger ones. Advise patients that reducing stress may accelerate ulcer healing.

## Ongoing Evaluation and Interventions

### Evaluating Therapeutic Effects
**Monitor for Relief of Pain.** Radiologic or endoscopic examination of the ulcer site may also be employed. Monitor gastric pH; treatment should increase pH to 5 or above. Educate patients about signs of GI bleeding (e.g., black, tarry stools, "coffee-ground" vomitus), and instruct them to notify the physician if these are observed.

**H. pylori.** If *H. pylori* was present at the onset of treatment, it may be useful to determine if the infection was eradicated.

### Minimizing Adverse Effects
**Antiandrogenic Effects.** *Cimetidine* can cause gynecomastia, reduced libido, and impotence. These effects reverse after drug withdrawal.

**CNS Effects.** *Cimetidine* can cause confusion, hallucinations, lethargy, somnolence, restlessness, and seizures. These responses are most likely in elderly patients who have renal or hepatic impairment. Inform patients about possible CNS effects, and instruct them to notify the physician if these occur. CNS effects are less likely with ranitidine, famotidine, and nizatidine.

### Minimizing Adverse Interactions
**Interactions Secondary to Inhibition of Drug Metabolism.** *Cimetidine* inhibits hepatic drug-metabolizing enzymes and can thereby increase levels of other drugs. Drugs of particular concern are *warfarin, phenytoin, theophylline*, and *lidocaine*. Dosages of these drugs may need to be reduced.

*Ranitidine* inhibits drug metabolism, but to a lesser degree than cimetidine. Famotidine and nizatidine do not inhibit drug metabolism.

**Antacids.** Antacids can decrease absorption of *cimetidine* and *ranitidine*. At least 1 hour should separate administration of these drugs.

## Antacids

> Aluminum hydroxide
> Magnesium hydroxide
> Calcium carbonate
> Sodium bicarbonate

## Preadministration Assessment

### Therapeutic Goal and Baseline Data
See Nursing Implications for H₂-receptor antagonists above.

### Identifying High-Risk Patients
Use all antacids with *caution* in patients with *hypertension* or *heart failure*. Use *magnesium-containing*

*antacids* with *caution* in patients with *renal insufficiency*.

## Implementation: Administration

### Route
Oral.

### Administration
Instruct patients to administer antacids 7 times a day: 1 and 3 hours after meals and at bedtime.

Instruct patients to take their medication on a regular schedule even after pain has subsided, since relief of pain does not necessarily indicate healing.

Instruct patients to shake liquid preparations before dispensing.

Instruct patients to chew antacid tablets thoroughly and to follow administration with a glass of water or milk.

## Ongoing Evaluation and Interventions

### Evaluating Therapeutic Effects
See Nursing Implications for H$_2$RAs above.

### Minimizing Adverse Effects
*Constipation and Diarrhea.* To minimize disruption of bowel function, a constipating antacid (aluminum hydroxide, calcium carbonate) is combined with a laxative antacid (magnesium hydroxide). Teach the patient to adjust the dosage of the constipating agent and laxative agent as needed to normalize bowel function.

*Sodium Loading.* Sodium in antacids can exacerbate hypertension and congestive heart failure. Patients with these disorders should use a low-sodium preparation.

### Minimizing Adverse Interactions
*Interactions Caused by Elevation of Gastric pH.* By raising gastric pH, antacids can reduce the availability of other drugs, including cimetidine and ranitidine, and can decrease the antiulcer effects of sucralfate. To minimize these interactions, instruct patients to allow 1 hour or more between antacid administration and administration of other drugs.

*Aluminum Hydroxide.* This antacid can bind to a variety of drugs (e.g., tetracyclines, warfarin, digoxin), thereby decreasing their availability. Increased doses of these agents may be needed.

# Laxatives

axatives are used to ease or stimulate defecation. These agents can soften the stool, increase stool volume, hasten fecal passage through the intestine, and facilitate evacuation from the rectum. When properly employed, laxatives are valuable medications. However, these agents are also subject to widespread abuse. Misuse of laxatives is largely the result of misconceptions about what constitutes normal bowel function.

Before we talk about laxatives, we need to distinguish between two terms: *laxative effect* and *catharsis*. The term *laxative effect* refers to production of a soft formed stool over a period of 1 or more days. In contrast, the term *catharsis* refers to a prompt, fluid evacuation of the bowel. Hence, a laxative effect is leisurely and relatively mild, whereas catharsis is fast and intense.

## General Considerations

### Function of the Colon

The principal function of the colon is to absorb water and electrolytes. Absorption of nutrients is minimal. Normally, about 1500 ml of fluid enters the colon each day, and approximately 90% gets absorbed. When intestinal function is healthy, the extent of fluid absorption is such that the resulting stool is soft (but formed) and capable of elimination without strain. However, when fluid absorption is excessive, as can happen when transport through the intestine is delayed, the resultant stool is dehydrated and hard. Conversely, if insufficient fluid is absorbed, watery stools result.

Frequency of bowel evacuation varies widely among individuals. For some people, bowel movements occur 2 or 3 times a day. For others, elimination may occur only 2 times a week. Because of this wide individual variation, we can't define a normal frequency for bowel movements. That is, although a daily bowel movement may be normal for many people, this timing may be abnormal for many others.

### Dietary Fiber

Proper function of the bowel is highly dependent on dietary fiber—the component of vegetable matter that escapes digestion in the stomach and small intestine. Fiber facilitates colonic function in two ways: (1) it can absorb water, thereby softening the feces and increasing their mass, and (2) it can be digested by colonic bacteria, whose subsequent growth increases fecal mass. The best source of fiber is bran. Fiber can also be obtained from fruits and vegetables. Ingestion of 20 to 60 gm of fiber a day should optimize intestinal function.

### Constipation

Constipation is determined primarily by stool *consistency* (degree of hardness); alterations in the *frequency* of bowel movements are of secondary importance. Hence, if the interval between bowel movements becomes prolonged, but the stool remains soft and hydrated, a diagnosis of constipation would be improper. Conversely, if bowel movements occur with regularity, but the feces are hard and dry, we would consider constipation to be present—despite the regular and frequent passage of stool.

The principal cause of constipation is poor diet—specifically, a diet deficient in fiber and fluid. Certain drugs (e.g., opioids, anticholinergics, some antacids) may also cause constipation.

In most cases, constipation can be readily corrected. Stools will become softer and more easily passed within days of increasing fiber and fluid in the diet. Mild exercise, especially after meals, will also help improve function of the bowel. If necessary, a laxative may be employed—but only briefly and only as an adjunct to diet and exercise.

## TABLE 72–1. CLASSIFICATION OF LAXATIVES BY PHARMACOLOGIC CATEGORY

| Class and Agent | Site of Action | Mechanism of Action |
|---|---|---|
| **Bulk-Forming Laxatives** | | |
| Methylcellulose<br>Psyllium<br>Polycarbophil | Small and large intestine | Absorb water, thereby softening and enlarging the fecal mass; fecal swelling promotes peristalsis |
| **Surfactant Laxatives** | | |
| Docusate sodium<br>Docusate calcium<br>Docusate potassium | Small and large intestine | Surfactant action softens stool by facilitating penetration of water; also cause secretion of water and electrolytes into intestine |
| **Stimulate Laxatives** | | |
| Bisacodyl<br>Senna<br>Cascara sagadra | Colon | 1) Stimulate peristalsis and (2) soften feces by increasing secretion of water and electrolytes into the intestine and decreasing water and electrolyte absorption |
| Castor oil | Small intestine | |
| **Osmotic Laxatives** | | |
| Magnesium hydroxide<br>Magnesium sulfate<br>Magnesium citrate<br>Magnesium phosphate | Small and large intestine | Osmotic action retains water and thereby softens the feces; fecal swelling promotes peristalsis |
| **Miscellaneous Laxatives** | | |
| Mineral oil | Colon | Lubricates and reduces water absorption |
| Glycerin suppository | Colon | Lubricates and causes reflex rectal contraction |
| Lactulose | Colon | Similar to osmotic laxatives |
| Polyethylene glycol-electrolyte solution | Small and large intestine | Similar to osmotic laxatives |

## Indications for Laxative Use

Laxatives can be highly beneficial when employed for valid indications. By softening the stool, laxatives can reduce the painful elimination that can be associated with episiotomy and with hemorrhoids and other anorectal lesions. In patients with cardiovascular diseases (e.g., aneurysm, myocardial infarction, disease of the cerebral or cardiac vasculature), softening of the stool decreases the amount of strain needed to defecate, thereby avoiding dangerous elevations of blood pressure. In geriatric patients, laxatives can help compensate for loss of tone in abdominal and perineal muscle. As an adjunct to anthelmintic therapy, laxatives can be used for (1) obtaining a fresh stool sample for diagnosis; (2) emptying the bowel prior to treatment (so as to increase parasitic exposure to anthelmintic medication); and (3) facilitating export of dead parasites following anthelmintic use. Additional applications of laxatives include (1) emptying of the bowel prior to surgery and diagnostic procedures (e.g., radiologic examination, proctosigmoidoscopy); (2) modification of the effluent from an ileostomy or colostomy; (3) prevention of fecal impaction in bedridden patients; (4) removal of ingested poisons; and (5) correction of constipation associated with pregnancy or use of certain drugs.

## Contraindications to Laxative Use

Laxatives are contraindicated for individuals with certain disorders of the bowel. Specifically, laxatives must be avoided by individuals experiencing abdominal pain, nausea, cramps, or other symptoms of appendicitis, regional enteritis, diverticulitis, and ulcerative colitis. Laxatives are also contraindicated for patients with acute surgical abdomen. In addition, laxatives should not be used in the presence of fecal impaction or obstruction of the bowel; under these conditions, increased peristalsis may cause bowel perforation. Lastly, laxatives should not be employed habitually for the treatment of constipation. Reasons for this last prohibition are discussed below under *Laxative Abuse*.

## Laxative Classification Schemes

Traditionally, laxatives have been classified according to general mechanism of action. This scheme has four

## TABLE 72-2. CLASSIFICATION OF LAXATIVES BY THERAPEUTIC RESPONSE

| Group I:<br>Produce Watery Stool<br>in 2–6 Hours | Group II:<br>Produce Semifluid Stool<br>in 6–12 Hours | Group III:<br>Produce Soft Stool<br>in 1–3 Days |
| --- | --- | --- |
| Osmotic laxatives (in high doses)<br>  Magnesium salts<br>  Sodium salts | Osmotic laxatives (in low doses)<br>  Magnesium salts<br>  Sodium salts | Bulk-forming laxatives<br>  Methylcellulose<br>  Psyllium<br>  Polycarbophil |
| Castor oil | Stimulant laxatives (except<br>  castor oil) | Surfactant laxatives<br>  Docusalt salts |
| Polyethylene glycol–electrolyte<br>  solution | Bisacodyl, oral*<br>  Phenolphthalein<br>  Senna<br>  Cascara | Lactulose |

*Bisacodyl suppositories act in 15 minutes.

major categories: (1) bulk-forming laxatives, (2) surfactant laxatives, (3) stimulant laxatives, and (4) osmotic laxatives. Representative drugs that belong to these classes are listed in Table 72-1.

From a clinical perspective, it can be helpful to classify laxatives according to therapeutic effect (time of onset and impact on stool consistency). When these properties are considered, most laxatives fall into one of three groups (labeled I, II, and III in this chapter). Group I agents act rapidly (within 2 to 6 hours) to impart a watery consistency to the stool. Laxatives in group I are especially useful when preparing the bowel for diagnostic procedures or surgery. Group II agents have an intermediate latency (6 to 12 hours) and produce a stool that is semifluid in texture. Group II agents are the ones most frequently abused by the general public. The group III laxatives act slowly (in 1 to 3 days) to produce a soft but formed stool. Uses for this group include treating constipation and preventing straining at stool. Representative members of groups I, II, and III are listed in Table 72-2.

# Basic Pharmacology of Laxatives

## Bulk-Forming Laxatives

The bulk-forming laxatives (e.g., methylcellulose, psyllium) have actions and effects much like those of dietary fiber. These agents consist of natural or semisynthetic polysaccharides and celluloses derived from grains and other plant material. With regard to clinical response, the bulk-forming agents belong to category III: these drugs produce a soft, formed stool 1 to 3 days after the onset of treatment.

***Mechanism of Action.*** The effects of bulk-forming agents on bowel function are identical to those of dietary fiber. Following ingestion, these agents, which are nondi-

gestible and nonabsorbable, swell in water to form a viscous solution or gel, thereby softening the fecal mass and increasing its bulk. Fecal volume may be further enlarged by growth of colonic bacteria, which can utilize these materials as nutrients. Transit through the intestine is hastened because swelling of the fecal mass stretches the intestinal wall, thereby stimulating peristalsis.

***Indications.*** Bulk-forming laxatives are the preferred agents for temporary treatment of constipation. Also, these drugs are widely used by patients with diverticulosis and irritable bowel syndrome. In addition, by altering fecal consistency, these agents can provide symptomatic relief of diarrhea and can reduce discomfort and inconvenience for patients with an ileostomy or colostomy.

***Adverse Effects.*** Untoward effects are minimal. Since the bulk-forming agents are not absorbed, systemic reactions are rare. *Esophageal obstruction* can occur if these agents are swallowed in the absence of sufficient fluid. To avoid this, bulk-forming laxatives should be administered with a full glass of water or juice. If their passage through the intestine is arrested, the bulk-forming agents may produce *intestinal obstruction* or *impaction.* Accordingly, these agents should be avoided if there is narrowing of the intestinal lumen.

***Preparations, Dosage, and Administration.*** *Psyllium* (prepared from *Plantago* seed), *methylcellulose,* and *polycarbophil* are the principal bulk-forming laxatives. All three preparations should be administered with a full glass of water or juice. Dosages for psyllium and methylcellulose are presented in Table 72-3.

## Surfactant Laxatives

***Actions.*** The surfactants (e.g., docusate sodium) are group III laxatives: these agents produce a soft stool several days after the onset of treatment. Surfactants alter stool consistency by lowering surface tension, which facilitates penetration of water into the feces. The surfactants may also act on the intestinal wall to (1) inhibit fluid absorption and (2) stimulate secretion of water and electrolytes into the intestinal lumen. In this respect, surfactants resemble the stimulant laxatives (see below).

**Preparations, Dosage, and Administration.** The surfactant family consists of three *docusate salts*: docusate sodium, docusate potassium, and docusate calcium. The dosage for docusate sodium [Colace, others], the prototype surfactant, is presented in Table 72–3. Administration of all surfactants should be accompanied by a full glass of water.

## Stimulant Laxatives

The stimulant laxatives (e.g., bisacodyl, castor oil) have two effects on the bowel. First, they stimulate intestinal motility—hence their name. Second, they act on the intestinal wall to produce a net increase of water and electrolytes within the intestinal lumen. This latter effect results from increasing the secretion of water and ions into the intestine, and reducing water and electrolyte absorption. Most stimulant laxatives act on the colon, producing a semifluid stool within 6 to 12 hours.

Stimulant laxatives are widely used—and abused—by the general public, and are of concern for this reason. They have few legitimate applications. Properties of individual agents are discussed below.

**Bisacodyl.** Bisacodyl [Dulcolax, others] is unique among the stimulant laxatives in that it can be administered by rectal suppository as well as by mouth. *Oral bisacodyl acts within 6 to 12 hours.* Hence tablets may be

### TABLE 72–3. REPRESENTATIVE LAXATIVES: TRADE NAMES, DOSAGE FORMS, AND DOSAGES

| Class and Generic Name | Trade Names | Dosage Forms | Dosage and Administration |
|---|---|---|---|
| *Bulk-Forming* | | | |
| Methylcellulose | Citrucel | Powder | *Powder:* 1 heaping tbsp in 8 oz cold water 1–3 times a day |
| Psyllium | Metamucil, Perdium Fiber, Reguloid, others | Granules, powder, effervescent powder, wafer | *Adults:* 1 rounded tsp (or 1 packet) mixed with water or other fluid, taken 1–3 times daily<br>*Children over 6 years:* 1/3 to 1/2 adult dose |
| *Surfactant* | | | |
| Docusate sodium | Colace, Modane Soft, others | Capsules, tablets, syrup, liquid | *Adults and children over 12 years:* 50–500 mg/day<br>*Children 6–12 years:* 40–120 mg/day<br>(All doses taken with a full glass of water) |
| *Stimulant* | | | |
| Bisacodyl | Dulcolax, others | Tablets, suppositories | *Adults:* 10–15 mg (tablets) or 10-mg suppository once daily<br>*Children:* 5-mg tablet or 5-mg suppository once daily |
| Phenolphthalein | Ex-Lax, Feen-a-Mint | Tablets, wafers, gum | *Adults:* 30–194 mg/day<br>*Children:* 6 years or older, 30–60 mg/day; 2–5 years, 15–20 mg/day |
| *Osmotic* | | | |
| Magnesium hydroxide (milk of magnesia) | | Liquid | *Low dose:* 15–30 ml<br>*High dose:* 30–60 ml |
| *Other* | | | |
| Mineral oil | Neo-Cultol, Milkinol, others | Liquid, jelly, emulsion | *Adults:* 45 ml PO bid<br>*Children:* 5–20 ml PO at bedtime |

given at bedtime to produce a response the following morning. Bisacodyl *suppositories* act rapidly (in 15 to 60 minutes). Dosages for bisacodyl are presented in Table 72–3.

Bisacodyl tablets are enteric coated to prevent gastric irritation. Accordingly, patients should be advised to swallow them intact, without chewing or crushing. Since milk and antacids accelerate dissolution of the enteric coating, the tablets should be administered no sooner than 1 hour after these substances.

Bisacodyl suppositories may cause a burning sensation and, with continued use, proctitis may develop. Accordingly, long-term use should be discouraged.

**Phenolphthalein.** Phenolphthalein is similar in structure and actions to bisacodyl. This agent acts on the colon to produce a semifluid stool in 6 to 8 hours. Because phenolphthalein undergoes enterohepatic recirculation, effects may persist for 3 to 4 days. The drug can impart a harmless pink tint to the urine; patients should be forewarned of this effect.  Phenolphthalein is the active ingredient in many over-the-counter (OTC) laxatives, including Ex-Lax and Feen-a-Mint. Dosage is shown in Table 72–3.

**Anthraquinones.** Anthraquinone compounds are the active ingredients in *Cascara sagadra* and *senna*, which are laxatives derived from plants. The actions and applications of these laxatives are similar to those of bisacodyl and phenolphthalein. The anthraquinones act on the colon to produce a soft or semifluid stool in 6 to 12 hours. Systemic absorption followed by renal secretion may be sufficient to impart a harmless yellowish-brown or pink color to the urine; patients should be forewarned of this effect.

**Castor Oil.** Castor oil is the only stimulant laxative that acts on the *small intestine*. As a result, this agent acts quickly (in 2 to 6 hours) to produce a watery stool. Hence, unlike the other stimulant laxatives, which are all group II agents, castor oil belongs to group I. Use of castor oil is limited to situations in which rapid and thorough evacuation of the bowel is desired (e.g., preparation for radiologic procedures). The drug is far too powerful to use routinely for constipation. Because of its relatively prompt action, castor oil should not be administered at bedtime. The drug has an unpleasant taste that can be improved by chilling and mixing with fruit juice.

## Osmotic Laxatives

**Actions and Uses.** The osmotic laxatives (e.g., magnesium hydroxide, sodium phosphate) are poorly absorbed salts whose osmotic action draws water into the intestinal lumen. Accumulation of water causes the fecal mass to soften and swell; swelling, in turn, stretches the intestinal wall and thereby stimulates peristalsis. When administered in low doses, the osmotic laxatives produce a soft or semifluid stool in 6 to 12 hours. In high doses, these agents act rapidly (in 2 to 6 hours) to cause a fluid evacuation of the bowel. High-dose therapy is employed to empty the bowel in preparation for diagnostic and surgical procedures. High doses are also employed to purge the bowel of ingested poisons, and to evacuate dead parasites following anthelmintic therapy.

**Preparations.** The osmotic laxatives include *magnesium salts* (magnesium hydroxide, magnesium citrate, and magnesium sulfate), *sodium salts* (sodium phosphate and sodium biphosphate), and *potassium salts* (potassium bitartrate and potassium phosphate). The dosage for magnesium hydroxide solution (also known as milk of magnesia) is presented in Table 72–3.

**Adverse Effects.** Osmotic laxatives can cause substantial loss of water. To avoid dehydration, treatment should be accompanied by augmented intake of fluids. Although the osmotic laxatives are poorly and slowly absorbed, some absorption does take place. In patients with renal dysfunction, magnesium and potassium can accumulate to toxic levels. Accordingly, osmotic laxatives that contain these elements are contraindicated in patients with kidney disease. Sodium absorption can cause fluid retention, which in turn can exacerbate heart failure, hypertension, and edema. Accordingly, sodium-containing laxatives are contraindicated for patients with these disorders.

### Miscellaneous Laxatives

**Mineral Oil.** Mineral oil is a mixture of indigestible and poorly absorbed hydrocarbons. Laxative action is produced by lubrication. Mineral oil is especially useful when administered by enema to treat fecal impaction.

Mineral oil can produce a variety of adverse effects. Aspiration of oil droplets can cause lipid pneumonia. Anal leakage can cause pruritus and soiling. Systemic absorption can produce deposition of mineral oil in the liver. Excessive dosing can decrease the absorption of fat-soluble vitamins.

**Lactulose.** Lactulose is a semisynthetic disaccharide composed of galactose and fructose. Lactulose is poorly absorbed and cannot be digested by intestinal enzymes. In the colon, resident bacteria metabolize lactulose to lactic, formic, and acetic acids. These acids exert a mild osmotic action, producing a soft, formed stool in 1 to 3 days. Although lactulose can relieve constipation, this agent is more expensive than therapeutically equivalent agents (bulk-forming laxatives) and also causes unpleasant side effects (flatulence and cramping are common). Accordingly, lactulose should be reserved for patients who do not respond adequately to bulk-forming laxatives.

In addition to its laxative action, lactulose can enhance intestinal excretion of ammonia. This property has been exploited to lower blood ammonia in patients with portal hypertension and hepatic encephalopathy occurring secondary to chronic liver disease.

**Glycerin Suppository.** Glycerin is an osmotic agent that softens and lubricates inspissated feces. The drug may also stimulate rectal contraction. Evacuation occurs about 30 minutes after suppository insertion. Glycerin suppositories have been useful for re-establishing normal bowel function following termination of chronic laxative use.

**Polyethylene Glycol–Electrolyte Solutions.** These bowel-cleansing solutions [CoLyte, GoLYTELY, others] contain a mixture of polyethylene glycol (a nonabsorbable osmotic agent) together with potassium chloride, sodium chloride, sodium sulfate, and sodium bicarbonate. The mixture is isosmotic with body fluids, and its composition is such that water and electrolytes are neither absorbed from nor secreted into the intestinal lumen. Hence, water is not lost and electrolyte balance is preserved. As a result, polyethylene glycol–electrolyte solutions can be used safely in patients who are dehydrated and in those who are especially sensitive to alterations in electrolyte levels (e.g., patients with renal impairment or cardiovascular disease). These preparations are indicated primarily for cleansing the bowel prior to diagnostic procedures. The volume of administration is huge (about 4 L). Patients must ingest 250 to 300 ml every 10 minutes for 2 to 3 hours. Bowel movements commence about 1 hour after initiation of treatment.

## Laxative Abuse

*Causes.* Many people believe that a daily and bountiful bowel movement is a requisite of good health, and that any deviation from this pattern merits correction. Such misconceptions are reinforced by aggressive marketing of OTC laxative preparations, of which there are literally hundreds. Not infrequently, the combination of tradition supported by advertising has led to habitual self-prescribing of laxatives by people for whom these agents are not indicated.

Laxatives can help perpetuate their own use. Strong laxatives can purge the entire bowel. When such overemptying occurs, spontaneous evacuation will be impossible until bowel content has been replenished, which may take 2 to 5 days. During the period of bowel refilling, the laxative user, having experienced no movement of the bowel, often becomes convinced that constipation has returned. In response, he or she takes yet another dose of laxative, thereby purging the bowel once more. In this manner, a vicious cycle of repeated laxative use and purging becomes established.

*Consequences.* Chronic exposure to laxatives can diminish defecatory reflexes, leading to further reliance on laxatives. Laxative abuse may also cause more serious pathologic changes, including electrolyte imbalance, dehydration, and colitis.

*Treatment.* The first step in breaking the laxative habit is abrupt cessation of laxative use. Following drug withdrawal, bowel movements will be absent for several days;

the patient should be informed of this fact. Any misconceptions that the patient has regarding bowel function should be corrected: the patient should be taught that a once-daily bowel movement may not be normal for him or her and that stool *quality* is more important than frequency and quantity. Instruction on bowel training (heeding the defecatory reflex, establishing a consistent time for bowel movements) should be provided. Increased consumption of fiber (bran, fruits, vegetables) should be stressed. The patient should be encouraged to exercise daily, especially after meals. Finally, the patient should be advised that, if a laxative must be used, it should be used only briefly and in the smallest effective dosage. Agents that produce catharsis must be avoided.

## KEY POINTS

- Laxatives are given to promote defecation.
- Constipation is determined primarily by stool *consistency*, not by *frequency* of bowel movements.
- Legitimate indications for laxatives include cardiovascular disorders, episiotomy, hemorrhoids, emptying the bowel before surgery and diagnostic procedures, ileostomy or colostomy, prevention of fecal impaction in bedridden patients, and constipation associated with pregnancy.
- Like dietary fiber, bulk-forming laxatives swell in water to form a viscous solution or gel, thereby softening the feces and increasing fecal mass. Increased mass stretches the bowel wall, thereby promoting peristalsis.
- Administer bulk-forming laxatives with fluid to avoid esophageal obstruction.
- Patients receiving osmotic laxatives must increase fluid intake to avoid dehydration.
- Because of their relatively rapid onset, Group I laxatives (castor oil, high-dose osmotic agents) should not be administered at bedtime.
- Laxatives—especially the stimulant type—are commonly misused (abused) by the public. To reduce abuse, educate clients about normal bowel function and about alternatives to laxatives (diet high in fiber and fluids, exercise, establishing regular bowel habits).

## Summary of Major Nursing Implications*

### Laxatives

## Implications That Apply to All Laxatives

### Identifying High-Risk Patients

Laxatives are *contraindicated* for individuals with *abdominal pain*, *nausea*, *cramps*, and other symptoms of

*appendicitis*, *regional enteritis*, *diverticulitis*, and *ulcerative colitis*. Laxatives are also *contraindicated* for patients with *acute surgical abdomen*, *fecal impaction*, and *obstruction of the bowel*.

### Reducing Laxative Abuse

Patient education is a key factor in reducing laxative abuse. Educate the patient about normal bowel function (to correct misconceptions), and provide instruction on establishing good bowel habits (heeding the defecatory reflex, establishing a consistent time for bowel movements). Advise the patient to exercise (especially after

*Patient education information is highlighted in color.

meals) and to increase consumption of fiber (bran, fruits, vegetables). Inform the patient that laxatives should be used only when clearly necessary and then only briefly in the lowest effective dosage. Warn the patient against using cathartics.

## Implications That Apply to Specific Laxatives

### Bulk-Forming Laxatives: Psyllium, Methylcellulose, and Polycarbophil

Instruct the patient to take bulk-forming agents with a full glass of water or juice to prevent esophageal obstruction.

Bulk-forming laxatives are contraindicated for individuals with narrowing of the intestinal lumen, a condition that increases the risk of intestinal obstruction and impaction.

### Surfactants: Docusate Salts

Instruct the patient to take surfactant agents with a full glass of water.

### Stimulant Laxatives

Stimulant agents are the laxatives most commonly abused by the general public. Discourage the patient from inappropriate use of these drugs.

***Bisacodyl.*** Administered PO and by rectal suppository. Instruct the patient to take oral bisacodyl no sooner than

1 hour after ingestion of milk or antacids. Instruct the patient to swallow tablets intact, without crushing or chewing.

Suppositories may cause a burning sensation; forewarn the patient. Warn the patient that prolonged use of bisacodyl suppositories can cause proctitis.

***Phenolphthalein.*** Forewarn the patient that phenolphthalein may impart a harmless pink tint to the urine.

***Anthraquinones: Cascara Sagadra and Senna.*** Forewarn the patient that anthraquinones can impart a harmless yellowish-brown or pink color to the urine.

***Castor Oil.*** Castor oil acts rapidly (in 2 to 6 hours); do not administer at bedtime. Advise the patient not to take castor oil late at night. Warn the patient that castor oil is a powerful laxative and should not be used to treat routine constipation. Administer in chilled fruit juice to improve palatability.

### Osmotic Laxatives: Magnesium Salts, Sodium Salts, and Potassium Salts

Effects are dose dependent. Low doses produce a soft or semifluid stool in 6 to 12 hours. Higher doses cause watery evacuation of the bowel in 2 to 6 hours.

To prevent dehydration, increase fluid intake during treatment.

*Magnesium salts* and *potassium salts* are contraindicated for patients with *renal dysfunction*.

*Sodium salts* are contraindicated for patients with *heart failure*, *hypertension*, or *edema*.

# CHAPTER 73

# Other Gastrointestinal Drugs

**Antiemetics**
    The Emetic Response
    Antiemetic Drugs
    Management of Chemotherapy-Induced Emesis
**Drugs for Motion Sickness**

**Antidiarrheal Agents**
    Nonspecific Antidiarrheal Agents
    Management of Infectious Diarrhea
**Drugs for Inflammatory Bowel Disease**
**Pancreatic Enzymes**
**Drugs Used to Dissolve Gallstones**
**Anorectal Preparations**

---

n this chapter we will discuss an assortment of gastrointestinal drugs whose indications range from emesis to colitis to gallstones. Two groups are emphasized: (1) antiemetics and (2) antidiarrheals.

## Antiemetics

The antiemetics are used to suppress vomiting. Our approach to these drugs is to review the emetic response, discuss the major antiemetic classes, and finish by considering the most important application of these drugs: management of chemotherapy-induced emesis.

Emesis is a complex reflex brought about by activation of the vomiting center, a nucleus of neurons located in the medulla oblongata. Some stimuli activate the vomiting center directly, whereas others act indirectly (Fig. 73-1). Direct-acting stimuli include signals from the cerebral cortex (anticipation, fear), signals from sensory organs (upsetting sights, noxious odors, pain), and signals from the vestibular apparatus of the inner ear. Indirect-acting stimuli first activate the chemoreceptor trigger zone (CTZ), which in turn activates the vomiting center. Activation of the CTZ occurs in two ways: (1) by signals from the stomach and small intestine (traveling along vagal afferents), and (2) by the direct action of emetogenic compounds (e.g., anticancer drugs, opioids, ipecac) that are carried to the CTZ in the blood. Once activated, the vomiting center signals the stomach, diaphragm, and abdominal muscles; the resulting coordinated response expels gastric contents.

Several types of receptors are involved in the vomiting response. Important among these are receptors for sero-

tonin, dopamine, acetylcholine, and histamine (see Fig. 73-1). Many antiemetics, including ondansetron [Zofran], prochlorperazine [Compazine], and dimenhydrinate [Dramamine], act by blocking one or more of these receptors.

### Antiemetic Drugs

A variety of antiemetics are available. Their classes, trade names, and dosages are summarized in Table 73-1. Uses and mechanisms are summarized in Table 73-2. Properties of the principal classes are discussed below.

#### Serotonin Antagonists

The serotonin antagonists are the most effective drugs available for suppressing nausea and vomiting caused by cisplatin and other highly emetogenic anticancer drugs. At this time, two serotonin antagonists are in use: ondansetron and granisetron.

*Ondansetron.* Ondansetron [Zofran] was the first serotonin antagonist approved for suppressing chemotherapy-induced emesis. This agent acts by blocking serotonin receptors (specifically, 5-HT$_3$ receptors) in the CTZ and on afferent vagal neurons in the upper GI tract. Ondansetron, which is very effective by itself, is even more effective when combined with dexamethasone. The drug's most common side effects are headache, diarrhea, and dizziness. Since ondansetron does not block dopamine receptors, it does not cause the extrapyramidal effects (e.g., akathisia, acute dystonia) seen with antiemetic phenothiazines.

Administration is intravenous or oral. The initial IV dose is 0.15 mg/kg infused slowly (over 15 minutes) beginning 30 minutes before chemotherapy; this dose is repeated 4 and 8 hours later. Alternatively, ondansetron can be given as a single 32-mg IV dose. The usual oral dosage is 8 mg 3 times a day.

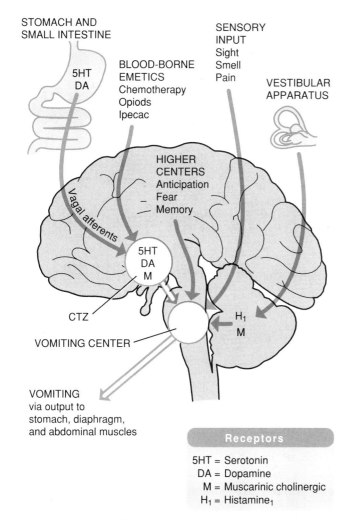

**Figure 73–1. The emetic response: stimuli, pathways, and receptors. CTZ** = chemoreceptor trigger zone.

STOMACH AND
SMALL INTESTINE

5HT
DA

BLOOD-BORNE
EMETICS
Chemotherapy
Opiods
Ipecac

SENSORY
INPUT
Sight
Smell
Pain

VESTIBULAR
APPARATUS

Vagal afferents

HIGHER
CENTERS
Anticipation
Fear
Memory

5HT
DA
M

$H_1$
M

CTZ

VOMITING CENTER

VOMITING
via output to
stomach, diaphragm,
and abdominal muscles

**Receptors**

5HT = Serotonin
DA = Dopamine
M = Muscarinic cholinergic
$H_1$ = Histamine$_1$

**Granisetron.** Like ondansetron, granisetron [Kytril] suppresses emesis by blocking serotonin receptors on afferent vagal neurons and in the CTZ. Principal adverse effects are headache (responsive to acetaminophen), weakness, tiredness, and diarrhea or constipation. Administration may be oral or IV. The recommended dosage is 10 μg/kg IV infused over 5 minutes, starting 30 minutes before chemotherapy.

## Dopamine Antagonists

**Phenothiazines.** The phenothiazines (e.g., prochlorperazine) suppress emesis by blocking dopamine$_2$ receptors in the CTZ. These drugs can help suppress emesis associated with surgery, cancer chemotherapy, toxins, and other causes. Side effects include extrapyramidal reactions, anticholinergic effects, hypotension, and sedation. The basic pharmacology of the phenothiazines is discussed in Chapter 29 (Antipsychotic Agents).

**Butyrophenones.** Two butyrophenones—*haloperidol* [Haldol] and *droperidol* [Inapsine]—are used as antiemetics. Like the phenothiazines, the butyrophenones suppress emesis by blocking dopamine$_2$ receptors in the CTZ. The butyrophenones are useful for postoperative nausea

and vomiting, and for emesis caused by cancer chemotherapy, radiation therapy, and toxins. Potential side effects are similar to those of the phenothiazines: extrapyramidal reactions, sedation, and hypotension. The pharmacology of the butyrophenones is discussed in Chapter 29.

**Metoclopramide.** *Actions.* Metoclopramide [Reglan] has two beneficial actions: (1) it suppresses emesis by blocking receptors for dopamine *and* serotonin in the CTZ, and (2) it increases upper GI motility (by enhancing the actions of acetylcholine).

*Therapeutic Uses.* Metoclopramide is a valuable drug for suppressing nausea and vomiting caused by highly emetogenic anticancer agents (e.g., cisplatin, dacarbazine). In addition, metoclopramide is given to suppress postoperative emesis and emesis caused by radiation therapy, toxins, and opioids. Other applications include relief of diabetic gastroparesis and suppression of gastroesophageal reflux.

*Adverse Effects.* With high-dose therapy, sedation and diarrhea are common. Like other dopamine antagonists, metoclopramide may cause extrapyramidal reactions, especially in children. These reactions can often be controlled by injection of diphenhydramine (a drug with prominent anticholinergic actions). Because of its ability to increase gastric and intestinal motility, metoclopramide is contraindicated in patients with obstruction, hemorrhage, or perforation of the GI tract.

*Preparations, Dosage, and Administration.* Metoclopramide [Reglan] is available in tablets (10 mg), as a syrup (5 mg/ml), and as an injection (5 mg/ml). Oral preparations are used for diabetic gastroparesis and gastroesophageal reflux.

For prophylaxis of chemotherapy-induced emesis, treatment is intravenous. Dosing is begun 30 minutes prior to chemotherapy. The initial dose is 1 to 2 mg/kg infused over 15 minutes or more. Additional doses of 1 to 2 mg/kg are administered 2, 4, 7, 10, and 13 hours after the first dose.

## Glucocorticoids

Two glucocorticoids—*methylprednisolone* [Solu-Medrol] and *dexamethasone* [Decadron]—are commonly used to suppress emesis caused by cancer chemotherapy (even though they are not FDA approved for this application). These drugs are effective alone and in combination with other antiemetics. The mechanism by which glucocorticoids suppress emesis is unknown. Both dexamethasone and methylprednisolone are administered intravenously. Since antiemetic use is intermittent and short term, serious side effects do not occur. The pharmacology of the glucocorticoids is discussed in Chapter 65.

## Cannabinoids

**Uses.** *Suppression of Emesis.* Two cannabinoids—*dronabinol* [Marinol] and *nabilone* [Cesamet]—are approved for treating nausea and vomiting associated with cancer chemotherapy. Dronabinol (delta-9-tetrahydrocannabinol; THC) is the principal psychoactive agent in *Cannabis sativa* (marijuana). Nabilone is a synthetic derivative of dronabinol. The mechanism by which cannabinoids sup-

## TABLE 73-1. ANTIEMETICS

| Class and Generic Name | Trade Name | Adult Dosage |
|---|---|---|
| SEROTONIN ANTAGONISTS | | |
| Ondansetron | Zofran | See Table 73-2 |
| Granisetron | Kytril | See Table 73-2 |
| DOPAMINE ANTAGONISTS | | |
| *Phenothiazines* | | |
| Chlorpromazine | Thorazine | 10-25 mg (PO, IM, IV) q 4-6 h PRN |
| Perphenazine | Trilafon | 8-30 mg/day in divided doses (PO, IM, IV) |
| Prochlorperazine | Compazine | 5-10 mg (PO, IM, IV) 3-4 times a day PRN |
| Promethazine | Phenergan | 12.5-25 mg (PO, IM, IV) q 4-6 h |
| Thiethylperazine | Torecan | 10 mg (PO) 3 times a day |
| *Butyrophenones* | | |
| Haloperidol | Haldol | 1-5 mg (PO, IM, IV) q 12 h PRN |
| Droperidol | Inapsine | 2.5-5 mg (IM, IV) q 4-6 h PRN |
| *Others* | | |
| Metoclopramide* | Reglan | See Table 73-2 |
| Domperidone | Motilium | 15 mg (IV), then 7.5 mg 2 q h × 7 |
| ANTICHOLINERGICS | | |
| *Antihistamines* | | |
| Buclizine | Bucladin-S | 50 mg (PO) q 4-6 h |
| Cyclizine | Marezine | 50 mg (PO, IM) q 4-6 h PRN |
| Dimenhydrinate | Dramamine | 50-100 mg (PO, IM, IV) q 4-6 h PRN |
| Diphenhydramine | Benadryl | 10-50 mg (PO, IM, IV) q 4-6 h PRN |
| Hydroxyzine | Vistaril, Atarax | 25-100 mg (PO, IM) q 6 h PRN |
| Meclizine | Bonine, Antivert | 25-50 mg (PO) q 24 h PRN |
| *Others* | | |
| Scopolamine | Transderm Scōp | 0.5 mg (transdermal) q 72 h PRN |
| GLUCOCORTICOIDS | | |
| Dexamethasone | Decadron | 10-20 mg (IV) before chemotherapy, then 4-8 mg |
| Methylprednisolone | Solu-Medrol | 2 doses of 125-500 mg (IV) 6 hr apart before chemotherapy |
| CANNABINOIDS | | |
| Dronabinol | Marinol | 5-7.5 mg/m² (PO) q 24 h PRN |
| Nabilone | Cesamet | 1-2 mg (PO) 3-4 times a day PRN |
| BENZODIAZEPINES | | |
| Lorazepam | Ativan | 1.0-1.5 mg (IV) before chemotherapy |
| Diazepam | Valium | 2-5 mg (PO) q 3 h |
| MISCELLANEOUS | | |
| Diphenidol | Vontrol | 25-50 mg (PO) q 4 h PRN |
| Benzquinamide | Emete-Con | 25-50 mg (IM, IV) q 3-4 h PRN |
| Phosphorated carbohydrate solution | Emetrol | 15-30 ml (PO) q 1-3 h PRN |

*Also blocks serotonin receptors.

press emesis is unknown. The basic pharmacology of the cannabinoids is discussed in Chapter 37.

*Appetite Stimulation. Dronabinol* is approved for stimulating appetite in patients with AIDS. The goal is to reduce AIDS-induced anorexia and prevent or reverse weight loss.

***Adverse Effects.*** When cannabinoids are used to prevent emesis or stimulate appetite, they can produce subjective effects identical to those elicited by smoking marijuana. Patients may experience temporal disintegration, dissociation, depersonalization, and dysphoria. Many people find these reactions intolerable. Because of their cen-

## TABLE 73-2. ANTIEMETICS: USES AND MECHANISM OF ACTION

| Class | Prototype | Antiemetic Use | Mechanism of Antiemetic Action |
|---|---|---|---|
| Serotonin antagonists | Ondansetron [Zofran] | Chemotherapy, radiation, postoperative | Blocks serotonin receptors on vagal afferents and in the CTZ |
| Dopamine antagonists | Prochlorperazine [Compazine] | Chemotherapy postoperative, general | Blocks dopamine receptors in the CTZ |
| Glucocorticoids | Dexamethasone [Decadron] | Chemotherapy | Unknown |
| Cannabinoids | Dronabinol [Marinol] | Chemotherapy | Unknown |
| Anticholinergics | Scopolamine [Transderm Scōp] | Motion sickness | Blocks muscarinic receptors in the pathway from the inner ear to the vomiting center |
| Antihistamines | Dimenhydrinate [Dramamine] | Motion sickness | Blocks $H_1$ receptors and muscarinic receptors in the pathway from the inner ear to the vomiting center |

tral nervous system (CNS) effects, cannabinoids are contraindicated for patients with psychiatric disorders. Dronabinol and nabilone have a high potential for abuse and are classified under Schedule II of the Controlled Substances Act. In addition to their subjective effects, cannabinoids can cause tachycardia and hypotension, and therefore must be used with caution in patients with cardiovascular disease.

***Preparations, Dosage, and Administration.*** Dronabinol [Marinol] and nabilone [Cesamet] are both dispensed in capsules for oral use. To *prevent emesis*, the dosage for dronabinol is 5 to 7.5 mg/m² every 2 hours as needed; the dosage for nabilone is 1 to 2 mg 3 or 4 times daily as needed.

Only *dronabinol* is approved for *stimulating appetite in patients with AIDS*. The recommended initial dosage is 2.5 mg twice daily, before lunch and supper. If this dosage is intolerable, 2.5 mg once daily may be tried. The maximum recommended daily dosage is 20 mg in divided doses.

### Benzodiazepines

*Lorazepam* [Ativan] is used in combination regimens to suppress nausea and vomiting caused by cancer chemotherapy. The drug has three principal benefits: sedation, suppression of anticipatory emesis, and production of anterograde amnesia. In addition, lorazepam may help control extrapyramidal reactions caused by phenothiazine antiemetics. The basic pharmacology of lorazepam and the other benzodiazepines is discussed in Chapter 32.

## Management of Chemotherapy-Induced Emesis

Many anticancer drugs cause severe nausea and vomiting. These reactions can be so intense that patients may discontinue chemotherapy rather than endure further discomfort. Fortunately, nausea and vomiting can be minimized with the antiemetics available today.

Chemotherapy is associated with three types of emesis: (1) anticipatory, (2) acute, and (3) delayed. *Anticipatory emesis* occurs before anticancer drugs are actually given; it is triggered by the memory of severe nausea and vomiting from a previous round of chemotherapy. *Acute emesis* happens shortly (1 to 2 hours) after chemotherapy is administered. In contrast, *delayed emesis* develops a day or more after drug administration.

Antiemetics are more effective at preventing emesis than at suppressing emesis that has already begun. For prevention, antiemetics are administered orally or parenterally. To suppress ongoing emesis, oral therapy won't work; hence parenteral administration is required.

For patients taking highly emetogenic drugs, antiemetic *combinations* are clearly more effective than single-drug therapy. A serotonin antagonist (e.g., ondansetron) plus dexamethasone is the current treatment of choice. Lorazepam may be added to reduce anxiety and anticipatory emesis, and to provide amnesia. The superior efficacy of combination therapy suggests that anticancer drugs may induce emesis by multiple mechanisms. Three combination regimens are shown in Table 73-3.

## Drugs for Motion Sickness

Motion sickness can be caused by sea, air, automobile, and space travel. Symptoms are nausea, vomiting, pallor, and cold sweats. The drugs used to treat motion sickness are most effective when given prophylactically, rather than after symptoms have begun.

### Scopolamine

Scopolamine, a muscarinic antagonist, is the most effective drug for prophylaxis and treatment of motion sick-

## TABLE 73-3. ANTIEMETIC COMBINATIONS FOR PATIENTS RECEIVING HIGHLY EMETOGENIC ANTICANCER DRUGS

| Regimen | Dosage |
| --- | --- |
| *Combination 1* | |
| Ondansetron | 32 mg IV once *or* 0.15 mg/kg IV q 4 h for 3 doses |
| Dexamethasone | 10–20 mg IV once |
| Lorazepam* | 1.0–1.5 mg IV once, or more |
| *Combination 2* | |
| Granisetron | 10 μg/kg IV once *or* 1 mg IV once |
| Dexamethasone | 10–20 mg IV once |
| Lorazepam* | 1.0–1.5 mg IV once, or more |
| *Combination 3* | |
| Metoclopramide | 3 mg/kg IV q 2–4 h for 3 doses |
| Dexamethasone | 10–20 mg IV once |
| Lorazepam | 1.0–1.5 mg IV once, or more |
| Diphenhydramine | 25–50 mg IV q 4-6 h |

*Lorazepam is optional.

ness. Benefits derive from suppressing nerve traffic in the neuronal pathway that connects the vestibular apparatus of the inner ear to the vomiting center (see Fig. 73-1). The most common side effects are dry mouth, blurred vision, and drowsiness. More severe but less common effects are urinary retention, constipation, and disorientation.

Scopolamine is available for oral, subcutaneous, and transdermal administration. The transdermal system [Transderm Scōp], an adhesive patch that contains scopolamine, is applied behind the ear. Anticholinergic side effects with transdermal administration may be less intense than with oral or subcutaneous administration.

### Antihistamines

The antihistamines used most often for motion sickness are dimenhydrinate [Dramamine], meclizine [Antivert], and cyclizine [Marezine]. Because these drugs block receptors for acetylcholine in addition to receptors for histamine, they appear in Table 73-1 as a subclass under *Anticholinergics*. Suppression of motion sickness is thought to result from blockade of histaminergic ($H_1$) and cholinergic (muscarinic) receptors in the neuronal pathway that leads from the inner ear to the vomiting center (see Fig. 73-1). The most important side effect of the antihistamines is sedation. In addition, these drugs can cause typical anticholinergic effects, including dry mouth, blurred vision, and urinary retention. Unfortunately, sedation limits their utility. For treatment of motion sickness, the antihistamines are less effective than scopolamine.

## Antidiarrheal Agents

Diarrhea is characterized by stools of excessive volume and fluidity, and by increased frequency of defecation. Diarrhea is a symptom of gastrointestinal disease and not a disease per se. Causes include infection, maldigestion, inflammation, and functional disorders of the bowel. The most serious complications of diarrhea are dehydration and depletion of electrolytes. Management is directed at the following: (1) diagnosis and treatment of the underlying disease, (2) replacement of lost water and salts, (3) relief of cramping, and (4) reducing the passage of unformed stools.

Antidiarrheal drugs fall into two major groups: (1) specific antidiarrheal drugs and (2) nonspecific antidiarrheal drugs. The specific agents are drugs that treat the underlying cause of diarrhea. Included in this group are anti-infective drugs and drugs used to correct malabsorption syndromes. Nonspecific antidiarrheals are agents that act on or within the bowel to provide symptomatic relief; these drugs do not influence the actual cause of diarrhea.

## Nonspecific Antidiarrheal Agents
### Opioids

Opioids are the most effective antidiarrheal drugs. By stimulating opioid receptors in the GI tract, these agents decrease intestinal motility, thereby slowing intestinal transit, which allows more time for absorption of fluid and electrolytes. In addition, stimulation of opioid receptors acts directly to decrease secretion of fluid into the small intestine and to increase absorption of fluid and salt. The net effect of these actions is to present the large intestine with less water. As a result, the fluidity and volume of stools are reduced, as is the frequency of defecation.

At the doses employed to relieve diarrhea, subjective effects and dependence do not occur. However, excessive doses can elicit typical morphine-like subjective effects. If severe overdose occurs, it should be treated with naloxone. In patients with inflammatory bowel disease, opioids may cause toxic megacolon.

## TABLE 73-4. OPIOIDS USED TO TREAT DIARRHEA

| Generic Name | Trade Name | CSA* Schedule | Antidiarrheal Dosage |
|---|---|---|---|
| Diphenoxylate (plus atropine)[†] | Lomotil, others | V | *Adults:* 5 mg, 4 times/day<br>*Children (initial dosage):*<br>    age 2-5 years—1 mg, 4 times/day<br>    age 5-8 years—1-2 mg, 4 times/day<br>    age 8-12 years—1-2 mg, 4 times/day |
| Difenoxin (plus atropine)[†] | Motofen | IV | *Adults:* 2 mg initially, then 1 mg after each loose stool |
| Loperamide | Imodium, others | NR[‡] | *Adults (initial dose):* 4 mg<br>*Children (initial dosage):*<br>    age 2-5 years—1 mg, 3 times/day<br>    age 5-8 years—2 mg, 2 times/day<br>    age 8-12 years—2 mg, 3 times/day |
| Paregoric (camphorated tincture of opium; contains 0.4 mg morphine/ml) | | III | *Adults:* 5-10 ml, 1-4 times/day<br>*Children:* 0.25-0.5 ml/kg, 1-4 times/day |
| Opium tincture (opioid content equivalent to 10 mg morphine/ml) | | II | 0.6 ml 4 times/day |

*Controlled Substances Act.
[†]Diphenoxylate and difenoxin are dispensed only in combination with atropine. The atropine dose is subtherapeutic and is present to discourage abuse.
[‡]Not regulated under the CSA.

Several opioid preparations—diphenoxylate, difenoxin, loperamide, paregoric, and opium tincture—are approved for treatment of diarrhea. Of these, diphenoxylate [Lomotil, others] and loperamide [Imodium, others] are the most frequently employed. Pharmacologic properties of these agents are discussed below. Dosages for diarrhea are summarized in Table 73-4.

**Diphenoxylate.** Diphenoxylate is an opioid whose only indication is diarrhea. The drug is insoluble in water, and hence cannot be abused by parenteral routes. When taken orally in antidiarrheal doses, diphenoxylate has no significant effect on the CNS. However, if taken in high doses, the drug can elicit typical morphine-like subjective responses.

Diphenoxylate is dispensed only in combination with atropine. The combination, whose most common trade name is *Lomotil*, is available in tablets and an oral liquid. Each tablet or 5 ml of liquid contains 2.5 mg of diphenoxylate and 25 μg of atropine sulfate. The atropine is present to discourage diphenoxylate abuse: doses of the combination that are sufficiently high to produce euphoria from the diphenoxylate would produce unpleasant side effects from the correspondingly high dose of atropine. Accordingly, the combination has a very low potential for abuse and is classified under Schedule V.

**Difenoxin.** Difenoxin is the major active metabolite of diphenoxylate. Like diphenoxylate, difenoxin can elicit morphine-like subjective effects if taken in high doses. To discourage excessive dosing, difenoxin, like diphenoxylate, is dispensed only in com-bination with atropine. The trade name for the combination is *Motofen*. Because its abuse potential is somewhat greater than that of diphenoxylate plus atropine, Motofen is classified as a Schedule IV preparation.

**Loperamide.** Loperamide [Imodium, others] is a structural analog of meperidine. The drug is employed to treat diarrhea and to reduce the volume of discharge from ileostomies. Beneficial effects result from suppression of bowel motility and from suppression of fluid secretion into the intestinal lumen. The drug is poorly absorbed and does not readily cross the blood-brain barrier. Very large oral doses fail to elicit morphine-like subjective effects. Loperamide has little or no potential for abuse, and is not classified under the Controlled Substances Act. The drug is dispensed in 2-mg capsules and in a liquid formulation (1 mg/5 ml).

**Paregoric.** Paregoric (camphorated tincture of opium) is a dilute solution of opium, containing morphine (0.4 mg/ml) as its main active ingredient. The primary indication for paregoric is diarrhea, although the preparation is also approved for the same indications as morphine. Antidiarrheal doses cause neither euphoria nor analgesia. Very high doses can cause typical morphine-like responses. Paregoric has a moderate potential for abuse and is classified as a Schedule III preparation.

**Opium Tincture.** Opium tincture is an alcohol-based solution that contains 10% opium by weight. The principal active ingredient—morphine—is present at 10 mg/ml. The primary indication for opium tincture is diarrhea. In addition, the preparation (in dilute form) may be given to suppress symptoms of withdrawal in opioid-dependent neonates. When administered in antidiarrheal doses, opium tincture does not produce analgesia or euphoria. However, high doses can cause typical opioid agonist effects. Opium tincture has a high potential for abuse and is classified as a Schedule II preparation.

#### Other Nonspecific Antidiarrheals

*Bulk-Forming Agents.* Paradoxically, methylcellulose, polycarbophil, and other bulk-forming laxatives are useful in the management of diarrhea. Benefits derive from giving the stool a more firm, less watery consistency. Stool volume is not decreased. The bulk-forming laxatives are discussed in Chapter 72.

*Anticholinergic Antispasmodics.* Muscarinic antagonists (e.g., atropine) can relieve cramping associated with diarrhea; these drugs do not alter fecal consistency or volume. Because of undesirable side effects (e.g., blurred vision, photophobia, dry mouth, urinary retention, tachycardia), anticholinergic drugs are of limited use. The pharmacology of the muscarinic blockers is discussed in Chapter 15.

### Management of Infectious Diarrhea

*General Considerations.* Infectious diarrhea may be produced by enteric infection with a variety of bacteria and protozoa. These infections are usually self-limited. Mild diarrhea can be managed with nonspecific antidiarrheals. However, in many cases, no treatment at all is required. Antibiotics should be administered only when clearly indicated. Indiscriminate use of antibiotics is undesirable in that it can promote emergence of antibiotic-resistant organisms, and can produce an asymptomatic carrier state by killing most, but not all, of the infectious agents. Conditions that do merit antibiotic treatment include severe infections with *Salmonella*, *Shigella*, *Campylobacter*, or *Clostridium*.

*Traveler's Diarrhea.* Tourists are often plagued by infectious diarrhea. This condition is known variously as Montezuma's revenge, the Aztec two-step, or Rangoon runs. In most cases, the causative organism is *Escherichia coli*. As a rule, treatment is unnecessary: infection with *E. coli* is self-limited and will run its course in 1 to 2 days.

However, if symptoms are especially severe, treatment with one of the fluoroquinolone antibiotics—*ciprofloxacin*, *ofloxacin*, or *norfloxacin*—is indicated. For milder symptoms, relief can be achieved with *loperamide*, a nonspecific antidiarrheal; however, by slowing peristalsis, this drug may delay export of the offending organism, and may thereby prolong the infection.

Prophylaxis is possible with *ciprofloxacin*, *ofloxacin*, or *norfloxacin*. However, since these drugs can cause serious side effects, prophylaxis is not recommended. The risk of traveler's diarrhea can be greatly reduced by avoiding local drinking water and by carefully washing foods.

## Drugs for Inflammatory Bowel Disease

Inflammatory bowel disease (IBD) has two forms: *Crohn's disease* and *ulcerative colitis*. Crohn's disease is characterized by transmural inflammation. The disease usually affects the terminal ileum, but can also affect any other part of the gastrointestinal tract. Ulcerative colitis is characterized by inflammation of the mucosa and submucosa of the colon and rectum. Both diseases produce abdominal cramps and diarrhea. Ulcerative colitis may produce rectal bleeding as well. About 15% of patients with ulcerative colitis eventually have an attack severe enough to require hospitalization for IV glucocorticoid therapy, which produces remission in 60% of patients; the remaining 40% usually require total colectomy. In the United States, IBD afflicts about 1 million people. Drug therapy of IBD is summarized in Table 73-5.

### TABLE 73-5. DRUGS FOR INFLAMMATORY BOWEL DISEASE

| Disease Intensity | Disease Form | | |
| --- | --- | --- | --- |
| | Ulcerative Colitis (Distal Only) | Ulcerative Colitis (Extensive) | Crohn's Disease |
| *Mild* | Aminosalicylate (PO or rectal) Glucocorticoid (rectal) | Aminosalicylate (PO) | Aminosalicylate (PO) Metronidazole |
| *Moderate* | Same as mild | Same as mild | Glucocorticoid (PO) Azathioprine (PO) Mercaptopurine (PO) |
| *Severe* | Glucocorticoid (PO or rectal) | Glucocorticoid (PO) | Glucocorticoid (IV) Cyclosporine (IV) |
| *Fulminant* | | Glucocorticoid (IV) Cyclosporine (IV) | |
| *Remission* | Aminosalicylate (PO or rectal) Azathioprine (PO) Mercaptopurine (PO) | Same as distal | Mesalamine (PO) Azathioprine (PO) Mercaptopurine (PO) |

Three classes of medications are employed: *aminosalicylates* (e.g., sulfasalazine), *glucocorticoids* (e.g., hydrocortisone), and *immunosuppressants* (e.g., azathioprine). None of these drugs is curative; at best they may control the disease process. Patients frequently require therapy with more than one agent.

## Aminosalicylates

Aminosalicylates (e.g., sulfasalazine, mesalamine) are used to treat mild or moderate ulcerative colitis and Crohn's disease, and to maintain remission after symptoms have subsided.

*Sulfasalazine.* Sulfasalazine [Azulfidine] belongs to the same chemical family as the sulfonamide antibiotics. However, although similar to the sulfonamides, sulfasalazine is not employed to treat infections; rather, the drug is approved only for IBD. In addition, the drug has been used on an investigational basis to treat rheumatoid arthritis (see Chapter 66).

*Actions.* Sulfasalazine is metabolized by intestinal bacteria into two compounds: 5-aminosalicylic acid (5-ASA) and sulfapyridine. 5-ASA is the component responsible for reducing inflammation in IBD; sulfapyridine is responsible for the adverse effects of treatment. Possible mechanisms by which 5-ASA reduces inflammation include suppression of prostaglandin synthesis and suppression of the migration of inflammatory cells into the affected region.

*Therapeutic Uses.* Sulfasalazine is most effective in the treatment of acute episodes of mild to moderate ulcerative colitis. Responses are less satisfactory when symptoms are severe. Sulfasalazine can also benefit patients with Crohn's disease.

*Adverse Effects.* Nausea, fever, rash, and arthralgia are common. Hematologic disorders (e.g., agranulocytosis, hemolytic anemia, macrocytic anemia) may also occur. Accordingly, complete blood counts should be obtained periodically. Sulfasalazine appears safe for use during pregnancy and lactation.

*Preparations, Dosage, and Administration.* Sulfasalazine [Azulfidine] is available in 500-mg tablets (plain and enteric coated) for oral administration. The *initial* adult dosage is 500 mg/day. *Maintenance* dosages range from 2 to 4 gm/day in divided doses.

*Mesalamine.* Mesalamine is the generic name for 5-ASA, the active agent in sulfasalazine. The drug is used for acute treatment of mild to moderate IBD and for maintenance therapy. Mesalamine can be administered by retention enema, by rectal suppository, and by mouth (in tablets that dissolve when they reach the terminal ileum). Side effects are less than with sulfasalazine. The most common side effects of oral therapy are headache and gastrointestinal upset. The adult dosage for oral mesalamine [Asacol] is 800 mg 3 times a day. The 60-mg rectal suppositories [Rowasa] are administered twice daily. The retention enema [Rowasa] is administered once daily (4 gm in 60 ml).

*Olsalazine.* Olsalazine [Dipentum] is a dimer composed of two molecules of 5-ASA, the active component of sulfasalazine. Olsalazine is approved for maintenance therapy of ulcerative colitis in patients unable to tolerate sulfasalazine. The drug's most common adverse effect is watery diarrhea, which occurs in 17% of those treated. Other side effects include abdominal pain, cramps, acne, rash, and joint pain. Olsalazine is dispensed in tablets for oral administration. The adult dosage is 500 mg twice daily with food.

## Glucocorticoids

The basic pharmacology of the glucocorticoids is presented in Chapters 56 and 65; discussion here is limited to the use of these drugs in IBD. Glucocorticoids (e.g., dexamethasone, budesonide) can relieve symptoms of ulcerative colitis and Crohn's disease. Benefits derive from anti-inflammatory actions. Glucocorticoids are indicated primarily for induction of remission, and not for long-term maintenance. Administration may be oral, IV, or rectal. Prolonged use of glucocorticoids can cause severe adverse effects, including adrenal suppression, osteoporosis, increased susceptibility to infection, and a cushingoid syndrome.

## Immunosuppressants

Immunosuppressants—azathioprine, mercaptopurine, cyclosporine, and methotrexate—are used for long-term therapy of selected patients with ulcerative colitis and Crohn's disease. Clinical experience is greatest with azathioprine and mercaptopurine.

*Azathioprine and Mercaptopurine.* These drugs are discussed together because one is the active form of the other. That is, azathioprine itself is inactive; once in the body, azathioprine is converted to mercaptopurine, a compound with pharmacologic activity.

Although not approved for IBD, azathioprine [Imuran] and mercaptopurine [Purinethol] have been employed with success to induce and maintain remission in both ulcerative colitis and Crohn's disease. Since onset of effects may be delayed for up to 6 months, these agents cannot be used for acute monotherapy. Furthermore, since these drugs are more toxic than aminosalicylates or glucocorticoids, they are generally reserved for patients who have not responded to traditional therapy. Major adverse effects are pancreatitis and neutropenia (secondary to bone marrow suppression). At the doses used for IBD, these drugs are neither carcinogenic nor teratogenic. The basic pharmacology of azathioprine and mercaptopurine is discussed in Chapters 67 and 96, respectively.

*Cyclosporine.* Cyclosporine [Sandimmune] is a stronger immunosuppressant than azathioprine or mercaptopurine, and is also faster acting. When used for IBD, the drug is generally reserved for patients with acute, severe ulcerative colitis or Crohn's disease that has not responded to glucocorticoids. For these patients, continuous IV infusion can rapidly induce remission. In addition to IV administration, the drug has been administered orally in low doses to maintain remission, but results have been inconsistent. Cyclosporine is a toxic compound that can cause renal dysfunction, neurotoxicity, and generalized suppression of the immune system. The basic pharmacology of cyclosporine is discussed in Chapter 67.

*Methotrexate.* In patients with Crohn's disease, methotrexate can promote short-term remission, and thereby reduce the need for glucocorticoids. Since the doses employed are low (25 mg once a week), the toxicity produced by high-dose therapy in cancer patients is avoided. The basic pharmacology of methotrexate is discussed in Chapter 96.

### Other Drugs

*Transdermal Nicotine.* It is well known that ulcerative colitis occurs mainly in *nonsmokers*, suggesting a possible protective action of nicotine. In support of this theory is the observation that transdermal nicotine (nicotine patches), combined with mesalamine, can reduce symptoms of active ulcerative colitis. When used alone to maintain remission, transdermal nicotine has been ineffective.

*Metronidazole.* In patients with mild or moderate Crohn's disease, metronidazole [Flagyl, Protostat] is as effective as sulfasalazine. Since relapse is likely if metronidazole is discontinued, long-term therapy is required. Unfortunately prolonged use of metronidazole poses a risk of peripheral neuropathy.

## Pancreatic Enzymes

The pancreas produces four digestive enzymes: *lipase, amylase, chymotrypsin,* and *trypsin.* These enzymes are secreted into the duodenum, where they help digest fats, carbohydrates, and proteins. To protect these enzymes from stomach acid and pepsin, the pancreas secretes bicarbonate. The bicarbonate neutralizes acid in the duodenum, and the resulting elevation in pH inactivates pepsin.

Deficiency of pancreatic enzymes can compromise digestion, especially the digestion of fats. Fatty stools are characteristic of the deficiency. When availability of pancreatic enzymes is reduced, replacement therapy is needed. Causes of deficiency include pancreatectomy, cystic fibrosis, pancreatitis, and obstruction of the pancreatic duct.

Pancreatic enzymes are available as two basic preparations: *pancreatin* and *pancrelipase.* Pancreatin is made from hog or beef pancreas. Pancrelipase is made from hog pancreas. Pancrelipase has enzyme activity far greater than that of pancreatin. As a result, pancrelipase is the preferred preparation. Trade names for pancrelipase include Viokase, Cotazym, and Pancrease MT.

Both pancreatin and pancrelipase are available in capsules that contain enteric-coated microspheres. The microsphere-containing preparations are preferred to conventional formulations (tablets, capsules) because the conventional formulations frequently fail to dissolve within the appropriate region of the intestine (i.e., the duodenum and upper jejunum).

Antacids and histamine$_2$-receptor blockers may be employed as adjuvants to pancreatic enzyme therapy. Their purpose is to reduce gastric pH, thereby protecting the enzymes from inactivation. However, these adjuvants are beneficial only when secretion of gastric acid is excessive.

Adverse reactions to pancreatic enzymes are rare. Allergic reactions occur occasionally. Large doses can cause diarrhea, nausea, and cramping.

Dosage is adjusted on an individual basis. Determining factors include the extent of enzyme deficiency, dietary fat content, and enzyme activity of the preparation selected. The efficacy of therapy can be evaluated by measuring the reduction in 24-hour fat excretion. Pancreatic enzymes should be taken with every meal and snack.

## Drugs Used to Dissolve Gallstones

The gallbladder serves as a repository for bile, a fluid composed of cholesterol, bile acids, and other substances. Following its production in the liver, bile may be secreted directly into the small intestine or it may be transferred to the gallbladder, where it is concentrated and stored.

Bile has two principal functions: (1) it aids in the digestion of fats, and (2) it serves as the only medium by which cholesterol is excreted from the body. The acids present in bile facilitate the absorption of fats. In addition, bile acids help solubilize cholesterol.

Cholelithiasis—development of gallstones—is the most common form of gallbladder disease. Most stones are formed from cholesterol. Stones made of cholesterol alone cannot be detected with x-rays, and hence are said to be *radiolucent.* In contrast, stones that contain calcium (in addition to cholesterol) are *radiopaque* (i.e., they absorb x-rays and therefore can be seen in a radiograph). Risk factors for cholelithiasis include obesity and high blood levels of cholesterol.

For many people, gallstones can be present for years without causing symptoms. When symptoms do develop, they can be much like those of indigestion (bloating, abdominal discomfort, gassiness). If a stone should lodge in the bile duct, severe pain and jaundice may result.

Cholelithiasis may be treated by cholecystectomy (surgical removal of the gallbladder) or with drugs. As a rule, when intervention is required, cholecystectomy is the preferred modality. In asymptomatic patients, more conservative measures (weight loss and reduced fat intake) may be indicated. Medications employed to dissolve gallstones are discussed below.

### Chenodiol (Chenodeoxycholic Acid)

*Actions.* Chenodiol [Chenix] is a naturally occurring bile acid that reduces hepatic production of cholesterol. Reduced cholesterol production lowers the cholesterol content of bile, which in turn facilitates the gradual dissolution of cholesterol gallstones. Chenodiol may also increase the amount of bile acid in bile, an effect that may enhance cholesterol solubility. It should be noted that chenodiol is useful only for dissolving *radiolucent* stones. *Radiopaque* stones (stones with significant calcium content) are not affected.

*Therapeutic Use.* Chenodiol is given to promote dissolution of cholesterol gallstones, but only in carefully selected patients. Success is most likely in women who have low cholesterol levels, stones of small size, and the ability to tolerate high doses of the drug. Complete disappearance of stones occurs in only 20% to 40% of patients. Therapy is usually prolonged; 2 years is common.

*Adverse Effects.* Diarrhea occurs in 30% to 40% of patients; dosage reduction will decrease this response. Of much greater concern, chenodiol can damage the liver. Hence, patients must have periodic tests of liver function. Because of its hepatotoxic effects, chenodiol is contraindicated for patients with pre-existing liver impairment. Chenodiol is also contraindicated during pregnancy (FDA Pregnancy Category X).

### Ursodiol (Ursodeoxycholic Acid)

Ursodiol [Actigall] is an analog of chenodiol. Like chenodiol, ursodiol reduces the cholesterol content of bile, thereby facilitating the gradual dissolution of cholesterol gallstones. In contrast to chenodiol, ursodiol does not increase production of bile acids. Like chenodiol, ursodiol promotes dissolution of *radiolucent* gallstones but not *radiopaque* gallstones. Ursodiol is indicated for dissolution of cholesterol gallstones in carefully selected patients.

Ursodiol is well tolerated. Significant adverse effects are rare. The drug is classified in FDA Pregnancy Category B.

Ursodiol is dispensed in 300-mg capsules for oral administration. The usual adult dosage is 4 to 5 mg/kg twice daily (1 capsule in the morning and 1 in the evening). Treatment lasts for months.

**Monooctanoin**

Monooctanoin [Moctanin] is a semisynthetic vegetable oil that can dissolve *cholesterol* gallstones; extended direct contact with the gallstones is required. The only use for monooctanoin is removal of stones that remain in the common bile duct following cholecystectomy. Administration is by continuous perfusion through a catheter placed directly in the common bile duct. Duration of perfusion is usually 2 to 10 days. Complete dissolution of stones occurs in approximately one third of those treated. Partial dissolution occurs in about 30% more. The most common side effects are gastrointestinal disturbances (abdominal pain, nausea, vomiting).

## Anorectal Preparations

Anorectal preparations can provide symptomatic relief from the discomfort of hemorrhoids and other anorectal disorders. The composition of these preparations varies widely. *Local anesthetics* (e.g., benzocaine, dibucaine) and *hydrocortisone* (a glucocorticoid) are common ingredients. Hydrocortisone suppresses inflammation, itching, and swelling. Local anesthetics reduce itching and pain. Anorectal preparations may also contain *emollients* (e.g., mineral oil, lanolin), whose lubricant properties reduce irritation, and *astringents* (e.g., bismuth subgallate, witch hazel, zinc oxide), which serve to reduce irritation and inflammation. Anorectal preparations are available in multiple formulations: suppositories, creams, ointments, foams, tissues, and pads.

## KEY POINTS

- Emesis results from activation of the vomiting center, which receives its principal stimulatory input from the chemoreceptor trigger zone, cerebral cortex, and inner ear.
- The serotonin antagonists, such as ondansetron [Zofran], are the most effective antiemetics available.
- To suppress chemotherapy-induced emesis, a combination of drugs is more effective than monotherapy. The current combination of choice is a serotonin antagonist (e.g., ondansetron) plus a glucocorticoid (e.g., dexamethasone), with or without lorazepam (a benzodiazepine).
- For management of chemotherapy-related emesis, antiemetics are more effective when given *before* chemotherapy (to *prevent* emesis) than when given after chemotherapy (in an effort to stop ongoing emesis).
- Opioids (e.g., diphenoxylate) are the most effective antidiarrheal agents available.
- Traveler's diarrhea can be treated with loperamide, a nonspecific antidiarrheal drug, or with a fluoroquinolone antibiotic (e.g., ciprofloxacin). The quinolones can also be used for prophylaxis.
- Sulfasalazine [Azulfidine] and the glucocorticoids (e.g., dexamethasone) are preferred drugs for treating inflammatory bowel disease (ulcerative colitis, Crohn's disease).

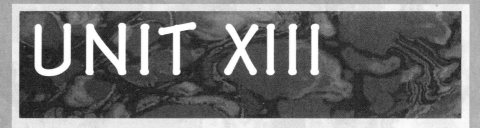

# UNIT XIII

# Metabolic Drugs

Vitamins

Drugs Affecting Calcium Levels and
Bone Mineralization

Enteral and Parenteral Nutrition

# Vitamins

itamins have the following defining characteristics: (1) they are *organic compounds*, (2) they are required in *minute amounts* for growth and maintenance of health, and (3) they do not serve as sources of energy (in contrast to fats, carbohydrates, and proteins), but rather are *essential for energy transformation and for the regulation of metabolic processes*. Several vitamins are inactive in their native form and must be converted into active compounds within the body.

## General Considerations

### Vitamin Allowances

#### Recommended Dietary Allowances

Recommended dietary allowances (RDAs) for vitamins are listed in Table 74-1. These values are established by the Food and Nutrition Board of the National Academy of Sciences and are intended to provide a standard for good nutrition. RDAs are revised periodically as new information becomes available. The values in Table 74-1 were released in 1989. It is important to note that RDAs apply only to individuals in good health. Vitamin requirements can be increased by illness, and therefore the allowances recommended in the table may not be appropriate for people who are sick. With the possible exception of the RDA for vitamin D, the values in the table represent a 100% *excess* of the vitamin intake considered necessary to avoid deficiency. Hence, RDAs should not be looked upon as minimum daily requirements.

For the vast majority of healthy people, diet alone can be relied upon to provide RDAs of all vitamins. Conse-

quently, although consumption of vitamin supplements is widespread, the practice is generally unnecessary and, in some cases, may even be harmful.

In the case of two vitamins—biotin and pantothenic acid—no RDAs have been set because we lack sufficient data. In lieu of RDAs, the Food and Nutrition Board has set established ranges of Estimated Safe and Adequate Daily Dietary Intakes for these vitamins. These values do not appear in Table 74-1, but they are given in the text.

#### Reference Daily Intakes

Official Reference Daily Intakes (RDIs), which are assigned by the U.S. Food and Drug Administration (FDA), serve as a legal standard for labeling foods with respect to nutritional content. RDIs appear on food packaging as *Percent Daily Intake* (based on a 2000 kcal/day diet). At this time, RDIs are the same as the former U.S. Recommended Daily Allowances (U.S. RDAs), which in turn are very similar to the RDAs shown in Table 74-1.

### Classification of Vitamins

The vitamins are divided into two major groups: *fat-soluble vitamins* and *water-soluble vitamins*. In the fat-soluble group are vitamins A, D, E, and K. The water-soluble group consists of vitamin C and members of the vitamin B complex (thiamine, riboflavin, niacin, pyridoxine, pantothenic acid, biotin, folic acid, cyanocobalamin). As a rule, storage of water-soluble vitamins is minimal; hence frequent ingestion is needed to avoid deficiency. In contrast, fat-soluble vitamins can be stored in massive amounts, which is good news and bad news. The good news is that extensive storage minimizes the risk of deficiency. The bad news is that extensive storage greatly increases the potential for toxicity in the event of excessive intake.

## TABLE 74–1. RECOMMENDED DAILY DIETARY ALLOWANCES[a]

| Age (years) | Fat-Soluble Vitamins | | | | | Water-Soluble Vitamins | | | | | |
|---|---|---|---|---|---|---|---|---|---|---|---|
|  | A (µg RE)[b] | D (µg)[c] | E (mg αTE)[d] | K (µg) | C (mg) | Thiamine (mg) | Riboflavin (mg) | Niacin (mg NE)[e] | B$_6$ (mg) | Folacin (µg) | B$_{12}$ (µg) |
| **Infants** 0.0–0.5 | 375 | 7.5 | 3 | 5 | 30 | 0.3 | 0.4 | 5 | 0.3 | 25 | 0.3 |
| 0.5–1.0 | 375 | 10 | 4 | 10 | 35 | 0.4 | 0.5 | 6 | 0.6 | 35 | 0.5 |
| **Children** 1–3 | 400 | 10 | 6 | 15 | 40 | 0.7 | 0.8 | 9 | 1.0 | 50 | 0.7 |
| 4–6 | 500 | 10 | 7 | 20 | 45 | 0.9 | 1.1 | 12 | 1.1 | 75 | 1.0 |
| 7–10 | 700 | 10 | 7 | 30 | 45 | 1.0 | 1.2 | 13 | 1.4 | 100 | 1.4 |
| **Males** 11–14 | 1000 | 10 | 10 | 45 | 50 | 1.3 | 1.5 | 17 | 1.7 | 150 | 2.0 |
| 15–18 | 1000 | 10 | 10 | 65 | 60 | 1.5 | 1.8 | 20 | 2.0 | 200 | 2.0 |
| 19–24 | 1000 | 10 | 10 | 70 | 60 | 1.5 | 1.7 | 19 | 2.0 | 200 | 2.0 |
| 25–50 | 1000 | 5 | 10 | 80 | 60 | 1.5 | 1.7 | 19 | 2.0 | 200 | 2.0 |
| 51+ | 1000 | 5 | 10 | 80 | 60 | 1.2 | 1.4 | 15 | 2.0 | 200 | 2.0 |
| **Females** 11–14 | 800 | 10 | 8 | 45 | 50 | 1.1 | 1.3 | 15 | 1.4 | 150 | 2.0 |
| 15–18 | 800 | 10 | 8 | 55 | 60 | 1.1 | 1.3 | 15 | 1.5 | 180[f] | 2.0 |
| 19–24 | 800 | 10 | 8 | 60 | 60 | 1.1 | 1.3 | 15 | 1.6 | 180[f] | 2.0 |
| 25–50 | 800 | 5 | 8 | 65 | 60 | 1.0 | 1.3 | 15 | 1.6 | 180[f] | 2.0 |
| 51+ | 800 | 5 | 8 | 65 | 60 | 1.0 | 1.2 | 13 | 1.6 | 180[f] | 2.0 |
| **Pregnant** | 800 | 10 | 10 | 65 | 70 | 1.5 | 1.6 | 17 | 2.2 | 400 | 2.2 |
| **Breast-feeding** 1st 6 months | 1300 | 10 | 12 | 65 | 95 | 1.6 | 1.8 | 20 | 2.1 | 280 | 2.6 |
| 2nd 6 months | 1200 | 10 | 11 | 65 | 90 | 1.6 | 1.7 | 20 | 2.1 | 260 | 2.6 |

[a]The allowances are intended to provide for individual variations among most normal persons as they live in the United States under usual environmental stresses.
[b]Retinol equivalents (1 RE = 1 µg retinol or 6 µg beta-carotene).
[c]As cholecalciferol (10 µg cholecalciferol = 400 IU vitamin D).
[d]Alpha-tocopherol equivalents (1 alpha-TE = 1 mg d-alpha-tocopherol).
[e]1 NE (niacin equivalent) is equal to 1 mg of niacin or 60 mg of dietary tryptophan.
[f]The U.S. Public Health Service recommends that all women who may become pregnant ingest 400 µg of folic acid each day.

Adapted with permission from Food and Nutrition Board. Recommended Dietary Allowances, 10th ed. Washington, DC, National Academy Press, 1989. Copyright 1989 by the National Academy of Sciences.

# Fat-Soluble Vitamins

## Vitamin A (Retinol)

**Actions.** Vitamin A, also known as retinol, has multiple functions. In the eyes, vitamin A plays an important role in adaptation to dim light. The vitamin is also needed to maintain the structural and functional integrity of the skin and mucous membranes.

**Sources.** Requirements for vitamin A can be met by (1) consuming foods that contain *preformed vitamin A* (retinol), and (2) consuming foods that contain *beta-carotene*, a compound that is converted to retinol by cells of the intestinal mucosa. Preformed vitamin A is present only in foods of animal origin. Good sources are butter, eggs, whole milk, and liver. Beta-carotene is a pigment food in many plants. Especially rich sources are carrots, spinach, tomatoes, and pumpkins.

**Units.** The unit employed to measure vitamin A activity is called the *retinol equivalent.* By definition, 1 retinol equivalent equals 1 µg of retinol or 6 µg of beta-carotene. The 1:6 ratio between retinol and beta-carotene reflects the fact that dietary beta-carotene is poorly absorbed and incompletely converted into retinol. Hence, 6 µg of dietary beta-carotene is required to produce the nutritional effect of 1 µg of retinol. In the past, vitamin A activity was measured in International Units (IU). One IU is equal to 0.3 retinol equivalents.

**Pharmacokinetics.** Under normal conditions, dietary vitamin A is readily absorbed and then stored in the liver. As a rule, liver reserves of vitamin A are large and will last for months if intake of retinol ceases. Normal plasma levels for retinol range between 30 and 70 µg/dl. In the absence of vitamin A intake, levels will be maintained through mobilization of liver reserves. As liver stores approach depletion, plasma levels will begin to decline. Signs and symptoms of deficiency appear when plasma levels fall below 20 µg/dl.

**Deficiency.** Because of the role of vitamin A in dark adaptation, night blindness is often the first indication of deficiency. With time, vitamin A deficiency may lead to *xerophthalmia* (a dry, thickened condition of the conjunctiva) and *keratomalacia* (degeneration of the cornea with keratinization of the corneal epithelium). When vitamin A deficiency is severe, blindness may occur. In addition to effects on the eye, deficiency can produce skin lesions and dysfunction of mucous membranes.

**Toxicity.** Vitamin A is highly teratogenic. As a result, excessive intake during pregnancy can cause *birth defects*, including defects of cranial–neural crest origin (e.g., craniofacial, central nervous system, thymus, and heart defects). Risk is highest among women taking vitamin A supplements. To avoid risk, women who are pregnant or considering becoming pregnant should limit vitamin A consumption to the RDA.

Excessive doses of vitamin A can cause a toxic state, referred to as hypervitaminosis A. Chronic intoxication affects multiple organ systems, especially the liver. Symptoms are diverse and may include vomiting, jaundice, hepatosplenomegaly, skin changes, hypomenorrhea, and elevation of intracranial pressure. Most symptoms disappear following vitamin A withdrawal. To avoid toxicity, it is recommended that routine consumption of vitamin A not exceed 7500 retinol equivalents/day.

***Therapeutic Uses.*** The only indication for vitamin A is prevention or correction of vitamin A deficiency. Contrary to earlier hopes, it is now clear that vitamin A, in the form of beta-carotene supplements, does not decrease the risk of cancer or cardiovascular disease. In fact, in a study comparing placebo with dietary supplements (beta-carotene plus vitamin A), subjects taking the supplements had a significantly *increased* risk of lung cancer and overall mortality. As discussed in Chapter 98, certain derivatives of vitamin A (tretinoin, isotretinoin, etretinate) are used to treat acne and other dermatologic disorders.

***Preparations, Dosage, and Administration.*** Vitamin A (retinol) is dispensed in the form of drops, tablets, and capsules for oral administration and as an injection for intramuscular use. Oral administration is generally preferred. For prevention of deficiency, dietary plus medicinal vitamin A should add up to the RDA (see Table 74–1). For treatment of deficiency, doses as high as 100 times the RDA may be required.

## Vitamin D

Vitamin D plays a critical role in the regulation of calcium and phosphorus metabolism. In children, deficiency causes *rickets.* In adults, deficiency causes *osteomalacia.* Excessive amounts of the vitamin are toxic. Symptoms result primarily from hypercalcemia. The pharmacology and physiology of vitamin D are discussed at length in Chapter 75.

## Vitamin E (Alpha-Tocopherol)

Vitamin E (alpha-tocopherol) is essential to the health of many species, but has no clearly established role in human nutrition. The vitamin has antioxidant properties, and these may help protect essential cellular components from oxidation. It may also protect red blood cells from hemolysis. In a recent study, consumption of vitamin E-rich foods—but not vitamin E supplements—was correlated with a decreased risk of mortality from coronary artery disease. In laboratory animals, vitamin E deficiency produces a variety of symptoms, some of which are severe. In humans, however, vitamin E deprivation has no obvious effect. The vitamin is also devoid of toxicity to humans. Since the nutritional role of vitamin E is uncertain, it is difficult to determine dietary requirements. The RDAs given in Table 74–1 are sufficient to maintain plasma content of the vitamin within the normal range. Although numerous uses for vitamin E have been proposed, the only established indication is the prevention or correction of deficiency. Vitamin E is present in fresh greens and many other vegetables. Seed oils and wheat germ are especially rich sources. In commercial preparations, vitamin E is present in multiple forms: *d,l*-alpha-tocopherol, *d*-alpha-tocopherol, *d,l*-alpha-tocopherol acetate, *d,l*-alpha-tocopherol acid succinate, *d*-alpha-tocopherol acid succinate, and *d*-alpha-tocopheryl acetate.

## Vitamin K

***Action.*** Vitamin K is required for synthesis of prothrombin and three other clotting factors (factors VII, IX, and X). All of these vitamin K–dependent factors are needed for coagulation of blood.

***Forms and Sources of Vitamin K.*** Vitamin K occurs in nature in two forms: (1) vitamin $K_1$, or phytonadione (phylloquinone) and (2) vitamin $K_2$. Phytonadione is present in a wide variety of foods. Vitamin $K_2$ is synthesized by the normal flora of the gut. Two other forms—vitamin $K_4$ (menadiol) and vitamin $K_3$ (menadione)—are produced synthetically. At this time, phytonadione is the only form of vitamin K available for therapeutic use.

***Requirements.*** Human requirements for vitamin K have not been precisely defined. The values established by the Food and Nutrition Board approximate 1 µg/kg of body weight. For most individuals, vitamin K requirements are readily met through dietary sources and through vitamin K synthesized by intestinal bacteria. Since bacterial colonization of the gut is not complete until several days after birth, levels of vitamin K may be low during the immediate postnatal period.

***Pharmacokinetics.*** Intestinal absorption of the natural forms of vitamin K (phytonadione and vitamin $K_2$) is adequate only in the presence of bile salts. Menadione and menadiol do not require bile salts for absorption. Following absorption, vitamin K is concentrated in the liver. Metabolism and secretion occur rapidly. Very little storage in tissues occurs.

***Deficiency.*** Vitamin K deficiency produces bleeding tendencies. If the deficiency is severe, spontaneous hemorrhage may occur. In newborns, intracranial hemorrhage is of particular concern.

An important cause of deficiency is reduced absorption. Since the natural forms of vitamin K require bile salts for their uptake, any condition that decreases availability of these salts (e.g., obstructive jaundice) can lead to deficiency. Malabsorption syndromes (sprue, celiac disease, cystic fibrosis of the pancreas) can also decrease vitamin K uptake. Other potential causes of impaired absorption are ulcerative colitis, regional enteritis, and surgical resection of the intestine.

Disruption of intestinal flora may result in deficiency by eliminating vitamin K–synthesizing bacteria. Hence deficiency may occur secondary to use of antibiotics. In infants, diarrhea may cause bacterial losses sufficient to result in deficiency.

The normal infant is born vitamin K deficient. Consequently, in order to rapidly elevate prothrombin levels, and thereby reduce the risk of neonatal hemorrhage, it is recommended that all infants receive a single injection of phytonadione (vitamin K₁) immediately after delivery.

As discussed in Chapter 50, the anticoagulant warfarin acts as an antagonist of vitamin K, and thereby decreases synthesis of vitamin K–dependent clotting actors. As a result, warfarin produces a state functionally equivalent to vitamin K deficiency. If the dosage of warfarin is excessive, hemorrhage can occur secondary to lack of prothrombin.

**Adverse Effects.** *Severe Hypersensitivity Reactions. Intravenous* administration of phytonadione can cause serious reactions (shock, respiratory arrest, cardiac arrest) that resemble anaphylaxis or hypersensitivity reactions. Death has occurred. Consequently, phytonadione should not be administered intravenously unless other routes are not feasible, and then only if the potential benefits clearly outweigh the risks.

*Hyperbilirubinemia.* When administered *parenterally* to newborns, vitamin K derivatives can elevate plasma levels of bilirubin, thereby posing a risk of *kernicterus*. The incidence of hyperbilirubinemia is greater among premature infants than full-term infants. Although all forms of vitamin K can elevate bilirubin levels, the risk is higher with menadione and menadiol than with phytonadione.

**Therapeutic Uses and Dosage.** Vitamin K has two major applications: (1) correction or prevention of hypoprothrombinemia and bleeding caused by vitamin K deficiency, and (2) control of hemorrhage caused by overdose with oral anticoagulants.

*Vitamin K Deficiency.* As discussed above, vitamin K deficiency can result from impaired vitamin absorption and from insufficient synthesis of the vitamin by intestinal flora. Rarely, deficiency results from inadequate diet. For children and adults, the usual dosage for correction of vitamin K deficiency ranges between 5 and 15 mg/day.

As noted above, infants are born vitamin K deficient. To prevent hemorrhagic disease in neonates, it is recommended that all newborns be given an injection of phytonadione (0.5 to 1 mg) immediately after delivery.

*Warfarin Overdose.* Vitamin K reverses hypoprothrombinemia and bleeding caused by excessive dosages of warfarin, an oral anticoagulant. Bleeding is controlled within hours of drug administration (see Chapter 50 for dosage).

**Preparations and Routes of Administration.** *Phytonadione* (vitamin K₁) is available in 5-mg tablets, marketed as Mephyton, and in two parenteral formulations, marketed as AquaMEPHYTON and Konakion. AquaMEPHYTON may be administered IM, SC, and IV. However, since IV administration is dangerous, this route should be used only when other routes are not feasible, and only if the perceived benefits outweigh the substantial risks. Konakion is intended for IM use only.

# Water-Soluble Vitamins

The group of water-soluble vitamins consists of vitamin C and members of the vitamin B complex (thiamine, ribo-

flavin, niacin, pyridoxine, pantothenic acid, biotin, folic acid, cyanocobalamin). The B vitamins differ widely from one another in both structure and function. They are grouped together because they were first isolated from the same sources (yeast and liver). Vitamin C is not found in the same foods as the B vitamins, and hence is classified by itself.

Two compounds—*pangamic acid* and *laetrile*—have been falsely promoted as B vitamins. Pangamic acid has been marketed as "vitamin B₁₅" and laetrile as "vitamin B₁₇." There is no proof that these compounds act as vitamins or have any other role in human nutrition.

## Vitamin C (Ascorbic Acid)

**Actions.** Vitamin C participates in multiple biochemical reactions. These include synthesis of adrenal steroids, conversion of folic acid to folinic acid, and regulation of the respiratory cycle in mitochondria. At the tissue level, vitamin C is required for production of collagen and other compounds that compose the intercellular matrix that binds cells together. In addition, vitamin C has antioxidant properties.

**Sources and Requirements.** The main dietary sources of ascorbic acid are citrus fruits and juices, tomatoes, potatoes, and other fruits and vegetables. Orange juice and lemon juice are especially rich in the vitamin. The RDA for adults is 60 mg. For women, the RDA increases to 70 mg during pregnancy and 95 mg during lactation. RDAs for children are shown in Table 74–1.

**Deficiency.** Deficiency of vitamin C can lead to *scurvy*, a disease that is rare in the United States. Symptoms include faulty bone and tooth development, loosening of the teeth, gingivitis, bleeding gums, poor wound healing, hemorrhage into muscles and joints, and ecchymoses (skin discoloration caused by leakage of blood into subcutaneous tissues). Many of these symptoms result from disruption of the intercellular matrix of capillaries and other tissues.

**Adverse Effects.** Ascorbic acid rarely causes adverse effects, even in huge doses. Very large amounts can induce diarrhea through direct irritation of the intestinal mucosa. Excessive doses may also promote formation of kidney stones by inducing excretion of large quantities of oxalic acid.

**Therapeutic Use.** The only established indication for vitamin C is prevention and treatment of scurvy. For severe, acute deficiency, parenteral administration is recommended. The usual adult dosage is 0.3 to 1 gm/day.

Vitamin C has been advocated for therapy of many conditions unrelated to deficiency, including cancers, asthma, osteoporosis, and the common cold. Claims of efficacy for several of these conditions have been definitively disproved. Other claims remain unproven. Studies have shown that large doses do not reduce the incidence of colds, although the intensity or duration of illness may be reduced slightly. Research has failed to show any benefit of vitamin C therapy for patients with advanced cancer, atherosclerosis, or schizophrenia. Vitamin C does not promote healing of wounds.

**Preparations and Routes of Administration.** Vitamin C is available in formulations for oral and parenteral administration. Oral products include tablets (ranging from 25 to 1500 mg), timed-release capsules (500 mg), and syrups (20 and 100 mg/ml). For parenteral use, vitamin C is available as ascorbic acid, sodium ascorbate, and calcium ascorbate. Administration may be SC, IM, or IV.

## Niacin (Nicotinic Acid)

Nicotinic acid is a vitamin and also has a role as a medicine. In its medicinal role, nicotinic acid is used to lower cholesterol levels; the doses required are *much* higher than those used to correct or prevent nutritional deficiency. Discussion in this chapter focuses on nicotinic acid as a vitamin. Use of nicotinic acid to reduce cholesterol is discussed in Chapter 49.

**Physiologic Actions.** Before it can exert physiologic effects, niacin must first be converted into NAD (nicotinamide-adenine dinucleotide) or NADP (nicotinamide-adenine dinucleotide phosphate). NAD and NADP then act as coenzymes in oxidation-reduction reactions essential for cellular respiration.

**Sources.** Nicotinic acid (or its nutritional equivalent, nicotinamide) is present in many foods of plant and animal origin. Particularly rich sources are liver, chicken, yeast, peanuts, cereal bran, and cereal germ.

In humans, the amino acid tryptophan can be converted to nicotinic acid; hence, proteins can be a source of the vitamin. About 60 mg of dietary tryptophan is required to produce 1 mg of nicotinic acid.

**Requirements.** RDAs for nicotinic acid are stated as niacin equivalents. By definition, 1 niacin equivalent is equal to 1 mg of niacin (nicotinic acid) or to 60 mg of tryptophan. RDAs are summarized in Table 74–1.

**Deficiency.** The syndrome caused by niacin deficiency is called *pellagra*, a term that is a condensation of the Italian words *pelle agra*, meaning "rough skin." As suggested by this name, a prominent symptom of pellagra is dermatitis, characterized by scaling and cracking of the skin in areas exposed to the sun. Other symptoms involve the gastrointestinal tract (abdominal pain, diarrhea, soreness of the tongue and mouth) and central nervous system (irritability, insomnia, memory loss, anxiety, dementia). All symptoms are readily reversed with niacin replacement therapy.

**Adverse Effects.** Nicotinic acid has very low toxicity. Small doses are completely devoid of adverse effects. When taken in large amounts to treat pellagra, nicotinic acid can cause vasodilation with resultant flushing, dizziness, and nausea. These reactions are temporary and harmless. Toxicity associated with high-dose therapy is discussed further in Chapter 49.

*Nicotinamide*, a compound that can substitute for nicotinic acid in the treatment of pellagra, is not a vasodilator, and hence does not produce the adverse effects associated with large doses of nicotinic acid. Accordingly, nicotinamide is often preferred to nicotinic acid for treating pellagra.

**Therapeutic Uses.** In its capacity as a vitamin, nicotinic acid is indicated only for the prevention or treatment of niacin deficiency. As noted, if given in large doses, nicotinic acid may also be used to lower cholesterol levels (see Chapter 49).

**Preparations, Dosage, and Administration.** *Nicotinic acid* (niacin) is available in tablets (20 to 500 mg), in capsules (125 to 500 mg), and as an elixir (10 mg/ml) for oral use. Niacin is also dispensed as an injection (100 mg/ml) for parenteral (SC, IM, and IV) administration. Dosages for mild deficiency range from 10 to 20 mg/day. For treatment of pellagra, daily doses may be as high as 500 mg. Dosages for treatment of hyperlipidemia are given in Chapter 49.

*Nicotinamide* (niacinamide) is dispensed in tablets (50 to 1000 mg) for oral administration and as an injection (100 mg/ml) for parenteral use. For treatment or prevention of pellagra, dosages range from 150 to 500 mg/day. Unlike nicotinic acid, nicotinamide has no effect on plasma lipoproteins and, hence, is not used to treat hyperlipidemias.

### Riboflavin (Vitamin B₂)

**Actions.** In order to exert its physiologic effects, riboflavin must first be converted into one of two active forms: flavin-adenine dinucleotide (FAD) or flavin mononucleotide (FMN). In the form of FAD and FMN, riboflavin acts as a coenzyme for a variety of oxidative reactions.

**Sources and Requirements.** Riboflavin is present in a variety of foods of animal and vegetable origin. Good sources are meats, chicken, eggs, and milk. Liver has an especially high riboflavin content. RDAs for riboflavin are summarized in Table 74–1.

**Toxicity.** Riboflavin appears devoid of toxicity to humans. When large doses are administered, the excess is rapidly excreted in the urine.

**Therapeutic Use: Riboflavin Deficiency.** Riboflavin is indicated only for prevention and correction of riboflavin deficiency, which usually occurs in conjunction with deficiency of other B vitamins. In its early state, riboflavin deficiency manifests as sore throat and angular stomatitis (cracks in the skin at the corners of the mouth). Symptoms that may appear later include cheilosis (painful cracks in the lips), glossitis (inflammation of the tongue), vascularization of the cornea, and itchy dermatitis of the scrotum or vulva. Oral riboflavin is used for treatment. The dosage is 5 to 10 mg/day.

## Thiamine (Vitamin B₁)

**Actions and Requirements.** The active form of thiamine (thiamine pyrophosphate) is an essential coenzyme for carbohydrate metabolism. Thiamine requirements are related to caloric intake, and are greatest when carbohydrates are the primary source of calories. For maintenance of good health, thiamine consumption should be at least 0.3 mg/1000 kcal in the diet. The RDAs in Table 74–1 represent approximately 0.5 mg of thiamine per 1000 kcal. Hence, these values allow about a twofold margin of safety. As indicated in Table 74–1, thiamine requirements increase markedly during pregnancy and lactation.

**Sources.** Thiamine is present in a variety of foods of plant and animal origin. Pork products are especially rich in the vitamin. Other good sources include peanuts, asparagus, and cereals (whole-grain and enriched).

**Deficiency.** Severe thiamine deficiency produces *beriberi*, a disorder having two distinct forms: *wet beriberi* and *dry beriberi*. *Wet beriberi* is so named because its primary symptom is fluid accumulation in the legs. Cardiovascular complications (palpitations, EKG abnormalities, high-output heart failure) are common and may progress rapidly to circulatory collapse and death. *Dry beriberi* is characterized by neurologic and motor deficits (e.g., anesthesia of the feet, ataxic gait, foot drop, and wrist drop); edema and cardiovascular symptoms are absent. Wet beriberi responds rapidly and dramatically to replacement therapy. In contrast, recovery from dry beriberi can be very slow.

In the United States, thiamine deficiency occurs most commonly among alcoholics. In this population, deficiency manifests as *Wernicke-Korsakoff syndrome* rather than frank beriberi. This syndrome is a serious disorder of the central nervous system, having neurologic and psychologic manifestations. Symptoms include nystagmus, diplopia, ataxia, and an inability to remember the recent past. Failure to correct the thiamine deficit may result in irreversible damage to the brain. Accordingly, if Wernicke-Korsakoff syndrome is suspected, parenteral thiamine should be administered immediately.

**Adverse Effects.** When taken orally, thiamine is devoid of adverse effects. Very rarely, parenteral administration produces anaphylactic reactions, which probably reflect hypersensitivity to thiamine.

**Therapeutic Use.** The only indication for thiamine is treatment and prevention of thiamine deficiency.

**Preparations, Dosage, and Administration.** Thiamine is dispensed in tablets (5 to 500 mg) for oral use and as an injection (100 and 200 mg/ml) for IM or IV administration. For mild deficiency, oral thiamine is preferred. Parenteral administration should be reserved for severe deficiency states (wet or dry beriberi, Wernicke-Korsakoff syndrome). The dosage for beriberi is 50 to 100 mg IM daily for 1 to 2 weeks, followed by 2.5 to 10 mg PO daily until recovery is complete.

## Pyridoxine (Vitamin B₆)

**Actions.** Before it can influence biologic processes, pyridoxine must first be converted to its active form: pyridoxal phosphate. As pyridoxal phosphate, the vitamin participates in the metabolism of amino acids and proteins.

**Requirements.** Pyridoxine requirements parallel intake of protein: as protein consumption increases, the need for pyridoxine increases as well. For the average adult male, 2.0 mg of pyridoxine daily will maintain good nutrition. The RDA for adult females is 1.6 mg per day. Pyridoxine requirements increase during pregnancy and lactation.

**Sources.** Pyridoxine is found in a variety of foods of animal and vegetable origin. Good sources include milk, meats (especially liver and kidney), soya beans, and whole-grain cereals.

**Deficiency.** Pyridoxine deficiency may result from poor diet, certain medications (especially isoniazid), and inborn errors of metabolism. Symptoms of deficiency include peripheral neuritis, seizures, glossitis, and skin lesions on the face.

In the United States, dietary deficiency of vitamin B₆ is rare, except among alcoholics. Within the alcoholic population, vitamin B₆ deficiency has an incidence of about 20% to 30% and occurs in combination with deficiency of other B vitamins.

Isoniazid (an antituberculous drug) prevents conversion of vitamin B₆ to its active form, and may thereby in-duce symptoms of deficiency (peripheral neuritis). Patients who are predisposed to this neuropathy (e.g., alcoholics, diabetics) should receive daily pyridoxine supplements.

Inborn errors of metabolism can prevent efficient utilization of vitamin B₆, resulting in greatly increased pyridoxine requirements. In the infant with such an inherited disorder, prominent symptoms are irritability, convulsions, and anemia. Unless treatment with vitamin B₆ is initiated early, permanent retardation may result.

**Adverse Effects.** At low doses, pyridoxine is devoid of adverse effects. However, if extremely large doses are taken (250 to 1000 times the RDA), neurologic injury may result. Symptoms include ataxia and numbness of the feet and hands.

**Drug Interactions.** Vitamin B₆ interferes with the utilization of levodopa by patients taking this drug for parkinsonism. Accordingly, patients receiving levodopa should be advised against taking vitamin B₆.

**Therapeutic Uses.** Pyridoxine is indicated for prevention and treatment of all vitamin B₆ deficiency states (dietary deficiency, isoniazid-induced deficiency, pyridoxine-dependency syndrome).

**Preparations, Dosage, and Administration.** Pyridoxine is dispensed in tablets (10 to 500 mg) for oral use and as an injection (100 mg/ml) for IM or IV administration. The dosage for correcting dietary deficiency is 10 to 20 mg/day for 3 weeks followed by 1.5 to 2.5 mg/day for maintenance. For treatment of deficiency induced by isoniazid, the dosage is 50 to 200 mg/day. For prophylaxis against isoniazid-induced deficiency, the dosage is 25 to 50 mg/day. Pyridoxine dependency syndrome may require initial doses up to 600 mg/day followed by 25 to 50 mg/day for life.

### Pantothenic Acid

The active form of pantothenic acid (coenzyme A) is an essential factor in a variety of biochemical processes. These include gluconeogenesis, intermediary metabolism of carbohydrates, and synthesis of steroid hormones, porphyrins, and acetylcholine. Pantothenic acid is present in numerous foods, and spontaneous deficiency has not been reported. No official RDA has been established. However, the Food and Nutrition Board has published "estimated safe and adequate daily dietary intake" levels. These are 2 to 3 mg for infants, 3 to 7 mg for children, and 4 to 7 mg for adults. Aside from minor gastrointestinal discomfort, no toxicity has been noted with doses 1000 times greater than these in adults. Pantothenic acid is available in single-ingredient tablets and in many multivitamin preparations. However, because deficiency does not occur, there is no indication for taking this vitamin.

### Biotin

Biotin is a cofactor for several reactions involved in the metabolism of carbohydrates and fats. This vitamin is present in a variety of foods. In addition, biotin is synthesized by intestinal bacteria in amounts sufficient to meet human nutritional needs. Consequently, biotin deficiency is extremely rare. When deficiency has been induced experimentally in volunteers, symptoms have included fatigue, depression, anorexia, muscle pain, and dermatitis. Biotin appears devoid of toxicity: subjects given large doses experienced no apparent ill effects. Because the amount of biotin produced by intestinal flora has not been quantified, the Food and Nutrition Board has been unable to establish an RDA for this vitamin. However, as with pantothenic acid, the Board has published "estimated safe and adequate daily dietary intake" levels. These are: 10 to 15 µg for infants, 20 to 30 µg for children ages 1 to 10 years, and 30 to 100 µg for children 11 years or older and for adults.

## Cyanocobalamin and Folic Acid

Cyanocobalamin (vitamin B₁₂) and folic acid (folacin) are essential factors in the synthesis of DNA. Deficiency of either vitamin manifests as megaloblastic anemia. Cyanocobalamin deficiency produces neurologic damage as well. Because deficiency presents as anemia, folic acid and cyanocobalamin are discussed in Chapter 51 (Drugs for Deficiency Anemias). The RDAs for these compounds are given in Table 74-1.

*Folic Acid Deficiency and Fetal Development.* Deficiency of folic acid during pregnancy can impair development of the central nervous system, resulting in neural tube defects: *anencephaly* and *spina bifida.* Anencephaly (failure of the brain to develop) is uniformly fatal. Spina bifida, a condition characterized by defective development of the bony encasement of the spinal cord, can result in nerve damage, paralysis, and other complications. Since the central nervous system develops early in pregnancy, it is essential that adequate levels of folic acid be present when pregnancy begins; if women wait until pregnancy is confirmed before increasing folic acid intake, it may be too late to prevent these disorders. Accordingly, the U.S. Public Health Service recommends that *all women who may become pregnant consume 400 µg of folic acid each day.* Since pregnancy can occur despite birth control measures, this recommendation applies even to women who don't *intend* to become pregnant. To help ensure adequate folic acid intake, the FDA now requires the addition of folic acid to enriched breads, flours, corn meals, pasta, grits, rice, and other grains.

## KEY POINTS

- Vitamins can be defined as organic compounds, required in minute amounts, that promote growth and maintenance of health by participating in energy transformation and regulation of metabolic processes.
- Recommended dietary allowances (RDAs) for vitamins, established by the Food and Nutrition Board of the National Academy of Sciences, represent a 100% *excess* of the vitamin intake considered necessary to avoid deficiency. Hence, RDAs should *not* be viewed as *minimum* daily requirements.
- For the vast majority of healthy people, diet alone can supply RDAs of all vitamins.
- Vitamins are divided into two major groups: fat-soluble vitamins (A, D, E, and K) and water-soluble vitamins (vitamin C and members of the vitamin B complex).
- Vitamin A deficiency can cause night blindness, xerophthalmia (a dry, thickened condition of the conjunctiva), and keratomalacia (degeneration of the cornea with keratinization of the corneal epithelium).
- High doses of vitamin A can cause birth defects. Accordingly, women who are pregnant or considering becoming pregnant should limit vitamin A intake to the RDA.
- Vitamin D plays a critical role in the regulation of calcium and phosphorus metabolism.
- In children, vitamin D deficiency causes rickets. In adults, deficiency causes osteomalacia.
- Vitamin K is required for synthesis of prothrombin and other clotting factors.
- Vitamin K deficiency causes bleeding tendencies. Severe deficiency can cause spontaneous hemorrhage.
- Vitamin K is used to treat vitamin K deficiency (including neonatal deficiency) and overdose with warfarin (an anticoagulant).
- Vitamin C deficiency can cause scurvy.
- Niacin (nicotinic acid) is both a vitamin and a drug.
- When niacin is used as a drug (to lower cholesterol levels), doses are much higher than when niacin is used to prevent or correct deficiency.
- Niacin deficiency results in pellagra.
- Severe thiamine deficiency produces beriberi.
- In the United States, thiamine deficiency occurs most commonly among alcoholics. In this population, deficiency manifests as Wernicke-Korsakoff syndrome rather than beriberi.
- Pyridoxine (vitamin B₆) deficiency can cause peripheral neuritis and other symptoms.
- Isoniazid, a drug for tuberculosis, prevents conversion of pyridoxine to its active form, and can thereby induce deficiency.
- Folic acid deficiency during early pregnancy can cause neural tube defects (anencephaly and spina bifida). To ensure folic acid sufficiency at the start of pregnancy, all women with the potential for becoming pregnant should consume 400 µg of folic acid every day.

# CHAPTER 75

# Drugs Affecting Calcium Levels and Bone Mineralization

I t is difficult to overemphasize the biologic importance of calcium, an element critical to the functional integrity of bone, nerve, muscle, the heart, and coagulation of blood. Since these calcium-dependent processes can be seriously disrupted by alterations in calcium availability, we must maintain calcium levels within narrow limits. To regulate calcium, three factors are employed: parathyroid hormone, vitamin D, and calcitonin. When these regulatory mechanisms fail, hypercalcemia or hypocalcemia results.

In approaching the drugs that influence calcium, we begin by reviewing calcium physiology. Next we discuss the syndromes produced by disruption of calcium metabolism. Having established this background, we discuss the pharmacologic agents used to treat calcium-related disorders. We complete the chapter with an in-depth discussion of osteoporosis, the most common calcium-related disorder.

## Calcium Physiology

### Functions and Daily Requirements

Calcium is critical to the function of the skeletal system, nervous system, muscular system, and cardiovascular system. In the skeletal system, calcium is required for the structural integrity of bone. In the nervous system, calcium helps regulate excitability and transmitter release. In the muscular system, calcium participates in excitation-contraction coupling and contraction itself. In the cardiovascular system, calcium plays a role in myocardial contraction, vascular contraction, and coagulation of blood.

Given the widespread functions of calcium, it is important that we have adequate calcium intake. Table 75-1 summarizes recommendations for calcium intake issued by the Food and Nutrition Board of the Institute of Medicine in 1997. With the exception of children less than four years old, no one should consume less than 800 mg of calcium each day, and most people need 1000 mg/day or more. However, in a survey reported in 1994, Americans, on average, consume less than 800 mg/day in their diets, indicating a need to increase dietary intake or use calcium supplements. Consuming sufficient calcium is especially important for reducing the risk of osteoporosis (see below).

### Body Stores

*Calcium in Bone.* The vast majority of calcium in the body (>98%) is present in bone. Calcium is deposited in bone in the form of hydroxyapatite crystals. It is important to appreciate that bone—and the calcium it contains—is not static. Rather, bone undergoes continuous *remodeling*, a process in which old bone is resorbed, after which new bone is deposited (Fig. 75-1). The cells that resorb old bone are called *osteoclasts* and the cells that deposit new bone are called *osteoblasts*. Both cell types originate in the bone marrow. In adults, about 25% of trabecular bone (the honeycomb-like material in the center of bones) is replaced each year. In contrast, only 3% of cortical bone (the dense material that surrounds trabecular bone) is replaced annually.

*Calcium in Blood.* The normal value for total serum calcium is 10 mg/dl (2.5 mM, 5 mEq/L). Of this total, about 50% is bound to proteins and other substances and, therefore, is unavailable for use. The remaining 50% is present as free, ionized calcium. It is the free calcium that participates in physiologic processes.

## TABLE 75–1. DAILY CALCIUM INTAKE BY LIFE-STAGE GROUP

| | Calcium Intake (mg/day) | |
| --- | --- | --- |
| Life-Stage Group[a] | Adequate Level[b] | Tolerable Upper Level[c] |
| 0 to 6 months | 210 | ND[d] |
| 6 to 12 months | 270 | ND |
| 1 through 3 years | 500 | 2500 |
| 4 through 8 years | 800 | 2500 |
| 9 through 18 years | 1300 | 2500 |
| 19 through 50 years | 1000 | 2500 |
| 51 years and older | 1200 | 2500 |

[a] Values apply to males and females. For females, there is no change during pregnancy or lactation.

[b] Values for Adequate Intake (AI) are derived through experimental or observational data that show a mean calcium intake that appears to sustain a desired indicator of health, such as calcium retention in bone, for most members of the population group. AI values are employed for calcium because there is insufficient data to derive an Estimated Average Requirement (EAR). AI values are *not* equivalent to Recommended Dietary Allowances (RDAs).

[c] The Tolerable Upper Intake Level (UI) is defined as the maximum intake that is not likely to pose a risk of adverse health effects in almost all healthy individuals in a specified group. The UI is not intended to be a recommended level of intake. There is no established benefit to consuming calcium above the AI.

[d] ND. Upper limit not determined owing to lack of data on adverse effects in this age group and concern regarding inability to handle excess calcium. To prevent excessive levels, calcium intake should be from food only.

Adapted from *Dietary Reference Intakes for Calcium, Phosphorous, Magnesium, Vitamin D and Fluoride,* Food and Nutrition Board, Institute of Medicine, National Academy Press, Washington, D.C., 1997.

## Absorption and Excretion

*Absorption.* Absorption of calcium takes place in the small intestine. Under normal conditions, about one third of ingested calcium is absorbed. Absorption is increased by parathyroid hormone and vitamin D (see below). In contrast, glucocorticoids decrease calcium absorption. Also, a variety of foods (e.g., spinach, whole grain cereals, bran) contain compounds that can interfere with calcium absorption.

*Excretion.* Excretion of calcium is primarily renal. The amount lost is determined by glomerular filtration and by the extent of tubular reabsorption. Excretion of calcium can be reduced by parathyroid hormone and vitamin D (see below). Excretion of calcium can be increased with loop diuretics (e.g., furosemide) and by loading with sodium. Calcitonin also augments calcium elimination (see below). In addition to renal excretion, substantial amounts of calcium can be lost through lactation.

## Physiologic Regulation of Calcium Levels

Blood levels of calcium are tightly controlled. The body maintains calcium levels by adjusting the rates of three processes: (1) absorption of calcium from the intestine, (2) excretion of calcium by the kidney, and (3) resorption or deposition of calcium in bone. Regulation of these processes is under the control of three factors: *parathyroid hormone, vitamin D,* and *calcitonin.* It should be noted that preservation of plasma calcium levels takes priority over the calcium requirements of bone. Hence, if serum calcium is low, calcium will be resorbed from bone and transferred to the blood—even if calcium resorption compromises the structural integrity of bone.

*Parathyroid Hormone.* Parathyroid hormone (PTH) is released from the parathyroid glands in response to low levels of plasma calcium. The effect of PTH is to restore calcium levels when they are low. PTH elevates serum calcium by three mechanisms: (1) it promotes calcium resorption from bone, (2) it promotes reabsorption of calcium that had been filtered by the glomerulus, and (3) it activates vitamin D, and thereby promotes absorption of calcium from the intestine. In addition to its effects on calcium, PTH reduces plasma levels of phosphate.

*Vitamin D.* Vitamin D is similar to PTH both in its effects on calcium levels and in the mechanisms by which these effects are produced. Like PTH, vitamin D increases plasma calcium content. Also like PTH, vitamin D elevates plasma calcium levels by (1) increasing calcium resorption from bone, (2) decreasing calcium excretion by the kidney, and (3) increasing calcium absorption from the intestine. In contrast to PTH, vitamin D elevates plasma levels of phosphate. The actions of vitamin D are discussed further below.

*Calcitonin.* Calcitonin, a hormone produced by the thyroid gland, decreases plasma levels of calcium. Hence, calcitonin acts in opposition to PTH and vitamin D. Calcitonin is released from the thyroid gland when calcium levels in blood rise too high. Calcitonin lowers calcium levels by inhibiting the resorption of calcium from bone and increasing calcium excretion by the kidney. Unlike PTH and vitamin D, calcitonin does not influence calcium absorption.

## Calcium-Related Pathophysiology

In this section, we review the majors disorders involving calcium—except for osteoporosis, which is discussed later.

### Hypercalcemia

*Clinical Presentation.* Hypercalcemia is usually asymptomatic. When symptoms are present, they often involve the kidney (damage to tubules and collecting ducts, resulting in polyuria, nocturia, and polydipsia), gastrointestinal tract (nausea, vomiting, constipation), and central nervous system (lethargy and depression). Hypercalcemia may also result in dysrhythmias and deposition of calcium in soft tissues.

*Causes.* Hypercalcemia may arise from a variety of causes. Life-threatening elevations in plasma calcium are associated most often with cancer. Hyperparathyroidism is another common cause of severe hypercalcemia (see below). Additional causes include vitamin D intoxication, sarcoidosis, and use of thiazide diuretics.

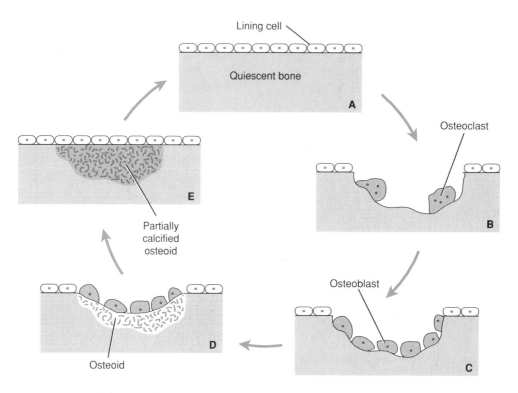

**Figure 75–1. Bone remodeling cycle.** *A*, Quiescent bone with *lining cells* covering the surface. *B*, Resorption of old bone by multinucleated *osteoclasts*. *C*, *Osteoblasts* migrate to the absorption site. *D*, Osteoblasts deposit *osteoid*, a matrix of collagen and other proteins. *E*, Osteoid undergoes *calcification*.

**Treatment.** Calcium levels can be lowered with drugs that (1) promote urinary excretion of calcium, (2) decrease mobilization of calcium from bone, (3) decrease intestinal absorption of calcium, and (4) form complexes with free calcium in blood. For severe hypercalcemia, initial therapy consists of replacing lost fluid with IV saline, followed by diuresis using IV saline and a loop diuretic (e.g., furosemide). Other agents for lowering calcium include inorganic phosphates (which promote calcium deposition in bone and reduce calcium absorption); EDTA (which binds calcium and promotes its excretion); glucocorticoids (which reduce intestinal absorption of calcium); and a group of drugs—calcitonin, bisphosphonates (e.g., pamidronate), plicamycin, inorganic phosphates, and gallium nitrate—that inhibit resorption of calcium from bone.

### Hypocalcemia

*Clinical Presentation and Cause.* Hypocalcemia enhances neuromuscular excitability. As a result, tetany, convulsions, and spasm of the pharynx and other muscles may occur. Hypocalcemia is caused most frequently by a deficiency of either parathyroid hormone, vitamin D, or dietary calcium.

*Treatment.* Severe hypocalcemia is corrected by infusing an intravenous calcium preparation (e.g., calcium gluconate). Once calcium levels have been restored, an oral calcium salt (e.g., calcium carbonate) can be given for maintenance. Vitamin D should be included in the regimen if there is a coexisting deficiency.

### Rickets

Rickets is a disease of childhood brought on by either insufficient dietary vitamin D or limited exposure to sunlight. The disease is extremely rare in the United States. Rickets is characterized by defective bone growth and skeletal deformities. Bone abnormalities are caused as follows: (1) vitamin D deficiency re-

sults in reduced calcium absorption; (2) in response to hypocalcemia, parathyroid hormone (PTH) is released; (3) PTH restores serum calcium by promoting calcium resorption from bone, thereby causing bones to soften; and (4) stress on the softened bones caused by weight bearing results in deformity. Treatment consists of vitamin D replacement therapy.

### Osteomalacia

Osteomalacia is the adult equivalent of rickets. Like rickets, this condition results from insufficient vitamin D. In the absence of vitamin D, mineralization of bone is impaired, resulting in back pain, bowing of the legs, fractures of the long bones, and kyphosis ("hunchback" curvature of the spine). Treatment consists of vitamin D replacement therapy.

### Paget's Disease of Bone

*Clinical Presentation.* Paget's disease of bone is a chronic condition seen most frequently in people over 40 years old. After osteoporosis, Paget's disease is the most common disorder of bone in the United States. The disease is characterized by increased bone resorption and replacement of the resorbed bone with abnormal bone. Increased bone turnover causes elevation in serum alkaline phosphatase (reflecting increased bone deposition) and increased urinary hydroxyproline (reflecting increased bone resorption). It is important to note that alterations in bone homeostasis do not occur evenly throughout the skeleton. Rather, alterations occur locally, most often in the pelvis, femur, spine, skull, and tibia. Although most people with Paget's disease are asymptomatic, about 10% experience bone pain and osteoarthritis; skeletal deformity may also occur. Weakening of bone may lead to fractures. Neurologic complications may occur secondary to compression of the spinal cord, spinal nerves, and cranial nerves. If bone associated with hearing is affected, deafness may result.

***Treatment.*** Asymptomatic patients are usually not treated. Mild pain can be managed with analgesics and anti-inflammatory agents. When the disease is more severe, a bisphosphonate (e.g., alendronate) is the treatment of choice; calcitonin is an alternative. Both agents suppress bone resorption.

## Hypoparathyroidism

Reductions in parathyroid hormone (PTH) usually result from inadvertent removal of the parathyroids during surgery on the thyroid gland. Lack of PTH causes hypocalcemia, which in turn may produce paresthesias, tetany, skeletal muscle spasm, laryngospasm, and convulsions. Symptoms can be relieved with calcium supplements (see *Hypocalcemia* above) and vitamin D.

## Hyperparathyroidism

***Clinical Presentation and Cause.*** Primary hyperparathyroidism usually results from parathyroid adenoma. The resulting increase in PTH secretion causes hypercalcemia and lowers serum phosphate. Hypercalcemia can cause skeletal muscle weakness, constipation (from decreased smooth muscle tone), and central nervous system (CNS) symptoms (lethargy, depression). Hypercalciuria and hyperphosphaturia are also present and may cause renal calculi. Loss of calcium and phosphate from bone may be sufficient to produce bone abnormalities.

***Treatment.*** Primary hyperparathyroidism is usually treated by surgical resection of the parathyroid glands. If surgery is contraindicated, hypercalcemia can be managed with the drugs discussed above under *Hypercalcemia*.

# Drugs for Disorders Involving Calcium

## Calcium Salts

Calcium salts are available in oral and parenteral formulations for treatment of hypocalcemic states. The various calcium salts differ in their percentage of elemental calcium. These differences must be accounted for when determining dosage.

## Oral Calcium Salts

***Therapeutic Uses.*** Oral calcium preparations are used to treat mild hypocalcemia. In addition, calcium salts are taken as dietary supplements. People who may need supplementary calcium include children, adolescents, the elderly, postmenopausal women, and women who are pregnant or breast-feeding.

***Adverse Effects.*** When calcium is taken chronically in high doses (3 to 4 gm/day), *hypercalcemia* can result. Hypercalcemia is most likely in patients who are also receiving large doses of vitamin D. Signs and symptoms include gastrointestinal disturbances (nausea, vomiting, constipation), renal dysfunction (polyuria, nephrolithiasis), and CNS effects (lethargy, depression). In addition, hypercalcemia may cause cardiac dysrhythmias and deposition of calcium in soft tissue. Hypercalcemia can be minimized with frequent monitoring of plasma calcium content.

***Drug Interactions.*** *Glucocorticoids* (e.g., prednisone) reduce absorption of oral calcium. Calcium binds to *tetracyclines*, thereby decreasing tetracycline absorption; to minimize this interaction, calcium and tetracyclines should be administered at least 1 hour apart. *Thiazide diuretics* decrease renal calcium excretion and may thereby cause hypercalcemia.

***Food Interactions.*** Certain foods contain substances that can suppress calcium absorption. One such substance —oxalic acid—is found in spinach, rhubarb, Swiss chard, and beets. Phytic acid, another depressant of calcium absorption, is present in bran and whole grain cereals. Oral calcium should not be administered with these foods.

***Preparations and Dosage.*** The calcium salts available for oral administration are listed in Table 75–2. Note that the dosage required to provide a particular amount of elemental calcium differs among preparations. Calcium carbonate, for example, has the highest percentage of calcium. Chewable tablets are preferred to standard tablets because of more consistent bioavailability. When calcium supplements are taken, total daily calcium intake (dietary plus supplemental) should equal the values in Table 75–1. To help ensure adequate absorption, no more than 600 mg should be consumed at one time.

## Parenteral Calcium Salts

***Therapeutic Use.*** Parenteral calcium salts are given to raise calcium levels rapidly in patients with symptoms of severe

## TABLE 75–2. ORAL CALCIUM SALTS

| Generic Name | Trade Names | Calcium Content | Dose providing 500 mg Calcium |
|---|---|---|---|
| Calcium acetate | Phos-Ex, PhosLo | 25% | 2.0 gm |
| Calcium carbonate | Various names | 40% | 1.3 gm |
| Calcium citrate | Citracal | 21% | 2.4 gm |
| Calcium glubionate | Neo-Calglucon | 6.6% | 7.6 gm |
| Calcium gluconate* | — | 9% | 5.5 gm |
| Calcium lactate | — | 13% | 3.8 gm |
| Dibasic calcium phosphate | — | 23% | 2.2 gm |
| Tricalcium phosphate | Posture | 39% | 1.3 gm |

*Also available in parenteral form (see Table 75–3).

## TABLE 75-3. CALCIUM SALTS FOR PARENTERAL ADMINISTRATION

| Generic Name | Dosage Form | Calcium per ml of Solution | Route | Usual Adult Dosage Range |
|---|---|---|---|---|
| Calcium chloride | 10% solution | 27 mg | IV | 5-10 ml (135-270 mg Ca) |
| Calcium gluconate* | 10% solution | 9 mg | IV | 5-20 ml (45-180 mg Ca) |
| Calcium gluceptate | 22% solution | 18 mg | IV | 5-20 ml (90-360 mg Ca) |
| | | | IM | 2-5 ml (36-90 mg Ca) |

*Also available in an oral formulation (see Table 75-2).

hypocalcemia (i.e., hypocalcemic tetany). Three parenteral preparations are available: *calcium chloride, calcium gluconate,* and *calcium gluceptate.* Intravenous calcium gluconate is the agent of choice.

**Adverse Effects.** *Calcium chloride* is highly irritating. Intramuscular injection may cause necrosis and sloughing; hence, this route must never be used. When the drug is administered IV, care must be taken to avoid extravasation, since local infiltration can produce severe injury. Although less of an irritant than calcium chloride, *calcium gluconate* can produce pain, sloughing, and abscess formation if administered IM. Overdose with any of the calcium salts can produce signs and symptoms of hypercalcemia (weakness, lethargy, nausea, vomiting, coma, death).

**Drug Interactions.** Parenteral calcium may cause severe bradycardia in patients taking *digoxin.* Accordingly, calcium infusions should be done slowly and cautiously in these patients. Several classes of compounds—*phosphates, carbonates, sulfates,* and *tartrates*—may cause calcium to precipitate, and hence should not be added to parenteral calcium solutions.

**Dosage and Administration.** All three parenteral calcium salts may be given IV; only calcium gluceptate can also be given IM. Solutions of calcium salts should be warmed to body temperature prior to administration. Intravenous injections should be done slowly (0.5 to 2 ml/min). Dosage forms and dosages are summarized in Table 75-3.

## Vitamin D

The term *vitamin D* refers to two compounds: *ergocalciferol* (vitamin $D_2$) and *cholecalciferol* (vitamin $D_3$). Vitamin $D_3$ is the form of vitamin D produced naturally in humans when the skin is exposed to sunlight. Vitamin $D_2$ is a form of vitamin D that occurs in the plant kingdom. Vitamin $D_2$ is used as a drug and to fortify foods. Both forms of vitamin D produce nearly identical effects. Therefore, rather than distinguishing between these compounds, we will use the term *vitamin D* to refer to vitamins $D_2$ and $D_3$ collectively.

### Physiologic Actions

Vitamin D is an important regulator of calcium and phosphorus homeostasis. Vitamin D increases blood levels of both elements, primarily by increasing their intestinal absorption and promoting their mobilization from bone. In addition, vitamin D reduces renal excretion of calcium and phosphate; however, the quantitative significance of this effect is not clear. With usual doses of vitamin D,

there is no net loss of calcium from bone; decalcification of bone occurs only when serum calcium concentrations cannot be maintained by increasing intestinal calcium absorption.

### Sources and Daily Requirements

Vitamin D is obtained through the diet and by exposure to sunlight. In the United States, vitamin D is present as an additive in a variety of foods, including milk, other dairy products, cereals, and candy. Because of these supplements, Americans rarely experience nutritional vitamin D deficiency.

In 1997, the Food and Nutrition Board of the Institute of Medicine issued new guidelines for Vitamin D intake. People 50 years old or younger should consume 200 international units (IU) per day; people ages 51 through 70 should consume 400 IU/day; and people older than 70 should consume 600 IU/day. Since substantial amounts of vitamin D may be present in the diet, and since vitamin D in excess can be harmful, supplements should not be taken unless the diet has first been evaluated and judged to be vitamin D deficient.

### Vitamin D Deficiency

Insufficient dietary vitamin D produces *rickets* in children and *osteomalacia* in adults. Signs and symptoms of these conditions are described above. Administration of vitamin D can completely reverse the symptoms of both conditions, unless permanent deformity has already developed.

#### Activation of Vitamin D

In order to affect calcium and phosphate metabolism, vitamin D must first undergo activation. The extent of this activation is carefully regulated, and is determined by calcium availability: when plasma calcium levels fall, activation of vitamin D is increased. The pathways for activating vitamins $D_2$ and $D_3$ are shown in Figure 75-2.

Let's begin consideration of vitamin D activation by focusing on the natural human vitamin (vitamin $D_3$). As shown in Figure 75-2, vitamin $D_3$ (cholecalciferol) is produced in the skin through the action of sunlight on provitamin $D_3$ (7-dehydrocholesterol). Neither provitamin $D_3$ nor vitamin $D_3$ itself possesses significant biologic activity. In the next reaction, enzymes in the liver convert cholecalciferol into calcifediol; calcifediol serves as a transport form of vitamin $D_3$ and possesses only slight biologic activity. In the final step of vitamin D activation, cal-

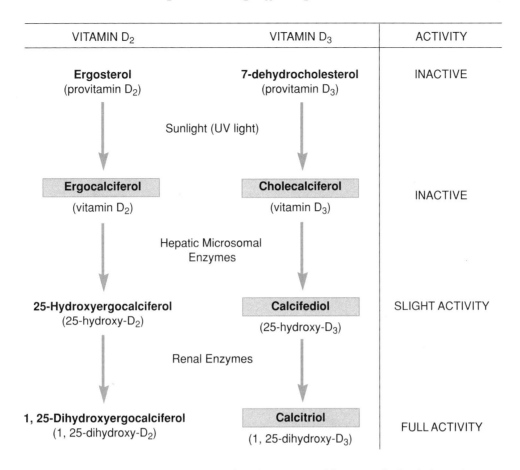

**Figure 75–2. Vitamin D activation.** Ergosterol is found in yeasts and fungi. 7-Dehydrocholesterol is present in the skin. (Colored boxes indicate forms of vitamin D used therapeutically.)

cifediol is converted into the highly active calcitriol. This reaction occurs in the kidney and can be stimulated by (1) parathyroid hormone, (2) reductions in dietary vitamin D, and (3) decline in plasma levels of calcium.

Vitamin $D_2$ is activated by the same enzymes that activate vitamin $D_3$. As we saw with vitamin $D_3$, only the last compound in the series (in this case 1,25-dihydroxyergocalciferol) displays significant biologic activity.

### Pharmacokinetics

Vitamin D is administered orally and absorbed from the small intestine. Bile is essential for absorption. Hence, in the absence of sufficient bile, IM administration may be required. Vitamin D is transported in the blood complexed with vitamin D–binding protein. Storage of vitamin D occurs primarily in the liver. As discussed above, vitamin D undergoes metabolic activation. Reactions that occur in the liver produce the major transport form of vitamin D. A later reaction in the kidney produces the fully active vitamin. Excretion of vitamin D is via the bile. Very little vitamin D leaves in urine.

### Viewing Vitamin D as a Hormone

Although referred to as a vitamin, vitamin D has all the characteristics of a hormone. With sufficient exposure to sunlight, the body can manufacture all the vitamin D it needs. Hence, under ideal conditions, external sources of vitamin D are probably unnecessary. Following its production in the skin, vitamin D travels to other locations (liver and kidney) for activation. Like other hormones, activated vitamin D then travels to various sites in the body (bone, intestine, kidney) to exert its regulatory ac-

tions. Also like other hormones, vitamin D undergoes feedback regulation: as plasma levels of calcium fall, activation of vitamin D increases; when plasma levels of calcium return to normal, the rate of vitamin D activation declines.

### Toxicity (Hypervitaminosis D)

Vitamin D toxicity (hypervitaminosis D) can be produced by doses of vitamin D in excess of 1000 IU/day in infants and 50,000 IU/day in adults. Poisoning occurs most commonly in children; causes include accidental ingestion and excessive administration of vitamin D by parents. Doses of potentially toxic magnitude are also encountered clinically. When these huge doses are used, the margin of safety is small, and patients should be monitored closely for signs of poisoning.

***Clinical Presentation.*** Most signs and symptoms of vitamin D toxicity occur secondary to hypercalcemia. Early responses include weakness, fatigue, nausea, vomiting, and constipation. With persistent hypercalcemia, kidney function is affected, resulting in polyuria, nocturia, and proteinuria. Calcium deposition in soft tissues can damage the heart, blood vessels, and lungs; calcium deposition in the kidneys can cause nephrolithiasis. Very large doses of vitamin D can cause decalcification of bone, resulting in osteoporosis; mobilization of bone calcium can occur despite the presence of high calcium concentrations in blood. In children, vitamin D poisoning can suppress growth for 6 months or longer.

***Treatment.*** Treatment consists of immediate discontinuation of vitamin D, high fluid intake, and institution of a low-calcium diet. Glucocorticoids may be given to suppress calcium absorption. If hypercalcemia is severe, renal excretion of calcium can be accelerated using a combination of intravenous saline and furosemide.

### Therapeutic Uses

The primary indications for vitamin D are nutritional rickets, osteomalacia, and hypoparathyroidism. Other applications include vitamin D-resistant rickets, vitamin D-dependent rickets, and renal osteodystrophy.

### Preparations, Dosage, and Administration

There are five preparations of vitamin D. Four of these—ergocalciferol, cholecalciferol, calcifediol, and calcitriol—are identical to forms of vitamin D that occur naturally. The fifth preparation—dihydrotachysterol—is a synthetic derivative of vitamin $D_2$. (The naturally occurring preparations are highlighted in colored boxes in Fig. 75-2.) Individual vitamin D preparations differ in their clinical applications. Indications for specific preparations are given below.

Vitamin D is usually administered by mouth. Intramuscular injections (of ergocalciferol) may also be used. Dosage is usually prescribed in international units (IU). (One IU is equivalent to the biologic activity in 0.025 μg of vitamin $D_3$.) Daily dosages of vitamin D range from 400 IU (for dietary supplementation) to as high as 500,000 IU (for vitamin D-resistant rickets).

*Ergocalciferol (Vitamin $D_2$).* Ergocalciferol [Calciferol, Drisdol] is used for hypoparathyroidism, vitamin D-resistant rickets, and familial hypophosphatemia. Ergocalciferol is dispensed in capsules (50,000 IU), tablets (50,000 IU), oral solution (8000 IU/ml), and as an injection (500,000 IU/ml). The dosage for vitamin D-resistant rickets ranges from 12,000 to 500,000 IU daily. The dosage for hypoparathyroidism ranges from 50,000 to 200,000 IU daily (together with 4 gm of calcium lactate given 6 times/day).

*Cholecalciferol (Vitamin $D_3$).* Vitamin $D_3$ [Delta-D] is given as a dietary supplement and for the prophylaxis and treatment of vitamin D deficiency. Cholecalciferol is available in tablets containing 400 IU and 1000 IU.

*Calcifediol (25-hydroxy-$D_3$).* Calcifediol [Calderol] is indicated for the management of metabolic bone disease and hypocalcemia in patients undergoing chronic renal dialysis. Calcifediol is available in capsules (20 and 50 μg) for oral use. The initial dosage is 300 to 350 μg/week (administered in divided doses on a daily or every-other-day schedule). For maintenance, daily doses of 50 to 100 μg are adequate for most patients.

*Calcitriol (1,25-dihydroxy-$D_3$).* Calcitriol [Rocaltrol, Calcijex] is indicated for treatment of hypoparathyroidism and for management of hypocalcemia in patients undergoing chronic renal dialysis. The drug is dispensed in capsules (0.25 and 0.5 μg) and as an injection (1 and 2 μg/ml). For dialysis patients, daily doses of 0.5 to 1.0 μg are usually adequate. The initial dosage for hypoparathyroidism is 0.25 μg/day.

*Dihydrotachysterol.* Dihydrotachysterol (DHT) is a synthetic derivative of vitamin $D_2$. DHT is interesting in that, unlike vitamins $D_2$ and $D_3$, it doesn't require renal enzymes for activation; metabolic conversation by the liver is all that is needed to render DHT fully active. DHT is indicated for hypoparathyroidism, postoperative tetany, and tetany of unknown cause. DHT is available in tablets (0.125, 0.2, and 0.4 mg), capsules (0.125 mg), and oral solutions (0.2 and 0.25 mg/ml). Preparations are marketed under the trade names DHT and Hytakerol.

## Calcitonin-Salmon

Calcitonin-salmon [Calcimar, Miacalcin], a form of calcitonin derived from salmon, is similar in structure to calci-

tonin synthesized by the human thyroid. Salmon calcitonin produces the same metabolic effects as human calcitonin but has a longer half-life and greater milligram potency. The drug is available for administration by injection and by nasal spray. Both forms of the drug are extremely safe.

### Actions

Calcitonin has two principal actions: (1) it inhibits the activity of osteoclasts, and thereby decreases bone resorption, and (2) it inhibits tubular resorption of calcium, and thereby increases calcium excretion. As a result of decreasing bone turnover, calcitonin decreases alkaline phosphatase in blood and increases hydroxyproline in urine.

### Therapeutic Uses

*Osteoporosis.* Calcitonin-salmon, administered by nasal spray, is indicated for *treatment* of established postmenopausal osteoporosis—but not for prevention. Benefits derive from suppressing bone resorption. The treatment program should include supplemental calcium and an adequate intake of vitamin D. Use of calcitonin for osteoporosis is discussed further under *Osteoporosis.*

*Paget's Disease of Bone.* Calcitonin is helpful in moderate to severe Paget's disease and is the drug of choice for rapid relief of pain associated with this disorder. Benefits occur secondary to inhibition of osteoclasts. Neurologic symptoms caused by spinal cord compression may be reduced.

*Hypercalcemia.* Calcitonin can lower plasma calcium levels in patients with hypercalcemia secondary to hyperparathyroidism, vitamin D toxicity, and cancer. Levels of calcium (and phosphorus) are lowered due to inhibition of bone resorption and increased excretion of calcium by the kidneys. Although calcitonin is effective against hypercalcemia, it is not a preferred treatment.

### Adverse Effects

Calcitonin is very safe. With intranasal administration, nasal dryness and irritation are the most common complaints. Following parenteral (IM, SC) administration, about 10% of patients experience nausea, which diminishes with time. An additional 10% have inflammatory reactions at the site of injection. Flushing of the face and hands may also occur. When salmon calcitonin is taken for a year or longer, neutralizing antibodies often develop; in some patients, these antibodies bind enough calcitonin to prevent therapeutic effects.

### Preparations, Dosage, and Administration

*Intranasal Spray.* Salmon calcitonin for intranasal use [Miacalcin] is available in a metered-dose dispenser that delivers 200 IU/activation. This formulation is approved only for *postmenopausal osteoporosis.* The dosage is 200 IU (1 spray) each day, alternating nostrils daily.

*Parenteral.* Salmon calcitonin for parenteral use [Calcimar, Miacalcin, Osteocalcin, Salmonine] is dispensed in 2-ml vials containing 200 IU/ml. Administration may be IM or SC. Dosages are the same for both routes. Dosages for specific indications are

- *Postmenopausal osteoporosis*—100 IU/day
- *Paget's disease of bone*—the initial dosage is 100 IU/day; the maintenance dosage is 50 IU daily or every other day
- *Hypercalcemia*—the initial dosage is 400 IU/kg every 12 hours; the maximal dosage is 8 IU/kg every 6 hours

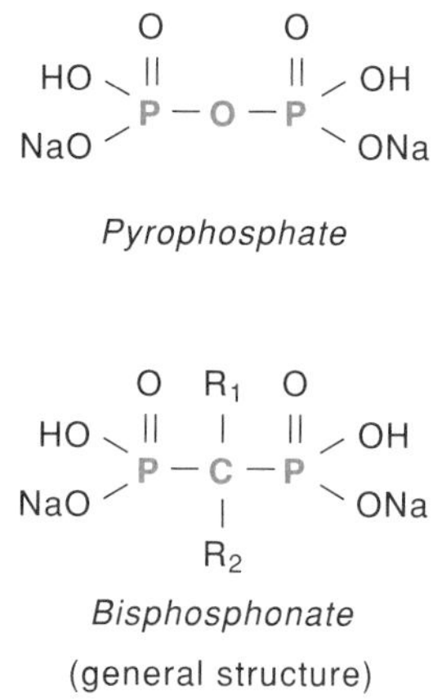

$$\begin{array}{ccc} & O & O \\ & \| & \| \\ HO-P-O-P-OH \\ NaO & & ONa \end{array}$$

*Pyrophosphate*

$$\begin{array}{cccc} & O & R_1 & O \\ & \| & | & \| \\ HO-P-C-P-OH \\ NaO & & | & ONa \\ & & R_2 \end{array}$$

*Bisphosphonate*
(general structure)

**Figure 75–3. Structure of pyrophosphate and bisphosphonates.**

## Bisphosphonates

Bisphosphonates are structural analogs of pyrophosphate (Fig. 75–3), a normal constituent of bone. These drugs undergo incorporation into bone, and then inhibit bone resorption by decreasing the activity of osteoclasts. Principal indications are osteoporosis, Paget's disease of bone, and hypercalcemia of malignancy. Although bisphosphonates are generally very safe, serious adverse effects can occur. All bisphosphonates are poorly absorbed from the GI tract, especially in the presence of food. At this time, four bisphosphonates are approved for use in the United States (Table 75-4). As shown in the Table, these drugs differ significantly in their relative potencies.

### Alendronate

Alendronate [Fosamax], a widely used biphosphonate, will serve as our prototype for the family. The drug is indicated for osteoporosis and Paget's disease of bone. Oral bioavailability is very low. Although alendronate is a generally safe drug, esophageal ulceration has occurred in some patients.

***Pharmacokinetics.*** Alendronate is administered orally, but bioavailability is very low (only 0.7%). If the drug is taken with solid food, essentially none is absorbed. Even coffee or orange juice can decrease absorption by 60%. Of the small fraction that is absorbed, about 50% is taken up rapidly by bone; the remaining 50% is excreted in the urine. Once alendronate has become incorporated into bone, it remains there for many years.

***Mechanism of Action.*** Alendronate suppresses resorption of bone by decreasing both the number and activity of osteoclasts. Several mechanisms are involved. As osteoclasts begin to resorb alendronate-containing bone, they ingest some of the drug, which then acts on the osteoclasts to inhibit their activity. In addition to inhibiting osteoclast activity, alendronate reduces the number of osteoclasts by (1) acting directly to decrease their recruitment and (2) acting on osteoblasts, which then produce an inhibitor of osteoclast formation.

***Therapeutic Use.*** *Postmenopausal Osteoporosis.* Alendronate is the only drug other than estrogen that is approved for the prevention and treatment of osteoporosis. In both cases, benefits derive from decreasing bone resorption by osteoclasts. The use of alendronate for osteoporosis is discussed further under *Osteoporosis.*

*Paget's Disease of Bone.* Alendronate is a first-line drug for treatment of Paget's disease. With continuous daily therapy for 3 months, the drug can produce a 50% decrease in serum alkaline phosphatase, indicating a substantial reduction in bone turnover. As in osteoporosis, benefits derive from inhibiting bone resorption by osteoclasts.

***Adverse Effects.*** With the exception of causing esophagitis, alendronate is devoid of serious adverse effects. When used in the low doses employed for osteoporosis, alendronate causes no more side effects than placebo. At the higher doses employed in Paget's disease, mild GI disturbances are common.

*Esophagitis*, sometimes resulting in ulceration, is alendronate's most serious adverse effect. Fortunately, esophagitis is rare, occurring in 1 of every 10,000 patients. The cause of injury is prolonged contact with the esophageal mucosa, which can occur if alendronate fails to pass completely through the esophagus. Reasons for incomplete passage include taking the drug with insuffi-

## TABLE 75–4. BISPHOSPHONATES: RELATIVE POTENCIES, ROUTES, AND USES

| Generic Name | Trade Name | Relative Potency | Route | Postmenopausal Osteoporosis | Paget's Disease | Hypercalcemia of Malignancy |
|---|---|---|---|---|---|---|
| Etidronate | Didronel | 1 | PO, IV | | A | A |
| Tiludronate | Skelid | 10 | PO | I | A | |
| Pamidronate | Aredia | 100 | IV | I | A | A |
| Alendronate | Fosamax | 1000 | PO | A | A | |

*A = FDA approved indication, I = investigational use.

cient water, taking the drug in a supine position, lying down after taking the drug, and having a pre-existing esophageal disorder that impedes drug passage. To promote complete passage, and thereby minimize risk of esophagitis, alendronate should be administered according to recommended guidelines (see below). Patients should be instructed to discontinue alendronate and contact the physician if they experience symptoms of esophageal injury (difficulty swallowing, pain upon swallowing, or new or worsening heartburn). Because of the risk of esophagitis, alendronate is contraindicated for patients with esophageal disorders that could prevent successful swallowing and for patients who are unable to sit or stand for at least 30 minutes.

In patient's with Paget's disease, alendronate can induce *hyperparathyroidism.* How? By inhibiting accelerated bone resorption, alendronate causes blood levels of calcium to fall. In response, secretion of parathyroid hormone is increased. To prevent hyperparathyroidism, patients should receive calcium supplements.

***Administration.*** Proper administration is necessary to maximize bioavailability and minimize the risk of esophagitis. To maximize bioavailability, alendronate should be taken in the morning before breakfast (i.e., on an empty stomach); no food, including orange juice or coffee, should be consumed for at least 30 minutes. To minimize the risk of esophagitis, patients should be instructed to

- Take alendronate with a full glass of water
- Remain upright (seated or standing) for at least 30 minutes and at least until completing their first meal of the day
- Avoid chewing or sucking the tablet

***Preparations and Dosage.*** Alendronate [Fosamax] is available in tablets (10 and 40 mg) for oral administration. Dosages for *postmenopausal osteoporosis* are 5 mg/day (for prevention) and 10 mg/day (for treatment). The dosage for *Paget's disease* is 40 mg once a day for 6 months.

### Etidronate

Etidronate [Didronel] is approved for *Paget's disease* and *hypercalcemia* of malignancy. The drug is not used for osteoporosis. In patients with highly active Paget's disease, etidronate can produce moderate clinical improvement. Unfortunately, when the drug is discontinued, relapse may occur rapidly. Side effects include abdominal cramps, diarrhea, nausea, and increased bone pain. In addition, etidronate causes defective mineralization of newly formed bone (osteomalacia), and can thereby increase the risk of fractures.

Etidronate is dispensed in 200- and 400-mg tablets for oral administration. As with all other bisphosphonates, bioavailability is low (less than 6%). To maximize absorption, food should be avoided for 2 hours after administration. For treatment of Paget's disease, the usual dosage is 5 mg/kg/day for no more than 6 months. Repeated treatments can be given, but not until 90 days have elapsed since the end of the prior course.

### Pamidronate

Pamidronate [Aredia] is an intravenous biphosphonate approved for *Paget's disease* and *hypercalcemia* of malignancy. Because of dose-related GI intolerance (e.g., mucosal erosion in the esophagus and stomach), pamidronate is not used orally.

***Therapeutic Use and Dosage.*** *Hypercalcemia of Malignancy.* When cancer cells metastasize to bone, they release factors that stimulate bone resorption by osteoclasts. The result is hypercalcemia, increased risk of fractures, and bone pain. By inhibiting osteoclasts, pamidronate can blunt cancer-mediated bone resorption. A typical dosage is 90 mg infused over 2 or 4 hours once every 4 weeks.

*Paget's Disease of Bone.* Like other bisphosphonates, pamidronate can decrease bone resorption in patients with Paget's disease. The dosage is 30 to 60 mg IV on three consecutive days. With this dosage, the mean duration of remission is 14 months.

***Adverse Effects.*** Intravenous pamidronate is devoid of serious adverse effects. In some patients, the first dose causes transient influenza-like symptoms. If pamidronate is not infused with sufficient fluid, venous irritation can occur. In contrast to etidronate, pamidronate does not interfere with bone mineralization. Because pamidronate inhibits accelerated bone resorption of Paget's disease, blood levels of calcium will fall, thereby triggering increased release of parathyroid hormone; to prevent hyperparathyroidism, patients should receive supplemental calcium.

### Tiludronate

***Actions and Uses.*** Tiludronate [Skelid] is a new, oral biphosphonate approved for *Paget's disease of bone.* In patients with this disease, the drug decreases abnormal bone growth and, unlike etidronate, does so without interfering with bone mineralization. Like other bisphosphonates, tiludronate becomes incorporated into bone and then ingested by osteoclasts; as a result, it inhibits the osteoclasts, and thereby prevents further bone resorption.

***Pharmacokinetics.*** Tiludronate is administered by mouth and bioavailability is low (6%). Food further decreases absorption. About 90% of the drug in blood is bound to serum proteins (mainly albumin). Tiludronate is eliminated largely unchanged in the urine.

***Adverse Effects.*** The most common side effects are nausea (9.3%), diarrhea (9.3%), and dyspepsia (5.3%). These are usually mild and rarely require discontinuation of treatment. Other side effects include chest pain, edema, paresthesias, hyperparathyroidism, vomiting, and flatulence.

***Preparations, Dosage, and Administration.*** Tiludronate is dispensed in 200 mg tablets for oral administration. The dosage is 400 mg once a day for 3 months. Patients should be instructed to take tiludronate with a full glass of water. Furthermore, they should not eat for 2 hours before or after taking the drug. Since calcium, aspirin, and aluminum- or magnesium-containing antacids greatly reduce tiludronate absorption, these drugs should not be administered within 2 hours of administering tiludronate.

## Slow-Release Sodium Fluoride

Slow-release sodium fluoride [Slow Fluoride] is under investigation for use in osteoporosis. The drug promotes formation of new bone by stimulating proliferation of osteoblasts. When given to postmenopausal women in a clinical trial, the drug increased spinal bone mass by 4% to 6% a year for each of 4 years and significantly decreased the rate of new vertebral fractures. Dosing was done in repeated cycles, each consisting of sodium fluoride (25 mg twice daily) for 12 months followed by 2 months without sodium fluoride; calcium citrate (400 mg twice daily) was taken continuously. To ensure healthy bone growth, it is critical that fluoride levels remain within the therapeutic range: 95 to 195 ng/ml. If levels are too low, benefits are lost. More importantly, if levels are too high, fluoride causes formation of abnormal bone that fractures easily. Slow-release sodium fluoride is considerably safer than standard sodium fluoride preparations, which can cause formation of fragile bone (secondary to excessive drug levels) as well as GI bleeding. Nausea, which occurs in about 10% of patients, can be prevented by ingesting slow-release fluoride with crackers or bread.

### Drugs for Hypercalcemia

*Furosemide.* Furosemide, a loop diuretic, promotes renal excretion of calcium. This action is useful for treating hypercalcemic emergencies. In managing such emergencies, isotonic saline (IV) must be given prior to furosemide. The dosage of furosemide for adults is 80 to 100 mg every 1 to 2 hours as needed; the infusion rate must not exceed 4 mg/min. To avoid fluid and electrolyte imbalance, urinary losses must be measured and replaced. The basic pharmacology of furosemide is discussed in Chapter 38 (Diuretics).

*Glucocorticoids.* Glucocorticoids reduce intestinal absorption of calcium. This action can be useful in the treatment of hypercalcemia. For severe hypercalcemia, parenteral glucocorticoid therapy is indicated (e.g., 100 to 500 mg hydrocortisone sodium succinate IV daily). Since glucocorticoids can produce serious adverse effects when used on a chronic basis, the risks of long-term treatment must be carefully weighed against the benefits. The basic pharmacology of the glucocorticoids is discussed in Chapter 65 (Glucocorticoids in Nonendocrine Diseases).

*Inorganic Phosphates.* Phosphates lower plasma levels of calcium and, therefore, can be employed to treat hypercalcemia. Suggested mechanisms for reducing plasma calcium include (1) decreased bone resorption, (2) increased bone formation, and (3) decreased intestinal absorption of calcium (secondary to decreased renal activation of vitamin D). Intravenous use of phosphates is hazardous and limited to treatment of life-threatening hypercalcemia. Oral administration is considerably safer.

Oral phosphates are given to treat mild to moderate hypercalcemia. These agents should not be given to patients with impaired kidney function or elevated levels of serum phosphate. Oral phosphates should not be combined with antacids that contain aluminum, magnesium, or calcium; all of these elements bind phosphate and will therefore prevent its absorption. Initial treatment should provide 1 to 2 gm of phosphorus/day. Doses are reduced when serum calcium levels normalize.

*Edetate Disodium.* Edetate disodium (EDTA) is a chelating agent that binds calcium in the blood; this interaction rapidly reduces the plasma concentration of free calcium. The EDTA-calcium complex is filtered by the glomerulus but not reabsorbed by the kidney tubules; hence, renal excretion of calcium is increased. Although EDTA is highly effective at reducing hypercalcemia, this agent is also very toxic: EDTA can cause profound hypocalcemia, resulting in tetany, convulsions, dysrhythmias, and death. Severe nephrotoxicity can also occur. Because of its toxicity, EDTA is used only for life-threatening hypercalcemic crisis. The usual adult dose is 40 mg/kg infused over 4 to 6 hours. The total daily dose must not exceed 3 gm.

*Plicamycin.* Plicamycin [Mithracin] is a cytotoxic antibiotic produced by several species of *Streptomyces*. Although used primarily for testicular cancer, plicamycin is also indicated for hypercalcemia. Plicamycin lowers plasma calcium levels by acting directly on bone to prevent calcium resorption. For management of hypercalcemia, relatively low doses are employed (e.g., 25 μg/kg/day for 3 to 4 days). Calcium-lowering effects may be visible within 1 to 2 days, and may persist for several days to 3 or more weeks. Plicamycin lowers platelet counts and reduces lev-

els of several clotting factors; both actions result in bleeding tendencies.

*Gallium Nitrate.* Gallium nitrate [Ganite] is used to treat hypercalcemia of malignancy. In addition, the drug is under investigation for use in Paget's disease of bone and postmenopausal osteoporosis. Gallium reduces calcium levels by preventing bone resorption; it may also increase bone formation. Gallium is highly nephrotoxic and must not be used with other nephrotoxic drugs, such as amphotericin B and the aminoglycosides. To minimize kidney damage, the patient must be hydrated with intravenous fluids before treatment. Renal function must be monitored. The usual single dose is 100 to 200 mg/M$^2$. This dose is diluted in 1 L of 5% dextrose or 0.9% sodium chloride and infused over 24 hours. The dose is repeated daily for 5 days.

*Bisphosphonates.* Pamidronate and etidronate are used for hypercalcemia of malignancy. The mechanism is suppression of bone resorption by osteoclasts. Use of pamidronate for hypercalcemia of malignancy is discussed above.

# Osteoporosis

## General Considerations

Osteoporosis is a serious medical problem characterized by low bone mass and increased bone fragility. Because of bone fragility, patients are susceptible to fractures from minor traumatic events, such as coughing, rolling over in bed, or falling from a standing position. In the United States, osteoporosis affects about 28 million people, most of them women, and leads to 1.5 million fractures each year. The most common fracture sites are the vertebrae, forearm (distal radius), and hip (femoral neck). Vertebral fractures can result in loss of height, spinal deformity, chronic back pain, and impaired breathing. Complications from hip fractures are a significant cause of mortality: of the 300,000 Americans who get hip fractures each year, about 50,000 die from complications. The cost of osteoporosis is high: in the United States, we spend about $10 billion a year to treat osteoporosis-related injury.

### Bone Mass

In men and women, bone mass changes across the life span. Bone mass peaks in the third decade, remains stable to age 50, and then slowly declines—at a rate that is usually less than 1% a year. In addition to this slow, aging-related decline, women go through a phase of *accelerated* bone loss (2% to 3% a year) that begins after menopause and continues for several years. In both the slow and accelerated phases of decline, bone is lost because resorption of old bone outpaces deposition of new bone.

### Primary Prevention: Calcium, Vitamin D, and Lifestyle

The risk of osteoporosis can be reduced by lifelong implementation of measures that can help maximize bone strength. Specifically, we need to (1) ensure a sufficiency of calcium and vitamin D and (2) adopt a lifestyle that promotes bone health. Calcium is needed to maximize bone growth early in life and to maintain bone integrity later in life. Vitamin D is needed to ensure calcium absorption. The amount of calcium needed for optimal bone health is indicated in Table 75-1. Note that, late in life, both men and women should take in 1200 mg of calcium daily. If the diet cannot provide this amount, supplements should be employed. Current recommendations for daily vitamin D intake are 200 IU prior to age 51, 400 IU from age 51 through age 70, and 600 IU thereafter. Lifestyle measures that promote bone health are

* Performing regular weight-bearing exercise (walking, jogging, dancing, racquet sports, team sports, stair climbing)
* Avoiding excessive alcohol
* Avoiding smoking

### Diagnosis and Monitoring

Osteoporosis is diagnosed by measuring bone mineral density (BMD), an important predictor of fracture risk. The technique used most often to measure BMD is called *dual-energy X-ray absorptiometry* (DEXA). Results of DEXA scans are reported in terms of *standard deviations* (SD) below mean BMD values in young adults. A BMD value that is 1 SD below the mean indicates 10% bone loss, a value that is 2 SD below the mean indicates 20% bone loss, and so forth. Using this system, the World Health Organization has defined *normal* BMD for women as being no more than 1 SD below the mean for young adults. BMD values between 1 SD below the mean and 2.5 SD below the mean define *osteopenia* (low bone mass). BMD values 2.5 SD below the mean or greater define *osteoporosis*.

Although we use BMD values to diagnose osteoporosis, it is important to note that low BMD is not the only predictor of fractures. Other important predictors are (1) a family history of osteoporotic fractures, (2) a personal history of fractures, and (3) a propensity to fall (e.g., because of Parkinsonism). Accordingly, if BMD is 2.3 SD below the mean (indicating osteopenia rather than osteoporosis), but the patient has a propensity to fall, then the patient may be at higher risk for fractures than an individual with a BMD 2.5 SD below the mean (indicating osteoporosis) but with no propensity to fall.

Although loss of bone at one site (e.g., forearm) can predict the risk of fractures at other sites (e.g., hip, spine), it is preferable to measure BMD at specific sites to predict specific risks. Accordingly, a thorough evaluation would include BMD measurements in the forearm, vertebrae, and femoral neck—the sites at which osteoporotic fractures occur most often.

Measurement of BMD is employed to monitor treatment as well as for diagnosis. If BMD stabilizes or increases, we can consider treatment a success. Conversely, if BMD continues to decline, treatment failure is indicated.

## Treating Osteoporosis in Women

The objective of treatment is to reduce fractures. To do this, we need to maintain or increase bone strength. In theory, two types of drugs can used for treatment: (1)

agents that decrease bone resorption and (2) agents that promote bone formation. Currently, the antiresorptive drugs—estrogen, bisphosphonates, and calcitonin—are the mainstays of treatment. Only one bone-forming drug—slow-release sodium fluoride—is available, and it has not been approved for routine use. Accordingly, since the primary treatment option is suppression of bone resorption (rather than promotion of bone formation), currently available drugs are most effective when given early to prevent bone from being lost. At this time, our ability to rebuild bone that has already been lost is very limited.

### Antiresorptive Therapy

Bone resorption can be reduced with estrogen, bisphosphonates (e.g., alendronate), and calcitonin, all of which inhibit osteoclasts. These antiresorptive agents can retard bone loss, but are largely unable to reverse loss that has already occurred. When these agents are used, bone density may increase slightly during the first year or two, but then levels off. With all antiresorptive drugs, success requires a sufficiency of calcium and vitamin D.

*Estrogen.* The basic pharmacology of estrogen as well as postmenopausal estrogen replacement therapy are discussed at length in Chapter 57 (Estrogens and Progestins). Discussion here focuses on the role of estrogen in osteoporosis.

Estrogen acts indirectly to suppress osteoclast proliferation, and thereby maintains a brake on bone resorption. Consequently, when estrogen levels decline, either because of natural menopause or surgical removal of the ovaries, osteoclasts increase in number, causing bone resorption to increase dramatically. Estrogen replacement therapy restores the brake on osteoclast proliferation, and thereby suppresses bone resorption.

Estrogen is the drug of choice for preventing and treating bone loss following menopause or surgical removal of the ovaries. Estrogen replacement decreases the risk of hip fractures by 50% and vertebral fractures by 70%. In addition, estrogen greatly decreases the risk of coronary artery disease, the major killer of postmenopausal women. Estrogen replacement therapy is most effective when initiated immediately after menopause. However, treatment begun at age 60 and even later can still offer significant protection. Since discontinuing estrogen will trigger a period of accelerated bone loss, estrogen therapy should continue late into life. Because of its well-established benefits, estrogen replacement therapy should be considered by all postmenopausal women—with the exception of women who have conditions that contraindicate estrogen use (e.g., breast cancer, endometrial cancer, thromboembolic disorders, undiagnosed abnormal uterine bleeding).

For replacement therapy, the usual estrogen dosage is 0.625 mg/day of conjugated equine estrogens [Premarin] or its equivalent. As discussed in Chapter 57, women with an intact uterus should also receive a progestin (e.g., medroxyprogesterone acetate) in order to minimize the risk of endometrial cancer. For women without a uterus, the progestin is unnecessary.

*Bisphosphonates: Alendronate.* At this time, alendronate [Fosamax] is the only biphosphonate approved for osteoporosis. The drug is safe and prevents fractures. Alendronate was approved initially only for *treating* existing osteoporosis, and was later approved for osteoporosis *prevention* as well. In both cases, benefits derive from inhibiting bone resorption by osteoclasts. To be effective, alendronate must be used in combination with adequate intake of calcium and vitamin D. The basic pharmacology of alendronate is discussed above.

When used to *treat* osteoporosis in postmenopausal women (average age 65), alendronate produced a modest increase in BMD in the spine and hip. More importantly, treatment decreased the rate of new fractures: compared with patients taking placebo, those taking alendronate experienced 51% fewer fractures of the hip, 47% fewer fractures of the spine, and 48% fewer fractures of the wrist. Furthermore, when spinal fractures did occur, loss of height was less than in women who had spinal fractures while taking placebo. The dosage for treatment of osteoporosis is 10 mg/day.

When given to *prevent* osteoporosis in postmenopausal women (ages 44 to 50), alendronate produced a small increase in BMD of the spine and hip. In contrast, women taking placebo *lost* BMD at those sites. The positive response to alendronate was basically the same as the response to estrogen. Currently, alendronate is the only alternative to estrogen for preventive therapy. However, since estrogen decreases the risk of cardiovascular disease, in addition to preventing osteoporosis, estrogen is still the preferred agent—except for women with conditions that contraindicate estrogen use. The dosage for prevention of osteoporosis is 5 mg/day—half the dosage used for treating osteoporosis.

***Calcitonin-Salmon Nasal Spray.*** Intranasal salmon calcitonin [Miacalcin] is used to treat established osteoporosis, but not to prevent osteoporosis. Benefits derive from inhibiting osteoclastic bone resorption. By doing so, the drug decreases bone loss and the risk of fractures. In women ages 68 to 72, two years of treatment with calcitonin increased BMD in the spine by 3%. In contrast, spinal BMD decreased by 1% in women taking placebo. In younger postmenopausal women (mean age 53), calcitonin increased average BMD by 2%, whereas average BMD decreased by 7% in women taking placebo. Not only is calcitonin moderately effective, it is very safe: the drug has been used for over 20 years with no long-term adverse effects. For management of osteoporosis, the dosage is one spray (200 IU) a day, alternating nostrils daily. The basic pharmacology of calcitonin is discussed above.

### Bone-Forming Therapy: Slow-Release Sodium Fluoride

Slow-release sodium fluoride [Slow Fluoride] is the only drug currently available for promoting bone growth, although it is not approved for this use. Unlike antiresorptive drugs, which act by suppressing bone resorption by osteoclasts, fluoride actively promotes bone growth by stimulating proliferation of osteoblasts. Fluoride treatment in postmenopausal women has increased vertebral mass by an average of 5% a year and significantly decreased the incidence of new vertebral fractures. Since excessive flu-

oride can increase bone fragility, dosing must be carefully controlled. The basic pharmacology of fluoride is discussed above.

## Treating Osteoporosis in Men

In the United States, about 2 million men have aging-related osteoporosis, and another 3 million are at risk. One of every 4 hip fractures occurs in men, as does 1 of every 3 spinal fractures. Although these rates are substantial, they are clearly much lower than rates in women. As noted above, bone mass in men peaks in the third decade, and begins progressive decline around age 50. The rate of decline in men is about equal to that in women, except for the accelerated phase of decline that occurs in women immediately after menopause. If men and women lose bone mass at similar rates, why do men experience less osteoporosis? The main reason is that bones in men, at their peak, are larger and stronger than bones in women. Hence, once decline begins, male bones can tolerate more loss than female bones before fractures are likely to occur. Factors that contribute to the risk of osteoporosis in men include low testosterone, use of glucocorticoids, white race, calcium deficiency, vitamin D deficiency, smoking, excessive alcohol consumption, and insufficient exercise.

Treatment of male osteoporosis is confounded by a lack of research. (Osteoporosis is one of the few areas of therapeutics in which research in women has greatly exceeded research in men.) Nonetheless, with the exception of estrogen, we can assume that the drugs used for osteoporosis in women will also be effective in men (although none are FDA approved for use in men). Accordingly, to decrease bone resorption, we could use either calcitonin or a bisphosphonate. To promote bone formation, we could employ slow-release sodium fluoride. In addition, if the patient is testosterone deficient, testosterone-replacement therapy would be appropriate, unless the patient has a disorder that contraindicates testosterone use (e.g., testicular cancer).

## KEY POINTS

* Calcium is critical to the function of the skeletal, nervous, muscular, and cardiovascular systems.
* More than 98% of calcium in the body is present in bone.
* Bone undergoes continuous remodeling, a process in which osteoclasts resorb old bone and then osteoblasts deposit new bone.
* The body maintains calcium levels by adjusting the rates of calcium resorption from bone, calcium absorption from the intestine, and calcium excretion by the kidney. These processes are regulated by parathyroid hormone, vitamin D, and calcitonin.
* Parathyroid hormone (PTH) elevates serum calcium by promoting resorption of calcium from bone, enhancing renal tubular resorption of calcium, and activating vitamin D, which then promotes absorption of calcium from the intestine.
* Like PTH, vitamin D increases serum calcium by increasing calcium resorption from bone, decreasing cal-

cium excretion by the kidney, and increasing calcium absorption from the intestine.

- Calcitonin lowers calcium levels by inhibiting calcium resorption from bone and increasing calcium excretion by the kidney.
- The various calcium salts used for therapy differ widely in their percentage of calcium.
- Of the oral calcium salts in use, calcium carbonate contains the most calcium per unit weight.
- Chewable calcium tablets are preferred to standard tablets because their bioavailability is more consistent.
- Glucocorticoids (e.g., prednisone) reduce absorption of oral calcium.
- Vitamin D is obtained through the diet and by exposure to sunlight.
- Vitamin D deficiency causes rickets in children and osteomalacia in adults.
- Calcitonin-salmon has the same metabolic effects as human calcitonin but has a longer half-life and greater milligram potency.
- Calcitonin-salmon is used primarily for osteoporosis. Benefits derive from inhibiting bone resorption by osteoclasts.
- Calcitonin-salmon is very safe.
- Alendronate, our prototype for the bisphosphonates, is used for prevention and treatment of osteoporosis and for treatment of Paget's disease of bone.
- Alendronate suppresses bone resorption by decreasing both the number and activity of osteoclasts.
- Bioavailability of alendronate is very low in the absence of food, and essentially zero in the presence of food. Accordingly, nothing should be eaten for at least 30 minutes after taking the drug.
- Alendronate can cause severe esophagitis if it stays in contact with the esophageal mucosa. Accordingly, patients should take the drug with a full glass of water and then remain upright for at least 30 minutes, and at least until completing their first meal of the day.
- Sodium fluoride promotes formation of new bone by stimulating proliferation of osteoblasts.
- Excessive sodium fluoride promotes formation of abnormal bone that is fragile and hence easily fractured.
- Osteoporosis is characterized by low bone mass and increased bone fragility, which renders patients vulnerable to fractures from minor trauma.
- The most common sites of osteoporotic fractures are the vertebrae, forearm (distal radius), and hip (femoral neck).

- Osteoporosis occurs mainly in the elderly. Why? Because after age 50, men and women experience aging-related bone loss that is slow but relentless. In addition, women experience several years of accelerated bone loss following menopause. In both cases, bone is lost because bone resorption by osteoclasts outpaces bone deposition by osteoblasts.
- To maximize bone strength, and thereby minimize the risk of osteoporosis, we all need to (1) ensure lifelong sufficiency of calcium and vitamin D and (2) adopt lifestyle measures that promote bone health (regular weight-bearing exercise and avoidance of smoking and excessive alcohol).
- Osteoporosis is diagnosed by measuring bone mineral density (BMD), which is done most commonly using dual-energy x-ray absorptiometry.
- The World Health Organization's diagnostic criterion for osteoporosis is BMD that is more than 2.5 standard deviations below the mean BMD for young adults.
- The objective of osteoporosis therapy is to reduce fractures.
- With currently available drugs, we are more able to prevent bone loss (using antiresorptive agents) than to rebuild bone that is already gone (using bone-forming agents).
- Antiresorptive drugs—estrogen, bisphosphonates (e.g., alendronate), and calcitonin—decrease bone loss by inhibiting the activity of osteoclasts.
- Because estrogen decreases the risk of osteoporosis *and* cardiovascular disease, it is considered the drug of choice for preventing and treating bone loss following menopause or surgical removal of the ovaries—except, of course, in women with conditions that contraindicate estrogen use (e.g., breast cancer).
- To be most effective, estrogen replacement therapy should begin soon after menopause and should continue late into life.
- In women with an intact uterus, estrogen replacement should be combined with a progestin so as to decrease the risk of endometrial cancer. A progestin is unnecessary if the uterus has been removed.
- For women who cannot, will not, or should not use estrogen to prevent or treat osteoporosis, alendronate is a good alternative.
- Calcitonin is perhaps the safest drug for osteoporosis, but is not as effective as estrogen or alendronate.
- Slow-release sodium fluoride can rebuild bone in people with osteoporosis, but is not yet approved for this use.

# Summary of Major Nursing Implications*

## Vitamin D

### Preadministration Assessment

#### Therapeutic Goal

Treatment of rickets, osteomalacia, and hypoparathyroidism.

### Baseline Data

The physician may order serum levels of vitamin D, calcium, phosphorus, and alkaline phosphatase as well as a 24-hour urinary calcium determination.

Assess dietary vitamin D and calcium content.

### Identifying High-Risk Patients

Vitamin D is *contraindicated* in the presence of *hypercalcemia*, *hypervitaminosis D*, and *malabsorption syndrome*. Exercise *caution* in patients taking *digoxin*.

*Patient education information is highlighted in color.

## Implementation: Administration

### Routes
Oral, IM.

### Administration
Instruct the patient to swallow oral preparations intact, without crushing or chewing.

Therapeutic responses to vitamin D require adequate calcium intake. Assess dietary calcium content and adjust to ensure calcium sufficiency.

## Ongoing Evaluation and Interventions

### Monitoring Summary
Monitor serum calcium, serum phosphorus, and urinary calcium.

### Minimizing Adverse Interactions
**Digoxin.** Vitamin D–induced hypercalcemia can cause dysrhythmias in patients taking digoxin. Monitor serum calcium and make certain it remains normal.

### Management of Toxicity
Large therapeutic doses may cause hypervitaminosis D, a syndrome characterized by hypercalcemia, hypercalciuria, decalcification of bone, and deposition of calcium in soft tissues. Monitor serum calcium content; levels should stay below 10 mg/dl. Monitor serum phosphorus and urinary calcium as well. If vitamin D toxicity develops, have the patient discontinue vitamin D immediately, increase fluid intake, and institute a low-calcium diet. In severe cases, calcium excretion can be accelerated with IV saline plus furosemide.

## Oral Calcium Salts

Calcium Acetate      Calcium Gluconate
Calcium Carbonate     Calcium Lactate
Calcium Citrate     Dibasic Calcium Phosphate
Calcium Glubionate

## Preadministration Assessment

### Therapeutic Goal
Treatment of mild hypocalcemia and supplementation of dietary calcium.

### Baseline Data
Obtain a serum calcium level.

### Identifying High-Risk Patients
Calcium salts are *contraindicated* for patients with *hypercalcemia*, *renal calculi*, and *hypophosphatemia*.

## Implementation: Administration

### Route
Oral.

### Dosage
Individual calcium salts differ from one another as to their percentage of elemental calcium. As a result, the dose required to provide a specific amount of calcium differs between the salts. Make certain that the patient does not switch arbitrarily to a different preparation.

### Administration
Advise the patient to take oral calcium salts with a large glass of water; administration with or after meals promotes absorption. Advise the patient to avoid foods that can suppress calcium absorption (e.g., spinach, Swiss chard, beets, bran, whole grain cereals).

## Ongoing Evaluation and Interventions

### Minimizing Adverse Effects
Prolonged therapy can cause hypercalcemia. Inform patients about signs of hypercalcemia (nausea, vomiting, constipation, frequent urination, lethargy, depression), and instruct them to notify the physician if these occur. Hypercalcemia can be minimized with frequent monitoring of serum calcium.

### Minimizing Adverse Interactions
**Glucocorticoids.** These drugs reduce calcium absorption; increased calcium dosage may be required.

**Tetracyclines.** Calcium binds to tetracyclines, thereby reducing tetracycline absorption. Instruct the patient to separate administration of tetracyclines and calcium by at least 1 hour.

**Thiazide Diuretics.** Thiazides decrease renal excretion of calcium. A reduction in calcium dosage may be needed to avoid hypercalcemia.

## Parenteral Calcium Salts

Calcium Chloride
Calcium Gluconate
Calcium Gluceptate

## Preadministration Assessment

### Therapeutic Goal
Reversal of clinical manifestations of hypocalcemia.

### Baseline Data
Assess for signs and symptoms of hypocalcemia (tetany, convulsions, laryngospasm, and spasm of other muscles). Obtain measurement of serum calcium.

### Identifying High-Risk Patients
Parenteral calcium is *contraindicated* for patients with *hypercalcemia* and *ventricular fibrillation*. Use with *extreme caution* in patients taking *digoxin*.

## Implementation: Administration

### Routes
IM, IV. *All* parenteral calcium salts may be given IV; only *calcium gluceptate* should be given IM.

### Administration
Warm solutions to body temperature prior to infusion or IM injection. Perform IV injections slowly (0.5 to 2 ml/min).

Drugs that contain phosphate, carbonate, sulfate, and tartrate groups can precipitate calcium; do not mix these drugs with parenteral calcium solutions.

*Calcium chloride* may cause necrosis and sloughing if solutions become extravasated. Monitor the infusion closely.

## Ongoing Evaluation and Interventions

### Evaluating Therapeutic Effects
Evaluate the patient for reductions in tetany, muscle spasm, laryngospasm, paresthesias, and other symptoms of severe hypocalcemia.

### Minimizing Adverse Effects
*Hypercalcemia.* Overdose can produce acute hypercalcemia, resulting in nausea, vomiting, weakness, lethargy, coma, and possibly death. Avoid hypercalcemia through careful control of dosage.

### Minimizing Adverse Interactions
*Digoxin.* Parenteral calcium may cause severe bradycardia in patients taking digoxin. Infuse calcium slowly and cautiously in these patients.

## Calcitonin-Salmon

## Preadministration Assessment

### Therapeutic Goal
Treatment of postmenopausal osteoporosis, Paget's disease of bone, and hypercalcemia.

### Baseline Data
The physician may order measurements of serum alkaline phosphatase, calcium, and phosphorus, as well as a 24-hour urinary hydroxyproline.

### Identifying High-Risk Patients
Salmon calcitonin is *contraindicated* for patients *allergic to this preparation.*

## Implementation: Administration

### Routes
*Intranasal.* For osteoporosis only.

*Parenteral (IM, SC).* For osteoporosis, Paget's disease, and hypercalcemia.

### Administration
*Intranasal.* Instruct patients to activate the metered-dose pump by holding the bottle upright and depressing the two white sidearms toward the bottle six times, which should produce a faint initial spray. The drug is then administered by placing the nozzle in the nostril and depressing the pump handle.

*Subcutaneous.* Teach patients how to inject calcitonin SC, and instruct them to rotate sites of injection.

## Ongoing Evaluation and Interventions

### Evaluating Therapeutic Effects
*Postmenopausal Osteoporosis.* Measurement of BMD should indicate retardation of bone loss (or perhaps a small increase in BMD).

*Paget's Disease of Bone.* Monitor for reductions in bone pain, serum alkaline phosphatase levels, and 24-hour urinary hydroxyproline value.

*Hypercalcemia.* Monitor for reductions in serum calcium and phosphorus levels.

## Alendronate (A Bisphosphonate)

## Preadministration Assessment

### Therapeutic Goals
Alendronate is taken to prevent or treat postmenopausal osteoporosis and to treat Paget's disease of bone.

### Baseline Data
*Postmenopausal Osteoporosis.* Obtain baseline values for bone mineral density (BMD) in the hip, vertebrae, and forearm.

*Paget's Disease.* Obtain a baseline value for serum alkaline phosphatase.

### Identifying High-Risk Patients
Alendronate is *contraindicated* for patients with *esophageal disorders that can impede swallowing* and for patients who *cannot sit or stand for at least 30 minutes.*

## Implementation: Administration

### Route
Oral.

### Administration
Proper administration is needed to maximize absorption and minimize the risk of esophagitis. Accordingly, you should instruct patients to

- Take alendronate in the morning before breakfast
- Take alendronate with a full glass of water

- Avoid chewing or sucking the tablet
- Remain upright (seated or standing) for at least 30 minutes and at least until completing breakfast
- Postpone eating anything, including orange juice or coffee, for at least 30 minutes after taking the drug

## Ongoing Evaluation and Interventions

### Evaluating Therapeutic Effects

*Postmenopausal Osteoporosis.* Obtain periodic determinations of BMD. If BMD increases, or at least remains constant, treatment is a success. Conversely, a significant decline in BMD indicates failure.

*Paget's Disease.* Obtain periodic measurements of serum alkaline phosphatase. A decline indicates that alendronate is working.

### Minimizing Adverse Effects

*Esophagitis.* Alendronate can cause severe esophagitis, sometimes resulting in ulceration. To minimize the risk, instruct patients to (1) administer the drug in accord with the guidelines described above, (2) avoid lying down after taking the drug, and (3) discontinue the drug and contact the physician if they experience symptoms of esophageal injury (difficulty swallowing, pain upon swallowing, or new or worsening heartburn). Avoid alendronate in patients with esophageal disorders that could impede swallowing and in patients who are unable to sit or stand for 30 minutes.

## Estrogen

Nursing implications for estrogen are summarized in Chapter 57.

# CHAPTER 76

# Enteral and Parenteral Nutrition

**Enteral Nutritional Therapy**
　Modes of Delivery
　Components of an Enteral Nutritional Regimen
　Complications of Treatment

**Parenteral Nutritional Therapy**
　Routes of Administration
　Components of a Parenteral Nutritional Regimen
　Preparation of Parenteral Nutrient Solutions
　Monitoring Treatment
　Complications of Treatment

Good nutrition is required to maintain health and permit healing at times of illness. As a rule, required nutrients—amino acids, carbohydrates, fats, vitamins, and minerals—can be obtained simply by ingestion of appropriate foods. However, this is not always the case; circumstances frequently arise in which nutritional needs cannot be fulfilled by eating. Under these conditions, nutritional support is required. Specific indications for nutritional support include (1) malnutrition; (2) coma; (3) bowel obstruction; (4) cancer chemotherapy (because of associated nausea and vomiting); and (5) trauma, major burns, and severe infection (because these disorders cause a hypermetabolic state). Nutritional support is also given to permit bowel rest for patients with inflammatory bowel disease and for those recovering from bowel surgery.

There are two major categories of nutritional support: *enteral* (via the gastrointestinal tract) and *parenteral* (intravenous). *Enteral* nutritional therapy is indicated for (1) patients who have a healthy digestive tract but are unable or unwilling to eat sufficient food, and (2) patients who have a digestive or absorptive disorder that cannot be overcome by diet modification. *Parenteral* nutritional support is indicated when nutrition cannot be maintained by eating or by enteral therapy.

## Enteral Nutritional Therapy

Enteral nutritional therapy is defined formally as provision of nutrients by way of the gastrointestinal tract. However, in everyday practice, enteral nutrition is taken to mean feeding by tube. In the discussion below, we will limit consideration to tube feeding.

Enteral therapy is indicated for two groups of patients: (1) those with a healthy digestive tract but who cannot or will not ingest sufficient food (e.g., anorectic patients, patients with an impaired ability to chew or swallow), and

(2) those with a digestive or absorptive disorder that cannot be compensated for by modification of diet. Depending on patient status, enteral therapy may be used as a supplement to oral feeding or to meet all nutritional needs. Contraindications to enteral therapy include total bowel obstruction, uncontrollable vomiting, paralytic ileus, and severe malabsorption.

## Modes of Delivery

### Tube Placement

For *short-term* therapy, a *nasogastric* tube is commonly used. When intragastric administration is contraindicated (e.g, poor gastric motility, no gag reflex) or when the risk of aspiration is high, a *nasoduodenal* or *nasojejunal* tube may be employed.

For *long-term* therapy (more than 1 to 3 months), feeding tubes may be surgically implanted directly into the esophagus, stomach, or jejunum.

### Schedule of Administration

Enteral nutritional support may be administered by four schedules: continuous infusion, cyclic infusion, intermittent infusion, and bolus administration. With *continuous infusion*, the total daily feeding is delivered at a constant rate over 24 hours. With *cyclic infusion*, the total daily feeding is delivered at a constant rate over several hours (rather than over 24 hours). With *intermittent infusion*, the total daily feeding is divided into three to six separate feedings that last 30 to 60 minutes each. *Bolus administration* is like intermittent infusion, except that the individual feedings last only a few minutes, rather than 30 to 60 minutes.

### Method of Administration

Enteral nutrition may be administered (1) by syringe, (2) by gravity using a drip chamber, and (3) by enteral pump. Use of a *syringe*, which is the least expensive method of delivery, is appropriate only for bolus administration or for short infusions. *Gravity feeding with a drip chamber* costs somewhat more than syringe administration, but is clearly easier for infusions that last for 30 minutes or more. When a drip chamber is employed, the rate of delivery must be adjusted manually when the patient changes position (e.g., sits up, stands, lies down). Use of an *enteral infusion pump* is the most expensive form of administration, but is also the most consistent. Furthermore, for administering infusion solutions that are too viscous to flow by gravity, a pump is the only instrument that will work.

## Components of an Enteral Nutritional Regimen

*Amino Acids.* All patients require an adequate supply of amino acids in order to conserve or rebuild lean body mass. Enteral solutions provide amino acids in various forms: intact proteins, hydrolyzed proteins, and free amino acids.

Specialized products are available to meet the unique amino acid needs of patients with renal failure, severe hepatic dysfunction, and other disorders. However, since proof of benefits for these formulas is generally lacking, their use is controversial.

*Carbohydrates.* Carbohydrates—in the form of dextrose, sucrose, lactose, starch, dextrin, and glucose oligosaccharides—are the primary source of calories in most enteral regimens. The simple sugars (dextrose, sucrose, and lactose) are absorbed more readily than complex carbohydrates (e.g., dextrin, starch). Hence, for patients with limited absorptive capacity, the simple sugars may be preferred. Because of their high osmolality, simple sugars can retain water in the intestinal lumen and can thereby promote diarrhea. Lactose intolerance (an inability to digest and absorb lactose) is common. Accordingly, most formulations in use today are lactose free.

*Fat.* Fats serve as a source of calories and are required to prevent and correct essential fatty acid deficiency. Most enteral formulations contain a high percentage of fat (in the form of polyunsaturated fats). However, the fat content of some formulas is quite low. The fats employed most frequently are corn oil, soybean oil, and safflower oil.

*Other Components.* Enteral formulations should provide required *electrolytes*, *vitamins*, and *trace elements*. As a rule, enteral fluids do not contain sufficient water to maintain adequate hydration; hence, supplemental water is often needed. Many oral formulations contain flavoring agents; the patient should be consulted regarding taste preference.

## Complications of Treatment

The most dangerous complication of enteral therapy is *aspiration pneumonitis*, a condition that can be fatal. To reduce the risk of aspiration, the upper body should be elevated (by raising the head of the bed to a 30-degree angle) during the infusion and for at least 1 hour after. High-risk patients (e.g., those prone to vomiting and those who lack a gag reflex) must not be given bolus feeding. For these people, feeding should be done by slow drip, and then only if the tip of the feeding tube has been placed into the duodenum or jejunum. If these tube placements are not possible, enteral therapy should be replaced with parenteral nutritional support.

About 10% of patients who are fed through a nasogastric tube experience adverse effects (e.g., diarrhea, vomiting, insufficient gastric emptying, gastrointestinal bleeding). These can be minimized by initiating therapy at a slow rate using a dilute nutrient solution. As the patient adjusts to therapy, the infusion rate and nutrient concentration can be increased.

Enteral therapy may be associated with metabolic disturbances (e.g., hyperglycemia, fluid and electrolyte imbalance, fatty acid deficiency). Monitoring serum glucose and electrolyte levels will help minimize metabolic disorders.

# Parenteral Nutritional Therapy

## Routes of Administration

Parenteral nutritional therapy may be administered through a *peripheral* vein or through a *central venous catheter* (which delivers nutrient solution directly into the superior vena cava). Peripheral infusion is indicated only for *short-term therapy* with relatively *dilute* nutrient solutions. If therapy is to be *prolonged* (i.e., lasting more than 10 to 12 days) or if *strongly hypertonic* solutions are to be given, central administration is required.

## Components of a Parenteral Nutritional Regimen

The core component of a parenteral nutritional regimen is a mixture of amino acids. Dextrose, fats, vitamins, and minerals are added as required.

### Amino Acids

*Nutritional Role.* Amino acids serve two purposes: (1) they foster conservation of existing lean body mass and (2) they promote wound healing and restoration of lean body mass. For healthy adults, the recommended dietary allowance (RDA) for amino acids is 0.9 gm/kg. The RDA for healthy infants and children ranges from 1.4 to 2.2 gm/kg. RDA values increase significantly in patients with malnutrition, trauma, burns, or infection.

*Complications of Therapy.* Blood urea nitrogen (BUN) may rise to dangerous levels, especially in patients with kidney dysfunction. If elevation of BUN exceeds normal limits, amino acid administration should be re-evaluated. In patients with liver disease, amino acid infusion may result in hepatic coma due to accumulation of nitrogenous compounds. Caution must be exercised in patients with cirrhosis, viral hepatitis, or cancer involving the liver.

**Formulations.** Amino acid solutions are available in general and specialized formulations. The general formulations consist of essential and nonessential amino acids; total amino acid concentrations range from 3.0% to 11.4%. Some mixtures also contain electrolytes. The general formulations will satisfy the nutritional requirements of most patients. Specialized products have been formulated to meet the unique needs of certain patients—specifically, patients in a state of high metabolic stress and patients experiencing liver failure or severe renal impairment. Special formulations are also available for pediatric patients.

**Administration.** The route of administration depends upon the amino acid concentration. Solutions whose amino acid content exceeds 4% are very hypertonic and, as a result, will cause phlebitis if administered peripherally. Accordingly, these concentrated solutions must be administered through a central venous catheter. Solutions composed of less than 4% amino acids may be administered peripherally.

### Dextrose

**Nutritional Role.** In order to utilize amino acids for conservation and synthesis of protein, the body requires a source of nonprotein calories. Dextrose (*D*-glucose) can provide these calories. For the average adult, daily requirements range from 25 to 35 kcal/kg, including those from protein.

**Complications of Therapy.** *Glucose intolerance* (hyperglycemia, glycosuria, osmotic diuresis) can occur. This response is most likely during the first few days of treatment. Glucose intolerance can be minimized by initiating therapy with low doses, followed by gradual dosage elevation. This progressive dosing permits the body to produce the extra amounts of insulin needed to process the abnormal glucose load. Glucose content of blood and urine should be measured every 6 hours until glucose tolerance has been demonstrated (usually within 2 to 3 days). If tolerance fails to develop, insulin can be added to the infusion mixture to control hyperglycemia. This IV insulin can be supplemented with subcutaneous insulin as needed. Special care must be exercised with the diabetic patient.

Hypertonic solutions of dextrose may cause *thrombosis* if administered via a peripheral vein. Consequently, solutions in excess of 10% dextrose should be infused via a central venous catheter.

Since insulin levels are elevated during dextrose therapy, and since insulin promotes cellular uptake of potassium, infusion of dextrose may be accompanied by *hypokalemia*. Hypokalemia can be avoided by monitoring plasma potassium content and administering potassium as required.

If dextrose is abruptly discontinued, *hypoglycemia* may develop (because of continued release of endogenous insulin). Accordingly, dextrose should be withdrawn slowly: when infusion of hypertonic dextrose is stopped, infusion of 10% dextrose should be instituted and maintained for 1 to 2 hours.

**Administration.** Depending on their concentrations, dextrose solutions may be administered through a peripheral vein or centrally. Hypertonic solutions (i.e., solutions containing more than 10% dextrose) can be administered safely only through a central venous catheter. More dilute solutions may be given by peripheral infusion. Dextrose solutions may be mixed with amino acid solutions prior to administration.

### Fat

**Nutritional Role.** Intravenous fat emulsions can serve two functions: (1) they can prevent or reverse essential fatty acid deficiency (EFAD) and (2) they can serve as a source of nonprotein calories. When the objective of treatment is avoidance or reversal of EFAD, fat emulsions are given in relatively small amounts (3% to 8% of total caloric intake). Much larger doses (up to 60% of total caloric intake) are used when fats are intended as a source of energy. When fats are administered for their caloric content, dextrose dosage must be reduced to keep total caloric intake constant.

Most fat emulsions are prepared from soybean oil. The principal components of these emulsions are linoleic, oleic, palmitic, linolenic, and stearic acids.

**Complications of Therapy.** Although fat emulsions are generally very safe, *death has occurred following administration to preterm infants*. Autopsy findings indicate fat accumulation within the blood vessels of the lungs. Intravenous fats should be administered slowly to preterm infants, and then only if the potential benefits clearly outweigh the risks.

The most common adverse effect of fat infusion is *hyperlipidemia*. This is especially likely in patients whose capacity to metabolize fats is impaired. Hyperlipidemia may also occur in patients with normal fat-metabolizing capacity if administration is too rapid or if too much dextrose is administered concurrently. Blood should be monitored for fat content to ensure that lipemia clears between infusions.

**Administration.** Fat emulsions are isotonic with plasma, and therefore may be administered safely through a peripheral vein. Central administration may be performed as well. Some preparations may be mixed with amino acid and dextrose solutions. Others must be administered separately. Fat emulsions may be infused in the same vein as dextrose–amino acid solutions. When this is done, the Y-connector through which the fat will flow should be placed *below* any in-line filter that may be present. This placement is needed because particles in fat emulsions are too large to pass through bacterial and particulate filters. Infusion of fat emulsion should be slow (0.5 to 1 ml/min) for the first 15 to 30 minutes. In the absence of adverse reactions (e.g., dyspnea, cyanosis, allergic responses), the infusion rate may then be increased.

### Electrolytes, Vitamins, and Trace Elements

In addition to amino acids, carbohydrates, and fats, patients receiving parenteral nutrition must be supplied with vitamins, electrolytes (sodium, potassium, calcium, magnesium, phosphate), and trace elements (copper, chromium, iodine, manganese, molybdenum, selenium, zinc). These nutrients should be incorporated into the regimen from the onset of treatment. The pharmacology of electrolytes and vitamins is discussed in Chapters 39 and 74, respectively.

## Preparation of Parenteral Nutrient Solutions

Parenteral nutrient solutions are prepared by mixing hypertonic dextrose with an amino acid solution. Vitamins, minerals, and electrolytes are added as indicated. Although a fat emulsion may also be added to this mixture, the usual practice is to administer fats separately. To prevent bacterial contamination, parenteral solutions should be prepared aseptically under a laminar-flow hood. Solutions should be stored under refrigeration and administered within 24 hours. Preparations that have become cloudy or darkened should be discarded. Drugs should not be added to solutions unless compatibility has been established.

## Monitoring Treatment

Nutritional therapy is assessed through bedside examination, determination of blood and urine chemistries, and daily monitoring of weight, intake, and output. Weight measurement provides the best overall index of the efficacy of treatment. However, although weight gain can be a measure of success, be aware that large increases in weight (greater than 0.5 kg/day) may indicate excessive fluid retention. This possibility should be evaluated.

Blood and urine chemistries should be determined prior to treatment and throughout the period of nutritional support. Serum should be measured frequently for BUN, electrolytes, and glucose. To assess the response to treatment, albumin, cholesterol, and triglycerides should be measured weekly. Prothrombin time, platelet counts, and serum osmolarity should also be determined weekly. Blood for laboratory tests should not be drawn from the vein being used to infuse nutrients.

## Complications of Treatment

The principal complications of parenteral nutritional therapy are infection and metabolic disturbances. Mechanical complications related to the catheter may also occur.

*Infection.* Patients receiving parenteral nutritional support are at constant risk of infection. This risk can be minimized by employing aseptic technique during catheter insertion and during preparation and administration of solutions. Use of a 0.22-micron filter can provide partial protection. A filter can hold back bacteria in the feeding solution, but cannot hold back bacterial endotoxins. Also, the filter can only retain bacteria that have entered the line at a site above the filter. In the event of fever, sepsis should be suspected. To assess for sepsis, blood for culture should be drawn from the tip of the intravenous line as well as from a separate venous site. If temperature remains elevated and no cause can be found, the catheter and nutrient solution should be replaced and the tip of the catheter should be cultured for bacterial contamination. If the fever does not drop rapidly, antibiotic therapy should be instituted.

*Metabolic Disturbances.* The principal metabolic complications of parenteral nutritional therapy have been discussed. These complications include hyperglycemia, hypoglycemia, hyperlipidemia, and elevation of BUN. In addition, the patient may experience overhydration, dehydration, acid-base imbalance, electrolyte imbalance, and deficiencies in trace elements and vitamins.

*Catheter-Related Complications.* Infusion into a peripheral vein may produce phlebitis at or near the site of catheter insertion. If this occurs, the catheter should be moved. The risk of phlebitis can be reduced by selecting a large peripheral vein and by infusing the nutrient solution slowly. Other catheter-related complications include pneumothorax (caused by insertion of a central catheter) and central venous thrombosis.

## KEY POINTS

- Enteral nutritional therapy can be defined as nutritional support administered via tube into the GI tract.
- For short-term therapy, enteral feeding tubes are inserted through the nose; for long-term therapy, tubes are surgically implanted directly into the esophagus, stomach, or jejunum.
- Enteral nutritional solutions may be delivered to the feeding tube with (1) a syringe, (2) a gravity method (employing a drip chamber or rate controller), or (3) an enteral infusion pump.
- The major complication of enteral nutritional therapy is aspiration pneumonitis.
- Parenteral nutrition is administered via either a central venous catheter (for long-term therapy or for hypertonic feeding solutions) or a peripheral vein (for short-term therapy or for dilute feeding solutions).
- With parenteral nutritional therapy, glucose intolerance may occur during the first few days (until the pancreas increases insulin release).
- The fat component of peripheral nutritional solutions can cause death in premature infants.
- Parenteral nutritional therapy poses a significant risk of infection.
- Enteral and parenteral nutritional solutions consist of amino acids, carbohydrates, fats, electrolytes, vitamins, and trace elements.

# UNIT XIV

# Chemotherapy of Infectious Diseases

# Basic Principles of Antimicrobial Therapy

With this chapter we begin our study of drugs used to treat infectious diseases. These drugs, which are given to about 30% of all hospitalized patients, constitute one of our most widely used families of medicines.

Modern antimicrobial agents had their debut in the 1930s and 1940s, and have greatly reduced morbidity and mortality from infection. As newer drugs are introduced, our ability to fight infections increases even more. However, despite impressive advances, continued progress is needed: there are organisms that respond poorly to available drugs; there are effective drugs whose use is limited by toxicity; and there is, because of evolving microbial resistance, the constant threat that currently effective antibiotics will be rendered useless.

In this introductory chapter, our discussion focuses on two principal themes. The first is microbial susceptibility to drugs, which includes special emphasis on microbial drug resistance. The second theme addresses how to use antimicrobial agents properly; this discussion includes criteria for drug selection, host factors that modify drug use, use of antimicrobial combinations, and use of antimicrobial agents for prophylaxis.

Before addressing our major topics, it will be helpful to clarify three terms: *chemotherapy*, *antibiotic*, and *antimicrobial agent*. Although we often think of *chemotherapy* as the use of drugs to kill or suppress cancer cells, this term was first defined as *the use of chemicals against invading organisms* (e.g., bacteria, viruses, fungi). Today, the word is applied both to treatment of cancer and treatment of infection. Hence, not only do we speak of cancer chemotherapy, we also speak of chemotherapy of infectious diseases.

It has become common practice to use the terms *antibiotic* and *antimicrobial drug* interchangeably. We will follow that practice. However, you should be aware that the formal definitions of these words are not identical. Strictly speaking, an *antibiotic* is a chemical that is produced by one microorganism and has the ability to harm other microbes. Under this definition, only those compounds that are actually made by microorganisms qualify as antibiotics; drugs such as the sulfonamides, which are produced in the laboratory, would not be considered antibiotics under the strict definition. In contrast, an *antimicrobial drug* is defined as any agent, natural or synthetic, that has the ability to kill or suppress microorganisms. Under this definition, no distinction is made between compounds produced by microbes and those made by chemists. From the perspective of therapeutics, there is no benefit to be gained from distinguishing between drugs made by microorganisms and drugs made by people; hence, the current practice is to use the terms *antibiotic* and *antimicrobial drug* as synonyms.

## Selective Toxicity

### What Is Selective Toxicity?

The term *selective toxicity* is defined as the ability of a drug to injure a target cell or target organism without injuring other cells or organisms that are in intimate contact with the target. As applied to antimicrobial drugs, selective toxicity indicates the ability of an antibiotic to kill or suppress infecting microbes without causing injury to the host. It is this property of selective toxicity that makes antibiotics the valuable drugs that they are. If it weren't for their selective toxicity—that is, if antibiotics were as harmful to the host as they are to infecting organisms—these drugs would have no therapeutic utility.

### How Is Selective Toxicity Achieved?

How is it that a drug can be highly toxic to microbes but benign to cells of the host? The answer to this question lies with differences in the cellular chemistry of mammals and microbes. There are biochemical processes critical to microbial well-being that do not take place in mammalian cells. Hence, drugs that selectively interfere with these unique microbial processes can cause serious injury to microorganisms while leaving mammalian cells intact. This concept is illustrated below.

***Disruption of the Bacterial Cell Wall.*** Unlike mammalian cells, bacteria are encased in a rigid cell wall. The protoplasm within this wall has a high concentration of solutes, making osmotic pressure within the bacterium high. If it were not for the cell wall, bacteria would absorb water, swell, and then burst. Several families of drugs (penicillins, cephalosporins, others) act to weaken the cell wall and thereby promote bacterial lysis. Since mammalian cells have no cell wall, drugs directed at this structure do not affect the host.

***Inhibition of an Enzyme Unique to Bacteria.*** The sulfonamides provide an excellent example of drugs whose selective toxicity derives from inhibition of an enzyme that is essential for bacterial growth but is not present in cells of the host. The enzyme that the sulfonamides inhibit is needed by bacteria for production of folic acid, a compound required by all cells—mammalian and bacterial—for synthesis of essential molecules (DNA, RNA, proteins). The folic acid used by mammalian cells is acquired directly from dietary sources. In contrast, bacteria lack the ability to take up folic acid from their environment. Hence, to meet their needs for this compound, bacteria first take up *para*-aminobenzoic acid (PABA), which is a precursor of folic acid, and then use the PABA to form folic acid. The sulfonamide drugs suppress bacterial growth by inhibiting an enzyme required to synthesize folic acid from PABA. Since mammalian cells do not synthesize folic acid, toxicity of sulfonamides is selective for microbes.

***Disruption of Bacterial Protein Synthesis.*** In bacteria as in mammalian cells, synthesis of proteins employs cellular components called ribosomes. However, although both cell types employ ribosomes, bacteria have ribosomes that differ in structure from those of mammals. Because of this structural difference, it is possible for drugs to disrupt the function of bacterial ribosomes while having little or no effect on ribosomes of the host. By doing so, drugs can alter protein synthesis in bacteria while leaving mammalian protein synthesis untouched. Hence, once again we see that biochemical differences between microbes and host cells can be exploited to produce selectively toxic effects.

# Classification of Antimicrobial Drugs

Various schemes are employed for classification of antimicrobial drugs. The two schemes most suited to our objectives are considered below.

## Classification by Susceptible Organism

Antibiotics differ widely in their antimicrobial activity. Some agents, called *narrow-spectrum antibiotics*, are

---

**TABLE 77–1. CLASSIFICATION OF ANTIMICROBIAL DRUGS BY SUSCEPTIBLE ORGANISMS\***

**ANTIBACTERIAL DRUGS**

***Narrow Spectrum***

  *Gram-positive cocci and gram-positive bacilli*
    Penicillin G and V
    Penicillinase-resistant penicillins: methicillin, nafcillin
    Vancomycin
    Erythromycin
    Clindamycin
  *Gram-negative aerobes*
    Aminoglycosides: gentamicin, others
    Cephalosporins (first and second generations)
  *Mycobacterium tuberculosis*
    Isoniazid
    Rifampin
    Ethambutol
    Pyrazinamide

***Broad Spectrum***

  *Gram-positive cocci and gram-negative bacilli*
    Broad-spectrum penicillins: ampicillin, others
    Extended-spectrum penicillins: carbenicillin, others
    Cephalosporins (third generation)
    Tetracyclines
    Imipenem
    Trimethoprim
    Sulfonamides: sulfisoxazole, sulfamethoxazole, others
    Fluoroquinolones: ciprofloxacin, norfloxacin, others

**ANTIVIRAL DRUGS**

    Acyclovir
    Azidothymidine
    Zidovudine
    Amantadine
    Saquinavir

**ANTIFUNGAL DRUGS**

    Amphotericin B
    Ketoconazole
    Itraconazole

---

\*The classification in this table is simplified. Table 77–3 presents a more comprehensive list of microorganisms and the drugs active against them.

---

active against only a few microorganisms. In contrast, *broad-spectrum antibiotics* are active against a wide variety of microbes. As we will see, narrow-spectrum drugs are generally preferred to broad-spectrum agents. Because of differences in antimicrobial spectra, not all drugs are appropriate for all patients: if therapy is to be successful, we must choose an antibiotic that is active against the specific organism responsible for the infection to be treated.

Table 77–1 classifies the major antimicrobial drugs according to susceptible organisms. The table shows three major groups: *antibacterial drugs*, *antifungal drugs*, and *antiviral drugs*. In addition, the table subdivides the antibacterial drugs into narrow-spectrum and broad-spectrum agents, and indicates the principal classes of bacteria against which these drugs are active.

## TABLE 77–2. CLASSIFICATION OF ANTIMICROBIAL DRUGS BY MECHANISM OF ACTION

| Drug Class | Antibiotics |
| --- | --- |
| Inhibitors of cell wall synthesis | Penicillins<br>Cephalosporins<br>Imipenem<br>Vancomycin |
| Drugs that disrupt the cell membrane | Amphotericin B<br>Ketoconazole |
| *Bactericidal* inhibitors of protein synthesis | Aminoglycosides |
| *Bacteriostatic* inhibitors of protein synthesis | Clindamycin<br>Erythromycin<br>Tetracyclines |
| Drugs that interfere with synthesis of bacterial DNA or RNA | Fluoroquinolones<br>Rifampin |
| Antimetabolites | Flucytosine<br>Sulfonamides<br>Trimethoprim |
| Drugs that inhibit viral enzymes | Acyclovir<br>Zidovudine<br>Saquinavir<br>Indinavir |
| Inhibitor of mycolic acid synthesis | Isoniazid |
| Drugs whose mechanism is unknown | Amantadine<br>Ethambutol<br>Pyrazinamide |

## Classification by Mechanism of Action

The antimicrobial drugs fall into seven major groups based on mechanisms of action. This classification is summarized in Table 77-2. Properties of the seven major classes are discussed briefly below.

- *Drugs that inhibit bacterial cell wall synthesis or activate enzymes that disrupt the cell wall.* These drugs (e.g., penicillins, cephalosporins) weaken the cell wall and thereby promote bacterial lysis and death.
- *Drugs that increase cell membrane permeability.* Drugs in this group (e.g., amphotericin B) increase the permeability of cell membranes, causing leakage of intracellular material.
- *Drugs that cause lethal inhibition of bacterial protein synthesis.* The aminoglycosides (e.g., gentamicin) are the only drugs in this group. It is not known why inhibition of protein synthesis by these agents results in cell death.
- *Drugs that cause nonlethal inhibition of protein synthesis.* Like the aminoglycosides, the drugs in this group (e.g., tetracyclines) inhibit bacterial protein synthesis. However, in contrast to the aminoglycosides, these agents only slow microbial growth; they do not kill bacteria at clinically achievable concentrations.

- *Drugs that inhibit bacterial synthesis of nucleic acids.* These drugs inhibit synthesis of DNA or RNA by binding directly to nucleic acids or by interacting with enzymes required for nucleic acid synthesis. Members of this group include rifampin and the fluoroquinolones (e.g., ciprofloxacin).
- *Antimetabolites.* These drugs disrupt specific biochemical reactions. The result is either a decrease in the synthesis of essential cell constituents or synthesis of nonfunctional analogs of normal metabolites. Examples of antimetabolites include trimethoprim and the sulfonamides.
- *Inhibitors of viral enzymes.* Two classes of drugs, protease inhibitors and nucleoside analogs, inhibit enzymes necessary for viral replication and infectivity. Examples are zidovudine, acyclovir, and saquinavir.

When considering the *antibacterial* drugs, it is useful to distinguish between agents that are *bactericidal* and those that are *bacteriostatic*. A *bactericidal* drug is one that is directly lethal to bacteria at clinically achievable concentrations. In contrast, *bacteriostatic* drugs are agents that can slow microbial growth but do not cause cell death. When a bacteriostatic drug is used, elimination of bacteria must ultimately be accomplished by host defenses (the immune system working in concert with phagocytic cells).

# Acquired Resistance to Antimicrobial Drugs

Over time, an organism that had once been highly responsive to an antibiotic may become less susceptible, or it may lose sensitivity to the drug entirely. In some cases, resistance to several drugs develops. Acquired resistance is of great concern in that it can render currently effective drugs useless, thereby creating a clinical crisis and a constant need for new antimicrobial agents. Organisms for which drug resistance is now a serious clinical problem include *Staphylococcus aureus*, *Enterococcus*, and *Mycobacterium tuberculosis*.

In the discussion that follows, we examine the mechanisms by which microbial drug resistance is acquired and the measures by which emergence of resistance can be delayed. As you read this section, please keep in mind that it is the *microbe* that becomes drug resistant—*not the patient*.

## Mechanisms of Microbial Drug Resistance

Microorganisms become drug resistant because of alterations in their function or structure. Four such alterations are described below.

- *Microbes may elaborate drug-metabolizing enzymes.* For example, many bacteria are now resistant to penicillin G because of increased production of penicillinase, an enzyme that converts penicillin into an inactive product. Through production of enzymes, some microorganisms are able to inactivate several different kinds of antibiotics.

- *Microbes may cease active uptake of certain drugs.* Since the site of action of many antibiotics is intracellular, reduced drug uptake will result in resistance. This mechanism is responsible for some cases of resistance to tetracyclines.
- *Microbial drug receptors may undergo change, resulting in decreased antibiotic binding and action.* For example, some bacteria are now resistant to streptomycin because of structural changes in bacterial ribosomes, the sites at which streptomycin acts to inhibit protein synthesis.
- *Microbes may synthesize compounds that antagonize drug actions.* For example, by acquiring the ability to synthesize increased quantities of PABA, some bacteria have developed resistance to sulfonamides.

## Mechanisms by Which Resistance Is Acquired

The alterations in structure and function discussed above are brought about by changes in the microbial genome. These genetic changes may result from spontaneous mutation or by acquisition of DNA from an external source. The most important mechanism by which bacteria obtain external DNA is conjugation with other bacteria.

**Spontaneous Mutation.** Spontaneous mutation results in random changes in a microbe's DNA. As a rule, spontaneous mutations confer resistance *to only one drug.* Development of multiple drug resistance would require multiple mutations, a phenomenon that is rare.

**Conjugation.** Conjugation is a process by which extrachromosomal DNA is transferred from one bacterium to another. In order to transfer resistance by conjugation, the donor organism must possess two unique DNA segments, one that codes for the mechanisms of drug resistance and one that codes for the "sexual" apparatus required for DNA transfer. Together, these two DNA segments constitute an *R factor* (resistance factor).

Conjugation takes place primarily between *gram-negative* bacteria. Genetic material may be transferred between members of the same species or between members of different species. Because transfer of R factors is not species specific, it is possible for pathogenic bacteria to acquire R factors from the normal flora of the body. Since R factors are becoming common in normal flora, the possibility of transferring resistance from normal flora to pathogens is of real clinical concern.

In contrast to spontaneous mutation, conjugation frequently results in *multiple drug resistance.* This can be achieved, for example, by transferring DNA that codes for several different drug-metabolizing enzymes. Hence, in a single event, a drug-sensitive bacterium can become highly drug resistant.

## Relationships between Antibiotic Use and the Emergence of Drug-Resistant Microbes

*Use of antibiotics promotes the emergence of drug-resistant microbes.* Please note, however, that although antibiotics promote drug resistance, these agents are not mutagenic and do not directly cause the genetic changes that underlie reduced drug sensitivity. Spontaneous mutation and conjugation are random events whose incidence is independent of drug use. Drugs simply serve to make conditions favorable for overgrowth of those microbes that possess mechanisms of drug resistance.

**How Do Antibiotics Promote Resistance?** To answer this question, we need to recall two aspects of microbial ecology: (1) microbes secrete compounds that are toxic to other microbes, and (2) microbes within a given ecologic niche (e.g., large intestine, urogenital tract, skin) compete with one another for available nutrients. Under drug-free conditions, the various microbes in a given location keep one another in check. Furthermore, if none of these organisms is drug resistant, introduction of antibiotics will be equally detrimental to all members of the population, and therefore will not promote the growth of any individual. However, *if a drug-resistant organism is present, antibiotics will create selection pressure favoring the growth of that microbe*: by killing off the sensitive organisms, the drug will eliminate toxins produced by those microbes, and thereby facilitate survival of the microbe that is drug resistant. Also, elimination of sensitive organisms will remove competition for available nutrients, thereby making conditions even more favorable for the drug-resistant microbe to flourish. Hence, although drug resistance is of no benefit to an organism when there are no antibiotics around, when antibiotics are used, these agents create selection pressure favoring overgrowth of those microbes that are resistant.

**Which Antibiotics Promote Resistance?** *All* antimicrobial drugs promote the emergence of drug-resistant organisms. However, some agents are more likely to promote resistance than others. Since *broad-spectrum* antibiotics kill off more competing organisms than do narrow-spectrum drugs, emergence of resistance is facilitated most by the broad-spectrum drugs.

**Does the Amount of Antibiotic Use Influence the Emergence of Resistance?** You bet! The more that antibiotics are used, the faster drug-resistant organisms will emerge. Not only do antibiotics promote emergence of resistant pathogens, these drugs also promote overgrowth of normal flora that possess mechanisms for resistance. Since drug use can increase resistance in normal flora, and since normal flora can transfer resistance to pathogens, every effort should be made to avoid use of antibiotics by individuals who don't actually need them (i.e., individuals who don't have a treatable infection). Because all use of antibiotics will further the emergence of resistance, there can be no excuse for casual or indiscriminate dispensing of antimicrobial drugs.

Since hospitals are sites of intensive antibiotic use, resident organisms can be extremely drug resistant. As a result, *nosocomial infections* (infections acquired in hospitals) are among the most difficult to treat.

### Suprainfection

Suprainfection is simply a special example of the emergence of drug resistance. A suprainfection is defined as a *new* infection that appears during the course of treatment for a primary infection. A new infection can develop because antibiotic use can eliminate the inhibitory influence of normal flora, thereby allowing a second infectious agent to flourish. Because broad-spectrum antibiotics kill off more normal flora than do narrow-spectrum drugs, suprainfections are more likely during use of broad-spectrum agents. Suprainfections can be difficult to treat, since they are, by definition, caused by microbes that are drug resistant. It should be noted that, in some texts, suprainfections are referred to as *superinfections*; this name may have been chosen to reflect the difficulties of treatment.

### Delaying the Emergence of Resistance

Several measures can help delay the emergence of resistance. First, antimicrobial agents should be used only when actually needed. (It is estimated that, in some settings, as much as 95% of antibiotic use is unnecessary.) Second, narrow-spectrum agents should be employed whenever possible; routine use of broad-spectrum drugs to compensate for diagnostic imprecision should be discouraged. Third, newer antibiotics should be reserved for situations in which older drugs are dangerous or no longer effective. Widespread use of the newer drugs will only hasten their obsolescence.

## Selection of Antibiotics

The therapeutic objective when treating infection is to produce maximal antimicrobial effects while causing minimal harm to the host. To achieve this goal, we must select the most appropriate antibiotic for the individual patient. When choosing this antibiotic, three principal factors must be considered: (1) the identity of the infecting organism, (2) drug sensitivity of the infecting organism, and (3) host factors, such as the site of infection and the status of host defenses.

For any given infection, several drugs may be effective. However, for most infections, there is usually one drug that is superior to the alternatives (Table 77–3). This drug of first choice may be preferred for several reasons, such as greater efficacy, lower toxicity, or narrower spectrum. Whenever possible, the drug of first choice should be employed. Alternative agents should be used only when the first-choice drug is inappropriate. Conditions that might rule out use of a first-choice agent include (1) allergy to the drug of choice, (2) inability of the drug of choice to penetrate to the site of infection, and (3) unusual susceptibility of the patient to a toxicity of the first-choice drug.

### Empiric Therapy Prior to Completion of Laboratory Tests

Optimal antimicrobial therapy requires identification of the infecting organism and determination of its drug sensitivity. However, when the patient has a severe infection, it may be necessary to begin treatment before test results are available. Under these conditions, drug selection must be based on clinical evaluation and knowledge of which microbes are most likely to cause infection at a particular site. If necessary, a broad-spectrum agent can be used for initial treatment. Then, once the identity and drug sensitivity of the infecting organism have been determined, we can switch to a more selective antibiotic. When conditions demand that we start therapy in the absence of laboratory data, it is essential that samples of exudates and body fluids be obtained for culture *prior to initiation of treatment*; if antibiotics are present at the time of sampling, these agents can suppress microbial growth in culture, thereby impeding identification.

### Identification of the Infecting Organism

The first rule of antimicrobial therapy is to *match the drug with the bug*. Hence, whenever possible, the infecting organism should be identified prior to initiation of therapy. If treatment is begun in the absence of a definitive diagnosis, positive identification should be established as soon as possible, since this will permit adjustment of the regimen to better conform with the drug sensitivity of the infecting organism.

The quickest, simplest, and most versatile technique for identifying microorganisms is microscopic examination of a *gram-stained preparation*. Samples for examination can be obtained from pus, sputum, urine, blood, and other body fluids. The most useful samples are direct aspirates from the site of infection.

In some cases, only a small number of infecting organisms will be present. Under these conditions, positive identification may require that the microbes be grown out in culture. As stressed above, material for culture should be obtained prior to initiating treatment. Furthermore, these samples should be taken in a fashion that minimizes contamination with normal body flora. Identification will be facilitated by avoiding exposure of samples to low temperature, antiseptics, and oxygen.

### Determination of Drug Susceptibility

Because of the emergence of drug-resistant organisms, testing for drug sensitivity is common. However, sensitivity testing is not always needed. Rather, testing is indicated only when the infecting organism is one in which resistance is likely. Hence, for microbes such as the group A streptococci, which have remained highly susceptible to penicillin, sensitivity testing is unnecessary. In contrast, when resistance is common, as it is with *Staphylococcus aureus* and the gram-negative bacilli, tests for drug sensitivity should be performed.

***Disk-Diffusion Test.*** The most widely used method for assessing drug sensitivity is the disk-diffusion test, also

## TABLE 77–3. ANTIMICROBIAL DRUGS OF CHOICE

| Organism | Drug of First Choice | Alternative Drugs |
|---|---|---|
| **GRAM-POSITIVE COCCI** | | |
| *Enterococcus* | | |
|   Endocarditis and other severe infections | Penicillin G *or* ampicillin with gentamicin | Vancomycin with gentamicin |
|   Uncomplicated urinary tract infection | Ampicillin *or* amoxicillin | Nitrofurantoin, a quinolone |
| *Staphylococcus aureus* | | |
|   Nonpenicillinase-producing | Penicillin G or V | Cefazolin, vancomycin, imipenem |
|   Penicillinase-producing | Nafcillin | Cefazolin, vancomycin, amoxicillin–clavulanic acid |
|   Methicillin-resistant | Vancomycin, with or without rifampin and/or gentamicin | Trimethoprim-sulfamethoxazole, minocycline |
| *Streptococcus pyogenes* (Group A) and groups C and G | Penicillin G or V | Clindamycin, vancomycin, erythromycin |
| *Streptococcus*, Group B | Penicillin G or ampicillin | Cefazolin, vancomycin, erythromycin |
| *Streptococcus viridans* group | Penicillin G with or without gentamicin | Cefazolin, vancomycin |
| *Streptococcus bovis* | Penicillin G | Cefazolin, vancomycin |
| *Streptococcus*, anaerobic | Penicillin G | Clindamycin, cefazolin, vancomycin |
| *Streptococcus pneumoniae* (pneumococcus) | Penicillin G or V | Erythromycin, cefazolin, vancomycin, chloramphenicol |
| **GRAM-NEGATIVE COCCI** | | |
| *Neisseria gonorrhoeae* (gonococcus) | Ceftriaxone or cefixime | Cefotaxime, penicillin G, spectinomycin, a fluoroquinolone |
| *Neisseria meningitidis* | Penicillin G | Cefotaxime, chloramphenicol |
| **GRAM-POSITIVE BACILLI** | | |
| *Bacillus anthracis* | Penicillin G | Erythromycin, a tetracycline |
| *Clostridium difficile* | Metronidazole | Bacitracin, vancomycin |
| *Clostridium perfringens* | Penicillin G | Metronidazole, chloramphenicol |
| *Clostridium tetani* | Penicillin G | A tetracycline |
| *Corynebacterium diphtheriae* | Erythromycin | Penicillin G |
| *Listeria monocytogenes* | Ampicillin with or without gentamicin | Trimethoprim-sulfamethoxazole |
| **ENTERIC GRAM-NEGATIVE BACILLI** | | |
| *Bacteroides* | | |
|   Oropharyngeal strains | Penicillin G or clindamycin | Metronidazole, cefoxitin |
|   Gastrointestinal strains | Metronidazole | Clindamycin, imipenem, ticarcillin–clavulanic acid |
| *Campylobacter jejuni* | Imipenem | Gentamicin |
| *Escherichia coli* | Cefotaxime, cefuroxime | Ampicillin with or without gentamicin, ticarcillin–clavulanic acid, trimethoprim–sulfamethoxazole |
| *Enterobacter* | Imipenem | Trimethoprim-sulfamethoxazole, a third-generation cephalosporin, a fluoroquinolone |
| *Helicobacter pylori* | Tetracycline plus metronidazole plus bismuth subsalicylate | Tetracycline plus clarithromycin plus bismuth subsalicylate |
| *Klebsiella pneumoniae* | Cefotaxime, ceftizoxime | Imipenem, gentamicin, tobramycin, amikacin |
| *Proteus*, indole positive (including *Providencia rettgeri* and *Morganella morganii*) | Cefotaxime, ceftizoxime, or ceftriaxone | Imipenem, gentamicin, a fluoroquinolone, trimethoprim–sulfamethoxazole |
| *Proteus mirabilis* | Ampicillin | A cephalosporin, trimethoprim–sulfamethoxazole |
| *Salmonella typhi* | Ceftriaxone or a fluoroquinolone | Trimethoprim-sulfamethoxazole, ampicillin, amoxicillin, chloramphenicol |
|   Other *Salmonella* | Ceftriaxone or cefotaxime or a fluoroquinolone | Trimethoprim-sulfamethoxazole, chloramphenicol, ampicillin, amoxicillin |
| *Serratia* | Cefotaxime, ceftizoxime, or ceftriaxone | Gentamicin, amikacin, imipenem |
| *Shigella* | A fluoroquinolone | Trimethoprim–sulfamethoxazole, ampicillin, ceftriaxone |
| *Yersinia enterocolitica* | Trimethoprim–sulfamethoxazole | A fluoroquinolone, gentamicin, tobramycin |

*Table continues on following page*

## TABLE 77-3. ANTIMICROBIAL DRUGS OF CHOICE *Continued*

| Organism | Drug of First Choice | Alternative Drugs |
|---|---|---|
| **OTHER GRAM-NEGATIVE BACILLI** | | |
| *Acinetobacter* | Imipenem | Trimethoprim-sulfamethoxazole, tobramycin, gentamicin |
| *Bordetella pertussis* (whooping cough) | Erythromycin | Trimethoprim-sulfamethoxazole, ampicillin |
| *Brucella* (brucellosis) | A tetracycline plus gentamicin | Rifampin plus a tetracycline, trimethoprim-sulfamethoxazole, chloramphenicol with or without streptomycin |
| *Calymmatobacterium granulomatis* | A tetracycline | Streptomycin, trimethoprim-sulfamethoxazole |
| *Francisella tularensis* (tularemia) | Streptomycin | Gentamicin, a tetracycline, chloramphenicol |
| *Gardnerella vaginalis* | Metronidazole (PO) | Topical clindamycin or metronidazole |
| *Haemophilus ducreyi* (chancroid) | Ceftriaxone or erythromycin | A fluoroquinolone |
| *Haemophilus influenzae* | | |
| Meningitis, epiglottitis, arthritis, and other serious infections | Cefotaxime or ceftriaxone | Cefuroxime, chloramphenicol |
| Upper respiratory infection and bronchitis | Trimethoprim-sulfamethoxazole | Cefuroxime, amoxicillin–clavulanic acid |
| *Legionella micdadei* | Erythromycin with or without rifampin | Clarithromycin, trimethoprim-sulfamethoxazole |
| *Legionella pneumophila* (legionnaires' disease) | Erythromycin plus rifampin | Clarithromycin, trimethoprim-sulfamethoxazole |
| *Pasteurella multocida* | Penicillin G | A tetracycline, a cephalosporin |
| *Pseudomonas aeruginosa* | | |
| Urinary tract infection | A fluoroquinolone | Piperacillin, ceftazidime, imipenem, carbenicillin, ticarcillin |
| Other infections | Ticarcillin, mezlocillin, or piperacillin plus tobramycin, gentamicin, or amikacin | Ceftazidime, gentamicin or amikacin, imipenem or aztreonam |
| *Pseudomonas mallei* (glanders) | Streptomycin plus a tetracycline | Streptomycin plus chloramphenicol |
| *Pseudomonas pseudomallei* (melioidosis) | Ceftazidime | Chloramphenicol plus doxycycline plus trimethoprim-sulfamethoxazole |
| *Spirillum minus* (rat bite fever) | Penicillin G | A tetracycline, streptomycin |
| *Streptobacillus moniliformis* (rat bite fever) | Penicillin G | A tetracycline, streptomycin |
| *Vibrio cholerae* (cholera) | A tetracycline | Trimethoprim-sulfamethoxazole, a fluoroquinolone |
| *Yersinia pestis* (plague) | Streptomycin | A tetracycline, chloramphenicol, gentamicin |
| **MYCOBACTERIA** | | |
| *Mycobacterium tuberculosis* | Isoniazid plus rifampin plus pyrazinamide with or without ethambutol or streptomycin | Cycloserine, ethionamide, kanamycin, capreomycin, ciprofloxacin, ofloxacin, aminosalicylic acid |
| *Mycobacterium leprae* (leprosy) | Dapsone plus rifampin with or without clofazimine | Minocycline, ofloxacin |
| *Mycobacterium avium* complex | Clarithromycin ± rifampin ± ethambutol ± clofazimine | Rifampin with ethambutol, ciprofloxacin, and clofazimine ± amikacin, capreomycin |
| **ACTINOMYCETES** | | |
| *Actinomycetes israelii* | Penicillin G | A tetracycline, erythromycin, clindamycin |
| *Nocardia* | Trimethoprim-sulfamethoxazole | Sulfisoxazole, imipenem, amikacin |
| **CHLAMYDIAE** | | |
| *Chlamydia psittaci* | A tetracycline | Chloramphenicol |
| *Chlamydia trachomatis* | | |
| Trachoma | Azithromycin | A tetracycline (oral plus topical) |
| Inclusion conjunctivitis | Erythromycin (oral or IV) | A sulfonamide |
| Pneumonia | Erythromycin | A sulfonamide |
| Urethritis, cervicitis | Doxycycline or azithromycin | Erythromycin, ofloxacin, sulfisoxazole |
| Lymphogranuloma venereum | Doxycycline | Erythromycin |
| **MYCOPLASMA** | | |
| *Mycoplasma pneumoniae* | Erythromycin or a tetracycline | Clarithromycin, azithromycin |
| *Ureaplasma urealyticum* | Erythromycin | A tetracycline, clarithromycin |

*Table continues on following page*

**TABLE 77-3. ANTIMICROBIAL DRUGS OF CHOICE** *Continued*

| Organism | Drug of First Choice | Alternative Drugs |
|---|---|---|
| **RICKETTSIA** | | |
| Rocky Mountain spotted fever, endemic typhus (murine), trench fever, typhus, scrub typhus Q fever | A tetracycline | Chloramphenicol, a fluoroquinolone |
| **SPIROCHETES** | | |
| *Borrelia burgdorferi* (Lyme disease) | Doxycycline or amoxicillin | Ceftriaxone, cefotaxime |
| *Borrelia recurrentis* (relapsing fever) | A tetracycline | Penicillin G |
| *Leptospira* | Penicillin G | A tetracycline |
| *Treponema pallidum* (syphilis) | Penicillin G | A tetracycline, ceftriaxone |
| *Treponema pertenue* (yaws) | Penicillin G | A tetracycline |
| **FUNGI** | | |
| *Aspergillus* species | Amphotericin B | Itraconazole |
| *Blastomyces dermatitidis* | Amphotericin B or itraconazole | Ketoconazole |
| *Candida* species (systemic) | Amphotericin B $\pm$ flucytosine | Fluconazole |
| *Coccidioides immitis* | Amphotericin B or fluconazole | Itraconazole, ketoconazole |
| *Cryptococcus neoformans* | Amphotericin B $\pm$ flucytosine | Itraconazole, fluconazole |
| *Histoplasma capsulatum* | Amphotericin B or itraconazole | Ketoconazole |
| *Mucor* | Amphotericin B | |
| *Paracoccidioides brasiliensis* | Amphotericin B or itraconazole | Ketoconazole |
| *Sporothrix schenckii* | Amphotericin B | Itraconazole |
| **VIRUSES** | | |
| Cytomegalovirus | Ganciclovir | Foscarnet |
| Herpes simplex virus | | |
| Keratitis | Trifluridine | Acyclovir, idoxuridine |
| Genital | Acyclovir | |
| Encephalitis | Acyclovir | |
| Neonatal | Acyclovir | |
| Disseminated, adult | Acyclovir | |
| Human immunodeficiency virus | See Chapter 88 | |
| Influenza A | Amantadine | Rimantadine |
| Respiratory syncytial virus | Ribavirin | |
| Varicella-zoster virus | Acyclovir | Foscarnet |

known as the Kirby-Bauer test. This test is performed by inoculating an agar plate with the infecting organism and then placing on that plate several small disks, each of which is impregnated with a different antibiotic. Because of diffusion, an antibiotic-containing zone becomes established around each of the disks. As the bacteria proliferate, growth will be inhibited around those disks that contain an antibiotic to which the bacteria are sensitive. The degree of drug sensitivity is proportional to the size of the bacteria-free zones. Hence, by measuring the diameter of these zones, we can determine the drugs to which the organism is more susceptible, as well as those to which it is highly resistant.

***Broth Dilution Procedure.*** An alternative method for assessing drug sensitivity is known as the broth dilution procedure. In this procedure, bacteria are grown in a series of tubes containing different concentrations of an antibiotic, thereby permitting assessment of antibacterial effects at specific drug concentrations. The advantage of this method over the disk-diffusion test is that it provides a more precise measure of drug sensitivity. By using the broth dilution procedure, we can establish close estimates of two clinically useful values: (1) the *minimum inhibitory concentration*, or *MIC* (defined as the lowest concentration of antibiotic that produces complete inhibition of bacterial growth); and (2) the *minimum bactericidal concentration*, or *MBC* (defined as the lowest concentration of drug that produces a 99.9% decline in the number of bacterial colonies). Because of the quantitative information provided, broth dilution procedures are especially useful for guiding therapy of infections that are especially difficult to treat.

## Host Factors That Modify Drug Choice, Route of Administration, or Dosage

In addition to matching the drug with the bug and determining the drug sensitivity of an infecting organism, we must consider host factors when prescribing an antimicrobial drug. Two host factors—host defenses and the site of infection—are unique to the selection of antibiotics. Other host factors, such as age, pregnancy, and previous drug reactions, are the same factors that must be considered when choosing any other drug.

## Host Defenses

Host defenses consist primarily of the immune system and phagocytic cells (macrophages, neutrophils). Without the contribution of these defenses, successful antimicrobial therapy would be rare. In most cases, the drugs we use to treat infection do not produce cure on their own. Rather, these agents work in concert with host defense systems to subdue infection. Accordingly, the usual objective of antibiotic treatment is not outright kill of infecting organisms. Rather, the goal is to suppress microbial growth to the point at which the balance is tipped in favor of the host. Underscoring the critical role of host defenses is the grim fact that people whose defenses are impaired, such as those with AIDS and those undergoing cancer chemotherapy, frequently die from infections that drugs alone are unable to control. When treating the immunocompromised host, our only hope lies with the use of drugs that are rapidly bactericidal, and even these agents may prove inadequate.

## Site of Infection

To be effective, an antibiotic must be present at the site of infection in a concentration greater than the MIC. At some sites, drug penetration may be hampered, making it difficult to achieve the MIC. For example, drug access can be impeded in meningitis (because of the blood-brain barrier), endocarditis (because bacterial vegetations in the heart are difficult to penetrate), and infected abscesses (because of poor vascularity and the presence of pus and other material). When treating meningitis, two approaches may be used to achieve the MIC: (1) we can select a drug that can readily cross the blood-brain barrier and (2) we can inject an antibiotic directly into the subarachnoid space. When pus and other fluids hinder drug access, surgical drainage is indicated.

Foreign materials (e.g., cardiac pacemakers, prosthetic joints and heart valves, synthetic vascular shunts) present a special local problem. Phagocytes react to these objects and attempt to destroy them. Because of this behavior, the phagocytes are less able to attack bacteria, thereby allowing microbes to flourish at the site. When attempts are made to treat these infections, relapse and failure are common. In many cases, the infection can be eliminated only by removing the foreign material.

## Other Host Factors

*Age.* Infants and the elderly are highly vulnerable to drug toxicity. In the elderly, heightened drug sensitivity is due in large part to reduced rates of drug metabolism and drug excretion, which can result in accumulation of antibiotics to toxic levels.

Multiple factors contribute to antibiotic sensitivity in infants. Because of poorly developed kidney and liver function, neonates eliminate drugs slowly. To avoid drug accumulation, many antibiotics must be used in low dosage.

The very young are also subject to special toxicities. For example, use of sulfonamides in newborns can produce kernicterus, a severe neurologic disorder caused by displacement of bilirubin from plasma proteins (see Chapter 82). The tetracyclines provide another example of a drug toxicity unique to the young: these antibiotics bind to developing teeth, causing discoloration.

*Pregnancy and Lactation.* Antimicrobial drugs can cross the placenta, posing a risk to the developing fetus. As noted above, tetracyclines can stain immature teeth. When gentamicin is used during pregnancy, irreversible hearing loss may result.

Antibiotic use during pregnancy may also pose a risk to the expectant mother. It has been shown, for example, that during pregnancy there is an increased incidence of toxicity from tetracycline, characterized by hepatic necrosis, pancreatitis, renal damage, and, in extreme cases, death.

Antibiotics can enter breast milk, possibly affecting the nursing infant. Sulfonamides, for example, can reach levels in milk that are sufficient to cause kernicterus in nursing newborns. As a general guideline, antibiotics and all other drugs should be avoided by women who are breast-feeding.

*Previous Allergic Reaction.* Severe allergic reactions are more common with the penicillins than with any other family of drugs. As a rule, patients with a history of allergy to the penicillins should not receive them again. The exception to this rule is treatment of a life-threatening infection for which no suitable alternative is available. In addition to the penicillins, other antibiotics (sulfonamides, trimethoprim, erythromycin) are associated with a high incidence of allergic responses. However, *severe* reactions to these agents are rare.

*Genetic Factors.* As with other drugs, responses to antibiotics can be influenced by the patient's genetic heritage. For example, some antibiotics (e.g., sulfonamides, nalidixic acid) can cause hemolysis in patients who, because of their genetic makeup, have red blood cells that are deficient in an enzyme called glucose-6-phosphate dehydrogenase. Clearly, people with this deficiency should not be given antibiotics that are likely to induce red cell lysis.

Genetic factors can also affect rates of metabolism. For example, hepatic inactivation of isoniazid is rapid in some people and slow in others. If the dosage is not adjusted accordingly, isoniazid may accumulate to toxic levels in the slow metabolizers, but may fail to achieve therapeutic levels in the rapid metabolizers.

# Dosage Size and Duration of Treatment

Successful therapy requires that the antibiotic be present at the site of infection in an effective concentration for a sufficient time. Dosages should be adjusted to produce drug concentrations that are equal to or greater than the

MIC for the infection being treated. Drug levels 4 to 8 times the MIC are often desirable.

Duration of therapy depends on a number of variables, including the status of host defenses, the site of the infection, and the identity of the infecting organism. *It is imperative that antibiotics not be discontinued prematurely. Patients should be instructed to take their medication for the entire prescribed course, even though symptoms may subside before the full course has been completed.* Early withdrawal is a common cause of recurrent infection, and the organisms responsible for relapse are likely to be more drug resistant than those that were present when therapy began.

# Therapy with Antibiotic Combinations

Therapy with a combination of antimicrobial agents is indicated *only in specific situations*. Under these well-defined conditions, use of multiple drugs may be life saving. However, it should be stressed that, although antibiotic combinations do have a valuable therapeutic role, routine use of two or more antibiotics should be discouraged. When an infection is caused by a single, identified microbe, treatment with just one drug is usually most appropriate.

## Antimicrobial Effects of Antibiotic Combinations

When two antibiotics are used together, the result may be *additive*, *potentiative*, or, in certain cases, *antagonistic*. An *additive* response is one in which the antimicrobial effect of the combination is equal to the sum of the effects of the two drugs alone. A *potentiative* interaction is one in which the effect of the combination is greater than the sum of the effects of the individual agents. A classic example of potentiation is produced by the combination of trimethoprim plus sulfamethoxazole, drugs that inhibit sequential steps in the synthesis of tetrahydrofolic acid (see Chapter 82).

In certain cases, a combination of two antibiotics may be less effective than one of the agents by itself. Such reduced responses indicate *antagonism* between the drugs. Antagonism is most likely when a *bacteriostatic* agent (e.g., tetracycline) is combined with a *bactericidal* drug (e.g., penicillin). Antagonism occurs because bactericidal drugs are usually effective only against organisms that are actively growing. Hence, when bacterial growth has been suppressed by a bacteriostatic drug, the effects of a bactericidal agent can be reduced. If host defenses are intact, antagonism between two antibiotics may be of little clinical significance. However, if host defenses are compromised, the consequences of antagonism can be dire.

## Indications for Antibiotic Combinations

***Initial Therapy of Severe Infection.*** The most common indication for use of multiple antibiotics is initial therapy of severe infection of unknown etiology, especially in the neutropenic host. Until the infecting organism has been identified, wide antimicrobial coverage is needed. Just how broad the coverage is will depend on the clinician's skill in narrowing the field of potential causative organisms. Once the identity of the infecting microbe is known, drug selection can be adjusted accordingly. As discussed above, samples for culture should be obtained before drug therapy is initiated.

***Mixed Infections.*** An infection may be caused by more than one microbe. Multiple infecting organisms are common in brain abscesses, pelvic infections, and infections resulting from perforation of abdominal organs. When the infecting microbes differ from one another in drug susceptibility, treatment with more than one antibiotic is required.

***Prevention of Resistance.*** Although use of multiple antibiotics is usually associated with *promotion* of drug resistance, there is one disease—*tuberculosis*—in which drug combinations are employed for the specific purpose of *suppressing* the emergence of resistant bacteria. Just why tuberculosis differs from other infections in this regard is discussed in Chapter 84.

***Decreased Toxicity.*** In some situations, an antibiotic combination can reduce the risk of toxicity to the host. For example, by combining flucytosine with amphotericin B in the treatment of fungal meningitis, the dosage of amphotericin B can be reduced, thereby decreasing the risk of amphotericin-induced damage to the kidneys.

***Enhanced Antibacterial Action.*** In specific infections, a combination of antibiotics can have greater antibacterial action than a single agent. This is true of the combined use of penicillin plus an aminoglycoside in the treatment of enterococcal endocarditis. Penicillin acts to weaken the bacterial cell wall; the aminoglycoside acts to suppress protein synthesis. The combination has enhanced antibacterial action because, by weakening the cell wall, penicillin facilitates penetration of the aminoglycoside to its intracellular site of action, thereby increasing the effects of the aminoglycoside.

## Disadvantages of Antibiotic Combinations

Use of multiple antibiotics has several drawbacks, including (1) increased risk of toxic and allergic reactions, (2) possible antagonism of antimicrobial effects, (3) increased risk of suprainfection, (4) selection of drug-resistant bacteria, and (5) increased cost. Because of these detriments, antimicrobial combinations should be employed only when clearly indicated.

# Prophylactic Use of Antimicrobial Drugs

It is estimated that between 30% and 50% of the antibiotics used in the United States are administered for prophylaxis. That is, these agents are given to prevent an infection from occurring rather than to treat an infection that is already established. Much of the prophylactic use of antibiotics is uncalled for. However, in certain situations, antimicrobial prophylaxis is both appropriate and effective. Whenever prophylaxis is attempted, the benefits must be weighed against the risks of toxicity, allergic reactions, suprainfection, and selection of drug-resistant organisms. Generally approved indications for prophylaxis are discussed below.

**Surgery.** Prophylactic use of antibiotics can decrease the incidence of infection in certain kinds of surgery. Procedures in which prophylactic efficacy has been documented include cardiac surgery, peripheral vascular surgery, orthopedic surgery, and surgery on the gastrointestinal tract (stomach, duodenum, colon, rectum, appendix). Prophylaxis is also beneficial for women undergoing a hysterectomy or an emergency cesarean section. In "dirty" surgery (operations performed on perforated abdominal organs, compound fractures, or lacerations from animal bites), the risk of infection is nearly 100%. For these operations, use of antibiotics is considered *treatment*, not prophylaxis. When antibiotics are given for prophylaxis, they should be administered before surgery has begun. If the procedure is unusually long, readministration during surgery may be indicated. As a rule, postoperative antibiotics are unnecessary. For most operations, a first-generation cephalosporin (e.g., cefazolin, cephalothin) will provide the needed protection.

**Bacterial Endocarditis.** Individuals with congenital or valvular heart disease and those with prosthetic heart valves are unusually susceptible to bacterial endocarditis. For these people, endocarditis can develop following surgery, dental procedures, and other procedures that may dislodge bacteria into the bloodstream. Hence, prior to undergoing such procedures, these patients should receive prophylactic antimicrobial medication.

**Neutropenia.** Severe neutropenia puts individuals at high risk of infection. There is some evidence that the incidence of bacterial infection may be reduced through antibiotic prophylaxis. However, prophylaxis may increase the risk of infection with fungi: by killing normal flora, whose presence helps suppress fungal growth, antibiotics can encourage fungal invasion.

**Other Indications for Antimicrobial Prophylaxis.** For young women with recurrent urinary tract infection, prophylaxis with trimethoprim-sulfamethoxazole may be helpful. Amantadine (an antiviral agent) may be employed for prophylaxis against type A influenza. For individuals who have had severe rheumatic carditis, lifelong prophylaxis with penicillin may be needed. Antimicrobial prophylaxis is indicated following exposure to organisms responsible for sexually transmitted diseases (e.g., syphilis, gonorrhea).

## Misuses of Antimicrobial Drugs

Throughout this chapter, we have focused on the proper use of antimicrobial medications. In this section, we consider important ways in which antibiotics are misused.

**Attempted Treatment of Untreatable Infection.** The majority of viral infections, including mumps, chickenpox, and the common cold, do not respond to currently available drugs. Hence, when drug therapy of these disorders is attempted, patients are exposed to all the risks of drug use without receiving any benefits.

**Treatment of Fever of Unknown Origin.** Although fever can be a sign of infection, it can also signify other diseases, including hepatitis, arthritis, and cancer. Unless the cause of a fever has been shown to be infection, antibiotics should not be employed. Reasons for this prohibition are the following: (1) if the fever is *not* due to an infection, antibiotics would not only be inappropriate, they would also expose the patient to unnecessary toxicity and would delay correct diagnosis of the fever's cause; and (2) if the fever *is* caused by infection, antibiotics could hamper later attempts to identify the infecting organism.

There is one situation in which fever, by itself, does constitute an indication for antibiotic use. That situation is fever in the severely immunocompromised host. Since fever may indicate infection, and since infection can be lethal to the immunocompromised patient, these patients should be given antibiotics when fever occurs—even if fever is the only indication that an infection may be present.

**Improper Dosage.** Like all other medications, antibiotics must be used in appropriate dosages. If the dosage is too low, the patient will be exposed to a risk of adverse effects without benefit of antibacterial effects. If the dosage is too high, the risks of suprainfection and adverse effects become unnecessarily high.

**Treatment in the Absence of Adequate Bacteriologic Information.** As stressed earlier, proper antimicrobial therapy requires information on the identity and drug sensitivity of the infecting organism. Except in life-threatening situations, therapy should not be undertaken in the absence of bacteriologic information. This important guideline is often ignored.

**Omission of Surgical Drainage.** Antibiotics may have limited efficacy in the presence of foreign material, necrotic tissue, or pus. Hence, when appropriate, surgical drainage and cleansing should be performed to promote antimicrobial effects.

## Monitoring Antimicrobial Therapy

Antimicrobial therapy is assessed by monitoring clinical responses and laboratory results. The frequency of monitoring is directly proportional to the severity of infection. Important clinical indicators of success are reduction of fever and resolution of signs and symptoms related to the affected organ system (e.g., improvement of breath sounds in patients with pneumonia).

Various laboratory tests are used to monitor treatment. Serum drug levels may be monitored for two reasons: (1)

to ensure that levels are sufficient for antimicrobial effects and (2) to avoid toxicity from excessive levels. Success of therapy is indicated by the disappearance of infectious organisms from post-treatment cultures; these cultures may become sterile within hours of the onset of treatment (as may happen with urinary tract infections), or they may not become sterile for weeks (as may happen with tuberculosis).

## KEY POINTS

- As applied to antibiotics, the term *selective toxicity* refers to the ability of a drug to injure invading microbes without injuring cells of the host.
- *Narrow-spectrum* antibiotics are active against only a few microorganisms, whereas *broad-spectrum* antibiotics are active against a wide array of microbes.
- *Bactericidal* drugs kill bacteria, whereas *bacteriostatic* drugs only suppress bacterial growth.
- Emergence of microbial resistance to drugs is a major concern in antimicrobial therapy.
- The principal method by which bacteria acquire resistance is *conjugation*, a process in which DNA coding for drug resistance is transferred from one bacterium to another.
- Although antibiotics do not directly create the genetic changes that make bacteria drug resistant, antibiotics do promote the emergence of drug-resistant organisms (by creating selection pressure that favors them).
- Broad-spectrum antibiotics promote the emergence of resistance more than narrow-spectrum antibiotics.
- We can delay the emergence of drug resistance by (1) using antibiotics only when clearly indicated, (2) using narrow-spectrum antibiotics whenever possible, and

(3) reserving newer antibiotics for situations in which older antibiotics are either ineffective or harmful.
- Effective antimicrobial therapy requires that we determine both the identity and drug sensitivity of the infecting organism.
- The *minimum inhibitory concentration* (MIC) of an antibiotic is defined as the lowest concentration needed to completely suppress bacterial growth. The *minimum bactericidal concentration* (MBC) is defined as the concentration that decreases the number of bacterial colonies by 99.9%.
- Host defenses—the immune system and phagocytic cells—are essential to the success of antimicrobial therapy.
- It is important that patients complete the prescribed course of antibiotic treatment, even though symptoms may abate before the full course is over.
- Although combinations of antibiotics should generally be avoided, they are appropriate in several situations, including (1) initial treatment of severe infections, (2) infection with more than one organism, (3) treatment of tuberculosis, and (4) treatment of an infection in which combination therapy can greatly enhance antibacterial effects.
- Appropriate indications for prophylactic antimicrobial treatment include (1) certain surgeries, (2) neutropenia, (3) recurrent urinary tract infections, and (4) patients at risk of bacterial endocarditis (e.g., those with prosthetic heart valves or congenital heart disease).
- Important *misuses* of antibiotics include (1) treatment of untreatable infections (e.g., the common cold and most other viral infections); (2) treatment of fever of unknown origin (except in the immunocompromised host); (3) treatment in the absence of adequate bacteriologic information; and (4) treatment in the absence of appropriate surgical drainage.

# CHAPTER 78

# Drugs That Weaken the Bacterial Cell Wall I: Penicillins

## Introduction to the Penicillins

The penicillins are practically ideal antibiotics. These drugs are active against a variety of bacteria and their direct toxicity is low. Allergic reactions constitute their principal adverse effects. Owing to their safety and efficacy, the penicillins are widely prescribed.

Because they have a beta-lactam ring in their structure (see Fig. 78–1), the penicillins are known as *beta-lactam antibiotics*. The beta-lactam family also includes the cephalosporins, aztreonam, and imipenem, which are discussed in Chapter 79. All of the beta-lactam antibiotics share the same mechanism of action: disruption of the bacterial cell wall.

## Mechanism of Action

To understand the actions of the penicillins, we must first understand the structure and function of the bacterial cell wall. The cell wall is a rigid, permeable, mesh-like structure that lies outside the cytoplasmic membrane. Within the cytoplasmic membrane, osmotic pressure is very high, creating a strong tendency for the bacterium to take up water and swell. If it were not for the rigid cell wall, which prevents the bacterium from expanding, water would be absorbed to such an extent that the bacterium would eventually burst.

The penicillins weaken the cell wall, causing the bacterium to take up excessive amounts of water and then rupture. As a result, the penicillins are usually bactericidal. For reasons that are not fully understood, penicillins are lethal only to bacteria undergoing active growth and division.

Penicillins weaken the cell wall by two actions: (1) *inhibition of transpeptidases* and (2) *disinhibition (activation) of autolysins. Transpeptidases* are enzymes critical to cell wall synthesis. Specifically, these enzymes catalyze the formation of cross-bridges between the peptidoglycan polymer strands that form the cell wall; these bridges give the cell wall its strength (see Figure 78–2). Autolysins are bacterial enzymes that cleave bonds in the cell wall. Bacteria employ these enzymes to break down segments of the cell wall to permit growth and division. By simultaneously inhibiting transpeptidases and activating autolysins, the penicillins (1) disrupt synthesis of the cell wall and (2) promote its active destruction. These combined actions result in cell lysis and death.

The molecular targets of the penicillins (transpeptidases, autolysins, other bacterial enzymes) are known collectively as *penicillin-binding proteins* (PBPs). These molecules are called PBPs because penicillins must bind to them to produce antibacterial effects. More than eight different PBPs have been identified. The PBPs that are most important in mediating the bactericidal actions of the penicillins are named PBP1 and PBP3. As indicated in Figure 78–3, PBPs are located on the outer surface of the cytoplasmic membrane.

Since mammalian cells lack a cell wall, and since penicillins act specifically on enzymes that affect cell wall integrity, the penicillins have virtually no *direct* effects on cells of the host. As a result, the penicillins are among our safest antibiotics.

## Mechanisms of Bacterial Resistance

Bacterial resistance to penicillins is determined primarily by two factors: (1) inability of penicillins to reach their tar-

PENICILLIN NUCLEUS

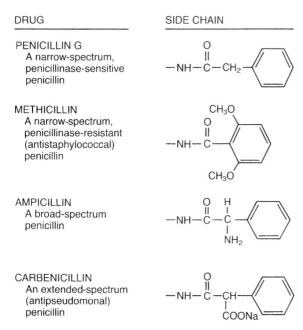

β-lactam ring

| DRUG | SIDE CHAIN |
|------|-----------|
| PENICILLIN G<br>A narrow-spectrum, penicillinase-sensitive penicillin | $-NH-\overset{\displaystyle O}{\overset{\|}{C}}-CH_2-$ (phenyl) |
| METHICILLIN<br>A narrow-spectrum, penicillinase-resistant (antistaphylococcal) penicillin | $-NH-\overset{\displaystyle O}{\overset{\|}{C}}-$ (phenyl with $CH_3O$ groups) |
| AMPICILLIN<br>A broad-spectrum penicillin | $-NH-\overset{\displaystyle O}{\overset{\|}{C}}-\overset{\displaystyle H}{\underset{\displaystyle NH_2}{C}}-$ (phenyl) |
| CARBENICILLIN<br>An extended-spectrum (antipseudomonal) penicillin | $-NH-\overset{\displaystyle O}{\overset{\|}{C}}-\underset{\displaystyle COONa}{CH}-$ (phenyl) |

**Figure 78–1. Structural formulas of representative penicillins.** The unique structure of individual penicillins is determined by the side chain coupled to the penicillin nucleus at the position labeled R. This side chain influences acid stability, pharmacokinetic properties, penicillinase resistance, and ability to bind specific penicillin-binding proteins.

gets (PBPs) and (2) inactivation of penicillins by bacterial enzymes.

## The Gram-Negative Cell Envelope

All bacteria are surrounded by a cell envelope. However, the cell envelope of gram-negative organisms differs from that of gram-positive organisms. Because of this difference, most penicillins are inactive against gram-negative bacteria.

As indicated in Figure 78–3, the cell envelope of *gram-positive* bacteria has only two layers: the cytoplasmic membrane plus a relatively thick cell wall. Despite its thickness, the cell wall can be readily penetrated by penicillins, giving them easy access to PBPs on the cytoplasmic membrane. As a result, penicillins are generally very active against gram-positive organisms.

The *gram-negative* cell envelope has three layers: the cytoplasmic membrane, a relatively thin cell wall, and an additional *outer membrane* (Fig. 78–3). Like the gram-positive cell wall, the gram-negative cell wall can be easily penetrated by penicillins. The outer membrane, in con-

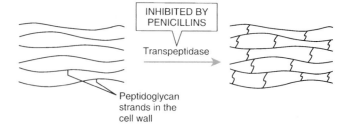

**Figure 78–2. Inhibition of transpeptidase by penicillins.** The bacterial cell wall is composed of long strands of a peptidoglycan polymer. As depicted, transpeptidase enzymes create cross-bridges between the peptidoglycan strands, giving the cell wall its strength. By inhibiting transpeptidases, penicillins prevent cross-bridge synthesis and thereby weaken the cell wall.

trast, is difficult to penetrate: only those penicillins that can pass through the small pores in the outer membrane are able to cross and reach PBPs on the cytoplasmic membrane. Since most penicillins cannot pass through the outer membrane, most penicillins are inactive against gram-negative bacteria.

## Penicillinases (Beta-Lactamases)

*Beta-lactamases* are enzymes that cleave the beta-lactam ring, and thereby render penicillins and other beta-lactam antibiotics inactive (Fig. 78–4). Bacteria produce a variety of beta-lactamases; some are specific for penicillins, some are specific for other beta-lactam antibiotics (e.g., cephalosporins), and some act on several kinds of beta-lactam antibiotics. Those beta-lactamases that act selectively on penicillins are referred to as *penicillinases*.

Penicillinases are synthesized by gram-positive and gram-negative bacteria. Gram-positive organisms produce large amounts of these enzymes, and then release them into the surrounding medium. In contrast, gram-negative bacteria produce penicillinases in relatively small amounts, and, rather than exporting them to the environment, secrete them into the periplasmic space (see Fig. 78–3).

The genes that code for synthesis of beta-lactamases are located on plasmids (extrachromosomal DNA) and chromosomes. Genes that are present on plasmids may be transferred from one bacterium to another, thereby promoting the spread of penicillin resistance.

Transfer of resistance is of special importance with *Staphylococcus aureus*. When penicillin was first introduced in the early 1940s, all strains of *Staph. aureus* were sensitive to the drug. However, by 1960, as many as 80% of *Staph. aureus* isolates in hospitals displayed penicillin resistance. Fortunately, a penicillin derivative (methicillin) that has resistance to the actions of beta-lactamases was introduced at this time. To date, no known strains of *Staph. aureus* produce beta-lactamases capable of inactivating methicillin or related penicillinase-resistant penicillins (although some strains of this organism are resistant to these drugs for other reasons).

GRAM-POSITIVE ENVELOPE                    GRAM-NEGATIVE ENVELOPE

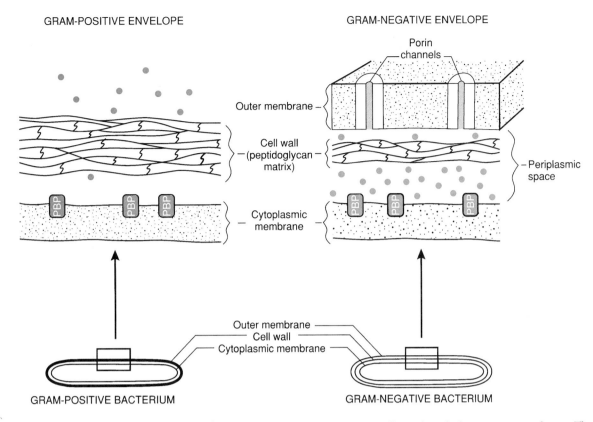

**Figure 78–3. The bacterial cell envelope.** Note that the gram-positive cell envelope lacks an outer membrane. The outer membrane of the gram-negative cell envelope prevents certain penicillins from reaching their target molecules. (PBP = penicillin-binding protein [transpeptidases and other penicillin target molecules]. Filled circles [•] represent beta-lactamases.)

## Chemistry

All of the penicillins are derived from a common nucleus: 6-aminopenicillanic acid. As shown in Figure 78–1, this nucleus contains a beta-lactam ring joined to a second ring. The beta-lactam ring is essential for antibacterial actions. Properties of individual penicillins are determined by additions made to the basic nucleus, primarily at the site labeled R. These modifications determine (1) affinity for PBPs, (2) resistance to penicillinases, (3) ability to penetrate the gram-negative cell envelope, (4) resistance to stomach acid, and (5) pharmacokinetic properties.

## Classification

The most useful classification of penicillins is based on antimicrobial spectrum. When classified according to spectrum, the penicillins fall into four major groups: (1) narrow-spectrum penicillins that are penicillinase sensitive, (2) narrow-spectrum penicillins that are penicillinase resistant (antistaphylococcal penicillins), (3) broad-spectrum penicillins (aminopenicillins), and (4) extended-spectrum penicillins (antipseudomonal penicillins). The individual agents that belong to these groups, together with their principal target organisms, are listed in Table 78–1.

## Properties of Individual Penicillins

### Penicillin G

Penicillin G (benzylpenicillin) was the first penicillin available and is the prototype for the penicillin family. This agent is often referred to simply as *penicillin*. Penicillin G is bactericidal to a number of gram-positive bacteria as well as to some gram-negative bacteria. Despite the introduction of newer antibiotics, penicillin G remains a drug of choice for many infections. The structure of penicillin G is shown in Figure 78–1.

#### Antimicrobial Spectrum

Penicillin G is active against most *gram-positive bacteria* (except penicillinase-producing staphylococci), gram-negative cocci (*Neisseria meningitidis* and nonpenicillinase-producing strains of *N. gonorrhoeae*), anaerobic bacteria, and spirochetes (including *Treponema pallidum*). With few exceptions, gram-negative bacilli are resistant. Although many organisms respond to penicillin G, the drug is considered a narrow-spectrum agent (as compared with other members of the penicillin family).

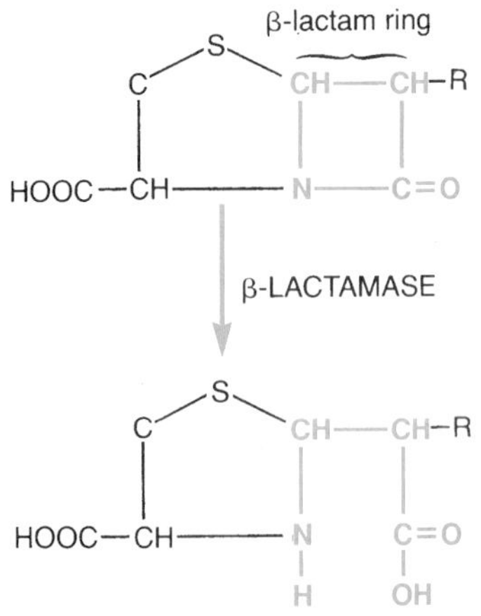

**Figure 78–4. The effect of beta-lactamase on the penicillin nucleus.**

### Therapeutic Uses

Penicillin G is a drug of first choice for infections caused by sensitive gram-positive cocci. Important among these infections are pneumonia and meningitis caused by *Streptococcus pneumoniae* (pneumococcus), pharyngitis caused by *Streptococcus pyogenes*, and infectious endocarditis caused by *Streptococcus viridans*. Penicillin is also the preferred drug for use against those few strains of *Staphylococcus aureus* that do not produce penicillinase.

Penicillin is a preferred agent for infections caused by several gram-positive bacilli. These infections are gas gangrene (caused by *Clostridium perfringens*), tetanus (caused by *Clostridium tetani*), and anthrax (caused by *Bacillus anthracis*).

Penicillin is the drug of first choice for meningitis caused by *Neisseria meningitidis* (meningococcus).

Although once the drug of choice for gonorrhea (caused by *Neisseria gonorrhoeae*), penicillin has been replaced by ceftriaxone as the primary treatment for this infection. Penicillin is now limited to treating infections caused by nonpenicillinase-producing strains of *N. gonorrhoeae*.

Penicillin is the drug of choice for syphilis, an infection caused by the spirochete *Treponema pallidum*.

In addition to treatment of active infections, penicillin G has important *prophylactic* applications. The drug is used to prevent syphilis in sexual partners of individuals known to have this infection. Benzathine penicillin G (administered monthly for life) is employed for prophylaxis against recurrent attacks of *rheumatic fever*; treatment is recommended for patients with a history of recurrent rheumatic fever and for those with clear evidence of rheumatic heart disease. Penicillin is also employed for *prophylaxis of bacterial endocarditis*; candidates for therapy include individuals with (1) prosthetic heart valves, (2) most congenital heart diseases, (3) acquired heart valvular disease, (4) mitral valve prolapse, and (5) previous history of bacterial endocarditis. For prevention of endocarditis, penicillin is administered prior to dental procedures and other procedures that are likely to produce temporary bacteremia.

### Pharmacokinetics

***Absorption.*** Penicillin G is available as four different salts: (1) *sodium* penicillin G, (2) *potassium* penicillin G, (3) *procaine* penicillin G, and (4) *benzathine* penicillin G. These salts differ with respect to route of administration and time course of action. With all four preparations, the salt dissociates to release penicillin G, the active form of these preparations.

*Oral.* Oral administration is rare. Penicillin G is unstable in acid, and the majority of an oral dose is destroyed in the stomach. Food delays gastric emptying and prolongs exposure of penicillin to gastric acid. Accordingly, to maximize oral absorption, penicillin G should be administered at least 1 hour before meals or 2 hours after. To produce equivalent blood levels, oral doses must be 4 to 5 times greater than parenteral doses.

*Intramuscular.* All forms of penicillin may be administered IM. However, it is important to note that the different salts are absorbed at very different rates. As indicated in Figure 78–5, absorption of *sodium* and *potassium* penicillin G is rapid; peak blood levels are achieved about 15

## TABLE 78–1. CLASSIFICATION OF THE PENICILLINS

| Penicillin Class | Drug | Clinically Useful Antimicrobial Spectrum |
|---|---|---|
| Narrow-spectrum penicillins: penicillinase sensitive | Penicillin G<br>Penicillin V | *Streptococcus* species, *Neisseria* species, many anaerobes, spirochetes, others |
| Narrow-spectrum penicillins: penicillinase resistant (antistaphylococcal penicillins) | Methicillin<br>Nafcillin<br>Oxacillin<br>Cloxacillin<br>Dicloxacillin | *Staphylococcus aureus* |
| Broad-spectrum penicillins: (aminopenicillins) | Ampicillin<br>Amoxicillin<br>Bacampicillin | *Haemophilus influenzae, Escherichia coli, Proteus mirabilis*, enterococci, *Neisseria gonorrhoeae* |
| Extended-spectrum penicillins: (antipseudomonal penicillins) | Carbenicillin indanyl<br>Ticarcillin<br>Mezlocillin<br>Piperacillin | Same as broad-spectrum penicillins plus *Pseudomonas aeruginosa, Enterobacter* species, *Proteus* (indole positive), *Bacteroides fragilis*, many *Klebsiella* |

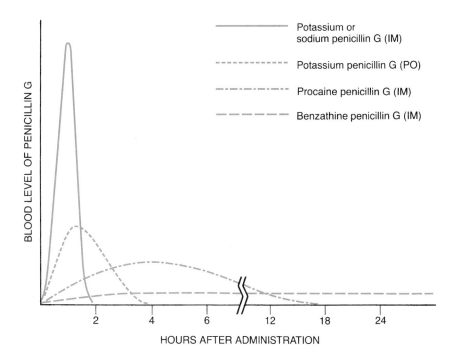

**Figure 78–5. Penicillin G blood levels following the administration of oral and intramuscular formulations of penicillin G.** (Adapted from Pratt, W.B., and Fekety, R. The Antimicrobial Drugs. New York, Oxford University Press, 1986.)

minutes after injection. In contrast, the *procaine* and *benzathine* salts are absorbed slowly. Because of their delayed absorption, these salts are referred to as *repository* forms of penicillin. When benzathine penicillin is injected IM, penicillin G is absorbed into the blood for weeks, but serum levels remain very low (see Fig. 78–5). Consequently, this preparation is useful only against highly sensitive organisms (e.g., *Treponema pallidum*, the bacterium that causes syphilis).

*Intravenous.* When high blood levels are needed rapidly, penicillin can be administered IV. Only the sodium and potassium salts should be given by this route. Procaine and benzathine salts must never be administered IV.

**Distribution.** Penicillin distributes well to most tissues and body fluids. In the absence of inflammation, penetration of the meninges and into fluids of joints and the eye is poor. However, in the *presence* of inflammation, entry into cerebrospinal fluid, joints, and the eye is enhanced, permitting treatment of infections caused by susceptible organisms.

**Elimination.** Penicillin is eliminated by the kidneys, primarily as the unchanged drug. Renal excretion of penicillin is accomplished mainly (90%) by active tubular secretion; the remaining 10% results from glomerular filtration. In older children and adults, the half-life of penicillin is very short (about 30 minutes). Kidney dysfunction causes the half-life to increase dramatically, and may necessitate a reduction in dosage. In patients at high risk of toxicity (those with renal impairment, the acutely ill, the elderly, the very young), kidney function should be monitored.

Renal excretion of penicillin can be delayed with *probenecid*, a compound that competes with penicillin for active tubular transport. Formerly, when penicillin was both scarce and expensive, probenecid was em-

ployed routinely to prolong the effects of the drug. Since penicillin is now available in abundance at low cost, concurrent use of probenecid is rarely indicated.

## Side Effects and Toxicities

Penicillin G is the least toxic of all antibiotics, and is among the safest of all medications. *Allergic reactions* are the principal concern; these reactions are discussed separately below. In addition to allergic reactions, penicillin G may cause *pain at sites of IM injection*, prolonged (but reversible) *sensory and motor dysfunction* following accidental injection into a peripheral nerve, and *neurotoxicity* (seizures, confusion, hallucinations) if blood levels are allowed to rise too high. Inadvertent *intra-arterial* injection can produce severe reactions (gangrene, necrosis, sloughing of tissue) and must be avoided.

Certain adverse effects may be caused by compounds coadministered with penicillin. For example, the procaine component of procaine penicillin G may cause bizarre behavioral effects when procaine penicillin is given in large doses. When large IV doses of potassium penicillin G are administered rapidly, hyperkalemia can result, possibly causing dysrhythmias and even cardiac arrest. Large intravenous doses of sodium penicillin G can cause sodium overload; exercise caution in patients with hypertension or cardiac disease.

## Penicillin Allergy

**General Considerations.** *Penicillins are the most common cause of drug allergy;* between 1% and 10% of patients who receive penicillins experience an allergic response. Reactions range in severity from minor rash to life-threatening anaphylaxis. Although allergic reactions can occur following administration of penicillins by any route, severe reactions are most likely with parenteral administration. As with most allergic reactions, there is no direct relationship between the size of the dose and the intensity of the allergic response. Although prior exposure to penicillins is required for an allergic reaction, responses may occur in the absence of prior penicillin use, since patients may have been exposed to penicillins produced by fungi or to penicillins present in foods of animal origin.

Because of cross-sensitivity, patients allergic to one penicillin should be considered allergic to all penicillins. In addition, about 5% to 10% of individuals allergic to penicillins display cross-sensitivity to *cephalosporins*. If at all possible, patients with penicillin allergy should not be treated with any member of the penicillin family; cephalosporins may be used cautiously in some patients.

Individuals allergic to penicillin should be encouraged to wear a Medic Alert bracelet or some other form of identification to alert health care personnel to their condition.

**Types of Allergic Reactions.** Penicillin reactions are classified as *immediate*, *accelerated*, and *late*. Immediate reactions occur 2 to 30 minutes after drug administration; accelerated reactions occur within 1 to 72 hours; and late reactions may take days or even weeks to develop.

*Anaphylaxis* (laryngeal edema, bronchoconstriction, severe hypotension) is an immediate hypersensitivity reaction, and is the reaction of greatest concern. Anaphylactic reactions occur more frequently with penicillins than with any other drugs. Fortunately, even with penicillins, the incidence of anaphylaxis is only about 0.02%. However, when these reactions occur, the risk of mortality is high (approximately 10%). The primary treatment for anaphylaxis is *epinephrine* (SC, IM, or IV) plus respiratory support. To ensure prompt treatment if anaphylaxis should develop, patients receiving parenteral penicillins should remain in the physician's office for at least 30 minutes after drug injection (i.e., until the risk of an anaphylactic reaction has passed).

**Development of Penicillin Allergy.** Before discussing penicillin allergy further, we need to review development of allergy to small molecules as a class. Drugs and other small molecules are unable to induce antibody formation directly. Therefore, in order to promote antibody formation, the small molecule must first bond covalently to a larger molecule (usually a protein). In these combinations, the small molecule is referred to as a hapten. The hapten-protein combination constitutes the complete *antigen* that stimulates antibody formation.

The hapten involved in development of penicillin antibodies is rarely intact penicillin itself. Rather, compounds formed from the degradation of penicillin are the actual haptens. As a result, most "penicillin antibodies" are not directed at penicillin itself. Instead, these antibodies are directed at various penicillin degradation products.

**Skin Tests for Penicillin Allergy.** Allergy to penicillin can decrease over time. Hence, an intense allergic reaction in the past does not necessarily indicate that such a reaction will occur again. In patients with a history of penicillin allergy, skin tests can be employed to assess the current risk of a severe reaction. These tests are performed by injecting a tiny amount of allergen intradermally and observing for an allergic response.

Two reagents can be employed to assess penicillin allergy. One of these, *benzylpenicilloyl-polylysine* (BPO-PL), tests primarily for *delayed* hypersensitivity. This reagent is referred to as a *major antigenic determinant*, a term indicating that the antibodies for which this reagent tests are relatively common. BPO-PL is a large polymeric molecule that is poorly absorbed. Hence, even in patients with severe penicillin allergy, a skin test with this compound carries little risk of a systemic reaction.

The second skin-test reagent, known as the *minor determinant mixture* (MDM), detects antibodies that mediate *immediate* allergic responses (e.g., anaphylaxis). The term *minor* indicates that the antibodies being tested for are relatively uncommon and not that the allergic response mediated by these antibodies is of minor significance. It is important to note that skin testing with MDM can be dangerous: in patients with severe penicillin allergy, the skin test itself can precipitate an anaphylactic reaction. Accordingly, the test should be performed only if epinephrine and facilities for respiratory support are immediately available.

For two reasons, penicillin itself is rarely employed for skin tests. First, skin testing with penicillin can elicit an anaphylactic reaction in highly sensitized individuals. Second, use of penicillin can produce a false-negative result. This second point is paradoxical and requires explanation. Recall that most antibodies that mediate penicillin allergy are directed against degradation products of penicillin, and not against penicillin itself. Nonetheless, intact penicillin is able to bind to the active site of these antibodies—but that binding will not trigger an immune response. As a result, when small amounts of degradation products are formed following intradermal injection of penicillin, the presence of large amounts of intact penicillin can compete with those products for antibody-binding sites, thereby preventing the degradation products from triggering an allergic reaction.

**Management of Patients with a History of Penicillin Allergy.** All patients who are candidates for penicillin therapy should be asked if they have experienced an allergic reaction to penicillin. For patients who indicate a history of penicillin allergy, the general rule is to avoid penicillins entirely. If the allergy is mild, a *cephalosporin* is often an appropriate alternative. However, if there is a history of anaphylaxis or some other severe allergic reaction, it is prudent to avoid cephalosporins as well (since there is a 5% to 10% risk of cross-sensitivity to cephalosporins). When a cephalosporin is indicated, an oral cephalosporin is preferred to a parenteral cephalosporin, since, as with the penicillins, the risk of severe allergic responses is lower with oral therapy. For many infections, *vancomycin* and *erythromycin* are effective and safe alternatives for patients with penicillin allergy.

Rarely, a patient with a history of anaphylaxis may have a life-threatening infection (e.g., enterococcal endocarditis) for which the alternatives to penicillins are ineffective. In these cases, the potential benefits of penicillin therapy outweigh the risks, and treatment should be instituted. To minimize the chances of an anaphylactic reaction, penicillin should be administered according to a desensitization schedule. In this procedure, an initial small dose is followed at 60-minute intervals by progressively larger doses until the full therapeutic dose has been achieved. It should be noted that the desensitization procedure is not without risk. Accordingly, epinephrine and facilities for respiratory support should be immediately available.

## Drug Interactions

*Aminoglycosides.* For some infections, penicillins are used in combination with an aminoglycoside (e.g., gentamicin). By weakening the cell wall, the penicillin facilitates access of the aminoglycoside to its intracellular site of action, thereby increasing bactericidal effects. Unfortunately, when penicillins are present in high concentrations, they interact chemically with aminoglycosides to cause inactivation of the aminoglycoside. Accordingly, *penicillins and aminoglycosides should not be mixed in the same intravenous solution.* Rather, these drugs should be administered separately. Once penicillins have been diluted in body fluids, the potential for inactivation of aminoglycosides is minimal.

*Probenecid.* As noted in the discussion of penicillin elimination, probenecid can delay renal excretion of penicillin, thereby prolonging antibacterial effects.

*Bacteriostatic Antibiotics.* Since penicillins are most effective against actively growing bacteria, concurrent use of a bacteriostatic antibiotic (e.g., tetracycline) could, in theory, reduce the bactericidal effects of the penicillin. However, the clinical significance of such interactions is not known. Moreover, there are infections for which combined therapy with a bacteriostatic agent and a penicillin is indicated. When such combined chemotherapy is employed, the penicillin should be administered a few hours before the bacteriostatic drug to minimize any reduction of penicillin's effects.

## Preparations, Dosage, and Administration

*Preparations and Routes of Administration.* Penicillin G is available as four different salts (sodium, potassium, procaine, and benzathine). These salts differ with respect to routes of administration: *potassium* penicillin G [Pentids, Pfizerpen] is administered PO, IM, and IV; *sodium* penicillin G is administered IM and IV; *benzathine* penicillin G [Bicillin, Permapen] is administered IM and PO; and *procaine* penicillin G [Crysticillin, Pfizerpen-AS, Wycillin] is administered IM. Check to ensure that the penicillin salt to be administered is appropriate for the intended route.

*Dosage.* Dosage of penicillin G is prescribed in units (1 unit equals 0.6 µg). Dosage ranges are summarized in Table 78-2. For any particular patient, the specific dosage will depend on the type and severity of infection. The dosage should be reduced in patients with severe renal impairment.

*Administration.* Oral penicillin G should be taken with a full glass of water at least 1 hour before meals or 2 hours after. Solutions for parenteral administration should be prepared according to the manufacturer's instructions. During IM administration, take care to avoid inadvertent injection into an artery or peripheral nerve.

## Penicillin V

Penicillin V is similar to penicillin G in most respects. These drugs differ primarily in their acid stability: penicillin V is stable in stomach acid, whereas penicillin G is not. As a result, when these two agents are administered orally in comparable doses, penicillin V achieves serum levels that are 2 to 5 times those of penicillin G. Accordingly, penicillin V is preferred to penicillin G for oral therapy. Penicillin V may be taken with meals. Dosages are summarized in Table 78-2. Trade names include Ledercillin VK, Pen-Vee K, and Veetids.

## Penicillinase-Resistant Penicillins (Antistaphylococcal Penicillins)

By altering the penicillin side chain, pharmaceutical chemists have created a group of penicillins that are highly resistant to inactivation by beta-lactamases. In the United States, five such drugs are available: *methicillin*, *nafcillin*, *oxacillin*, *cloxacillin*, and *dicloxacillin*. These agents have a very narrow antimicrobial spectrum and are used only against penicillinase-producing strains of staphylococcus (*Staphylococcus aureus* and *Staphylococcus epidermidis*). Since most strains of staphylococci produce penicillinase, the penicillinase-resistant penicillins are drugs of choice for the majority of staphylococcal infections. It should be noted that these agents should not be used against infections caused by nonpenicillinase-producing staphylococci, since these drugs are less active than penicillin G against these bacteria.

An increasing clinical problem is the emergence of staphylococcal strains referred to as *methicillin resistant*, a term used to indicate *lack of susceptibility to methicillin and all other penicillinase-resistant penicillins*. This resistance to methicillin appears to result from production of altered PBPs to which the penicillinase-resistant penicillins are unable to bind. Currently, vancomycin (alone or combined with rifampin) is the treatment of choice for infections caused by methicillin-resistant staphylococci.

### Methicillin

Methicillin [Staphcillin] is the oldest of the penicillinase-resistant penicillins and is no longer widely employed. In addition to causing allergic reactions typical of all penicillins, methicillin may produce interstitial nephritis, an adverse effect that is usually reversible but sometimes progresses to complete renal failure. Methicillin may be administered IM and IV, but, because of acid lability, cannot be taken by mouth. The structure of methicillin is shown in Figure 78-1. Dosages are summarized in Table 78-2.

### Nafcillin

Nafcillin is usually administered IM or IV. Although the drug is also available in a formulation for oral use, absorption from the gastrointestinal tract is incomplete and erratic; consequently, oral administration is not recommended. Trade names are Nafcil, Nallpen, and Unipen. Dosages are summarized in Table 78-2.

### Oxacillin, Cloxacillin, and Dicloxacillin

These three drugs are similar in structure and pharmacokinetic properties. All are acid stable and available for oral administration; oxacillin may also be administered parenterally (IM and IV). Oral administration of all three drugs may be done with meals. Dosages and trade names are summarized in Table 78-2.

## Broad-Spectrum Penicillins (Aminopenicillins)

The family of broad-spectrum penicillins consists of *ampicillin*, *amoxicillin*, and *bacampicillin*. These drugs have the same antimicrobial spectrum as penicillin G, *plus* increased activity against certain gram-negative bacilli, including *Haemophilus influenzae*, *Escherichia coli*, *Salmonella*, and *Shigella*. This broadened spectrum is due in large part to an increased ability to penetrate the gram-negative cell envelope. All of the broad-spectrum penicillins are readily inactivated by beta-lactamases. Hence,

### TABLE 78-2. DOSAGES FOR PENICILLIN

| Generic Name | Trade Name | Route | Dosing Interval (hr) | Total Daily Dosage[a] | |
| --- | --- | --- | --- | --- | --- |
| | | | | Adults | Children |
| *Narrow-Spectrum Pencillins: Penicillinase-Sensitive* | | | | | |
| Penicillin G | Many trade names | PO | 6 | 1.6–3.2 million units[b] | 40,000–80,000 units/kg[b] |
| | | IM, IV | 4 | 1.2–2.4 million units[b] | 100,000–250,000 units/kg[b] |
| Pencillin V | Ledercillin VK, Veetids, Pen-Vee K, others | PO | 4–6 | 0.5–2 g | 25–50 mg/kg |
| *Narrow-Spectrum Pencillins: Penicillinase-Resistant (Antistaphylococcal Penicillins)* | | | | | |
| Methicillin | Staphcillin | IM, IV | 4–6 | 4–12 gm | 100–200 mg/kg |
| Nafcillin | Nafcil, Nallpen, Unipen | PO | 6 | 2–4 gm | 50–100 mg/kg |
| | | IM, IV | 4–6 | 2–9 gm | 100–200 mg/kg |
| Oxacillin | Bactocill, Prostaphlin | PO | 6 | 2–4 gm | 50–100 mg/kg |
| | | IM, IV | 4–6 | 2–12 gm | 100–200 mg/kg |
| Cloxacillin | Cloxapen, Tegopen | PO | 6 | 2–4 gm | 50–100 mg/kg |
| Dicloxacillin | Dycill, Dynapen, Pathocil | PO | 6 | 1–2 gm | 12.5–25 mg/kg |
| *Broad-Spectrum Pencillins: (Aminopenicillins)* | | | | | |
| Ampicillin | D-Amp, Omnipen, Principen, Polycillin, Totacillin | PO | 6–8 | 2–4 gm | 50–100 mg/kg |
| | | IM, IV | 6–8 | 2–12 gm | 10–200 mg/kg |
| Ampicillin-sulbactam | Unasyn | IM, IV | 6 | 4–8 gm[c] | — |
| Amoxicillin | Amoxil, Biomox, Trimox, Polymox, Wymox | PO | 8 | 0.75–1.5 gm | 20–40 mg/kg |
| Amoxicillin-clavulanate | Augmentin | PO | 8 | 250–500 mg[d] | 20–40 mg/kg[d] |
| Bacampicillin | Spectrobid | PO | 12 | 0.8–1.6 gm | 25–50 mg/kg |
| *Extended-Spectrum Pencillins: (Antipseudomonal Penicillins)* | | | | | |
| Carbenicillin Indanyl | Geocillin | PO | 4–6 | 1.5–3 gm | — |
| | | IM | 6 | 4–8 gm | 50–200 mg/kg |
| | | IV | 4–6 | 30–40 gm | 100–600 mg/kg |
| Ticarcillin | Ticar | IM | 6 | 4 gm | 50–100 mg/kg |
| | | IV | 4–6 | 200–300 mg/kg | 200–300 mg/kg |
| Ticarcillin-clavulanate | Timentin | IV | 4–6 | 200–300 mg/kg[e] | — |
| Mezlocillin | Mezlin | IM | 6 | 4–8 gm | — |
| | | IV | 4–6 | 6–18 gm | 300 mg/kg |
| Piperacillin | Pipracil | IM | 6–12 | 6–8 gm | — |
| | | IV | 4–6 | 12–24 gm | 200–300 mg/kg |
| Piperacillin-tazobactam | Zosyn | IV | 6 | 12 g[f] | — |

[a]Doses vary widely, depending upon the type and severity of infection; doses and dosing intervals presented here may not be appropriate for all patients.
[b]10,000 units = 6 mg.
[c]Dose based on ampicillin content.
[d]Dose based on amoxicillin content.
[e]Dose based on ticarcillin content.
[f]Dose based on piperacillin content.

these drugs are ineffective against most infections caused by *Staphylococcus aureus*.

Properties of individual broad-spectrum penicillins are discussed below. Dosages are summarized in Table 78-2.

## Ampicillin

Ampicillin was the first broad-spectrum penicillin available for clinical use. The agent is a preferred or alternative drug for infections caused by *Streptococcus faecalis*, *Bordetella pertussis*, *Proteus mirabilis*, *E. coli*, *Salmonella*, *Shigella*, and *Haemophilus influenzae*. The drug's most common side effects are rash and diarrhea; both reactions occur more frequently with ampicillin than with any other penicillin. Administration may be parenteral or by mouth. It should be noted, however, that for oral therapy, amoxicillin is preferred (see below). Trade names are D-Amp, Omnipen, Polycillin, Principen, and Totacillin. Routes and usual dosages are summarized in Table 78-2. Dosages must be reduced in patients with renal impairment. As discussed below, ampicillin is available in a fixed-dose combination with sulbactam, an inhibitor of bacterial beta-lactamases.

## Amoxicillin

Amoxicillin is similar to ampicillin in structure and actions. These drugs differ primarily in acid stability, amoxicillin being the more acid resistant. Hence, when the two drugs are administered orally in equivalent doses, blood levels of amoxicillin are greater than those of ampicillin. Accordingly, when oral therapy is indicated, amoxicillin is preferred. Amoxicillin produces less diarrhea than ampicillin, perhaps because less amoxicillin remains unabsorbed in the intestine. Trade names are Amoxil, Biomox, Polymox, Trimox, and Wymox. As discussed below, amoxicillin is also available in a fixed-dose combination with clavulanic acid, an inhibitor of bacterial beta-lactamases. Amoxicillin itself is the most frequently prescribed antibiotic in the United States.

## Bacampicillin

Bacampicillin [Spectrobid] is a prodrug form of ampicillin; once in the body, bacampicillin is rapidly converted to ampicillin, its active form. Bacampicillin is acid stable and administration is oral. The drug may be taken with meals. Because of its resistance to acid, bacampicillin produces blood levels of ampicillin that are 2 times greater than those achieved with equivalent oral doses of ampicillin itself. Despite this difference, bacampicillin offers no clinical advantage over ampicillin or amoxicillin, and is usually more expensive.

# Extended-Spectrum Penicillins (Antipseudomonal Penicillins)

The family of extended-spectrum penicillins consists of four drugs: *ticarcillin*, *carbenicillin indanyl*, *mezlocillin*, and *piperacillin*. The antimicrobial spectrum of these drugs includes organisms that are susceptible to the aminopenicillins plus *Pseudomonas aeruginosa*, *Enterobacter* species, *Proteus* (indole positive), *Bacteroides fragilis*, and many *Klebsiella*. All of the extended-spec-trum penicillins are susceptible to beta-lactamases, and hence are ineffective against most strains of *Staphylococcus aureus*.

The extended-spectrum penicillins are used primarily for infections with *Pseudomonas aeruginosa*. These infections often occur in the immunocompromised host and can be very difficult to eradicate. To increase killing of *Pseudomonas*, an antipseudomonal aminoglycoside (gentamicin, tobramycin, amikacin, netilmicin) is almost always added to the regimen. When these combinations are employed, the penicillin and the aminoglycoside should not be mixed in the same IV solution, since high concentrations of penicillins can inactivate aminoglycosides.

Properties of individual extended-spectrum penicillins are discussed below. Dosages are summarized in Table 78-2.

## Ticarcillin

***Antimicrobial Spectrum and Therapeutic Use.*** Ticarcillin [Ticar] has one of the broadest antimicrobial spectra of all penicillins. However, like other extended-spectrum penicillins, the drug is susceptible to destruction by penicillinase.

The primary indication for ticarcillin is infection caused by *Pseudomonas aeruginosa*. When used against *Pseudomonas*, the drug is usually employed in combination with an aminoglycoside.

***Adverse Effects.*** In addition to promoting the allergic reactions typical of all penicillins, ticarcillin can cause unique adverse effects. Since the drug is administered as the *disodium salt*, and since large intravenous doses are often required, symptoms of *sodium overload* (e.g., congestive heart failure) may develop. Also, ticarcillin interferes with platelet function and can thereby promote *bleeding*.

***Preparations and Administration.*** Ticarcillin is unstable in acid, and hence must be given parenterally (IM or IV). When ticarcillin is used in combination with an aminoglycoside, the two drugs should be administered separately.

As discussed later in the chapter, ticarcillin is available in a fixed-dose combination with clavulanic acid, a beta-lactamase inhibitor. The combination [Timentin] is administered intravenously.

Dosages for patients with normal kidney function are summarized in Table 78-2. Dosages must be reduced in patients with renal impairment.

## Carbenicillin Indanyl

Carbenicillin indanyl [Geocillin] is acid stable and administered orally. Once absorbed, the drug is converted to carbenicillin, its active form. Excretion is renal, and the drug becomes concentrated in urine. Carbenicillin indanyl is indicated only for urinary tract infections caused by *Pseudomonas aeruginosa* or indole-positive *Proteus*. Drug levels at sites outside the urinary tract are too low for clinically significant antibacterial effects. Oral carbenicillin should not be taken with meals.

## Newer Antipseudomonal Penicillins: Mezlocillin and Piperacillin

Mezlocillin [Mezlin] and piperacillin [Pipracil] have broad antimicrobial spectra. However, like other extended-spectrum penicillins, these drugs are penicillinase sensitive. Both drugs are highly active against *Pseudomonas aeruginosa*, and their principal indication is infection with this organism. Like ticarcillin, mezlocillin and piperacillin can cause bleeding secondary to disruption of platelet function. Both drugs are acid labile and must be administered parenterally (IM or IV). The risk of sodium overload with IV mezlocillin or IV piperacillin is much less than with IV ticarcillin. When these drugs are used in combination with an aminoglycoside, they should not be mixed in the same IV solution. Dosages of mezlocillin and piperacillin for patients with normal kidney function are shown in Table 78-2. Dosages of both drugs should be reduced in patients with renal dysfunction. As discussed below, piperacillin is also available in a fixed-dose combination with tazobactam, a beta-lactamase inhibitor.

## Penicillins Combined With a Beta-Lactamase Inhibitor

As their name indicates, beta-lactamase inhibitors are drugs that inhibit bacterial beta-lactamases. By combining a beta-lactamase inhibitor with a penicillinase-sensitive penicillin, we can extend the antimicrobial spectrum of the penicillin. In the United States, three beta-lactamase inhibitors are used: *clavulanic acid*, *tazobactam*, and *sulbactam*. These agents are not dispensed alone. Rather, they are dispensed in fixed-dose combinations with a penicillin. Four such combination products are available:

- Ampicillin + sulbactam = [Unasyn]
- Amoxicillin + clavulanic acid = [Augmentin]
- Ticarcillin + clavulanic acid = [Timentin]
- Piperacillin + tazobactam = [Zosyn]

Since beta-lactamase inhibitors have minimal toxicity, adverse effects seen with the combination products are those caused by the penicillin. Routes of administration and dosages for these products are summarized in Table 78-2.

## KEY POINTS

- Penicillins weaken the bacterial cell wall, causing lysis and death.

- Some bacteria resist penicillins by producing penicillinases (beta-lactamases), enzymes that inactivate penicillins.
- Gram-negative bacteria are resistant to most penicillins because most penicillins are unable to penetrate the gram-negative cell envelope.
- Penicillins are the safest antibiotics available.
- The principal adverse effect of penicillins is production of allergic reactions, which can range in intensity from rash to life-threatening anaphylaxis.
- Patients allergic to one penicillin should be considered cross-allergic to all other penicillins. In addition, they have a 5% to 10% chance of cross-allergy to cephalosporins.
- Vancomycin and erythromycin are safe and effective alternatives to penicillins for patients with penicillin allergy.
- Penicillins are normally eliminated rapidly by the kidney, but can accumulate to harmful levels if renal function is severely impaired.
- The principal differences among the penicillins relate to antibacterial spectrum, stability in stomach acid, and duration of action.
- Penicillin G has a narrow antibacterial spectrum and is unstable in stomach acid.
- *Benzathine* penicillin G is released very slowly following IM injection, and thereby produces prolonged antibacterial effects.
- The penicillinase-resistant penicillins, such as methicillin and nafcillin, are used primarily against penicillinase-producing strains of *Staphylococcus aureus*.
- In contrast to penicillin G, the broad-spectrum penicillins, such as ampicillin and amoxicillin, have useful activity against gram-negative bacilli.
- Extended-spectrum penicillins, such as ticarcillin, are useful against *Pseudomonas aeruginosa*.
- Beta-lactamase inhibitors, such as clavulanic acid, are combined with certain penicillins to increase their activity against beta-lactamase–producing bacteria.
- Penicillins should not be combined with aminoglycosides (e.g., gentamicin) in the same IV solution.

# Summary of Major Nursing Implications*

## Penicillins

Except where indicated otherwise, the implications summarized below apply to all members of the penicillin family.

## Preadministration Assessment

### Therapeutic Goal
Treatment of infections caused by sensitive bacteria.

### Baseline Data
The physician may order tests to identify the infecting organism and its drug sensitivity. Take samples for microbiologic culture prior to initiation of treatment.

In patients with a history of penicillin allergy, a skin test may be performed to determine current allergic status.

### Identifying High-Risk Patients
Penicillins are *contraindicated* for patients with a *history of severe allergic reactions to penicillins, cephalosporins*, or *imipenem*.

## Implementation: Administration

### Routes
Penicillins are administered orally, IV, and IM. Routes for individual agents are summarized in Table 78-2. Before giving a penicillin, check to ensure that the preparation is appropriate for the intended route.

---

*Patient education information is highlighted in color.

## Dosage

Doses for penicillin G are prescribed in units (1 unit equals 0.6 µg). Doses for all other penicillins are prescribed by weight.

Dosages for individual penicillins are summarized in Table 78-2.

## Administration

During IM injection, aspirate to avoid injection into an artery. Take care to avoid injection into a nerve.

Instruct the patient to take oral penicillins with a full glass of water 1 hour before meals or 2 hours after. *Penicillin V, amoxicillin, amoxicillin-clavulanate,* and *bacampicillin* may be taken with meals.

Instruct the patient to complete the prescribed course of treatment, even though symptoms may abate before the full course is over.

Probenecid may be administered with penicillins to delay penicillin excretion.

## Ongoing Evaluation and Interventions

### Evaluating Therapeutic Effects

Monitor the patient for indications of antimicrobial effects (e.g., reduction in fever, pain, or inflammation; improved appetite or sense of well-being).

### Monitoring Kidney Function

Renal impairment can cause penicillins to accumulate to toxic levels; monitoring of kidney function can help avoid injury. Measurement of intake and output is of particular value in patients with kidney disease, in acutely ill patients, and in the very old and very young. Notify the physician if a significant change in intake-output ratio develops.

### Minimizing Adverse Effects

*Allergic Reactions.* Penicillin allergy is common. Rarely, life-threatening anaphylaxis occurs. Interview the patient for a history of penicillin allergy.

For patients with prior allergic responses, a skin test may be ordered to assess current allergic status. Exercise caution: the skin test itself can cause a severe reaction. When skin tests are performed, epinephrine and facilities for respiratory support should be immediately available.

Advise the patient with penicillin allergy to wear some form of identification (e.g., Medic Alert bracelet) to alert emergency health care personnel.

Instruct outpatients to report any signs of an allergic response (e.g., skin rash, itching, hives).

Whenever a parenteral penicillin is used, keep the patient under observation for at least 30 minutes. If anaphylaxis occurs, treatment consists of *epinephrine* (SC, IM, or IV) plus respiratory support.

As a rule, patients with a history of penicillin allergy should not receive penicillins again. If previous reactions have been mild, a cephalosporin (preferably oral) may be an appropriate alternative. However, if severe immediate reactions have occurred, cephalosporins should be avoided too.

Rarely, a patient with a history of anaphylaxis nonetheless requires penicillin. To minimize the risk of a severe reaction, administer penicillin according to a desensitization schedule. Be aware, however, that the procedure does not guarantee that anaphylaxis will not occur. Accordingly, have epinephrine and facilities for respiratory support immediately available.

*Sodium Loading.* High intravenous doses of *sodium penicillin G, carbenicillin,* or *ticarcillin* can produce sodium overload. Exercise caution in patients under sodium restriction (e.g., cardiac patients, those with hypertension). Monitor electrolytes and cardiac status.

*Hyperkalemia.* High doses of intravenous *potassium penicillin G* may cause hyperkalemia, possibly resulting in dysrhythmias or cardiac arrest. Monitor electrolyte and cardiac status.

*Effects Resulting from Incorrect Injection.* Take care to avoid intra-arterial injection or injection into peripheral nerves, since serious injury can result.

### Minimizing Adverse Interactions

*Aminoglycosides.* When present in high concentration, penicillins can inactivate aminoglycosides (e.g., gentamicin). Do not mix penicillins and aminoglycosides in the same IV solution.

*Bacteriostatic Antibiotics.* Suppression of bacterial growth with a bacteriostatic agent can, in theory, decrease the effectiveness of penicillins. When a bacteriostatic drug is combined with a penicillin, administer the penicillin a few hours before the bacteriostatic drug.

# CHAPTER 79

# Drugs That Weaken the Bacterial Cell Wall II: Cephalosporins, Imipenem, Aztreonam, Vancomycin, and Teicoplanin

**Cephalosporins**
**Other Inhibitors of Cell Wall Synthesis**
  Imipenem
  Meropenem
  Aztreonam
  Vancomycin
  Teicoplanin

Like the penicillins, the drugs discussed in this chapter are inhibitors of cell wall synthesis. By disrupting the cell wall, these drugs produce bacterial lysis and death. Most of the chapter focuses on the cephalosporins, our most extensively used antibacterial drugs. With only two exceptions—vancomycin and teicoplanin—the drugs addressed in this chapter belong to the beta-lactam family.

## Cephalosporins

The cephalosporins are beta-lactam antibiotics similar in structure and actions to the penicillins. These drugs are bactericidal, often resistant to beta-lactamases, and active against a broad spectrum of pathogens. Toxicity is low. Because of these attributes, the cephalosporins are popular therapeutic agents and constitute our most widely used group of antibiotics. Hospitals in the United States spend more money on cephalosporins than on all other antibiotics combined.

### Chemistry

All of the cephalosporins are derived from the same nucleus. As shown in Figure 79–1, this nucleus contains a *beta-lactam ring* fused to a second ring. The beta-lactam ring is required for antibacterial activity. Unique properties of individual cephalosporins are determined by additions made to the nucleus at the sites labeled $R_1$, $R_2$, and $R_3$. Structures of three representative cephalosporins are shown.

### Mechanism of Action

The cephalosporins are bactericidal drugs with a mechanism of action like that of the penicillins. These agents bind to penicillin-binding proteins (PBPs) and thereby (1) disrupt cell wall synthesis and (2) activate autolysins (enzymes that cleave bonds in the cell wall). The resultant damage to the cell wall causes death by lysis. Like the penicillins, cephalosporins are most effective against cells undergoing active growth and division.

### Resistance

The principal cause of cephalosporin resistance is production of beta-lactamases, enzymes that cleave the beta-lactam ring of cephalosporins, and thereby render these drugs inactive. The beta-lactamases that act on cephalosporins are sometimes referred to as *cephalosporinases*. Some of the beta-lactamases that act on cephalosporins can also cleave the beta-lactam ring of penicillins.

Not all cephalosporins are equally susceptible to beta-lactamases. Most *first-generation* cephalosporins are destroyed by beta-lactamases; *second-generation* cephalosporins are less sensitive to destruction; and *third-* and *fourth-generation* cephalosporins are highly resistant to beta-lactamases.

In some cases, bacterial resistance results from production of altered PBPs that have a low affinity for cephalosporins. Methicillin-resistant staphylococci produce these unusual PBPs and are resistant to cephalosporins as a result.

### Classification and Antimicrobial Spectra

The cephalosporins have been grouped into four "generations" based on the order of their introduction to clinical use. The generations differ significantly with respect to

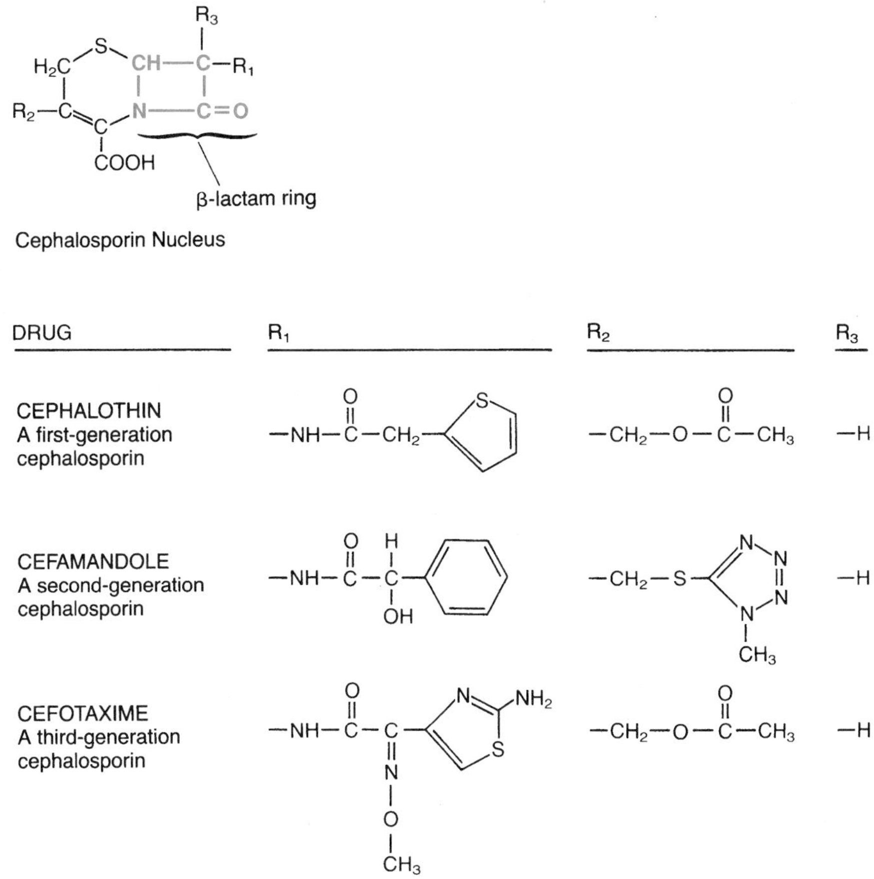

**Figure 79–1. Structural formulas of representative cephalosporins.** The unique structure and pharmacologic properties of individual cephalosporins are determined by additions made to the cephalosporin nucleus at the positions labeled $R_1$, $R_2$, and $R_3$.

antimicrobial spectra and susceptibility to beta-lactamases. In general, *as we progress from first-generation agents to fourth-generation agents, there is (1) increasing activity against gram-negative bacteria and anaerobes, (2) increasing resistance to destruction by beta-lactamases, and (3) increasing ability to reach the cerebrospinal fluid (CSF)*. These differences are summarized in Table 79–1.

*First-generation* cephalosporins, represented by cephalothin, are highly active against gram-positive bacteria. These drugs are the most active of all cephalosporins against staphylococci and nonenterococcal streptococci. However, those staphylococci that are resistant to methicillin are also resistant to first-generation cephalosporins (and to most other cephalosporins as well). The first-generation drugs have only modest activity against gram-negative bacteria. These drugs do not reach effective concentrations in CSF.

*Second-generation* cephalosporins (e.g., cefamandole) have enhanced activity against gram-negative bacteria. The increase is due to a combination of factors: (1) increased affinity for PBPs of gram-negative bacteria, (2) increased ability to penetrate the gram-negative cell envelope, and (3) increased resistance to beta-lactamases produced by gram-negative organisms. However, none of the second-generation agents is active against *Pseudomonas aeruginosa*. These drugs do not reach effective concentrations in CSF.

*Third-generation* cephalosporins (e.g., cefotaxime) have a broad spectrum of antimicrobial activity. Because of increased resistance to beta-lactamases, these agents are considerably more active against gram-negative aerobes than are the first- and second-generation drugs. Some third-generation cephalosporins (e.g., ceftazidime) have important activity against *Pseudomonas aeruginosa*. Others (e.g., cefixime) lack such activity. In contrast to first- and second-generation cephalosporins, the third-generation agents are able to reach clinically effective concentrations in CSF.

Cefepime, the first *fourth-generation* cephalosporin, is highly resistant to beta-lactamases and has a very broad antibacterial spectrum. Activity against *Pseudomonas aeruginosa* is equal to that of ceftazidime. Penetration to the CSF is good.

## Pharmacokinetics

***Absorption.*** Because of poor absorption from the gastrointestinal tract, *most cephalosporins must be administered parenterally* (IM or IV). Of the 26 cephalosporins used in the United States, only 10 can be administered by mouth (see Table 79–2). Of these, only two (cephradine and cefuroxime) can be administered orally and by injection.

***Distribution.*** Cephalosporins distribute well to most body fluids and tissues. Therapeutic concentrations are achieved in pleural, pericardial, and peritoneal fluids.

## TABLE 79-1. MAJOR DIFFERENCES BETWEEN CEPHALOSPORIN GENERATIONS

| Class | Activity against Gram-Negative Bacteria | Resistance to Beta-Lactamases | Distribution to Cerebrospinal Fluid |
|---|---|---|---|
| *First Generation* (e.g., cephalothin) | Low | Low | Poor |
| *Second Generation* (e.g., cefamandole) | Higher | Higher | Poor |
| *Third Generation* (e.g., cefotaxime) | Higher | Higher | Good |
| *Fourth Generation* (e.g., cefepime) | Highest | Highest | Good |

Concentrations in ocular fluids are generally low. Penetration to the CSF by first- and second-generation drugs is unreliable, and these drugs should not be used to treat bacterial meningitis. In contrast, CSF levels achieved with third- and fourth-generation drugs are generally sufficient for bactericidal effects.

**Elimination.** Practically all cephalosporins are eliminated by the *kidney*; excretion is by a combination of glomerular filtration and active tubular secretion. Probenecid can decrease tubular secretion of some cephalosporins, thereby prolonging their effects. In patients with renal insufficiency, dosages of most cephalosporins must be reduced to prevent accumulation to toxic levels.

Two cephalosporins—*cefoperazone* and *ceftriaxone*—are eliminated largely by nonrenal routes. Consequently, there is no need to reduce their dosage in patients with kidney dysfunction.

## Adverse Effects

The cephalosporins are generally well tolerated and constitute one of our safest groups of antimicrobial drugs. Serious adverse effects are rare.

**Allergic Reactions.** Hypersensitivity reactions are the most frequent adverse effects. Maculopapular rash that develops several days after the onset of treatment is most common. Severe, immediate reactions (e.g., bronchospasm, anaphylaxis) are rare. If, during the course of treatment, signs of allergy appear (e.g., urticaria, rash, hypotension, difficulty in breathing), the drug should be discontinued immediately. Anaphylaxis is treated with respiratory support and parenteral epinephrine. Patients with a history of cephalosporin allergy should not be given these drugs.

Because of structural similarities between penicillins and cephalosporins, patients allergic to one type of drug may experience cross-reactivity with the other. In clinical practice, the incidence of cross-reactivity has been low: only about 5% to 10% of penicillin-allergic patients experience an allergic reaction if given a cephalosporin. For patients with *mild* penicillin allergy, cephalosporins can be used with minimal concern about allergic responses. However, because of the potential for fatal anaphylaxis, *cephalosporins should not be given to patients with a history of severe allergic reactions to penicillins.*

**Bleeding.** Five cephalosporins—*cefamandole, cefmetazole, cefoperazone, cefotetan,* and *moxalactam*—cause bleeding tendencies. Two mechanisms are involved: (1) reduction of prothrombin levels (through interference with vitamin K metabolism), and (2) impairment of platelet aggregation. All five drugs share the first mechanism; only *moxalactam* damages platelets. Because moxalactam suppresses hemostasis in two ways, bleeding can be considerably more severe than with the other four drugs. Consequently, moxalactam should be avoided.

Several measures can reduce the risk of hemorrhage. During prolonged treatment, patients should be monitored for prothrombin time, bleeding time, or both. Parenteral vitamin K can correct an abnormal prothrombin time. Patients should be observed for signs of bleeding, and, if bleeding develops, the cephalosporin should be withdrawn. Caution should be exercised during concurrent use of anticoagulants or thrombolytic agents. Because of their antiplatelet effects, aspirin and other nonsteroidal anti-inflammatory drugs should be used with care. Caution should be exercised in patients with a history of bleeding disorders.

**Thrombophlebitis.** Thrombophlebitis may develop during IV infusion. This reaction can be minimized by rotating the infusion site and by administering cephalosporins slowly and in dilute solution. Patients should be observed for phlebitis; if the reaction develops, the infusion site should be changed.

**Other Adverse Effects.** Cephalosporins may cause *pain at sites of IM injection*; patients should be forewarned of this possibility. Rarely, cephalosporins may be the cause of *antibiotic-associated pseudomembranous colitis* due to overgrowth with *Clostridium difficile.* If this suprainfection develops, the cephalosporin should be discontinued and, if necessary, oral vancomycin or metronidazole should be given. *Nephrotoxicity* has been associated with cephalothin.

## TABLE 79-2. PHARMACOKINETIC PROPERTIES OF THE CEPHALOSPORINS

| Class | Drug | Routes of Administration | Major Route of Elimination | Half-life (hr) Normal Renal Function | Half-life (hr) Severe Renal Impairment |
|---|---|---|---|---|---|
| *First Generation* | Cefadroxil | PO | Renal | 1.2-1.3 | 20-25 |
| | Cefazolin | IM, IV | Renal | 1.5-2.2 | 24-50 |
| | Cephalexin | PO | Renal | 0.4-1.0 | 10-20 |
| | Cephalothin | IM, IV | Renal | 0.4-1.0 | 3-18 |
| | Cephapirin | IM, IV | Renal | 0.3-0.7 | 2.4 |
| | Cephradine | PO, IM, IV | Renal | 0.8-2.0 | 8-15 |
| *Second Generation* | Cefaclor | PO | Renal | 0.6-0.9 | 2-3 |
| | Cefamandole | IM, IV | Renal | 0.5-1.0 | 8-14 |
| | Cefmetazole | IV | Renal | 1.2 | — |
| | Cefonicid | IM, IV | Renal | 3.5-4.9 | 17-56 |
| | Ceforanide | IM, IV | Renal | 2.5-3.5 | 25-30 |
| | Cefotetan | IM, IV | Renal | 3.0-4.5 | 13-35 |
| | Cefoxitin | IM, IV | Renal | 0.7-1.0 | 13-22 |
| | Cefprozil | PO | Renal | 1.3 | 5-6 |
| | Cefuroxime | PO, IM, IV | Renal | 1.0-1.9 | 15-22 |
| | Loracarbef | PO | Renal | 1 | 32 |
| *Third Generation* | Cefixime | PO | Renal | 3-4 | 11.5 |
| | Cefoperazone | IM, IV | Biliary | 1.7-2.6 | 2.2 |
| | Cefotaxime | IM, IV | Renal | 0.9-1.4 | 3-11 |
| | Cefpodoxime | PO | Renal | 2-3 | 9.8 |
| | Ceftazidime | IM, IV | Renal | 1.9-2.0 | — |
| | Ceftibuten | PO | Renal | 2 | increased |
| | Ceftizoxime | IM, IV | Renal | 1.1-2.3 | 30 |
| | Ceftriaxone | IM, IV | Hepatic | 5.8-8.7 | 15.7 |
| | Moxalactam | IM, IV | Renal | 1.9-3.5 | 19-30 |
| *Fourth Generation* | Cefepime | IM, IV | Renal | 2 | increased |

## Drug Interactions

***Probenecid.*** Probenecid delays renal excretion of some cephalosporins and can thereby prolong their effects. This is the same interaction that occurs between probenecid and the penicillins.

***Alcohol.*** Five cephalosporins—*cefamandole, cefmetazole, cefoperazone, cefotetan,* and *moxalactam*—induce a state of alcohol intolerance. If a patient receiving one of these drugs were to ingest alcohol, a ***disulfiram-like reaction*** could occur. As discussed in Chapter 36, the disulfiram effect is brought on by accumulation of acetaldehyde and can be extremely dangerous. Accordingly, patients taking these cephalosporins must not consume alcohol in any form.

***Drugs That Promote Bleeding.*** As noted above, five cephalosporins—*cefamandole, cefmetazole, cefoperazone, cefotetan,* and *moxalactam*—promote bleeding tendencies. Caution should be exercised if these drugs are used in combination with other drugs that promote bleeding (nonsteroidal anti-inflammatory drugs, anticoagulants, thrombolytics).

## Therapeutic Uses

The therapeutic role of the cephalosporins is continually evolving as new agents are introduced and as more experience is gained with older ones. Only general recommendations are considered here.

The cephalosporins are broad-spectrum, bactericidal drugs with a high therapeutic index. These agents have been employed widely and successfully against a variety of infections. Cephalosporins can be useful alternatives for patients with mild penicillin allergy.

The four generations of cephalosporins differ significantly in their applications. The *first- and second-generation cephalosporins are rarely drugs of choice for active infections.* In most cases, equally effective and less expensive alternatives are available. In contrast, *the third-generation agents have qualities that make them the preferred therapy for several infections.* The role of fourth-generation agents is yet to be established.

***First-Generation Cephalosporins.*** When a cephalosporin is indicated for a *gram-positive infection,* a first-generation drug should be used; these agents are the most active of the cephalosporins against gram-positive organisms and are less expensive than other cephalosporins. First-generation agents are frequently employed as alternatives to penicillins to treat infections caused by staphylococci or streptococci (except enterococci) in patients with penicillin allergy. However, it is important to note that cephalosporins should be given only to patients with a history of *mild* penicillin allergy—not to those who have experienced severe, immediate hypersensitivity reactions.

The first-generation agents have been employed widely for *prophylaxis against infection in surgical patients.* First-generation agents are preferred to second- or third-generation cephalosporins for surgical prophylaxis because they are as effective as the newer drugs, less expensive, and have a narrower antimicrobial spectrum.

### Second-Generation Cephalosporins.
Specific indications for second-generation cephalosporins are limited. *Cefuroxime*, a prototype for the group, has been used with success against pneumonia caused by *Haemophilus influenzae, Klebsiella*, pneumococci, and staphylococci. Oral cefuroxime is useful for otitis, sinusitis, and respiratory tract infections. *Cefoxitin* is useful for abdominal and pelvic infections.

### Third-Generation Cephalosporins.
Because of their high activity against gram-negative organisms, and because of their ability to penetrate to the CSF, third-generation cephalosporins are drugs of choice for meningitis caused by enteric, gram-negative bacilli. *Ceftazidime* is of special utility for treating meningitis caused by *Pseudomonas aeruginosa. Nosocomial infections* caused by gram-negative bacilli, which are often resistant to first- and second-generation cephalosporins and most other commonly used antibiotics, are appropriate indications for the third-generation drugs. Two third-generation agents—*ceftriaxone* and *cefotaxime*—are drugs of choice for infections caused by *Neisseria gonorrhoeae* (gonorrhea), *Haemophilus influenzae, Proteus, Salmonella, Klebsiella,* and *Serratia*.

The third-generation cephalosporins should not be used routinely. Rather, these agents should be given only when conditions demand, since in this way emergence of organisms resistant to these drugs will be delayed.

## Drug Selection

Over two dozen cephalosporins are currently employed in the United States, and selection among them can be a challenge. Within each generation, the similarities among cephalosporins are more pronounced than the differences. Hence, aside from cost, there is frequently no rational basis for choosing one drug over another. However, there *are* some differences between cephalosporins, and these differences may render one agent preferable to another for treating a specific infection in a specific patient. The differences that do exist can be grouped into three main categories: (1) antimicrobial spectrum, (2) adverse effects, and (3) pharmacokinetics (e.g., route of administration, penetration to the CSF, time course, mode of elimination). Drug selection based on consideration of these differences is discussed below.

### Antimicrobial Spectrum.
A prime rule of antimicrobial therapy is to match the drug with the bug: the drug should be active against known or suspected pathogens, but its spectrum should be no broader than required. When a cephalosporin is appropriate, we should select from among those drugs known to have good activity against the causative pathogen. The third- and fourth-generation agents, with their very broad antimicrobial spectra, should be avoided in situations where a narrower spectrum, first- or second-generation drug would suffice.

For some infections, one cephalosporin may be decidedly more effective than all others, and should be selected on this basis. For example, *ceftazidime* (a third-generation drug) is the most effective of all cephalosporins against *Pseudomonas aeruginosa* and is clearly the preferred cephalosporin for treating infections caused by this microbe.

### Adverse Effects.
Although most cephalosporins produce the same spectrum of adverse effects, a few agents can cause unique reactions. In particular, five cephalosporins—*cefamandole, cefmetazole, cefoperazone, cefotetan,* and *moxalactam*—produce bleeding tendencies and intolerance to alcohol. When an equally effective alternative is available, it would be prudent to avoid these five drugs.

### Pharmacokinetics.
Four pharmacokinetic properties are of interest: (1) route of administration, (2) duration of action, (3) distribution to CSF, and (4) route of elimination. The relationship of these properties to drug selection is discussed below.

*Route of Administration.* Nine cephalosporins can be administered orally. These drugs may be preferred for treating mild to moderate infections in patients who can't tolerate parenteral agents.

*Duration of Action.* In patients with normal renal function, the half-lives of the cephalosporins range from about 30 minutes to 9 hours (see Table 79-2). Because they require fewer administrations per day, drugs with a long half-life are frequently preferred to those with a short half-life. The drugs with the longest half-lives in each generation are as follows: first generation, *cefazolin* (1.5 to 2 hours); second generation, *cefonicid* (4.5 hours); and third generation, *ceftriaxone* (6 to 9 hours).

*Distribution to Cerebrospinal Fluid.* Only the third- and fourth-generation agents produce CSF levels sufficient for bactericidal effects. Hence, for treatment of meningitis caused by susceptible organisms, these drugs are preferred over first- and second-generation cephalosporins. One third-generation drug—*cefoperazone*—is notable for its *inability* to achieve therapeutic concentrations in the CSF.

*Route of Elimination.* Most cephalosporins are eliminated by the kidneys and, if dosage is not carefully adjusted, may accumulate to toxic levels in patients with kidney dysfunction. Only two agents—*cefoperazone* and *ceftriaxone*—are eliminated in significant amounts by nonrenal routes, and hence can be used with relative safety in patients with renal impairment.

## Dosage and Administration

### Routes of Administration.
The majority of cephalosporins cannot be absorbed from the gastrointestinal tract and must therefore be administered parenterally (IM or IV). As shown in Table 79-3, only 10 cephalosporins can be given orally. Two drugs—*cephradine* and *cefuroxime*—can be administered both orally and by injection.

### Dosage.
Dosages are summarized in Table 79-3. For most cephalosporins (*cefoperazone* and *ceftriaxone* excepted), the dosage should be reduced in patients with significant renal impairment.

### Administration.
*Oral.* If oral cephalosporins produce nausea, administration with food can reduce the response. Oral suspensions should be stored under refrigeration.

*Intramuscular.* Intramuscular injections should be made deep into a large muscle. Intramuscular injection of cephalosporins is frequently painful; the patient should be forewarned. The injection site should be checked for induration, tenderness, and redness; the physician should be informed if these reactions occur.

*Intravenous.* For intravenous therapy, cephalosporins may be administered by three techniques: (1) bolus injection, (2) slow injection (over a 3- to 5-minute period), and (3) continuous infusion. The physician's order should state which method is to be used. If there is uncertainty as to method of administration, clarification should be requested. Solutions for parenteral adminis-

## TABLE 79-3. CEPHALOSPORIN DOSAGES

| Drug | Trade Name | Route | Dosing Interval (hr) | Total Daily Dosage* Adults (gm) | Total Daily Dosage* Children (mg/kg) |
|---|---|---|---|---|---|
| *First Generation* | | | | | |
| Cefadroxil | Duricef | PO | 12, 24 | 1-2 | 30 |
| Cefazolin | Ancef, Kefzol, Zolicef | IM, IV | 6, 8 | 2-12 | 80-160 |
| Cephalexin | Biocef, Keflex, Keftab | PO | 6 | 1-4 | 25-50 |
| Cephalothin | Keflin | IM, IV | 4, 6 | 2-12 | 80-160 |
| Cephapirin | Cefadyl | IM, IV | 4, 6 | 2-12 | 40-80 |
| Cephradine | Velosef | IM, IV | 4, 6 | 2-12 | 50-100 |
| | | PO | 6 | 1-4 | 25-50 |
| *Second Generation* | | | | | |
| Cefaclor | Ceclor | PO | 8 | 0.75-1.5 | 20-40 |
| Cefamandole | Mandol | IM, IV | 4, 8 | 1.5-12 | 50-150 |
| Cefmetazole | Zefazone | IV | 6, 12 | 4-8 | — |
| Cefonicid | Monocid | IM, IV | 24 | 0.5-2 | — |
| Ceforanide | Precef | IM, IV | 12 | 1-2 | 20-40 |
| Cefotetan | Cefotan | IM, IV | 12 | 2-6 | — |
| Cefoxitin | Mefoxin | IM, IV | 4, 8 | 3-12 | 80-160 |
| Cefprozil | Cefzil | PO | 12, 24 | 05.-1 | 30 |
| Cefuroxime | Ceftin, Kefurox, Zinacef | IM, IV | 8 | 2.25-9 | 50-100 |
| | | PO | 12 | 0.5-1 | 250-500 |
| Loracarbef | Lorabid | PO | 12, 24 | 0.5-1 | 30 |
| *Third Generation* | | | | | |
| Cefixime | Suprax | PO | 24 | 0.4 | 8 |
| Cefoperazone | Cefobid | IM, IV | 6, 8 | 2-12 | 100-150 |
| Cefotaxime | Claforan | IM, IV | 4, 8 | 2-12 | 100-200 |
| Cefpodoxime | Vantin | PO | 12 | 0.2-0.4 | 10 |
| Ceftazidime | Ceptaz, Fortaz, Tazidime, Tazicef | IM, IV | 8, 12 | 0.5-6 | 90-150 |
| Ceftibuten | Cedax | PO | 24 | 0.4 | 9 |
| Ceftizoxime | Cefizox | IM, IV | 6, 12 | 2-12 | 150-200 |
| Ceftriaxone | Rocephin | IM, IV | 12, 24 | 1-4 | 50-100 |
| Moxalactam | Moxam | IM, IV | 8 | 2-12 | 150-200 |
| *Fourth Generation* | | | | | |
| Cefepime | Maxipime | IM, IV | 12 | 1-2 | — |

*With the exceptions of cefoperazone and ceftriaxone, cephalosporins require a reduction of dosage for patients with severe kidney dysfunction

tration should be prepared according to the manufacturer's recommendations.

# Other Inhibitors of Cell Wall Synthesis

## Imipenem

Imipenem [Primaxin], a relatively new beta-lactam antibiotic, has the broadest antimicrobial spectrum of any drug. Because of its broad spectrum, imipenem may be of special use for treating mixed infections in which anaerobes, *Staphylococcus aureus*, and gram-negative bacilli may all be involved. Imipenem is dispensed in fixed-dose combination with cilastatin, a compound that inhibits destruction of imipenem by renal enzymes.

*Chemistry.* Imipenem belongs to a new class of beta-lactam antibiotics known as *carbapenems*. At this time, imipenem is the only carbapenem employed clinically. The structure of imipenem is shown in Figure 79-2.

*Mechanism of Action.* Imipenem binds to two penicillin-binding proteins (PBP1 and PBP2), causing weakening of the bacterial cell wall with subsequent lysis and death. Antimicrobial effects are enhanced by the drug's resistance to practically all beta-lactamases, and by its ability to penetrate the gram-negative cell envelope.

*Antimicrobial Spectrum.* Imipenem is active against most bacterial pathogens, including organisms resistant to other antibiotics. The drug is highly active against gram-

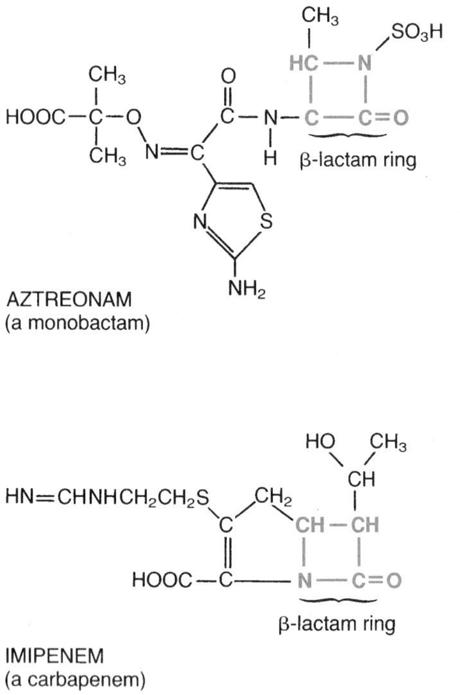

**AZTREONAM**
(a monobactam)

**IMIPENEM**
(a carbapenem)

**Figure 79–2. Miscellaneous beta-lactam antibiotics.**

positive cocci and most gram-negative cocci and bacilli. In addition, imipenem is the most effective beta-lactam antibiotic for use against anaerobic bacteria.

*Pharmacokinetics.* Imipenem is not absorbed from the gastrointestinal tract and hence must be given parenterally (IV or IM). The drug is well distributed to body fluids and tissues. Imipenem penetrates the meninges to produce therapeutic concentrations in the CSF.

Elimination is primarily renal. When employed alone, imipenem is inactivated by an enzyme (dipeptidase) present in the kidney; as a result, drug levels in urine are low. To increase urinary concentrations, imipenem is administered in combination with *cilastatin*, a dipeptidase inhibitor. When the combination is used, about 70% of imipenem is excreted unchanged in the urine.

*Adverse Effects.* Imipenem is generally well tolerated. *Gastrointestinal effects* (nausea, vomiting, diarrhea) are most common. *Hypersensitivity reactions* (rashes, pruritus, drug fever) have occurred; patients allergic to other beta-lactam antibiotics may have an allergic reaction if given imipenem. *Suprainfections* with bacteria or fungi develop in about 4% of patients. Rarely, *seizures* have occurred.

*Therapeutic Use.* Because of its broad spectrum and low toxicity, imipenem has been used widely. The drug has proved effective for serious infections caused by gram-positive cocci, gram-negative cocci, gram-negative bacilli, and anaerobic bacteria. This broad antimicrobial spectrum gives imipenem special utility for chemotherapy of mixed infections (e.g., simultaneous infection with aerobic and anaerobic bacteria). When imipenem has been given alone to treat infections caused by *Pseudomonas aerugi-*

*nosa*, resistant organisms have emerged. Consequently, imipenem should be combined with another antipseudomonal drug for use against this microbe.

*Preparations, Dosage, and Administration.* Imipenem is dispensed in 1:1 fixed-dose combinations with cilastatin. The combination products are marketed under the trade name Primaxin. Two formulations are available: Primaxin I.V. and Primaxin I.M., for intravenous and intramuscular use, respectively. These products are dispensed in powder form and must be reconstituted in accord with the manufacturer's instructions. The usual adult dosage (based on imipenem content) is 250 to 500 mg every 6 hours. Dosage should be reduced in patients with renal impairment.

## Meropenem

*Actions and Uses.* Meropenem [Merrem IV] is an expensive new intravenous antibiotic similar to imipenem-cilastatin. The drug is active against most clinically important gram-positive and gram-negative aerobes and anaerobes. Approved indications are (1) bacterial meningitis in children age 3 months or older and (2) complicated intra-abdominal infections in children and adults. Meropenem may prove especially useful for nosocomial infections caused by organisms resistant to other antibiotics.

*Pharmacokinetics.* Meropenem is administered IV and distributes to all body fluids and tissues. The drug has a plasma half-life of 1 hour and is eliminated primarily unchanged in the urine. In contrast to imipenem, meropenem is not degraded by renal dipeptidases, and hence does not need to be given with cilastatin.

*Adverse Effects.* Like other beta-lactam antibiotics, meropenem is generally well tolerated. Principal adverse effects are rashes, diarrhea, nausea, and vomiting. As with imipenem, seizures occur rarely. The risk of seizures is highest in patients with CNS disorders (e.g., brain lesions, history of seizures) and bacterial meningitis.

*Preparations, Dosage, and Administration.* Meropenem [Merrem IV] is dispensed in powdered form to be reconstituted for IV administration. Depending on the volume employed, the drug may be (1) infused over 15 to 30 minutes or (2) injected as a bolus over 3 to 5 minutes. The dosage for adults is 1 g every 8 hours. The dosage for pediatric patients is 20 mg/kg every 8 hours (for intra-abdominal infections) and 40 mg/kg every 8 hours (for bacterial meningitis). Adult and pediatric dosages must be reduced for patients with significant renal impairment (creatinine clearance <50 ml/min).

## Aztreonam

*Chemistry.* Aztreonam [Azactam] belongs to a new class of beta-lactam antibiotics known as *monobactams*. These agents contain a beta-lactam ring, but the ring is not fused with a second ring. The structure of aztreonam is shown in Figure 79–2.

*Mechanism of Action.* Aztreonam binds to PBP3. Hence, like most beta-lactam antibiotics, the drug inhibits bacterial cell wall synthesis, ultimately causing the cell to rupture and die. The drug does not bind to PBPs produced by anaerobes or gram-positive bacteria.

*Antimicrobial Spectrum and Therapeutic Use.* Aztreonam has a narrow antimicrobial spectrum: the drug is active only against gram-negative aerobic bacteria. Susceptible organisms include *Neisseria* species, *Haemophilus influenzae*, *Pseudomonas aeruginosa*, and Enterobacteriaceae (e.g., *E. coli*, *Klebsiella*, *Proteus*, *Serratia*, *Salmonella*, *Shigella*). Aztreonam is highly resistant to beta-lactamases, and therefore is active against many gram-negative aerobes that produce these enzymes. The drug is not active against gram-positive bacteria and anaerobes.

*Pharmacokinetics.* Aztreonam is not absorbed from the gastrointestinal tract and must therefore be administered parenterally (IM or IV). Once in the bloodstream, the drug distributes widely to most body fluids and tissues. Therapeutic concentrations can be achieved in the CSF. Aztreonam is eliminated by the kidneys, primarily as the unchanged drug.

*Adverse Effects.* Aztreonam is generally well tolerated. Adverse effects are like those of other beta-lactam antibiotics. The most common side effects are pain and thrombophlebitis at sites of injection. Because aztreonam differs greatly in structure from penicillins and cephalosporins, there is little cross-allergenicity between these drugs. Hence, it appears that aztreonam is safe for patients with allergies to other beta-lactam antibiotics.

*Preparations, Dosage, and Administration.* Aztreonam [Azactam] is dispensed in powdered form to be reconstituted for IM or IV administration. The usual adult dosage is 1 to 2 gm every 8 to 12 hours. Dosage should be reduced in patients with kidney dysfunction.

## Vancomycin

Vancomycin [Lyphocin, Vancoled, Vancocin] is a potentially toxic drug used only for serious infections. Principal indications are antibiotic-associated pseudomembranous colitis (caused by *Clostridium difficile*), infection with methicillin-resistant *Staphylococcus aureus*, and treatment of serious infections by susceptible organisms in patients allergic to penicillins. Unlike most other drugs discussed in this chapter, vancomycin does not contain a beta-lactam ring.

*Mechanism of Action.* Like the other drugs discussed in this chapter, vancomycin inhibits cell wall synthesis and thereby promotes bacterial lysis and death. However, in contrast to the beta-lactam antibiotics, vancomycin does not interact with penicillin-binding proteins. Instead, vancomycin disrupts the cell wall by binding to molecules that serve as precursors for cell wall biosynthesis.

*Antimicrobial Spectrum.* Vancomycin is active only against gram-positive bacteria. The drug is especially active against *Staphylococcus aureus* and *Staph. epidermidis*, including strains of both species that are methicillin resistant. Other susceptible organisms include streptococci and *Clostridium difficile*.

*Pharmacokinetics.* Absorption from the gastrointestinal tract is poor. Hence, for most infections, vancomycin is given parenterally (by slow intravenous infusion). Oral administration is employed only for infections of the intestine.

Vancomycin is well distributed to most body fluids and tissues. Although the drug enters the CSF, levels may be insufficient to treat meningitis. Hence, if meningeal infection fails to respond to IV therapy, concurrent intrathecal administration may be required.

Vancomycin is eliminated unchanged by the kidneys. In patients with kidney dysfunction, dosage must be reduced.

*Therapeutic Use.* Vancomycin should be reserved for treatment of serious infections. This agent is the drug of choice for infections caused by methicillin-resistant *Staph. aureus* or *Staph. epidermidis*; most strains of these bacteria remain vancomycin sensitive. Oral vancomycin is the treatment of choice for antibiotic-associated pseudomembranous colitis caused by suprainfection with *Clostridium difficile*. The drug is also employed as an alternative to penicillins and cephalosporins to treat severe infections (e.g., staphylococcal and streptococcal endocarditis) in patients allergic to the beta-lactam antibiotics.

*Adverse Effects.* The most serious adverse effect is *ototoxicity*. Although hearing impairment is often reversible, permanent impairment can occur. Ototoxicity is most likely when plasma levels of vancomycin exceed 30 µg/ml. The risk of hearing loss is increased by high dosage, prolonged treatment, renal impairment, and concurrent use of other ototoxic drugs (e.g., aminoglycosides, ethacrynic acid).

Rapid infusion of vancomycin can cause a variety of disturbing effects, including rashes, flushing, tachycardia, and hypotension. These effects, which are thought to result from release of histamine, can be avoided by infusing vancomycin slowly (over 60 minutes or more).

*Thrombophlebitis* is common. This reaction can be minimized by administering vancomycin in dilute solution and by changing the infusion site frequently.

Patients who are allergic to penicillins are not cross-allergic to vancomycin. Accordingly, vancomycin is an alternative to these beta-lactam antibiotics in patients allergic to them.

*Preparations, Dosage, and Administration.* For treatment of *systemic infection*, vancomycin is administered by intermittent infusion over 60 minutes or more. The usual adult dosage is 2 gm/day administered in divided doses at 6- or 12-hour intervals. The dosage for children is 44 mg/kg/day administered in divided doses at 6- or 12-hour intervals. In patients with renal impairment, dosages must be reduced. Serum drug levels should be monitored to ensure that dosage is appropriate. Blood for measuring drug levels should be drawn 1.5 to 2.5 hours after completing the IV infusion. Peak levels of 30 to 40 µg/ml are generally acceptable.

For treatment of *antibiotic-associated pseudomembranous colitis*, vancomycin is given orally. The adult dosage is 125 to 500 mg every 6 hours. The dosage for children is 11 mg/kg every 6 hours. Since vancomycin is not absorbed from the gastrointestinal tract, there is no need to decrease oral doses in patients with renal impairment.

### Teicoplanin

*Chemistry and Actions.* Teicoplanin [Targocid] is an investigational drug similar in actions and structure to vancomycin. Both drugs disrupt cell wall synthesis to cause lysis and death, and both are active only against gram-positive bacteria. Sensitive organisms include methicillin-resistant *Staph. aureus*, enterococci, and *Clostridium difficile*. Like vancomycin—and unlike the other drugs discussed in the chapter—teicoplanin does not have a beta-lactam ring.

*Pharmacokinetics.* The kinetics of teicoplanin are much like those of vancomycin—except that teicoplanin can be administered IM as well as IV. Neither drug is absorbed from the GI tract, so oral administration is reserved for infections of the intestine. Following parenteral administration, teicoplanin is well distributed to tissues and most body fluids, but not to the CSF. Teicoplanin has a long half-life (up to 100 hours) and is eliminated intact by the kidneys.

*Adverse Effects.* Teicoplanin is largely devoid of adverse effects. In contrast to vancomycin, teicoplanin does not promote histamine release, and hence does not cause infusion-related reactions (flushing, tachycardia, hypotension). Ototoxicity may occur but is rare. Not surprisingly, patients allergic to beta-lactam antibiotics are *not* cross-allergic to teicoplanin.

*Therapeutic Use.* Teicoplanin has been used with success against an array of infections, but its therapeutic niche is yet to be established. Potential applications include osteomyelitis and endocarditis caused by methicillin-resistant staphylococci, streptococci, and enterococci. Combining the drug with gentamicin can increase bactericidal actions.

Teicoplanin represents a safe and effective alternative to vancomycin, and offers several advantages. These are (1) the option of IM administration, (2) shorter infusion time with IV administration (30 minutes versus 60), (3) once-a-day dosing, and (4) the absence of serious adverse effects, including infusion-related reactions.

***Dosage and Administration.*** Teicoplanin may be given parenterally or orally. Parenteral administration is done by IM injection, IV injection, or 30-minute IV infusion. For parenteral therapy, the usual adult dosage is 6 mg/kg initially followed by 3 mg/kg every 24 hours. Dosage should be reduced in patients with renal impairment. As noted above, oral therapy is used only for intestinal infections.

## KEY POINTS

- Cephalosporins are beta-lactam antibiotics that weaken the bacterial cell wall, causing lysis and death.
- The major cause of cephalosporin resistance is production of beta-lactamases.
- Cephalosporins can be grouped into four "generations." As we progress from first- to fourth-generation drugs, there is (1) increasing activity against gram-negative bacteria, (2) increasing resistance to destruction by beta-lactamases, and (3) increasing ability to reach CSF.

- The majority of cephalosporins must be administered parenterally; only 10 of the 24 available in the United States can be administered orally.
- Except for cefoperazone and ceftriaxone, all cephalosporins are eliminated by the kidneys, and therefore must be given in reduced dosage in patients with renal insufficiency.
- The most common adverse effects of cephalosporins are allergic reactions. Patients allergic to penicillins have a 5% to 10% risk of cross-reactivity with cephalosporins.
- Five cephalosporins—cefamandole, cefmetazole, cefoperazone, cefotetan, and moxalactam—cause bleeding tendencies and disulfiram-like reactions.
- Imipenem, a beta-lactam antibiotic, has the broadest antimicrobial spectrum of any drug.
- Vancomycin is an important but potentially toxic drug generally reserved for (1) antibiotic-associated pseudomembranous colitis (caused by *C. difficile*), (2) infections with methicillin-resistant *Staph. aureus*, and (3) serious infections by susceptible organisms in patients allergic to penicillins.

# Summary of Major Nursing Implications*

## Cephalosporins

Except where indicated, the implications summarized below apply to all members of the cephalosporin family.

## Preadministration Assessment

### Therapeutic Goal
Treatment of infections caused by susceptible organisms.

### Baseline Data
The physician may order tests to determine the identity and drug sensitivity of the infecting organism. Take samples for culture prior to initiating treatment.

### Identifying High-Risk Patients
Cephalosporins are *contraindicated* for patients with a *history of allergic reactions to cephalosporins or severe allergic reactions to penicillins.*

## Implementation: Administration

### Routes
Most cephalosporins are administered parenterally (IM or IV). Ten are administered orally; of these, two—*cephradine* and *cefuroxime*—can also be administered parenter-

ally. Routes for individual cephalosporins are given in Table 79-3.

### Dosage
Dosages are summarized in Table 79-3. Dosages for all cephalosporins except cefoperazone and ceftriaxone should be reduced in patients with significant renal impairment.

### Administration
***Oral.*** Advise the patient to take oral cephalosporins with food if gastric upset occurs. Instruct the patient to refrigerate oral suspensions.

Instruct the patient to complete the prescribed course of therapy even though symptoms may abate before the full course is over.

***Intramuscular.*** Make IM injections deep into a large muscle. These injections are frequently painful; forewarn the patient. Check the injection site for induration, tenderness, and redness; notify the physician if these occur.

***Intravenous.*** Techniques for IV administration are bolus injection, slow injection (over 3 to 5 minutes), and continuous infusion. The physician's order should specify which method to use; request clarification if the order is unclear.

## Ongoing Evaluation and Interventions

### Evaluating Therapeutic Effects
Monitor for indications of antimicrobial effects (e.g., reduction in fever, pain, or inflammation; improved appetite or sense of well-being).

---

*Patient education information is highlighted in color.

## Minimizing Adverse Effects

*Allergic Reactions.* Hypersensitivity reactions are relatively common; life-threatening anaphylaxis has occurred. Avoid cephalosporins in patients with a history of cephalosporin allergy or *severe* penicillin allergy. If penicillin allergy is *mild*, cephalosporins can be used with relative safety. Instruct the patient to report any signs of allergy (e.g., skin rash, itching, hives). If anaphylaxis occurs, administer parenteral epinephrine and provide respiratory support.

*Bleeding. Cefamandole, cefmetazole, cefoperazone, cefotetan,* and *moxalactam* can promote bleeding. Severe bleeding is most likely with moxalactam; this drug should be avoided. Monitor prothrombin time, bleeding time, or both. Parenteral vitamin K can correct abnormal prothrombin time. Observe patients for signs of bleeding; if bleeding develops, discontinue drug use. Exercise caution in patients with a history of bleeding disorders and in patients receiving drugs that can interfere with hemostasis (aspirin and other nonsteroidal anti-inflammatory drugs, anticoagulants, thrombolytics).

*Thrombophlebitis.* Intravenous cephalosporins may cause thrombophlebitis. To minimize this reaction, rotate the injection site and inject cephalosporins slowly and in dilute solution. Observe the patient for phlebitis; change the infusion site if phlebitis develops.

*Antibiotic-Associated Pseudomembranous Colitis.* Colitis may develop, especially with use of broad-spectrum cephalosporins. Notify the physician if diarrhea develops (a possible indication of colitis). If antibiotic-associated pseudomembranous colitis is diagnosed, discontinue the cephalosporin. Oral vancomycin or metronidazole may be needed.

## Minimizing Adverse Interactions

*Alcohol. Cefamandole, cefmetazole, cefoperazone, cefotetan,* and *moxalactam* can cause alcohol intolerance, causing a serious disulfiram-like reaction if alcohol is consumed. Inform patients about alcohol intolerance and warn them not to drink alcoholic beverages.

*Drugs That Promote Bleeding.* Drugs that interfere with hemostasis—*aspirin and other nonsteroidal anti-inflammatory drugs, anticoagulants, thrombolytics*—can intensify bleeding tendencies caused by *Cefamandole, cefmetazole, cefoperazone, cefotetan,* and *moxalactam.* These drugs should not be used in combination.

# CHAPTER 80

# Bacteriostatic Inhibitors of Protein Synthesis: Tetracyclines, Macrolides, Clindamycin, Chloramphenicol, and Spectinomycin

**Tetracyclines**
**Macrolides**
   Erythromycin
   Clarithromycin
   Azithromycin
   Dirithromycin

**Clindamycin**
**Chloramphenicol**
**Spectinomycin**

All of the drugs discussed in this chapter are inhibitors of bacterial protein synthesis. Unlike the aminoglycosides, whose effects on protein synthesis produce microbial death, the drugs considered here are bacteriostatic. That is, these agents suppress bacterial growth and replication but do not produce outright kill. In general, the drugs presented here are second-line agents, primarily because of emerging resistance or toxicity.

## Tetracyclines

The tetracyclines are *broad-spectrum* antibiotics. Six members of the family are available for systemic therapy in the United States. All six—tetracycline, oxytetracycline, demeclocycline, methacycline, doxycycline, and minocycline—are similar in structure, antimicrobial actions, and adverse effects. Principal differences among the tetracyclines are pharmacokinetic. Since the similarities among these drugs are more pronounced than the differences, we will discuss the tetracyclines as a group, rather than focusing on a prototype. Unique properties of individual tetracyclines are indicated where appropriate.

### Mechanism of Action

The tetracyclines suppress bacterial growth by inhibiting protein synthesis. These drugs block protein synthesis by binding to the 30S ribosomal subunit, thereby inhibiting binding of transfer RNA to the messenger RNA–ribosome complex. As a result, addition of amino acids to the growing peptide chain is prevented. At the concen-

trations achieved clinically, the tetracyclines are bacteriostatic.

Selective toxicity of the tetracyclines is determined in large part by the relative inability of these drugs to cross mammalian cell membranes. In order to influence protein synthesis, tetracyclines must first gain access to the cell interior. Entry into bacteria is accomplished by way of an energy-dependent transport process. Mammalian cells lack such a transport system, and therefore do not actively accumulate the drug. Consequently, although tetracyclines are inherently capable of inhibiting protein synthesis in mammalian cells, drug levels within host cells remain too low to suppress protein production.

### Microbial Resistance

Bacterial resistance to the tetracyclines results from reduced drug accumulation, increased drug inactivation, and decreased access of drug to ribosomes caused by the presence of ribosome protection proteins. Regarding reduced accumulation, two mechanisms are involved: (1) decreased uptake and (2) acquisition of the ability to actively extrude tetracyclines.

### Antimicrobial Spectrum

The tetracyclines are broad-spectrum antibiotics. These agents are active against a wide variety of gram-positive and gram-negative bacteria. Sensitive organisms include *Rickettsia*, spirochetes, *Brucella*, *Chlamydia*, *Mycoplasma*, *Helicobacter pylori*, and *Vibrio cholerae*.

### Therapeutic Uses

*Treatment of Infectious Diseases.* Extensive use of tetracyclines has resulted in increasing bacterial resistance. Because of microbial resistance, and because antibiotics with greater selectivity and less toxicity are now available, use of tetracyclines has declined. Today, tetracyclines are rarely drugs of first choice. Disorders for which tetracyclines *are* considered first-line drugs include (1) rickettsial diseases (e.g., Rocky Mountain spotted fever, typhus fever, Q fever); (2) infections caused by *Chlamydia trachomatis* (trachoma, lymphogranuloma venereum, urethritis, cervicitis); (3) brucellosis; (4) cholera; (5) pneumonia caused by *Mycoplasma pneumoniae*; (6) Lyme disease; and (7) gastric infection with *H. pylori.*

**Treatment of Acne.** Tetracyclines are used topically and orally for severe acne vulgaris. Beneficial effects derive from suppressing the growth and metabolic activity of *Propionibacterium acnes*, causing the organism to reduce secretion of inflammatory chemicals. Oral doses of tetracyclines employed in acne are relatively low. As a result, adverse effects are minimal. Treatment of acne is discussed further in Chapter 98 (Drugs for the Skin).

**Peptic Ulcer Disease.** *Helicobacter pylori*, a bacterium that lives in the stomach, is a major contributing factor to peptic ulcer disease. Tetracyclines, in combination with metronidazole and bismuth subsalicylate, are the current treatment of choice for eradicating this organism. The role of *H. pylori* in ulcer formation is discussed in Chapter 71 (Drugs for Peptic Ulcer Disease).

**Rheumatoid Arthritis.** Minocycline can reduce symptoms in patients with rheumatoid arthritis, suggesting a possible infectious component to the disease.

## Pharmacokinetics

Individual tetracyclines differ significantly in their pharmacokinetic properties. Of particular significance are differences in half-life and route of elimination. Also of clinical importance are differences in the extent to which food decreases absorption. The pharmacokinetic properties of individual tetracyclines are summarized in Table 80-1.

**Duration of Action.** The tetracyclines can be divided into three groups: short acting, intermediate acting, and long acting (see Table 80-1). These differences in time course are related to differences in lipid solubility: the short-acting tetracyclines (tetracycline, oxytetracycline) have relatively low lipid solubility, whereas the long-acting agents (doxycycline, minocycline) have relatively high lipid solubility.

**Absorption.** All of the tetracyclines are orally effective, although the extent of absorption differs among individual agents (see Table 80-1). Absorption of the short-acting and intermediate-acting tetracyclines is reduced in the presence of food. In contrast, food does not reduce absorption of the long-acting agents.

The tetracyclines form insoluble chelates with calcium, iron, magnesium, aluminum, and zinc. Formation of such chelates decreases absorption. Accordingly, *tetracyclines should not be administered together with (1) calcium supplements, (2) milk products (because they contain calcium), (3) iron supplements, (4) magnesium-containing laxatives,* and *(5) most antacids* (because they contain magnesium, aluminum, or both).

**Distribution.** Tetracyclines are widely distributed to most tissues and body fluids. However, penetration to the cerebrospinal fluid (CSF) is poor, and levels achieved in the CSF are inadequate for treating meningeal infections. Tetracyclines readily cross the placenta and enter the fetal circulation.

**Elimination.** Tetracyclines are eliminated via renal and hepatic routes. All tetracyclines are excreted by the liver into the bile. After the bile enters the intestine, most tetracyclines are reabsorbed.

Ultimate elimination of short-acting and intermediate-acting tetracyclines is in the urine, largely as the unchanged drug (see Table 80-1). Because these agents undergo renal excretion, they can accumulate to toxic levels if kidney function fails. Consequently, *short-acting and intermediate-acting tetracyclines should not be administered to patients with renal failure.*

The long-acting tetracyclines are eliminated by the liver, primarily as metabolites. Because these agents are excreted by the liver, their half-lives are unaffected by kidney dysfunction. Accordingly, *the long-acting agents are drugs of choice for tetracycline-responsive infections in patients with renal impairment.*

## TABLE 80-1. PHARMACOKINETIC PROPERTIES OF THE TETRACYCLINES

| Class | Drug | Lipid Solubility | Percent of Oral Dose Absorbed | Effect of Food on Absorption | Principal Route of Elimination | Half-life Normal (hr) | Half-life Anuric (hr) |
|---|---|---|---|---|---|---|---|
| *Short Acting* | Tetracycline | Low | 76 | Decrease | Renal | 8 | 57–108* |
| | Oxytetracycline | Low | 58 | Decrease | Renal | 9 | 47–66* |
| *Intermediate Acting* | Demeclocycline | Moderate | 66 | Decrease | Renal | 12 | 40–60* |
| | Methacycline | Moderate | 58 | Decrease | Renal | 14 | 44* |
| *Long Acting* | Doxycycline | High | 93 | No change | Hepatic | 18 | 12–22 |
| | Minocycline | High | 95 | No change | Hepatic | 16 | 11–23 |

*Because of greatly prolonged half-life and potential for accumulation to toxic levels, this drug should not be employed in patients with kidney dysfunction.

## Adverse Effects

*Gastrointestinal Irritation.* Tetracyclines irritate the gastrointestinal tract. As a result, oral therapy is frequently associated with epigastric burning, cramps, nausea, vomiting, and diarrhea. These reactions can be reduced by giving tetracyclines with meals—although food may decrease absorption. Occasionally, tetracyclines have caused esophageal ulceration. This reaction can be minimized by avoiding administration at bedtime. Since diarrhea may result from suprainfection of the bowel (in addition to nonspecific irritation), it is important that the cause of diarrhea be determined.

*Effects on Bones and Teeth.* Tetracyclines bind to calcium in developing teeth, resulting in yellow or brown discoloration; hypoplasia of the enamel may also occur. The intensity of tooth discoloration is related to the total cumulative dose; staining is darker with prolonged and repeated treatment. When taken after the fourth month of gestation, tetracyclines can cause staining of *deciduous* teeth. However, use of these drugs during pregnancy will not affect the *permanent* teeth. Discoloration of permanent teeth occurs when tetracyclines are taken by patients ages 4 months to 5 years, the interval during which tooth enamel is being formed. Accordingly, these drugs should be avoided if at all possible by children under the age of 5 years. The risk of tooth discoloration with *doxycycline* and *oxytetracycline* may be less than with other tetracyclines.

Tetracyclines can suppress long-bone growth in premature infants. This effect is reversible upon discontinuation of treatment.

*Suprainfection.* As discussed in Chapter 77, a suprainfection is an overgrowth with drug-resistant microbes. This overgrowth occurs secondary to suppression of drug-sensitive organisms. Because the tetracyclines are broad-spectrum agents, and therefore can decrease viability of a wide variety of microbes, the risk of suprainfection is greater than with antibiotics that have a more narrow antimicrobial spectrum.

Suprainfection of the bowel with staphylococci or with *Clostridium difficile* produces severe diarrhea and can be life threatening. The infection caused by *C. difficile* is known as *antibiotic-associated pseudomembranous colitis.* Patients should be instructed to notify the physician if significant diarrhea occurs so that the possibility of bacterial suprainfection can be evaluated. If a diagnosis of supra-infection with staphylococci or *C. difficile* is made, tetracyclines should be discontinued immediately. Treatment consists of oral *vancomycin* or *metronidazole* plus vigorous fluid and electrolyte replacement therapy.

Overgrowth with fungi (commonly *Candida albicans*) may occur in the mouth, pharynx, vagina, and bowel. Symptoms include vaginal or anal itching; inflammatory lesions of the anogenital region; and a black, furry appearance of the tongue. Suprainfection with *Candida* can be managed by discontinuing tetracycline use. When this is not possible, treatment with an antifungal drug is indicated.

*Hepatotoxicity.* Tetracyclines can cause fatty infiltration of the liver. Hepatotoxicity manifests clinically as lethargy and jaundice. Rarely, the condition progresses to massive liver failure. Liver damage is most likely when tetracyclines are administered intravenously in high dosage (greater than 2 gm/day). Pregnant and postpartum women who have kidney disease are at particularly high risk.

*Renal Toxicity.* Tetracyclines may exacerbate renal dysfunction in patients with pre-existing kidney disease. Since most tetracyclines are excreted by the kidneys, these agents should not be given to patients with renal impairment. Exceptions to this rule are *doxycycline* and perhaps *minocycline*; since these two agents are eliminated primarily by the liver, decreased kidney function does not cause them to accumulate.

*Photosensitivity.* All of the tetracyclines can increase the sensitivity of the skin to ultraviolet light. The most common result is exaggerated sunburn. Patients should be advised to avoid prolonged exposure to sunlight, wear protective clothing, and apply a sunscreen to exposed skin.

*Other Adverse Effects.* *Vestibular toxicity*, manifesting as dizziness, lightheadedness, and unsteadiness, has occurred with *minocycline*. Rarely, tetracyclines have produced *pseudotumor cerebri* (a benign elevation in intracranial pressure). In a few patients, demeclocycline has produced *nephrogenic diabetes insipidus*, a syndrome characterized by thirst, increased frequency of urination, and unusual weakness or tiredness. Because of their irritant properties, tetracyclines can cause *pain at sites of IM injection* and *thrombophlebitis when administered IV.*

## Drug and Food Interactions

As noted above, tetracyclines can form nonabsorbable chelates with certain metal ions (calcium, iron, magnesium, aluminum, zinc). Substances that contain these ions include *milk products, calcium supplements, iron supplements, magnesium-containing laxatives,* and *most antacids.* If a tetracycline is administered with these agents, absorption of the tetracycline will be decreased. To minimize interference with tetracycline absorption, *tetracyclines should be administered at least 2 hours before or 2 hours after ingestion of chelating agents.*

## Dosage and Administration

*Administration.* Tetracyclines may be administered orally, intravenously, and by intramuscular injection. Oral administration is preferred, and all tetracyclines are available in oral formulations. As a rule, oral tetracyclines should be taken on an empty stomach (1 hour before or 2 hours after meals) and with a full glass of water. An interval of at least 2 hours should separate administration of oral tetracyclines and ingestion of products capable of chelating these drugs (e.g., milk, calcium or iron supplements, antacids). Several tetracyclines can be given intravenously (Table 80–2), but this route should be employed only when oral therapy cannot be tolerated or has proved inadequate. Intramuscular injection is extremely painful and used only rarely.

*Dosage.* Dosage is determined by the nature and intensity of the infection being treated. Typical systemic doses for adults and children over the age of 8 years are summarized in Table 80–2.

**TABLE 80-2. TETRACYCLINES: ROUTES OF ADMINISTRATION, DOSAGE INTERVAL, AND DOSAGE**

| Class | Drug | Trade Names | Route | Usual Dosing Interval (hr) | Total Daily Dose — Adult (mg) | Total Daily Dose — Pediatric (mg/kg)[a] |
|---|---|---|---|---|---|---|
| *Short Acting* | Tetracycline | Achromycin, Sumycin others | PO | 6 | 1000-2000 | 25-50 |
| | | | IV[b] | 12 | 500-1000 | 10-20 |
| | | | IM[c] | 12 | 300 | 15-25 |
| | Oxytetracycline | Terramycin, Uri-Tet | PO | 6 | 1000-2000 | 25-50 |
| | | | IM[c] | 12 | 300 | 15-25 |
| *Intermediate Acting* | Demeclocycline | Declomycin | PO | 12 | 600 | 6-12 |
| | Methacycline | Rondomycin | PO | 12 | 600 | 6-12 |
| *Long Acting* | Doxycycline | Vibramycin, others | PO | 24 | 100[d] | 2.2[e] |
| | | | IV[b] | 24 | 100-200[f] | 2.2-4.4[g] |
| | Minocycline | Minocin | PO | 12 | 200[h] | 4[i] |
| | | | IV[b] | 12 | 200[h] | 4[i] |

[a]Doses presented are for children over the age of 8 years; use in children below this age may cause permanent staining of teeth.
[b]The intravenous route is used only if oral therapy cannot be tolerated or is inadequate.
[c]Intramuscular injection is extremely painful and used only rarely
[d]First-day regimen is 100 mg initially followed by 100 mg 12 hours later.
[e]First-day regimen is 2.2 mg/kg initially followed by 2.2 mg/kg 12 hours later.
[f]First-day regimen is 200 mg in one or two slow infusions (1 to 4 hours).
[g]First-day regimen is 4.4 mg/kg in one or two slow infusions (1 to 4 hours).
[h]First-day regimen is 200 mg initially followed by 100 mg 12 hours later.
[i]First-day regimen is 4 mg/kg initially followed by 2 mg/kg 12 hours later.

## Summary of Major Precautions

With the exceptions of doxycycline and minocycline, the tetracyclines are eliminated primarily in the urine, and will accumulate to toxic levels in the presence of kidney disease; accordingly, most tetracyclines should not be administered to patients with renal failure. Tetracyclines can cause discoloration of deciduous and permanent teeth; tooth discoloration can be avoided by withholding these drugs from pregnant women and from children under the age of 5 years. Diarrhea may indicate a potentially life-threatening suprainfection of the bowel; advise patients to notify the physician if diarrhea occurs. High-dose intravenous therapy has been associated with severe liver damage, particularly in pregnant and postpartum women who have kidney disease; as a rule, women in these categories should not receive tetracyclines.

### Summary of Unique Properties of Individual Tetracyclines

**Tetracycline.** Tetracycline hydrochloride [Achromycin, Sumycin, others] is the least expensive and most widely used member of the tetracycline family. This drug has the indications, pharmacokinetics, adverse effects, and drug interactions described above for the tetracyclines as a group. Like most tetracyclines, tetracycline hydrochloride should not be administered with food, and is contraindicated for patients with kidney dysfunction. This agent and all other tetracyclines should not be given to pregnant women or to children under the age of 8 years.

**Oxytetracycline.** Oxytetracycline [Terramycin, others] is a short-acting agent similar to tetracycline in most respects. The principal difference between these drugs is cost: brand-name preparations of oxytetracycline are more expensive than brand-name preparations of tetracycline.

**Demeclocycline.** Demeclocycline [Declomycin] shares the actions, indications, and adverse effects described above for the tetracyclines as a group. Because of its intermediate duration of action, demeclocycline can be administered at dosing intervals that are longer than those used for tetracycline. Demeclocycline is a relatively new drug, and treatment can be expensive.

Demeclocycline is unique among the tetracyclines in its ability to stimulate urine flow. This side effect can lead to excessive urination, thirst, and tiredness. Because of its effect on renal function, demeclocycline has been employed therapeutically to promote urine production in patients suffering from the syndrome of inappropriate (excessive) secretion of antidiuretic hormone.

**Methacycline.** Methacycline [Rondomycin] shares the actions, indications, and adverse effects described above for the tetracyclines as a group. Like demeclocycline, methacycline is an intermediate-acting agent, and hence administration can be less frequent than with tetracycline. The cost of methacycline is even greater than that of demeclocycline.

**Doxycycline.** Doxycycline [Vibramycin, others] is a long-acting agent that shares the actions and adverse effects described above for the tetracyclines as a group. Because of its extended half-life, doxycycline can be administered once daily. Absorption of oral doxycycline is greater than that of tetracycline, and is not diminished by food or milk; thus, the drug may be administered with meals. Doxycycline is eliminated primarily by nonrenal mechanisms. As a result, this agent is safe for patients with renal failure. Doxycycline is a first-line drug for Lyme disease and chlamydial infections (urethritis, cervicitis, lymphogranuloma venereum).

***Minocycline.*** Minocycline [Minocin] is a long-acting agent similar in most respects to doxycycline. Like doxycycline, minocycline can be taken with food. Minocycline is safe for patients with kidney disease. Minocycline is unique among the tetracyclines in that it can damage the vestibular system, causing unsteadiness, lightheadedness, and dizziness; vestibular toxicity limits the use of this drug. Minocycline is expensive; treatment costs significantly more than with tetracycline.

# Macrolides

The macrolides are broad-spectrum antibiotics that act by inhibiting bacterial protein synthesis. These drugs are called macrolides because of their large size. Erythromycin is the oldest member of the family. The newer members—azithromycin, clarithromycin, and dirithromycin—are derivatives of erythromycin. When used alone, the macrolides are devoid of serious toxicity. However, when combined with certain other drugs, two of the macrolides—erythromycin and clarithromycin—can cause serious toxicity.

## Erythromycin

Erythromycin has a relatively broad spectrum of antimicrobial action and is a preferred or alternative treatment for a number of infectious diseases. The drug is one of our safest antibiotics and will serve as our prototype for the macrolide family.

### Mechanism of Action

Antibacterial effects result from inhibition of protein synthesis: erythromycin binds to the 50S ribosomal subunit and thereby blocks addition of new amino acids to the growing peptide chain. Erythromycin is usually bacteriostatic, but can be bactericidal against highly susceptible organisms or when present at high concentrations. The drug is selectively toxic to bacteria because ribosomes in the cytoplasm of mammalian cells do not bind the drug. Also, in contrast to chloramphenicol (see below), erythromycin cannot cross the mitochondrial membrane, and therefore does not inhibit protein synthesis in host mitochondria.

### Antimicrobial Spectrum

Erythromycin's antibacterial spectrum is *similar* to that of *penicillin*. The drug is active against most gram-positive bacteria as well as some gram-negative microbes. Bacterial sensitivity is determined in large part by the ability of erythromycin to gain access to the cell interior.

### Therapeutic Uses

Erythromycin is a commonly used antimicrobial agent. *This drug is the treatment of first choice for several infections and is employed as an alternative to penicillin G in patients allergic to penicillins.*

Erythromycin is the preferred treatment for pneumonia caused by *Legionella pneumophila* (legionnaires' disease). The regimen for this infection also includes rifampin.

Erythromycin is considered the drug of first choice for individuals infected with *Bordetella pertussis*, the causative agent of *whooping cough*. Since symptoms are caused by a toxin, erythromycin does little to alter the course of the disease. However, by eliminating *B. pertussis* from the nasopharynx, treatment does lower infectivity.

*Corynebacterium diphtheriae* is highly sensitive to erythromycin. Accordingly, erythromycin is the treatment of choice for *acute diphtheria* and eliminating the diphtheria carrier state.

Several infections respond equally well to erythromycin and to tetracyclines. Both agents are drugs of first choice for certain chlamydial infections (urethritis, cervicitis) and for pneumonia caused by *Mycoplasma pneumoniae*.

Erythromycin is commonly employed as an alternative to penicillin G in patients with penicillin allergy. The drug is used most frequently as a substitute for penicillin to treat respiratory tract infections caused by *Streptococcus pneumoniae* and by group A *Streptococcus pyogenes*. Erythromycin can also be employed as an alternative to penicillin for preventing recurrences of rheumatic fever and bacterial endocarditis.

### Pharmacokinetics

***Absorption and Bioavailability.*** Erythromycin for oral administration is available in four forms: *erythromycin base* and three derivatives of the base, *erythromycin estolate, erythromycin stearate,* and *erythromycin ethylsuccinate.* The base is unstable in stomach acid, and absorption can be variable; the derivatives were synthesized to improve bioavailability. Bioavailability has also been enhanced by use of acid-resistant coatings. These coatings protect erythromycin while in the stomach and then dissolve in the duodenum, thereby permitting absorption of erythromycin from the small intestine. As a rule, *food decreases the absorption of erythromycin base and erythromycin stearate,* whereas absorption of the estolate and ethylsuccinate forms is not affected. Only erythromycin base is biologically active; the derivatives must be converted to the base (either in the intestine or following absorption) in order to exert antibacterial effects. When used properly (i.e., when dosage is correct and the effects of food are accounted for), all of the oral erythromycins produce equivalent therapeutic effects.

In addition to its oral forms, erythromycin is available as *erythromycin lactobionate* for intravenous use. This IV preparation produces plasma drug levels that are higher than those achieved with oral erythromycins.

***Distribution.*** Erythromycin is readily distributed to most tissues and body fluids. Penetration to the CSF, however, is poor. Erythromycin crosses the placenta, but adverse effects on the fetus have not been observed.

***Elimination.*** Erythromycin is eliminated primarily by hepatic mechanisms. The drug is concentrated in the liver and then excreted in the bile. A small amount (10% to 15%) is excreted unchanged in the urine. Since elimination is primarily hepatic, the dosage need not be reduced in patients with renal dysfunction.

## Adverse Effects

Erythromycin is generally free of serious toxicity and is one of the safest antibiotics available. The toxicity of principal concern is occasional liver injury with *erythromycin estolate*.

*Gastrointestinal Effects.* Gastrointestinal disturbances (epigastric pain, nausea, vomiting, diarrhea) are the most common adverse effects. These can be reduced by administering erythromycin with meals. However, this should be done only when using those forms of erythromycin whose absorption is unaffected by food (erythromycin estolate, erythromycin ethylsuccinate, certain enteric-coated formulations of erythromycin base). Patients who experience persistent or severe gastrointestinal reactions should notify the physician.

*Liver Injury.* The most serious toxicity of erythromycin is *cholestatic hepatitis*. This reaction occurs almost exclusively in adults, and is caused by *erythromycin estolate* and not by other forms of the drug. Symptoms include nausea, vomiting, abdominal pain, jaundice, and elevations in plasma levels of bilirubin and liver transaminases. Hepatic injury usually develops 10 to 20 days after initiation of treatment. However, the reaction can occur in a few hours if erythromycin is administered to patients who experienced hepatotoxicity in the past. Because of its capacity for injuring the liver, erythromycin estolate should be avoided by patients with pre-existing hepatic disease. Patients should be instructed to report signs of liver injury (e.g., severe abdominal pain, yellow discoloration of the skin or eyes, darkened urine, pale stools). Symptoms reverse following drug withdrawal.

*Other Adverse Effects.* By killing off sensitive gut flora, erythromycin can promote *suprainfection of the bowel*. *Thrombophlebitis* can occur with intravenous administration; this reaction can be minimized by slow infusion of dilute drug solution. Rarely, high-dose therapy has caused *transient loss of hearing*.

## Drug Interactions

Erythromycin can increase the plasma levels and half-lives of several drugs, thereby posing a risk of toxicity. Erythromycin raises drug levels by inhibiting hepatic drug-metabolizing enzymes that employ cytochrome P-450. Elevation of levels is a particular concern with *astemizole* and *terfenadine*, two antihistamines that can cause fatal dysrhythmias when present in excessive amounts. Accordingly, erythromycin should never be combined with these drugs. Elevated levels are also a concern with *theophylline* (used to treat asthma), *carbamazepine* (an anticonvulsant), and *warfarin* (an anticoagulant); when these agents are combined with erythromycin, the patient should be monitored closely for signs of toxicity.

Erythromycin prevents binding of *chloramphenicol* and *clindamycin* to bacterial ribosomes, thereby antagonizing the effects of these antibiotics. Accordingly, concurrent use of erythromycin with these two drugs is not recommended.

## Preparations, Dosage, and Administration

*Preparations.* Erythromycin is available in formulations for oral and intravenous administration. All preparations have the same antimicrobial spectrum and indications. Adverse effects are also similar, except that cholestatic hepatitis occurs only with erythromycin estolate.

*Oral Dosage and Administration.* Oral erythromycins should be administered on an empty stomach and with a full glass of water. If necessary, some preparations (erythromycin estolate, erythromycin ethylsuccinate, certain enteric-coated preparations of erythromycin base) can be administered with food to decrease gastrointestinal reactions. The usual *adult* dosage for *erythromycin base, estolate,* and *stearate* is 250 to 500 mg every 6 hours; the adult dosage for *erythromycin ethylsuccinate* is 400 to 800 mg every 6 hours. The usual *pediatric* dosage for all oral erythromycins is 7.5 to 12.5 mg/kg every 6 hours.

Trade names for oral erythromycins include E-Mycin, Eryc, and PCE Dispertab (for erythromycin base); Ilosone (for erythromycin estolate); E.E.S. and EryPed (for erythromycin ethylsuccinate); and Eramycin, Erythrocin, and Wyamycin S (for erythromycin stearate).

*Intravenous Dosage and Administration.* Intravenous administration is reserved for severe infections and is used only rarely. Continuous infusion is preferred to intermittent administration. Only *erythromycin lactobionate* is given IV. The usual *adult* dosage is 1 to 4 gm daily. The usual *pediatric* dosage is 15 to 50 mg/kg/day. Erythromycin should be infused slowly and in dilute solution to minimize the risk of thrombophlebitis. For instruction on preparation and storage of IV solutions, consult the manufacturer's literature.

## Clarithromycin

*Actions and Therapeutic Uses.* Like erythromycin, clarithromycin [Biaxin] binds the 50S subunit of bacterial ribosomes, causing inhibition of protein synthesis. The drug is approved for respiratory tract infections, uncomplicated infections of the skin and skin structures, and prevention of disseminated *Mycobacterium avium* complex infections in patients with advanced HIV infection.

*Pharmacokinetics.* Clarithromycin is well absorbed following oral administration, regardless of the presence of food. The drug is widely distributed and readily penetrates cells. Elimination is by hepatic metabolism and renal excretion. A reduction in dosage may be needed in patients with severe renal dysfunction.

*Adverse Effects and Interactions.* Clarithromycin is well tolerated and does not produce the intense nausea seen with erythromycin. The most common reactions (3%) have been diarrhea, nausea, and distorted taste; all have been described as mild to moderate. In clinical trials, only 3% of patients withdrew because of side effects, compared with 20% who withdrew when taking erythromycin. High doses of clarithromycin have caused fetal abnormalities in laboratory animals; possible effects on the human fetus are unknown.

Like erythromycin, clarithromycin can elevate blood levels of other drugs by inhibiting their hepatic metabolism. Clarithromycin must not be combined with *terfenadine* or *astemizole*, since the combination would increase the risk of fatal dysrhythmias. Like erythromycin, clarithromycin can elevate levels of *warfarin, carbamazepine,* and *theophylline*; dosages of these drugs may need to be reduced.

*Preparations, Dosage, and Administration.* Clarithromycin [Biaxin] is dispensed in two oral formulations: tablets (250 and 500 mg) and granules for oral suspension (25 and 50 mg/ml). The recommended dosage is 250 or 500 mg every 12 hours for 7 to 14 days; the exact dosage size and duration depend on the infection being treated. The drug may be taken without regard to meals.

### Azithromycin

***Actions and Therapeutic Uses.*** Like erythromycin, azithromycin [Zithromax] binds the 50S subunit of bacterial ribosomes, causing inhibition of protein synthesis. The drug is approved for respiratory tract infections, uncomplicated infections of the skin and skin structures, and nongonococcal urethritis caused by *Chlamydia trachomatis*, for which it is a drug of first choice. Like clarithromycin, azithromycin is under investigation as treatment for disseminated *Mycobacterium avium* complex infections and other infections associated with AIDS.

***Pharmacokinetics.*** Absorption of azithromycin is reduced by 50% in the presence of food. Accordingly, the drug should not be administered with meals. Following absorption, azithromycin is widely distributed to tissues and becomes concentrated in cells. The drug is eliminated in the bile, both as metabolites and as parent drug.

***Adverse Effects and Interactions.*** Like clarithromycin, azithromycin is well tolerated and does not produce the intense nausea seen with erythromycin. The most common reactions have been diarrhea (5%) and nausea and abdominal pain (3%). In one clinical trial, only 0.7% of patients withdrew because of drug-induced side effects. Aluminum- and magnesium-containing antacids reduce the rate (but not the extent) of azithromycin absorption. In contrast to erythromycin and clarithromycin, azithromycin does not inhibit the metabolism of other drugs, and hence can be used safely with terfenadine and astemizole.

***Preparations, Dosage, and Administration.*** Azithromycin [Zithromax] is dispensed in two oral formulations: 250-mg capsules and a suspension (20 and 40 mg/ml). The usual dosing schedule is 500 mg once on the first day, followed by 250 mg once daily on the following 4 days. The drug should be taken 1 hour before meals or 2 hours after. It must not be taken with food or with aluminum- or magnesium-containing antacids.

### Dirithromycin

***Actions and Therapeutic Uses.*** Dirithromycin [Dynabac] is the newest member of the macrolide family. The drug's mechanism of action, antimicrobial spectrum, and clinical effects are much like those of erythromycin. Approved indications include bronchitis caused by *Streptococcus pneumoniae* (but not by *H. influenzae*); community-acquired pneumonia caused by pneumococci, *Mycoplasma pneumoniae*, or *Legionella pneumophila*; and skin and soft tissue infections caused by *Staphylococcus aureus*.

***Pharmacokinetics.*** Following oral administration, dirithromy-cin is absorbed from the GI tract and converted by nonenzymatic hydrolysis into erythromycylamine, an active metabolite. The drug reaches high concentrations in tissues, although serum concentrations may be low. Dirithromycin and its metabolite are eliminated slowly in the bile, with a half-life of about 40 hours. Because of this extended half-life, once-daily dosing is sufficient.

***Adverse Effects and Interactions.*** As with erythromycin, nausea and abdominal pain are common; the reported incidence is about 10%, but the actual incidence may be higher. In contrast to erythromycin and clarithromycin, dirithromycin does not inhibit the metabolism of other drugs, and hence appears safe for patients taking terfenadine or astemizole.

***Preparations, Dosage, and Administration.*** Dirithromycin [Dynabac] is dispensed in 250-mg enteric-coated tablets for oral use. The usual dosage is 500 mg once daily for 7 to 14 days.

Dirithromycin should be taken with meals or within 1 hour after eating. Food does not reduce absorption.

---

# Clindamycin

Clindamycin [Cleocin] can promote severe *antibiotic-associated pseudomembranous* colitis, a condition that can be fatal. Because of the risk of colitis, indications for clindamycin are limited. Currently, the drug is indicated only for certain anaerobic infections located outside the central nervous system (CNS).

## Mechanism of Action

Clindamycin binds to the 50S subunit of bacterial ribosomes and thereby inhibits protein synthesis. The ribosomal site at which clindamycin binds overlaps the binding sites for erythromycin and chloramphenicol. As a result, these agents may antagonize one another's effects. Accordingly, there are no indications for concurrent use of clindamycin with these other antibiotics.

## Antimicrobial Spectrum

Clindamycin is active against most anaerobic bacteria (gram positive and gram negative) and most gram-positive aerobes. Gram-negative aerobes are generally resistant. Susceptible anaerobes include *Bacteroides fragilis*, *Fusobacterium*, *Clostridium perfringens*, and anaerobic streptococci. Clindamycin is usually bacteriostatic; however, bactericidal effects may occur if the target organism is especially sensitive. Resistance can be a significant clinical problem with *B. fragilis*.

## Therapeutic Use

Because of its efficacy against gram-positive cocci, clindamycin was once used widely as an alternative to penicillin. However, following the discovery that clindamycin can promote antibiotic-associated pseudomembranous colitis (see below), use of this drug has declined. Today, clindamycin is employed primarily for anaerobic infections outside the CNS (the drug does not cross the blood-brain barrier). Clindamycin is a preferred drug for abdominal and pelvic infections caused by *Bacteroides fragilis*. In addition, it can be used as a substitute for penicillin G to treat severe infections with other anaerobes (e.g., *Clostridium perfringens*, *Fusobacterium nucleatum*, anaerobic streptococci).

### Pharmacokinetics

***Absorption and Distribution.*** Clindamycin may be administered orally, IM, and IV. Absorption from the gastrointestinal tract is nearly complete and is not affected by food. The drug is widely distributed to most body fluids and tissues, including synovial fluid and bone. Penetration to the cerebrospinal fluid is poor.

***Elimination.*** Clindamycin undergoes hepatic metabolism to active and inactive products. These metabolites are excreted in the urine and bile. Only 10% of the drug is eliminated unchanged by the kidneys. In normal individuals, the half-life of clindamycin is approximately 3 hours; this value is increased only slightly in patients with substantial reductions in liver or kidney function. Hence, dosage need not be reduced in such patients. However, the drug may accumulate to toxic levels in the presence of *combined* renal and hepatic disease. Under these conditions, a reduction in dosage is indicated.

## Adverse Effects

*Antibiotic-Associated Pseudomembranous Colitis.* The most severe toxicity associated with clindamycin is a condition known as *antibiotic-associated pseudomembranous colitis* (AAPMC). The cause is suprainfection of the bowel with *Clostridium difficile*, an anaerobic grampositive bacillus. AAPMC is characterized by profuse, watery diarrhea (10 to 20 stools per day), abdominal pain, fever, and leukocytosis. Stools often contain mucus and blood. Symptoms usually begin during the first week of treatment; however, they may also develop as much as 4 to 6 weeks after clindamycin withdrawal. Left untreated, the condition can be fatal. AAPMC occurs with parenteral and oral therapy. Because of the risk of colitis, patients should be instructed to report significant diarrhea (more than 5 watery stools per day). If suprainfection with *C. difficile* is diagnosed, clindamycin should be discontinued and the patient should be given oral vancomycin or metronidazole, which are drugs of choice for eliminating *C. difficile* from the bowel. Diarrhea usually ceases 3 to 5 days after initiation of vancomycin treatment. Vigorous replacement therapy with fluids and electrolytes is usually indicated. Drugs that decrease bowel motility (e.g., opioids, anticholinergics) may worsen symptoms and should not be used.

*Other Adverse Effects.* Diarrhea (unrelated to AAPMC) is relatively common. *Hypersensitivity reactions* (especially rashes) occur frequently. *Hepatotoxicity* and *blood dyscrasias* (agranulocytosis, leukopenia, thrombocytopenia) develop rarely. Rapid intravenous administration can cause *electrocardiographic changes*, *hypotension*, and *cardiac arrest.*

## Preparations, Dosage, and Administration

*Preparations.* Clindamycin is available as *clindamycin hydrochloride* and *clindamycin palmitate hydrochloride* for oral use and as *clindamycin phosphate* for IM or IV use. Clindamycin hydrochloride [Cleocin] is dispensed in capsules (75, 150, and 300 mg). Clindamycin palmitate hydrochloride [Cleocin Pediatric] is dispensed as flavored granules, which are reconstituted with fluid to make an oral solution containing 15 mg of clindamycin per milliliter. Clindamycin phosphate [Cleocin Phosphate] is dispensed in solution (150 mg/ml).

*Oral Dosage and Administration.* For *clindamycin hydrochloride*, the adult dosage ranges from 150 to 450 mg every 6 hours; the pediatric dosage ranges from 8 to 20 mg/kg daily in three or four divided doses. For *clindamycin palmitate hydrochloride*, adult and pediatric dosages range from 8 to 25 mg/kg/day administered in three or four divided doses. Oral clindamycin should be taken with a full glass of water. The drug may be administered with meals.

*Parenteral Dosage and Administration.* For parenteral (IM or IV) therapy, *clindamycin phosphate* is employed. Intramuscular and IV dosages are the same. The usual adult dosage is 0.6 to 3.6 gm/day administered in three or four divided doses. The usual pediatric dosage is 15 to 40 mg/kg/day in three or four divided doses.

# Chloramphenicol

Chloramphenicol [Chloromycetin] is a broad-spectrum antibiotic with the potential for causing *fatal aplastic anemia* and other blood dyscrasias. Because of the risk of severe blood disorders, use of chloramphenicol is limited to treatment of serious infections for which less toxic drugs are ineffective.

## Mechanism of Action

Chloramphenicol inhibits bacterial protein synthesis. The drug binds reversibly to the 50S subunit of bacterial ribosomes and thereby prevents addition of new amino acids to the growing peptide chain. Chloramphenicol is usually bacteriostatic, but can be bactericidal against highly susceptible organisms or if drug concentrations are high.

Since most protein synthesis in mammalian cells is carried out in the cytoplasm employing ribosomes that are insensitive to chloramphenicol, toxic effects of chloramphenicol are restricted largely to bacteria. However, since the ribosomes of mammalian *mitochondria* are very similar to the ribosomes of bacteria, chloramphenicol is capable of decreasing mitochondrial protein synthesis in the host. This action may underlie certain adverse effects of the drug (e.g., dose-dependent bone marrow depression, gray syndrome in infants).

## Antimicrobial Spectrum

Chloramphenicol is active against a broad spectrum of bacteria. A large number of gram-positive and gram-negative aerobic organisms are sensitive. Included in this group are *Salmonella typhi*, *Haemophilus influenzae*, *Neisseria meningitidis*, and *Streptococcus pneumoniae*. Most anaerobic bacteria (e.g., *Bacteroides fragilis*) are also susceptible. In addition, chloramphenicol is active against rickettsiae, chlamydiae, mycoplasmas, and treponemas.

## Resistance

Resistance among gram-negative bacteria results from acquisition of an R factor that codes for acetyltransferase, an enzyme that inactivates chloramphenicol. This same R factor also codes for resistance to tetracyclines, and frequently confers resistance to penicillins as well.

## Pharmacokinetics

Chloramphenicol is available in three forms: chloramphenicol *base*, chloramphenicol *palmitate*, and chloramphenicol *succinate*. The base and palmitate are administered orally; the succinate is administered IV. The palmitate and succinate esters are prodrugs that must be hydrolyzed to yield free chloramphenicol before they can act.

*Absorption.* Chloramphenicol base is readily absorbed following oral administration. For absorption of the *palmitate* to take place, the molecule must first be hydrolyzed to chloramphenicol base by pancreatic lipases in the duodenum. When the palmitate is administered to newborns, blood levels of chloramphenicol are highly variable.

Following IV administration, chloramphenicol *succinate* must be hydrolyzed to chloramphenicol before it can exert antibacterial effects. This conversion is variable and incomplete. Production of active drug is especially erratic in newborns, infants, and young children.

**Distribution.** Chloramphenicol is highly lipid soluble and widely distributed to body tissues and fluids. Therapeutic concentrations are readily achieved in the CSF, and drug levels in the brain may be as much as 9 times those in plasma. As a result, chloramphenicol is of special value for treating meningitis and brain abscesses caused by susceptible bacteria. The drug crosses the placenta and is secreted in breast milk.

**Metabolism and Excretion.** Chloramphenicol is eliminated primarily by hepatic metabolism. Inactive metabolites are excreted in the urine. In patients with liver dysfunction, the half-life of chloramphenicol is prolonged and drug accumulation can occur. Accordingly, the dosage should be reduced in the presence of liver disease. Because the kidneys serve only to excrete inactive metabolites, there is no need for dosage reduction in patients with renal dysfunction. In neonates, hepatic metabolism is not fully developed and the half-life of chloramphenicol is prolonged.

**Monitoring Chloramphenicol Serum Levels.** Because chloramphenicol has a low therapeutic index, and because serum levels of the drug can vary substantially among patients, monitoring of drug levels is frequently indicated. Monitoring is especially important for neonates, infants, and young children, since chloramphenicol levels in these patients can be highly variable. Monitoring is also important for patients with liver disease and for patients receiving certain drugs (e.g., phenytoin, phenobarbital, rifampin) that can alter the rate of chloramphenicol metabolism. For most infections, effective therapy is achieved with peak serum drug levels of 10 to 20 µg/ml and trough levels of 5 to 10 µg/ml. The risk of dose-dependent bone marrow depression is significantly increased when peak levels rise above 25 µg/ml.

### Therapeutic Use

Chloramphenicol was once employed widely; however, awareness that the drug can cause fatal aplastic anemia has led to sharp restrictions in its use. Currently, chloramphenicol is indicated only for severe (life-threatening) infections for which safer drugs are either ineffective or contraindicated.

Chloramphenicol is a drug of choice for acute typhoid fever caused by sensitive strains of *Salmonella typhi.* However, chloramphenicol is not recommended for routine therapy of the typhoid carrier state.

Chloramphenicol is lethal to *Haemophilus influenzae,* an organism that can infect the meninges and other sites. At one time, chloramphenicol plus ampicillin was considered the regimen of choice for initial treatment of meningitis caused by this microbe. However, the advent of third-generation cephalosporins that readily penetrate the meninges has reduced the use of chloramphenicol for this infection.

### Adverse Effects

The most important adverse effects of chloramphenicol are gray syndrome and toxicities related to the blood. It is because of these adverse effects that indications for chloramphenicol are limited.

**Gray Syndrome.** Gray syndrome is a potentially fatal toxicity observed most commonly in newborns. Initial symptoms are vomiting, abdominal distention, cyanosis, and gray discoloration of the skin. These may be followed by vasomotor collapse and death. The syndrome results from accumulation of chloramphenicol to high levels. Newborns are especially vulnerable to the gray syndrome because (1) hepatic function is insufficient to detoxify chloramphenicol and (2) renal function is insufficient to

excrete active drug. Although the gray syndrome is usually observed in neonates, it can occur in older children and adults if dosage is excessive. If drug use is discontinued immediately upon appearance of early symptoms, the syndrome is usually reversible. The risk of gray syndrome in infants can be reduced by using appropriately low doses and monitoring chloramphenicol levels in serum.

**Reversible Bone Marrow Depression.** Chloramphenicol can produce dose-related depression of the bone marrow, resulting in anemia and sometimes leukopenia and thrombocytopenia. Marrow depression is a toxic reaction to chloramphenicol and occurs most commonly when plasma drug levels exceed 25 µg/ml. The cause of bone marrow depression appears to be inhibition of protein synthesis in host mitochondria. To promote early detection of bone marrow depression, complete blood counts should be performed prior to therapy and every 2 days during the period of treatment. Patients should be advised to notify the physician if signs of blood disorders develop (e.g., sore throat, fever, unusual bleeding or bruising). Chloramphenicol should be withdrawn if evidence of bone marrow depression is detected. Depression of bone marrow usually reverses within 1 to 3 weeks following discontinuation of drug use. The anemia associated with toxic bone marrow depression is not related to aplastic anemia (see below).

**Aplastic Anemia.** Rarely, chloramphenicol produces aplastic anemia, a condition characterized by pancytopenia and bone marrow aplasia. This reaction is usually fatal. Aplastic anemia occurs with an incidence of approximately 1 in 35,000, and is not related to chloramphenicol dosage. As a rule, the reaction develops weeks or months after termination of treatment. Aplastic anemia can occur with oral, intravenous, or even topical (ophthalmic) use of the drug. The mechanism underlying aplastic anemia has not been determined, but toxicity may result from a genetic predisposition. Unfortunately, aplastic anemia cannot be predicted by monitoring the blood.

**Other Adverse Effects.** *Gastrointestinal effects* (vomiting, diarrhea, glossitis) occur occasionally. *Herxheimer reactions* have occurred during treatment of typhoid fever. *Neurologic effects* (peripheral neuropathy, optic neuritis, confusion, delirium) develop rarely, usually in association with prolonged treatment. Other rare toxicities include *suprainfection of the bowel, allergic reactions,* and *fever.*

### Drug Interactions

Chloramphenicol can inhibit hepatic drug-metabolizing enzymes, thereby prolonging the half-lives of a variety of drugs. Agents whose metabolism may be affected include *phenytoin* (an anticonvulsant), *warfarin* (an anticoagulant), and two oral hypoglycemics, *tolbutamide* and *chlorpropamide*. If these drugs are taken concurrently with chloramphenicol, their dosages should be reduced to avoid accumulation to toxic levels.

### Preparations, Dosage, and Administration

**General Considerations Regarding Route of Administration and Dosage.** For treatment of systemic infections, chloramphenicol may be administered orally or IV. For initial therapy of serious infections, IV administration is generally preferred; oral therapy may be substituted later if conditions warrant.

As a rule, the dosing objective is to produce peak chloramphenicol plasma levels that range between 10 and 20 µg/ml. This objective can be achieved by monitoring serum levels of the drug. Monitoring is especially important in newborns, patients with liver disease, and patients receiving drugs that can alter chloramphenicol disposition (e.g., phenytoin).

**Preparations.** *Chloramphenicol base* [Chloromycetin Kapseals] is dispensed in 250-mg capsules for oral administration.

*Chloramphenicol palmitate* [Chloromycetin Palmitate] is available as an oral suspension (30 mg/ml). *Chloramphenicol sodium succinate* [Chloromycetin Sodium Succinate] is dispensed as a powder to be reconstituted for IV infusion.

**Dosage and Administration.** Recommended dosages for oral and intravenous administration are the same. As a rule, oral doses should be taken on an empty stomach at least 1 hour before meals or 2 hours after. If gastric upset occurs, discomfort may be reduced by taking chloramphenicol with food. The usual dosage for adults and children is 12.5 to 25 mg/kg every 6 hours. For infants 7 days old or less, the usual dosage is 25 mg/kg once a day. For infants more than 7 days old, the recommended dosage is 25 mg/kg every 12 hours. The dosage should be reduced for patients with liver dysfunction.

## Spectinomycin

**Mechanism of Action and Antimicrobial Spectrum.** Spectinomycin [Trobicin] binds to the 30S ribosomal subunit and thereby suppresses bacterial protein synthesis. The drug is active against a number of gram-negative bacteria. Resistance develops frequently.

**Therapeutic Use.** Because resistant organisms emerge rapidly, use of spectinomycin is limited. The principal indication for the drug is anogenital *gonorrhea* in patients who cannot tolerate ceftriaxone, the drug of choice for this infection.

**Pharmacokinetics.** Spectinomycin is administered only by IM injection; the drug is not absorbed from the gastrointestinal tract and cannot be used orally. Most of the drug is excreted unchanged in the urine. The plasma half-life is approximately 2 hours.

**Adverse Effects.** Spectinomycin is generally well tolerated. Adverse effects seen occasionally include soreness at the site of injection, dizziness, nausea, urticaria, pruritus, chills, fever, and insomnia.

**Preparations, Dosage, and Administration.** Spectinomycin [Trobicin] is dispensed as a sterile powder together with sufficient diluent to produce a 400 mg/ml solution upon reconstitution. For treatment of uncomplicated gonorrhea of the rectum or genitalia, the usual adult dose is 2 gm administered as a single IM (intragluteal) injection. For children weighing less than 45 kg, a single injection of 40 mg/kg is given. For disseminated gonococcal infection, the adult dosage is 2 gm twice a day for 3 days.

## KEY POINTS

• Tetracyclines are broad-spectrum, bacteriostatic antibiotics that act by inhibiting bacterial protein synthesis.

• Tetracyclines are first-choice drugs for only a few infections. These include infections caused by *Chlamydia trachomatis*, rickettsia (e.g., Rocky Mountain spotted fever), *H. pylori* (i.e., peptic ulcer disease), and *Mycoplasma pneumoniae.*

• Tetracyclines form insoluble chelates with calcium, iron, magnesium, aluminum, and zinc. Accordingly, they must not be administered with calcium supplements, milk products, iron supplements, magnesium-containing laxatives, and most antacids.

• Except for doxycycline and minocycline, tetracyclines should not be given to patients with renal failure.

• Except for doxycycline and minocycline, tetracyclines should not be administered with food.

• Tetracyclines can stain developing teeth, and therefore should not be given to pregnant women or children under 5 years.

• Because they are broad spectrum antibiotics, tetracyclines can cause suprainfections—especially antibiotic-associated pseudomembranous colitis and overgrowth of the mouth, pharynx, vagina, or bowel with *Candida albicans.*

• High doses of tetracyclines can cause severe liver damage, especially in pregnant and postpartum women who have kidney impairment.

• Erythromycin, the prototype of the macrolide antibiotics, is a bacteriostatic drug that acts by inhibiting bacterial protein synthesis.

• Erythromycin has an antimicrobial spectrum similar to that of penicillin G, and hence can be used in place of penicillin G in patients with penicillin allergy.

• Although erythromycin is generally very safe, one form of the drug—erythromycin estolate—can cause serious liver injury.

• Erythromycin can raise levels of terfenadine, astemizole, and other drugs by inhibiting hepatic drug-metabolizing enzymes. Erythromycin should never be combined with terfenadine or astemizole, since raising their levels can result in fatal dysrhythmias.

• Clindamycin causes a high incidence of antibiotic-associated pseudomembranous colitis, and hence has limited uses.

• Chloramphenicol can cause fatal aplastic anemia and other serious blood dyscrasias. As a result, the drug should be used only when clearly indicated.

# Summary of Major Nursing Implications*

## Tetracyclines

Demeclocycline    Minocycline
Doxycycline       Oxytetracycline
Methacycline      Tetracycline

Except where stated otherwise, the implications summarized below pertain to all members of the tetracycline family.

## Preadministration Assessment

### Therapeutic Goal
Treatment of tetracycline-sensitive infections and acne.

*Patient education information is highlighted in color.

### Identifying High-Risk Patients

Tetracyclines should not be used during *pregnancy* or *by children under the age of 5 years.* Except for *doxycycline* and *minocycline,* tetracyclines must be used with great *caution* in patients with significant *renal impairment.*

## Implementation: Administration

### Routes

Oral, IM, IV. For routes applicable to specific agents, see Table 80-2.

### Administration

*Oral.* Advise patients to take oral tetracyclines on an empty stomach (1 hour before meals or 2 hours after) and with a full glass of water. *Doxycycline* and *minocycline* may be taken with food.

Absorption of tetracyclines will be reduced by certain chelating agents: *milk products, calcium supplements, iron supplements, magnesium-containing laxatives,* and most *antacids.* Instruct the patient to separate ingestion of tetracyclines and these chelators by at least 2 hours.

Instruct the patient to complete the prescribed course of treatment, even though symptoms may abate before the full course is over.

*Parenteral. Intravenous* administration is performed only when oral administration is ineffective or cannot be tolerated. *Intramuscular* injection is painful and used only rarely.

## Ongoing Evaluation and Interventions

### Minimizing Adverse Effects

*Gastrointestinal Irritation.* Inform the patient that GI distress (epigastric burning, cramps, nausea, vomiting, diarrhea) can be reduced by taking tetracyclines with meals.

*Effects on Teeth.* Tetracyclines can discolor developing teeth. To prevent this effect, avoid use of tetracyclines by pregnant women and by children under the age of 5 years.

*Suprainfection.* Tetracyclines can promote bacterial suprainfection of the bowel, resulting in severe diarrhea. Instruct the patient to notify the physician if significant diarrhea develops. If suprainfection is diagnosed, discontinue tetracyclines immediately; treatment consists of oral vancomycin or metronidazole plus vigorous fluid and electrolyte replacement therapy.

Fungal overgrowth may occur in the mouth, pharynx, vagina, and bowel. Inform patients about symptoms of fungal infection (vaginal or anal itching; inflammatory lesions of the anogenital region; black, furry appearance of the tongue), and advise them to notify the physician if these occur. Suprainfection caused by *Candida* can be managed by discontinuing the tetracycline or by giving an antifungal drug.

*Hepatotoxicity.* Tetracyclines can cause fatty infiltration of the liver, resulting in jaundice and, rarely, massive liver failure. The risk of liver injury can be reduced by (1) avoiding high-dose intravenous therapy and (2) withholding tetracyclines from pregnant and postpartum women who have kidney disease.

*Renal Toxicity.* Tetracyclines can exacerbate pre-existing renal impairment. With the exception of *doxycycline* and perhaps *minocycline,* tetracyclines should not be used by patients with kidney disease.

*Photosensitivity.* Tetracyclines can increase the sensitivity of the skin to ultraviolet light, thereby increasing the risk of sunburn. Advise the patient to avoid prolonged exposure to sunlight, wear protective clothing, and apply a sunscreen to exposed skin.

# Erythromycin

The implications summarized below pertain to all forms of erythromycin, except where noted otherwise.

## Preadministration Assessment

### Therapeutic Goal

Erythromycin is indicated for legionnaires' disease, whooping cough, diphtheria, urethritis and cervicitis caused by *Chlamydia trachomatis,* and other infections caused by erythromycin-sensitive organisms. The drug is also used as a substitute for penicillin G in penicillin-allergic patients.

### Identifying High-Risk Patients

*All erythromycins* are *contraindicated* in patients taking *astemizole* or *terfenadine. Erythromycin estolate* is *contraindicated* for patients with *liver disease.*

## Implementation: Administration

### Routes

*Oral.* Erythromycin base, erythromycin estolate, erythromycin ethylsuccinate, and erythromycin stearate.

*Intravenous.* Erythromycin lactobionate.

### Administration

*Oral.* Advise the patient to take oral preparations on an empty stomach (1 hour before meals or 2 hours after) and with a full glass of water. However, if GI upset occurs, administration may be done with meals.

Inform patients using *erythromycin estolate, erythromycin ethylsuccinate,* and *enteric-coated formulations of erythromycin base* that these preparations may be taken without regard to meals.

Instruct the patient to complete the prescribed course of treatment, even though symptoms may abate before the full course is over.

*Intravenous.* Administer by slow infusion and in dilute solution to minimize thrombophlebitis.

## Ongoing Evaluation and Interventions

### Minimizing Adverse Effects

*Gastrointestinal Effects.* Gastrointestinal disturbances (epigastric pain, nausea, vomiting, diarrhea) can be reduced by administering erythromycin with meals. Advise the patient to notify the physician if gastrointestinal reactions are severe or persistent.

*Liver Injury.* *Erythromycin estolate* may cause *cholestatic hepatitis.* Inform patients about signs of liver injury (e.g., severe abdominal pain, yellow discoloration of skin or eyes, darkened urine, pale stools), and advise them to notify the physician if these develop. If cholestatic hepatitis occurs, erythromycin estolate should be withdrawn. Do not give erythromycin estolate to patients with liver dysfunction.

### Minimizing Adverse Interactions

Erythromycin can increase the half-lives and plasma levels of several drugs. Since raising the levels of *astemizole* or *terfenadine* can cause fatal dysrhythmias, these drugs must never be combined with erythromycin. When erythromycin is combined with *theophylline, carbamazepine,* or *warfarin,* patients should be monitored closely for toxicity.

Erythromycin can antagonize the antibacterial actions of *clindamycin* and *chloramphenicol.* Concurrent use of erythromycin with these agents is not recommended.

## Clindamycin

## Preadministration Assessment

### Therapeutic Goal

Treatment of anaerobic infections outside the CNS.

## Implementation: Administration

### Routes

Oral, IM, IV.

### Administration

Instruct the patient to take oral clindamycin with a full glass of water.

Instruct the patient to complete the prescribed course of treatment, even though symptoms may abate before the full course is over.

## Ongoing Evaluation and Interventions

### Minimizing Adverse Effects

*Antibiotic-Associated Pseudomembranous Colitis.* Clindamycin can promote AAPMC, a potentially fatal suprainfection. Prominent symptoms are profuse watery diarrhea, abdominal pain, fever, and leukocytosis. Stools often contain mucus and blood. Instruct the patient to report significant diarrhea (more than five watery stools per day). If AAPMC is diagnosed, discontinue clindamycin. Treat with oral vancomycin or metronidazole and vigorous replacement of fluids and electrolytes. Drugs that decrease bowel motility (e.g., opioids, anticholinergics) may worsen symptoms and should be avoided.

## Chloramphenicol

## Preadministration Assessment

### Therapeutic Use

Treatment of severe (life-threatening) infections for which safer drugs are ineffective or contraindicated.

### Baseline Data

Obtain blood cell counts.

### Identifying High-Risk Patients

Chloramphenicol is *contraindicated* for patients with a *history of toxic reactions to chloramphenicol.* The drug should be used *cautiously* in patients with *liver disease* and *during pregnancy and lactation.*

## Implementation: Administration

### Routes

Oral, intravenous. Dosage is the same by both routes.

### Administration

Instruct patients to take chloramphenicol on an empty stomach at least 1 hour before meals or 2 hours after. If GI upset occurs, the drug may be taken with meals.

Instruct the patient to complete the prescribed course of treatment, even though symptoms may abate before the full course is over.

## Ongoing Evaluation and Interventions

### Monitoring Drug Levels

Knowledge of plasma drug levels is particularly valuable in patients with liver disease, the young (newborns, infants, young children), and patients receiving drugs that can alter chloramphenicol disposition (e.g., phenobarbital, phenytoin, rifampin). The dosage is adjusted to produce peak plasma levels of 10 to 20 µg/ml and trough levels of 5 to 10 µg/ml.

### Minimizing Adverse Effects

*Gray Syndrome.* The gray syndrome usually occurs in newborns. Manifestations include vomiting, abdominal distention, cyanosis, and gray discoloration of the skin; vasomotor collapse and death can occur. Observe the patient for symptoms and terminate therapy if they occur. The risk of gray syndrome can be reduced by giving appropriately low doses and monitoring chloramphenicol levels.

**Reversible Bone Marrow Depression.** Chloramphenicol can produce reversible dose-related depression of bone marrow, manifesting as anemia, leukopenia, and thrombocytopenia. Blood cell counts should be obtained prior to therapy and every 2 days during therapy. Inform patients about early signs of hematologic toxicity (e.g., sore throat, fever, unusual bleeding or bruising), and instruct them to notify the physician if these occur. If bone marrow depression is diagnosed, chloramphenicol should be withdrawn immediately. The risk of bone marrow depression can be minimized by keeping peak plasma drug levels below 25 µg/ml.

**Aplastic Anemia.** Very rarely, chloramphenicol causes aplastic anemia, a condition with a high rate of mortality. The risk of aplastic anemia can be minimized by using chloramphenicol only when clearly indicated.

## Minimizing Adverse Interactions

Chloramphenicol can prolong the half-lives of a variety of drugs, including *phenytoin*, *warfarin*, and *oral hypoglycemics*. If these drugs are combined with chloramphenicol, their dosages should be reduced.

# CHAPTER 81

# Aminoglycosides: Bactericidal Inhibitors of Protein Synthesis

**Basic Pharmacology of the Aminoglycosides**
**Properties of Individual Aminoglycosides**
    Gentamicin
    Tobramycin
    Amikacin
    Other Aminoglycosides

The aminoglycosides are narrow-spectrum antibiotics, used primarily against aerobic gram-negative bacilli. These drugs disrupt protein synthesis and cause bacterial death. The aminoglycosides can cause serious injury to the kidney and inner ear. Because of these toxicities, indications for the aminoglycosides are limited. All of the aminoglycosides carry multiple positive charges. As a result, these agents are not absorbed from the gastrointestinal tract, and hence must be administered parenterally to treat systemic infections. In the United States, eight aminoglycosides are approved for clinical use. The agents employed most commonly are *gentamicin, tobramycin,* and *amikacin.* In approaching the aminoglycosides, we will first discuss the properties shared by these drugs as a group. After this, we will consider the unique characteristics of individual aminoglycosides.

## Basic Pharmacology of the Aminoglycosides

### Chemistry

The aminoglycosides are composed of two or more amino sugars connected by a glycoside linkage, hence the family name. At physiologic pH, these drugs are polycations (i.e., they carry several positive charges), and therefore cannot readily cross membranes. As a result, aminoglycosides are not absorbed from the gastrointestinal tract, do not enter the cerebrospinal fluid, and are rapidly excreted by the kidneys. Structural formulas for the three major aminoglycosides are shown in Figure 81–1.

### Mechanism of Action

The aminoglycosides disrupt bacterial protein synthesis. These drugs bind to the 30S ribosomal subunit, caus-

ing (1) inhibition of protein synthesis and (2) production of abnormal proteins (secondary to misreading of the genetic code). The aminoglycosides are rapidly *bactericidal.*

Bacterial kill appears to result from production of abnormal proteins rather than from simple inhibition of protein synthesis. Data suggest that abnormal proteins become inserted in the bacterial cell membrane, causing it to leak. The resultant loss of cell contents causes death. Inhibition of protein synthesis per se does not seem the likely cause of bacterial death. This statement is based on the observation that complete blockade of protein synthesis by other antibiotics (e.g., tetracyclines, chloramphenicol) is usually only bacteriostatic.

### Microbial Resistance

The principal cause for bacterial resistance is production of enzymes that can inactivate aminoglycosides. Among gram-negative bacteria, the genetic information needed to synthesize these enzymes is acquired by transfer of R factors. To date, more than 20 different aminoglycoside-inactivating enzymes have been identified. Since each of the aminoglycosides can be modified by more than one of these enzymes, and since each enzyme can act on more than one aminoglycoside, patterns of bacterial resistance to the aminoglycosides can be complex.

Of all the aminoglycosides, *amikacin* is *least* susceptible to inactivation by bacterial enzymes. As a result, resistance to amikacin is uncommon. To minimize emergence of bacteria resistant to amikacin, it is recommended that the drug be reserved for infections that are unresponsive to other aminoglycosides.

### Antimicrobial Spectrum

Bactericidal effects of the aminoglycosides are limited almost exclusively to *aerobic gram-negative bacilli.* Sensitive organisms include *Escherichia coli, Klebsiella*

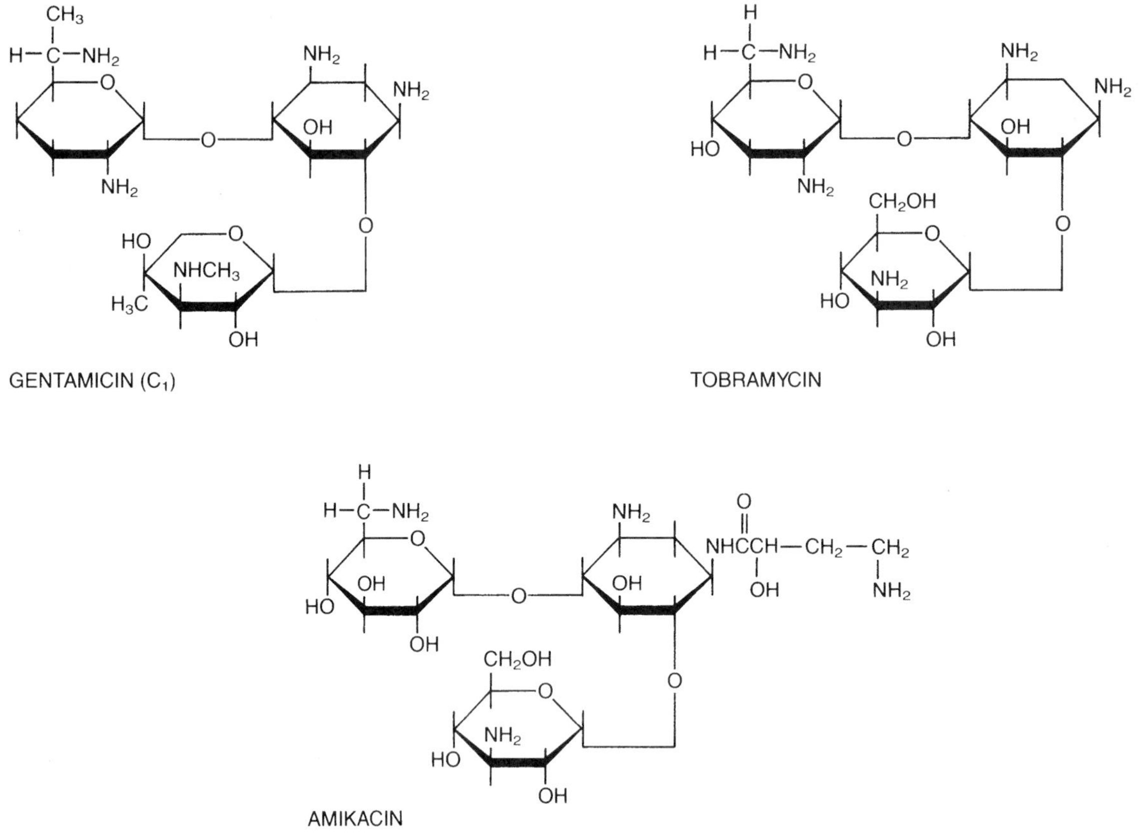

**Figure 81–1. Structural formulas of the major aminoglycosides.**

*pneumoniae, Serratia marcescens, Proteus mirabilis,* and *Pseudomonas aeruginosa.* Aminoglycosides are inactive against most gram-positive bacteria.

Aminoglycosides are *ineffective* against *anaerobes.* To produce their antibacterial effects, aminoglycosides must be transported across the bacterial cell membrane, a process that is oxygen dependent. Since, by definition, anaerobic organisms live in the absence of oxygen, these microbes cannot take up the aminoglycosides, and therefore are drug resistant. For the same reason, aminoglycosides are inactive against facultative bacteria when these organisms are living under anaerobic conditions.

## Therapeutic Use

*Parenteral Therapy.* The principal use for parenteral aminoglycosides is treatment of *serious infections due to aerobic gram-negative bacilli.* Primary target organisms are *Pseudomonas aeruginosa* and the Enterobacteriaceae (e.g., *E. coli, Klebsiella, Serratia, Proteus mirabilis*).

The aminoglycosides used most for parenteral therapy are gentamicin, tobramycin, and amikacin. Selection among these three drugs depends in large part on patterns of resistance in a given community or hospital. In settings where resistance to aminoglycosides is uncommon, either gentamicin or tobramycin is usually preferred. Of these two drugs, gentamicin is less costly and may be selected on this basis. Organisms resistant to both gentamicin and tobramycin are usually sensitive to amikacin. Accordingly, in settings where resistance to gentamicin and tobramycin is common, amikacin may be preferred for initial therapy.

*Oral Therapy.* Aminoglycosides are not absorbed from the gastrointestinal tract; hence, oral administration is used only for local effects within the intestine. In patients anticipating elective colorectal surgery, oral aminoglycosides have been given prophylactically to suppress bacterial growth in the bowel. One aminoglycoside (paromomycin) is used to treat intestinal amebiasis and tapeworm infestation.

*Topical Therapy. Neomycin* is available in formulations for application to the eyes, ears, and skin. Topical preparations of *gentamicin* and *tobramycin* are used to treat conjunctivitis caused by susceptible gram-negative bacilli. *Gentamicin* is also available in a formulation intended for application to the skin. However, because gentamicin-resistant organisms emerge rapidly, this preparation is not recommended.

## Pharmacokinetics

All of the aminoglycosides have similar pharmacokinetic profiles. Pharmacokinetic properties of the principal aminoglycosides are summarized in Table 81–1.

*Absorption.* Because they are polycations, the aminoglycosides cross membranes poorly. As a result, very little (about 1%) of an oral dose is absorbed. Hence, for treatment of systemic infections, aminoglycosides must be given parenterally (IM or IV). Absorption following application to the intact skin is minimal. However, when used for wound irrigation, aminoglycosides may be absorbed in amounts sufficient to produce systemic toxicity.

*Distribution.* Distribution of aminoglycosides is limited largely to extracellular fluid. Entry into the cerebrospi-

**TABLE 81–1. DOSAGES AND PHARMACOKINETIC PROPERTIES OF THE MAJOR AMINOGLYCOSIDES**

| Drug | Route | Total Daily Dosage (mg/kg)* | | Half-life in Adults (hr) | | Therapeutic Level, peak (µg/ml) | Toxic Level (µg/ml) | |
| | | Adults | Children | Normal | Anuric | | Peak[†] | Trough[‡] |
|---|---|---|---|---|---|---|---|---|
| Amikacin | IM, IV | 15 | 15 | 2–3 | 24–60 | 16–32 | >35 | >10 |
| Gentamicin | IM, IV | 3–5 | 6–7.5 | 2 | 24–60 | 4–8 | >12 | >2 |
| Tobramycin | IM, IV | 3–5 | 6–7.5 | 2–2.5 | 24–60 | 4–8 | >12 | >2 |
| Netilmicin | IM, IV | 4–6.5 | 5.5–8 | 2–2.7 | 40 | 6–10 | >16 | >4 |

*Because of interpatient variability, standard doses cannot be relied upon to produce appropriate serum drug levels; dosages should be adjusted on the basis of serum drug measurements.
†Measured 1 hour after IM injection or 30 minutes after a 30-minute infusion.
‡Measured just before the next dose.

nal fluid is insufficient to treat meningitis in adults. Aminoglycosides bind tightly to renal tissue, achieving levels in the kidney up to 50 times higher than levels in serum. These high levels correlate with production of nephrotoxicity (see below). Aminoglycosides penetrate readily to the perilymph and endolymph of the inner ear, and there is a direct relationship between levels achieved in these fluids and production of ototoxicity (see below). Aminoglycosides can cross the placenta and may have toxic effects on the fetus.

**Elimination.** The aminoglycosides are eliminated primarily by the kidneys. These drugs are not metabolized. In patients with normal renal function, the half-lives of the aminoglycosides range from 2 to 3 hours. However, since elimination is almost exclusively renal, half-lives increase dramatically in patients with kidney dysfunction (see Table 81-1). *Accordingly, if serious toxicity is to be avoided, it is essential to reduce the dosage or increase the dosing interval in patients with kidney disease.*

**Interpatient Variation.** Different patients receiving the same aminoglycoside dosage (in milligrams per kilogram of body weight) can achieve widely different serum levels of drug. This interpatient variation is caused by a number of factors, including age, percentage body fat, and pathophysiology (e.g., kidney dysfunction, fever, edema, dehydration). Because of variability among patients, aminoglycoside dosage must be individualized. As dramatic evidence of this need, in one clinical study it was observed that, in order to produce equivalent serum drug levels, the required doses of aminoglycosides ranged from as little as 0.5 mg/kg in one patient to a high of 25.8 mg/kg in another—a difference in dosage of more than 50-fold.

### Maintaining Appropriate Serum Drug Levels

For therapy with aminoglycosides to be both safe and effective, serum drug levels should be maintained within a narrow range. This is necessary because the levels that cause toxicity are only slightly greater than those required for bactericidal effects. In order to keep aminoglycoside levels within an acceptable range, dosage must be carefully adjusted for each patient.

Monitoring of serum drug levels provides the best basis for adjustment of aminoglycoside dosage. To produce bacterial kill while minimizing the risk of toxicity, it is necessary to keep peak and trough levels within an appropriate range. Dosage should be adjusted so that peak levels are high enough to kill bacteria but not so high as to be toxic. Since excessive trough levels correlate with increased toxicity, high trough levels must be avoided. When using gentamicin, for example, the dosage should be adjusted so that peak serum levels do not exceed 12 µg/ml while trough levels do not exceed 2 µg/ml. Therapeutic and toxic levels for gentamicin and the other aminoglycosides are summarized in Table 81-1.

When drawing blood samples for determination of aminoglycoside levels, timing is important. Samples for measurement of peak levels should be taken 1 hour after IM injection and 30 minutes after completion of a 30-minute IV infusion. Blood for trough measurements should be taken just prior to the next dose.

### Adverse Effects

The aminoglycosides can produce serious toxicity, especially to the inner ear and kidney. These toxicities limit the clinical utility of these drugs.

**Ototoxicity.** All the aminoglycosides can damage the inner ear, thereby impairing balance and hearing. Hearing loss results from damage to hair cells within the cochlea; disruption of balance results from damage to hair cells of the vestibular apparatus. The biochemical basis of these effects is not known. Factors that increase the risk of ototoxicity include (1) kidney dysfunction, (2) concurrent use of ethacrynic acid (a drug that has ototoxic properties of its own), and (3) administration of aminoglycosides in excessive doses or for more than 10 days.

Patients should be monitored for ototoxicity. Hearing loss begins with decreased acuity in the high-frequency range. This initial effect can be detected only through audiometric testing. Auditory toxicity may also manifest as tinnitus or a sense of fullness in the ears. Symptoms of vestibular damage include nausea, unsteadiness, dizziness, and vertigo. Patients should be informed about the symptoms of ototoxicity and instructed to report them.

If ototoxicity is detected, aminoglycosides should be withdrawn or given in reduced dosage. If impairment of hearing or balance is only moderate, symptoms usually reverse following discontinuation of drug use. However, if ototoxicity is extensive, the patient may suffer permanent hearing impairment or even complete hearing loss.

The risk of ototoxicity can be minimized in several ways. Dosages should be adjusted so that *trough* serum drug levels do not exceed recommended values. (Aminoglycosides diffuse out of the endolymph and perilymph during the trough time, thereby decreasing exposure of sensitive cells to these drugs.) Special care should be exercised to ensure safe levels in patients with kidney dysfunction. When possible, aminoglycosides should be used for no more than 10 days. Concurrent use of ethacrynic acid should be avoided. Patients should be monitored for early signs of cochlear and vestibular damage.

*Nephrotoxicity.* Aminoglycosides can injure cells of the proximal renal tubules. These drugs are taken up by tubular cells and achieve high intracellular concentrations. There is a direct correlation between intracellular levels and renal injury. Aminoglycoside-induced nephrotoxicity usually manifests as acute tubular necrosis. Prominent symptoms are proteinuria, casts in the urine, production of dilute urine, and elevations in serum creatinine and blood urea nitrogen (BUN). Serum creatinine and BUN should be monitored. The risk of nephrotoxicity is especially high in the elderly, in patients with pre-existing kidney disease, and in patients receiving other nephrotoxic drugs (e.g., amphotericin B, cephalothin). Fortunately, cells of the proximal tubule regenerate readily. As a result, injury to the kidney usually reverses following cessation of aminoglycoside use.

*Neuromuscular Blockade.* Aminoglycosides can inhibit neuromuscular transmission, causing flaccid paralysis and potentially fatal depression of respiration. Most episodes of neuromuscular blockade have occurred following intraperitoneal or intrapleural instillation of aminoglycosides. However, neuromuscular blockade has also occurred following intravenous and intramuscular administration. The risk of paralysis is increased by concurrent use of neuromuscular blocking agents and general anesthetics. Myasthenia gravis constitutes an additional risk. Neuromuscular blockade can be reversed by calcium; IV infusion of a calcium salt (e.g., calcium gluconate) is the treatment of choice. Because of increased physician awareness, aminoglycoside-induced neuromuscular blockade is now a clinical rarity.

*Other Adverse Effects.* Hypersensitivity reactions (e.g., rash, pruritus, urticaria) occur occasionally. Blood dyscrasias (neutropenia, agranulocytosis, aplastic anemia) are rare. Streptomycin has been associated with neurologic disorders (optic nerve dysfunction, peripheral neuritis, paresthesias of the face and hands). Oral neomycin has caused suprainfection of the bowel and intestinal malabsorption; topical neomycin may cause contact dermatitis.

### Drug Interactions

*Penicillins.* Penicillins and aminoglycosides are frequently employed in combination to enhance bacterial kill. (By disrupting the cell wall, penicillins facilitate access of aminoglycosides to their site of action.) When present in high concentrations, penicillins can inactivate aminoglycosides by direct chemical interaction. Accordingly, *penicillins and aminoglycosides should not be mixed together in the same intravenous solution.* (Inactivation is not likely to occur within the body, since drug concentrations are usually too low for significant chemical interaction.)

*Ototoxic Drugs.* The risk of injury to the inner ear is significantly increased by concurrent use of *ethacrynic acid*, a loop diuretic that has ototoxic actions of its own. The combination of an aminoglycoside with two other loop diuretics, furosemide and bumetanide, appears to cause no more ototoxicity than the aminoglycoside alone.

*Nephrotoxic Drugs.* The risk of renal damage is increased by concurrent therapy with other nephrotoxic agents. Additive or potentiative nephrotoxicity has been observed with *methoxyflurane, amphotericin B, cephalosporins, polymyxins,* and *vancomycin.*

*Skeletal Muscle Relaxants.* Aminoglycosides can intensify neuromuscular blockade induced by tubocurarine, pancuronium, and other skeletal muscle relaxants. If aminoglycosides are used with these agents, caution must be exercised to avoid respiratory arrest.

# Properties of Individual Aminoglycosides

## Gentamicin

*Therapeutic Use.* Gentamicin [Garamycin, Jenamicin] is used to treat serious infections caused by aerobic gram-negative bacilli. Primary target organisms are *Pseudomonas aeruginosa* and the Enterobacteriaceae (e.g., *E. coli, Klebsiella, Serratia, Proteus mirabilis*). In hospitals where resistance is not a problem, gentamicin is often the preferred aminoglycoside for use against these bacteria. The principal advantage of gentamicin over the other major aminoglycosides (tobramycin and amikacin) is low cost. Unfortunately, resistance to gentamicin is increasing, and cross-resistance to tobramycin is common. For infections that are resistant to gentamicin and tobramycin, amikacin is usually effective. In addition to its use against gram-negative bacilli, gentamicin can be combined with ampicillin or penicillin to treat enterococcal endocarditis.

*Adverse Effects and Interactions.* Like all other aminoglycosides, gentamicin is toxic to the kidney and inner ear. Caution must be exercised when combining gentamicin with other nephrotoxic or ototoxic drugs. Gentamicin is inactivated by penicillins and should not be mixed with these drugs in the same IV solution.

*Preparations, Dosage, and Administration.* Gentamicin sulfate [Garamycin, Jenamicin] is dispensed in several concentrations for IM and IV administration. The usual adult dosage is 1 to 1.7 mg/kg every 8 hours. The usual pediatric dosage is 2 to 2.5

mg/kg every 8 hours. Because of substantial interpatient variation, it is desirable to monitor serum drug levels and to adjust dosage accordingly: peak levels should range from 4 to 8 µg/ml and trough levels should not exceed 2 µg/ml. In patients with renal dysfunction, the dosage should be reduced or the dosing interval increased. For intravenous administration, the drug should be diluted in either sodium chloride for injection or 5% dextrose and infused over 30 minutes or more. Gentamicin should not be mixed with penicillins in the same IV solution. Duration of treatment is usually 7 to 10 days.

## Tobramycin

***Uses, Adverse Effects, and Interactions.*** Tobramycin [Nebcin] is similar to gentamicin in its uses, adverse effects, and interactions. The drug is more active than gentamicin against *Pseudomonas aeruginosa*, but less active against enterococci and *Serratia*. Like all other aminoglycosides, tobramycin can injure the inner ear and kidney. If possible, concurrent therapy with other ototoxic or nephrotoxic drugs should be avoided.

***Preparations, Dosage, and Administration.*** Tobramycin sulfate [Nebcin] is dispensed in solution (10 and 40 mg/ml) and as a powder (30 mg/ml after reconstitution) for IM and IV administration. The usual adult dosage is 1 to 1.7 mg/kg every 8 hours. The usual pediatric dosage is 2 to 2.5 mg/kg every 8 hours. Ideally, dosages should be individualized to produce peak and trough levels within the ranges indicated in Table 81–1. In patients with renal dysfunction, dosage should be reduced or the dosing interval increased. For intravenous administration, the drug should be diluted in either 0.9% Sodium Chloride for Injection or 5% dextrose and infused over 30 minutes or more. Tobramycin should not be mixed with penicillins in the same IV solution. Duration of treatment is usually 7 to 10 days.

## Amikacin

***Uses, Adverse Effects, and Interactions.*** Amikacin [Amikin] has two outstanding features: (1) of all the aminoglycosides, amikacin has the broadest spectrum of action against gram-negative bacilli, and (2) of all the aminoglycosides, amikacin is the least vulnerable to inactivation by bacterial enzymes. Because most aminoglycoside-inactivating enzymes do not affect amikacin, the incidence of bacterial resistance to this agent is lower than with other aminoglycosides. As a result, amikacin is often effective against bacteria that are resistant to the other major aminoglycosides (gentamicin and tobramycin). In hospitals where resistance to gentamicin and tobramycin is common, amikacin is the preferred agent for initial treatment of infections caused by aerobic gram-negative bacilli. However, in settings where resistance to the other aminoglycosides is infrequent, amikacin should be reserved for infections of proven aminoglycoside resistance; this practice will delay emergence of organisms resistant to amikacin. Like all other aminoglycosides, amikacin is toxic to the kidney and inner ear. Caution should be ex-

ercised if amikacin is used in combination with other ototoxic or nephrotoxic drugs.

***Preparations, Dosage, and Administration.*** Amikacin sulfate [Amikin] is available in solution (50 and 250 mg/ml) for parenteral (IM and IV) administration. For intravenous use, amikacin should be diluted in sodium chloride or 5% dextrose for injection; infusion time should be 30 to 60 minutes in adults and 1 to 2 hours in infants. The recommended dosage for adults and children is 15 mg/kg/day administered in equally divided doses at 8- or 12-hour intervals. In patients with kidney dysfunction, dosage should be reduced or the dosing interval increased; dosage adjustments should be based on measurements of serum drug levels. As a rule, duration of treatment should not exceed 10 days.

## Other Aminoglycosides

### Netilmicin

Netilmicin [Netromycin] has an antibacterial spectrum similar to that of gentamicin. Netilmicin has some resistance to the bacterial enzymes that inactivate gentamicin and tobramycin. However, netilmicin is more vulnerable to inactivation than amikacin. Like other aminoglycosides, netilmicin is ototoxic and nephrotoxic, although ototoxicity may be less than with other aminoglycosides. Administration is IM or IV. The dosage for adults is 1.3 to 2.2 mg/kg every 8 hours; the dosage for children is 1.8 to 2.7 mg/kg every 8 hours. Duration of treatment ranges from 7 to 14 days.

### Neomycin

Neomycin is the most toxic of the aminoglycosides; the drug can cause severe damage to the kidneys and inner ear. Because of its toxicity, neomycin is not administered parenterally. Neomycin is employed primarily for topical treatment of infections of the eye, ear, and skin. The drug is also administered orally to suppress bowel flora prior to surgery of the intestine. Since aminoglycosides are not absorbed from the gastrointestinal tract, oral administration constitutes a local (nonsystemic) use of the drug. Oral neomycin can cause suprainfection of the bowel as well as an intestinal malabsorption syndrome.

### Kanamycin

Kanamycin [Kantrex] is an older aminoglycoside to which bacterial resistance is common. The drug is still active against some gram-negative bacilli, but *Serratia* and *Pseudomonas aeruginosa* are resistant. Because of resistance, systemic use of the drug has sharply declined; for treatment of systemic infections, gentamicin, tobramycin, and amikacin are preferred. Like neomycin, kanamycin is employed to suppress bacterial flora of the bowel prior to elective colorectal surgery. Kanamycin is dispensed in capsules for oral use and as an injection for IM and IV administration.

### Streptomycin

Streptomycin, discovered in 1943, was the first aminoglycoside drug. Although once employed widely, streptomycin has been largely replaced by safer or more effective medications. As discussed in Chapter 84, streptomycin can be used in combination with other drugs to treat tuberculosis, but newer and safer agents (rifampin, isoniazid, ethambutol) are generally preferred. Streptomycin is also indicated for several uncommon infections (plague, tularemia, glanders, brucellosis). When combined with ampicillin or penicillin G, streptomycin may be used for enterococcal endocarditis.

### Paromomycin

Paromomycin [Humatin] is an aminoglycoside employed only for local effects within the intestine. The drug is administered orally to treat intestinal amebiasis and tapeworm infestations.

The dosage for both indications is 8 to 12 mg/kg 3 times daily for 5 to 10 days. Principal adverse effects are nausea, cramps, and diarrhea. Paromomycin is dispensed in 250-mg capsules.

## KEY POINTS

- Aminoglycosides are narrow-spectrum antibiotics, used primarily against aerobic gram-negative bacilli.
- Aminoglycosides disrupt protein synthesis and cause bacterial death.
- Because aminoglycosides carry multiple positive charges, these agents are not absorbed from the gastrointestinal tract, do not cross the blood-brain barrier, and are excreted rapidly by the kidney.
- Aminoglycosides can cause irreversible injury to sensory cells of the inner ear, resulting in hearing loss and disturbance of balance.
- Aminoglycosides are nephrotoxic, but injury to the kidney is usually reversible.
- Because aminoglycosides have a narrow therapeutic range, monitoring of serum drug levels is common. *Peak* levels must be high enough to cause bacterial kill; *trough* levels must be low enough to minimize toxicity.

# Summary of Major Nursing Implications*

## Aminoglycosides

| | |
|---|---|
| Amikacin | Kanamycin |
| Gentamicin | Neomycin |
| Tobramycin | Paromomycin |
| Netilmicin | |

Except where noted, the implications summarized below apply to all of the aminoglycosides.

## Preadministration Assessment

### Therapeutic Goal
*Parenteral Therapy.* Treatment of serious infections caused by gram-negative aerobic bacilli.

*Oral Therapy.* Suppression of bowel flora prior to elective colorectal surgery.

*Topical Therapy.* Treatment of local infections of the eyes, ears, and skin.

### Identifying High-Risk Patients
Aminoglycosides must be used with *caution* in patients with *renal impairment*, *pre-existing hearing impairment*, and *myasthenia gravis*, and in *patients receiving ototoxic drugs* (especially ethacrynic acid), *nephrotoxic drugs* (e.g., amphotericin B, cephalosporins, vancomycin), and *neuromuscular blocking agents*.

## Implementation: Administration

### Routes
*Intramuscular and Intravenous.* Gentamicin, tobramycin, amikacin, netilmicin, kanamycin.

*Oral.* Neomycin, kanamycin, paromomycin.

*Topical.* Neomycin, gentamicin, tobramycin.

### Administration
Aminoglycosides must be given parenterally (IV, IM) to treat systemic infections. Intravenous infusions should be done slowly (over 30 minutes or more). Do not mix aminoglycosides and penicillins in the same IV solution.

When possible, adjust the dosage on the basis of plasma drug levels. Draw blood samples for measurement of peak levels 1 hour after IM injection and 30 minutes after completion of an IV infusion; draw samples for trough levels just prior to the next dose.

In patients with renal dysfunction, the dosage should be reduced or the dosing interval increased.

## Ongoing Evaluation and Interventions

### Monitoring Summary
Monitor aminoglycoside levels (peaks and troughs), inner ear function (hearing and balance), creatinine clearance, BUN, and urine output.

### Minimizing Adverse Effects
*Ototoxicity.* Aminoglycosides can damage the inner ear, thereby impairing hearing and balance. Monitor for ototoxicity; use audiometry in high-risk patients. Instruct patients to report symptoms of ototoxicity (hearing loss, tinnitus, nausea, unsteadiness, dizziness, vertigo). If ototoxicity is detected, aminoglycosides should be discontinued or used in reduced dosage.

*Nephrotoxicity.* Aminoglycosides can cause acute tubular necrosis. To evaluate renal injury, monitor serum creatinine and BUN. If oliguria or anuria develops, withhold the aminoglycoside and notify the physician.

*Neuromuscular Blockade.* Aminoglycosides can inhibit neuromuscular transmission, causing potentially fatal respiratory depression. Carefully observe patients with myasthenia gravis and patients receiving skeletal muscle relaxants or general anesthetics. Aminoglycoside-induced neuromuscular blockade can be reversed with intravenous *calcium gluconate*.

### Minimizing Adverse Interactions
*Penicillins.* Aminoglycosides can be inactivated by high concentrations of penicillins. Never mix penicillins and aminoglycosides in the same intravenous solution.

---

*Patient education information is highlighted in color.

**Ototoxic and Nephrotoxic Drugs.** Exercise caution when using aminoglycosides in combination with other nephrotoxic or ototoxic drugs. Increased nephrotoxicity has been observed with *methoxyflurane, amphotericin B, cephalosporins, polymyxins,* and *vancomycin.* The risk of ototoxicity is increased by *ethacrynic acid.*

**Skeletal Muscle Relaxants.** Aminoglycosides can intensify neuromuscular blockade induced by tubocurarine, pancuronium, and other skeletal muscle relaxants. When aminoglycosides are used concurrently with these agents, exercise caution to avoid respiratory arrest.

# CHAPTER 82

# Sulfonamides and Trimethoprim

**Sulfonamides**
 Basic Pharmacology
 Sulfonamide Preparations
**Trimethoprim**
**Trimethoprim-Sulfamethoxazole**

The sulfonamides and trimethoprim are broad-spectrum antimicrobial drugs that have closely related mechanisms of action: they all disrupt the synthesis of tetrahydrofolic acid. In approaching these drugs, we will begin with the sulfonamides, followed by trimethoprim. We will conclude with trimethoprim-sulfamethoxazole, an important fixed-dose combination product.

## Sulfonamides

The sulfonamides were the first drugs available for systemic treatment of bacterial infections. The introduction and subsequent widespread use of these drugs produced a sharp decline in morbidity and mortality from susceptible infections. Until the penicillins became generally available, sulfonamides remained the mainstay of antibacterial chemotherapy. With the advent of newer antimicrobial drugs, use of the sulfonamides has greatly declined. However, the sulfonamides still have an important therapeutic role, primarily in the treatment of urinary tract infections. With the introduction of trimethoprim-sulfamethoxazole in the 1970s, indications for the sulfonamides have expanded.

### Basic Pharmacology

Similarities among the sulfonamides are more striking than differences. Accordingly, rather than focusing on a representative prototype, we will discuss the sulfonamides as a group.

### Chemistry

The general structural formula for the sulfonamides is shown in Figure 82-1. As you can see, sulfonamides are structural analogs of *para-aminobenzoic acid* (PABA). The antimicrobial actions of sulfonamides are based on this structural similarity.

Individual sulfonamides vary greatly with respect to solubility in water. The older sulfonamides have low solubility; as a result, these agents often crystallized out in the urine, causing injury to the kidneys. The sulfonamides in current use have relatively high water solubility; hence, the risk of renal damage is now low.

### Mechanism of Action

Sulfonamides suppress bacterial growth by inhibiting synthesis of *folic acid* (folate), a compound required by all cells for biosynthesis of DNA, RNA, and proteins. The steps in folate synthesis are shown in Figure 82-2. As indicated, sulfonamides block the step in which PABA is combined with pteridine to form dihydropteroic acid. Because of their structural similarity to PABA, sulfonamides act as competitive inhibitors of this reaction. Sulfonamides are usually bacteriostatic. Hence, host defenses are essential for complete elimination of infection.

If all cells require folate, why don't sulfonamides harm the host? To answer this question, we need to understand how bacteria and mammalian cells acquire folic acid. Bacteria are unable to take up folate from their environment. Consequently, they must synthesize folic acid from precursors. It is this process that sulfonamides disrupt. In contrast to bacteria, mammalian cells do not manufacture their own folate. Rather, they simply take up folic acid obtained from the diet, using a specialized transport system for uptake. Since mammalian cells use preformed folic acid rather than synthesizing it, sulfonamides are harmless to the host.

### Microbial Resistance

Many bacterial species have developed resistance to sulfonamides, thereby decreasing the utility of these drugs. Resistance is especially high among gonococci, meningococci, staphylococci, streptococci, and shigellae. Resistance may be acquired by spontaneous mutation or by transfer of R factors. Principal mechanisms of resistance are (1) synthesis of PABA in amounts sufficient to overcome sulfonamide-mediated inhibition of dihydropteroate synthetase, (2) alteration in the structure of dihydropteroate synthetase such that binding and inhibition by sulfonamides is reduced, and (3) reduced sulfonamide uptake.

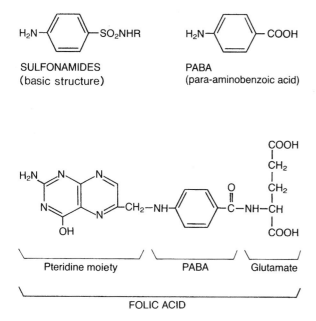

**Figure 82–1. Structural relationships among sulfon-amides, PABA, and folic acid.**

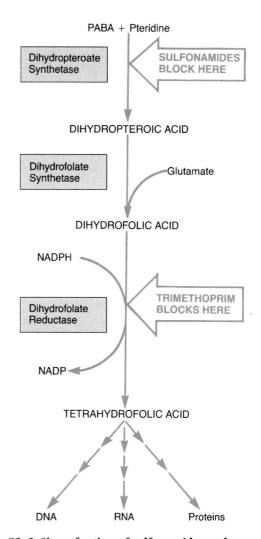

**Figure 82–2. Sites of action of sulfonamides and trimethoprim.** Sulfonamides and trimethoprim inhibit sequential steps in the synthesis of tetrahydrofolic acid (FAH$_4$). In the absence of FAH$_4$, bacteria are unable to synthesize DNA, RNA, and proteins.

## Antimicrobial Spectrum

The sulfonamides are active against a broad spectrum of microbes. Susceptible organisms include gram-positive cocci, gram-negative bacilli, actinomycetes (e.g., *Nocardia*), chlamydiae (e.g., *Chlamydia trachomatis*), and some protozoa (e.g., *Toxoplasma*, plasmodia).

## Therapeutic Uses

Although the sulfonamides were once employed widely, applications are now limited. Sulfonamide use has declined for two reasons: (1) introduction of bactericidal antibiotics that have less toxicity than sulfonamides and (2) development of bacterial resistance to sulfonamides. Today, urinary tract infection is the principal indication for sulfonamides. In addition, sulfonamides are drugs of choice for nocardiosis.

*Urinary Tract Infection.* Sulfonamides are often preferred drugs for acute infections of the urinary tract. About 90% of these infections are due to *Escherichia coli*, a bacterium that is usually sulfonamide sensitive. Of the sulfonamides available, *sulfisoxazole* is generally favored. This drug has high solubility in urine, achieves effective concentrations within the urinary tract, and is less expensive than other sulfonamides. When infection is recurrent, or when urinary tract obstruction is present, treatment with a sulfonamide alone may not be sufficient. Treatment of urinary tract infections is discussed further in Chapter 83.

*Other Uses.* Sulfonamides are drugs of choice for nocardiosis (infection with *Nocardia asteroides*). In addition, sulfonamides are alternatives to doxycycline and erythromycin for infections caused by *Chlamydia trachomatis* (trachoma, inclusion conjunctivitis, urethritis, lymphogranuloma venereum). Sulfonamides may be combined with erythromycin or penicillin to treat otitis media caused by amoxicillin-resistant strains of *Haemo-*

*philus influenzae*. For patients allergic to penicillin, sulfonamides are alternative drugs for prophylaxis of rheumatic fever. Sulfonamides are used in conjunction with pyrimethamine to treat two protozoal infections: toxoplasmosis and malaria caused by chloroquine-resistant *Plasmodium falciparum*.

One sulfonamide preparation—sulfasalazine—is used to treat ulcerative colitis. The benefits of sulfasalazine in this disorder are not due to suppression of microbial growth. Treatment of ulcerative colitis is considered in Chapter 73.

### Pharmacokinetics

*Absorption.* Sulfonamides are well absorbed following oral administration. When applied topically to the skin or mucous membranes, sulfonamides may be absorbed in amounts sufficient to cause systemic effects.

*Distribution.* Sulfonamides are well distributed to all tissues. Concentrations in pleural, peritoneal, ocular, and similar body fluids may be as much as 80% of the concentration in blood. Sulfonamides readily cross the placenta, and levels achieved in the fetus are sufficient to produce antimicrobial effects and toxicity.

***Metabolism.*** Sulfonamides are metabolized in the liver; the principal reaction is acetylation. Acetylated derivatives of sulfonamides lack antimicrobial activity, but are just as toxic as the parent compounds. Acetylation may decrease sulfonamide solubility, thereby increasing the risk of renal damage from crystal formation.

***Excretion.*** Sulfonamides are excreted primarily by the kidneys. Hence, the rate of renal excretion is the principal determinant of sulfonamide half-life. Sulfonamides that are excreted slowly have a longer duration of action than those that are excreted rapidly.

## Adverse Effects

Sulfonamides can cause multiple adverse effects. Prominent among these are hypersensitivity reactions, blood dyscrasias, and kernicterus (in newborn infants). Renal damage from crystalluria had been a problem with older sulfonamides but is of minimal concern with the drugs available today.

***Hypersensitivity Reactions.*** Sulfonamides can induce a variety of hypersensitivity reactions. Mild reactions—rash, drug fever, photosensitivity—are relatively common. To minimize photosensitivity reactions, patients should avoid prolonged exposure to sunlight, wear protective clothing, and apply a sunscreen to exposed skin.

Hypersensitivity reactions are especially frequent with topical sulfonamides. As a result, these preparations are no longer employed routinely. Rather, their use is restricted to ophthalmic infections, burns, and vaginitis caused by *Gardnerella vaginalis*.

The most severe hypersensitivity response to sulfonamides is *Stevens-Johnson syndrome*, a rare reaction that has a mortality rate of about 25%. Symptoms include widespread lesions of the skin and mucous membranes, together with fever, malaise, and toxemia. The reaction is most likely with long-acting sulfonamides, agents that have been banned in the United States. Shorter acting sulfonamides may also induce the syndrome, but the incidence with these drugs is low. To minimize the risk of severe reactions, sulfonamides should be discontinued as soon as skin rash of any sort is observed. In addition, sulfonamides should not be given to patients with a history of hypersensitivity to the sulfonamides or to chemically related drugs, including sulfonylureas (oral hypoglycemic drugs), thiazide diuretics, and loop diuretics.

***Hematologic Effects.*** Sulfonamides can cause *hemolytic anemia* in patients whose red blood cells have a genetically determined deficiency in glucose-6-phosphate dehydrogenase (G-6-PD). This inherited trait is most common among African Americans and people of Mediterranean origin. Rarely, hemolysis occurs in the absence of G-6-PD deficiency. Red cell lysis can produce fever, pallor, and jaundice; patients should be observed for these signs. In addition to hemolytic anemia, sulfonamides can cause agranulocytosis, leukopenia, thrombocytopenia, and, very rarely, aplastic anemia. When sulfonamides are used for a long time, periodic blood tests should be obtained.

***Kernicterus.*** Kernicterus is a disorder in newborns caused by deposition of bilirubin in the brain. Bilirubin is neurotoxic and can cause severe neurologic deficits and even death. Under normal conditions, infants are not vulnerable to kernicterus because any bilirubin present in the blood is tightly bound to plasma proteins, and therefore is not free to enter the central nervous system (CNS). Sulfonamides promote kernicterus by displacing bilirubin from plasma proteins. Since the blood-brain barrier of infants is poorly developed, the newly freed bilirubin has easy access to sites within the brain. *Because of the risk of kernicterus, sulfonamides should not be administered to infants under the age of 2 months. In addition, sulfonamides should not be given to pregnant women near term or to mothers who are breast-feeding.*

***Renal Damage from Crystalluria.*** Because of their low solubility, older sulfonamides tended to come out of solution in the urine, forming crystalline aggregates in the kidneys, ureters, and bladder. These aggregates caused irritation and obstruction, sometimes resulting in anuria and even death. Renal damage is uncommon with today's sulfonamides because their solubility is relatively high. To minimize the risk of renal damage, adults should maintain a daily urine output of 1200 ml. This can be accomplished by consuming 8 to 10 glasses of water each day. Since the solubility of sulfonamides is highest at elevated pH, alkalinization of the urine (e.g., with sodium bicarbonate) can further decrease the chances of crystalluria.

## Drug Interactions

Sulfonamides can intensify the effects of warfarin, phenytoin, and oral hypoglycemics (e.g., tolbutamide). The principal mechanism is inhibition of hepatic metabolism. When combined with sulfonamides, these drugs may require a reduction in dosage to prevent toxicity.

## Sulfonamide Preparations

The sulfonamides fall into two major categories: (1) systemic sulfonamides and (2) sulfonamides used for local effects. The sulfonamides employed for systemic therapy are more widely used.

### Systemic Sulfonamides

The systemic sulfonamides can be subdivided based on duration of action. As indicated in Table 82-1, two groups are available in the United States: (1) short-acting agents and (2) intermediate-acting agents. Long-acting sulfonamides produce a high incidence of Stevens-Johnson syndrome and have been withdrawn from the American market. The short-acting sulfonamides are used primarily to treat infections of the urinary tract. Except where noted below, the adverse effects and drug interactions of individual sulfonamides are the same as those discussed above. Dosages and trade names for systemic sulfonamides are summarized in Table 82-1.

***Sulfisoxazole.*** Sulfisoxazole [Gantrisin], a short-acting sulfonamide, can be considered the prototype of the sulfonamide family. This drug is the preferred sulfonamide for chemotherapy of urinary tract infections. Sulfisoxazole

## TABLE 82-1. SYSTEMIC SULFONAMIDES

| Class* | Generic Name | Trade Name | Usual Adult Oral Maintenance Dosage |
|---|---|---|---|
| *Short Acting* | Sulfisoxazole | Gantrisin | 1 gm ever 4–6 hr |
| | Sulfacytine | Renoquid | 250 mg every 6 hr |
| | Sulfadiazine | — | 1 gm every 4–6 hr |
| | Sulfamethizole | Thiosulfil Forte | 0.5 to 1 gm every 6 hr |
| | Trisulfapyrimidines:<br>    Sulfadiazine plus<br>    Sulfamerazine plus<br>    Sulfamethazine | Triple Sulfa No. 2 | 1 gm every 6 hr |
| *Intermediate Acting* | Sulfamethoxazole | Gantanol, Urobak | 1 gm every 12 hr |

*Long-acting sulfonamides (e.g., sulfamethoxypyridazine, sulfameter) are no longer available in the United States.

is just as effective as other sulfonamides and less expensive. Moreover, because of its high water solubility, sulfisoxazole poses a minimal risk of crystalluria. Since high plasma concentrations of sulfisoxazole can be achieved, the drug is useful against a variety of systemic infections (e.g., nocardiosis, melioidosis, chancroid). In addition, sulfisoxazole can be combined with penicillin or erythromycin to treat otitis media caused by amoxicillin-resistant *H. influenzae*. The drug is also used for prophylaxis of rheumatic fever in patients allergic to penicillin. Sulfisoxazole may be administered orally or by injection (IV, SC, IM). Oral administration is preferred.

**Sulfamethoxazole.** Sulfamethoxazole [Gantanol, Urobak] is the only intermediate-acting sulfonamide available. Indications for this drug are the same as for sulfisoxazole. Because of its prolonged duration of action, sulfamethoxazole can be administered less frequently than the short-acting sulfonamides. This drug has lower water solubility than sulfisoxazole, and hence presents a greater risk of injury to the kidneys. The risk of renal damage can be minimized by maintaining adequate hydration. Sulfamethoxazole is employed primarily in fixed-dose combination with trimethoprim. This combination is discussed later in the chapter. Administration is oral.

**Sulfadiazine.** Sulfadiazine is a short-acting sulfonamide. The drug is less soluble than other short-acting agents. Hence, if renal damage is to be avoided, high urine flow must be maintained. Sulfadiazine crosses the blood-brain barrier with ease, and therefore is the best sulfonamide for prophylaxis of meningitis. Sulfadiazine is also a preferred agent for chemotherapy of nocardiosis. When combined with pyrimethamine, sulfadiazine is useful against toxoplasmosis. The drug is dispensed in tablets for oral administration.

**Sulfacytine.** Sulfacytine [Renoquid] is a newer sulfonamide. The drug is short acting and has high water solubility. The only indication for this agent is acute infection of the urinary tract. Sulfacytine is more expensive than the older sulfonamides. Administration is oral.

**Sulfamethizole.** Sulfamethizole [Thiosulfil Forte] is a short-acting sulfonamide. The drug is used only for urinary tract infections. Sulfamethizole is dispensed in tablets for oral administration.

**Trisulfapyrimidines.** Trisulfapyrimidines [Triple Sulfa No. 2] is a preparation containing relatively low amounts of three poorly soluble sulfonamides: *sulfadiazine*, *sulfamerazine*, and *sulfamethazine*. Before the more soluble sulfonamides became available, combination preparations such as trisulfapyrimidines were employed in efforts to decrease sulfonamide-induced damage to the kidneys. The rationale for these combinations is as follows. First, by combining three sulfonamides in low dosage, powerful antibacterial action can be achieved because the effects of the individual drugs are additive. Second, since the presence of one sulfonamide does not influence the solubility of the others, it is possible for the total urinary concentration of sulfonamide to be high without risking formation of crystals, provided the concentration of the individual agents remains below each drug's level of saturation. With the advent of more soluble sulfonamides, multiple sulfonamide preparations have become obsolete. Trisulfapyrimidines is the only such combination that remains on the market.

### Topical Sulfonamides

Topical sulfonamides have been associated with a high incidence of hypersensitivity reactions and are not used routinely. The preparations discussed below have proven utility and a relatively low incidence of hypersensitivity.

**Sulfacetamide.** Sulfacetamide is widely used for superficial infections of the eye (e.g., conjunctivitis, corneal ulcer). The drug may cause blurred vision, sensitivity to bright light, headache, browache, and local irritation. Hypersensitivity is rare, but severe reactions have occurred. Accordingly, sulfacetamide should not be used by patients with a history of hypersensitivity to sulfonamides, sulfonylureas, or thiazide or loop diuretics. Sulfacetamide is available in solution and ointment formulations for local application to the eye. Trade names include Isopto Cetamide and Sodium Sulamyd.

**Silver Sulfadiazine and Mafenide.** Both of these sulfonamides are employed to prevent bacterial colonization in patients with second- and third-degree burns. Mafenide acts by the same mechanism as other sulfonamides. In contrast, antibacterial effects of silver sulfadiazine are due primarily to release of free silver—and not to the sulfonamide portion of the molecule. Local application of mafenide is frequently painful. In contrast, application of silver sulfadiazine is usually pain free. Following topical application, both agents can be absorbed in amounts sufficient to produce systemic effects. Mafenide, but not silver sulfadiazine, is metabolized to a compound that can suppress renal excretion of acid, thereby causing acidosis. Accordingly, patients receiving mafenide should be monitored for acid-base status. If acidosis becomes severe, mafenide should be discontinued for 1 to 2 days. Mafenide is marketed under the trade name Sulfamylon. The trade names for silver sulfadiazine are Silvadene, Thermazene, and SSD Cream.

# Trimethoprim

Like the sulfonamides, trimethoprim [Proloprim, Trimpex] suppresses production of tetrahydrofolic acid. Trimethoprim is active against a broad spectrum of microbes.

## Mechanism of Action

As indicated in Figure 82–2, trimethoprim is an *inhibitor of dihydrofolate reductase*, the enzyme that converts dihydrofolic acid to its active form: tetrahydrofolic acid. Hence, like the sulfonamides, trimethoprim suppresses bacterial synthesis of DNA, RNA, and proteins. Depending upon conditions at the site of infection, trimethoprim may be bactericidal or bacteriostatic.

Although mammalian cells also contain dihydrofolate reductase, trimethoprim is selectively toxic to bacteria. This selectivity is based on structural differences between bacterial dihydrofolate reductase and the enzyme found in mammalian cells. Because of these structural differences, trimethoprim inhibits the bacterial enzyme at concentrations about 40,000 times lower than those required to inhibit mammalian dihydrofolate reductase. As a result, we can suppress bacterial growth with doses that have essentially no effect on the host.

### Microbial Resistance

Bacteria acquire resistance to trimethoprim by three mechanisms: (1) synthesis of increased amounts of dihydrofolate reductase, (2) production of an altered dihydrofolate reductase that has a low affinity for trimethoprim, and (3) reduced cellular permeability to trimethoprim. Resistance has resulted from spontaneous mutation and from transfer of R factors. In the United States, bacterial resistance is uncommon.

### Antimicrobial Spectrum

Trimethoprim is active against many gram-positive bacilli and some gram-negative bacilli (e.g., *Corynebacterium diphtheriae*, *Listeria monocytogenes*). Most aerobic gram-negative bacilli of clinical importance are also sensitive, including *E. coli*, *Klebsiella*, *Proteus mirabilis*, *Serratia marcescens*, *Salmonella*, *Shigella*, and *H. influenzae*. In addition, trimethoprim is active against some pathogenic protozoa (e.g., *Pneumocystis carinii*, *Toxoplasma gondii*, and the protozoa responsible for malaria).

## Therapeutic Uses

Trimethoprim is approved only for initial therapy of acute, uncomplicated urinary tract infections due to susceptible organisms (e.g., *E. coli*, *Proteus mirabilis*, *Enterobacter* species, and *Staphylococcus saprophyticus*). When combined with sulfamethoxazole, trimethoprim has considerably more applications; these are discussed later in the chapter.

## Pharmacokinetics

Trimethoprim is absorbed rapidly and completely from the gastrointestinal tract. The drug is quite lipid soluble, and therefore undergoes wide distribution to body fluids and tissues. Trimethoprim readily crosses the placenta. Most of an administered dose is excreted unchanged by the kidneys. Hence, in the presence of renal dysfunction, the half-life of trimethoprim is prolonged. The concentration of trimethoprim achieved in urine is considerably higher than the concurrent concentration in blood.

## Adverse Effects

Trimethoprim is generally well tolerated. The most frequent adverse effects are itching and rash. Gastrointestinal reactions (e.g., epigastric distress, nausea, vomiting, glossitis, stomatitis) occur occasionally.

***Hematologic Effects.*** Since mammalian dihydrofolate reductase is relatively insensitive to trimethoprim, toxicities related to suppression of tetrahydrofolate production are rare. These rare effects—*megaloblastic anemia*, *thrombocytopenia*, and *neutropenia*—occur only in individuals with pre-existing folic acid deficiency. Accordingly, caution should be exercised when administering trimethoprim to patients in whom folate deficiency might be likely (e.g., alcoholics, pregnant women, debilitated patients). If early signs of bone marrow suppression occur (e.g., sore throat, fever, pallor), complete blood counts should be performed. If a significant reduction in blood cell counts is observed, trimethoprim should be discontinued. Administration of folinic acid (leucovorin) will restore normal hematopoiesis.

***Use in Pregnancy and Lactation.*** Large doses of trimethoprim have caused fetal malformations in animals. To date, no developmental abnormalities have been observed in humans. However, since trimethoprim readily crosses the placenta, prudence dictates that the drug not be used routinely during pregnancy. The risk of exacerbating pregnancy-related folate deficiency is an additional reason not to use the drug at this time.

Trimethoprim is excreted in breast milk and may interfere with folic acid utilization by the nursing infant. The drug should be administered with caution to women who are breast-feeding.

### Preparations, Dosage, and Administration

Trimethoprim [Proloprim, Trimpex] is dispensed in 100- and 200-mg tablets for oral use. For urinary tract infections, the usual dosage is 100 mg every 12 hours or 200 mg every 24 hours. Duration of treatment is 10 days. Dosage should be reduced in patients with renal dysfunction.

# Trimethoprim-Sulfamethoxazole

Trimethoprim (TMP) and sulfamethoxazole (SMZ) are marketed together in a fixed-dose combination product. This combination (TMP-SMZ) is a powerful antimicrobial preparation whose components act in concert to inhibit sequential steps in tetrahydrofolic acid synthesis. Trade names for TMP-SMZ are Bactrim, Cotrim, and Septra. In many countries the combination is known generically as *co-trimoxazole*.

## Mechanism of Action

The antimicrobial effects of TMP-SMZ result from inhibiting consecutive steps in the synthesis of tetrahydrofolic acid: SMZ acts first to inhibit incorporation of PABA into folic acid; TMP then inhibits dihydrofolate reductase, the enzyme that converts dihydrofolic acid into tetrahydrofolate (see Fig. 82–2). As a result of these actions, the ability of the target organism to produce nucleic acids and proteins is greatly suppressed. By inhibiting two reactions required for synthesis of tetrahydrofolate, TMP and SMZ potentiate each other's effects. That is, the antimicrobial effect of the combination is more powerful than the sum of the effects of TMP and SMZ alone. TMP-SMZ is selectively toxic to microbes because (1) mammalian cells use preformed folic acid, and therefore are not affected by SMZ, and (2) dihydrofolate reductases of mammalian cells are relatively insensitive to inhibition by TMP.

### Microbial Resistance

Resistance to the combination of TMP plus SMZ is less than to either drug alone. This is logical since the chances of an organism acquiring resistance to both drugs are less than its chances of developing resistance to just one or the other. Specific mechanisms of resistance to sulfonamides and TMP are discussed earlier in the chapter.

### Antimicrobial Spectrum

TMP-SMZ is active against a wide range of gram-positive and gram-negative bacteria. This should be no surprise since TMP and SMZ by themselves are broad-spectrum antimicrobial drugs. Most urinary tract pathogens are susceptible. Specific bacteria against which TMP-SMZ is consistently effective include *E. coli*, *Proteus mirabilis*, *Salmonella typhi*, *Shigella* species, *Vibrio cholerae*, *H. influenzae*, and *Yersinia pestis*. TMP-SMZ is also active against *Nocardia* and certain protozoa (*Pneumocystis carinii* and *Plasmodium* species).

## Therapeutic Uses

TMP-SMZ is a preferred or alternative medication for a variety of infectious diseases. The combination is especially valuable for urinary tract infections, otitis media, bronchitis, shigellosis, and pneumonia and other infections caused by *Pneumocystis carinii*.

### Urinary Tract Infection.
TMP-SMZ is indicated for chemotherapy of uncomplicated urinary tract infection caused by susceptible strains of *E. coli*, *Klebsiella*, *Enterobacter*, *Proteus mirabilis*, *P. vulgaris*, and *Morga-*

*nella morganii*. The combination is particularly useful for chronic and recurrent infections.

### Pneumocystis carinii Infections.
TMP-SMZ is the treatment of choice for pneumonia and other infections caused by *Pneumocystis carinii*, an opportunistic organism that thrives in immunocompromised hosts (e.g., cancer patients, organ transplant recipients, individuals with AIDS). When given to AIDS patients, TMP-SMZ produces a high incidence of adverse effects. The dosage for treating *Pneumocystis carinii* infections in AIDS patients is given in Chapter 88.

### Gastrointestinal Infections.
TMP-SMZ is a treatment of choice for shigellosis caused by susceptible strains of *Shigella flexneri* and *S. sonnei*. In addition, the combination is an alternative to chloramphenicol and ampicillin for typhoid fever.

### Other Infections.
TMP-SMZ can be used for otitis media and acute exacerbations of chronic bronchitis when these infections are due to susceptible strains of *H. influenzae* or *Streptococcus pneumoniae*. The preparation is also useful against urethritis and pharyngeal infection caused by penicillinase-producing *Neisseria gonorrhoeae*. Other infections that can be treated with TMP-SMZ include whooping cough, nocardiosis, brucellosis, melioidosis, and chancroid.

## Pharmacokinetics

### Absorption and Distribution.
TMP-SMZ may be administered orally or by IV infusion. Both components of TMP-SMZ are well distributed throughout the body. Therapeutic concentrations are achieved in tissues and body fluids (e.g., vaginal secretions, cerebrospinal fluid, pleural effusions, bile, aqueous humor). Both TMP and SMZ readily cross the placenta, and both enter breast milk.

### Plasma Drug Levels.
Optimal antibacterial effects are produced when the ratio of TMP to SMZ is 1:20. To achieve this 1:20 ratio in plasma, TMP and SMZ must be administered in a ratio of 1:5. Hence, standard tablets contain 80 mg of TMP and 400 mg of SMZ. Because the plasma half-lives of TMP and SMZ are similar (10 hours for TMP and 11 hours for SMZ), levels of both drugs decline in parallel, and the 1:20 ratio is maintained as the drugs undergo elimination.

### Elimination.
Both TMP and SMZ are excreted primarily by the kidneys. About 70% of urinary SMZ is present as inactive metabolites. In contrast, TMP undergoes little hepatic metabolism prior to excretion. Both agents are concentrated in the urine. Hence levels of active drug are higher in the urine than in plasma, despite some conversion to inactive products.

## Adverse Effects

TMP-SMZ is generally well tolerated; toxicity from routine use is rare. The most common adverse effects are nausea, vomiting, and rash. However, although infrequent, all of the serious toxicities associated with sulfonamides can occur with TMP-SMZ. That is, the combination can cause hypersensitivity reactions (including Stevens-Johnson syndrome), blood dyscrasias (hemolytic anemia, agranulocytosis, leukopenia, thrombocytopenia, aplastic anemia), kernicterus, and renal damage. Primarily because of its TMP component, TMP-SMZ can induce megaloblastic anemia, but only in patients who are folate deficient. TMP-SMZ may also cause adverse CNS effects (headache, depression, hallucinations). Hyperkalemia is a potential complication of TMP-SMZ therapy, especially when the dosage is high. Patients suffering from AIDS are unusually susceptible to TMP-SMZ toxicity. In this group, the incidence of adverse effects (rash, recurrent fever, leukopenia) is about 55%.

Several measures can reduce the incidence and severity of adverse effects. Crystalluria can be avoided by maintaining adequate hydration. Periodic blood tests permit early detection of hematologic disorders. To avoid kernicterus, TMP-SMZ should be withheld from pregnant women near term, nursing mothers, and infants under the age of 2 months. The risk of megaloblastic anemia can be reduced by withholding sulfonamides from individuals likely to be folate deficient (e.g., debilitated patients, pregnant women, alcoholics). Hypersensitivity reactions can be minimized by avoiding TMP-SMZ in patients with a history of hypersensitivity to sulfonamides or to chemically related drugs, including thiazide diuretics, loop diuretics, and oral hypoglycemics (sulfonylureas).

### Drug Interactions

Interactions of TMP-SMZ with other drugs are due primarily to the presence of SMZ. Hence, like sulfonamides used alone, SMZ in the combination can intensify the effects of warfarin, phenytoin, and oral hypoglycemics (e.g., tolbutamide). Accordingly, when these drugs are combined with TMP-SMZ, a reduction in their dosage may be needed.

### Preparations, Dosage, and Administration

**Preparations.** Trimethoprim-sulfamethoxazole [Bactrim, Cotrim, Septra] is dispensed in tablets and a suspension for oral use, and in solution for IV infusion. The ratio of TMP to SMZ in all preparations is 1:5. Two strengths of tablets are available: *standard tablets* contain 80 mg TMP and 400 mg SMZ; *double-strength tablets* contain 160 mg TMP and 800 mg SMZ. Each milliliter of the *oral suspension* contains 8 mg TMP and 40 mg SMZ. Each milliliter of the *IV infusion solution* contains 16 mg TMP and 80 mg SMZ.

**Oral Dosing.** For management of most infections, the usual *adult* dosage is 160 mg TMP plus 800 mg SMZ administered every 12 hours for 10 to 14 days. To treat shigellosis or traveler's diarrhea, the same dose is administered every 12 hours for 5 days. In the presence of renal impairment (creatinine clearance 15 to 30 ml/min), the dosage should be reduced by 50%. If cre-

atinine clearance is below 15 ml/minute, TMP-SMZ should not be used.

To treat urinary tract infections and acute otitis media in *children*, the usual dosage is 4 mg/kg TMP plus 20 mg/kg SMZ administered every 12 hours for 10 days. The same dose, administered every 12 hours for 5 days, is used to treat shigellosis. As in adults, the dosage should be reduced in patients with renal dysfunction.

**Intravenous Dosing.** Intravenous TMP-SMZ is used for severe infections. The following dosages are for adults and children, and are based on the TMP component of TMP-SMZ. For urinary tract infection or shigellosis, the total daily dose is 8 to 10 mg/kg. This total dose is administered in two to four divided doses given at equally spaced intervals. Duration of treatment is 14 days for urinary tract infection and 5 days for shigellosis. For treatment of *Pneumocystis carinii* pneumonia, the total daily dose is 15 to 20 mg/kg. This dose is administered in three or four divided doses given at equally spaced intervals. Duration of treatment is 2 weeks or less. Dosage for all indications should be reduced in patients with renal impairment.

## KEY POINTS

- The sulfonamides and trimethoprim act by inhibiting bacterial synthesis of folic acid.
- Sulfonamides are used primarily to treat urinary tract infections.
- The principal adverse effects of sulfonamides are (1) hypersensitivity reactions, ranging from mild (rash, photosensitivity) to severe (Stevens-Johnson syndrome); (2) hemolytic anemia; (3) kernicterus; and (4) renal damage.
- The combination product TMP-SMZ inhibits sequential steps in bacterial folic acid synthesis, and therefore is much more powerful than either TMP or SMZ alone.
- TMP-SMZ is a preferred drug for treating urinary tract infections and is the drug of choice for *Pneumocystis carinii* infections in patients with AIDS and other immunodeficiency states.
- The principal adverse effects of TMP-SMZ are like those caused by sulfonamides (i.e., hypersensitivity reactions, hemolytic anemia, kernicterus, and renal injury).

## Summary of Major Nursing Implications*

## Sulfonamides

| | |
|---|---|
| Sulfacytine | Sulfamethoxazole |
| Sulfadiazine | Sulfisoxazole |
| Sulfamethizole | Trisulfapyrimidines |

The nursing implications summarized here apply to *systemic* sulfonamides. Implications specific to topical sulfonamides are not summarized.

## Preadministration Assessment

### Therapeutic Goal

Sulfonamides are used primarily for urinary tract infections caused by *E. coli* and other susceptible organisms.

### Identifying High-Risk Patients

Sulfonamides are *contraindicated* during *pregnancy* and *lactation*, for *infants under the age of 2 months*, and for patients with a *history of hypersensitivity to sulfonamides and chemically related drugs, including thiazide diuretics, loop diuretics, and oral hypoglycemics (sulfonylureas)*. Exercise *caution* in patients with *renal impairment*.

---

*Patient education information is highlighted in color.

## Implementation: Administration

### Routes

All systemic sulfonamides can be administered orally. *Sulfisoxazole* can also be administered parenterally (IV, SC, IM).

### Administration

Advise patients to take oral sulfonamides on an empty stomach and with a full glass of water.

Instruct patients to complete the prescribed course of treatment, even though symptoms may abate before the full course is over.

Administer IV *sulfisoxazole* by slow injection or IV drip.

## Ongoing Evaluation and Interventions

### Minimizing Adverse Effects

*Hypersensitivity Reactions.* Sulfonamides can induce *severe hypersensitivity reactions* (e.g., Stevens-Johnson syndrome). Do not give sulfonamides to patients with a history of hypersensitivity to sulfonamides or to chemically related drugs, including sulfonylureas, thiazide diuretics, and loop diuretics. Instruct the patient to discontinue drug use immediately at the first sign of hypersensitivity (e.g., rash).

*Photosensitivity reactions* may occur. Advise the patient to avoid prolonged exposure to sunlight, wear protective clothing, and apply a sunscreen to exposed skin.

*Hematologic Effects.* Sulfonamides can cause hemolytic anemia and other blood dyscrasias (agranulocytosis, leukopenia, thrombocytopenia, aplastic anemia). Observe patients for signs of hemolysis (fever, pallor, jaundice). When sulfonamide therapy is prolonged, periodic blood cell counts should be made.

*Kernicterus.* Sulfonamides can cause kernicterus in newborns. Do not give these drugs to pregnant women near term, nursing mothers, or infants under the age of 2 months.

*Renal Damage.* Deposition of sulfonamide crystals can injure the kidney. To minimize crystalluria, maintain hydration sufficient to produce a daily urine flow of 1200 ml in adults. Alkalinization of urine (e.g., with sodium bicarbonate) can also be beneficial. Advise outpatients to consume 8 to 10 glasses of water per day.

### Minimizing Adverse Interactions

Sulfonamides can intensify the effects of *warfarin, phenytoin,* and *oral hypoglycemics* (e.g., tolbutamide). When combined with sulfonamides, these drugs may require a reduction in dosage.

## Trimethoprim

## Preadministration Assessment

### Therapeutic Goal

Initial treatment of uncomplicated urinary tract infections caused by *E. coli* and other susceptible organisms.

### Identifying High-Risk Patients

Trimethoprim is *contraindicated* in patients with *folate deficiency* (manifested as megaloblastic anemia). When possible, the drug should be avoided during *pregnancy* and *lactation.*

## Implementation: Administration

### Route

Oral.

### Dosage and Administration

Instruct patients to complete the prescribed course of treatment, even though symptoms may abate before the full course is over.

Reduce the dosage in patients with renal dysfunction.

## Ongoing Evaluation and Interventions

### Minimizing Adverse Effects

*Hematologic Effects.* Trimethoprim can cause blood dyscrasias (megaloblastic anemia, thrombocytopenia, neutropenia) by exacerbating pre-existing folic acid deficiency. Avoid trimethoprim when folate deficiency is likely (e.g., in alcoholics, pregnant women, debilitated patients). Inform patients about early signs of blood disorders (e.g., sore throat, fever, pallor), and instruct them to notify the physician if these occur. Complete blood counts should be performed. If a significant reduction in counts is observed, discontinue trimethoprim. Normal hematopoiesis can be restored with folinic acid (leucovorin).

*Use in Pregnancy and Lactation.* Trimethoprim should be avoided during pregnancy and lactation. The drug can exacerbate folate deficiency in pregnant women and cause folate deficiency in the nursing infant whose mother is taking trimethoprim.

## Trimethoprim-Sulfamethoxazole

## Preadministration Assessment

### Therapeutic Goal

Indications include urinary tract infections caused by *E. coli* and other susceptible organisms, shigellosis, pneumonia and other infections caused by *Pneumocystis carinii*, and otitis media caused by susceptible strains of *H. influenzae.*

### Identifying High-Risk Patients

TMP-SMZ is *contraindicated* during *pregnancy and lactation,* for *infants under the age of 2 months,* in patients with *folate deficiency* (manifested as megaloblastic anemia), and for patients with a *history of hypersensitivity to sulfonamides and chemically related drugs, including thiazide diuretics, loop diuretics, and oral hypoglycemics (sulfonylureas).*

## Implementation: Administration

### Routes

Oral, intravenous (for severe infections).

### Dosage Adjustment

In patients with renal impairment (creatinine clearance of 15 to 30 ml/min), decrease dosage by 50%. If creatinine clearance falls below 15 ml/min, discontinue drug use.

### Administration

Instruct the patient to complete the prescribed course of treatment, even though symptoms may abate before the full course is over.

## Ongoing Evaluation and Interventions

### Minimizing Adverse Effects

Although serious adverse reactions are rare, TMP-SMZ can nonetheless cause all of the toxicities associated with sulfonamides and trimethoprim used alone. Hence, the nursing implications summarized above regarding adverse effects of the sulfonamides alone and trimethoprim alone apply to the combination of TMP-SMZ.

### Minimizing Adverse Interactions

TMP-SMZ has the same drug interactions as sulfonamides used alone. That is, TMP-SMZ can increase the effects of *warfarin*, *phenytoin*, and *oral hypoglycemics*. When combined with TMP-SMZ, these drugs may require a reduction in dosage.

# CHAPTER 83

# Drug Therapy of Urinary Tract Infections

rinary tract infections (UTIs) are the most common infections encountered today. Estimates indicate that between 10% and 20% of all females experience at least one UTI, and many experience recurrent infections. UTIs occur much less frequently in males, but are more likely to be associated with complications (e.g., septicemia, pyelonephritis).

Infections may be limited to bacterial colonization of the urine, or bacteria may invade tissues of the urinary tract. When bacteria invade tissues, characteristic inflammatory syndromes result: *urethritis* (inflammation of the urethra), *cystitis* (inflammation of the urinary bladder), *pyelonephritis* (inflammation of the kidney and its pelvis), and *prostatitis* (inflammation of the prostate).

UTIs may be classified according to their location—in either the lower urinary tract or the upper urinary tract. Within this classification scheme, *cystitis* and *urethritis* are considered *lower tract infections*, whereas *pyelonephritis* is considered an *upper tract infection.*

UTIs are referred to as being *complicated* or *uncomplicated.* Complicated UTIs occur in males and females and are associated with some predisposing factor, such as calculi (stones), prostatic hypertrophy, an indwelling catheter, or an impediment to the flow of urine (e.g., physical obstruction). *Uncomplicated* UTIs occur primarily in women of child-bearing age and are not associated with any particular predisposing factor.

## Organisms That Cause Urinary Tract Infections

The bacteria that cause UTIs differ between community-acquired infections and hospital-acquired (nosocomial) infections. The majority (>80%) of uncomplicated, commu-

nity-acquired UTIs are caused by *Escherichia coli.* Rarely, other gram-negative bacilli—*Klebsiella, Enterobacter, Proteus, Providencia, Pseudomonas*—are the cause. Gram-positive cocci, especially *Staphylococcus saprophyticus*, account for 10% to 15% of community-acquired infections. Hospital-acquired UTIs are frequently caused by *Klebsiella, Proteus, Enterobacter, Pseudomonas*, staphylococci, and enterococci; *E. coli* is responsible for less than 50% of nosocomial infections. Although most UTIs involve only one organism, infection with multiple organisms may occur, especially in patients with an indwelling urinary catheter, renal stones, or chronic renal abscesses.

## Overview of the Drugs Used to Treat Urinary Tract Infections

Several classes of antibiotics are used to treat UTIs. These include sulfonamides, trimethoprim, penicillins, aminoglycosides, cephalosporins, tetracyclines, and fluoroquinolones. The drugs employed for *oral* therapy of UTIs are summarized in Table 83–1. Those employed for *parenteral* therapy are summarized in Table 83-2. With the exception of the urinary tract antiseptics noted in Table 83–1, all of these antibiotics are discussed at length in other chapters. The basic pharmacology of the urinary tract antiseptics is presented in this chapter.

## Specific Urinary Tract Infections and Their Treatment

In this section, we consider the characteristics and treatment of the major UTIs: acute cystitis, acute urethral syn-

## TABLE 83–1. DRUGS FOR ORAL THERAPY OF URINARY TRACT INFECTIONS

| Drugs | Comments |
|---|---|
| *Sulfonamides*<br>Sulfisoxazole<br>Sulfamethoxazole | Sulfonamides are useful for the first episodes of infection. They have generally been replaced by more active agents due to development of bacterial resistance. Their only advantage is low cost. |
| *Trimethoprim-<br>Sulfamethoxazole* | This combination is highly effective against most aerobic enteric bacteria, except *Pseudomonas.* High urinary tract tissue levels and urine levels are achieved, which may be important in treatment of complicated infections. Also effective as prophylaxis for recurrent infection. |
| *Penicillins*<br>Ampicillin<br>Amoxicillin<br>Amoxicillin-clavulanate | Ampicillin, the standard broad-spectrum penicillin, is active against most enteric bacteria that cause UTI, but reports of *E. coli* resistance are increasing. Amoxicillin is better absorbed and has fewer side effects. Amoxicillin-clavulanate is preferred for resistance problems. |
| *Cephalosporins*<br>Cephalexin<br>Cephradine<br>Cefadroxil | These drugs offer no major advantage over other drugs for UTI and are more expensive. They may be useful in cases of resistance to amoxicillin and trimethoprim-sulfamethoxazole. These drugs are not as effective for single-dose therapy. |
| *Tetracyclines*<br>Tetracycline<br>Doxycycline<br>Oxytetracycline<br>Minocycline | These drugs are effective for initial episodes of UTI. However, resistance develops rapidly, and therefore treatment should be guided by sensitivity testing. Use can result in candidal overgrowth. Tetracyclines are useful primarily for chlamydial infections. |
| *Fluoroquinolones*<br>Ciprofloxacin<br>Norfloxacin<br>Ofloxacin | These broad-spectrum antibiotics are active against most organisms that cause UTI, including *Proteus, E. coli,* and other Enterobacteriaceae. Ciprofloxacin and ofloxacin are used parenterally as well as orally. |
| *Urinary Tract Antiseptics*<br>Methenamine<br>Nalidixic acid<br>Cinoxacin<br>Nitrofurantoin | Methenamine is reserved for prophylactic therapy and suppressive use between episodes of infection. Nalidixic acid and cinoxacin are effective for initial episodes of infection due to *E. coli* and other Enterobacteriaceae, but not *Proteus.* Nitrofurantoin is effective as both a therapeutic and a prophylactic agent in patients with recurrent urinary tract infections; the drug's main advantage is lack of resistance, even after prolonged therapy. |

Modified from Mullinex, T., Casabar, E., and Price, R. A. *In* DePiro, J.T. (ed.). Pharmacotherapy: A Pathophysiologic Approach, 2nd ed., p. 1706. Norwalk, CT, Appleton & Lange, 1992.

drome, acute pyelonephritis, acute bacterial prostatitis, and recurrent UTIs. Most of these infections can be treated with oral therapy on an outpatient basis. The principal exception to this rule is severe pyelonephritis, which requires intravenous therapy in a hospital setting. Drugs and dosages for outpatient therapy are summarized in Table 83–3.

## Acute Cystitis

Acute cystitis is a lower urinary tract infection that occurs most often in women of child-bearing age. Clinical manifestations are dysuria, urinary urgency, urinary frequency, suprapubic discomfort, pyuria, and bacteriuria (more than 100,000 bacteria/ml of urine). It is important to note that many women (30% or more) with symptoms of acute cystitis also have asymptomatic upper urinary tract infection (subclinical pyelonephritis). In uncomplicated, community-acquired cystitis, the principal causative organisms are *Escherichia coli* (80%), *Staphylococcus saprophyticus* (11%), and *Streptococcus faecalis.*

For community-acquired infections, three types of oral therapy can be employed: (1) single-dose therapy, (2) short-course therapy (3 to 5 days), and (3) conventional therapy (7 to 14 days). *Single-dose* therapy and *short-course* therapy are recommended only for uncomplicated, community-acquired infections in women who are not pregnant and whose symptoms began less than 7 days before starting treatment. Short-course therapy is more effective than single-dose therapy and is preferred.

## TABLE 83–2. DRUGS FOR PARENTERAL THERAPY OF URINARY TRACT INFECTIONS

| Drugs | Comments |
|---|---|
| *Aminoglycosides*<br>Gentamicin<br>Tobramycin<br>Amikacin | Gentamicin and tobramycin are equally effective, and gentamicin is less expensive. Tobramycin is more active against *Pseudomonas*, which may be important in serious systemic infections. Amikacin is generally reserved for multiresistant bacteria. |
| *Pencillins*<br>Ampicillin<br>Ticarcillin<br>Mezlocillin<br>Piperacillin | These agents are generally equally effective for susceptible bacteria. The extended-spectrum penicillins are more active against *Pseudomonas* and enterococci, and are often preferred over cephalosporins. Penicillins are very useful in renally impaired patients or when an aminoglycoside is to be avoided. |
| *Cephalosporins*<br>Cefonicid<br>Ceforanide<br>Cefotaxime<br>Ceftizoxime | Second- and third-generation cephalosporins have a broad spectrum of activity against gram-negative bacteria but are not active against enterococci and have limited activity against *Pseudomonas*. They are useful for nosocomial infections and urosepsis due to susceptible pathogens. |
| *Imipenem-Cilastatin* | This combination has a very broad spectrum of activity, including gram-positive, gram-negative, and anaerobic bacteria. It is active against enterococci and *Pseudomonas*, but may be associated with candidal suprainfection. |
| *Aztreonam* | This monobactam is active only against gram-negative bacteria, including *Pseudomonas*. Generally useful for nosocomial infections when aminoglycosides are to be avoided, and in penicillin-allergic patients. |
| *Fluoroquinolones*<br>Ciprofloxacin<br>Ofloxacin | These broad-spectrum antibiotics are active against most organisms that cause UTI, including *Proteus, E. coli*, and other Enterobacteriaceae. |

Modified from Mullinex, T., Casabar, E., and Price, R. A. *In* DePiro, J.T. (ed.). Pharmacotherapy: A Pathophysiologic Approach, 2nd ed., p. 1706. Norwalk, CT, Appleton & Lange, 1992.

Advantages of short-course therapy over conventional therapy are lower cost, greater compliance, fewer side effects, and less potential for promoting emergence of bacterial resistance. *Conventional* therapy is indicated for all patients who do not meet the criteria for short-course therapy; these patients include males, children, pregnant women, and women with suspected upper tract involvement. Drugs and dosing regimens for oral therapy of acute cystitis are summarized in Table 83–3.

## Acute Urethral Syndrome

Acute urethral syndrome occurs in females. Clinical manifestations are dysuria, urinary frequency, urinary urgency, and pyuria. There is no significant bacteriuria (i.e., bacterial counts are less than 100,000/ml). The syndrome is usually caused by *E. coli, Staphylococcus saprophyticus*, or *Chlamydia trachomatis*. It may also be caused by *Neisseria gonorrhoeae, Gardnerella vaginalis*, and *Ureaplasma urealyticum*.

Treatment depends on the causative organisms. For infections caused by *E. coli* or staphylococci, a single dose of two double-strength tablets of trimethoprim-sulfamethoxazole is often curative. If this is ineffective, or if the infection is due to *Chlamydia, Ureaplasma*, or *Trichomonas*, doxycycline should be used (100 mg twice daily for 10 to 14 days). Doxycycline is also effective against gonococcal urethritis, but ceftriaxone is preferred.

## Recurrent Urinary Tract Infections

Recurrent urinary tract infections result from *relapse* or from *reinfection*. *Relapse* is caused by recolonization with the same organism responsible for the initial infection, whereas *reinfection* is caused by colonization with a new organism.

**Reinfection.** More than 80% of recurrent UTIs in females are due to reinfection. These usually involve the lower urinary tract and may be related to sexual intercourse or use of a contraceptive diaphragm. If reinfections are *infrequent* (only one or two a year), each episode should be treated as a separate infection. Single-dose or short-course therapy can be used.

When reinfections are *frequent* (three or more a year), long-term prophylaxis may be indicated. Prophylaxis can

## TABLE 83–3. ORAL THERAPY OF URINARY TRACT INFECTIONS IN ADULTS

*Acute Cystitis*

| | |
|---|---|
| Trimethoprim-sulfamethoxazole (double-strength tablets) | 2 tablets once *or*<br>1 tablet twice daily for 3 days *or*<br>1 tablet twice daily for 10–14 days |
| Trimethoprim | 400 mg once *or*<br>200 mg twice daily for 3 days *or*<br>100 mg twice daily for 10–14 days |
| Sulfisoxazole | 2 gm once *or*<br>1 gm every 6 hours for 10–14 days |
| Amoxicillin | 3 gm once *or*<br>250 mg twice daily for 10–14 days |
| Norfloxacin | 400 mg twice daily for 10–14 days |
| Ciprofloxacin | 500 mg twice daily for 10–14 days |
| Ofloxacin | 200 mg twice daily for 7–10 days |
| Nitroflurantoin | 200 mg once *or*<br>100 mg every 6 hours for 3 days |

*Acute Urethral Syndrome: Initial Therapy*

| | |
|---|---|
| Trimethoprim-sulfamethoxazole | 2 double-strength tablets once |
| Amoxicillin | 3 gm once |

*Acute Urethral Syndrome: If Initial Therapy Fails*

| | |
|---|---|
| Doxycycline | 100 mg twice daily for 10–14 days |

*Long-Term Prophylaxis of Recurrent Infection*

| | |
|---|---|
| Trimethoprim-sulfamethoxazole | 1/2 single-strength tablet daily for 6 months |
| Nitrofurantoin | 50 mg once daily for 6 months |
| Trimethoprim | 100 mg once daily for 6 months |

*Acute Pyelonephritis (mild)*

| | |
|---|---|
| Trimethoprim-sulfamethoxazole | 1 double-strength tablet twice daily for 2 weeks or longer |

*Acute Bacterial Prostatitis*

| | |
|---|---|
| Trimethoprim-sulfamethoxazole | 1 double-strength tablet twice daily for 30 days |

be achieved with low daily doses of trimethoprim (100 mg), nitrofurantoin (50 or 100 mg), or trimethoprim-sulfamethoxazole (one half of a single-strength tablet). Prophylaxis should continue for 6 to 12 months. During this time, periodic urine cultures should be obtained. If a symptomatic episode occurs, standard therapy for acute cystitis should be given. If reinfection is associated with sexual intercourse, the risk can be decreased by voiding after intercourse and by single-dose prophylaxis (e.g., 2 double-strength tablets of trimethoprim-sulfamethoxazole taken after intercourse).

*Relapse.* Recolonization with the original infecting organism accounts for 20% of recurrent UTIs. Symptoms that reappear shortly after completion of a course of therapy suggest either a structural abnormality of the urinary tract, involvement of the kidneys, or chronic bacterial prostatitis (the most common cause of recurrent UTIs in

males). If obstruction of the urinary tract is present, it should be corrected surgically. If renal calculi are the cause of relapse, they should be removed.

Drug therapy is progressive. When relapse occurs in women after short-course therapy, a 2-week course of therapy should be tried. If this fails, an additional 4 to 6 weeks of therapy should be tried. If this too is unsuccessful, long-term therapy (6 months) may be indicated. Drugs employed for long-term therapy of relapse include trimethoprim-sulfamethoxazole, norfloxacin, and ciprofloxacin.

## Acute Pyelonephritis

Acute pyelonephritis is an infection of the kidney. This disorder is common in young children, the elderly, and women of child-bearing age. Clinical manifestations include fever, chills, severe flank pain, dysuria, urinary frequency, urinary urgency, pyuria, and usually bacteriuria (more than 100,000 bacteria/ml of urine). *E. coli* is the causative organism in 90% of initial, community-acquired infections. *Mild to moderate infection* can be treated on an outpatient basis with oral trimethoprim-sulfamethoxazole (1 double-strength tablet twice daily for 2 weeks or longer). Severe infection requires hospitalization and intravenous antibiotics; the preferred therapy is an aminoglycoside (e.g., gentamicin, amikacin) combined with ampicillin. Once the infection has been controlled with IV antibiotics, therapy with oral antibiotics can be instituted.

## Acute Bacterial Prostatitis

Acute bacterial prostatitis is defined as inflammation of the prostate caused by local bacterial infection. Clinical manifestations include high fever, chills, malaise, myalgia, localized pain, and various urinary tract symptoms (dysuria, nocturia, urinary urgency, urinary frequency, urinary retention). In most cases (80%), *E. coli* is the causative organism. Infection is frequently associated with an indwelling urethral catheter, urethral instrumentation, or transurethral prostatic resection. However, in many patients the infection has no obvious cause. Bacterial prostatitis responds well to antimicrobial therapy. Drugs for oral therapy include trimethoprim-sulfamethoxazole and the fluoroquinolones (e.g., ciprofloxacin, norfloxacin). Aminoglycosides (e.g., gentamicin, amikacin) are used for parenteral therapy.

# Urinary Tract Antiseptics

The urinary tract antiseptics are drugs whose use is restricted to the treatment of UTIs. The major urinary tract antiseptics are *nitrofurantoin, methenamine, nalidixic acid,* and *cinoxacin.* All four drugs become concentrated in the urine, and are active against the common urinary tract pathogens. These drugs do not achieve effective antibacterial concentrations in blood or tissues, and therefore cannot be used for infections at sites outside the urinary tract. As a rule, the urinary tract antiseptics are second-choice drugs for treatment and prophylaxis of UTIs.

### Nitrofurantoin

Nitrofurantoin [Furadantin, Macrodantin, Macrobid] is a broad-spectrum antimicrobial drug. The agent is bacteriostatic in low concentrations and bactericidal in high concentrations. Therapeutic levels are achieved only in the urine. Hence the drug is useful only against infections of the urinary tract. Nitrofurantoin can cause a variety of serious adverse effects.

Nitrofurantoin injures cells by causing damage to DNA. However, in order to damage DNA, the drug must first be converted to a reactive form. Nitrofurantoin is selectively toxic to bacteria because they, unlike mammalian cells, possess relatively high levels of the enzyme that activates the drug

#### Antimicrobial Spectrum

Nitrofurantoin is active against a large number of gram-positive and gram-negative bacteria. Susceptible organisms include staphylococci, streptococci, *Neisseria, Bacteroides,* and most strains of *Escherichia coli.* These sensitive bacteria rarely acquire resistance. Organisms that are frequently insensitive include *Proteus, Pseudomonas, Enterobacter,* and *Klebsiella.*

#### Therapeutic Use

Nitrofurantoin is indicated for acute infections of the lower urinary tract that are caused by susceptible organisms. In addition, nitrofurantoin can be used for prophylaxis of recurrent lower UTI. The drug is not recommended for infections of the upper urinary tract.

#### Pharmacokinetics

*Absorption and Distribution.* Nitrofurantoin is available in two oral formulations: *macrocrystalline* and *microcrystalline.* The macrocrystalline preparation is absorbed relatively slowly, and produces less gastrointestinal distress than the microcrystalline form. Both formulations produce equivalent therapeutic effects. Nitrofurantoin is distributed to tissues, but only in small amounts. Therapeutic concentrations are achieved only in the urine.

*Metabolism and Excretion.* About two thirds of each dose undergoes metabolic degradation, primarily in the liver; the remaining third is excreted intact in the urine. Nitrofurantoin achieves a urinary concentration of about 200 µg/ml (compared with less than 2 µg/ml in the plasma). The drug imparts a harmless brown color to the urine; patients should be forewarned of this effect.

For two reasons, the drug should not be administered to individuals with kidney impairment (creatinine clearance less than 40 ml/minute). First, in the absence of proper renal function, levels of nitrofurantoin in the urine are too low to be effective. Second, renal dysfunction reduces nitrofurantoin excretion, causing plasma drug levels to rise, thereby presenting a risk of systemic toxicity.

#### Adverse Effects

*Gastrointestinal Effects.* The most frequent adverse reactions are gastrointestinal disturbances (e.g., anorexia, nausea, vomiting, diarrhea). These can be minimized by administering nitrofurantoin with milk or with meals, by reducing the dosage, and by using the macrocrystalline formulation.

*Pulmonary Reactions.* Nitrofurantoin can induce two kinds of pulmonary reactions: acute and subacute. Acute reactions, which are most common, are manifested by dyspnea, chest pain, chills, fever, cough, and alveolar infiltrates. These symptoms resolve in 2 to 4 days following cessation of treatment. Acute pulmonary responses are thought to be hypersensitivity reactions. Patients with a history of such responses should not receive nitrofurantoin again. Subacute reactions are rare and occur during prolonged treatment. Symptoms (e.g., dyspnea, cough, malaise) usually regress over weeks to months after nitrofurantoin withdrawal. However, in some patients permanent lung damage may occur.

*Hematologic Effects.* Nitrofurantoin can cause a variety of hematologic reactions, including agranulocytosis, leukopenia, thrombocytopenia, and megaloblastic anemia. In addition, hemolytic anemia may occur in infants and patients whose red blood cells have an inherited deficiency in glucose-6-phosphate dehydrogenase. Because of the potential for hemolytic anemia in newborns, nitrofurantoin is contraindicated for pregnant women near term and for infants under the age of 1 month.

*Peripheral Neuropathy.* Damage to sensory and motor nerves is a serious concern. Demyelination and nerve degeneration can occur and may be irreversible. Early symptoms include muscle weakness, tingling sensations, and numbness. The patient should be informed of these symptoms and instructed to report them. Neuropathy is most likely in patients with renal impairment and in those taking nitrofurantoin chronically.

*Other Adverse Effects.* Nitrofurantoin can cause multiple neurologic effects (e.g., headache, vertigo, drowsiness, nystagmus); all are readily reversible. Hepatotoxicity (cholestatic jaundice, chronic hepatitis, hepatocellular damage) occurs rarely.

### Preparations, Dosage, and Administration

*Preparations.* Microcrystalline nitrofurantoin [Furadantin] is dispensed in a 5-mg/ml oral suspension. Macrocrystalline nitrofurantoin [Macrodantin, Macrobid] is dispensed in 25-, 50-, and 100-mg capsules.

*Dosage and Administration.* For *treatment* of acute UTI, the *adult* dosage is 50 mg 3 to 4 times a day; the *pediatric* dosage is 5 to 7 mg/kg/day administered in four divided doses. For *prophylaxis* of recurrent UTI, low doses are employed (e.g., 50 to 100 mg at bedtime for adults and 1 mg/kg/day in one or two doses for children). Nitrofurantoin can be administered with meals and milk to reduce gastrointestinal distress.

## Methenamine

### Mechanism of Action

Under acidic conditions, methenamine [Mandelamine, Hiprex, Urex] decomposes into ammonia and formaldehyde. The formaldehyde denatures bacterial proteins, causing death. For formaldehyde to be released, the urine must be acidic (pH 5.5 or less). Since formaldehyde is not formed at physiologic systemic pH, methenamine is devoid of systemic toxicity.

### Antimicrobial Spectrum

Virtually all bacteria are susceptible to formaldehyde; resistance does not exist. Certain bacteria (e.g., *Proteus* species) can elevate urinary pH (by splitting urea to form ammonia). Since formaldehyde is not released under alkaline conditions, infections with these urea-splitting organisms are often unresponsive to methenamine.

### Therapeutic Uses

Methenamine is used for *chronic* UTI, but is *not* recommended for *acute* infection. The drug can suppress recurrent UTI in females, but trimethoprim-sulfamethoxazole is preferred for this indication. Methenamine is not active against infections of the upper urinary tract, since there is insufficient time for formaldehyde to be formed as the drug traverses the kidney. Methenamine does not prevent UTIs associated with catheters.

### Pharmacokinetics

*Absorption and Distribution.* Methenamine is rapidly absorbed after oral administration. However, approximately 30% of each dose may be converted to ammonia and formaldehyde in the acidic environment of the stomach. This reaction can be minimized by using enteric-coated preparations. The drug is distributed throughout total body water.

*Excretion.* Methenamine is eliminated by the kidneys. Within the urinary tract, about 20% of the drug decomposes to form formaldehyde. Levels of formaldehyde are highest within the bladder. Since formaldehyde generation takes place slowly, and since transit time through the kidney is brief, formaldehyde levels in the *kidney* remain subtherapeutic. Ingestion of large amounts of fluid will reduce antibacterial effects by diluting methenamine and raising urinary pH. Poorly metabolized acids (e.g., hippuric acid, mandelic acid, ascorbic acid) have been administered with methenamine in attempts to acidify the urine, and thereby increase formaldehyde formation; however, there is no evidence that these acids enhance therapeutic effects.

### Adverse Effects and Precautions

Methenamine is relatively safe and generally well tolerated. Gastric distress occurs occasionally, presumably from formaldehyde release in the stomach. Use of enteric-coated preparations may reduce this response. Chronic high-dose therapy can cause bladder irritation, manifested as dysuria, frequent voiding, urinary urgency, proteinuria, and hematuria. Since decomposition of methenamine generates ammonia (in addition to formaldehyde), the drug is contraindicated for patients with liver dysfunction. Methenamine salts (methenamine mandelate, methenamine hippurate) should not be used by patients with renal impairment, since crystalluria may be caused by precipitation of the mandelate or hippurate moiety.

### Drug Interactions

*Urinary Alkalinizers.* Drugs that elevate urinary pH (e.g., acetazolamide, sodium bicarbonate) inhibit formaldehyde production, and can thereby reduce the antibacterial effects of methenamine. Patients taking methenamine should not be given alkalinizing agents.

*Sulfonamides.* Methenamine should not be combined with sulfonamides: formaldehyde forms an insoluble complex with sulfonamides, thereby posing a risk of urinary tract injury from crystalluria.

### Preparations, Dosage, and Administration

Methenamine is available as two salts: methenamine mandelate and methenamine hippurate.

*Methenamine mandelate* [Mandelamine] is dispensed in enteric-coated tablets (0.5 and 1 gm) and a suspension (0.1 gm/ml) for oral use. The usual adult dosage is 1 gm 4 times a day. The dosage for children 6 to 12 years old is 0.5 gm 4 times a day. For children under the age of 6, the dosage is 0.25 gm/30 lb 4 times a day.

*Methenamine hippurate* [Hiprex, Urex] is dispensed in 1-gm tablets for oral administration. The dosage for adults and for children over the age of 12 years is 1 gm twice a day. For children ages 6 to 12 years, the dosage is 500 mg to 1 gm twice a day.

## Nalidixic Acid

### Mechanism of Action

Nalidixic acid [NegGram], which is a chemical relative of the fluoroquinolones, inhibits replication of bacterial DNA, thereby causing DNA degradation and cell death. The precise target of nalidixic acid is *DNA gyrase*, the bacterial enzyme that converts closed circular DNA into a supercoiled configuration; if supercoiling does not occur, DNA replication cannot take place.

### Microbial Resistance

Resistant bacteria often emerge during treatment. Two mechanisms for resistance have been described: (1) production of an altered DNA gyrase that has reduced sensitivity to nalidixic acid and (2) reduced bacterial uptake of nalidixic acid. Cross-resistance with cinoxacin is common. A frequent factor in resistance is treatment with suboptimal doses. (Low levels of nalidixic acid favor overgrowth with drug-resistant organisms.) Fortunately, resistance to nalidixic acid is not carried on R factors, and therefore is not transferable.

### Antimicrobial Spectrum

Nalidixic acid is active against most gram-negative urinary tract pathogens, including *E. coli*, *Klebsiella*, *Enterobacter*, and *Proteus* species. *Pseudomonas aeruginosa* is resistant, as are most gram-positive aerobic cocci.

### Therapeutic Uses

Nalidixic acid is approved only for treatment of UTIs. This drug has been used for control of acute infection and for prophylaxis against recurrent UTI. However, for both applications, other drugs are preferred. Nalidixic acid is not useful against infections outside the urinary tract.

## Pharmacokinetics

Nalidixic acid is well absorbed from the gastrointestinal tract, and then undergoes rapid hepatic metabolism. Only one metabolite—hydroxynalidixic acid—has antibacterial actions. Nalidixic acid and its metabolites are excreted in the urine. The concentration of active drug in urine is about 10 times greater than in plasma. Therapeutic levels are achieved in urine even in patients with moderate to severe renal impairment. Drug concentrations outside the urinary tract are too low for antibacterial effects.

## Adverse Effects

Although nalidixic acid can cause multiple untoward effects, the incidence of severe reactions is low. The most common effects are gastrointestinal disturbances (nausea, vomiting, abdominal discomfort), rash, and visual disturbances (blurred vision, diplopia, poor accommodation, photophobia, altered color perception). Patients experiencing reduced visual acuity should exercise appropriate caution. Photosensitivity reactions can occur; patients should be advised to avoid excessive exposure to sunlight, wear protective clothing, and apply a sunscreen to exposed skin. Convulsions have occurred on occasion; accordingly, nalidixic acid is contraindicated for individuals with a history of convulsive disorders. Nalidixic acid may produce intracranial hypertension in pediatric patients; the drug should not be administered to children under the age of 3 months. Blood dyscrasias (thrombocytopenia, leukopenia, hemolytic anemia) and jaundice are rare; however, when nalidixic acid is used for more than 2 weeks, blood cell counts and liver function tests should be performed.

## Drug Interactions

Nalidixic acid can intensify the effects of oral anticoagulants (e.g., warfarin) by displacing these agents from binding sites on plasma proteins. Accordingly, when an oral anticoagulant is combined with nalidixic acid, a reduction in anticoagulant dosage may be needed.

## Preparations, Dosage, and Administration

Nalidixic acid [NegGram] is dispensed in tablets (250 mg, 500 mg, 1 gm) and in suspension (50 mg/ml) for oral use. The adult dosage is 1 gm 4 times a day for 1 week. For children under the age of 12 years, the dosage is 55 mg/kg/day in four divided doses. Nalidixic acid should not be given to children less than 3 months old.

## Cinoxacin

Cinoxacin [Cinobac] is a close chemical relative of nalidixic acid. Both drugs have the same mechanism of action, antimicrobial spectrum, and indications. Furthermore, organisms that are resistant to nalidixic acid are often resistant to cinoxacin. As with other urinary tract antiseptics, therapeutic levels of cinoxacin are achieved only in the urine. Adverse effects are like those of nalidixic acid, but their incidence is relatively low. Cinoxacin is excreted by the kidneys, primarily as the unchanged drug. The drug is dispensed in 250- and 500-mg capsules for oral use. The usual adult dosage is 1 gm/day administered in two or four divided doses. The dosage should be reduced in patients with renal impairment; failure to do so could result in accumulation of cinoxacin to toxic levels.

# KEY POINTS

- *E. coli* is the most common cause of uncomplicated, community-acquired UTIs.
- Except for pyelonephritis, most UTIs can be treated with oral therapy on an outpatient basis.
- Trimethoprim-sulfamethoxazole is frequently the treatment of choice for oral therapy of UTIs.
- Many drugs, including penicillins, cephalosporins, and fluoroquinolones, may be used for parenteral therapy of UTIs.
- Prophylaxis of recurrent UTI can be achieved with daily low doses of trimethoprim alone, trimethoprim-sulfamethoxazole, or nitrofurantoin.
- As a rule, the urinary tract antiseptics—nitrofurantoin, methenamine, nalidixic acid, and cinoxacin—are second-choice drugs for treating UTIs.

# CHAPTER 84

# Antimycobacterial Agents: Drugs for Tuberculosis, Leprosy, and *Mycobacterium avium* Complex Infection

---

---

O ur focus in this chapter is on infections caused by three mycobacteria: *Mycobacterium tuberculosis, Mycobacterium avium* complex, and *Mycobacterium leprae.* The mycobacteria are slow-growing microbes, and the infections they cause require prolonged treatment. Because therapy is prolonged, drug toxicity and poor patient compliance are significant clinical problems. In addition, prolonged treatment promotes the emergence of drug-resistant bacteria.

Tuberculosis—the principal topic of this chapter—is a global public health problem. Worldwide, tuberculosis kills more adults than any other infectious disease. The death rate around the world is 3 million per year; the death rate among Americans is 2000 a year.

Although new cases of tuberculosis in the United States declined slightly between 1993 and 1995 (from 25,300 to 22,800), new cases increased in the rest of the world. The estimated worldwide incidence of new cases is 9 million a year. Of these, the vast majority (95%) occur in developing countries. There are two reasons for the resurgence of tuberculosis: AIDS and the emergence of multidrug-resistant mycobacteria.

## Tuberculosis I: Clinical Considerations

### Pathogenesis

Tuberculosis is caused by *Mycobacterium tuberculosis,* an organism also known as the *tubercle bacillus.* Infections may be limited to the lungs or may become disseminated. In most cases, the bacteria are quiescent, and the infected individual is free of symptoms. However, when the disease is active, morbidity can be significant. In the United States, approximately 10 million people harbor tubercle bacilli; however, only a small fraction of these people have symptomatic disease.

#### Primary Infection

Infection with *M. tuberculosis* is transmitted from person to person by inhaling infected sputum that has been aerosolized by coughing or sneezing. Hence, initial infection is in the lung. Once in the lung, tubercle bacilli are taken up by phagocytic cells (macrophages and neutrophils). At first the bacilli are resistant to the destructive activity of phagocytes and multiply freely within them. Infection can spread from the lungs to other organs via the lymphatic and circulatory systems.

In most cases, immunity to *M. tuberculosis* develops within a few weeks, and the infection is brought under complete control. The immune system facilitates control by increasing the ability of phagocytes to suppress multiplication of tubercle bacilli. Because of this rapid response by the immune system, most (90%) individuals with primary infection never develop clinical or radiologic evidence of disease. However, even though symptoms are absent and the progression of infection is halted, the infected individual is likely to harbor tubercle bacilli lifelong (unless drugs are given to eliminate quiescent bacilli). Hence, in the absence of treatment, the threat of reactivation is ever present.

If the immune system fails to control the primary infection, clinical disease (tuberculosis) develops. The result is necrosis and cavitation of lung tissue. Lung tissue may also become caseous (cheese-like in appearance). Since phagocytes do not function at sites of necrosis, cellular immunity is unable to suppress the active infection. In the absence of treatment, tissue destruction progresses, and death may result.

### Reactivation

The term *reactivation* refers to renewed multiplication of tubercle bacilli that had been dormant following control of a primary infection. Until recently, it was assumed that most new cases of symptomatic tuberculosis resulted from reactivation of an old infection. However, new data indicate that, among some groups, reactivation may be responsible for only 60% of new infections—the remaining 40% resulting from recent person-to-person transmission.

### Screening

In order to reduce the incidence of tuberculosis, we must detect and treat individuals with asymptomatic infection. Detection is accomplished by screen testing. It is recommended that all high-risk persons undergo screening. In this group are those with HIV infection, health care workers, and those with other risk factors for tuberculosis, such as chronic renal failure, hematologic malignancy, and use of immunosuppressive drugs.

The screen employed most commonly is the *tuberculin skin test*. The test is performed by giving an intradermal injection of a protein derived from *M. tuberculosis*. The protein is referred to as *purified protein derivative*, or *PPD*. The test is read 48 to 72 hours after injection. In people harboring tubercle bacilli, injection of PPD can elicit a local hypersensitivity reaction. A positive reaction is indicated by the size of the zone of induration (hardness)—not the zone of erythema (redness). It should be noted that false-negative results are common, and can be as high as 70% in patients with AIDS.

## Diagnosis

If an individual has a positive tuberculin skin test or clinical manifestations that suggest tuberculosis, diagnostic testing for tuberculosis should be done. A definitive diagnosis is made with chest x-rays and microbiologic evaluation of sputum. A chest x-ray should be ordered for all persons suspected of active infection.

Sputum is evaluated in two ways: (1) by microscopic examination of sputum smears and (2) by culturing sputum samples. Microscopic examination cannot provide a definitive diagnosis. This is because direct observation cannot distinguish between *Mycobacterium tuberculosis* and other mycobacteria. Furthermore, microscopic examination is much less sensitive than culturing. Accordingly, sputum cultures are required for definitive diagnosis. Because *M. tuberculosis* grows very slowly, results of sputum cultures are often delayed by as long as 3 to 6 weeks. However, with newer culturing techniques, results have been obtained in less than 1 week. In addition to providing positive identification of *M. tuberculosis*, cultures are necessary to determine drug sensitivity.

## Treatment of Active Disease

The availability of modern chemotherapeutic agents has dramatically altered the treatment of tuberculosis. Whereas patients once faced lengthy hospitalization, therapy can now be performed on an outpatient basis for most patients. Prolonged bed rest is not required, nor is it recommended. To reduce emergence of resistance, treatment is always done with two or more drugs. In addition, many authorities recommend direct observation of drug administration to ensure compliance.

The goal of treatment is to eliminate symptoms and prevent relapse. To accomplish this, treatment must kill tubercle bacilli that are actively dividing as well as those that are "resting." Success is indicated by an absence of observable mycobacteria in sputum and by the failure of sputum cultures to yield colonies of *M. tuberculosis*.

### Drug Resistance

Drug resistance is a major impediment to successful therapy. Some infecting bacilli are inherently resistant; others develop resistance over the course of treatment. Some bacilli are resistant to just one drug; others are resistant to multiple drugs. Infection with a resistant organism may be acquired in two ways: (1) through contact with someone who harbors resistant bacteria and (2) through repeated ineffectual courses of therapy (see below).

*Multidrug* resistance is a recent and ominous development. Resistance to isoniazid and rifampin—two mainstays of therapy—is of particular concern. Infection with multidrug-resistant organisms greatly increases the risk of death, especially among patients with AIDS. In addition, multidrug resistance is expensive: the cost of treating one case of resistant tuberculosis is about $180,000, compared with $12,000 per case for nonresistant tuberculosis.

The incidence of drug resistance is increasing. Thirty years ago, primary resistance to isoniazid occurred in less than 2% of patients; today the incidence is 9%. The incidence of multidrug resistance varies among communities. Nationwide, the average is 1 of every 10 patients. The highest incidence of multidrug resistance is found in New York City, where fully two thirds of all cases occur.

*The principal cause underlying the emergence of resistance is inadequate drug therapy.* Treatment may be too short; dosage may be too low; patient compliance may be erratic; and, perhaps most importantly, the regimen may contain too few drugs (see below).

### The Prime Directive: Always Treat Tuberculosis with Two or More Drugs

*Antituberculous regimens must always contain two or more drugs to which the infecting organism is sensitive.* To understand why this is so, we need to begin with five facts: (1) resistance in *M. tuberculosis* occurs because of spontaneous mutations; (2) each mutational event confers resistance to only one drug; (3) mutations conferring resistance to a single drug occur in about 1 of every 100 million ($10^8$) bacteria; (4) the bacterial burden in active tuberculosis is well above $10^8$ organisms but far below $10^{16}$; and (5) *M. tuberculosis* grows slowly, hence treatment is prolonged. Now, let's assume we initiate therapy with a *single* drug, and that all bacteria in our patient are sensitive at the start of treatment. What will happen? Over time, at least one of the more than $10^8$ bacteria in our patient will mutate to a resistant form. Hence, as we proceed with treatment, we will kill all sensitive bacteria, but the descendants of the newly resistant bacterium will continue to flourish, thereby causing treatment failure. In contrast, if we initiate therapy with *two* drugs, treatment will succeed. Why? Because failure would require that at least one bacterium undergo two resistance-conferring mutations, one for each drug. Since two such mutations occur in only 1 of every $10^{16}$ bacteria ($10^{16}$ is the product of the probabilities for each mutation), and since the total bacterial load is much less than $10^{16}$, the chances of the two events occurring in one of the bacteria in our patient are nil.

Not only do drug combinations decrease the risk of resistance, combination therapy can reduce the incidence of relapse. Since some drugs (e.g., isoniazid, rifampin) are especially effective against actively dividing bacilli, whereas other drugs (e.g., pyrazinamide) are most active against intracellular (quiescent) bacilli, by using certain combinations of antituberculous agents we can increase the chances of killing all tubercle bacilli present, whether they are actively multiplying or resting. Hence, the risk of relapse is lowered.

In Chapter 77 (Basic Principles of Antimicrobial Therapy), we noted that treatment with multiple antibiotics broadens the spectrum of antimicrobial coverage, thereby increasing the risk of suprainfection. This is not the case with multiple drug therapy of tuberculosis. The major drugs used against *M. tuberculosis* are selective for this organism. As a result, these drugs, even when used in combination, do not kill off other microorganisms, and there-fore do not create the conditions that lead to suprainfection.

In summary, because treatment is prolonged, there is a high risk that drug-resistant bacilli will emerge if only one antituberculous agent is employed. Since the chances of a bacterium developing resistance to two drugs is very low, treatment with two or more drugs minimizes the risk of drug resistance. Accordingly, when treating tuberculosis, we must always use two or more drugs to which the organism is sensitive.

### Determining Drug Sensitivity

Because resistance to one or more antituberculous drugs is common, and because many patterns of resistance are possible, it is essential that we determine drug sensitivity in isolates from each patient at the onset of treatment. Unfortunately, sensitivity tests often take several weeks to complete. Until test results are available, drug selection must be empiric, based on patterns of drug resistance in the community and the immunocompetence of the patient. However, once test results are available, the regimen should be adjusted accordingly. In the event of treatment failure, sensitivity tests should be repeated.

### Treatment Regimens

A variety of regimens are employed for active tuberculosis. Drug selection is based largely on the susceptibility of the infecting organism and the immunocompetence of the host. Therapy is usually initiated with a four-drug regimen; isoniazid and rifampin are almost always included. In the event of suspected or proved resistance, more drugs are added; the total may be as high as seven. Representative regimens are shown in Table 84–1 and discussed below.

Treatment can be divided into two phases. The goal of the initial phase is to eliminate actively dividing extracellular tubercle bacilli, and thereby render the sputum noninfectious. The goal of the second phase is to eliminate intracellular "persisters."

*Drug-Sensitive Tubercle Bacilli.* If the infecting organism is not resistant to isoniazid, rifampin, and other antituberculous drugs, treatment can be relatively simple. The two regimens used most frequently are summarized in Table 84–1. The first regimen has two phases. The initial phase, which lasts 2 months, consists of daily therapy with *isoniazid*, *rifampin*, and *pyrazinamide*. The second phase, which lasts 4 months, consists of daily or biweekly therapy with just *isoniazid* and *rifampin*. The second regimen consists of just two drugs: *isoniazid* and *rifampin*. These are taken daily for 1 month and then either daily or biweekly for another 8 months. Note that both regimens are prolonged, making compliance a significant problem.

*Possibly Resistant Tubercle Bacilli.* In communities where the incidence of drug resistance is greater than 4%, initial therapy should consist of four drugs: *isoniazid*, *rifampin*, and *pyrazinamide*, combined with either *ethambutol* or *streptomycin*. If susceptibility tests indicate lack of resistance, therapy should continue with just isoniazid, rifampin, and pyrazinamide for the remainder of

## TABLE 84–1. REPRESENTATIVE ANTITUBERCULOUS REGIMENS

**HIV-Negative Patients**

| Drug-Sensitive TB | Possibly Resistant TB | Multidrug-Resistant TB | **HIV-Positive Patients** |
|---|---|---|---|
| *Initial therapy:* INH + RIF + PYR daily for 2 months *Then:* INH + RIF daily or biweekly for 4 months *OR* *Initial therapy:* INH + RIF daily for 1 month *Then:* INH + RIF daily or biweekly for 8 months | *Initial therapy:* INH + RIF + PYR + either EMB or SM *Then:* If tests reveal full sensitivity, switch to INH + RIF + PYR for remainder of first 2 months, followed by INH + RIF for 4 months | Treatment should consist of at least three drugs to which the organism is sensitive, and should continue for 12 to 24 months. Initial empiric therapy might include INH + RIF + PYR + EMB + kanamycin, amikacin, or capreomycin + ciproflaxin or ofloxacin + cycloserine, ethionamide, or *p*-aminosalicyclic acid | The treatment options for HIV-negative patients can be used, but treatment should continue for at least 9 months, and for at least 6 months after sputum conversion |

TB = tuberculosis, INH = isoniazid, RIF = rifampin, PYR = pyrazinamide, EMB = ethambutol, SM = streptomycin.

the first 2 months, and then with just isoniazid and rifampin for another 4 months.

***Multidrug-Resistant Tubercle Bacilli.*** Multidrug resistance is defined as resistance to at least isoniazid and rifampin. Treatment requires at least three drugs to which the organism is sensitive, and should continue for 12 to 24 months after sputum conversion. Initial therapy may consist of five, six, or even seven drugs. Hence, an initial regimen might include (1) isoniazid; (2) rifampin; (3) pyrazinamide; (4) ethambutol; (5) kanamycin, amikacin, or capreomycin; (6) ciprofloxacin or ofloxacin; and (7) cycloserine, ethionamide, or *para*-aminosalicylic acid.

***Therapy in Patients with AIDS.*** Between 2% and 20% of patients with AIDS develop active tuberculosis. Because of their reduced ability to fight infection, these patients require more aggressive therapy than immunocompetent patients. In general, the regimens described above can be used; however, treatment should continue for at least 9 months, and for at least 6 months after sputum cultures have become negative.

### Duration of Treatment

The ideal duration of treatment has not been established. For patients with drug-sensitive tuberculosis, the minimum duration is 6 months. For patients with multidrug-resistant infection, and for patients with HIV or AIDS, treatment may last as long as 24 months after sputum cultures have become negative.

### Evaluating Treatment

Three modes are employed to evaluate therapy: bacteriologic evaluation of sputum, clinical evaluation, and chest x-rays.

In patients with positive pretreatment sputum tests, sputum should be evaluated every 2 to 4 weeks initially,

and then monthly after sputum cultures become negative. With proper drug selection and good compliance, sputum cultures become negative in over 90% of patients after 3 months of treatment.

Treatment failures should be evaluated for drug resistance and patient compliance. In the absence of demonstrated drug resistance, treatment with the same regimen should continue, using direct observation of drug administration to ensure that medication is being taken as prescribed. In patients with drug-resistant tuberculosis, *two* effective drugs should be added to the regimen.

In patients with negative pretreatment sputum tests, treatment is monitored by chest x-rays and clinical evaluation. In most patients, clinical manifestations (e.g., fever, malaise, anorexia, cough) should decrease markedly within 2 weeks. The x-ray should show improvement within 3 months.

After completion of therapy, patients should be examined every 3 to 6 months for signs and symptoms of relapse.

## Preventive Therapy

*Isoniazid* is the only antituberculous drug proved effective for preventive therapy. Following contact with an individual who has active tuberculosis, isoniazid is given to prevent development of active tuberculosis and to prevent transmission of infection to others. When used for prophylaxis, isoniazid is usually administered daily for 6 to 12 months.

Candidates for prophylaxis include (1) HIV-infected individuals with significant reactions to a tuberculin test, (2) individuals in close contact with tuberculosis patients, and (3) newly infected individuals. Since the chance of developing serious disease is especially high among infants,

1. HIV-infected persons with a significant reaction to a tuberculin text

2. Household members and other close contacts of patients with active pulmonary tuberculosis

3. Newly infected persons (i.e., those who have had a tuberculin skin test conversion during the previous 2 years)

4. Persons with a history of tuberculosis and inadequate chemotherapy.

5. Persons with a positive tuberculin skin test and an abnormal chest x-ray consistent with previous (nonprogressive) tuberculous disease. These patients have a negative bacteriology and stable parenchymal lesions

6. Persons with significant reactions to a tuberculin skin test and who are at special risk of developing active tuberculosis. These include patients with

   • Silicosis
   • Diabetes mellitus
   • Certain hematologic and reticuloendothelial diseases (leukemia, Hodgkin's disease)
   • End-stage renal disease
   • Clinical conditions associated with substantial weight loss or chronic undernutrition, including the postgastrectomy state, intestinal bypass surgery, chronic peptic ulcer disease, chronic malabsorption syndromes, and carcinomas of the oropharynx and upper gastrointestinal tract that inhibit adequate nutritional intake

   and patients undergoing

   • Prolonged therapy with glucocorticoids
   • Immunosuppressive therapy

7. All tuberculin skin test reactors under age 35

Adapted from Drug Evaluations Annual 1993, p. 1600, Table 4. Chicago, American Medical Association, 1992.

adolescents, and patients undergoing immunosuppressive therapy, these people should almost always be treated. A comprehensive list of candidates for isoniazid prophylaxis is given in Table 84–2.

As a rule, the potential benefits of preventive therapy outweigh the risks of liver damage, which is the principal toxicity of isoniazid. However, because prophylaxis does carry some risk of hepatotoxicity, not everyone who has been exposed to tuberculosis is a candidate. Prophylaxis is contraindicated for individuals with liver disease and for those who have had serious adverse reactions to isoniazid in the past. Since the risk of isoniazid-induced liver damage increases significantly with advancing age, people over age 35 should not be treated routinely; rather, preventive therapy should be reserved for tuberculin-positive patients in whom other risk factors are present, such as diabetes, leukemia, or drug-induced immunosuppression. In the event of pregnancy, prophylaxis should be postponed until after delivery.

Drugs other than isoniazid should be used following exposure to drug-resistant tubercle bacilli. If the organism is resistant solely to isoniazid, preventive treatment should consist of rifampin with or without ethambutol. If the organism is resistant to multiple drugs, the regimen should consist of pyrazinamide combined with either ethambutol, ciprofloxacin, or ofloxacin.

# Tuberculosis II: Pharmacology of Individual Antituberculous Drugs

Based on their clinical utility, the antituberculous drugs can be divided into two groups: first-line drugs and second-line drugs. The first-line drugs are *isoniazid, rifampin, pyrazinamide, ethambutol,* and *streptomycin.* Of these, isoniazid and rifampin are the most important. The second-line drugs—*para-aminosalicylic acid (PAS), kanamycin, amikacin, capreomycin, ethionamide, cycloserine, ciprofloxacin,* and *ofloxacin*—are generally less effective and more toxic than the primary drugs. The second-line agents are used in combination with the primary drugs to treat disseminated tuberculosis and tuberculosis caused by organisms resistant to the first-line drugs. Adverse effects and routes of administration of the antituberculous drugs are summarized in Table 84–3.

## Isoniazid

Isoniazid [Laniazid, Nydrazid] is the primary agent for treatment and prophylaxis of tuberculosis. This drug is superior to alternative drugs with regard to efficacy, toxicity, ease of use, patient acceptance, and affordability. With the exception of patients who cannot tolerate the drug, isoniazid should be taken by all individuals infected with isoniazid-sensitive strains of *M. tuberculosis.*

### Antimicrobial Spectrum and Mechanism of Action

Isoniazid is highly selective for mycobacteria. The drug can kill tubercle bacilli at concentrations 10,000 times lower than those needed to affect gram-positive and gram-negative bacteria. Isoniazid is bactericidal to mycobacteria that are actively dividing, but is only bacteriostatic to "resting" organisms.

Although the mechanism by which isoniazid acts is not known with certainty, available data suggest that the drug suppresses bacterial growth by inhibiting synthesis of mycolic acid, a component of the mycobacterial cell wall. Since mycolic acid is not produced by other bacteria or by cells of the host, this mechanism would explain why isoniazid is so selective for mycobacteria.

### Resistance

Tubercle bacilli can develop resistance to isoniazid during treatment. Acquired resistance results from spontaneous mutation—not from transfer of R factors. The precise mechanism underlying resistance has not been

**TABLE 84–3. ANTITUBERCULOUS DRUGS: ROUTES AND MAJOR ADVERSE EFFECTS**

| Drug | Route | Major Adverse Effects |
|---|---|---|
| *First-Line Drugs* | | |
| Isoniazid | PO, IM | Hepatoxicity, peripheral neuritis |
| Rifampin | PO, IV | Hepatoxicity |
| Pyrazinamide | PO | Hepatoxicity |
| Ethambutol | PO | Optic neuritis |
| Streptomycin | IM | Eighth nerve damage, nephrotoxicity |
| *Second-Line Drugs* | | |
| Capreomycin | IM | Eighth nerve damage, nephrotoxicity |
| Kanamycin | IM, IV | Eighth nerve damage, nephrotoxicity |
| Amikacin | IM, IV | Eighth nerve damage, nephrotoxicity |
| Cycloserine | PO | Psychoses, seizure, rash |
| Ethionamide | PO | GI intolerance, hepatotoxicity |
| Ciprofloxacin | PO | GI intolerance |
| Ofloxacin | PO | GI intolerance |
| *p*-Aminosalicylc acid | PO | GI intolerance |

established. Emergence of resistance can be decreased through multiple-drug therapy. Organisms resistant to isoniazid are cross-resistant to ethionamide, but not to other drugs used for tuberculosis.

### Pharmacokinetics

*Absorption and Distribution.* Isoniazid is administered orally and by IM injection. The drug is well absorbed with either route. Once in the blood, isoniazid is widely distributed to tissues and body fluids. Concentrations in cerebrospinal fluid (CSF) are about 20% of those in plasma.

*Metabolism.* Isoniazid is inactivated in the liver, primarily by *acetylation.* The ability to acetylate isoniazid is genetically determined: about 50% of people in the United States are *rapid* acetylators and the other 50% are *slow* acetylators. The half-life of isoniazid in rapid acetylators is approximately 1 hour. The half-life in slow acetylators is about 3 hours. It is important to note that differences in rates of acetylation generally have little impact on the *efficacy* of isoniazid, provided patients are taking the drug daily. However, *nonhepatic toxicities* may be more likely in slow acetylators, since drug accumulation is greater in these patients.

*Excretion.* Isoniazid is excreted in the urine, primarily as inactive metabolites. In patients who are slow acetylators and who also have renal insufficiency, the drug may accumulate to toxic levels.

### Therapeutic Use

Isoniazid is indicated only for treatment and prophylaxis of tuberculosis. When taken for prophylaxis, isoniazid is administered alone. When employed for treatment, the drug must be taken in combination with at least one other antituberculous agent (e.g., rifampin).

### Adverse Effects

*Peripheral Neuropathy.* Dose-related peripheral neuropathy is the drug's most common adverse effect. Principal symptoms are symmetric paresthesias (tingling, numbness, burning, pain) of the hands and feet. Clumsi-

ness, unsteadiness, and muscle aches may also develop. Peripheral neuropathy results from isoniazid-induced deficiency in pyridoxine (vitamin B$_6$). If peripheral neuropathy develops, it can be reversed by administering pyridoxine (50 to 200 mg daily). In patients predisposed to neuropathy (e.g., alcoholics, diabetics), small doses of pyridoxine (6 to 50 mg/day) can be administered with isoniazid as prophylaxis against peripheral neuritis. This practice reduces the risk of neuropathy from 20% down to less than 1%.

*Hepatotoxicity.* Isoniazid can cause hepatocellular injury and multilobular necrosis. Death has occurred. Liver injury is thought to result from production of a toxic isoniazid metabolite. The greatest risk factor for liver damage is advancing age: the incidence of hepatotoxicity is nil in patients under 20 years; 1.2% in those ages 35 to 49; 2.3% in those ages 50 to 64; and 8% in those over 65. Patients should be informed about signs of hepatitis (anorexia, malaise, fatigue, nausea, yellowing of the skin or eyes) and instructed to notify the physician if these develop. Patients should also undergo monthly evaluation for these signs. Some clinicians perform monthly determinations of serum aspartate transaminase (AST) activity, since elevation of AST activity is indicative of liver injury. However, since AST levels may rise and then return to normal, despite continued isoniazid use, increases in AST may not be predictive of clinical hepatitis. It is recommended that isoniazid be withdrawn if signs of hepatitis develop or if AST activity rises to a level 3 times greater than the pretreatment baseline. Caution should be exercised when giving isoniazid to alcoholics and individuals with pre-existing disorders of the liver.

*Other Adverse Effects.* A variety of *CNS effects* can occur, including optic neuritis, seizures, dizziness, ataxia, and psychologic disturbances (depression, agitation, impairment of memory, hallucinations, toxic psychosis). *Anemia* may result from isoniazid-induced deficiency in pyridoxine. *Gastrointestinal distress*, *dry mouth*, and *urinary retention* occur on occasion. *Allergy* to isoniazid can produce fever, rashes, and a syndrome resembling lupus erythematosus.

## Drug Interactions

*Phenytoin.* Isoniazid can interfere with the metabolism of phenytoin, thereby causing the anticonvulsant to accumulate to toxic levels. Signs of phenytoin excess include ataxia and incoordination. Plasma levels of phenytoin should be monitored, and phenytoin dosage should be reduced as appropriate. Dosage of isoniazid should not be changed.

*Alcohol, Rifampin, and Pyrazinamide.* Daily ingestion of alcohol or concurrent therapy with rifampin or pyrazinamide increases the risk of hepatotoxicity. Patients should be encouraged to reduce or eliminate consumption of alcohol.

### Preparations, Dosage, and Administration

*Preparations.* Isoniazid [Laniazid, Nydrazid] is dispensed in tablets (50, 100, and 300 mg) and a syrup (10 mg/ml) for oral use, and in solution (100 mg/ml in 10-ml vials) for IM injection. Isoniazid is also available in fixed-dose combinations: capsules sold as *Rifamate* contain 150 mg of isoniazid and 300 mg of rifampin; tablets sold as *Rifater* contain 50 mg of isoniazid, 120 mg of rifampin, and 300 mg of pyrazinamide.

*Oral Dosage.* For treatment of active tuberculosis, the usual adult dosage is 300 mg/day. Alternatively, a dosage of 15 mg/kg twice a week can be employed. The pediatric dosage for active tuberculosis is 10 to 20 mg/kg/day. For prophylaxis of tuberculosis, the adult dosage is 300 mg/day and the pediatric dosage is 10 mg/kg/day.

*Intramuscular Dosage.* Parenteral therapy is administered in critical situations when oral treatment is not possible. The dosage is 300 mg daily.

## Rifampin

Rifampin [Rifadin, Rimactane] is equal to isoniazid in importance as an antituberculous drug. Prior to the appearance of resistant tubercle bacilli, the combination of rifampin plus isoniazid was the most frequently prescribed regimen for uncomplicated pulmonary tuberculosis.

## Antimicrobial Spectrum

Rifampin is a broad-spectrum antibiotic. The drug is active against most gram-positive bacteria as well as many gram-negative organisms. The drug is bactericidal to *Mycobacterium tuberculosis* and *M. leprae*. Other bacteria that are highly sensitive include *Neisseria meningitidis*, *Haemophilus influenzae*, *Staphylococcus aureus*, and *Legionella* species.

## Mechanism of Action and Bacterial Resistance

Rifampin inhibits bacterial DNA-dependent RNA polymerase, and thereby suppresses RNA synthesis and, consequently, protein synthesis. The results are bactericidal. Since mammalian RNA polymerases are not affected by the drug, rifampin is selectively toxic to microbes. Bacterial resistance to rifampin results from production of an altered form of RNA polymerase.

## Pharmacokinetics

*Absorption and Distribution.* Rifampin is well absorbed if taken on an empty stomach. However, if the drug is taken with or shortly after a meal, both the rate and extent of absorption can be significantly reduced. Rifampin is distributed widely to tissues and body fluids, including the cerebrospinal fluid. The drug is lipid soluble, and hence has ready access to intracellular bacteria.

*Elimination.* Rifampin is eliminated primarily by hepatic metabolism. Only about 20% of the drug leaves the body in the urine. Rifampin induces hepatic drug-metabolizing enzymes, including those responsible for its own inactivation. As a result, the rate at which rifampin is metabolized increases over the first weeks of therapy, causing the half-life of the drug to decrease—from an initial value of about 4 hours down to 2 hours at the end of 2 weeks. Because rifampin is eliminated by hepatic metabolism, patients with liver dysfunction require a reduction in dosage. No change in dosage is needed in patients with kidney disease.

## Therapeutic Use

*Tuberculosis.* Rifampin is one of our most effective antituberculous drugs. This agent is bactericidal to tubercle bacilli at extracellular and intracellular sites. Rifampin is a drug of choice for treating pulmonary tuberculosis and disseminated disease. Because resistance can develop rapidly when rifampin is employed alone, the drug is always employed in combination with at least one other antituberculous agent. Despite the capacity of rifampin to produce a variety of adverse effects, toxicity rarely requires discontinuation of treatment.

*Leprosy.* Rifampin is bactericidal to *Mycobacterium leprae* and has become an important agent for the treatment of leprosy.

*Meningococcus Carriers.* Rifampin is highly active against *Neisseria meningitidis* and is indicated for short-term therapy to eliminate this bacterium from the nasopharynx of asymptomatic carriers. Because resistant organisms emerge rapidly, rifampin should not be used to treat active meningococcal disease.

## Adverse Effects

Rifampin is generally well tolerated. When employed at recommended dosages, the drug rarely causes significant toxicity. The most common adverse effect of concern is hepatitis.

*Hepatotoxicity.* Rifampin is toxic to the liver and may cause jaundice and even hepatitis. Asymptomatic elevation of liver enzymes occurs in about 14% of patients. The incidence of hepatitis is less than 1%. Hepatotoxicity is most likely in alcoholics and patients with pre-existing liver disease. These individuals should be monitored closely for signs of liver dysfunction. Tests of liver function (serum transaminase levels) should be made prior to treatment and every 2 to 4 weeks thereafter. Patients should be informed about signs of hepatitis (jaundice, anorexia, malaise, fatigue, nausea) and instructed to notify the physician if these develop.

*Discoloration of Body Fluids.* Rifampin frequently imparts a red-orange color to urine, sweat, saliva, and tears.

Patients should be forewarned of this harmless effect. Permanent staining of soft contact lenses has occurred on occasion; the patient should consult an ophthalmologist regarding the advisability of contact lens use.

*Other Adverse Effects.* *Gastrointestinal disturbances* (anorexia, nausea, abdominal discomfort) and *cutaneous reactions* (flushing, itching, rash) occur occasionally. Rarely, intermittent high-dose therapy has produced a *flu-like syndrome*, characterized by fever, chills, muscle aches, headache, and dizziness. This reaction appears to have an immunologic basis. In some patients, high-dose therapy has been associated with *shortness of breath*, *hemolytic anemia*, *shock*, and *acute renal failure*.

### Drug Interactions

*Accelerated Metabolism of Other Drugs.* Because of its ability to induce hepatic drug-metabolizing enzymes, rifampin can increase the rate at which many drugs are metabolized. This action can reduce the effects of a variety of medicines, including *oral contraceptives*, *warfarin*, and *methadone*. When these drugs are used in conjunction with rifampin, an increase in their dosages may be required.

*Isoniazid and Pyrazinamide.* Rifampin, isoniazid, and pyrazinamide are all hepatotoxic. Hence, when these drugs are used in combination, as they often are, the risk of liver injury may be greater than when they are used alone.

#### Preparations, Dosage, and Administration

*Preparations.* Rifampin [Rifadin, Rimactane] is dispensed in capsules (150 and 300 mg) for oral administration. Oral rifampin is also available in two fixed-dose combinations: the capsules, sold as *Rifamate*, contain 300 mg of rifampin and 150 mg of isoniazid; the tablets, sold as *Rifater*, contain 120 mg of rifampin, 50 mg of isoniazid, and 300 mg of pyrazinamide. Rifampin [Rifadin] is also available in powder form to be reconstituted for IV infusion.

*Oral Dosage and Administration.* For treatment of tuberculosis, the usual adult dosage is 600 mg or 10 mg/kg daily. The pediatric dosage is 10 to 20 mg/kg/day. Rifampin is administered as a single daily dose 1 hour before a meal or 2 hours after. The dosage should be reduced in the presence of liver dysfunction.

*Intravenous Administration.* Dissolve 600 mg of powdered rifampin in 10 ml of Sterile Water for Injection to make a concentrated solution (60 mg/ml). Dilute an appropriate dose of the concentrate in 500 ml of 5% dextrose and infuse over 3 hours.

## Pyrazinamide

### Antimicrobial Activity and Therapeutic Use

Pyrazinamide is bactericidal to *Mycobacterium tuberculosis.* The mechanism of antibacterial action is not known. Currently, the combination of pyrazinamide with rifampin and isoniazid is considered the regimen of choice for tuberculosis caused by nonresistant bacteria. In this regimen, pyrazinamide is discontinued after 2 months, while the other two agents are continued for an additional 4 months (see Table 84–1).

### Pharmacokinetics

Pyrazinamide is well absorbed following oral administration and is widely distributed to tissues and body fluids. In the liver, the drug is converted to pyrazinoic acid, an active metabolite,

and then to 5-hydroxypyrazinoic acid, which is inactive. Excretion is renal, primarily as inactive metabolites.

### Adverse Effects

*Hepatotoxicity.* Liver injury is the principal adverse effect. High-dose therapy has caused hepatitis, and, rarely, fatal hepatic necrosis. Fortunately, these reactions are relatively uncommon with the low-dose, short-term therapy employed currently. The earliest manifestations of liver damage are elevations in serum levels of transaminases (aspartate aminotransferase [AST] and alanine aminotransferase [ALT]). Levels of these enzymes should be measured prior to treatment and every 2 to 4 weeks thereafter. Patients should be informed about signs of hepatitis (e.g., malaise, anorexia, nausea, vomiting, yellowish discoloration of the skin and eyes) and instructed to notify the physician if these develop. Pyrazinamide should be discontinued if significant injury to the liver occurs. The drug should not be used by patients with pre-existing liver dysfunction. The risk of liver injury is increased by concurrent therapy with isoniazid and rifampin, both of which are hepatotoxic.

*Other Adverse Effects.* Pyrazinamide and its metabolites can inhibit renal excretion of uric acid, thereby causing *hyperuricemia*; although usually asymptomatic, pyrazinamide-induced hyperuricemia has resulted in *gouty arthritis* rarely. Additional adverse effects include *arthralgia*, *gastrointestinal disturbances* (nausea, vomiting, diarrhea), *rashes*, and *photosensitivity.*

#### Preparations, Dosage, and Administration

Pyrazinamide is dispensed in 500-mg tablets for oral administration. The usual adult dosage is 20 to 30 mg/kg administered once a day. The maximum daily dosage should not exceed 2 gm. Pyrazinamide is also available in a fixed-dose combination with isoniazid and rifampin, sold under the trade name *Rifater.*

## Ethambutol

### Antimicrobial Action

Ethambutol [Myambutol] is active only against mycobacteria; nearly all strains of *M. tuberculosis* are sensitive. The drug is bacteriostatic, not bactericidal. Ethambutol is usually active against tubercle bacilli that are resistant to isoniazid and rifampin. Although ethambutol is known to suppress incorporation of mycolic acid in the wall, the precise mechanism by which ethambutol suppresses bacterial growth has not been established.

### Therapeutic Use

Ethambutol is an important antituberculous drug. This agent is employed for initial treatment of tuberculosis and for retreatment of patients who have received therapy previously. Like other drugs for tuberculosis, ethambutol is always employed as part of a multidrug regimen.

#### Pharmacokinetics

Ethambutol is readily absorbed following oral administration. The drug is widely distributed to most tissues and body fluids; levels in cerebrospinal fluid, however, remain low. Ethambutol undergoes little hepatic metabolism and is excreted primarily in the urine. In patients with normal kidney function, the drug's half-life is 3 to 4 hours; the half-life increases to 8 hours in patients with renal impairment.

## Adverse Effects

Ethambutol is generally well tolerated. The only significant adverse effect is optic neuritis.

*Optic Neuritis.* Ethambutol can produce dose-related optic neuritis, resulting in blurred vision, constriction of the visual field, and disturbance of color discrimination. The mechanism underlying these effects is not known. Symptoms usually resolve upon discontinuation of treatment; however, for some patients, visual disturbance may persist. Color discrimination and visual acuity should be assessed prior to treatment and monthly thereafter. Patients should be advised to report any alteration in vision. If ocular toxicity develops, ethambutol should be withdrawn immediately. Because visual changes can be difficult to monitor in pediatric patients, ethambutol is not recommended for children less than 13 years old.

*Other Adverse Effects.* Ethambutol can produce *allergic reactions* (dermatitis, pruritus), *gastrointestinal upset*, and *confusion*. The drug inhibits renal excretion of uric acid, causing *asymptomatic hyperuricemia* in about 50% of patients; occasionally, elevation of uric acid levels results in *acute gouty arthritis*. Rare adverse effects include *peripheral neuropathy*, *renal damage*, and *thrombocytopenia*.

## Preparations, Dosage, and Administration

Ethambutol [Myambutol] is dispensed in 100- and 400-mg tablets for oral administration. For *initial* therapy of tuberculosis, the usual dosage for adults and children is 15 mg/kg once a day. For *retreatment* therapy, the usual dosage is 25 mg/kg/day for the first 60 days and 15 mg/kg/day thereafter; all doses are given once a day. Ethambutol may be taken with food if GI upset occurs.

## Streptomycin

Streptomycin, an aminoglycoside antibiotic, was our first effective antituberculous drug. The basic pharmacology of streptomycin and the other aminoglycosides is discussed in Chapter 81. Consideration here is limited to the use of streptomycin for tuberculosis.

*Antibacterial Activity.* Streptomycin is bactericidal to tubercle bacilli *in vitro*; however, the drug has relatively low sterilizing activity *in vivo*. This discrepancy is explained by the inability of streptomycin to penetrate mammalian cells; since tubercle bacilli are frequently present at intracellular sites, many escape exposure to the drug.

*Adverse Effects.* The most characteristic toxicity is *injury to the eighth cranial nerve, resulting in hearing loss and disturbance of balance.* However, when the drug is prescribed properly, effects on auditory and vestibular function are rare. The risk of eighth nerve toxicity is increased by advanced age and kidney dysfunction. Tests of hearing and balance should be performed periodically during the course of treatment. Special care should be taken to adjust the dosage in patients with renal impairment. Additional adverse effects include *nephrotoxicity*, *facial paresthesias*, and *rash*.

*Therapeutic Status, Dosage, and Administration.* Streptomycin must be administered by IM injection. Because it cannot be used orally, and because of its potential for eighth nerve toxicity, streptomycin is considerably less attractive than the newer antituberculous drugs (rifampin, isoniazid, pyrazinamide, etham-

butol) for initial treatment. Accordingly, use of this once-popular agent has sharply declined. Today, streptomycin is employed primarily in three-drug regimens for chemotherapy of severe mycobacterial infection. The usual adult dosage is 15 mg/kg 5 days a week. The recommended dosage for children is 20 to 40 mg/kg/day.

## Second-Line Antituberculous Drugs

The group of second-line antituberculous drugs consists of *para-aminosalicylic acid (PAS)*, *kanamycin*, *capreomycin*, *ethionamide*, *cycloserine*, *ofloxacin*, and *ciprofloxacin*. In general, these drugs are less effective and more toxic than the first-line antituberculous drugs. As a result, the principal use of second-line drugs is treatment of tuberculosis caused by organisms that have proved resistant to the first-line agents. In addition, the second-line drugs are used to treat severe pulmonary tuberculosis as well as disseminated (extrapulmonary) infection. The second-line drugs are always employed in conjunction with a major antituberculous drug. Principal toxicities are summarized in Table 84–3.

### Para-Aminosalicylic Acid

*Actions and Uses.* PAS is similar in structure and actions to the sulfonamides. Like the sulfonamides, PAS exerts its antibacterial effects by inhibiting synthesis of folic acid. However, in contrast to the sulfonamides, which are broad-spectrum antibiotics, PAS is active only against mycobacteria. In the United States, PAS has been employed primarily as a substitute for ethambutol in pediatric patients. The drug is always used in combination with other antituberculous agents.

*Pharmacokinetics.* PAS is administered orally and is well absorbed from the gastrointestinal tract. The drug is distributed widely to most tissues and body fluids; however, levels in CSF remain low. PAS undergoes extensive hepatic metabolism. Metabolites and parent drug are excreted in the urine.

*Adverse Effects.* PAS is poorly tolerated by adults; children accept the drug somewhat better. The most frequent adverse effects are gastrointestinal disturbances (nausea, vomiting, diarrhea). Because PAS is administered in large doses as a sodium salt, substantial sodium loading may occur. Additional adverse effects are allergic reactions, hepatotoxicity, and goiter.

*Preparations, Dosage, and Administration.* Aminosalicylate sodium [Sodium P.A.S.] is dispensed in 500-mg tablets for oral administration. Tablets that are discolored (brown, purple) should not be used. The drug loses its effectiveness if exposed to sunlight, extreme heat, or moisture. Accordingly, it should not be stored in kitchen or bathroom cabinets. If stomach upset occurs, the drug may be administered with food. The daily dosage for adults is 14 to 16 gm in two or three divided doses. The daily dosage for children is 275 to 420 mg/kg in three to four divided doses.

### Ethionamide

*Actions and Uses.* Ethionamide [Trecator-SC], a relative of isoniazid, is active against mycobacteria, but less so than isoniazid. Ethionamide is administered with other antituberculous drugs to treat tuberculosis that is resistant to first-line agents. Gastrointestinal disturbances limit patient acceptance of the drug. Ethionamide is the least well tolerated of all antituberculous drugs, and hence should be used only when there are no alternatives.

*Pharmacokinetics.* Ethionamide is readily absorbed following oral administration. The drug is widely distributed to tissues and body fluids, including the CSF. Ethionamide undergoes extensive metabolism and is excreted in the urine, primarily as metabolites.

**Adverse Effects.** Gastrointestinal effects (anorexia, nausea, vomiting, diarrhea, metallic taste) occur often; intolerance of these effects frequently leads to discontinuation. Ethionamide is toxic to the liver. Hepatotoxicity is assessed by measuring serum transaminases (AST, ALT) prior to treatment and periodically thereafter. Additional adverse effects include peripheral neuropathy, central nervous system (CNS) effects (convulsions, mental disturbance), and allergic reactions.

**Preparations, Dosage, and Administration.** Ethionamide [Trecator-SC] is dispensed in 250-mg tablets for oral administration. The usual adult dosage is 0.5 to 1 gm/day in divided doses. The recommended pediatric dosage is 15 to 20 mg/kg/day (maximum of 1 gm).

### Cycloserine

**Actions and Uses.** Cycloserine [Seromycin Pulvules] is an antibiotic produced by a species of *Streptomyces*. The drug is bacteriostatic and acts by inhibiting synthesis of the cell wall. Cycloserine is used to treat tuberculosis that is resistant to first-line drugs.

**Pharmacokinetics.** Cycloserine is rapidly absorbed following oral administration. The drug is widely distributed to tissues and body fluids, including the CSF. Elimination is by hepatic metabolism and renal excretion; about 50% of the drug leaves the body unchanged in the urine. Cycloserine may accumulate to toxic levels in patients with renal impairment.

**Adverse Effects.** CNS effects occur frequently and can be severe. Possible reactions include anxiety, depression, confusion, hallucinations, paranoia, hyperreflexia, and seizures. Psychotic episodes occur in approximately 10% of patients; symptoms usually subside within 2 weeks following drug withdrawal. Pyridoxine may prevent neurotoxic effects. Other adverse effects include peripheral neuropathy, hepatotoxicity, and folate deficiency. To minimize the risk of adverse effects, serum concentrations should be measured regularly; peak concentrations, measured 2 hours after dosing, should be 25 to 35 µg/ml.

**Preparations, Dosage, and Administration.** Cycloserine [Seromycin Pulvules] is dispensed in 250-mg capsules for oral administration. The initial dosage for adults is 250 mg twice daily for 2 weeks; the maintenance dosage is 500 mg to 1 gm daily in divided doses. The dosage for children is 10 to 20 mg/kg/day.

### Capreomycin

Capreomycin [Capastat Sulfate] is an antibiotic derived from a species of *Streptomyces*. Antibacterial effects are probably due to inhibition of protein synthesis. The drug is bacteriostatic to *Mycobacterium tuberculosis*. Capreomycin is used only for tuberculosis resistant to primary agents. The drug's principal toxicity is renal damage; accordingly, it should not be taken by patients with kidney disease. Capreomycin may also cause eighth nerve damage, resulting in hearing loss, tinnitus, and disturbance of balance. Administration is by deep IM injection (the drug is not absorbed from the GI tract, and hence cannot be administered orally). The usual dosage for adults is 1 gm/day for 60 to 120 days, followed by 1-gm doses 2 to 3 times a week. The dosage for children is 15 mg/kg/day (up to a maximum of 1 gm).

### Kanamycin and Amikacin

Kanamycin [Kantrex, others] and amikacin [Amikin] are aminoglycoside antibiotics that have good activity against *M. tuberculosis*. Like streptomycin and other aminoglycosides, kanamycin and amikacin are nephrotoxic and may damage the eighth cranial nerve. Neither drug is absorbed from the GI tract, hence administration is IM or IV. The adult dosage for both drugs is 15 mg/kg/day; the pediatric dosage is 15 to 30 mg/kg/day. The pharmacology of kanamycin, amikacin, and the other aminoglycosides is discussed in Chapter 81.

### Ofloxacin and Ciprofloxacin

Ofloxacin [Floxin] and ciprofloxacin [Cipro] are fluoroquinolone antibiotics indicated for a wide variety of bacterial infections (see Chapter 85). Both drugs have good activity against *M. tuberculosis*. As therapy for tuberculosis, these agents are reserved for prophylaxis and treatment of infection caused by multidrug-resistant organisms. Both agents are generally well tolerated, although gastrointestinal disturbances are relatively common. Tendon rupture occurs rarely. The adult dosage for ofloxacin is 600 to 800 mg daily, given in one or two doses. The adult dosage for ciprofloxacin is 500 to 750 mg twice a day. Neither drug is recommended for children.

## Drugs for *Mycobacterium avium* Complex Infection

*Mycobacterium avium* complex (MAC) consists of two nearly indistinguishable organisms: *Mycobacterium avium* and *Mycobacterium intracellulare*. Colonization with MAC begins in the lungs or gastrointestinal tract, but then may spread to the blood, bone marrow, liver, spleen, lymph nodes, brain, kidneys, and skin. Disseminated infection is common in patients with HIV infection; the incidence at autopsy is 50%. In patients without HIV infection, symptomatic MAC infection is usually limited to the lungs. Signs and symptoms of disseminated MAC infection include fever, night sweats, weight loss, lethargy, anemia, and abnormal liver function tests. The preferred agents for *prophylaxis* of disseminated infection are *azithromycin* and *clarithromycin*. Regimens for treating *active infection* should include either *azithromycin* or *clarithromycin*, plus at least one other drug—usually *ethambutol*. Additional drugs may be added as needed; options include rifabutin, rifampin, ciprofloxacin, clofazimine, and amikacin.

### Rifabutin

**Actions and Use.** Rifabutin [Mycobutin] is a close chemical relative of rifampin. Like rifampin, rifabutin inhibits mycobacterial DNA-dependent RNA polymerase, and thereby suppresses protein synthesis. The drug is approved for prevention of disseminated MAC disease in patients with advanced HIV infection (CD4 lymphocyte counts below 200 cells/mm$^3$). In addition to this approved application, rifabutin is used to treat active MAC disease.

In patients with MAC infection who are also infected with *M. tuberculosis*, treatment with rifabutin can encourage emergence of *rifampin* resistance in *M. tuberculosis*. Accordingly, if *M. tuberculosis* is present, patients should receive concurrent prophylaxis with isoniazid.

**Pharmacokinetics.** Rifabutin is administered orally. Absorption is unaffected by food. Peak plasma levels are reached in 2 to 3 hours. The drug is widely distributed and achieves high concentrations in the lungs. Rifabutin is metabolized in the liver and excreted in the urine, bile, and feces. The half-life is 45 hours.

**Adverse Effects.** Rifabutin is generally well tolerated. The most common side effects are *rash* (4%), *gastroin-*

*testinal disturbances* (3%), and *neutropenia* (2%). Like rifampin, rifabutin can impart a *harmless brown-orange discoloration to urine, sweat, saliva, and tears*; soft contact lenses may be permanently stained. Rifabutin poses a risk of *uveitis*, and hence should be discontinued if ocular pain or blurred vision develops. Other adverse effects include *myositis, hepatitis, arthralgia, chest pain with dyspnea*, and a *flu-like syndrome*.

**Drug Interactions.** Like rifampin, rifabutin *induces hepatic drug metabolizing enzymes*, although to a lesser extent. By increasing enzyme activity, rifabutin can decrease blood levels of *zidovudine*, an important drug for treatment of HIV infection. In addition, rifabutin can reduce levels of *oral contraceptives*; hence, patients should be advised to use a nonhormonal method of birth control.

**Preparations, Dosage, and Administration.** Rifabutin [Mycobutin] is dispensed in 150-mg capsules for oral administration. The usual dosage is 300 mg once a day. To reduce gastrointestinal upset, an alternative dosing schedule of 150 mg twice daily may be used.

## Other Drugs for *M. avium* Complex Infection

**Macrolide Antibiotics: Azithromycin and Clarithromycin.** The basic pharmacology of azithromycin [Zithromax] and clarithromycin [Biaxin] is discussed in Chapter 80. Consideration here is limited to the use of these drugs against MAC.

Azithromycin and clarithromycin are drugs of choice for prophylaxis and treatment of MAC infection. All patients with active disease should receive one of these drugs. To prevent emergence of resistance, azithromycin or clarithromycin should be combined with at least one other agent; many authorities recommend ethambutol. The most common side effects of the macrolides are gastrointestinal disturbances (nausea, diarrhea, vomiting, abdominal pain). For treatment of MAC infection, the dosage of azithromycin is 500 daily; the dosage for clarithromycin is 500 to 2000 mg twice daily.

**Ethambutol.** Ethambutol is combined with either azithromycin or clarithromycin to treat disseminated MAC infection. The toxicity of greatest concern is optic neuritis. The dosage for MAC disease is 15 to 25 mg/kg/day. The basic pharmacology of ethambutol is discussed above.

**Additional Agents.** If a macrolide plus ethambutol is insufficient to control disseminated MAC infection, one or more of the following may be added: rifabutin (450 to 600 mg/day), rifampin (600 mg/day), ciprofloxacin (750 mg twice daily), clofazimine (100 to 300 mg/day), and amikacin (7.5 to 15 mg/kg/day). All of these drugs are administered orally, except amikacin, which is administered IM or IV.

## Drugs for Leprosy

Leprosy (Hansen's disease) is caused by *Mycobacterium leprae*. Worldwide, leprosy constitutes a major public health problem; about 12 million people are estimated to have the disease. In the United States, the number of cases is approximately 4000.

Leprosy is acquired through exposure to individuals who have the infection. Bacilli are transmitted from the respiratory tract of the infected person to the respiratory tract of the noninfected person. Fortunately, when leprosy is properly treated, infectivity is essentially nil. Accordingly, for patients who are receiving adequate chemotherapy, isolation is not required.

Treatment of leprosy has three major objectives: (1) conversion of the patient to a noninfectious state, (2) prevention of bacterial multiplication, and (3) avoidance or reduction of complications of leprosy. To achieve these objectives, the World Health Organization recommends that all patients receive treatment with multiple drugs. *Dapsone* has been and remains a mainstay of therapy. Other important agents are *rifampin* and *clofazimine*. Therapy is prolonged, lasting from several months to many years.

### Dapsone

**Actions and Uses.** Dapsone is a primary drug for treatment of leprosy. This agent is effective, low in toxicity, and inexpensive. Dapsone is chemically related to the sulfonamides and probably shares their mechanism of action: inhibition of folic acid synthesis. Depending on its concentration, dapsone can be bactericidal or bacteriostatic. Although once employed alone to treat leprosy, dapsone is now employed in combination with other antileprosy drugs, usually rifampin and clofazimine.

**Pharmacokinetics.** Dapsone is absorbed slowly but completely from the GI tract. Once in the blood, the drug is widely distributed to tissues and body fluids. Dapsone is acetylated in the liver and has a plasma half-life of 10 to 50 hours. Excretion is renal, primarily as metabolites.

**Adverse Effects.** Dapsone is generally well tolerated; the drug may be taken for years without significant untoward effects. The most common adverse effects are gastrointestinal disturbances, headache, rash, and a syndrome that resembles mononucleosis. Hemolytic anemia occurs occasionally; severe reactions are usually limited to patients with profound glucose-6-phosphate dehydrogenase deficiency. Rare reactions include agranulocytosis, exfoliative dermatitis, and hepatitis.

**Preparations, Dosage, and Administration.** Dapsone is dispensed in 25- and 100-mg tablets for oral administration. The usual dosage for adults is 100 mg/day; the daily dosage for children is 1 mg/kg. As a rule, dapsone is administered in combination with rifampin and clofazimine.

### Clofazimine

**Actions and Uses.** Clofazimine [Lamprene] is weakly bactericidal to *Mycobacterium leprae*. The mechanism of antibacterial effects has not been determined. In treatment of leprosy, clofazimine is combined with dapsone and rifampin. In addition to its antibacterial action, clofazimine has anti-inflammatory actions.

**Pharmacokinetics.** Clofazimine is administered orally and undergoes partial absorption. Absorbed drug is retained in tissues. Because of tissue retention, the half-life of clofazimine is extremely long—about 70 days.

**Adverse Effects.** Dangerous reactions are uncommon. However, clofazimine frequently imparts a red-brown color to the skin and conjunctiva. The drug may also discolor urine, sweat, saliva, and tears. Because of these effects on pigmentation, patients with light-colored skin often find clofazimine unacceptable. Pigmentation usually clears 6 to 12 months after completing treatment. Deposition of clofazimine in the small intestine produces the drug's most serious effects: intestinal obstruction, pain, and bleeding.

**Preparations, Dosage, and Administration.** Clofazimine [Lamprene] is dispensed in 50- and 100-mg capsules for oral use. The usual adult dosage is 50 to 100 mg daily.

### Rifampin

Rifampin is bactericidal to *Mycobacterium leprae*. For treatment of leprosy, the drug is combined with dapsone, with or without clofazimine. The usual adult dosage is 600 mg daily; the dosage for children is 10 to 20 mg/kg/day (but no more than 600 mg/day). For leprosy control programs in developing countries, where the cost of *daily* rifampin is prohibitive, the World Health Organization recommends supervised *monthly* treatment with a single 600-mg dose, which has been shown equivalent to daily dosing. The basic pharmacology of rifampin is discussed above under *Pharmacology of Individual Antituberculous Drugs.*

## KEY POINTS

- Most people infected with *M. tuberculosis* remain asymptomatic, although they will harbor dormant bacteria for life (in the absence of drug therapy).
- Symptomatic tuberculosis can result from reactivation of an old infection or from recent person-to-person transmission.
- The *tuberculin skin test*—used to screen for tuberculosis—is performed by giving an intradermal injection of PPD (purified protein derivative) and then assessing for a zone of induration (hardness) at the site.
- Drug resistance, and especially multidrug resistance, is a serious impediment to successful therapy of tuberculosis.
- The principal cause of drug resistance in tuberculosis is inadequate drug therapy, which kills sensitive bacteria while allowing resistant mutants to flourish.
- To prevent emergence of resistance, tuberculosis must always be treated with at least two drugs to which the infecting organism is sensitive. Accordingly, isolates from all patients must be tested for resistance.
- Therapy of tuberculosis is prolonged, lasting from a minimum of 6 months to 2 years or even longer.
- The first-line drugs for tuberculosis are isoniazid, rifampin, pyrazinamide, ethambutol, and streptomycin.

- In communities where resistance is likely, the regimen for initial therapy of tuberculosis consists of four drugs: isoniazid, rifampin, and pyrazinamide, plus either ethambutol or streptomycin.
- Initial therapy of multidrug-resistant tuberculosis may require as many as seven drugs.
- Tuberculosis in HIV-positive patients can be treated with the same regimens used for HIV-negative patients, although the duration of treatment is longer.
- Three methods are employed to evaluate therapy: bacteriologic evaluation of sputum, clinical evaluation, and chest x-rays.
- Isoniazid can cause peripheral neuropathy by depleting pyridoxine (vitamin $B_6$). Peripheral neuropathy can be reversed or prevented with pyridoxine supplements.
- Isoniazid can injure the liver. The greatest risk factor is advancing age.
- Isoniazid is the only drug proved effective for preventive therapy of tuberculosis.
- Rifampin induces hepatic drug-metabolizing enzymes, and can thereby increase the metabolism of other drugs; important among these are oral contraceptives, warfarin, and methadone.
- Like isoniazid, rifampin and pyrazinamide are hepatotoxic. Accordingly, when these three drugs are combined, as they often are, the risk of liver injury can be significant.
- Ethambutol can cause optic neuritis.
- Azithromycin and clarithromycin are the drugs of choice for preventing disseminated MAC infection in patients with advanced HIV infection.
- Rifabutin, a drug for MAC infection, can induce hepatic drug metabolizing enzymes, thereby decreasing the effects of other drugs.
- All patients with disseminated MAC infection should receive azithromycin or clarithromycin, combined with ethambutol (or another appropriate drug) to prevent emergence of resistance.

## Summary of Major Nursing Implications*

The nursing implications summarized below are limited to the drug therapy of tuberculosis.

## Implications That Apply to All Antituberculous Drugs

### Promoting Compliance

Treatment of active tuberculosis is prolonged and demands concurrent use of two or more drugs; as a result, compliance can be a significant problem. To promote compliance, educate the patient about the rationale for multidrug therapy and the need for long-term treatment. Encourage patients to take their medication exactly as pre-

scribed, and to continue treatment until the infection has resolved. Some authorities recommend directly observed administration to ensure compliance.

### Evaluating Treatment

Success is indicated by (1) reductions in fever, malaise, anorexia, cough, and other clinical manifestations of tuberculosis (usually within weeks), (2) radiographic evidence of improvement (usually in 3 months), and (3) an absence of *M. tuberculosis* in sputum cultures (usually after 3 to 6 months).

## Isoniazid

In addition to the implications summarized below, see above for implications on *promoting compliance* and

---

*Patient education information is highlighted in color.

*evaluating treatment* that apply to all antituberculous drugs.

## Preadministration Assessment

### Therapeutic Goal

Treatment or prophylaxis of infection with *Mycobacterium tuberculosis*.

### Baseline Data

Obtain a chest x-ray, microbiologic tests of sputum, and baseline tests of liver function.

### Identifying High-Risk Patients

Isoniazid is *contraindicated* for patients with *acute liver disease* or a *history of isoniazid-induced hepatotoxicity*. Use the drug with *caution* in alcoholics, *diabetics, patients with vitamin B₆ deficiency, patients over the age of 50*, and *patients who are taking phenytoin, rifampin*, or *pyrazinamide*.

## Implementation: Administration

### Routes

Oral, IM.

### Administration

Advise the patient to take isoniazid on an empty stomach, either 1 hour before meals or 2 hours after. Advise the patient to take the drug with meals if GI upset occurs.

## Ongoing Evaluation and Interventions

### Minimizing Adverse Effects

*Peripheral Neuropathy.* Inform patients about symptoms of peripheral neuropathy (tingling, numbing, burning, or pain in the hands or feet), and instruct them to notify the physician if these occur. Peripheral neuritis can be reversed with small daily doses of pyridoxine (vitamin B₆). In patients at high risk of neuropathy (e.g., alcoholics, diabetics), give pyridoxine prophylactically.

*Hepatotoxicity.* Isoniazid can cause hepatocellular damage and multilobular hepatic necrosis. Inform patients about signs of hepatitis (jaundice, anorexia, malaise, fatigue, nausea), and instruct them to notify the physician if these develop. Evaluate patients monthly for signs of hepatitis. Monthly determinations of AST activity may be ordered. If clinical signs of hepatitis appear, or if AST activity exceeds 3 times the pretreatment baseline, isoniazid should be withdrawn. Daily ingestion of alcohol increases the risk of liver injury; urge the patient to minimize or eliminate alcohol consumption.

### Minimizing Adverse Interactions

*Phenytoin.* Isoniazid can suppress the metabolism of phenytoin, thereby causing phenytoin levels to rise. Plasma content of phenytoin should be monitored. If necessary, phenytoin dosage should be reduced.

## Rifampin

In addition to the implications summarized below, see above for implications on *promoting compliance* and *evaluating treatment* that apply to all antituberculous drugs.

## Preadministration Assessment

### Therapeutic Goal

Treatment of tuberculosis or leprosy.

### Baseline Data

Obtain a chest x-ray, microbiologic tests of sputum, and baseline tests of liver function.

### Identifying High-Risk Patients

Use with *caution* in patients with *liver disease* and in *alcoholics*.

## Implementation: Administration

### Routes

Oral, IV.

### Dosage

Reduce the dosage in patients with liver dysfunction.

### Administration

Instruct the patient to take oral rifampin once a day, either 1 hour before a meal or 2 hours after.

Administer IV rifampin by slow infusion (over 3 hours).

## Ongoing Evaluation and Interventions

### Minimizing Adverse Effects

*Hepatotoxicity.* Rifampin may cause jaundice or hepatitis. Inform patients about signs of liver dysfunction (anorexia, darkened urine, pale stools, yellow discoloration of eyes or skin) and instruct them to notify the physician if these develop. Monitor patients for signs of liver dysfunction. Tests of liver function should be made prior to treatment and every 2 to 4 weeks thereafter.

*Discoloration of Body Fluids.* Forewarn patients that rifampin may impart a harmless red-orange color to urine, sweat, saliva, and tears. Warn patients that soft contact lenses may undergo permanent staining; advise them to consult an ophthalmologist about continued use of these lenses.

### Minimizing Adverse Interactions

*Accelerated Metabolism of Other Drugs.* Rifampin can accelerate the metabolism of many drugs, thereby reducing their therapeutic effects. This action is of particular concern with *oral contraceptives, warfarin*, and *methadone*. When these agents are used in conjunction with rifampin, an increase in their dosage may be required.

*Pyrazinamide and Isoniazid.* These hepatotoxic antituberculous drugs can increase the risk of liver injury when used with rifampin.

# Pyrazinamide

In addition to the implications summarized below, see above for implications on *promoting compliance* and *evaluating treatment* that apply to all antituberculous drugs.

## Preadministration Assessment

### Therapeutic Goal
Treatment of tuberculosis.

### Baseline Data
Obtain a chest x-ray, microbiologic tests of sputum, and baseline tests of liver function.

### Identifying High-Risk Patients
Pyrazinamide is *contraindicated* for patients with *severe liver dysfunction* or *acute gout*. Use with *caution* in *alcoholics*.

## Implementation: Administration

### Route
Oral.

### Administration
Usually administered once a day.

## Ongoing Evaluation and Interventions

### Minimizing Adverse Effects
Hepatotoxicity. Inform patients about symptoms of hepatitis (malaise, anorexia, nausea, vomiting, yellowish discoloration of the skin and eyes), and instruct them to notify the physician if these develop. Levels of AST and ALT should be measured prior to treatment and every 2 to 4 weeks thereafter. If severe liver injury occurs, pyrazinamide should be withdrawn. The risk of liver injury is increased by concurrent therapy with isoniazid and rifampin, both of which are hepatotoxic.

# Ethambutol

In addition to the implications summarized below, see above for implications on *promoting compliance* and *evaluating treatment* that apply to all antituberculous drugs.

## Preadministration Assessment

### Therapeutic Goal
Treatment of tuberculosis.

### Baseline Data
Obtain a chest x-ray, microbiologic tests of sputum, and baseline vision tests.

### Identifying High-Risk Patients
Ethambutol is *contraindicated* for patients with *optic neuritis*.

## Implementation: Administration

### Route
Oral.

### Administration
Usually administered once a day. Advise the patient to take ethambutol with food if GI upset occurs.

## Ongoing Evaluation and Interventions

### Minimizing Adverse Effects
*Optic Neuritis.* Ethambutol can cause dose-related optic neuritis. Symptoms include blurred vision, altered color discrimination, and constriction of visual fields. Baseline vision tests are required. Instruct the patient to report any alteration in vision (e.g., blurring of vision, reduced color discrimination). If ocular toxicity develops, ethambutol should be withdrawn at once.

# CHAPTER 85

# Miscellaneous Antibacterial Drugs: Fluoroquinolones, Rifampin, Metronidazole, Polymyxins, and Bacitracin

**Fluoroquinolones**
Ciprofloxacin
Norfloxacin
Newer Fluoroquinolones

**Additional Antibacterial Drugs**
Metronidazole
Rifampin
Bacitracin
Polymyxin B

## Fluoroquinolones

The fluoroquinolones are close chemical relatives of nalidixic acid, a narrow-spectrum antibiotic used only for urinary tract infections. However, in contrast to nalidixic acid, the fluoroquinolones have a broad antimicrobial spectrum and a variety of clinical applications. Side effects are generally mild, and resistance develops slowly.

## Ciprofloxacin

Ciprofloxacin [Cipro] was among the first fluoroquinolones available and will serve as our prototype for the family. This drug can be administered orally and is active against a broad spectrum of bacterial pathogens. The drug has been used as an alternative to parenteral antibiotics for treatment of several serious infections. Because it can be administered by mouth, ciprofloxacin allows easy treatment on an outpatient basis rather than requiring hospitalization for parenteral antibacterial therapy.

### Mechanism of Action

Like nalidixic acid, ciprofloxacin *inhibits bacterial DNA gyrase*, an enzyme that converts closed circular DNA into a supercoiled configuration. In the absence of supercoiling, DNA replication cannot take place. The drug is rapidly bactericidal. However, the precise mechanism of cell death is not understood. Since the mammalian equivalent of DNA gyrase is relatively insensitive to fluoroquinolones, cells of the host are not affected.

### Antimicrobial Spectrum

Ciprofloxacin is active against a broad spectrum of bacteria, including most aerobic gram-negative bacteria and some gram-positive bacteria. Most urinary tract pathogens, including

*Escherichia coli* and *Klebsiella*, are sensitive. The drug is also highly active against most bacteria that cause enteritis (e.g., *Salmonella*, *Shigella*, *Campylobacter jejuni*, *E. coli*). Other sensitive organisms include *Pseudomonas aeruginosa*, *Haemophilus influenzae*, gonococci, meningococci, and many streptococci. Activity against anaerobes is fair to poor. *Clostridium difficile* is resistant.

### Bacterial Resistance

Resistance to fluoroquinolones has developed during treatment of infections with *Staphylococcus aureus*, *Serratia marcescens*, *Campylobacter jejuni*, and *Pseudomonas aeruginosa*. Two mechanisms appear responsible: (1) alterations in DNA gyrase and (2) reduced ability of the drug to cross bacterial membranes. There have been no reports of transfer of resistance via R factors.

### Pharmacokinetics

Ciprofloxacin may be administered orally or IV. Following oral administration, the drug is rapidly but incompletely absorbed. High concentrations are achieved in urine, stool, bile, saliva, bone, and prostate tissue. Drug levels in cerebrospinal fluid remain low. Ciprofloxacin has a plasma half-life of about 4 hours. Elimination is by a combination of hepatic metabolism and renal excretion.

### Therapeutic Uses

Ciprofloxacin is approved for a wide variety of infections. These include infections of the respiratory tract, urinary tract, gastrointestinal tract, bones, joints, skin, and soft tissues. Because it is active against a variety of pathogens and can be given orally, ciprofloxacin represents an alternative to parenteral treatment for many serious infections. The drug is not useful against infections caused by anaerobes.

### Adverse Effects

Ciprofloxacin can induce a variety of mild adverse effects, including gastrointestinal reactions (nausea, vomit-

920

ing, diarrhea, abdominal pain) and central nervous system (CNS) effects (dizziness, headache, restlessness, confusion). *Candida* infections of the pharynx and vagina may develop as a result of treatment. Very rarely, seizures have occurred.

Rarely, ciprofloxacin and other fluoroquinolones have caused *tendon rupture*—usually of the Achilles tendon. When given to immature animals, fluoroquinolones disrupt the extracellular matrix of cartilage; a similar mechanism may underlie tendon rupture in humans. Since tendon injury is reversible if diagnosed early, fluoroquinolones should be discontinued at the first sign of tendon pain or inflammation. In addition, the patient should refrain from exercise until tendinitis has been ruled out. Because of the risk of tendon rupture, ciprofloxacin is not recommended for children under 18 years of age or for women who are pregnant or breast-feeding.

## Drug and Food Interactions

***Drugs That Reduce Absorption.*** Absorption of ciprofloxacin can be reduced by (1) aluminum- or magnesium-containing antacids, (2) iron salts, (3) zinc salts, and (4) sucralfate. These agents should be administered at least 4 hours before or 2 hours after ciprofloxacin.

***Theophylline.*** Ciprofloxacin can increase plasma levels of the asthma drug theophylline. Theophylline levels should be monitored and the dosage adjusted accordingly.

***Warfarin.*** Ciprofloxacin can elevate levels of warfarin. Prothrombin time should be monitored and the dosage of warfarin reduced as appropriate.

***Milk.*** Milk can reduce absorption of ciprofloxacin. Accordingly, the drug should not be taken with milk.

### Preparations, Dosage, and Administration

***Oral.*** Ciprofloxacin [Cipro] is dispensed in tablets (250, 500, and 750 mg) for oral administration. The dosage for urinary tract infections is 250 or 500 mg 2 times a day, usually for 7 to 14 days. For other infections, dosages range from 500 to 750 mg 2 times a day. Dosage should be reduced for patients with renal impairment.

***Intravenous.*** Ciprofloxacin [Cipro I.V.] is dispensed in solution (2 and 10 mg/ml) for IV administration. The infusion should be done slowly (over 60 minutes). Intravenous dosages range from 200 to 400 mg every 12 hours.

## Norfloxacin

Norfloxacin [Noroxin] is a fluoroquinolone antibiotic with an antimicrobial spectrum like that of ciprofloxacin. The drug is used orally and labeled only for urinary tract infections (UTIs). However, despite the limits of the labeling, norfloxacin has proved useful for bacterial gastroenteritis, gonorrhea, and gonococcal urethritis.

***Pharmacokinetics.*** Norfloxacin undergoes rapid but incomplete absorption following oral administration. The drug is widely distributed to body tissues and fluids. Excretion is primarily renal, and high concentrations are achieved in the urine. About 30% of the drug is eliminated in the bile and feces. In patients with normal kidney function, the half-life is approximately 4 hours; this value doubles in patients with renal impairment.

***Therapeutic Uses.*** *Urinary Tract Infections.* Norfloxacin was originally approved only for UTIs. The drug has proved effective

against UTIs caused by *Pseudomonas aeruginosa* and other gram-negative bacteria that can display multiple drug resistance.

*Other Uses.* Norfloxacin is now approved for prostatitis caused by *E. coli*, and for uncomplicated urethral and cervical gonorrhea. In addition to these labeled uses, norfloxacin is employed to treat bacterial gastroenteritis (caused by *Escherichia coli*, *Shigella*, *Salmonella*, and other pathogens).

***Adverse Effects.*** Norfloxacin is generally well tolerated. Gastrointestinal effects (nausea, vomiting, anorexia) have been most frequent. The drug has produced a variety of CNS reactions, including headache, dizziness, drowsiness, lightheadedness, depression, and disturbance of vision. Skin rash develops occasionally. Like ciprofloxacin, norfloxacin poses a risk of tendon rupture. Accordingly, norfloxacin is not recommended for children under 18 years of age or for women who are pregnant or breast-feeding.

***Drug and Food Interactions.*** Norfloxacin shares the same interactions as ciprofloxacin. Absorption is suppressed by milk, aluminum- and magnesium-containing antacids, iron and zinc salts, and sucralfate. The drug can elevate levels of theophylline and intensify effects of warfarin.

***Preparations, Dosage, and Administration.*** Norfloxacin [Noroxin] is dispensed in 400-mg tablets for oral administration. The drug should be taken on an empty stomach with a full glass of water. For uncomplicated urinary tract infections, the usual dosage is 400 mg twice daily for 3 days. Prolonged treatment (10 days to 3 weeks) is employed for patients with complicated infections of the urinary tract. Dosage should be reduced in the presence of kidney dysfunction.

## Newer Fluoroquinolones

### Ofloxacin

***Basic Pharmacology.*** Ofloxacin [Floxin] is similar to ciprofloxacin in mechanism of action, antimicrobial spectrum, therapeutic applications, and adverse effects. Like ciprofloxacin, the drug may be administered orally or IV. In the absence of food, bioavailability of oral ofloxacin is 90%; food greatly reduces availability. Ofloxacin is widely distributed to tissues and excreted in the urine. Like ciprofloxacin, ofloxacin can cause a variety of mild adverse effects, including nausea, vomiting, headache, and dizziness. Serious reactions are rare. Like other fluoroquinolones, ofloxacin poses a risk of tendon rupture and should not be used by children under 18 years or by women who are pregnant or breast-feeding. Ofloxacin elevates plasma levels of warfarin, but, in contrast to ciprofloxacin, does not elevate levels of theophylline. Absorption of oral ofloxacin is reduced by sucralfate, iron and zinc salts, and magnesium- and aluminum-containing antacids.

***Preparations, Dosage, and Administration.*** Ofloxacin is available in tablets (200, 300, and 400 mg) for oral administration and in solution (4, 10, and 20 mg/ml) for slow IV infusion; concentrated solutions must be diluted prior to administration. The usual *oral* dosage is 200 to 400 mg every 12 hours; duration of treatment may last 1 day to 6 weeks. Dosage should be reduced in patients with renal impairment. Oral ofloxacin should not be taken with food.

### Lomefloxacin

***Basic Pharmacology.*** Lomefloxacin [Maxaquin] is similar to ciprofloxacin with regard to mechanism, antimicrobial spectrum, and adverse effects. Approved indications are limited to UTIs and to acute bronchitis caused by *Haemophilus influenzae* or *Moraxella catarrhalis*. Administration is oral and bioavailability is high (98%), even in the presence of food. The drug is widely distributed to tissues and eliminated by the kidney. Lomefloxacin has a prolonged half-life that permits once-a-day dosing. Like ciprofloxacin, lomefloxacin can cause various mild adverse effects, including nausea, vomiting, headache, and dizziness. Serious reactions are rare. Like other fluoroquinolones, lomefloxacin poses a risk of tendon rupture and therefore should not be used by children under the age of 18 or by women who are pregnant or breast-feeding. Absorption of lomefloxacin is reduced by magnesium- and aluminum-containing antacids, iron and zinc salts, and sucralfate. In contrast to ciprofloxacin, lomefloxacin does not elevate plasma levels of theophylline.

***Preparations, Dosage, and Administration.*** Lomefloxacin is available in 400-mg tablets for oral administration. The drug may be taken without regard to meals. The usual dosage is 400 mg once a day for 10 to 14 days. Dosage should be reduced in patients with renal impairment.

### Enoxacin

***Basic Pharmacology.*** Enoxacin [Penetrex] is similar to ciprofloxacin in mechanism of action and adverse effects. The drug's antimicrobial spectrum is narrower than that of ciprofloxacin. Approved indications are limited to UTIs and to uncomplicated urethral and cervical gonorrhea. Administration is oral and bioavailability is high (90%); food reduces availability. The drug is widely distributed to tissues and eliminated by the kidney. Like ciprofloxacin, enoxacin can cause a variety of mild adverse effects, including nausea, vomiting, headache, and dizziness. Serious reactions are rare. Like other fluoroquinolones, enoxacin poses a risk of tendon rupture, and therefore should not be used by children under the age of 18 or by women who are pregnant or nursing. Absorption of enoxacin is reduced by magnesium- and aluminum-containing antacids, iron and zinc salts, and sucralfate. Like ciprofloxacin, enoxacin can elevate plasma levels of theophylline and warfarin.

***Preparations, Dosage, and Administration.*** Enoxacin is available in tablets (200 and 400 mg) for oral administration. The drug should be taken 1 hour before meals or 2 hours after. The dosage for urinary tract infections is 200 or 400 mg every 12 hours for 7 to 14 days. The dosage for uncomplicated gonorrhea is 400 mg once. Doses should be reduced in patients with renal impairment.

### Sparfloxacin

Sparfloxacin [Zagam] is a new oral fluoroquinolone approved for treating community acquired pneumonia (CAP) and acute bacterial exacerbations of chronic bronchitis. The drug is active against virtually all common respiratory tract pathogens, including drug-resistant strains of *Streptococcus pneumoniae*, a major cause of CAP.

Sparfloxacin is generally well tolerated. The most common side effect is increased sensitivity to sunlight. In addition, the drug can cause tendonitis, GI disturbances (nausea, diarrhea, abdominal discomfort), headache, dizziness, and insomnia.

Sparfloxacin is available in 200-mg tablets for oral use. The dosage is 400-mg on day 1, followed by 200 mg once a day on days 2 through 10.

### Levofloxacin

Levofloxacin [Levaquin] is a new fluoroquinolone approved for respiratory tract infections (acute maxillary sinusitis, community acquired pneumonia, acute bacterial exacerbations of chronic bronchitis), complicated urinary tract infections, and uncomplicated infections of the skin. Susceptible pathogens include *Streptococcus pneumoniae*, *Haemophilus influenzae*, and *Staphylococcus aureus*. Administration is oral or intravenous. The usual dosage is 500 mg once a day for 7 to 14 days. In patients with renal impairment, the dosage is 500 mg every 48 hours.

# Additional Antibacterial Drugs

## Metronidazole

Metronidazole [Flagyl, Protostat, Metro I.V.] is used for protozoal infections and infections caused by obligate anaerobic bacteria. The basic pharmacology of metronidazole is discussed in Chapter 93, as is the drug's use against protozoal infections. Consideration here is limited to antibacterial applications.

***Mechanism of Antibacterial Action.*** Metronidazole is lethal to anaerobic organisms only. To exert its bactericidal effects, metronidazole must first be taken up by cells and then converted into its active form; only anaerobes are capable of performing the conversion. The active form of metronidazole interacts with DNA to cause strand breakage and loss of helical structure, effects that result in inhibition of nucleic acid synthesis and cell death. Since aerobic bacteria are unable to activate metronidazole, these organisms are insensitive to the drug.

***Antibacterial Spectrum.*** Metronidazole is active against obligate anaerobes only. Sensitive bacterial pathogens include *Bacteroides fragilis* (and other *Bacteroides* species), *Clostridium difficile* (and other *Clostridium* species), *Fusobacterium* species, *Gardnerella vaginalis*, *Peptococcus* species, and *Peptostreptococcus* species.

***Therapeutic Uses.*** Metronidazole is active against a variety of *anaerobic* bacterial infections, including infections of the central nervous system, abdominal organs, bones and joints, skin and soft tissues, and genitourinary tract. Frequently, such infections also involve aerobic bacteria, and therapy must include a drug that is active against them. Metronidazole is employed for prophylaxis in surgical procedures associated with a high risk of infection by anaerobes (e.g., colorectal surgery, abdominal surgery, vaginal surgery). In addition, the drug is used in combination with a tetracycline and bismuth subsalicylate to eradicate *Helicobacter pylori* in people with peptic ulcer disease. Development of resistance to metronidazole is rare.

***Preparations, Dosage, and Administration.*** For initial treatment of serious bacterial infections, metronidazole is administered by IV infusion. Under appropriate conditions, the patient may be transferred to oral therapy.

*Intravenous Formulations.* Metronidazole is available in two formulations—powder and solution—for IV use. The powdered form [Flagyl IV] is dispensed in 500-mg vials and must be reconstituted prior to use (see below). The IV solution [Flagyl I.V. RTU, Metronidazole Redi-Infusion, Metro I.V.] contains 5 mg of metronidazole per milliliter and is ready to use.

*Preparation of Powdered Metronidazole for IV Infusion.* The powder is readied for infusion in three steps: (1) reconstitution, (2) dilution in IV solution, and (3) neutralization. These steps must be performed in the order given. The powder is reconstituted using 4.4 ml of any of the following liquids: Sterile Water for Injection, Bacteriostatic Water for Injection, 0.9% Sodium Chloride Injection, or Bacteriostatic 0.9% Sodium Chloride Injection. The resulting concentrated solution contains approximately 100 mg of metronidazole per milliliter. This solution is then diluted to a concentration of 8 mg/ml (or less) using any of the following IV solutions: 0.9% Sodium Chloride Injection, 5% Dextrose Injection, or Lactated Ringer's Injection. Neutralization of the diluted solution is accomplished by adding 5 mEq of sodium bicarbonate injection for each 500 mg of metronidazole present; this procedure should elevate pH to a value between 6.0 and 7.0. Neutralized solutions should not be refrigerated, since cooling may cause metronidazole to precipitate.

*Intravenous Dosage and Administration.* Infusions must be done slowly (over a 1-hour interval). Therapy of anaerobic infections in adults is initiated with a loading dose of 15 mg/kg. After this, maintenance doses of 7.5 mg/kg are administered every 6 to 8 hours. Duration of treatment is usually 1 to 2 weeks. Patients who have kidney dysfunction and are receiving prolonged treatment may need a reduced dosage to avoid accumulation of the drug to toxic levels.

*Oral Preparations and Dosage.* Metronidazole [Flagyl, Protostat] is dispensed in tablets (250 and 500 mg) for oral administration. The adult dosage for anaerobic infections is 7.5 mg/kg every 6 hours. For bacterial vaginosis in adults, a dosage of 500 mg twice daily for 7 days is effective. Pseudomembranous colitis caused by *Clostridium difficile* is treated with 500 mg 3 times a day for 7 to 15 days.

## Rifampin

Rifampin [Rifadin, Rimactane] is a broad-spectrum antibacterial drug employed primarily for tuberculosis (see Chapter 84). However, the drug is also used against several nontuberculous infections. Rifampin is useful for treating *asymptomatic carriers of Neisseria meningitidis*, but is not given to treat active meningococcal infection. Unlabeled uses include treatment of leprosy, gram-negative bacteremia in infancy, and infections caused by *Staphylococcus aureus* and *S. epidermidis* (e.g., endocarditis, osteomyelitis, prostatitis). Rifampin has also been employed for prophylaxis of meningitis due to *Haemophilus influenzae*. Because resistance can develop rapidly, established bacterial infections should not be treated with rifampin alone. The basic pharmacology of rifampin and the use of this agent in tuberculosis are presented in Chapter 84.

## Bacitracin

Bacitracin is a polypeptide antibiotic produced by a strain of *Bacillus subtilis.* The drug is almost always employed topically. Since parenteral administration can cause serious toxicity, and since superior agents are available, bacitracin is no longer used for systemic infections.

*Mechanism of Action and Antimicrobial Spectrum.* Bacitracin inhibits synthesis of the bacterial cell wall, thereby causing cell lysis and death. The drug is active against most gram-positive bacteria, including staphylococci, streptococci, and *Clostridium difficile. Neisseria* species and *Haemophilus influenzae* are also susceptible, but most other gram-negative bacteria are resistant. Acquisition of resistance by sensitive organisms is uncommon.

*Adverse Effects.* Rarely, topical bacitracin causes local hypersensitivity reactions. Parenteral (IM) administration can produce severe nephrotoxicity.

*Therapeutic Uses.* Bacitracin is used for topical treatment of bacterial infections. The drug is very active against staphylococci and group A streptococci, the pathogens that cause most acute infections of the skin. Because of this activity, bacitracin has been marketed in a variety of topical preparations for treatment of skin infections. Many of these preparations contain additional antibiotics, usually polymyxin B, neomycin, or both.

## Polymyxin B

Polymyxin B is a bactericidal drug employed primarily for local effects. Because of serious systemic toxicity, parenteral administration is rare.

*Antibacterial Spectrum and Mechanism of Action.* Polymyxin B is bactericidal to a broad spectrum of aerobic, gram-negative bacilli. Gram-positive bacteria and most anaerobes are resistant.

Bactericidal effects result from binding of polymyxin B to the bacterial cell membrane, an action that disrupts membrane structure and thereby increases membrane permeability. The increase in permeability leads to inhibition of cellular respiration and cell death. The resistance displayed by gram-positive bacteria has been attributed to the thick gram-positive cell wall, a structure that may prevent access of polymyxin B to the cell membrane.

*Therapeutic Uses.* Polymyxin B is used most commonly for topical treatment of the eyes, ears, and skin. Preparations designed for application to the skin frequently contain other antibiotics, such as bacitracin and neomycin. In addition to its topical uses, polymyxin B (together with neomycin) has been employed as a bladder irrigant to prevent infection in patients with indwelling catheters.

Parenteral use is extremely limited; polymyxin B is not a drug of choice for any systemic infection. The primary indication for parenteral polymyxin B is serious infection caused by *Pseudomonas aeruginosa.* Polymyxin may be given when preferred drugs have been ineffective or intolerable.

*Adverse Effects.* The major adverse effects associated with parenteral therapy are neurotoxicity and nephrotoxicity. Both occur frequently and limit the systemic use of this drug. Polymyxin B is not absorbed from sites of topical application; hence topical use does not cause systemic effects. Rarely, topical polymyxin B produces hypersensitivity.

## KEY POINTS

- Fluoroquinolones are broad-spectrum antibiotics with a wide variety of clinical applications.
- Patients who might otherwise require hospitalization for parenteral antibacterial therapy can often be treated as outpatients with oral ciprofloxacin.
- Fluoroquinolones act by inhibiting bacterial DNA gyrase.
- Because fluoroquinolones can cause tendon rupture, they should be discontinued at the first sign of tendon pain or inflammation. Also, the patient should not exercise until tendinitis has been ruled out.
- Absorption of ciprofloxacin can be reduced by milk, aluminum- and magnesium-containing antacids, iron and zinc salts, and sucralfate.
- In addition to its use against protozoa, metronidazole is used against infections caused by obligate anaerobic bacteria (e.g., *Bacteroides fragilis, Clostridium difficile*).

# Antifungal Agents

The antifungal agents fall into two major groups: (1) drugs for systemic mycoses (i.e., systemic fungal infections), and (2) drugs for superficial mycoses. Some drugs are used for both. Systemic infections occur much less frequently than superficial infections, but are considerably more dangerous. Accordingly, therapy of systemic mycoses is the primary focus of this chapter.

## Drugs for Systemic Mycoses

Systemic mycoses can be subdivided into two categories: (1) opportunistic infections and (2) nonopportunistic infections. The opportunistic mycoses—*candidiasis, aspergillosis, cryptococcosis,* and *mucormycosis*—are seen primarily in the debilitated or immunocompromised host. Nonopportunistic infections can occur in any host. These latter mycoses, which are relatively uncommon, include *sporotrichosis, blastomycosis, histoplasmosis,* and *coccidioidomycosis.* Treating systemic mycoses can be difficult: these infections often resist treatment, and hence may require prolonged therapy with drugs that frequently prove toxic.

### Amphotericin B

Amphotericin B [Fungizone Intravenous, Abelcet, Amphotec] is an important but dangerous drug. This agent is active against a broad spectrum of pathogenic fungi and is a drug of choice for most systemic mycoses (see Table 86-1). Unfortunately, amphotericin B is highly toxic; renal damage is of particular concern. Because of its potential for harm, amphotericin B should be employed only against infections that are progressive and potentially fatal. For treatment of systemic mycoses, amphotericin B is almost always administered by IV infusion. Intrathecal injection has been used for fungal meningitis. For most systemic infections, administration must be performed daily or every other day for several months.

### Chemistry

Amphotericin B belongs to a group of drugs known as *polyene antibiotics,* agents that are so named because their structures contain a series of conjugated double bonds. Nystatin, another antifungal drug, also belongs to this family.

### Mechanism of Action

Amphotericin B binds to components of the fungal cell membrane, thereby increasing permeability. The resultant leakage of intracellular cations (especially potassium) reduces viability. Depending on the concentration of amphotericin B and the susceptibility of the fungus, the drug may be fungicidal or fungistatic.

The component of the fungal membrane to which amphotericin B binds is called *ergosterol,* a member of the *sterol* family of compounds. For a cell to be susceptible, its cytoplasmic membrane must contain sterols. Since bacterial membranes lack sterols, bacteria are not affected.

Much of the toxicity of amphotericin is attributable to the presence of sterols (principally cholesterol) in mammalian cell membranes. By binding to cholesterol in mammalian membranes, amphotericin is thought to affect host cells in much the same way it affects fungi. There is some selective toxicity for fungi because amphotericin binds more strongly to ergosterol (the major sterol in fungal membranes) than it does to cholesterol (the principal sterol of mammalian cell membranes).

### Microbial Susceptibility and Resistance

Amphotericin B is active against a broad spectrum of fungi. Some protozoa (e.g., *Leishmania braziliensis*) are also susceptible. As noted, bacteria are resistant to the drug.

## TABLE 86–1. DRUGS OF CHOICE FOR SYSTEMIC MYCOSES

| Infection | Causative Organism | Drugs of Choice | Alternative Drugs |
|---|---|---|---|
| Aspergillosis | *Aspergillus* species | Amphotericin B | Itraconazole |
| Blastomycosis | *Blastomyces dermatitidis* | Amphotericin B *or* itraconazole | Ketoconazole |
| Candidiasis | *Candida* species | Amphotericin B ± flucytosine | Fluconazole |
| Coccidiodomycosis Chronic suppression | *Coccidioides immitis* | Amphotericin B *or* fluconazole Fluconazole | Itraconazole, ketoconazole Amphotericin B |
| Cryptococcosis | *Cryptococcus neoformans* | Amphotericin B ± flucytosine | Itraconazole, fluconazole |
| Histoplasmosis Chronic suppression | *Histoplasma capsulatum* | Amphotericin B *or* itraconazole Itraconazole | Ketoconazole Amphotericin B |
| Mucormycosis | *Mucor* | Amphotericin B | No dependable alternative |
| Paracoccidioidomycosis | *Paracoccidioides brasiliensis* | Amphotericin B *or* itraconazole | Ketoconazole |
| Sporotrichosis | *Sporothrix schenckii* | Amphotericin B | Itraconazole |

Emergence of resistant fungi during amphotericin therapy is extremely rare. On occasion, resistance has been observed during long-term treatment. In all cases in which resistance has developed, the resistant fungi had membranes whose ergosterol content was reduced or absent.

### Therapeutic Uses

*Amphotericin B is a drug of choice for most systemic mycoses* (see Table 86-1). Prior to the availability of this agent, systemic fungal infections usually proved fatal. Treatment is prolonged; 6 to 8 weeks is common. In some cases, treatment may last for 3 or 4 months. In addition to its systemic use, amphotericin is employed topically.

### Pharmacokinetics

**Absorption and Distribution.** Absorption of amphotericin B from the gastrointestinal tract is poor, and oral therapy of systemic infection is not effective. Hence, for treatment of deep mycoses, the drug must be administered IV. Most of the amphotericin in the body is bound to sterol-containing membranes in various tissues. Levels about half those in plasma are achieved in aqueous humor and in peritoneal, pleural, and joint fluids. The drug does not readily penetrate to the cerebrospinal fluid (CSF).

**Metabolism and Excretion.** Little is known about the elimination of amphotericin B. We do not know whether the drug is metabolized or how the majority of this compound is removed from the body. Renal excretion of unchanged drug is minimal. Accordingly, there is no need to reduce the dosage in patients with pre-existing kidney dysfunction. Complete elimination of amphotericin takes a long time; the drug has been detected in tissues more than a year after cessation of treatment.

### Adverse Effects

Amphotericin can induce a variety of serious adverse effects. Patients should be under close supervision, preferably in a hospital.

**Effects Associated with Intravenous Infusion.** Intravenous infusion of amphotericin frequently produces fever, chills, rigors, nausea, and headache. Mild reactions can be reduced by pretreatment with diphenhydramine plus aspirin or acetaminophen. Meperidine can be administered if rigors occur. If other measures fail, hydrocortisone (a glucocorticoid) can be used to decrease fever and chills. However, since glucocorticoids can reduce the patient's ability to fight infection, routine use of hydrocortisone should be avoided. In addition to the above effects, infusion of amphotericin is associated with a high incidence of phlebitis; this can be minimized by frequently changing peripheral venous sites or by administration through a larger central vein.

**Nephrotoxicity.** Amphotericin exerts direct toxicity on cells of the kidney; renal impairment occurs in practically all patients. The extent of kidney damage is related to the total dose administered during the full course of treatment. In most cases, renal function returns to normal following cessation of drug use. However, if the total dose exceeds 4 gm, residual impairment is likely. Kidney damage can be minimized by infusing 1 L of saline on the day of amphotericin administration. Other nephrotoxic drugs (e.g., aminoglycosides) should be avoided. To evaluate renal injury, tests of kidney function should be performed weekly; intake and output should be monitored. If plasma creatinine content rises above 3.5 mg/dl, amphotericin dosage should be reduced.

**Hypokalemia.** Damage to the kidneys often causes hypokalemia. Potassium supplements may be needed to correct hypokalemia. Patients should undergo frequent determinations of potassium levels and serum creatinine content.

**Effects Associated with Intrathecal Injection.** Intrathecal administration may cause nausea, vomiting, headache, and pain in the back, legs, and abdomen. Rare reactions include visual disturbances, impairment of hearing, and paresthesias (tingling, numbness, or pain in the hands and feet).

**Other Adverse Effects.** Infusion of amphotericin may be associated with delirium, hypotension, hypertension, wheezing, and hypoxia. Bone marrow depression has occurred, resulting in normocytic, normochromic anemia; for evaluation, hematocrit determinations should be performed. Rarely, amphotericin has caused rash, convulsions, anaphylaxis, dysrhythmias, acute liver failure, and nephrogenic diabetes insipidus.

## Drug Interactions

**Nephrotoxic Drugs.** Use of amphotericin with other nephrotoxic drugs (e.g., aminoglycosides, cyclosporine) increases the risk of injury to the kidneys. Accordingly, these combinations should be avoided if at all possible.

**Flucytosine.** Amphotericin potentiates the antifungal actions of flucytosine, apparently by enhancing entry of flucytosine into fungal cells. Because of this potentiative interaction, the combination of flucytosine with a relatively low dose of amphotericin can produce antifungal effects equivalent to those of a high dose of amphotericin alone. By allowing a reduction in amphotericin dosage, the combination decreases the risk of amphotericin-induced toxicity.

### Dosage and Administration

**Preparations.** Amphotericin B is available in three forms: *amphotericin B deoxycholate* [Fungizone Intravenous], *liposomal amphotericin B* [Abelcet], and *amphotericin B cholesteryl* [Amphotec]. The deoxycholate form is considered conventional. The liposomal form is indicated only for invasive fungal infections in patients who are refractory to or intolerant of conventional therapy. Similarly, the cholesteryl form is indicated only for invasive aspergillosis in patients with renal impairment or intolerance of conventional amphotericin B.

**Routes.** For treatment of systemic mycoses, amphotericin B is almost always administered by IV infusion. Infusions should be performed slowly (over 2 to 4 hours) to minimize phlebitis and cardiovascular reactions. Alternate-day dosing can reduce adverse effects. As a rule, several months of therapy are required. Since amphotericin B does not readily enter the CSF, intrathecal injection is used to treat fungal meningitis.

**IV Dosage and Administration.** Dosage is individualized based on the severity of the disease and the patient's ability to tolerate the drug. Optimal dosage has not been established. A small (1-mg) test dose is often given to assess patient reaction. After this, therapy is initiated with a dosage of 0.25 mg/kg/day. Maintenance dosages range from 1.5 to 6.0 mg/kg/day, depending on the severity of the infection and the form of amphotericin being used. Dosage should be reduced in patients with renal impairment. The infusion solution should be checked periodically for a precipitate and, if a precipitate is seen, administration should be discontinued immediately. Because the treatment period is prolonged, the administration site should be rotated; this will reduce the risk of phlebitis and help ensure continued availability of a suitable vein.

## Ketoconazole

Ketoconazole [Nizoral] is an oral alternative to amphotericin B for treatment of less severe systemic mycoses. The drug is safer than amphotericin B and has the additional advantage of being orally usable.

Ketoconazole belongs to the azole family of antifungal agents, for which it can be considered the prototype. Other family members are fluconazole, itraconazole, miconazole, clotrimazole, and econazole. All are active against a broad spectrum of fungi. Some are used for systemic mycoses, some for superficial mycoses, and some for both types of infection.

### Mechanism of Action

Ketoconazole inhibits the synthesis of ergosterol, an essential component of the fungal cytoplasmic membrane. This results in increased membrane permeability and leakage of cellular components. Accumulation of ergosterol precursors may also contribute to antifungal actions. Ketoconazole is fungistatic at lower concentrations and fungicidal at higher concentrations.

### Antifungal Spectrum

Most of the fungi that cause systemic mycoses are susceptible. Ketoconazole is also active against the fungi that cause superficial infections (dermatophytes and *Candida* species). Emergence of resistance is rare.

### Therapeutic Uses

Ketoconazole is an alternative to amphotericin B for treatment of systemic mycoses. The drug is much less toxic than amphotericin and only somewhat less effective. Specific indications are listed in Table 86-1. Responses to ketoconazole are slow. Accordingly, the drug is less useful for severe, acute infections than for long-term suppression of chronic mycoses. Ketoconazole is also a valuable drug for treating superficial mycoses; these applications are considered later in the chapter.

### Pharmacokinetics

**Absorption.** Ketoconazole is a weak base and requires an acidic environment for dissolution and absorption. Oral ketoconazole is well absorbed from the gastrointestinal tract, provided that gastric acid levels are normal. In patients with achlorhydria (absence of gastric acid), absorption is low. Drugs that reduce gastric acidity (e.g., antacids, $H_2$ blocking agents, proton pump inhibitors) decrease ketoconazole absorption.

**Distribution.** Most of the ketoconazole present in the blood is bound to plasma proteins. The drug crosses the blood-brain barrier poorly and concentrations in cerebrospinal fluid remain low. In contrast, high levels of ketoconazole are achieved in the skin, making oral ketoconazole useful against superficial mycoses.

**Elimination.** Ketoconazole is eliminated by hepatic metabolism. Its half-life is approximately 3 hours. In the presence of liver dysfunction, the half-life can be substantially prolonged. Since elimination is hepatic, renal impairment does not influence the intensity or duration of action. Hence, no dosage adjustment is needed in patients with kidney disease.

### Adverse Effects

Ketoconazole is generally well tolerated. The most common adverse reactions—nausea and vomiting—can be reduced by giving the drug with food. The most serious effects involve the liver.

**Hepatotoxicity.** Effects of ketoconazole on the liver are rare but potentially severe; fatal hepatic necrosis has occurred. Liver function should be evaluated prior to treatment and at least monthly thereafter. Ketoconazole should be discontinued at the first sign of liver injury. The drug should be employed with caution in patients with a history of hepatic disease. Patients should be advised to notify the physician if symptoms suggesting liver dysfunction develop (e.g., unusual fatigue, anorexia, nausea, vomiting, jaundice, dark urine, pale stools).

**Endocrine Effects.** Just as ketoconazole inhibits steroid synthesis in fungi, the drug can inhibit steroid synthesis in humans. In males, inhibition of testosterone synthesis has caused gynecomastia, decreased libido, and reduced potency; reversible sterility has occurred with high doses. In females, reduction of estradiol synthesis has caused menstrual irregularities.

***Other Adverse Effects.*** Ketoconazole can produce a variety of relatively mild adverse effects, including rash, itching, dizziness, fever, chills, constipation, diarrhea, photophobia, and headache. Rarely, ketoconazole has caused anaphylaxis, severe epigastric pain, and altered function of the adrenals.

## Drug Interactions

***Drugs That Raise Gastric pH.*** Drugs that decrease gastric acidity—antacids, $H_2$ antagonists, proton pump inhibitors, anticholinergic drugs—can greatly reduce ketoconazole absorption. To minimize reductions in absorption, these agents should be administered no sooner than 2 hours after ingestion of ketoconazole. (Since proton pump inhibitors have a prolonged duration of action, patients using these agents may have insufficient stomach acid for ketoconazole absorption, regardless of when the proton pump inhibitor is administered.)

***Terfenadine and Astemizole.*** Ketoconazole inhibits drug metabolizing enzymes, and can thereby increase levels of certain drugs. The most important of these are terfenadine [Seldane] and astemizole [Hismanal]—widely used nonsedating antihistamines. When present at excessive levels, these drugs can cause potentially fatal cardiac dysrhythmias. Accordingly, concurrent use of terfenadine or astemizole with ketoconazole is contraindicated.

***Rifampin.*** Rifampin reduces plasma levels of ketoconazole, apparently by enhancing hepatic metabolism. If these drugs are used concurrently, ketoconazole dosage should be increased—and even then it may be impossible to achieve therapeutic levels of the drug.

## Preparations, Dosage, and Administration

Ketoconazole [Nizoral] is dispensed in 200-mg tablets for oral administration. The recommended adult dosage is 200 mg once a day. For chemotherapy of severe infection, daily doses of 400 to 800 mg may be required. The dosage for children over 2 years of age is 3.3 to 6.6 mg/kg/day in a single dose. Duration of treatment is 6 months or longer. Since an acidic environment is needed for ketoconazole absorption, patients with achlorhydria should dissolve the tablets in 4 ml of 0.2 N hydrochloric acid; the solution should be sipped through a plastic or glass straw to avoid damage to the teeth.

## Itraconazole

***Actions and Uses.*** Itraconazole [Sporanox], a member of the azole family of antifungal agents, is active against a broad spectrum of fungal pathogens. Like ketoconazole, the drug inhibits synthesis of ergosterol, causing the fungal cell membrane to leak. Approved indications are blastomycosis (pulmonary and extrapulmonary), histoplasmosis, aspergillosis, and onychomycosis. However, because of its broad antifungal spectrum, the drug has been used for other systemic fungal infections (coccidioidomycosis, cryptococcosis, paracoccidioidomycosis, sporotrichosis) and for superficial fungal infections.

***Pharmacokinetics.*** Itraconazole is administered orally, and absorption is greatly enhanced by the presence of food. The drug is widely distributed to lipophilic tissues. In contrast, concentrations in aqueous fluids (e.g., saliva, CSF) are negligible.

The drug undergoes extensive hepatic metabolism. About 40% of each dose is excreted in the urine as inactive metabolites.

***Adverse Effects.*** Itraconazole is well tolerated in usual doses. Gastrointestinal reactions (nausea, vomiting, diarrhea) are most common, occurring in about 10% of those treated. Other common reactions include rash (8.6%), headache (3.8%), abdominal pain (3.3%), and edema (3.5%). Hepatitis has occurred rarely, and the involvement of itraconazole is not clear. Liver function should be monitored in patients with pre-existing liver disease.

***Drug Interactions.*** Itraconazole can elevate plasma levels of several drugs, including cyclosporine, digoxin, sulfonylureas, warfarin, terfenadine, astemizole, and cisapride. In patients taking cyclosporine or digoxin, levels of these drugs should be monitored; in patients taking sulfonylureas, blood glucose levels should be monitored; and in patients taking warfarin, prothrombin time should be monitored. Since the combination of itraconazole with terfenadine or astemizole can result in potentially fatal cardiac dysrhythmias, itraconazole should not be used with these drugs. Similarly, the combination of cisapride with itraconazole can cause ventricular dysrhythmias, torsades de pointes, and death; accordingly, the combination is contraindicated.

Phenytoin, isoniazid, and rifampin can reduce plasma levels of itraconazole. The dosage of itraconazole may need to be increased.

***Preparations, Dosage, and Administration.*** Itraconazole [Sporanox] is dispensed in 100-mg capsules for oral administration. The drug should be taken with food to increase absorption. The recommended dosage is 200 mg once a day. If needed, the daily dosage may be increased to 400 mg (administered in two divided doses).

## Fluconazole

***Actions and Uses.*** Fluconazole [Diflucan] belongs to the azole group of antifungal agents. The drug has the same mechanism of action as ketoconazole: inhibition of ergosterol synthesis with resultant damage to the cytoplasmic membrane and accumulation of ergosterol precursors. The drug is primarily fungistatic. Fluconazole is used to treat oropharyngeal and esophageal *Candida* infections and meningitis caused by *Cryptococcus neoformans* and *Coccidioides immitis*. In addition, it was recently approved for single-dose oral therapy of vaginal candidiasis.

***Pharmacokinetics.*** Fluconazole is well absorbed (90%) following oral administration. The drug is widely distributed to tissues and body fluids, including the cerebrospinal fluid (CSF). Most of the drug is eliminated unchanged in the urine. Fluconazole has a half-life of 30 hours, making once-a-day dosing sufficient.

***Adverse Effects and Interactions.*** Fluconazole is less toxic than ketoconazole and is generally well tolerated. The most common reactions are nausea (3.7%), headache (1.9%), rash (1.8%), vomiting (1.7%), abdominal pain (1.7%), and diarrhea (1.5%). Rarely, treatment has been associated with hepatic necrosis, Stevens-Johnson syndrome, and anaphylaxis. Fluconazole can inhibit hepatic drug-metabolizing enzymes, thereby increasing the levels of other drugs, including warfarin, phenytoin, and cyclosporine.

***Preparations, Dosage, and Administration.*** Fluconazole [Diflucan] is dispensed in tablets (50, 100, and 200 mg) for oral administration and in solution (2 mg/ml) for intravenous infusion. Since oral absorption is rapid and nearly complete, oral and IV dosages are the same. For treatment of oropharyngeal and esophageal candidiasis, the usual dosage is 200 mg on the first day, followed by 100 mg once daily thereafter. For treatment of systemic candidiasis and cryptococcal meningitis, the usual dosage is 400 mg on the first day, followed by 200 mg once daily thereafter. Duration of treatment ranges from 3 weeks to more than 3 months, depending on the infection being treated.

## Miconazole

Miconazole, like ketoconazole, belongs to the azole family of compounds. The antifungal actions of both drugs are similar. Miconazole is employed primarily for topical treatment of superficial mycoses. Because of toxicity, miconazole is rarely employed to treat systemic infections. When used for systemic therapy, the drug must be given IV. Administration by this route is associated with a high incidence of adverse effects, including phlebitis, thrombocytosis, nausea, vomiting, pruritus, rash, and fever. Miconazole enhances the actions of warfarin; hence warfarin dosage must be reduced. Miconazole can antagonize the effects of amphotericin B in the treatment of candidiasis.

Miconazole for intravenous use [Monistat i.v.] is dispensed as a 10 mg/ml solution in 20-ml ampuls. The drug is diluted in 0.9% saline plus 5% dextrose and infused slowly (over 30 to 60 minutes). The daily dosage for adults is 200 mg to 3.6 gm administered in three or four divided doses at equally spaced intervals. Duration of treatment is 2 to 20 weeks.

## Flucytosine

Flucytosine [Ancobon] is employed to treat serious infections caused by *Candida* species and *Cryptococcus neoformans*. Because development of resistance is common, flucytosine is almost always used in combination with amphotericin B. Caution must be exercised in patients with renal impairment and hematologic disorders.

### Mechanism of Action

The antifungal effects of flucytosine derive from disruption of DNA and RNA synthesis. Flucytosine is taken up by fungal cells and converted to 5-fluorouracil, the active form of the drug. The enzyme responsible for conversion is cytosine deaminase. Fungi that lack cytosine deaminase are not susceptible to the drug. Since mammalian cells lack cytosine deaminase, flucytosine has relatively low toxicity to the host.

### Fungal Resistance

Development of resistance to flucytosine during therapy is common and constitutes a serious clinical problem. Several mechanisms of resistance have been described, including (1) a reduction in fungal cytosine permease, the enzyme required for uptake of flucytosine, and (2) loss of cytosine deaminase, the enzyme required to convert flucytosine to its active form.

### Antifungal Spectrum and Therapeutic Uses

Flucytosine has a narrow antifungal spectrum. Fungicidal activity is highest against *Candida* species and *Cryptococcus neoformans*. Most other fungi are resistant. Because of this narrow spectrum, flucytosine is indicated only for candidiasis and cryptococcosis. For treatment of serious infections (e.g., cryptococcal meningitis, systemic candidiasis), flucytosine should be combined with amphotericin B. This combination offers two advantages over the use of flucytosine alone: (1) antifungal activity is enhanced and (2) emergence of resistant fungi is reduced.

### Pharmacokinetics

Flucytosine is readily absorbed from the gastrointestinal tract and is well distributed throughout the body. The drug has good access to the central nervous system; levels in cerebrospinal fluid are about 80% of those in plasma. Flucytosine is eliminated by the kidneys, principally as the unchanged drug. The half-life of flucytosine is about 4 hours in patients with normal renal function. However, in the presence of renal insufficiency, the half-life is greatly prolonged. Accordingly, dosages must be reduced in patients with kidney dysfunction.

### Adverse Effects

*Hematologic Effects.* Bone marrow depression is the most serious complication of treatment. Marrow depression usually manifests as reversible neutropenia or thrombocytopenia. Rarely, fatal agranulocytosis has developed. Platelet and leukocyte counts should be obtained weekly. Adverse hematologic effects are most likely when plasma levels of flucytosine exceed 100 µg/ml; the dosage should be adjusted to keep drug levels below this value. Flucytosine should be used with caution in patients with pre-existing bone marrow depression.

*Hepatotoxicity.* Mild and reversible liver dysfunction occurs frequently, but severe hepatic injury is rare. Effects on liver function should be monitored by making weekly determinations of serum transaminase and alkaline phosphatase levels.

### Drug Interactions

Flucytosine is often combined with *amphotericin B*. As noted, this combination offers several advantages. However, use of the combination can also be detrimental. Since amphotericin B is nephrotoxic, and since flucytosine is eliminated by the kidneys, amphotericin B–induced kidney damage may suppress flucytosine excretion, and may thereby promote flucytosine toxicity. Accordingly, *it is important to monitor renal function and flucytosine levels when amphotericin B and flucytosine are employed concurrently.*

### Preparations, Dosage, and Administration

Flucytosine [Ancobon] is dispensed in 250- and 500-mg capsules for oral administration. The usual dosage for patients with normal kidney function is 50 to 150 mg/kg/day administered in divided doses at 6-hour intervals. At this dosage, some patients must ingest 10 or more capsules 4 times each day. Dosages must be reduced for patients with renal insufficiency. Nausea and vomiting associated with drug administration can be decreased by taking flucytosine capsules over a 15-minute interval.

# Drugs for Superficial Mycoses

The superficial mycoses are caused by two groups of organisms: (1) *Candida* species and (2) dermatophytes (species of *Epidermophyton*, *Trichophyton*, and *Microsporum*). *Candida* infections usually occur in mucous membranes and moist skin; chronic infections may involve the scalp, skin, and nails. Dermatophytoses are generally confined to the skin, hair, and nails. Superficial infections with dermatophytes are more common than superficial infections with *Candida*.

## Overview of Drug Therapy

Superficial mycoses can be treated with a variety of topical and oral drugs. For mild to moderate infections, topical agents are generally preferred. Specific indications for the drugs used against superficial mycoses are summarized in Tables 86–2 and 86–3. Some of these drugs are also used for systemic infections.

### Dermatophytic Infections (Ringworm)

Dermatophytic infections are commonly referred to as ringworm (because of characteristic ring-shaped lesions). There are four principal dermatophytic infections, de-

## TABLE 86-2. DRUGS FOR SUPERFICIAL FUNGAL INFECTIONS

| Drug | Route | Ringworm[†] | Candida infection* Skin | Candida infection* Mouth | Onychomycosis[‡] |
|---|---|---|---|---|---|
| **Azoles** | | | | | |
| Clotrimazole | Topical | ✔ | ✔ | ✔ | |
| Econazole | Topical | ✔ | ✔ | | |
| Fluconazole | Oral | | | ✔ | ✔ |
| Itraconazole | Oral | ✔ | | | ✔ |
| Ketoconazole | Oral | ✔ | | ✔ | ✔ |
| | Topical | ✔ | ✔ | | |
| Miconazole | Topical | ✔ | ✔ | | |
| Oxiconazole | Topical | ✔ | | | |
| Sulconazole | Topical | ✔ | | | |
| **Others** | | | | | |
| Amphotericin B | Topical | | ✔ | | |
| Ciclopirox | Topical | ✔ | ✔ | | |
| Griseofulvin | Oral | ✔ | | | ✔ |
| Haloprogin | Topical | ✔ | | | |
| Naftifine | Topical | ✔ | | | |
| Nystatin | Topical | | ✔ | ✔ | |
| Terbinafine | Oral | | | | ✔ |
| | Topical | ✔ | | | |
| Tolnaftate | Topical | ✔ | | | |
| Undecylenate | Topical | ✔ | | | |

*Vulvovaginal candidiasis is addressed in Table 86–3.
[†]Ringworm is a popular term for dermatophytic infections, including tinea pedis (ringworm of the foot, "athlete's foot"), tinea cruris (ringworm of the groin, "jock itch"), and tinea corporis (ringworm of the body).
[‡]Onychomycosis is a clinical term for fungal infection of the toenails and fingernails.

fined by their location: (1) tinea pedis (ringworm of the foot, or "athlete's foot"), (2) tinea corporis (ringworm of the body), (3) tinea cruris (ringworm of the groin, or "jock itch"), and (4) tinea capitis (ringworm of the scalp).

**Tinea Pedis.** Tinea pedis, the most common fungal infection, generally responds well to topical therapy. Agents are listed in Table 86-2. Patients should be advised to wear absorbent cotton socks, change their shoes often, and dry their feet after bathing.

**Tinea Corporis.** Tinea corporis usually responds to the drugs listed in Table 86-2. Treatment should continue for at least 1 week after symptoms have cleared. Severe infection may require a systemic antifungal agent (e.g., griseofulvin).

## TABLE 86-3. DRUGS FOR VULVOVAGINAL CANDIDIASIS

| Generic Name | Trade Name | Formulation | Dosage |
|---|---|---|---|
| *Oral Preparation* | | | |
| Fluconazole | Diflucan | 150-mg oral tablet | 1 tablet PO once |
| *Topical Preparations* | | | |
| Butoconazole | Femstat | 2% vaginal cream | 5 gm at HS × 6 days (pregnant) or 3 days (not pregnant) |
| Clotrimazole | Femcare | 100-mg vaginal tablet | 1 tablet at HS × 7 days |
| | | 1% vaginal cream | 5 gm at HS × 7 days |
| | Gyne-Lotrimin | 100-mg vaginal tablet | 1 tablet at HS × 7 days |
| | | 500-mg vaginal tablet | 1 tablet at HS once |
| | | 1% vaginal cream | 5 gm at HS × 7 days |
| | Mycelex-7 | 100-mg vaginal tablet | 1 tablet at HS × 7 days |
| | | 1% vaginal cream | 5 gm at HS × 7 days |
| | Mycelex-G | 500-mg vaginal tablet | 1 tablet at HS once |
| Miconazole | Monistat 3 | 200-mg vaginal suppository | 1 suppository at HS × 3 days |
| | Monistat 7 | 100-mg vaginal suppository | 1 suppository at HS × 7 days |
| | | 2% vaginal cream | 5 gm at HS × 7 days |
| Terconazole | Terazol 3 | 80-mg vaginal suppository | 1 suppository at HS × 3 days |
| | | 0.8% vaginal cream | 5 gm at HS × 3 days |
| Tioconazole | Vagistat | 6.5% vaginal ointment | 4.6 gm at HS once |
| Nystatin | Mycostatin | 100,000-U vaginal tablet | 1 tablet at HS × 14 day |

**Tinea Cruris.** Tinea cruris responds well to topical therapy. Treatment should continue for at least 1 week after symptoms have abated. If the infection is severely inflamed, a systemic antifungal drug (e.g., clotrimazole) may be needed; topical or systemic glucocorticoids may be needed as well.

**Tinea Capitis.** Tinea capitis is difficult to treat. Topical drugs are not likely to work. Oral griseofulvin is a preferred therapy. Treatment should continue for at least 2 to 3 months. If griseofulvin is not effective, itraconazole may be tried.

## Candidiasis

**Vulvovaginal.** Vulvovaginal candidiasis is very common. About 25% of women of reproductive age develop this infection. Predisposing factors include pregnancy, obesity, diabetes, debilitation, HIV infection, and use of certain drugs, including oral contraceptives, systemic glucocorticoids, anticancer agents, immunosuppressants, and systemic antibiotics. In the past, most regimens required daily application of a topical drug for 1 to 2 weeks. When higher doses of newer drugs are employed, the infection can often be eliminated with just 1 to 3 days of topical therapy. Most recently, *oral* fluconazole has been employed; a single 150-mg dose can be curative—but causes more side effects than topical agents. The drugs employed for vulvovaginal candidiasis are summarized in Table 86-3. All appear equally effective. The longer regimens have no demonstrated advantage over the shorter regimens.

**Oral.** Oral candidiasis, also known as *thrush*, is seen often. Topical therapy with nystatin or clotrimazole is generally effective. In the immunocompromised host, systemic therapy with oral fluconazole or ketoconazole is generally required.

## Onychomycosis (Fungal Infection of the Nails)

Fungal infection of the nails, known as onychomycosis, is difficult to eradicate and requires prolonged therapy with systemic drugs. Infections may be caused by dermatophytes or by *Candida* species. Topical therapy is not effective. With systemic therapy, antifungal drugs become incorporated into keratin as the nails grow. Some drugs also diffuse into the nails from below. Since onychomycosis is largely a cosmetic problem, treatment is usually optional.

For years, oral griseofulvin was the only treatment available. The drug is active against dermatophytes, but not against *Candida*. Treatment generally lasts 6 to 12 months.

Recently, several new drugs have been employed. These include terbinafine and three azoles: fluconazole, itraconazole, and ketoconazole. In contrast to griseofulvin, these drugs are active against *Candida* species as well as dermatophytes. All of these drugs cause adverse effects, including gastrointestinal reactions (e.g., nausea, vomiting, abdominal pain), headache, and skin reactions (e.g., itching, rash). Treatment generally lasts 6 to 12 weeks, but more prolonged treatment may be required.

# Azoles: Clotrimazole, Ketoconazole, Others

Ten members of the azole family are used for superficial mycoses (see Tables 86-2 and 86-3). The usual route is topical. Three of the azoles—fluconazole, miconazole, and ketoconazole—are used for systemic mycoses in addition to superficial mycoses.

The azoles are active against a broad spectrum of pathogenic fungi, including dermatophytes and *Candida* species. Antifungal effects result from inhibiting the biosynthesis of ergosterol, an essential component of the fungal cytoplasmic membrane.

## Clotrimazole

*Therapeutic Uses.* Topical clotrimazole is a drug of choice for dermatophytic infections and candidiasis of the skin, mouth, and vagina.

*Adverse Effects.* When applied to the skin, clotrimazole can cause stinging, erythema, edema, urticaria, pruritus, and peeling. However, the incidence of these reactions is low. Intravaginal administration is occasionally associated with burning sensations and lower abdominal cramps. The oral formulation can cause gastrointestinal distress.

*Preparations, Dosage, and Administration.* Clotrimazole is available as an oral troche, as a cream or tablet for intravaginal use, and in three formulations for application to the skin (cream, lotion, solution). For fungal infections of the skin, the drug is applied twice daily for 1 week or longer. Several dosing schedules have been employed for vulvovaginal candidiasis, including (1) intravaginal insertion of one 250-mg tablet nightly for 7 days, (2) intravaginal insertion of one 500-mg tablet once at bedtime, and (3) intravaginal application of 5 gm of 1% cream once a day for 1 week. Trade names for clotrimazole include Femcare, Gyne-Lotrimin, Lotrimin, and Mycelex.

## Ketoconazole

Ketoconazole [Nizoral] is approved for both oral and topical therapy of superficial mycoses. Oral ketoconazole provides effective treatment of dermatophytic infections as well as candidiasis of the skin, mouth, and vagina. However, because of the toxicity associated with oral use, this route should be reserved for infections that have failed to respond to topical agents (e.g., clotrimazole, miconazole). Ketoconazole is available in cream and shampoo formulations for topical therapy of dermatophytic infections and for candidiasis of the skin. The basic pharmacology of ketoconazole is discussed in the section on systemic mycoses.

## Miconazole

*Therapeutic Uses.* Miconazole is an azole antifungal drug available for topical and systemic administration. Topical miconazole is a drug of choice for dermatophytic infections as well as for cutaneous and vaginal candidiasis. Systemic uses are discussed above.

*Adverse Effects.* Untoward effects of topical miconazole are generally mild. Intravaginal administration causes burning, itching, and irritation in about 7% of patients. When applied to the skin, miconazole occasionally causes irritation, burning, and maceration. Topical application is not associated with systemic toxicity.

*Preparations, Dosage, and Administration.* Miconazole is available in cream, liquid, and powder formulations for application to the skin, and in cream and suppository formulations for intravaginal application. Cutaneous mycoses are treated with twice-daily applications for 2 to 4 weeks. For vaginal candidiasis, 2% miconazole cream or a 100-mg suppository is administered nightly for 1 week. Alternatively, a 200-mg suppository can be administered nightly for 3 days. Trade names for topical miconazole are Micatin, Monistat-Derm, Monistat 3, and Monistat 7.

## Fluconazole

Fluconazole [Diflucan] can be used for *oral* therapy of vulvovaginal candidiasis, oropharyngeal candidiasis, and onychomycosis. The dosage for vulvovaginal candidiasis is 150 mg taken once. The dosage for oropharyngeal candidiasis is 200 mg on day 1 followed by 100 mg daily for 2 weeks. The dosage for onychomycosis is 100 mg daily for 3 to 12 weeks. The basic pharmacology of fluconazole is discussed above under *Drugs for Systemic Mycoses*.

### Newer Azole Drugs

*Econazole.* Econazole [Spectazole] is available for topical application only. The drug is indicated for ringworm infections and superficial candidiasis. Local adverse effects (burning, erythema, stinging, itching) occur in about 3% of patients. Less than 1% of topical econazole is absorbed, and systemic toxicity has not been reported. Econazole, dispensed in a 1% cream, is applied twice daily for 2 to 4 weeks.

*Oxiconazole and Sulconazole.* Oxiconazole [Oxistat] and sulconazole [Exelderm] are broad-spectrum antifungal drugs. Both are approved for topical treatment of tinea infections. Local adverse effects (itching, burning, irritation, erythema) occur in less than 3% of those treated. Neither drug is absorbed to a significant degree, and systemic toxicity has not been reported. Oxiconazole is dispensed as a cream, and sulconazole is dispensed as a cream and in solution. Both drugs are applied once daily for 2 to 4 weeks.

*Butoconazole, Terconazole, and Tioconazole.* These azole drugs are approved only for topical treatment of vulvovaginal candidiasis. All three are fungicidal. Local adverse effects (burning, itching) occur in 2% to 6% of those treated. Absorption following intravaginal administration is low, and systemic reactions are rare (except for headache from terconazole). Because of a small risk of fetal injury, these drugs are not recommended for use during the first trimester of pregnancy. Trade names, formulations, and dosages are presented in Table 86-3.

# Griseofulvin

Griseofulvin is administered orally for treatment of superficial mycoses. The drug is inactive against organisms that cause systemic fungal infections.

*Mechanism of Action.* Following absorption, griseofulvin is deposited in the keratin precursor cells of skin, hair, and nails. Because of the presence of griseofulvin, newly formed keratin is resistant to fungal invasion. Hence, as infected keratin is shed, it is replaced by fungus-free tissue.

Griseofulvin produces its fungicidal effects by inhibiting fungal mitosis. The drug inhibits mitosis by binding to components of microtubules, the structures that form the mitotic spindle. Because griseofulvin acts by disrupting mitosis, the drug only affects fungi that are actively growing.

*Pharmacokinetics.* Griseofulvin is administered orally. Absorption can be enhanced by taking the drug with a fatty meal. As noted, griseofulvin is deposited in the keratin precursor cells of skin, hair, and nails. Elimination is by hepatic metabolism and renal excretion.

***Therapeutic Uses.*** Griseofulvin is employed orally to treat dermatophytic infections of the skin, hair, and nails. The drug is not active against *Candida* species, nor is it useful for treating systemic mycoses. Dermatophytic infections of the skin respond relatively quickly (in 3 to 8 weeks). However, infections of the palms may require 2 to 3 months of treatment, and a year or more may be needed to eliminate infections of the toenails.

***Adverse Effects.*** Most untoward effects are not serious. Transient headache is common, occurring in about 15% of patients. Other mild reactions include rash, insomnia, tiredness, and gastrointestinal effects (nausea, vomiting, diarrhea). Griseofulvin may cause hepatotoxicity and photosensitivity in patients with porphyria. The drug is contraindicated for individuals with a history of porphyria or hepatocellular disease.

***Drug Interactions.*** Griseofulvin induces hepatic drug-metabolizing enzymes and can thereby decrease the effects of *warfarin*. When this combination is used, the dosage of warfarin may need to be increased.

***Preparations, Dosage, and Administration.*** Griseofulvin is prepared in two particle sizes: microsized and ultramicrosized. The microcrystalline form [Fulvicin-U/F, Fulvicin V, Grifulvin V, Grisactin] is dispensed in tablets (250 and 500 mg), capsules (125 and 250 mg), and a suspension (125 mg/5 ml). The ultramicrocrystalline form [Fulvicin P/G, Grisactin Ultra, Gris-PEG] is dispensed in tablets, ranging in size from 125 to 330 mg.

Dosage depends to some degree upon which formulation (microsized or ultramicrosized) is being used. With the microsized formulations, the usual adult dosage is 500 mg to 1 gm per day; the usual dosage for children is 11 mg/kg/day. The ultramicrosized particles are better absorbed than the microsized particles. As a result, doses of ultramicrocrystalline griseofulvin are about 30% lower than doses of the microcrystalline form.

## Polyene Antibiotics

### Amphotericin B

Amphotericin B [Fungizone] is a broad-spectrum antifungal drug available for intravenous and topical use. As discussed above, intravenous amphotericin B is a drug of choice for most systemic mycoses. In contrast, topical amphotericin is limited to treatment of candidiasis of the skin. The drug is not employed to treat vaginal candidiasis, and is ineffective against dermatophytic infections. Adverse effects (burning, itching, erythema) from topical application occur occasionally. Absorption following topical application is minimal, and does not result in systemic toxicity. Topical amphotericin B is dispensed in cream, lotion, and ointment formulations. The drug is applied 2 to 4 times each day. Duration of treatment is 1 to 4 weeks.

### Nystatin

***Actions, Uses, and Adverse Effects.*** Nystatin is a polyene antibiotic. Use is limited to treatment of candidiasis. This agent is the drug of choice for chemotherapy of intestinal candidiasis, and is also employed to treat candidal infections of the skin, mouth, esophagus, and vagina. Nystatin can be administered orally and topically. There is no significant absorption associated with either route.

Oral nystatin occasionally causes gastrointestinal disturbance (nausea, vomiting, diarrhea). Topical application may produce local irritation.

***Preparations, Dosage, and Administration.*** For oral administration, nystatin is dispensed as a suspension and in tablets and lozenges; dosages range from 100,000 units to 1 million units 3 to 4 times a day. Vaginal tablets are employed for vaginal candidiasis; the usual dosage is 100,000 units once a day for 2 weeks. Nystatin is dispensed as a cream, ointment, and powder to treat candidiasis of the skin. The cream and ointment formulations are applied twice daily; the powder is applied 3 times daily. Trade names for nystatin include Mycostatin, Nilstat, and Nystex.

## Other Drugs for Superficial Mycoses

### Tolnaftate

Tolnaftate is employed topically to treat a variety of superficial mycoses. The drug is active against dermatophytes, but not against *Candida* species. The mechanism of antifungal action is unknown. Adverse effects (sensitization, irritation) are extremely rare. Tolnaftate is available in several formulations. Creams, gels, and solutions are most effective; powders are used adjunctively. The drug is applied twice daily for 2 to 3 weeks. Trade names include Aftate, Tinactin, Ting, and Zeasorb-AF.

### Haloprogin

Haloprogin [Halotex] is a topical antifungal agent that is active against dermatophytes and *Candida* species. The primary indication for the drug is tinea pedis (athlete's foot). Principal side effects are irritation, burning sensations, and peeling of skin. The drug is dispensed as a cream and in solution. Treatment consists of twice-daily application for 2 to 3 weeks.

### Undecylenic Acid

Undecylenic acid [Desenex, Cruex, others] is a topical agent used to treat superficial mycoses. The drug is active against dermatophytes but not *Candida* species. The major indication for this agent is tinea pedis (athlete's foot). However, other drugs (tolnaftate, haloprogin, the azoles) are more effective.

### Ciclopirox Olamine

Ciclopirox olamine [Loprox], a broad-spectrum antifungal drug, is active against dermatophytes and *Candida* species. This agent is applied topically to treat superficial candidiasis and tinea pedis, tinea cruris, and tinea corporis. The drug penetrates the epidermis to the dermis, but absorption is minimal and no significant systemic accumulation occurs. There is no toxicity from local application. Ciclopirox olamine is dispensed in cream and lotion formulations. Treatment consists of twice-daily application for 2 to 4 weeks.

### Naftifine

Naftifine [Naftin] is the first representative of a new class of antifungal drugs, the allylamines. Although approved only for topical treatment of dermatophytic infections, naftifine is active against a broad spectrum of pathogenic fungi. The drug acts primarily by inhibiting squalene epoxidase, thereby causing squalene to accumulate within fungi to toxic levels. In addition, naftifine inhibits synthesis of ergosterol. The most common adverse effects are burning and stinging. Absorption following topical administration is low (about 6%), and systemic effects have not been reported. Naftifine is dispensed in two formulations: 1% cream and 1% gel. The cream is applied once daily; the gel is applied twice daily. The usual duration of treatment is 4 weeks.

### Terbinafine

Terbinafine [Lamisil] belongs to the same chemical family as naftifine and has the same mechanism of action: inhibition of both squalene epoxidase and synthesis of ergosterol. The drug is highly active against dermatophytes, and less active against *Candida* species. Terbinafine is available in topical and oral formulations. Topical therapy is used for ringworm infections (e.g., tinea corporis, tinea cruris, tinea pedis). Oral therapy is used for onychomycosis (fungal infection of the nails). Adverse effects with topical therapy are minimal. The most common side effects with oral therapy are headache, diarrhea, dyspepsia, and abdominal pain. Oral terbinafine may also cause skin reactions, liver injury, and disturbance of taste. For topical therapy, terbinafine 1% cream is applied twice daily for 1 to 4 weeks. For oral therapy of nail infections, the dosage is 250 mg/day for 6 to 12 weeks.

## KEY POINTS

- Amphotericin B is a drug of choice for most systemic mycoses—despite its potential for serious harm.
- Amphotericin B binds to ergosterol in the fungal cell membrane, thereby making the membrane more permeable. The resultant leakage of intracellular cations reduces viability.
- Much of the toxicity of amphotericin B results from binding to cholesterol in host cell membranes.
- Because oral absorption of amphotericin B is poor, the drug must be administered IV to treat systemic mycoses.
- Amphotericin B infusion frequently causes fever, chills, rigors, nausea, and headache. Pretreatment with diphenhydramine plus an analgesic (aspirin or acetaminophen) can reduce mild symptoms. A glucocorticoid can be used for severe reactions. Meperidine can reduce rigors.
- Amphotericin B causes renal injury in most patients. Kidney damage can be minimized by infusing 1 L of saline on the day of amphotericin administration.

- If possible, amphotericin B should not be combined with other nephrotoxic drugs (e.g., aminoglycosides, cyclosporine).
- Ketoconazole, the prototype of the azole family of antifungal agents, is active against a broad spectrum of fungi.
- Ketoconazole inhibits synthesis of ergosterol, and thereby increases cell membrane permeability, which in turn causes leakage of cellular components.
- Ketoconazole is an alternative to IV amphotericin for many fungal infections. Advantages are less toxicity and oral usability.
- Ketoconazole requires an acidic environment for dissolution and absorption. Accordingly, antacids, $H_2$ blocking agents, proton pump inhibitors, and other drugs that reduce gastric acidity will decrease ketoconazole absorption.
- Ketoconazole is hepatotoxic. Liver function must be monitored.
- Ketoconazole inhibits metabolism of terfenadine and astemizole, and can thereby cause them to accumulate to toxic levels; fatal dysrhythmias may result. Accordingly, concurrent use of ketoconazole with these drugs is contraindicated.
- Topical clotrimazole, a member of the azole family of antifungals, is a drug of choice for many superficial mycoses caused by dermatophytes and *Candida* species.
- Onychomycosis (fungal infection of the fingernails and toenails) is difficult to treat and requires prolonged therapy. Agents employed include griseofulvin, terbinafine, and several azoles (e.g., ketoconazole).
- Vulvovaginal candidiasis can be treated with a single oral dose of fluconazole or with short-term topical therapy (e.g., one 500-mg vaginal tablet of clotrimazole).

# Summary of Major Nursing Implications*

The implications summarized below pertain only to use of antifungal drugs in the treatment of systemic mycoses.

## Amphotericin B

### Preadministration Assessment

#### Therapeutic Goal
Treatment of progressive and potentially fatal systemic fungal infections. Flucytosine may be given to enhance therapeutic effects.

#### Identifying High-Risk Patients
When used as it should be (i.e., for life-threatening infections) amphotericin has no contraindications.

## Implementation: Administration

### Routes
Intravenous, intrathecal.

### Intravenous Administration
Use aseptic technique when preparing infusion solutions. Infuse slowly (over 2 to 4 hours). Check the solution periodically for a precipitate; if a precipitate forms, discontinue the infusion immediately. Therapy lasts for several months; rotate the infusion site to reduce phlebitis and ensure availability of a usable vein. Dosages must be individualized. Alternate-day dosing may be ordered to reduce adverse effects.

## Ongoing Evaluation and Interventions

### Minimizing Adverse Effects
*General Considerations.* Amphotericin can produce serious adverse effects. The patient should be under close supervision, preferably in a hospital.

*Effects Associated with Intravenous Infusion.* Infusion of amphotericin can cause fever, chills, rigors, nausea, and headache. Pretreatment with diphenhydramine plus aspirin or acetaminophen can minimize these reactions. Give meperidine if rigors develop. If other measures fail, give hydrocortisone to suppress symptoms. Rotate the infusion site to avoid phlebitis.

*Nephrotoxicity.* Almost all patients experience renal impairment. Monitor and record intake and output. Kidney function should be tested weekly; if plasma creatinine content rises above 3.5 mg/dl, amphotericin dosage should be reduced. The risk of renal damage can be decreased by infusing 1 L of saline on the day of amphotericin administration and by avoiding other nephrotoxic drugs (e.g., aminoglycosides, cyclosporine).

*Hypokalemia.* Renal injury may cause hypokalemia. Serum potassium should be measured frequently. Correct hypokalemia with potassium supplements.

*Hematologic Effects.* Normocytic, normochromic anemia has occurred secondary to amphotericin-induced depression of bone marrow. Hematocrit determinations should be performed to monitor for this anemia.

### Minimizing Adverse Interactions

*Nephrotoxic Drugs.* Unless clearly required, amphotericin should not be combined with other nephrotoxic drugs, such as the aminoglycosides and cyclosporine.

## Ketoconazole

### Preadministration Assessment

#### Therapeutic Use
Treatment of systemic and superficial mycoses. Because of its slow onset, ketoconazole is best suited for long-term therapy of chronic fungal infections.

#### Baseline Data
Obtain baseline tests of liver function.

#### Identifying High-Risk Patients
Ketoconazole is *contraindicated* for patients taking *terfenadine* or *astemizole*. Use with *caution* in patients with liver disease.

### Implementation: Administration

#### Route
Oral.

#### Administration
Advise patients to take ketoconazole with food to minimize nausea and vomiting.

An acidic environment is needed for absorption. Instruct patients with achlorhydria to dissolve ketoconazole tablets in 4 ml of 0.2 N HCl and to sip this solution through a glass or plastic straw (to protect the teeth), and to follow drug administration with a glass of water.

## Ongoing Evaluation and Interventions

### Minimizing Adverse Effects

*Hepatotoxicity.* Hepatotoxicity is rare but potentially serious; fatal hepatic necrosis has occurred. Tests of liver function should be obtained prior to treatment and at intervals of 1 month or less thereafter. At the first indication of liver injury, ketoconazole should be withdrawn. Inform patients about symptoms of liver dysfunction (e.g., unusual fatigue, anorexia, nausea, vomiting, jaundice, dark urine, pale stools), and advise them to notify the physician if these occur.

### Minimizing Adverse Interactions

*Drugs That Raise Gastric pH.* Antacids, $H_2$ antagonists, anticholinergic drugs, and proton pump inhibitors can reduce ketoconazole absorption. These drugs should be administered no sooner than 2 hours after ingestion of ketoconazole. (Since proton pump inhibitors have a prolonged duration of action, patients using these agents may have insufficient stomach acid for ketoconazole absorption, regardless of when the proton pump inhibitor is administered.)

*Rifampin.* This drug reduces plasma levels of ketoconazole. Ketoconazole dosage should be increased if these agents are used concurrently.

*Terfenadine and Astemizole.* Concurrent use of terfenadine or astemizole with ketoconazole is contraindicated because of the risk of potentially fatal cardiac dysrhythmias.

## Flucytosine

### Preadministration Assessment

#### Therapeutic Use
Treatment of serious infections caused by *Candida* species and *Cryptococcus neoformans*. Flucytosine is usually combined with amphotericin B.

#### Baseline Data
Obtain baseline tests of renal function, hematologic status, and serum electrolytes.

#### Identifying High-Risk Patients
Use with *extreme caution* in patients with *kidney disease* or *bone marrow depression*.

### Implementation: Administration

#### Route
Oral.

#### Dosage and Administration
Treatment may require ingestion of 10 or more capsules 4 times a day; advise patients to take capsules a few at a time over a 15-minute interval to minimize nausea and vomiting. Dosage must be reduced in patients with renal impairment.

## Ongoing Evaluation and Interventions

### Monitoring Summary

Obtain weekly tests of liver function (serum transaminase and alkaline phosphatase levels) and hematologic status (leukocyte counts). In patients receiving amphotericin B concurrently, and in those with pre-existing renal impairment, monitor kidney function and flucytosine levels.

### Minimizing Adverse Effects

*Hematologic Effects.* Flucytosine-induced bone marrow depression can cause neutropenia, thrombocytopenia, and fatal agranulocytosis. The risk of these effects can be minimized by adjusting the dosage to keep plasma flucytosine levels below 100 μg/ml. Obtain weekly leukocyte counts to monitor hematologic effects.

*Hepatotoxicity.* Mild and reversible liver dysfunction occurs frequently; severe hepatic damage is rare. Obtain weekly determinations of serum transaminase and alkaline phosphatase levels to evaluate liver function.

### Minimizing Adverse Interactions

*Amphotericin B.* Kidney damage from amphotericin B may decrease flucytosine excretion, thereby increasing toxicity secondary to flucytosine accumulation. When these drugs are combined, renal function and flucytosine levels must be monitored.

# CHAPTER 87

# Antiviral Agents I: Drugs for Non-HIV Viral Infections

**Systemic Antiviral Agents**
Acyclovir
Ganciclovir
Famciclovir
Valacyclovir
Cidofovir
Foscarnet
Ribavirin
Amantadine
Rimantadine
Interferon Alfa

**Ophthalmic Antiviral Agents**
Trifluridine
Vidarabine
Idoxuridine

A ntiviral drugs are discussed in this chapter and the one that follows. In this chapter, we consider drugs used to treat infections caused by viruses other than HIV. In Chapter 88, we consider drugs used against HIV infection. Although several new antiviral drugs have been introduced in the last decade, our ability to treat viral infections remains limited. Compared with the dramatic advances made in antibacterial therapy over the past half-century, efforts to develop safe and effective antiviral drugs have been much less successful. A major reason for this lack of success resides in the process of viral replication: viruses are obligate intracellular parasites that use the biochemical machinery of host cells to reproduce. Because the viral growth cycle employs host-cell enzymes and substrates, it is difficult to suppress viral replication without also doing significant harm to the host. The useful antiviral drugs that have been developed act by affecting biochemical processes unique to viral reproduction. As our knowledge of viral molecular biology advances, additional virus-specific processes will surely be discovered, thereby giving us new targets against which to direct drugs.

At this time, 15 drugs are available in the United States for treating non-HIV viral infections. These drugs are active against a narrow spectrum of viruses, and hence their utility is limited to a few types of infections. Twelve of these drugs are employed to treat systemic infections. Three are applied topically to treat infections of the eye. Drugs of first choice for systemic infections are listed in Table 87-1.

## Systemic Antiviral Agents

### Acyclovir

Acyclovir [Zovirax] is the agent of first choice for infections caused by herpes simplex viruses and varicella-zoster virus. The drug can be administered topically, orally, and intravenously. Serious side effects are uncommon.

#### Antiviral Spectrum

Acyclovir is active only against members of the herpesvirus family, a group that includes *herpes simplex viruses* (HSV), *varicella-zoster virus* (VZV), and *cytomegalovirus* (CMV). Of these viruses, HSV are most sensitive, VZV is moderately sensitive, and most strains of CMV are resistant.

#### Mechanism of Action

Acyclovir inhibits viral replication by suppressing synthesis of viral DNA. To exert its antiviral effects, acyclovir must first be activated. The critical step in activation is conversion of acyclovir to acyclo-GMP by thymidine kinase. Once formed, acyclo-GMP is converted to acyclo-GTP, the compound directly responsible for inhibiting DNA synthesis. Acyclo-GTP suppresses DNA synthesis by (1) inhibiting viral DNA polymerase and (2) becoming incorporated into the growing strand of viral DNA, which blocks further strand growth.

## TABLE 87–1. DRUGS OF CHOICE FOR NON-HIV VIRAL INFECTIONS

| Virus and Infection | Drug of Choice |
| --- | --- |
| **Herpes Simplex Virus** | |
| Genital herpes | Acyclovir |
| Encephalitis | Acyclovir |
| Mucocutaneous disease in the immunocompromised host | Acyclovir |
| Neonatal | Acyclovir |
| Acyclovir-resistent | Foscarnet |
| Keratoconjunctivitis | Trifluridine |
| **Varicella-Zoster Virus** | |
| Varicella (chicken pox) | Acyclovir |
| Herpes zoster (shingles) | Acyclovir |
| Varicella or zoster in the immunocompromised host | Acyclovir |
| Acyclovir-resistent | Foscarnet |
| **Cytomegalovirus** | |
| Retinitis | Ganciclovir *or* foscarnet |
| **Influenza A Virus** | |
| Respiratory tract infection | Amantadine *or* rimantadine |
| **Respiratory Syncytial Virus** | |
| Bronchiolitis, pneumonia | Ribavirin |
| **Hepatitis Viruses B and C** | |
| Chronic hepatitis | Interferon alfa-2b |

The selectivity of acyclovir is based in large part on the ability of certain viruses to activate the drug. Herpes simplex viruses are especially sensitive to acyclovir because the drug is a much better substrate for thymidine kinase produced by HSV than it is for mammalian thymidine kinase. Hence, formation of acyclo-GMP, the limiting step in the activation of acyclovir, occurs almost exclusively in cells infected with HSV. Cytomegalovirus is inherently resistant to the drug because acyclovir is a poor substrate for the form of thymidine kinase produced by this virus.

### Resistance

Herpesviruses develop resistance to acyclovir by three mechanisms: decreased production of thymidine kinase, alteration of thymidine kinase such that it no longer converts acyclovir to acyclo-GMP, and alteration of viral DNA polymerase such that it is less sensitive to inhibition. Of these mechanisms, thymidine kinase deficiency is by far the most common. Resistance is rare in immunocompetent patients, but many cases have been reported in transplant patients and patients with AIDS. Lesions caused by resistant HSV can be extensive and severe, progressing despite continued acyclovir therapy. Acyclovir-resistant HSV and VZV usually respond to intravenous foscarnet.

### Therapeutic Uses

**Herpes Simplex Genitalis.** Genital herpes infections are caused by *type 2 HSV* (HSV-2). For patients with ini-

tial infection, *topical* acyclovir reduces the duration of viral shedding, but does not accelerate healing. Topical acyclovir is not effective for *recurrent* genital infections. *Oral* acyclovir is superior to topical therapy for initial genital infections and recurrent infections. For patients with initial infection, oral therapy decreases formation of additional lesions and decreases the duration and severity of the initial episode. For patients with recurrent herpes genitalis, continuous oral therapy reduces the frequency at which lesions appear. When initial genital infection is especially severe, *intravenous* acyclovir may be indicated. Patients with primary or recurrent herpes genitalis should be informed that, although acyclovir can decrease symptoms, the drug does not eliminate the virus and does not produce cure. Also, patients should be advised to avoid sexual contact when lesions are present.

**Mucocutaneous Herpes Simplex Infections.** Herpes infections of the face and oropharynx are usually caused by HSV-2. For immunocompetent patients, *oral* acyclovir can be used to treat primary infections of the gums and mouth. Oral acyclovir can also be taken *prophylactically* to prevent episodes of *recurrent* herpes labialis (fever blisters). However, there is no effective treatment for active herpes labialis. Mucocutaneous herpes infections can be especially severe in immunocompromised patients. For these people, *intravenous* acyclovir is the treatment of choice.

**Varicella-Zoster Infections.** High-dose *oral* acyclovir is effective therapy for herpes zoster (shingles) in older adults. Oral therapy is also effective for varicella (chickenpox) in children, adolescents, and adults, provided that dosing is begun early (within 24 hours of rash onset). *Intravenous* acyclovir is the treatment of choice for varicella-zoster infection in the immunocompromised host.

### Pharmacokinetics

Acyclovir is administered topically, orally, and intravenously. Oral bioavailability is low, ranging from 15% to 30%. No significant absorption occurs with topical use. Once in the blood, acyclovir is distributed widely to body fluids and tissues. Levels achieved in cerebrospinal fluid are 50% of those in plasma. Elimination is renal, primarily as the unchanged drug. In patients with normal kidney function, acyclovir has a half-life of 2.5 hours. The half-life is prolonged by renal impairment, reaching 20 hours in anuric patients. Accordingly, dosages should be reduced in patients with kidney disease.

### Adverse Effects

**Intravenous Therapy.** Intravenous acyclovir is generally well tolerated. The most common reactions are *phlebitis* and *inflammation* at the site of infusion. Reversible *nephrotoxicity*, manifested as elevations in serum creatinine and blood urea nitrogen (BUN), occurs in some patients. The cause of nephrotoxicity is deposition of acyclovir in renal tubules. The risk of renal injury is increased by dehydration and by use of other nephrotoxic drugs. Kidney damage can be minimized by infusing acyclovir slowly (over 1 hour) and by ensuring adequate hydration during the infusion and for 2 hours after.

*Oral and Topical Therapy.* Oral acyclovir is devoid of serious adverse effects. Renal impairment has not been reported. The most common reactions to oral therapy are nausea, vomiting, diarrhea, headache, and vertigo. Topical acyclovir frequently causes transient burning or stinging sensations; systemic reactions do not occur.

### Preparations, Dosage, and Administration

*Topical.* Acyclovir [Zovirax] is dispensed as a 5% ointment for topical use. This formulation is indicated for initial episodes of herpes genitalis and for mild mucocutaneous herpes simplex infections in the immunocompromised host. The drug is applied six times a day at 3-hour intervals. Patients should be advised to apply the drug with a finger cot or rubber glove to avoid viral transfer to other body sites or other people.

*Oral.* Oral acyclovir [Zovirax] is available in capsules (200 mg), tablets (400 and 800 mg), and a suspension (200 mg/5 ml). Dosages for patients with normal kidney function are given below. Dosages must be reduced for patients with renal impairment.

- For initial episodes of herpes genitalis, the usual dosage is 200 mg 5 times a day (at 4-hour intervals) for 10 days.
- For long-term suppressive therapy of recurrent genital infections, the usual dosage is 400 mg twice daily for up to 12 months. Alternative dosages range from 200 mg 3 times a day to 200 mg 5 times a day.
- For acute therapy of herpes zoster, the dosage is 800 mg 5 times a day (at 4-hour intervals) for 7 to 10 days.
- For varicella (chickenpox), the dosage is 20 mg/kg (but no more than 800 mg) 4 times a day for 5 days. Treatment should begin at the earliest sign of rash.

*Intravenous.* Acyclovir [Zovirax] is dispensed as a powder (500 mg/10-ml vial, 1000 mg/20-ml vial) to be reconstituted for IV administration. The drug is administered by slow IV infusion (over 1 hour or more). It must not be given as an IV bolus or by IM or SC injection. To minimize the risk of renal damage, hydrate the patient during the infusion and for 2 hours after. Dosages for patients with normal kidney function are given below. Dosages should be reduced for patients with renal impairment.

- For mucocutaneous herpes simplex infection in the immunocompromised host, the adult dosage is 5 mg/kg infused every 8 hours for 7 days. The dosage for children under 12 years is 250 mg/m$^2$ infused every 8 hours for 7 days.
- For varicella-zoster infection in the immunocompromised host, the adult dosage is 10 mg/kg infused every 8 hours for 7 days. The dosage for children under 12 years is 500 mg/m$^2$ infused every 8 hours for 7 days.
- For severe initial episodes of herpes genitalis in the immunocompetent host, the adult dosage is 5 mg/kg infused every 8 hours for 5 days. The dosage for children under 12 years is 250 mg/m$^2$ infused every 8 hours for 5 days.

## Ganciclovir

Ganciclovir [Cytovene, Vitrasert] is a synthetic antiviral agent with activity against herpesviruses, including cytomegalovirus (CMV). Because the drug can cause serious adverse effects, especially granulocytopenia and thrombo-

cytopenia, use should be restricted to prevention and treatment of CMV infection in the immunocompromised host.

*Mechanism of Action.* Ganciclovir is converted to its active form, ganciclovir triphosphate, within infected cells. As ganciclovir triphosphate, it suppresses replication of viral DNA by (1) inhibiting viral DNA polymerase and (2) undergoing incorporation into the growing DNA chain, which causes premature chain termination.

*Pharmacokinetics.* Bioavailability of oral ganciclovir is low: only 5% under fasting conditions and 9% when taken with food. Once in the blood, the drug is widely distributed to body fluids and tissues. Ganciclovir is excreted unchanged in the urine. In patients with normal renal function, the half-life is about 3 hours. In patients with renal impairment, the half-life is prolonged. Accordingly, dosages should be reduced in patients with kidney disease.

*Therapeutic Use.* Ganciclovir has two approved indications: (1) treatment of CMV retinitis in immunocompromised patients, including those with AIDS; and (2) prevention of CMV infection in transplant patients considered at risk. In patients with AIDS; CMV retinitis has an incidence of 15% to 40%. Although most AIDS patients respond initially, the relapse rate is high, even with continued maintenance therapy. To reduce the risk of relapse, patients with AIDS must continue maintenance therapy for life. The risk of relapse is higher with oral ganciclovir than with IV ganciclovir. Since viral resistance can develop during treatment, this possibility should be considered if the patient responds poorly.

*Adverse Effects.* *Granulocytopenia and Thrombocytopenia.* The adverse effect of greatest concern is bone marrow suppression, which can result in granulocytopenia (40%) and thrombocytopenia (20%). These hematologic responses can be exacerbated by concurrent therapy with zidovudine. Conversely, granulocytopenia can be reduced with granulocyte colony-stimulating factors (see Chapter 52). Because of the risk of adverse hematologic effects, blood cell counts must be monitored. Treatment should be interrupted if the absolute neutrophil count falls below 500/mm$^3$ or if the platelet counts falls below 25,000/mm$^3$. Cell counts usually begin to recover within 3 to 5 days. Ganciclovir should be used with caution in patients with pre-existing cytopenias and in those with a history of cytopenic reactions to other drugs.

*Reproductive Toxicity.* Ganciclovir is teratogenic and embryotoxic in laboratory animals and probably in humans. Women should be advised to avoid pregnancy during therapy and for 90 days after ceasing treatment. At doses equivalent to those used therapeutically, ganciclovir inhibits spermatogenesis in mice; sterility is reversible with low doses and irreversible with high doses. Female infertility may also occur. Patients should be forewarned of these effects.

*Other Adverse Effects.* Incidental effects include *nausea, fever, rash, anemia, liver dysfunction,* and *confusion and other central nervous system (CNS) symptoms.*

***Preparations, Dosage, and Administration.*** *Intravenous.* Ganciclovir [Cytovene] is available as a powder to be reconstituted for IV infusion. Solutions are alkaline and must be infused into a freely flowing vein to avoid local injury. For treatment of CMV retinitis, the initial dosage for adults with normal renal function is 5 mg/kg (infused over 1 hour) every 12 hours for 14 to 21 days. Two maintenance dosages can be used: (1) 5 mg/kg infused over 1 hour once every day, or (2) 6 mg/kg infused over 1 hour once a day, 5 days each week. Dosages must be reduced for patients with renal impairment. Since patients with AIDS must continue maintenance therapy for life, they need a permanent IV line and equipment for home infusion. Adequate hydration must be maintained in all patients to ensure the drug's renal excretion.

*Oral.* Oral ganciclovir [Cytovene] is indicated for maintenance therapy in patients with CMV retinitis. The dosage is 1000 mg 3 times daily with food.

*Intraocular.* The ganciclovir intraocular implant [Vitraset] is indicated for CMV retinitis in patients with AIDS. Surgical implantation, which takes about 1 hour, is performed under local anesthesia on an outpatient basis. Vision is usually blurred for 2 to 4 weeks after the procedure. The implant must be replaced every 5 to 8 months. Clinical trials indicate that CMV retinitis progresses more slowly in patients who receive intraocular ganciclovir compared with those on IV ganciclovir.

## Famciclovir

Famciclovir [Famvir] is a prodrug used to treat acute herpes zoster. Benefits are equivalent to those of acyclovir. Adverse effects are minimal.

***Pharmacokinetics.*** Famciclovir undergoes rapid absorption from the GI tract followed by enzymatic conversion to *penciclovir*, its active form. Food decreases the rate of famciclovir absorption but not the extent. As a result, the amount of penciclovir produced is the same whether famciclovir is taken with or without food. Penciclovir is excreted in the urine, largely unchanged. The plasma half-life of penciclovir is about 2.5 hours. However, the half-life of penciclovir within cells is much longer. In patients with renal impairment, the plasma half-life of penciclovir is prolonged.

***Mechanism of Action and Antiviral Spectrum.*** Penciclovir undergoes intracellular conversion to penciclovir triphosphate, a compound that inhibits viral DNA polymerase, and thereby prevents replication of viral DNA. Under clinical conditions, formation of penciclovir triphosphate requires viral thymidine kinase. As a result, inhibition of DNA synthesis is limited to cells that are infected, leaving the vast majority of host cells unharmed. *In vitro*, penciclovir is active against HSV-1, HSV-2, and VZV.

***Therapeutic Use.*** At this time, famciclovir is approved only for acute herpes zoster (shingles). In a clinical trial comparing famciclovir with placebo, the drug decreased the time to full crusting from 7 days to 5 days. Famciclovir did not decrease the *incidence* of postherpetic neuralgia, but did decrease the *duration* from 112 days to 61 days. In a trial comparing famciclovir with acyclovir, both drugs had equivalent effects.

***Adverse Effects.*** Famciclovir is very well tolerated. In clinical trials, the incidence of side effects was the same as in patients taking a placebo. Safety for use during pregnancy or breast feeding and in children under the age of 18 has not been established.

***Preparations, Dosage, and Administration.*** Famciclovir [Famvir] is dispensed in 500-mg tablets for oral administration. The recommended dosage is 500 mg every 8 hours, beginning no more than 72 hours after onset of herpes zoster symptoms. In patients with renal impairment, the interval between doses should be increased to 12 hours or 24 hours, depending on the degree of impairment. Famciclovir can be taken without regard to meals.

## Valacyclovir

***Actions and Uses.*** Valacyclovir [Valtrex], a prodrug form of acyclovir, is approved for oral therapy of herpes zoster (shingles) in the immunocompetent host. Benefits depend on conversion of valacyclovir to acyclovir, the active form. In a clinical trial in patients with *herpes zoster*, valacyclovir (1000 mg 3 times a day for 7 or 14 days) was somewhat more effective than acyclovir (800 mg 5 times a day for 7 days) in reducing the duration of pain and the duration of postherpetic neuralgia. In clinical trials in patients with initial or recurrent *genital herpes*, valacyclovir (1000 mg twice a day) and acyclovir (200 mg 5 times a day) produced similar results.

***Pharmacokinetics.*** After oral administration, valacyclovir undergoes rapid absorption followed by rapid and essentially complete conversion of acyclovir. When acyclovir itself is given orally, bioavailability is only 15% to 30%. In contrast, when valacyclovir is given orally, the effective availability of acyclovir is greatly increased—to about 55%. Hence, valacyclovir represents a more efficient way of getting acyclovir into the body. Following conversion of valacyclovir to acyclovir, the kinetics are the same as if acyclovir itself had been given.

***Adverse Effects.*** In some immunocompromised patients, valacyclovir has produced a condition known as *thrombotic thrombocytopenic purpura/hemolytic uremic syndrome* (TTP/HUS). This syndrome, which is potentially fatal, has not occurred in immunocompetent patients. Valacyclovir is not approved for use in immunocompromised hosts. Aside from causing TTP/HUS, valacyclovir is generally well tolerated, producing the same side effects seen with oral acyclovir (e.g., nausea, vomiting, diarrhea, headache, vertigo).

***Preparations, Dosage, and Administration.*** Valacyclovir [Valtrex] is available in 500-mg capsules for oral use. The drug may be given without regard to meals. For treatment of herpes zoster, the recommended dosage is 1000 mg 3 times a day for 7 days. Therapy should begin as soon as possible after onset of symptoms. Dosage should be reduced in patients with renal impairment.

## Cidofovir

Cidofovir [Vistide] is a new IV drug for treating CMV retinitis in patients with AIDS. Alternative drugs for this infection are foscarnet, which is given IV, and ganciclovir, which may be administered IV, PO, or by ocular insert. Compared with IV foscarnet or IV ganciclovir, cidofovir has the distinct advantage of needing fewer infusions: whereas foscarnet and ganciclovir must be infused daily, cidofovir is infused just once a week or every other week. The major adverse effect of cidofovir is kidney damage.

***Mechanism of Action.*** Once inside cells, cidofovir is converted to cidofovir diphosphate, its active form. As the diphosphate, cidofovir causes selective inhibition of viral DNA polymerase, and thereby inhibits viral DNA synthesis. Intracellular concentrations of cidofovir diphosphate are too low to inhibit human DNA polymerases, hence host cells are spared.

***Antiviral Spectrum and Therapeutic Use.*** Cidofovir is active against herpesviruses, including CMV, HSV-1, HSV-2, and VZV. At this time, the drug is approved only for treating CMV retinitis in patients with AIDS. Whether the drug is active against CMV infections in other patients or at other sites (e.g., GI tract, lungs) is not known. In clinical trials in patients with AIDS and established CMV retinitis, cidofovir significantly delayed progression of retinitis.

***Pharmacokinetics.*** Cidofovir is administered by IV infusion and is excreted by the kidneys. Probenecid competes with cidofovir for renal tubular secretion, and thereby delays elimination. Cidofovir has a prolonged *intracellular* half-life (17 to 65 hours), and therefore long intervals can separate doses. In contrast, intravenous foscarnet and ganciclovir must be infused daily.

**Adverse Effects.** The principal adverse effect is *kidney damage*. To reduce the risk of injury, all patients must receive probenecid and IV hydration therapy with each cidofovir infusion. Also, they should be monitored for signs of renal damage (proteinuria, elevation of serum creatinine). If injury is indicated, cidofovir should be withheld or the dosage reduced, depending on the degree of damage. In addition to kidney damage, cidofovir can cause *granulocytopenia*; accordingly, neutrophil counts should be monitored.

**Preparations, Dosage, and Administration.** Cidofovir [Vistide] is dispensed in solution (75 mg/ml) in 5-ml ampules. To reduce the risk of renal injury, cidofovir infusions must be accompanied by IV hydration therapy and PO probenecid.

Each cidofovir dose—for induction or for maintenance—consists of 5 mg/kg infused IV over 1 hour. For induction, two doses are given 1 week apart. For maintenance, one dose is given every 2 weeks. The size of each dose must be reduced for patients with renal impairment. If impairment is severe, cidofovir should not be administered.

Oral probenecid must accompany each infusion. The dosage is 2 gm 3 hours before the infusion, 1 gm 1 hour after the infusion, and 1 gm more 8 hours after that. Ingesting food before each dose can decrease probenecid-induced nausea and vomiting. An antiemetic may also be used.

Hydration is accomplished by infusing 1 L of 0.9% saline solution over 1 to 2 hours immediately before infusing cidofovir. For patients who can tolerate it, 1 L more can be infused over 1 to 3 hours, beginning when the cidofovir infusion begins or as soon as it is over.

## Foscarnet

Foscarnet [Foscavir] is active against all known herpesviruses, including CMV, HSV-1, HSV-2, and VZV. Compared with ganciclovir, foscarnet is more difficult to administer, less well tolerated, and much more expensive (the cost to the pharmacy is about $20,000 a year). The major adverse effect is renal injury.

**Mechanism of Action.** Foscarnet is an analog of pyrophosphate that inhibits viral DNA polymerases and reverse transcriptases, and thereby inhibits synthesis of viral nucleic acids. At the concentrations achieved clinically, the drug does not inhibit host DNA replication. Unlike many other antiviral drugs, which must undergo conversion to an active form, foscarnet is active as administered.

**Therapeutic Use.** Foscarnet has two approved indications: (1) CMV retinitis in patients with AIDS and (2) acyclovir-resistant mucocutaneous HSV infection in the immunocompromised host. CMV retinitis resistant to ganciclovir may respond to foscarnet.

**Pharmacokinetics.** Foscarnet has low oral bioavailability and must be administered intravenously. The drug is poorly soluble in water and does not penetrate cells easily. As a result, it must be given in large doses with large volumes of fluid. Between 10% and 28% of each dose is deposited in bone; the remainder is excreted unchanged in the urine. Because foscarnet is eliminated by the kidneys, dosages must be reduced in patients with renal impairment. The plasma half-life is 3 to 5 hours.

**Adverse Effects and Interactions.** Foscarnet is generally less well tolerated than ganciclovir. However, unlike ganciclovir, foscarnet does not cause granulocytopenia or thrombocytopenia.

*Nephrotoxicity.* Renal injury, as evidenced by a rise in serum creatinine concentration, is the most common dose-limiting toxicity. Most patients develop some degree of renal impairment. Renal injury occurs most often during the second week of therapy. The risk of nephrotoxicity is increased by concurrent use of other nephrotoxic drugs, including amphotericin B, aminoglycosides (e.g., gentamicin), and pentamidine. Prehydration with intravenous saline may reduce the risk of renal injury. Renal function (creatinine clearance) should be monitored closely and the dosage should be reduced if renal impairment develops.

*Electrolyte and Mineral Imbalances.* Foscarnet frequently causes hypocalcemia, hypokalemia, hypomagnesemia, and hypo- or hyperphosphatemia. Ionized serum calcium may be reduced despite normal levels of total serum calcium. Patients should be informed about symptoms of low ionized calcium (e.g., paresthesias, numbness in the extremities, perioral tingling) and instructed to report these. Severe hypocalcemia can result in dysrhythmias, tetany, and seizures. Serum levels of calcium, magnesium, potassium, and phosphorus should be measured frequently. Special caution is required in patients with pre-existing electrolyte, cardiac, or neurologic abnormalities. The risk of hypocalcemia is increased by concurrent use of pentamidine.

*Other Adverse Effects.* Common reactions include fever (65%), nausea (47%), anemia (33%), diarrhea (30%), vomiting (26%), and headache (26%). In addition, foscarnet can cause fatigue, tremor, irritability, genital ulceration, abnormal liver function tests, neutropenia, anemia, and seizures.

**Preparations, Dosage, and Administration.** Foscarnet [Foscavir] is dispensed in solution (24 mg/ml) for IV infusion. An infusion pump is essential to reduce the risk of accidental overdosage. Infusions may be administered through a central venous line or a peripheral vein. When a central venous line is used, a concentrated (24 mg/ml) solution may be given. When a peripheral vein is used, the solution should be diluted to 12 mg/ml. For patients with normal kidney function, the *initial* dosage is 60 mg/kg (for CMV infection) or 40 mg/kg (for HSV infection) infused over 1 hour (or longer) every 8 hours for 2 to 3 weeks. The *maintenance* dosage (for CMV or HSV infection) is 90 to 120 mg/kg infused over 2 hours once daily. All dosages must be reduced for patients with renal impairment.

## Ribavirin

**Antiviral Actions.** Ribavirin [Virazole] is virustatic. The drug is active against respiratory syncytial virus (RSV), influenza virus (types A and B), and herpes simplex virus. Although several biochemical actions of the drug have been described, it is not known which (if any) of these are responsible for antiviral effects.

**Therapeutic Uses.** Ribavirin is labeled only for severe viral pneumonia caused by RSV in carefully selected, hospitalized infants and young children. Unfortunately, benefits of treatment are usually minimal—and the cost is high (over $1300/day). Ribavirin should not be used for mild RSV infections.

Ribavirin has been employed investigationally to treat influenza A and B. Administration should be initiated within 24 hours of the onset of symptoms. Additional unlabeled uses include measles, herpes genitalis, acute and chronic hepatitis, Lassa fever, and Korean hemorrhagic fever.

**Pharmacokinetics.** Ribavirin is administered by oral inhalation. The drug is absorbed from the lungs and achieves high concentrations in respiratory tract secretions and erythrocytes. Concentrations in plasma remain low. The drug is metabolized to active and inactive products. Excretion is via the urine (30% to 55%) and feces (15%). Ribavirin that is sequestered in erythrocytes remains in the body for weeks.

**Adverse Effects.** Inhalation of ribavirin produces little or no systemic toxicity. However, although generally safe, inhaled ribavirin does pose a hazard to infants undergoing mechanical assistance of ventilation: the drug can precipitate in the respiratory apparatus, thereby interfering with safe and effective respiratory support. Consequently, ribavirin should not be administered to infants who need respiratory assistance. In some infants and in adults who have asthma or chronic obstructive lung disease, ribavirin has caused deterioration of pulmonary function. Accordingly, respiratory function should be carefully monitored. If deterioration occurs, ribavirin should be discontinued. When administered systemically (orally or IV), ribavirin frequently causes anemia. This has not been reported with inhalational therapy.

***Use in Pregnancy.*** Ribavirin is contraindicated for use during pregnancy. Although studies in primates indicate no effect on the developing fetus, ribavirin has proved either teratogenic or embryolethal in nearly all other species tested. No studies in humans have been performed. Ribavirin is classified under FDA Pregnancy Category X: the risk of use during pregnancy clearly outweighs any potential benefits. Because of the risk of significant drug exposure, pregnant women should not directly care for patients undergoing ribavirin aerosol therapy.

***Preparations, Dosage, and Administration.*** Ribavirin [Virazole] is dispensed as a powder (6 gm/100-ml vial) to be reconstituted for aerosol administration. According to the manufacturer, only one device—the Viratek Small Particle Aerosol Generator (SPAG) Model SPAG-2—should be employed for ribavirin administration. The SPAG-2 is used to deliver ribavirin to an infant oxygen hood. Treatment is given 12 to 18 hours a day for no less than 3 days and no more than 1 week. The drug should not be administered to patients who require ventilatory assistance. To reconstitute powdered ribavirin, dissolve 6 gm of the drug in sterile water for injection or inhalation, transfer this concentrated solution to the SPAG-2 reservoir, and dilute to a final volume of 300 ml using sterile water for injection or inhalation. The final concentration of ribavirin is 20 mg/ml. This solution is aerosolized and inhaled by the patient.

## Amantadine

Amantadine [Symmetrel, Symadine] is an antiviral drug employed for prophylaxis and treatment of infections caused by type A influenza virus. As discussed in Chapter 22, the drug is also used to treat Parkinson's disease.

***Mechanism of Antiviral Action.*** Just how amantadine suppresses viral growth is not completely understood. The drug can prevent penetration of influenza A virus into host cells and can inhibit viral uncoating. In addition, it inhibits an early step in replication of viral components.

***Therapeutic Use.*** Antiviral applications of amantadine are limited to prophylaxis and treatment of respiratory tract infections caused by *type A influenza virus* strains. The drug is not active against type B influenza. Prophylaxis should be instituted only in the presence of a documented influenza A epidemic. Candidates for prophylaxis include (1) individuals at high risk of developing complications from influenza (e.g., elderly patients and those with cardiopulmonary disease) and (2) health care workers and family members who make extensive contact with patients at risk. Prophylaxis is continued until the epidemic abates (usually in 5 to 6 weeks). It should be noted that immunization against influenza A is preferred to prophylaxis with amantadine. Since amantadine does not impede the immune response to influenza A vaccine, individuals at risk can be vaccinated while receiving amantadine for prophylaxis. Amantadine can be discontinued 2 weeks after vaccination. For treatment of active influenza

A infection, amantadine is most effective when therapy is instituted early (within 48 hours of the onset of symptoms).

***Pharmacokinetics.*** Amantadine is well absorbed following oral administration and is distributed widely to body fluids and tissues. The drug crosses the blood-brain barrier and the placenta. It also appears in saliva, nasal secretions, and breast milk. Amantadine is not metabolized. Excretion is via the kidneys. In patients with renal impairment, amantadine will accumulate to high levels if the dosage is not reduced.

***Adverse Effects.*** Amantadine is generally well tolerated when given in the doses employed for prophylaxis and treatment of influenza.

*Central Nervous System Effects.* CNS effects occur in 10% to 30% of patients. Reactions include dizziness, nervousness, insomnia, and difficulty in concentrating. Individuals involved in hazardous activities should exercise appropriate caution. More serious CNS effects (depression, hallucinations, seizures) have occurred. Accordingly, care should be exercised in patients with a history of epilepsy or psychosis.

*Cardiovascular Effects.* Rarely, amantadine has caused congestive heart failure (CHF). The drug should be used with caution in patients with CHF or peripheral edema. Patients should be instructed to contact their physician if they experience shortness of breath or swelling of the extremities.

Orthostatic hypotension has occurred. Patients should be advised to move slowly when assuming an upright position. Also, they should be advised to sit or lie down if dizziness or lightheadedness occurs.

*Use in Pregnancy and Lactation.* Amantadine is teratogenic and embryotoxic in rats. Adequate studies during human pregnancy have not been performed. The drug crosses the placenta and is classified in FDA Pregnancy Category C. It should be avoided by pregnant women unless the benefits of treatment are deemed to outweigh the potential risks to the fetus. Amantadine is secreted in breast milk and should not be used by nursing mothers.

***Drug Interactions.*** Amantadine can intensify the peripheral and CNS effects of anticholinergic drugs. When amantadine has been combined with anticholinergic drugs, psychotic reactions resembling those associated with atropine poisoning have occurred. Such responses can be reduced by lowering the dosage of amantadine or the anticholinergic agent.

***Preparations, Dosage, and Administration.*** Amantadine [Symmetrel, Symadine] is dispensed in 100-mg capsules and a syrup (10 mg/ml) for oral use. For treatment or prophylaxis of influenza A, the dosage for patients older than 9 years is 100 mg twice daily. For children ages 1 to 9 years, the dosage is 4.4 to 8.8 mg/kg/day in 2 or 3 divided doses. The dosage must be reduced in patients with kidney dysfunction. Prophylactic administration should commence prior to anticipated viral exposure and should continue for as long as the influenza A epidemic lasts. For treatment of active influenza A infection, therapy should begin within 48 hours of the onset of symptoms and should continue for 4 to 5 days.

### Rimantadine

Rimantadine [Flumadine] is very similar to amantadine in structure, actions, and uses. Like amantadine, rimantadine is indicated only for prophylaxis and treatment of *influenza A* virus infections. Administration is oral and bioavailability appears to be greater than 90%. In contrast to amantadine, which is not metabolized, rimantadine undergoes extensive metabolism prior to excretion in the urine. Primary adverse effects are nervousness, lightheadedness, difficulty in concentration, sleep disturbances, and fatigue. However, these occur less frequently with rimantadine than with amantadine (3% versus up to 30%). The *adult* dosage for *treatment* or *prophylaxis* is 100 mg twice daily; the duration of therapy is 5 days for treatment of active infection and up to 6 weeks for prophylaxis. The dosage for *prophylaxis* in *children* is 5 mg/kg/day. Rimantadine is not approved for treating active infection in children. Rimantadine is available in 100-mg capsules and a 10 mg/ml syrup.

### Interferon Alfa

Human interferons are naturally occurring compounds with complex antiviral, immunomodulatory, and antineoplastic actions. The interferon family has three major classes, designated alfa (alpha), beta, and gamma. Currently, all interferons employed clinically belong to the alfa class. Three forms of interferon alfa are available: alfa-2a [Roferon-A], alfa-2b [Intron A], and alfa-n3 [Alferon N]. In the discussion below, these compounds are referred to collectively as interferon alfa. Commercial production is by recombinant DNA technology. Interferons are used to treat a variety of viral infections (see below) and neoplastic diseases (Chapter 96).

***Mechanism of Antiviral Action.*** Interferon alfa has multiple effects on the viral replication cycle. After binding to receptors on host cell membranes, the drug blocks (1) viral entry into cells, (2) synthesis of viral messenger RNA and viral proteins, and (3) viral assembly and release.

***Pharmacokinetics.*** Interferon alfa is not absorbed orally, hence administration is parenteral (IM and SC). Plasma drug levels peak in 4 to 8 hours. Inactivation occurs rapidly in body fluids and tissues. No intact drug appears in the urine.

***Adverse Effects.*** Interferon alfa causes multiple adverse effects. The most common is a flu-like syndrome characterized by fever (74% to 98%), fatigue (89% to 98%), myalgia (69% to 73%), headache (66% to 71%), and chills (41% to 64%). Symptoms tend to diminish with continued therapy. Some symptoms (fever, headache, myalgia) can be reduced with acetaminophen. Other common adverse effects include anorexia, weight loss, diarrhea, abdominal pain, dizziness, and cough. Prolonged or high-dose therapy can cause bone marrow suppression; neurotoxicity, including profound fatigue and depression; hair loss; thyroid dysfunction; and, possibly, cardiotoxicity.

***Antiviral Uses and Dosages.*** Principal systemic antiviral applications are *chronic hepatitis B* and *chronic hepatitis C.* In patients with chronic hepatitis B, parenteral interferon alfa-2b (5 million IU/day for 4 months) has produced biochemical and histologic improvement in about 40% of recipients. Remissions have been prolonged. In patients with chronic hepatitis C, interferon alfa-2b (2 or 3 million IU 3 times a week for 6 months) has caused biochemical and histologic improvement in about 50% of recipients. Unfortunately, approximately half of responders relapse when treatment is stopped. There is some indication that giving interferon alfa during acute hepatitis C decreases the risk of progression to chronic disease. Additional antiviral applications include *cytomegalovirus, herpes simplex, varicella-zoster, herpes keratoconjunctivitis,* and *condylomata acuminata* (genital warts).

### Ophthalmic Antiviral Agents

### Trifluridine

Trifluridine [Viroptic] is indicated only for topical treatment of ocular infections caused by HSV types 1 and 2. The drug is given to treat acute keratoconjunctivitis and recurrent epithelial keratitis. Antiviral actions result from inhibiting DNA synthesis. The most common side effects are localized burning and sting-

ing. Edema of the eyelid occurs in about 3% of patients. Systemic absorption is minimal following topical administration. Hence, the drug is devoid of systemic toxicity. Trifluridine is dispensed in a 1% ophthalmic solution. Treatment consists of placing 1 drop on the cornea every 2 hours (while the patient is awake) for a maximum of 9 drops/day. Once re-epithelialization of the cornea has occurred, the dosage is reduced to 5 drops/day administered one at a time every 4 hours. Treatment continues for 7 days.

### Vidarabine

Like trifluridine, topical vidarabine [Vira-A] is indicated for acute keratoconjunctivitis and recurrent epithelial keratitis caused by HSV types 1 and 2. Antiviral effects result from inhibition of viral DNA polymerase and from premature termination of the growing viral DNA chain. The most frequent side effects are burning sensations, photophobia, and lacrimation. Absorption of topical vidarabine is insignificant, and systemic toxicity has not been reported. Vidarabine is available in a 3% ointment for application to the eye. About one-half inch of ointment is administered into the lower conjunctival sac five times a day at 3-hour intervals. As a rule, treatment lasts for no more than 3 weeks.

### Idoxuridine

Idoxuridine [Herplex Liquifilm, Stoxil] was the first effective antiviral drug for use in humans. Antiviral effects result from incorporation of a metabolite of idoxuridine into viral DNA. Idoxuridine is indicated only for keratitis caused by type 1 HSV. The drug is inactive against type 2 HSV. Because vidarabine and trifluridine are more effective and less toxic than idoxuridine, these newer agents have largely replaced idoxuridine for treating herpes simplex keratitis. Side effects of idoxuridine include inflammation, itching, photophobia, edema of the eyelid, lacrimal duct occlusion, and punctate defects in the corneal epithelium. Topical application has not been associated with systemic toxicity. Idoxuridine is dispensed in a 0.5% ointment and a 0.1% solution.

## KEY POINTS

- Because viruses use host-cell enzymes and substrates to reproduce, it is difficult to suppress viral reproduction without also harming the host.
- Acyclovir is the drug of choice for infections caused by herpes simplex viruses and varicella-zoster virus.
- Following conversion to its active form, acyclovir suppresses viral reproduction by inhibiting viral DNA polymerase and causing premature termination of viral DNA strand growth. Since the active form of acyclovir is not a good inhibitor of human DNA polymerase, cells of the host are spared.
- In patients with genital herpes infections, oral acyclovir can decrease the duration and severity of the initial episode and the frequency of lesion recurrence.
- Although acyclovir reduces symptoms of genital herpes, the drug does not produce cure (i.e., it does not eliminate the virus) and does not prevent transmission to sexual partners when lesions are present.
- Acyclovir is eliminated unchanged by the kidneys, hence the dosage must be reduced in patients with renal impairment.

- Intravenous acyclovir can injure the kidneys. Renal damage can be minimized by infusing acyclovir slowly and ensuring adequate hydration during and after the infusion.
- Ganciclovir is the drug of choice for prophylaxis and treatment of CMV infection in immunocompromised hosts, including those with AIDS.
- Ganciclovir does not cure CMV retinitis in patients with AIDS, hence treatment must continue for life.
- Like acyclovir, ganciclovir becomes activated within in-

fected cells, after which it inhibits viral DNA polymerase and causes premature termination of viral DNA strand growth.
- Like acyclovir, ganciclovir is excreted unchanged in the urine, hence the dosage must be reduced in patients with renal impairment.
- The major adverse effects of ganciclovir are granulocytopenia and thrombocytopenia.
- Amantadine is used for prophylaxis and treatment of influenza A infections, but not influenza B.

# Summary of Major Nursing Implications*

## Acyclivor

### Preadminstration Assessment

#### Therapeutic Goal
Treatment of infections caused by herpes simplex viruses and varicella-zoster virus.

#### Identifying High-Risk Patients
Use with *caution* in patients who are *dehydrated*, have *renal impairment*, or are taking other *nephrotoxic drugs.*

### Implementation: Administration

#### Routes
Topical, oral, IV.

#### Dosage
Oral and IV dosages must be reduced in patients with renal impairment.

#### Administration
*Topical.* Advise patients to apply the drug with a finger cot or rubber glove to avoid viral transfer to other body sites and other people.

*Oral.* Dosages vary widely for different indications.

*Intravenous.* Give by slow IV infusion (over 1 hour or more). Never administer by IV bolus.

### Implementation: Measures to Enhance Therapeutic Effects
Inform patients with herpes simplex genitalis that acyclovir only decreases symptoms; the drug does not eliminate the virus and does not produce cure. Advise patients to

cleanse the affected area with soap and water three to four times a day, drying thoroughly after each wash. Advise patients to avoid sexual contact while lesions are present.

### Ongoing Evaluation and Interventions

#### Evaluating Therapeutic Effects
Observe for decreased clinical manifestations of herpes simplex and varicella-zoster infection. Virologic testing may also be performed.

#### Minimizing Adverse Effects
*Nephrotoxicity.* Intravenous acyclovir can precipitate in renal tubules, causing reversible kidney damage. To minimize the risk of injury, infuse acyclovir slowly and ensure adequate hydration during the infusion and for 2 hours after. Exercise caution in patients with pre-existing renal impairment and in those who are dehydrated or taking other nephrotoxic drugs.

## Ganciclovir

### Preadministration Assessment

#### Therapeutic Goal
Treatment and prevention of CMV infection in immunocompromised patients, including those with AIDS and those taking immunosuppressive drugs following organ transplantation.

#### Baseline Data
Obtain a complete blood count and platelet count.

#### Identifying High-Risk Patients
Ganciclovir is *contraindicated* during *pregnancy* and for patients with *neutrophil counts below 500/mm³* or *platelet counts below 25,000/mm³.* Use with *caution* in patients taking *zidovudine* or *nephrotoxic drugs* (e.g., amphotericin B, cyclosporine) and in patients with a *history of cytopenic reactions to other drugs.*

---

*Patient education information is highlighted in color.

## Implementation: Administration

### Routes

Oral, IV, intraocular.

### Dosage

Oral and IV dosages must be reduced in patients with renal impairment. AIDS patients with CMV retinitis must take ganciclovir for life.

### Administration

*Intravenous.* Give by slow IV infusion (over 1 hour or more). Ensure adequate hydration to promote renal excretion.

*Oral.* Administer with food.

*Intraocular Implants.* Surgical implants are replaced every 5 to 8 months.

## Ongoing Evaluation and Interventions

### Minimizing Adverse Effects

*Granulocytopenia and Thrombocytopenia.* Ganciclovir suppresses bone marrow function when given IV or PO. Obtain complete blood counts and platelet counts frequently. Discontinue ganciclovir if the neutrophil count falls below 500/mm$^3$ or the platelet count falls below 25,000/mm$^3$. The risk of granulocytopenia can be reduced by giving granulocyte colony-stimulating factors. The risk of granulocytopenia is increased by concurrent therapy with zidovudine (a drug for AIDS).

*Reproductive Toxicity.* In animals, ganciclovir is teratogenic and embryotoxic and suppresses spermatogenesis. Warn female patients against becoming pregnant. Inform males about possible sterility.

# CHAPTER 88

# Antiviral Agents II: Drugs for HIV Infection and Related Opportunistic Infections

Our topic for this chapter is drug therapy of infection with the *human immunodeficiency virus* (HIV), the microbe that causes *acquired immunodeficiency syndrome* (AIDS). HIV promotes immunodeficiency by killing CD4 T lymphocytes (CD4 T cells), which are needed to mount an immune response (see Chapter 62). As a result of immunodeficiency, patients are at risk of opportunistic infections and certain neoplasms.

It is important to understand that HIV infection is not synonymous with AIDS, which develops years after the infection was first acquired. The current definition of AIDS, established by the Centers for Disease Control and Prevention (CDC) in 1993, is a syndrome in which the individual is HIV positive and has either (1) CD4 T cell counts below 200 cells/$\mu$l or (2) an AIDS-defining illness. Included in the CDC's long list of AIDS-defining illnesses are *Pneumocystis carinii* pneumonia, cytomegalovirus retinitis, disseminated histoplasmosis, tuberculosis, and Kaposi's sarcoma.

Since being identified as a new disease in 1981, AIDS has become a global epidemic. In the United States, between 650,000 and 900,000 people are infected. Worldwide, the figure is over 20 million. The cost of caring for AIDS patients is staggering—estimated at $15 billion for 1995 in the United States alone. The personal and social costs are incalculable.

Over the past few years, therapy of HIV infection has made dramatic advances. Notable among these are the development of protease inhibitors and their use in triple-drug therapy. As a result of these advances, we can now decrease plasma HIV to levels that are undetectable with current assays, and can thereby slow loss of immune function, preserve health, and prolong life. However, these benefits do not come without a price: treatment is complex and expensive, poses a risk of toxicity and serious drug interactions, and must continue indefinitely. Accordingly, if treatment is to succeed, patients must be highly motivated and well informed about all aspects of the treatment program.

To date, we do not have a cure for HIV. Although treatment can greatly reduce HIV levels—often rendering the virus undetectable with current technology—discontinuation of treatment has always been associated with a rebound in HIV replication. Whether long-term treatment with triple therapy can actually eradicate HIV is unknown. Because treatment does not eliminate the virus, patients must considered infectious and be warned to avoid behaviors that can transmit HIV to others.

Since understanding this chapter requires a basic understanding of the immune system, you may find it helpful to read Chapter 62 (Review of the Immune System) before proceeding.

# Pathophysiology

## Characteristics of HIV

HIV is a *retrovirus*. Like all other viruses, retroviruses lack the machinery needed for self-replication, and hence are obligate intracellular parasites. However, in contrast to other viruses, retroviruses have positive-sense single-stranded RNA as their genetic material. Accordingly, in order to replicate, retroviruses must first transcribe their RNA into DNA. The enzyme employed for this process is viral *RNA-dependent DNA polymerase*, commonly known as *reverse transcriptase*. (The enzyme is called reverse transcriptase to distinguish it from DNA-dependent RNA polymerase, the host enzyme that transcribes DNA into RNA, which is the usual ["forward"] transcription process.) The name *retrovirus* is derived from the first two letters of *reverse* and *transcriptase*.

There are two types of HIV, referred to as HIV-1 and HIV-2. HIV-1 is found worldwide, whereas HIV-2 is found mainly in West Africa. Although HIV-1 and HIV-2 differ with respect to genetic makeup and antigenicity, they both cause similar disease syndromes. Not all drugs that are effective against HIV-1 are also effective against HIV-2.

### Target Cells

The principal cells attacked by HIV are *CD4 T cells* (helper T lymphocytes). As discussed in Chapter 62, these cells are essential components of the immune system. They are required for production of antibodies by B lymphocytes and for activation of cytolytic T lymphocytes. Accordingly, as HIV kills CD4 T cells, the immune system undergoes progressive decline. As a result of immune decline, infected individuals become increasingly vulnerable to opportunistic infections, the major cause of death among people with AIDS. HIV targets CD4 T cells because the CD4 proteins on the surface of these cells provide points of attachment for HIV (see below); without such a receptor, HIV would be unable to connect with and penetrate these cells. Once HIV has infected a CD4 T cell, the cell dies in about 1.25 days. It is important to appreciate that only a few percent of CD4 T cells circulate in the blood; the vast majority reside in lymph nodes and other lymphoid tissues.

In addition to infecting CD4 T cells, HIV infects *macrophages* and *microglial cells* (the central nervous system counterparts of macrophages), both of which carry CD4 proteins. Since macrophages and microglial cells are resistant to destruction by HIV, they can survive despite being infected. As a result, they serve as a reservoir of HIV during chronic infection.

### Structure of HIV

The structure of HIV, like that of all viruses, is very simple. As shown in Figure 88–1, the major components of the HIV *virion* (i.e., the entire virus particle) are *nucleic acid* (RNA), surrounded by *core proteins*, which in turn are surrounded by a *capsid* (protein shell), which in turn is surrounded by a *lipid bilayer envelope* (derived from the membrane of the host cell).

The central core contains two separate but identical single strands of RNA, each with its own molecule of reverse transcriptase attached. The RNA serves as the template for DNA synthesis.

The outer envelope of HIV contains *glycoproteins* that are needed for attachment to host cells. Each glycoprotein consists of two subunits, known as *gp 41* and *gp 120*. The smaller protein (gp 41) is embedded in the lipid bilayer of the viral envelope; the larger protein (gp 120) is connected firmly to gp 41. (The numbers 41 and 120 simply indicate the mass of these glycoproteins in thousands of daltons.)

## Replication Cycle of HIV

The replication cycle of HIV is depicted in Figure 88–2. The numbers below correspond to the steps in the figure.

- *Step 1.* The cycle begins with attachment of HIV to the host cell. The primary connection takes place between *gp120* on the HIV envelope and a *CD4 protein* on the host cell membrane. Several other host proteins act in concert with CD4 to tighten the bond with HIV. Two of these co-receptors—known as CCR5 and CXCR4—are of particular importance.
- In *step 2*, the lipid bilayer envelope of HIV fuses with the lipid bilayer of the host cell membrane. Fusion is followed by release of HIV RNA into the host cell.
- In *step 3*, HIV RNA is transcribed into single-stranded DNA by HIV *reverse transcriptase*. This enzyme is the target of several important drugs.
- In *step 4*, reverse transcriptase converts the single strand of HIV DNA into double-stranded HIV DNA.
- In *step 5*, the double-stranded HIV DNA becomes integrated into the host's DNA.
- In *step 6*, the HIV DNA undergoes transcription into RNA. Some of the resulting RNA becomes the genome for daughter HIV virions (step 6a). The rest of the RNA is messenger RNA that codes HIV proteins (step 6b).
- In *step 7*, messenger RNA is translated into HIV glycoproteins (step 7a) and HIV enzymes and structural proteins (step 7b).
- In *step 8*, the components of HIV migrate to the cell surface and assemble into a new virus. Prior to virus assembly, HIV glycoproteins become incorporated into the host cell membrane (step 8a). In steps 8b and 8c, the other components of the virion migrate to the cell surface, where they undergo assembly into the new virus.
- In *step 9*, the newly formed virus buds off from the host cell. As indicated, the outer envelope of the virion is derived from the cell membrane of the host.
- In *step 10*, which occurs either during or immediately after budding off, HIV undergoes final maturation under the influence of *protease*, an enzyme that cleaves certain large polyproteins into their smaller, functional forms. If protease fails to

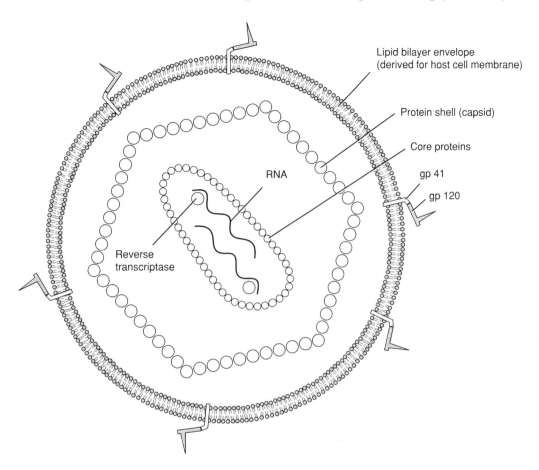

**Figure 88–1. Structure of the human immunodeficiency virus.** gp41 = glycoprotein 41, gp120 = glycoprotein 120. Note that HIV has two single strands of RNA, and that each strand is associated with a molecule of reverse transcriptase.

cleave these proteins, HIV will remain immature and noninfectious.

## Replication Rate

HIV replicates rapidly during *all* stages of the infection. During the initial phase of infection, replication is massive. This is because (1) the population of CD4 cells is still large, thereby providing a large breeding ground for the virus, and (2) the host has not yet mounted an immune response against HIV, hence replication can proceed unopposed. As a result of massive replication, plasma levels of HIV can exceed 10 million virions/ml. During this stage of high viral load, patients often experience an *acute retroviral syndrome* (see below).

Over the next few months, as the immune system begins to attack HIV, plasma levels of HIV undergo a sharp decline and then level off. A typical steady-state level is between 1000 and 100,000 virions/ml. Please note, however, that steady state numbers can be deceptive. The plasma half-life of HIV is only 6 hours; that is, every 6 hours, half of the HIV virions in plasma are lost. Accordingly, in order to maintain the steady state levels typically seen during chronic HIV infection, the actual rate of *replication* is between 1 and 10 *billion* virions/day. Despite this high rate of ongoing replication, infected in-

dividuals may remain asymptomatic for about 10 years, after which symptoms of advanced HIV disease appear.

## Mutation and Drug Resistance

HIV mutates rapidly. The reason is that HIV reverse transcriptase is an error-prone enzyme. Hence, whenever the enzyme transcribes HIV RNA into single-stranded DNA and then into double-stranded DNA, there is a high probability of introducing base-pair errors. In fact, according to one estimate, up to 10 incorrect bases may be incorporated into HIV DNA during each round of replication. Because of these errors, HIV can rapidly mutate from a drug-sensitive form into a drug-resistant form. The probability of developing drug resistance in the individual patient is directly related to the total viral load. That is, the more virions the patient harbors, the greater the likelihood that at least one will become drug resistant. To minimize the emergence of drug resistance, patients should be treated with a combination of antiretroviral drugs. This is the same strategy we employ to prevent emergence of resistance when treating tuberculosis (see Chapter 84).

## Transmission of HIV

HIV is transmitted sexually and by other means. The virus is present in all body fluids of infected individuals.

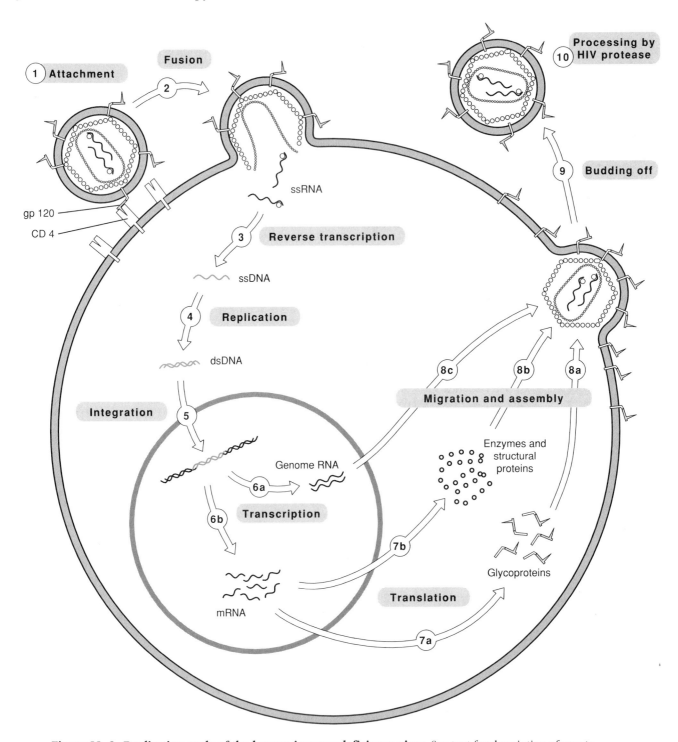

**Figure 88–2. Replication cycle of the human immunodeficiency virus.** See text for description of events. ssRNA = single-stranded RNA, ssDNA = single-stranded DNA, dsDNA = double-stranded DNA, mRNA = messenger RNA.

Transmission can be via intimate contact with semen, vaginal secretions, and blood. The disease can be transmitted by sexual contact, transfusion, sharing IV needles, and accidental needle sticks. In addition, it can be transmitted to the fetus by an infected mother, usually during the perinatal period. Initially, HIV infection was limited largely to homosexual males, injection drug users, and hemophiliacs. However, the disease can now be found routinely in the population at large. The risk of contract-

ing HIV can be greatly reduced by use of condoms and by screening blood supplies for HIV.

## Clinical Course of HIV Infection

HIV infection follows a triphasic clinical course. During the initial phase, HIV undergoes massive replication, causing blood levels of HIV to rise very high. As a result, between 50% and 90% of patients experience a flu-like *acute*

- Fever
- Lymphadenopathy
- Pharyngitis
- Rash–Erythematous maculopapular rash with lesions on face and trunk and sometimes extremities, including palm and soles
- Mucocutaneous ulceration involving mouth, esophagus, or genitals
- Myalgia or arthralgia
- Diarrhea
- Headache
- Nausea and vomiting
- Hepatosplenomegaly
- Thrush
- Weight loss
- Neurologic symptoms
  Meningoencephalitis or aseptic meningitis
  Peripheral neuropathy or radiculopathy
  Facial palsy
  Guillain-Barré neuritis
  Brachial neuritis
  Cognitive impairment or psychosis

*retroviral syndrome.* Signs and symptoms include fever, lymphadenopathy, pharyngitis, rash, myalgia, and headache (see Table 88-1). Soon, however, the immune system mounts a counterattack, causing HIV levels to fall. As a result, symptoms of the acute syndrome fade. Very often, the acute retroviral syndrome is perceived as influenza, and hence goes unrecognized for what it really is.

The middle phase of HIV infection is characterized by prolonged *clinical latency.* Blood levels of HIV remain relatively low, and most patients are asymptomatic. How-

ever, as noted above, HIV continues to replicate despite apparent dormancy. Because of persistent HIV replication, CD4 T cells undergo progressive decline. The average duration of clinical latency is 10 years.

During the late phase of HIV infection, CD4 T cells drop below a critical level (200 cells/µl), rendering the patient highly vulnerable to opportunistic infections and certain neoplasms (e.g., Kaposi's sarcoma).

Many patients with HIV infection experience neurologic complications. Both the peripheral and central nervous systems may be involved. *Peripheral neuropathies* affect 20% to 40% of patients and may develop at any time in the course of HIV infection. In contrast, *CNS complications* usually occur late in the disease. Symptoms of CNS injury include decreased cognition, reduced concentration, memory loss, mental slowness, and motor complaints (e.g., ataxia, tremors). Neuronal injury may be the direct result of HIV infection or may develop secondary to an opportunistic CNS infection.

# Classification of Antiretroviral Drugs

At this time, we have two major classes of antiretroviral drugs: *reverse transcriptase inhibitors* and *protease inhibitors.* The reverse transcriptase inhibitors are subdivided into (1) agents that are structural analogs of nucleosides, referred to as *nucleoside reverse transcriptase inhibitors* and (2) agents that are not analogs of nucleosides, referred to as *non-nucleoside reverse transcriptase inhibitors.* Drugs that belong to these classes are listed in Table 88-2. All antiretroviral drugs are administered orally.

**TABLE 88-2. CLASSIFICATION OF ANTIRETROVIRAL DRUGS**

| Generic Name | Trade Name | Chemical Name/Abbreviation |
|---|---|---|
| *Nucleoside Reverse Transcriptase Inhibitors* | | |
| Didanosine | Videx | Dideoxyinosine, ddI |
| Lamivudine | Epivir | 3TC |
| Stavudine | Zerit | d4T |
| Zalcitabine | Hivid | Dideoxycytidine, ddC |
| Zidovudine | Retrovir | Azidothymidine, AZT, ZDV |
| *Non-nucleoside Reverse Transcriptase Inhibitors* | | |
| Delavirdine | Rescriptor | |
| Nevirapine | Viramune | |
| *Protease Inhibitors* | | |
| Indinavir | Crixivan | |
| Nelfinavir | Viracept | |
| Ritonavir | Norvir | |
| Saquinavir | Invirase | |

# Nucleoside Reverse Transcriptase Inhibitors

The nucleoside reverse transcriptase inhibitors (NRTIs) were the first drugs used against HIV infection and remain mainstays of treatment. As their name suggests, the NRTIs are chemical relatives of naturally occurring nucleosides, the building blocks of DNA. Antiretroviral effects derive from suppressing synthesis of viral DNA by reverse transcriptase. In order to be effective, all of the NRTIs must first undergo intracellular conversion to their active (triphosphate) forms. At this time, five NRTIs are approved for general use. Major properties of these drugs are summarized in Table 88-3.

## Zidovudine

Zidovudine [Retrovir] was the first NRTI available and will serve as our prototype for the group. The drug is an analog of thymidine, a naturally occurring nucleoside. When employed in combination with other antiretroviral drugs, zidovudine can decrease viral load, increase CD4 T cell counts, delay onset of disease symptoms, and reduce symptom severity. The drug's principal dose-limiting toxicities are *severe anemia* and *neutropenia*. Abbreviations for this agent are ZDV (for zidovudine) and AZT (for azidothymidine, its original name).

## Mechanism of Antiviral Action

Zidovudine inhibits HIV replication by suppressing synthesis of viral DNA. To do this, zidovudine must first undergo intracellular conversion to its active form, zidovudine triphosphate (ZTP). In the form of ZTP, the drug acts as a substrate for reverse transcriptase. However, when ZTP becomes incorporated into the growing DNA strand, it prevents reverse transcriptase from adding more bases; hence, further growth of the strand is blocked. In addition to causing premature strand termination, ZTP competes with natural nucleoside triphosphates for binding to the active site of reverse transcriptase; the result is competitive inhibition of the enzyme.

## Therapeutic Use

Zidovudine is indicated for HIV infection. This agent penetrates to the CNS better than most antiretroviral drugs, and hence can be especially valuable for relieving cognitive symptoms. Because monotherapy with any antiretroviral drug can rapidly lead to resistance, zidovudine should always be combined with at least one other antiretroviral agent. The role of zidovudine and other agents in the management of HIV infection is discussed at length later in the chapter.

### Pharmacokinetics

Zidovudine is readily absorbed following oral administration and distributes to all body tissues, including the CNS. After entering the blood, some of the drug is taken up by cells and converted to ZTP, the active form. The remainder undergoes rapid

## TABLE 88-3. PROPERTIES OF NUCLEOSIDE REVERSE TRANSCRIPTASE INHIBITORS

| | Zidovudine (AZT, ZDV) | Didanosine (ddI) | Zalcitabine (ddC) | Stavudine (d4T) | Lamivudine (3TC) |
|---|---|---|---|---|---|
| **Trade name** | Retrovir | Videx | Hivid | Zerit | Epivir |
| **Dosage** | 300 mg bid | >60 kg: 200 mg bid<br><60 kg: 125 mg bid | 0.75 mg tid | >60 kg: 40 mg bid<br><60 kg: 30 mg bid | 150 mg bid |
| **Bioavailability** | 60% | Tablet: 40%<br>Powder: 30% | 85% | 86% | 86% |
| **Serum half-life** | 1.1 hr | 1.6 hr | 1.2 hr | 1.0 hr | 3–6 hr |
| **Intracellular half-life** | 3 hr | 12 hr | 3 hr | 3.5 hr | 12 hr |
| **Elimination** | Hepatic metabolism followed by renal excretion | Partial metabolism followed by renal excretion | Partial metabolism followed by renal excretion | Partial metabolism followed by renal excretion | Renal excretion (unchanged) |
| **Major toxicity** | • Bone marrow depression: anemia, neutropenia<br>• GI intolerance<br>• Headache<br>• Insomnia<br>• Myopathy | • Pancreatitis<br>• Peripheral neuropathy<br>• GI: nausea, diarrhea | • Peripheral neuropathy<br>• Pancreatitis (rarely)<br>• Stomatitis | • Peripheral neuropathy<br>• Pancreatitis (rarely) | • Minimal toxicity |

Adapted from *Guidelines for the Use of Antiretroviral Agents in HIV-Infected Adults and Adolescents*, prepared by the Panel on Clinical Practices for Treatment of HIV Infection convened by the Department of Health and Human Services and the Henry J. Kaiser Family Foundation, 1997.

hepatic conversion to an inactive metabolite. Both zidovudine and its inactive metabolite are eliminated by renal excretion. The *plasma* half-life of the drug is approximately 1 hour. The *intracellular* half-life is 3 hours.

## Adverse Effects

*Anemia and Neutropenia.* Severe anemia and neutropenia are zidovudine's principal toxic effects. Multiple transfusions may be required. The risk of hematologic toxicity is increased by high-dose therapy, advanced HIV infection, deficiencies in vitamin $B_{12}$ and folic acid, and concurrent use of drugs that are myelosuppressive, nephrotoxic, or directly toxic to circulating blood cells. Anemia and neutropenia generally resolve following zidovudine withdrawal.

Hematologic status (hemoglobin concentration and neutrophil counts) should be determined before treatment and at least every 4 weeks thereafter. Hemoglobin levels may fall significantly within 2 to 4 weeks; neutrophil counts may not fall until after week 6. For patients who develop severe anemia (hemoglobin <5 gm/dl or down 25% from the pretreatment baseline) or severe neutropenia (neutrophil count <750 cells/μl or down 50% from the pretreatment baseline), zidovudine should be interrupted until there is evidence of bone marrow recovery. If neutropenia and anemia are less severe, a reduction in dosage may be sufficient. Transfusions may permit some patients to continue drug use.

*Granulocyte colony-stimulating factors* may be given to reverse zidovudine-induced neutropenia. Also, if erythropoietin levels are not already elevated, *epoetin alfa* (recombinant erythropoietin) can be given to reduce transfusion requirements in patients with anemia. Granulocyte colony-stimulating factors and epoetin alfa are discussed in Chapter 52.

*Other Adverse Effects.* *Gastrointestinal effects* (anorexia, nausea, vomiting, diarrhea, abdominal pain, stomach upset) occur on occasion. Possible *CNS reactions* include headache, insomnia, confusion, anxiety, nervousness, and seizures. *Myopathy* (damage to muscle fibers) may also occur.

## Drug Interactions

Drugs that are myelosuppressive, nephrotoxic, or directly toxic to circulating blood cells can increase the risk of zidovudine-induced hematologic toxicity. Notable among these drugs is *ganciclovir*, an antiviral agent used to treat cytomegalovirus retinitis, a common infection in patients with AIDS. Other drugs of concern include *dapsone*, *pentamidine*, *pyrimethamine*, *trimethoprim-sulfamethoxazole*, *amphotericin B*, *flucytosine*, *vincristine*, *vinblastine*, and *doxorubicin*.

### Preparations, Dosage, and Administration

*Preparations.* Zidovudine [Retrovir] is available in capsules (100 mg), tablets (300 mg), and a syrup (10 mg/ml) for oral therapy and in solution (10 mg/ml) for IV use.

*Oral Therapy.* The recommended dosage is 300 mg twice a day or 200 mg 3 times a day. The dosage for treating CNS effects (cognitive slowing, motor slowing, dementia) is 1200 mg/day (i.e., twice the normal dosage).

Hematologic monitoring should be done every 2 weeks. If severe anemia or severe neutropenia develops, treatment should be interrupted until there is evidence of bone marrow recovery. If anemia or neutropenia is mild, a reduction in dosage may be sufficient.

*Intravenous Therapy.* Intravenous zidovudine is indicated for adults with AIDS who have a history of cytologically confirmed *Pneumocystis carinii* pneumonia or a CD4 T cell count below 200 cells/μl. The IV dosage is 1 to 2 mg/kg (infused over 1 hour) every 4 hours around the clock. Rapid infusion and bolus injection must be avoided. Intravenous therapy should be stopped as soon as oral therapy is appropriate.

Intravenous solutions are prepared by withdrawing the calculated dose from the stock vial and diluting it to 4 mg/ml (or less) in 5% dextrose for injection. The solution should not be mixed with biologic or colloidal fluids (e.g., blood products, protein solutions) and should be administered within 8 hours (if held at room temperature) or within 24 hours (if held under refrigeration).

### Didanosine

*Actions and Uses.* Didanosine [Videx], also known as dideoxyinosine (ddI), is an analog of inosine, a naturally occurring nucleoside. The drug is taken up by host cells where it undergoes conversion to its active form, dideoxyadenosine triphosphate (ddATP). Like the active form of zidovudine, ddATP suppresses viral replication primarily by causing premature termination of the growing DNA strand. In addition, it competes with natural nucleoside triphosphates for binding to the active center of reverse transcriptase, and thereby further suppresses DNA synthesis. In clinical trials, didanosine increased CD4 T cell counts, decreased viremia, and reduced symptoms in patients with AIDS.

Didanosine is approved only for HIV infection. Because monotherapy with any antiretroviral drug can rapidly lead to resistance, didanosine should always be used in combination with at least one other antiretroviral agent.

*Pharmacokinetics.* Didanosine is administered orally and bioavailability is low (about 35%). Absorption is greatly reduced by food and gastric acidity. To decrease gastric acidity, and thereby enhance absorption, didanosine is formulated with buffering agents. Didanosine crosses the blood-brain barrier poorly; levels in cerebrospinal fluid are only 20% of those in plasma. Much of the drug (35% to 60%) is excreted unchanged in the urine. The plasma half-life in patients with normal renal function is 1.6 hours, but is three times longer in patients with renal failure. The intracellular half-life is 12 hours.

*Adverse Effects.* *Pancreatitis*, which can be fatal, is the major dose-limiting toxicity. The incidence is 3% to 17%. Patients should be monitored for indications of developing pancreatitis (increased serum amylase in association with increased serum triglycerides, decreased serum calcium, and nausea, vomiting, or abdominal pain). If evolving pancreatitis is diagnosed, didanosine should be withdrawn. The risk of pancreatitis is increased by a history of pancreatitis or alcoholism and by use of intravenous pentamidine. Caution should be exercised with these patients. Additional adverse effects include *diarrhea* (28%), *peripheral neuropathy* (20%), *chills or fever* (12%), and *rash or pruritus* (9%). In contrast to zidovudine, didanosine causes minimal bone marrow suppression.

*Drug Interactions.* Like didanosine, *zalcitabine* and *stavudine* both cause peripheral neuropathy and pancreatitis. Accordingly, any combination of these agents should be used with great caution, if at all.

*Preparations, Dosage, and Administration.* Didanosine [Videx] is available in three formulations: chewable buffered tablets

(25, 50, 100, and 150 mg), buffered powder for oral solution (100, 167, 250, and 375 mg in single-dose packets), and pediatric powder for oral solution (in 2-gm and 4-gm bottles). Bioavailability of the tablets is about 20% greater than that of the oral solution. Since absorption is greatly reduced by food, administration should be done 1 hour before meals or 2 hours after. Instruct patients using the tablets to either (1) chew them thoroughly, or (2) manually crush or disperse them in at least 1 ounce of water. Instruct patients using powdered didanosine to (1) pour the contents of one packet into 4 ounces of water (not fruit juice or any other acid-containing beverage); (2) stir the mixture until the drug dissolves (about 2 to 3 minutes); and (3) drink the solution immediately.

Dosage is based on body weight. For adults over 60 kg, the dosage is 200 mg twice daily. For adults under 60 kg, the dosage is 125 mg twice daily. Dosages should be reduced in patients with renal impairment. To ensure adequate buffering of gastric acid, patients using didanosine tablets must take two tablets (of appropriate size) for each dose.

### Zalcitabine

***Actions and Uses.*** Zalcitabine [Hivid], also known as dideoxycytidine (ddC), is an analog of cytidine, a naturally occurring nucleoside. Zalcitabine is a prodrug that undergoes conversion to its active form (ddC triphosphate) within host cells. The active form inhibits viral DNA synthesis by (1) causing premature termination of the growing DNA strand and (2) competing with natural nucleoside triphosphates for binding to reverse transcriptase. Toxicity of zalcitabine results in part from inhibiting mitochondrial DNA polymerase in host cells.

Zalcitabine is approved only for HIV infection. Like all other drugs used to treat HIV, zalcitabine should be used in combination with at least one other antiretroviral drug so as to reduce the risk of resistance.

***Pharmacokinetics.*** Zalcitabine is administered orally and bioavailability is 85%. Food delays absorption and reduces the amount absorbed by 14%. The drug crosses the blood-brain barrier poorly; levels in cerebrospinal fluid are only 20% of those in blood. Elimination is primarily by renal excretion; hepatic metabolism is minimal. The plasma half-life is 1.2 hours. The intracellular half-life is 3 hours.

***Adverse Effects.*** *Peripheral neuropathy*, which develops in 10% to 30% of patients, manifests initially as numbness and burning sensations in the extremities. These symptoms may progress to sharp shooting pain and severe continuous burning if the drug is not withdrawn. Pain of severe neuropathy requires opioid (narcotic) analgesics for control. Patients should be informed about the early symptoms of neuropathy and instructed to report them immediately. Neuropathy reverses slowly if zalcitabine is withdrawn early, but may become irreversible if the drug is continued.

*Pancreatitis* from zalcitabine is uncommon (<1% incidence), but can be fatal. Patients should be monitored for indications of impending pancreatitis (rising serum amylase in association with rising serum triglycerides, decreasing serum calcium, and nausea, vomiting, or abdominal pain). If evolving pancreatitis is diagnosed, zalcitabine should be withdrawn. Caution is required in patients with a history of pancreatitis or alcoholism and in those receiving intravenous pentamidine.

Severe *stomatitis* (oral ulcers) occurred in 3% of patients in two clinical trials. In other trials, the incidence was even higher but the severity was lower.

***Drug Interactions.*** Like zalcitabine, *didanosine* and *stavudine* both cause peripheral neuropathy and pancreatitis. Accordingly, any combination of these agents should be used with great caution, if at all. *Alcohol* and *intravenous pentamidine* increase the risk of pancreatitis.

***Preparations, Dosage, and Administration.*** Zalcitabine [Hivid] is available in tablets (0.375 and 0.75 mg) for oral administration. The recommended dosage is 0.75 mg every 8 hours.

### Stavudine

***Actions and Uses.*** Stavudine [Zerit], also known as d4T, is an analog of thymidine, a naturally occurring nucleoside. Following uptake by cells, stavudine is converted to its active form, stavudine triphosphate. The active drug then suppresses HIV replication by (1) causing premature termination of the growing DNA strand and (2) competing with natural nucleoside triphosphates for binding to reverse transcriptase.

Stavudine is approved only for HIV infection. Like all other drugs used against HIV, stavudine should be combined with at least one other antiretroviral agent to decrease the risk of resistance.

***Pharmacokinetics.*** Stavudine is administered orally and bioavailability is 86%. Food has little or no effect on absorption. Penetration to the CNS is good. Elimination is by a combination of hepatic metabolism and renal excretion. The plasma half-life is 1.0 hours. The intracellular half-life is 3.5 hours.

***Adverse Effects.*** Like didanosine and zalcitabine, stavudine causes *peripheral neuropathy*. In clinical trials, neuropathy developed in 15% to 21% of patients. Patients should be informed about early symptoms of neuropathy (numbness, tingling, or pain in hands and feet) and instructed to report them immediately. Neuropathy may resolve if the drug is withdrawn. If symptoms resolve completely, resumption of treatment may be considered, but the dosage should be reduced.

Stavudine can cause *pancreatitis*. Although the incidence is low (1%), pancreatitis can be fatal. Patients should be monitored for indications of pancreatitis, and if evolving pancreatitis is diagnosed, stavudine should be withdrawn.

***Drug Interactions.*** Like stavudine, *didanosine* and *zalcitabine* both cause peripheral neuropathy and pancreatitis. Accordingly, any combination of these agents should be used with great caution, if at all.

***Preparations, Dosage, and Administration.*** Stavudine [Zerit] is available in capsules (15, 20, 30, and 40 mg) for oral administration. The recommended dosage is 40 mg twice a day (for patients >60 kg) and 30 mg twice a day (for patients <60 kg). Stavudine may be administered with or without food.

### Lamivudine

Lamivudine [Epivir], also known as 3TC, is an analog of cytidine, a naturally occurring nucleoside. Following uptake by cells, the drug is converted to its active form, lamivudine triphosphate, which then suppresses HIV replication by (1) causing premature termination of the growing DNA strand and (2) competing with natural nucleoside triphosphates for binding to reverse transcriptase.

Lamivudine is approved only for HIV infection. Like all other drugs used against HIV, lamivudine should be combined with at least one other antiretroviral agent so as to decrease the risk of resistance.

Lamivudine is administered orally and bioavailability is high (86%). Food slows the rate of absorption but does not decrease the extent. The drug is eliminated intact in the urine. The plasma half-life is 3 to 6 hours and the intracellular half-life is 12 hours.

Side effects of lamivudine are minimal. Some patients experience insomnia and headache, but these usually fade in a few weeks.

Lamivudine is available in 150-mg tablets and a 10 mg/ml oral solution. The usual adult dosage is 150 mg twice daily. The pediatric dosage is 4 mg/kg twice daily. In patients with renal dysfunction, dosages should be reduced. Lamivudine may be administered with or without food.

# Non-nucleoside Reverse Transcriptase Inhibitors

The non-nucleoside reverse transcriptase inhibitors (NNRTIs) differ from the NRTIs in structure and mechanism of action. As their name suggests, the NNRTIs are not structurally related to naturally occurring nucleosides—and, in contrast to the NRTIs, which inhibit synthesis of HIV DNA primarily by causing premature termination of the growing DNA strand, the NNRTIs bind to active center of reverse transcriptase, and thereby cause direct inhibition. In addition, whereas NRTIs must undergo intracellular conversion to their active forms, the NNRTIs are active as administered. At this time, two NNRTIs are available: nevirapine [Viramune] and delavirdine [Rescriptor]. The principal adverse effect of both drugs is rash, which is sometimes severe. Pharmacologic properties of these drugs are summarized in Table 88–4.

## Nevirapine

*Mechanism of Action.* Nevirapine [Viramune] binds directly to HIV reverse transcriptase and thereby disrupts the active center of the enzyme. As a result, enzyme activity is suppressed. Nevirapine only inhibits reverse transcriptase of HIV-1; the drug not inhibit the reverse transcriptase of HIV-2. In addition, nevirapine does not inhibit human DNA polymerase, and hence is harmless to us.

*Pharmacokinetics.* Nevirapine is well absorbed (90%) following oral administration, both in the presence and absence of food. The drug is very lipid soluble, and hence can cross both the placenta and blood-brain barrier and can enter breast milk with ease. Concentrations achieved in cerebrospinal fluid are about 45% of those in plasma. Elimination of nevirapine is the result of hepatic metabolism followed by excretion in the urine (80%) and feces.

*Resistance.* Resistance to nevirapine develops rapidly if the drug is used alone. Accordingly, nevirapine should always be combined with other antiretroviral drugs.

*Therapeutic Use.* Nevirapine is approved only for treating infection with HIV-1; the drug is not active against HIV-2. To reduce the risk of resistance, nevirapine should never be used alone. Rather it should always be combined with at least one other antiretroviral drug, and preferably with two.

*Adverse Effects.* The most common adverse effect is *rash*, which usually occurs early in therapy and can be severe or even life-threatening. For most patients, the rash is benign, and, if needed, can be managed with an antihistamine or topical glucocorticoid. However, if the patient experiences severe rash or rash associated with fever, blistering, oral lesions, conjunctivitis, muscle pain, or joint pain, nevirapine should be withdrawn, since these symp-

## TABLE 88-4. PROPERTIES OF NON-NUCLEOSIDE REVERSE TRANSCRIPTASE INHIBITORS

| | **Nevirapine** | **Delavirdine** |
|---|---|---|
| **Trade name** | Viramune | Rescriptor |
| **Dosage** | 200 mg once a day for 14 days, then 200 mg twice a day | 400 mg tid (mix four 100-mg tabs in 3 or more ounces of water to produce a slurry) |
| **Bioavailability** | >90% | 85% |
| **Serum half-life** | 25–30 hr | 5.6 hr |
| **Elimination** | Metabolized by P-450, followed by excretion in urine (80%) and feces | Metabolized by P-450, followed by excretion in urine (51%) and feces |
| **Major toxicity** | Rash | Rash |
| **Drug interactions** | • *Induces* P-450 and may thereby *decrease* levels of other drugs; effects on protease inhibitors and oral contraceptives are of particular concern<br>• Rifampin and rifabutin also induce P-450, and may thereby decrease levels of nevirapine | • *Inhibits* P-450 and may thereby *increase* levels of other drugs<br>• Because of P-450 inhibition, the following drugs are *contraindicated*: astemizole, terfenadine, alprazolam, midazolam, triazolam, and cisapride<br>• Because of P-450 inhibition, the following drugs should be used with *caution*: indinavir, saquinavir, clarithromycin, dapsone, ergot alkaloids, dihydropyridine calcium channel blockers, quinidine, and warfarin<br>• Antacids and didanosine decrease absorption of delavirdine; do not administer within 1 hr of delavirdine |

toms may indicate the patient is developing *erythema multiforme* or *Stevens-Johnson syndrome*. Rash can be minimized by using a low dosage initially and then increasing the dosage if no rash occurs.

**Drug Interactions.** Nevirapine induces the activity of hepatic cytochrome P-450 drug-metabolizing enzymes, and can thereby increase the metabolism of other drugs, causing their levels to decline. The ability to decrease levels of *protease inhibitors* and *oral contraceptives* is of particular concern. Like nevirapine, *rifampin* and *rifabutin* can also induce cytochrome P-450; hence, combining these agents with nevirapine could greatly accelerate drug metabolism.

**Preparations, Dosage, and Administration.** Nevirapine [Viramune] is available in 200-mg tablets for oral administration. The initial dosage is 200 mg once a day for 14 days. If no rash develops, the dosage is increased to 200 mg twice a day.

### Delavirdine

**Actions, Resistance, and Use.** Delavirdine [Rescriptor] is similar to nevirapine in actions and uses. Like nevirapine, delavirdine is a non-nucleoside that acts directly to inhibit reverse transcriptase, thereby suppressing HIV replication. Because resistant forms of HIV rapidly emerge when delavirdine is used alone, the drug should always be combined with at least one other antiretroviral agent. Like nevirapine, delavirdine is active only against HIV-1.

**Adverse Effects.** Like nevirapine, delavirdine causes potentially serious *rash*. In clinical trials, rash developed in up to 50% of patients; erythema multiforme and Stevens-Johnson syndrome have been reported. If severe rash develops, the drug should be withdrawn. Other common side effects include headache, fatigue, GI intolerance (nausea, vomiting, diarrhea), and elevation of liver enzymes.

**Drug Interactions.** In contrast to nevirapine, which induces cytochrome P-450, delavirdine *inhibits* cytochrome P-450. As a result, levels of drugs taken concurrently may rise. To avoid toxicity from excessive drug levels, patients taking delavirdine should not take astemizole, terfenadine, alprazolam, midazolam, triazolam, or cisapride. Other drugs whose levels may be increased include indinavir, saquinavir, clarithromycin, dapsone, warfarin, quinidine, ergot alkaloids, and the dihydropyridine-type calcium channel blockers; all of these agents should be used with caution. Drugs that induce P-450 (e.g., rifampin, rifabutin, phenytoin, phenobarbital, carbamazepine) may decrease levels of delavirdine, and may thereby reduce its efficacy. Antacids and didanosine can decrease levels of delavirdine; accordingly, at least 1 hour should separate administration of delavirdine and administration of these drugs.

**Preparations, Dosage, and Administration.** Delavirdine [Rescriptor] is available in 100-mg tablets for oral administration. The recommended dosage is 400 mg (4 tablets) 3 times a day, taken with or without food. Patients who are unable to swallow the tablets whole can mix them with water (at least 3 ounces) and swallow the resulting suspension. Acidity enhances absorption. Accordingly, patients with achlorhydria (lack of stomach acid) should administer delavirdine with an acidic beverage (e.g., orange juice, cranberry juice).

## Protease Inhibitors

The protease inhibitors are the most effective antiretroviral drugs available. When used in combination with re-

verse transcriptase inhibitors, these agents can reduce viral load to a level that is undetectable by current assays. As a rule, adverse effects of the protease inhibitors are moderate and relatively easy to manage. In contrast, since all of the available agents inhibit cytochrome P-450, managing drug interactions can be a challenge.

As with other antiretroviral drugs, HIV resistance can be a significant problem. Mutant strains of HIV that are resistant to one protease inhibitor are likely to be cross-resistant with other protease inhibitors. In contrast, since protease inhibitors do not share the same mechanism as the reverse transcriptase inhibitors, cross-resistance between protease inhibitors and reverse transcriptase inhibitors is unlikely. To reduce the risk of resistance, protease inhibitors should never be used alone; rather, they should always be combined with at least one reverse transcriptase inhibitor, and preferably two.

Four protease inhibitors are now approved for general use. To date, studies comparing these drugs have not been conducted. Accordingly, selection among them cannot be based on relative efficacy. Until data on relative efficacy are available, drug selection can be based on side-effect profiles, drug interactions, and patient acceptance. The major properties of the protease inhibitors are summarized in Table 88–5.

### Saquinavir

Saquinavir [Invirase] was the first protease inhibitor to receive FDA approval and will serve as our prototype for the group. In the test tube, saquinavir appears more potent than the other protease inhibitors. However, because of low bioavailability of the current formulation (hard gelatin capsule), saquinavir is much less effective than the other protease inhibitors *in vivo*. A new formulation with improved bioavailability should be available soon. However, until the new formulation is released, saquinavir should be considered a second-choice drug.

**Mechanism of Action.** To understand the effects of saquinavir and the other protease inhibitors, we must first understand the function of HIV protease. As noted above, protease catalyzes the final step in HIV maturation. When the various enzymes and structural proteins of HIV are synthesized, they are not produced as separate entities; rather, they are strung together in large polyproteins. The role of protease is to cleave bonds in the polyproteins, thereby freeing the individual enzymes and structural proteins. Once these components have been freed, HIV can complete its maturation.

Protease inhibitors bind to the active site of HIV protease and thereby prevent the enzyme from cleaving HIV polyproteins. As a result, the structural proteins and enzymes of HIV are unable to function, and hence the virus remains immature and noninfectious.

**Pharmacokinetics.** Saquinavir is administered orally and *bioavailability is low*. Low bioavailability appears to result from a combination of poor absorption and extensive first-pass metabolism. With the current formulation, only 4% of each dose reaches the systemic circulation. Food increases bioavailability, and hence saquinavir

## TABLE 88-5. PROPERTIES OF PROTEASE INHIBITORS

| | Indinavir | Ritonavir | Saquinavir | Nelfinavir |
|---|---|---|---|---|
| **Trade name** | Crixivan | Norvir | Invirase | Viracept |
| **Maintenance dosage** | 800 mg q 8 h | 600 mg q 12 h | 600 mg q 8 h | 750 mg q 8 h |
| **Administration** | Take 1 hour before meals or 2 hours after; may take with skim milk or a low-fat meal | Take with food | Take with a high-fat meal | Take with food |
| **Storage** | Room temperature, protected from moisture | Refrigerate | Room temperature | Room temperature |
| **Bioavailability** | 30% | Adequate | Hard gelatin capsule: low (4%) and erratic | 20%–80% |
| **Plasma half-life** | 1.5–2 hr | 3–5 hr | 1–2 hr | 3.5–5 hr |
| **Adverse effects** | • Nephrolithiasis<br>• GI intolerance<br>• Misc.: headache, asthenia, blurred vision, dizziness, rash, metallic taste, thrombocytopenia | • GI: nausea, vomiting, diarrhea<br>• Paresthesias (circumoral and peripheral)<br>• Asthenia (weakness)<br>• Taste perversion | • Very well tolerated; nausea, diarrhea, and headache occur rarely | • GI: diarrhea |
| **Drug interactions** | • Inhibits P-450 (but less than ritonavir does)<br>• Because of P-450 inhibition, do not combine with astemizole, terfenadine, cisapride, triazolam, midazolam, or ergot alkaloids<br>• Indinavir levels reduced by rifampin and rifabutin<br>• Indinavir levels increased by ketoconazole<br>• Absorption reduced by didanosine, unless taken at least 1 hr apart | • Inhibits P-450 powerfully<br>• P-450 inhibition increases levels of many drugs, hence concurrent use is contraindicated*<br>• Ritonavir decreases levels of ethinyl estradiol (found in many oral contraceptives), theophylline, clarithromycin, sulfamethoxazole, and zidovudine<br>• Absorption reduced by didanosine, unless taken at least 2 hr apart | • Inhibits P-450 (but less than ritonavir does)<br>• Because of P-450 inhibition, do not combine with astemizole, terfenadine, cisapride, midazolam, triazolam, or ergot alkaloids<br>• Saquinavir levels reduced by rifampin and rifabutin, and possibly by phenobarbital, phenytoin, dexamethasone, and carbamazepine<br>• Saquinavir levels increased by ritonavir, ketoconazole, and grapefruit juice | • Inhibits P-450 (but less than ritonavir does)<br>• Because of P-450 inhibition, do not combine with astemizole, terfenadine, cisapride, midazolam, triazolam, or ergot alkaloids<br>• Nelfinavir levels reduced by rifampin and rifabutin<br>• Nelfinavir decreases levels of ethinyl estradiol and norethindrone (both found in many oral contraceptives)<br>• Nelfinavir increases levels of ketoconazole |

*Drugs contraindicated for concurrent use with ritonavir are alprazolam, amiodarone, astemizole, bepridil, bupropion, cisapride, clorazepate, clozapine, diazepam, encainide, estazolam, flecainide, flurazepam, meperidine, midazolam, piroxicam, propoxyphene, propafenone, quinidine, terfenadine, triazolam, zolpidem, and ergot alkaloids.
Adapted from *Guidelines for the Use of Antiretroviral Agents in HIV-Infected Adults and Adolescents*, prepared by the Panel on Clinical Practices for Treatment of HIV Infection convened by the Department of Health and Human Services and the Henry J. Kaiser Family Foundation, 1997.

should always be taken with a meal. In the blood, saquinavir is highly (98%) bound to plasma proteins. Elimination results from metabolism by cytochrome P-450 enzymes, followed by excretion primarily in the feces; urinary excretion is minimal. The plasma half-life of saquinavir is 1 to 2 hours.

**Therapeutic Use.** Saquinavir is approved only for treatment of HIV infection. To reduce emergence of resistance, the drug should always be combined with at least one inhibitor of reverse transcriptase. Because of low bioavailability of the current formulation, saquinavir should not be used as a first-line drug.

**Adverse Effects.** Saquinavir is very well tolerated. The most common side effects are *headache, nausea, diarrhea*, and *abdominal pain*—and even these occur only rarely.

Recent circumstantial evidence suggests that saquinavir and the other protease inhibitors may cause *diabetes*, although a definitive link has not been established. At this time, protease inhibitors have been associated with 83 cases of either new-onset diabetes or abrupt exacerbation of existing diabetes. What the underlying mechanism might be is not obvious. Because of the possible risk of diabetes, patients should be instructed to report signs of the disease (e.g., increased thirst, increased urination, unexplained weight loss) should they occur.

**Drug and Food Interactions.** Saquinavir *inhibits cytochrome P-450 drug-metabolizing enzymes*, and can thereby decrease the metabolism of other drugs, causing their levels to rise. The result can be serious toxicity. For example, *terfenadine* and *astemizole* (two nonsedating antihistamines) can cause fatal cardiac dysrhythmias when present in excessive amounts. Accordingly, these agents should never be combined with saquinavir. Other drugs to avoid include *cisapride* and *ergot alkaloids.*

*Rifampin, rifabutin*, and other drugs that *induce* cytochrome P-450 can accelerate metabolism of saquinavir, thereby decreasing its levels. Given that levels of saquinavir are low to start with, any further reduction would seriously compromise therapy. Accordingly, P-450-inducing agents should be avoided.

Agents that *inhibit* P-450 can slow the metabolism of saquinavir, thereby increasing its levels. Inhibitors of P-450 include *ritonavir* (another protease inhibitor), *ketoconazole* (an antifungal agent), and *grapefruit juice*. Combining any of these agents with saquinavir can enhance therapeutic effects.

**Preparations, Dosage, and Administration.** Saquinavir [Invirase] is available in 200-mg hard gel capsules for oral administration. The recommended dosage is 600 mg every 8 hours. To ensure adequate absorption, the drug should always be taken with food.

## Indinavir

**Actions and Use.** Indinavir [Crixivan] inhibits HIV protease and thereby prevents the cleavage of large HIV polyproteins into their smaller, functional forms. As a result, HIV particles remain immature and noninfectious. Indinavir is approved only for treatment of HIV infection. To reduce the risk of resistance, indinavir should be combined with at least one inhibitor of reverse transcriptase.

**Pharmacokinetics.** When administered on an empty stomach, indinavir has moderate (30%) bioavailability. Administration with a meal high in fat, protein, or calories can decrease absorption by 70%. Indinavir undergoes metabolism by hepatic cytochrome P-450 followed by excretion in the feces (83%) and urine (19%). The plasma half-life of the drug is 1.5 to 2 hours. In patients with liver dysfunction, indinavir levels may increase and the half-life may be prolonged.

**Adverse Effects.** Indinavir is generally well tolerated. The major adverse effect of note is *nephrolithiasis* (kidney stones), manifested by flank pain with or without hematuria. As a rule, indinavir-induced nephrolithiasis does not compromise kidney

function and resolves following hydration and interruption of therapy for 1 to 3 days. To decrease the risk of nephrolithiasis, patients should consume at least 48 ounces (1.5 L) of water daily. Like other protease inhibitors, indinavir may pose a risk of *diabetes*; hence patients should watch for symptoms (e.g., increased thirst and urination, unexplained weight loss). Other side effects include *GI intolerance, headache, asthenia* (weakness), *blurred vision, dizziness, rash, metallic taste*, and *thrombocytopenia*.

**Drug Interactions.** Indinavir *inhibits cytochrome P-450*, and can thereby decrease the metabolism of other drugs. As a result, drugs may accumulate to dangerous or even life-threatening levels. Agents that can produce serious toxicity because of this interaction include *astemizole, terfenadine, cisapride, triazolam, midazolam*, and *ergot alkaloids*. Accordingly, patients taking indinavir must not be given these drugs.

*Didanosine* can decrease absorption of indinavir. The mechanism is reduction of acidity. Let me explain. Didanosine and indinavir differ in their acidity requirements: whereas indinavir needs acidity for absorption, acidity decreases absorption of didanosine. Because acidity decreases absorption of didanosine, the drug is formulated with a buffering agent to neutralize gastric acid. Hence, if didanosine and indinavir were administered together, the buffering agent in didanosine would reduce absorption of indinavir. To prevent this interaction, indinavir and didanosine should be administered at least 1 hour apart.

*Rifampin* and *rifabutin* can induce cytochrome P-450. As a result, these drugs can accelerate metabolism of indinavir, thereby decreasing its levels. In contrast, levels of indinavir can be increased by *ketoconazole*.

**Preparations, Dosage, Administration, and Storage.** Indinavir [Crixivan] is available in 200- and 400-mg capsules for oral administration. The recommended dosage is 800 mg every 8 hours. To maximize absorption, administer the drug either (1) with water but on an empty stomach (i.e., 1 hour before a meal or 2 hours after) or (2) with skim milk, coffee, tea, or a low-fat meal (e.g., corn flakes with skim milk and sugar). Do not administer with a large meal. If the regimen includes didanosine, indinavir and didanosine should be administered at least 1 hour apart.

Indinavir should be stored at room temperature and protected from moisture, since moisture can degrade the drug. To protect indinavir from moisture, store tightly sealed in the vesicant-containing package supplied by the manufacturer.

## Ritonavir

**Actions and Uses.** Ritonavir [Norvir] inhibits HIV protease, and thereby prevents maturation of HIV. The drug is active against HIV-1 and HIV-2. Ritonavir is approved for treatment of HIV infection in adults and children. To reduce emergence of resistance, the ritonavir should always be combined with at least one reverse transcriptase inhibitor.

**Pharmacokinetics.** Ritonavir is well absorbed following administration in capsules or oral solution. Food increases absorption of ritonavir in capsules by 15%. Dilution of the oral solution in chocolate milk, Ensure, or Advera has no impact on absorption, but does improve its taste (which is otherwise unpleasant). Ritonavir undergoes metabolism by the hepatic cytochrome P-450 system, followed by excretion in the feces (84%) and urine (11%). The drug's plasma half-life is 3 to 5 hours.

**Adverse Effects.** Adverse effects are common during the initial weeks of therapy and then tend to fade. The effects seen most often are nausea (25%), diarrhea (16%), vomiting (14%), muscle weakness (12%), altered taste (8%), and paresthesias (tingling or numbness) around the mouth and in the extremities. These effects can be reduced by initiating therapy at a low dosage and then gradually titrating up to the maintenance dosage. Like other protease inhibitors, ritonavir may pose a risk of *diabetes*; hence patients should watch for symptoms (e.g., increased thirst and urination, unexplained weight loss).

**Drug Interactions.** Ritonavir is a *powerful inhibitor of cytochrome P-450 drug-metabolizing enzymes*, and can thereby decrease the metabolism of other drugs, causing their levels to rise. Because drug accumulation can result in serious adverse effects, ritonavir is contraindicated for use with a large number of agents, including terfenadine and astemizole, which can cause fatal dysrhythmias when present at excessive levels. A complete list of contraindicated drugs is given in the second footnote of Table 88–5.

In some cases, ritonavir *decreases* levels of other drugs. Among these are *ethinyl estradiol* (a component of many oral contraceptives), *zidovudine, clarithromycin, sulfamethoxazole,* and *theophylline.* Care must be taken to ensure that concentrations of these drugs do not fall to subtherapeutic levels.

**Preparations, Dosage, Administration, and Storage.** Ritonavir [Norvir] is available in 100-mg capsules and an 80-mg/ml oral solution. The maintenance dosage for adults is 600 mg every 12 hours. The maintenance dosage for children is 400 mg/m$^2$ every 12 hours. Adverse effects can be minimized by starting therapy with a low dosage and then titrating up to the maintenance dosage. If possible, ritonavir should be administered with food. Palatability of the oral solution can be improved by mixing it with chocolate milk, Ensure, or Advera within 1 hour of administration. Ritonavir should be stored refrigerated (36˚F to 46{F) and protected from light.

### Nelfinavir

**Actions and Uses.** Nelfinavir [Viracept] is the fourth protease inhibitor to become available in the United States. The drug inhibits HIV protease, and thereby prevents maturation of HIV. Nelfinavir is approved for treatment of HIV infection in adults and children as young as 2 years old. To reduce emergence of resistance, the drug should always be combined with at least one reverse transcriptase inhibitor.

**Pharmacokinetics.** Nelfinavir is administered orally, and food increases absorption greatly (two- to threefold). In plasma, more than 98% of the drug is protein bound. Nelfinavir undergoes extensive hepatic metabolism followed by excretion in the feces. Only 1% of the drug is excreted in the urine. The plasma half-life of nelfinavir is 3.5 to 5 hours.

**Adverse Effects.** *Diarrhea* is the only adverse effect of note. During clinical trials, 20% to 32% of patients developed moderate to severe diarrhea. In most cases, diarrhea can be managed with an over-the-counter antidiarrheal drug (e.g., loperamide).

Like other protease inhibitors, nelfinavir may pose a risk of *diabetes.* Accordingly, patients should be instructed to watch for symptoms (e.g., increased thirst and urination, unexplained weight loss).

**Drug Interactions.** Nelfinavir *inhibits cytochrome P-450 drug-metabolizing enzymes*, and can thereby decrease the metabolism of other drugs, causing their levels to rise. Accumulation of several drugs, including *astemizole, terfenadine, midazolam, triazolam, cisapride,* and *ergot alkaloids,* can result in serious adverse effects. Accordingly, these agents are contraindicated for patients taking nelfinavir.

Nelfinavir *decreases* levels of *ethinyl estradiol* and *norethindrone,* a combination found in many oral contraceptives. Women taking oral contraceptives should be advised to use an alternative or additional form of contraception.

*Rifampin* and *rifabutin* induce hepatic drug-metabolizing enzymes, and can thereby decrease levels of nelfinavir. Accordingly, patients receiving nelfinavir should avoid antibiotics.

**Preparations, Dosage, and Administration.** Nelfinavir [Viracept] is available in 250-mg tablets and a 50-mg/g powder for oral administration. The powder should be mixed with a small amount of water, milk, formula, soy formula, soy milk, or dietary supplement; it should *not* be mixed with acidic foods or juices (e.g., applesauce, apple juice, orange juice) because the resulting combination may have a bitter taste. The recommended adult dosage is 750 mg every 8 hours. The pediatric dosage is 20 to 30 mg/kg every 8 hours. Nelfinavir should be administered with food to enhance absorption.

## Management of HIV Infection

Management of HIV infection has changed dramatically in the recent past. The reason is the now well-established efficacy of multidrug therapy—usually, a protease inhibitor plus two NRTIs.

As we shall see, therapy of HIV disease is complex. Patients typically take three drugs for HIV itself, and may take additional drugs for opportunistic infections. As a result, the potential for adverse effects and drug interactions is large. Also, among the drugs used for HIV, resistance is a common complication. Because of these complexities, management is best done by clinicians with extensive experience in treating HIV disease.

In the summer of 1997, two agencies of the U.S. government released reports related to the management of HIV infection. The first report—*Guidelines for the Use of Antiretroviral Agents in HIV-Infected Adults and Adolescents*—was prepared by the Panel on Clinical Practices for Treatment of HIV Infection, convened by the Department of Health and Human Services and the Henry J. Kaiser Family Foundation. The second document—*Report of the NIH Panel to Define Principles of Therapy of HIV Infection*—is a companion to the first, and was sponsored by the Office of AIDS Research of the National Institutes of Health. Both reports are available on the Internet at *www.hivatis.org/guidelin.html.* Much of the discussion that follows is based on these reports. A summary of treatment principles, as found in the second report, is presented in Table 88–6.

### Laboratory Monitoring

The principal laboratory tests employed to monitor HIV infection and guide therapy are *plasma HIV RNA* (viral load) *assays* and *CD4 T cell counts.* Measurement of viral load indicates the magnitude of HIV replication and predicts the rate of CD4 T cell destruction. In contrast, CD4 T cell counts indicate how much damage the immune system has already suffered.

#### Viral Load (Plasma HIV RNA)

*Treatment of HIV infection is guided primarily by monitoring viral load, which is determined by measuring HIV RNA in plasma.* The source of the RNA is intact HIV virions (virus particles), each of which has two copies

## TABLE 88-6. PRINCIPLES OF THERAPY OF HIV INFECTION

1. Ongoing HIV infection leads to immune system damage and progression to AIDS. HIV infection is always harmful, and true long-term survival free of clinically significant immune dysfunction is unusual.

2. Plasma HIV RNA levels reflect the magnitude of HIV replication and its associated rate of CD4 T cell destruction, whereas CD4 T cell counts indicate the extent of HIV-induced immune damage already suffered. Periodic measurement of plasma HIV RNA levels and CD4 T cell counts is necessary to determine the risk of disease progression in an HIV-infected individual and to determine when to initiate or modify antiretroviral regimens.

3. Because rates of disease progression differ among individuals, treatment decisions should be based on the individual's risk, as indicated by plasma HIV RNA levels and CD4 T cell counts.

4. Combination therapy with potent antiretroviral drugs that greatly suppresses HIV replication—as evidenced by reduction of plasma HIV RNA to levels that cannot be detected by sensitive assays—limits the potential for selection of drug-resistant HIV variants, which is the major cause of treatment failure. Accordingly, the goal of therapy should be to achieve maximum suppression of HIV replication.

5. The most effective way to achieve lasting suppression of HIV replication is to treat the patient with a combination of effective anti-HIV drugs that (1) the patient has not been treated with before and (2) are not cross-resistant with drugs the patient has been treated with before.

6. For each antiretroviral drug in a combination regimen, the dosage and dosing schedule should be optimal.

7. The available effective antiretroviral drugs are limited as to number and mechanism of action. In addition, cross-resistance between specific drugs has been documented. As a result, any change in antiretroviral therapy increases future therapeutic constraints.

8. Women should receive optimal antiretroviral therapy regardless of whether they are pregnant.

9. The same principles of antiretroviral therapy that apply to adults also apply to children, although the treatment of children involves unique pharmacologic, virologic, and immunologic considerations.

10. Acute primary HIV infection should be treated with a combination of antiretroviral drugs that reduces the viral load to a level that cannot be detected by sensitive plasma HIV RNA assays.

11. HIV-infected persons, even those with viral loads below detectable limits, should be considered infectious, and hence should be counseled to avoid sexual and drug-use behaviors that are associated with transmission or acquisition of HIV and other infectious pathogens.

Adapted from the *Report of the NIH Panel to Define Principles of Therapy of HIV Infection*, sponsored by the Office of AIDS Research of the National Institutes of Health, 1997.

---

of HIV RNA. Guidelines regarding when to measure HIV RNA are summarized in Table 88-7.

The principal tests employed to measure HIV RNA are (1) the reverse transcriptase polymerase chain reaction (RT-PCR) assay and (2) the branched-chain DNA amplification (bDNA) assay. With both tests, results are expressed as either (1) the number of copies of HIV RNA/ml or (2) the log of the number of copies of HIV RNA/ml. It is important to note, however, that values obtained using the RT-PCR assay may be as much as twofold higher than values obtained using the bDNA assay. Accordingly, in order to interpret test results, the clinician must know which test was employed. Also, to obtain reliable test results, it is essential that blood for HIV RNA determinations be collected and preserved according to recommended procedures.

Given that the vast majority of HIV in the body is present in lymphoid tissues rather than in the blood, you might ask whether measurement of HIV RNA in *plasma* is a true reflection of the *total body* load of HIV. The answer is "Yes." The reason is that, when HIV in lymphoid tissues replicates, many of the new virions are released into the blood. As a result, levels of HIV in blood parallel levels of HIV in lymphoid tissues. Accordingly, measurement of HIV RNA in blood gives us an accurate picture of the total HIV load.

Plasma HIV RNA is the best measurement available for predicting clinical outcome. If HIV RNA is high (e.g., 100,000 copies/ml), the prognosis is poor. Conversely, if HIV RNA is low (e.g., 5000 copies/ml), the risk of disease progression and death is greatly reduced. Accordingly, the goal of HIV therapy is to decrease plasma HIV RNA as much as possible—preferably to levels that are undetectable with current assays (i.e., below 500 to 1000 copies/ml). It is important to appreciate, however, that, even when plasma HIV RNA is below the current limits of detection, the patient may still be at risk of disease progression, and may still be able to transmit HIV to others.

With triple-drug therapy (see below), levels of HIV RNA should decline measurably within 10 days of the onset of treatment, and should fall to 1% of baseline within 2 weeks of the onset of treatment. After 8 weeks of treatment, HIV RNA should reach its minimum level. Hopefully, HIV RNA will be undetectable at this time.

## CD4 T Cell Counts

Before assays for HIV RNA were available, CD4 T cell counts were the primary laboratory test for monitoring therapy. Although CD4 T cell counts remain important, they lack the predictive power of viral load measurements. However, CD4 T cell counts can still tell us how much damage HIV has already caused. By knowing the ex-

## TABLE 88-7. TIMES WHEN PLASMA HIV RNA SHOULD BE MEASURED

| When to Measure Plasma HIV RNA | Information Obtained | Use of the Information |
|---|---|---|
| When a patient presents with a syndrome consistent with acute HIV infection | Establishes presence of HIV when HIV antibody test is negative or indeterminate | Diagnosis of HIV infection |
| Following initial diagnosis of HIV infection | Establishes baseline viral load | Decision to start or defer therapy |
| Every 3-4 months in patients with diagnosed HIV infection but who are not on antiretroviral therapy | Extent to which viral load has increased | Decision to initiate therapy |
| 4 weeks after starting antiretroviral therapy | Initial assessment of drug efficacy | Decision to continue or change therapy |
| 3-4 months after starting antiretroviral therapy | Maximal effect of therapy | Decision to continue or change therapy |
| Every 3-4 months in patients on antiretroviral therapy | Durability of drug effects | Decision to continue or change therapy |
| When a clinical event or a decline in CD4 T cells occurs | Establishes whether the clinical event or decline in CD4 T cells occurred in association with an increase in viral load | Decision to initiate, continue, or change therapy |

Adapted from *Guidelines for the Use of Antiretroviral Agents in HIV-Infected Adults and Adolescents*, prepared by the Panel on Clinical Practices for Treatment of HIV Infection convened by the Department of Health and Human Services and the Henry J. Kaiser Family Foundation, 1997.

tent of immunodeficiency, we can assess the risk of opportunistic infection, and hence can initiate timely prophylactic therapy.

As antiretroviral therapy takes effect, CD4 T cell counts will begin to rise, indicating some return of immune function. Increases of 100 to 250 cells/µl have been observed. It is not clear, however, whether restoration of CD4 T cell counts produces complete immunocompetency. Until this question has been resolved, prophylactic therapy against opportunistic infections should continue, despite a substantial rise in CD4 T cells.

Measurement of CD4 T cells should be done when HIV infection is diagnosed and every 3 to 6 months thereafter. A healthy range for CD4 T cells is 800 to 1200 cells/µl. A 30% reduction is considered significant. Among people with HIV infection, a CD4 T cell count above 500 cells/µl is considered relatively high. In contrast, a count below 50 cells/µl indicates very advanced HIV disease.

## Treatment of Adult Patients

As discussed above, HIV disease has three basic phases, an initial acute phase, followed by a prolonged asymptomatic phase, followed in turn by a late symptomatic phase, during which AIDS occurs. We will consider drug therapy for each phase separately. However, to facilitate discussion, we will not discuss them in the sequence in which they actually occur. Rather, we will discuss symptomatic HIV disease first, then asymptomatic HIV disease, and then acute HIV disease. For patients with symptomatic HIV dis-

ease or acute HIV disease, the benefits of treatment clearly outweigh the risks; hence immediate treatment is recommended. In contrast, for patients with asymptomatic HIV disease, the benefits of immediate treatment may not outweigh the risks; hence, in some cases, it may be appropriate to delay initiation of treatment.

### Symptomatic HIV Disease

*All patients with symptomatic (advanced) HIV disease should receive maximally effective antiretroviral therapy.* The preferred regimen consists of three drugs: *one protease inhibitor plus two NRTIs* (see Table 88-8). An alternative regimen also consists of three drugs: *one NNRTI plus two NRTIs* (Table 88-8). However, this regimen is less effective than the preferred regimen. Two-drug combinations are not generally recommended, and monotherapy should always be avoided (except during pregnancy, as discussed below).

When treating symptomatic HIV disease, *the goal is to achieve maximal and sustained suppression of HIV replication, as evidenced by reduction of plasma HIV RNA to levels that cannot be detected with sensitive assays.* We employ a combination of drugs to achieve this goal, in part because combination therapy suppresses viral replication better than monotherapy. More importantly, *combination therapy reduces the risk of resistance.* Why? Because the probability that HIV will undergo a mutation that confers simultaneous resistance to three drugs is much smaller than the probability of undergoing a mutation that confers resistance to just one drug.

## TABLE 88-8. REGIMENS FOR INITIAL THERAPY OF HIV INFECTION

### PREFERRED REGIMEN: 1 PI + 2 NRTIs

A three-drug regimen containing one PI and two NRTIs produces clinical benefits and a sustained reduction of plasma HIV RNA below detectable levels in the majority of patients who comply with the regimen.

| *Protease Inhibitors* | *NRTI Combinations* |
| --- | --- |
| Indinavir | Zidovudine + didanosine |
| Nelfinavir | Zidovudine + zalcitabine |
| Ritonavir | Zidovudine + lamivudine[†] |
| Saquinavir* | Stavudine + lamivudine[†] |
| | Stavudine + didanosine |

### ALTERNATIVE REGIMEN: 1 NNRTI + 2 NRTIs

A three-drug regimen containing one NNRTI and two NRTIs can decrease plasma HIV RNA to undetectable levels in many patients, but the antiviral effect may not be sustained as long as with the preferred regimen.

| *NNRTIs[‡]* | *NRTI Combinations* |
| --- | --- |
| Nevirapine | Same as in the preferred regimen |
| Delavirdine | |

NNRTI = non-nucleoside reverse transcriptase inhibitor, NRTI = nucleoside reverse transcriptase inhibitor, PI = protease inhibitor.
*The hard-gelatin capsule formulation of saquinavir in current use is not recommended due to poor bioavailability. Until an improved formulation is available, saquinavir should be considered a second-choice drug.
[†]High-level resistance to lamivudine develops within 2 to 4 weeks in partially suppressive regimens; optimal use is in antiretroviral combinations that reduce viral load to <500 copies/ml.
[‡]Of the two NNRTIs in current use, only nevirapine has been shown effective in combination with NRTIs. Data for delavirdine are not available.

Accordingly, if our patient is taking three drugs, and a virion mutates to a form that is resistant to one of those drugs, the other two drugs will continue to be effective against the resistant virion, and hence suppression of replication will be sustained. On the other hand, if our patient were only taking the single drug to which HIV had developed resistance, then treatment would obviously fail. Because of concerns about resistance, when a patient who began treatment with monotherapy is switched to multidrug therapy, we should employ drugs that (1) the patient has not used before and (2) are not cross-resistant with drugs the patient has used before.

Plasma HIV RNA should be monitored to assess the impact of treatment. With triple-drug therapy, levels of HIV RNA should decline measurably within 10 days of the onset of treatment, and should fall to 1% of baseline within 2 weeks of the onset of treatment. After 8 weeks of treatment, HIV RNA should reach its minimum level. Hopefully, HIV RNA will be undetectable at this time.

It is important to appreciate that reducing plasma HIV RNA to undetectable levels does not mean that HIV has been eradicated, nor does it mean the patient has been cured. It only means that the amount of HIV in plasma is too low for us to measure with current assays. Whether long-term treatment with multiple drugs can actually *eliminate* HIV is yet to be proved. Accordingly, until more is known, we must assume that, despite maximally effective treatment, patients still harbor HIV and therefore are still infectious. Because patients still harbor HIV, treatment should continue indefinitely. Because patients remain infectious, they should be counseled to avoid behaviors that can transmit HIV.

A combination of factors—complex regimens, adverse effects, drug-drug and drug-food interactions—make safe and effective triple-drug therapy difficult. The following examples illustrate the extent of the problem.

- *Complexity of the regimen*—A typical regimen might include ritonavir, zidovudine, and didanosine. The dosage for ritonavir is 600 mg (6 tablets) taken every 12 hours with food; the dosage for zidovudine is 300 mg (1 tablet or 3 capsules) taken every 8 hours without regard to meals; and the dosage for didanosine is 200 mg (2 tablets) taken twice daily, 1 hour before meals or 2 hours after—for a total of 19 to 25 tablets or capsules a day. In addition to these antiretroviral drugs, the patient may be taking medications to treat opportunistic infections, as well as medication to promote appetite.

- *Adverse effects*—In the regimen described above, the patient is at risk of multiple adverse effects. Ritonavir can cause GI disturbances, paresthesias, weakness, and altered taste; zidovudine can cause neutropenia and anemia; and didanosine can cause pancreatitis and peripheral neuropathy. Drugs for opportunistic infections will increase the potential for side effects. To decrease the risk of serious injury, drugs with overlapping toxicities should be avoided.

- *Drug-drug interactions*—The potential for significant drug interactions is huge. Ritonavir inhibits cytochrome P-450, and can thereby suppress metabolism of many other drugs, causing their levels to rise. In addition, ritonavir can *reduce* levels of a few drugs, including ethinyl estradiol, a component of many oral contraceptives. Didanosine can reduce absorption of ritonavir, unless the drugs are administered 2 hours apart. Drugs that depress bone marrow function can increase the risk of anemia and neutropenia from zidovudine. One such bone-marrow depressant—ganciclovir—is encountered often because of its use against cytomegalovirus retinitis, a common opportunistic infection in people with AIDS.

- *Drug-food interactions*—Food decreases absorption of didanosine, and hence the drug should be taken on an empty stomach. In contrast, food enhances absorption of ritonavir, and hence the drug should be administered with meals. Since patients with AIDS are frequently anorectic, administration with meals may be problematic.

Because of these multiple difficulties, extensive patient education is essential. Accordingly, patients should be counseled about the importance of strict adherence to the regimen, timing of dosing with regard to meals, and adverse effects and interactions to be alert for.

## Asymptomatic HIV Disease

Making the decision to treat patients during the asymptomatic phase of HIV disease is more complex than during the symptomatic phase. During the symptomatic phase, the benefits of treatment clearly outweigh the risks for all patients, and hence all patients should receive treatment. However, during the asymptomatic phase, the risks of treatment may outweigh the benefits for some patients. Accordingly, when asymptomatic patients and their physicians are deciding whether or not to initiate antiretroviral therapy, they must take multiple factors into account. Specifically, they must consider the potential benefits and risks of treatment, as well as factors unique to each patient. These are summarized in Table 88–9.

Early intervention offers several benefits, the most obvious being reduction of viral load. As a result, progression of immunodeficiency is slowed, progression to AIDS is delayed, and life may be prolonged. In addition, suppression of replication decreases the rate of HIV mutation, and can

---

### TABLE 88-9. FACTORS TO CONSIDER WHEN DECIDING TO INITIATE ANTIRETROVIRAL THERAPY DURING THE ASYMPTOMATIC PHASE OF HIV DISEASE

*Potential Benefits*

- Reduction of viral load
- Control of viral replication decreases rate of mutation, and can thereby decrease production of drug-resistant mutants
- Prevention of progressive immunodeficiency; potential preservation of a normal immune system
- Delayed progression to AIDS and prolongation of life
- Treatment while the patient is still healthy allows better tolerance of drug side effects

*Potential Risks*

- Reduction in quality of life owing to adverse drug effects and the constraints imposed by a complex dosing schedule
- Exposure of HIV to antiretroviral drugs can lead to earlier emergence of drug-resistant mutants
- If resistance develops, drug options for future therapy will be limited
- If resistance develops, the risk of transmitting resistant mutants will be increased
- Long-term toxicity of certain antiretroviral drugs is not yet known
- Long-term efficacy of current antiretroviral therapies is not yet known

*Factors Unique to the Patient*

- Willingness to start therapy
- Likelihood of adhering to the regimen
- Degree of immunodeficiency, as indicated by CD4 T cell count; in general, offer treatment to all patients with <500 CD4 T cells/μl, regardless of HIV RNA level
- Risk of disease progression, as indicated by plasma HIV RNA; in general, offer treatment to all patients with >10,000 copies/ml (by bDNA assay) or >20,000 copies/ml (by RT-PCR assay)

---

thereby decrease production of drug-resistant mutants. Finally, when therapy is begun while the patient is still relatively healthy, the patient will be better able to tolerate drug toxicity.

Unfortunately, early intervention does have drawbacks. Drug therapy will *decrease* quality of life by (1) exposing an otherwise symptom-free person to adverse effects and (2) creating the need to rigidly follow a complex regimen. In addition, neither the long-term efficacy nor the long-term toxicity of current drugs is known. Hence, the patient is facing a potential risk of losing benefits as well as experiencing adverse effects of which we are currently unaware. Finally, although it is true that decreasing viral load and replication will decrease spontaneous production of resistant mutants, if resistant mutants *are* produced, the presence of drugs will create selection pressure favoring their emergence. Hence, it is possible that drug therapy will allow resistance to develop sooner than it would have in the absence of drugs. This is especially true if the patient fails to adhere to the regimen. Furthermore, if resistance does develop, drug options for future therapy will be limited, and the risk of transmitting resistance will be increased.

In addition to balancing benefits versus risks, factors unique to the patient must be considered before initiating therapy. Obviously, the patient must want treatment. Also, the patient must be prepared to adhere to a demanding dosing schedule. Finally, the patient's HIV status must be considered. Specifically, we must consider (1) the degree of immunodeficiency, as evidenced by CD4 T cell counts, and (2) the risk of disease progression, as evidenced by plasma HIV RNA level. As a rule, treatment should be offered to all patients with low CD4 T cell counts (i.e., <500 cells/μl) and to all patients with a high viral load (i.e., >10,000 copies of HIV RNA/ml [as measured by bDNA assay] or >20,000 copies/ml [as measured by RT-PCR assay). For patients at lower risk (i.e., >500 CD4 T cells/μl and less than 10,000 to 20,000 copies of HIV RNA/ml), it may be safe to temporarily postpone treatment. However, if treatment is delayed, HIV status should be re-evaluated every 3 to 4 months.

If the patient and physician do agree to initiate treatment, the goal is the same as with symptomatic patients: reduction of HIV RNA to levels that are undetectable with sensitive assays. As with symptomatic patients, the preferred regimen consists of three drugs: a protease inhibitor plus two NRTIs (Table 88–8).

## Acute HIV Disease

*All patients with primary acute HIV disease should receive maximally effective antiretroviral therapy.* As with symptomatic HIV disease, the preferred regimen consists of three drugs: one protease inhibitor plus two NRTIs.

Early and aggressive intervention offers multiple potential benefits. Of greatest interest is the possibility of eradicating HIV before it gets firmly established, although eradication has not yet been demonstrated. However, even if we can't clear HIV from the body, early treatment still offers the following benefits:

- By suppressing the initial burst of viral replication, treatment may decrease the extent to which HIV disseminates throughout the body.
- By reducing viral load, treatment can preserve immune system function, and may also slow the progression of HIV disease.
- By reducing viral load and the rate of replication, treatment can decrease the rate of mutation, and hence can decrease the risk that a drug-resistant virion will emerge.

As with asymptomatic HIV disease, treatment of acute HIV infection does have potential drawbacks. These include

- Reduction in quality of life because of drug toxicity and the constraints imposed by a complex dosing schedule.
- Possible blunting of the early immune response to HIV because of reduced viral presence.
- Emergence of drug-resistant HIV if treatment fails.

Nonetheless, given the potential benefits of treatment, these drawbacks do not comprise a compelling reason to postpone therapy.

### Changing the Regimen

There are four basic reasons for changing antiretroviral therapy: treatment failure, drug toxicity, patient noncompliance, and use of a suboptimal regimen. Guidelines for altering the regimen under these four conditions are discussed below. Unfortunately, only nine antiretroviral drugs are currently available; hence options for changing the regimen are clearly limited.

**Treatment Failure.** Treatment failure is arguably the most compelling reason for changing the regimen. Failure is indicated if

- Plasma HIV RNA fails to drop by 10-fold within the first 4 weeks of treatment
- Plasma HIV RNA fails to drop to undetectable levels within the first 4 to 6 months of treatment
- Plasma HIV RNA rebounds after falling to an undetectable level
- CD4 T cell counts continue to drop despite antiretroviral treatment
- Clinical disease progresses despite antiretroviral treatment.

Of these five signs of failure, the first three are the most meaningful, in that they represent a direct measurement of antiretroviral effects.

When treatment failure occurs, the reason must be determined. Possibilities include patient noncompliance, poor drug absorption, accelerated drug metabolism owing to drug interactions, and viral resistance. If noncompliance is the cause, patient education may help (see below). If poor absorption is the cause, changing the timing of administration with respect to meals or increasing the dosage may help. If accelerated metabolism is the cause, increasing the dosage may help; alternatively, it may be appropriate to substitute a different drug for the one that is causing metabolism to increase.

When failure is the result of resistance, the preferred response is to change *all* drugs in the regimen. This makes sense in that failure means that HIV is replicating despite current treatment, indicating the presence of at least one HIV strain that is resistant to all drugs in the regimen. If we were to add or change just one drug, resistance would quickly develop to that agent, and failure would occur again. The risk of renewed resistance is substantially lower if we change at least two drugs, and even lower if we change three. When we change the regimen, the new drugs should be agents that (1) the patient has not taken previously and (2) are not cross-resistant with drugs the patient has taken before. Ideally, if the patient has been taking a protease inhibitor and two NRTIs, the replacement regimen would consist of a new protease inhibitor and two new NRTIs. Unfortunately, some patients are already resistant to nearly all of the available drugs; hence their options are limited. In such cases, it is rational to continue with the current regimen, which may at least provide partial suppression. To date, there is limited experience with regimens that consist of either two protease inhibitors or a protease inhibitor plus an NNRTI. Nonetheless, for patients who have no other choice, these combinations are potential options. Because cross-resistance is common between ritonavir and indinavir (two protease inhibitors), these drugs should not be substituted for each other. Likewise, because cross-resistance is common between nevirapine and delavirdine (two NNRTIs), these drugs should not be substituted for each other.

**Treatment with a Suboptimal Regimen.** Suboptimal therapy is indicated by a failure to suppress plasma HIV RNA to an undetectable level. In addition to this laboratory definition of suboptimal, treatment with a single NRTI is always considered suboptimal, and treatment with two NRTIs is generally considered suboptimal. For patients taking either a single NRTI or two NRTIs, substituting two new NRTIs and a protease inhibitor would be appropriate. Note that the new drugs *replace* the old drugs; they are not taken in addition to the old ones.

**Drug Toxicity.** If a patient experiences toxicity typical of a particular drug in the regimen, that drug should be withdrawn and replaced with a drug that is (1) from the same class and (2) of equal efficacy. For example, if a patient taking zidovudine were to develop anemia and neutropenia, zidovudine should be discontinued and replaced with another NRTI (e.g., lamivudine). Note that, when toxicity is the reason for altering the regimen, changing just one drug is proper, whereas, when resistance or suboptimal treatment is the reason, *all* of the drugs should be changed.

**Noncompliance.** Noncompliance can occur for multiple reasons. Among these are lack of understanding, adverse effects, and complexity of the regimen. Accordingly, the reason for noncompliance must be explored. If lack of understanding is the cause, then intensive education may correct the problem. If adverse effects are the cause, then replacing the offending drug is indicated. As noted above, the new drug should be from the same class as the old one, and should also have similar efficacy. If complexity of the regimen is the reason for noncompliance, simplification may be appropriate. Although a more simple regimen may have less intrinsic ability to suppress viral replication, it may nonetheless be more effective—since drugs that are actually taken work infinitely better than drugs that remain on the shelf.

## Treatment of Pregnant Patients

In general, *management of HIV infection in pregnant women should follow the same guidelines for managing HIV infection in nonpregnant adults.* That is, women should receive optimal antiretroviral therapy, regardless of their pregnancy status. When treating HIV infection in pregnant women, the goal is to balance the benefits of treatment (reducing viral load, thereby promoting the health of the mother and decreasing the risk of HIV transmission to the fetus) against the risks of treatment (causing teratogenic harm to the fetus). As a rule, the benefits of treatment outweigh the risks. Accordingly, the primary determinants of therapy are the clinical, virologic, and immunologic status of the mother; pregnancy is a secondary consideration. Nonetheless, pregnancy should not be ignored. Since the risk of teratogenesis is greatest during the first trimester (i.e., first 14 weeks of pregnancy), it might be appropriate to interrupt therapy until the first trimester is over, especially if the maternal risk is low (i.e., CD4 T cell count exceeds 500 cells/μl and plasma HIV RNA is below 10,000 to 20,000 copies/ml). The drawback, of course, is that viral load will increase, and may thereby potentiate HIV disease in the mother and enhance transmission to the fetus. Accordingly, many experts recommend continuation of maximally effective treatment even during the first trimester. If the mother *does* decide to interrupt treatment, *all* antiretroviral drugs should be stopped. (This is necessary because continuing treatment with just one or two drugs would increase the risk of resistance, and would thereby render those drugs ineffective for current or future use by the patient.) When treatment resumes, the full regimen should be reinstituted.

Drug selection is problematic in that information on pharmacokinetics and safety during pregnancy is largely lacking. Except for didanosine, all of the available NRTIs showed some fetal risk in animal studies. Of the two NNRTIs in current use, only nevirapine has been tested in women. As for the protease inhibitors, we have no data on their safety in pregnancy.

To date, zidovudine is the only drug proved to reduce the risk of perinatal HIV transmission. When used as recommended, the drug decreases the risk of HIV transmission by 70% to 80%. Accordingly, if the mother is being treated with multiple antiretroviral drugs, zidovudine should be part of the regimen. If HIV infection is in its early stage, thereby allowing the mother to postpone therapy until pregnancy is over, she might still elect to undergo time-limited monotherapy with zidovudine to protect the fetus.

## Treatment of Pediatric Patients

*The same principles that guide antiretroviral therapy in adults also apply to children.* Most studies on HIV replication and antiretroviral therapy have been conducted in adults. However, it is unlikely that HIV behaves any differently in children or that the fundamentals of antiretroviral therapy differ either. In fact, the few studies that have been conducted indicate that the virology of HIV is the same in children and adults, suggesting that optimal antiretroviral therapy should be similar. Accordingly, like adults, children should be treated with a combination of antiretroviral drugs that produces lasting suppression of plasma HIV RNA to levels that cannot be detected by current assays.

At this time, information on the pharmacokinetics of antiretroviral drugs in children is limited. As a result, pediatric dosages for some drugs have not been determined. Hence, if these agents were to be used, the resulting plasma levels might be too low to be effective or too high to be safe. Therefore, to ensure maximal efficacy and minimal harm, children should be treated only with drugs for which pediatric dosages have been established.

## Postexposure Prophylaxis

One-time exposure to HIV carries a very small, but nonetheless real, risk of becoming infected. Exposure may result from unprotected vaginal or anal intercourse, receptive oral intercourse, sharing a contaminated needle, or an accidental needle stick.

The risk of developing HIV disease after a single exposure can be reduced—but not eliminated—with prophylactic drugs. The recommended regimen is two NRTIs—*zidovudine* (200 mg tid) plus *lamivudine* (150 mg bid)—for 4 weeks. If the source of HIV had advanced AIDS or had been treated with NRTIs, a *protease inhibitor* (e.g., indinavir, 800 mg tid) should be taken as well. Prophylactic therapy is based on the premise that early treatment may prevent initial cellular infection and local propagation of HIV, thereby allowing host immune defenses to eliminate the virus before it can become established. Accordingly, prophylaxis is likely to be most effective when initiated within *hours* of HIV exposure; initiation beyond 72 hours is not recommended.

## Management of Opportunistic Infections

Individuals with advanced HIV disease are vulnerable to infections caused by opportunistic organisms (i.e., organisms that rarely cause serious disease, except when host defenses are compromised). The risk is greatest among patients with fewer than 200 CD4 T cells/µl. In the United States, between 200,000 and 250,000 HIV-infected people are in this group. Prophylaxis and treatment of common opportunistic infections are discussed below.

### *Pneumocystis carinii* Pneumonia

Among people with AIDS, *Pneumocystis carinii* pneumonia (PCP) is the most common opportunistic infection and the leading cause of death. PCP occurs in up to 80% of HIV-infected individuals and kills about 20%. Following control of an initial infection, the rate of recurrence is 60% within the first year.

Clinical manifestations of PCP are generally nonspecific. Early symptoms include fever, cough, dyspnea, chest discomfort, pallor, and cyanosis. In advanced infection, lung morphology is altered. Left untreated, PCP has a mortality rate of 90%.

**Treatment of Active PCP.** The treatment of choice for PCP is *trimethoprim plus sulfamethoxazole* (TMP-SMZ), marketed as Bactrim, Cotrim, and Septra. TMP-SMZ is effective in 90% of patients; nothing works better. As a rule, clinical improvement is seen in 4 to 8 days. For patients who are severely immunocompromised, intravenous *pentamidine* [Pentam 300] may be preferred. Alternatives to TMP-SMZ or pentamidine include *atovaquone* [Mepron], *trimethoprim plus dapsone*, *trimetrexate plus folinic acid*, and *primaquine plus clindamycin.* All of these agents are less effective than TMP-SMZ or pentamidine, but may be better tolerated. Treatment of PCP with TMP-SMZ, pentamidine, and atovaquone is discussed further in Chapter 93; dosages for PCP appear there as well.

**Prophylaxis of PCP.** Prophylactic therapy is recommended for all patients with a CD4 T cell count below 200 cells/µl and for all patients who have had a previous bout of PCP. The preferred medication for prophylaxis is *trimethoprim plus sulfamethoxazole*, given as one double-strength tablet each day. For patients who cannot tolerate TMP-SMZ, *aerosolized pentamidine* [NebuPent] may be used instead. Unfortunately, although aerosolized pentamidine is better tolerated than TMP-SMZ, it is not as effective. The dosage is 300 mg once a month.

### Cytomegalovirus Retinitis

Cytomegalovirus (CMV) retinitis is among the most common complications in people with AIDS, affecting about one-third of patients in United States. Individuals with CD4 T cell counts below 50 cells/µl are most vulnerable. Left untreated, CMV retinitis invariably leads to retinal necrosis and loss of vision.

Drug therapy of CMV retinitis proceeds in two stages: induction followed by maintenance. The induction phase reduces the viral load and greatly slows the rate of disease progression. However, induction does not eliminate the virus. Accordingly, maintenance therapy, which must continue for life, is given to reduce the risk of relapse. Unfortunately, even with maintenance therapy, progressive loss of vision often occurs.

CMV retinitis can be treated with three agents: *ganciclovir*, *cidofovir*, and *foscarnet.* The basic pharmacology of these drugs is discussed in Chapter 87. All three drugs may be given intravenously. In addition, ganciclovir may be given orally, by intraocular implant, and by direct injection into the eye. Like ganciclovir, foscarnet may also be injected directly into the eye.

Maintenance therapy is very expensive. Current *wholesale* prices for a year's supply are $8891 for IV ganciclovir, $17,082 for PO ganciclovir, $5000 for ganciclovir implants, $17,670 for IV cidofovir, and between $27,800 and $32,200 for IV foscarnet!

**Ganciclovir.** Ganciclovir [Cytovene] is the drug of choice for CMV retinitis. For induction, intravenous administration is traditional, although intraocular implants or direct intraocular injections may also be used. For maintenance therapy, intraocular implants or daily IV infusions are the preferred treatments. The implants are more effective than the infusions and cause fewer side effects. However, patients receiving the implants are at greater risk of developing a systemic CMV infection. The dose-limiting toxicities of IV ganciclovir are neutropenia and thrombocytopenia secondary to bone marrow depression. In addition, there is a risk of infection in the central venous catheter employed for the infusions.

**Foscarnet.** Foscarnet [Foscavir] is less well tolerated than ganciclovir and much more expensive. As a rule, the drug is administered by IV infusion—twice daily for induction and once daily for maintenance. To receive infusions daily, patients require an indwelling central venous catheter, and hence face a risk of the catheter becoming infected. Dose-limiting toxicities of foscarnet are nephrotoxicity, electrolyte imbalance (especially hypocalcemia), genital ulceration, and fluid overload.

**Cidofovir.** Cidofovir [Vistide] is a new IV drug for CMV retinitis. This agent has a longer effective half-life than either ganciclovir or foscarnet, and hence can be administered less frequently. Specifically, whereas ganciclovir and foscarnet must be infused daily for maintenance therapy, cidofovir is infused just once every 2 weeks. Because cidofovir infusions are infrequent, patients do not require an indwelling central catheter, and hence do not face a risk of catheter infection. The major dose-limiting toxicities of cidofovir are kidney damage and neutropenia. To reduce the risk of kidney injury, all patients must be given probenecid and IV hydration therapy with each infusion.

### *Mycobacterium tuberculosis* and *Mycobacterium avium* Complex

*Mycobacterium tuberculosis* and *Mycobacterium avium* complex are slow-growing microbes that require prolonged drug exposure to be eradicated. Because therapy is prolonged, emergence of resistance is a significant concern. To reduce the risk of resistance, these infections are always treated with multiple drugs—just like HIV itself. Mycobacterial infections and their treatment are discussed at length in Chapter 84. A brief summary of treatment is presented here.

***Mycobacterium tuberculosis.*** Between 2% and 20% of people with AIDS become infected with *M. tuberculosis*. If the infection is caused by drug-sensitive mycobacteria, treatment is relatively simple. In one protocol, treatment is initiated with a three-drug regimen—*isoniazid plus rifampin plus pyrazinamide*—and then switched to a two-drug regimen—*isonizazid plus rifampin*—2 months later. Treatment should last for at least 9 months, and for at least 3 months after sputum tests for *M. tuberculosis* have become negative. Treatment of drug-resistant infections can be very difficult, sometimes requiring as many as seven drugs. Specific regimens for drug-sensitive and drug-resistant tuberculosis are summarized in Table 84-1.

***Mycobacterium avium Complex.*** *Mycobacterium avium* complex (MAC) consists of two nearly identical microbes: *Mycobacterium avium* and *Mycobacterium intracellulare*. Infection with MAC begins in the lungs or GI tract, but can then disseminate to the blood, bone marrow, liver, spleen, lymph nodes, brain, kidneys, and skin. Among people with AIDS, disseminated infection is common, being present in 50% at autopsy. Signs and symptoms of disseminated MAC infection include fever, night sweats, weight loss, lethargy, anemia, and abnormal liver function tests. For *treatment* of disseminated infection, the regimen should include either *azithromycin* or *clarithromycin*, plus at least one other drug, typically *ethambutol*. If needed, more drugs may be added; options include *rifabutin, rifampin, ciprofloxacin, clofazimine,* and *amikacin*. For *prophylaxis* of MAC infection, either *azithromycin* or *clarithromycin* should be used. (Until recently, rifabutin was preferred for prophylaxis; however, rifabutin is now considered a second-choice agent.)

### *Toxoplasma* Encephalitis

*Toxoplasma gondii* is a protozoan of the sporozoa class. In the immunocompetent host, infection with *T. gondii* is generally benign. However, in the immunocompromised host, infection can be lethal. Among patients with AIDS, toxoplasmosis usually manifests as *encephalitis* (inflammation of the brain or brainstem). Symptoms include fever, headache, seizures, aphasia (loss of speech), lethargy, confusion, dementia, focal neurologic deficits, and progression to coma. *Toxoplasma* encephalitis is most likely late in HIV disease, usually after CD4 T cell counts fall below 100 cells/μl. In the United States, the incidence of *Toxoplasma* encephalitis among AIDS patients is 3% to 10%, making this the most common opportunistic infection of the CNS in this group.

The treatment of choice for *Toxoplasma* encephalitis is *pyrimethamine plus sulfadiazine*. The sulfadiazine component can cause rash and crystalluria. For patients who cannot tolerate sulfadiazine, alternative regimens include *pyrimethamine plus clindamycin, pyrimethamine plus atovaquone,* and single-drug therapy with either *clarithromycin* or *azithromycin*.

Once toxoplasmosis has been controlled, lifelong maintenance therapy is needed to reduce the risk of relapse. The preferred maintenance regimen is *trimethoprim plus sulfamethoxazole*, given as one double-strength tablet daily. Unfortunately, even with maintenance therapy, most patients eventually relapse.

### Cryptococcal Meningitis

*Cryptococcus neoformans* is a fungus that infects 9% to 13% of patients with AIDS. In 80% of these patients, cryptococcosis manifests as meningitis (inflammation of the meninges). The most common symptoms are fever and headache. Other symptoms include nausea, vomiting, photophobia, and altered mental status. Cryptococcal meningitis typically occurs late in HIV disease, usually after CD4 T cell counts fall below 100 cells/μl. In addition to infecting the meninges, *C. neoformans* can infect the blood, lungs, skin, and prostate.

The treatment of choice for cryptococcal meningitis is *amphotericin B* infused daily, usually for 2 weeks or longer. Oral *flucytosine* may be combined with the amphotericin. The major adverse effect of amphotericin is kidney damage, whereas the principal concern with flucytosine is bone marrow depression (neutropenia, thrombocytopenia). Compared with amphotericin B alone, the combination of amphotericin plus flucytosine decreases rates of treatment failure and relapse. However, mortality rates with both treatments are similar. Because bone-marrow depression is a significant concern for patients with AIDS, those taking flucytosine should be monitored closely.

After the initial infection has been controlled, patients should continue maintenance therapy indefinitely. The treatment of choice is oral *fluconazole* daily. In the absence of maintenance therapy, patients are at increased risk of relapse and death.

The pharmacology of amphotericin B, flucytosine, and fluconazole is discussed at length in Chapter 86.

### Varicella-Zoster Virus Infection

Varicella-zoster virus (VZV) can cause *chickenpox* and *herpes zoster*, also known as *shingles* or simply *zoster*. Among adults with AIDS, VZV infection usually manifests as shingles, which results from reactivation of latent VZV infection. The preferred treatment for shingles is high-dose *oral acyclovir* (800 mg 5 times daily for 7 to 10 days). *Oral famciclovir* and *intravenous foscarnet* are alternatives. For patients with disseminated VZV infection, the preferred treatment is *intravenous acyclovir* (10 mg/kg every 8 hours for 1 to 2 weeks); intravenous foscarnet is an alternative. The pharmacology of acyclovir, famciclovir, and foscarnet is discussed at length in Chapter 87.

### Herpes Simplex Virus Infection

Infection with herpes simplex virus (HSV) is common among patients with HIV disease. Lesions may occur at multiple sites, including the lips, tongue, oral cavity, genitals, and perianal region. In patients with advanced HIV disease, HSV may infect the esophagus, colon, lungs, eyes, and CNS. For infection at all sites, *acyclovir* is the drug of choice. Administration may be oral or IV. Responses usually occur within 3 to 10 days. Duration of treatment ranges from 7 to 21 days. For patients with acyclovir-resistant HSV, intravenous *foscarnet* is the treatment of choice.

## Candidiasis

HIV-infected patients frequently develop infection with *Candida* species, usually *Candida albicans.* The most common sites are the oropharynx and esophagus. Up to 75% of patients experience oral candidiasis (thrush), which often responds to topical therapy (e.g., "swishing and swallowing" a *nystatin suspension* or sucking *miconazole troches*). As an alternative, patients may be given systemic therapy with an oral azole (*fluconazole, ketoconazole,* or *itraconazole*). Oral azoles are more convenient than topical therapy and probably more effective; however, they are also more expensive. Prophylaxis of recurrent oral candidiasis is not always needed. However, if recurrences are frequent or severe, chronic intermittent therapy with an oral azole may be considered.

For esophageal candidiasis, systemic therapy is required. Options include oral *ketoconazole,* oral *fluconazole,* and intravenous *amphotericin B.* All patients with a documented history of esophageal candidiasis should be considered for chronic suppressive therapy with oral fluconazole.

## KEY POINTS

- HIV is a retrovirus that, like all other retroviruses, has RNA as its genetic material.
- HIV uses reverse transcriptase to convert its RNA into DNA.
- HIV uses protease to break large HIV polyproteins into their smaller, functional forms.
- The principal target of HIV is CD4 T cells (helper T lymphocytes). These cells are attacked by HIV because they carry CD4 proteins on their surface, thereby providing HIV with a required point of attachment.
- Because of errors made by reverse transcriptase, HIV can mutate rapidly from a drug-sensitive form into a drug-resistant form.
- HIV infection has three phases. During the initial phase, many patients experience a flu-like acute retroviral syndrome. During the prolonged middle phase, patients are asymptomatic, although CD4 T cells undergo progressive decline. During the late phase, CD4 T cells drop below a critical level (200 cells/μl), rendering the patient vulnerable to opportunistic infections and certain neoplasms.
- HIV replicates rapidly during all phases of HIV infection, including the prolonged phase of clinical latency.
- We have three classes of antiretroviral drugs: nucleoside reverse transcriptase inhibitors (NRTIs), nonnucleoside reverse transcriptase inhibitors (NNRTIs), and protease inhibitors.
- NRTIs suppress HIV replication in two ways: (1) they become incorporated into the growing strand of viral DNA by reverse transcriptase, and thereby prevent further strand growth; and (2) they compete with natural nucleoside triphosphates for binding to the active center of reverse transcriptase, and thereby competitively inhibit the enzyme.
- In order to interact with reverse transcriptase, NRTIs must first undergo conversion to their active (triphosphate) forms.
- Zidovudine (an NRTI) can cause severe anemia and neutropenia.
- Didanosine, stavudine, and zalcitabine (all NRTIs) can cause pancreatitis and peripheral neuropathy. Accordingly, any combination of these drugs should be used with great caution, if at all.
- NNRTIs (e.g., nevirapine) differ from NRTIs in that they are not analogs of natural nucleosides, are active as administered, and cause direct noncompetitive inhibition of reverse transcriptase by binding to its active center.
- NNRTIs frequently cause rash, which can be severe and even life-threatening.
- Protease inhibitors (e.g., saquinavir) are the most effective antiretroviral drugs available.
- Protease inhibitors bind to HIV protease and thereby prevent the enzyme from cleaving HIV polyproteins. As a result, enzymes and structural proteins of HIV remain nonfunctional, and hence the virus remains immature and noninfectious.
- Circumstantial evidence suggests that protease inhibitors may cause diabetes, although a definitive link has not been established.
- All protease inhibitors inhibit cytochrome P-450, and can thereby suppress metabolism of other drugs, causing their levels to rise. Accordingly, patients should avoid astemizole, terfenadine, and certain other drugs whose accumulation could lead to serious toxicity.
- Resistance to antiretroviral drugs is a major problem. To reduce emergence of resistance, these drugs should never be used alone; rather, they should always combined with at least one other antiretroviral drug, and preferably with two.
- The principal laboratory tests employed to monitor HIV infection and guide therapy are plasma HIV RNA (viral load) and CD4 T cell counts. Plasma HIV RNA levels indicate the magnitude of HIV replication and predict the rate of CD4 T cell destruction, whereas CD4 T cell counts indicate how much damage the immune system has already suffered.
- Plasma HIV RNA is the best measurement for predicting clinical outcome: if HIV RNA is high, the prognosis is poor; conversely, if HIV RNA is low, the risk of disease progression and death is greatly reduced. Accordingly, the goal of antiretroviral therapy is to decrease plasma HIV RNA to levels that are undetectable with current assays.
- Reducing plasma HIV RNA to undetectable levels does not mean that HIV has been eradicated. It only means that there is too little HIV present for us to measure. Until more is known, we must assume that, despite maximally effective treatment, patients still harbor HIV

and are still infectious. Accordingly, treatment should continue indefinitely and patients should be warned to avoid behaviors that can transmit HIV.

- All patients with acute primary HIV disease or advanced (symptomatic) HIV disease should receive maximally effective antiretroviral therapy. The preferred regimen consists of three drugs: one protease inhibitor plus two NRTIs.

- For some patients with asymptomatic HIV disease, it may be appropriate to temporarily postpone antiretroviral therapy.

- In general, the principles that guide antiretroviral therapy in nonpregnant adults also apply during pregnancy. Put another way, women should receive optimal antiretroviral therapy, regardless of their pregnancy status.

- Zidovudine is the only drug proved to reduce the risk of perinatal HIV transmission. Accordingly, if a pregnant woman is being treated with multiple antiretroviral drugs, zidovudine should be part of the regimen.

- In general, the principles that guide antiretroviral therapy in adults also apply to children.

- An important reason for changing an antiretroviral regimen is treatment failure, as indicated by (1) failure of plasma HIV RNA to drop to an undetectable level, (2) a rebound in plasma HIV RNA after falling to an undetectable level, (3) continued decline of CD4 T cell counts, and (4) progression of clinical disease.

- When treatment failure is the result of drug resistance, the preferred response is to change *all* drugs in the regimen. Furthermore, the new drugs should be agents that the patient has not taken before and are not cross-resistant with drugs the patient has taken before.

- Because of declining CD4 T cell counts, individuals with advanced HIV disease are at risk for opportunistic infections.

- Among people with AIDS, *Pneumocystis carinii* pneumonia (PCP) is the most common opportunistic infection and the leading cause of death.

- The preferred regimen for prophylaxis and treatment of PCP is trimethoprim plus sulfamethoxazole.

- Ganciclovir is the drug of choice for cytomegalovirus retinitis in people with advanced HIV disease.

# Summary of Major Nursing Implications*

## Nucleoside Reverse Transcriptase Inhibitors

| | |
|---|---|
| Didanosine | Zalcitabine |
| Lamivudine | Zidovudine |
| Stavudine | |

### Preadministration Assessment

#### Therapeutic Goal

The treatment goal is to reduce plasma HIV RNA to undetectable levels, and thereby preserve the health and prolong the life of the HIV-infected patient.

#### Baseline Data

*All NRTIs.* Assess the patient's clinical status and obtain a plasma HIV RNA level and CD4 T cell count.

*Zidovudine.* Obtain a hemoglobin value and granulocyte count.

#### Identifying High-Risk Patients

*Didanosine, Stavudine, and Zalcitabine.* The risk of pancreatitis is increased by a history of alcoholism or pancreatitis and by use of intravenous pentamidine.

*Zidovudine.* The risk of hematologic toxicity is increased by a low granulocyte count, hemoglobin level, vitamin $B_{12}$ level, or folic acid level, and by concurrent use of drugs that are myelosuppressive, nephrotoxic, or toxic to circulating blood cells.

## Implementation: Adminstration

### Routes

*All NRTIs.* Oral.

*Zidovudine.* Oral and intravenous.

### Administration

*All NRTIs.* Instruct the patient to adhere closely to the prescribed dosing schedule.

*Didanosine.* Instruct patients to take didanosine 1 hour before meals or 2 hours after.

Instruct patients taking didanosine *tablets* to either (1) chew them thoroughly or (2) manually crush them or disperse them in at least 1 ounce of water.

Instruct patients taking *powdered* didanosine to pour the contents of one packet into 4 ounces of water (not fruit juice or any other acid-containing beverage), stir the mixture until the drug dissolves (about 2 to 3 minutes), and then drink the solution immediately.

*Lamivudine and Stavudine.* Inform patients that these drugs may be taken with or without food.

*Zidovudine.* Administer IV zidovudine slowly (over 1 hour). Do not mix the solution with biologic or colloidal fluids (e.g., blood products, protein solutions). Administer within 8 hours (if stored at room temperature) or within 24 hours (if stored under refrigeration).

### Ongoing Evaluation and Interventions

#### Evaluating Therapeutic Effects

*Plasma HIV RNA.* Success is indicated by a reduction in plasma HIV RNA. With triple-drug therapy, plasma HIV RNA should fall to 1% of baseline within 2 weeks, and

---

*Patient education information is highlighted in color.

reach a minimum by 8 weeks. Ideally, the minimum will be undetectable with sensitive assays.

*CD4 T Cell Counts.* As viral load decreases, CD4 T cell counts may rise, indicating some restoration of immune function.

### Minimizing Adverse Effects

*Anemia and Neutropenia. Zidovudine* can cause severe anemia and neutropenia. Determine hematologic status before treatment and at least every 4 weeks thereafter. In the event of severe anemia (hemoglobin <7.5 gm/dl or down 25% from the pretreatment baseline) or severe neutropenia (granulocyte count <750 cells/µl or down 50% from the pretreatment baseline), interrupt treatment until there is evidence of bone marrow recovery. If neutropenia and anemia are less severe, a reduction in dosage may be sufficient. Some patients may require multiple transfusions. Granulocyte colony-stimulating factors can be used to reverse neutropenia. Epoetin alfa (recombinant erythropoietin) can be given to reduce transfusion requirements in patients with anemia, provided endogenous erythropoietin levels are not already elevated.

*Pancreatitis. Didanosine, stavudine,* and *zalcitabine* can cause potentially fatal pancreatitis. Monitor patients for signs of developing pancreatitis (elevated serum amylase in association with elevated serum triglycerides, decreased serum calcium, and nausea, vomiting, or abdominal pain). If evolving pancreatitis is diagnosed, these drugs should be withdrawn.

*Peripheral Neuropathy. Didanosine, stavudine,* and *zalcitabine* can cause painful peripheral neuropathy. Inform patients about early signs of neuropathy (numbness, tingling, or pain in hands and feet) and instruct them to report these immediately. Treat pain of severe neuropathy with opioid analgesics. Neuropathy may reverse if these drugs are withdrawn early.

*HIV Transmission.* Reduction of plasma HIV RNA may create a false sense of safety. Accordingly, inform patients that, even when HIV RNA is undetectable, they may still be infectious, and hence should avoid behaviors that can transmit HIV.

### Minimizing Adverse Interactions

*Didanosine, Stavudine, and Zalcitabine.* All three drugs can cause pancreatitis and peripheral neuritis. Accordingly, any combination of these agents must be used with great caution.

*Zidovudine.* Drugs that are myelosuppressive, nephrotoxic, or directly toxic to circulating blood cells can increase the risk of hematologic toxicity. Drugs of concern include ganciclovir, dapsone, pentamidine, pyrimethamine, trimethoprim-sulfamethoxazole, amphotericin B, flucytosine, vincristine, vinblastine, and doxorubicin.

## Non-Nucleoside Reverse Transcriptase Inhibitors

Delavirdine        Nevirapine

### Preadministration Assessment

#### Therapeutic Goal

The treatment goal is to reduce plasma HIV RNA to undetectable levels, and thereby preserve the health and prolong the life of the HIV-infected patient.

#### Baseline Data

Assess the patient's clinical status and obtain a plasma HIV RNA level and CD4 T cell count.

### Implementation: Administration

#### Route

Oral

#### Administration

*Delavirdine.* Administer with or without food. Advise patients who cannot swallow delavirdine tablets whole to mix them with 3 or more ounces of water. Advise patients with achlorhydria to take delavirdine with an acidic beverage, such as orange or cranberry juice.

*Nevirapine.* Administer with or without food.

### Ongoing Evaluation and Interventions

#### Evaluating Therapeutic Effects

*Plasma HIV RNA.* Success is indicated by a reduction in plasma HIV RNA. With triple-drug therapy, plasma HIV RNA should fall to 1% of baseline within 2 weeks, and reach a minimum by 8 weeks. Ideally, the minimum will be undetectable with sensitive assays.

*CD4 T Cell Counts.* As viral load decreases, CD4 T cell counts may rise, indicating some restoration of immune function.

#### Minimizing Adverse Effects

*Rash.* Rash is common and may range from mild to severe to life-threatening. If rash is mild, treat with an antihistamine or topical glucocorticoid. If rash is severe or associated with signs of erythema multiforme or Stevens-Johnson syndrome (fever, blistering, oral lesions, conjunctivitis, muscle pain, joint pain), the NNRTI should be withdrawn. To minimize rash, use a low dosage initially and then increase it if no rash occurs.

*HIV Transmission.* Reduction of plasma HIV RNA may create a false sense of safety. Accordingly, inform patients that, even when HIV RNA is undetectable, they may still be infectious, and hence should avoid behaviors that can transmit HIV.

#### Minimizing Adverse Interactions

*Nevirapine.* Nevirapine *induces* cytochrome P-450 and can thereby decrease levels of other drugs. Effects on *protease inhibitors* and *oral contraceptives* are of particular concern. Combining nevirapine with *rifampin* or *rifabutin*, which also induce P-450, could greatly accelerate drug metabolism.

*Delavirdine.* Delavirdine *inhibits* P-450, and can thereby increase levels of other drugs. To avoid toxicity from excessive drug levels, the patient must not take *astemizole, terfenadine, alprazolam, midazolam, triazolam,* or *cisapride.* In addition the following drugs should be used with caution: indinavir, saquinavir, clarithromycin, dapsone, warfarin, quinidine, ergot alkaloids, and the dihydropyridine-type calcium channel blockers.

*Antacids* and *didanosine* can decrease levels of delavirdine. To minimize this effect, instruct patients not to administer these drugs at least 1 hour before or 1 hour after delavirdine.

## Protease Inhibitors

| | |
|---|---|
| Indinavir | Ritonavir |
| Nelfinavir | Saquinavir |

## Preadministration: Assessment

### Therapeutic Goal
The treatment goal is to reduce plasma HIV RNA to undetectable levels, and thereby preserve the health and prolong the life of the HIV-infected patient.

### Baseline Data
Assess the patient's clinical status and obtain a plasma HIV RNA level and CD4 T cell count.

## Implementation: Administration

### Routes
All protease inhibitors are taken orally.

### Administration and Storage
*All Protease Inhibitors.* Instruct patients to adhere closely to the prescribed dosing schedule.

*Saquinavir.* Instruct patients to take saquinavir with food.

*Indinavir.* Instruct patients to administer indinavir (1) with water but on an empty stomach (i.e., 1 hour before a meal or 2 hours after) or (2) with skim milk, coffee, tea, or a low-fat meal (e.g., corn flakes with skim milk and sugar), but not with a large meal. Instruct patients to store indinavir at room temperature in the package supplied by the manufacturer.

*Ritonavir.* Advise patients to take ritonavir with food. Instruct patients to mix the oral solution formulation with chocolate milk, Ensure, or Advera (within 1 hour of administration) to improve the taste. Instruct patients to store ritonavir refrigerated (36°F to 46°F) and protected from light.

*Nelfinavir.* Instruct patients to take nelfinavir with food. Instruct patients to mix the powder formulation with a small amount of water, milk, formula, soy formula, soy milk, or dietary supplement, but *not* with acidic foods or juices (e.g., applesauce, apple juice, orange juice).

## Ongoing Evaluation and Interventions

### Evaluating Therapeutic Effects
*Plasma HIV RNA.* Success is indicated by a reduction in plasma HIV RNA. With triple-drug therapy, plasma HIV RNA should fall to 1% of baseline within 2 weeks, and reach a minimum by 8 weeks. Ideally, the minimum will be undetectable with sensitive assays.

*CD4 T Cell Counts.* As viral load decreases, CD4 T cell counts may rise, indicating some restoration of immune function.

### Minimizing Adverse Effects
*Diabetes.* All protease inhibitors may pose a risk of diabetes. Inform patients about symptoms of diabetes (e.g., increased thirst, increased urination, unexplained weight loss), and instruct them to report these should they occur.

*Nephrolithiasis. Indinavir* can cause nephrolithiasis. Management consists of hydration and interruption of indinavir for 1 to 3 days. To decrease the risk of nephrolithiasis, instruct patients to consume at least 48 ounces (1.5 L) of water daily.

*Diarrhea. Nelfinavir* causes diarrhea in 20% to 32% of patients. Diarrhea can usually be managed with loperamide or some other over-the-counter antidiarrheal drug.

*HIV Transmission.* Reduction of plasma HIV RNA may create a false sense of safety. Accordingly, inform patients that, even when HIV RNA is undetectable, they may still be infectious, and hence should avoid behaviors that can transmit HIV.

### Minimizing Adverse Interactions
*Interactions Secondary to Inhibition of Cytochrome P-450.* All protease inhibitors inhibit cytochrome P-450, and can thereby increase levels of other drugs. To avoid serious toxicity from excessive drug levels, patients must not take *astemizole, terfenadine, cisapride, triazolam, midazolam,* and *ergot alkaloids.* Additional drugs to avoid are listed in Table 88-5.

*Didanosine.* Didanosine reduces absorption of *indinavir* and *ritonavir.* To minimize this problem, didanosine should be administered 1 or 2 hours apart from these drugs.

*Rifampin and Rifabutin.* These antimycobacterial drugs induce cytochrome P-450, and can thereby reduce levels of the protease inhibitors, possibly compromising therapeutic effects.

*Oral Contraceptives. Ritonavir* and *nelfinavir* can reduce levels of ethinyl estradiol, a component of many oral contraceptives. Advise patients to use an alternative or additional form of contraception.

# CHAPTER 89

# Drug Therapy of Sexually Transmitted Diseases

Chlamydia trachomatis Infections
Gonococcal Infections
Nongonococcal Urethritis
Pelvic Inflammatory Disease
Acute Epididymitis
Syphilis
Acquired Immunodeficiency Syndrome

Chancroid
Trichomoniasis
Bacterial Vaginosis
Herpes Simplex Infections
Genital and Anal Warts (Condyloma Acuminatum)
Pediculosis Pubis and Scabies

Sexually transmitted diseases (STDs) are defined as infectious or parasitic diseases that are transmitted primarily through sexual contact. STDs are common in the United States and constitute a major public health problem; according to the Centers for Disease Control and Prevention, Americans have a 25% lifetime risk of contracting an STD. Our objective in this chapter is to describe the principal STDs and provide an overview of their drug therapy. Table 89-1 presents a summary of the common STDs, their causative organisms, and the drugs of choice for treatment. The basic pharmacology of these drugs is discussed in previous chapters.

## Chlamydia Trachomatis Infections

Chlamydia trachomatis is the most common cause of bacterial STD in the United States, infecting about 4 million people annually. The various strains of this organism can cause genital tract infections, proctitis, conjunctivitis, lymphogranuloma venereum, and neonatal ophthalmia and pneumonia. Drugs of choice for these infections are summarized in Table 89-1.

**Genital Tract Infections.** Genital tract infections (e.g., urethritis, cervicitis, epididymitis) with C. trachomatis are common. About 3 million new cases develop each year. One reason for this explosive spread is the mild nature of symptoms, especially in women. Unfortunately, although symptoms are mild, infection is not benign: the Centers for Disease Control and Prevention (CDC) estimates that these infections cause sterility in up to 50,000 women each year, primarily from fallopian tube scarring.

For uncomplicated urethral, cervical, or rectal infections in adults, two treatments are recommended: (1) a single 1-gm oral dose of *azithromycin* [Zithromax], or (2) 100 mg of *doxycycline* [Vibramycin, others] twice daily PO for 7 days. *Ofloxacin* [Floxin] is an alternative.

**Infection in Pregnancy.** The drug of choice for C. trachomatis infections during pregnancy is *erythromycin* (500 mg PO for 7 days). Either of three preparations may be used: erythromycin base, erythromycin stearate, or erythromycin ethylsuccinate. Erythromycin *estolate* is contraindicated during pregnancy because of the risk of maternal liver injury. For women who cannot take erythromycin, *amoxicillin* [Amoxil, others] can be used as a substitute. Although doxycycline and other tetracyclines are active against C. trachomatis, these drugs are contraindicated because they can damage fetal teeth and bones. Similarly, sulfisoxazole and other sulfonamides are active, but these drugs are contraindicated near term because they can cause kernicterus in the infant. When attempting to control C. trachomatis infection in pregnancy, concurrent therapy of the male sexual partner is essential.

**Neonatal Ophthalmia and Pneumonia.** About half the infants born to women with cervical C. trachomatis acquire the infection during the birth process. These infants are at risk for conjunctivitis and pneumonia. Pneumonia is generally not severe and lasts about 6 weeks. Conjunctivitis does not result in blindness and spontaneously resolves in 6 months. The preferred treatment for both infections is systemic *erythromycin*, 12.5 mg/kg (PO or IV) 4 times daily for 2 weeks. Although topical erythromycin, tetracycline, or silver nitrate may be given to prevent conjunctivitis, none of these treatments is completely effective.

**Lymphogranuloma Venereum.** Lymphogranuloma venereum (LGV) is caused by a unique strain of C. trachomatis. Transmission is strictly by sexual contact. LGV is most common in tropical countries, but does occur in the United States, especially in the South. Infection begins as a small erosion or papule in the genital region. From

## TABLE 89-1. SEXUALLY TRANSMITTED DISEASES: CAUSATIVE ORGANISMS AND DRUGS OF CHOICE

| Disease or Syndrome | Drug(s) of Choice | Causative Organism(s) |
|---|---|---|
| *Chlamydia trachomatis Infections* | | *Chlamydia trachomatis* |
| Urethris Cervicitis Proctitis Conjunctivitis | Azithromycin (PO) *or* doxycycline (PO) | |
| Infection in pregnancy | Erythromycin (PO) | |
| Neonatal infections: Ophthalmia Pneumonia | Erythromycin (PO or IV) | |
| Lymphogranuloma Venereum | Doxycycline (PO) | |
| *Gonococcal Infections (Gonorrhea)* | | *Neisseria gonorrhoeae* |
| Urethral Cervical Rectal Pharyngeal Ophthalmia (adults) | Ceftriaxone (IM) | |
| Bacteremia Arthritis Meningitis | Ceftriaxone (IV) with or without cefixime (IV) | |
| Neonatal ophthalmia | Ceftriaxone (IM) *or* cefotaxime (IM or IV) | |
| *Nongonococcal Urethritis* | Doxycycline (PO) | *Chlamydia trachomatis, Ureaplasma urealyticum, Trichomonas vaginalis* |
| *Pelvic Inflammatory Disease (PID)* | | *Neisseria gonorrhoeae, Chlamydia trachomatis* |
| Inpatients | *Initial therapy:* Cefoxitin (IV) *or* cefotetan (IV), either one plus doxycycline (IV) | |
| Outpatients | *Initial therapy:* Cefoxin (IM) combined with probenecid (PO) *or* ceftriaxone (IM) *Followed by:* Doxycycline (PO) | |
| *Sexually Acquired Epididymitis* | Ofloxacin (PO) | *Chlamydia trachomatis, Neisseria gonorrhoeae* |
| *Syphilis* | | *Treponema pallidum* |
| Early stage (primary, secondary, or latent syphilis of less than 1 year's duration) Late stage (syphilis of more than 1 year's duration) | Benzathine penicillin G (IM) | |
| Neurosyphilis | Penicillin G (IV) | |
| Congenital syphilis | Penicillin G (IM or IV) *or* procaine penicillin G (IM) | |

**TABLE 89–1. SEXUALLY TRANSMITTED DISEASES: CAUSATIVE ORGANISMS AND DRUGS OF CHOICE Continued**

| Disease or Syndrome | Drug(s) of Choice | Causative Organism(s) |
|---|---|---|
| Acquired Immunodeficiency Syndrome (AIDS) | See Chapter 88 | Human immunodeficiency virus |
| Bacterial Vaginosis | Metronidazole (PO) | Gardnerella vaginalis, Mycoplasma hominis, various anaerobes |
| Trichomoniasis | Metronidazole (PO) | Trichomonas vaginalis |
| Chancroid | Erythromycin (PO) or ceftriaxone (IM) or azithromycin | Haemophilus ducreyi |
| Herpes simplex | Acyclovir (PO or IV) | Herpes simplex virus |
| Genital and Anal Warts | Preferred treatment: Cryotherapy Alternative treatments: Podophyllum resin or trichloroacetic acid (both topical) | Human papillomavirus |
| Pediculosis Pubis | 1% permethrin (topical) | Phthirus pubis (pubic lice) |
| Scabies | 5% permethrin (topical) | Sarcoptes scabiei |

this site, the organism migrates to regional lymph nodes, causing swelling, tenderness, and blockage of lymphatic flow. Tremendous enlargement of the genitalia may result. The enlarged nodes, called buboes, may break open and drain. The treatment of choice for genital, inguinal, and anorectal LGV is *doxycycline* [Vibramycin, others], 100 mg PO twice daily for 3 weeks. *Erythromycin* may be used as a substitute.

## Gonococcal Infections

**Gonorrhea.** This infection is caused by *Neisseria gonorrhoeae*, a gram-negative diplococcus frequently referred to as the gonococcus. The incidence of gonorrhea is high: about 1.1 million Americans acquire the infection each year. Gonorrhea is transmitted primarily by sexual contact, although it can also be transmitted by contact with infected exudates.

The intensity of symptoms differs between men and women. In men, the main symptoms are a burning sensation while urinating and a pus-like discharge from the penis. In contrast, gonorrhea in women is commonly asymptomatic. However, serious infection of female reproductive structures (vagina, urethra, cervix, ovaries, fallopian tubes) can occur, ultimately resulting in sterility. Among people who engage in oral sex, the mouth and throat can become infected, causing a sore throat and tonsillitis. Among people who engage in receptive anal sex, the rectum can become infected, causing a purulent discharge and constant urge to move the bowels. Bacteremia can develop in both sexes, causing cutaneous lesions, arthritis, and, rarely, meningitis and endocarditis.

Because of antibiotic resistance, treatment of gonorrhea has changed over the years—and undoubtedly will continue to evolve. In the 1930s, virtually all strains of the gonococcus were sensitive to sulfonamides. However, within a decade, sulfonamide resistance had become common. Fortunately, by that time penicillin had become available, and the drug was active against all gonococcal strains. However, in 1976, organisms resistant to penicillin began to emerge. Currently, about 10% of gonococci in the United States are penicillin resistant. Tetracycline resistance has also been noted.

At this time, the drug of choice for uncomplicated gonorrhea is *ceftriaxone* [Rocephin], administered as a single IM dose (125 to 250 mg). For patients who cannot use ceftriaxone, alternatives are *cefixime* [Suprax], *ciprofloxacin* [Cipro], and *ofloxacin* [Floxin]. Since patients infected with *N. gonorrhoeae* very frequently are co-infected with *C. trachomatis*, treatment should always include oral doxycycline or azithromycin.

For disseminated gonorrhea (bacteremia, arthritis, meningitis), parenteral therapy is required. Options include (1) *ceftriaxone* (1 gm IV daily for 7 to 10 days), or (2) *ceftriaxone* (1 gm IV daily for 3 days) followed by *cefixime* (400 mg PO twice daily for 7 days).

**Gonococcal Neonatal Ophthalmia.** This infection is acquired from an infected mother during the birthing process. The initial symptom is conjunctivitis. Over time, other structures of the eye become involved. Blindness can result. Gonococcal ophthalmia is prevented by applying a topical drug to the conjunctival sac immediately postpartum. Any of three agents is effective: *0.5% erythromycin, 1% tetracycline,* or *1% silver nitrate.* For infants with active ophthalmia, parenteral therapy with ceftriaxone (IM) or cefotaxime (IM or IV) is indicated.

# Nongonococcal Urethritis

Nongonococcal urethritis (NGU) is defined as urethritis caused by any organism other than *Neisseria gonorrhoeae,* the gonococcus. The most common infectious agents are *Chlamydia trachomatis* (25% to 40%), *Ureaplasma urealyticum* (about 20%), and *Trichomonas vaginalis* (<5%). NGU is diagnosed by the presence of polymorphonuclear leukocytes and a negative culture for *N. gonorrhoeae.* The infection is especially prevalent among sexually active adolescent girls. The drug of choice for NGU is *doxycycline* [Vibramycin]. Dosage is 100 mg twice daily for 7 days. In patients for whom doxycycline is contraindicated (pregnant women, young children), *erythromycin* can be used instead.

# Pelvic Inflammatory Disease

Acute pelvic inflammatory disease (PID) is a syndrome that includes endometritis, pelvic peritonitis, tubo-ovarian abscess, and inflammation of the fallopian tubes. Infertility can result. Prominent symptoms are abdominal pain, vaginal discharge, and fever. Most frequently, PID is caused by *Neisseria gonorrhoeae* and/or *Chlamydia trachomatis.* However, *Mycoplasma hominis* as well as assorted anaerobic and facultative bacteria may also be involved.

Because multiple organisms are likely to be involved, drug therapy must provide broad coverage. Since no single drug can do this, combination therapy is required. For the hospitalized patient, treatment can be initiated with *cefotaxime* (IV) or *cefotetan* (IV), with either one followed by *doxycycline* (IV). This initial therapy is followed by oral *doxycycline.* The entire course of treatment takes 14 days.

For the outpatient, treatment can be initiated either with *cefoxitin* (IM) combined with probenecid (PO), or with *ceftriaxone* (IM) by itself. This initial therapy is followed by oral *doxycycline* for 14 days. Since PID can be difficult to treat, and since the consequences of failure can be severe (e.g., sterility), many experts recommend that all patients receive intravenous antibiotics in a hospital.

# Acute Epididymitis

Epididymitis may be acquired by sexual contact or nonsexually. Sexually acquired epididymitis is usually caused by *Neisseria gonorrhoeae* and/or *Chlamydia trachomatis.* This syndrome occurs primarily in young adults (under 35 years) and may be associated with urethritis. Primary symptoms are fever accompanied by pain in the back of the testicles that develops over the course of several hours. The infection can be treated with *ofloxacin* [Floxin], 300 mg PO twice daily for 10 days. Testicular pain can be managed with analgesics, bed rest, and ice packs.

Nonsexually transmitted epididymitis generally occurs in older men and men who have had urinary tract instrumentation. Causative organisms are gram-negative enteric bacilli and *Pseudomonas.* Ofloxacin can be used for treatment.

# Syphilis

Syphilis is caused by the spirochete *Treponema pallidum.* The incidence of syphilis has increased steadily over the past decade to reach its highest rate in over 40 years. In the United States, about 120,000 people are infected each year. Fortunately, *T. pallidum* has remained highly responsive to penicillin, the drug of choice for treatment.

**Characteristics.** Syphilis develops in three stages, termed primary, secondary, and tertiary. *T. pallidum* enters the body by penetrating the mucous membranes of the mouth, vagina, or urethra of the penis. After an incubation period of 1 to 4 weeks, a primary lesion, called a chancre, develops at the site of entry. The chancre is a hard, red, protruding, painless sore. Nearby lymph nodes may become swollen. Within a few weeks the chancre heals spontaneously, although *T. pallidum* is still present.

Two to 6 weeks after the chancre heals, secondary syphilis develops. Symptoms result from spread of *T. pallidum* via the bloodstream. Skin lesions and flu-like symptoms (fever, headache, reduced appetite, general malaise) are typical. Enlarged lymph nodes and joint pain may also be present. The symptoms of secondary syphilis resolve in 4 to 8 weeks—but may recur episodically over the next 3 to 4 years.

Tertiary syphilis develops 5 to 40 years after the initial infection. Almost any organ can be involved. Infection of the brain—neurosyphilis—is common, and can cause senility, paralysis, and severe psychiatric symptoms. The heart valves and aorta may be damaged. Lesions may also occur in the skin, bones, joints, and eyes. The risk of neurosyphilis is increased in individuals who are infected with HIV.

Infants exposed to *T. pallidum in utero* can be born with syphilis. Signs of congenital syphilis include sores, rhinitis, severe tenderness over bones, and deafness.

**Treatment.** *Penicillin G* is the drug of choice for all stages of syphilis. The form and dosage of penicillin G depend on the disease stage. *Early syphilis* (primary, secondary, or latent syphilis of less than 1 year's duration) is treated with a single IM dose (2.4 million units) of benzathine penicillin G. *Late syphilis* (more than 1 year's duration) is also treated with IM benzathine penicillin G, but the dosage is increased (2.4 million units once a week for 3 weeks). *Neurosyphilis* requires more aggressive therapy. The recommended treatment is 2 to 4 million units of *intravenous* penicillin G every 4 hours for 10 to 14 days. For *congenital syphilis*, two regimens have been recommended: (1) penicillin G (IM or IV), 50,000 units/kg every 8 to 12 hours for 10 to 14 days, or (2) IM procaine penicillin G, 50,000 units/kg once daily for 10 to 14 days. *Syphilis in pregnancy* should be treated with penicillin G, using a dosage appropriate to the stage of the disease. If a pregnant woman is allergic to penicillins, the U.S. Public Health Service recommends that she go through a penicillin-allergy desensitization protocol to permit penicillin use, rather than substituting another drug for penicillin.

# Acquired Immunodeficiency Syndrome

Acquired immunodeficiency syndrome (AIDS) is caused by the human immunodeficiency virus (HIV). Since the last edition of this book, treatment options for HIV infection have advanced significantly. To accommodate this new information, HIV infection and AIDS-related opportunistic infections have been assigned their own chapter (see Chapter 88).

# Chancroid

Chancroid, also known as soft chancre, is caused by *Haemophilus ducreyi*. Transmission is primarily by sexual contact. The infection is characterized by a painful, ragged ulcer at the site of inoculation, usually the external genitalia. Regional lymph nodes may be swollen. Multiple secondary lesions may develop. Although primarily a tropical disease, chancroid has become an important STD in the United States. Recommended treatments are (1) *erythromycin*, 500 mg PO 4 times daily for 7 days; (2) *ceftriaxone* [Rocephin], 250 mg IM once; and (3) *azithromycin* [Zithromax], 1 gm PO once.

# Trichomoniasis

Trichomoniasis is an STD caused by *Trichomonas vaginalis*. In women, the infection may be asymptomatic or may cause a thin, watery vaginal discharge, along with burning and itching sensations. In men, the infection is usually symptom free. Most infections can be eliminated with a single, 2-gm dose of *metronidazole* [Flagyl, others]. This dose can be repeated in the event of treatment failure. Metronidazole is contraindicated during the first trimester of pregnancy, but can be taken during the sec-

ond and third trimesters. Male partners of infected women should always be treated, even if they are asymptomatic.

# Bacterial Vaginosis

Bacterial vaginosis results from an alteration in vaginal microflora. Organisms responsible for the syndrome include *Gardnerella vaginalis* (also known as *Haemophilus vaginalis*), *Mycoplasma hominis*, and various anaerobes. The syndrome occurs most commonly in sexually active women, but may not actually be transmitted sexually. Bacterial vaginosis is characterized by a malodorous vaginal discharge, elevation of vaginal pH (above 4.5), and generation of a fishy odor when vaginal secretions are mixed with 10% potassium hydroxide.

Treatment may be oral or intravaginal. The recommended oral therapy is *metronidazole* [Flagyl], 500 mg twice a day for 7 days. Two intravaginal options are available: (1) metronidazole (0.75% gel), 5 gm twice daily for 5 days, and (2) *clindamycin* (2% cream), 5 gm every evening for 7 days.

# Herpes Simplex Infections

***Characteristics.*** Most genital herpes infections are caused by herpes simplex virus type 2 (HSV-2). A few genital infections are caused by herpes simplex virus type 1, the herpesvirus that causes cold sores. Genital herpes is transmitted primarily by sexual contact. In the United States, the infection has reached epidemic proportions, afflicting over 20 million people. About 500,000 new cases occur annually. There is no cure.

Symptoms of primary infection develop 6 to 8 days after contact. In females, blisters or vesicles can appear on the perianal skin, labia, vagina, cervix, and foreskin of the clitoris. In males, vesicles develop on the penis and occasionally on the testicles. Painful urination and a watery discharge can occur in both sexes. Also, the patient may experience systemic symptoms: fever, headache, myalgia, and tender, swollen lymph nodes in the affected region. Within days, the original blisters can evolve into large, painful, ulcer-like sores. Over the next 2 to 3 weeks, all symptoms resolve spontaneously. However, this does not indicate cure: the virus remains present in a latent state and can cause recurrence. Since we can't eliminate the virus, symptoms may recur for life. Fortunately, subsequent episodes become progressively shorter and less severe, and in some cases cease entirely. Transmission of HSV-2 can occur during the symptomatic period and for 1 week after. Infected individuals should avoid sexual contact during this time. Use of a condom reduces the risk of transmission.

***Neonatal Infection.*** Genital herpes in pregnant women can be transmitted to the infant. The infant can acquire the virus *in utero* or during delivery. Infection acquired *in utero* can result in spontaneous abortion or fetal malformation. Infection acquired during delivery can cause severe neurologic damage and even death. To protect the infant during delivery, birth should be accomplished by cesarean section if the mother has an active infection.

**Treatment.** *Acyclovir* [Zovirax] is the drug of choice for genital herpes. Although this drug cannot eliminate the virus, it can reduce systemic symptoms and shorten the duration of pain and viral shedding. When taken continuously, it can decrease the rate of recurrence. Depending on the intensity of symptoms, administration may be oral or intravenous. Topical administration may also be used but is not very effective. Patients should be warned that acyclovir will not protect against transmission of HSV-2 when infections are active and that sexual intimacy should be avoided at these times. The pharmacology of acyclovir is discussed in Chapter 87.

## Genital and Anal Warts (Condyloma Acuminatum)

Genital and perianal warts are caused by human papillomaviruses (HPVs), of which there are 40 different types. Although warts caused by most types of HPV are benign, warts caused by a few types have been strongly associated with genital carcinoma. Accordingly, a wart biopsy may be appropriate.

HPV can be transmitted by sexual contact. Individuals with anogenital warts should be warned that they can transmit the infection to sexual partners. Partners of infected individuals should be examined for warts. Use of a condom can minimize the risk of transmission.

Several forms of therapy are used to remove venereal warts. However, no form of therapy has been shown to eradicate the virus. Hence, even after successful wart removal, the virus is likely to remain.

For most patients with external genital or perianal warts, cryotherapy (freezing) is the treatment of choice.

This can be done with liquid nitrogen or a cryoprobe. Alternatives to cryotherapy include topical drugs, electrodesiccation, electrocautery, laser surgery, and conventional surgery.

Of the drugs used to treat venereal warts, *podophyllum resin* (podophyllin) is employed most widely. Podophyllum resin is a mixture of resins from the May apple or mandrake (*Podophyllum peltatum Linne*). The active ingredient in the resin is podophyllotoxin. Formulations used to remove warts contain 25% podophyllum resin. These formulations are highly caustic and should be applied only by a trained physician. To minimize the risk of toxicity from systemic absorption, the resin should be washed off with alcohol or soap and water within 1 to 4 hours of its application. Each treatment should be limited to a small surface area and to a small number of warts. A similar but less caustic preparation (0.5% podofilox), marketed under the trade name Condylox, is available for use at home. Topical *trichloroacetic acid* is an alternative to podophyllin.

## Pediculosis Pubis and Scabies

Pediculosis pubis and scabies are skin infestations caused by lice and mites, respectively. Both infestations produce intense itching, and both can be transmitted by sexual contact. Topical *permethrin* can eliminate both organisms: 1% permethrin [Nix] is used for pubic lice; 5% permethrin [RID] is used for scabies. Pediculosis, scabies, and their treatment are discussed fully in Chapter 94 (Ectoparasiticides).

## KEY POINTS

- All of the drugs used to treat STDs have been introduced in previous chapters. Key points for these drugs are presented in those chapters.

# CHAPTER 90

# Antiseptics and Disinfectants

A ntiseptics and disinfectants are locally acting drugs that are toxic to microorganisms. These agents are used to reduce acquisition and transmission of infection. Drugs suitable for antisepsis and disinfection cannot be used internally because of toxicity.

## General Considerations

### Terminology

The terms *antiseptic* and *disinfectant* are not synonymous. In common usage, the term *antiseptic* is reserved for agents *applied to living tissue*. *Disinfectants* are preparations *applied to inanimate objects*. As a rule, agents used as disinfectants are too harsh for application to living tissue. Disinfectants are employed most frequently to decontaminate surgical instruments and to cleanse hospitals and other medical facilities. Most uses of antiseptics are prophylactic. For example, antiseptics are used to cleanse the hands of medical personnel; they are applied to the patient's skin prior to invasive procedures (surgery, insertion of needles); and they are used to bathe neonates. Rarely, antiseptics are employed to treat an existing local infection. However, in most cases, established infections are best treated with a systemic antimicrobial drug.

Several related terms may need clarification. *Sterilization* indicates complete destruction of all microorganisms. In contrast, *sanitization* implies only that contamination has been reduced to a level compatible with public health standards. A *germicide* is a drug that *kills* microorganisms. Germicides may be divided into subcategories: *bactericides*, *virucides*, *fungicides*, and *amebicides*. In contrast to a germicide, a *germistatic drug* is one that *de-creases* the growth and replication of microorganisms but does not produce kill.

### Properties of an Ideal Antiseptic

The ideal antiseptic, like any other ideal drug, should be safe, effective, and selective. The preparation should be germicidal (rather than germistatic) and should have a broad spectrum of antimicrobial activity: the drug should kill bacteria and their spores, and also viruses, protozoa, yeasts, and fungi. Drug actions should be rapid and sustained. Development of microbial resistance should be low. The drug should have no harmful effects on humans: it should not produce local injury, impair healing, or produce systemic toxicity following topical application. Lastly, the drug should not cause stains, and should be devoid of offensive odor. No antiseptic has all of these characteristics.

### Time Course of Action

Toxicity to microorganisms is determined in part by duration of exposure to an antiseptic or disinfectant. Some agents act much more quickly than others. For example, ethanol (70% solution) reduces the cutaneous bacterial count by 50% in just 36 seconds. In contrast, benzalkonium chloride (at a dilution of 1:1000) requires 7 minutes to produce an equivalent effect. Because such differences in time course exist, effective use of antiseptics and disinfectants requires that health care personnel acquaint themselves with the exposure requirements of these agents.

### Use of Antiseptics to Treat Established Local Infection

In the past, topical agents were used routinely to treat established local infection. Today, *systemic* anti-infective drugs are the treatment of choice. Systemic agents are preferred for two reasons: systemic agents are more effective than topical drugs, and they are less damaging to inflamed or abraded tissue. Experience has shown that antiseptics do little to reduce infection in wounds, cuts, and abrasions. This lack of efficacy is attributed to poor penetration into the site of infection, and to diminished activity in the presence of wound exudates. Although of limited value for *established* local infection, antiseptics are quite useful as *prophylaxis*: when applied properly, antiseptics can help cleanse wounds and decrease microbial contamination.

## Using Antiseptics and Disinfectants Most Effectively

The principal value of antiseptics and disinfectants derives from their ability to prevent contamination of the patient by microorganisms present in the *environment*; it appears that antiseptics applied directly to the *patient* contribute relatively little to prophylaxis against infection. A number of clinical studies support this conclusion. In one study, over 5000 preoperative patients were bathed with hexachlorophene. Although this treatment greatly reduced the concentration of surface bacteria, it had no effect on the incidence of postoperative infection. Similarly, in a study of patients who had undergone cardiothoracic surgery, it was found that most postoperative infections were caused by organisms not present at the site of the incision. From these studies and others, we can conclude that infections are caused primarily by environmental microorganisms rather than by organisms living on the skin of the patient. Consequently, use of antiseptics by nurses, physicians, and others who contact the patient is of much greater importance than application of antiseptics to the patient. Patients also benefit greatly by the rigorous use of disinfectants to decontaminate surgical supplies and medical buildings.

# Properties of Individual Antiseptics and Disinfectants

Antiseptics and disinfectants belong to a variety of chemical families, ranging from alcohols to iodine compounds to phenols. The various antiseptics and disinfectants differ from one another with respect to mechanism of action, time course of effects, and antimicrobial spectra. In almost all cases, the drugs employed as disinfectants are not used for antisepsis and vice versa. The more commonly employed antiseptics and disinfectants are listed in Table 90-1. For each drug, the table indicates chemical family and clinical use (antisepsis, disinfection, or both). The pharmacology of individual antiseptics and disinfectants is discussed below.

## Alcohols

### Ethanol

Ethanol (ethyl alcohol) is an effective virucide and also kills most common pathogenic bacteria. The drug is inactive against bacterial spores, and its activity against

## TABLE 90-1. ANTISEPTICS AND DISINFECTANTS: CHEMICAL CATEGORY AND APPLICATION

| Chemical Category | Drug | Application | |
|---|---|:---:|:---:|
| | | Antisepsis | Disinfection |
| *Alcohols* | Ethanol | ✔ | |
| | Isopropanol | ✔ | |
| *Aldehydes* | Glutaraldehyde | | ✔ |
| | Formaldehyde | | ✔ |
| *Iodine Compounds* | Iodine tincture | ✔ | |
| | Iodine solution | ✔ | |
| | Povidone iodine | ✔ | ✔ |
| *Chlorine Compounds* | Oxychlorosene | ✔ | |
| | Sodium hypochlorite | ✔ | ✔ |
| *Phenolic Compound* | Hexachlorophene | ✔ | |
| *Miscellaneous Agents* | Chlorhexidine | ✔ | |
| | Thimerosal | ✔ | |
| | Hydrogen peroxide | | ✔ |
| | Benzalkonium chloride | ✔ | ✔ |

fungi is erratic. Bactericidal effects result from precipitation of bacterial protein and from dissolution of membranes. Ethanol can enhance the effects of several other antimicrobial preparations (e.g., chlorhexidine, hexachlorophene, benzalkonium chloride).

Ethanol is employed almost exclusively for antisepsis. The most frequent use is cleansing of the skin prior to needle insertion and minor surgery. Because of its limited activity against bacterial spores and fungi, ethanol is poorly suited for use as a disinfectant.

Optimal bacterial kill requires that ethanol be present in the proper concentration and for sufficient time. The drug is most effective at a concentration of 70%. Higher concentrations are *less* active. To produce 90% kill of surface bacteria, the skin must be kept moist with ethanol for 2 minutes. This extended exposure can be accomplished by use of ethanol foam. Exposure is prolonged because evaporation from this formulation is slower than from ethanol solution.

Ethanol should not be applied to open wounds. The drug can increase tissue damage and, by causing coagulation of proteins, can form a mass under which bacteria can multiply.

### Isopropanol

Isopropanol (isopropyl alcohol) is employed primarily as an antiseptic. When applied in concentrations greater than 70%, isopropanol is somewhat more germicidal than ethanol. Like ethanol, isopropanol can increase the effects of other antiseptics. Isopropanol promotes local vasodilation and can thereby increase bleeding from needle punctures and incisions. Isopropanol is available in concentrations ranging from 70% to 100%.

## Aldehydes
### Glutaraldehyde

Glutaraldehyde [Cidex] is lethal to all microorganisms; the drug kills bacteria, bacterial spores, viruses, and fungi. Antimicrobial effects result from cross-linking and precipitation of proteins. Glutaraldehyde is used to disinfect and sterilize surgical instruments and other medical supplies, including respiratory and anesthetic equipment, catheters, and thermometers. The drug is too harsh for use as an antiseptic. To completely eliminate bacterial spores, instruments and equipment must be immersed in glutaraldehyde for at least 10 hours. Glutaraldehyde is most active at alkaline pH. However, under alkaline conditions, glutaraldehyde eventually becomes inactive because of gradual polymerization. Consequently, alkaline solutions of glutaraldehyde are active for only 2 to 4 weeks. Glutaraldehyde should be used with adequate ventilation, since fumes can irritate the respiratory tract.

### Formaldehyde

Formaldehyde kills bacteria, bacterial spores, viruses, and fungi. Like glutaraldehyde, formaldehyde is too harsh for application to the skin. Accordingly, use is limited to disinfection and sterilization of equipment and instruments. For two reasons, formaldehyde is less desirable than glutaraldehyde. First, formaldehyde acts slowly: destruction of bacterial spores may take 2 to 4 days. Second, because of its greater volatility, formaldehyde tends to cause more respiratory irritation than glutaraldehyde.

## Iodine Compounds
### Iodine Solution and Iodine Tincture

Iodine was first employed as an antiseptic more than 150 years ago. Despite the introduction of numerous other drugs, iodine remains one of our most widely used germicidal agents. The drug is extremely effective, having the ability to kill all known bacteria, fungi, protozoa, viruses, and yeasts. Additional assets are low cost and relative lack of toxicity.

The composition of iodine solution and iodine tincture is very similar. Iodine *solution* consists of 2% elemental iodine and 2.4% sodium iodide in water. Iodine *tincture* contains the same amounts of elemental iodine and sodium iodide and also contains 47% ethanol. The ethanol enhances the antimicrobial activity of iodine tincture.

The germicidal activity of iodine tincture and iodine solution is due only to *free* (dissolved) elemental iodine. In both the tincture and the solution, the concentration of free elemental iodine is only about 0.15%. This low figure reflects the poor solubility of iodine. Since only free iodine is active, most of the elemental iodine and all of the sodium iodide present in iodine tincture and iodine solution do not contribute *directly* to microbicidal activity. However, these components do contribute *indirectly* by serving as reservoirs from which free elemental iodine can be released.

Iodine tincture and iodine solution are employed primarily for antisepsis of the skin, a use for which these drugs are the most effective agents available. When the skin is *intact*, iodine *tincture* is preferred. This preparation is commonly employed to cleanse the skin prior to intravenous injection and to withdrawal of blood for microbial culture. For treatment of *wounds* and *abrasions*, iodine *solution* should be employed. (Because of the irritant properties of alcohol, iodine tincture is less appropriate for application to broken skin.)

### Povidone-Iodine

Povidone-iodine is a complex composed of elemental iodine with povidone (an organic polymer). Povidone-iodine has no antimicrobial activity of its own, but rather serves as a reservoir from which elemental iodine can be released. Free elemental iodine is the active germicide. The concentration of free iodine achieved through application of povidone-iodine is lower than that produced with iodine tincture or iodine solution. Hence, povidone-iodine is less effective than these other iodine preparations. Povidone-iodine is employed primarily for prophylaxis against postoperative infection. Additional uses include hand washing, surgical scrubbing, and preparation of the skin prior to invasive procedures (e.g., surgery, aspiration, injection). In addition, povidone-iodine is employed to sterilize equipment; however, superior disinfectants are available. The drug is dispensed in a variety of formulations (ointments, solutions, aerosols, gels). It is also available impregnated in swabs, sponges, and wipes. Trade names include ACU-dyne, Betadine, and Operand.

## Chlorine Compounds

Chlorine is lethal to a wide variety of microbes. Chlorine is active both as elemental chlorine and as hypochlorous acid, which is formed by reaction of chlorine with water. Chlorine is used extensively to sanitize water supplies and swimming pools. However, because of physical properties that make working with chlorine difficult, chlorine itself is rarely used clinically. Instead, chlorine-containing compounds with the ability to release hypochlorous acid are employed.

## Oxychlorosene Sodium

Oxychlorosene sodium [Clorpactin] is a complex mixture of hypochlorous acid with alkylphenyl sulfonates. Antimicrobial effects derive from the release of hypochlorous acid. Oxychlorosene is lethal to bacteria, yeast, fungi, viruses, molds, and spores. This agent is employed as a topical antiseptic and can be especially useful for treating localized infection caused by drug-resistant microbes. Oxychlorosene is also employed to irrigate and cleanse fistulas, sinus tracts, wounds, and empyemas (pus-filled cavities).

### Sodium Hypochlorite

Sodium hypochlorite kills bacteria, spores, fungi, protozoa, and viruses. Undiluted (5%) solutions are employed commonly as household bleach. These concentrated solutions are too irritating for application to human tissue. For antiseptic use, dilute solutions (0.5%) are employed. These dilute preparations can be used to irrigate wounds and to cleanse and deodorize necrotic tissue. To minimize local irritation, solutions of sodium hypochlorite should be rinsed off promptly. A 1% solution can be used to sterilize equipment. Solutions of sodium hypochlorite are unstable and must be prepared fresh for each use.

## Phenols

The family of phenolic compounds consists of phenol itself and several phenol derivatives. Following its introduction in 1867, phenol rapidly became both the antiseptic and disinfectant of choice. Today, use of phenol for antiseptic purposes is rare. However, the drug is still employed in some hospitals as a disinfectant. Three phenol derivatives are discussed below.

## Hexachlorophene

**Actions.** Hexachlorophene is *bacteriostatic*, not bactericidal. The drug is quite active against gram-positive bacteria—the bacteria found most frequently on the skin. However, hexachlorophene has little or no effect on gram-negative bacteria. In fact, when used on a regular basis, hexachlorophene encourages overgrowth with gram-negative organisms. (By killing off gram-positive bacteria, hexachlorophene makes conditions more conducive to gram-negative growth.)

**Uses.** Hexachlorophene is employed most commonly as a hand-washing preparation for health care personnel. Although the effects of a single wash are minimal, with repeated use hexachlorophene can produce significant reductions in the population of cutaneous gram-positive bacteria. This cumulative effect results from residual hexachlorophene retained on the skin. Hexachlorophene has been employed to prepare the skin prior to surgery. However, availability of superior antiseptics (e.g., chlorhexidine) makes this use inappropriate.

**Adverse Effects.** Hexachlorophene can be absorbed through intact skin and mucous membranes. Absorption through denuded areas can be especially great. If absorbed in sufficient amounts, hexachlorophene causes central nervous system stimulation. Responses range from confusion to twitching to seizures. Deaths have occurred. To minimize systemic toxicity, hexachlorophene should not be applied extensively to burns, wounds, cuts, or mucous membranes. In addition, total body bathing, especially of infants, should be avoided. For bathing infants, chlorhexidine is safer and more effective.

**Preparations.** Hexachlorophene is available only by prescription. The drug is dispensed in solution and as a foam. Trade names are pHisoHex and Septisol.

## Miscellaneous Agents

### Chlorhexidine

**Actions.** Chlorhexidine is an important surgical antiseptic. The drug is fast acting and lethal to most gram-positive and gram-negative bacteria. Virucidal activity is lacking. Antibacterial effects are reduced somewhat in the presence of soap, blood, and pus. Chlorhexidine that remains on the skin after rinsing is sufficient to exert continuing germicidal effects.

**Uses.** Chlorhexidine is used for preoperative preparation of the skin and as a surgical scrub, hand-wash preparation, and wound cleanser.

**Adverse Effects.** Chlorhexidine is very safe. Routine preoperative use only rarely causes local adverse effects. Inadvertent IV injection has been reported twice: in one patient, hemolysis occurred; in the other, no ill effects were observed.

**Preparations.** Chlorhexidine gluconate (0.5%, 2%, 4%) is dispensed in combination with isopropanol (4% or 70%). Trade names include Exidine-2 Scrub, Dyna-Hex Skin Cleanser, Hibistat Germicidal Hand Rinse, and Hibiclens.

### Hydrogen Peroxide

Hydrogen peroxide is an excellent disinfectant and sterilizing agent, but is useless as an antiseptic. The entity in hydrogen peroxide solution responsible for antimicrobial effects is the hydroxyl free radical. These free radicals are destroyed when hydrogen peroxide is acted upon by catalase, an enzyme found in all tissues. Hence, contact with tissue terminates hydrogen peroxide's germicidal actions. The only benefit resulting from application of hydrogen peroxide to wounds derives from liberation of oxygen (by the reaction with catalase), which causes frothing that is sufficient to loosen debris and thereby facilitate cleansing. The principal use of hydrogen peroxide is disinfection and sterilization of instruments. A 3% to 6% solution is employed.

### Thimerosal

Thimerosal is an organic compound that contains 49% mercury, the active antimicrobial factor. Thimerosal has only weak bacteriostatic and fungistatic properties; it does not kill bacteria or fungi. Antimicrobial actions are reduced in the presence of blood and tissue proteins. Thimerosal is less effective than ethanol. Use on large areas of denuded skin may yield systemic toxicity from absorption of mercury. Poisoning from thimerosal ingestion can be treated with dimercaprol (see Chapter 100). Thimerosal has been employed to irrigate wounds and to prepare the skin prior to surgery. It has also been employed as an antiseptic for the eyes, nose, throat, and genitourinary tract. Trade names are Mersol and AeroAid.

### Benzalkonium Chloride

*Actions.* Benzalkonium chloride (BAC) is an organic quaternary ammonium compound that has antimicrobial and detergent properties. BAC is active against many gram-positive and gram-negative bacteria as well as some fungi, protozoa, and viruses. The drug is relatively inactive against *Mycobacterium tuberculosis*, *Clostridium*, and other spore-forming bacteria. Germicidal effects result from disruption of membranes, and are enhanced in the presence of ethanol. BAC is inactivated by soaps and organic material. The actions of BAC are slow compared with those of iodine.

*Antiseptic Uses.* BAC is employed for preoperative preparation of the skin and mucous membranes; as a surgical scrub; as an antiseptic for abrasions and minor wounds; as a vaginal douche; and for irrigation of the eyes, body cavities, and genitourinary tract. Since BAC is inactivated by soap, all soap must be removed by rinsing with water and 70% alcohol prior to BAC application. Concentrated solutions of BAC can cause severe local damage. Hence, care must be taken to use solutions of appropriate dilution. For several reasons (limited antimicrobial spectrum, lack of rapid action, potential for toxicity, availability of superior agents), there seems to be little to recommend BAC for antiseptic use.

*Disinfectant Use.* Immersion in BAC solution is employed for sterile storage of instruments and supplies. Adsorption of BAC onto porous material can significantly reduce the concentration of BAC in solutions. To ensure continuing efficacy, solutions should be changed or at least replenished with BAC on a regular basis.

*Preparations and Dosage.* BAC is dispensed in concentrated (17%) and diluted (1:750) solution. Trade names are Benza and Zephiran. Recommended dilutions are 1:750 (for application to intact skin and to minor wounds and abrasions); 1:2000 to 1:5000 (for application to mucous membranes and diseased or seriously damaged skin); and 1:750 to 1:5000 (for storage of instruments and supplies).

## KEY POINTS

- Because the various antiseptics and disinfectants require different durations of exposure to be effective, you must know the time course of action of the specific agent you are working with.
- Although antiseptics can help prevent *development* of a local infection, systemic anti-infective drugs are preferred for treating an *established* local infection.
- Washing with antiseptics by nurses, physicians, and others who contact the patient will do more to protect patients from infection than will application of antiseptics to patients themselves.

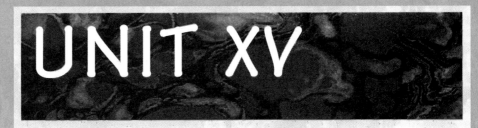

# UNIT XV

# Chemotherapy of Parasitic Diseases

Anthelmintics

Antiprotozoal Drugs I: Antimalarial Agents

Antiprotozoal Drugs II: Miscellaneous Agents

Ectoparasiticides

# CHAPTER 91

# Anthelmintics

**Classification of Parasitic Worms**
**Helminthic Infestations**
    Nematode Infestations (Intestinal)
    Nematode Infestations (Extraintestinal)
    Cestode Infestations
    Trematode Infestations

**Drugs of Choice for Helminthiasis**
    Mebendazole
    Thiabendazole
    Pyrantel
    Praziquantel
    Diethylcarbamazine
    Albendazole
    Ivermectin

Helminths are parasitic worms; *anthelmintics* are the drugs used against them. Helminthiasis (worm infestation) is the most common affliction of humans, affecting more than 2 billion people worldwide. The intestine is a frequent site of infestation. Other sites include the liver, lymphatic system, and blood vessels. Infestation is frequently asymptomatic. However, infestation with some parasites can cause severe complications. Helminthiasis is most prevalent where sanitation is poor. Cleanliness greatly reduces the risk of infestation.

Treatment of helminthiasis is not always indicated. Most parasitic worms do not reproduce within the human body. Hence, in the absence of reinfestation, many infections subside on their own as adult worms die. Since many infestations abate spontaneously, treatment may be optional. In countries where physicians and medication are readily available, drug therapy is definitely indicated. However, in less fortunate locales, several factors—cost of medication, limited medical facilities, high probability of reinfestation—may render individual treatment impractical. In these places, preventative measures, such as improved hygiene and elimination of carriers, may be the most valuable means of controlling infestation.

In approaching the anthelmintic drugs, we will begin by reviewing classification of the parasitic worms. Next we will briefly discuss the characteristics of the more common helminthic infestations. After this, we will discuss the drugs of choice for treating helminthiasis.

## Classification of Parasitic Worms

The most common parasitic worms belong to three classes: Nematoda (roundworms), Cestoda (tapeworms), and Trematoda (flukes). Nematodes belong to the phylum Nemathelminthes. Cestodes and trematodes belong to the phylum Platyhelminthes (flat worms).

### Nematodes (Roundworms)

Parasitic nematodes can be subdivided into two groups: (1) those that infest the intestinal lumen and (2) those that inhabit tissues. There are five major species of intestinal nematodes. Common names for these organisms are giant roundworm, pinworm, hookworm, whipworm, and threadworm. Official names of these parasites are listed in Table 91–1. Two types of nematodes invade tissues: (1) pork roundworms (responsible for trichinosis) and (2) filariae. The three species of filariae encountered most commonly are listed in Table 91–1.

### Cestodes (Tapeworms)

Three species of cestodes infest humans. Common names for these parasites are beef tapeworm, pork tapeworm, and fish tapeworm. Official names of these organisms appear in Table 91–1.

### Trematodes (Flukes)

Five species of trematodes infest humans. These organisms fall into four groups having the following common names: blood fluke, liver fluke, intestinal fluke, and lung fluke. Official names of the five species belonging to these groups are given in Table 91–1.

## Helminthic Infestations

This section describes the major characteristics of infestation by specific helminths. These infestations can differ with respect to anatomic site and danger to the host. Infestations also differ with respect to the drugs employed for treatment (see Table 91–1 for a summary).

## TABLE 91–1. DRUGS OF CHOICE FOR PARASITIC WORMS

| Worm Class | Parasitic Organism | | Drugs of Choice |
| | Common Name | Official Name | |
| --- | --- | --- | --- |
| Nematodes (roundworms): Intestinal | Giant roundworm<br>Pinworm<br>Hookworm | *Ascaris lumbricoides*<br>*Enterobius vermicularis*<br>*Ancylostoma duodenale,*<br>*Necator americanus* | Mebendazole or pyrantel |
| | Whipworm | *Trichuris trichiura* | Mebendazole |
| | Threadworm | *Strongyloides stercoralis* | Thiabendazole |
| Nematodes: Tissue invading | Pork roundworm | *Trichinella spiralis* | Mebendazole* |
| | Filariae | *Wuchereria bancrofti,*<br>*Brugia malayi, Loa loa* | Diethylcarbamazine |
| Cestodes (tapeworms) | Beef tapeworm<br>Pork tapeworm<br>Fish tapeworm | *Taenia saginata*<br>*Taenia solium*<br>*Diphyllobothrium latum* | Praziquantel |
| Trematodes (flukes) | Blood fluke<br>Intestinal fluke<br>Lung fluke | *Schistosoma* species<br>*Fasciolopsis buski*<br>*Paragonimus westermani* | Praziquantel |
| | Liver fluke | *Fasciola hepatica,*<br>*Clonorchis sinensis* | Bithionol† |

*Not FDA approved for this indication.
†Available from the Centers for Disease Control and Prevention.

The name applied to an infestation is based on the official name of the invading organism. For example, infestation with the giant roundworm, whose official name is *Ascaris lumbricoides*, is referred to as *ascariasis*.

In the discussion below, the helminthic infestations are grouped in four categories: (1) nematode infestations of the intestine, (2) nematode infestations at extraintestinal sites, (3) cestode infestations, and (4) trematode infestations.

### Nematode Infestations (Intestinal)

*Ascariasis (Giant Roundworm Infestation).* Ascariasis is the most prevalent helminthic infestation. Worldwide, one of every three people is affected. Adult worms inhabit the small intestine. Ascariasis is usually asymptomatic. However, serious complications can result if worms migrate into the pancreatic duct, bile duct, gallbladder, or liver. In addition, if infestation is extremely heavy, intestinal blockage may occur. Because of these potential hazards, ascariasis should always be treated. Drugs of choice are *mebendazole* and *pyrantel.*

*Enterobiasis (Pinworm Infestation).* Enterobiasis is the most common helminthic infestation in the United States. Adult pinworms inhabit the ileum and large intestine. Their life span is approximately 2 months. Although usually asymptomatic, enterobiasis may cause intense perineal itching in some patients. Serious complications are rare. Drugs of choice are *mebendazole* and *pyrantel.* Because enterobiasis is readily transmitted, all family members of an infected individual should be treated simultaneously.

*Ancylostomiasis and Necatoriasis (Hookworm Infestation).* Hookworm infestation is most common in rural areas where hygiene is poor and people go barefoot. Adult hookworms attach to the wall of the small intestine and suck blood. As a result, infestation is associated with chronic blood loss and progressive anemia. Symptomatic anemia is most likely in menstruating women and undernourished individuals. Nausea, vomiting, and abdominal pain may accompany the infestation. *Mebendazole* and *pyrantel* are the treatments of choice.

*Trichuriasis (Whipworm Infestation).* Trichuriasis is extremely common, affecting about 1 billion people worldwide. Larvae and adult worms inhabit the large intestine. Mature worms may live for 10 or more years. The disease is usually devoid of symptoms. However, when the worm burden is very large, rectal prolapse may occur. Patients with severe infestation require therapy. *Mebendazole* is the treatment of choice.

*Strongyloidiasis (Threadworm Infestation).* Strongyloidiasis is common in the southern United States. Larval and adult threadworms inhabit the small intestine. The disease can be very dangerous, although symptoms are usually absent. Mild infestation may cause abdominal pain and occasional diarrhea. Severe infestation can cause vomiting, massive diarrhea, dehydration, electrolyte imbalance, and secondary bacteremia. Deaths have occurred. Affected individuals should always be treated. *Thiabendazole* is the agent of choice. *Ivermectin* is an alternative.

### Nematode Infestations (Extraintestinal)

*Trichinosis (Pork Roundworm Infestation).* Trichinosis is acquired by eating undercooked pork that is infested with encysted larvae of *Trichinella spiralis*. Adult worms reside in the intestine, whereas larvae migrate to skeletal muscle and become encysted. Some encysted larvae live for years; others die and calcify within months. Symptoms of trichinosis include gastrointestinal upset, fever, muscle pain, and sore throat. Potentially lethal complications (heart failure, meningitis, neuritis) arise in some patients. *Mebendazole* is the drug of choice for killing adult worms and migrating larvae. However, this agent may not be active against larvae that have become encysted. *Prednisone* (a glucocorticoid) is given to reduce inflammation during larval migration.

**Wuchereriasis and Brugiasis (Lymphatic Filarial Infestation).** *Wuchereria bancrofti* and *Brugia malayi* are filarial nematodes that invade the lymphatic system. Infestation with either organism can cause severe complications. When infestation is heavy, lymphatic obstruction occurs, resulting in *elephantiasis* (usually of the scrotum or legs). In addition, "filarial fever" may develop. Symptoms include chills, fever, headache, nausea, vomiting, constipation, and lymphadenitis. The drug of choice for use against both filarial species is *diethylcarbamazine.*

## Cestode Infestations

**Taeniasis (Beef and Pork Tapeworm Infestation).** Taeniasis is acquired by eating undercooked beef or pork that contains tapeworm larvae. Adult tapeworms live attached to the wall of the small intestine. Infestation is usually asymptomatic. Taeniasis is treated with *praziquantel.*

**Diphyllobothriasis (Fish Tapeworm Infestation).** Diphyllobothriasis is acquired by ingestion of undercooked fish that is infested with tapeworm larvae. Adult worms inhabit the ileum. Infestation is usually devoid of symptoms. Worms can be killed with *praziquantel.*

## Trematode Infestations

**Schistosomiasis (Blood Fluke Infestations).** The term *schistosomiasis* refers to infestation with blood flukes of any species (e.g., *Schistosoma mansoni, S. japonicum*). Specific snails serve as intermediate hosts for these flukes. Schistosomiasis cannot be acquired in the continental United States because the appropriate snails are not indigenous.

Schistosomiasis has an acute and a chronic phase. The acute phase subsides in 3 to 4 months. Symptoms that accompany this phase include lymphadenopathy, fever, anorexia, malaise, muscle pain, and rash. During the chronic phase, schistosomes take up residence in the vascular system, primarily in the veins of the intestines and liver. This late infestation can produce intestinal polyposis, hepatosplenomegaly, and portal hypertension. For either the acute or the chronic stage, *praziquantel* is the treatment of choice.

**Fascioliasis (Liver Fluke Infestation).** Fascioliasis is the only fluke infestation indigenous to the United States. These parasites inhabit the biliary tract. Symptoms (anorexia, mild fever, fatigue, aching in the region of the liver) are delayed for 1 to 3 months.

*Bithionol* [Bitin, Lorothidol] is the treatment of choice for liver flukes. The most frequent adverse effects of the drug are photosensitivity reactions, vomiting, diarrhea, abdominal pain, and urticaria. Leukopenia and toxic hepatitis occur rarely. The recommended dosage for adults and children is 30 to 50 mg on alternate days for 10 to 15 doses. Bithionol, an investigational drug in the United States, is available from the Centers for Disease Control and Prevention.

**Fasciolopsiasis (Intestinal Fluke Infestation).** Fasciolopsiasis is most common in Southeast Asia. Adult worms inhabit the small intestine. The disease is usually asymptomatic. In some people, ulcer-like pain is experienced. Disruption of bowel function (constipation or diarrhea) may occur. In the presence of massive infestation, bowel obstruction may develop; clearance may require surgery. *Praziquantel* is the treatment of choice.

# Drugs of Choice for Helminthiasis

The five most commonly employed anthelmintic drugs are considered below. These agents differ from one another in antiparasitic spectra: some agents are active against several worms; others are more selective. Because of these differences, it is important to identify the invading organism so that the most appropriate therapeutic agent can be chosen. Table 91–2 lists the major anthelmintic drugs and indicates the parasites against which each is most effective. Although the discussion that follows is limited to drugs of choice, be aware that additional anthelmintics are available.

## Mebendazole

**Target Organisms.** Mebendazole [Vermox] is a drug of choice for most *intestinal roundworms*. This agent clears infestation with *pinworms, hookworms, whipworms,* and *giant roundworms*. Because of its relatively broad spectrum of action, mebendazole is especially useful for treatment of mixed infestations. In addition to its use against intestinal roundworms, mebendazole is the drug of choice for *pork roundworms,* the cause of trichinosis.

**Mechanism of Action.** Mebendazole prevents uptake of glucose by susceptible intestinal worms. Lack of glucose results in immobilization followed by slow death. Since the worms die slowly, up to 3 days may elapse between initiation of treatment and complete clearance of parasites. Mebendazole does not influence glucose uptake or utilization by humans.

**Pharmacokinetics.** Only a small fraction (5% to 10%) of orally administered mebendazole is absorbed, and this fraction undergoes rapid metabolism. Consequently, plasma levels of mebendazole remain low.

**Adverse Effects.** Systemic effects are rare at usual doses, perhaps because the drug is so poorly absorbed. In patients with massive parasitic infestations, transient abdominal pain and diarrhea may occur.

Relatively low doses of mebendazole are embryotoxic and teratogenic in rats. However, these effects have not been observed in dogs, sheep, or horses. Limited experience with mebendazole in pregnant women has shown no increase in spontaneous abortion or fetal malformation. Nonetheless, *it is recommended that pregnant women avoid this drug, especially during the first trimester.*

**Preparations, Dosage, and Administration.** Mebendazole [Vermox] is available in 100-mg tablets for oral administration. The tablets may be chewed, crushed, or swallowed whole. Dosages are summarized in Table 91–2.

## Thiabendazole

**Target Organisms.** Thiabendazole [Mintezol] is the drug of choice for *threadworms*. Although the drug is also active against pork roundworm, mebendazole is preferred.

**Mechanism of Action.** Thiabendazole can inhibit helminth-specific fumarate reductase, but the contribution of this action to therapeutic effects is not known. Symptomatic improvement in patients with trichinosis may result in part from the analgesic, antipyretic, and anti-inflammatory actions of thiabendazole.

## TABLE 91–2. FIRST CHOICE ANTHELMINTIC DRUGS: TARGET ORGANISMS AND DOSAGES

| Generic Name [Trade Name] | Target Organism | Adult Dosage | Pediatric Dosage |
|---|---|---|---|
| Mebendazole [Vermox] | Giant roundworm Whipworm Hookworm | 100 mg bid for 3 days | Same as adult |
| | Pork roundworm | 200–400 mg tid for 3 days, then 400–500 mg tid for 10 days | Same as adult |
| | Pinworm | 100 mg; repeat in 2 weeks | Same as adult |
| Thiabenzadole [Mintezol] | Threadworm | 25 mg/kg bid for 2 days | Same as adult |
| Pyrantel [Antiminth] | Giant roundworm | 11 mg/kg (once) | Same as adult |
| | Hookworm | 11 mg/kg for 3 days | Same as adult |
| | Pinworm | 11 mg/kg; repeat in 2 weeks | Same as adult |
| Praziquantel [Biltricide] | Beef tapeworm Pork tapeworm Fish tapeworm | 5–10 mg/kg (once) | Same as adult |
| | Blood flukes | 20 mg/kg tid for 1 day | Same as adult |
| | Intestinal fluke | 25 mg/kg tid for 1 day | Same as adult |
| | Lung fluke | 25 mg/kg tid for 2 days | Same as adult |
| Diethylcarbamazine [Hetrazan] | Filariae | Day 1: 50 mg Day 2: 50 mg tid Day 3: 100 mg tid Days 4–21: 2 mg/kg tid | Day 1: 1 mg/kg Day 2: 1 mg/kg tid Day 3: 1–2 mg/kg tid Days 4–21: 2 mg/kg tid |
| Bithionol* [Bitin, Lorothidol] | Liver fluke | 30–50 mg on alternate days for 10–15 doses | Same as adult |

*Available from the Centers for Disease Control and Prevention.

**Pharmacokinetics.** Thiabendazole undergoes rapid absorption and metabolism. Most of each dose is excreted in the urine as metabolites within 24 hours.

**Adverse Effects.** The incidence of adverse reactions is high: as many as one third of those treated become incapacitated for several hours. The most common effects are gastrointestinal (anorexia, nausea, vomiting) and neurologic (dizziness, drowsiness). Because of the potential for reduced alertness, patients should avoid hazardous activities (e.g., driving). Hepatotoxicity with jaundice has been reported. Accordingly, thiabendazole should be avoided in patients with liver dysfunction.

**Preparations, Dosage, and Administration.** Thiabendazole [Mintezol] is available in 500-mg chewable tablets and an oral suspension (100 mg/ml). Patients should be instructed to chew the tablets thoroughly. Gastrointestinal discomfort can be reduced by administering thiabendazole with food. The adult and pediatric dosage for threadworm infestation is 25 mg/kg twice daily for 2 days.

### Pyrantel

**Target Organisms.** Pyrantel is active against *intestinal nematodes*. The drug is an alternative to mebendazole for infestations with *hookworms, pinworms,* and *giant roundworms*.

**Mechanism of Action.** Pyrantel is a depolarizing neuromuscular blocking agent that causes spastic paralysis of intestinal parasites. The paralyzed worms are cleared in the feces.

**Pharmacokinetics.** Pyrantel is poorly absorbed, and plasma levels remain low. Most of an administered dose is excreted unchanged in the feces.

**Adverse Effects.** Serious reactions are rare. The most common effects are gastrointestinal reactions (nausea, vomiting, diarrhea, stomach pain, cramps). Possible central nervous system effects include dizziness, drowsiness, headache, and insomnia.

**Preparations, Dosage, and Administration.** Pyrantel pamoate [Antiminth, Reese's Pinworm] is dispensed in liquid formulations (50 mg/ml) for oral use. The entire prescribed dose should be taken at one time. Dosages for intestinal nematodes are given in Table 91–2.

### Praziquantel

**Target Organisms.** Praziquantel [Biltricide] is very active against *nematodes* (flukes) and *cestodes* (tapeworms). This agent is a drug of choice for *tapeworms, schistosomiasis,* and other *fluke infestations*.

**Mechanism of Action.** Praziquantel is readily absorbed by helminths. At low therapeutic concentrations, the drug produces spastic paralysis, causing detachment of worms from body tissues. At high therapeutic concentrations, praziquantel disrupts the integument of the worms, rendering the parasites vulnerable to lethal attack by host defenses.

***Pharmacokinetics.*** Praziquantel is rapidly absorbed from the GI tract. The drug undergoes extensive hepatic metabolism. Metabolites are excreted in the urine.

***Adverse Effects.*** Praziquantel is relatively free of toxicity. Transient headache and abdominal discomfort are the most frequent reactions. Drowsiness may occur, and patients should avoid driving and other hazardous activities.

***Preparations, Dosage, and Administration.*** Praziquantel [Biltricide] is available in 600-mg tablets for oral administration. Tablets should be swallowed intact. Dosages for tapeworm and fluke infestations are presented in Table 91–2.

### Diethylcarbamazine

***Target Organisms.*** Diethylcarbamazine [Hetrazan] is the drug of choice for *filarial infestations*. The drug destroys microfilariae of *Wuchereria bancrofti*, *Brugia malayi*, and *Loa loa*. In addition, it kills adult females of these species.

***Mechanism of Action.*** Diethylcarbamazine has two antifilarial actions. First, the drug reduces muscular activity, thereby causing parasites to be dislodged from their site of attachment. Second, by altering the surface properties of the parasites, the drug renders the organisms more vulnerable to attack by host defenses.

***Pharmacokinetics.*** Diethylcarbamazine is readily absorbed and undergoes rapid and extensive metabolism. Metabolites are excreted in the urine.

***Adverse Effects.*** Reactions caused directly by diethylcarbamazine are minor (headache, weakness, dizziness, nausea, vomiting). Indirect effects, occurring secondary to death of the parasites, can be more serious. These include rashes, intense itching, encephalitis, fever, tachycardia, lymphadenitis, leukocytosis, and proteinuria. Fortunately, these reactions are transient, lasting only a few days, and they can be minimized by pretreatment with glucocorticoids.

***Preparations, Dosage, and Administration.*** Diethylcarbamazine citrate [Hetrazan] is dispensed in 50-mg tablets for oral use. The drug is available without charge from Lederle Laboratories. Dosages for filarial infestations are presented in Table 91–2.

### Albendazole

***Target Organisms.*** Albendazole [Albenza] is active against many cestode and nematode parasites, including larval forms of *Taenia solium* and *Echinococcus granulosus*. In the United States, the drug is approved for (1) parenchymal *neurocysticercosis* caused by larval forms of the pork tapeworm, *T. Solium*, and (2) *cystic hydatid disease* of the liver, lung, and peritoneum caused by larval form of the dog tapeworm, *E. granulosus*. Albendazole can also be used to treat *ascariasis*, *trichuriasis*, *enterobiasis*, and *strongyloidiasis*, although it is not approved for these helminthic infestations.

***Mechanism of Action.*** Albendazole inhibits polymerization of tubulin, and thereby prevents formation of cytoplasmic microtubules. As a result, microtubule-dependent uptake of glucose is prevented.

***Pharmacokinetics.*** Albendazole is poorly absorbed from the GI tract, owing largely to low solubility in water. Absorption is enhanced by administration with a fatty meal. Following absorption, albendazole is rapidly converted to albendazole sulfoxide, its active form. Albendazole sulfoxide is distributed widely to body fluids and tissues, and is excreted in the bile. The drug's half-life is 8 to 12 hours.

***Adverse Effects.*** Albendazole is generally well tolerated. Mild to moderate *liver impairment* has occurred in 16% of patients, as indicated by elevation of liver transaminases in plasma. Liver function should be assessed before treatment and periodically thereafter. Albendazole is teratogenic in animals and hence *should not be used during pregnancy*. If pregnancy occurs, the drug should be discontinued immediately.

***Preparations, Dosage, and Administration.*** Albendazole [Albenza] is dispensed in 200-mg tablets for oral use. Each dose (for neurocysticercosis or cystic hydatid disease) is 400 mg (for patients >60 kg) or 7.5 mg/kg (for patients <60 kg). The dosing schedule for cystic hydatid disease is 2 doses twice daily with meals for 8 to 30 days. Dosing for neurocysticercosis is done in three consecutive cycles, each consisting of 2 doses twice daily with meals for 28 days followed by 14 days with no drug.

### Ivermectin

In 1997, ivermectin [Stromectol] was approved by the Food and Drug Administration for treatment of two helminthic infestations: *onchocerciasis* (a major cause of blindness worldwide) and intestinal *strongyloidiasis*. The drug has been used in other parts of the world since 1987, where it has been taken by over 6 million people. Ivermectin is a structural analog of the macrolide antibiotics (e.g., erythromycin) but lacks antibacterial activity. Anthelmintic effects appear to result from promoting opening of chloride channels. In patients with onchocerciasis, ivermectin greatly reduces the number of microfilariae in the skin and eyes following a single oral dose (150 µg/kg). In patients with intestinal strongyloidiasis, the cure rate is 64% to 100% following a single dose (200 µg/kg).

The most common adverse effects are diarrhea, nausea, dizziness, rashes, and pruritus. Recent studies indicate that ivermectin can also cure *scabies*, an infestation discussed in Chapter 94. In addition to its use in humans, ivermectin is used widely to treat parasitic infections in animals.

## KEY POINTS

- Since each anthelmintic drug is active against a limited range of worms, we must take care to select the appropriate drug for the infestation to be treated.
- With the exception of thiabendazole, the drugs discussed in this chapter are generally devoid of serious adverse effects.
- Since many worm infestations are asymptomatic and self-limited, drug therapy can be optional. When cost is no issue, treatment is clearly indicated; however, in countries where health care funds are very limited, preventative public health measures directed at improved hygiene and elimination of carriers may be more cost-effective than treating each infested individual

# Antiprotozoal Drugs I: Antimalarial Agents

alaria is a parasitic disease caused by protozoa of the genus *Plasmodium*. With the exception of tuberculosis, malaria kills more people than any other infectious disease. Between 270 million and 490 million people are afflicted, and more than 2 million die each year. Seventy-five percent of deaths occur in Africa, primarily among children. In the United States, about 1000 cases are reported annually.

Large-scale attempts to eradicate the disease have achieved only partial success. Eradication programs have been directed at the malarial parasite as well as the *Anopheles* mosquito, the insect that transmits malaria to humans. Failure to produce complete control has resulted largely from development of drug resistance by both the parasite and the mosquito. The incidence of malaria is now rising in regions where it had once been suppressed. There remains a great need for safe, effective, and affordable agents capable of killing the malaria parasite and its mosquito carrier.

In approaching the antimalarial drugs, we will begin by reviewing the life cycle of the malaria parasite. After that we will discuss the two major subtypes of malaria: falciparum malaria and vivax malaria. Next, we will consider basic principles of treatment, focusing on therapeutic objectives and drug selection. Having established this background, we will discuss the pharmacology of the major antimalarial drugs.

## Life Cycle of the Malaria Parasite

In order to understand the actions and specific applications of antimalarial drugs, we must first understand the life cycle of the malaria parasite. As indicated in Figure 92–1, this cycle takes place in two hosts: humans and the female *Anopheles* mosquito. In the human host, the parasite undergoes asexual reproduction. In the mosquito, the parasite undergoes sexual reproduction.

The human phase of the life cycle begins when sporozoites are injected into the bloodstream by a feeding *Anopheles* mosquito. These sporozoites invade parenchymal cells of the liver, where they multiply and transform into merozoites. This process, which takes from 12 to 26 days, depending upon the species of parasite, is referred to as the pre-erythrocytic or exoerythrocytic phase of the life cycle. Upon release from the liver, merozoites infect erythrocytes. Within the erythrocyte, each parasite differentiates and divides, becoming first a trophozoite and then a multinucleated schizont. The schizont then evolves into new merozoites. This process of asexual reproduction takes 2 to 3 days, after which red blood cells burst and release the new merozoites into the blood. These new merozoites then infect fresh erythrocytes, thereby establishing an escalating cycle of red cell invasion and lysis. Each time the erythrocytes rupture, they release pyrogenic agents. These substances induce the repeating episodes of fever that characterize malaria. After several cycles of asexual repro-duction, a few parasites differentiate into male and female gametocytes.

Sexual reproduction occurs following ingestion of gametocyte-containing blood by a female *Anopheles* mosquito. Within the mosquito, the gametocytes differentiate into mature forms, after which fertilization takes place. The resulting zygote then produces sporozoites, thus completing sexual reproduction.

## Types of Malaria

Malaria is caused by four different species of *Plasmodium*. We will limit discussion to the two species en-

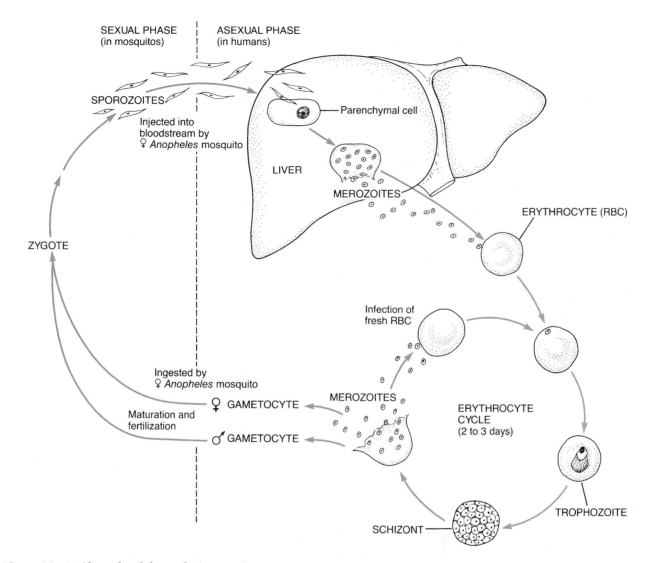

**Figure 92–1. Life cycle of the malaria parasite.**

countered most frequently: *Plasmodium vivax* and *Plasmodium falciparum*. Malaria caused by either species is characterized by high fever, chills, and profuse sweating. However, despite similarity of symptoms, these two forms of malaria are very different. They differ most with regard to severity of symptoms, occurrence of relapse, and drug resistance. These and other differences are summarized in Table 92–1.

## Vivax Malaria

Vivax malaria, caused by *P. vivax*, is the most common form of malaria. Fortunately, the disease is relatively mild and usually self-limiting. Since drug resistance by *P. vivax* is still uncommon, symptoms can be readily suppressed with medication.

Infection begins when the host is inoculated with *P. vivax* sporozoites. After 26 days, merozoites emerge from the liver and begin their attack on erythrocytes. Symptoms of malaria (chills, fever, sweating) commence as infected erythrocytes rupture, releasing pyrogens and

other substances into the blood. Symptoms peak, decline, and peak again every 48 hours in response to cyclic reinfection and lysis of red cells. This cycle continues until terminated by drugs or by acquired immunity. Unfortunately, relapse is likely following termination of the acute attack. Relapse is possible because dormant forms of *P. vivax* remain in the liver. These dormant forms periodically evolve into merozoites, emerge from the liver, and start the erythrocytic cycle anew. Relapse becomes less frequent with the passage of time, and, after 2 or more years, ceases entirely. Relapse can be stopped with drugs capable of killing the dormant hepatic parasites.

## Falciparum Malaria

Malaria caused by *P. falciparum* is less common than malaria caused by *P. vivax*, but is much more severe. In the absence of treatment, the disease is lethal to about 10% of its victims. This infection is made even more dangerous by the emergence of drug-resistant strains of *P. falciparum*. Unlike the symptoms of vivax malaria, which

**TABLE 92-1. COMPARISON OF VIVAX MALARIA AND FALCIPARUM MALARIA**

| Characteristics | Type of Malaria | |
| --- | --- | --- |
| | Vivax Malaria | Falciparum Malaria |
| Causative organism | *Plasmodium vivax* | *Plasmodium falciparum* |
| Frequency of infection | More common | Less common |
| Latency of symptoms | 26 days | 12 days |
| Intensity of symptoms | Mild | Severe |
| Timing of febrile paroxysms | Every 2 days | Irregular |
| Probability of relapse | High | None |
| Drug resistance | Uncommon | Common |

peak every 48 hours, the symptoms of falciparum malaria occur at irregular intervals. The erythrocyte cycle of *P. falciparum* can destroy up to 60% of circulating red blood cells, resulting in profound anemia and weakness. The hemoglobin released from these cells causes the urine to darken, giving rise to the term *blackwater fever*. Falciparum malaria can produce serious complications, including pulmonary edema, hypoglycemia, and toxic encephalopathy, characterized by confusion, coma, and convulsions. When treated early, falciparum malaria usually responds well. However, if treatment is delayed, the disease may progress rapidly to irreversible shock and death. In contrast to infection with *P. vivax*, infection with *P. falciparum* does not relapse. This is because there are no dormant forms of *P. falciparum* in the liver. Hence, once the erythrocytic forms have been eliminated, the patient is free of the infection.

# Principles of Antimalarial Therapy

## Therapeutic Objectives

Drug responsiveness of the malaria parasite changes as the parasite goes through its life cycle. The *erythrocytic* stages are killed most easily, whereas the *exoerythrocytic* (hepatic) stages are more difficult to kill. *Sporozoites* do not respond to drugs at all. Because of these differences in drug sensitivity, antimalarial therapy has three separate objectives: (1) treatment of an acute attack (clinical cure), (2) prevention of relapse (radical cure), and (3) prophylaxis (suppressive therapy). Because sporozoites are insensitive to drugs, therapy cannot prevent primary infection of the liver.

**Treatment of Acute Attack.** Clinical cure is accomplished with drugs that are active against erythrocytic forms of the malaria parasite. By eliminating parasites from red blood cells, the erythrocytic cycle is stopped and symptoms cease. For patients with vivax malaria, clinical cure will not prevent relapse, since dormant parasites re-

main in the liver. However, for patients with falciparum malaria, successful treatment of the acute attack will prevent further episodes (unless the patient is reinoculated by another infected mosquito).

**Prevention of Relapse.** People infected with *P. vivax* harbor dormant parasites in the liver. In order to prevent relapse, a drug capable of killing these hepatic forms must be taken. The use of drugs to eradicate hepatic *P. vivax* is referred to as radical cure. Since reinfection by a mosquito bite is a virtual certainty as long as one remains in a region where malaria is endemic, radical cure is usually postponed until departure from the region.

**Prophylaxis.** Persons anticipating travel to an area where malaria is endemic should take antimalarial medication for prophylaxis. Although drugs cannot prevent primary infection of the liver, they *can* prevent infection of erythrocytes. Hence, although the parasite may be present, symptoms of malaria are avoided. Since prophylactic treatment prevents only symptoms and not invasion of the liver, such treatment is often referred to as *suppressive therapy*.

Nondrug measures can help greatly to prevent infection. Since *Anopheles* mosquitoes only bite between dusk and dawn, clothing that covers as much skin as possible should be worn during this time; a DEET-containing insect repellent should be applied to skin that remains exposed. Sleeping under mosquito netting that has been impregnated with permethrin (an insecticide) further reduces the risk of a bite.

## Drug Selection

Selection of antimalarial drugs is based largely on two factors: (1) the goal of treatment and (2) drug resistance of the causative strain of *Plasmodium*. Drugs of choice for treatment and prophylaxis are discussed below and summarized in Table 92–2.

**Treatment of Acute Attacks.** Chloroquine is the drug of choice for an acute attack of malaria caused by either *P. vivax* or by chloroquine-sensitive strains of *P. falciparum*. As a rule, a 3-day course of treatment produces clinical cure. For strains of *P. falciparum* that are resistant to chloroquine—and most are—quinine is the drug of

## TABLE 92-2. DRUGS OF CHOICE FOR MALARIA*

| Therapeutic Objective | Plasmodium strain | | |
| --- | --- | --- | --- |
| | *P. vivax* | *P. falciparum:* Chloroquine Sensitive | *P. falciparum:* Chloroquine Resistant |
| *Treatment of Acute Attack* | Chloroquine[†] | Chloroquine[†] | Quinine[†] *plus either* tetracycline, Fansidar,[‡] or clindamycin |
| *Prevention of Relapse* | Primaquine | NA[§] | NA[§] |
| *Prophylaxis* | Chloroquine | Chloroquine | Mefloquine or doxycycline[‖] |

*All drugs are administered orally except where noted.
[†] For severe attacks, treat parenterally with either quinidine gluconate or quinine dihydrochloride.
[‡] Fansidar = pyrimethamine plus sulfadoxine.
[§] Not applicable. Malaria caused by *P. falciparum* does not relapse following successful treatment of the acute attack.
[‖] Doxycycline is used in regions of mefloquine resistance.

choice, combined with either tetracycline, clindamycin, or Fansidar (pyrimethamine plus sulfadoxine).

**Prevention of Relapse.** The drug of choice for preventing relapse of vivax malaria is primaquine, a drug that is highly active against the hepatic stages of *P. vivax.* For falciparum malaria, no treatment is needed, since relapse does not occur following clinical cure of this form of malaria.

**Prophylaxis.** Selection of drugs for prophylaxis is based on the drug sensitivity of the plasmodial species found in the region to which travel is intended. In regions where chloroquine-sensitive strains are found, chloroquine is the preferred drug for prophylaxis. In regions of chloroquine-resistant *P. falciparum,* mefloquine is the preferred prophylactic agent. Alternatively, the traveler can take chloroquine for prophylaxis and then take Fansidar (pyrimethamine plus sulfadoxine) if febrile symptoms of malaria develop.

# Pharmacology of the Major Antimalarial Drugs

## Chloroquine

**Actions and Use.** Chloroquine [Aralen] is the most generally useful of the antimalarial drugs. This agent is highly active against erythrocytic forms of the malaria parasite. Consequently, chloroquine is the drug of choice for treating acute attacks caused by *P. vivax* and by chloroquine-sensitive strains of *P. falciparum.* Chloroquine is also the drug of first choice for prophylaxis (suppressive therapy).

Chloroquine is not active against *exoerythrocytic* forms of the malaria parasite. Hence, the drug is unable to prevent primary infection by *P. vivax* or *P. falciparum.* Nor

is it able to prevent relapse of vivax malaria, which is caused by emergence of dormant hepatic parasites.

Several mechanisms have been proposed to explain the lethal effects of chloroquine on erythrocytic stages of the malaria parasite. The most likely is that chloroquine prevents the organism from converting heme to nontoxic metabolites. (Heme, a potentially toxic compound, is produced by the parasite as it digests hemoglobin in the host's red blood cells.) Chloroquine concentrates in parasitized erythrocytes, and this may explain the selective actions against erythrocytic forms of *Plasmodium.*

**Pharmacokinetics.** Chloroquine is rapidly and completely absorbed from the gastrointestinal tract. A substantial fraction of absorbed drug is deposited in certain tissues (e.g., lung, spleen, liver, kidney). Slow release from these sites helps maintain therapeutic plasma levels. Hence, when used for prophylaxis, chloroquine can be administered just once a week. Excretion is primarily nonrenal.

**Adverse Effects.** Since the doses required for prophylaxis are low, and since the higher doses required for treatment are taken only briefly, chloroquine rarely causes serious adverse effects. When employed to treat an acute malarial attack, chloroquine may cause visual disturbances, pruritus, headache, and gastrointestinal effects (abdominal discomfort, nausea, diarrhea). Gastrointestinal effects can be minimized by taking the drug with meals. Because chloroquine concentrates in the liver, it should be used with caution in patients with hepatic disease.

**Routes of Administration.** Chloroquine may be administered orally or IM. Oral therapy is preferred. Intramuscular administration is employed only when emesis precludes oral treatment or when infection is especially severe.

**Preparations and Dosage.** *Chloroquine phosphate* [Aralen] is dispensed in tablets (250 and 500 mg) for oral administration.

*Chloroquine hydrochloride* (50 mg/ml in 5-ml ampules) is employed for IM injection.

For *prophylaxis* of malaria, the adult dosage is 500 mg of chloroquine phosphate once a week. The pediatric dosage is 8.3 mg/kg once a week. Treatment should commence 1 week before expected exposure to malaria and should continue for 4 weeks after leaving the endemic region.

To *treat an acute attack*, the adult dosage is 1 gm of chloroquine phosphate (PO) initially followed in 6 hours by a dose of 500 mg. Additional 500-mg doses are given on days 2 and 3.

## Primaquine

**Actions and Use.** Primaquine is highly active against *hepatic* forms of *P. vivax*. Effects against *erythrocytic* forms are less profound. The drug is used to eradicate *P. vivax* from the liver, thereby preventing relapse. Primaquine is similar to chloroquine in structure, and may act by the same mechanism: promotion of heme accumulation to toxic levels within the parasite.

**Pharmacokinetics.** Primaquine is well absorbed following oral administration. Absorbed drug is rapidly metabolized to products of low antimalarial activity. Metabolites are excreted in the urine.

**Adverse Effects.** The most serious and frequent response to primaquine is hemolysis. This reaction develops in patients whose red blood cells are deficient in an enzyme named glucose-6-phosphate dehydrogenase (G-6-PD). Deficiency of G-6-PD is an inherited trait, occurring most commonly in black populations and in darker-skinned whites (e.g., Sardinians, Greeks, Iranians, Sephardic Jews). When possible, patients suspected of G-6-PD deficiency should be screened for this trait before treatment. During primaquine therapy, periodic blood counts should be performed. Also, the urine should be monitored (darkening indicates the presence of hemoglobin). If severe hemolysis develops, primaquine should be discontinued.

**Preparations, Dosage, and Administration.** Primaquine phosphate is dispensed in 26.3-mg tablets. Administration is oral. For radical cure (prevention of relapse) of vivax malaria, the usual adult dosage is 26.3 mg/day for 2 weeks. The pediatric dosage is 0.53 mg/kg/day for 2 weeks.

## Quinine

At one time, quinine was the only drug available to treat malaria. Today, quinine has been largely replaced by more effective and less toxic agents (e.g., chloroquine). However, quinine still has an important role: treatment of chloroquine-resistant falciparum malaria. Quinine occurs naturally in the bark of the cinchona tree. Commercial preparations are derived from this source.

**Actions and Use.** Quinine is active against erythrocytic forms of *Plasmodium* but has little effect on sporozoites and hepatic forms. Like chloroquine, quinine concentrates in parasitized red blood cells and may be selective against erythrocytic parasites for this reason. Also like chloroquine, quinine kills plasmodia by causing heme to accumulate within the parasites to toxic levels.

The principal application of quinine is malaria caused by chloroquine-resistant *P. falciparum*. Because quinine is not highly active, adjunctive therapy with another agent is common. Drugs employed for adjunctive therapy include tetracycline, Fansidar (pyrimethamine plus sulfadoxine), and clindamycin.

**Pharmacokinetics.** Quinine is well absorbed from the gastrointestinal tract, even in the presence of diarrhea. The drug is metabolized by the liver, and metabolites are excreted in the urine. Plasma levels of quinine fall rapidly upon discontinuation of drug use.

**Adverse Effects.** At usual therapeutic doses, quinine frequently causes mild *cinchonism*, a syndrome characterized by tinnitus (ringing in the ears), headache, visual disturbances, nausea, and diarrhea. The physician should be notified if these symptoms develop. Because of its adverse effects on vision and hearing, quinine is contraindicated for patients with optic neuritis or tinnitus.

Like primaquine, quinine can cause *hemolysis* in patients whose red blood cells are deficient in G-6-PD. Patients using the drug should be monitored for hemolytic anemia. Quinine is contraindicated in the presence of G-6-PD deficiency.

Intravenous administration may cause *hypotension* and *acute circulatory failure*. To minimize these responses, IV quinine should be diluted and injected slowly. Patients should be transferred to oral medication as soon as possible.

Quinine has *quinidine-like effects on the heart* and must be used cautiously in patients with atrial fibrillation: by enhancing atrioventricular conduction, quinine can increase passage of atrial impulses to the ventricles, thereby causing a dangerous increase in ventricular rate.

Quinine can cause profound *hypoglycemia*. The mechanism is stimulation of pancreatic beta cells, which results in hyperinsulinemia. Quinine-induced hypoglycemia can be difficult to treat, even with glucose infusions.

*Quinine is classified in FDA Pregnancy Category X: the risks of use during pregnancy clearly outweigh any possible benefits.* The drug has caused fetal abnormalities, the most common being deafness from damage to the auditory nerve. Quinine can stimulate the uterus, and might thereby induce premature labor. *The drug must not be taken by pregnant women.*

**Preparations, Dosage, and Administration.** Quinine is available as two salts: *quinine sulfate*, for oral administration, and *quinine dihydrochloride*,* for intravenous administration.

For chloroquine-resistant falciparum malaria, the adult oral dosage is 650 mg every 8 hours for 3 to 7 days. The pediatric oral dosage is 8 mg/kg every 8 hours for 3 to 7 days.

## Pyrimethamine

**Therapeutic Use.** Pyrimethamine is used against chloroquine-resistant *P. falciparum*. It is a drug of choice for acute attacks and an alternative to mefloquine and doxycycline for prophylaxis. When taken for *prophylaxis*, pyrimethamine is combined with a sulfonamide (e.g., sulfadoxine). When used for *treatment*, pyrimethamine is combined with quinine as well as a sulfonamide.

In addition to its antimalarial use, pyrimethamine is the drug of first choice for toxoplasmosis (see Chapter 93).

*No longer available in the United States.

**Mechanism of Action.** Pyrimethamine inhibits dihydrofolate reductase, an enzyme that converts folic acid to its active form. Without active folic acid, cells are unable to synthesize DNA, RNA, and proteins. Pyrimethamine rarely disrupts host biochemistry because the concentration of pyrimethamine required to inhibit human dihydrofolate reductase is about 1000 times greater than the concentration needed to inhibit plasmodial dihydrofolate reductase.

The effects of pyrimethamine are potentiated by concurrent use of a sulfonamide. Unlike humans, the malaria parasite is unable to take up preformed folic acid from its environment. Consequently, the parasite must synthesize folic acid of its own. Sulfonamides inhibit this synthesis. Hence, the combination of a sulfonamide with pyrimethamine produces a *sequential block* in a critical biochemical pathway. In step one, sulfonamides inhibit folic acid synthesis, thereby reducing folic acid levels. In step two, pyrimethamine prevents conversion of the reduced pool of folic acid into an active form. This sequential block has devastating effects on the parasite.

**Pharmacokinetics.** Pyrimethamine is well absorbed following oral administration. The drug is highly bound to plasma proteins, and is therefore eliminated slowly. The plasma half-life of the drug is approximately 4 days. Pyrimethamine undergoes limited hepatic metabolism. Metabolites and parent drug are excreted in the urine.

**Adverse Effects.** At the doses employed for treatment or prophylaxis of malaria, pyrimethamine produces few adverse effects. However, at high doses, such as those used to treat toxoplasmosis, pyrimethamine can produce symptoms of *folic acid deficiency*. Symptoms result from effects on the bone marrow and the gastrointestinal mucosa, tissues that have a high percentage of cells undergoing division. Effects on the bone marrow manifest as leukopenia, thrombocytopenia, and anemia. Effects on the gastrointestinal mucosa manifest as ulcerative stomatitis, atrophic glossitis, pharyngitis, and diarrhea. These responses reverse upon discontinuation of treatment, and can be prevented by giving folic acid or folinic acid.

**Preparations.** Pyrimethamine is dispensed alone and in combination with sulfadoxine. The combination preparation, known as *Fansidar*, contains 25 mg of pyrimethamine and 500 mg of sulfadoxine. Tablets containing pyrimethamine alone (25 mg) are marketed under the trade name *Daraprim*.

**Dosage and Administration.** Administration is oral. When used to treat malaria, pyrimethamine is almost always taken in combination with a sulfonamide. The doses presented here refer to the combination of pyrimethamine with sulfadoxine [Fansidar]. To treat an acute attack of chloroquine-resistant falciparum malaria, Fansidar is administered as a single dose in the following amounts: for adults, 3 tablets; for children ages 9 to 14 years, 2 tablets; for children ages 4 to 8 years, 1 tablet; for children 1 to 3 years, one-half tablet, and for children under 1 year, one-quarter tablet.

The dosage for toxoplasmosis is given in Chapter 93.

## Mefloquine

**Actions and Uses.** Mefloquine [Lariam] kills erythrocytic forms of *P. vivax* and *P. falciparum*. The mechanism of action is unknown. Currently, mefloquine is the drug of choice for prophylactic therapy of chloroquine-resistant *P. falciparum* infections. It can also be used to treat an acute attack. Unfortunately, resistance to mefloquine may emerge rapidly. The mechanism of resistance is not known.

**Pharmacokinetics.** Mefloquine is well absorbed following oral administration. The drug undergoes hepatic metabolism and is excreted in the bile and feces. Mefloquine has a prolonged half-life, ranging from 1 to 4 weeks.

**Adverse Effects.** Adverse effects are dose related. At the low doses employed for prophylaxis, reactions are generally mild (nausea, dizziness, syncope). At the higher doses used for treatment of acute attacks, more intense reactions may occur, including gastrointestinal disturbances, nightmares, altered vision, and headache. Some of these effects may be indistinguishable from symptoms of malaria.

Toxicity to the central nervous system is a concern. The drug can cause vertigo, confusion, psychosis, and convulsions. The incidence of these neuropsychiatric effects is about 1 in 13,000 at the low doses used for prophylaxis, but increases to 1 in 250 at the doses used to treat an ongoing attack. Mefloquine should not be given to people with epilepsy or psychiatric disorders.

**Preparations, Dosage, and Administration.** Mefloquine [Lariam] is available in 250-mg tablets for oral administration.

For *prophylaxis*, the adult dosage is 250 mg once a week. Treatment should begin 1 week prior to travel to an endemic region and should continue for 4 weeks after leaving.

The adult dose for *acute treatment* of *P. falciparum* malaria is 1250 mg (5 tablets) taken all at once with at least 8 ounces of water.

### Halofantrine

Halofantrine [Halfan] is used for acute therapy of malaria caused by multidrug-resistant *P. falciparum*. This agent kills the erythrocytic stage of *Plasmodium* species. The mechanism is unknown. Development of resistance may be a problem. Administration is oral and absorption is low and variable, but can be greatly increased by fatty foods. Because absorption is so variable, clinical responses vary as well. Adverse effects include pruritus, abdominal pain, diarrhea, and slowing of cardiac conduction, which poses a risk of ventricular dysrhythmias.

### Antibacterial Drugs

**Tetracyclines.** Two members of the tetracycline family—*doxycycline* and *tetracycline* itself—are used to treat malaria. Both drugs kill the erythrocytic stage of the malaria parasite, although the rate of kill is slow. Tetracycline is used to treat acute attacks by multidrug-resistant *P. falciparum*. Because of its slow action, tetracycline must be combined with quinine, which acts more quickly. Doxycycline is used for short-term prophylaxis against *P. falciparum* in regions where the organism is resistant to mefloquine. Both tetracycline and doxycycline are contraindicated for pregnant women and for children less than 8 years old.

**Sulfonamides.** Like the tetracyclines, sulfonamides act slowly to kill the erythrocytic stage of the malaria parasite. For antimalarial therapy, sulfonamides are combined with pyrimethamine. The combination used most often is pyrimethamine plus sulfadoxine, available under the trade name Fansidar. Fansidar is combined with quinine to treat acute attacks caused by chloroquine-resistant *P. falciparum*.

**Clindamycin.** Clindamycin is active against the erythrocytic stage of the malaria parasite. The drug is used as an adjunct to quinine to treat malaria caused by chloroquine-resistant *P. falciparum*. The principal adverse effect of clindamycin is colitis secondary to overgrowth of the bowel with *Clostridium difficile*.

## KEY POINTS

- There are two principal forms of malaria, one caused by *Plasmodium vivax* and the other by *Plasmodium falciparum*.
- Vivax malaria is more common than falciparum malaria, but falciparum malaria is more severe.
- Drug resistance is common with *P. falciparum* and uncommon with *P. vivax*.
- Plasmodia reside in the liver and in erythrocytes. Those in the liver are harder to kill.
- Clinical cure of malaria (i.e., elimination of symptoms) results from killing plasmodia in erythrocytes.
- Vivax malaria relapses after clinical cure (because dormant parasites remain in the liver); falciparum malaria does not relapse.

- Chloroquine is the drug of choice for treatment and prophylaxis of malaria caused by *P. vivax* and by sensitive strains of *P. falciparum*.
- Quinine, combined with an adjunctive drug (e.g., tetracycline), is the drug of choice for treatment of malaria caused by chloroquine-resistant *P. falciparum*. Mefloquine is the drug of choice for prophylaxis.
- Primaquine, which kills dormant *P. vivax* in the liver, is the drug of choice for preventing relapse of vivax malaria.
- The principal adverse effect of primaquine is hemolytic anemia, which occurs in patients whose red blood cells have a genetically determined deficiency in glucose-6-phosphate dehydrogenase.
- The principal adverse effects of quinine are cinchonism (tinnitus, headache, visual disturbances, nausea, vomiting), hemolytic anemia (like primaquine), and birth defects (if given to pregnant women).
- High therapeutic doses of mefloquine can cause neuropsychiatric reactions, and hence should be avoided in patients with epilepsy or psychiatric disorders.

# CHAPTER 93

# Antiprotozoal Drugs II: Miscellaneous Agents

**Protozoal Infections**
**Drugs of Choice for Protozoal Infections**
    Iodoquinol
    Metronidazole
    Trimethoprim Plus Sulfamethoxazole
    Pentamidine
    Atovaquone

    Melarsoprol
    Eflornithine
    Nifurtimox
    Pyrimethamine
    Sodium Stibogluconate
    Suramin

Because of increasing world travel by Americans, and because of increased immigration by individuals from regions where infectious protozoa are endemic (South America, Asia, Africa), the incidence of protozoal infection in the United States is rising. The organisms encountered most frequently are *Entamoeba histolytica*, *Trichomonas vaginalis*, and *Giardia lamblia*. Infections with most other protozoa (e.g., *Leishmania* species, trypanosomes) are rare in North America. In approaching the antiprotozoal drugs, we will begin by discussing the diseases that protozoa produce. After that we will discuss the drugs used for treatment.

## Protozoal Infections

Our goal in this section is to describe the major protozoal infections (except for malaria, which is the subject of Chapter 92). Discussion focuses on causative organisms, sites of infection, symptoms of disease, and preferred drug therapy. Causative organisms and drugs of choice are summarized in Table 93-1.

### Amebiasis

Amebiasis is an infestation with *Entamoeba histolytica*. In the United States, the disease affects between 2% and 4% of the population. Worldwide, about 10% of the population is infected. The principal site of infestation is the intestine. However, amebas may migrate to other tissues, most commonly the liver, where abscesses may form. Amebiasis is usually asymptomatic. When symptoms are present, the most characteristic are diarrhea, abdominal pain, and weight loss.

Drugs of choice for amebiasis are *iodoquinol* and *metronidazole*. Iodoquinol is active only against amebas residing in the intestine. Metronidazole is active against amebas that inhabit the intestine, liver, and all other sites. For patients with asymptomatic intestinal infection, therapy with iodoquinol alone is sufficient. For patients with severe intestinal disease or with liver abscesses, metronidazole is given initially, followed by iodoquinol.

### Giardiasis

Giardiasis is an infection with *Giardia lamblia*. In the United States, giardiasis has an incidence of 2% to 10%. Infestation usually occurs by contact with contaminated objects or by drinking contaminated water. The primary habitat of *Giardia lamblia* is the upper small intestine. Occasionally, organisms migrate to the bile ducts and gallbladder. As many as 50% of affected individuals remain free of symptoms. However, symptoms that are both unpleasant and uncomfortable can develop. These include profound malaise; heartburn; vomiting; colicky pain after eating; and malodorous belching, flatulence, and diarrhea. The pain associated with giardiasis may mimic that of gallstones, appendicitis, peptic ulcers, or hiatal hernia. For treatment, the current drug of choice is *metronidazole*. (Quinacrine, the former drug of choice, is more effective than metronidazole but is no longer available in the United States.)

### Leishmaniasis

The term *leishmaniasis* refers to infestation by certain protozoal species belonging to the genus *Leishmania*. Worldwide, the incidence of leishmaniasis is estimated at 10 million. The disease is acquired through the bite of sand flies indigenous to tropical and subtropical regions. In the human host, the parasites take up residence inside cells of the reticuloendothelial system.

Leishmaniasis has three different forms: *cutaneous*, *mucocutaneous*, and *visceral*. The particular form acquired is determined by the species of *Leishmania* involved. The forms of leishmaniasis vary greatly in severity, ranging from mild (cutaneous leishmaniasis) to potentially fatal (visceral leishmaniasis). In *cutaneous* leishmaniasis, a nodule forms at the site of inoculation; later, this nodule may evolve into an ulcer that is very slow to heal. *Mucocutaneous* leishmaniasis is characterized by ulceration in the mucosa of the mouth, nose, and pharynx. Symptoms of *visceral* leishmaniasis include fever, hepatosplenomegaly, liver dysfunction, hypoalbuminemia, pancytopenia, lymphadenopathy, and hemorrhage. If left untreated, the disease is frequently fatal. For all forms of leishmaniasis, *sodium stibogluconate* is the treatment of choice. *Amphotericin B*, a drug used for fungal infections (see Chapter 86), is

## TABLE 93-1. DRUGS OF CHOICE FOR PROTOZOAL INFECTION

| Disease | Causative Protozoan | Drugs of Choice |
|---|---|---|
| Amebiasis | *Entamoeba histolytica* | Iodoquinol Metronidazole |
| Giardiasis | *Giardia lamblia* | Metronidazole |
| Leishmaniasis | *Leishmania* species | Sodium stibogluconate |
| *Pneumocystis carinii* pneumonia | *Pneumocystis carinii* | Trimethoprim plus sulfamethoxazole; pentamidine |
| Toxoplasmosis | *Toxoplasma gondii* | Pyrimethamine plus sulfadiazine |
| Trichomoniasis | *Trichomonas vaginalis* | Metronidazole |
| Trypanosomiasis, African (sleeping sickness) | *Trypanosoma brucei gambiense, Trypanosoma brucei rhodesiense* | Suramin Melarsoprol Eflornithine |
| Trypanosomiasis, American (Chagas' disease) | *Trypanosoma cruzi* | Nifurtimox |

more effective than sodium stibogluconate, but costs more and must be administered in a hospital.

### *Pneumocystis carinii* Pneumonia

*Pneumocystis carinii* pneumonia (PCP) is caused by *Pneumocystis carinii*, an organism that was until recently classified as a protozoan, but is now classified as a fungus. Although *P. carinii* is now considered a fungus, treatment is nonetheless discussed here, rather than in Chapter 86, because the drugs employed are primarily antiprotozoal.

In people with AIDS, PCP is the most common opportunistic infection and the leading cause of death. PCP occurs in up to 80% of HIV-infected individuals and kills 15% to 20%. Following control of an initial infection, the rate of recurrence is 60% within the first year. Because of the high risk of PCP in people with AIDS, prophylactic therapy is recommended.

Clinical manifestations of PCP are generally nonspecific. Early symptoms include cough, dyspnea, chest discomfort, pallor, and cyanosis. In advanced infection, lung morphology is altered. Left untreated, the disease has a mortality rate of 90%.

The treatment of choice for PCP is *trimethoprim plus sulfamethoxazole*. For patients who are severely immunocompromised, *pentamidine* may be preferred. Alternative treatments include *atovaquone*, *trimethoprim plus dapsone*, *trimethrexate plus folinic acid*, and *primaquine plus clindamycin*. For prophylaxis of PCP, *trimethoprim plus sulfamethoxazole* is the medication of choice. Alternative prophylactic drugs are *aerosolized pentamidine* and *dapsone*.

### Toxoplasmosis

Toxoplasmosis is caused by infection with *Toxoplasma gondii*, a protozoan of the class Sporozoa. The parasite is harbored by many animals as well as by humans. Infection is acquired most commonly by eating undercooked meat. However, toxoplasmosis may also be congenital. Congenital infection can damage the brain, eyes, liver, and other organs. Extensive disease is usually fatal. In immunocompetent adults, infection is usually asymptomatic. However, in immunocompromised hosts, such as those with AIDS, the disease may progress to encephalitis and death. The treatment of choice is *pyrimethamine plus sulfadiazine*.

### Trichomoniasis

Trichomoniasis is caused by *Trichomonas vaginalis*, a flagellated protozoan. Trichomoniasis is a common disease, affecting about 200 million people worldwide. The usual site of infestation is the genitourinary tract. Parasites may also inhabit the rectum. In females, infection results in vaginitis. In males, infection causes urethritis. The disease is usually transmitted sexually but can also be acquired by contact with contaminated objects (e.g., toilet seats). Oral *metronidazole* is the treatment of choice.

### Trypanosomiasis

There are two major forms of trypanosomiasis: African trypanosomiasis and American trypanosomiasis. Both forms are caused by protozoal species belonging to the genus *Trypanosoma*.

***African Trypanosomiasis (Sleeping Sickness).*** African trypanosomiasis, transmitted by the bite of the tsetse fly, is caused by two subspecies of *Trypanosoma brucei*: *T. brucei rhodesiense* and *T. brucei gambiense*. Trypanosomiasis caused by either subspecies has similar symptoms. Early symptoms include fever, lymphadenopathy, hepatosplenomegaly, dyspnea, and tachycardia. Late symptoms, which result from involvement of the central nervous system (CNS), include mental dullness, incoordination, and apathy. As CNS involvement advances, sleep becomes constant and death may eventually follow. During the early phase of African trypanosomiasis, *suramin* and *eflornithine* are the agents of choice. During the late (CNS) stage, *melarsoprol* and *eflornithine* are the agents of choice. All three drugs—suramin, eflornithine, and melarsoprol—can produce serious side effects, and all three require prolonged use. Treatment is difficult and frequently unsuccessful.

***American Trypanosomiasis (Chagas' Disease).*** Chagas' disease is caused by infection with *Trypanosoma cruzi*, a protozoan of the class Sporozoa. The disease is prevalent in South America and the Caribbean, where it affects some 10 million people. The parasites are harbored in the digestive tract of certain blood-sucking bugs, and are transmitted as follows: the bug bites a sleeping person (usually on the face) and also defecates; the parasites, which are contained in the bug's feces, are then forced into the bite wound by rubbing or scratching. An early sign of the disease is swelling and severe inflammation at the site of inoculation. Over time, parasites invade cardiac cells and neurons of the myenteric plexus. Destruction of these cells can cause cardiomyopathy, megaesophagus, and megacolon. Deaths have occurred, usually secondary to cardiac injury. In its early phase, Chagas' disease can be treated with *nifurtimox.* Unfortunately, neither this drug nor any other is very effective against chronic infection.

# Drugs of Choice for Protozoal Infections

The major antiprotozoal drugs are discussed below. With the exception of metronidazole, each of these agents is active against only one organism. Although consideration here is limited to drugs of choice, be aware that additional antiprotozoal drugs are available.

## Iodoquinol

***Actions and Use.*** Iodoquinol [Yodoxin] is the drug of choice for asymptomatic intestinal amebiasis. In addition, the drug is employed in conjunction with metronidazole to treat symptomatic intestinal infection and systemic amebiasis. In these last two cases, iodoquinol is administered after treatment with metronidazole to eliminate any surviving intestinal parasites. The mechanism of amebicidal action is unknown.

***Pharmacokinetics.*** Only a small fraction (5% to 8%) of oral iodoquinol is absorbed. The fraction absorbed is excreted as metabolites in the urine.

***Adverse Effects.*** Mild reactions occur occasionally. These include rash, acne, slight thyroid enlargement, and gastrointestinal effects (nausea, vomiting, diarrhea, cramps, pruritus ani). Rarely, prolonged therapy at very high doses has caused optic atrophy with permanent loss of vision.

***Preparations, Dosage, and Administration.*** Iodoquinol [Yodoxin] is available in tablets (210 and 650 mg) and as a powder for oral administration. The usual adult dosage is 650 mg 3 times a day for 20 days. The dosage for children is 10 to 13 mg/kg 3 times a day for 20 days.

## Metronidazole

***Therapeutic Uses.*** Metronidazole [Flagyl, Metizol, Protostat] is the drug of choice for symptomatic intestinal amebiasis and systemic amebiasis. Because most of an administered dose is absorbed in the small intestine, concentrations in the colon remain low. Consequently, for treatment of amebiasis, metronidazole is followed by iodoquinol, an amebicidal drug that achieves high colonic levels. As a result, iodoquinol kills those intestinal parasites that may have survived therapy with metronidazole.

Metronidazole is the agent of choice for infection with *Trichomonas vaginalis.* The drug is effective against trichomoniasis in males as well as in females.

Metronidazole is the drug of choice for giardiasis. Quinacrine, the former drug of choice, is more effective but has been withdrawn from the U.S. market.

Many anaerobic bacteria are sensitive to metronidazole. Antibacterial applications are discussed in Chapter 85.

***Mechanism of Action.*** To be effective, metronidazole must first be converted to a more chemically reactive form. This reactive form interacts with DNA, causing strand breakage and loss of helical structure. The resulting impairment of DNA function is thought responsible for the antimicrobial and mutagenic actions of the drug.

***Pharmacokinetics.*** Metronidazole is readily absorbed from the GI tract. The drug undergoes extensive hepatic metabolism. Metabolites and unchanged drug are excreted in the urine.

***Adverse Effects.*** Metronidazole produces a variety of untoward effects, but these rarely require termination of treatment. The most common side effects are nausea, headache, dry mouth, and an unpleasant metallic taste. Other common responses include stomatitis, vomiting, diarrhea, insomnia, vertigo, and weakness. Harmless darkening of the urine may occur; patients should be forewarned of this effect. Certain neurologic effects (numbness in the extremities, ataxia, convulsions) occur rarely; metronidazole should be withdrawn if these develop. Metronidazole should not be used by patients with active disease of the CNS. Carcinogenic effects have been observed in rodents; however, there is no evidence for increased incidence of cancer in humans.

***Use in Pregnancy.*** Metronidazole readily crosses the placenta, and is mutagenic in bacteria. However, experience to date has shown no effect on the developing fetus following treatment of pregnant women. Nonetheless, it is recommended that metronidazole be avoided during the first trimester, and employed with caution throughout the rest of pregnancy.

***Drug Interactions.*** Metronidazole has disulfiram-like effects and can therefore produce unpleasant or dangerous reactions if taken in conjunction with *alcohol.* Accordingly, patients must be warned against alcohol consumption.

Metronidazole inhibits inactivation of *warfarin,* an anticoagulant. Dosages of warfarin must be lowered.

***Preparations, Dosage, and Administration.*** Metronidazole [Flagyl, Metizol, Protostat] is available in tablets (250 and 500 mg), as a powder (to be reconstituted for injection), and as a ready-to-use injection. For treatment of protozoal infections, the oral tablets are used. Antibacterial therapy usually requires IV administration. Dosages for antiprotozoal therapy are given below. Dosages for antibacterial therapy are presented in Chapter 85.

*Amebiasis.* The usual adult dosage is 750 mg 3 times daily for 10 days. The pediatric dosage is 12 to 17 mg/kg 3 times daily for 10 days. Following treatment with metronidazole, iodoquinol is given for 20 days.

*Trichomoniasis.* Treatment for adults consists of either (1) a single 2-gm dose, (2) 250 mg 3 times a day for 7 days, or (3) 375 mg twice a day for 7 days. The pediatric dosage is 5 mg/kg 3 times daily for 7 days.

*Giardiasis.* The adult dosage is 250 mg 3 times daily for 5 days. The pediatric dosage is 5 mg/kg 3 times daily for 5 days.

## Trimethoprim Plus Sulfamethoxazole

The combination of trimethoprim plus sulfamethoxazole, sold under the trade names Bactrim, Cotrim, and Septra, is the treatment of choice for active *Pneumocystis carinii* pneumonia (PCP) and for prophylaxis of PCP. This combination is also important for bacterial infections. The pharmacology of trimethoprim plus sulfamethoxazole is discussed at length in Chapter 82.

For therapy of PCP, the *total daily* dose for adults and children is 15 mg/kg of trimethoprim and 75 mg/kg of sulfamethoxazole. The total daily dose is given in three or four divided doses. Treatment lasts for 2 to 3 weeks. Administration may be oral or intravenous.

For prophylaxis of PCP, the adult dose—160 mg trimethoprim plus 800 mg sulfamethoxazole—is administered once a day, 3 days a week. The pediatric dose—150 mg/m$^2$ trimethoprim plus 750 mg/m$^2$ sulfamethoxazole—is administered twice a day, 3 days a week.

## Pentamidine

**Actions.** Pentamidine [Pentam 300, NebuPent] is active against *Pneumocystis carinii.* The drug disrupts synthesis of DNA, RNA, phospholipids, and proteins. We do not know if these actions underlie its antiprotozoal effects.

**Uses.** Pentamidine is given by injection (IM or IV) and by inhalation. Pentamidine injection is used to treat active *Pneumocystis carinii* pneumonia. *Inhaled* pentamidine is used to prevent PCP in high-risk, HIV-positive patients. High-risk patients are those with (1) a history of one or more episodes of PCP or (2) peripheral CD4 lymphocyte counts less than 200 cells/mm$^3$. In addition to treatment of PCP, pentamidine has been used on an investigational basis to treat leishmaniasis and trypanosomiasis.

**Pharmacokinetics.** For treatment of active PCP, pentamidine is administered IM or IV. Equivalent blood levels are achieved with both routes. The drug is extensively bound in tissues. Penetration to the brain and cerebrospinal fluid is poor. Between 50% and 65% of each dose is excreted rapidly in the urine. The remaining drug is excreted slowly, over a month or more.

**Adverse Effects Associated with Parenteral Administration.** Pentamidine can produce serious side effects when given IM or IV. Caution must be exercised.

Sudden and severe *hypotension* occurs in about 1% of patients. The fall in blood pressure may cause tachycardia, dizziness, and fainting. To minimize hypotensive responses, patients should receive the drug while lying down. Blood pressure should be monitored closely.

*Hypoglycemia* and *hyperglycemia* have occurred. Hypoglycemia has been associated with necrosis of pancreatic islet cells and excessive insulin levels. The cause of hyperglycemia is unknown. Because of possible fluctuations in glucose levels, blood glucose should be monitored daily.

Intramuscular administration is painful. Necrosis at the injection site followed by formation of a sterile abscess is common.

Some adverse effects can be life threatening when severe. These reactions and their incidences are leukopenia (2.8%), thrombocytopenia (1.7%), acute renal failure (0.5%), hypocalcemia (0.2%), and dysrhythmias (0.2%).

**Adverse Effects Associated with Aerosolized Pentamidine.** Inhaled pentamidine does not cause the severe adverse effects associated with parenteral pentamidine. The most common reactions are cough (38%) and bronchospasm (15%). These are more pronounced in patients with asthma or a history of smoking. Both reactions can be controlled with an inhaled bronchodilator, and rarely necessitate pentamidine withdrawal.

**Preparations, Dosage, and Administration.** Pentamidine isethionate *for injection* [Pentam 300] is dispensed in 300-mg single-dose vials. Administration is IM or IV. For treatment of active PCP, the dosage for adults and children is 3 to 4 mg/kg daily for 2 to 3 weeks. Intravenous administration must be done slowly (over 60 minutes).

Pentamidine isethionate *aerosol* [NebuPent] is used for prophylaxis of PCP in patients with AIDS. The dosage is 300 mg once every 4 weeks. Administration is performed with a Respirgard II nebulizer by Marquest. Solutions should be freshly prepared.

## Atovaquone

**Actions and Use.** Atovaquone [Mepron] is a new drug approved for mild to moderate PCP in patients who cannot tolerate trimethoprim-sulfamethoxazole or parenteral pentamidine. Atovaquone is less effective than the first-line drugs but is better tolerated. A mechanism of action has not been determined.

**Pharmacokinetics.** Atovaquone was initially formulated in tablets, but is now formulated as a suspension. This change was made because absorption of the tablets was poor and erratic. Absorption of the suspension is more complete and is greatly enhanced by food, especially fatty food. Atovaquone is 99% bound to plasma proteins, has a prolonged half-life (2 to 3 days), and is excreted unchanged in the feces.

**Adverse Effects and Interactions.** The principal adverse effect is rash, which occurs in 20% to 40% of patients. Other adverse effects include nausea (21%), diarrhea (16%), headache (16%), vomiting (14%), fever (14%), and insomnia (10%). Safety for use by children or by women who are pregnant or breast-feeding has not been established. Because of its high protein binding, atovaquone should not be combined with other drugs that are highly protein bound.

**Preparations, Dosage, and Administration.** Atova-quone [Mepron] is dispensed as a suspension (150 mg/ml) for oral use. The adult dosage is 750 mg twice daily for 21 days. Because absorption is poor in the absence of food, the drug must be administered with meals.

## Melarsoprol

**Therapeutic Use.** Melarsoprol [Arsobal] is a drug of choice for African trypanosomiasis (sleeping sickness). The drug is employed during the *late* stage of the disease (i.e., after CNS involvement has developed). For earlier stages of the disease, suramin, which is less toxic, is the treatment of choice.

**Mechanism of Action.** Melarsoprol is an organic arsenical compound that reacts with sulfhydryl groups of proteins. Antiparasitic effects result from inactivation of enzymes. This same action appears to underlie the serious toxicity of the drug. Melarsoprol is more toxic to parasites than to humans because it penetrates parasitic membranes more easily than human cells.

**Adverse Effects.** Melarsoprol is quite toxic, and adverse reactions are common. Frequent responses include hypertension, albuminuria, peripheral neuropathy, myocardial damage, and Herxheimer-type reactions. Reactive encephalopathy may develop during the first course of treatment. Although fatalities have occurred, they are much less common than in the past.

**Preparations, Dosage, and Administration.** Melarsoprol [Arsobal] is administered by slow IV injection. The drug is highly irritating to tissues, and care must be taken to avoid extravasation. Because of its toxicity, melarsoprol should be administered in a hospital setting. Treatment for adults begins with 2 to 3.6 mg/kg IV daily for 3 days. Seven days later a second course (3.6 mg/kg IV daily for 3 days) is given. This is repeated once more after 10 to 21 days. Melarsoprol can be obtained through the Centers for Disease Control and Prevention. The drug is not available commercially.

## Eflornithine

**Actions and Use.** Eflornithine [Ornidyl] is a new drug for treating African trypanosomiasis (sleeping sickness) caused by *T. brucei gambiense*. The drug is effective in both the early and late (CNS) stages of the disease. Benefits result from irreversible inhibition of ornithine decarboxylase, an enzyme needed for biosynthesis of polyamines, compounds required by all cells for division and differentiation. Parasites weakened by eflornithine become highly vulnerable to lethal attack by host defenses. Since cells of the host can readily synthesize more ornithine decarboxylase to replace inhibited enzyme, cells of the host are spared.

**Pharmacokinetics.** Eflornithine may be administered orally or IV. Once in the blood, the drug is well distributed to body fluids and tissues, including the CNS. Eflornithine has a half-life of 100 minutes and is eliminated largely unchanged in the urine.

**Adverse Effects.** The most common adverse effects are anemia (48%), diarrhea (39%), and leukopenia (27%). Seizures may occur early in therapy but then subside, despite continued treatment. Since IV administration of eflornithine requires large volumes of fluid, fluid overload may develop over the course of treatment.

**Preparations, Dosage, and Administration.** Eflornithine may be administered orally or intravenously; IV therapy is more effective and preferred. The dosage for adults is 100 mg/kg IV 4 times daily for 14 days. Higher doses may be needed in children. Eflornithine is dispensed as a concentrated solution (200 mg/ml in 100-ml vials) and must be diluted for IV infusion.

## Nifurtimox

**Therapeutic Use.** Nifurtimox [Lampit] is the drug of choice for American trypanosomiasis (Chagas' disease). The drug is most effective in the acute stage of the disease, curing about 80% of patients. Chronic disease is less responsive.

**Pharmacokinetics.** Nifurtimox is well absorbed from the GI tract and undergoes rapid and extensive metabolism. Metabolites are excreted in the urine.

**Adverse Effects.** Therapy is prolonged, and significant untoward effects occur frequently. Gastrointestinal effects (anorexia, nausea, vomiting, abdominal pain) and peripheral neuropathy

are especially common. Weight loss resulting from GI effects may require discontinuation of treatment. Additional common reactions include rash and CNS effects (memory loss, insomnia, vertigo, headache).

**Preparations, Dosage, and Administration.** Nifurtimox [Lampit] is dispensed in 100-mg tablets. In the United States, the drug is available only from the Centers for Disease Control and Prevention. The adult dosage is 2 to 2.5 mg/kg 4 times daily for 120 days. For young children (ages 1 through 10 years), the usual dosage is 4 to 5 mg/kg 4 times daily for 90 days. For older children (ages 11 to 16 years), the usual dosage is 3 to 4 mg/kg 4 times daily for 90 days.

## Pyrimethamine

Pyrimethamine [Daraprim], combined with sulfadiazine, is the treatment of choice for toxoplasmosis. Pyrimethamine is also important for treating malaria (Chapter 92). For toxoplasmosis, the adult dosage is 25 to 100 mg daily for 3 to 4 weeks. The pediatric dosage is 2 mg/kg/day for 3 days followed by 1 mg/kg/day for 4 weeks. For adults and children, each dose of pyrimethamine should be accompanied by 10 mg of folinic acid to reduce side effects. In addition, the regimen must include sulfadiazine: for adults, 1 to 1.5 gm 4 times a day for 3 to 4 weeks; for children, 100 to 200 mg/kg/day for 3 to 4 weeks. The basic pharmacology of pyrimethamine is discussed in Chapter 92.

## Sodium Stibogluconate

Sodium stibogluconate [Pentostam] is the drug of choice for leishmaniasis. The mechanism of action is unknown. The drug is poorly absorbed from the GI tract, and hence must be administered parenterally (IM or IV). Sodium stibogluconate undergoes little metabolism and is excreted rapidly in the urine. Although severe side effects can occur, the drug is generally well tolerated. The most frequent untoward reactions are muscle pain, joint stiffness, and bradycardia. Changes in the electrocardiogram are common and occasionally precede serious dysrhythmias. Liver and renal dysfunction, shock, and sudden death occur rarely. Sodium stibogluconate is dispensed in aqueous solution for IM and IV injection. For leishmaniasis, the usual adult and pediatric dosage is 20 mg/kg/day (IM or IV) for 20 to 28 days. In the United States, the drug is available only from the Centers for Disease Control and Prevention.

## Suramin

**Actions and Uses.** Suramin sodium [Germanin] is a drug of choice for treating the early phase of African trypanosomiasis (sleeping sickness); for the late phase of the disease (i.e., the stage of CNS involvement), melarsoprol and eflornithine are preferred treatments. Suramin is known to inhibit many trypanosomal enzymes; however, its primary mechanism of action has not been established.

**Pharmacokinetics.** The drug is poorly absorbed from the GI tract, and therefore must be administered parenterally (IV). Suramin binds tightly to plasma proteins and remains in the bloodstream for months. Penetration into cells is low. Excretion is renal.

**Adverse Effects.** Side effects can be severe, hence treatment should take place in a hospital. Frequent reactions include vomiting, itching, rash, paresthesias, photophobia, and hyperesthesia of the palms and soles. Suramin concentrates in the kidney and can cause local damage, resulting in the appearance of protein, blood cells, and casts in the urine. If urinary casts are observed, treatment should cease. Rarely, a shock-like syndrome develops after IV administration. To minimize the risk of this reaction, a small test dose (200 mg) is administered; in the absence of a severe reaction, full doses may follow.

***Preparations, Dosage, and Administration.*** Suramin sodium [Germanin] is available from the Centers for Disease Control and Prevention. The drug is dispensed in 1-gm ampules. Administration is by slow IV infusion. Suramin is unstable, hence fresh solutions must be made daily. The adult dosage is 1 gm IV on days 1, 3, 7, 14, and 21. The pediatric dosage is 20 mg/kg IV administered by the same schedule employed for adults.

## KEY POINTS

- The principal protozoal infections seen in the United States are trichomoniasis, giardiasis, and amebiasis.
- Metronidazole is the drug of choice for trichomoniasis, giardiasis, and symptomatic or systemic amebiasis.
- Iodoquinol is the drug of choice for asymptomatic amebiasis.
- Patients taking metronidazole should be warned against consuming alcohol because of the risk of a disulfiram-like reaction.
- *Pneumocystis carinii* pneumonia (PCP), which is now classified as a fungal infection, is the most common opportunistic infection, and the leading cause of death, in people with AIDS.
- Trimethoprim plus sulfamethoxazole is the preparation of choice for prophylaxis and treatment of PCP.
- *Parenteral* pentamidine is an alternative to trimethoprim-sulfamethoxazole for treatment of PCP, and *aerosolized* pentamidine is an alternative for prophylaxis.

# CHAPTER 94

# Ectoparasiticides

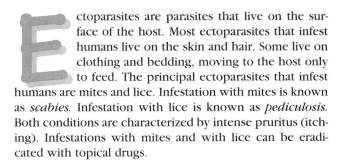ctoparasites are parasites that live on the surface of the host. Most ectoparasites that infest humans live on the skin and hair. Some live on clothing and bedding, moving to the host only to feed. The principal ectoparasites that infest humans are mites and lice. Infestation with mites is known as *scabies*. Infestation with lice is known as *pediculosis*. Both conditions are characterized by intense pruritus (itching). Infestations with mites and with lice can be eradicated with topical drugs.

## Ectoparasitic Infestations

### Scabies

Scabies is caused by infestation with *Sarcoptes scabiei*, an organism known commonly as the itch mite. Irritation results from the female mite burrowing beneath the skin to lay eggs. Burrows may be visible as small ridges or dotted lines. In adults, the most common sites of infestation are the wrists, elbows, nipples, navel, genital region, and webs of the fingers. In children, infestation is most likely on the head, neck, and buttocks.

The primary symptom of scabies is pruritus. Itching is most intense just after going to bed. Scratching may result in abrasion and secondary infection.

Transmission of scabies is usually by direct contact. This contact may be sexual or of a less intimate nature. Scabies may also be transmitted through contact with infested linen, towels, or clothing.

Scabies is best treated using a pesticide-containing lotion or cream. To eradicate mites, the entire body surface must be treated (excluding the face and scalp in adults). To prevent reinfestation, bedding and intimate clothing should be machine washed and dried.

Several drugs can kill mites. *Permethrin* (5% cream formulation) is the drug of choice. This preparation is effec-

tive in just one application. *Crotamiton* and *lindane* are alternatives. Recent studies indicate that a single oral dose (200 µg/kg) of *ivermectin* [Stromectol] can cure scabies, although the drug is not yet approved for this indication.

### Pediculosis

Pediculosis is a general term referring to infestation with any of several kinds of lice. The types of lice encountered most frequently are *Pediculus humanus capitis* (head louse), *Pediculus humanus corporis* (body louse), and *Phthirus pubis* (pubic or crab louse). Infestation with any of these insects causes pruritus. Infestations with head, pubic, and body lice differ with regard to method of treatment and mode of acquisition.

### Pubic Lice

Pubic lice, commonly known as crabs, usually reside on the skin and hair of the pubic region. However, pubic lice may also be found on the eyelashes and other parts of the body. As a rule, infestation is transmitted through sexual contact. Consequently, crabs are most common among people who have multiple sexual partners. Two preparations—*permethrin* (1% liquid) and *malathion* (0.5% lotion)—are drugs of choice for eliminating crabs. Infestation of the eyelashes is treated with petrolatum ophthalmic ointment. Clothing and linen should be disinfected by washing in very hot water, followed by machine drying at high temperature.

### Head Lice

Head lice reside on the scalp and lay their nits (eggs) on the hair. Adult lice may be difficult to observe. Nits, however, are usually visible. Infestation may be associated with hives, boils, impetigo, and other skin disorders. The head louse is more democratic than the pubic or body louse and can be found infesting people from all socio-economic groups. Head lice may be transmitted by close personal contact and by contact with infested clothing, hairbrushes, furniture, and other objects. Treatments of choice are *permethrin* and *malathion.* Both drugs kill adult lice as well as nits. Eradication of head lice does not require shaving or cutting the hair.

### Body Lice

Despite their name, body lice reside not on the body but on clothing. These lice move to the body only to feed. Consequently, body lice are rarely seen on the skin. Rather, these insects can be found in bed linens and the seams of garments. Transmission of body lice is by contact with infested clothing or bedding. Body lice are relatively uncommon in the United States, where regular laundering precludes infestation. Infestation is most likely among vagrants and other people whose clothes may not be frequently washed. The majority of body lice can be removed from the host simply by removal of clothing. Those lice that remain on the body can be killed by applying a pesticide; *permethrin* and *malathion* are drugs of choice. Clothing and bedding should be disinfected by washing and drying at high temperature.

# Pharmacology of Ectoparasiticides

Ectoparasitic infestations are treated with topical drugs. These agents are dispensed in the form of creams, gels, lotions, and shampoos. The pharmacology of scabicides and pediculicides is discussed below. Properties of the five major ectoparasiticides are summarized in Table 94-1.

## Permethrin

### Basic Pharmacology

*Actions and Uses.* Permethrin [Nix, Elimite] is toxic to mites, lice, and their ova. The drug kills adult insects by disrupting nerve traffic, thereby causing paralysis. In addition to killing mites and lice, permethrin is active against fleas and ticks. The 1% formulation [Nix] is a drug of choice for lice. The 5% formulation [Elimite] has replaced lindane as the drug of choice for scabies. As a rule, only one application is required.

*Pharmacokinetics.* Very little (about 2%) of topically applied permethrin is absorbed. The fraction absorbed is rapidly inactivated and excreted in the urine.

*Adverse Effects.* Topical permethrin is devoid of serious adverse effects. The drug may cause some exacerbation of the itching, erythema, and edema normally associated with pediculosis. Other reactions include temporary sensations of burning, stinging, and numbness.

### Preparations and Administration

*Preparations.* Permethrin is dispensed in two concentrations: (1) a 1% liquid [Nix] used for lice and (2) a 5% cream [Elimite] used for scabies.

*Administration. Head Lice.* Before applying permethrin (1% liquid) to remove head lice, the hair should be washed, rinsed, and towel dried. Permethrin is then applied in an amount sufficient to saturate the hair and scalp. After 10 minutes, permethrin should be removed with a warm-water rinse. If needed, retreatment can be performed in 7 days. However, reapplication is required in less than 1% of cases.

*Scabies.* The 5% cream [Elimite] is massaged into the skin, from the head to the soles of the feet. After 8 to 14 hours, the cream is removed by washing. Thirty grams is sufficient for the average adult. Only one application is needed.

## TABLE 94–1. ECTOPARASITICIDES: TRADE NAMES, INDICATIONS, DOSAGE FORMS, AND ADVERSE EFFECTS

| Generic Name | Trade Names | Indications Scabies (Mites) | Pediculosis (Lice) | Dosage Forms | Adverse Effects |
|---|---|---|---|---|---|
| Permethrin | Nix Elimite | ✔ | ✔ | Liquid: 1% Cream: 5% | Occasional: burning, stinging, itching, numbness, pain, rash, erythema, edema |
| Crotamiton | Eurax | ✔ | | Cream: 10% Lotion: 10% | Occasional: rash, conjunctivitis |
| Malathion | Ovide | | ✔ | Lotion: 0.5% | Occasional: local irritation |
| Pyrethrins plus piperonyl butoxide | RID, others | | ✔ | Gel Liquid Shampoo | Occasional: irritation to eyes and mucous membranes following inadvertent contact |
| Lindane | Kwell, others | ✔ | ✔ | Cream: 1% Lotion: 1% Shampoo: 1% | Occasional: rash, conjunctivitis Rare: convulsions, aplastic anemia |

## Malathion

***Actions and Uses.*** Malathion [Ovide] is an organophosphate cholinesterase inhibitor (see Chapter 16). The drug kills lice and their ova. Humans and other mammals are not harmed because an enzyme in their blood converts malathion to nontoxic metabolites. The drug is approved for treatment of head lice. It is also used widely as an insecticide.

***Adverse Effects and Interactions.*** The preparation used topically for head lice is devoid of significant adverse effects. Scalp irritation occurs occasionally. No systemic toxicity has been reported. Likewise, no drug interactions have been reported.

***Preparations and Administration.*** Malathion [Ovide] is dispensed in a 5% lotion. The preparation is applied to dry hair, gently massaged until the scalp is moist, and allowed to dry naturally. (The lotion is flammable because of its 78% alcohol content. Hence, hair dryers and other sources of heat should be avoided until the alcohol has dried.) Eight to 12 hours after application, malathion is washed off with shampoo. Dead lice and ova can then be removed with a fine-tooth comb. Treatment may be repeated in 7 to 9 days if needed.

### Crotamiton

Crotamiton [Eurax] is used to treat scabies. The drug is not indicated for pediculosis. This agent has scabicidal actions and may also relieve itching by an independent mechanism. Mild adverse reactions (dermatitis, conjunctivitis) occur occasionally. Crotamiton is dispensed in cream and lotion formulations.

To treat scabies, crotamiton is massaged into the skin of the entire body, starting with the chin and working down. The head and face are treated only if needed. Special attention should be given to skin folds and creases. Contact with the eyes, mucous membranes, and any regions of inflammation should be avoided. A second application is made 24 hours after the first. A cleansing bath should be taken 48 hours after the second application. If needed, treatment can be repeated in 7 days.

### Pyrethrins Plus Piperonyl Butoxide

The combination of pyrethrins with piperonyl butoxide is used to remove pubic and head lice. Pyrethrins are the components of this preparation that are toxic to lice. The piperonyl butoxide enhances pyrethrins' action by decreasing the ability of insects to metabolize pyrethrins to inactive products. Pyrethrins undergo little transcutaneous absorption and are one of the safest insecticides available. Principal adverse effects are irritation to the eyes and mucous membranes. Accordingly, contact with these areas should be avoided. Pharmaceutical preparations vary in their content of pyrethrins (0.18% to 0.33%) as well as in their content of piperonyl butoxide (2% to 4%). Treatment consists of applying the preparation (gel, liquid, shampoo) to the infested region, followed later by a warm-water rinse. The procedure should be repeated in a week. Nits are removed by combing.

### Lindane

#### Actions and Uses

Lindane [Kwell, others] is absorbed through the chitin shell of adult mites and lice and causes death by inducing convulsions. The drug is also lethal to the eggs. At one time, lindane had been a drug of choice for pediculosis and scabies; however, the FDA now recommends that lindane be reserved for patients who fail to respond to preferred drugs, such as permethrin. Because of the risk of convulsions, pediatric use of lindane should be avoided.

#### Adverse Effects

***Irritation.*** Lindane is irritating to the eyes and mucous membranes. Application to the face should be avoided. If contact occurs, the affected area should be flushed with water.

***Convulsions.*** Lindane can penetrate the intact skin and, if absorbed in sufficient amounts, can cause convulsions. Convulsions can also result from lindane ingestion. Fortunately, convulsions are rare, resulting most often from drug ingestion or from inappropriate administration. If a seizure develops, it can be controlled with an IV barbiturate (e.g., phenobarbital) or IV diazepam.

Patients at highest risk for convulsions are premature infants, children, and patients with pre-existing seizure disorders. Premature infants are especially vulnerable because lindane can penetrate their skin with relative ease, and because limited liver function prevents premature infants from detoxifying absorbed drug. As noted above, lindane should not be used on pediatric patients unless safer drugs have failed to control infestation.

#### Preparations and Administration

***Preparations.*** Lindane [Kwell, Scabene, G-well] is dispensed as a lotion, cream, and shampoo. The concentration of lindane in all formulations is 1%.

***Administration.*** *Scabies.* To treat scabies, a thin layer of cream or lotion is applied to the entire body below the head. No more than 30 gm (1 oz) should be used. The drug is removed by washing 8 to 12 hours later. As a rule, only one application is required. Pruritus may persist because of residual insect products. This itching does not indicate a need for additional treatment.

*Head Lice.* To kill head lice and their nits, lindane shampoo (30 to 60 gm) should be worked into dry hair and left in place for 4 minutes. After this, the shampoo should be rinsed off with warm water. Dead nits can be removed with a comb or tweezers. Lindane cream can be employed to treat head lice, but this formulation is less convenient than the shampoo.

*Pubic Lice.* The affected region should receive the same treatment employed for the removal of head lice. Shampoo is preferred to lotion. Although one treatment is usually sufficient, a second application in 7 days may be required. Sexual partners should be treated concurrently. Lindane should not be used to treat infestation of the eyelashes by the pubic louse. For this condition, petrolatum ophthalmic ointment is employed.

*Body Lice.* Body lice can be killed by applying a thin layer of lindane ointment or cream to affected areas. The drug should be washed off 8 to 12 hours after application.

## KEY POINTS

- Pediculosis (lice) and scabies (mites) can be treated effectively and safely with topical drugs.
- Permethrin is the drug of choice for both mites and lice. The 5% cream [Elimite] is for mites; the 1% solution [Nix] is for lice.

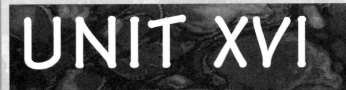

# UNIT XVI

# Cancer Chemotherapy

**Basic Principles of Cancer Chemotherapy**

**Anticancer Drugs**

# CHAPTER 95

# Basic Principles of Cancer Chemotherapy

As mortality from infectious diseases has declined, thanks to the development of antimicrobial drugs, cancer has emerged as a leading cause of death. In the United States the number of deaths from cancer is about 550,000 a year—second only to deaths from heart disease. Among women ages 30 to 74, neoplastic diseases lead all other causes of mortality. Among children ages 1 to 14 years, cancer is the leading nonaccidental cause of death. As shown in Table 95-1, the three most common cancers in women are breast, lung, and colorectal cancers. In men, the most common are prostate, lung, and colorectal cancers.

We have three major modalities for treating cancer: *surgery*, *radiotherapy*, and *chemotherapy* (drug therapy). Surgery and/or irradiation are preferred for most solid cancers. Drug therapy is the treatment of choice for *disseminated* cancers (leukemias, disseminated lymphomas, widespread metastases) and a few localized cancers (e.g., choriocarcinoma, testicular carcinoma). Drug therapy also has an important role as an adjunct to surgery and irradiation: by killing malignant cells that surgery and irradiation leave behind, adjuvant chemotherapy can significantly prolong life.

The modern era of cancer chemotherapy dates from 1942, the year in which "nitrogen mustards" were first used to treat cancer. Since the introduction of nitrogen mustards, chemotherapy has made significant advances. Patients with some neoplastic diseases now have a good chance of being cured (Table 95-2). Cancers with a high cure rate include Hodgkin's disease, Ewing's sarcoma, and acute lymphocytic leukemia. For many patients whose cancer is not yet curable, chemotherapy can still be of value, offering realistic hopes of palliation and prolongation of useful life. However, although progress in chemotherapy has been encouraging, the ability to cure most cancers with drugs remains elusive. At this time, the major impediment to successful chemotherapy is toxicity of anticancer drugs to normal tissues.

Our principal objectives in this chapter are to examine the major obstacles confronting success in chemotherapy, the strategies being employed to overcome those obstacles, and the major toxicities of the anticancer drugs and the steps that can be taken to minimize their harm and discomfort. As preparation for addressing these issues, we will begin the chapter by discussing (1) the nature of cancer itself and (2) the tissue growth fraction and its relationship to cancer chemotherapy.

## What Is Cancer?

In the discussion below, we consider properties shared by neoplastic cells as a group. However, although the discussion addresses cancers in general, be aware that the term *cancer* refers to a group of disorders and not to a single disease. The various forms of cancer differ in both phenotype and aggressiveness. In addition, they differ in responsiveness to drugs.

**TABLE 95–1. ESTIMATED NEW CANCER CASES AND DEATHS, UNITED STATES, 1996**

| Type of Cancer | Females | | Males | |
| --- | --- | --- | --- | --- |
| | New Cases | Deaths | New Cases | Deaths |
| All types | 594,850 | 262,440 | 764,300 | 292,300 |
| Prostate | | | 317,100 | 41,400 |
| Breast | 184,300 | 44,300 | 1,400 | 260 |
| Lung | 78,100 | 64,300 | 98,900 | 94,400 |
| Colorectal | 65,900 | 27,500 | 67,600 | 27,400 |
| Uterus | 49,700 | 10,900 | | |
| Leukemias and lymphomas | 45,300 | 25,060 | 56,900 | 30,150 |
| Urinary tract | 26,700 | 8,600 | 56,800 | 15,100 |
| Ovary | 26,700 | 14,800 | | |
| Melanoma of skin | 16,500 | 2,700 | 21,800 | 4,600 |
| Pancreas | 13,900 | 14,200 | 12,400 | 13,600 |
| Oral cavity and pharnyx | 9,390 | 2,800 | 20,100 | 5,380 |
| Liver | 9,100 | 6,800 | 10,800 | 8,400 |
| Stomach | 8,800 | 5,700 | 14,000 | 8,300 |
| Brain and other CNS | 7,500 | 6,100 | 10,400 | 7,200 |

Data from *Facts and Figures* in the American Cancer Society site on the World Wide Web (http://www.cancer.org).

## Characteristics of Neoplastic Cells

*Persistent Proliferation.* Unlike normal cells, whose proliferation is carefully controlled, cancer cells undergo unrestrained growth and division. This capacity for persistent proliferation is the most distinguishing property of malignant cells. In the absence of intervention, cancerous tissues will continue to grow until they cause death.

It was once believed that cancer cells divided more rapidly than normal cells and that this excessive rate of division was responsible for the abnormal growth patterns of cancerous tissues. We now know that this concept is not correct. Division of neoplastic cells is not necessarily rapid: although some cancers are composed of cells that divide rapidly, others are composed of cells that divide slowly. The correct explanation for the relentless growth of tumors is that *malignant cells are unresponsive to the feedback mechanisms that regulate cellular proliferation in healthy tissue.* Hence, cancer cells are able to continue multiplying under conditions that would suppress further growth and division of normal cells.

*Invasive Growth.* In the absence of malignancy, the various types of cells that compose a tissue remain segregated from one another; cells of one type do not invade territory that belongs to cells of a different type. In contrast, malignant cells are free of the constraints that inhibit invasive growth. As a result, cells of a solid tumor can penetrate adjacent tissues, thereby allowing the cancer to spread.

*Formation of Metastases.* Metastases are secondary tumors that appear at sites distant from the primary tumor. Metastases result from the unique ability of malignant cells to break away from their site of origin, migrate to other parts of the body (via the lymphatic and circulatory systems), and then reimplant to form a new tumor.

## Etiology of Cancer

The abnormal behavior of cancer cells results from alterations in their DNA. Specifically, malignant transformation results from a combination of activation of oncogenes (cancer-causing genes) and inactivation of tumor suppressor genes (genes that prevent replication of cells that have become cancerous). These genetic alterations are caused by chemical carcinogens, viruses, and radiation (x-rays, ultraviolet light, radioisotopes). Malignant transformation occurs in three major stages, called initiation, promotion, and progression. These stages suggest that DNA in cancer cells undergoes a series of modifications, rather than just a single change.

## The Growth Fraction and Its Relationship to Chemotherapy

The growth fraction of a tissue is a major determinant of its responsiveness to chemotherapy. Consequently, before we discuss the anticancer drugs, we must first understand the growth fraction. In order to define the growth fraction, we need to review the cell cycle.

### The Cell Cycle

The cell cycle is the sequence of events that a cell goes through from one mitotic division to the next. As shown in Figure 95–1, the cell cycle consists of four major

## TABLE 95-2. SOME CANCERS FOR WHICH DRUGS MAY BE CURATIVE

| Type of Cancer | Drug Therapy |
| --- | --- |
| Hodgkin's lymphoma | Doxorubicin + bleomycin + vinblastine + dacarbazine |
| Burkitt's lymphoma | Cyclophosphamide + vincristine + methotrexate + doxorubicin + prednisone |
| Choriocarcinoma | Methotrexate ± leucovorin |
| Small cell cancer of lung | Etoposide + cisplatin |
| Testicular cancer | Cisplatin + etoposide ± bleomycin |
| Wilms' tumor* | Dactinomycin + vincristine ± doxorubicin ± cyclophosphamide |
| Ewing's sarcoma* | Cyclophosphamide + doxorubicin + vincristine alternating with etoposide + ifosfamide (with mesna) |
| Acute lymphocytic leukemia | Vincristine + prednisone + asparaginase + daunorubicin or doxorubicin ± cyclophosphamide |

*Chemotherapy is combined with surgery and/or radiotherapy in these cancers.

phases, named $G_1$, S, $G_2$, and M. (The length of the arrows in the figure is proportional to the time spent in each phase.) For purposes of discussion, we can imagine the cycle as beginning with $G_1$, the phase in which the cell prepares to make DNA. Following $G_1$, the cell enters S phase, the phase in which DNA synthesis actually takes place. Once synthesis of DNA is complete, the cell enters $G_2$ and prepares for mitosis. Mitosis (cell division) occurs next during M phase. Upon completion of mitosis, the resulting daughter cells have two options: they can enter $G_1$ and repeat the cycle, or they can enter the phase known as $G_0$. Cells that enter $G_0$ become mitotically dormant; these cells do not replicate and are not considered to be participating in the cell cycle. Cells may remain in $G_0$ for days, weeks, or even years. Under appropriate conditions, resting cells may leave $G_0$ and resume active participation in the cycle.

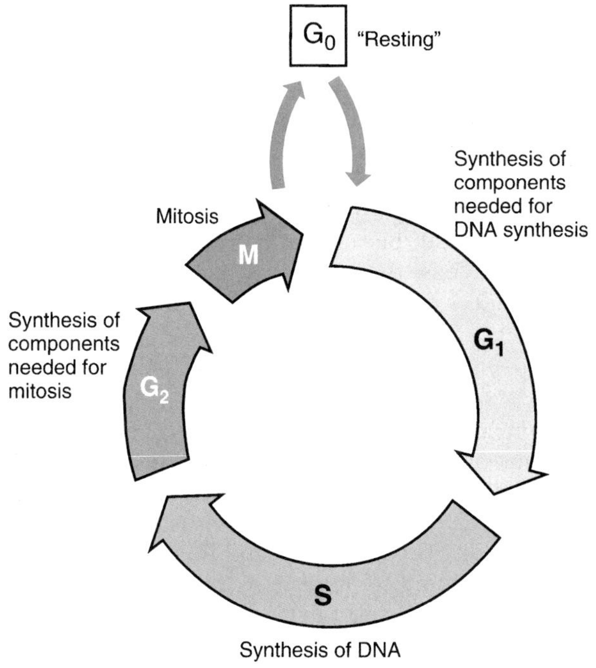

### The Growth Fraction

If we were to examine any tissue, we would observe that some cells are going through the cell cycle, whereas others are "resting" in $G_0$. The ratio of proliferating cells to $G_0$ cells is called the *growth fraction*. A tissue with a large percentage of proliferating cells and few cells in $G_0$ would have a *high* growth fraction. Conversely, a tissue composed mostly of $G_0$ cells would have a *low* growth fraction.

### Impact of Tissue Growth Fraction on Responsiveness to Anticancer Drugs

As a rule, *anticancer drugs are much more toxic to tissues that have a high growth fraction than to tissues that have a low growth fraction*. This is because most anticancer agents are more active against proliferating cells than they are against cells in $G_0$. Proliferating cells are especially sensitive to chemotherapy because anticancer drugs usually act by disrupting DNA synthesis or mitosis—activities that only proliferating cells carry out. Unfortunately, toxicity of anticancer drugs is not restricted to *cancers* that have a high growth fraction: these drugs are also toxic to *normal tissues* whose growth fraction is high (e.g., bone marrow, gastrointestinal epithelium, hair follicles, sperm-forming cells).

Having established the relationship between growth fraction and drug sensitivity, we can apply this knowledge to predict how specific cancers will respond to chemotherapy. As a rule, *solid tumors* have a *low* growth frac-

Figure 95-1. The cell cycle.

tion, and hence tend to respond poorly. In contrast, *disseminated cancers* have a *high* growth fraction and generally respond *well*. In practical terms, this means that the leukemias and lymphomas, which are disseminated forms of cancer, represent the majority of cancers that can be successfully treated with drugs. Conversely, and unfortunately, the most common cancers—solid tumors of the breast, lung, prostate, colon, and rectum—are much less responsive to drugs.

# Obstacles to Successful Chemotherapy

Our objective in this section is to examine the major factors that make success in cancer chemotherapy difficult. Foremost among these is the serious and unavoidable toxicity to normal cells caused by currently available anticancer drugs.

## Toxicity to Normal Cells

Toxicity to normal cells is the principal barrier to success in chemotherapy. Injury to normal cells occurs primarily in tissues whose growth fraction is high (bone marrow, gastrointestinal epithelium, hair follicles, germinal epithelium of the testes). Drug-induced injury to each of these tissues is discussed in detail later in the chapter. For now we will consider injury to normal cells as a group.

*Toxicity to normal cells is dose limiting.* That is, dosage cannot exceed an amount that produces the maximally tolerated degree of injury to normal cells. Hence, although very large doses of anticancer agents might be able to produce 100% kill of malignant cells, such doses cannot be given because of the very real risk of killing the patient.

Why is it that anticancer drugs are so harmful to normal tissues? These drugs injure normal tissue because they lack *selective toxicity*, a property that can be defined as *the ability to kill one kind of cell* (target cell) *without killing other cells with which the target cell is in intimate contact.* We first encountered this concept in Chapter 77 (Basic Principles of Antimicrobial Therapy). In that chapter we noted that the great success that has been achieved in antimicrobial therapy has been possible because antimicrobial drugs are highly selective in their toxicity. Penicillin, for example, can readily kill invading bacteria while being virtually harmless to cells of the host. This high degree of selective toxicity stands in sharp contrast to the lack of selectivity displayed by most anticancer drugs.

Why have we been unable to develop drugs that are selectively toxic to neoplastic cells? Achieving selective toxicity has been elusive because normal cells and malignant cells are very much alike. Production of a selectively toxic drug requires that the target cell have some biochemical feature that normal cells lack. By way of illustration, let's consider how penicillin achieves its selectively toxic effects. Penicillin kills bacteria by disrupting the bacterial cell wall. Since our cells have no cell wall, penicillin can't hurt us. Our current understanding of cancer cells offers no such basis for creating selectively toxic anticancer drugs: we have yet to identify a unique biochemical characteristic of cancer cells that would render them vulnerable to selective attack with chemotherapeutic agents. Thus, until means of selective attack are discovered, we will remain unable to kill or injure malignant cells without causing harm to many noncancer cells.

## Cure Requires 100% Cell Kill

To cure a patient of cancer we must eliminate virtually every malignant cell from the body; just one remaining cell can proliferate and cause relapse. For most patients, 100% cell kill cannot be achieved. Factors that make it difficult to produce complete cell kill include (1) the kinetics of drug-induced cell kill, (2) minimal participation of the immune system in eliminating malignant cells, and (3) disappearance of symptoms before all cancer cells are gone.

*Kinetics of Drug-Induced Cell Kill.* Killing of cancer cells follows *first-order kinetics.* That is, at any given dose, a drug will kill a *constant percentage* of malignant cells, *regardless of how many cells are actually present.* This means that the dose required to shrink a cancer from $10^3$ cells down to 10 cells will be just as big, for example, as the dose required to reduce that cancer from $10^9$ cells down to $10^7$ cells. Hence, with each successive round of chemotherapy, drug dosage must remain the same, even though the cancer is getting progressively smaller. This means that, if treatment is to continue, the patient must be able to tolerate the same degree of toxicity late in therapy as he or she could tolerate when therapy began. For many patients, this is not possible.

*Nonparticipation of Host Defenses in Cell Kill.* In contrast to the antimicrobial drugs, anticancer agents receive very little help from host defenses. Accordingly, anticancer agents must produce cell kill almost entirely on their own. There are two reasons why host defenses contribute so little. First, because of their immunosuppressant actions, anticancer drugs seriously compromise immune function. Second, because malignant cells are so much like normal cells, the immune system generally fails to identify cancer cells as appropriate for attack.

*When Should Treatment Stop?* We have no way of knowing when 100% cell kill has been achieved. As a result, there is no definitive method for deciding just when chemotherapy should stop. As indicated in Figure 95-2, symptoms disappear long before the last malignant cell has been eliminated. Once a cancer has been reduced to less than 1 million cells, it becomes virtually undetectable; all signs of disease are absent, and the patient is considered to be in complete remission. It is obvious, however, that a patient harboring a million malignant cells is by no means cured. It is also obvious that further chemotherapy is indicated. However, what is not so obvious is just how long therapy should last: since the patient is already

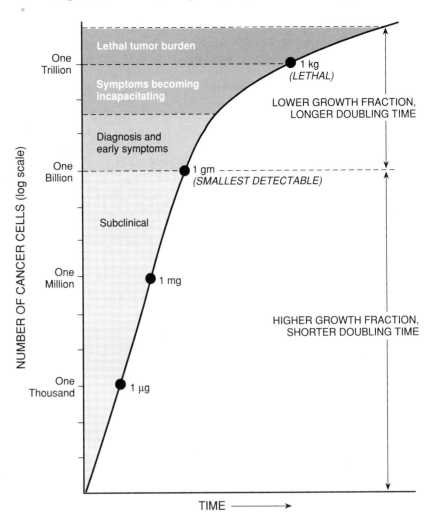

**Figure 95–2. Gompertzian tumor growth curve showing the relationship between tumor size and clinical status.**

asymptomatic, we have no objective means of determining when to discontinue drug use. The clinical dilemma is this: if therapy is continued too long, the patient will be needlessly exposed to serious toxicity; conversely, if drugs are withdrawn prematurely, relapse will occur.

## Failure of Early Detection

Early detection of cancer is rare. At this time, cancer of the cervix, which can be diagnosed with a Pap smear, is the only neoplastic disease capable of truly early detection. All other forms of cancer are significantly advanced by the time they have grown large enough for discovery. The smallest detectable cancers are about 1 cm in diameter, have a mass of 1 gm, and consist of about 1 billion cells (see Fig. 95-2). Detection at this stage cannot be considered early.

Late detection has three important consequences. First, by the time the primary tumor is discovered, metastases may have formed. Second, the tumor will be less responsive to drugs than it would have been at an earlier stage (see below). Third, since cancer has been present for a long time, the patient may be debilitated by the disease, and therefore less able to tolerate treatment.

## Solid Tumors Respond Poorly

As noted earlier, solid tumors have a low growth fraction (high percentage of $G_0$ cells) and are generally unresponsive to chemotherapy. There are two reasons for this low responsiveness. First, $G_0$ cells do not perform the activities that most anticancer drugs are designed to disrupt. Second, because $G_0$ cells are not active participants in the cell cycle, they have time to repair drug-induced damage before that damage can do them serious harm.

Not all solid tumors are equally unresponsive: as a rule, *large tumors are even less responsive than small tumors.* This difference occurs because, as solid tumors increase in size, many of their cells leave the cell cycle and enter $G_0$, causing the growth fraction to decline. Tumor growth slows, in large part, because blood flow in the tumor core is low, depriving cells of nutrients and oxygen. The decrease in growth fraction in older tumors is a major reason that therapeutic success is more likely when cancers are detected early. Because the rate of growth declines as a tumor gets larger, the tumor growth curve is said to follow *Gompertzian kinetics* (see Fig. 95-2).

The drug sensitivity of a solid tumor can be enhanced by *debulking.* When a solid tumor is reduced in size by surgery or irradiation, many of the remaining cells leave

$G_0$ and re-enter the cell cycle, thereby increasing their sensitivity to chemotherapy. This phenomenon is known as recruitment. It is because of recruitment that chemotherapy can be very useful as an adjunct to surgery or irradiation even though drugs may have been largely ineffective before debulking was done.

## Drug Resistance

During the course of chemotherapy, cancer cells can develop resistance to the drugs used against them. Drug resistance can be a significant cause of therapeutic failure. Mechanisms of resistance include reduced drug uptake, increased drug efflux, reduced drug activation, reduced target molecule sensitivity to a drug, and increased repair of drug-induced damage to DNA.

Cellular production of a drug transport molecule, known as *P-glycoprotein*, can confer *multiple drug resistance* upon cells. P-glycoprotein is a large molecule that spans the cytoplasmic membrane and serves to pump drugs out of the cell. Induction of P-glycoprotein synthesis following exposure to a single anticancer drug produces cross-resistance to many structurally unrelated agents. Several drugs, including calcium channel blockers, have been used investigationally to inhibit the P-glycoprotein pump and reverse multiple drug resistance.

Drug resistance usually results from a change in DNA. Mutation to a drug-resistant form is a spontaneous event and is not caused by the anticancer drugs themselves. However, although drugs do not *cause* the mutations that render cells resistant, drugs do *create selection pressure* favoring the drug-resistant mutants. That is, by killing drug-sensitive cells, anticancer agents create a competition-free environment in which drug-resistant mutants can flourish.

Since the presence of anticancer agents favors the growth of drug-resistant cells, as therapy proceeds, the number of resistant cells will increase. Because resistant cells cannot be killed with drugs, the risk of therapeutic failure becomes greater with each course of therapy. Since patients are usually exposed to drugs over an extended time, therapeutic failure owing to drug resistance is a significant problem.

## Heterogeneity of Tumor Cells

Tumors do not consist of a single population of identical cells. Rather, because of ongoing mutation, tumors are composed of subpopulations of dissimilar cells. These subpopulations can differ in morphology, growth rate, and metastatic ability. More importantly, they can differ in responsiveness to drugs (primarily because of increased resistance). As a tumor ages, cellular heterogeneity increases.

## Limited Drug Access to Tumor Cells

Because of a tumor's location or blood supply, drugs may have limited access to its cells. Large solid tumors have poor vascularization, especially near the core. Hence, cells within these tumors are difficult to reach with drugs. Similarly, tumors of the central nervous system (CNS) are difficult to reach because most anticancer drugs have difficulty crossing the blood-brain barrier.

# Strategies for Achieving Maximum Benefits from Chemotherapy

## Intermittent Chemotherapy

The ultimate goal of chemotherapy is to produce 100% kill of neoplastic cells while causing limited injury to normal tissues (especially the bone marrow and gastrointestinal epithelium). Intermittent therapy is the primary technique for achieving this goal. When anticancer drugs are administered on an intermittent schedule, normal cells are given the opportunity to repopulate between rounds of therapy. However, for this approach to succeed, one obvious requirement must be met: *normal cells must repopulate faster than the malignant cells*. If the malignant cells grow back faster than normal cells, there can be no reduction in tumor burden between rounds of treatment. The successful use of intermittent therapy is depicted in Figure 95–3.

## Combination Chemotherapy

Chemotherapy employing a combination of drugs is generally much more effective than therapy with just one drug. Accordingly, most patients are now treated with two or more agents.

### Benefits of Drug Combinations

Combination chemotherapy offers three major advantages: (1) suppression of drug resistance, (2) increased cancer cell kill, and (3) reduced injury to normal cells (at any given level of anticancer effect).

*Suppression of Drug Resistance.* Drug resistance occurs less frequently with multiple-drug therapy than with single-drug therapy. To understand why, we need to recall that resistance is acquired through random mutational events. The probability of a cell undergoing two or more mutations, and therefore developing resistance to a combination of drugs, is smaller than the probability of a cell undergoing the single mutation needed to develop resistance to one drug. Because drug resistance is reduced with combination chemotherapy, the chances of therapeutic success are increased.

*Increased Cancer Cell Kill.* If we administer several anticancer drugs, each with a different mechanism of action, we will kill more malignant cells than if we use only one drug. Therapeutic effects are enhanced because the combination attacks the cancer in several ways instead of just one. Greater cell kill is especially likely if a drug-resistant subpopulation of cells is present. The superiority of drug

(Arrows indicate times of drug administration)

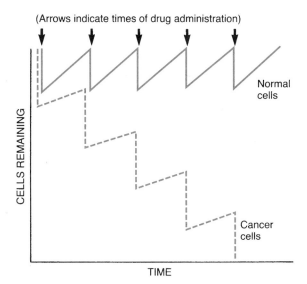

**Figure 95–3. Recovery of critical normal cells during intermittent chemotherapy.** Cancer cells and normal cells (e.g., cells of the bone marrow) are killed with each drug administration. In the intervals between doses, both types of cells proliferate. Since, in this example, normal cells repopulate faster than cancer cells, normal cells are able to recover entirely between doses, whereas regrowth of the cancer cells is only partial. Hence, with each succeeding round of treatment, the total number of cancer cells becomes smaller, whereas the number of normal cells remains within a tolerable range. Note that differential loss of malignant cells is possible only if these cells repopulate more slowly than normal cells. If cancer cells grow back as fast as normal cells, intermittent chemotherapy will fail.

combinations over single-drug therapy is illustrated by the data in Table 95–3.

***Reduced Injury to Normal Cells.*** By using a combination of drugs *that do not have overlapping toxicities*, we can achieve a greater anticancer effect than we could *safely* achieve using any of the agents alone. Why this is so is illustrated by the data in Table 95–4. This table summarizes responses to two drugs—vincristine and cyclophosphamide—when given individually and in combination. Both drugs kill malignant cells, but they act by different mechanisms: cyclophosphamide damages DNA whereas vincristine blocks mitosis. Furthermore, these drugs have different toxicities: cyclophosphamide causes *neutropenia*, whereas vincristine is *neurotoxic*. In the table, the intensity of effects is indicated by plus (+) symbols; the more plusses, the more intense the response. With either drug, 2+ represents the maximum degree of toxicity that can be tolerated. When administered alone in doses that produce 2+ toxicity, each drug produces an anticancer effect of 2+ intensity; this is the greatest therapeutic effect that we can safely achieve with either drug by itself. Now let's consider the effect of combining these drugs, giving each in its maximally tolerated dose. The total anticancer effect of the combination is 4+, twice the effect that could be achieved safely with either agent alone. Since the toxicities of these agents do not overlap,

overall toxicity of the combination remains at a tolerable level—although the patient is now exposed to two kinds of toxicity rather than one.

### Guidelines for Drug Selection

From the preceding discussion, we can extract three guidelines for selecting drugs for use in combination: (1) each drug should be effective by itself, (2) each drug should have a different mechanism of action, and (3) the drugs should have minimally overlapping toxicities.

## Optimizing Dosing Schedules

The schedule by which an anticancer drug is administered is an important determinant of the outcome of treatment. The experiment summarized in Table 95–5 provides a dramatic illustration of this point. In this experiment, two groups of mice were inoculated with cancer cells and then treated with cytarabine. Mice in group I received a *single large dose* of cytarabine on days 2, 6, 10, and 14 after being inoculated with cancer cells. The mice in group II were treated on the same days as the group I mice but, rather than receiving one large dose of cytarabine, they were given *eight small doses*, one every 3 hours. By the end of the study, all of the group II mice were cured. In stark contrast, all of the group I mice were dead. Since the two groups had the same disease and were given the same drug, we must conclude that the life-and-death difference in outcome was due to the dosing schedules employed.

To understand these results, we need to know two properties of cytarabine: (1) the drug kills cells by disrupting DNA synthesis, and (2) it undergoes rapid inactivation. Since cytarabine acts by disrupting DNA synthesis, it can only affect cells while they are in the S phase of the cell cycle. Since the drug is rapidly inactivated, and since many cells will not be in S phase during the short time before inactivation occurs, many cells will escape injury following each dose. The group I mice died because administration of just one large dose every 4 days did not maintain active drug in the body for a time sufficient to catch all cancer cells as they cycled through S phase. Since the group II mice received multiple doses over a 24-hour period on each of 4 days, the presence of active drug was sustained. Hence, the chance of cancer cells being in S phase while active drug was present was greatly increased, thereby leading to enhanced cell kill with resultant cure.

The message from this experiment is that selection of the right drugs for cancer therapy is only one of the requirements for success; those drugs must also be administered according to schedules that will maximize their effects. Dosing schedules are especially critical for drugs that, like cytarabine, act during a specific phase of the cell cycle.

## Regional Drug Delivery

By using special techniques for drug delivery, we can increase drug access to tumors, and can thereby increase cell kill and reduce systemic toxicity.

**TABLE 95-3. SINGLE-DRUG TREATMENT VERSUS COMBINATION CHEMOTHERAPY**

| Type of Cancer | Method of Treatment and Drugs Employed | Percentage of Patients with Complete Remission |
|---|---|---|
| Acute lymphocytic leukemia of childhood | *Single-Drug Therapy* | |
| | Daunorubicin | 38 |
| | Prednisone | 63 |
| | Vincristine | 57 |
| | *Combination Chemotherapy* | |
| | Prednisone + vincristine | 90 |
| | Prednisone + vincristine + daunorubicin | 97 |
| Hodgkin's disease | *Single-Drug Therapy* | |
| | Vincristine | <10 |
| | Prednisone | <5 |
| | Procarbazine | <10 |
| | Mechlorethamine | 20 |
| | *Combination Chemotherapy* | |
| | Vincristine + prednisone + mechlorethamine + procarbazine | 81 |

Data from DeVita, V. T., Young, R. C., and Canellos, G. P. Combination versus single agent chemotherapy: A review of the basis for selection of drug treatment of cancer. Cancer 35:98, 1975.

***Intra-arterial Delivery.*** Local intra-arterial infusion can be used to treat solid tumors. This technique has the advantage of establishing a high concentration of drug in the vicinity of the tumor while minimizing toxicity to the rest of the body. Specific routes include carotid artery delivery (for brain tumors) and hepatic artery delivery (for liver metastases). Clearly, intra-arterial therapy is suitable only for localized cancers.

***Intrathecal Delivery.*** As noted previously, many anticancer agents are unable to cross the blood-brain barrier, and therefore cannot reach malignant cells within the CNS. To enhance therapy of CNS cancers, drugs can be administered intrathecally (by injection directly into the subarachnoid space). This technique bypasses the blood-brain barrier, thereby giving drugs better access to cells within the CNS.

***Other Specialized Routes.*** Anticancer agents can be administered via the portal vein to treat liver metastases, and directly into the bladder to treat bladder cancer. Neoplasms located in the pleural and peritoneal cavities can be treated by direct intracavitary drug administration. As discussed in Chapter 96, carmustine, a drug for brain tumors, is now available in a wafer that is implanted in the brain to kill cancer cells left behind following surgical removal of a tumor.

# Major Toxicities of Anticancer Drugs and Their Management

The anticancer drugs constitute our most toxic group of medicines. Serious injury occurs most often to tissues that have a high growth fraction (bone marrow, gastrointestinal epithelium, hair follicles, and sperm-forming cells). In the discussion below, we consider the more common tox-

**TABLE 95-4. RESPONSES TO CYCLOPHOSPHAMIDE AND VINCRISTINE ALONE AND IN COMBINATION**

| Therapeutic Regimen | Anticancer Effect | Toxicity | |
|---|---|---|---|
| | | Neutropenia | Neurotoxicity |
| Cyclophosphamide | ++ | ++ | 0 |
| Vincristine | ++ | 0 | ++ |
| Cyclophosphamide + vincristine | ++++ | ++ | ++ |

**TABLE 95-5. EFFECT OF DOSING SCHEDULE ON THERAPEUTIC RESPONSE**

**TABLE 95-5. EFFECT OF DOSING SCHEDULE ON THERAPEUTIC RESPONSE**

| Experimental Group | Dosage Size | Dosing Schedule | Mice Surviving |
|---|---|---|---|
| I | 240 mg/kg | 1 dose/day* | None |
| II | 15 mg/kg | 8 doses/day* | 100% |

*Cytarabine was administered on days 2, 6, 10, and 14 after mice were inoculated with leukemia cells. See text for further details.

icities of the anticancer drugs along with steps that can be taken to minimize harm and discomfort.

## Bone Marrow Suppression

Anticancer drugs are highly toxic to the bone marrow, a tissue with a high proportion of proliferating cells. Myelosuppression reduces the number of circulating neutrophils, thrombocytes, and erythrocytes. Loss of these cells has three major consequences: (1) infection (from loss of neutrophils), (2) bleeding (from loss of thrombocytes), and (3) anemia (from loss of erythrocytes).

### Neutropenia

Neutrophils (neutrophilic granulocytes) are white blood cells that play an essential role in fighting infection. In patients with neutropenia (a reduction in circulating neutrophils), both the incidence and severity of infection are increased. Infections that are normally benign (e.g., candidiasis) can become life-threatening. There is no question that infection secondary to neutropenia is the most serious complication of cancer chemotherapy. The grim reality of this problem cannot be stressed too much.

With most anticancer drugs, onset of neutropenia is *rapid* and recovery develops relatively *quickly*. Neutropenia begins to develop a few days after drug administration, and the lowest neutrophil count, called the *nadir*, occurs between days 10 and 14. Neutrophil counts then recover in 3 to 4 weeks. Patients are at highest risk during the nadir; hence special care should be taken to avoid contagion during this time.

With some anticancer drugs, neutropenia is *delayed*. Neutrophil counts begin to fall in 1 to 2 weeks, and reach their nadir between weeks 3 and 4. Full recovery may not occur until after 7 weeks.

Monitoring of neutrophil counts is essential. Normal counts range from 2500 to 7000 cells/mm$^3$. If neutropenia is substantial (absolute neutrophil count below 500/mm$^3$), the next round of chemotherapy should be delayed until neutrophil counts return toward normal.

Lack of neutrophils confounds the diagnosis of infection. This is because the usual signs of infection (e.g., pus, abscesses, infiltrates on the chest x-ray) depend on having neutrophils present. In the absence of neutrophils, *fever* is the principal early sign of infection.

Patients must be their own first line of defense against infection. They should be made aware of the serious risk they face and should be taught how to minimize contagion. They should be informed that fever may be the only indication of infection and instructed to notify the physician immediately if fever develops. Since infection is commonly acquired through contact with other people, hospitalized patients should be instructed to refuse direct contact with anyone who has not washed his or her hands in the patient's presence. This rule applies not only to visiting friends and relatives but also to nurses, physicians, and all other hospital staff. The normal flora of the body are a major source of infection; the risk of acquiring an infection with these microbes can be reduced by daily examination and cleansing of the skin and oral cavity.

Hospitalization of the infection-free neutropenic patient is controversial. Some physicians feel that hospitalization *increases* the risk of acquiring a serious infection. This is because hospitals harbor drug-resistant microbes, which can make hospital-acquired (nosocomial) infections especially difficult to treat. Accordingly, these physicians recommend that neutropenic patients stay at home as long as they remain infection-free.

If neutropenic patients are hospitalized, every precaution must be taken to prevent them from acquiring a nosocomial infection. They should be given an isolation room and monitored frequently for fever. Certain foods (e.g., salads) abound in pathogenic bacteria and must be avoided.

When a neutropenic patient develops an infection, immediate and vigorous intervention is required. Specimens for culture should be taken to determine the identity and drug sensitivity of the infecting organism. While awaiting reports on the cultures, empiric therapy with intravenous antibiotics should be instituted. The drugs selected should cover all likely pathogens.

In recent years, *colony-stimulating factors* have been employed to minimize neutropenia. Two preparations are available: *granulocyte colony-stimulating factor* (G-CSF, filgrastim) and *granulocyte-macrophage colony-stimulating factor* (GM-CSF, sargramostim). Both drugs act on the bone marrow to enhance granulocyte (neutrophil) production. Colony-stimulating factors can decrease the incidence, magnitude, and duration of neutropenia. As a result, they can decrease the incidence and severity of infection as well as the need for IV antibiotics and hospitalization. The basic pharmacology of G-CSF and GM-CSF is discussed in Chapter 52 (Hematopoietic Growth Factors).

### Thrombocytopenia

Bone marrow suppression can cause thrombocytopenia (a reduction in circulating platelets), thereby increasing the risk of serious bleeding. Bleeding from the nose and gums is relatively common. Bleeding from the gums can be reduced by avoiding vigorous tooth brushing. Drugs that promote bleeding (e.g., aspirin, anticoagulants) should not be used. When a mild analgesic is required, acetaminophen, which does not promote bleeding, is preferred to aspirin. For patients with severe thrombocytopenia, platelet infusion is the mainstay of treatment.

Caution should be exercised when performing procedures that might promote bleeding. Intravenous needles should be inserted with special care. Intramuscular injections should be avoided if possible. Blood pressure cuffs should be applied cautiously, since overinflation may cause bruising or bleeding.

### Anemia

Anemia is defined as a reduction in the number of circulating erythrocytes (red blood cells). Although anticancer drugs can suppress erythrocyte production, anemia is much less common than neutropenia or thrombocytopenia. This is because circulating erythrocytes have a long life span (120 days), which usually allows erythrocyte production to recover before levels of existing erythrocytes decline.

If anemia does develop, it can be treated with a transfusion or with epoetin (erythropoietin), a hormone that stimulates production of red blood cells. Since transfusions require hospitalization, whereas epoetin can be administered at home, epoetin therapy can spare the patient inconvenience. However, epoetin has the drawback of being expensive. In addition, epoetin cannot be used in patients with leukemias and other myeloid malignancies, since it may stimulate proliferation of these cancers. The basic pharmacology of epoetin is discussed in Chapter 52.

### Digestive Tract Injury

The epithelial lining of the gastrointestinal tract has a very high growth fraction, and hence is exquisitely sensitive to cytotoxic drugs. Stomatitis and diarrhea are common. Severe gastrointestinal injury can be life threatening.

**Stomatitis.** Stomatitis (inflammation of the oral mucosa) often develops a few days after the onset of chemotherapy and may persist for 2 or more weeks after treatment has ceased. Inflammation can progress to denudation and ulceration, and is often complicated by in-

### TABLE 95-6. EMETOGENIC POTENTIAL OF SELECTED CYTOTOXIC ANTICANCER DRUGS

| *Severe* | *Moderate* |
|---|---|
| Cisplatin | Cytarabine |
| Dacarbazine | Procarbazine |
| Nitrogen mustard | Mitomycin |
| Streptozocin | Methotrexate (high doses) |
| *Moderately Severe* | *Mild* |
| Cyclophosphamide | Etoposide |
| Ifosfamide | Fluorouracil |
| Doxorubicin | Hydroxyurea |
| Nitrosourea | Bleomycin |
| Dactinomycin | Vinblastine |
| | Vincristine |
| | Chlorambucil |
| | Methotrexate (low doses) |

fection. Pain can be severe, inhibiting eating, speaking, and swallowing. Management measures include good oral hygiene and a bland diet. A combination of topical anesthetics and systemic analgesics may be required to relieve pain. Topical antifungal drugs may be needed to control infection with *Candida albicans.* Inflammation can be reduced with a glucocorticoid and diphenhydramine (an antihistamine). Severe stomatitis may necessitate interrupting chemotherapy.

**Diarrhea.** By injuring the epithelial lining of the intestine, anticancer drugs can impair absorption of fluids and other nutrients, thereby causing diarrhea. Diarrhea can be reduced with a diet high in fiber (which gives the stool a more firm consistency) and by eating constipating foods (e.g., cheeses).

### Nausea and Vomiting

Nausea and vomiting are common sequelae of cancer chemotherapy. These responses, which result in part from stimulation of the chemoreceptor trigger zone, can be both immediate and dramatic, and may persist for hours. In some cases, discomfort is so great as to prompt refusal of further treatment.

It is important to appreciate that the nausea and vomiting associated with anticancer drugs are typically much more severe than with most other medicines. Hence, whereas these reactions are generally unremarkable with most drugs, they must be considered major and characteristic side effects of cancer chemotherapy. The emetogenic potential of several anticancer drugs is indicated in Table 95-6.

Nausea and vomiting can be reduced by premedication with antiemetics. These drugs offer three benefits: (1) reduction of anticipatory nausea and vomiting, (2) prevention of dehydration and malnutrition secondary to frequent nausea and vomiting, and (3) promotion of compliance with anticancer therapy by reducing discomfort. Of the antiemetics in use, *ondansetron* [Zofran] in combination with *dexamethasone* is unusually effective. Other antiemetics employed during chemotherapy include *metoclopramide* [Reglan], *prochlorperazine*, *methylprednisolone*, and *lorazepam* [Ativan]. In addition, two cannabinoids (marijuana-like drugs) are available: *dronabinol* [Marinol] and *nabilone* [Cesamet]. Combinations of antiemetics are more effective than single-drug therapy. The antiemetic drugs and their use in chemotherapy are discussed further in Chapter 73.

### Other Important Toxicities

**Alopecia.** Reversible alopecia (hair loss) results from injury to hair follicles. Alopecia can occur with most cytotoxic anticancer drugs. Hair loss begins 7 to 10 days after the onset of treatment and becomes maximal in 1 to 2 months. Regeneration begins 1 to 2 months after the last course of treatment.

While alopecia is not dangerous, it is nonetheless very upsetting. In fact, for many cancer patients, alopecia is second only to vomiting as their greatest treatment-related fear. If treatment is expected to cause hair loss, the patient should be forewarned. For patients who wish to wear a hairpiece, it should be selected before hair loss occurs. Hairpieces are tax-deductible as medical expenses and are covered by some health insurance plans.

***Reproductive Toxicity.*** The developing fetus and the germinal epithelium of the testes have high growth fractions. As a result, both are highly susceptible to injury by anticancer drugs. These drugs can interfere with embryogenesis, causing death of the early embryo. They may also cause fetal malformation. Accordingly, women undergoing chemotherapy should be warned against becoming pregnant. If pregnancy occurs, the possibility of terminating the pregnancy should be discussed. Drug effects on the ovaries may result in amenorrhea, menopausal symptoms, and atrophy of the vaginal epithelium.

Anticancer drugs can cause irreversible sterility in males. Men should be forewarned of this effect and counseled about sperm banking.

***Hyperuricemia.*** Hyperuricemia is defined as an excessive level of uric acid in the blood. Uric acid, a compound with low solubility, is formed by the breakdown of DNA following cell death. Hyperuricemia is especially common following treatment for leukemias and lymphomas, since therapy results in massive cell kill. The major concern with hyperuricemia is injury to the kidneys secondary to deposition of uric acid crystals in renal tubules. The risk of crystal formation can be reduced by increasing fluid intake. If necessary, uric acid levels can be lowered with *allopurinol*, a drug that suppresses uric acid formation. The basic pharmacology of allopurinol is discussed in Chapter 66.

***Local Injury from Extravasation of Vesicants.*** Certain anticancer drugs, known as *vesicants*, are highly chemically reactive. These drugs can cause severe local injury if they make direct contact with tissues. Vesicants are administered intravenously, since rapid dilution in venous blood minimizes the risk of injury. Administration is usually by injection (IV push) through a sidearm in a freely flowing IV line. Sites of previous irradiation should be avoided. Extreme care must be exercised to prevent extravasation, since leakage can produce high local concentrations, resulting in prolonged pain, infection, and loss of mobility. Severe injury can lead to necrosis and sloughing, requiring surgical debridement and skin grafting. If extravasation occurs, the infusion should be stopped immediately. Vesicants should be administered only by clinicians specially trained in their safe handling and use.

***Unique Toxicities.*** In addition to the toxicities discussed above, most of which apply to the anticancer drugs as a group, some agents produce unique toxicities. For example, daunorubicin can cause serious harm to the heart, cisplatin can injure the kidneys, and vincristine can injure peripheral nerves. Special toxicities of individual drugs are considered in Chapter 96.

***Carcinogenesis.*** Along with their other adverse actions, anticancer drugs have one final and ironic toxicity:

these drugs, which are used to treat cancer, have *caused* cancer in some patients. Cancer results from drug-induced damage to DNA. Cancers caused by anticancer drugs may take many years to appear.

## Making the Decision to Treat

From the preceding discussion of toxicities, it is clear that anticancer drugs can cause great harm. Given the known dangers of these drugs, we must ask ourselves why such toxic substances are administered to sick people at all. The answer to this question lies with the primary dictum of therapeutics, which states that the benefits of therapy must outweigh the risks. For most patients undergoing chemotherapy, the conditions of this rule are met. That is, although the toxicities of the anticancer drugs can be very bad, the potential benefits (cure, prolonged life, palliation) justify the risks. However, the desirability of treating cancer with drugs is not always obvious. There are patients whose chances of being helped by chemotherapy may be very remote, while their chances of experiencing serious injury remain ever present. Since the potential benefits for some patients are small and the risks are large, the decision to institute chemotherapy must be made with careful deliberation.

Before the decision to treat can be made, the patient must be given some idea of the probable benefits that the proposed therapy has to offer. There are three basic benefits that chemotherapy can provide: cure, palliation, and prolongation of useful life. For treatment to be justified, there should be reason to believe that at least one of these benefits may be forthcoming. If a patient cannot be offered some reasonable hope of cure, palliation, or prolongation of useful life, it would be difficult to justify treatment.

The most important factors for predicting the outcome of chemotherapy are (1) the general health status of the patient and (2) the responsiveness of the particular cancer the patient has. General health status can be assessed with the Karnofsky Performance Scale (Table 95-7). A Karnofsky rating of less than 40 indicates that the patient is very debilitated and not likely to tolerate the additional stress of chemotherapy. Patients with a low Karnofsky rating should receive anticancer drugs only if the type of cancer they have is known to be especially responsive.

The responsiveness of some common cancers is indicated in Table 95-8. Patients with highly responsive types of cancer should almost always be treated, regardless of their Karnofsky rating. In contrast, patients with minimally responsive types of cancer should be treated only after careful consideration. It may well be that such patients are better off limiting their problems to the cancer itself, without adding the dangers and discomforts of a course of treatment that has little to offer.

An important requirement for deciding in favor of chemotherapy is that the impact of treatment be measurable. That is, there must be some objective means of de-

## TABLE 95-7. KARNOFSKY PERFORMANCE SCALE

| Definition | Percentage | Criteria |
|---|---|---|
| Able to carry on normal activity and work; no special care needed | 100 | Normal; no complaints; no evidence of disease |
| | 90 | Able to carry on normal activity; minor signs or symptoms of disease |
| | 80 | Normal activity with effort; some signs or symptoms of disease |
| Unable to work; able to live at home and care for most personal needs; a varying amount of assistance needed | 70 | Cares for self; unable to carry on normal activity or do active work |
| | 60 | Requires occasional assistance; able to care for most needs |
| | 50 | Requires considerable assistance and frequent medical care |
| Unable to care for self; requires equivalent of institutional or hospital care; disease may be progressing rapidly | 40 | Disabled; requires special care and assistance |
| | 30 | Severely disabled; hospitalization is indicated although death not imminent |
| | 20 | Very sick, hospitalization necessary; active supportive treatment necessary |
| | 10 | Moribund; fatal processes progressing rapidly |
| | 0 | Dead |

termining the cancer's response to therapy. For solid tumors, we should be able to measure a decrease in tumor size. For hematologic cancers, we should be able to measure a decrease in the number of circulating neoplastic cells. If we have no way to measure the response of a cancer, then we have no way of knowing if treatment has done any good. If we cannot determine that drugs are doing something beneficial, there is little justification for giving them.

Clearly, not all patients are candidates for chemotherapy. The decision to institute treatment must be made on an individual basis. Patients should be informed as accurately as possible about the potential risks and benefits of the therapy under consideration. When the decision to

## TABLE 95-8. RESPONSIVENESS OF SOME CANCERS TO CHEMOTHERAPY

| Responsiveness to Chemotherapy | Type of Cancer | Probable Benefits of Chemotherapy |
|---|---|---|
| High | Hodgkin's disease<br>Burkitt's lymphoma<br>Acute lymphocytic leukemia<br>Choriocarcinoma<br>Wilms' tumor<br>Ewing's sarcoma | Cure or substantial prolongation of life |
| Moderate | Breast cancer<br>Cervical carcinoma<br>Chronic lymphocytic leukemia<br>Bladder cancer<br>Multiple myeloma<br>Prostate carcinoma | Prolongation of life; palliation |
| Minimal | Colorectal cancer<br>Hepatocellular<br>Melanoma<br>Pancreatic cancer<br>Renal cancer<br>Osteogenic sarcoma | Palliation; minimal prolongation of life |

treat is made, it should be the result of collaboration between the patient, family, and physician, and should reflect a conviction on the part of the patient that, within his or her set of values, the potential benefits outweigh the inherent risks.

# Looking Ahead

Does the future offer hope of developing chemotherapeutic cures for all forms of cancer? This question can be cautiously answered in the affirmative. There is no theoretical reason to believe that cancers are inherently incapable of cure. On the contrary, there is good reason to believe that cancers are in fact curable diseases. We have discussed the issue of selective toxicity and concluded that the absence of selectively toxic anticancer drugs constitutes the primary obstacle to truly curative therapy. We currently lack selectively toxic drugs because we have yet to identify biochemical characteristics of cancer cells that would render them vulnerable to selective attack. However, although we have yet to discover a chink in cancer's biochemical armor, it is not unreasonable to think that one nonetheless exists. Cancer cells are, after all, different from normal cells. This difference, manifested as unrestrained growth, must have a biochemical basis. That biochemical basis, when it is finally understood, may well provide the basis for making chemotherapeutic agents that are truly selective in their toxicity—drugs that are as selective for cancer cells as, for example, penicillin G is for gram-positive bacteria. Drugs with this degree of selectivity will offer a cure for neoplastic diseases. It is not completely naive to believe that such drugs will eventually be developed.

## KEY POINTS

- Cancer cells are characterized by persistent proliferation, invasive growth, and the ability to form metastases.
- Cancer can be treated with three modalities: surgery, radiotherapy, and chemotherapy.
- Surgery and/or irradiation are the treatments of choice for most *solid* cancers.
- Drugs are the treatment of choice for *disseminated* cancers (leukemias, disseminated lymphomas, widespread metastases). Drugs are also used as adjuvants to surgery and irradiation to kill malignant cells that surgery and irradiation leave behind.
- The cell cycle has four major phases: $G_1$, in which cells prepare to synthesize DNA; S, in which cells synthesize DNA; $G_2$, in which cells prepare for mitosis; and M, in which cells undergo mitosis (division). Following mitosis, the resulting daughter cells may either enter $G_1$ and repeat the cycle, or enter $G_0$ and become mitotically dormant.
- The growth fraction is defined as the ratio of proliferating cells to $G_0$ cells in a tissue.

- Tissues with a large percentage of proliferating cells and few cells in $G_0$ have a high growth fraction. Conversely, tissues composed mostly of $G_0$ cells have a low growth fraction.
- Most anticancer drugs are much more toxic to cancers that have a high growth fraction than to cancers that have a low growth fraction. This is because most anticancer drugs are more active against proliferating cells than against cells in $G_0$.
- As a rule, solid tumors have a low growth fraction, and hence tend to respond poorly to drugs. In contrast, disseminated cancers have a high growth fraction and generally respond well.
- To cure a patient of cancer, we must produce 100% cell kill, which is usually impossible.
- Killing of cancer cells follows first-order kinetics. That is, at any given dose, drugs kill a constant *percentage* of malignant cells, regardless of how many cells are actually present.
- Over the course of chemotherapy, cancer cells often become drug resistant, thereby decreasing the chances of success.
- The purpose of intermittent chemotherapy is to allow normal cells to repopulate between rounds of chemotherapy. Unfortunately, if the cancer cells repopulate as rapidly as (or more rapidly than) the normal cells, there will be no reduction in tumor burden with each round of treatment, and hence treatment will fail.
- Combination chemotherapy is generally much more effective than single-drug therapy. This is because combination therapy can (1) suppress drug resistance, (2) increase cell kill, and (3) reduce injury to normal cells (at any given level of anticancer effect).
- Ideally, the drugs used in combination therapy should have (1) different mechanisms of action, (2) minimally overlapping toxicities, and (3) good efficacy when used alone.
- For drugs that act during a specific phase of the cell cycle, selecting the right dosing schedule is critical to the success of treatment.
- Toxicity to normal tissues is the major obstacle to successful chemotherapy.
- Anticancer drugs injure normal tissue because they lack selective toxicity.
- Serious toxicity occurs most often to normal tissues that have a high growth fraction (i.e., bone marrow, gastrointestinal epithelium, hair follicles, and sperm-forming cells).
- Myelosuppression (toxicity to bone marrow) can reduce the number of neutrophils, thrombocytes, and erythrocytes, thereby posing a risk of infection (from loss of neutrophils), bleeding (from loss of thrombocytes), and anemia (from loss of erythrocytes).
- Loss of neutrophils and thrombocytes during chemotherapy is common; loss of erythrocytes is rare.
- In patients taking myelosuppressive drugs, neutrophil counts must be monitored. If neutropenia is substantial (absolute neutrophil count below $500/mm^3$), the next round of chemotherapy should be postponed.
- When a neutropenic patient develops an infection, immediate and vigorous intervention is required. Until lab

reports on the identity and drug sensitivity of the infecting organism are available, empiric therapy with intravenous antibiotics should be instituted.

- Neutropenia can be minimized by treatment with granulocyte colony-stimulating factor or granulocyte-macrophage colony-stimulating factor, both of which act on the bone marrow to increase neutrophil production.
- By injuring the epithelial lining of the GI tract, anticancer drugs often cause stomatitis and diarrhea.
- Many anticancer drugs cause moderate to severe nausea and vomiting, in part by stimulating the chemoreceptor trigger zone.
- Nausea and vomiting can be reduced by premedication with antiemetics. The combination of ondansetron plus dexamethasone is especially effective.
- Anticancer drugs often injure hair follicles, thereby causing alopecia (hair loss). Patients who may want to wear a hairpiece should select one before hair loss occurs.

- Anticancer drugs can cause fetal malformation and embryonic death. Accordingly, women undergoing chemotherapy should be warned against becoming pregnant.
- Anticancer drugs can cause irreversible sterility in men. Accordingly, men undergoing chemotherapy should be counseled about possible sperm banking.
- Chemotherapy can cause hyperuricemia as a result of DNA degradation secondary to massive cell death.
- Renal injury from hyperuricemia can be minimized by giving fluids and allopurinol, a drug that blocks formation of uric acid.
- Anticancer drugs with vesicant properties can cause severe local injury if the IV line through which they are being administered becomes extravasated.
- Cancer chemotherapy has three possible benefits: cure, palliation, and prolongation of useful life. For treatment to be justified, there should be reason to believe that at least one of these benefits will be forthcoming.

# Anticancer Drugs

The family of anticancer drugs is large and diverse. We will not attempt to consider all of these agents in detail. Rather, discussion focuses on selected representative drugs. Basic principles of cancer chemotherapy are considered in Chapter 95.

## Introduction to the Anticancer Drugs

### Drug Classification

The anticancer drugs fall into three major classes: (1) cytotoxic agents, (2) hormones and hormone antagonists, and (3) biologic response modifiers. The cytotoxic agents, which constitute the largest group of anticancer drugs, can be subclassified as follows: (1) alkylating agents, (2) antimetabolites, (3) antitumor antibiotics, (4) mitotic inhibitors, (5) topoisomerase inhibitors, and (6) miscellaneous cytotoxic drugs. Individual cytotoxic agents are listed in Table 96-1.

### Mechanisms of Cytotoxic Action

Table 96-2 summarizes the principal mechanisms by which the *cytotoxic* anticancer drugs act. As the table shows, most cytotoxic agents disrupt processes related to synthesis of DNA or its precursors. In addition, some

agents (e.g., vinblastine, vincristine) act specifically to block mitosis, and one drug—asparaginase—disrupts synthesis of proteins. Note that, with the exception of asparaginase, all of these drugs disrupt processes carried out exclusively by cells that are undergoing proliferation. This explains why anticancer drugs are most toxic to tissues that have a high growth fraction (i.e., a high proportion of proliferating cells).

### Cell-Cycle Phase Specificity

As we discussed in Chapter 95, the cell cycle is the sequence of events that a cell goes through from one mitotic division to the next. Some anticancer agents, known as *cell-cycle phase specific drugs*, are effective only during a specific phase of the cell cycle. Other anticancer agents, known as *cell-cycle phase nonspecific drugs*, can affect cells during any phase of the cell cycle. All of the hormones, hormone antagonists, and biologic response modifiers are phase nonspecific. In contrast, about half of the cytotoxic anticancer drugs are phase nonspecific, whereas the other half are phase specific. The phase specificity of individual cytotoxic agents is summarized in Table 96-1.

*Cell-Cycle Phase Specific Drugs.* Phase-specific agents are toxic only to cells that are passing through a particular phase of the cell cycle. Vincristine, for example, acts by causing mitotic arrest; hence, the drug is effective only during M phase. Other agents act by disrupting DNA synthesis; hence, they are effective only during S phase. Because of their phase specificity, these drugs are toxic only

**TABLE 96-1. CYTOTOXIC ANTICANCER DRUGS**

| Generic Name | Trade Name | Cell-Cycle Phase Specificity | Route* | Dose-Limiting Toxicity |
|---|---|---|---|---|
| **ALKYLATING AGENTS** | | | | |
| *Nitrogen Mustards* | | | | |
| Cyclophosphamide | Cytoxan, Neosar | Phase nonspecific | PO, IV | Bone marrow depression |
| Chlorambucil | Leukeran | Phase nonspecific | PO | Bone marrow depression |
| Ifosfamide | Ifex | Phase nonspecific | IV | Bone marrow depression |
| Melphalan | Alkeran | Phase nonspecific | PO, IV | Bone marrow depression |
| Mechlorethamine | Mustargen | Phase nonspecific, but M and $G_1$ most sensitive | IV, IC, T | Bone marrow depression |
| *Nitrosoureas* | | | | |
| Carmustine | BiCNU | Phase nonspecific | IV, T | Bone marrow depression |
| Lomustine | CeeNU, Gliadel | Phase nonspecific | PO | Bone marrow depression |
| Streptozocin | Zanosar | Phase nonspecific | IV | Nephrotoxicity |
| *Others* | | | | |
| Busulfan | Myleran | Phase nonspecific | PO | Bone marrow depression |
| Carboplatin | Paraplatin | Phase nonspecific | IV | Bone marrow depression |
| Cisplatin | Platinol | Phase nonspecific | IV | Nephrotoxocity |
| **ANTIMETABOLITES** | | | | |
| *Folic Acid Analogs* | | | | |
| Methotrexate | Folex | S-phase specific | IV, IM, PO, IT | Bone marrow depression, oral and GI ulceration |
| *Pyrimidine Analogs* | | | | |
| Cytarabine | Cytosar-U | S-phase specific | IV, SC, IT | Bone marrow depression |
| Fluorouracil | Adrucil | Phase nonspecific, but cell must be cycling | IV | Bone marrow depression, oral and GI ulceration |
| Floxuridine | FUDR | Phase nonspecific, but cell must be cycling | IA | Bone marrow depression, oral and GI ulceration |
| Gemcitabine | Gemzar | S-phase specific | IV | Bone marrow depression |
| *Purine Analogs* | | | | |
| Mercaptopurine | Purinethol | S-phase specific | PO | Bone marrow depression |
| Thioguanine | Generic only | S-phase specific | PO, IV | Bone marrow depression |
| Fludarabine | Fludara | S-phase specific | IV | Bone marrow depression |
| Pentostatin | Nipent | S-phase specific | IV | Bone marrow depression, CNS depression |
| Cladribine | Leustatin | Phase nonspecific | IV | Bone marrow depression |
| **ANTITUMOR ANTIBIOTICS** | | | | |
| Bleomycin | Blenoxane | $G_2$-phase specific | IV, IM, SC | Pneumonitis and pulmonary fibrosis |
| Dactinomycin | Cosmegen | Phase nonspecific | IV | Bone marrow depression, oral ulceration |
| Daunorubicin | Cerubidine | Phase nonspecific | IV | Bone marrow depression, cardiotoxicity |
| Doxorubicin | Adriamycin, Rubex | Phase nonspecific | IV | Bone marrow depression, cardiotoxocity |
| Idarubicin | Idamycin | Phase nonspecific, but S phase most sensitive | IV | Bone marrow depression |
| Mitomycin | Mutamycin | Phase nonspecific | IV | Bone marrow depression |
| Mitoxantrone | Novantrone | Phase nonspecific | IV | Bone marrow depression |
| Plicamycin | Mithracin | Phase nonspecific | IV | Bone marrow depression, bleeding disorders |
| **MITOTIC INHIBITORS** | | | | |
| Vinblastine | Navelbine | M-phase specific | IV | Bone marrow depression |
| Vincristine | Velban, others | M-phase specific | IV | Peripheral neuropathy |
| Vinorelbine | Oncovin, Vincasar | M-phase specific | IV | Bone marrow depression |

*Key: IA = intra-arterial, IC = intracavitary, IM = intramuscular, IT = intrathecal, IV = intravenous, PO = oral, SC = subcutaneous, T = topical.

**TABLE 96-1.** *Continued*

| Generic Name | Trade Name | Cell-Cycle Phase Specificity | Route* | Dose-Limiting Toxicity |
|---|---|---|---|---|
| **TOPOISOMERASE INHIBITORS** | | | | |
| Etoposide | VePesid | $G_2$-phase specific | IV | Bone marrow depression |
| Teniposide | Vumon | $G_2$-phase specific | IV | Bone marrow depression |
| Irinotecan | Camptosar | S-phase specific | IV | Late diarrhea |
| Topotecan | Hycamtin | S-phase specific | IV | Bone marrow depression |
| **MISCELLANEOUS** | | | | |
| Altretamine | Hexalen | Mechanism unknown | PO | Bone marrow depression |
| Asparaginase | Elspar | $G_1$-phase specific | IV, IM | None |
| Pegaspargase | Oncaspar | $G_1$-phase specific | IV, IM | None |
| Dacarbazine | DTIC-Dome | Phase nonspecific | IV | Bone marrow depression |
| Hydroxyurea | Hydrea | S-phase nonspecific | PO | Bone marrow depression |
| Procarbazine | Matulane | Phase nonspecific | PO | Bone marrow depression |
| Mitotane | Lysodren | Phase nonspecific | PO | CNS depression |
| Docetaxel | Taxotere | $G_2$-phase specific | IV | Bone marrow depression |
| Paclitaxel | Taxol | $G_2$-phase specific | IV | Bone marrow depression |

to cells that are active participants in the cell cycle; cells that are "resting" in $G_0$ will not be harmed. Obviously, if these drugs are to be effective, they must be present as neoplastic cells cycle through the specific phase in which they act. This means that these drugs must be present for an extended time. To accomplish this, phase-specific drugs are often administered by prolonged infusion. Alternatively, they can be given in multiple small doses at short intervals over an extended time. Because the dosing schedule is so critical to therapeutic response, phase-specific drugs are also known as *schedule-dependent drugs.*

***Cell-Cycle Phase Nonspecific Drugs.*** The phase-nonspecific drugs can act during any phase of the cell cycle, including $G_0$. Among the phase-nonspecific drugs are the alkylating agents and most antitumor antibiotics. Since phase-

**TABLE 96-2. ACTIONS OF REPRESENTATIVE CYTOTOXIC ANTICANCER DRUGS**

| Drug | Drug Action | Cellular Process Disrupted |
|---|---|---|
| Cyclophosphamide, cisplatin | Alkylates DNA, causing cross-links and strand breakage | DNA and RNA synthesis |
| Methotrexate | Inhibits one-carbon transfer reactions | Synthesis of DNA precursors (purines, dTMP) |
| Hydroxyurea | Inhibits ribonucleotide reductase | Synthesis of DNA precursors (blocks conversion of ribonecleotides into deoxyribonecleotides) |
| Thioguanine, mercaptopurine | Inhibits purine ring synthesis and nucleotide interconversion | Synthesis of DNA precursors (purines, pyrimidines, ribonucleotides, and deoxyribonucleotides) |
| Fluorouracil | Inhibits thymidylate synthetase | Synthesis of dTMP, a DNA precursor |
| Cytarabine | Inhibits DNA polymerase | DNA synthesis |
| Bleomycin | Breaks DNA strands and prevents their repair | DNA synthesis |
| Plicamycin | Binds to DNA | DNA and RNA synthesis |
| Dactinomycin, daunorubicin | Intercalates between base pairs of DNA | DNA and RNA synthesis |
| Vinblastine, vincristine | Blocks microtubule assembly | Mitosis |
| Asparaginase | Deaminates asparagine, depriving cells of this amino acid | Protein synthesis |
| Topotecan | Inhibits topoisomerase I | Impairs DNA replication |
| Etoposide | Inhibits topoisomerase II | Prevents resealing of DNA strand breaks |

nonspecific drugs can injure $G_0$ cells, whereas phase-specific drugs cannot, phase-nonspecific drugs can increase cell kill when used together with phase-specific drugs.

Although the phase-nonspecific drugs can inflict biochemical lesions at any time during the cell cycle, *as a rule these drugs are more toxic to proliferating cells than to cells in $G_0$*. There are two reasons for the greater sensitivity of proliferating cells. First, cells in $G_0$ often have time to repair drug-induced damage before it can result in significant harm. In contrast, proliferating cells lack time for repair. Second, toxicity may not become manifest until the cell attempts to proliferate. For example, many alkylating agents act by producing cross-links between DNA strands. Although these biochemical lesions can be made at any time, they are largely without effect until cells attempt to replicate DNA. This is much like inflicting a flat tire on an automobile: the tire can be deflated at any time; however, loss of air is consequential only if the car is moving. Carrying the analogy further, if the flat occurs while the car is stopped, and is repaired before travel is attempted, the flat will have no functional impact at all.

## Toxicity

As discussed in Chapter 95, many anticancer drugs are toxic to normal tissues—especially tissues that have a high percentage of proliferating cells (bone marrow, hair follicles, gastrointestinal epithelium, and germinal epithelium). The common major toxicities of the anticancer drugs, together with management procedures, are discussed at length in Chapter 95. Accordingly, as we consider individual anticancer agents in this chapter, discussion of most toxicities will be brief.

## Dosage, Handling, and Administration

*Dosage and Administration.* Cancer chemotherapy is a highly specialized field. Accordingly, in a general text such as this, presentation of detailed information on dosage and administration of specific agents would be inappropriate. However, you should be aware that dosages for anticancer agents must be individualized and that timing of administration may vary with the particular protocol being followed. Also, because of the complex and hazardous nature of cancer chemotherapy, anticancer drugs should be administered under the direct supervision of a physician experienced in their use.

*Handling of Cytotoxic Drugs.* Antineoplastic drugs are often mutagenic, teratogenic, and carcinogenic. In addition, direct contact with the skin, eyes, and mucous membranes can result in local injury. Accordingly, it is imperative that health care personnel involved in the preparation and administration of these drugs follow safe handling procedures. Risks of injury from contact with parenteral chemotherapeutic drugs can be minimized by use of containment equipment and approved technique.

*Administration of Vesicants.* As we discussed in Chapter 95, extravasation of vesicants can cause severe local injury, sometimes requiring surgical debridement and skin grafting. Drugs with strong vesicant properties include carmustine, dacarbazine, dactinomycin, daunorubicin, doxorubicin, mechlorethamine, mitomycin, plicamycin, streptozocin, vinblastine, and vincristine. To minimize the risk of injury, IV administration should be performed only into veins with good flow. Sites of previous irradiation should be avoided. If extravasation occurs, administration should be discontinued immediately.

# Alkylating Agents

The family of alkylating agents consists of nitrogen mustards, nitrosoureas, and other compounds. Before considering the properties of individual alkylating agents, we will discuss the characteristics of the group as a whole. The alkylating agents are listed in Table 96–1.

## Shared Properties

*Mechanism of Action.* The alkylating agents are highly reactive compounds that have the ability to transfer an alkyl group to a variety of cell constituents. Cell kill results primarily from alkylation of DNA. As a rule, alkylating agents interact with DNA by forming a covalent bond with a specific nitrogen atom in guanine (Fig. 96–1).

Some alkylating agents have two reactive sites, whereas others have only one. Alkylating agents with two reactive sites (*bifunctional* agents) are able to bind DNA in two places to form *cross-links*. These bridges may be formed within a single strand of DNA or between parallel DNA strands. Figure 96–1 illustrates the production of interstrand cross-links by nitrogen mustard. Alkylating agents with only one reative site (*monofunctional* agents) lack the ability to form cross-links, but can still bind to a single guanine in DNA.

The consequences of guanine alkylation are miscoding, scission of DNA strands, and, if cross-links have been formed, inhibition of DNA replication. Since cross-linking of DNA is especially injurious, cell death is more likely with bifunctional agents than with monofunctional agents.

Because alkylation reactions can take place at any time during the cell cycle, alkylating agents are considered *cell-cycle phase nonspecific*. However, *most of these drugs are more toxic to proliferating cells than to cells in $G_0$*. This is because (1) alkylation of DNA produces its most detrimental effects when cells attempt to replicate DNA, and because (2) resting cells are often able to repair damage to DNA before it can affect cell function. Because alkylating agents are phase nonspecific, they needn't be present over an extended time. Accordingly, they can be administered in a single bolus dose.

*Resistance.* Development of resistance to alkylating agents is common. A major cause is increased production of enzymes that perform DNA repair. Resistance may also result from decreased uptake of alkylating agents and from increased production of nucleophiles (compounds that act as substitute targets for alkylation).

*Toxicities.* Alkylating agents are toxic to tissues that have a high growth fraction. Hence, these drugs may in-

A

B

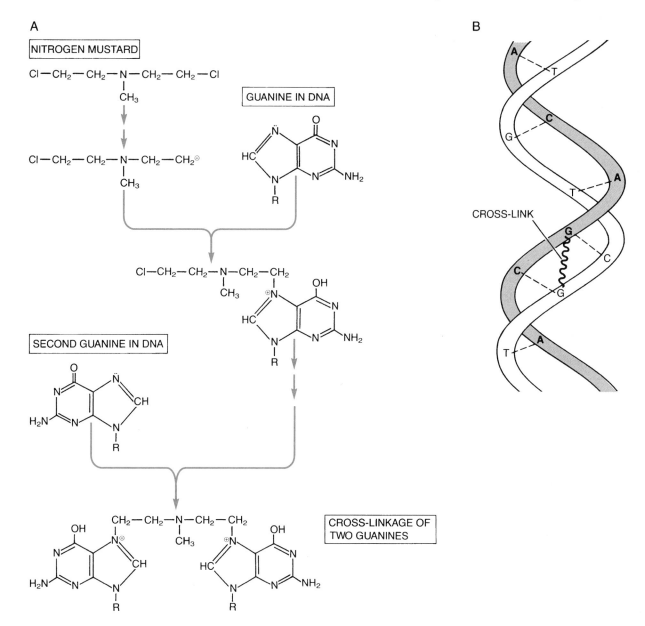

**Figure 96–1. Cross-linking of DNA by an alkylating agent.** *A*, Reactions leading to cross-linkage between guanine moieties in DNA. *B*, Schematic representation of interstrand cross-linking within the DNA double helix. (A = adenine, C = cytosine, G = guanine, T = thymine.)

jure cells of the bone marrow, hair follicles, gastrointestinal mucosa, and germinal epithelium. Blood dyscrasias (neutropenia, thrombocytopenia, anemia) caused by bone marrow depression are of greatest concern. Nausea and vomiting occur with all alkylating agents, and can be especially severe with cisplatin. Practically all of these drugs are vesicants and, therefore, must be administered intravenously.

## Properties of Individual Alkylating Agents
### Nitrogen Mustards

*Cyclophosphamide.* Cyclophosphamide [Cytoxan, Neosar] is a bifunctional agent active against a *broad spectrum* of neoplastic diseases. Indications include *Hodgkin's dis-*

*ease, non-Hodgkin's lymphomas, multiple myeloma,* and *solid tumors of the head, neck, ovary,* and *breast.* Of all the alkylating agents, cyclophosphamide is the most widely employed.

Cyclophosphamide is a prodrug that undergoes conversion to its active form in the liver. Because activation is required, onset of effects is delayed. In contrast to most other alkylating agents, cyclophosphamide is not a vesicant, and hence can be administered orally as well as IV. Oral doses should be administered with food.

The major dose-limiting toxicity is bone marrow depression. Severe nausea, vomiting, and alopecia are also common. In addition, the drug can cause acute hemorrhagic cystitis; renal damage can be minimized by maintaining adequate hydration. Other adverse effects include sterility, immunosuppression, and hypersensitivity reactions.

**Mechlorethamine.** Mechlorethamine [Mustargen], a bifunctional compound, was the first alkylating agent employed clinically. Applications include *Hodgkin's disease* and *non-Hodgkin's lymphomas*. Mechlorethamine is a powerful vesicant and can cause severe local injury. Accordingly, for systemic therapy, the drug must be administered intravenously. Caution must be exercised to avoid both extravasation and direct contact with the skin. Once in the bloodstream, mechlorethamine undergoes rapid conversion to inactive compounds. The dose-limiting toxicity is bone marrow depression. Other major toxicities include nausea, vomiting, alopecia, diarrhea, stomatitis, amenorrhea, and sterility.

**Chlorambucil.** Chlorambucil [Leukeran] is the safest nitrogen mustard available. Bone marrow depression is the major dose-limiting toxicity. Other adverse effects include hepatotoxicity, sterility, pulmonary infiltrates, and pulmonary fibrosis. Nausea and vomiting are usually mild. Chlorambucil is a drug of choice for *chronic lymphocytic leukemia*. The drug is also used to treat *Hodgkin's disease, non-Hodgkin's lymphomas,* and *ovarian cancers.* Administration is oral.

**Melphalan.** Melphalan [Alkeran], a bifunctional agent, is generally well tolerated. Bone marrow depression is the major dose-limiting toxicity. The drug has caused leukemia and may also be mutagenic. Melphalan is not a vesicant. Severe nausea and vomiting are rare. Administration is oral and IV. Melphalan is a drug of choice for palliative therapy of *multiple myeloma.* The drug is also active against *carcinoma of the ovary and breast.*

**Ifosfamide.** Ifosfamide [Ifex], a derivative of cyclophosphamide, is approved only for refractory *germ-cell cancer of the testes.* Dose-limiting toxicities are bone marrow depression and hemorrhagic cystitis. The risk of cystitis is minimized by concurrent therapy with *mesna* [Mesnex] and by extensive hydration (at least 2 L of oral or IV fluid daily). Because of the risk of cystitis, urinalysis should be performed before each dose. If the analysis reveals microscopic hematuria, dosing should be postponed until the hematuria resolves. Additional adverse effects include nausea, vomiting, metabolic acidosis, and central nervous system (CNS) toxicity (confusion, hallucinations, blurred vision, coma). Administration is intravenous.

## Nitrosoureas

The nitrosoureas, which are bifunctional alkylating agents, are active against a broad spectrum of neoplastic diseases. Cell kill results from cross-linking of DNA. Unlike most anticancer drugs, the nitrosoureas are highly lipophilic, and hence can readily penetrate the blood-brain barrier. As a result, these drugs are especially useful against *cancers of the CNS.* The major dose-limiting toxicity is *delayed bone marrow depression.*

**Carmustine (BCNU).** Carmustine [BiCNU, Gliadel] was the first nitrosourea to undergo extensive clinical testing and can be considered the prototype for the group. Because of its ability to cross the blood-brain barrier, carmustine is used frequently to treat *primary and metastatic tumors of the brain.* Other indications include *Hodgkin's disease, non-Hodgkin's lymphomas, multiple myeloma, malignant melanoma, hepatoma,* and *adenocarcinoma of the stomach, colon, and rectum.* The principal dose-limiting toxicity is delayed bone marrow depression; leukocyte and thrombocyte nadirs occur 4 to 6 weeks after treatment. Nausea and vomiting can be severe. Injury to the liver, kidneys, and lungs has been reported.

Administration may be topical or intravenous. Topical administration is done by implanting a biodegradable, carmustine-impregnated wafer [Gliadel] into the cavity created by surgical removal of a brain tumor. This technique has the obvious benefit of concentrating the drug in the place where it is most needed. When administered IV, carmustine can cause local phlebitis, even though it is not a vesicant.

**Lomustine (CCNU).** Lomustine [CeeNU] is similar to carmustine in actions and uses. Like carmustine, lomustine crosses the blood-brain barrier and can be used to treat *CNS cancers.* The drug also has activity against *lymphomas, melanomas,* and *carcinomas of the breast, lung, and colon.* As with carmustine, the major dose-limiting toxicity is delayed bone marrow depression. Additional toxicities include nausea and vomiting, renal and hepatic toxicity, pulmonary fibrosis, and neurologic reactions. Administration is oral.

**Streptozocin.** Streptozocin [Zanosar] differs significantly from the other nitrosoureas. The drug contains a glucose moiety that causes selective drug uptake by islet cells of the pancreas. This selective uptake underlies the drug's principal use: *metastatic islet-cell tumors.* The major dose-limiting toxicity is kidney damage. Accordingly, renal function should be monitored in all patients. As with other nitrosoureas, nausea and vomiting can be severe. Additional toxicities include hypoglycemia, hyperglycemia, diarrhea, chills, and fever. In contrast to other nitrosoureas, streptozocin causes minimal bone marrow depression. Administration is intravenous.

## Additional Alkylating Agents

**Cisplatin.** Although not a true alkylating agent, cisplatin [Platinol] is discussed in this section because, like the true alkylating agents, the drug kills cells primarily by forming cross-links between and within strands of DNA. Cisplatin's principal indication is *testicular cancer.* Other indications include *carcinomas of the ovary, bladder, head,* and *neck.* The major dose-limiting toxicity is damage to the kidney, which can be minimized by extensive hydration coupled with diuretic therapy and *amifostine* [Ethyol]. Nausea and vomiting are severe, beginning about 1 hour after administration and persisting for 1 to 2 days. Other adverse effects include neurotoxicity, bone marrow depression, and toxicity to the ear, which manifests tinnitus and high-frequency hearing loss. Administration is by IV infusion.

**Carboplatin.** Carboplatin [Paraplatin] is an analog of cisplatin. Cell kill appears to result from cross-linking of DNA. The drug's only approved indications are initial and palliative therapy of *ovarian cancer.* Unlabeled uses include *small cell cancer of the lung, squamous cell cancer of the head and neck,* and *endometrial cancer.* The major dose-limiting toxicity is bone marrow depression. Nausea and vomiting occur, but are less severe than with cisplatin. Similarly, nephrotoxicity, neurotoxicity, and hearing loss are less frequent than with cisplatin. Carboplatin is administered by intravenous infusion. Anaphylactic reactions have occurred minutes after administration; symptoms can be managed with epinephrine, glucocorticoids, and antihistamines.

**Busulfan.** Busulfan [Myleran] is a bifunctional agent whose cytotoxic effects are limited almost exclusively to the bone marrow. Because it causes selective attack on the bone marrow, busulfan is a drug of choice for *chronic myelogenous leukemia.* The remission rate is 90% with one course of therapy. Dose-limiting toxicities are bone marrow depression, pulmonary infiltrates, and pulmonary fibrosis. Other toxicities include nausea, vomiting, alopecia, gynecomastia, male and female sterility, skin hyperpigmentation, cataracts, and hepatitis. Administration is oral.

# Antimetabolites

Antimetabolites are structural analogs of important natural metabolites. Because they resemble natural metabolites, these drugs are able to disrupt critical metabolic processes. Some antimetabolites inhibit enzymes that synthesize essential cellular constituents. Others undergo incorporation into DNA, thereby disrupting DNA replication and function.

Antimetabolites are effective only against cells that are active participants in the cell cycle. Most antimetabolites are S-phase specific. Some can act during any phase of the cycle except $G_0$. To be effective, agents that are S-phase specific must be present for an extended time.

There are three classes of antimetabolites: (1) folic acid analogs, (2) purine analogs, and (3) pyrimidine analogs. Members of each class are listed in Table 96–1.

## Folic Acid Analog: Methotrexate

Folic acid, in its active form, is needed for several essential biochemical reactions. The folic acid analogs act by preventing the conversion of folic acid to its active form. At this time, methotrexate is the only folate analog employed in cancer chemotherapy. Other folate analogs are used to treat bacterial infections (trimethoprim) and malaria (pyrimethamine).

*Mechanism of Action.* As shown in Figure 96–2, methotrexate [Folex] *inhibits dihydrofolate reductase*, the enzyme that converts dihydrofolic acid ($FH_2$) into tetrahydrofolic acid ($FH_4$). Since production of $FH_4$ is a necessary step in the activation of folic acid, and since activated folic acid is required for biosynthesis of essential cellular constituents (DNA, RNA, proteins), inhibition of $FH_4$ production has multiple effects on the cell. Of all the processes that are suppressed by methotrexate, biosynthesis of thymidylate appears to be most critical. Suppression of thymidylate synthesis is critical because, in the absence of thymidylate, cells are unable to make DNA. Since cell kill results primarily from disruption of DNA synthesis, methotrexate is considered S-phase specific.

A technique known as *leucovorin rescue* can be employed to enhance the effects of methotrexate. Some neoplastic cells are unresponsive to methotrexate because they lack the transport system required for active uptake of the drug. By giving massive doses of methotrexate, the drug can be forced into these cells by passive diffusion. However, since this process also exposes normal cells to extremely high concentrations of methotrexate, these cells are also at risk. To save normal cells, leucovorin (citrovorum factor, folinic acid) is given. As shown in Figure 96–2, leucovorin bypasses the metabolic block caused by methotrexate, thereby permitting normal cells to synthe-

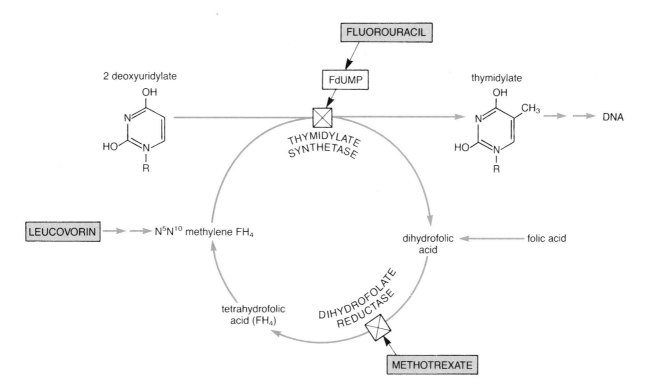

**Figure 96–2. Actions of methotrexate, leucovorin, and fluorouracil.** (FdUMP = 5-fluoro-2′-deoxyuridine-5′-monophosphate, □ = blockade of reaction.)

size thymidylate and other compounds. Malignant cells are not saved because leucovorin uptake requires the same transport system employed for methotrexate uptake, a transport system that these cells lack. It should be noted that leucovorin rescue is potentially hazardous: *failure to administer leucovorin in the right dose at the right time can be fatal.*

**Resistance.** Acquired resistance to methotrexate can result from three mechanisms: (1) decreased uptake of methotrexate, (2) increased synthesis of dihydrofolate reductase (the target enzyme for methotrexate), and (3) synthesis of a modified form of dihydrofolate reductase that has a reduced affinity for methotrexate.

**Pharmacokinetics.** Methotrexate can be administered orally, IM, IV, and intrathecally. For most cancers of the CNS, intrathecal administration is employed. Metabolism of methotrexate is minimal. Most of each dose is excreted intact in the urine. Because elimination is renal, methotrexate can accumulate to dangerous levels in patients with kidney dysfunction; hence, the dosage must be reduced to minimize injury.

**Therapeutic Uses.** *Neoplastic Diseases.* Methotrexate is curative for women with *choriocarcinoma.* The drug is also active against *non-Hodgkin's lymphomas* and *acute lymphocytic leukemia of childhood.* Very large doses coupled with leucovorin rescue have been employed to treat *head and neck sarcomas* and *osteogenic sarcoma.*

*Other Indications.* Low doses are used to control *severe psoriasis* (see Chapter 98). Higher doses are used to treat severe *rheumatoid arthritis* (see Chapter 66).

**Toxicity.** The usual dose-limiting toxicities are bone marrow depression, pulmonary infiltrates and fibrosis, and oral and gastrointestinal ulceration. Death may result from intestinal perforation and hemorrhagic enteritis. Nausea and vomiting may occur shortly after administration. High doses can cause direct injury to the kidneys. To promote drug excretion, and thereby minimize renal damage, the urine should be alkalinized and adequate hydration should be maintained. Methotrexate has been associated with fetal malformation and death. Accordingly, pregnancy should be avoided until at least 6 months after completing treatment.

## Pyrimidine Analogs

Pyrimidines (cytosine, thymine, uracil) are bases employed in the biosynthesis of DNA and RNA. The pyrimidine analogs, because of their structural similarity to naturally occurring pyrimidines, can act in several ways: (1) they can inhibit biosynthesis of pyrimidines, (2) they can inhibit biosynthesis of DNA and RNA, and (3) they can undergo incorporation into DNA and RNA, thereby disrupting nucleic acid function. All of the pyrimidine analogs are prodrugs that must be converted to their active forms within the body.

### Cytarabine

Cytarabine [Cytosar-U], also known as *cytosine arabinoside* and *Ara C,* is an analog of deoxycytidine. The drug has an established role in treating *acute myelogenous leukemia.*

**Mechanism of Action.** Cytarabine is converted to its active form—Ara-CTP—within the body. As Ara-CTP, the drug becomes incorporated into DNA. By a mechanism that is not fully understood, this incorporation suppresses further DNA synthesis. Ara-CTP may also impede DNA synthesis by a second mechanism: inhibition of DNA polymerase. Cytarabine is highly S-phase specific.

**Resistance.** Decreased conversion of cytarabine to Ara-CTP is a major cause of resistance. Other mechanisms include decreased uptake of cytarabine, increased conversion of cytarabine to an inactive product, and increased production of dCTP (the natural metabolite with which Ara-CTP competes for incorporation into DNA).

**Pharmacokinetics.** Administration may be IV, SC, or intrathecal. Cytarabine is not active orally. Drug that is not taken up by cells undergoes rapid deamination in the liver. Metabolites are excreted in the urine.

**Therapeutic Uses.** The principal indication for cytarabine is *acute myelogenous leukemia.* The drug has been combined with thioguanine and daunorubicin or doxorubicin to treat this disease. Other applications include *acute lymphocytic leukemia, chronic myelogenous leukemia,* and *non-Hodgkin's lymphomas.*

**Toxicity.** Bone marrow suppression (neutropenia, thrombocytopenia) is the usual dose-limiting toxicity. Nausea, vomiting, and fever may develop, especially after bolus IV injection. Other toxicities include stomatitis, liver injury, and conjunctivitis. High doses may cause pulmonary edema and central and peripheral neurotoxicity.

### Fluorouracil

Fluorouracil [Adrucil] is a fluorinated derivative of uracil. The drug is employed extensively to treat solid tumors.

**Mechanism of Action.** In order to exert cytotoxic effects, fluorouracil must be converted to its active form, 5-fluoro-2'-deoxyuridine-5'-monophosphate (FdUMP). As shown in Figure 96–2, FdUMP inhibits thymidylate synthetase, thereby depriving cells of thymidylate needed to make DNA. Fluorouracil is active only against cells that are going through the cell cycle. However, the drug lacks phase specificity.

**Resistance.** Potential mechanisms for resistance are (1) decreased activation of fluorouracil and (2) production of altered thymidylate synthetase that has a low affinity for FdUMP. The clinical significance of these mechanisms has not been established.

**Therapeutic Uses.** Chemotherapeutic use of fluorouracil is limited to solid tumors. The drug is employed for palliative therapy of *carcinomas of the colon, rectum, breast, stomach,* and *pancreas.* In addition to therapy of cancer, fluorouracil is employed topically to treat *premalignant keratoses* (see Chapter 98).

**Pharmacokinetics.** Administration is intravenous. Continuous infusion is more effective and less toxic than bolus administration. Fluorouracil is distributed widely and enters the CNS with ease. Elimination is by rapid hepatic metabolism.

**Toxicity.** The usual dose-limiting toxicities are bone marrow depression (neutropenia) and oral and GI ulceration. To minimize GI injury (e.g., ulceration of the oropharynx or bowel), fluorouracil should be discontinued as soon as mild reactions (stomatitis, diarrhea) occur. Other adverse effects include alopecia, hyperpigmentation, and neurologic deficits.

### Floxuridine

Floxuridine [FUDR], like fluorouracil, is converted to FdUMP within the body. Hence, the pharmacologic effects of floxuridine and fluorouracil are nearly identical. Floxuridine is used most for *metastatic carcinoma of the colon.* The drug is administered only by intra-arterial infusion.

### Gemcitabine

*Mechanism of Action.* Gemcitabine [Gemzar] is a nucleoside analog that inhibits DNA synthesis. Hence, the drug is S-phase specific. Following uptake by cells, gemcitabine is converted to two active forms: gemcitabine diphosphate and gemcitabine triphosphate. Gemcitabine diphosphate inhibits ribonucleotide reductase, an enzyme needed to form deoxynucleoside triphosphates, which are required for DNA synthesis. Gemcitabine triphosphate undergoes incorporation into DNA, where it inhibits further strand elongation.

*Therapeutic Use.* Gemcitabine is indicated for *adenocarcinoma of the pancreas,* a cancer that is highly resistant to treatment. The drug may be used for (1) first-line therapy in patients with locally advanced or metastatic pancreatic cancer, and (2) patients previously treated with fluorouracil. In clinical trials, gemcitabine reduced pain, improved functional status, and prolonged life slightly. The recommended dosage is 1000 mg/m$^2$ infused IV over 30 minutes once a week for up to 7 weeks. After a 1-week hiatus, treatment is resumed, but dosing is reduced to one infusion every 3 to 4 weeks.

*Toxicity.* Although gemcitabine can cause a wide variety of adverse effects, the drug is fairly well tolerated. Myelosuppression is the dose-limiting toxicity. Nausea and vomiting are common (70%) but usually mild to moderate. Other common reactions include elevation of serum transaminases (75%), proteinuria (45%), hematuria (35%), pain (45%), and fever (41%). Less common reactions include diarrhea, constipation, stomatitis, dyspnea, paresthesias, edema, alopecia, and rash.

## Purine Analogs

Like the pyrimidines, the purines (adenine, guanine, hypoxanthine) are bases employed for biosynthesis of nucleic acids. The purine analogs discussed in this chapter are used primarily in the treatment of cancer. Purine analogs discussed in other chapters are used for immunosuppression, antiviral therapy, and gout.

### Mercaptopurine

*Mechanisms of Action and Resistance.* Mercaptopurine [Purinethol] is a prodrug that undergoes conversion to its active form within cells. Following activation, the drug can disrupt multiple biochemical processes, including purine biosynthesis, nucleotide interconversion, and biosynthesis of nucleic acids. All of these actions probably contribute to cytotoxic effects. Mercaptopurine is S-phase specific. Mechanisms of resistance include reduced activation of the drug and accelerated deactivation.

*Pharmacokinetics.* Mercaptopurine is administered orally and undergoes erratic absorption. Absorbed drug is distributed widely, but not to the CNS. Extensive metabolism occurs in the liver; an important reaction is catalyzed by xanthine oxidase. Accordingly, for patients receiving allopurinol (an inhibitor of xanthine oxidase), mercaptopurine dosage should be reduced.

*Therapeutic Uses.* The principal indication for mercaptopurine is *acute lymphocytic leukemia* in children and adults.

The drug may also be of some benefit in *acute and chronic myelogenous leukemia* in adults.

*Toxicity.* Bone marrow depression (neutropenia, thrombocytopenia, anemia) is the principal dose-limiting toxicity. Hepatic dysfunction, which usually manifests as cholestatic jaundice, occurs in about 30% of patients. Other adverse effects include nausea, vomiting, and oral and intestinal ulceration. Concurrent use of allopurinol increases the overall risk of toxicity. Mercaptopurine is mutagenic; hence women using the drug should be warned against becoming pregnant.

### Thioguanine

*Actions and Uses.* Thioguanine acts much like mercaptopurine. Following conversion to its active form, thioguanine inhibits purine synthesis and the interconversion of nucleotides. DNA synthesis is also inhibited. Like mercaptopurine, thioguanine is S-phase specific. The drug is used primarily for *acute lymphocytic and myelogenous leukemias.*

*Pharmacokinetics.* Administration is oral; absorption is erratic and incomplete. Thioguanine does not distribute to the CNS. Inactivation is by hepatic metabolism. In contrast to mercaptopurine, thioguanine is not degraded by xanthine oxidase. Thus, the drug can be employed concurrently with allopurinol without a reduction in dosage.

*Toxicity.* The usual dose-limiting toxicity is bone marrow depression. Gastrointestinal reactions (nausea, vomiting, diarrhea) may develop, but these are less severe than with mercaptopurine. Liver injury, manifesting as cholestatic jaundice, may occur.

### Pentostatin

Pentostatin [Nipent] is an analog of adenosine. The drug inhibits adenosine deaminase and thereby suppresses synthesis of DNA. The only approved indication for pentostatin is *hairy cell leukemia* that has not responded to interferon alfa. The major dose-limiting toxicities are bone marrow depression and CNS depression. Other toxicities include nausea, vomiting, rash, and fever. Administration is by IV bolus or IV infusion. Pentostatin is expensive; the cost to the pharmacist for a single course of therapy is approximately $1400.

### Fludarabine

Fludarabine [Fludara] is an analog of adenosine. The drug is approved only for *chronic lymphocytic leukemia.* Following IV infusion, fludarabine undergoes rapid conversion to its active form, 2-fluoro-ara-ATP. Cell kill appears to result from inhibition of DNA replication. Thus, the drug is probably S-phase specific. The major dose-limiting toxicity is bone marrow depression (neutropenia, thrombocytopenia, anemia). Other common toxicities include nausea, vomiting, and chills. When given in especially high doses during clinical trials, fludarabine caused severe neurologic effects, including blindness, coma, and death. However, neurologic effects are rare (0.2%) at maximal recommended therapeutic doses.

### Cladribine

Cladribine [Leustatin] is an adenosine analog with a unique combination of actions. Unlike other purine analogs, which inhibit DNA synthesis only, cladribine inhibits both DNA synthesis and DNA repair. As a result, the drug is active against quiescent cells as well as those that are actively dividing. Cladribine is highly active against *hairy cell leukemia* (HCL) and is considered a drug of choice for this cancer. The drug is also active against *chronic lymphocytic leukemia, non-Hodgkin's lymphomas, acute myeloid leukemia,* and *mycosis fungoides.* The major dose-limiting toxicity is myelosuppression. Very high doses (four to nine times normal) have caused acute nephrotoxicity and delayed-onset neurotoxicity. For patients with HCL, cladribine is administered as a continuous IV infusion over 7 consecutive days.

# Antitumor Antibiotics

The antitumor antibiotics are cytotoxic drugs originally isolated from cultures of *Streptomyces*. In this section, we consider five antitumor antibiotics along with three of their derivatives. The antitumor antibiotics and their derivatives are used only to treat cancer; they are not used to treat infections. All of these drugs injure cells through direct interaction with DNA. Because of poor gastrointestinal absorption, they are all administered parenterally (usually IV).

## Dactinomycin (Actinomycin D)

**Mechanism of Action.** Dactinomycin [Cosmegen] is a planar molecule that kills cells through *intercalation* with DNA. We can understand intercalation by envisioning the stacked base pairs of DNA as having a structure like that of a stack of coins. Having a coin-like shape itself, dactinomycin is able to slip between base pairs of DNA, after which the drug becomes bound to DNA. This process (intercalation) distorts DNA structure. Because of this distortion, RNA polymerase is unable to use DNA as a template. Hence, synthesis of RNA and, consequently, proteins is inhibited. Unlike RNA polymerase, DNA polymerase is relatively insensitive to the change in DNA. Consequently, DNA synthesis is not suppressed. Dactinomycin is *phase nonspecific.*

**Pharmacokinetics.** Administration is by intravenous infusion. Because of tissue uptake and binding to DNA, dactinomycin is rapidly cleared from the blood. The drug does not cross the blood-brain barrier. Elimination occurs slowly by biliary and renal excretion.

**Therapeutic Uses.** Major indications for dactinomycin are *Wilms' tumor* and *rhabdomyosarcoma*. Other indications include *choriocarcinoma, Ewing's sarcoma, Kaposi's sarcoma,* and *testicular cancer.*

**Toxicity.** Dose-limiting toxicities are bone marrow depression and oral and gastrointestinal mucositis. Other toxicities include nausea, vomiting, diarrhea, alopecia, folliculitis, and, in previously irradiated areas, dermatitis. Dactinomycin is extremely corrosive to soft tissue. Hence, extravasation will cause severe local injury.

## Doxorubicin

Doxorubicin [Adriamycin, Rubex] is active against a broad spectrum of neoplastic diseases. Unfortunately, cardiotoxicity limits the drug's utility.

**Mechanism of Action.** Like dactinomycin, doxorubicin intercalates with DNA, causing distortion of DNA structure. As a result, DNA is unable to function as a template for synthesis of DNA and RNA. Doxorubicin also acts on DNA to cause strand scission.

**Pharmacokinetics.** Doxorubicin is administered by intravenous infusion and undergoes rapid uptake by tissues. The drug does not cross the blood-brain barrier. Much of each dose is metabolized in the liver. Hence, dosages must be reduced for patients with hepatic impairment. Doxorubicin and its metabolites are eliminated primarily by biliary excretion.

**Therapeutic Uses.** Doxorubicin is active against many neoplastic diseases. The drug is employed to treat solid tumors and disseminated cancers. Specific indications include *Hodgkin's and non-Hodgkin's lymphomas, acute lymphoblastic and myeloblastic leukemias, sarcomas of soft tissue and bone,* and *various carcinomas,* including *carcinoma of the lung, stomach, breast, ovary, testes, and thyroid.*

**Toxicity.** *Cardiotoxicity.* Doxorubicin can cause acute and delayed injury to the heart. Acute effects (dysrhythmias, EKG changes) can develop within minutes of administration. As a rule, these reactions are usually transient, lasting no more than 2 weeks.

*Delayed cardiotoxicity* manifests as congestive heart failure secondary to diffuse cardiomyopathy (myofibril degeneration). The condition is often unresponsive to treatment. Delayed cardiac injury is directly related to the total cumulative dose of doxorubicin: the risk of heart failure increases significantly as the cumulative lifetime dose rises above 550 mg/m². Accordingly, the total dose should not exceed this amount. Doxorubicin causes cardiotoxicity by forming an intracellular complex with iron that catalyzes the formation of oxygen free radicals.

A new drug—dexrazoxane [Zinecard]—can protect the heart from doxorubicin. To do so, dexrazoxane must first undergo conversion to a chelating agent within the body; in this active form, the drug binds intracellular iron, thereby preventing the iron from interacting with doxorubicin. In clinical trials, dexrazoxane significantly decreased the incidence of doxorubicin-induced heart failure. However, treatment did have two complications: (1) the drug appeared to intensify myelosuppression, and (2) it may have reduced the anticancer effects of doxorubicin. To ensure that the benefits of chemotherapy are not compromised, dexrazoxane is approved only for patients who have already received 300 mg/m² of doxorubicin. Furthermore, the drug is approved only for patients receiving doxorubicin for *breast cancer* (even though doxorubicin is used to treat other malignancies). The reason for this second restriction is that intensification of myelosuppression may be greater in patients with tumors other than breast cancer.

*Other Toxicities.* Acute toxicity usually manifests as nausea and vomiting. Because of its vesicant properties, doxorubicin can cause severe local injury if extravasation occurs. In addition, the drug imparts a harmless red coloration to urine and sweat; patients should be forewarned. The usual dose-limiting toxicity is bone marrow depression. Neutropenia develops in about 70% of patients. Thrombocytopenia and anemia may occur also. Additional delayed toxicities include alopecia, stomatitis, anorexia, conjunctivitis, and pigmentation in the extremities.

## Daunorubicin, Liposomal

Liposomal daunorubicin [DaunoXome] is a new formulation of daunorubicin designed to increase delivery of the drug to tumor cells and decrease its uptake by normal cells. The preparation consists of an aqueous solution of daunorubicin encapsulated within minuscule lipid vesicles (liposomes). Once the liposomes are in the vicinity of the tumor, they release daunorubicin over time. Liposomal daunorubicin is administered as a 1-hour IV infusion.

Daunorubicin is nearly identical in structure to doxorubicin, and shares many of that drug's properties. Like doxorubicin, daunorubicin intercalates with DNA and thereby inhibits DNA and RNA synthesis. The drug can act during all phases of the cell cycle, but cytotoxicity is greatest during S phase. The only indication for liposomal daunorubicin is *HIV-related Kaposi's sarcoma*. As with doxorubicin, the major dose-limiting toxicities are bone marrow depression and congestive heart failure. In addition, daunorubicin may cause nausea, vomiting, stomatitis, and alopecia. Like doxorubicin, daunorubicin imparts a harmless red coloration to urine and tears; patients should be forewarned.

### Idarubicin

Idarubicin [Idamycin] is a structural analog of daunorubicin and doxorubicin. The drug's only approved indication is *acute myelogenous leukemia* in adults. Cell kill results from intercalation with DNA and subsequent inhibition of nucleic acid synthesis. Idarubicin is most effective during S phase, but is not considered phase specific. Following IV infusion, the drug undergoes rapid and widespread distribution. Elimination is by hepatic metabolism followed by biliary excretion. The principal dose-limiting toxicity is bone marrow depression. Like daunorubicin and doxorubicin, idarubicin is cardiotoxic, but the maximal cumulative dose has not been determined. Additional toxicities include nausea, vomiting, alopecia, and stomatitis. Idarubicin is a vesicant and can cause severe local injury upon extravasation.

### Mitoxantrone

Mitoxantrone [Novantrone] is a structural analog of doxorubicin and daunorubicin but is less toxic than those drugs. Mitoxantrone appears to act by two mechanisms: (1) intercalation of DNA and (2) promotion of DNA strand breakage secondary to activation of topoisomerase II. The drug is cell-cycle phase nonspecific. Principal applications are *acute nonlymphocytic leukemias*, *lymphomas*, and *breast cancer*. Mitoxantrone is administered intravenously and undergoes rapid and widespread distribution. Elimination occurs slowly, primarily by hepatic metabolism and biliary excretion. The major dose-limiting toxicity is bone marrow depression. Other important toxicities—nausea, vomiting, alopecia, mucositis, and cardiotoxicity—are less severe than with doxorubicin. Mitoxantrone imparts a harmless blue-green tint to the urine, skin, and sclera; patients should be forewarned.

### Bleomycin

The preparation of bleomycin [Blenoxane] used clinically contains a mixture of glycopeptides. The major components of the mixture are bleomycin $A_2$ and bleomycin $B_2$. Bleomycin is unusual among the anticancer drugs in that it causes very little bone marrow suppression. However, it can cause severe injury to the lungs. Because myelosuppression is minimal, bleomycin is especially useful in combination chemotherapy. Bleomycin binds to DNA, causing chain scission and fragmentation. The drug is most effective during $G_2$.

Bleomycin is approved for palliative therapy of a broad spectrum of tumors. Specific indications include *testicular carcinomas* (embryonal cell, choriocarcinoma, teratocarcinoma), *lymphomas* (Hodgkin's, reticulum cell sarcoma, lymphosarcoma), and *squamous cell carcinomas* (head, neck, larynx, cervix, penis, vulva, and skin).

Administration is parenteral (IM, IV, and SC). High concentrations are achieved in the skin and lungs. The drug does not enter the CNS. Most tissues contain large amounts of bleomycin hydrolase, an enzyme that renders the drug inactive. However, cells of the skin and lungs, which are sites of toxicity, lack this enzyme. Most of each dose is excreted unchanged in the urine.

The major dose-limiting toxicity is injury to the lungs, which occurs in about 10% of patients. Injury manifests initially as pneumonitis. In about 1% of patients, pneumonitis progresses to severe pulmonary fibrosis and death. Pulmonary function should be monitored and bleomycin be discontinued at the first sign of adverse changes.

Additional toxicities include stomatitis, alopecia, and skin reactions (hyperpigmentation, hyperkeratosis, pruritus erythema, ulceration, vesiculation). Nausea and vomiting are usually mild. Unlike most other anticancer agents, bleomycin exerts minimal toxicity to bone marrow. About 1% of patients with lymphomas experience a unique hypersensitivity reaction, characterized by fever, chills, confusion, hypotension, and wheezing.

### Mitomycin

Mitomycin [Mutamycin] is a prodrug that is converted to its active form within cells. Following activation, the drug functions as a bifunctional or trifunctional alkylating agent. Cell death is caused by cross-linking of DNA with resultant blockade of DNA synthesis. Mitomycin may also induce strand scission. The drug is active during all phases of the cell cycle, but toxicity is greatest during late $G_1$ and early S phase.

Mitomycin is labeled for *adenocarcinoma of the stomach and pancreas*. Unlabeled uses include *carcinomas of the colon, rectum, esophagus, lung, breast, cervix,* and *bladder*.

Mitomycin is administered by intravenous infusion and is distributed widely, but not to the CNS. The drug is rapidly metabolized by the liver. Metabolites are excreted in the urine.

The major dose-limiting toxicity is delayed bone marrow depression; nadirs for neutropenia and thrombocytopenia usually occur 3 to 4 weeks after treatment. Other toxicities include nausea, vomiting, stomatitis, alopecia, renal toxicity, and pulmonary toxicity. Mitomycin is a vesicant and can cause severe local injury upon extravasation.

### Plicamycin (Mithramycin)

Plicamycin [Mithracin] is a highly toxic drug whose use in cancer chemotherapy is restricted to *testicular carcinoma*. Cell kill results from binding to DNA with subsequent inhibition of DNA and RNA synthesis. The drug is cell-cycle phase nonspecific. Dose-related bleeding is the most serious toxicity. Bleeding results from thrombocytopenia and deficiencies of several clotting factors. Because of the risk of hemorrhage, plicamycin should be used only in a hospital setting. Patients with coagulation disorders and pre-existing thrombocytopenia should not receive the drug. Additional toxicities include nausea, vomiting, stomatitis, renal injury, and disruption of calcium metabolism. Plicamycin is administered intravenously, and little is known about its fate. Elimination is renal. In addition to management of testicular cancer, plicamycin is used to manage *hypercalcemia of malignancy*. This application is considered in Chapter 75 (Drugs Affecting Calcium Levels and Bone Mineralization).

## Mitotic Inhibitors

Mitotic inhibitors are drugs that act during M phase to prevent cell division. The principal mitotic inhibitors are *vincristine* and *vinblastine*. Both drugs are derived from *Vinca rosea* (the periwinkle plant), and hence are known as *vinca alkaloids*. Vincristine and vinblastine have nearly identical structures and share the same mechanism of action. However, these drugs have quite different toxicities. Vincristine is toxic to peripheral nerves, but does little damage to bone marrow. Conversely, vinblastine can cause significant bone marrow depression, but is relatively harmless to nerves. Vincristine and vinblastine do not share the same indications.

## Vincristine

**Mechanism of Action.** Vincristine [Oncovin, Vincasar] blocks mitosis during metaphase. The drug does this by preventing the assembly of microtubules (the filaments that move chromosomes during cell division). In the absence of microtubules, distribution of chromosomes to daughter cells becomes random. This failure to correctly allocate chromosomes is the presumed cause of cell death. Vincristine disrupts microtubule assembly by binding to *tubulin*, the major protein of which microtubules are composed. The drug is M-phase specific.

**Pharmacokinetics.** Because of low and erratic oral absorption, vincristine must be given intravenously. The drug leaves the blood rapidly and enters tissues, where it becomes tightly but reversibly bound. Penetration to the CNS is poor. Most of each dose undergoes hepatic metabolism followed by biliary excretion. Only 12% of the drug is eliminated in the urine.

**Therapeutic Uses.** Vincristine is bone marrow sparing. Accordingly, the drug is ideal for combination chemotherapy. Indications include *Hodgkin's and non-Hodgkin's lymphomas, acute lymphocytic leukemia, Wilms' tumor, rhabdomyosarcoma, Kaposi's sarcoma, breast cancer*, and *bladder cancer.*

**Toxicity.** *Peripheral neuropathy* is the major dose-limiting toxicity. Vincristine injures neurons by disrupting neurotubules, structures that are required for axonal transport of enzymes and organelles. Injury to neurotubules results from binding to tubulin, the same protein found in microtubules. Nearly all patients experience symptoms of sensory or motor nerve injury (e.g., decreased reflexes, weakness, paresthesias, sensory loss). Symptoms of injury to autonomic nerves (e.g., constipation, urinary hesitancy) are less common, occurring in 30% to 50% of those treated. Since vincristine does not readily enter the CNS, injury to the brain is minimal.

In contrast to most anticancer drugs, *vincristine causes little toxicity to bone marrow.* As a result, the drug is especially desirable for combined therapy with other anticancer drugs.

Vincristine is a powerful irritant and can cause severe local injury if extravasation occurs. Alopecia develops in about 20% of patients. Nausea and vomiting are rare.

## Vinblastine

Vinblastine [Velban, Velsar, Alkaban] is a structural analog of vincristine. The two drugs share the same mechanism of action: production of metaphase arrest through blockade of microtubule assembly. Like vincristine, vinblastine is administered intravenously, does not cross the blood-brain barrier, and is eliminated by biliary and urinary excretion. Indications for vinblastine include *Kaposi's sarcoma, Hodgkin's and non-Hodgkin's lymphomas*, and *carcinoma of the breast and testes.* The major

dose-limiting toxicity is bone marrow depression. (Note that vinblastine differs markedly from vincristine in this action.) Neurotoxicity can occur but is much less severe than with vincristine. Additional adverse effects include nausea, vomiting, alopecia, stomatitis, and severe local injury if extravasation should occur.

## Vinorelbine

Vinorelbine [Navelbine] is a semisynthetic vinca alkaloid similar in structure and actions to vincristine and vinblastine. The drug is approved only for *non-small-cell lung cancer*. Investigational uses include *breast cancer, ovarian cancer*, and *Hodgkin's disease*. Benefits derive from causing metaphase arrest through inhibition of microtubule assembly. Vinorelbine is administered IV, undergoes hepatic metabolism, and is eliminated primarily in the bile. Like vinblastine, and unlike vincristine, vinorelbine can cause profound bone marrow depression; neutropenia develops in about 50% of those treated. Peripheral neuropathy occurs, but is less severe than with vincristine. Other adverse effects include alopecia, constipation, nausea, and vomiting, all of which are generally mild to moderate. Like vincristine and vinblastine, vinorelbine can cause local tissue necrosis if extravasation occurs.

## Topoisomerase Inhibitors

### Topotecan

**Mechanism of Action.** Topotecan [Hycamtin] inhibits topoisomerase I, an enzyme that relieves torsional strain in DNA by creating *reversible* single-strand breaks. Topotecan binds to the DNA–topoisomerase I complex, and thereby prevents repair of the strand breaks caused by topoisomerase. Cytotoxicity is believed to result from impaired DNA replication. Hence, effects become manifest during S phase of the cell cycle.

**Therapeutic Use.** Topotecan is approved only for *metastatic cancer of the ovary* that is refractory to cisplatin and other more traditional drugs. In clinical trials, topotecan was modestly effective. A single course of treatment consists of 1.5 mg/mm$^3$ infused IV over 30 minutes on 5 consecutive days. Courses can be repeated after a 16-day hiatus. At least four courses are recommended. Treatment is expensive: each course costs over $2500 for the drug, plus additional fees for giving the infusions.

**Toxicity.** Bone marrow suppression is the dose-limiting toxicity. Neutropenia occurs in 98% of patients, thereby posing a risk of serious infection. Anemia and thrombocytopenia are also common, and frequently require transfusion of platelets and red blood cells. Because of myelosuppression, frequent counts of peripheral blood cells should be performed. If the neutrophil count is below 1500 cells/mm$^3$, topotecan should be withheld. In addition to causing myelosuppression, topotecan can cause alopecia, nausea, vomiting, diarrhea, stomatitis, abdominal pain, and headache.

### Irinotecan

**Actions and Uses.** Like topotecan, irinotecan [Camptosar] and its active metabolite (SN-38) inhibit topoisomerase I. As a result, DNA replication is impaired. Cytotoxic effects become apparent during the S phase of the cell cycle. Irinotecan is approved for *metastatic cancer of the colon or rectum* that has progressed despite treatment with fluorouracil. Investigational uses include *advanced cancer of the breast, ovary, lung*, and *stomach*. For colorectal cancer, the recommended dosage is 125 mg/m$^2$ infused IV over 90 minutes once weekly for 4 weeks. In clinical trials, this dosage produced an objective response (complete or partial) in 15% of patients. The average response duration was 5.8 months. Irinotecan is expensive: for a 4-week course of treatment, the price is $4000 for irinotecan itself, plus the cost of administration.

***Adverse Effects.*** Two types of *severe diarrhea* can occur: early and late. Early diarrhea occurs in 50% of patients; late diarrhea occurs in 88%. Early and late diarrhea differ with respect to cause and treatment. Early diarrhea occurs within 24 hours of infusion onset. The cause is excessive cholinergic stimulation of the GI tract. Accordingly, early diarrhea can be suppressed with IV atropine. Late diarrhea develops 24 hours or more after the infusion. It can be prolonged, causing severe dehydration and electrolyte imbalance, and can thereby pose a threat to life. Late diarrhea should be treated immediately with loperamide. Fluid and electrolytes should be replaced as needed.

Myelosuppression can result in neutropenia (54%) and anemia (61%). Serious thrombocytopenia is uncommon. Sepsis secondary to neutropenia has resulted in death. If the neutrophil count falls below 500 cells/mm$^3$, irinotecan should be temporarily withheld.

In addition to diarrhea and myelosuppression, irinotecan can cause nausea (86%), vomiting (67%), asthenia (76%), alopecia (61%), abdominal discomfort (57%), anorexia (55%), fever (45%), and weight loss (30%). Less common side effects include stomatitis, dyspepsia, headache, cough, rhinitis, insomnia, and rash.

### Etoposide

Etoposide [VePesid] is derived from podophyllotoxin, a naturally occurring plant alkaloid. The drug inhibits DNA topoisomerase II, and thereby prevents resealing of DNA strand breaks. The resultant damage to DNA arrests the cell cycle in G$_2$ phase. Etoposide is approved only for *refractory testicular cancer* and *small-cell cancer of the lung.*

Administration is oral and intravenous. Penetration to the CNS is low. Most of the drug is eliminated intact in the urine. Hence, dosages must be reduced in patients with renal impairment.

The major dose-limiting toxicity is bone marrow depression. Other toxicities include alopecia, peripheral neuropathy, and mucositis. Early adverse effects include nausea, vomiting, diarrhea, and fever. Hypotension can occur with rapid IV administration.

### Teniposide

Teniposide [Vumon] is an analog of etoposide and shares that drug's mechanism of action: inhibition of DNA topoisomerase II with resultant DNA strand scission and G$_2$ arrest. The only approved indication for teniposide is *refractory acute lymphoblastic leukemia* of childhood.

Administration is by slow IV infusion. Most of each dose becomes bound to plasma proteins. Penetration to the CNS is poor. Elimination is by hepatic metabolism and renal excretion.

The major dose-limiting toxicity is bone marrow depression (neutropenia, thrombocytopenia, anemia). Severe hypersensitivity reactions (urticaria, angioedema, bronchospasm, hypotension) occur in about 5% of patients; symptoms can be suppressed with epinephrine. Secondary leukemias have developed within 8 years of initial drug exposure. Other toxicities include nausea, vomiting, diarrhea, and alopecia.

# Miscellaneous Cytotoxic Drugs

## Asparaginase

***Mechanism of Action.*** Asparaginase [Elspar] is an enzyme that converts asparagine, an essential amino acid, into aspartic acid. By converting asparagine to aspartic acid, the drug deprives cells of asparagine needed to synthesize proteins. However, not all cells are affected. In fact, toxicity from asparaginase is limited almost exclusively to leukemic lymphoblasts. The reason is that these cells are unable to manufacture their own asparagine, whereas normal cells can, which allows them to replace the asparagine that asparaginase took away. Asparaginase appears to act selectively during G$_1$.

***Pharmacokinetics.*** Administration is parenteral (IM and IV). Distribution is restricted to the vascular system. The drug does not cross the blood-brain barrier. Asparaginase is inactivated by serum proteases.

***Therapeutic Use.*** The only indication for asparaginase is *acute* lymphocytic leukemia. For induction of remission, asparaginase is usually combined with prednisone and vincristine, and perhaps daunorubicin or doxorubicin.

***Toxicity.*** Asparaginase can cause severe adverse effects. However, the spectrum of toxicities differs from that of other anticancer drugs. By inhibiting protein synthesis, the drug can cause coagulation deficiencies and injury to the liver, pancreas, and kidneys. Symptoms of CNS depression, ranging from confusion to coma, develop in about 30% of patients. Nausea and vomiting can be intense and may limit the dose that can be tolerated. Since asparaginase is a foreign protein, hypersensitivity reactions are common; fatal anaphylaxis can occur, and facilities for resuscitation should be immediately available. In contrast to most other anticancer drugs, asparaginase does not depress the bone marrow, nor does it cause alopecia, oral ulceration, or intestinal ulceration.

### Pegaspargase

Pegaspargase [Oncaspar] is a modified form of asparaginase that causes fewer hypersensitivity reactions. Otherwise, the drugs are very similar. They have the same mechanism of action (destruction of asparagine) and produce the same spectrum of adverse effects (hypersensitivity reactions, pancreatitis, coagulopathy, and liver and kidney dysfunction). Of the patients who had hypersensitivity reactions to asparaginase, about 30% also have them with pegaspargase. Pegaspargase is indicated only for *acute lymphocytic leukemia*, and only in patients who had a hypersensitivity reaction to asparaginase. Administration is IM or IV.

### Paclitaxel

***Actions and Uses.*** Paclitaxel [Taxol] is a mitotic spindle poison originally prepared from the bark of the Western yew tree. The drug acts during late G$_2$ to promote formation of stable microtubule bundles, thereby inhibiting cell replication. Paclitaxel is approved for *metastatic ovarian and breast cancers* that have not responded to first-line drugs. Investigational uses include advanced lung cancer (small-cell and non-small-cell), advanced head and neck cancer, adenocarcinoma of the upper GI tract, and leukemias.

***Pharmacokinetics.*** Paclitaxel is administered by 24-hour infusion. The drug undergoes wide distribution, but not to the CNS. Very little is known about how paclitaxel is eliminated; small amounts appear in the urine and bile, but the fate of the remainder is unknown.

***Toxicity.*** Severe hypersensitivity reactions (hypotension, dyspnea, angioedema, urticaria) have occurred during the infusion, probably in response to the vehicle (polysorbate 80) rather than to paclitaxel itself. The risk of severe hypersensitivity reactions can be minimized by performing the infusion slowly and by pretreatment with a glucocorticoid (dexamethasone), histamine$_1$-receptor antagonist (diphenhydramine), and histamine$_2$-receptor antagonist (cimetidine).

The major dose-limiting toxicity is bone marrow depression (neutropenia). Peripheral neuropathy develops with repeated infusions and may also be dose limiting. Paclitaxel can affect the heart, causing bradycardia, second- and third-degree heart block, and even fatal myocardial infarction. Muscle and joint pain have occurred. Practically all patients experience sudden but reversible alopecia, which frequently involves the body as well as the scalp. Gastrointestinal reactions (nausea, vomiting, diarrhea, mucositis) are generally mild.

### Docetaxel

*Actions, Use, and Source.* Docetaxel [Taxotere] is similar in structure and actions to paclitaxel. Like paclitaxel, docetaxel stabilizes microtubules, and thereby inhibits mitosis. At this time, docetaxel is approved only for locally advanced or metastatic *breast cancer* that has progressed or relapsed despite ongoing treatment with doxorubicin or another anthracycline anticancer drug. In clinical trials, docetaxel produced objective responses in over 40% of patients. The recommended dosage is 60 or 100 mg/m$^2$ infused IV over 1 hour every 3 weeks. Like paclitaxel, docetaxel is expensive: the price of a single dose is $1500 to $1900, plus the cost of administration. Docetaxel is manufactured by a semisynthetic process that begins with a compound extracted from needles of the European yew tree.

*Toxicity.* Significant *neutropenia* develops in virtually all patients. Docetaxel should be withheld if neutrophil counts fall below 1500 cells/mm$^3$. In clinical trials, death from sepsis occurred in 1% of patients with normal liver function and 11% of patients with abnormal liver function. Since liver dysfunction increases the risk of death, docetaxel should be avoided if signs of liver disease are present (i.e., plasma aminotransferase activity more than 1.5 times normal and alkaline phosphatase activity more than 2.5 times normal).

Severe *hypersensitivity* can occur. Manifestations include hypotension, bronchospasm, and generalized rash or erythema. Docetaxel should be avoided in patients who reacted strongly to a previous dose or to any drug containing polysorbate 80 (the vehicle docetaxel is supplied in). To reduce hypersensitivity reactions, patients should be treated with an oral glucocorticoid for 5 days, beginning 1 day before each infusion.

Severe *fluid retention* can occur, especially in patients with abnormal liver function. Possible manifestations include generalized edema, dyspnea at rest, cardiac tamponade, pleural effusion requiring urgent drainage, and pronounced abdominal distention (from ascites). As with hypersensitivity reactions, fluid retention can be reduced by treatment with oral glucocorticoids.

Additional common toxicities are anemia, nausea, diarrhea, stomatitis, fever, and neurosensory symptoms (paresthesias, pain).

### Hydroxyurea

*Mechanism of Action.* Hydroxyurea [Hydrea] inhibits DNA replication by suppressing synthesis of DNA precursors. Specifically, the drug inhibits ribonucleoside diphosphate reductase, the enzyme that converts ribonucleotides into their corresponding deoxyribonucleotides. In the absence of deoxyribonucleotides, DNA cannot be made. Hydroxyurea is S-phase specific.

*Pharmacokinetics.* Hydroxyurea is rapidly absorbed following oral administration. Unlike most anticancer agents, hydroxyurea crosses the blood-brain barrier with ease. Part of each dose is metabolized in the liver. Parent drug and metabolites are eliminated primarily in the urine.

*Therapeutic Uses.* The principal indication for hydroxyurea is *chronic myelocytic leukemia.* The drug is also used for recurrent, metastatic, or inoperable *carcinoma of the ovary.* Re-

cently, hydroxyurea was shown to relieve symptoms of *sickle-cell disease.*

*Toxicity.* The principal dose-limiting toxicity is bone marrow depression. The drug also causes nausea, vomiting, and dysuria. Neurologic deficits and stomatitis may occur, but these are rare. Hydroxyurea is teratogenic in experimental animals. Hence, like most other anticancer agents, the drug should be avoided during pregnancy.

### Mitotane

*Chemistry, Actions, and Uses.* Mitotane [Lysodren] is a structural analog of two insecticides: DDD and DDT. For reasons that are not understood, the drug is selectively toxic to cells of the adrenal cortex; normal cells and neoplastic adrenal cells are both injured. The only indication for mitotane is palliative therapy of inoperable *adrenocortical carcinoma.*

*Pharmacokinetics.* Mitotane is administered orally, and about 40% of each dose is absorbed. The drug is distributed widely, but not to the CNS. Because of storage in tissues (primarily fat), active drug remains in the body for weeks after administration has ceased. Elimination is by hepatic metabolism and renal excretion.

*Toxicity.* The principal dose-limiting toxicities are CNS depression, nausea, and vomiting. Because mitotane injures the adrenal cortex, adrenal insufficiency is likely. Accordingly, patients will require supplemental glucocorticoids, especially at times of stress. Dermatitis is common. Other adverse effects include visual disturbances, orthostatic hypotension, and renal damage, manifested as hematuria, hemorrhagic cystitis, and albuminuria. Mitotane does not cause the toxicities associated with most other anticancer drugs (bone marrow depression, alopecia, oral and gastrointestinal ulceration).

### Procarbazine

*Mechanism of Action.* Procarbazine [Matulane] is a prodrug that is converted to active metabolites in the liver. The metabolites cause chromosomal damage and suppress synthesis of DNA, RNA, and proteins. The precise cause of cell death is not known. Procarbazine is cell-cycle phase nonspecific.

*Pharmacokinetics.* Procarbazine is readily absorbed following oral administration, but undergoes rapid and extensive hepatic metabolism. Active metabolites are highly lipid soluble and cross the blood-brain barrier with ease. Procarbazine and its metabolites are excreted primarily in the urine.

*Therapeutic Uses.* The major indication for procarbazine is *advanced Hodgkin's disease.* Other uses include *non-Hodgkin's lymphomas* and *brain tumors.* For treating Hodgkin's disease, procarbazine is combined with mechlorethamine, vincristine [Oncovin], and prednisone, in the so-called MOPP regimen.

*Toxicity.* The usual dose-limiting toxicity is bone marrow depression. Nausea and vomiting may also be dose limiting. Other adverse effects include peripheral neuropathy, CNS depression, secondary leukemias, and sterility, especially in males.

Procarbazine can interact with other drugs. Because of its CNS effects, procarbazine should not be combined with CNS depressants (e.g., barbiturates, phenothiazines, opioids). Ingestion of alcohol can induce a disulfiram-like response. Because procarbazine inhibits monoamine oxidase, there is a risk of severe hypertension in response to sympathomimetic drugs, tricyclic antidepressants, and tyramine-rich foods.

### Dacarbazine

*Actions and Uses.* Dacarbazine [DTIC-Dome] is a prodrug that is activated by the liver. Although the precise mechanism of cell kill is not known, there is evidence for alkylation of DNA, inhibition of DNA and RNA synthesis, and interaction with sulfhydryl groups on proteins. Dacarbazine is considered cell-cycle phase nonspecific. The principal indication for the drug is *metastatic malignant melanoma*, but the response rate is low (about 20%).

*Pharmacokinetics.* Since gastrointestinal absorption is erratic, procarbazine is administered IV. Penetration to the CNS is poor. Elimination is by hepatic metabolism and renal excretion.

*Toxicity.* Bone marrow depression is the usual dose-limiting toxicity. Nausea and vomiting occur in most patients, occasionally requiring cessation of treatment. Other toxicities include a flu-like syndrome, hepatic necrosis, photosensitivity, and burning pain along the injection site.

### Altretamine (Hexamethylmelamine)

Altretamine [Hexalen], formerly known as hexamethylmelamine, is indicated for palliative therapy of persistent or recurrent *ovarian cancer*. Altretamine is a prodrug that is converted to active metabolites in the body. The mechanism by which the metabolites act is not known. Altretamine is well absorbed following oral administration, but undergoes rapid and extensive hepatic metabolism. The metabolites are excreted in the urine. The principal dose-limiting toxicity is bone marrow depression. Nausea and vomiting can also be dose limiting. Peripheral sensory neuropathy is common. Central neurotoxicity (tremors, ataxia, vertigo, hallucinations, seizures, depression) is less common. Because of peripheral and central neurotoxicity, patients should receive regular neurologic evaluations.

# Hormones and Hormone Antagonists

The hormones and hormone antagonists are the least toxic of all anticancer drugs. Because these agents act through specific hormone receptors on target tissues, their actions are highly selective. As a result, these drugs are devoid of the severe cytotoxic effects that characterize most anticancer agents. The hormonal anticancer drugs fall into five basic categories: (5) glucocorticoids, (2) androgens and antiandrogens, (3) estrogens and antiestrogens, (4) progestins, and (5) gonadotropin-releasing hormone analogs. The principal indications for these drugs are cancers of the breast, endometrium, and prostate. In addition, the glucocorticoids are used against lymphomas and certain leukemias. Trade names, routes of administration, and indications are summarized in Table 96–3.

## TABLE 96–3. HORMONES AND HORMONE ANTAGONISTS

| Generic Name | Trade Name | Route | Indications |
|---|---|---|---|
| *Androgens* | | | |
| Fluoxymesterone | Halotestin | PO | Breast cancer |
| Testosterone | Generic only | PO | Breast cancer |
| *Gn-RH\* Agonists* | | | |
| Leuprolide | Lupron | IM, SC | Prostate cancer |
| Goserelin | Zoladex | SC | Prostate cancer |
| *Androgen Receptor Blockers* | | | |
| Flutamide | Eulexin | PO | Prostate cancer |
| Bicalutamide | Casodex | PO | Prostate cancer |
| Nilutamide | Nilandron | PO | Prostate cancer |
| *Estrogens* | | | |
| Diethylstilbestrol diphosphate | Stilphostrol | PO, IV | Prostate cancer |
| Ethinyl estradiol | Estinyl | PO | Prostate cancer |
| *Estrogen Mustard* | | | |
| Estramustine | Emcyt | PO | Prostate cancer |
| *Antiestrogens* | | | |
| Tamoxifen | Nolvadex | PO | Breast cancer |
| Anastrozole | Arimidex | PO | Breast cancer |
| *Progestins* | | | |
| Medroxyprogesterone acetate | Depo-Provera | PO, IM | Endometrial cancer |
| Megestrol acetate | Megace | PO | Breast and endometrial cancer |
| *Glucocorticoid* | | | |
| Prednisone | Deltasone, others | PO | Acute and chronic lymphocytic leukemias, Hodgkin's and non-Hodgkin's lymphomas |

\*Gonadotropin-releasing hormone analogs.

## Glucocorticoids

The basic pharmacology of the glucocorticoids is discussed in Chapter 65 (Glucocorticoids in Nonendocrine Diseases). Discussion here is limited to their the use in cancer.

Glucocorticoids (e.g., *prednisone*) are used in combination with other agents to treat cancers arising from lymphoid tissue. Specific indications are *acute and chronic lymphocytic leukemias, Hodgkin's disease,* and *non-Hodgkin's lymphomas.* Glucocorticoids are beneficial in these cancers because of their direct toxicity to lymphoid tissues: high-dose therapy causes suppression of mitosis, dissolution of lymphocytes, regression of lymphatic tissue, and cell death. When used acutely, glucocorticoids are devoid of significant adverse effects. However, with prolonged treatment, these drugs can cause a broad spectrum of serious toxicities, including osteoporosis, adrenal insufficiency, increased susceptibility to infection, peptic ulcers, fluid and electrolyte disturbances, myopathy, growth retardation, and cutaneous atrophy.

In addition to their use against lymphoid-derived cancers, glucocorticoids are used to manage complications of cancer and cancer therapy. Specific benefits include suppression of chemotherapy-induced nausea and vomiting, reduction of cerebral edema secondary to irradiation of the cranium, reduction of pain secondary to nerve compression or edema, and suppression of hypercalcemia in steroid-responsive tumors. In addition, glucocorticoids can improve appetite, promote weight gain, and impart a generalized sense of well-being.

## Antiestrogens

### Tamoxifen

Tamoxifen [Nolvadex] is the most widely prescribe anticancer agent in the world. The drug is an *antiestrogen* approved for adjunctive therapy of *breast cancer* following total or segmental mastectomy. In addition, it is under investigation for *preventing* breast cancer in high-risk women. The drug works by binding to estrogen receptors, thereby preventing their activation by estradiol, the principal naturally occurring estrogen. If tamoxifen is to be of benefit, target cells must be estrogen-receptor (ER) positive. That is, they must possess receptors for estrogens. In the United States, the usual dosage is 10 mg PO twice a day.

The most common adverse effects of tamoxifen are nausea, vomiting, hot flushes, and menstrual irregularities. In bone, tamoxifen acts like a weak estrogen, and hence does not promote osteoporosis. In fact, in postmenopausal women, the drug helps *preserve* bone mineral density.

Tamoxifen appears to increase the risk of endometrial cancer. In women taking the drug to *treat* breast cancer, the benefits probably outweigh this risk. However, in women taking the drug to *prevent* breast cancer, the risk of endometrial cancer may outweigh any protective benefits.

### Anastrozole

*Mechanism and Use.* Anastrozole [Arimidex] is an oral drug approved for treating postmenopausal women with advanced *breast cancer* that has progressed despite use of tamoxifen, the preferred treatment for the disease. Anastrozole works by depriving the cancer of estrogen. In postmenopausal women, the major source of estrogen is adrenal androgens, which are converted to estrogen by the enzyme *aromatase* in peripheral tissues. Anastrozole inhibits aromatase, and thereby reduces estrogen production. With regular use, the drug lowers estrogen to clinically undetectable levels. In women with estrogen-dependent tumors, estrogen deprivation can arrest tumor growth and may also kill tumor cells. In clinical trials, anastrozole was not effective in women with ER-negative tumors and in women who did not respond initially to tamoxifen. The recommended dosage is 1 mg PO once a day.

*Adverse Effects.* Anastrozole is generally well tolerated. In clinical trials, only 3.3.% of patients withdrew because of adverse effects. At a dose of 1 mg, the most common adverse effects are asthenia (16%), nausea (16%), headache (13%), and hot flushes (12%). Other reactions include anorexia, vomiting, diarrhea, constipation, dyspnea, peripheral edema, vaginal hemorrhage, hypertension, and pain (including bone, back, pelvic, and abdominal pain).

## Drugs for Prostate Cancer

### Gonadotropin-Releasing Hormone Agonists

The gonadotropin-releasing hormone (Gn-RH) agonists suppress production of androgens by the testes. Hence, they can be looked on as indirect-acting antiandrogens. At this time, two Gn-RH agonists are available: leuprolide and goserelin. Both drugs are used to treat cancer of the prostate. In addition, leuprolide is used for endometriosis (see Chapter 59).

*Leuprolide. Therapeutic Use.* Leuprolide [Lupron, Lupron Depot] is a synthetic analog of gonadotropin-releasing hormone (Gn-RH), also known as *luteinizing hormone-releasing hormone* (LH-RH). Leuprolide is indicated for *advanced carcinoma of the prostate.* Palliation is the primary benefit. For patients with prostate cancer, leuprolide represents an alternative to orchiectomy (surgical castration). Leuprolide may be administered daily (SC), monthly (IM), or every 3 months (IM).

*Mechanism of Action.* Cells of the prostate, both normal and neoplastic, are androgen dependent. Leuprolide provides palliation by suppressing androgen production in the *testes.* During the initial phase of treatment, leuprolide *mimics* Gn-RH. That is, the drug acts on the pituitary to *stimulate* release of interstitial cell–stimulating hormone (ICSH), which acts on the testes to *increase* production of testosterone. As a result, there may be a transient "flare" in cancer symptoms. However, with con- tinuous exposure to leuprolide, pituitary Gn-RH receptors become desensitized. As a result, release of ICSH *declines,* causing testosterone production to decline as well. After several weeks of treatment, testosterone levels are equivalent to those seen after surgical castration. Because leuprolide therapy mimics the effects of orchiectomy, treatment is often referred to as "chemical castration."

It is important to note that leuprolide does *not* decrease production of *adrenal* androgens, which account for about 9% of the androgens in circulation. Hence, even though production of testicular androgens is essentially eliminated, adrenal androgens can provide some support for prostate cancer cells. To offset the effects of adrenal androgens, leuprolide is often combined with an androgen receptor blocker (e.g., flutamide). The androgen receptor blocker has the additional benefit of preventing the symptom flare that can occur early in treatment.

*Adverse Effects.* Leuprolide is generally well tolerated. Hot flushes are the most common adverse effect, but these usually decline as treatment progresses. Impotence and loss of libido may occur. During the initial weeks of treatment, elevation of testosterone levels may aggravate bone pain and urinary obstruction caused by prostate cancer. As a result, patients with vertebral metastases or pre-existing obstruction of the urinary tract may find treatment intolerable. As noted above, concurrent treatment with an androgen receptor blocker can minimize these problems.

**Goserelin.** Goserelin [Zoladex], like leuprolide, is a Gn-RH analog used for advanced prostate cancer. Both drugs share the same mechanism of action and adverse effects. Administration of goserelin is unique. The drug is formulated as a pellet that is dispensed in a syringe with a 16-gauge needle. The pellet is implanted by SC injection in the upper abdominal wall. Local anesthesia may be used prior to the injection.

## Androgen Receptor Blockers

Three androgen receptor blockers are available: flutamide, bicalutamide, and nilutamide. The only indication for these drugs is cancer of the prostate. Furthermore, when used to treat prostate cancer, these drugs should be combined with either surgical castration (orchiectomy) or chemical castration (Gn-RH agonist therapy).

**Flutamide.** Flutamide [Eulexin] was the first androgen receptor antagonist available. The drug is indicated only for *metastatic prostate cancer*, and then only in patients taking a Gn-RH agonist (e.g., leuprolide). Benefits derive from blocking androgen receptors within tumor cells, thereby depriving them of needed androgenic stimulation. In patients taking a Gn-RH agonist, flutamide serves two purposes: (1) it prevents cancer cells from undergoing increased stimulation during the initial phase of Gn-RH therapy, when androgen production is increased (see discussion of leuprolide above); and (2) it blocks the effects of adrenal androgens, whose production is not affected by Gn-RH agonists. In one clinical study, patients receiving flutamide plus leuprolide had a mean survival time of nearly 3 years, compared with 2.3 years for those receiving leuprolide alone.

Flutamide is administered orally and undergoes rapid and complete absorption. Most of each dose is converted to an active metabolite on the first pass through the liver. Parent drug and metabolites are excreted in the urine.

The most common adverse effect is gynecomastia. Nausea, vomiting, and diarrhea occur less frequently. Rarely, toxic hepatitis has occurred. The risk of serious injury can be reduced by monitoring liver function.

**Bicalutamide.** Like flutamide, bicalutamide [Casodex] is an androgen receptor blocker used to treat *advanced prostate cancer* in men undergoing therapy with a Gn-RH agonist (e.g., leuprolide). The rationale for this combination therapy is explained in the discussion of flutamide. When bicalutamide was used alone in clinical trials, the most common side effects were breast pain (38%) and gynecomastia (39%). When the drug is combined with leuprolide, the most common side effect is hot flushes (49%). The incidence of significant diarrhea with bicalutamide (6%) is much higher than with flutamide (0.5%).

**Nilutamide.** Like flutamide and bicalutamide, nilutamide [Nilandron] blocks intracellular receptors for androgens. The drug is approved for treatment of *metastatic prostate cancer* in men who have undergone orchiectomy (surgical castration). Benefits derive from blocking the actions of adrenal androgens, which are not reduced by castration. In clinical trials, nilutamide reduced bone pain, prolonged progression-free survival, and increased median survival time. The recommended dosage is 300 mg once daily PO for 30 days followed by 150 mg once daily thereafter. Dosing should commence within 24 hour of surgical castration.

Although nilutamide is structurally similar to flutamide, the drug is not as well tolerated. The most common adverse effects are hot flushes (67%), delayed adaptation to darkness (57%), nausea (24%), constipation (20%), insomnia (16%), and gynecomastia (11%). Other reactions occur less frequently, but are more dangerous. About 2% of patients experience dyspnea secondary to interstitial pneumonitis; if this develops, nilutamide should be withdrawn. About 1% of patients develop hepatitis. To ensure early diagnosis, liver function should be monitored.

## Estrogens

*Diethylstilbestrol diphosphate* [Stilphostrol] and other estrogens are second-line drugs for treating *prostate cancer*. Benefits derive from suppressing production of androgens, which prostate cells need to thrive. Estrogens suppress androgen production acting in the pituitary to suppress release of interstitial cell–stimulating hormone (ICSH); in the absence of ICSH, production of androgens by the testes declines. Adverse effects of estrogens include nausea, fluid retention, hypercalcemia, depression, thromboembolic disorders, and gynecomastia. The basic pharmacology of the estrogens is discussed in Chapter 57.

## Estramustine (An Estrogen Mustard)

Estramustine [Emcyt] is a hybrid molecule composed of estradiol (an estrogen) coupled to nor-nitrogen mustard (an alkylating agent). The only indication for the drug is palliative therapy of *advanced prostate cancer*. Following oral administration, estramustine becomes concentrated in prostate cells, apparently through the actions of a unique "estramustine-binding protein." Injury to prostate cells appears to result from two mechanisms. First, estramustine acts as a weak alkylating agent. Second, hydrolysis of estramustine releases free estradiol, which suppresses ICSH release by the pituitary, thereby depriving prostate cells of hormonal support.

Adverse effects are caused primarily by free estradiol. Gynecomastia is common. The most serious effect is increased risk of thrombosis, with resultant myocardial infarction and stroke. Other adverse effects include fluid retention, nausea, vomiting, diarrhea, and hypercalcemia.

## Androgens

The basic pharmacology of the androgens is discussed in Chapter 61. Consideration here is limited to therapy of cancer.

*Therapeutic Use.* Androgens are employed for palliative therapy in women with advanced or metastatic *carcinoma of the breast.* It should be noted, however, that tamoxifen is the preferred drug for this indication. Androgen therapy should be instituted only if surgery and irradiation are deemed inappropriate. After a delay of several weeks, objective responses are obtained in 50% to 60% of those treated. Beneficial effects persist for 12 to 14 months. The androgens employed most frequently are *fluoxymesterone* [Halotestin] and *testosterone*.

**Adverse Effects.** The doses used for breast cancer are high, making virilization a common side effect. Symptoms include clitoral enlargement, proliferation of facial and body hair, deepening of the voice, increased libido, and male-pattern baldness.

The effects of androgens coupled with the effects of osteolytic metastases can result in severe hypercalcemia. Principal dangers are ectopic calcification (especially in the urinary tract) and disruption of calcium-dependent physiologic processes. If hypercalcemia develops, androgen therapy should be temporarily withheld and large volumes of fluids should be administered. Androgen therapy may resume after calcium levels normalize.

### Progestins

Two progestins are employed to treat cancers: *medroxyprogesterone acetate* [Depo-Provera] and *megestrol acetate* [Megace]. Both drugs are indicated for *advanced endometrial carcinoma*. Megestrol is also indicated for *advanced breast cancer*. In women with metastatic endometrial cancer, progestins promote palliation and tumor regression. About 30% of patients have objective responses. Among those who respond, survival time is increased to about 2 years. This compares with survival times of 6 months among nonresponders. Patients with tumors that test positive for progesterone receptors are more likely to respond. However, the exact mechanism by which progestins suppress tumor growth is not known. The principal adverse effects of progestins are fluid retention and nonfluid weight gain. Hypercalcemia may occur if bone metastases are present. Progestins are teratogens, and therefore should be avoided during the first 4 months of pregnancy. The basic pharmacology of the progestins is discussed in Chapter 57.

# Biologic Response Modifiers: Immunostimulants

Biologic response modifiers are drugs that alter host responses to cancer. Many of these drugs are immunostimulants, some can render cancer cells nonmalignant by causing them to differentiate into nonproliferative forms, and some (hematopoietic growth factors) enable the host to better tolerate the myelosuppressive actions of anticancer drugs (see Chapter 52). In this chapter, all of the biologic response modifiers discussed are immunostimulants. Their trade names, indications, and routes of administration are summarized in Table 96–4.

## Interferon Alfa-2a and Interferon Alfa-2b

Interferons are naturally occurring proteins with complex antiviral, anticancer, and immunomodulatory actions. Release of endogenous interferons is triggered by viral infections and other stimuli. Interferons are active against a variety of solid tumors and hematologic malignancies. They are also active against several viruses (see Chapter 87).

**Description.** Interferon alfa-2a [Roferon-A] and interferon alfa-2b [Intron A] are glycoproteins that contain 165 amino acids. These two drugs, referred to collectively as interferon alfa-2, are identical except for one amino acid. Commercial production is by recombinant DNA technology.

**Mechanism of Action.** Anticancer effects are thought to result from two basic processes: (1) enhancement of host immune responses and (2) direct antiproliferative effects on cancer cells. Both processes are mediated by binding of interferons to cell-surface receptors, with resultant increased expression of certain genes and reduced expression of other genes. Interferons can cause $G_0$ cells to remain dormant, thereby preventing their proliferation. In addition, interferons can cause proliferating cells to differentiate into nonproliferative mature forms.

**Antineoplastic Uses.** Interferons alfa-2a and alfa-2b are approved for *hairy cell leukemia*, *chronic myelogenous leukemia*, *malignant melanoma*, and *AIDS-related Kaposi's sarcoma*. Investigational uses include *acute leukemias* and *cancers of the bladder*, *ovary*, and *kidney*. Response rates are generally higher with hematologic cancers than with solid tumors.

**TABLE 96–4. BIOLOGIC RESPONSE MODIFIERS: IMMUNOSTIMULANTS**

| Generic Name | Trade Name | Route | Indications |
|---|---|---|---|
| Interferon alfa-2a<br>Interferon alfa-2b | Roferon-A<br>Intron A | IM, IV, SC | Hairy cell leukemia, chronic myelogenous leukemia, malignant melanoma, AIDS-related Kaposi's sarcoma* |
| Aldesleukin (interleukin-2) | Proleukin | IV | Metastatic renal cell cancer |
| Levamisole | Ergamisol | PO | Stage II colon cancer (combination therapy with fluorouracil) |
| BCG vaccine | TheraCys, TICE BCG | Intravesical | *In situ* bladder cancer |

*In addition to these approved indications, interferons have been used to treat many other cancers, including acute leukemias and cancers of the bladder, ovary, and kidney.

**Pharmacokinetics.** Interferon alfa-2 is administered by IM or SC injection. Plasma drug levels peak in 4 to 8 hours. Inactivation occurs rapidly in body fluids and tissues. No intact drug appears in the urine.

**Adverse Effects.** Interferon alfa-2 causes multiple adverse effects. The most common is a flu-like syndrome characterized by fever, fatigue, myalgia, headache, and chills. Symptoms tend to diminish with continued therapy. Some symptoms (fever, headache, myalgia) can be reduced with acetaminophen. Other common effects include anorexia, weight loss, diarrhea, abdominal pain, dizziness, and cough. Prolonged or high-dose therapy can cause bone marrow depression, thyroid dysfunction, alopecia, cardiotoxicity, and neurotoxicity, which can cause profound fatigue and depression.

### Aldesleukin (Interleukin-2)

Aldesleukin [Proleukin], also known as interleukin-2, is an immunostimulant used for advanced renal carcinoma. Because severe adverse effects are very common, the drug must be administered in a hospital that has an intensive care facility; a specialist in cardiopulmonary or intensive care medicine must be available.

**Description and Actions.** Aldesleukin is a large glycoprotein nearly identical in structure and actions to human interleukin-2. The drug is produced by recombinant DNA technology. Like interleukin-2, aldesleukin stimulates immune function. Specific responses include increased production and cytotoxicity of lymphocytes; increased production of interleukin-1, interferon gamma, and tumor necrosis factor; and induction of lymphokine-activated killer (LAK) cell activity. The exact mechanism of antitumor action is not known.

**Therapeutic Use.** Aldesleukin is approved only for *metastatic renal cell cancer* in adults. Objective responses occur in about 15% of patients (4% respond completely and 11% partially). The median duration of responses (complete and partial) is approximately 2 years. Investigational uses include *Kaposi's sarcoma, melanoma,* and *colorectal cancer.*

**Pharmacokinetics.** Aldesleukin is administered by intravenous infusion and distributes throughout the extracellular space. About 70% of each dose undergoes preferential uptake by the liver, kidneys, and lungs. Renal enzymes convert the drug into inactive metabolites, which are then excreted in the urine. Aldesleukin has an elimination half-life of just 85 minutes.

**Adverse Effects.** Practically all patients experience significant toxicity, and the fatality rate is high (4%). Effects seen most frequently are fever and chills (89%), nausea and vomiting (87%), hypotension (85%), anemia (77%), diarrhea (76%), altered mental status (76%), sinus tachycardia (70%), impaired renal function (61%), impaired liver function (56%), pulmonary congestion (54%), dyspnea (52%), and pruritus (48%).

Capillary leak syndrome (CLS) is of particular concern. This potentially fatal reaction is characterized by hypotension and reduced organ perfusion secondary to loss of vascular tone and extravasation of plasma proteins and fluid. Symptoms begin to develop immediately after treatment. CLS may be associated with angina pectoris, cardiac dysrhythmias, myocardial infarction, pronounced respiratory insufficiency, renal insufficiency, GI bleeding, and altered mental status. Because of the risk of CLS, aldesleukin must not be given to patients with cardiac, pulmonary, renal, hepatic, or CNS impairment. Careful monitoring is essential.

### Levamisole

**Actions.** Levamisole [Ergamisol] is an immunostimulant. The drug can help restore immune responses that are depressed, but does not enhance responses that are normal. Specific effects include increased antibody formation, increased proliferation and activity of T cells, and increased function of neutrophils, monocytes, and macrophages. The precise mechanism underlying these effects is not known.

**Therapeutic Use.** Levamisole, in combination with fluorouracil, is approved only for adjuvant therapy following surgical resection of stage III *colon cancer.* Although levamisole alone or fluorouracil alone has little effect, the combination produces a 41% decrease in the risk of cancer recurrence and a 33% decrease in mortality (as compared with surgical controls who received no adjuvant therapy).

**Pharmacokinetics.** Levamisole is administered orally and is rapidly absorbed. The drug undergoes extensive hepatic metabolism followed by urinary excretion. Fluorouracil, which is used together with levamisole, is administered IV.

**Adverse Effects.** Reactions to levamisole alone are infrequent and mild. In contrast, reactions to levamisole plus fluorouracil can be severe, but these are due primarily to the fluorouracil. The principal dose-limiting toxicity of the combination is bone marrow suppression. The most common responses to the combination are nausea, vomiting, and diarrhea. Other reactions include alopecia, oral and GI ulceration, flulike symptoms, metallic taste, dizziness, and arthralgia.

### BCG Vaccine

**Description and Therapeutic Use.** BCG vaccine [TheraCys, TICE BCG] is a freeze-dried preparation of attenuated *Mycobacterium bovis* (bacillus of Calmette and Guerin). The vaccine is approved for primary and relapsed *carcinoma in situ of the bladder,* both in the presence and absence of associated papillary tumors. However, the vaccine should not be used for papillary tumors alone. To treat bladder cancers, BCG is administered intravesically (i.e., directly into the bladder through a urethral catheter).

**Mechanism of Action.** BCG is a nonspecific immunostimulant. Instillation in the bladder produces a local inflammatory response that, by an unknown mechanism, promotes regression of tumor lesions in the urothelial lining.

**Adverse Effects.** The most common adverse effects, which result from bladder irritation, are dysuria, urinary frequency, urinary urgency, and hematuria. Urinary status should be monitored closely. The most common systemic reactions are malaise, fatigue, fever, and chills.

Since BCG vaccine consists of live *Mycobacterium bovis,* therapy carries a risk of systemic infection, including fatal septic shock. Accordingly, the vaccine is contraindicated for (1) immunocompromised patients (e.g., those taking immunosuppressant drugs, those with symptomatic or asymptomatic HIV infection); (2) patients with fever of unknown origin (since it may signify infection); and (3) patients with urinary tract infections (since there is an increased risk of systemic absorption of BCG).

Since BCG vaccine is infectious, it must be handled using aseptic technique. All materials employed during administration should be disposed of in plastic bags labeled "Infectious Waste." Urine voided within 6 hours of BCG instillation should be disinfected with an equal volume of 5% hypochlorite before flushing.

## KEY POINTS

- Anticancer drugs fall into three major classes: (1) cytotoxic agents (which kill cancer cells), (2) hormones and hormone antagonists (most of which deprive cancers needed hormonal support), and (3) biologic response modifiers (which enhance immune system responses to neoplasms).

- *Cell-cycle phase specific drugs* are effective only during a specific phase of the cell cycle (e.g., S phase, M phase). Accordingly, these drugs are only active against cells that are participating in the cell cycle. Cells in $G_0$ are spared.

- To be effective, cell-cycle phase specific drugs must be present as neoplastic cells cycle through the phase in which the drugs act. In practical terms, this means that phase-specific drugs must be in the blood continuously over a long time.

- *Cell-cycle phase nonspecific drugs* can affect cells during any phase of the cell cycle, including $G_0$.

- Although phase-nonspecific drugs can inflict biochemical lesions at any time during the cell cycle, they usually are more toxic to proliferating cells than to cells in $G_0$. This is because (1) $G_0$ cells often have time to repair drug-induced damage before it can result in significant harm, and (2) toxicity may not become manifest until the cells attempts to divide.

- About 50% of the *cytotoxic* anticancer drugs are phase specific; the other 50% are phase nonspecific.

- All of the hormones, hormone antagonists, and biologic response modifiers are phase nonspecific.

- Alkylating agents injure cells primarily by forming covalent bonds with DNA.

- *Bifunctional* alkylating agents form *cross-links* in DNA, and thereby prevent DNA replication. Bifunctional agents are more effective than monofunctional agents.

- Because alkylation reactions can take place at any time during the cell cycle, alkylating agents are considered cell-cycle phase nonspecific.

- Cyclophosphamide, the most widely used alkylating agent, is active against a broad spectrum of neoplastic diseases.

- Carmustine (an alkylating agent) is available in a wafer for implantation into the cavity created by surgical excision of a brain tumor. This unique delivery system provides high local concentrations of the drug.

- Antimetabolites are analogs of important natural metabolites, and hence are able to disrupt critical metabolic processes, especially DNA replication.

- Most antimetabolites are S-phase specific.

- Methotrexate, a folic acid analog, prevents conversion of folic acid to its active form. Cell kill results primarily from inhibition of DNA synthesis.

- High-doses of methotrexate coupled with *leucovorin rescue* can be used to treat methotrexate-resistant tumors. This technique can be very dangerous in that failure to give sufficient leucovorin at the right time can be lethal.

- Cytarabine, a pyrimidine analog, undergoes intracellular activation followed by incorporation into DNA, where it acts to inhibit DNA synthesis.

- Fluorouracil, an analog of uracil, undergoes intracellular activation, after which it inhibits thymidylate synthetase, thereby depriving cells of thymidylate needed to make DNA.

- Antitumor antibiotics are used to treat cancer, not infections.

- Dactinomycin (Actinomycin D) intercalates DNA, thereby distorting its structure. As a result, RNA polymerase is unable to use DNA as a template, and therefore protein synthesis is disrupted. Interestingly, DNA synthesis is not affected.

- Doxorubicin is cardiotoxic. To reduce the risk of heart failure, the cumulative lifetime dose should be kept below 550 mg/m$^2$. The risk can be further reduced with dexrazoxane, a drug that helps protect the heart from doxorubicin.

- Vincristine and vinblastine block assembly of the microtubules that move chromosomes during cell division. Accordingly, the drugs are M-phase specific.

- *Vincristine* is toxic to *peripheral nerves*, but does *not* significantly depress bone marrow function. Because it spares bone marrow, vincristine can be safely combined with drugs that depress bone marrow.

- In contrast to vincristine, vinblastine causes significant bone marrow depression, but is relatively harmless to peripheral nerves.

- Asparaginase converts asparagine into aspartic acid, and thereby deprives cells of asparagine needed to make proteins. Cytotoxicity is limited primarily to leukemic lymphoblasts. Why? Because these cells are unable to manufacture their own asparagine, whereas normal cells can.

- Hormonal anticancer drugs act through specific hormone receptors on target tissues; hence their actions are highly selective. As a result, these drugs are devoid of the severe cytotoxic effects that characterize most anticancer agents.

- Glucocorticoids are toxic to cancers of lymphoid origin (e.g., acute and chronic lymphocytic leukemias, Hodgkin's disease, non-Hodgkin's lymphomas.)

- In addition to their use against lymphoid-derived cancers, glucocorticoids are used to manage complications of cancer and cancer therapy. Specific benefits include suppression of chemotherapy-induced nausea and vomiting, reduction of cerebral edema secondary to irradiation of the cranium, reduction of pain secondary to nerve compression or edema, and suppression of hypercalcemia in steroid-responsive tumors. Also, glucocorticoids can improve appetite, promote weight gain, and impart a generalized sense of well-being.

- When used acutely, glucocorticoids are devoid of significant adverse effects. However, with prolonged use, these drugs can cause a broad spectrum of serious toxicities, including osteoporosis, adrenal insufficiency, increased susceptibility to infection, and peptic ulcers.

- Tamoxifen is an antiestrogen (estrogen receptor blocker) used for adjunctive therapy of breast cancer following mastectomy. For tamoxifen to work, target cells must be ER positive (i.e., they must have estrogen receptors).

- Tamoxifen appears to *increase* the risk of endometrial cancer. In women taking the drug to *treat* breast cancer, the benefits probably outweigh this risk. However, in women taking the drug to *prevent* breast cancer, the risk of endometrial cancer may outweigh any protective benefits.

• Prostate cancer can be treated with gonadotropin-releasing hormone (Gn-RH) agonists and androgen receptor blockers. Benefits derive from reducing the stimulation of prostate cells by androgens.

• Leuprolide, a Gn-RH agonist, has a biphasic mechanism of action. During the initial phase, the drug *stimulates* release of interstitial cell–stimulating hormone (ICSH) from the pituitary, and thereby *increases* production of testosterone by the testes. As a result, there may be a transient "flare" in prostate cancer symptoms. With continuous use, the drug suppresses ICSH release, and thereby causes testosterone production to fall. It is important to note that the drug does not decrease production of *adrenal* androgens.

• Flutamide, an androgen receptor blocker, is used in combination with a Gn-RH agonist to treat prostate cancer. Benefits derive from (1) preventing cancer cells from undergoing increased stimulation during the initial phase of Gn-RH therapy, and (2) blocking the effects of adrenal androgens on prostate cells.

• Interferon alfa benefits cancer patients by enhancing immune responses and by suppressing proliferation of cancer cells.

# UNIT XVII

## Additional Important Drugs

Drugs for the Eye
Drugs for the Skin
Miscellaneous Noteworthy Drugs

# Drugs for the Eye

The drugs addressed in this chapter are used to diagnose and treat ophthalmic disorders. Our primary interest is glaucoma. Many of the drugs used for disorders of the eye are discussed at length in other chapters; accordingly, discussion here is limited to their ophthalmologic applications.

## Glaucoma and Its Treatment

The term *glaucoma* refers to a group of diseases characterized by visual field loss secondary to optic nerve damage. The most common forms of glaucoma are *primary open-angle glaucoma* and *acute angle-closure glaucoma*. These forms of glaucoma differ with respect to underlying pathology and treatment. With either form, irreversible blindness can result.

Before proceeding, we need to review the roll of aqueous humor in maintaining intraocular pressure (IOP). As indicated in Figure 97–1, aqueous humor is produced by the ciliary body and secreted into the posterior chamber of the eye. From there it circulates around the iris into the anterior chamber, and then exits the anterior chamber via the trabecular meshwork and canal of Schlemm. If outflow from the anterior chamber is impeded, backpressure will develop, and IOP will rise. Conversely, if production of aqueous humor falls, IOP will decline.

### Primary Open-Angle Glaucoma

#### Characteristics

Primary open-angle glaucoma (POAG) is the most common form of glaucoma in the United States. About 90% of people with glaucoma have this type. POAG is the leading cause of blindness among African Americans and the third leading cause among whites. Over 2 million Americans have POAG, and 80,000 of them have some degree of visual impairment.

POAG is characterized by progressive optic nerve damage with eventual visual field loss. The pathologic process that leads to optic nerve damage is not understood. Intraocular pressure (IOP) is often elevated, but it may also be normal. POAG is a painless, insidious disease in which optic nerve injury develops over a period of years. Symptoms are absent until extensive optic nerve damage has been produced. The disease has a genetic basis and is most common in people over 40.

#### Risk Factors

Risk factors for POAG include elevation of IOP, African American heritage, family history of POAG, advancing age, myopia, diabetes, and hypertension. Since POAG is devoid of symptoms (until significant and irreversible optic nerve damage has occurred), individuals with risk factors should undergo periodic testing for early POAG. Diagnosis is based on glaucomatous optic nerve atrophy in association with characteristic reduction in peripheral vision.

The primary risk factor for glaucoma is elevated IOP. However, it is important to note that glaucomatous optic nerve damage can develop even though IOP is normal (i.e., below 20 mm Hg). Furthermore, some individuals can have very high IOP (e.g., 30 mm Hg) with no optic nerve injury. These individuals are said to have *ocular hypertension*. We do not know whether early intervention to reduce IOP in these people will prevent eventual development of glaucoma.

The incidence of POAG in African Americans is more than 3 times the incidence in whites. In addition, the age of onset is lower and the course of the disease is more aggressive. Because African Americans are at increased risk for POAG, they should be diligent about receiving periodic tests for the disease.

#### Management

POAG is managed primarily by chronic drug therapy directed at reducing IOP, the major risk factor for POAG. Drugs reduce IOP by either (1) facilitating aqueous humor outflow or (2) reducing aqueous humor production. The

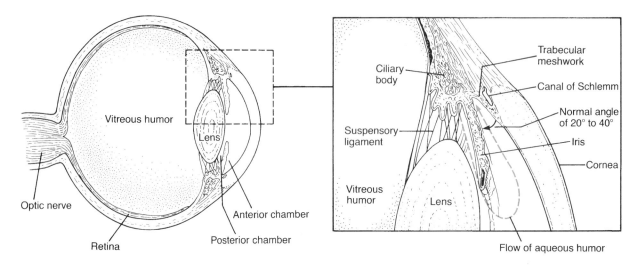

**Figure 97–1. Anatomy of the normal eye.**

principal agents employed are *beta-adrenergic blocking drug*s (e.g., timolol, betaxolol) and *pilocarpine* (a muscarinic cholinergic agonist). Other medications include adrenergic agonists (e.g., epinephrine, dipivefrin), prostaglandins, cholinesterase inhibitors, and carbonic anhydrase inhibitors. The carbonic anhydrase inhibitors are available in oral and topical formulations. All of the other drugs are administered topically only. Because most antiglaucoma agents are applied locally, systemic effects are relatively uncommon. However, serious systemic reactions can occur if sufficient absorption takes place. The drugs employed in glaucoma are summarized in Table 97–1.

If drugs are unable to reduce IOP to an acceptable level, surgical intervention to promote outflow of aqueous humor is indicated. The most common procedure is trabeculectomy, which creates a shunt that allows aqueous humor to exit the anterior chamber. Unfortunately, scarring may cause the shunt to close.

## Angle-Closure Glaucoma

Angle-closure glaucoma is precipitated by displacement of the iris such that it covers the trabecular meshwork, thereby preventing exit of aqueous humor from the anterior chamber. As a result, IOP increases rapidly to dangerous levels. This disorder is referred to as angle-closure or narrow-angle glaucoma because the angle between the cornea and the iris is greatly reduced (Fig. 97–2). Angle-closure glaucoma develops suddenly and is extremely painful. In the absence of treatment, irreversible loss of vision occurs in 1 to 2 days. This disorder is much less common than open-angle glaucoma.

Treatment consists of *drug therapy* (to control the acute attack) followed by *corrective surgery*. A combination of drugs (osmotic agents, short-acting miotics, carbonic anhydrase inhibitors, topical beta-adrenergic blocking agents) is employed to suppress symptoms. Once IOP has been reduced with drugs, definitive treatment can be rendered with surgery. Two surgical procedures are employed: laser *iridotomy* and *iridectomy* performed by

conventional surgery. Both procedures alter the iris to permit unimpeded outflow of aqueous humor.

## Drugs Used to Treat Glaucoma

### Beta-Adrenergic Blocking Agents

Five beta blockers—*betaxolol, carteolol, metipranolol, levobunolol,* and *timolol*—are approved for treating glaucoma. These agents cause less disturbance of vision than pilocarpine (see below) and are first-line drugs for glaucoma. The basic pharmacology of the beta blockers is discussed in Chapter 19. Consideration here is limited to their use in glaucoma.

***Mechanism of Action.*** The beta-adrenergic blockers lower IOP by decreasing production of aqueous humor. Reductions in IOP occur with "nonselective" beta blockers (drugs that block beta₁ *and* beta₂ receptors) as well as with "cardioselective" beta blockers (drugs that block beta₁ receptors only). It is not certain that the beneficial effects of the beta-receptor antagonists are actually due to beta-receptor blockade. This uncertainty stems from the observation that beta-adrenergic *agonists* (e.g., isoproterenol) can also lower IOP.

***Use in Glaucoma.*** Beta blockers are used primarily for open-angle glaucoma. These drugs are suitable for initial therapy and maintenance therapy. Efficacy of the beta blockers is equivalent to that of pilocarpine. In addition to their use in open-angle glaucoma, beta blockers may be employed in combination with other drugs for emergency management of acute angle-closure glaucoma.

***Adverse Effects.*** Local effects are generally minimal, although patients commonly complain of transient ocular stinging. Beta blockers occasionally cause conjunctivitis, blurred vision, photophobia, and dry eyes.

Beta blockers can be absorbed in amounts sufficient to cause *systemic effects.* These reactions are more important than local effects. Effects on the heart and lungs are of greatest concern.

Blockade of cardiac beta₁ receptors can produce bradycardia and atrioventricular (AV) heart block. Pulse rate

## TABLE 97–1. DRUGS FOR GLAUCOMA

| Class | Drugs | Mechanism | Adverse Effects |
|---|---|---|---|
| *Beta Blockers* | | | |
| Nonselective | Timolol Carteolol Levobunolol Metipranolol | Decreased aqueous formation | Heart block, bradycardia, bronchospasm |
| Beta₁ selective | Betaxolol | | Heart block, bradycardia, hypotension |
| *Cholinergic Agonists* | | | |
| Direct acting | Pilocarpine | Increased aqueous outflow | Miosis, blurred vision |
| AChE inhibitors | Echothiophate | | Miosis, blurred vision |
| *Epinephrine* | Epinephrine Dipivefrin* | Increased aqueous outflow | Mydriasis, tachycardia, increased blood pressure |
| *Prostaglandins* | Latanoprost | Increased aqueous outflow | Heightened brown pigmentation of the iris |
| *Carbonic Anhydrase Inhibitors* | | | |
| Systemic | Acetazolamide | Decreased aqueous formation | Malaise, anorexia, fatigue, paresthesias, acid-base disturbances, electrolyte imbalance, nephrolithiasis |
| Topical | Dorzolamide | | Ocular stinging, bitter taste, conjunctivitis, lid reactions |
| *Alpha₂ Agonists* | Apraclonidine | Decreased aqueous formation | Headache, dry mouth, dry nose, altered taste, conjunctivitis, lid reactions, pruritus, tearing, blurred vision |

*Dipivefrin is converted to epinephrine in the eye.

should be monitored. Because of their ability to depress cardiac function, beta blockers are contraindicated for patients with heart failure, AV heart block, sinus bradycardia, and cardiogenic shock. The risk of cardiac effects is about equal with all of the ophthalmic beta blockers.

Blockade of beta₂ receptors in the lung can cause bronchospasm. Constriction of the bronchi can occur with "beta₁-selective" antagonists as well as with "nonselective" beta-adrenergic blockers—although the risk is greatest with the nonselective agents. Only one ophthalmic beta blocker is beta₁ selective. This agent—*betaxolol*—is the preferred beta blocker for patients with asthma or chronic obstructive pulmonary disease.

***Preparations, Dosage, and Administration.*** The ophthalmic beta blockers are listed in Table 97–2. As shown in the table, these drugs differ from one another in two important ways: receptor selectivity and frequency of dosing.

### Pilocarpine

Pilocarpine is a direct-acting muscarinic agonist (parasympathomimetic agent). The basic pharmacology of the muscarinic agonists is discussed in Chapter 15.

Consideration here is limited to the use of pilocarpine in glaucoma.

***Effects on the Eye.*** By stimulating cholinergic receptors in the eye, pilocarpine produces two direct effects: (1) *miosis* (constriction of the pupil secondary to contraction of the iris sphincter), and (2) *contraction of the ciliary muscle* (an action that focuses the lens for near vision). IOP is lowered indirectly. In patients with *open-angle glaucoma*, IOP is reduced because the tension generated by contracting the ciliary muscle promotes widening of the spaces within the trabecular meshwork, thereby facilitating outflow of aqueous humor. In *angle-closure glaucoma*, contraction of the iris sphincter pulls the iris away from the pores of the trabecular meshwork, thereby removing the impediment to aqueous humor outflow.

***Therapeutic Uses.*** Pilocarpine is a first-line drug for initial and maintenance therapy of open-angle glaucoma. Although cholinesterase inhibitors act in much the same manner as pilocarpine (see below), pilocarpine is preferred. In addition to its applications in open-angle glaucoma, pilocarpine can be used for emergency treatment of acute angle-closure glaucoma.

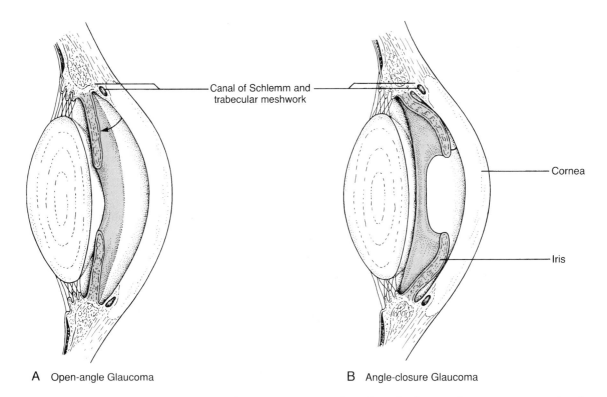

A   Open-angle Glaucoma                    B   Angle-closure Glaucoma

**Figure 97–2. Comparative anatomy of the eye in open-angle and angle-closure glaucoma.** *A*, Note that the angle between the iris and cornea is open in open-angle glaucoma, permitting unimpeded outflow of aqueous humor through the canal of Schlemm and trabecular meshwork. *B*, Note that the angle between the iris and cornea is constricted in angle-closure glaucoma, thereby blocking outflow of aqueous humor through the canal of Schlemm and trabecular meshwork.

**Adverse Effects.** The major side effects of pilocarpine concern the eye. Contraction of the ciliary muscle focuses the lens for near vision; corrective lenses can provide partial compensation for this problem. Occasionally, sustained contraction of the ciliary muscle causes retinal detachment. Constriction of the pupil, caused by contraction of the iris sphincter, may decrease visual acuity.

Pilocarpine may also produce local irritation, eye pain, and brow ache.

Rarely, pilocarpine is absorbed in amounts sufficient to cause systemic effects. Stimulation of muscarinic receptors throughout the body can produce a variety of responses, including bradycardia, bronchospasm, hypotension, urinary urgency, diarrhea, hypersalivation, and

## TABLE 97-2. BETA-ADRENERGIC BLOCKING AGENTS USED IN GLAUCOMA

| Drug | Receptor Specificity | Formulation | Usual Dosage |
|---|---|---|---|
| Betaxolol [Betoptic] | Beta$_1$ | 0.25% suspension<br>0.5% solution | 1 drop twice a day<br>1 drop twice a day |
| Carteolol [Ocupress] | Beta$_1$, beta$_2$ | 1% solution | 1 drop twice a day |
| Levobunolol [Betagan Liquifilm, AKBeta] | Beta$_1$, beta$_2$ | 0.25% solution<br>0.5% solution | 1 drop twice a day<br>1 drop once or twice a day |
| Metipranolol [OptiPranolol] | Beta$_1$, beta$_2$ | 0.3% solution | 1 drop twice a day |
| Timolol [Timoptic] | Beta$_1$, beta$_2$ | 0.25% solution<br>0.5% solution<br>0.25% gel<br>0.5% gel | 1 drop once or twice a day<br>1 drop once or twice a day<br>1 drop once daily<br>1 drop once daily |

sweating. Caution should be exercised in patients with asthma or bradycardia. Systemic toxicity can be reversed with a muscarinic antagonist (e.g., atropine).

***Preparations, Dosage, and Administration.*** Pilocarpine is available in solution, a gel, and an "ocular system." With all three formulations, administration is topical. Pilocarpine solutions have a relatively short duration of action and must be administered more frequently than the gel or ocular system.

*Pilocarpine Solutions. Pilocarpine hydrochloride* [Adsorbocarpine, Akarpine, Isopto Carpine, Ocu-Carpine, Pilocar, Piloptic, Pilostat] and *pilocarpine nitrate* [Pilagan] are dispensed in solution for topical application to the conjunctiva. Concentrations range from 0.25% to 10%. For maintenance therapy of open-angle glaucoma, the usual dosage is 1 drop of solution (0.5% to 4%) applied 4 times a day. For patients with acute angle-closure glaucoma, the drug is applied much more frequently (e.g., every 5 to 10 minutes for three to six doses, then 1 drop every 1 to 3 hours).

*Pilocarpine Gel.* Pilocarpine ophthalmic gel [Pilopine HS] consists of 4% pilocarpine hydrochloride in an aqueous gel base. The preparation has a long duration of action, making once-a-day dosing sufficient. For chronic open-angle glaucoma, the usual dosage is one-half inch of gel applied to the conjunctiva at bedtime.

*Pilocarpine Ocular System.* The pilocarpine ocular system [Ocusert Pilo-20, Ocusert Pilo-40] consists of a bilayered membrane surrounding a reservoir of pilocarpine solution. The tiny unit is placed in the conjunctival sac, after which pilocarpine is slowly released. A replacement unit should be installed once a week. The ocular system is indicated for chronic open-angle glaucoma. Since the unit may fall out during sleep, patients should be advised to check each morning for its presence. Occasionally, the ocular system may migrate to the cornea, causing discomfort and disturbance of vision. Conjunctival irritation may also occur.

## Epinephrine and Dipivefrin

*Epinephrine* is an adrenergic agonist that acts at alpha- and beta-adrenergic receptors. The basic pharmacology of epinephrine is discussed in Chapter 18. Consideration here is limited to its use in glaucoma.

*Dipivefrin* is a prodrug form of epinephrine. Because of its high lipid solubility, dipivefrin penetrates the cornea more readily than epinephrine. Once in the eye, dipivefrin is converted to epinephrine by ocular enzymes.

***Actions and Uses in Glaucoma.*** Epinephrine is used for open-angle glaucoma. The drug reduces IOP apparently by increasing aqueous humor outflow. The mechanism by which outflow is enhanced is not understood. Epinephrine may be used alone and in combination with beta blockers, carbonic anhydrase inhibitors, osmotic agents, and miotics (pilocarpine, cholinesterase inhibitors).

***Adverse Effects.*** Mild reactions—headache, brow ache, blurred vision, ocular irritation—are relatively common. By contracting the radial muscle of the iris, epinephrine can cause mydriasis (pupil dilation) and thereby aggravate angle-closure glaucoma. Accordingly, epinephrine is contraindicated for patients with this disorder. In the patient whose lens has been removed, epinephrine can cause an unusual edema of the retina. This reaction is reversible upon discontinuation of treatment. Systemic absorption can cause tachycardia and elevation of blood pressure;

caution should be exercised in patients with hypertension, dysrhythmias, and hyperthyroidism (hyperthyroidism sensitizes the heart to stimulation by catecholamines).

***Preparations, Dosage, and Administration.*** Ophthalmic solutions of epinephrine contain one of two salts: *epinephrine hydrochloride* [Epifrin, Glaucon] or *epinephrine borate* [Epinal]. For treatment of open-angle glaucoma, 1 drop of solution (0.25% to 2%) is instilled into the conjunctival sac once or twice daily.

*Dipivefrin* [Propine] is dispensed in a 0.1% solution. For treatment of open-angle glaucoma, 1 drop is instilled into the conjunctival sac every 12 hours.

## Latanoprost

Latanoprost [Xalatan], an analog of prostaglandin $F_2$ alpha, is a new topical drug used to lower IOP in patients with open-angle glaucoma and ocular hypertension. Latanoprost lowers IOP by facilitating aqueous humor outflow. The recommended dosage is 1 drop (0.005% solution) applied once daily in the evening. In clinical trials, latanoprost applied once daily was equivalent to timolol applied twice daily.

Latanoprost is generally well tolerated and systemic reactions are rare. The most significant side effect is heightened brown pigmentation of the iris. The effect is most noticeable in patients whose irides are green-brown, yellow-brown, or blue/gray-brown. The effect is rare in patients whose irides are blue, green, or blue-green. Heightened pigmentation stops progressing when latanoprost is discontinued, but does not regress. Other side effects include blurred vision, burning, stinging, conjunctival hyperemia, and punctate keratopathy.

### Long-Acting Cholinesterase Inhibitors: Echothiophate, Demecarium, and Physostigmine

The basic pharmacology of the cholinesterase inhibitors is discussed in Chapter 16. Consideration here is limited to their use in glaucoma.

***Effects on the Eye.*** The cholinesterase inhibitors inhibit breakdown of acetylcholine (ACh), thereby promoting accumulation of ACh at muscarinic receptors. By doing so, cholinesterase inhibitors can produce the same ocular effects as pilocarpine (i.e., miosis, focusing of the lens for near vision, reduction of IOP).

***Use in Glaucoma.*** The cholinesterase inhibitors are indicated for POAG. However, because of concerns about adverse effects (see below), these agents are not drugs of first choice. Rather, they are reserved for patients who have responded poorly to preferred medications (e.g., beta blockers, pilocarpine, epinephrine).

***Adverse Effects.*** Like pilocarpine, cholinesterase inhibitors can cause *myopia* (secondary to contraction of the ciliary muscle) and excessive pupillary constriction. However, of much greater concern is the association between long-acting cholinesterase inhibitors and development of *cataracts*. Absorption of cholinesterase inhibitors into the systemic circulation can produce typical *parasympathomimetic responses*, including bradycardia, bronchospasm, sweating, salivation, urinary urgency, and diarrhea.

***Preparations, Dosage, and Administration.*** *Echothiophate iodide* [Phospholine Iodide] is dispensed as a powder for reconstitution to solutions that range in strength from 0.03% to 0.25%. For treatment of open-angle glaucoma, the 0.03% solution is commonly employed. Administration into the conjunctival sac may be done once daily, twice daily, or every other day.

*Demecarium bromide* [Humorsol] is dispensed in sterile solution (0.125%, 0.25%) for topical application to the eye. For initial treatment of open-angle glaucoma, 1 drop is instilled into the conjunctival sac every 12 to 48 hours.

*Physostigmine* [Eserine] is dispensed in a 0.25% ointment for topical use. The ointment is applied to the lower fornix up to 3 times a day. Chronic treatment with physostigmine is associated with a high incidence of conjunctivitis.

### Systemic Carbonic Anhydrase Inhibitors

Three carbonic anhydrase inhibitors—*acetazolamide, dichlorphenamide*, and *methazolamide*—are used systemically to treat glaucoma. Acetazolamide is the most frequently employed.

***Actions and Uses in Glaucoma.*** The carbonic anhydrase inhibitors lower IOP by decreasing production of aqueous humor. Maximally effective doses reduce flow of aqueous humor by 50%. Administration is oral.

Carbonic anhydrase inhibitors are employed primarily for long-term treatment of open-angle glaucoma. These agents are not drugs of first choice. Rather, they should be reserved for patients who have been refractory to preferred medications (e.g., beta blockers, pilocarpine, epinephrine, cholinesterase inhibitors). Carbonic anhydrase inhibitors may also be given (in combination with other antiglaucoma drugs) to produce rapid lowering of IOP in patients with angle-closure glaucoma.

***Adverse Effects.*** Carbonic anhydrase inhibitors can produce a variety of adverse effects. Effects on the nervous system, which are relatively common, include malaise, anorexia, fatigue, and paresthesias. The sense of malaise causes many patients to discontinue drug use. Reduced appetite, coupled with gastrointestinal disturbances (nausea, vomiting, diarrhea) may result in weight loss. Carbonic anhydrase inhibitors are teratogenic in animals and should be avoided by women who are pregnant, especially during the first trimester. Additional concerns are acid-base disturbances, electrolyte imbalance, and nephrolithiasis (formation of renal calculi).

***Preparations, Dosage, and Administration.*** *Acetazolamide* [Diamox, Diamox Sequels, Dazamide] is dispensed in tablets (125 and 250 mg) and sustained-release capsules (500 mg) for oral use, and as an injection (500 mg/vial) for IM and IV administration. The usual dosage range is 250 mg to 1 gm per day in divided doses.

*Dichlorphenamide* [Daranide] is dispensed in 50-mg tablets for oral use. The usual dosage is 25 to 50 mg 1 to 3 times a day.

*Methazolamide* [Neptazane] is dispensed in 25- and 50-mg tablets for oral use. The usual dosage is 50 to 100 mg 2 or 3 times a day.

### Topical Carbonic Anhydrase Inhibitor: Dorzolamide

Dorzolamide [Trusopt], the first topical carbonic anhydrase inhibitor, is indicated for lowering IOP in patients with open-angle glaucoma and ocular hypertension. The drug lowers IOP by decreasing aqueous humor production. The recommended dosage is 1 drop (2% solution) 3 times a day. In clinical trials, responses to dorzolamide were similar to those produced with beta blockers (betaxolol and timolol).

Dorzolamide is generally well tolerated. The most common side effects are ocular stinging and bitter taste immediately after dosing. Between 10% and 15% of patients experience allergic reactions, primarily conjunctivitis and lid reactions. If these occur, the patient should stop using dorzolamide and contact the physician. Additional reactions include blurred vision, tearing, eye dryness, and photophobia. In contrast to systemic carbonic anhydrase inhibitors, dorzolamide does not produce acidosis or electrolyte imbalance.

### Alpha₂ Agonist: Apraclonidine

Apraclonidine [Iodipine], a topical alpha$_2$-adrenergic agonist, lowers IOP by reducing aqueous humor production. The drug is indicated for (1) short-term therapy of open-angle glaucoma in patients who have not responded adequately to maximal doses of other IOP-lowering drugs, and (2) preoperative medication prior to laser trabeculoplasty or iridotomy. Side effects include headache, dry mouth, dry nose, altered taste, conjunctivitis, lid reactions, pruritus, tearing, and blurred vision. For short-term therapy of glaucoma, the dosage is 1 or 2 drops (0.5% solution) 3 times a day.

### Osmotic Agents

Four osmotic agents—*mannitol, urea, glycerin*, and *isosorbide*—are employed in the treatment of glaucoma. These preparations render the plasma hypertonic to intraocular fluid and thereby draw water from the eye. This action results in a rapid and marked reduction of IOP. The principal indication for osmotic agents is emergency treatment of acute angle-closure glaucoma. Use in open-angle glaucoma is limited to the perioperative period. Glycerin and isosorbide are administered orally; mannitol and urea are administered by IV infusion. Doses for these drugs range from 0.5 to 2 gm/kg. Common side effects are headache, nausea, and vomiting. The use of mannitol for osmotic diuresis is discussed in Chapter 38.

# Cycloplegics and Mydriatics

*Cycloplegics* are drugs that cause paralysis of the ciliary muscle, whereas *mydriatics* are drugs that dilate the pupil. Cycloplegics and mydriatics are employed primarily to facilitate diagnosis and surgery of ophthalmic disorders. Agents used to produce cycloplegia, mydriasis, or both fall into two classes: (1) *anticholinergic agents* (muscarinic antagonists) and (2) *adrenergic agonists.*

## Anticholinergic Agents

Several muscarinic antagonists (Table 97–3) are employed topically for diagnosis and treatment of ophthalmic disorders. The basic pharmacology of the anticholinergic drugs is discussed in Chapter 15. Consideration here is limited to their ophthalmic applications.

### Effects on the Eye

The anticholinergic drugs produce mydriasis and cycloplegia. Mydriasis results from blockade of the muscarinic receptors that promote contraction of the iris sphincter; cycloplegia results from blockade of muscarinic receptors that promote contraction of the ciliary muscle. As discussed below, relaxation of the iris can lead to elevation of IOP.

### Ophthalmic Applications

***Adjunct to Measurement of Refraction.*** The term *refraction* refers to the bending of light by the cornea and lens. When ocular refraction is proper, incoming light is bent such that a sharp image is formed on the retina. Errors in refraction can produce nearsightedness, farsightedness, and astigmatism (a visual disturbance caused by irregularities in the curvature of the cornea).

## TABLE 97-3. MUSCARINIC ANTAGONISTS USED FOR MYDRIASIS AND CYCLOPLEGIA

| Generic Name | Trade Names | Strength of Solution (%) | Mydriasis Peak (min) | Mydriasis Recovery (days) | Cycloplegia Peak (min) | Cycloplegia Recovery (days) |
|---|---|---|---|---|---|---|
| Atropine | Atropisol Isopto Atropine Atropine Care | 0.5-2 | 30-40 | 7-12 | 60-180 | 6-12 |
| Cyclopentolate | AK-Pentolate Cyclogyl Pentolair | 0.5-2 | 30-60 | 1 | 25-75 | 0.25-1 |
| Homatropine | Isopto Homatropine | 2-5 | 40-60 | 1-3 | 30-60 | 1-3 |
| Scopolamine | Isopto Hyoscine | 0.25 | 20-30 | 3-7 | 30-60 | 3-7 |
| Tropicamide | Mydriacyl Tropicacyl Opticyl | 0.5-1 | 20-40 | 0.25 | 20-35 | <0.25 |

Both the mydriatic and cycloplegic properties of the muscarinic antagonists can be of use in evaluating errors of refraction. Mydriasis (widening of the pupil) facilitates observation of the eye's interior. Cycloplegia (paralysis of the ciliary muscle) prevents the lens from undergoing changes in configuration during the assessment.

***Intraocular Examination.*** Dilatation of the pupil with an anticholinergic agent facilitates observation of the inside of the eye. In addition, by paralyzing the iris sphincter, muscarinic antagonists prevent reflexive constriction of the pupil in response to the light from an ophthalmoscope (the hand-held device used to view the eye's interior). Since adrenergic agonists (e.g., phenylephrine) also dilate the pupil, but by a mechanism different from that of the anticholinergic drugs, an adrenergic agonist can be combined with a muscarinic antagonist to increase the degree of mydriasis.

***Intraocular Surgery.*** Anticholinergic agents may be employed to facilitate ocular surgery and reduce postoperative complications. Mydriasis induced by these drugs can aid in cataract extraction and procedures to correct retinal detachment. For these operations, the muscarinic antagonist may be combined with an adrenergic agonist to maximize pupillary dilatation. In certain postoperative patients, mydriatics are employed to prevent development of synechiae (adhesions of the iris to neighboring structures in the eye).

***Treatment of Anterior Uveitis.*** Uveitis is an inflammation of the uvea (the vascular layer of the eye). Symptoms include ocular pain and photophobia. Uveitis is treated with a glucocorticoid (to reduce inflammation) plus an anticholinergic agent. By promoting relaxation of the ciliary muscle and the iris sphincter, anticholinergic drugs help relieve pain and prevent adhesion of the iris to the lens.

### Adverse Effects

***Blurred Vision and Photophobia.*** The most common side effects of topical anticholinergic drugs are photophobia and blurred vision. Photophobia occurs because paralysis of the iris sphincter prevents the pupil from constricting in response to bright light. Vision is blurred because paralysis of the ciliary muscle prevents focusing for near vision.

***Precipitation of Angle-Closure Glaucoma.*** By relaxing the iris sphincter, anticholinergic drugs can induce closure of the filtration angle in individuals whose eyes have a narrow angle to begin with. Angle closure occurs as follows: (1) partial dilatation of the pupil maximizes contact between the iris and the lens, thereby impeding exit of aqueous humor from the posterior chamber, and (2) the resultant increase in pressure within the posterior chamber pushes the iris forward, causing blockage of the trabecular meshwork. Caution must be exercised in patients predisposed to angle closure.

***Systemic Effects.*** Topically applied anticholinergic drugs can be absorbed in amounts sufficient to produce systemic toxicity. Symptoms include dry mouth, blurred vision, photophobia, constipation, fever, tachycardia, and CNS effects (confusion, hallucinations, delirium, coma); death can occur. Muscarinic poisoning can be treated with physostigmine (see Chapter 15).

## Adrenergic Agonists

Adrenergic agonists are mydriatic agents; pupillary dilatation results from stimulation of alpha-adrenergic receptors located on the radial (dilator) muscle of the iris. The adrenergic agonists do not cause cycloplegia. Of the adrenergic agents given to induce mydriasis, phenylephrine is the most frequently employed. The adrenergic agonists are considered at length in Chapter 18. Discussion here is limited to the mydriatic use of *phenylephrine*.

### Therapeutic and Diagnostic Applications

The mydriatic applications of phenylephrine are much like those of the anticholinergic drugs. Phenylephrine-induced mydriasis is used as an aid to intraocular surgery, measurement of refraction, and ophthalmoscopic examination. In patients with anterior uveitis, phenylephrine is given to dilate the pupil as part of an overall program of treatment.

## Adverse Effects

*Effects on the Eye.* Like the anticholinergic drugs, phenylephrine can precipitate angle-closure glaucoma secondary to production of mydriasis; caution must be exercised in patients whose filtration angle is naturally narrow. Contraction of the dilator muscle may dislodge pigment granules from degenerating cells of the iris; these granules, which appear as "floaters" in the anterior chamber, are usually cleared from the eye within a day. Phenylephrine may also cause ocular pain, corneal clouding, and brow ache.

*Systemic Effects.* Rarely, topical phenylephrine is absorbed in amounts sufficient to produce systemic toxicity. Cardiovascular responses (e.g., hypertension, ventricular dysrhythmias, cardiac arrest) are of greatest concern. Other systemic reactions include sweating, blanching, tremor, agitation, and confusion.

## Additional Ophthalmic Drugs

### Demulcents (Artificial Tears)

Ophthalmic demulcents are isotonic solutions employed as substitutes for natural tears. Most preparations contain *polyvinyl alcohol*, *cellulose esters*, or both. Artificial tears are indicated for treatment of dry-eye syndromes and relief of discomfort and dryness caused by irritants, wind, and sun. In addition, demulcents may be used to lubricate artificial eyes. Artificial tears are devoid of adverse effects, and hence may be administered as frequently and as long as desired.

### Ocular Decongestants

Ocular decongestants are weak solutions of adrenergic agonists applied topically to constrict dilated conjunctival blood vessels. These preparations are used to reduce redness of the eye caused by minor irritation. The adrenergic agents employed as decongestants are *phenylephrine*, *naphazoline*, and *tetrahydrozoline*. When applied to the eye in the low concentrations found in decongestant products, adrenergic agonists rarely cause adverse effects. Local reactions (stinging, burning, reactive hyperemia) may occur with overuse. The adrenergic agonists are discussed at length in Chapter 18.

### Glucocorticoids

Glucocorticoids (anti-inflammatory corticosteroids) are used for inflammatory disorders of the eye (e.g., uveitis, iritis, conjunctivitis). Administration may be topical or by local injection. Short-term therapy is generally devoid of adverse effects. In contrast, prolonged therapy may cause cataracts, reduced visual acuity, and glaucoma. In addition, there is an increased risk of infection secondary to corticosteroid-induced suppression of host defenses. The glucocorticoids are discussed at length in Chapter 65.

### Dyes

*Fluorescein* is a water-soluble dye that produces an intense green color. This agent is applied to the surface of the eye to detect lesions of the corneal epithelium; intact areas of the cornea

remain uncolored while abrasions and other defects turn bright green. Intravenous fluorescein is used to facilitate visualization of retinal blood vessels; IV fluorescein has been employed as an aid for evaluating diabetic retinopathy and other abnormalities of the retinal vasculature. Fluorescein can also be used topically and IV to assess flow of aqueous humor. Adverse effects from systemic administration include nausea, vomiting, paresthesias, and pruritus; severe reactions (anaphylaxis, pulmonary edema, cardiac arrest) are rare.

*Rose bengal* is applied topically to visualize abrasions of the corneal and conjunctival epithelium. Injured tissue appears rose colored when viewed with a slit lamp. The dye is employed for diagnosis of superficial injury to corneal and conjunctival tissue.

### Corneal Dehydrating Agents

*Anhydrous glycerin* [Ophthalgan], *hypertonic sodium chloride* [Adsorbonac, AK-NaCl, Muro-128, Muroptic-5], and *hypertonic glucose* [Glucose-40] are used topically to reduce edema of the cornea. When applied to the surface of the eye, these agents create a hypertonic film that extracts water from the corneal epithelium. Topical glycerin is painful and therefore unsuited for long-term use. Hypertonic sodium chloride may cause transient stinging and burning.

### Chymotrypsin

Chymotrypsin [Catarase 1:500] is a proteolytic enzyme employed during surgery of intracapsular cataracts; the enzyme is given to dissolve the ciliary zonules (i.e., the suspensory structures that support the lens). Chymotrypsin is administered by injection behind the iris into the posterior chamber. Adverse effects include elevation of intraocular pressure, corneal edema, and uveitis. Also, healing of incisions may be delayed.

### Antiviral Agents

Three drugs—*trifluridine*, *vidarabine*, and *idoxuridine*—are used topically to treat viral infections of the eye. The pharmacology and applications of these drugs are discussed in Chapter 87.

## KEY POINTS

- The glaucomas are a group of diseases characterized by visual field loss secondary to optic nerve damage.
- In open-angle glaucoma, optic nerve injury develops gradually over a period of years. The cause of nerve damage is not known.
- In angle-closure glaucoma, there is blockage of aqueous humor outflow, which causes an abrupt rise in IOP. In the absence of treatment, irreversible damage to the optic nerve occurs within 1 or 2 days.
- Drug therapy of open-angle glaucoma is directed at reducing elevated IOP, the major risk factor for this disease.
- Angle-closure glaucoma is treated with drugs to rapidly reduce IOP and then with corrective surgery to allow aqueous humor outflow.
- Drugs reduce IOP by either facilitating aqueous humor outflow or reducing aqueous humor production.
- Timolol and other topical beta blockers lower IOP by decreasing aqueous humor production.
- Topical beta blockers can be absorbed in amounts sufficient to cause bronchospasm, bradycardia, and AV heart block.

- Pilocarpine, a muscarinic agonist, lowers IOP by contracting the ciliary muscle and the iris sphincter. In open-angle glaucoma, contraction of the ciliary muscle widens the spaces within the trabecular meshwork, and thereby facilitates aqueous humor outflow. In angle-closure glaucoma, contraction of the iris sphincter pulls the iris away from the pores of the trabecular meshwork, and thereby removes the impediment to aqueous humor outflow.
- By contracting the ciliary muscle, pilocarpine focuses the lens for near vision. Corrective lenses can help restore far vision.
- By contracting the iris sphincter, pilocarpine can reduce visual acuity.
- Epinephrine, an adrenergic agonist, reduces IOP by increasing aqueous humor outflow.
- Topical epinephrine can be absorbed in amounts sufficient to cause tachycardia and elevation of blood pressure.
- By contracting the radial muscle of the iris, epinephrine dilates the pupil and can thereby aggravate angle-closure glaucoma. Accordingly, epinephrine is contraindicated for this disorder.
- Latanoprost, an analog of prostaglandin $F_2$ alpha, lowers IOP by facilitating aqueous humor outflow.
- Latanoprost can intensify brown pigmentation of the iris.
- Cycloplegics are drugs that paralyze the ciliary muscle.
- Mydriatics are drugs that dilate the pupil.
- Atropine and other anticholinergic drugs cause cycloplegia by blocking muscarinic receptors on the ciliary muscle and mydriasis by blocking muscarinic receptors on the iris sphincter.
- By paralyzing the ciliary muscle, anticholinergic drugs prevent the eye from focusing for near vision.
- By paralyzing the iris sphincter, anticholinergic drugs prevent the pupil from constricting in response to bright light; photophobia results.
- Phenylephrine, an adrenergic agonist, causes mydriasis by stimulating alpha-adrenergic receptors on the radial (dilator) muscle of the iris.

# CHAPTER 98

# Drugs for the Skin

Our objective in this chapter is to discuss some of the more frequently encountered dermatologic drugs. Most are employed topically; some are given systemically. Before discussing the dermatologic drugs, we will review the anatomy of the skin.

## Anatomy of the Skin

The skin is composed of three distinct layers: the epidermis, the dermis, and a layer of subcutaneous fat. These layers and other features of the skin are depicted in Figure 98-1.

*Epidermis.* The epidermis is the outermost layer of the skin and is composed almost entirely of closely packed cells. As indicated in Figure 98-1B, the epidermis itself consists of several layers. The deepest, known as the *basal cell layer* or *stratum germinativum*, contains the only epidermal cells that are mitotically active. All cells of the epidermis arise from this layer. Production of new cells within the basal layer pushes older cells outward. During their migration, these cells become smaller and flatter. As epidermal cells near the surface of the skin, they die and their cytoplasm is converted to *keratin*, a hard, proteinaceous material. Because of its high content of keratin, the outer layer of the epidermis has a rough, horny texture. Because of its texture, this layer is referred to as the *cornified layer* or *stratum corneum*. By a process that is not fully understood, the surface of the stratum corneum undergoes continuous exfoliation (shedding). This shedding completes the growth cycle of the epidermis.

In addition to germinal cells, the basal layer of the epidermis contains *melanocytes*. These cells, which are few in number, produce *melanin*, the pigment that determines skin color. Following its synthesis within melanocytes, melanin is transferred to other cells of the epidermis. Melanin protects the skin against ultraviolet radiation, which is the principal stimulus for melanin production.

*Dermis.* The dermis underlies the epidermis and is composed largely of connective tissue, primarily *collagen*. A major function of the dermis is to provide support and nourishment for the epidermis. Structures found in the dermis include blood vessels, nerves, and muscle. The dermis also contains *sweat glands*, *sebaceous glands*, and *hair follicles*. Sebaceous glands secrete an oily composite known as *sebum*. Almost all sebaceous glands are associated hair follicles (see Fig. 98-1).

*Subcutaneous Tissue.* Subcutaneous tissue consists largely of fat. This fatty layer provides protection and insulation. In addition, the stored fat constitutes a reserve source of calories.

## Topical Glucocorticoids

The basic pharmacology of the glucocorticoids (anti-inflammatory corticosteroids) is discussed in Chapter 65. Consideration here is limited to the use of glucocorticoids for disorders of the skin.

*Actions and Uses.* Topical glucocorticoids are employed to relieve inflammation and itching associated with a variety of dermatologic disorders (e.g., insect bites,

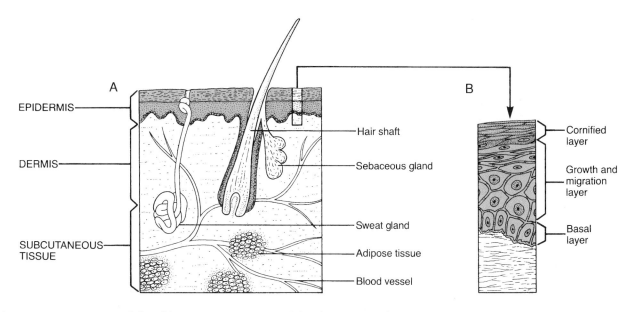

**Figure 98–1. Anatomy of the skin.** *A*, Major structures of the skin. *B*, Growth layers of the epidermis.

minor burns, seborrheic dermatitis, psoriasis, eczema, pemphigus). The mechanisms by which glucocorticoids suppress inflammation and other symptoms are discussed in Chapter 65.

The vehicle in which a glucocorticoid is dispersed (e.g., cream, ointment, gel) can enhance the therapeutic response by facilitating penetration of the glucocorticoid to its site of action. The vehicle may provide additional benefits by acting as a drying agent or as an emollient.

***Relative Potency.*** Glucocorticoid preparations vary widely in potency. As indicated in Table 98–1, steroid preparations can be assigned to four groups, which range from low potency to super-high potency. Preparations within each group are of approximately equal potency.

It is important to note that the intensity of the response to topical glucocorticoids depends not only on the concentration and inherent activity of the glucocorticoid, but also on the vehicle employed and the method of application. Occlusive dressings can enhance percutaneous absorption by as much as 10-fold, thereby greatly increasing pharmacologic effects.

***Absorption.*** Topical glucocorticoids can be absorbed into the systemic circulation. The extent of absorption is proportional to the duration of use and the amount of surface covered. Absorption is higher from regions where the skin is especially permeable (scalp, axilla, face, eyelids, neck, perineum, genitalia) and lower from regions where penetrability is poor (back, palms, soles). Absorption through intact skin is less than through inflamed skin. As noted above, absorption is influenced by the vehicle, and can be greatly increased by use of an occlusive dressing.

***Adverse Effects.*** Adverse effects may be local or systemic. Factors that increase the risk of adverse effects include use of high-potency glucocorticoids, use of occlu-

sive dressings, prolonged therapy, and application over a large surface area.

*Local Reactions.* Glucocorticoids increase the risk of local infection, and may also produce irritation. With prolonged use, glucocorticoids can cause atrophy of the dermis and epidermis, resulting in thinning of the skin, striae (stretch marks), purpura (red spots caused by local hemorrhage), and telangiectasia (red, wart-like lesions caused by capillary dilation). Long-term therapy may induce acne and hypertrichosis (excessive growth of hair, especially on the face).

*Systemic Toxicity.* Topical glucocorticoids can be absorbed in amounts sufficient to produce systemic toxicity. Principal concerns are growth retardation (in children) and adrenal suppression (in all age groups). Systemic toxicity is more likely under extreme conditions of use (prolonged therapy in which extensive surfaces are treated with large doses of high-potency agents in conjunction with occlusive dressings). When these conditions are present, monitoring of the hypothalamic-pituitary-adrenal axis is indicated. Systemic toxicity of the glucocorticoids is discussed at length in Chapter 65.

***Administration.*** Topical glucocorticoids should be applied in a thin film and gently rubbed into the skin. Patients should be advised not to use occlusive dressings (bandages, plastic wraps) unless the physician tells them to. Tight-fitting diapers and plastic pants can act as occlusive dressings and should not be worn when glucocorticoids are applied to the diaper region of infants.

## Keratolytic Agents

Keratolytic agents are drugs that promote shedding of the horny layer of the skin. Effects range from peeling to ex-

## TABLE 98-1. RELATIVE POTENCY OF TOPICAL GLUCOCORTICOID PREPARATIONS

| Potency Class and Drug | Formulation | Concentration |
| --- | --- | --- |
| *Super-High Potency* | | |
| Betamethasone dipropionate [Diprolene] | Cream, ointment, lotion | 0.05% |
| Clobetasol propionate [Temovate] | Cream, ointment | 0.05% |
| Diflorasone diacetate [Psorcon, Maxiflor, Florone] | Ointment | 0.05% |
| Halobetasol propionate [Ultravate] | Cream, ointment | 0.05% |
| *High Potency* | | |
| Amcinonide [Cyclocort] | Cream, ointment, lotion | 0.1% |
| Betamethasone dipropionate [Diprosone] | Cream, ointment | 0.05% |
| Desoximetasone [Topicort] | Cream, ointment | 0.25% |
| Diflorasone diacetate [Florone, Maxiflor] | Cream, ointment | 0.05% |
| Fluocinolone acetonide [Synalar-HP] | Cream | 0.2% |
| Fluocinonide [Fluonex, Lidex] | Cream, ointment, gel | 0.05% |
| Halcinonide [Halog] | Cream, ointment | 0.1% |
| Triamcinolone acetonide [Aristocort, others] | Ointment | 0.1% |
| *Medium Potency* | | |
| Betamethasone benzoate [Uticort] | Lotion | 0.025% |
| Betamethasone dipropionate [Diprosone, others] | Lotion | 0.05% |
| Betamethasone valerate [Valisone, Betatrex] | Cream, ointment, lotion | 0.1% |
| Clocortolone pivalate [Cloderm] | Cream | 0.1% |
| Desoximetasone [Topicort] | Cream | 0.05% |
| Fluocinolone acetonide [Flurosyn, Synalar] | Cream, ointment | 0.025% |
| Flurandrenolide [Cordran] | Cream, ointment, lotion | 0.05% |
| Fluticasone propionate [Cutivate] | Ointment | 0.005% |
| | Cream | 0.05% |
| Halcinonide [Halog] | Cream | 0.025% |
| Hydrocortisone valerate [Westcort] | Cream, ointment | 0.2% |
| Mometasone furoate [Elocon] | Cream, ointment, lotion | 0.1% |
| Triamcinolone acetonide [Aristocort, Kenalog] | Cream, ointment, lotion | 0.1% |
| *Low Potency* | | |
| Alclometasone dipropionate [Aclovate] | Cream, ointment | 0.05% |
| Desonide [DesOwen, Tridesilon] | Cream | 0.05% |
| Dexamethasone [Decaspray] | Aerosol | 0.04% |
| Dexamethasone sodium phosphate [Decadron phosphate] | Cream | 0.1% |
| Fluocinolone acetonide [Flurosyn, Synalar] | Cream, solution | 0.01% |
| Hydrocortisone [Cortizone-10, Hycort] | Cream, ointment, lotion | 1% |

tensive desquamation of the stratum corneum. Three keratolytic compounds—*salicylic acid, resorcinol,* and *sulfur*—are considered below. A fourth agent—*benzoyl peroxide*—is discussed later under *Drugs Used to Treat Acne.*

**Salicylic Acid.** Salicylic acid promotes desquamation by dissolving the intracellular cement that binds scales to the stratum corneum. Keratolytic effects are achieved with drug concentrations ranging from 3% to 6%. At concentrations above 6%, tissue injury is likely. Low (3% to 6%) concentrations are used to treat dandruff, seborrheic dermatitis, acne, and psoriasis. Higher concentrations (up to 40%) are used to remove warts and corns.

Salicylic acid is readily absorbed through the skin and systemic toxicity (salicylism) can result. Symptoms include tinnitus, hyperpnea, and psychologic disturbances. Systemic effects can be minimized by avoiding prolonged use of high concentrations over a large surface.

**Resorcinol.** Resorcinol has mild keratolytic and antimicrobial activity. The drug is used to treat acne, eczema, psoriasis, and seborrheic dermatitis. Resorcinol is available in a variety of formulations, including shampoos, ointments, lotions, and creams. Usual concentrations range from 1% to 10%.

**Sulfur.** Sulfur promotes peeling and drying. The compound has been used to treat acne, dandruff, psoriasis, and seborrheic dermatitis. Sulfur is available in lotions, gels, and shampoos. Concentrations range from 2% to 10%.

## Acne and Its Treatment

### Pathophysiology

Acne is a skin disorder common in adolescents and young adults. Lesions usually develop on the face, neck, chest, shoulders, and back. In mild acne, *open comedones* (blackheads) are the most common lesion. A comedo forms when sebum combines with keratin to form a plug within a pore (oxidation of the sebum causes the exposed surface of the plug to turn black). *Closed comedones* (whiteheads) develop when pores become stuffed with sebum and scales below the skin surface. In its most severe form, acne is characterized by abscesses and inflammatory cysts.

Onset of acne is initiated by increased production of androgens during adolescence. Under the influence of androgens, sebum production and turnover of follicular epithelial cells are increased, leading to plugging of pores. Symptoms are intensified by the activity of *Propionibacterium acnes*, a microbe that converts sebum into irritant fatty acids. This bacterium also releases chemotactic factors that promote inflammation. Oily skin and a genetic predisposition are additional contributing factors.

## Overview of Treatment

### Nondrug Therapy

Nondrug measures can help minimize lesions, especially in patients with milder acne. Surface oiliness should be reduced by gentle cleansing 2 or 3 times a day. Care should be taken to avoid irritation from vigorous scrubbing and use of abrasives. Oil-based moisturizing products should be avoided. Additional nondrug measures (e.g., comedo extraction, dermabrasion, collagen injection) may be indicated for some individuals. Dietary measures don't help.

### Drug Therapy

Drug selection is based on severity of symptoms. *Mild* acne can be managed with cleansers, drying agents (acetone, alcohol), and keratolytics (sulfur, resorcinol, salicylic acid, and 2.5% or 5% benzoyl peroxide). Topical agents for *moderate* acne include 10% benzoyl peroxide, tretinoin, adapalene, azelaic acid, and antibiotics (e.g., clindamycin, erythromycin). Drugs for *severe* acne include systemic antibiotics (usually tetracycline), isotretinoin, and intralesional glucocorticoids.

## Drugs Used to Treat Acne

### Benzoyl Peroxide

*Actions and Uses.* Benzoyl peroxide is employed topically to treat mild to moderate acne. The drug decreases symptoms by (1) promoting keratolysis (peeling of the horny layer of the epidermis), and (2) suppressing growth of *P. acnes.* (Antibacterial effects are caused by release of active oxygen.)

*Adverse Effects.* Benzoyl peroxide may produce drying and peeling of the skin. If signs of severe local irritation occur (e.g., burning, blistering, scaling, swelling), the frequency of application should be reduced. The drug is absorbed through the skin, but systemic toxicity has not been reported.

*Preparations, Dosage, and Administration.* Benzoyl peroxide is available in a variety of formulations (e.g., lotions, creams, gels) for topical use. Concentrations range from 2.5% to 10%. For

initial therapy, once-a-day application is recommended. Later, the frequency of administration can be increased to 4 times a day as tolerance permits. Patients should be advised to avoid application to the eyes, mouth, and mucous membranes, and to inflamed or denuded skin.

### Antibiotics

*Topical.* Topical antibiotics are indicated for moderate acne. The objective is to suppress growth of *P. acnes.* The antibiotics used most are *clindamycin* and *erythromycin.* Either drug may be employed alone or in combination with other topical antiacne drugs (e.g., benzoyl peroxide, tretinoin). With prolonged use, bacterial resistance may develop. A fixed-dose combination of 3% erythromycin with 5% benzoyl peroxide is available under the trade name Benzamycin.

*Oral.* When acne is severe enough to warrant systemic antibiotic therapy, oral *tetracycline* is the treatment of choice. Tetracycline is effective, inexpensive, and has low toxicity. Treatment reduces the population of *P. acnes*, the amount of keratin in sebaceous follicles, and the percentage of free fatty acids in surface lipids. A satisfactory alternative to tetracycline is *erythromycin.*

Although tetracycline is the most frequently used *oral* antibiotic for acne, it is rarely used *topically.* Topical use is limited because tetracycline has relatively low efficacy when applied topically and because topical application turns the skin yellow.

### Tretinoin

*Uses and Mechanisms.* Tretinoin [Retin-A, Renova], a derivative of vitamin A, is a topical drug used for acne and removal of fine wrinkles. Formulations for acne are marketed under the trade name Retin-A. The formulation for wrinkles, which is nearly identical to one of the formulations for acne, is marketed under the trade name Renova. Tretinoin should not be confused with isotretinoin, an *oral* antiacne medicine (see below).

*Acne.* Tretinoin is approved for topical treatment of mild to moderate acne. Therapeutic effects can be enhanced by using the drug in combination with benzoyl peroxide and oral antibiotics.

Although the mechanism for clearing acne is unknown, tretinoin is thought to help at least in part by increasing the turnover and reducing the cohesiveness of epithelial cells within hair follicles. These actions may promote removal of existing comedones and may suppress formation of new plugs. In addition, by reducing the thickness of the stratum corneum, tretinoin can enhance penetration of other antiacne drugs.

*Fine Wrinkles.* Tretinoin was recently approved for mitigating (reducing) fine wrinkles, tactile roughness, and mottled hyperpigmentation (liver spots, age spots) in facial skin. Benefits may derive from suppressing genes that code for specific proteases that break down collagen and elastin. In clinical trials, responses to tretinoin were modest. In fact, many patients achieved equivalent effects with a program of comprehensive skin care and sun protection. It is important to note that tretinoin does *not* repair deep, coarse wrinkles and other damage caused by chronic sun exposure. Furthermore, the drug does not eliminate wrinkles, repair sun-damaged skin, reverse photoaging, or restore the microscopic structure of skin to a more youthful pattern. Lastly, benefits in patients over the age of 50 have not been established.

**Adverse Effects.** Tretinoin can cause localized reactions, but absorption is insufficient to cause systemic toxicity. In patients with sensitive skin, tretinoin may induce blistering, peeling, crusting, burning, and edema. These effects can be intensified by concurrent use of abrasive soaps and keratolytic agents (e.g., sulfur, resorcinol, benzoyl peroxide, salicylic acid). Accordingly, these preparations should be discontinued prior to tretinoin therapy.

Tretinoin increases susceptibility to sunburn. Patients should be warned to apply a sunscreen (SPF 15 or greater) and wear protective clothing. Patients with existing sunburn should not use the drug.

**Preparations, Dosage, and Administration.** *For Acne.* Tretinoin [Retin-A] is available in three formulations for acne: cream (0.025%, 0.05%, 0.1%), gel (0.01%, 0.025%), and liquid (0.05%). Administration is topical, usually once daily at bedtime. Before application, the skin should be washed, toweled dry, and allowed to dry fully for 15 to 30 minutes. The drug should not be applied to open wounds or to areas of sunburn or windburn. Contact with the eyes, nose, and mouth should be avoided.

*For Fine Wrinkles.* Tretinoin [Renova] is available in a 0.05% cream for treating fine wrinkles of the face. The drug is applied once daily at bedtime. Cosmetics should be washed off before use. Up to 6 months of treatment may be needed to see a response.

## Adapalene

Adapalene [Differin] is a new topical antiacne drug similar to tretinoin. Through actions exerted in the cell nucleus, adapalene modulates inflammation, epithelial keratinization, and differentiation of follicular cells. As a result, the drug reduces formation of comedones and inflammatory lesions. Benefits take 8 to 12 weeks to develop. During the early weeks of treatment, adapalene may appear to exacerbate acne because of effects on previously invisible lesions. In clinical trials, 0.1% adapalene gel was as effective as 0.025% tretinoin gel in reducing the total number of comedones, and was more effective than tretinoin in reducing the total number of acne lesions and inflammatory lesions.

Adverse effects are limited to sites of application. The drug is not absorbed, and hence systemic effects are absent. Common effects include burning (10%–40%), pruritus or burning immediately after application (20%), erythema, dryness, and scaling. These are most likely during the first 2 to 4 weeks of treatment and tend to subside as treatment continues.

Adapalene increases the risk of developing sunburn and can intensify existing sunburn. Accordingly, all patients should apply a sunscreen and wear protective clothing prior to extended sun exposure. In addition, adapalene should not be used until existing sunburn has resolved.

## Azelaic Acid

Azelaic acid [Azelex] is a new topical drug for mild to moderate acne. It appears to work by suppressing growth of *P. acnes* and by decreasing proliferation of keratinocytes, which decreases the thickness of the stratum corneum. In clinical trials, topical azelaic acid (20% cream) was as effective as 5% topical benzoyl peroxide, 0.05% topical tretinoin, or 2% topical erythromycin. For severe acne, azelaic acid was much less effective than oral isotretinoin. Adverse effects—which are uncommon and less intense than with tretinoin or benzoyl peroxide—include pruritus, burning, stinging, tingling, and erythema. Azelaic acid may decrease pigmentation in patients with dark complexions; hence these people should be monitored for hypopigmentation. Azelaic acid is applied twice daily by gently massaging a thin film into the affected area. Contact with the eyes, nose, and mouth should be avoided. Before application, the skin should be washed and dried.

## Isotretinoin

**Actions and Use.** Isotretinoin, a derivative of vitamin A, is used to treat *severe* acne vulgaris, a condition for which the drug is highly effective. For most patients, a single course of therapy can produce complete and prolonged remission. However, because the risk of serious side effects is high, isotretinoin should be reserved for patients who have failed to respond to more conventional agents, including oral antibiotics.

Isotretinoin has several actions that may contribute to its antiacne effects. The drug decreases sebum production, sebaceous gland size, inflammation, and keratinization. In addition, by decreasing availability of sebum, a nutrient for *P. acnes*, isotretinoin lowers the skin population of this microbe.

**Pharmacokinetics.** Absorption from the gastrointestinal tract is rapid but incomplete. In the blood, isotretinoin is nearly 100% bound to plasma albumin. The drug undergoes metabolism in the liver and possibly in cells of the intestinal wall. Excretion is by a combination of renal and biliary processes. The drug's half-life is 10 to 20 hours.

**Adverse Effects.** The most common reactions are nosebleeds (80%), inflammation of the lips (90%), inflammation of the eyes (40%), and dryness or itching of the skin, nose, and mouth (80%). About 15% of patients experience pain, tenderness, or stiffness in muscles, bones, and joints. Less common reactions include skin rash, headache, hair loss, and peeling of skin from the palms and soles. Reductions in night vision have occurred, sometimes with sudden onset. The skin may become sensitized to ultraviolet light; patients should be advised to wear protective clothing or a sunscreen if responses to sunlight become exaggerated. Rarely, isotretinoin causes optic neuritis, cataracts, papilledema (edema of the optic disk), and pseudotumor cerebri (benign elevation of intracranial pressure).

Triglyceride levels may become elevated. Blood triglyceride content should be measured prior to treatment and periodically thereafter until effects on triglycerides have been evaluated. Alcohol can potentiate hypertriglyceridemia and should be avoided.

Although adverse effects occur frequently, most reverse upon discontinuing the drug. Teratogenic effects are the major and obvious exception to this rule.

***Contraindication: Pregnancy.*** *Isotretinoin is terato-genic and must not be used during pregnancy.* The drug is classified in FDA Pregnancy Category X: the risks of use during pregnancy clearly outweigh any possible benefits. Major fetal abnormalities that have occurred include hydrocephalus, microcephaly, facial malformation, cleft palate, cardiovascular defects, and abnormal formation of the outer ear.

Before isotretinoin is given to women of reproductive age, pregnancy should be ruled out and a method of contraception implemented. Contraception should be initiated at least 1 month prior to the onset of treatment and should continue for at least 1 month after treatment has ceased. Women should be thoroughly counseled about the potential for fetal harm if pregnancy should occur. If pregnancy does occur, isotretinoin should be discontinued immediately, and possible termination of pregnancy should be discussed.

***Drug Interactions.*** Adverse effects of isotretinoin can be increased by *tetracyclines* and *vitamin A*. Tetracyclines increase the risk of pseudotumor cerebri and papilledema. Vitamin A, being a relative of isotretinoin, can produce generalized intensification of isotretinoin toxicity. Because of the potential for increased toxicity, tetracyclines and vitamin A supplements should be discontinued prior to isotretinoin therapy.

***Preparations, Dosage, and Administration.*** Isotretinoin [Accutane] is dispensed in capsules (10, 20, and 40 mg) for oral administration. The usual course of treatment is 0.5 to 1 mg/kg/day (in two divided doses) for 15 to 20 weeks. If needed, a second course may be given, but not until 2 months have elapsed after completing the first course.

## Psoriasis and Its Treatment

### Pathophysiology

Psoriasis is a chronic disorder that follows an erratic course. The initial episode usually develops in early adulthood. Subsequent attacks may occur spontaneously or may be triggered by emotional stress, streptococcal pharyngitis (sore throat), and certain drugs (e.g., propranolol, indomethacin). There is no cure for psoriasis, but symptoms can usually be controlled with medication. Drug-induced remission is common and may last from a few weeks to many years.

Psoriasis has varying degrees of severity. Mild disease manifests as red patches covered with silvery scales; lesions typically appear on the scalp, elbows, knees, palms, and soles. Severe disease may involve the entire skin surface and mucous membranes; patients may develop superficial pustules, high fever, leukocytosis, and painful fissuring of the skin. The primary defect in psoriasis is accelerated maturation of the epidermis: in people with psoriasis, epidermal cells complete their growth cycle in 3 to 4 days, rather than the 26 to 28 days required for maturation in healthy skin.

### Overview of Treatment

Drug selection is based on the severity of symptoms. For mild psoriasis, topical glucocorticoids are usually adequate; keratolytic agents (e.g., sulfur, salicylic acid) may be useful adjuncts to steroid therapy. Calcipotriene may also be tried. For patients with moderate symptoms, coal tar or anthralin may be added to the regimen. Topical therapy with tar and anthralin can be enhanced by exposing the skin to ultraviolet B light. Treatment options for severe psoriasis include phototherapy or systemic treatment with methotrexate or etretinate.

### Topical Drugs for Psoriasis

#### Glucocorticoids

In the United States, glucocorticoids are the most commonly used topical drugs for psoriasis. Preparations of super-high-potency are employed where plaques are thickest. However, super-high-potency agents should not be applied to the face, groin, axilla, or genitalia because skin in these regions is especially vulnerable to glucocorticoid-induced atrophy.

#### Anthralin

Anthralin is indicated only for topical treatment of psoriasis. The drug inhibits DNA synthesis and thereby suppresses proliferation of hyperplastic epidermal cells.

Anthralin may cause local irritation, especially when applied in concentrations exceeding 1%. Erythema (redness) may develop in normal skin adjacent to areas of treatment. Severe conjunctivitis can develop following contact with the eyes. Systemic toxicity has not been documented. Anthralin preparations can stain clothing, skin, and hair.

Anthralin is dispensed in ointments and creams, with concentrations ranging from 0.1% to 1%. In conventional therapy, the drug is applied to lesions at bedtime and allowed to remain in place overnight. Stains can be avoided by wearing old clothing and by covering treated areas with a dressing. Trade names for anthralin products are Anthra-Derm, Lasan, Drithocreme, and Dritho-Scalp.

#### Tars

Tars suppress DNA synthesis, mitotic activity, and cell proliferation. Coal tar is the tar employed most frequently. Preparations that contain juniper tar, birch tar, and pine tar are also available. Tar-containing products (e.g., shampoos, lotions, creams) are used to treat psoriasis and other chronic disorders of the skin. Tars have an unpleasant odor and can cause irritation, stinging, and burning. They may also stain the skin and hair. Systemic toxicity does not occur.

#### Calcipotriene

Calcipotriene [Dovonex], an analog of vitamin $D_3$, is the newest topical preparation for mild to moderate psoriasis. Responses are equal to those achieved with medium-potency topical glucocorticoids. Benefits may derive from the drug's ability to suppress cell differentiation and proliferation. The most common adverse effect is local skin irritation. Unlike glucocorticoids, calcipotriene does not cause thinning of the skin. At doses twice the weekly recommended maximum of 100 gm, calcipotriene has caused hypercalcemia. Long-term safety has not been established.

### Systemic Drugs for Psoriasis

#### Methotrexate

The basic pharmacology of methotrexate [Folex, Rheumatrex] is discussed in Chapter 96 (Anticancer Drugs). Consideration here is limited to the use of methotrexate for psoriasis.

***Actions and Use in Psoriasis.*** Methotrexate is a cytotoxic agent that shows some selectivity for tissues with a high growth fraction (i.e., tissues with a large percentage of actively dividing cells). Benefits in psoriasis result from reduced proliferation of epidermal cells. The biochemical mechanisms underlying suppression of cell growth and division are discussed in Chapter 96. Methotrexate is highly toxic (see below) and should be used only in patients with severe, debilitating psoriasis that has not responded to safer therapy.

*Adverse Effects.* Methotrexate is administered systemically, and toxicity can be severe. Death has occurred. Patients should be fully informed of the risks of treatment. Close medical supervision is required. Gastrointestinal effects (diarrhea, ulcerative stomatitis) are the most frequent reasons for interrupting therapy. Blood dyscrasias (anemia, leukopenia, thrombocytopenia) from bone marrow depression are an additional major concern. With prolonged use, even at relatively low doses, methotrexate can cause significant harm to the liver; hepatic function must be monitored. A liver biopsy is the best method for assessing injury. Methotrexate can cause congenital anomalies and fetal death. Accordingly, the drug is contraindicated during pregnancy.

*Dosage and Administration.* Methotrexate may be administered PO, IM, or IV. Various dosing schedules have been developed. In one schedule, the drug is administered once a week as a single large dose (10 to 25 mg). In an alternative schedule, three smaller doses (2.5 to 5 mg) are administered at 12-hour intervals; this dosing sequence is repeated weekly. Regardless of the schedule chosen, dosages must be individualized.

### Etretinate

*Therapeutic Use.* Oral etretinate [Tegison] is indicated for severe pustular and erythrodermic psoriasis. Side effects can be severe; hence, the drug should be reserved for patients who have not responded to safer treatments. Initial responses develop in many patients after 4 to 6 weeks of treatment. However, other patients may require 6 months of treatment before a clinical response is evident. Long-term maintenance therapy is sometimes required.

*Mechanism of Action.* Etretinate acts on epithelial cells to inhibit keratinization, proliferation, and differentiation. These actions probably contribute to the drug's beneficial effects. Benefits may also derive from anti-inflammatory and immunomodulatory actions.

*Adverse Effects.* Adverse effects are extremely common. Dermatologic effects (hair loss; peeling of palms, soles, and fingertips) occur in 75% of patients. Mucous membranes are affected, causing dry nose (75%), thirst and sore mouth (50-75%), and nose bleed (25%). Other very common reactions include bone and joint pain (50-75%), muscle cramps (25-50%), fatigue (50-75%), headache (25-50%), and eye irritation (50-75%). In addition, etretinate can elevate plasma concentrations of cholesterol and triglycerides, and can reduce levels of high-density lipoproteins.

*Contraindication: Pregnancy. Etretinate can cause severe fetal malformations and must not be used during pregnancy.* The drug is classified in FDA Pregnancy Category X: the risks to the developing fetus outweigh any possible benefits of treatment. Pregnancy must be ruled out before etretinate is given. Women of child-bearing age should be instructed to use some form of contraception before starting treatment, during treatment, and for an indefinite period after treatment has stopped (etretinate can be measured in the blood up to 3 years after terminating treatment). If pregnancy occurs during treatment, etretinate should be discontinued immediately, and termination of pregnancy should be considered.

*Preparations, Dosage, and Administration.* Etretinate [Tegison] is dispensed in capsules (10 and 25 mg) for oral administration. The usual initial adult dosage is 0.75 to 1 mg/kg/day in divided doses. The maximum dosage is 1.5 mg/kg/day.

### Glucocorticoids

Systemic glucocorticoids are effective against psoriasis, but cause Cushing's syndrome and other serious side effects. In addition, psoriasis may worsen when glucocorticoids are discontinued. Most specialists do not use these drugs. If systemic glu-cocorticoids must be employed, they should be reserved for short-term therapy of patients with severe symptoms.

## Phototherapy

### Ultraviolet B Irradiation Plus Coal Tar

In this procedure, affected regions are covered with 1% coal tar ointment and then exposed to short-wave ultraviolet radiation (ultraviolet B, UVB). This form of treatment is very safe and produces remission in 80% of patients. Unfortunately, the procedure is expensive and time consuming (up to 30 treatments are needed), and patients dislike being coated with smelly coal tar.

### Photochemotherapy (PUVA Therapy)

Photochemotherapy combines the use of long-wave ultraviolet radiation (ultraviolet A, UVA) with *methoxsalen*, an orally administered photosensitive drug. Methoxsalen belongs to a chemical family known as psoralens. In response to UVA light shined on the skin, methoxsalen is thought to undergo a photochemical reaction with DNA, resulting in the formation of a DNA-psoralen complex. This alteration in DNA structure is thought to underlie the ability of photochemotherapy to decrease proliferation of epidermal cells. Adverse effects associated with the procedure include pruritus, nausea, and erythema. In addition, the process may accelerate aging of the skin and may increase the risk of skin cancer. Photochemotherapy is indicated for patients with extensive, active psoriasis who have not responded adequately to more conventional therapy. An alternative name for photochemotherapy is *PUVA therapy*; PUVA is an abbreviation derived from *psoralen* and *ultraviolet A.*

---

## Miscellaneous Dermatologic Drugs

### Agents Used to Remove Warts

The common wart (*verruca vulgaris*) is a virally induced skin disease that manifests as a hard, horny nodule. Warts may appear anywhere on the body but are most common on the hands and feet. It should be noted that warts are benign lesions and their presence is no threat to health.

Warts may be removed by physical procedures and by application of drugs. The physical methods of wart removal are freezing, electrodesiccation (destruction with an electric current), and curettage (surgical removal with a loop-shaped cutting tool). The principal pharmacologic agents employed are *salicylic acid, podophyllum resin*, and *cantharidin*. Salicylic acid is discussed above; podophyllum, and cantharidin are discussed below.

### Podophyllum Resin

*Actions and Uses.* Podophyllum resin is indicated primarily for condylomata acuminata (venereal warts). The drug is not very effective against common warts. The major active component of podophyllum resin is *podophyllotoxin*, a compound that inhibits synthesis of DNA and mitosis. These actions eventually lead to cell death and erosion of warty tissue.

*Adverse Effects.* Podophyllum can be absorbed in amounts sufficient to cause systemic toxicity. Systemic effects are most likely when the drug is applied to large areas in excessive amounts. Potential systemic reactions include central and peripheral neuropathy, kidney damage, and blood dyscrasias. Podophyllum is teratogenic and must not be used during pregnancy.

*Preparations and Administration.* Podophyllum resin [Podocon-25, Podofin] is available in a 25% solution for topical use. Application should be limited to small areas. The drug should not be applied to moles or birthmarks, nor should it be applied to warts that are bleeding or friable (easily crumbled) or that have undergone recent biopsy. When used to remove venereal warts, podophyllum resin should be washed off 1 to 6 hours after application. Treatment may be repeated at weekly intervals for up to 4 weeks.

**Cantharidin**

Cantharidin [Cantharone, Verr-Canth] is a topical agent used to remove common warts and the nodules associated with molluscum contagiosum, a benign, virally induced skin disease. Clearance of these growths results from acantholysis (dissolution of intercellular bridges within the epidermis). Lower layers of the skin are not affected. For treatment of common warts, cantharidin is applied to the lesion, allowed to dry, and covered with nonporous tape. The tape should be removed in 24 hours. If needed, this procedure may be repeated in 1 to 2 weeks. Cantharidin is harmful to normal skin. In the event of accidental exposure, the affected area should be cleansed immediately with acetone or alcohol.

## Antiperspirants and Deodorants

Perspiration is produced by two types of sweat glands: *eccrine glands* and *apocrine glands.* The eccrine glands secrete profuse, watery perspiration. The output of apocrine glands is low in volume and rich in organic compounds. The unpleasant odor associated with sweating results from chemical and bacterial degradation of the compounds in apocrine sweat. Eccrine glands contribute to odor formation by creating a moist environment that favors growth of bacteria. Perspiration odor can be reduced with *antiperspirants* (agents that decrease flow of eccrine sweat) and *deodorants* (antiseptics that suppress growth of skin-dwelling bacteria).

**Antiperspirants.** The principal compounds employed as antiperspirants are *aluminum chlorohydrate, aluminum zirconium chlorohydrate, aluminum chloride,* and *buffered aluminum sulfate.* These agents can decrease flow of eccrine sweat by 20% to 50%. The reduction in flow is thought to result from inhibition of sweat production and from partial occlusion of sweat glands. Topical antiperspirants can cause stinging, burning, itching, and irritation. Dermatitis and ulceration occur rarely.

**Deodorants.** Deodorants inhibit growth of the surface bacteria that degrade components of apocrine sweat into malodorous products; deodorants do not suppress sweat formation. Agents employed as deodorants include *carbanilide, triclocarban,* and *triclosan.* These antiseptics are the active ingredients in deodorant soaps, such as Dial, Lifebuoy, Safeguard, and Zest.

## Drugs for Seborrheic Dermatitis and Dandruff

Seborrheic dermatitis is characterized by inflammation and scaling of the scalp and face. Skin of the underarms, chest, and anogenital region may also be affected. Symptoms result from an inflammatory reaction to infection with *Pityrosporum ovale,* a microbe in the yeast family.

Symptoms respond rapidly to topical treatment with *ketoconazole* [Nizoral], a drug with activity against yeast (see Chapter 86). For treatment of seborrhea, ketoconazole is available in cream and shampoo formulations. Concurrent use of topical glucocorticoids can accelerate initial responses. Once the yeast infection has been controlled, remission can be maintained by periodic use of a shampoo that contains a yeast-suppressing drug, such as *ketoconazole, pyrithione zinc,* or *selenium sulfide.*

## Topical Minoxidil for Baldness

Minoxidil is a direct-acting vasodilator used primarily for severe hypertension. The basic pharmacology of minoxidil is discussed in Chapter 40. Consideration here is limited to the use of minoxidil to promote hair growth.

**Actions, Uses, and Dosage.** A 2% minoxidil solution [Rogaine] is approved for topical treatment of male-pattern baldness. The usual dosage is 1 ml applied 2 times a day. Topical minoxidil increases cutaneous blood flow (by inducing vasodilation), and may also stimulate resting hair follicles to enter a state of active growth. These actions may explain the ability of minoxidil to promote hair growth.

**Clinical Response.** Minoxidil can retard loss of hair and stimulate hair growth. Beneficial effects take several months to develop. Unfortunately, response rates have been somewhat disappointing: only about one third of patients experience significant restoration of hair to regions of baldness. Hair regrowth is most likely when baldness has developed recently and has been limited to a small area. Upon discontinuation of minoxidil, newly gained hair is lost in 3 to 4 months, and the natural progression of hair loss resumes. In some cases, beneficial effects may decline even with uninterrupted treatment.

**Adverse Effects.** Topical minoxidil is generally devoid of adverse effects. A few patients have experienced pruritus and local allergic responses (e.g., rash, swelling, burning sensation). Absorption is low (about 1.5%), and systemic reactions (e.g., hypotension, headache, flushing) are rare.

## Debriding Enzymes

Topical enzymes can be applied to burns and wounds to facilitate debridement (removal of foreign material and necrotic tissue). Three such debriding preparations—*collagenase, sutilains,* and a *fibrinolysin-desoxyribonuclease combination*—are discussed below.

**Collagenase.** Collagenase [Santyl] digests native and denatured collagen, the compound that composes 75% of the dry weight of skin. By dissolving collagen, the enzyme can facilitate loosening and removal of tissue debris. Collagenase is used to promote debridement of dermal lesions and severe burns. The enzyme is inactivated by detergents, certain antiseptics (hexachlorophene, nitrofurazone, benzalkonium chloride, iodine), and heavy metals (e.g., mercury, silver). Accordingly, these compounds must be removed by careful washing prior to collagenase use. Collagenase ointment is applied once daily and covered with a sterile dressing. Side effects are limited to transient erythema in surrounding tissue. Allergic and toxic reactions have not been reported.

**Sutilains.** Sutilains [Travase] is a proteolytic enzyme that digests necrotic material but has no effect on viable tissue. The enzyme is used as an aid to debridement of decubitus ulcers, second- or third-degree burns, and other skin lesions. Like collagenase, sutilains can be inactivated by detergents and certain antiseptics (e.g., hexachlorophene, nitrofurazone, benzalkonium chloride, iodine); hence, these agents must be removed by washing prior to sutilains application. Sutilains ointment should be applied to the site of injury and to adjacent healthy skin, and the treated area should be covered with a wet dressing. Application may be repeated 3 or 4 times each day. Mild local reactions (transient pain, paresthesias) are benign. In the event of more serious local toxicity (hemorrhage, dermatitis), sutilains should be discontinued. Systemic toxicity has not been reported.

**Fibrinolysin Plus Desoxyribonuclease.** Fibrinolysin is an enzyme that digests fibrin, a major component of clots; desoxyribonuclease digests deoxyribonucleic acid (DNA). The rationale for the combined use of these enzymes derives from the observation that purulent exudates are composed largely of fibrin and nucleic acids. The enzyme combination is indicated for debridement of surgical wounds, ulcerative lesions, and second- or third-degree burns. Side effects include local irritation and erythema.

The combination of fibrinolysin plus desoxyribonuclease is dispensed in two forms: an ointment, and a powder for reconstitution to solution. These products are marketed under the trade name Elase.

### Fluorouracil

The basic pharmacology of fluorouracil is discussed in Chapter 96 (Anticancer Drugs). Discussion here is limited to the use of fluorouracil for dermatologic disorders.

***Actions and Uses in Dermatology.*** Fluorouracil is indicated for topical treatment of *multiple actinic keratoses* and *superficial basal cell carcinoma*. Cytotoxic effects result from disruption of DNA and RNA synthesis. A course of topical treatment elicits the following sequence of responses: (1) mild inflammation; (2) severe inflammation, often with burning, stinging, and vesicle formation; (3) tissue disintegration, characterized by erosion, ulceration, and necrosis; and (4) healing. Although fluorouracil is only applied for 2 to 6 weeks, the process just described may require 3 or more months for completion.

***Adverse Effects.*** Among the more frequent reactions to fluorouracil are itching, burning, rash, inflammation, and increased sensitivity to sunlight. Intense, burning pain develops occasionally. Darkening of the skin is rare. Absorption is insufficient to cause systemic toxicity.

***Preparations and Administration.*** Fluorouracil [Efudex, Fluoroplex] is dispensed in a cream (1% and 5%) and solution (1%, 2%, and 5%) for topical use. For treatment of actinic keratoses, the drug is applied twice daily until a stage-three response (tissue disintegration) develops, usually within 2 to 6 weeks. Complete healing may not occur for another 1 to 2 months.

### Sunscreens

Sunlight has multiple effects on the skin. In addition to promoting tanning, solar radiation can cause burns, premature aging of the skin, and skin cancer. Sun exposure can also cause photosensitivity reactions to drugs. All of these effects are due to ultraviolet light. Sunburn, carcinogenesis, and premature aging of the skin are caused primarily by ultraviolet (UV) radiation in the B range (wavelengths of 290 to 320 nm). In contrast, tanning and most drug-related photosensitivity reactions are triggered by UV light in the A range (wavelengths of 320 to 400 nm).

***Therapeutic Uses of Sunscreens.*** Sunscreens impede penetration of solar radiation to viable cells of the skin. These preparations are used primarily to prevent sunburn. Sunscreens are also used to prevent skin cancer, delay premature aging of the skin, and prevent photosensitivity reactions to certain drugs (e.g., tricyclic antidepressants, phenothiazines, sulfonamides, sulfonylureas).

***Compounds Employed as Sunscreens.*** Most compounds employed as sunscreens act by absorbing UV light. The agents used to absorb UV radiation fall into five major groups: (1) *para*-aminobenzoic acid (PABA) and its esters, (2) cinnamates, (3) salicylates, (4) benzophenones, and (5) anthranilates. All of these compounds absorb UV radiation in the B range; only the benzophenones and anthranilates have the additional ability to absorb some UVA light.

Two sunscreen formulations—Photoplex and Shade UVA Guard—offer extended protection against UVA radiation. Photoplex has two active ingredients: padimate O, which provides UVB protection, and avobenzone, which provides extended UVA protection. Shade UVA Guard has three active ingredients: octyl methoxycinnamate, which provides UVB protection, and avobenzone and oxybenzone, which provide extended UVA protection. Because they protect against UVA, Photoplex and Shade UVA Guard may be superior to other sunscreens for preventing photosensitivity reactions to drugs.

Some sunscreens act as physical barriers to the sun's rays. Hence, rather than absorbing solar radiation, these compounds reflect and scatter sunlight, thereby preventing its penetration to the skin. The agents employed as physical sunblocks include *titanium dioxide*, *zinc oxide*, and *talc*. Preparations containing these compounds are especially useful for protecting limited areas (e.g., nose, lips, tips of ears).

***Sun Protection Factor.*** Commercial sunscreen products are labeled with a sun protection factor (SPF). The SPF is determined by shining UV light on adjacent regions of protected and unprotected skin and recording the time required for erythema (redness) to develop in both areas. The SPF is calculated by dividing the time required for erythema to develop in the protected region by the time required for erythema to develop in the unprotected region. For example, if the unprotected region developed erythema in 15 minutes, whereas 150 minutes were required for burn to appear in the protected region, the sunscreen would have an SPF of 10 (150 divided by 15). The SPF for sunscreens ranges from 1 (lowest protection) to 50 (highest protection). An SPF of 15 or greater is recommended. It should be noted that the methods for determining the SPF are not highly precise; hence, all products labeled with the same SPF may not provide an equal degree of protection.

***Using Sunscreens to Prevent Sunburn.*** Sunscreens must be used properly to achieve maximum benefit. Individuals who have skin that burns easily should choose a preparation with a high SPF. For all people, protection is greatest when a sunscreen has been allowed to penetrate the skin in advance of exposure to the sun. Accordingly, it is recommended that sunscreens be applied 30 minutes to 1 hour prior to going outdoors. The amount applied is an important determinant of protection; 2 $mg/cm^2$ is considered adequate. Sunscreens should be reapplied after swimming and profuse sweating; failure to do so reduces the duration of protection. However, it is important to note that reapplication will not extend the period of protection beyond that indicated by the SPF. That is, if treated skin can be expected to burn when sun exposure exceeds 2 hours, no amount of reapplication can prevent burning if the duration of exposure exceeds the limit.

Environmental factors play a part in sunscreen use. The intensity of UVB radiation is greatest between the hours of 10 AM and 3 PM. Accordingly, the need for a sunscreen is correspondingly high during this time. Ultraviolet radiation can be reflected by painted surfaces, white sand, and snow, thereby augmenting total UV exposure; the contribution of reflected radiation should be considered when choosing a sunscreen. Clouds can filter out UV radiation. However, it should be appreciated that the amount of UV light reaching the ground on a bright day with thin cloud cover can be as much as 80% of that reaching the ground on days that are sunny and clear. Ultraviolet radiation can penetrate at least several centimeters of clear water; swimmers should be made aware of this fact.

***Adverse Effects of Sunscreens.*** Sunscreens are generally well tolerated. Contact sensitivity and photosensitivity reactions occur in a few individuals. These reactions can be elicited by almost all sunscreen products. However, for most people, a nonsensitizing preparation can be found.

### Local Anesthetics

Local anesthetics (e.g., benzocaine, dibucaine) can be applied topically to relieve pain and itching associated with various skin disorders, including sunburn, plant poisoning, fungal infections, diaper rash, and eczema. Selection of a topical anesthetic is based on required duration of action, desired vehicle (cream, ointment, solution, gel), and prior history of hypersensitivity reactions. The pharmacology of the local anesthetics is discussed in Chapter 26. Table 26-2 lists the agents available for application to the skin.

## Anti-Infective Agents

The skin is subject to fungal, viral, and bacterial infections. Some of these infections respond to topical treatment; others require systemic treatment. *Antibacterial* drugs are discussed in Chapters 78 through 82. *Antifungal* and *antiviral* drugs are discussed in Chapters 86 and 87, respectively. Topical drugs for prophylaxis against infection (antiseptics) are discussed in Chapter 90.

## KEY POINTS

- Topical glucocorticoids are employed to relieve inflammation and itching associated with a variety of dermatologic disorders.
- Preparations of topical glucocorticoids are classified into four potency groups: low, medium, high, and super-high.
- Prolonged use of topical glucocorticoids can cause atrophy of the dermis and epidermis.
- Topical glucocorticoids can be absorbed in amounts sufficient to cause systemic toxicity. Principal concerns are growth retardation and adrenal suppression.

- Keratolytic agents—salicylic acid, resorcinol, sulfur, and benzoyl peroxide—promote shedding of the horny layer of the skin.
- Topical antibiotics, such as clindamycin or erythromycin, help clear mild to moderate acne by suppressing growth of *P. acnes*.
- Tetracycline is the most frequently used oral antibiotic for acne.
- Tretinoin, a derivative of vitamin A, is a topical drug used for acne and for removing fine wrinkles from the face.
- Topical tretinoin increases susceptibility to sunburn. Patients should use a sunscreen (SPF 15 or greater) and wear protective clothing.
- Azelaic acid, a topical drug for mild to moderate acne, appears to work by suppressing growth of *P. acnes* and by decreasing proliferation of keratinocytes.
- Isotretinoin is an oral drug for severe acne.
- Isotretinoin causes multiple adverse effects, including nosebleeds, inflammation of the lips and eyes, and pain, tenderness, or stiffness in muscles, bones, and joints.
- Isotretinoin is teratogenic and must not be used during pregnancy.

# CHAPTER 99

# Miscellaneous Noteworthy Drugs

**Drugs for Obesity**
    Assessment of Health Risk
    Treatment Options
    Appetite-Suppressant Drugs

**Drugs for Respiratory Distress Syndrome**
**Drugs for Benign Prostatic Hyperplasia**
**Drugs for Cystic Fibrosis**
**Riluzole for Amyotropic Lateral Sclerosis**

## Drugs for Obesity

Obesity, defined as an excess of body fat, is a major public health problem. The condition increases the risk of hypertension, heart disease, diabetes mellitus, and some cancers. In the United States, 58 million adults (35% of women and 31% of men) are obese or overweight, as are 25% of children ages 6 to 17. Obesity-related disorders kill about 300,000 Americans each year, which makes obesity the second leading cause of preventable death. (Smoking, which kills about 500,000 Americans each year, is the leading cause.)

Obesity is now viewed as a chronic disease, much like hypertension and diabetes. Despite intensive research, the underlying cause remains incompletely understood. Contributing factors include genetics, metabolism, and appetite regulation in the brain, along with environmental, psychosocial, and cultural factors. Although obese people can lose weight, the tendency to regain weight cannot be eliminated. Put another way, obesity cannot yet be cured. Accordingly, for most patients, lifelong management is required.

Much of the discussion that follows is based on recommendations in *Guidance for Treatment of Adult Obesity*, published in 1996 by two not-for-profit organizations: Shape Up America! and the American Obesity Association.

### Assessment of Health Risk

Health risk is determined by (1) the degree of obesity (as reflected in the body mass index) and (2) the presence of comorbid conditions (e.g., hypertension, heart disease) and other risk factors (e.g., family history of obesity, pattern of fat distribution, smoking, lack of physical activity).

***Body Mass Index.*** The body mass index (BMI), which is based on the patient's height and weight, is a simple way to estimate weight-related health risk. BMI is calculated by dividing weight (in kilograms) by the square of height (in meters). Hence, BMI is expressed in units of

$kg/m^2$. As shown in Figure 99–1, BMI can also be calculated using the patient's weight in *pounds* and height in *inches*. To facilitate BMI determination, Figure 99–1 also contains a BMI chart. Values in the chart apply only to individuals ages 19 to 70. The values do *not* apply to growing children, elderly patients who are frail and sedentary, women who are pregnant or lactating, and competitive athletes or body builders (i.e., individuals who are heavy because of muscle mass rather than excess fat).

***Comorbid Conditions.*** Comorbid conditions are disorders that get worse with increasing weight gain and improve with weight loss. Major comorbid conditions include hypertension, coronary artery disease, heart failure, elevated low-density lipoprotein (LDL) cholesterol, noninsulin-dependent diabetes (type II diabetes), sleep apnea (obesity is the primary cause), and osteoarthritis. Comorbid conditions increase the health risk over that associated with an elevated BMI alone.

***BMI-Related Health Risk.*** As indicated in Table 99–1, health risk rises as BMI gets larger. In addition, the risk is increased by the presence of comorbid conditions and other risk factors. In the *absence* of comorbid conditions, health risk is minimal for individuals with a BMI below 25, and low for individuals with a BMI below 27. Conversely, a BMI of 27 or more indicates significant risk. In the *presence* of comorbid conditions, health risk is low for individuals with a BMI below 25, and significant at a BMI of 25 or higher.

### Treatment Options

Treatment options are based on BMI-related health risk (Table 99–1). Options are summarized in Table 99–2 and discussed below.

***Minimal Health Risk.*** Individuals in this health risk category are at minimal risk for all-cause mortality. Accordingly, there is no health-associated reason for them to lose weight. Nonetheless, discussion of ways to prevent weight gain may be appropriate.

## BMI CHART

WEIGHT (pounds)

| HEIGHT | 120 | 125 | 130 | 135 | 140 | 145 | 150 | 155 | 160 | 165 | 170 | 175 | 180 | 185 | 190 | 195 | 200 | 205 | 210 | 215 | 220 | 225 |
|---|---|---|---|---|---|---|---|---|---|---|---|---|---|---|---|---|---|---|---|---|---|---|
| 5' 0" | 23 | 24 | 25 | 26 | 27 | 28 | 29 | 30 | 31 | 32 | 33 | 34 | 35 | 36 | 37 | 38 | 39 | 40 | 41 | 42 | 43 | 44 |
| 5' 1" | 23 | 24 | 25 | 26 | 26 | 27 | 28 | 29 | 30 | 31 | 32 | 33 | 34 | 35 | 36 | 37 | 38 | 39 | 40 | 41 | 42 | 43 |
| 5' 2" | 22 | 23 | 24 | 25 | 26 | 27 | 27 | 28 | 29 | 30 | 31 | 32 | 33 | 34 | 35 | 36 | 37 | 37 | 38 | 39 | 40 | 41 |
| 5' 3" | 21 | 22 | 23 | 24 | 25 | 26 | 27 | 27 | 28 | 29 | 30 | 31 | 32 | 33 | 34 | 35 | 35 | 36 | 37 | 38 | 39 | 40 |
| 5' 4" | 21 | 21 | 22 | 23 | 24 | 25 | 26 | 27 | 27 | 28 | 29 | 30 | 31 | 32 | 33 | 33 | 34 | 35 | 36 | 37 | 38 | 39 |
| 5' 5" | 20 | 21 | 22 | 22 | 23 | 24 | 25 | 26 | 27 | 27 | 28 | 29 | 30 | 31 | 32 | 32 | 33 | 34 | 35 | 36 | 37 | 37 |
| 5' 6" | 19 | 20 | 21 | 22 | 23 | 23 | 24 | 25 | 26 | 27 | 27 | 28 | 29 | 30 | 31 | 31 | 32 | 33 | 34 | 35 | 36 | 36 |
| 5' 7" | 19 | 20 | 20 | 21 | 22 | 23 | 23 | 24 | 25 | 26 | 27 | 27 | 28 | 29 | 30 | 31 | 31 | 32 | 33 | 34 | 34 | 35 |
| 5' 8" | 18 | 19 | 20 | 21 | 21 | 22 | 23 | 24 | 24 | 25 | 26 | 27 | 27 | 28 | 29 | 30 | 30 | 31 | 32 | 33 | 33 | 34 |
| 5' 9" | 18 | 18 | 19 | 20 | 21 | 21 | 22 | 23 | 24 | 24 | 25 | 26 | 27 | 27 | 28 | 29 | 30 | 30 | 31 | 32 | 33 | 33 |
| 5'10" | 17 | 18 | 19 | 19 | 20 | 21 | 22 | 22 | 23 | 24 | 24 | 25 | 26 | 27 | 27 | 28 | 29 | 29 | 30 | 31 | 32 | 32 |
| 5'11" | 17 | 17 | 18 | 19 | 20 | 20 | 21 | 22 | 22 | 23 | 24 | 24 | 25 | 26 | 26 | 27 | 28 | 29 | 29 | 30 | 31 | 31 |
| 6' 0" | 16 | 17 | 18 | 18 | 19 | 20 | 20 | 21 | 22 | 22 | 23 | 24 | 24 | 25 | 26 | 26 | 27 | 28 | 28 | 29 | 30 | 31 |
| 6' 1" | 16 | 16 | 17 | 18 | 18 | 19 | 20 | 20 | 21 | 22 | 22 | 23 | 24 | 24 | 25 | 26 | 26 | 27 | 28 | 28 | 29 | 30 |
| 6' 2" | 15 | 16 | 17 | 17 | 18 | 19 | 19 | 20 | 21 | 21 | 22 | 22 | 23 | 24 | 24 | 25 | 26 | 26 | 27 | 28 | 28 | 29 |
| 6' 3" | 15 | 16 | 16 | 17 | 17 | 18 | 19 | 19 | 20 | 21 | 21 | 22 | 22 | 23 | 24 | 24 | 25 | 26 | 26 | 27 | 27 | 28 |
| 6' 4" | 15 | 15 | 16 | 16 | 17 | 18 | 18 | 19 | 19 | 20 | 21 | 21 | 22 | 23 | 23 | 24 | 24 | 25 | 26 | 26 | 27 | 27 |

## CALCULATING YOUR BMI

To calculate your BMI, all you need to know is your height (in inches) and weight (in pounds). You can then calculate your BMI as follows:

Step 1) Multiply your weight by 703
Step 2) Multiply your height by your height (square the height)
Step 3) Divide the result in step 1 by the result in step 2.

*Example:* For a person 5'7" (67") tall weighing 142 pounds.

Step 1) 142 x 703 = 99826
Step 2) 67 x 67 = 4489
Step 3) 99286 •/• 4489 = 22.2   (Rounded off, BMI = 22)

**Figure 99–1. BMI chart and method for calculating BMI.** Shading in the BMI chart indicates degree of health risk. For individuals *without* comorbid conditions, no shading indicates *minimal* risk, light shading indicates *low* risk, and dark shading indicates risk that is *moderate or greater*. For individuals *with* comorbid conditions, light shading indicates *moderate* risk and dark shading indicates risk that is *high or greater*. (Adapted from Guidance for Treatment of Adult Obesity, published jointly by Shape Up America! and American Obesity Association, 1996.)

***Low Health Risk.*** People in this category are at slightly increased risk for all-cause mortality. Accordingly, further weight gain should be avoided. If the patient desires, a plan for modest weight reduction should be offered.

***Moderate Health Risk.*** People in this category are at increased risk for hypertension, coronary artery disease, heart failure, noninsulin-dependent diabetes, stroke, and some types of cancer. As a result, their risk of early death is elevated. Ideally, treatment should include a reduced-calorie diet and increased physical activity. If the patient does not want to lose weight, the clinician should at least discuss a plan to prevent further gain.

***High or Very High Health Risk.*** Weight reduction is clearly indicated. The treatment plan should include a reduced-calorie diet, increased physical activity (as appropriate), and drug therapy. At this time, all of the drugs used to treat obesity act by suppressing appetite. Drugs that act by other mechanisms, such as reducing fat absorption or increasing energy metabolism, are under development.

***Extremely High Health Risk.*** For people in this category, obesity and comorbidity decrease both the quality of life and life expectancy. Accordingly, weight reduction is strongly recommended. Treatment options include a

| BMI Category | Health Risk Based Only on BMI | Health Risk Adjusted for Presence of Comorbid Conditions and/or Other Risk Factors* |
|---|---|---|
| <25 | Minimal | Low |
| 25 to <27 | Low | Moderate |
| 27 to <30 | Moderate | High |
| 30 to <35 | High | Very high |
| 35 to <40 | Very high | Extremely high |
| 40 or more | Extremely high | Extremely high |

*Comorbid conditions and risk factors include hypertension, coronary artery disease, heart failure, elevated LDL-cholesterol, noninsulin-dependent diabetes (type II diabetes), sleep apnea, osteoarthritis, personal or family history of obesity, smoking, and lack of physical activity.

Adapted from Guidance for Treatment of Adult Obesity, published jointly by Shape Up America! and American Obesity Association, 1996.

**TABLE 99–2. OBESITY TREATMENT BASED ON BMI-BASED HEALTH RISK**

| BMI-Based Health Risk | Suggested Treatment |
|---|---|
| Minimal or low | Healthful eating and/or moderate-deficit diet<br>Increased physical activity<br>Lifestyle change strategies |
| Moderate | The above plus *low-calorie diet* |
| High or very high | All of the above plus *drug therapy* and *very-low calorie diet* |
| Extremely high | All of the above plus *surgical intervention* |

Adapted from Guidance for Treatment of Adult Obesity, published jointly by Shape Up America! and American Obesity Association, 1996.

reduced-calorie diet and drug therapy. In addition, for patients with a BMI of 40 or more (in the absence of co-morbidity), or 35 or more (in the presence of comorbidity), surgical intervention should be considered. The two most widely accepted procedures are known as *vertical banded gastroplasty* and *Roux-en-Y gastric bypass*.

## Appetite-Suppressant Drugs

Appetite suppressants, also known as *anorexiants*, are intended for use in the context of a comprehensive weight reduction program—one that includes exercise, behavior modification, and a reduced-calorie diet. Drugs are not indicated as the sole means of controlling caloric intake. Furthermore, they should be reserved for patients whose BMI-related health risk is high, very high, or extremely high (see Table 99–2). Drugs are not appropriate for patients whose BMI-related health risk is low or minimal.

To remain effective, anorexiant drugs must be taken indefinitely. The reason is that the majority of patients regain lost weight when drugs are discontinued. (This is analogous to the return of high blood pressure when antihypertensive drugs are withdrawn.) Unfortunately, none of the available appetite suppressants are approved for long-term use. However, although anorexiants are not approved for prolonged use, such use is nonetheless common. (Until recently, dexfenfluramine was approved for prolonged use, but the drug was withdrawn because of concerns about causing valvular heart disease.)

Patients should lose at least 4 pounds during the first 4 weeks of drug treatment. If this initial response is absent, further drug use should be questioned. With prolonged treatment, the greatest weight loss occurs during the first 6 months. After that, continued treatment helps maintain the loss. In most cases, weight is regained when long-term treatment is discontinued.

Appetite suppressants fall into two major categories: serotonergic drugs and catecholaminergic drugs. Members of both groups are listed in Table 99–3, along with their trade names and dosages.

### Serotonergic Agents

Until recently, two serotonergic agents were available: dexfenfluramine and fenfluramine. However, in 1997 both drugs were withdrawn from the market because they appear to injure valves of the heart. In addition to causing valvular heart disease, both drugs carry a small risk of primary pulmonary hypertension, a potentially fatal disease. In contrast to the catecholaminergic agents, which all cause central nervous system (CNS) stimulation, the serotonergic drugs cause mild CNS depression.

*Dexfenfluramine.* *Therapeutic Use.* Prior to being withdrawn, dexfenfluramine [Redux] was the only anorexiant approved by the FDA for long-term use. Benefits derive from suppressing appetite for carbohydrates. Initial therapy facilitates weight loss, whereas maintenance therapy helps prevent weight from being regained. Compared with patients taking placebo, those taking dexfenfluramine lost more weight and were better able to maintain weight loss. However, when treatment is discontinued, weight loss among those receiving placebo and those receiving dexfenfluramine became equal within months. This observation underscores the need for continuous treatment.

When dexfenfluramine was available, it was indicated only for individuals who were significantly overweight. Candidates should have a BMI of 30 or more (in the absence of comorbid conditions) or 27 or more (in the presence of comorbid conditions). Dexfenfluramine was never considered appropriate for slightly overweight people looking for an easy way to drop a few pounds.

*Mechanism of Action.* Dexfenfluramine reduces appetite by increasing stimulation of serotonin receptors in the brain. Two mechanisms are involved. (1) the drug promotes serotonin release and inhibits serotonin reuptake, thereby increasing serotonin availability at receptors, and

## TABLE 99-3. APPETITE-SUPPRESSANT DRUG

| Generic Name | Trade Name | Adult Dosage* | CSA[†] Schedule |
|---|---|---|---|
| *Serotonergic Agents* | | | |
| Dexfenfluramine[§] | Redux | 15 mg 2 times/day | IV |
| Fenfluramine[§] | Pondimin | 20 mg 3 times/day | IV |
| *Catecholaminergic Agents* | | | |
| Benzphetamine | Didrex | 25–50 mg 1–3 times/day | III |
| Diethylpropion | Tenuate, Tepanil | 25 mg 3 times/day SR: 75 mg once/day | IV |
| Mazindol | Mazanor, Sanorex | 1 mg 3 times/day or 2 mg once/day | IV |
| Phendimetrazine | Bontril, Prelu-2, Plegine, X-Trozine | 35 mg 2–3 times/day SR: 105 mg once/day | III |
| Phenmetrazine | Preludin | 75 mg once a day | II |
| Phentermine | Adipex-P, Fastin, Ionamin, Obenix, Oby-Cap, Oby-Trim, Zantryl | 8 mg 3 times/day or 15–37.5 mg once/day | IV |
| Phenylpropanolamine | Dexatrim, Acutrim | 25 mg 3 times/day SR: 75 mg once/day | NR[‡] |

*SR = sustained release.
[†]CSA = Controlled Substance Act.
[‡]NR = Not regulated under CSA.
[§]Withdrawn from the market in 1997.

(2) a metabolite of dexfenfluramine (d-norfenfluramine) activates serotonin receptors directly.

*Pharmacokinetics.* Dexfenfluramine is administered by mouth and undergoes slow but complete absorption in the intestines. Plasma drug levels peak about three hours after dosing. Hepatic metabolism converts some of each dose to inactive metabolites and some to *d*-norfenfluramine, an active metabolite. All metabolites are excreted in the urine. The half-life of fenfluramine itself is about 17 hours, compared with 32 hours for *d*-norfenfluramine.

*Adverse Effects.* Common side effects include *diarrhea* (17.5%), *dry mouth* (12.5%), and *drowsiness* (7.1%). In contrast to the catecholaminergic drugs, dexfenfluramine does not cause CNS stimulation, and therefore has a low potential for abuse. Accordingly, the drug is classified under Schedule IV of the Controlled Substances Act.

Studies reported in 1997 suggest that dexfenfluramine can cause *valvular heart disease*. Echocardiographic examination of patients taking the drug indicates a 30% incidence of regurgitation involving the mitral, aortic, and/or tricuspid valves. Although most patients with valve injury have been asymptomatic, some have displayed symptoms of heart failure (dyspnea, fatigue, edema). In a few cases, surgery has been required to correct valve leakage. At this time, we do not know if asymptomatic valve injury is reversible. Because of the association between dexfenfluramine and valvular heart disease, the drug has been withdrawn from the market. Individuals who have taken dexfenfluramine should consult their physicians about appropriate follow-up

Rarely, patients taking dexfenfluramine have developed *primary pulmonary hypertension* (PPH), a potentially fatal disorder characterized by elevated pulmonary artery pressure. The 4-year survival rate is only 55%. To improve chances of survival, patients should be instructed to report early signs of PPH, such as fatigue, dyspnea, reduced exercise tolerance, chest pain, fainting, and swollen ankles. It should be noted that a risk of PPH is not limited to dexfenfluramine: fenfluramine, phendimetrazine, and other anorexiants have also been implicated. Fortunately, the incidence of PPH is extremely low: the disorder develops in about 28 patients per million patients-years of drug use. By way of comparison, the risk of dying from dexfenfluramine-induced PPH is about equal to the risk of dying from penicillin-induced anaphylaxis or oral contraceptive-induced cardiovascular complications.

*Drug Interactions.* Because of the risk of serotonin syndrome (see Chapter 30), dexfenfluramine should not be taken with fluoxetine [Prozac] and other *selective serotonin reuptake inhibitors* (SSRIs). In addition, the drug should not be combined with selegiline [Eldepryl], phenelzine [Nardil], and other *monoamine oxidase inhibitors* (MAOIs). MAOIs should be withdrawn at least 2 weeks before giving dexfenfluramine, and dexfenfluramine should be withdrawn at least 3 weeks before giving an MAOI.

*Preparations, Dosage, and Administration.* Prior to being withdrawn, dexfenfluramine [Redux] was available in 15-mg tablets for oral use. The recommended dosage was 15 mg twice daily with meals.

**Fenfluramine.** Fenfluramine [Pondimin] is a racemic mixture of *d*-fenfluramine (dexfenfluramine) and *l*-fenfluramine. Only the *d*-isomer is active. Accordingly, the pharmacologic profile of fenfluramine is nearly identical to that of dexfenfluramine. Like dexfenfluramine, fenfluramine carries a high risk of valvular heart disease, and hence has been withdrawn from the market. Prior to being withdrawn, fenfluramine was frequently prescribed in combination with phentermine (see below).

### Catecholaminergic Agents

Catecholaminergic agents act primarily by increasing availability of norepinephrine at receptors in the brain. The result is a decrease in appetite. Catecholaminergic anorexiants fall into two major groups: amphetamines and nonamphetamines. In general, the amphetamines have a higher abuse potential than the nonamphetamines. Accordingly, nonamphetamines are generally preferred.

**Amphetamines.** Because of their ability to suppress appetite, the amphetamines have been employed as adjunctive aids in programs for weight loss. However, because of their high abuse potential, and because they offer no advantages over less dangerous drugs, amphetamines are not usually recommended for weight reduction. In fact, in some states, the use of amphetamines for weight reduction is prohibited by law. When deciding to employ amphetamines to promote weight loss, the risks of abuse must be carefully weighed against the potential benefits. Prescriptions for weight control should be short term. Amphetamines should not be provided when overeating is the result of psychologic factors, since amphetamines are ineffective for these people.

Dosage depends on the amphetamine preparation. For *dextroamphetamine* [Dexedrine, others] and *amphetamine sulfate*, the dosage is 5 to 30 mg/day. For *methamphetamine* [Desoxyn], the dosage is 10 to 15 mg/day. For *amphetamine complex* [Biphetamine], the dosage is 10 to 15 mg/day.

The basic pharmacology of the amphetamines is discussed in Chapter 33.

**Nonamphetamines.** The nonamphetamine catecholaminergic agents are listed in Table 99–3. None of these drugs is more effective than the amphetamines at suppressing appetite. However, in most cases, these agents cause fewer adverse effects than the amphetamines and have a lower potential for abuse. Hence, these drugs are generally preferred to amphetamines for promoting weight loss.

All of these drugs are CNS stimulants. Consequently, like the amphetamines, they can increase alertness, decrease fatigue, and induce nervousness and insomnia. Because of their potential to interfere with sleep, they should be administered no later than 4 PM. Upon discontinuation of treatment, fatigue and depression may replace CNS stimulation.

Like the amphetamines, most of the nonamphetamine catecholaminergic agents have effects in the periphery as well the CNS. Peripheral effects of greatest significance are tachycardia, anginal pain, and hypertension. Accordingly, these drugs should be used with caution in patients with cardiovascular disease.

Although the abuse potential of the nonamphetamine anorexiants is generally lower than that of the amphetamines, abuse can nonetheless occur. As shown in Table 99–3, classification of these drugs under the Controlled Substances Act ranges from Schedule II to Schedule IV; only phenylpropanolamine is unregulated. To reduce the risk of abuse, an attempt should be made to identify abuse-prone patients prior to treatment.

Tolerance is common and may be seen in 6 to 12 weeks. Tolerance to the anorexiant effects of one agent produces cross-tolerance to the others. If tolerance develops, the appropriate response is to discontinue the drug rather than increase the dosage.

For two reasons, these drugs are not recommended for use during pregnancy. First, they are not very effective during preg-

nancy; hence there is little point in taking them. Second, *in utero* exposure to these agents poses an increased risk of cleft palate and congenital heart defects.

## Combination Therapy: Fenfluramine plus Phentermine (Fen-Phen)

Prior to 1997, when fenfluramine was withdrawn from the market, it was common practice to treat patients with a combination of fenfluramine (a serotonergic agent) and phentermine (a catecholaminergic agent)—although the combination, commonly known as "fen-phen," was never approved by the FDA. In theory, fen-phen has two potential benefits. First, since fenfluramine and phentermine act by different mechanisms, the combination might suppress appetite while allowing both drugs to be given in reduced dosages, thereby decreasing side effects. Second, since fenfluramine and phentermine have opposing effects on arousal (fenfluramine causes drowsiness whereas phentermine causes stimulation), combined use might neutralize both effects. As discussed above, fenfluramine has been associated with valvular heart disease, and hence is no longer available. In contrast, phentermine, by itself, does *not* appear to injure the heart, and hence may still be purchased for use alone.

# Drugs for Respiratory Distress Syndrome

Respiratory distress syndrome (RDS) is the primary cause of morbidity and mortality in premature infants. The underlying cause is deficiency of lung surfactant, a complex mixture of phospholipids and apoproteins that lowers surface tension on alveolar surfaces. Consequences of surfactant deficiency include alveolar collapse, pulmonary edema, reduced lung compliance, small airway epithelial damage, hypoxia, and, ultimately, respiratory failure.

Increased production of cortisol during weeks 30 to 32 of gestation initiates production of lung surfactant. However, surfactant production is not fully adequate until weeks 34 to 36. As a result, the earlier the premature infant is delivered, the greater the risk of RDS. Among infants born during weeks 26 to 28, the incidence of RDS is 60% to 80%; by weeks 30 to 32, the incidence drops to only 20%.

## Antenatal Glucocorticoids

When preterm delivery cannot be prevented, injecting the mother with glucocorticoids can accelerate fetal lung maturation, and thereby decrease the incidence and severity of RDS. Glucocorticoids act by stimulating production of fibroblast pneumocyte factor, which in turn stimulates production of surfactant by fetal pneumocytes. Glucocorticoids are effective when used during weeks 24 to 34 of gestation. Beyond week 34, fetal lungs are sufficiently mature that no benefit is gained by giving glucocorticoids. Common regimens include (1) dexamethasone, 4 mg IM or IV every 8 hours for 6 doses; and (2) betamethasone, two 12-mg doses injected IM, 12 or 24 hours apart. To be effective, the last glucocorticoid dose must be administered at least 24 hours before delivery, but no more than 7 days before. Accordingly, if delivery does not take place within 7 days of the last dose, and if tests of amniotic fluid do not indicate lung maturation, glucocorticoid dosing should be repeated. The basic pharmacology of the glucocorticoids is discussed in Chapters 56 and 65.

## Lung Surfactant

Lung surfactant, administered by direct intratracheal instillation, is indicated for prevention and treatment (rescue therapy) of RDS. Surfactant therapy rapidly improves oxygenation and lung compliance, reduces the need for supplemental oxygen and mechanical ventilation, and decreases neonatal mortality by 33%.

In the United States, two surfactant preparations are available: *beractant* [Survanta] and *colfosceril palmitate* [Exosurf Neonatal]. Both contain dipalmitoylphosphatidylcholine (aka colfosceril or lecithin), the major surface-active compound in natural surfactant. At this time, there is insufficient data to recommend one drug over the other. For prevention or treatment of RDS, the dosage is 67.5 mg/kg for colfosceril and 100 mg/kg for beractant. Since the effects of a single dose are often transient, administration may need to be repeated.

Adverse effects result primarily from the administration process. Bradycardia and oxygen desaturation, which occur secondary to vagal stimulation and airway obstruction, are most common. If these occur, it may be necessary to temporarily suspend administration. Other adverse effects include pulmonary hemorrhage, mucous plugging, and endotracheal tube reflux.

# Drugs for Benign Prostatic Hyperplasia

## Pathophysiology and Overview of Treatment

*Pathophysiology.* Benign prostatic hyperplasia (BPH) is a nonmalignant enlargement of the prostate caused by excessive growth of epithelial (glandular) and smooth muscle cells. Overgrowth of epithelial cells causes *mechanical obstruction* of the urethra, whereas overgrowth of smooth muscle causes *dynamic obstruction* of the urethra. In men with BPH, the ratio of epithelium to smooth muscle varies from 1:3 to 4:1—in general, the larger the prostate, the higher the percentage of epithelium. Signs and symptoms of BPH include urinary hesitancy, urinary urgency, increased frequency of urination, dysuria, nocturia, straining to void, postvoid dribbling, decreased force and caliber of the urinary stream, and a sensation of incomplete bladder emptying. There is no direct correlation between symptoms and prostate size. Hence, some men with only moderate enlargement may be highly symptomatic, whereas others with substantial enlargement may have no symptoms at all. BPH is a very common condition that develops in more than 50% of men by age 60 and 90% by age 85. Although BPH and prostate cancer can co-exist, there is no evidence that one disorder predisposes to the other.

*Treatment Modalities.* BPH can be managed in three ways: drug therapy, surgery, and "watchful waiting." Surgical options include transurethral resection of the prostate, transurethral electrovaporization of the prostate, and laser prostatectomy. These procedures are most appropriate for men with severe symptoms or complications (urinary tract infection, uremia due to obstruction, bladder stones). Watchful waiting, which consists of reassurance and annual re-evaluation, is appropriate for men with minimal symptoms.

## Drug Therapy

BPH can be treated with *finasteride* and with *alpha₁-adrenergic antagonists*. The goal of treatment is to relieve bothersome urinary symptoms. As discussed below, finasteride may be most appropriate for patients with very large prostates, whereas alpha blockers may be preferred for patients with relatively small prostates.

*Finasteride.* Finasteride [Proscar] promotes shrinkage of the prostate. Benefits of treatment develop slowly, over 6 to 12 months. Finasteride works by preventing conversion of testosterone to dihydrotestosterone (DHT), the active form of testosterone in the prostate. By decreasing DHT availability, finasteride promotes regression of prostate epithelial tissue, and thereby decreases *mechanical obstruction* of the urethra. Since the percentage of epithelial tissue is highest in very large prostates, finasteride is most effective in men whose prostates are highly enlarged. Conversely, the drug has little or no effect if the degree of prostate enlargement is small. Finasteride is generally well tolerated. However, it does decrease ejaculate volume and libido in 5% to 10% of patients. In addition, gynecomastia (breast enlargement) develops in some men. The usual dosage is 5 mg/day. Treatment continues for life.

Finasteride decreases serum levels of prostate-specific antigen (PSA), a marker for prostate cancer. The expected decline is 30% to 50%. PSA levels should be determined prior to treatment and 6 months later. If PSA levels do not fall as expected, the patient should be evaluated for cancer of the prostate.

*Alpha₁-Adrenergic Antagonists.* Alpha₁ antagonists, such as *terazosin* [Hytrin], *doxazosin* [Cardura], and tamsulosin [Flomax], relax smooth muscle in the prostate capsule, prostatic urethra, and bladder neck, and thereby decrease *dynamic obstruction* of the urethra. Improvement in symptoms and urinary flow develops rapidly. Since dynamic obstruction is the major contributor to symptoms in patients with relatively mild prostatic enlargement, alpha blockers are preferred to finasteride for these men. Since alpha blockers are indicated for hypertension as well as BPH, these drugs are especially well suited for patients with both disorders. Adverse effects include hypotension, fainting, dizziness, somnolence, nasal congestion, impotence, and retrograde ejaculation (secondary to relaxation of smooth muscle in the bladder neck). Unlike finasteride, alpha blockers do not decrease levels of PSA. To maintain benefits, alpha blockers must be taken lifelong. The basic pharmacology of alpha blockers is discussed in Chapter 19.

# Drugs for Cystic Fibrosis

Cystic fibrosis (CF) is an inherited disorder that results in damage to the lungs, pancreas, and other organs. Thirty years ago, 50% of children diagnosed with CF died before the age of 5. Today, the mean survival is 30 years. Drugs cannot cure CF, but they can reduce symptoms and slow progression of injury.

## Pathophysiology

The underlying cause of CF is mutation of the gene that codes for a particular type of chloride channel, referred to as the cystic fibrosis transmembrane regulator (CFTR). In cells that have defective CFTRs, the normal transmembrane flow of chloride ions, sodium ions, and water is disrupted. In the lungs, exocrine glands (e.g., pancreas), and other structures, disruption of ion and water flux alters secretions.

*Pancreas.* Disruption of chloride transport in the pancreas impairs secretion of bicarbonate and digestive enzymes into the small intestine. The immediate result is maldigestion and malabsorption of fats and other nutrients. Absorption of fat-soluble vitamins, especially vitamins A and E, is reduced secondary to malabsorption of fats. Over time, accumulation of digestive enzymes within pancreatic cells leads to cellular destruction. At autopsy, the pancreas appears scarred and fibrotic, which led pathologists to name this illness fibrocystic disease of the pancreas—later shortened to cystic fibrosis. Until replacement therapy with pancreatic enzymes became possible, malabsorption of nutrients was the major cause of death for patients with CF.

*Lungs.* Today, destruction of lung tissue is the major cause of morbidity and mortality among patients with CF. In the cells that line the airway, defective CFTRs impair secretion of chloride and enhance reabsorption of water and sodium. As a result, mucus becomes thick and viscous, causing plugging of the airway and promoting chronic bacterial colonization. All patients eventually develop active pulmonary infection; the most common pathogens are *Staphylococcus aureus*, *Haemophilus influenzae*, and *Pseudomonas aeruginosa*. Infection elicits an inflammatory response that is mediated primarily by neutrophils. Accumulation of DNA from dead neutrophils further increases the viscosity of sputum. Over time, chronic bronchitis and associated inflammation cause progressive destruction of lung tissue. In 95% of patients, death from cardiorespiratory failure ultimately ensues.

*Reproductive Organs.* Among patients with CF, 98% of males and 70% to 80% of females are infertile. In males,

the usual cause is *in utero* obstruction of the vas deferens. In females, the cause appears to be production of thick, sticky cervical mucus, which impedes penetration of sperm.

## Drug Therapy

Drugs are used to alleviate symptoms of CF and delay progression of injury to the lungs. Agents employed include pancreatic enzymes, fat-soluble vitamins, antibiotics, dornase alfa, and ibuprofen. Gene therapy is under investigation.

*Pancreatic Enzymes.* These enzymes are given as replacement therapy. All preparations contain lipase, protease, and amylase. The most effective formulations deliver the enzymes in enteric-coated microspheres, which are designed to (1) protect the enzymes from stomach acid and (2) ensure dissolution in the duodenum, the site where the enzymes act. Pancreatic enzymes are discussed further in Chapter 73.

*Fat-Soluble Vitamins.* There are four fat-soluble vitamins: A, D, E, and K. Among patients with CF, deficiencies in vitamins A and E are relatively common, whereas deficiency in vitamin K is uncommon and deficiency in vitamin D is rare. Since vitamins are safe and relatively inexpensive, supplementation with all four is common practice.

*Antibiotics.* Antibiotics are used to manage acute exacerbations of chronic lung infection. Agents employed include aminoglycosides (e.g., gentamicin, tobramycin), penicillins (e.g., carbenicillin, ticarcillin), and third-generation cephalosporins (e.g., ceftazidime). Selection among these agents is often empiric. The usual duration of therapy is 14 to 21 days. Success is indicated by improvement in pulmonary function, decreased sputum production, decreased dyspnea, normalization of the white blood cell count, and improvement in overall sense of well being.

*Dornase Alfa.* Dornase alfa [Pulmozyme], a purified preparation of recombinant human deoxyribonuclease, decreases the viscosity of sputum in patients with CF. Dornase alfa is administered by inhalation, using an approved nebulizer. Benefits derive from breaking down extracellular DNA that has accumulated in the lungs secondary to death of neutrophils. With daily use, dornase alfa can improve pulmonary function and decrease infection in some patients. The drug is generally well tolerated. Adverse effects include hoarseness, pharyngitis, laryngitis, rash, chest pain, and conjunctivitis. Dosing is begun at 2.5 mg once daily and may be increased to 2.5 mg twice daily if needed. To remain effective, dornase alfa must be administered daily for life. Unfortunately, treatment is expensive. A year's supply of dornase alfa costs over $12,000. The nebulizer costs another $2000.

*Ibuprofen.* High-dose ibuprofen can slow progression of pulmonary damage in patients with mild lung disease caused by CF. Benefits derive from suppressing the inflammatory response that underlies destruction of lung tissue. Ibuprofen dosage should be sufficient to produce peak plasma drug levels of 50 to 100 µg/ml. Side effects attributable to ibuprofen include conjunctivitis and epistaxis (nosebleed).

# Riluzole for Amyotropic Lateral Sclerosis

Amyotrophic lateral sclerosis (ALS, Lou Gehrig's disease) is a neuromuscular disorder characterized by progressive muscle wasting and loss of strength. The underlying cause is degeneration of motor neurons, especially in the outside (lateral) portion of the spinal cord. Why motor neurons degenerate is unknown. Initial symptoms typically include weakness in the hands and legs, muscle cramps, stiffness, and twitching. Over time, the patient becomes weaker and weaker. Eventually, all skeletal muscles, including the muscles of respiration, become paralyzed. Intellectual function, eye movement, bladder function, and sensation are not affected. Most patients die within 3 to 5 years, although some survive for a decade or longer. In the United states, ALS strikes about 5000 people each year. At this time, the disease has no cure.

*Riluzole* [Rilutek], the only drug currently available for treating ALS, may offer modest benefits to some patients. In clinical trials, the drug prolonged life or delayed the need for a tracheostomy by a few months. However, benefits were limited to patients whose nerve degeneration began in the *medulla*; riluzole did not help patients whose nerve degeneration began in the *spinal cord*. The reason for this difference is unknown. Riluzole is generally well tolerated. The most common adverse effects are asthenia (decreased strength), GI reactions (nausea, vomiting, diarrhea, abdominal pain), CNS effects (dizziness, vertigo, somnolence), and decreased lung function. Riluzole is available in 50-mg tablets for oral administration. The recommended dosage is 50 mg every 12 hours. Increasing the dosage does not increase benefits, but does increase the risk of adverse effects. Riluzole should be taken 1 hour before meals or 2 hours after so as to increase bioavailability.

## KEY POINTS

- Obesity (excessive body fat) is a chronic disease that requires lifelong treatment.
- The body mass index (BMI), expressed in $kg/m^2$, is a measure of weight-related health risk.
- Comorbid conditions, such as hypertension, heart disease, and type II diabetes, increase weight-related health risk.
- Weight-related health risk is significant when BMI is 27 or above (or 25 or above in the presence of comorbid conditions).

- Appetite-suppressant drugs (anorexiants) should be used in the context of a comprehensive weight reduction program that includes exercise, behavior modification, and a reduced-calorie diet.
- Most patients regain lost weight when anorexiants are discontinued. Hence, to remain effective, these drugs must be taken indefinitely.
- Serotonergic anorexiants are CNS depressants, whereas catecholaminergic anorexiants are CNS stimulants.
- Dexfenfluramine and fenfluramine, two serotonergic anorexiants, are associated with valvular heart disease and hence have been withdrawn.
- Respiratory distress syndrome (RDS), the primary cause of morbidity and mortality in premature infants, results from a deficiency in lung surfactant.
- When preterm birth is unavoidable, injecting the mother with glucocorticoids can accelerate fetal lung maturation, and can thereby decrease the risk of RDS.
- Lung surfactant—beractant or colfosceril palmitate—is given to preterm infants to prevent or treat RDS.
- Symptoms of benign prostatic hyperplasia (BPH) result from (1) mechanical obstruction of the urethra (secondary to overgrowth of epithelial cells), and (2) dynamic obstruction of the urethra (secondary to overgrowth of smooth muscle).
- Finasteride [Proscar] promotes regression of prostate epithelial tissue, and thereby decreases mechanical obstruction of the urethra. Since the percentage of epithelial tissue is highest in very large prostates, finasteride is most effective in men whose prostates are highly enlarged.
- Alpha$_1$ antagonists (e.g., terazosin [Hytrin], doxazosin [Cardura]) relax smooth muscle in the prostate capsule, prostatic urethra, and bladder neck, and thereby decrease dynamic obstruction of the urethra.
- Cystic fibrosis (CF) is an inherited disorder that results in damage to the lungs, pancreas, and other organs.
- Dornase alfa [Pulmozyme] can improve pulmonary function and decrease infection in some patients with CF. The drug decreases the viscosity of sputum by breaking down extracellular DNA that has accumulated secondary to death of neutrophils.
- In patients with CF, high-dose ibuprofen can slow progression of pulmonary damage. Benefits derive from suppressing the inflammatory response that underlies destruction of lung tissue.
- In patients with CF, supplemental pancreatic enzymes promote digestion and absorption of nutrients. All preparations contain lipase, protease, and amylase.
- In patients with amyotrophic lateral sclerosis (Lou Gehrig's disease), Riluzole [Rilutek] can prolong life or delay the need for a tracheostomy by a few months.

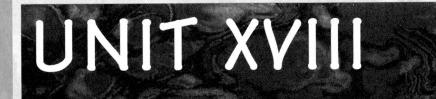

# UNIT XVIII

# Toxicology

Management of Poisoning

# Management of Poisoning

oisoning is defined as a pathologic state caused by a toxic agent. Sources of poisoning include medications, plants, environmental pollutants, and drugs of abuse. These toxicants may enter the body orally, by inhalation, or by absorption through the skin. Poisoning may be accidental or intentional. Symptoms of poisoning often mimic those of disease; hence, the possibility of poisoning should be considered whenever a diagnosis is made.

Poisonings occur at an estimated rate of 5 million per year, and about 5000 deaths result. Approximately 60% of these fatalities are due to ingestion of drugs, either prescription medicines or over-the-counter (OTC) preparations. The remaining deaths are caused by other chemicals. The *incidence* of poisoning is highest in young children; however, the *mortality rate* in this group is low. Most poisoning-related hospital admissions result from suicide attempts by adults.

## Fundamentals of Treatment

Poisoning is a medical emergency and requires rapid treatment. Management has five basic elements: (1) supportive care, (2) identification of the poison, (3) prevention of further absorption, (4) promotion of poison removal, and (5) use of specific antidotes. These essentials are discussed below.

### Supportive Care

Supportive care is the most important element in managing acute poisoning. Support is based on the clinical status of the patient and requires no knowledge specific to the poison involved. Maintenance of respiration and circulation are the primary concerns. Measures for support of breathing include insertion of an airway, administration of humidified oxygen, and mechanical ventilation. Volume depletion (resulting from vomiting, diarrhea, or sweating) can compromise circulation. Volume should be restored by administering normal saline or Ringer's solution. Severe hypoglycemia may occur, resulting in coma. Levels of blood glucose should be monitored. For coma of unknown etiology, IV dextrose should be given immediately—even if information on blood glucose is lacking. Acid-base disturbances may occur; determination of arterial blood gases will facilitate diagnosis and management. If convulsions develop, IV diazepam is the treatment of choice.

### Poison Identification

Treatment of poisoning is facilitated by knowing the identity and dosage of the toxicant. Efforts to obtain this information should proceed concurrently with medical management.

A history is one means by which a toxic agent may be identified. However, experience has shown that histories taken at times of poisoning are frequently inaccurate. That is, statements about the nature or quantity of poison may be incorrect.

Positive identification can be made using analytic techniques. A gas chromatograph/mass spectrometer can provide qualitative and quantitative information. Analyses can be performed on specimens of blood, urine, and gastric contents. To determine whether poison levels are rising or falling, analyses should be performed on sequential blood samples taken about 2 hours apart.

### Prevention of Further Absorption

By reducing the absorption of a poison, we can minimize its blood levels, and thereby significantly decrease morbidity and mortality. Five procedures are available to reduce absorption: (1) induction of emesis (usually with syrup of ipecac), (2) gastric lavage, (3) administration of activated charcoal, (4) purgation (with a saline cathartic), and (5) surface decontamination when exposure is topical. Details of these procedures are discussed in the next section.

## Promotion of Poison Removal

Measures that help eliminate poison from the body shorten the duration of exposure and, if implemented before plasma levels have peaked, can reduce the maximal level of poison achieved. By shortening exposure and reducing maximal poison levels, these measures can decrease the severity of symptoms.

Removal of poison can be promoted with drugs and with nonpharmacologic techniques. The drugs used for poison removal act by increasing renal excretion of toxic agents. The nonpharmacologic methods of poison removal include peritoneal dialysis, hemodialysis, and exchange transfusion. Details on methods of poison removal are presented later.

## Use of Specific Antidotes

An antidote is an agent administered to counteract the effects of a poison. Examples include naloxone (used to reverse poisoning by heroin and other opioids) and physostigmine (used to treat poisoning by atropine and other anticholinergic drugs). Several specific antidotes are discussed later in this chapter. Unfortunately, although antidotes can be extremely valuable, these agents are rare: for most poisons, we have no specific antidote. Hence, for most patients, treatment is limited to the general measures described above.

# Drugs and Procedures Used to Minimize Poison Absorption

## Syrup of Ipecac

*Actions and Uses.* Syrup of ipecac is the drug of choice for induction of emesis. Ipecac is indicated following ingestion of practically all poisons. Emesis is caused by stimulation of the chemoreceptor trigger zone of the medulla and by an irritant action exerted in the stomach. Vomiting usually occurs 20 to 30 minutes after drug administration. After vomiting is over, activated charcoal can be administered to remove residual poison from the stomach and intestine. (Charcoal should not be administered prior to emesis since it can adsorb the ipecac and may thereby reduce ipecac's effects.) If ipecac fails to provoke vomiting, gastric lavage can be used to empty the stomach of poison (see below). The most common side effects of ipecac are sedation and diarrhea.

*Contraindications.* Although generally indicated in cases of poison ingestion, induction of vomiting can be hazardous in some situations. Ipecac is contraindicated following ingestion of strong acids or bases. Under these circumstances, regurgitation increases the risk of gastric perforation and esophageal necrosis. Ipecac is also contraindicated for patients who are comatose, delirious, or experiencing convulsions. Under these conditions, induction of vomiting may result in aspiration of gastric contents.

*Preparations, Dosage, and Administration.* Ipecac syrup is dispensed in 15- and 30-ml containers. The drug is available without prescription and should be kept in all households that have children older than 1 year. The presence of fluid in the stomach increases the effects of ipecac. Hence, administration should be accompanied by an appropriate volume of water. The dose of ipecac syrup for children under 1 year of age is 5 to 10 ml followed by one-half to 1 glass of water. The dose for older children and adults is 15 ml followed by 1 to 2 glasses of water. If vomiting does not occur within 20 minutes, dosing should be repeated.

## Activated Charcoal

Activated charcoal is an inert substance that adsorbs drugs and other chemicals. Binding of toxicants to charcoal is essentially irreversible. Since the charcoal particles cannot be absorbed into the blood, adsorption of poisons onto charcoal prevents toxicity. The charcoal-poison complex is eliminated in the stool. Patients should be advised that charcoal will turn the feces black. When ipecac is being used, charcoal should be administered only after vomiting has taken place. Charcoal is nontoxic and there are no contraindications to its use.

Since charcoal can adsorb antidotes, and thereby neutralize their benefits, antidotes should not be administered immediately before, with, or shortly after the charcoal.

Activated charcoal has the consistency of a fine powder and is mixed with water for oral administration. The adult dose is 50 to 100 gm. Pediatric doses range from 25 to 50 gm. For toxicants that are slowly absorbed, and for ones that undergo enterohepatic recirculation or secretion from the blood into the stomach, sequential doses can be beneficial. Since charcoal is devoid of toxicity, there is no upper limit to the amount that may be given.

## Saline Cathartics

Cathartics hasten passage of toxicants through the intestine, and thereby minimize absorption. Saline cathartics (e.g., sodium sulfate, magnesium sulfate) are the agents of choice. These preparations act rapidly and have little toxicity. For patients on a low-sodium regimen (e.g., patients with hypertension or heart failure), magnesium sulfate (Epsom salt) is preferred to sodium sulfate. Cathartics do not reduce adsorption onto charcoal, and will accelerate charcoal elimination. When a cathartic is administered simultaneously with charcoal, the interval between administration and the appearance of black stool provides an index of intestinal transit time.

## Gastric Lavage

Gastric lavage (irrigation of the stomach) is indicated in cases of significant poisoning when induction of emesis cannot be performed. Since emesis is more effective than lavage, ipecac is preferred to lavage except when emesis is contraindicated. Although early use of lavage or ipecac is desirable, these procedures can still be beneficial hours after poison has been ingested.

Lavage is accomplished using a large-bore orogastric tube (No. 36 to 42 French for adults, No. 22 to 28 French for children). Smaller tubes should be avoided since they may not permit removal of solids (food, pills, capsules, tablets) and because their small diameter will impede flow of the lavage fluid. If the patient is comatose, an endotracheal tube with an inflatable cuff should be installed to protect the airway. Because of the anatomy of the stomach, the patient should be placed on the left side with the head down. Prior to initiation of lavage, stomach contents should be aspirated and sent for toxicologic analysis. Lavage may be performed employing tap water or saline solution. Multiple washes are instilled using 150 to 200 ml/wash (for adults and older children) or 50 to 100 ml/wash (for children under 5 years). Larger volumes should be avoided since they may push stomach contents into the small intestine. Washes should be repeated until the fluid retrieved from the stomach is clear. About 10 to 12 washes are required.

## Surface Decontamination

Topical exposure to toxicants can cause local and systemic injury. To minimize injury, contaminated clothing should be removed, and the poison should be washed from the victim. The recommended procedure is to alternate soap-and-water washes with alcohol washes. Health personnel performing these washes should take precautions to avoid becoming contaminated themselves. If the eyes have been exposed, they should be flushed with water for at least 15 minutes. Shampoo should be employed to remove toxic agents from the hair and scalp.

# Drugs and Procedures Used for Poison Removal

## Drugs That Enhance Renal Excretion

Drugs that alter the pH of urine can accelerate the excretion of organic acids and bases. Agents that *elevate* urinary pH (i.e., make the urine more alkaline) will promote the excretion of *acids*. Drugs that *lower* urinary pH will promote the excretion of *bases*. The mechanism underlying these effects is called *ion trapping* (see Chapter 5).

The drugs employed most frequently to alter urinary pH are *sodium bicarbonate* and *ammonium chloride*. Both are administered IV. Sodium bicarbonate renders the urine more alkaline, which decreases the passive reabsorption of acids (e.g., aspirin, phenobarbital), and thereby accelerates their excretion. Ammonium chloride acidifies the urine, and thereby increases the excretion of bases (e.g., amphetamines, phencyclidine). Because of the buffer systems present in blood, sodium bicarbonate and ammonium chloride have a relatively small effect on the pH of blood.

## Nondrug Methods of Poison Removal

Several nondrug procedures—peritoneal dialysis, hemodialysis, hemoperfusion, exchange transfusion—can be employed to remove toxicants from the body. Although these procedures are usually of limited value, they can be lifesaving in some situations. Nondrug procedures are most effective (1) when binding of toxicants to plasma proteins is low, and (2) when blood levels of toxicants are high (i.e., when distribution of the toxic agent is restricted to the blood and extracellular fluid).

Each of the nondrug methods of poison removal has its benefits and drawbacks. *Peritoneal dialysis* has two advantages: the procedure is relatively simple and it occupies a minimum of staff time. *Hemodialysis*, although more difficult than peritoneal dialysis, is about 20 times more effective. *Hemoperfusion* is a process in which blood is passed over a column of charcoal or absorbent resin. If the affinity of the resin for a particular poison is high, this procedure can strip a toxicant from binding sites on plasma proteins. The principal disadvantage of hemoperfusion is loss of platelets. When binding of a poison to plasma proteins is particularly avid, *exchange transfusion* can be an effective method of removal.

# Specific Antidotes

## Heavy Metal Antagonists

The heavy metals most frequently responsible for poisoning are lead, iron, mercury, arsenic, gold, and copper. These metals cause injury by forming complexes with enzymes and other physiologically important molecules. Poisoning may result from environmental exposure, intentional overdosage, or therapeutic use of heavy metals.

The drugs given to treat heavy metal poisoning are called *chelating agents* or *chelators*. These agents interact with metals to form *chelates*—ring structures in which the metal and the chelating agent form two or more points of attachment. The chelate formed by mercury and dimercaprol illustrates this concept (Fig. 100–1).

Useful chelating agents have a high affinity for heavy metals, and can therefore compete successfully with endogenous molecules for metal binding. By preventing initial binding of metals to endogenous molecules, chelators can prevent injury; by stripping metals that have already become bound, chelators can enhance their excretion.

The selectivity of a heavy metal antagonist is determined by its affinity for specific metals. Some antagonists are selective for only one metal, whereas others can form

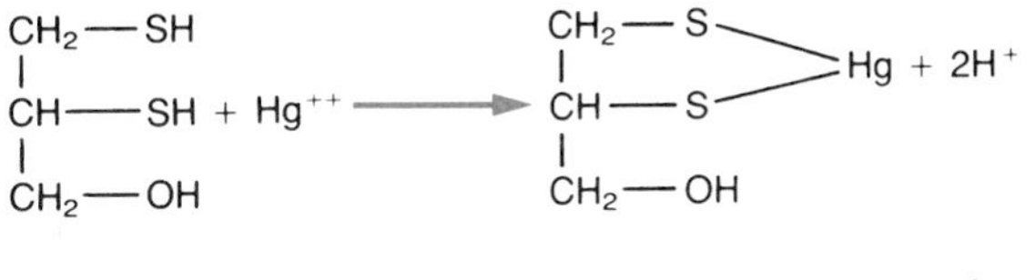

**Figure 100–1. Chelation of mercury by dimercaprol.**

chelates with several metals. Deferoxamine, for example, binds selectively to iron. In contrast, dimercaprol is relatively nonselective, binding tightly with arsenic, mercury salts, and gold.

Properties desirable in a heavy metal antagonist include (1) high affinity for a toxic metal, (2) low affinity for essential endogenous metals (e.g., magnesium, zinc), (3) an ability to reach sites of metal storage, (4) high activity at physiologic pH, (5) formation of chelates that are less toxic than the free metal, and (6) formation of chelates that are easily excreted.

### Deferoxamine

*Actions and Uses.* Deferoxamine has a high affinity for ferric iron. The drug chelates free iron and can also strip iron bound to ferritin and hemosiderin. In contrast, iron present in hemoglobin and cytochromes is not affected. Deferoxamine is employed to treat acute and chronic iron toxicity.

*Pharmacokinetics.* Deferoxamine is poorly absorbed from the gastrointestinal tract; hence, administration is parenteral. The chelate formed between deferoxamine and iron is excreted primarily in the urine.

*Adverse Effects.* Deferoxamine is generally well tolerated. Pain may occur at the site of injection. Rapid IV infusion may cause hypotension, tachycardia, erythema, and urticaria. Prolonged therapy may be associated with allergic reactions, abdominal discomfort, leg cramps, fever, and dysuria.

*Contraindications.* Because deferoxamine is excreted by the kidneys, the drug should not be given to patients with renal insufficiency. Deferoxamine has caused fetal malformation in experimental animals, and therefore is not recommended for pregnant women.

*Preparations, Dosage, and Administration.* Deferoxamine mesylate [Desferal Mesylate] is dispensed as a powder to be reconstituted for injection. The drug can be administered by IM injection and by IV or SC infusion. Intramuscular injection is preferred for most patients. Intravenous infusion is usually reserved for patients in shock. The dosage for IM or IV administration is the same. The initial dose for adults and children is 1 gm. This is followed 4 and 8 hours later with 0.5-gm doses. For IV administration, the maximum rate of infusion is 15 mg/kg/hr.

### Dimercaprol

*Actions and Uses.* Dimercaprol binds with arsenic, gold, and mercury. The resulting chelates are excreted in the urine. The drug is used as the sole chelator to rid the body of arsenic, mercury, or gold. In addition, dimercaprol can be combined with edetate calcium disodium to treat poisoning with lead. Since dimercaprol is more effective at *preventing* binding of metals to endogenous molecules than it is at reversing binding that has already taken place, benefits are greatest when the drug is administered early (within 1 to 2 hours after metal ingestion).

*Pharmacokinetics.* Administration is by deep IM injection. Dimercaprol cannot be used orally. The drug has a short plasma half-life; complete elimination occurs in approximately 4 hours.

*Adverse Effects.* At recommended doses, dimercaprol is generally well tolerated. Tachycardia and elevation of blood pressure occur frequently; blood pressure returns to normal within hours. Pain and sterile abscesses may occur at sites of injection. Fever is common in children. High doses produce a broad spectrum of untoward effects.

Chelates formed with dimercaprol are unstable at acidic pH. Hence, if the urine is acidic, heavy metals may dissociate from dimercaprol, resulting in renal toxicity. To protect the kidneys, the urine should be kept alkaline.

*Preparations, Dosage, and Administration.* Dimercaprol [BAL In Oil] is dispensed in ampules containing 300 mg of the drug in 3 ml of peanut oil. The preparation is administered by deep IM injection. For *mild poisoning with gold or arsenic*, doses of 2.5 mg/kg are administered according to the following schedule: 4 times daily on days 1 and 2, twice daily on day 3, and once daily on days 4 through 13. For *acute poisoning with mercury*, the initial dose is 5 mg/kg. Subsequent doses of 2.5 mg/kg are administered 1 or 2 times daily for 10 days.

### Edetate Calcium Disodium (Calcium EDTA)

*Actions and Uses.* Calcium EDTA is used primarily for lead poisoning. The drug combines with lead to form a stable chelate that is excreted in the urine.

*Pharmacokinetics.* Calcium EDTA may be administered IV or IM. The drug is poorly absorbed from the GI tract and is not administered orally. Elimination is by glomerular filtration. Because calcium EDTA is excreted by the kidneys, the drug should be employed only if urine flow is adequate. If urine flow is insufficient, it should be restored with IV fluids prior to administration of the chelator. If anuria develops during the course of treatment, administration of calcium EDTA should cease.

*Adverse Effects.* The principal toxicity of calcium EDTA is renal tubular necrosis. Signs of renal damage include hematuria and proteinuria. Daily urinalysis should be performed to monitor for these effects. If renal toxicity develops, the drug should be discontinued immediately.

*Preparations, Dosage, and Administration.* Calcium EDTA [Calcium Disodium Versenate] is dispensed in 5-ml ampules containing 1000 mg of drug. Administration may be IV or IM. The IV route is preferred for adults, whereas IM is preferred for children.

For IV use, the contents of 1 ampule are diluted in 250 to 500 ml of 5% dextrose solution or normal saline. Infusion should be done slowly (over 1 hour or more). The adult dosage is 1 gm twice daily for 5 days. After a 2-day hiatus, a second course may be given if needed.

The IM dosage for children is 35 mg/kg (or less) administered twice daily for 3 to 5 days. After a pause of 4 days or more, a second course is given.

### Penicillamine

*Actions.* Penicillamine is a breakdown product of penicillin. Commercial preparations are made synthetically. Penicillamine forms water-soluble chelates with copper, iron, lead, arsenic, gold, and mercury. These complexes are excreted in the urine.

*Therapeutic Uses.* The principal indication for penicillamine is *Wilson's disease*, a disorder of copper metabolism. Individuals with this disease are deficient in ceruloplasmin, a plasma protein that serves as a carrier for copper. Symptoms result from deposition of copper in the liver, brain, kidneys, eyes, and other organs. Penicillamine relieves symptoms by promoting copper excretion. Therapeutic effects may take several months to develop. Additional uses are *rheumatoid arthritis* and *cystinuria*. Beneficial effects in these disorders are not related to chelation of heavy metals.

*Pharmacokinetics.* Penicillamine is well absorbed following oral administration. Food greatly reduces the extent of absorption. Once absorbed, penicillamine is rapidly excreted in the urine.

*Adverse Effects.* With prolonged use, penicillamine can cause varied and serious toxicities. Deaths have occurred. The drug

## TABLE 100-1. SPECIFIC ANTIDOTES DISCUSSED IN PREVIOUS CHAPTERS

| Antidote | | Toxic/Overdosed Substance | Chapter |
|---|---|---|---|
| Generic Name | Trade Name | | |
| Atropine | | Muscarinic agonists, cholinesterase inhibitors | 15 |
| Physostigmine | Antilirium | Anticholinergic drugs | 16 |
| Neostigmine | Prostigmin | Nondepolarizing neuromuscular blockers | 16 |
| Pralidoxime | Protopam | Organophosphate cholinesterase inhibitors | 16 |
| Naloxone | Narcan | Opioids | 25 |
| Flumazenil | Romazicon | Benzodiazepines | 32 |
| Digoxin immune fab | Digibind | Digoxin, digitoxin | 46 |
| Vitamin K | | Warfarin | 50 |
| Protamine sulfate | | Heparin | 50 |
| Glucagon | | Insulin-induced hypoglycemia | 53 |
| Acetylcysteine | Mucomyst | Acetaminophen | 64 |
| Leucovorin | Wellcovorin | Methotrexate and other folate antagonists | 96 |

should be employed only with close medical supervision. Possible cutaneous reactions include urticaria, maculopapular and morbilliform rashes, pemphigoid lesions, and pruritus. Bone marrow suppression can result in leukopenia, agranulocytosis, and aplastic anemia—reactions that can be fatal. Autoimmune and immune complex disorders have been associated with penicillamine; these include dermatomyositis, polymyositis, lupus erythematosus, alveolitis, and myasthenia gravis. Renal toxicity may occur.

**Contraindications.** Penicillamine is contraindicated for patients who have experienced agranulocytosis or aplastic anemia when receiving penicillamine in the past. The drug is also contraindicated for patients with rheumatoid arthritis who also are pregnant or have renal insufficiency.

**Preparations, Dosage, and Administration.** Penicillamine [Cuprimine, Depen] is dispensed in 125-mg capsules and 250-mg tablets for oral administration. For Wilson's disease, the usual dosage is 250 mg 4 times a day. Doses should be administered 1 hour before meals and at bedtime. Dosage is adjusted on the basis of untoward effects and urinary copper content. Treatment is long term.

### Succimer

**Actions and Uses.** Succimer binds avidly with lead, mercury, and arsenic. Binding is less avid with copper and zinc. Binding to iron, calcium, and magnesium is minimal; hence succimer presents no risk of depleting these essential minerals.

Succimer is approved for treatment of lead poisoning in children. The drug may also be useful against poisoning with arsenic, mercury, and other heavy metals.

**Pharmacokinetics.** Succimer is rapidly but variably absorbed following oral administration. The drug undergoes extensive metabolism. Metabolites and parent drug are eliminated slowly in the urine.

**Adverse Effects.** Adverse effects appear to be mild. About 10% of patients experience gastrointestinal reactions (nausea, diarrhea, cramps). Other moderate reactions include nasal congestion, muscle pain, and rash. Succimer has caused temporary ele-

vations in serum transaminases, indicating possible liver injury. Accordingly, serum transaminases should be monitored before treatment and weekly thereafter. In addition, caution should be exercised in patients with liver disease. In mice the drug is teratogenic and fetotoxic. Since succimer is a relatively new drug, it may also cause as-yet unreported adverse effects.

**Preparations, Dosage, and Administration.** Succimer [Chemet] is dispensed in 100-mg capsules for oral use. For children over 1 year, treatment consists of 10 mg/kg or 350 mg/m² every 8 hours for 5 days, and then every 12 hours for 14 more days. If needed, this entire course can be repeated after a minimum hiatus of 2 weeks.

## Other Important Antidotes

Throughout this text we have considered the toxic effects of various drugs. Where appropriate, we have discussed specific antidotes used for treatment. For example, when discussing the adverse effects of opioids, we also discussed treatment of opioid overdosage with naloxone. Similarly, when discussing heparin toxicity, we discussed the use of protamine sulfate as treatment. The major specific antidotes presented in previous chapters are summarized in Table 100-1.

## Poison Control Centers

In the United States there are more than 500 local poison control centers and over 40 certified regional centers. These centers are accessible by phone and can provide immediate instruction on the management of acute poisoning. In the majority of cases, the information supplied will permit successful treatment at home. By facilitating rapid treatment, poison control centers can decrease morbidity and mortality, and can help reduce the cost of emergency care. Phone numbers for regional poison control centers are given in Appendix F.

## KEY POINTS

- Management of poisoning has five basic components: supportive care, poison identification, prevention of further absorption, promotion of poison removal, and use of specific antidotes.
- Absorption of toxicants can be reduced in five ways: induction of vomiting with *syrup of ipecac*, adsorption onto *activated charcoal*, removal by *gastric lavage*, acceleration of intestinal transit with *cathartics*, and *surface decontamination* (if exposure is topical).
- Removal of absorbed poisons can be accelerated by using drugs to *enhance renal excretion* and by nondrug methods, such as *hemodialysis* and *exchange transfusion*.
- For most poisons we do not have specific antidotes.
- Heavy metal poisoning can be treated with *chelating agents*.
- Poison control centers can offer immediate, expert assistance over the phone.

# Appendix A

# Guide to Gender-Related Drugs

Because this book is structured largely on the basis of pharmacologic drug classes, discussions of drugs for gender-related therapy are scattered throughout the book. The purpose of this guide is to help you locate gender-specific content. Chapter numbers are in **bold** type and page numbers are in parentheses.

# APPENDIX B

# Weights and Measures

## Volume Equivalents

| | | | |
|---|---|---|---|
| 1 milliliter | = | 0.034 | fluid ounce |
| | = | 0.271 | fluid dram |
| | = | 16.2 | minims |
| 1 liter | = | 1000 | milliliters |
| | = | 33.8 | fluid ounces |
| | = | 2.11 | pints |
| | = | 1.06 | quarts |
| | = | 0.26 | gallon |
| 1 cubic centimeter | = | 1 | milliliter |
| 1 minim | = | 0.062 | milliliter |
| 1 fluid dram | = | 3.70 | milliliters |
| | = | 60 | minims |
| 1 fluid ounce | = | 29.6 | milliliters |
| | = | 2 | tablespoons |
| | = | 8 | fluid drams |
| 1 teaspoon | = | 5 | milliliters |
| 1 tablespoon | = | 15 | milliliters |
| | = | 3 | teaspoons |
| 1 cup | = | 237 | milliliters |
| | = | 8 | fluid ounces |
| | = | 16 | tablespoons |
| 1 pint | = | 473 | milliliters |
| | = | 16 | fluid ounces |
| | = | 2 | cups |
| 1 quart | = | 946 | milliliters |
| | = | 32 | fluid ounces |
| | = | 2 | pints |
| 1 gallon | = | 3785 | milliliters |
| | = | 128 | fluid ounces |
| | = | 4 | quarts |

## Mass Equivalents

| | | | |
|---|---|---|---|
| 1 milligram | = | 0.0154 | grain (apothecaries') |
| | = | 1000 | micrograms |
| 1 gram | = | 15.4 | grains (apothecaries') |
| | = | 0.0322 | ounce (apothecaries') |
| | = | 0.0353 | ounce (avoirdupois) |
| | = | 0.257 | dram (apothecaries') |
| 1 grain (apothecaries') | = | 64.8 | milligrams |
| | = | 0.0021 | ounce (apothecaries') |
| | = | 0.0023 | ounce (avoirdupois) |
| | = | 0.0167 | dram (apothecaries') |
| 1 dram (apothecaries') | = | 3.89 | grams |
| 1 ounce (apothecaries') | = | 31.1 | grams |
| 1 ounce (avoirdupois) | = | 28.4 | grams |
| 1 pound (avoirdupois) | = | 454 | grams |
| | = | 0.454 | kilogram |
| | = | 16 | ounces (avoirdupois) |
| 1 kilogram | = | 2.20 | pounds (avoirdupois) |

## Temperature Conversion

(Celsius degrees × 9/5) + 32 = Fahrenheit degrees
(Fahrenheit degrees − 32) × 5/9 = Celsius degrees

# APPENDIX C

# Normal Laboratory Values

## Part I.  Hematology

| Measurement | Normal Laboratory Values* | |
|---|---|---|
| | Traditional Units | SI Units[†] |
| ***Cell Counts*** | | |
| Erythrocytes | | |
|     Adult female | 4.2-5.4 million/mm$^3$ | 4.2-5.4 × 10$^{12}$/L |
|     Adult male | 4.2-6.2 million/mm$^3$ | 4.2-6.2 × 10$^{12}$/L |
|     Newborn | 4.8-7.2 million/mm$^3$ | 4.8-7.2 × 10$^{12}$/L |
|     Child | 3.8-5.5 million/mm$^3$ | 3.8-5.5 × 10$^{12}$/L |
| Leukocytes | | |
|   Total | | |
|     Adult | 5000-10,000/mm$^3$ | 5-10 × 10$^9$/L |
|     Newborn | 9000-30,000/mm$^3$ | 9-30 × 10$^9$/L |
|   Differential | | |
|     Neutrophils | 50%-70% | 0.50-0.70 |
|      Segments | 50%-65% | 0.50-0.65 |
|      Bands | 0%-5% | 0.0-0.05 |
|     Eosinophils | 0%-3% | 0.0-0.03 |
|     Basophils | 1%-3% | 0.01-0.03 |
|     Lymphocytes | 25%-35% | 0.25-0.35 |
|     Monocytes | 2%-6% | 0.02-0.06 |
| Platelets | | |
|     Adult | 150,000-400,000/mm$^3$ | 150-400 × 10$^9$/L |
|     Newborn | 150,000-300,000/mm$^3$ | 150-300 × 10$^9$/L |
|     Infant | 200,000-475,000/mm$^3$ | 200-475 × 10$^9$/L |
| Reticulocytes | | |
|     Adult | 10,000-75,000/mm$^3$ (0.1%-2.4% of all RBCs) | 10-75 × 10$^9$/L |
|     Newborn | 2.5%-6.5% of all RBCs | 2.5%-6.5% of all RBCs |
|     Infant | 0.5%-3.5% of all RBCs | 0.5%-3.5% of all RBCs |
| ***Coagulation-Related Tests*** | | |
| Bleeding time | 3-9.5 min | 180-570 sec |
| Activated partial thromboplastin time (APTT) | 25-35 sec | 25-35 sec |
| Prothrombin time | <2 sec from control | <2 sec from control |
| ***Corpuscular Values of Erythrocytes*** | | |
| Mean corpuscular volume (MCV) | | |
|     Adult | 80-96 μm$^3$ | 80-96 fl |
|     Newborn | 96-108 μm$^3$ | 96-108 fl |
|     Child | 82-92 μm$^3$ | 82-92 fl |
| Mean corpuscular hemoglobin (MCH) | | |
|     Adult | 27-31 pg/RBC | 27-31 pg/RBC |
|     Newborn | 32-34 pg/RBC | 32-34 pg/RBC |
|     Child | 27-31 pg/RBC | 27-31 pg/RBC |
| Mean corpuscular hemoglobin concentration (MCHC) | 32-36 gm/dl | 320-360 gm/L |

*Table continued on following page*

# Part I. Hematology *(Continued)*

| Measurement | Normal Laboratory Values* | |
| --- | --- | --- |
| | Traditional Units | SI Units† |
| ***Erythrocyte Sedimentation Rate*** | | |
| Wintrobe method | | |
| Adult female | 0-15 mm/hr | 0-15 mm/hr |
| Adult male | 0-7 mm/hr | 0-7 mm/hr |
| Newborn | 0-2 mm/hr | 0-2 mm/hr |
| Westergren method | | |
| Female | 0-20 mm/hr | 0-20 mm/hr |
| Male | 0-15 mm/hr | 0-15 mm/hr |
| ***Hematocrit*** | | |
| Adult female | 36%-48% | 0.36-0.48 |
| Adult male | 42%-53% | 0.42-0.53 |
| Newborn | 42%-54% | 0.42-0.54 |
| Child (1-3 yr) | 29%-40% | 0.29-0.40 |
| Child (4-10 yr) | 36%-48% | 0.36-0.48 |
| ***Hemoglobin Concentration*** | | |
| Adult female | 12-16 gm/dl | 120-160 gm/L |
| Adult male | 13-18 gm/dl | 130-180 gm/L |
| Newborn | 14-24 gm/dl | 140-240 gm/L |

# Part II. Blood Chemistry

| Measurement | Normal Laboratory Values* | |
| --- | --- | --- |
| | Traditional Units | SI Units† |
| Adrenocorticotropichormone (ACTH) | | |
| 6 AM | 10-80 pg/ml | 2-16 pmol/ml |
| 6 PM | <50 pg/ml | <10 pmol/ml |
| Aldosterone | | |
| Normal sodium diet | 8.1-15.5 ng/dl | 220-430 pmol/L |
| Restricted sodium diet | 20.8-44.4 ng/dl | 580-1240 pmol/L |
| Ammonia | 10-80 µg/dl | 5-50 µmol/L |
| Amylase | 0-125 U/L | 0-2.17 µkat/L |
| Bicarbonate | 22-26 mEq/L | 22-26 mEq/L |
| Bilirubin | | |
| Adult | | |
| Direct | 0.1-0.4 mg/dl | 1.7-6.8 µmol/L |
| Indirect | 0.2-0.7 mg/dl | 3.4-12.0 µmol/L |
| Total | 0.3-1.1 mg/dl | 5.1-18.8 µmol/L |
| Newborn (total) | 1-12 mg/dl | 17-205 µmol/L |
| Child (total) | 0.2-0.8 mg/dl | 3.4-13.7 µmol/L |
| Calcitonin | | |
| Female | 0-28 pg/ml | 0-8.2 pmol/L |
| Male | 0-14 pg/ml | 0-4.1 pmol/L |
| Calcium | 8.8-10.3 mg/dl | 2.2-2.6 mmol/L |
| Carbon dioxide content | | |
| Adult | 24-40 mEq/L | 24-40 mmol/L |
| Infant | 20-28 mEq/L | 20-28 mmol/L |
| Chloride | 96-106 mEq/L | 96-106 mmol/L |
| Cholesterol | See Table 49-2 | |
| Cholinesterase, plasma | 620-1370 U/L | 10.3-22.8 µkat/L |
| Copper, total | | |
| Adult female | 70-140 µg/dl | 11-22 µmol/L |
| Adult male | 85-155 µg/dl | 13-24 µmol/L |
| Newborn | 20-70 µg/dl | 3-11 µmol/L |
| Child | 30-150 µg/dl | 5-24 µmol/L |

## Part II. Blood Chemistry *(Continued)*

| | Normal Laboratory Values* | |
|---|---|---|
| **Measurement** | **Traditional Units** | **SI Units**[†] |
| Cortisol | | |
| Adult | | |
| 8 AM | 4-19 µg/dl | 110-520 nmol/L |
| 4 PM | 2-25 µg/dl | 50-410 nmol/L |
| 10 PM | <50% of AM value | <50% of AM value |
| Child | | |
| 8 AM | 10-25 µg/dl | 280-700 nmol/L |
| 4 PM | 5-10 µg/dl | 140-280 nmol/L |
| Creatine phosphokinase (CK, CPK) | | |
| Female | 10-55 U/L (30°) | 10-55 U/L (30°) |
| | 30-135 U/L (37°) | 30-135 U/L (37°) |
| Male | 12-80 U/L (30°) | 12-80 U/L (30°) |
| | 55-170 U/L (37°) | 55-170 U/L (37°) |
| Creatinine | 0.6-1.2 mg/dl | 50-110 µmol/L |
| Ferritin (serum) | | |
| Iron deficiency | 0-12 ng/ml | 0-4.8 nmol/L |
| Borderline | 13-20 ng/ml | 5.2-8 nmol/L |
| Iron excess | >400 ng/ml | >160 nmol/L |
| Fibrinogen | 200-400 mg/dl | 2.0-4.0 gm/L |
| Folic acid | 2-10 ng/ml | 4-22 nmol/L |
| Follicle-stimulating hormone (FSH) | | |
| Female | 2-15 IU/L | 2-15 IU/L |
| Peak production | 20-50 IU/L | 20-50 IU/L |
| Male | 1-10 IU/L | 1-10 IU/L |
| Free fatty acids | 8-20 mg/dl | 80-200 mg/L |
| Gases | | |
| $pCO_2$ | 33-44 mm Hg | 4.4-5.9 kPa |
| $pO_2$ | 75-105 mm Hg | 10-14 kPa |
| Glucose, fasting | | |
| Adult | 60-115 mg/dl | 3.4-6.6 mmol/L |
| Newborn | 30-80 mg/dl | 1.7-4.6 mmol/L |
| Child | 60-100 mg/dl | 3.4-5.7 mmol/L |
| Glucose-6-phosphate dehydrogenase (G-6-PD) | 5-15 U/gm hemoglobin | 5-15 U/gm hemoglobin |
| Insulin (fasting) | 5-20 mU/L | 35-145 pmol/L |
| Iron | | |
| Adult female | 60-160 µg/dl | 11-29 µmol/L |
| Adult male | 80-180 µg/dl | 14-32 µmol/L |
| Newborn | 100-200 µg/dl | 18-36 µmol/L |
| Child (6 months–2 years) | 40-100 µg/dl | 7-18 µmol/L |
| Iron-binding capacity | | |
| Adult | 250-450 µg/dl | 45-80 µmol/L |
| Newborn | 60-175 µg/dl | 11-31 µmol/L |
| Child (6 months–2 years) | 100-300 µg/dl | 17-53 µmol/L |
| Lactate dehydrogenase (LDH) | 50-150 U/L | 0.82-2.66 µkat/L |
| Lipoprotein cholesterol | | |
| LDL cholesterol | See Table 49-2 | |
| HDL cholesterol | See Table 49-2 | |
| Magnesium | 1.6-2.4 mEq/L | 0.8-1.2 mmol/L |
| Osmolality | 280-300 mOsm/kg of serum water | 280-300 mmol/kg |
| pH | 7.35-7.45 | 7.35-7.45 |
| Phosphatase | | |
| Acid | 0-5.5 U/L | 0-90 µkat/L |
| Alkaline | 30-120 U/L | 0.5-2.0 µkat/L |
| Potassium | | |
| Adult | 3.5-5.0 mEq/L | 3.5-5.0 mmol/L |
| Infant | 3.6-5.8 mEq/L | 3.6-5.8 mmol/L |
| Child | 3.5-5.5 mEq/L | 3.5-5.5 mmol/L |

*Table continued on following page*

## Part II. Blood Chemistry *(Continued)*

| Measurement | Normal Laboratory Values* | |
|---|---|---|
| | Traditional Units | SI Units[†] |
| Progesterone | | |
|   Follicular phase | <2 ng/ml | <6 nmol/L |
|   Luteal phase | 2–20 ng/ml | 6–64 nmol/L |
| Prolactin | 2–15 ng/ml | 80–600 pmol/L |
| Protein | | |
|   Total | 6.0–8.0 gm/dl | 60–80 gm/L |
|   Albumin | 3.5–5.5 gm/dl | 35–55 gm/L |
|   Globulin | | |
|     Alpha$_1$ | 0.2–0.4 gm/dl | 2–4 gm/L |
|     Alpha$_2$ | 0.5–0.9 gm/dl | 5–9 gm/L |
|     Beta | 0.6–1.1 gm/dl | 6–11 gm/L |
|     Gamma | 0.7–1.7 gm/dl | 7–17 gm/L |
| Renin activity | | |
|   Normal sodium diet | 1.1–4.1 ng/ml/hr | 0.3–1.1 ng/(L-s) |
|   Restricted sodium diet | 6.2–12.4 ng/ml/hr | 1.7–3.4 ng/(L-s) |
| Sodium | 135–145 mEq/L | 135–145 mmol/L |
| Testosterone | | |
|   Female | 0.6 ng/ml | 2 nmol/L |
|   Male | 4.6–8 ng/ml | 14–28 nmol/L |
| Thyroid function tests | | |
|   Thyroid-stimulating hormone | 2–11 µU/ml | 2–11 mU/L |
|   Thyroxine (T$_4$) | | |
|     Adult | 4.4–9.9 µg/dl | 57–127 nmol/L |
|     Newborn | 11–23 µg/dl | 142–296 nmol/L |
|     1–4 months | 7.5–16.5 µg/dl | 97–212 nmol/L |
|     4–12 months | 5.5–14.5 µg/dl | 71–187 nmol/L |
|     1–6 years | 5.5–13.5 µg/dl | 71–174 nmol/L |
|     6–10 years | 5–12.5 µg/dl | 64–161 nmol/L |
|   Thyroxine binding globulin | 12–28 µg/dl | 150–360 nmol/L |
|   Triiodothyronine (T$_3$) | 75–220 µg/dl | 1.2–3.4 nmol/L |
|   T$_3$ resin uptake | 25%–38% | 0.25–0.35 |
| Transaminases | | |
|   AST (aspartate aminotransferase) | | |
|     Adult | 8–20 U/L (30°) | 0.13–0.33 µkat/L (30°) |
| | 7–40 U/L (37°) | 0.12–0.67 µkat/L (37°) |
|     Newborn | 4 times adult value | 4 times adult value |
|   ALT (alanine aminotransferase) | 8–20 U/L (30°) | 0.13–0.33 µkat/L (30°) |
| | 5–37 U/L (37°) | 0.08–0.62 µkat/L (37°) |
| Triglycerides | 40–150 mg/dl | 0.4–1.5 g/L |
| Urea nitrogen, blood (BUN) | | |
|   Adult female | 8–20 mg/dl | 2.9–7.1 mmol/L |
|   Adult male | 10–25 mg/dl | 3.6–8.9 mmol/L |
|   Infant | 5–15 mg/dl | 1.8–5.4 mmol/L |
|   Child | 5–20 mg/dl | 1.8–7.1 mmol/L |
| Uric acid | 2–7 mg/dl | 120–420 µmol/L |
| Vitamin B$_{12}$ | 205–876 pg/ml | 150–674 pmol/L |

## Part III. Urine Chemistry

| Measurement | Normal Laboratory Values* | |
|---|---|---|
| | Traditional Units | SI Units[†] |
| Aldosterone | 3–20 µg/24 hr | 8.3–55.5 nmol/day |
| Calcium | <250 mg/24 hr | <6.2 mmol/day |
| Catecholamines | | |
|   Epinephrine | <20 µg/24 hr | <109 nmol/day |
|   Norepinephrine | <100 µg/24 hr | <590 nmol/day |
| Cortisol | 10–100 µg/24 hr | 30–300 nmol/day |

# Part III. Urine Chemistry *(Continued)*

| Measurement | Normal Laboratory Values* | |
|---|---|---|
| | Traditional Units | SI Units[†] |
| Creatine | | |
| Female | 0–80 mg/24 hr | 0–600 µmol/day |
| Male | 0–40 mg/24 hr | 0–3000 µmol/day |
| Creatinine | 15–25 mg/kg/24 hr | 0.13–0.22 nmol/kg/day |
| Creatinine clearance | | |
| Female | 105–132 ml/min | 1.2–2.2 ml/sec |
| Male | 110–150 ml/min | 1.8–2.5 ml/sec |
| 17-Hydroxycorticosteroids | | |
| Female | 2–8 mg/24 hr | 2–25 µmol/day |
| Male | 3–10 mg/24 hr | 10–30 µmol/day |
| 17-Ketosteroids | | |
| Female | | |
| 10 yr | 1–4 mg/24 hr | 3.5–14 µmol/day |
| 20 yr | 4–16 mg/24 hr | 14–56 µmol/day |
| 30 yr | 4–14 mg/24 hr | 14–49 µmol/day |
| 50 yr | 3–9 mg/24 hr | 10–32 µmol/day |
| 70 yr | 1–7 mg/24 hr | 3.5–25 µmol/day |
| Male | | |
| 10 yr | 1–4 mg/24 hr | 3.5–14 µmol/day |
| 20 yr | 6–21 mg/24 hr | 21–74 µmol/day |
| 30 yr | 8–26 mg/24 hr | 28–91 µmol/day |
| 50 yr | 5–18 mg/24 hr | 18–63 µmol/day |
| 70 yr | 2–10 mg/24 hr | 7–35 µmol/day |
| Potassium | 25–100 mEq/24 hr | 25–100 mmol/day |
| Sodium | (diet dependent) | (diet dependent) |

*The values presented are intended as guidelines only. Laboratory values may vary with the method employed and among different laboratories using the same method. When a laboratory issues a report, the report will include normal values for that laboratory.
[†]Système International d'Unités (International System of Units).

# APPENDIX D

# Commonly Used Abbreviations

| | | | |
|---|---|---|---|
| ac | before meals (*ante cibum*) | DNA | deoxyribonucleic acid |
| ACh | acetylcholine | DPI | dry-powder inhaler |
| ad lib | freely as desired (*ad libitum*) | DS | double strength |
| ADHD | attention-deficit/hyperactivity disorder | ECG (EKG) | electrocardiogram |
| ADL | activities of daily living | ECT | electroconvulsive therapy |
| ADP | adenosine diphosphate | EEG | electroencephalogram |
| AED | antiepileptic drug | EKG (ECG) | electrocardiogram |
| AIDS | acquired immunodeficiency syndrome | F | Fahrenheit |
| ALT | alanine aminotransferase (also known as SGPT) | FDA | Food and Drug Administration |
| | | FEV | forced expiratory volume |
| AMI | acute myocardial infarction | FFA | free fatty acid |
| AMP | adenosine monophosphate | g (gm) | gram |
| ANA | antinuclear antibodies | G-6-PD | glucose-6-phosphate dehydrogenase |
| ARC | AIDS-related complex | GABA | gamma-aminobutyric acid |
| ASA | acetylsalicylic acid (aspirin) | GFR | glomerular filtration rate |
| AST | aspartate aminotransferase (also known as SGOT) | GI | gastrointestinal |
| | | gm (g) | gram |
| ATP | adenosine triphosphate | GMP | guanosine monophosphate |
| AV | atrioventricular | gr | grain |
| bid | two times a day (*bis in die*) | GTP | guanosine triphosphate |
| bin | two times a night (*bis in nocte*) | GU | genitourinary |
| bol | bolus | h, hr | hour |
| BP | blood pressure | $H_2RA$ | histamine$_2$-receptor antagonist |
| BPH | benign prostatic hyperplasia | HBGM | home blood glucose monitoring |
| BUN | blood urea nitrogen | HDL | high-density lipoprotein |
| C | Celsius (centigrade) | HIV | human immunodeficiency virus |
| CABG | coronary artery bypass graft | HRT | hormone replacement therapy |
| CAD | coronary artery disease | hs | at bedtime (hour of sleep; *hora somni*) |
| cAMP | cyclic adenosine 3′,5′- monophosphate | HSV | herpes simplex virus |
| CAT | computerized axial tomography | IBD | inflammatory bowel disease |
| CBC | complete blood count | ICP | intracranial pressure |
| cc | cubic centimeter (milliliter) | IDDM | insulin-dependent diabetes mellitus |
| CDC | Centers for Disease Control and Prevention | IM | intramuscular, intramuscularly |
| | | INR | international normalized ratio |
| CHF | congestive heart failure | IOP | intraocular pressure |
| CMV | cytomegalovirus | IPV | inactivated polio vaccine |
| CNS | central nervous system | ISA | intrinsic sympathomimetic activity |
| COMT | catechol-*o*-methyltransferase | IU | international unit |
| COPD | chronic obstructive pulmonary disease | IUD | intrauterine device |
| CPK | creatine phosphokinase | IV | intravenous, intravenously |
| CSF | cerebrospinal fluid | kg | kilogram |
| CTZ | chemoreceptor trigger zone | KVO | keep vein open |
| CVA | cerebrovascular accident | L | liter |
| DBP | diastolic blood pressure | LD | lethal dose |
| DC | direct current | LDL | low-density lipoprotein |
| DKA | diabetic ketoacidosis | LGV | lymphogranuloma venereum |
| dl | deciliter (100 ml) | LSD | D-lysergic acid diethylamide |
| DMARD | disease-modifying antirheumatic drug | m | minim |

| | | | |
|---|---|---|---|
| MAC | minimum alveolar concentration; *Mycobacterium avium* complex | PMS | premenstrual syndrome |
| MAO | monoamine oxidase | PO | by mouth (*per os*) |
| MAOI | monoamine oxidase inhibitor | PPD | purified protein derivative (tuberculin) |
| MAP | mean arterial pressure | PR | by the rectum (*per rectum*) |
| MBC | minimum bactericidal concentration | PRN | as needed (*pro re nata*) |
| mcg (µg) | microgram | PT | prothrombin time |
| MDI | metered-dose inhaler | PTCA | percutaneous transluminal coronary angioplasty |
| MEC | minimum effective concentration | PTT | partial thromboplastin time |
| mEq | milliequivalent | PVC | premature ventricular complex |
| MHC | major histocompatibility complex | qd | every day (*quaque die*) |
| mg | milligram | qh | every hour (*quaque hora*) |
| MI | myocardial infarction | qid | four times a day (*quater in die*) |
| MIC | minimum inhibitory concentration | qod | every other day |
| ml | milliliter | RA | rheumatoid arthritis |
| mM | millimole | RBC | red blood cell (erythrocyte) |
| MMR | measles, mumps, rubella | RDA | recommended dietary allowance |
| mOsm | milliosmole | REM | rapid eye movement |
| MRI | magnetic resonance imaging | RNA | ribonucleic acid |
| ng | nanogram | SA | sinoatrial |
| NGU | nongonococcal urethritis | SAARD | slow-acting antirheumatic drug |
| NIDDM | noninsulin-dependent diabetes mellitus | SBP | systolic blood pressure |
| | | SC (SQ) | subcutaneous, subcutaneously |
| NNRTI | non-nucleoside reverse transcriptase inhibitor | SGOT | serum glutamic-oxaloacetic transaminase (also known as AST) |
| npo | nothing by mouth (*nil per os*) | SGPT | serum glutamic-pyruvic transaminase (also known as ALT) |
| NRTI | nucleoside reverse transcriptase inhibitor | sl | sublingual |
| NSAID | nonsteroidal anti-inflammatory drug | SLE | systemic lupus erythematosus |
| OC | oral contraceptive | SPF | sun protection factor |
| OD | right eye (*oculus dexter*) | SQ (SC) | subcutaneous, subcutaneously |
| OPV | oral polio vaccine | SR | sarcoplasmic reticulum; sustained release |
| OS | left eye (*oculus sinister*) | | |
| OTC | over-the-counter | SSRI | selective serotonin reuptake inhibitor |
| OU | both eyes (*oculus uterque*) | stat | immediately |
| PABA | *para*-aminobenzoic acid | STD | sexually transmitted disease |
| pc | after meals (*post cibum*) | SVT | supraventricular tachycardia |
| PCP | *Pneumocystis carinii* pneumonia | TIA | transient ischemic attack |
| PEFR | peak expiratory flow rate | tid | three times a day (*ter in die*) |
| PET | positron emission tomography | UTI | urinary tract infection |
| pg | picogram | VLDL | very-low-density lipoprotein |
| PG | prostaglandin | VSM | vascular smooth muscle |
| PID | pelvic inflammatory disease | WBC | white blood cell (leukocyte) |

# APPENDIX E

# Techniques of Drug Administration

*Linda A. Moore, M.S.N., Ed.D., R.N.*

| Type of Administration | Technique to Be Used |
| --- | --- |

## Oral

**Liquids**

### General Considerations

1. Perform any required dilution using appropriate liquid. Avoid liquids that can reduce drug absorption (e.g., milk will decrease absorption of tetracyclines).
2. Measure using medicine cup or device supplied with medication.
3. Pour medication away from label/directions.
4. Read amount at bottom of meniscus (see diagram).

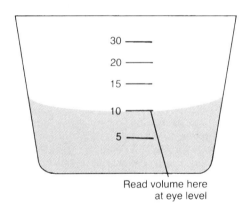

5. Do not leave patient before medication is taken.

### Infants

Do not mix medication with formula or juice in bottle (you cannot be sure of amount taken if all of the liquid is not swallowed).

### Nasogastric Tube Administration

1. Ensure correct location of the tube.
2. Follow directions for diluting (e.g., Metamucil becomes thick rapidly and should be mixed at time of administration, not before).
3. Follow with sufficient liquid to clear the tube (stay within fluid restrictions).

**Tablets, Capsules**

1. If possible, have the patient in a sitting position to facilitate swallowing.
2. Check requirement for administration with food or liquids (e.g., medications that irritate often need to be given with food; some medications may have decreased absorption with food).
3. Provide proper liquid for swallowing (stay within fluid restrictions, or, if patient needs increased fluids, this is a good time to provide extra fluid).

**Chewable Tables**

Be sure tablet is completely chewed before it is swallowed.

## Sublingual and Buccal

Sublingual
1. Place tablet under tongue, and instruct patient to hold it there until dissolved.
2. Swallowing of residual should then occur.

Buccal
1. Instruct patient to hold medication between teeth and cheek until it is dissolved.
2. Residual can then be swallowed.

## Rectal (Suppository)

1. Patient is to lie in left lateral Sims' position.
2. Nurse to wear gloves during procedure.
3. Lubricate suppository and glove fingertip with water-soluble lubricant.
4. Insert suppository when rectal sphincter is relaxed (see diagram).

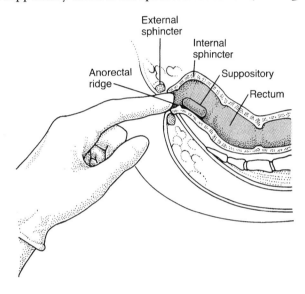

5. Instruct patient as to length of time to retain medication (about 20 to 30 minutes for defecation stimulation and about 60 minutes for systemic absorption).

## Vaginal

1. Wear gloves during procedure.
2. Insert foam or suppository into vagina.
3. Instruct patient as to length of time to remain lying down.

## Topical

1. Wear gloves when applying *any* topical ointment.
2. Apply with applicator, gauze, or gloved hand.
3. Apply a thin layer by patting, not rubbing.
4. Take care to protect the patient's clothing.
5. Certain medications require plastic wrap to increase absorption (e.g., nitroglycerin ointment).

## Otic

1. Medication should be at body temperature.
2. Patient should lie on side with appropriate ear up.

3. Instill drops toward auditory canal wall, not on eardrum. Procedure varies for adults and children. *Adults:* The auricle is pulled back and posteriorly. *Infants:* The auricle is pulled down and posteriorly (see diagram).

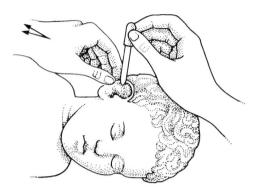

4. Rest hand administering drops lightly against the patient's head to prevent injury from dropper should the patient suddenly move.
5. Patient should remain in this position for about 15 minutes.

## Optic

1. Have patient lying on back with eyes facing up.
2. Do not touch tip of dropper to patient or to any object.

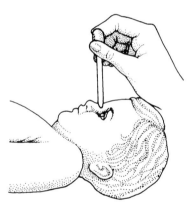

3. Have tissues available to blot any overflow from eyes (use separate tissue for each eye).
4. Rest hand instilling drops on patient's forehead to stabilize dropper and to prevent injury due to sudden patient movement.
5. Instill drops into conjunctival pouch while patient looks upward (see diagram).
6. To decrease systemic absorption, light pressure may be applied to lacrimal sac for about a minute.
7. *Ointment* is applied as a thin "ribbon" along inner aspect of lower lid. Do not touch tube to eye or other surface.

## Intradermal

1. Select an appropriate site. (Usual sites for *skin testing* are shown in the diagram.)

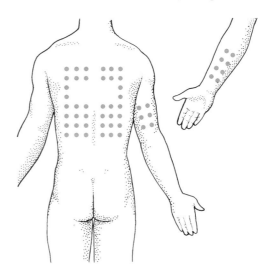

2. Use a short-bevel (26-gauge, ⅜-in) needle.
3. Amount of medication is limited to 1 ml or less.
4. If skin testing is being done, have emergency medication (epinephrine) available.
5. With bevel of needle pointed up, inject medication into layers of the skin (see diagram).

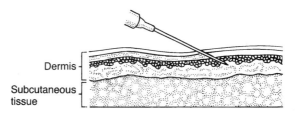

6. Use dry wipe to wipe area following injection.

## Subcutaneous

1. Select a needle size (usually 25- to 27-gauge, ½- to ⅝-in).
2. Select a site that has adequate subcutaneous tissue and that is away from bony prominences, major nerves, and blood vessels (see diagram).

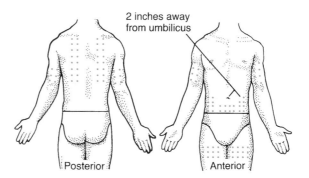

3. Angle of needle insertion depends on size of the individual. Obese people will require needle inserted at 90° angle, whereas very thin people will require pinching of the skin, with insertion at a 90° angle to the pocket pinched. Individuals who are neither fat nor very thin require a 45° angle for needle insertion (see diagram).

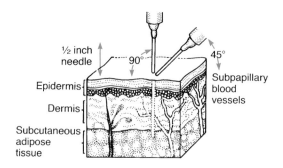

4. Aspiration for blood depends on substance being injected. Follow protocol.
5. Do not rub most SC injection sites.

## Intramuscular

1. Select a needle length appropriate to size of patient. The needle should be long enough to reach to the middle of the muscle. Measure the circumference of the arm and select appropriate needle length. The average person requires a 1½- to 2-inch needle. Muscular males require 2- to 3-inch needles or as long as 3- to 5-inches in some cases.
2. Select technique of injection.
   a. *Standard*—insert needle at 90° angle to the muscle after area is cleaned.
   b. *Z-track method*—pull tissue to one side, insert needle, inject medication, and allow tissue to return to original position as needle is removed. (Used for medications that damage tissue and as method to decrease pain of injection.)
3. Select site of injection:
   a. *Dorsogluteal*—to locate, draw a diagonal line between the superior iliac spine and the greater trochanter of the femur (see diagram). Patient should be prone with toes turned inward. *Do not use this site for children less than 2 years of age or for children who are emaciated.*
   b. *Ventrogluteal*—to locate, place palm of hand over the greater trochanter of the femur with thumb pointing to patient's abdomen, index finger placed over the anterior iliac spine, and middle finger spread back toward the iliac crest. The V-shaped area between the fingers is the ventrogluteal site. Direct needle toward largest muscle mass (see diagram).

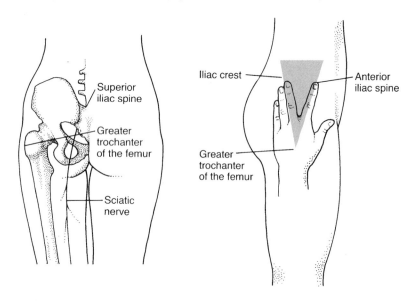

c. *Anteriolateral thigh*—to locate, area is one third the distance from the greater trochanter and the knee and is between the midline of the anterior and lateral thighs (see diagram). *This is a good site for infants and children.*

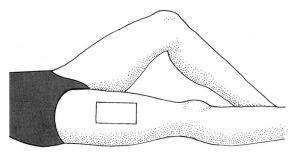

d. *Deltoid*—to locate, bordered above by 2 fingerbreadths below the acromion process and below by 2 fingerbreadths above the insertion of the deltoid (see diagram). Injection site must be in lateral aspect of the arm.

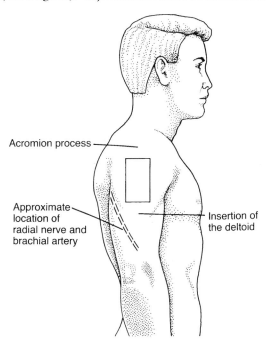

Acromion process

Approximate location of radial nerve and brachial artery

Insertion of the deltoid

4. Insert needle at 90° angle. Aspirate to be sure the needle is not in a blood vessel. Inject slowly. Withdraw needle, and apply pressure to site.

## Intravenous

1. Only clinicians with specific training should inject medication intravenously.
2. Medications can be administered into a continuous IV or a heparin lock designed for intermittent administration. Be sure medication is compatible with solution being infused. Check for infiltration prior to administering medication.
3. Do not administer medications that have precipitates or discoloration.
4. Dilute according to directions. Certain medications are not to be diluted. Be sure to check specifics.
5. If "piggybacking" medication, set drip rate for proper infusion time. Note drop rate on IV tubing package.
6. Tape IV securely but with some flexibility in the tubing.
7. Check IV frequently for correct infusion rate. Discontinue when complete dose has been delivered.
8. Record the name of the medication and volume of fluid administered.

# Certified Regional Poison Control Centers

Regional poison centers certified by the American Association of Poison Control Centers are accessible 24 hours a day; have a specially trained, full-time staff (usually nurses, pharmacists, or both); are directed by a board-certified physician-toxicologist; and are associated with a medical center that has laboratory facilities and personnel needed for the diagnosis and management of poisoning. In addition, certified poison centers participate in the toxic exposure surveillance system, and offer poison-prevention education to the public and poison-treatment education to health professionals. (This list was updated in November 1996.)

## Alabama

### Alabama Poison Center, Tuscaloosa
408-A Paul Bryant Drive
Tuscaloosa, AL 35401
Emergency Phone:
(800) 462-0800 (AL only)
(205) 345-0600

### Regional Poison Control Center
The Children's Hospital of Alabama
1600 Seventh Avenue South
Birmingham, AL 35233-1711
Emergency Phone:
(205) 939-9201
(800) 292-6678 (AL only)
(205) 933-4050

## Arizona

### Arizona Poison and Drug Information Center
Arizona Health Sciences Center, Room #1156
1501 North Campbell Avenue
Tucson, AZ 85724
Emergency Phone:
(800) 362-0101 (AZ only)
(520) 626-6016

### Samaritan Regional Poison Center
Good Samaritan Regional Medical Center, Ancillary-1
1111 East McDowell Road
Phoenix, AZ 85006
Emergency Phone:
(602) 253-3334

## California

### Central California Regional Poison Control Center
Valley Children's Hospital
3151 North Millbrook, IN31
Fresno, CA 93703
Emergency Phone:
(800) 346-5922 (Central CA only)
(209) 445-1222

### San Diego Regional Poison Center
UCSD Medical Center
200 West Arbor Drive
San Diego, CA 92103-8925
Emergency Phone:
(619) 543-6000
(800) 876-4766 (in 619 area code only)

### University of California, Davis, Medical Center
Regional Poison Control Center
2315 Stockton Boulevard
Sacramento, CA 95817
Emergency Phone:
(916) 734-3692
(800) 342-9293
(Northern CA only)

## Colorado

### Rocky Mountain Poison and Drug Center
8802 East Ninth Avenue
Denver, CO 80220-6800
Emergency Phone:
(303) 629-1123

# Connecticut

**Connecticut Regional Poison Center**
University of Connecticut Health Center
263 Farmington Avenue
Farmington, CT 06030
Emergency Phone:
(800) 343-2722 (CT only)
(203) 679-3056

# District of Columbia

**National Capital Poison Center**
3201 New Mexico Avenue N.W., Suite 310
Washington, DC 20016
Emergency Phone:
(202) 625-3333,
(202) 362-8563 (TTY)

# Florida

**Florida Poison Information Center–Miami**
University of Miami School of Medicine
Department of Pediatrics
P.O. Box 016960 (R-131)
Miami, FL 33101
Emergency Phone:
(800) 282-3171 (FL only)

**Florida Poison Information Center–Jacksonville**
University Medical Center
University of Florida Health Science
  Center–Jacksonville
655 West 8th Street
Jacksonville, FL 32209
Emergency Phone:
(904) 549-4480
(800) 282-3170 (FL only)

**The Florida Poison Information and
  Toxicology Resource Center**
Tampa General Hospital
P.O. Box 1289
Tampa, FL 33601
Emergency Phone:
(813) 253-4444 (Tampa)
(800) 282-3171 (Florida)

# Georgia

**Georgia Poison Center**
Grady Memorial Hospital
80 Butler Street S.E.
P.O. Box 26066
Atlanta, GA 30335-3801
Emergency Phone:
(800) 282-5846 (GA only)
(404) 616-9000

# Indiana

**Indiana Poison Center**
Methodist Hospital of Indiana
1701 North Senate Boulevard
P.O. Box 1367
Indianapolis, IN 46206-1367
Emergency Phone:
(800) 382-9097 (IN only)
(317) 929-2323

# Kentucky

**Kentucky Regional Poison Center of Kosair's
  Children's Hospital**
Medical Towers South, Suite 572
P.O. Box 35070
Louisville, KY 40232-5070
Emergency Phone:
(502) 629-7275
(800) 722-5725 (KY only)

# Louisiana

**Louisiana Drug and Poison Information Center**
Northeast Louisiana University
Sugar Hall
Monroe, LA 71209-6430
Emergency Phone:
(800) 256-9822
(318) 362-5393

# Maryland

**Maryland Poison Center**
20 North Pine Street
Baltimore, MD 21201
Emergency Phone:
(410) 528-7701
(800) 492-2414 (MD only)

**National Capital Poison Center
(D.C. suburbs only)**
3201 New Mexico Avenue N.W., Suite 310
Washington, DC 20016
Emergency Phone:
(202) 625-3333
(202) 362-8563 (TTY)

## Massachusetts

**Massachusetts Poison Control System**
300 Longwood Avenue
Boston, MA 02115
Emergency Phone:
(617) 232-2120
(800) 682-9211

## Michigan

**Poison Control Center**
Children's Hospital of Michigan
4160 John R., Suite 425
Detroit, MI 48201
Emergency Phone:
(313) 745-5711

## Minnesota

**Hennepin Regional Poison Center**
Hennepin County Medical Center
701 Park Avenue
Minneapolis, MN 55415
Emergency Phone:
(612) 347-3141
Petline: (612) 337-7387
TDD: (612) 337-7474

**Minnesota Regional Poison Center**
8100 34th Avenue South
P.O. Box 1309
Minneapolis, MN 55440-1309
Emergency Phone:
(612) 221-2113

## Missouri

**Cardinal Glennon Children's Hospital Regional
Poison Center**
1465 South Grand Boulevard
St. Louis, MO 63104
Emergency Phone:
(314) 772-5200
(800) 366-8888

## Montana

**Rocky Mountain Poison and Drug Center**
8802 East Ninth Avenue
Denver, CO 80220
Emergency Phone:
(303) 629-1123

## Nebraska

**The Poison Center**
8301 Dodge Street
Omaha, NE 68114
Emergency Phone:
(402) 390-5555 (Omaha)
(800) 955-9119 (NE & WY)

## New Jersey

**New Jersey Poison Information
and Education System**
201 Lyons Avenue
Newark, NJ 07112
Emergency Phone:
(800) 962-1253

## New Mexico

**New Mexico Poison and Drug Information Center**
University of New Mexico
Health Sciences Library, Room 125
Albuquerque, NM 87131-1076
Emergency Phone:
(505) 843-2551
(800) 432-6866 (NM only)

## New York

**Central New York Poison Control Center**
SUNY Health Science Center
750 East Adams Street
Syracuse, NY 13203
Emergency Phone:
(315) 476-4766
(800) 252-5655 (NY only)

**Finger Lakes Regional Poison Center**
University of Rochester Medical Center
601 Elmwood Avenue
Box 321, Room G-3275
Rochester, NY 14642
Emergency Phone:
(800) 333-0542
(716) 275-5151

**Hudson Valley Regional Poison Center**
Phelps Memorial Hospital Center
701 North Broadway
North Tarrytown, NY 10591
Emergency Phone:
(800) 336-6997
(914) 366-3030

**Long Island Regional Poison Control Center**
Winthrop University Hospital
259 First Street
Mineola, NY 11501
Emergency Phones:
(516) 542-2323, 542-2324
(516) 542-2325, 542-3813

**New York City Poison Control Center**
N.Y.C. Department of Health
455 First Avenue, Room 123
New York, NY 10016
Emergency Phone:
(212) 340-4494
(212) P-O-I-S-O-N-S
TDD (212) 689-9014

## North Carolina

**Carolinas Poison Center**
1012 South Kings Drive, Suite 206
P.O. Box 32861
Charlotte, NC 28232-2861
Emergency Phone:
(704) 355-4000
(800) 84-TOXIN
(800) 848-6946

## Ohio

**Central Ohio Poison Center**
700 Children's Drive
Columbus, OH 43205-2696
Emergency Phone:
(614) 228-1323
(800) 682-7625
(614) 228-2272 (TTY)
(614) 461-2012

**Cincinnati Drug & Poison Information Center and Regional Poison Control System**
P.O. Box 670144
Cincinnati, OH 45267-0144
Emergency Phone:
(513) 558-5111
(800) 872-5111 (OH only)

## Oregon

**Oregon Poison Center**
Oregon Health Sciences University
3181 S. W. Sam Jackson Park Road CB550
Portland, OR 97201
Emergency Room:
(503) 494-8968
(800) 452-7165 (OR only)

## Pennsylvania

**Central Pennsylvania Poison Center**
University Hospital
Milton S. Hershey Medical Center
Hershey, PA 17033
Emergency Phone:
(800) 521-6110

**The Poison Control Center**
3600 Sciences Center, Suite 220
Philadelphia, PA 19104-2641
Emergency Phone:
(215) 386-2100

**Pittsburgh Poison Center**
3705 Fifth Avenue
Pittsburgh, PA 15213
Emergency Phone:
(412) 681-6669

## Rhode Island

**Rhode Island Poison Center**
593 Eddy Street
Providence, RI 02903
Emergency Phone:
(401) 444-5727

# Tennessee

### Middle Tennessee Poison Center
The Center for Clinical Toxicology
Vanderbilt University Medical Center
1161 21st Avenue South
501 Oxford House
Nashville, TN 37232-4632
Emergency Phone:
(800) 288-9999
(615) 936-2034

# Texas

### Central Texas Poison Center
Scott & White Memorial Hospital
2401 South 31st Street
Temple, TX 76508
Emergency Phone:
(800) 764-7661

### North Texas Poison Center
5201 Harry Hines Boulevard
P.O. Box 35926
Dallas, TX 75235
Emergency Phone:
(800) 764-7661
Texas Watts (800) 441-0040

### Southeast Texas Poison Center
The University of Texas Medical Branch
301 University Avenue
Galveston, TX 77550-2780
Emergency Phone:
(409) 765-1420 (Galveston)
(713) 654-1701 (Houston)
(800) 764-7661

# Utah

### Utah Poison Control Center
410 Chipeta Way, Suite 230
Salt Lake City, UT 84108
Emergency Phone:
(801) 581-2151
(800) 456-7707 (UT only)

# Virginia

### Blue Ridge Poison Center
P.O. Box 67, Blue Ridge
University of Virginia Medical Center
Charlottesville, VA 22901
Emergency Phone:
(804) 924-5543
(800) 451-1428

### National Capital Poison Center
### (Northern VA only)
3201 New Mexico Avenue N.W., Suite 310
Washington, DC 20016
Emergency Phone:
(202) 625-3333
(202) 362-8563 (TTY)

# Washington

### Washington Poison Center
155 N.E. 100th Street, Suite #400
Seattle, WA 98125
Emergency Phone:
(206) 526-2121
(800) 732-6985
(800) 572-0638 (TDD only)
(206) 517-2394

# West Virginia

### West Virginia Poison Center
3110 MacCorkle Avenue S.E.
Charleston, WV 25304
Emergency Phone:
(800) 642-3625 (WV only)
(304) 348-4211

# Wyoming

### The Poison Center
8301 Dodge Street
Omaha, NE 68114
Emergency Phone:
(402) 390-5555 (Omaha)
(800) 955-9119 (NE & WY)

# Canadian Drug Information

*Alfred J. Rémillard, PharmD*

## International System of Units

In an attempt to standardize the large number of different units used worldwide and thus improve communication, the *Système International d'Unités* (International System of Units; SI) was recommended in 1954. In 1971, the mole (mol) was adopted as the standard for designating the amount of substance present, and the liter (L) was adopted as the standard for designating volume. The World Health Organization recommended the adoption of SI units in 1977. However, Canada had already implemented an equivalent system in 1971.

In therapeutics, the major change caused by adopting the SI was to express drug concentrations present in body fluids in molar units (e.g., mmol/L) rather than in mass units (e.g., mg/L). This allows us to better compare the pharmacologic and pharmacodynamic effects of different drugs, since these effects are now related to the number of molecules (e.g., mmol) of drug present rather than to the number of mass units (e.g., mg).

## Drug Serum Concentrations

Many drugs have known therapeutic or toxic levels that are monitored in patients to ensure safety and efficacy. In Canada, clinical laboratories report these levels in SI units. Levels traditionally reported as milligrams per milliliter (mg/ml) can be converted to millimoles per liter (mmol/L) once the conversion factor (CF) is calculated:

$$CF = \frac{1000}{\text{molecular weight of the drug}}$$

To convert from micrograms per milliliter to SI units, the following equation is used:

$$\mu g/ml \times CF = \mu mol/L$$

To convert from SI units to micrograms per milliliter, the following equation is used:

$$\frac{\mu mol/L}{CF} = \mu g/ml$$

Table G-1 lists some important drugs for which therapeutic or toxic levels have been established. For most of these drugs, the levels presented are *trough* (minimum) values, which are measured in blood samples drawn just prior to the next dose. For the aminoglycosides and vancomycin, two levels are listed: a *trough* level and a *peak* (maximum) level. Levels must remain between the peak and trough to maintain efficacy of these drugs and minimize toxicity.

## Canadian Drug Legislation

In Canada, two acts form the basis of drug laws. The Food and Drug Act, which was amended in 1953, controls the manufacture, distribution, and sale of all drugs except narcotics. The Narcotic Control Act (1961) controls the manufacture, distribution, and sale of narcotic drugs. The responsibility for administering these Acts rests with the Health Protection Branch, Department of National Health and Welfare. Both acts contain general statements relating to the safety and efficacy of drugs. Detailed requirements are outlined in the Food and Drug Regulations.

### Prescription Drugs (Schedule F)

The Food and Drug Regulations separate drugs sold in Canada into several categories, referred to as Schedules. Schedule F lists all prescription drugs, and includes diverse classes such as antihypertensives, hormonal preparations, and psychotropic medications. These drugs are available to the general public only with a prescription from a medical practitioner. Prescriptions for Schedule F medications may be written or verbal (i.e., telephone order to the pharmacist) and can be refilled as often as indicated by the physician. More than 350 drugs are listed in Schedule F, which is subject to frequent changes. The symbol Pr must appear on all manufacturing labels. Although some drugs may be classified *federally* as nonprescription, the *provinces* may nonetheless require a prescription, as occurs with digoxin, for example.

## TABLE G-1.  THERAPEUTIC SERUM DRUG CONCENTRATIONS

| Drugs | SI Reference Interval | SI Unit | Conversion Factor | Traditional Reference Interval | Traditional Reference Unit |
|---|---|---|---|---|---|
| Acetaminophen | 13–40 | μmol/L | 66.16 | 0.2–0.6 | mg/dl |
| Acetylsalicylic acid | 7.2–21.7 | μmol/L | 0.0724 | 100–300 | mg/dl |
| Amikacin* | — | — | — | 15–25[†]; <8[‡] | μg/ml |
| Amitriptyline | 430–900[§] | nmol/L | 3.605 | 120–250[§] | ng/ml |
| Carbamazepine | 17–42 | μmol/L | 4.233 | 4–10 | μg/ml |
| Desipramine | 430–750 | nmol/L | 3.754 | 115–200 | ng/ml |
| Digoxin | 0.6–2.8 | nmol/L | 1.282 | 0.5–2.2 | ng/ml |
| Disopyramide | 6–18 | μmol/L | 2.946 | 2–6 | μg/ml |
| Gentamicin* | — | — | — | 6–10[†]; <2[‡] | μg/ml |
| Imipramine | 640–1070[§] | nmol/L | 3.566 | 180–300[§] | ng/ml |
| Lidocaine | 4.5–21.5 | μmol/L | 4.267 | 1–5 | μg/ml |
| Lithium | 0.4–1.2 | mmol/L | 1.0 | 0.4–1.2 | mEq/L |
| Netilmicin | — | — | — | 6–10[†]; <2[‡] | μg/ml |
| Nortriptyline | 190–570 | nmol/L | 3.797 | 50–150 | ng/ml |
| Phenobarbital | 65–170 | μmol/L | 4.306 | 15–40 | μg/ml |
| Phenytoin | 40–80 | μmol/L | 3.964 | 10–20 | μg/ml |
| Primidone | 25–46 | μmol/L | 4.582 | 6–10 | μg/ml |
| Procainamide | 17–34[§] | μmol/L | 4.249 | 4–8[§] | μg/ml |
| Quinidine | 4.6–9.2 | μmol/L | 3.082 | 1.5–3 | μg/ml |
| Theophylline | 55–110 | μmol/L | 5.55 | 10–20 | μg/ml |
| Tobramycin* | — | — | — | 6–10[†]; <2[‡] | μg/ml |
| Valproic acid | 300–700 | μmol/L | 6.934 | 50–100 | μg/ml |
| Vancomycin* | — | — | — | 25–40[†]; <10[‡] | μg/ml |

*Aminoglycosides (amikacin, gentamicin, netilmicin, tobramycin) and vancomycin are not reported in SI units because of the variability of their molecular weights
[†]Peak drug level.
[‡]Trough drug level.
[§]Drug level reported as the total of the parent drug and its active metabolite.

## Controlled Drugs (Schedule G)

Controlled drugs, listed in Schedule G of the Food and Drug Act, have a moderate potential for abuse. Accordingly, these agents require greater control than Schedule F drugs (prescription drugs), which have essentially no potential for abuse. Schedule G contains about 14 drugs, including potent analgesics (nalbuphine, butorphanol), amphetamine and its congeners, and the barbiturates (phenobarbital, amobarbital, secobarbital). The distribution of controlled substances is more restricted than the distribution of Schedule F drugs. Schedule G drugs can be obtained by a written or verbal prescription, but refills are only allowed with a written order. The symbol Ⓒ must appear on the labels of these drugs. Schedule G is similar to Schedule III of the Controlled Substances Act in the United States.

## Restricted Drugs (Schedule H)

These agents are hallucinogenic, potentially dangerous, and have no recognized medical use. Examples include LSD, peyote, and mescaline. These chemicals are available legally only to medical institutions involved in specialized research. This category is similar to Schedule I of the Controlled Substances Act in the United States.

## Narcotic Drugs

Narcotic drugs are controlled by the Narcotic Control Act and Regulations. Examples include coca leaves (cocaine), opium, codeine, morphine, phencyclidine, and *Cannabis* (marijuana). The major clinical use for these drugs is strong analgesia. However, they all have potent psychotropic effects and addictive potential. As a result, their availability must be strictly controlled. Narcotic agents can be dispensed only with a written prescription. No refills are allowed. The letter N must appear on all labels and professional advertisements.

An exception to the narcotic drug regulations is low-dose codeine (8-mg tablets and 20 mg/30 ml solution), which can be purchased without a prescription. The codeine must be in a preparation that contains at least two additional medicinal ingredients (acetylsalicylic acid and caffeine) and can be sold only by a pharmacist.

## Nonprescription Drugs

Nonprescription drugs, also known as over-the-counter (OTC) medications, can be purchased without a prescription. Familiar drugs that have been available for years without prescription include mild analgesics (e.g., aspirin, acetaminophen), nasal decongestants (e.g., phenylephrine, phenylpropanolamine), antacids (e.g., calcium carbonate), and laxatives (e.g., magnesium hydroxide).

Many established prescription drugs are now being transferred to the OTC category. Experience has shown that drugs that become available as OTC products have strong consumer acceptance and increased sales. To be considered for OTC status, prescription products should have an established record of safety and efficacy. Since many older prescription drugs are being replaced by newer, superior prescription drugs, manufacturers have a strong incentive to promote the transfer of their older prescription drugs to the OTC category. In general, this transfer has proceeded more slowly in Canada than in the United States. However, certain agents, such as pediculocides and antihistamines, made the transfer in Canada first. Very often, when drugs are given OTC status, formulations are not as strong as their prescription counterparts. Examples include ibuprofen [Motrin] in 200-mg tablets, hydrocortisone in 0.5% topical preparations, and low-dose histamine$_2$-receptor antagonists, such as cimetidine [Tagamet].

### Schedules of Nonprescription Drugs

Although the Food and Drug Act and Regulations place no restrictions on how OTC drugs are sold, most provinces have drug schedules—administered by their respective Pharmacy Acts—to determine the conditions and place of sale. Because federal regulations are lacking, regulations on the sales of nonprescription drugs differ from province to province. To rectify this problem, the Health Protection Branch (HPB), working with provincial regulatory bodies, appointed the Canadian Drug Advisory Committee, whose mandate is to make recommendations to provincial regulators about drug scheduling. After establishing scientific criteria to determine the degree of professional involvement required for the sale and judicious use of drug products, this committee proposed a harmonized drug schedule to be implemented across Canada. This model has four drug categories:

- Schedule I—Prescription
- Schedule II—Pharmacist monitored
- Schedule III—Pharmacy-only sales
- Unscheduled

Drugs in Schedules I, II, and III are available only in pharmacies, whereas drugs in the Unscheduled category are available in pharmacies and in other outlets, such as grocery stores. The committee's recommendations were accepted by the National Association of Pharmacy Regulatory Authorities, and now each province is gradually implementing the new schedules. Also, a newly appointed National Drug Scheduling Advisory Committee will advise the federal government and provincial regulators as to which schedule a nonprescription drug should be assigned to.

**Schedule I.** This schedule includes all prescription products (Schedules F and G and Narcotics). Under the new system, provinces retain the authority to assign prescription status to a nonprescription drug. Nitroglycerin is a drug that might be regulated in this manner.

**Schedule II.** Drugs in this category are available only from the pharmacist, and only after consultation with the pharmacist. Schedule II agents must be kept in a place to which public access is restricted and in which there is no opportunity for patients to select the drug without assistance. Examples of Schedule II drugs include insulin, antihistamines associated with significant drug interactions (e.g., terfenadine, astemizole), and low-dose combination products containing codeine.

**Schedule III.** These drugs are sold from the self-selection area of the pharmacy. However, since these agents may present risks, a pharmacist must be available to assist the patient in making an appropriate selection. Examples of Schedule III drugs include low-dose formulations of ibuprofen, traditional antihistamines, and histamine$_2$ antagonists (e.g., famotidine).

**Unscheduled.** These drugs have proven safety and the public is considered familiar with their use. Examples include medicated shampoos, mild analgesics (e.g., aspirin), and cough drops. Unscheduled drugs are available through grocery stores and other retail outlets.

## New Drug Development in Canada

The process for approving a new drug in Canada is very similar, if not identical, to the process in the United States. The same drug data that are required for approval by the Food and Drug Administration in the United States are required by the Health Protection Branch in Canada. The principal difference between Canada and the United States is one of nomenclature: once preclinical testing is completed, the manufacturer in Canada applies for a *Preclinical New Drug Submission*, versus an Investigational New Drug in the United States; at the end of clinical testing, the manufacturer in Canada seeks a *New Drug Submission* (NDS), versus a New Drug Application in the United States.

After all the information on a new drug has been submitted—including results of preclinical and clinical testing, method of manufacturing, packaging, labeling, and results of stability testing—the pharmaceutical company receives a *Notice of Compliance* (NOC) from the HPB, and the drug enters the market.

Although data collection for a new drug is thorough, there is no guarantee that all adverse reactions are known, especially when the drug is used concurrently with other drugs. Also, long-term effects are not fully appreciated. For these reasons, postmarketing surveillance plays a major role in monitoring new drugs. The manufacturer must immediately report any new clinical findings, unexpected adverse effects, or therapeutic failures to the HPB.

## Patent Laws

Patent laws in Canada continue to evolve. In 1969, the Patent Act was changed to include compulsory licensing. This new provision allowed generic drug companies to manufacture and distribute patented drugs in Canada, provided that a minimal 4% royalty fee was paid to the patent holder. This system was introduced to help control drug prices. Unfortunately, the system caused a decline in revenue to "innovative" pharmaceutical companies, with a resultant decline in research on new drug development. After much debate, and retroactive to June 1987, the Patent Act was amended to give patent holders market exclusivity either (1) for 7 to 10 years or (2) until the 17-year patent (from date of filing) expires, whichever comes first. The Patent Act was then further amended to "make Canada's intellectual property legislation more in line with that of the major industrialized countries."

In response to provisions of the North American Free Trade Agreement (NAFTA) and the General Agreement on Tariffs and Trade (GATT), Bill C-91 was introduced in 1993. This bill (1) eliminated compulsory licensing and (2) extended patent protection on brand name drugs to 20 years, thereby making Canadian patent laws consistent with those of the United States and other industrialized nations. Section 14 of Bill C-91 calls for a Parliamentary Review of legislation in 1997. A special committee will review the impact of Bill C-91 on such factors as drug prices, drug research and development, and job creation.

In order to respond to concerns arising from changes in the Patent Act, a Patented Medicine Prices Review Board was created. Its mandate is to (1) ensure that prices of patented medicines are not excessive and (2) report on the ratios of research and development expenditures relative to sales for individual patentees and for the pharmaceutical industry as a whole.

## Some Important Canadian Trade Names

The list below contains common trade names used in Canada, many of which are the same as those used in the United States. In this list, trade names are presented in SMALL CAPITAL LETTERS and generic names are presented in standard type. Trade names that are formed by simply affixing a manufacturer's prefix to a generic name are not included; examples of such names are APO-FLURAZEPAM (flurazepam), NOVO-DIGOXIN (digoxin), PMS-ISONIAZID (isoniazid), and SYN-DILTIAZEM (diltiazem). An asterisk (*) indicates a drug that is available in Canada but not in the United States; these drugs are not discussed in the text.

3TC, lamivudine

5-Aminosalicylic acid, ASACOL, MESASAL, PENTASA, QUINTASA, SALOFALK

ABBOKINASE, urokinase

ABENOL, acetaminophen

ACCUPRIL, quinapril

ACCUTANE, isotretinoin

Acebutolol, MONITAN, RHOTRAL, SECTRAL

Acetaminophen, ABENOL, ATASOL, PANADOL, TYLENOL

ACETAZOLAM, acetazolamide

Acetazolamide, ACETAZOLAM, DIAMOX, NOVO-ZOLAMIDE

Acetohexamide, DIMELOR

ACETOXYL, benzoyl peroxide

Acetylcysteine, MUCOMYST, PARVOLEX

Acetylsalicylic acid, ECOTRIN, ENTROPHEN

ACHROMYCIN, tetracycline

ACILAC, lactulose

Acitretin, SORIATANE

ACTIFED, tripolidine

ACTIPROFEN, ibuprofen

ACTIVASE, alteplase

ACULAR, ketorolac

Acyclovir, AVIRAX, ZOVIRAX

ADALAT, nifedipine

ADENOCARD, adenosine

Adenosine, ADENOCARD

ADRIAMYCIN, doxorubicin

ADVIL, ibuprofen

AEROSPORIN, polymyxin B

AK-CON, naphazoline

AK-PENTOLATE, cyclopentolate

AK-SULF, sulfacetamide

AKARPINE, pilocarpine

AKINETON, biperiden

ALBERT TIAFEN, tiaprofenic acid* (NSAID)

Albuterol, *see* Salbutamol

ALDACTONE, spironolactone

ALDOMET, methyldopa

Alfacalcidol, ONE-ALPHA

ALFENTA, alfentanil

Alfentanil, ALFENTA

ALLERDRYL, diphenhydramine

Allopurinol, NOVO-PUROL, PURINOL, ZYLOPRIM

ALOMIDE, lodoxamide (antiallergy eye drops)

ALOPHEN, phenolphthalein

Alpha$_1$ proteinase inhibitor, PROLASTIN

Alprazolam, APO-ALPRAZ, NOVO-ALPRAZOL, NU-ALPRAZ, XANAX

Alprostadil, CAVERJECT, PROSTIN VR

ALTACE, ramipril

Alteplase, ACTIVASE

Altretamine, HEXALEN

ALUPENT, metaproterenol

Amantadine, EDANTADINE, SYMMETREL

AMATINE, midodrine

Ambenonium, MYTELASE

Amcinonide, CYCLOCORT

AMERSOL, ibuprofen

AMICAR, aminocaproic acid

Amikacin, AMIKIN
AMIKIN, amikacin
Amiloride, MIDAMOR
Aminobenzoate, POTABA
Aminocaproic acid, AMICAR
Aminoglutethimide, CYTADREN
Aminophylline, PHYLLOCONTIN
Amitriptyline, ELAVIL, LEVATE, NOVOTRIPTYN
Amlodipine, NORVASC
Amobarbital, AMYTAL
Amoxapine, ASENDIN
Amoxicillin, AMOXIL, APO-AMOXI, NOVAMOXIN, NU-AMOXI
Amoxicillin-clavulanate, CLAVULIN
AMOXIL, amoxicillin
Amphotericin B, FUNGIZONE
Ampicillin, AMPICIN, APO-AMPI, NU-AMPI, PENBRITIN
AMPICIN, ampicillin
Amrinone, INOCOR
AMYTAL, amobarbital
ANAFRANIL, clomipramine
ANANDRON, nilutamide
ANAPOLON 50, oxymetholone
ANAPROX, naproxen
ANCEF, cefazolin
ANCOTIL, flucytosine
Ancrod* (anticoagulant), ARVIN
ANDROCUR, cyproterone* (antiandrogen)
ANEXATE, flumazenil
Anileridine* (narcotic), LERITINE
ANSAID, flurbiprofen
ANTABUSE, disulfiram
ANTHRANOL, dithranol
ANTILURIUM, physostigmine
ANTIVERT, meclizine
ANTURAN, sulfinpyrazone
APARKANE, trihexyphenidyl
APO-ALPRAZ, alprazolam
APO-AMOXI, amoxicillin
APO-AMPI, ampicillin
APO-ATENOL, atenolol
APO-CAPTO, captopril
APO-CHLORAX, clidinium
APO-CLOXI, cloxacillin
APO-DICLO, diclofenac
APO-DILTIAZ, diltiazem
APO-DOXY, doxycycline
APO-ERYTHRO, erythromycin
APO-GAIN, minoxidil
APO-HYDRO, hydrochlorothiazide
APO-IPRAVENT, ipratropium
APO-ISDN, isosorbide dinitrate
APO-KETO, ketoprofen
APO-LEVOCARD, levodopa-carbidopa
APO-METOCLOP, metoclopramide
APO-NADOL, nadolol
APO-NIFED, nifedipine
APO-PEN-VK, penicillin V
APO-PINDOL, pindolol

APO-PRAZO, prazosin
APO-SALVENT, salbutamol (albuterol in United States)
APO-SULFATRIM, trimethoprim-sulfamethoxazole
APO-SULIN, sulindac
APO-TAMOX, tamoxifen
APO-TETRA, tetracycline
APO-TRIAZO, triazolam
APO-TRIHEX, trihexyphenidyl
APO-TRIMIP, trimipramine
APO-VERAP, verapamil
Apraclonidine, IOPIDINE
APRESOLINE, hydralazine
Aprotinin, TRASYLOL
ARALEN, chloroquine
AREDIA, pamidronate
ARISTOCORT, triamcinolone
ARLIDIN, nylidrin
ARTANE, trihexyphenidyl
ARVIN, ancrod* (anticoagulant)
ASACOL, 5-aminosalicyclic acid
ASENDIN, amoxapine
Asparaginase, KIDROLASE
Astemizole, HISMANAL
ATARAX, hydroxyzine
ATASOL, acetaminophen
Atenolol, APO-ATENOL, NOVO-ATENOL, TENORMIN
ATIVAN, lorazepam
Atorvastatin, LIPITOR
Atovaquone, MEPRON
Atracurium, TRACRIUM
ATROMID-S, clofibrate
Atropine, ATROPISOL
ATROPISOL, atropine
ATROVENT, ipratropium
Auranofin, RIDAURA
AUREOMYCIN, chlortetracycline
AVENTYL, nortriptyline
AVIRAX, acyclovir
AVLOSULFON, dapsone
AXID, nizatidine
Azatadine, OPTIMINE
Azathioprine, IMURAN
Azithromycin, ZITHROMAX
Bacampicillin, PENGLOBE
BACIGUENT, bacitracin
BACITIN, bacitracin
Bacitracin, BACIGUENT, BACITIN
Baclofen, LIORESAL, NU-BACLO
BACTRIM, trimethoprim-sulfamethoxazole
BACTROBAN, mupirocin (antibiotic)
BANLIN, propantheline
BCG, IMMUCYST
BECLOFORTE, beclomethasone
Beclomethasone, BECLOFORTE, BECLOVENT, BECONASE,
    VANCENASE, VANCERIL
BECLOVENT, beclomethasone
BECONASE, beclomethasone
BENADRYL, diphenhydramine

Benazepril, LOTESIN
Bendroflumethiazide, NATURETIN
BENEMID, probenecid
BENOXYL, benzoyl peroxide
Benserazide, PROLOPA
BENTYLOL, dicyclomine
BENURYL, probenecid
BENYLIN, dextromethorphan
Benzafibrate* (antihyperlipidemic), BEZALIP
Benzoyl peroxide, ACETOXYL, BENOXYL
Benztropine, COGENTIN
BEROTEC, fenoterol
BETAGAN, levobunolol
BETALOC, metoprolol
Betamethasone, CELESTONE, DIPROSONE
Betaxolol, BETOPTIC
Bethanechol, DUVOID, MYOTONACHOL, URECHOLINE
BETOPTIC, betaxolol
BEZALIP, benzafibrate* (antihyperlipidemic)
BIAXIN, clarithromycin
BICILLIN, penicillin G
BICNU, carmustine
Biperiden, AKINETON
BIQUIN, quinidine
Bisacodyl, DULCOLAX
BLOCADREN, timolol
BONAMINE, meclizine
BONEFOS, clodronate* (for hypercalcemia)
BRETYLATE, bretylium
Bretylium, BRETYLATE
BREVIBLOC, esmolol
BRICANYL, terbutaline
BRIETAL, methohexital
Bromazepam* (benzodiazepine), LECTOPAM
Bromocriptine, PARLODEL
Brompheniramine, DIMETANE, DIMETAPP
BRONALIDE, flunisolide
BRONKAID, epinephrine
Budesonide, ENTOCORT, PULMICORT, RHINOCORT
Bufexamac* (NSAID, topical), NORFEMAC
Bumetadine, BURINEX
BURINEX, bumetadine
Buserelin* (LH-RH analog), SUPREFACT
BUSPAR, buspirone
Buspirone, BUSPAR
Busulfan, MYLERAN
Butabarbital, BUTISOL
BUTISOL, butabarbital
Butorphanol, STADOL NS
CALCIJEX, calcitriol
CALCIMAR, calcitonin
Calcitonin, CALCIMAR, CALTINE
Calcitriol, CALCIJEX, ROCALTROL
CALTINE, calcitonin
CANESTEN, clotrimazole
CANTHACUR, cantharidin
Cantharidin, CANTHACUR, CANTHARONE
CANTHARONE, cantharidin
CAPOTEN, captopril

Capsaicin, ZOSTRIX
Captopril, APO-CAPTO, CAPOTEN, NU-CAPTO
Carbamazepine, NOVO-CARBAMAZ, TEGRETOL
CARBOCAINE, mepivacaine
CARBOLITH, lithium carbonate
Carboplatin, PARAPLATIN
CARDENE, nicardipine
CARDIZEM, diltiazem
CARDURA, doxazosin
Carmustine, BICNU
CATAPRES, clonidine
CATARASE, chymotrypsin
CECLOR, cefaclor
CEDOCARD, isosorbide
CEDOCARD-SR, isosorbide dinitrate
Cefaclor, CECLOR
Cefadroxil, DURICEF
Cefamandole, MANDOL
Cefazolin, ANCEF, KEFZOL
Cefepime, MAXIPIME
Cefixime, SOPRAX
CEFIZOX, ceftriaxone
CEFOMONIL, cefsulodin
CEFOTAN, cefotetan
Cefotaxime, CLAFORAN
Cefotetan, CEFOTAN
Cefoxitin, MEFOXIN
Cefprozil, CEFZIL
Cefsulodin, CEFOMONIL
Ceftazidime, CEPTAZ, FORTAZ, TAZIDIME
CEFTIN, cefuroxime
Ceftriaxone, CEFIZOX
Cefuroxime, CEFTIN, KEFUROX, ZINACEF
CEFZIL, cefprozil
CELESTONE, betamethasone
CELONTIN, methsuximide
Cephalexin, KEFLEX, NOVO-LEXIN
CEPHULAC, lactulose
CEPTAZ, ceftazidime
CEREVON, ferrous succinate
CERUBIDINE, daunorubicin
CESAMET, nabilone
Cetirizine, REACTINE
CHLOR-TRIPOLON, chlorpheniramine
Chlorambucil, LEUKERAN
Chloramphenicol, CHLOROMYCETIN, PENTAMYCETIN
Chlordiazepoxide, CORAX, LIBRIUM, NOVO-POXIDE
CHLOROMYCETIN, chloramphenicol
Chloroquine, ARALEN
Chlorothiazide, SUPRES
Chlorphenesin, MYCIL
Chlorpheniramine, CHLOR-TRIPOLON
CHLORPROM, chlorpromazine
CHLORPROMANYL, chlorpromazine
Chlorpromazine, CHLORPROM, CHLORPROMANYL, LARGACTIL
Chlorpropamide, DIABINESE, NOVO-PROPAMIDE
Chlortetracycline, AUREOMYCIN
Chlorthalidone, HYGROTON, NOVO-THALIDONE, URIDON
Cholecalciferol, D-TABS

CHOLEDYL, oxtriphylline
Cholestyramine, NOVO-CHOLAMINE, QUESTRAN
Choline magnesium trisalicylate, TRILISATE
Choline salicylate, TEEJEL, TRILISATE
CHOLOXIN, dextrothyroxine
CHRONULAC, lactulose
CHYMODIACTIN, chymopapain
Chymopapain, CHYMODIACTIN
Chymotrypsin, CATARASE, ZONULYN
CIDOMYCIN, gentamicin
Cilazapril* (ACE inhibitor), INHIBACE
CILOXAN, ciprofloxacin
Cimetidine, NU-CIMET, PEPTOL, TAGAMET
CIPRO, ciprofloxacin
Ciprofloxacin, CILOXAN, CIPRO
Cisapride, PROPULSID
Cisplatin, PLATINOL
CITANEST, prilocaine
Cladribine, LEUSTATIN
CLAFORAN, cefotaxime
CLARIPEX, clofibrate
Clarithromycin, BIAXIN
CLARITIN, loratadine
CLAVULIN, amoxicillin-clavulanate
Clemastine, TAVIST
Clidinium, APO-CHLORAX, CORIUM, LIBRAX
Clindamycin, DALACIN C
CLINORIL, sulindac
Clobazam* (benzodiazepine, anticonvulsant), FRISIUM
Clobetasol, DERMASONE, DERMOVATE
Clodronate* (bisphosphonate), BONEFOS, OSTAC
Clofibrate, ATROMID-S, CLARIPEX, NOVO-FIBRATE
Clomipramine, ANAFRANIL, NOVO-CLOPAMINE
Clonazepam, RIVOTRIL
Clonidine, CATAPRES, DIXARIT
CLOPIXOL, zuclopenthixol* (antipsychotic)
Clorazepate, NOVO-CLOPATE, TRANXENE
CLOTRIMADERM, clotrimazole
Clotrimazole, CANESTEN, CLOTRIMADERM, MYCLO-DERM, NEO-ZOL
Cloxacillin, APO-CLOXI, NOVO-CLOXIN, NU-CLOXI, ORBENIN, TEGOPEN
Clozapine, CLOZARIL
CLOZARIL, clozapine
COGENTIN, benztropine
COLACE, ducosate sodium
COLESTID, colestipol
Colestipol, COLESTID
COMBANTRIN, pyrantel
CORADUR, isosorbide dinitrate
CORAMINE, nikethamide
CORAX, chlordiazepoxide
CORGARD, nadolol
CORIUM, clindinium
CORONEX, isosorbide dinitrate
CORTATE, hydrocortisone
CORTEF, hydrocortisone
Cortisone, CORTONE
CORTONE, cortisone
CORTROSYN, cosyntropin

COSMEGEN, dactinomycin
Cosyntropin, CORTROSYN, SYNACTHEN DEPOT
COZAAR, losartan
CRIXIVAN, indinavir
Cromolyn, INTAL, NALCROM, OPTICROM, RYNACROM
CUPRIMINE, penicillamine
Cyanocobalamin, RUBION, RUBRAMIN
Cyclizine, MARZINE
Cyclobenzaprine, FLEXERIL, NOVO-CYCLOPRINE
CYCLOCORT, amcinonide
CYCLOGYL, cyclopentolate
CYCLOMEN, danazol
Cyclopentolate, AK-PENTOLATE, CYCLOGYL, DIOPENTOLATE
Cyclophosphamide, CYTOXAN, PROCYTOX
Cycloserine, SANDIMMUNE
CYKLOKAPRON, tranexamic acid* (hemostatic)
CYLERT, pemoline
Cyproheptadine, PERIACTIN
Cyproterone* (antiandrogen), ANDROCUR
CYTADREN, aminoglutethimide
Cytarabine, CYTOSAR
CYTOMEL, liothyronine
CYTOSAR, cytarabine
CYTOTEC, misoprostol
CYTOVENE, ganciclovir
CYTOXAN, cyclophosphamide
D-TABS, cholecalciferol
Dacarbazine, DTIC
Dactinomycin, COSMEGEN
DALACIN C, clindamycin
DALMANE, flurazepam
Danazol, CYCLOMEN
DANTRIUM, dantrolene
Dantrolene, DANTRIUM
Dapsone, AVLOSULFON
DARBID, isopropamide
DARVON, propoxyphene
Daunorubicin, CERUBIDINE
DDAVP, desmopressin
DECADRON, dexamethasone
Deferoxamine, DESFERAL
DEHYDRAL, methenamine
DELALUTIN, hydroxyprogesterone
DELATESTRYL, testosterone
Delavirdine, RESCRIPTOR
DELSYM, dextromethorphan
DELTASONE, prednisone
DEMADREX, torsemide
DEPAKENE, valproic acid
DEPEN, penicillamine
DEPO-MEDROL, methylprednisolone
DEPO-PROVERA, medroxyprogesterone
DERMASONE, clobetasol
DERMOVATE, clobetasol
DESFERAL, deferoxamine
Desipramine, NORPRAMIN, PERTOFRANE
Desmopressin, DDAVP
DESYREL, trazodone
Dexamethasone, DECADRON, DEXASONE, MAXIDEX

Dexamphetamine, DEXEDRINE
DEXASONE, dexamethasone
Dexbrompheniramine, DRIXORAL, DRIXTAB
Dexchlorpheniramine, POLARAMINE
DEXEDRINE, dexamphetamine
Dextromethorphan, BENYLIN, DELSYM, ROBIDEX, ROBITUSSIN
Dextrothyroxine, CHOLOXIN
DIABETA, glyburide
DIABINESE, chlorpropamide
DIAMICRON, glicazide*
DIAMOX, acetazolamide
DIAZEMULS, diazepam
Diazepam, DIAZEMULS, E-PAM, NOVO-DIPAM, VALIUM, VIVOL
Diazoxide, HYPERSTAT, PROGLYCEM
DICLECTIN, doxylamine
Diclofenac, APO-DICLO, NOVO-DIFENAC, NU-DICLO, VOLTAREN
Dicyclomine, BENTYLOL, FORMULEX
Didanosine, VIDEX
DIDRONEL, etidronate
Dienestrol, ORTHO DIENESTROL
Diethylcarbamazine, HETRAZAN
Diethylpropion, NOBESINE, TENUATE
Diethylstilbestrol, HONVOL
DIFLUCAN, fluconazole
Diflunisal, DOLOBID
DIGIBIND, digoxin immune Fab
DIGITALINE, digitoxin
Digitoxin, DIGITALINE
Digoxin immune Fab, DIGIBIND
Digoxin, LANOXIN
DILANTIN, phenytoin
DILAUDID, hydromorphone
DILOSYN, methdilazine
Diltiazem, APO-DILTIAZ, CARDIZEM, NU-DILTIAZ
DIMELOR, acetohexamide
Dimenhydrinate, GRAVOL, NAUSEATOL, TRAVEL AID
DIMETANE, brompheniramine
DIMETAPP, brompheniramine
Dinoprostone, PREPIDIL, PROSTIN
DIOPENTOLATE, cyclopentolate
DIOTROPE, tropicamide
DIPENTUM, olsalazine
Diphenhydramine, ALLERDRYL, BENADRYL
DIPROSONE, betamethasone
Dipyridamole, NOVO-DIPIRADOL, PERSANTINE
DISALCID, salsalate
DISIPAL, orphenadrine
Disopyramide, NORPACE, RYTHMODAN
Disulfiram, ANTABUSE
Dithranol, ANTHRANOL
DITROPAN, oxybutynin* (urinary antispasmotic)
Divalproex, EPIVAL
DIXARIT, clonidine
Dobutamine, DOBUTREX
DOBUTREX, dobutamine
Docusate calcium, SURFAK
Docusate sodium, COLACE, SELAX, SOFLAX
DOLOBID, diflunisal
DOLORAL, morphine

Domperidone, MOTILIUM
DOPAMET, methyldopa
Dopamine, INTROPIN
Dornase alfa, PULMOZYME
Doxacurium, NUROMAX
Doxazosin, CARDURA
Doxepin, SINEQUAN, TRIADAPIN
DOXIDAN, phenolphthalein
Doxorubicin, ADRIAMYCIN
DOXYCIN, doxycycline
Doxycycline, APO-DOXY, DOXYCIN, NOVO-DOXYLIN, VIBRAMYCIN
Doxylamine, DICLECTIN
DRISDOL, ergocalciferol
DRIXORAL, dexbrompheniramine* (antihistamine)
DRIXTAB, dexbrompheniramine* (antihistamine)
DTIC, dacarbazine
DULCOLAX, bisacodyl
DURABOLIN, nandrolone
DURAGESIC, fentanyl
DURALITH, lithium carbonate
DURETIC, methyclothiazide
DURICEF, cefadroxil
DUVOID, bethanechol
DYRENIUM, triamterene
E-MYCIN, erythromycin
E-PAM, diazepam
Echothiophate, PHOSPHOLINE IODIDE
Econazole, ECOSTATIN
ECOSTATIN, econazole
ECOTRIN, acetylsalicylic acid
EDANTADINE, amantadine
EDECRIN, ethacrynic acid
Edoxudine* (antiviral), VIROSTAT
Edrophonium, ENLON, TENSILON
EFFEXOR, venlafaxine
ELDEPRYL, selegiline
ELDISINE, vindesine
ELTOR, pseudoephedrine
ELTROXIN, levothyroxine
Enalapril, VASOTEC
Enalaprilat, VASOTEC IV
ENDOCET, oxycodone-acetaminophen
ENLON, edrophonium
Enoxaparin, LOVENOX
ENTOCORT, budesonide
ENTROPHEN, acetylsalicylic acid
Epinephrine, BRONKAID, SUS-PHRINE
EPIVAL, divalproex
Epoetin alfa, EPREX
EPREX, epoetin alfa
EQUANIL, meprobamate
ERGAMISOL, levamisole
Ergocalciferol, DRISDOL, OSTOFORTE
Ergoloid mesylates, HYDERGINE
ERGOMAR, ergotamine
Ergotamine, ERGOMAR, ERGOTRATE, GYNERGEN
ERGOTRATE, ergotamine
ERYC, erythromycin
ERYTHROMID, erythromycin

Erythromycin, APO-ERYTHRO, E-MYCIN, ERYC, ERYTHROMID, NOVO-RYTHRO
Esmolol, BREVIBLOC
ESTINYL, ethinyl estradiol
Estrone, FEMOGEN
Estropipate, OGEN
Ethacrynic acid, EDECRIN
Ethambutol, ETIBI, MYAMBUTOL
Ethinyl estradiol, ESTINYL
Ethopropazine, PARSITAN
Ethosuximide, ZARONTIN
ETIBI, ethambutol
Etidronate, DIDRONEL
Etodolac, ULTRADOL
EUFLEX, flutamide
EUGLUCON, glyburide
FACTREL, gonadorelin
Famciclovir, FAMVIR
Famotidine, PEPCID
FAMVIR, famciclovir
FASTIN, phentermine
FELDENE, piroxicam
Felodipine, PLENDIL, RENEDIL
FEMOGEN, estrone
Fenfluramine, PONDERAL, PONDIMIN
Fenofibrate* (antihyperlipidemic), LIPIDIL MICRO
Fenoprofen, NALFON
Fenoterol, BEROTEC
Fentanyl, DURAGESIC, SUBLIMAZE
FER-IN-SOL, ferrous sulfate
Ferrous fumarate, PALAFER
Ferrous succinate, CEREVON
Ferrous sulfate, FER-IN-SOL, SLOW-FE
Feverfew* (antimigraine), TANACET 125
FIBREPUR, psyllium
Filgrastim, NEUPOGEN
Finasteride, PROSCAR
FLAGYL, metronidazole
FLAMAZINE, silver sulfadiazine
Flavoxate* (antispasmotic), URISPAS
FLAXEDIL, gallamine
Flecainide, TAMBOCOR
FLEXERIL, cyclobenzaprine
Floctafenine* (NSAID), IDARAC
FLORINEF, fludrocortisone
FLOXIN, ofloxacin
FLUANXOL, flupenthixol
FLUCLOX, flucloxacillin* (antibiotic)
Flucloxacillin* (antibiotic), FLUCLOX
Fluconazole, DIFLUCAN
Flucytosine, ANCOTIL
FLUDARA, fludarabine
Fludarabine, FLUDARA
Fludrocortisone, FLORINEF
Flumazenil, ANEXATE
Flunarizine, SIBELIUM
Flunisolide, BRONALIDE, RHINALAR
FLUOR-I-STRIP, fluorescein
Fluorescein, FLUORESCITE, FLUOR-I-STRIP

FLUORESCITE, fluorescein
FLUOTHANE, halothane
Fluoxetine, PROZAC
Flupenthixol, FLUANXOL
Fluphenazine, MODECATE, MODITEN
Flurazepam, DALMANE, NOVO-FLUPAM, SOMNOL, SOMPAM
Flurbiprofen, ANSAID, FROBEN
Fluspirilene* (antipsychotic), IMAP
Flutamide, EUFLEX
Fluvastatin, LESCOL
Fluvoxamine, LUVOX
Folic acid, NOVO-FOLACID
FORANE, isoflurane
FORMULEX, dicyclomine
FORTAZ, ceftazidime
Fosinopril, MONOPRIL
FRISIUM, clobazam* (benzodiazepine, anticonvulsant)
FROBEN, flurbiprofen
FULVICIN, griseofulvin
FUNGIZONE, amphotericin B
Furosemide, FUROSIDE, LASIX, NOVO-SEMIDE, URITOL
FUROSIDE, furosemide
Gabapentin, NEURONTIN
Gallamine, FLAXEDIL
Ganciclovir, CYTOVENE
GARAMYCIN, gentamicin
GASTROZEPIN, pirenzepine
Gemfibrozil, LOPID
GEN-GLYBE, glyburide
GENT-AK, gentamicin
GENTACIDIN, gentamicin
Gentamicin, CIDOMYCIN, GARAMYCIN, GENTACIDIN, GENT-AK, GENTRASUL
GENTRASUL, gentamicin
GESTEROL, progesterone
Glicazide*, DIAMICRON
GLUCOPHAGE, metformin
Glyburide, DIABETA, EUGLUCON, GEN-GLYBE
Gonadorelin, FACTREL, LUTREPULSE, RELISORM
Goserelin, ZOLADREX
GRAVOL, dimenhydrinate
Griseofulvin, FULVICIN, GRISOVIN-FP
GRISOVIN-FP, griseofulvin
Guanethidine, ISMELIN
GYNECURE, tioconazole
GYNERGEN, ergotamine
HALCION, triazolam
HALDOL, haloperidol
Haloperidol, HALDOL, NOVO-PERIDOL, PERIDOL
Halothane, FLUOTHANE
HEPALEAN, heparin
Heparin, HEPALEAN
HERPLEX, idoxuridine
HETRAZAN, diethylcarbamazine
HEXALEN, altretamine
HISMANAL, astemizole
HISTANTIL, promethazine
HIVID, zalcitabine
HONVOL, diethylstilbestrol

HUMATROPE, somatropin
HYCODAN, hydrocodone
HYCORT, hydrocortisone
HYDERGINE, ergoloid mesylates
Hydralazine, APRESOLINE, NOVO-HYLAZIN, NU-HYDRAL
Hydrochlorothiazide, APO-HYDRO, HYDRODIURIL, NOVO-HYDRAZIDE
Hydrocodone, HYCODAN
Hydrocortisone, CORTATE, CORTEF, HYCORT
HYDRODIURIL, hydrochlorothiazide
HYDROMORPH CONTIN, hydromorphone
Hydromorphone, DILAUDID, HYDROMORPH CONTIN
Hydroxychloroquine, PLAQUENIL
Hydroxyprogesterone, DELALUTIN
Hydroxyzine, ATARAX, MULTIPAX
HYGROTON, chlorthalidone
HYPERSTAT, diazoxide
HYPRHO-D, RhO (D) immune globulin
HYTRIN, terazosin
Ibuprofen, ACTIPROFEN, ADVIL, AMERSOL, MEDIPREN, MOTRIN, NOVO-PROFEN
IDARAC, floctafenine* (NSAID)
Idoxuridine, HERPLEX, STOXIL
IMAP, fluspirilene* (antipsychotic)
IMFERON, iron dextran
Imipenem-cilastatin, PRIMAXIN
Imipramine, IMPRIL, NOVO-PRAMINE, TOFRANIL
IMITREX, sumatriptan
IMMUCYST, BCG
IMODIUM, loperamide
IMOVANE, zopiclone* (hypnotic)
IMPRIL, imipramine
IMURAN, azathioprine
Indapamide, LOZIDE
INDERAL, propranolol
Indinavir, CRIXIVAN
INDOCID, indomethacin
Indomethacin, INDOCID, INDOTEC, NOVO-METHACIN, NU-INDO
INDOTEC, indomethacin
INDUR, isosorbide mononitrate
INHIBACE, cilazapril* (ACE inhibitor)
INOCOR, amrinone
INTAL, cromolyn
Interferon alfa-n1, WELLFERON
INTROPIN, dopamine
INVIRASE, saquinavir
IONAMIN, phentermine
IOPIDINE, apraclonidine
Ipratropium, APO-IPRAVENT, ATROVENT, NOVO-IPRAMIDE
Iron dextran, IMFERON
Iron sorbitex, JECTOFER
ISMELIN, guanethidine
ISMO, isosorbide mononitrate
Isoflurane, FORANE
Isoniazid, ISOTAMINE
Isoproterenol, ISUPREL
ISOPTIN, verapamil
ISOPTO-CARPINE, pilocarpine
ISORDIL, isosorbide dinitrate

Isosorbide dinitrate, APO-ISDN, CEDOCARD-SR, CORADUR, CORONEX, ISORDIL
Isosorbide mononitrate, INDUR, ISMO
ISOTAMINE, isoniazid
Isotretinoin, ACCUTANE, ISOTREX
ISOTREX, isotretinoin
Isoxsuprine, VASODILAN
ISUPREL, isoproterenol
Itraconazole, SPORANOX
JECTOFER, iron sorbitex
KABIKINASE, streptokinase
KEFLEX, cephalexin
KEFUROX, cefuroxime
KEFZOL, cefazolin
KEMADRIN, procyclidine
Ketazolam* (benzodiazepine), LOFTRAN
Ketoconazole, NIZORAL
Ketoprofen, APO-KETO, NOVO-KETO, ORUDIS, ORUVAIL, RHODIS
Ketorolac, ACULAR, TORADOL
Ketotifen* (antiallergy), ZADITEN
KIDROLASE, asparaginase
KONAKION, phytomenadione
KWELLADA, lindane
*l*-Tryptophan, TRYPTAN
Labetalol, TRANDATE
Lactulose, ACILAC, CEPHULAC, CHRONULAC, RHODIALOSE
LAMICTAL, lamotrigine
Lamivudine, 3TC
Lamotrigine, LAMICTAL
LANOXIN, digoxin
LANVIS, thioguanine
LARGACTIL, chlorpromazine
LASIX, furosemide
LECTOPAM, bromazepam* (benzodiazepine)
LERITINE, anileridine* (narcotic)
LESCOL, fluvastatin
LEUKERAN, chlorambucil
Leuprolide, LUPRON
LEUSTATIN, cladribine
Levamisole, ERGAMISOL
Levarterenol, *see* Norepinephrine
LEVATE, amitriptyline
LEVO T, levothyroxine
LEVO-DROMORAN, levorphanol
Levobunolol, BETAGAN
Levocabastine, LIVOSTIN
Levodopa-benserazide* (antiparkinson), PROLOPA
Levodopa-carbidopa, APO-LEVOCARD, SINEMET
LEVOPHED, norephinephrine
Levorphanol, LEVO-DROMORAN
Levothyroxine, ELTROXIN, LEVO T, SYNTHROID
LIBRAX, clidinium
LIBRIUM, chlordiazepoxide
Lidocaine, XYLOCARD
LINCOCIN, lincomycin
Lincomycin, LINCOCIN
Lindane, KWELLADA
LIORESAL, baclofen
Liothyronine, CYTOMEL

LIPIDIL MICRO, fenofibrate* (antihyperlipidemic)
LIPITOR, atrovastatin
Lisinopril, PRINIVIL, ZESTRIL
Lithium carbonate, CARBOLITH, DURALITH, LITHIZINE
LITHIZINE, lithium carbonate
LIVOSTIN, levocabastine
Lodoxamide* (antiallergy eye drops), ALOMIDE
LOFTRAN, ketazolam* (benzodiazepine)
LONITEN, minoxidil
Loperamide, IMODIUM
LOPID, gemfibrozil
LOPRESSOR, metoprolol
Loratadine, CLARITIN
Lorazepam, ATIVAN, NOVO-LORAZEM, NU-LORAZ
Losartan, COZAAR
LOSEC, omeprazole
LOTENSIN, benazepril
Lovastatin, MEVACOR
LOVENOX, enoxaparin
LOXAPAC, loxapine
Loxapine, LOXAPAC
LOZIDE, indapamide
LUDIOMIL, maprotiline
LUPRON, leuprolide
LUTREPULSE, gonadorelin
LUVOX, fluvoxamine
M.O.S., morphine
MACRODANTIN, nitrofurantoin
MAJEPTIL, thioproperazine* (antipsychotic)
MANDELAMINE, methenamine
MANDOL, cefamandole
MANERIX, moclobemide* (MAOI)
Maprotiline, LUDIOMIL
MARZINE, cyclizine
MAXERAN, metoclopramide
MAXIDEX, dexamethasone
MAXIPIME, cefepime
Mazindol, SANOREX
MEBARAL, mephobarbital
Mebendazole, VERMOX
Meclizine, ANTIVERT, BONAMINE
MEDIPREN, ibuprofen
MEDROL, methylprednisolone
Medroxyprogesterone, DEPO-PROVERA, PROVERA
Mefenamic acid, PONSTAN
MEFOXIN, cefoxitin
MEGACILLIN, penicillin G
MELLARIL, thioridazine
Menadiol, SYNKAVITE
Mephenytoin, MESANTOIN
Mephobarbital, MEBARAL
Mepivacaine, CARBOCAINE
Meprobamate, EQUANIL, NOVO-MEPRO
MEPRON, atovaquone
MESANTOIN, mephenytoin
MESASAL, 5-aminosalicylic acid
Mesna, UROMITEXAN
Mesoridazine, SERENTIL
MESTINON, pyridostigmine

METAMUCIL, psyllium
METANDREN, methyltestosterone
Metaproterenol, ALUPENT
Metformin, GLUCOPHAGE
Methazolamide, NEPTAZANE
Methdilazine, DILOSYN
Methenamine, DEHYDRAL, MANDELAMINE, URASAL
Methimazole, TAPAZOLE
Methocarbamol-ASA, ROBAXIN, ROBAXISAL
Methohexital, BRIETAL
Methotrimeprazine, NOVO-MEPRAZINE, NOZINAN
Methoxamine, VASOXYL
Methsuximide, CELONTIN
Methyclothiazide, DURETIC
Methyldopa, ALDOMET, DOPAMET, NOVO-MEDOPA, NU-MEDOPA
Methylphenidate, RITALIN
Methylprednisolone, DEPO-MEDROL, MEDROL
Methyltestosterone, METANDREN
Methylsergide, SANSERT
Metoclopramide, APO-METOCLOP, MAXERAN, REGLAN
Metolazone, ZAROXOLYN
Metoprolol, BETALOC, LOPRESSOR, NOVO-METOPROL,
    NU-METOP
Metronidazole, FLAGYL, NOVO-NIDAZOL, TRIKACIDE
MEVACOR, lovastatin
Mexiletine, MEXITIL
MEXITIL, mexiletine
MICATIN, miconazole
Miconazole, MICATIN, MONISTAT
MICRONOR, norethindrone
MIDAMOR, amiloride
Midazolam, VERSED
Midodrine, AMATINE
Milrinone, PRIMACOR
MINIPRESS, prazosin
MINOCIN, minocycline
Minocycline, MINOCIN
Minoxidil, APO-GAIN, LONITEN, ROGAINE
MINTEZOL, thiabendazole
MIOCARPINE, pilocarpine
Misoprostol, CYTOTEC
MOBENOL, tolbutamide
MOBIFLEX, tenoxicam* (NSAID)
Moclobemide* (MAOI), MANERIX
MODECATE, fluphenazine
MODITEN, fluphenazine
MOGADON, nitrazepam
MONISTAT, miconazole
MONITAN, acebutolol
MONOPRIL, fosinopril
Morphine, DOLORAL, MS CONTIN, M.O.S.
MOTILIUM, domperidone
MOTRIN, ibuprofen
MS CONTIN, morphine
MUCOMYST, acetylcysteine
MULTIPAX, hydroxyzine
Mupirocin (antibiotic), BACTROBAN
Muromonab-CD3, OKT3, ORTHOCLONE
MYAMBUTOL, ethambutol

MYCIFRADIN, neomycin
MYCIGUENT, neomycin
MYCIL, chlorphenesin
MYCLO-DERM, clotrimazole
MYDFRIN, phenylephrine
MYDRIACYL, tropicamide
MYLERAN, busulfan
MYOTONACHOL, bethanechol
MYSOLINE, primidone
MYTELASE, ambenonium
Nabilone, CESAMET
Nadolol, APO-NADOL, CORGARD
Nafarelin, SYNAREL
Nafcillin, UNIPEN
NAFRINE, oxymetazoline
Nalbuphine, NUBAIN
NALCROM, cromolyn
NALFON, fenoprofen
Nalidixic acid, NEGGRAM
Naloxone, NARCAN
Naltrexone, REVIA
Nandrolone, DURABOLIN
Naphazoline, AK-CON, PRIVINE, RHINO-MEX-N, VASOCON
NAPROSYN, naproxen
Naproxen, ANAPROX, NAPROSYN, NAXEN, NEOPROX,
    NOVO-NAPROX, NU-NAPROX
NARCAN, naloxone
NARDIL, phenelzine
NASACORT, triamcinolone
NATULAN, procarbazine
NATURETIN, bendroflumethiazide
NAUSEATOL, dimenhydrinate
NAVANE, thiothixene
NAXEN, naproxen
NEBCIN, tobramycin
Nedocromil, TILADE
Nefazodone, SERZONE
NEGGRAM, nalidixic acid
Nelfinavir, VIRACEPT
NEMBUTAL, pentobarbital
NEO-PAUSE, testosterone/estradiol
NEO-PROX, naproxen
NEO-SYNEPHRINE, phenylephrine
NEO-ZOL, clotrimazole
Neomycin, MYCIFRADIN, MYCIGUENT
Neostigmine, PROSTIGMIN
NEPTAZANE, methazolamide
Netilmicin, NETROMYCIN
NETROMYCIN, netilmicin
NEULEPTIL, pericyazine* (antipsychotic)
NEUPOGEN, filgrastim
NEURONTIN, gabapentin
Nevirapine, VIRAMUNE
Nicardipine, CARDENE
NICODERM, nicotine
NICORETTE, nicotine
Nicotine, NICODERM, NICORETTE, NICOTROL
Nicotinyl alcohol tartrate, RONIACOL
NICOTROL, nicotine

Nifedipine, ADALAT, APO-NIFED, NOVO-NIFEDIN, NU-NIFED
Nikethamide, CORAMINE
NILSTAT, nystatin
Nilutamide, ANANDRON
Nimodipine, NIMOTOP
NIMOTOP, nimodipine
Nitrazepam, MOGADON
Nitrofurantoin, MACRODANTIN, NOVO-FURAN
Nitroglycerin, NITROL, NITROSTAT, TRANSDERM-NITRO
NITROL, nitroglycerin
NITROSTAT, nitroglycerin (intravenous)
Nizatidine, AXID
NIZORAL, ketoconazole
NOBESINE, diethylpropion
NOLVADEX, tamoxifen
Norepinephrine, LEVOPHED
Norethindrone, MICRONOR, NORLUTATE
NORFEMAC, bufexamac* (NSAID, topical)
NORFLEX, orphenadrine
Norfloxacin, NOROXIN
NORLUTATE, norethindrone
NOROXIN, norfloxacin
NORPACE, disopyramide
NORPRAMIN, desipramine
Nortriptyline, AVENTYL
NORVASC, amlodipine
NORVIR, ritonavir
NOVA-RECTAL, pentobarbital
NOVAMOXIN, amoxicillin
NOVO-ALPRAZOL, alprazolam
NOVO-ATENOL, atenolol
novo-AZT, zidovudine
NOVO-BUTAMIDE, tolbutamide
NOVO-BUTAZONE, phenylbutazone
NOVO-CARBAMAZ, carbamazepine
NOVO-CHOLAMINE, cholestyramine
NOVO-CLOPAMINE, clomipramine
NOVO-CLOPATE, clorazepate
NOVO-CLOXIN, cloxacillin
NOVO-CYCLOPRINE, cyclobenzaprine
NOVO-DIFENAC, diclofenac
NOVO-DIPAM, diazepam
NOVO-DIPIRADOL, dipyridamole
NOVO-DOXYLIN, doxycycline
NOVO-FIBRATE, clofibrate
NOVO-FLUPAM, flurazepam
NOVO-FLURAZINE, trifluoperazine
NOVO-FOLACID, folic acid
NOVO-FURAN, nitrofurantoin
NOVO-HEXIDYL, trihexyphenidyl
NOVO-HYDRAZIDE, hydrochlorothiazide
NOVO-HYLAZIN, hydralazine
NOVO-IPRAMIDE, ipratropium
NOVO-KETO, ketoprofen
NOVO-LEXIN, cephalexin
NOVO-LORAZEM, lorazepam
NOVO-MEDOPA, methyldopa
NOVO-MEPRAZINE, methotrimeprazine
NOVO-MEPRO, meprobamate

NOVO-METHACIN, indomethacin
NOVO-METOPROL, metoprolol
NOVO-MUCILAX, psyllium
NOVO-NAPROX, naproxen
NOVO-NIDAZOL, metronidazole
NOVO-NEFEDIN, nifedipine
NOVO-PEN-VK, penicillin V
NOVO-PERIDOL, haloperidol
NOVO-PINDOL, pindolol
NOVO-PIROCAM, piroxicam
NOVO-POXIDE, chlordiazepoxide
NOVO-PRANOL, propranolol
NOVO-PRAZIN, prazosin
NOVO-PRED, prednisolone
NOVO-PROFEN, ibuprofen
NOVO-PROPAMIDE, chlorpropamide
NOVO-PUROL, allopurinol
NOVO-PYRAZONE, sulfinpyrazone
NOVO-RANIDINE, ranitidine
NOVO-RIDAZINE, thioridazine
NOVO-RYTHRO, erythromycin
NOVO-SALMOL, salbutamol (albuterol in United States)
NOVO-SECOBARB, secobarbital
NOVO-SEMIDE, furosemide
NOVO-SPIROTON, spironolactone
NOVO-SUNDAC, sulindac
NOVO-TETRA, tetracycline
NOVO-THALIDONE, chlorthalidone
NOVO-TIMOL, timolol
NOVO-TRIMEL, trimethoprim-sulfamethoxazole
NOVO-TRIOLAM, triazolam
NOVO-TRIPRAMINE, trimipramine
NOVO-VERAMIL, verapamil
NOVO-ZOLAMIDE, acetazolamide
NOVOTRIPHYL, oxtriphylline
NOZINAN, methotrimeprazine or levomepromazine
NU-ALPRAZ, alprazolam
NU-AMOXI, amoxicillin
NU-AMPI, ampicillin
NU-BACLO, baclofen
NU-CAPTO, captopril
NU-CIMET, cimetidine
NU-CLOXI, cloxacillin
NU-DICLO, diclofenac
NU-DILTIAZ, diltiazem
NU-HYDRAL, hydralazine
NU-INDO, indomethacin
NU-LORAZ, lorazepam
NU-MEDOPA, methyldopa
NU-METOP, metoprolol
NU-NAPROX, naproxen
NU-NIFED, nifedipine
NU-PEN-VK, penicillin V
NU-PINDOL, pindolol
NU-PIROX, piroxicam
NU-PRAZO, prazosin
NU-RANIT, ranitidine
NU-TETRA, tetracycline
NU-TRIAZO, triazolam

NU-VERAP, verapamil
NUBAIN, nalbuphine
NUMORPHAN, oxymorphone
NUPROCHLOR, prochlorperazine
NUROMAX, doxacurium
NYADERM, nystatin
Nylidrin, ARLIDIN
Nystatin, MYCOSTATIN, NILSTAT, NYADERM
Octreotide, SANDOSTATIN
OCUCLEAR, oxymetazoline
OCUFLOX, ofloxacin
Ofloxacin, FLOXIN, OCUFLOX
OGEN, estropipate
OKT3, muronomab-CD3
Olanzepine, ZYPREXA
Omeprazole, LOSEC
ONCOVIN, vincristine
Ondansetron, ZOFRAN
ONE-ALPHA, alfacalcidol
OPHTHO-SULF, sulfacetamide
OPTICROM, cromolyn
OPTIMINE, azatadine
ORAP, pimozide
ORBENIN, cloxacillin
Orciprenaline, *see* Metaproterenol
ORFENACE, orphenadrine
ORINASE, tolbutamide
ORNADE, phenylpropanolamine
Orphenadrine, DISIPAL, NORFLEX, ORFENACE
ORTHO DIENESTROL, dienestrol
ORTHOCLONE, muromonab-CD3
ORUDIS, ketoprofen
ORUVAIL, ketoprofen
Olsalazine, DIPENTUM
OSTAC, clodronate* (bisphosphonate)
OSTOFORTE, ergocalciferol
OTRIVIN, xylometazoline
OVOL, simethicone
Oxazepam, OXPAM, SERAX
OXPAM, oxazepam
Oxprenolol, TRASICOR
Oxtriphylline, CHOLEDYL, NOVO-TRIPHYL
OXYBUTAZONE, oxyphenbutazone
Oxybutynin* (urinary antispasmotic), DITROPAN
OXYCOCET, oxycodone-acetaminophen
Oxycodone-acetaminophen, ENDOCET, OXYCOCET, PERCOCET, ROXICET
Oxymetazoline, NAFRINE, OCUCLEAR
Oxymetholone, ANAPOLON 50
Oxymorphone, NUMORPHAN
Oxyphenbutazone, OXYBUTAZONE, TANDEARIL
Paclitaxel, TAXOL
PALAFER, ferrous fumarate
Pamidronate, AREDIA
PANADOL, acetaminophen
PANECTYL, trimeprazine
PARAPLATIN, carboplatin
PARLODEL, bromocriptine
PARNATE, tranylcypromine

Paroxetine, PAXIL

PARSITAN, ethopropazine

PARVOLEX, acetylcysteine

PAXIL, paroxetine

Pemoline, CYLERT

PEN-VEE, penicillin V

PENBRITIN, ampicillin

PENGLOBE, bacampicillin

Penicillamine, CUPRIMINE, DEPEN

Penicillin G, BICILLIN, MEGACILLIN

Penicillin V, APO-PEN-VK, NOVO-PEN-VK, NU-PEN-VK, PEN-VEE, PVF

PENTACARINAT, pentamidine

Pentaerythritol tetranitrate, PERITRATE

Pentamidine, PENTACARINATE, PNEUMOPENT

PENTAMYCETIN, chloramphenicol

PENTASA, 5-aminosalicylic acid

Pentazocine, TALWIN

Pentobarbital, NOVA-RECTAL, NEMBUTAL

Pentoxifylline, TRENTAL

PEPCID, famotidine

PEPTOL, cimetidine

PERCOCET, oxycodone-acetaminophen

Pergolide, PERMAX

PERIACTIN, cyproheptadine

Pericyazine* (antipsychotic), NEULEPTIL

PERIDOL, haloperidol

PERITRATE, pentaerythritol tetranitrate

PERMAX, pergolide

Perphenazine, PHENAZINE, TRILAFON

PERSANTINE, dipyridamole

PERTOFRANE, desipramine

PHENAZINE, perphenazine

PHENAZO, phenazopyridine* (urinary analgesic)

Phenazopyridine* (urinary analgesic), PHENAZO, PYRIDIUM, PYRONIUM

PHENERGAN, promethazine

Phenolphthalein, ALOPHEN, DOXIDAN

Phentermine, FASTIN, IONAMIN

Phentolamine, ROGITINE

Phenylbutazine, NOVO-BUTAZONE

Phenylephrine, MYDFRIN, NEO-SYNEPHRINE

Phenylpropanolamine, ORNADE, SINE-OFF

Phenylzine, NARDIL

Phenytoin, DILANTIN

PHOSPHOLINE IODIDE, echothiophate

PHYLLOCONTIN, aminophylline

Physostigmine, ANTILURIUM

Phytomenadione, KONAKION

Pilocarpine, AKARPINE, ISOPTOCARPINE, MIOCARPINE, PILOPINE

PILOPINE, pilocarpine

Pimozide, ORAP

Pindolol, APO-PINDOL, NOVO-PINDOL, NU-PINDOL, VISKEN

Piperacillin, PIPRACIL

Pipericillin-tazobactam, TAZOCIN

PIPORTIL-L4, pipotiazine* (antipsychotic)

Pipotiazine* (antipsychotic), PIPORTIL-L4

PIPRACIL, piperacillin

Pirenzepine, GASTROZEPIN

Piroxicam, FELDENE, NOVO-PIROCAM, NU-PIROX

PITRESSIN, vasopressin

Pivampicillin* (antibacterial), PONDOCILLIN

Pizotifen* (antimigraine), SANDOMIGRAN

PLAQUENIL, hydroxychloroquine

PLATINOL, cisplatin

PLENDIL, felodipine

PNEUMOPENT, pentamidine

PODOFILM, podophyllum resin

Podophyllum resin, PODOFILM

POLARAMINE, dexchlorpheniramine

Polymyxin B, AEROSPORIN

PONDERAL, fenfluramine

PONDIMIN, fenfluramine

PONDOCILLIN, pivampicillin* (antibacterial)

PONSTAN, mefenamic acid

POTABA, aminobenzoate

Pramoxine, TRONOTHANE

PRAVACHOL, pravastatin

Pravastatin, PRAVACHOL

Prazosin, APO-PRAZO, MINIPRESS, NOVO-PRAZIN, NU-PRAZO

Prednisolone, NOVO-PRED

Prednisone, DELTASONE, WINPRED

PREPIDIL, dinoprostone

PRESSYN, vasopressin

Prilocaine, CITANEST

PRIMACOR, milrinone

PRIMAXIN, imipenem-cilastatin

Primidone, MYSOLINE, SERTAN

PRINIVIL, lisinopril

PRIVINE, naphazoline

PRO-BANTHINE, propantheline

Probenecid, BENEMID, BENURYL

Procainamide, PROCAN SR, PRONESTYL

PROCAN SR, procainamide

Procarbazine, NATULAN

Prochlorperazine, NU-PROCHLOR, STEMETIL

PROCYCLID, procyclidine

Procyclidine, KEMADRIN, PROCYCLID

PROCYTOX, cyclophosphamide

PRODIEM, psyllium

Progesterone, GESTEROL

PROGLYCEM, diazoxide

PROLASTIN, alpha$_1$ proteinase inhibitor

PROLOPA, levodopa-benserazide* (antiparkinson)

PROLOPRIM, trimethoprim

Promethazine, HISTANTIL, PHENERGAN

PRONESTYL, procainamide

Propafenone, RYTHMOL

PROPANTHEL, propantheline

Propantheline, PRO-BANTHINE, PROPANTHEL

Propoxyphene, DARVON

Propranolol, INDERAL, NOVO-PRANOL

PROPULSID, cisapride

PROPYL-THYRACIL, propylthiouracil

Propylthiouracil, PROPYL-THYRACIL

PROSCAR, finasteride

PROSTIGMIN, neostigmine

PROSTIN, dinoprostone

Protriptyline, TRIPTIL
PROVERA, medroxyprogesterone
PROZAC, fluoxetine
Pseudoephedrine, ELTOR, SUDAFED
Psyllium, FIBREPUR, METAMUCIL, NOVO-MUCILAX, PRODIEM
PULMICORT, budesonide
PULMOPHYLLINE, theophylline
PULMOZYME, dornase alfa
PURINOL, allopurinol
PVF, penicillin V
Pyrantel, COMBANTRIN
Pyrazinamide, TEBRAZID
PYRIBENZAMINE, tripelennamine
PYRIDIUM, phenazopyridine* (urinary analgesic)
Pyridostigmine, MESTINON, REGONOL
PYRONIUM, phenazopyridine
Pyrvinium pamoate, VANQUIN
QUESTRAN, cholestyramine
Quinapril, ACCUPRIL
QUINIDEX, quinidine
Quinidine, BIQUIN, QUINIDEX
Ramipril, ALTACE
Ranitidine, NOVO-RANIDINE, NU-RANIT, ZANTAC
REACTINE, cetirizine
RECTOVALONE, tixocotrol* (mineralocorticoid)
REGLAN, metoclopramide
REGONOL, pyridostigmine
RELISORM, gonadorelin
RENEDIL, felodipine
RESCRIPTOR, delavirdine
Reserpine, SERPASIL
RESTORIL, temazepam
RETROVIR, zidovudine
REVERIN, rolitetracycline* (antibiotic)
REVIA, naltrexone
RHINALAR, flunisolide
RHINO-MEX-N, naphazoline
RHINOCORT, budesonide
RhO (D) immune globulin, HYPRHO-D, WIN-RHO
RHODIALOSE, lactulose
RHODIS, ketoprofen
RHOTRAL, acebutolol
RHOTRIMINE, trimipramine
RHOVANE, zopiclone* (hypnotic)
Ribavirin, VIRAZOLE
RIDAURA, auranofin
RIFADIN, rifampin
Rifampin, RIFADIN, RIMACTANE, ROFACT
RIMACTANE, rifampin
RIOPAN, simethicone
RISPERDAL, risperidone
Risperidone, RISPERDAL
RITALIN, methylphenidate
Ritonavir, NORVIR
RIVOTRIL, clonazepam
ROBAXIN, methocarbamol-ASA
ROBAXISAL, methocarbamol-ASA
ROBIDEX, dextromethorphan
ROBITUSSIN, dextromethorphan

ROCALTROL, calcitriol
ROFACT, rifampin
ROGAINE, minoxidil
ROGITINE, phentolamine
Rolitetracycline* (antibiotic), REVERIN
RONIACOL, nicotinyl alcohol tartrate
ROVAMYCINE, spiramycin* (antibiotic)
ROXICET, oxycodone-acetaminophen
RUBION, cyanocobalamin
RUBRAMIN, cyanocobalamin
RYNACROM, cromolyn
RYTHMODAN, disopyramide
RYTHMOL, propafenone
S.A.S., sulfasalazine
SABRIL, vigabatrin
SALAZOPYRIN, sulfasalazine
Salbutamol (albuterol in United States), APO-SALVENT,
    NOVO-SALMOL, VENTOLIN
Salmeterol, SEREVENT
SALOFALK, 5-aminosalicylic acid
Salsalate, DISALCID
SANDIMMUNE, cycloserine
SANDOMIGRAN, pizotifen* (antimigraine)
SANDOSTATIN, octreotide
SANOREX, mazindol
SANSERT, methysergide
Saquinavir, INVIRASE
Scopolamine, TRANSDERM-V
Secobarbital, NOVO-SECOBARB, SECONAL
SECONAL, secobarbital
SECTRAL, acebutolol
SELAX, docusate sodium
SELDANE, terfenadine
Selegiline, ELDEPRYL
SENNATAB, sennosides*
Sennosides*, SENNATAB, SENOKOT
SENOKOT, sennosides*
SEPTRA, trimethoprim-sulfamethoxazole
SERAX, oxazepam
SERENTIL, mesoridazine
SEREVENT, salmeterol
SERPASIL, reserpine
SERTAN, primidone
Sertraline, ZOLOFT
SERZONE, nefazodone
SIBELIUM, flunarizine
Silver sulfadiazine, FLAMAZINE
Simethicone, OVOL, RIOPAN
Simvastatin, ZOCOR
SINE-OFF, phenylpropanolamine
SINEMET, levodopa-carbidopa
SINEQUAN, doxepin
SLO-BID, theophylline
SLOW-FE, ferrous sulfate
SOFLAX, docusate sodium
Somatostatin, STILAMIN
Somatropin, HUMATROPE
SOMNOL, flurazepam
SOMOPHYLLIN, theophylline

SOMPAM, flurazepam
SOPRAX, cefixime
SORIATANE, acitretin
SOTACOR, sotalol
Sotalol, SOTACOR
Spectinomycin, TROBICIN
SPERSACARPINE, pilocarpine
Spiramycin* (antibiotic), ROVAMYCINE
Spironolactone, ALDACTONE, NOVO-SPIROTON
SPORANOX, itraconazole
STADOL NS, butorphanol
Stanozolol, WINSTROL
Stavudine, ZERIT
STELAZINE, trifluoperazine
STEMETIL, prochlorperazine
STIEVAA, tretinoin
STILAMIN, somatostatin
STOXIL, idoxuridine
STREPTASE, streptokinase
Streptokinase, STREPTASE, KABIKINASE
Streptozocin, ZANOSAR
SUBLIMAZE, fentanyl
SUDAFED, pseudoephedrine
SULAMYD, sulfacetamide
SULCRATE, sucralfate
Sulfacetamide, AK-SULF, OPHTHO-SULF, SULAMYD, SULFEX
Sulfasalazine, SALAZOPYRIN, S.A.S.
SULFEX, sulfacetamide
Sulfinpyrazone, ANTURAN, NOVO-PYRAZONE
Sulfisoxazole, NOVO-SOXAZOLE, SULFIZOLE
SULFIZOLE, sulfisoxazole
Sulindac, APO-SULIN, CLINORIL, NOVO-SUNDAC
Sumatriptan, IMITREX
SUPREFACT, buserelin* (LH-RH analog)
SUPRES, chlorothiazide
SURFAK, docusate calcium
SURGAM, tiaprofenic acid* (NSAID)
SURMONTIL, trimipramine
SUS-PHRINE, epinephrine
SYMMETREL, amantadine
SYNACTHEN DEPOT, cosyntropin
SYNAREL, nafarelin
SYNKAVITE, menadiol
SYNTHROID, levothyroxine
TAGAMET, cimetidine
TALWIN, pentazocine
TAMBOCOR, flecainide
TAMONE, tamoxifen
Tamoxifen, APO-TAMOX, NOLVADEX, TAMONE
TANACET 125, feverfew* (antimigraine)
TANDERIL, oxyphenbutazone
TAPAZOLE, methimazole
TAVIST, clemastine
TAXOL, paclitaxel
TAZIDIME, ceftazidime
TAZOCIN, piperacillin-tazobactam
TEBRAZID, pyrazinamide
TEEJEL, choline salicylate
TEGOPEN, cloxacillin

TEGRETOL, carbamazepine
Temazepam, RESTORIL
TENORMIN, atenolol
Tenoxicam* (NSAID), MOBIFLEX
TENSILON, edrophonium
TENUATE, diethylpropion
TERAZOL, terconazole
Terazosin, HYTRIN
Terbutaline, BRICANYL
Terconazole, TERAZOL
Terfenadine, SELDANE
TERFLUZINE, trifluoperazine
Testosterone, DELATESTRYL
Testosterone-estradiol, NEO-PAUSE
Tetracycline, ACHROMYCIN, APO-TETRA, NOVO-TETRA, NU-TETRA, TETRACYN
TETRACYN, tetracycline
THEO-DUR, theophylline
THEOLAIR, theophylline
Theophylline, PULMOPHYLLINE, SLO-BID, SOMOPHYLLIN, THEO-DUR, THEOLAIR
Thiabendazole, MINTEZOL
Thiethylperazine, TORECAN
Thioguanine, LANVIS
Thioproperazine* (antipsychotic), MAJEPTIL
Thioridazine, MELLARIL, NOVO-RIDAZINE
Thiothixene, NAVANE
Tiaprofenic acid* (NSAID), ALBERT TIAFEN, SURGAM
TICAR, ticarcillin
Ticarcillin, TICAR
Ticarcillin-clavulanate, TIMENTIN
TICLID, ticlopidine
Ticlopidine, TICLID
TILADE, nedocromil
TIMENTIN, ticarcillin-clavulanate
Timolol, BLOCADREN, NOVO-TIMOL, TIMOPTIC
TIMOPTIC, timolol
Tioconazole, GYNECURE, TROSYD
Tixocotrol* (mineralocorticoid), RECTOVALONE
Tobramycin, NEBCIN
Tocainide, TONOCARD
TOFRANIL, imipramine
Tolbutamide, MOBENOL, NOVO-BUTAMIDE, ORINASE
TOLECTIN, tolmetin
Tolmetin, TOLECTIN
TONOCARD, tocainide
TORADOL, ketorolac
TORECAN, thiethylperazine
Torsemide, DEMADREX
TRACRIUM, atracurium
TRANDATE, labetalol
Tranexamic acid* (hemostatic), CYCLOKAPRON
TRANSDERM-NITRO, nitroglycerin
TRANSDERM-V, scopolamine
TRANXENE, clorazepate
Tranylcypromine, PARNATE
TRASICOR, oxprenolol
TRASYLOL, aprotinin
TRAVEL AID, dimenhydrinate

Trazodone, DESYREL
TRENTAL, pentoxifylline
Tretinoin, STIEVAA, VITAMIN A ACID
TRIADAPIN, doxepin
Triamcinolone, ARISTOCORT, NASACORT
Triamterene, APO-TRIAZIDE, DYRENIUM
Triazolam, APO-TRIAZO, HALCION, NOVO-TRIOLAM, NU-TRIAZO
Trifluoperazine, NOVO-FLURAZINE, STELAZINE, TERFLUZINE
Trihexyphenidyl, APARKANE, APO-TRIHEX, ARTANE, NOVO-HEXIDYL
TRIKACIDE, metronidazole
TRILAFON, perphenazine
TRILISATE, choline magnesium trisalicyate, choline salicylate
Trimeprazine, PANECTYL
Trimethoprim, PROLOPRIM
Trimethoprim-sulfamethoxazole, APO-SULFATRIM, BACTRIM, NOVO-TRIMEL, SEPTRA
Trimipramine, APO-TRIMIP, NOVO-TRIPRAMINE, RHOTRIMINE, SURMONTIL
Tripelennamine, PYRIBENZAMINE
Triprolidine, ACTIFED
TRIPTIL, protriptyline
TROBICIN, spectinomycin
TRONOTHANE, pramoxine
TROPICACYL, tropicamide
Tropicamide, DIOTROPE, MYDRIACYL, TROPICACYL
TROSYD, tioconazole
TRYPTAN, *l*-tryptophan
TUBARINE, tubocurarine
Tubocurarine, TUBARINE
TYLENOL, acetaminophen
ULTRADOL, etodolac
UNIPEN, nafcillin
URASAL, methenamine
URECHOLINE, bethanechol
URIDON, chlorthalidone
URISPAS, flavoxate* (antispasmodic)
URITOL, furosemide
Urokinase, ABBOKINASE
UROMITEXAN, mesna
Ursodiol, URSOFALK
URSOFALK, ursodiol
VALIUM, diazepam
Valporic acid, DEPAKENE
VANCENASE, beclomethasone
VANCERIL, beclomethasone
VANCOCIN, vancomycin
Vancomycin, VANCOCIN
VANQUIN, pyrvinium pamoate
VASOCON, naphazoline
VASODILAN, isoxsuprine
Vasopressin, PITRESSIN, PRESSYN
VASOTEC, enalapril
VASOTEC IV, enalaprilat
VASOXYL, methoxamine

VELBE, vinblastine
Venlafaxine, EFFEXOR
VENTOLIN, salbutamol (albuterol in United States)
Verapamil, APO-VERAP, ISOPTIN, NOVO-VERAMIL, NU-VERAP
VERMOX, mebendazole
VERSED, midazolam
VIBRAMYCIN, doxycycline
Vidarabine, VIRA-A
VIDEX, didanosine
Vigabatrin, SABRIL
Vinblastine, VELBE
Vincristine, ONCOVIN
Vindesine, ELDISINE
VIRA-A, vidarabine
VIRACEPT, nelfinavir
VIRAMUNE, nevirapine
VIRAZOLE, ribavirin
VIROSTAT, edoxudine* (antiviral)
VISKEN, pindolol
VITAMIN A ACID, tretinoin
VIVOL, diazepam
VOLTAREN, diclofenac
Warfarin, WARFILONE
WARFILONE, warfarin
WELLFERON, interferon alfa-n1
WIN-RHO, RhO (D) immune globulin
WINPRED, prednisone
WINSTROL, stanozolol
XYLOCARD, lidocaine
Xylometazoline, OTRIVIN
YOCON, yohimbine
Yohimbine, YOCON
ZADITEN, ketotifen* (antiallergy)
Zalcitabine, HIVID
ZANOSAR, streptozocin
ZANTAC, ranitidine
ZARONTIN, ethosuximide
ZAROXOLYN, metolazone
ZERIT, stavudine
ZESTRIL, lisinopril
Zidovudine, NOVO-AZT, RETROVIR
ZINACEF, cefuroxime
ZITHROMAX, azithromycin
ZOCOR, simvastatin
ZOFRAN, ondansetron
ZOLADEX, goserelin
ZOLOFT, sertraline
ZONULYN, chymotrypsin
Zopiclone* (hypnotic), IMOVANE, RHOVANE
ZOSTRIX, capsaicin
ZOVIRAX, acyclovir
Zuclopenthixol* (antipsychotic), CLOPIXOL
ZYLOPRIM, allopurinol
ZYPREXA, olanzepine

# References

Anon. To the Year 2000: The Changing Roles of Nonprescription Medicines and the Practice of Pharmacy. Ottawa, Nonprescription Drug Manufacturers Association of Canada, 1992.

Bachynsky, J. Nonprescription drugs in health care. *In* Nonprescription Drug Reference for Health Professionals. Ottawa, Canadian Pharmaceutical Association, 1996.

Evans, W.E., Schentag, J.J., and Jusko, W.J. (eds.). Applied Pharmacokinetics: Principles of Therapeutic Drug Monitoring. Spokane, WA, Applied Therapeutics, Inc., 1992.

Health Protection and Drug Laws. Ottawa, Health and Welfare Canada, Canadian Publishing Center, 1988.

Health Protection Branch, Information Newsletter. Issue No. 798, September 9, 1991.

Johnson, G.E., Hannah, K.J., and Zerr, S.R. Pharmacology and the Nursing Process, 3rd ed. Philadelphia, W.B. Saunders, 1992.

Mailhot, R. The Canadian drug regulatory process. J. Clin. Pharmacol. 26:232, 1986.

McLeod, D.C. SI units in drug therapeutics. Drug Intell. Clin. Pharm. 22:990, 1988.

Subcommittee of Metric Commission Canada, Sector 9.10. SI Manual in Health Care, 2nd ed. Ottawa, Health and Welfare, Canada, 1982.

Sullivan, P. CMA to support increased patent protection for drugs but will attach strong qualifications. Can. Med. Assoc. J. 147:1669, 1992.

# Appendix H

# Drug- and Health-Related Resources on the Internet

*Theodore G. Tong, PharmD*

If you know of a good site to add to this collection, please contact Dr. Tong via e-mail at *tong@Pharmacy. Arizona.EDU*

## General Internet Resources

Learn the Net
*http://www.learnthenet.com*
(Comprehensive; A necessary tourist information stop for anyone starting out on the information highway!)

Life On the Internet
*http://www.pbs.org/internet/*
(Examines the ways people use this new medium.)

Critical Evaluation Skills for Web Resources
*http://www.science.widener.edu/~withers/webeval.htm*
(Offers materials to evaluate the informational content of Web resources.)

## Search Engines

Search engines are popular tools for locating Web sites that have content of interest to the searcher. Among the most popular search engines are

Yahoo: *http://www.yahoo.com/health*
AltaVista: *http://www.altavista.digital.com*
Magellan: *http://www.mckinley.com*
Lycos: *http://www.lycos.com*
Infoseek: *http://www.infoseek.com*
WebCrawler: *http://www.webcrawler.com*
Excite: *http://www.excite.com*

## Drug- and Health-Related Sites

### United States Government Sites

Healthfinder, U.S. Health Human Services Office
*http://www.healthfinder.gov/*

(Healthfinder brings together under one umbrella the broad range of consumer health information resources produced by the federal government and its many partners. The site has hyperlinks to over 550 Web sites, including more than 200 federal sites and 350 state, local, not-for-profit, university, and other consumer health resources. The site also includes links to (1) nearly 500 selected on-line documents, (2) FAQs (frequently asked questions) on health issues of concern to the American public, and (3) data bases and Web search engines, catalogued by topic and agency. Healthfinder combats "information overload" and endless searches by organizing these resources in a subject index, which allows consumers to quickly locate the health information they want. Future plans for the site include a full-text index, health risk appraisals, and expanded publication ordering.)

The Food and Drug Administration Home Page
*http://www.fda.gov/fdahomepage.html*

Center for Food Safety and Nutrition (CFSN)
*http://vm.cfsan.fda.gov/*

Centers for Disease Control and Prevention (CDC)
*http://www.cdc.gov/cdc.html*

CDC Morbidity Mortality Weekly Report
*http://www.cdc.gov/epo/mmwr/mmwr.html*

National Institutes of Health
*http://www.nih.gov/*

National Institute of Drug Abuse
*http://www.nida.nih.gov/*

National Library of Medicine
*http://www.nlm.nih.gov/*

### General Health-Related Sites

World Health Organization
*http://www.who.ch/*

Pharmaceutical Information Network
*http://www.pharminfo.com*
(Comprehensive Directory of links, forums, data bases.)

*http://www.pharminfo.com/drg_mnu.html*
(More quick reference on drug interactions, side effects, dosage.)

University of Oklahoma's Virtual Pharmacy Library
*http://www.cph.uokhsc.edu/pharmacy*

PharmWeb's Home Page
*http://www.mcc.ac.uk/pharmacy/*
(Comprehensive list of pharmacy Internet resources.)

Martindale's Health Science Guide
*http://www-sci.lib.uci.edu/HSG/HSGuide.html*
*http://www-sci.lib.uci.edu/HSG/Pharmacy.html*
(Access to "virtual" Pharmacy Center and numerous health-related links.)

University of California Irvine Health Promotion Center
*http://www.socecol.uci.edu/!soc...art/research/hpc/
hpc-links.html*
(Strategies of health promotion [health risk appraisal, prevention, protective behavior, lifestyle changes] are extensively listed and linked with other internet resources. Described as keeping an interdisciplinary, ecological view of community health.)

The Institute for Safe Medical Practices
*http://www.geohealthweb.com/smp/*

Agency for Health Care Policy and Research Guidelines
*http://www.ahcpr.gov/*
(Has clinical practice guidelines for 18 disorders, including depression, cancer pain, heart failure, and prostatic hyperplasia.)

Health Information Management Society
*http://www.himss.org*

Medical/Health Sciences Libraries on the Web
*http://www.arcade.uiowa.edu/hardin-www/hslibs.html*
(Links to many medical and health sciences libraries grouped by state.)

Hospital Web
*http://neuro-www.mgh.harvard.edu/hospitalweb.nclk*
(Links to hospital home pages worldwide.)

## Professional Health Organizations

American Pharmaceutical Association
*http://www.aphanet.org/*

National Community Pharmacists Association
*http://www.ncpanet.org/*

American Medical Association
*http://www.ama-assn.org/*
(View selected text from JAMA.)

American College of Clinical Pharmacy
*http://www.accp.com/*

American College of Physicians
*http://www.acponline.org/*
(Contains items from Annals of Internal Medicine.)

Massachusetts Medical Society
*http://www.nejm.org/*
(View published materials from New England Journal of Medicine.)

British Medical Journal
*http://www.bmj.com/bmj/index.htm*

American Society of Health Systems Pharmacy
*http://www.ashp.com/pub/ashp*

California Pharmacists Association (CPhA)
*http://www.cpha.com/#top*
(Carries national calendar of pharmacy events, California Pharmacist, WWW pharmacy links, CPhA's job market, CPhA publications, and other interesting sites and pages.)

## Sites for Pharmacists and Other Health Professionals

Drug Topics
*http://www.drugtopics.com*

Pharmacy Times
*http://www.pharmacytimes.com*

U.S. Pharmacist
*http://www.uspharmacist.com*

For The Pharmacist
*http://www.forthepharmacists.com*
(Serves day-to-day information needs of pharmacists. Updated daily. Provides a variety of news and information, including information on new drugs and natural/homeopathic medicines.)

Institute for Safe Medication Practices (ISMP)
*http://www.ismp.org*
(When you have trouble dealing with a serious medication error and need advice on how to address such incidents and to prevent repetition.)

Material Safety Data Information
*http://hazard.com/msds*
(Allows searches for product name or producer, and provides links to other Internet sites with MSDS information.)

Medis
*http://www.docnet.org.uk/medis/search.html*
(A search page for abstracts and articles from major medical sites.)

Medscape
*http://www5.medscape.com*
(Peer-reviewed articles, medical news, and access to Medline.)

## Resources for Patients

AIDSLINE
*http://amas.nlm.nih.gov/aidsline.html*

JAMA HIV/AIDS Information Center
*http:ama-assn.org/special/hiv*

Alzheimer's Association
*http://www.alz.org*

NIMH Anxiety Disorders Information Center
*http://nimh.nih.gov/anxiety*

Your Health Daily
*http://yourhealthdaily.com/*
  (Daily health and medical news from material published
  by Medical Tribune News Service and the New York
  Times.)

Arizona Poison and Drug Information Center
*http://www.pharmacy.arizona.edu/poison-html*

Poison Prevention Web Site
*http://www.ipl.org/youth/poisonsafe/*
  (Interactive educational experience for young children
  designed to be completed with a parent or an adult.)

American Association of Poison Control Centers
*http://www.nlu.edu/aapcc*

USP Public Access to Elements for Useful Patient Information
*http://www.usp.org/did/elements.htm*
  (Has patient information for the 200 most commonly
  prescribed medicines.)

Healthtouch
*http://www.healthtouch.com/*
  (Search for uses and side effects of prescription and
  OTC medicines.)

HealthAnswers
*http://healthanswers.com/*
  (Consumer health care information site.)

Internet Drug Index
*http://www.rxlist.com/*
  (Search engine allows user to search for any drug by
  trade or generic name. Extensive drug information,
  including drug interactions.)

Top 200 Prescribed Medicines
*http://www.rxlist.com.top200.htm*
*http://www.rxlist.com/interact.htm*

Foodborne Illnesses
*http://www.cdc.gov/ncidod/diseases/foodborn/
  foodborn.htm*

Ask Dr. Weil
*http://www.drweil.com/*
  (Visit his virtual clinic for information on natural remedies, diet/nutrition, drugs, disease prevention, Chinese
  medicine, and more.)

American Academy of Allergy, Asthma, and Immunology
*http://www.aaaai.org/*
  (Patient and professional resources, include treatment
  guidelines.)

American Diabetes Association
*http://www.diabetes.org/*

American Heart Association
*http://www.amhrt.org/*
  (Resources and links concerning heart health, heart
  attacks, stroke, and vessel  disease.)

CancerNet
*http://icic.nci.nih.gov/*
  (National Cancer Institute's information resources.)

OncoLink
*http://www.oncolink.upenn.edu/*

National Institute of Arthritis and Musculoskeletal and Skin
  Diseases
*http://www.nih.gov/niams*

Women's Health America
*http://www.womenshealth.com/*

Women's Health Interactive
*http://www.womens-health.com/main.html*

## Natural and Alternative Medicine

ALGY's Herb Page
*http://www.algy.com/herb/medcat.html*

Acupuncture and Asian Medicine Resource
*http://www.acupuncture.com*

Alternative Medicine, Shiffman Medical Library, Wayne
  State University
*http://www.libraries.wayne.edu/shiffman/altmed/
  altmed.html*

Alternative Medicine Home Page
*http://www.pitt.edu/~cbw/altm.html*

Alternative and Complementary Medicines
*http://www.altmedicine.com/altmed.htm*
  (Caution: has a link to the Alternative Medicine home
  page at *http://www.ptt.edu/~cbw/altm.html*, a site
  that includes unorthodox, unproven, unconventional,
  or alternative, complementary, innovative, integrative
  therapies.)

NIH, Office of Alternative Medicine (OAM)
*http://www.altmed.od.nih.gov*

American Botanical Council: Herbalgram
*http://www.herbalgram.org*

Cyberbotanica
*http://biotech.chem.indiana.edu/botany*

Dr. Bower's Complimentary and Alternative Medicine Home
  Page
*http://galen.med.virginia.edu*

Get Well-Natural Health Advice for You and Your Family
*http://www.moreinfo.com.au/getwell*

Health Care Information Resources Alternative Medicine
*http://www-hsl.mcmaster.ca/tomflem/altmed.html*

Herbal Encyclopedia
*http://www.wic.net/waltzark/herbenc.htm*

Herb Web
*http://www.herbweb.com*

Herb Research Foundation
*http://www.herbs.org/*

Herbs by Symptom
*http://www.mothernature.com/herb.htm*

Herbal Materia Medica
*http://www.healthy.net/clinic/therapy/herbal/herbic/
herbs/index.html*

Herbal Information Center
*http://www.healthy.net/clinic/therapy/herbal/herbic/
index.html*

Index of Herbs
*http://www.chatlink.com/~herbseed/herbindx.htm*

Natural Medicine Q & A Page
*http://www.pharmacytimes.com/natmed.html*

New York Online Access to Health (NOAH)
*http://www.noah.cuny.edu/alternative/alternative.html*

Phytochemical and Ethnobotanical Databases: Agricultural
  Research Service
*http://www.ars-grin.gov/~ngrisb/*

Southwest School of Botanical Medicine
*http://www.rt66.com/hrbmoore/HOMEPAGE/
HomePage.html*

# INDEX

Note: **Boldface** page numbers indicate prototypes, other important drugs, and major topics. *Italic* page numbers indicate figures. Page numbers followed by t indicate tables. Trade names appear in SMALL CAPITAL LETTERS followed by the generic name in parentheses; check for further information under the generic name.

## A

ABBOKINASE (urokinase), 545t, 546
Abbreviations, table of, 1088-1089
Abciximab, 544
Abdominal distention, bethanechol in, 122
ABELCET (amphotericin B), 924, 926
Abortion. *See also* Emergency postcoital contraception
  carboprost in, 646, 661-662
  dinoprostone in, 646, 661-662
  methotrexate plus misoprostol in, 645-646
  mifepristone (RU 486) in, 645
  misoprostol in, 645
  oxytocin in, 660
Absence seizures
  characteristics, 205
  drug therapy
    clonazepam in, 213
    ethosuximide in, 213
    summary, 205t
    valproic acid in, 212
Absorption of drugs, **33-38**
  definition, 33
  factors influencing, 33-34
  in infants, 86
  variability in, 74-75
Abuse of drugs. *See* Drug abuse
Acapulco gold (marijuana), 380-382
Acarbose, **589-590**
ACCOLATE (zafirlukast), 751t, 757
ACCUPRIL (quinapril), 426t
ACCUTANE (isotretinoin), 1059
ACE. *See* Angiotensin-converting enzyme
ACE inhibitors. *See* Angiotensin-converting enzyme inhibitors
Acebutolol. *See also* Beta-adrenergic antagonists
  clinical pharmacology, summary, 172t
  nursing implications, 174-175
  uses
    cardiac dysrhythmias, 509
    summary, 173t
ACEL-IMMUNE (diphtheria and tetanus toxoids and acellular pertussis vaccine), 740t
Acetaminophen, **705-706**
  nursing implications, 708
  pharmacokinetics, 705, *705*
  in premenstrual syndrome, 632
Acetazolamide, in glaucoma, 1050
Acetohexamide. *See also* Sulfonylureas
  nursing implications, 595
  time course and dosage, 588t
Acetone, abuse of, 385
Acetophenazine. *See also* Antipsychotic agents
  major side effects, 282t

Acetophenazine (*Continued*)
  nursing implications, 293-295
  routes and dosage, 283t
Acetylcholine. *See also* Autonomic nervous system
  hydrolysis of, *130*
  life cycle, 113-114, *114*
  limitations on clinical use, 123
  peripheral locations of, 106, *107*
  receptors for
    functions, peripheral, 110-111, 111t
    locations, peripheral, *110*
    structure, *53*
  role in parkinsonism, 193, *194*
  structure, *114*
Acetylcholinesterase, 114
Acetylcholinesterase inhibitors. *See* Cholinesterase inhibitors
Acetylcysteine
  for acetaminophen overdose, 706
  mucolytic use, 769
Acetyl-L-carnitine, 354
Acetylsalicylic acid. *See* Aspirin
ACHROMYCIN (tetracycline), 873, 873t
ACHROMYCIN V (tetracycline), 775t
Acid-base disturbances, **407-408**
  effects on drug distribution, 72, *72*
  types and treatment
    metabolic acidosis, 408
    metabolic alkalosis, 408
    respiratory acidosis, 407-408
    respiratory alkalosis, 407
Acid-neutralizing capacity
  of common antacids, 782t
  definition, 782
Acidosis
  metabolic, 408
  respiratory, 407-408
*Acinetobacter* infections, drugs of choice in, 843t
ACLOVATE (alclometasone dipropionate), 1056t
Acne, **1056-1059**
  drug therapy, 1057-1059
    adapalene in, 1058
    antibiotics in, 1057
    azelaic acid in, 1058
    benzoyl peroxide in, 1057
    isotretinoin in, 1058-1059
    overview of, 1057
    tretinoin in, 1057-1958
  nondrug therapy, 1057
  pathophysiology, 1056-1057
Acquired immunodeficiency syndrome. *See* Human immunodeficiency virus infection
Acravistine, in allergic rhinitis, 768t

Acromegaly, 611
  octreotide in, 611
ACTH. *See* Adrenocorticotropic hormone
ACTHAR (corticotropin), 622
ACTIDIL (triprolidine), 692t
ACTIFED (triprolidine/pseudoephedrine), 768t
ACTIGALL (ursodiol), 802
Actinic keratosis, fluorouracil in, 1062
*Actinomyces israelii* infections, drugs of choice in, 843t
Actinomycin D, 1030
ACTIVASE (alteplase), 545t, 546
Activated charcoal, use in poisoning, 1076
Activated partial thromboplastin time, 537
ACTRON CAPLETS (ketoprofen), 702
ACU-DYNE (povidone-iodine), 978
Acute retroviral syndrome, 948-949, 949t
ACUTRIM (phenylpropanolamine), 1067t
Acyclovir, **936-938**
  in genital herpes virus infections, 975
  in HSV infection in AIDS, 965-966
  nursing implications, 943
ADALAT CC (nifedipine), 434
ADALAT (nifedipine), 432, 434, 457, 663
Adapalene, 1058
ADD. *See* Attention-deficit/hyperactivity disorder
ADDERALL (amphetamine mixture), 342
Addiction, definition, 360
Addison's disease, 619
ADENOCARD (adenosine), 501t, 512
Adenohypophyseal hormones. *See* Anterior pituitary hormones
Adenosine, **512**
ADH (antidiuretic hormone), 612-614
ADHD. *See* Attention-deficit/hyperactivity disorder
ADIPEX-P (phentermine), 1067t
Administration of drugs
  enteral, definition, 34-35
  major routes, properties of, 34-38
    intramuscular, 36-37
    intravenous, 35-36
    oral, 37
    subcutaneous, 37
  parenteral, definition, 35
  techniques of administration, 1090-1095
    buccal, 1091
    intradermal, 1092-1093
    intramuscular, 1094-1095
    intravenous, 1095-1096
    optic, 1092
    oral, 1090
    otic, 1091-1092
    rectal, 1091
    subcutaneous, 1093-1094

# Major Drug Classes and Their Prototypes

## Endocrine Drugs

### Drugs for Diabetes
*Insulin Preparations*
  Regular insulin (insulin injection)
  Lispro insulin
  Lente insulins
*Sulfonylureas*
  Tolbutamide
*Biguanides*
  Metformin
*Alpha-Glucosidase Inhibitors*
  Acarbose
*Thiazolidinediones*
  Troglitazone
### Drugs for Thyroid Disorders
*Drugs for Hypothyroidism*
  Levothyroxine ($T_4$)
*Drugs for Hyperthyroidism*
  Propylthiouracil
### Estrogens
  Conjugated estrogens [Premarin]
  Estradiol
### Contraceptive Agents
*Combination Oral Contraceptives*
  Ethinyl estradiol plus norethindrone
*Progestin-Only Oral Contraceptives*
  Norethindrone
*Long-Acting Contraceptives*
  Subdermal progestin implant [Norplant]
  Depot medroxyprogesterone acetate
*Emergency Postcoital Contraceptives*
  Ethinyl estradiol plus norgestrel
### Uterine Stimulants and Relaxants
*Uterine Stimulants*
  Oxytocin
  Ergonovine
*Uterine Relaxants*
  Ritodrine

## Anti-Inflammatory, Antiallergic, and Immunologic Drugs

### Antihistamines ($H_1$ Antagonists)
*First-Generation $H_1$ Antagonists*
  Diphenhydramine
*Second-Generation (Nonsedating) $H_1$ Antagonists*
  Terfenadine
### Aspirin-Like Drugs
*Nonsteroidal Anti-inflammatory Drugs*
  Aspirin
  Ibuprofen
*Drugs That Lack Anti-inflammatory Actions*
  Acetaminophen

### Glucocorticoids
  Hydrocortisone
  Prednisone
### Drugs for Rheumatoid Arthritis
*Nonsteroidal Anti-inflammatory Drugs*
  Aspirin (salicylate)
  Naproxen (nonsalicylate)
*Glucocorticoids*
  Prednisone
*Disease-Modifying Antirheumatic Drugs*
  Methotrexate
  Hydroxychloroquine
### Immunosuppressants
*First-line agents*
  Cyclosporine
  Tacrolimus
*Glucocorticoids*
  Prednisone

## Respiratory Tract Drugs

### Drugs for Asthma
*Anti-inflammatory Drugs: Glucocorticoids*
  Beclomethasone (inhaled)
  Prednisone (oral)
*Anti-inflammatory Drugs: Others*
  Cromolyn
  Zafirlukast (leukotriene antagonist)
*Bronchodilators: Beta$_2$-Adrenergic Agonists*
  Terbutaline (inhaled, short acting)
  Salmeterol (inhaled, long acting)
  Albuterol (oral)
*Bronchodilators: Others*
  Theophylline (methylxanthine)
  Ipratropium (muscarinic antagonist)

## Gastrointestinal Drugs

### Drugs for Peptic Ulcer Disease
*Antibiotics (for Helicobacter pylori)*
  Metronidazole plus tetracycline plus amoxicillin
*$H_2$ Antagonists*
  Cimetidine
*Proton Pump Inhibitors*
  Omeprazole
*Mucosal Protectants*
  Sucralfate
*Muscarinic Antagonists*
  Pirenzepine
*Antacids*
  Aluminum hydroxide/magnesium hydroxide
*Drug for NSAID-Induced Ulcers*
  Misoprostol

*Continued*

# Major Drug Classes and Their Prototypes
*(Continued)*